PHARMACOLOGY
FOR HEALTH PROFESSIONALS

— 6th Edition —

PHARMACOLOGY
FOR HEALTH PROFESSIONALS

6th Edition

Kathleen Knights, Shaunagh Darroch, Andrew Rowland, Mary Bushell

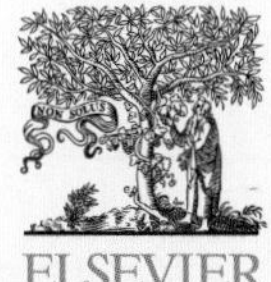

ELSEVIER

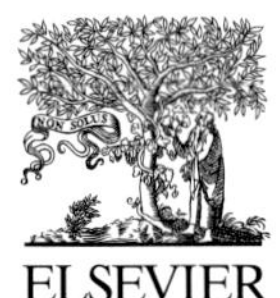

Elsevier Australia. ACN 001 002 357
(a division of Reed International Books Australia Pty Ltd)
Tower 1, 475 Victoria Avenue, Chatswood, NSW 2067

ISBN: 978-0-7295-4390-3

National Library of Australia Cataloguing-in-Publication Data

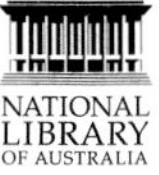

A catalogue record for this book is available from the National Library of Australia

Senior Content Strategist: Melinda McEvoy
Content Project Manager: Shruti Raj
Edited by Matt Davies
Proofread by Tim Learner
Copyrights Coordinator: Arun Prasad Kandasamy
Cover and internal design by Georgette Hall

Typeset by GW Tech

Printed in Singapore by KHL Printing Co Pte Ltd

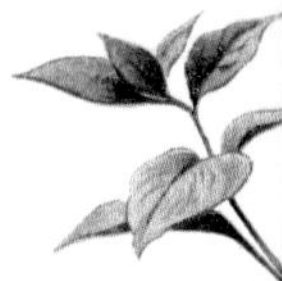

CONTENTS

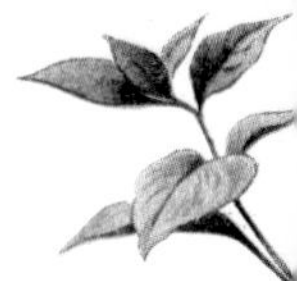

ORGANISATION OF CONTENT

Book Structure

As with previous editions, this book is divided into units. Units 1 and 2 introduce general aspects of the clinical use of drugs and the principles of pharmacology; Units 3–10 consider drugs acting on the major systems of the body, from the autonomic nervous system through to the reproductive system; Units 11–13 cover drugs affecting general pathological conditions, including neoplasia, infections and inflammations; and Unit 14 includes a range of special topics including drugs affecting the skin, eye and ear, pharmacotherapy of obesity as well as new chapters on drugs in aged care, vaccines and complementary therapies.

To enhance learning, chapters begin with a Critical Thinking Scenario that lays the foundation for applying the key physiological, biochemical and pathological processes that underpin the subsequent discussions of pharmacology. We consider that this integrated approach facilitates an understanding of the cellular and molecular aspects of drug action, the rationales for the clinical use of drugs in particular disease processes and their therapeutic and adverse effects and drug interactions. Throughout each chapter, snapshots of key information are provided in the Key Points boxes, the new humanoid models and the comprehensive Drugs at a Glance tables. Application to the clinical situation is enhanced through new Clinical Focus Boxes.

In some chapters, information is based on drug groups, with relevant details of the diseases for which they may be indicated, whereas in others the flow of information starts with the diseases or conditions and leads on to a discussion of the drug groups relevant to treatment. Drug Monographs give detailed information on commonly used drugs. It should be noted that specific pharmacokinetic data, drug dosage and formulation, individual adverse effects and drug interactions vary between drugs in the same group; current evidence-based drug information resources should always be consulted before administering any drug.

Terms and spelling

It is inevitable that with harmonisation many spellings and terminologies about which people feel strongly will change. We have agreed on the following usages, and apologise to those we offend:

- Although the terms 'adverse effect', 'adverse reaction' and 'adverse event' are often used (mistakenly) interchangeably, we have standardised the use of these terms throughout the book. Simply stated, a drug causes an *adverse effect*, a person suffers an *adverse reaction* to a drug, and an *adverse event* occurs while a person is taking a drug, but it is not necessarily due to the drug (see Ch 7 for full explanations).
- Drugs affecting (a system): we have used this term purposely at times – for example, in 'Drugs Affecting the Skin' (Ch 39) – to include not only drugs used to treat conditions of the organ or system but also drugs that may have adverse effects particularly in that system or may be administered to that tissue to have an action elsewhere in the body.
- Drug names: throughout the text, Australian-approved (generic) drug names are used. However, in line with recommendations from the Therapeutic Goods Administration (2016), drug names have been updated consistent with International Non-Proprietary Names (INNs). When these are markedly different from American and/or Canadian names, this may be noted for clarity such as 'paracetamol, known as acetaminophen in the United States'. As drugs may be marketed under multiple trade names that are subject to frequent changes or deletions, we have not included trade names except in instances where readers may be so familiar with a trade name as to identify most readily with it – for example, diazepam, marketed as Valium; paracetamol, marketed as Panadol; or sildenafil, marketed as Viagra.
- Dysrhythmia: although the terms 'arrhythmia' and 'antiarrhythmic drugs' occur frequently in the literature, we have chosen to use the terms 'dysrhythmia' and 'antidysrhythmic drugs'. The prefix 'a' means 'without' and, in that regard, the only arrhythmia is asystole.
- We have now adopted the generally accepted spelling 'fetus' rather than 'foetus' and 'estrogen' instead of 'oestrogen'.
- Gonadotrophin (for example): the suffix 'trophic' means bringing nourishment, whereas 'tropic' means turning or moving in response to a stimulus; they appear to have become interchangeable in words such as gonadotrophin. There is an understanding that the English term is '-trophin', whereas '-tropin' is American usage. We have standardised on the form -trophin except where the approved name for a hormone or drug is otherwise, as in somatropin and follitropin.
- Receptor: because many drugs interact with molecular targets (e.g. enzymes, ion channels and receptors), we have chosen to standardise use of the term 'receptor' in accordance with the IUPHAR Committee on Receptor

Nomenclature and Drug Classification 2003 (see Ch 4).

- 5-hydroxytryptamine: in line with accepted terminology, the term '5-hydroxytryptamine', abbreviated as 5-HT, is used throughout this book. Use of the term 'serotonin' is restricted to the first mention of 5-HT in a chapter (as a reminder that this is synonymous with 5-HT) and in reference to specific drug groups – for example, selective serotonin reuptake inhibitors.

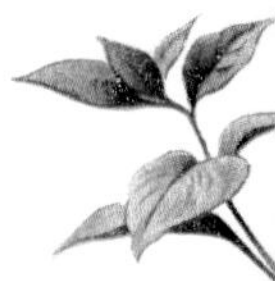

GUIDE TO TEXT

Get the most out of your textbook by familiarising yourself with the key features of this new edition of *Pharmacology for Health Professionals*.

Chapter Opening Features

Chapters have been carefully structured to aid learning. Chapter openings are designed to help you focus and mentally organise content.

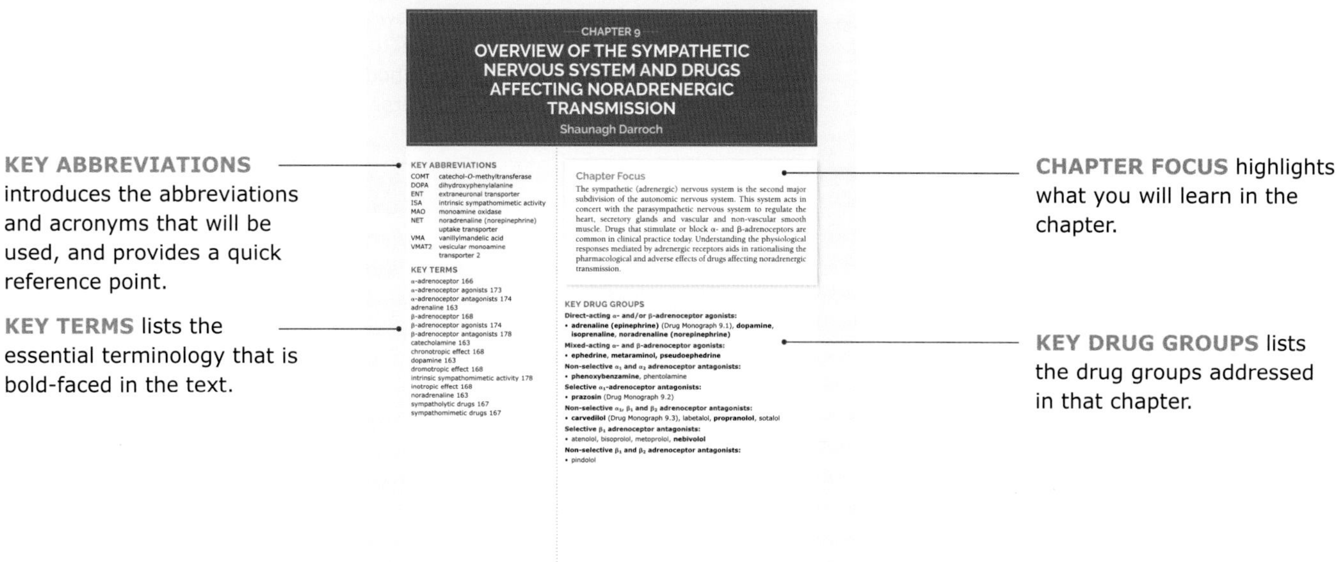

CHAPTER 9

OVERVIEW OF THE SYMPATHETIC NERVOUS SYSTEM AND DRUGS AFFECTING NORADRENERGIC TRANSMISSION

Shaunagh Darroch

KEY ABBREVIATIONS

COMT catechol-O-methyltransferase
DOPA dihydroxyphenylalanine
ENT extraneuronal transporter
ISA intrinsic sympathomimetic activity
MAO monoamine oxidase
NET noradrenaline (norepinephrine) uptake transporter
VMA vanillylmandelic acid
VMAT2 vesicular monoamine transporter 2

KEY TERMS

α-adrenoceptor 166
α-adrenoceptor agonists 173
α-adrenoceptor antagonists 174
adrenaline 163
β-adrenoceptor 168
β-adrenoceptor agonists 174
β-adrenoceptor antagonists 178
catecholamine 163
chronotropic effect 168
dopamine 163
dromotropic effect 168
intrinsic sympathomimetic activity 178
inotropic effect 168
noradrenaline 163
sympatholytic drugs 167
sympathomimetic drugs 167

Chapter Focus

The sympathetic (adrenergic) nervous system is the second major subdivision of the autonomic nervous system. This system acts in concert with the parasympathetic nervous system to regulate the heart, secretory glands and vascular and non-vascular smooth muscle. Drugs that stimulate or block α- and β-adrenoceptors are common in clinical practice today. Understanding the physiological responses mediated by adrenergic receptors aids in rationalising the pharmacological and adverse effects of drugs affecting noradrenergic transmission.

KEY DRUG GROUPS

Direct-acting α- and/or β-adrenoceptor agonists:
- **adrenaline (epinephrine)** (Drug Monograph 9.1), **dopamine**, **isoprenaline**, **noradrenaline (norepinephrine)**

Mixed-acting α- and β-adrenoceptor agonists:
- **ephedrine**, **metaraminol**, **pseudoephedrine**

Non-selective α_1 and α_2 adrenoceptor antagonists:
- **phenoxybenzamine**, phentolamine

Selective α_1-adrenoceptor antagonists:
- **prazosin** (Drug Monograph 9.2)

Non-selective α_1, β_1 and β_2 adrenoceptor antagonists:
- **carvedilol** (Drug Monograph 9.3), labetalol, **propranolol**, sotalol

Selective β_1 adrenoceptor antagonists:
- atenolol, bisoprolol, metoprolol, **nebivolol**

Non-selective β_1 and β_2 adrenoceptor antagonists:
- pindolol

KEY ABBREVIATIONS introduces the abbreviations and acronyms that will be used, and provides a quick reference point.

KEY TERMS lists the essential terminology that is bold-faced in the text.

CHAPTER FOCUS highlights what you will learn in the chapter.

KEY DRUG GROUPS lists the drug groups addressed in that chapter.

Tables and Boxes

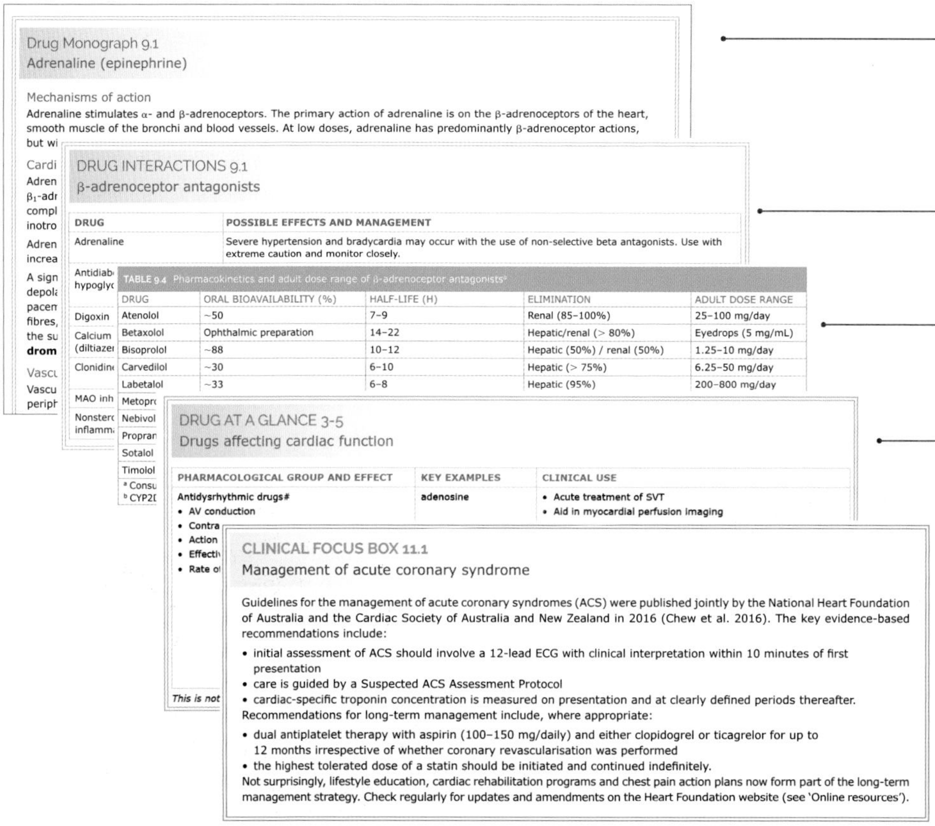

Drug Monograph 9.1
Adrenaline (epinephrine)

Mechanisms of action
Adrenaline stimulates α- and β-adrenoceptors. The primary action of adrenaline is on the β-adrenoceptors of the heart, smooth muscle of the bronchi and blood vessels. At low doses, adrenaline has predominantly β-adrenoceptor actions, but wi…

DRUG INTERACTIONS 9.1
β-adrenoceptor antagonists

DRUG	POSSIBLE EFFECTS AND MANAGEMENT
Adrenaline	Severe hypertension and bradycardia may occur with the use of non-selective beta antagonists. Use with extreme caution and monitor closely.

TABLE 9.4 Pharmacokinetics and adult dose range of β-adrenoceptor antagonists[a]

DRUG	ORAL BIOAVAILABILITY (%)	HALF-LIFE (H)	ELIMINATION	ADULT DOSE RANGE
Atenolol	~50	7–9	Renal (85–100%)	25–100 mg/day
Betaxolol	Ophthalmic preparation	14–22	Hepatic/renal (> 80%)	Eyedrops (5 mg/mL)
Bisoprolol	~88	10–12	Hepatic (50%) / renal (50%)	1.25–10 mg/day
Carvedilol	~30	6–10	Hepatic (> 75%)	6.25–50 mg/day
Labetalol	~33	6–8	Hepatic (95%)	200–800 mg/day

DRUG AT A GLANCE 3-5
Drugs affecting cardiac function

PHARMACOLOGICAL GROUP AND EFFECT	KEY EXAMPLES	CLINICAL USE
Antidysrhythmic drugs# • AV conduction	adenosine	• Acute treatment of SVT • Aid in myocardial perfusion imaging

CLINICAL FOCUS BOX 11.1
Management of acute coronary syndrome

Guidelines for the management of acute coronary syndromes (ACS) were published jointly by the National Heart Foundation of Australia and the Cardiac Society of Australia and New Zealand in 2016 (Chew et al. 2016). The key evidence-based recommendations include:

- initial assessment of ACS should involve a 12-lead ECG with clinical interpretation within 10 minutes of first presentation
- care is guided by a Suspected ACS Assessment Protocol
- cardiac-specific troponin concentration is measured on presentation and at clearly defined periods thereafter.

Recommendations for long-term management include, where appropriate:

- dual antiplatelet therapy with aspirin (100–150 mg/daily) and either clopidogrel or ticagrelor for up to 12 months irrespective of whether coronary revascularisation was performed
- the highest tolerated dose of a statin should be initiated and continued indefinitely.

Not surprisingly, lifestyle education, cardiac rehabilitation programs and chest pain action plans now form part of the long-term management strategy. Check regularly for updates and amendments on the Heart Foundation website (see 'Online resources').

DRUG MONOGRAPHS describe important aspects of either the prototype of a drug group or the most commonly prescribed drug of a group.

DRUG INTERACTIONS TABLES highlight drug interactions of clinical relevance.

TABLES AND BOXES provide additional information and summaries on a range of topics.

DRUGS AT A GLANCE TABLES summarise the main therapeutic groups and effects and give examples of key drugs and their clinical use.

CLINICAL FOCUS BOXES provide descriptions of items of special relevance to Australasia and details of evidence based pharmacological management of common diseases and conditions

CRITICAL THINKING SCENARIO

Terry, a 61-year-old male, was diagnosed with renal cell cancer 2 years ago and has been taking 50 mg of sunitinib (a cancer medicine) daily without any complications ever since. Last week Terry contracted COVID-19. Fearing that he is quite frail, Terry's doctor prescribed a 5-day course of Paxlovid (nirmatrelvir/ritonavir) to help minimise his symptoms. What, if any, impact is Paxlovid likely to have on Terry's cancer medicine and how might this be addressed?

CRITICAL THINKING SCENARIO for each chapter allows application of the key physiological, biochemical and pathological processes that underpin the pharmacological use of a particular drug.

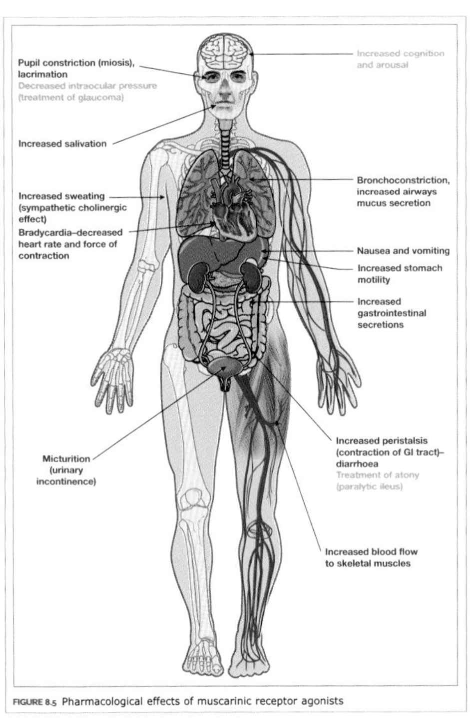

FIGURE 8.5 Pharmacological effects of muscarinic receptor agonists

HUMANOID MODEL are a new addition to the book. For illustrative purposes these models use selected organs, tissues, body parts etc. to explain pharmacological/adverse effects of various drugs or drug groups.

KEY POINTS

Pharmacodynamics

- An agonist binds to the orthosteric site of the receptor (governed by affinity) and activates the receptor (governed by efficacy) to produce the same response as the endogenous ligand.
- Partial agonists produce less than the maximal effect caused by the endogenous ligand, even when all receptors are occupied.
- An antagonist binds to a receptor and blocks access of the endogenous ligand, diminishing the normal response.
- When a drug is administered, the response usually increases in proportion to the dose until the receptors

KEY POINTS reinforce your learning and help you to review material.

REVIEW EXERCISES

1 Ms FG, a 14-year-old, presents to the emergency department after an allergic reaction after eating peanuts at a party. She first experienced breathing difficulties and swelling of her lips and hands. As she is being triaged, she collapses. She is administered adrenaline 1:1000 IM injection into her thigh. Explain the effect of adrenaline on the cardiovascular and respiratory systems. Explain why this drug is useful in treating anaphylactic shock.

2 Ms MC has recently been diagnosed with moderate heart failure. She has been prescribed an ACE inhibitor to reduce fluid load and now her cardiologist has prescribed the beta-blocker nebivolol. She has now titrated her dose from 1.25 mg to a 5 mg dose. She returns to the clinic in 2 weeks complaining of tiredness, insomnia and vivid dreams. What is your explanation as to why these symptoms have occurred? Should she stop taking nebivolol immediately?

REVIEW EXERCISES are given for every chapter to help you master the material in manageable parts.

REFERENCES

Brunton LL, Chabner BA, Knollmann BC, editors: Goodman & Gilman's the pharmacological basis of therapeutics, ed 13, New York, 2017, McGraw-Hill.

Salerno E: Pharmacology for health professionals, St Louis, 1999, Mosby.

Schena G, Caplan MJ. Everything You Always Wanted to Know about β3-AR * (* But Were Afraid to Ask). Cells. 2019 Apr 16;8(4):357. doi: 10.3390/cells8040357. PMID: 30995798; PMCID: PMC6523418.

Therapeutic Goods Administration 2021. Changes to adrenaline and noradrenaline labels [online] Available at: <https://www.tga.gov.au/changes-adrenaline-and-noradrenaline-labels [Accessed 9 Oct 2021].

ONLINE RESOURCES

Australasian Society of Clinical Immunology and Allergy: https://www.allergy.org.au/ (accessed 24 February 2022)

Australian Resuscitation Council: https://www.resus.org.au/ (accessed 24 February 2022)

More weblinks at: http://evolve.elsevier.com/AU/Knights/pharmacology/.

REFERENCES is an up-to-date bibliography at the end of each chapter, with references relevant to all health professionals.

ONLINE RESOURCES lists key websites where you can find additional information. Further web links are also supplied on the Evolve site for this text.

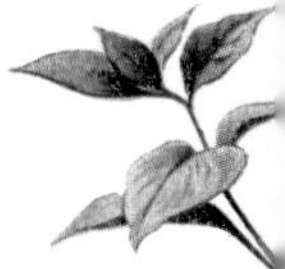

PREFACE

Pharmacology is a universal discipline, but the availability of drugs and the patterns of their use differ between countries. Most pharmacology texts are written for health professionals and students in the northern hemisphere; this 6th edition continues to be ideally suited to the needs of all health professionals practising in Australia and New Zealand. The discussion of drugs reflects the names used and their availability and clinical use within the Australasian region, and the material on drug legislation and ethical principles focuses on regional aspects. To complement and enhance this regional flavour, information on traditional medicinal plants and patterns of use of medicines by Indigenous peoples is interspersed in relevant chapters. We acknowledge that paramedics and practitioners of some other professions, such as nursing, midwifery, podiatry, physiotherapy, optometry and orthoptics, are increasingly being granted limited prescribing rights, and additional information relevant to these emerging roles has been incorporated throughout the 6th edition.

As much of pharmacology is predicated on an understanding of physiology and biochemistry, the 6th edition showcases fully updated, revised and condensed chapters that reduce the overlap of material. The content is more concise and reflects recent epidemiological data, research findings, the introduction of new drugs, withdrawals of old drugs and changes in recommendations and guidelines from learned bodies on the pharmacological management of disease conditions. Many of the figures have been redrawn and new figures (e.g. humanoid models) included to enhance understanding and interest. This edition also features:

- new chapters on vaccines and drugs in aged care
- Key Points boxes that provide a snapshot of important information
- new and updated Drug Monographs using either the prototype of a drug group or the most commonly prescribed drug of a group, or drugs that have gained 'drug of first choice' status
- tables containing more details of drug interactions occurring with major drug groups
- new comprehensive Drugs at a Glance tables
- information on recent changes in the pharmacological management of major conditions, including asthma, cardiac failure, cancers, stroke, dementia, diabetes mellitus, epilepsy, HIV, hypertension, osteoporosis, rheumatoid arthritis, macular degeneration, otitis media, endometriosis, common complications of pregnancy and childbirth, and on anaesthesia in surgery and analgesia and sedation for children
- new Clinical Focus Boxes, including descriptions of items of special interest specific to Australasia and of typical pharmacological treatment of common diseases and conditions
- enhanced information on the use of complementary and alternative medicine modalities and on interactions between drugs and these therapies
- a full-colour treatment to distinguish the text elements and make navigating the text easy.

With advances in drug development, drugs in clinical use continue to have a high rate of obsolescence. The facts learned for a particular drug may therefore become irrelevant when each year brings new drugs with differing modes of action. With an emphasis on personalised or precision medicine, the challenge for health professionals is to stay up to date with advances in the field of pharmacology and their impact on the quality use of medicines. We have retained both a scientific and a clinical approach, founded on evidence-based medicine and always emphasising the clinical use and therapeutic/adverse effects of drugs. Information on the clinical use of drugs is based especially on data in the *Australian Medicines Handbook*, the *Therapeutic Guidelines* series and reviews in *Drugs*, the *Medical Journal of Australia*, *Australian Family Physician* and *Australian Prescriber*. We are confident that this 6th edition will continue to fulfil the needs of students and academics in all health professions and will make the study of pharmacology logical, enjoyable, easy and, above all, interesting.

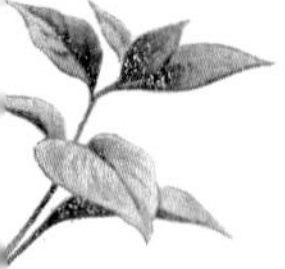

ACKNOWLEDGEMENTS

The authors of the 6th edition of *Pharmacology for Health Professionals* would like to express their gratitude to Bronwen Bryant for the integral role she played in the first five editions. As one of the original authors, her drive, enthusiasm and passion for pharmacology helped to lay the foundations of the hybrid physiology/pharmacology/clinical pharmacology focus of the text. The 6th edition continues her legacy.

The authors thank all readers (students, academics and colleagues) who have provided helpful and constructive comments, which we have addressed in this edition.

The authors also thank and acknowledge the invaluable assistance of the following people, whose time and expertise contributed to the accuracy and clarity of the information:

Dr Gordon Baker
Professorial Fellow
The University of Melbourne
Melbourne, Victoria

Dr Alison Bryant-Smith, MBBS/BA, MPH, MSurgEd, MRCOG, FRANZCOG
Consultant obstetrician/gynaecologist
Melbourne, Victoria

Rosemary Bryant-Smith, BA, LLB(Hons)
Director, HR Governance, Risk and Policy
Office of the Provost, The University of Melbourne
Melbourne, Victoria

Dr Alan Ch'ng, BPharm, MBBS, FANZCA
Consultant Anaesthetist
Fiona Stanley and Fremantle Hospitals Group
Perth, Western Australia

Maxine Cuskelly, BA, GradDipLib, GradDipEdit&Publ
Library Manager
CL Butchers Pharmacy Library
Monash University
Melbourne, Victoria

Sylvia Pilz, BArt, GDipMuseumSt, MInfoSt
Subject Librarian
Monash University
Melbourne, Victoria

Dr Philippa Shilson, MBBS(Hons), FRACP
Paediatrician
Geelong, Victoria

For valuable discussions, with thanks to:

Dr Antony Sutherland, MBBS
Neurology Advanced Trainee
St Vincent's Hospital Melbourne – Neuroscience Department
Monash University
Melbourne, Victoria

Dr Yiying (Sally) Tsang, MBBS(Hons), BA, MEpi(Distinct), AMusA, FANZCA
Anaesthetist
Melbourne, Victoria

Dr Melanie S Van Twest, BA, BLitt(Hons), MBBS, MA, FACRRM
Rural Generalist and GP anaesthetist
Melbourne, Victoria

The authors acknowledge use of information from the *New Zealand Universal List of Medicines*, which uses information from Medsafe, PHARMAC and the Pharmacy Guild of New Zealand.

Reviewers

The authors and Elsevier Australia are grateful to the following reviewers for their insightful observations and recommendations, which greatly assisted us in developing the 6th edition:

Arduino A Mangoni, MD(Hons), PhD, FRCP, MRCP, FRACP
Professor of Clinical Pharmacology
College of Medicine and Public Health
Flinders University
Adelaide, South Australia

Lori J Delaney, RN, BN, PGDip CritCare, PGCertEd, MN, MIHM
Lecturer in Nursing
Faculty of Health
Queensland University of Technology
Brisbane, Queensland

Sam Kosari, BPharm(Hons), PhD
Associate Professor
University of Canberra
Canberra, Australian Capital Territory

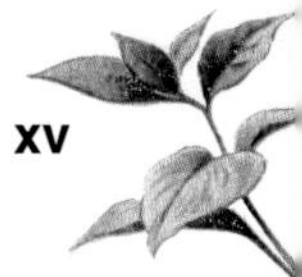

Kalpana Raghunathan, RN, BNurs, BA, GradDipDevStudies, MNurs(Education), MHumanResourceMgt, MDevStudies, DipCommunityDev, DipBusinessMgt

Education Strategy and Curriculum Development Consultant
Caramar Educational Design
Melbourne, Victoria

Maree Donna Simpson, BPharm, BSc(Hons), PhD, MPS, GradCertUnivTeach&Learn

SFHEA Discipline Leader
Pharmacy and Health Studies Group
School of Biomedical Sciences
Charles Sturt University
Orange, New South Wales

Jordan Irwin

Health Medical & Applied Sci
New Pharmacology Unit for Echo Program
Central Queensland University

Michael J McGivern

School of Nursing
Northtec

Amy Shepherd

Mater Education Ltd
Diploma of Nursing Pharmacology
Mater Edu

Hemant Mehta

ACU Canberra-Nursing, Midwifery & Paramedicine
BIOL122-Human Biological Science 2
Australian Catholic University

Robert Batterbee

School of Health Professions
NUR231 - Complexities of health and Illness Across the Lifespan 1
Murdoch

Sandra Leathwick

Nursing Midwifery & Paramedicine (McAuley)
Grad Cert in Clinical Nursing
Australian Catholic University

Jessie Johnson-Cash

Schl Nursing Midwifery & Paramed
HLT201 Therapeutics in Midwifery
Central Queensland University

Gudrun Dannenfeldt

Healthcare & Social Practice
HCBN5106 Nursing the person with long term health needs
Unitec

Adeniyi Adeleye

Nursing, Midwifery & Soc Sci
NURS12154 Pharmacology for Nursing Practice
Central Queensland University

Peta Winters-Chang

Nursing, Midwifery & SocWk
MIDW1101 Introduction Midwifery Practice
University of Queensland

Samira Kerbage

Nursing- Swinburne
Bachelor of Nursing
Swinburne

Mohammed Salahudeen

Pharmacy UniTas
CSA236 - Pharmacology in Paramedic Practice (Hobart)
University of Tasmania

Technical Reviewers

Jerry Perkins, B.Pharm (Syd); B.Sc. (UNSW)

Lynne Perkins, B.Pharm (Syd); BVA (Syd)

Colleagues and Editors

We would like to acknowledge the support of our colleagues at Flinders University (KK, AR), Victoria University (SD), University of Canberra (MB) and the authors who previously kindly gave permission to use or adapt their work for our purposes, in particular Professors John Murtagh, George Sweeney and the late Bill Bowman.

Our role as authors has again been challenging, and we record our thanks to staff and associates of Elsevier, especially Melinda McEvoy (Senior Content Strategist) and Shruti Raj (Content Project Manager) for their stimulus, guidance and patience; editor Matt Davies for his editorial rigour; and pharmacists Jerry Perkins and Lynne Mackinnon for their careful technical checking. It is inevitable that recommendations for drug indications, availability, scheduling and dosage will change, and current evidence-based drug information sources should always be consulted prior to drug administration. We apologise for any errors and welcome comments and feedback on the 6th edition of *Pharmacology for Health Professionals.*

Kathleen Knights

Emeritus Professor
Discipline of Clinical Pharmacology
College of Medicine and Public Health
Flinders University
Adelaide, South Australia

Shaunagh Darroch

Freelance Pharmacologist
Melbourne, Victoria

Andrew Rowland
Associate Professor
Discipline of Clinical Pharmacology
College of Medicine and Public Health
Flinders University
Adelaide, South Australia

Mary Bushell
Clinical Assistant Professor
Discipline of Pharmacy
Faculty of Health
University of Canberra
Canberra, Australian Capital Territory

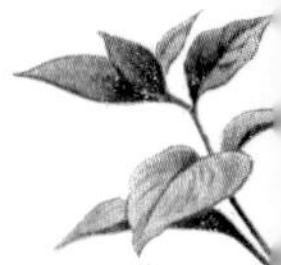

ABOUT THE AUTHORS

Kathleen Knights

Kathie completed a Bachelor of Science (Honours) degree at North East London Polytechnic, majoring in pharmacology, while working as a research assistant at Guy's Hospital, London. On returning home to Adelaide, she accepted a research position in the Department of Anaesthesia and Intensive Care in the School of Medicine at Flinders University, where she also completed a PhD investigating the hepatotoxicity of the inhalational anaesthetic agent halothane.

Kathie's academic career developed throughout her time at Flinders, progressing from her initial appointment as Lecturer to Professor in Clinical Pharmacology. Her teaching crossed discipline boundaries, covering medicine, nursing, nutrition and dietetics, optometry and paramedic sciences. She was a recipient of a Carrick Award in 2007 and the ASCEPT Teaching Excellence Award in 2010, both awards recognising her outstanding contribution to student learning. Her research interests centred on drug metabolism, specifically the metabolism of non-steroidal anti-inflammatory drugs and their mechanisms of renal toxicity. An invited speaker at national and international conferences, Kathie has published extensively in peer-reviewed international journals and books.

Kathie retired in 2014 and is now an Emeritus Professor in the Department of Clinical Pharmacology in the College of Medicine and Public Health, Flinders University. In 2020 she was awarded a Fellowship of ASCEPT, which recognised her significant contribution to the discipline and to the society. She remains a passionate advocate of the discipline of pharmacology.

Shaunagh Darroch

Shaunagh completed a Bachelor of Science degree at Monash University, majoring in pharmacology and physiology. She subsequently moved to the Victorian College of Pharmacy (now Monash University), where she completed a Master of Pharmacy degree in the field of cholinergic pharmacology.

Shaunagh's academic career has involved lecturing and tutoring positions, including at Monash University, La Trobe University and Victoria University within the disciplines of pharmacy, paramedicine, nursing and midwifery, podiatry, physiotherapy, and health and biomedical sciences. She has been involved in course and curriculum development, as well as face-to-face and online teaching of basic, advanced and clinical pharmacology, physiology and pathophysiology. She has been a visiting lecturer at the University of Hong Kong (School of Professional and Continuing Education) and the Fiji School of Medicine.

Alongside her many research publications and communications, Shaunagh has been a contributor to several Australian and international textbooks including the previous editions of *Pharmacology for Health Professionals*. Her research interests have ranged from G protein-coupled receptors through to paramedic clinical practice.

Shaunagh continues to be an enthusiastic educator and communicator. She is currently involved in curriculum design and development across several universities, in addition to writing and editing consultancies in various disciplines.

Andrew Rowland

Andrew completed a PhD investigating better ways to use in vitro models to predict drug metabolism in humans in 2009. He then spent two years as a post-doctoral researcher before taking up an academic position in the School of Medicine at Flinders University. Now Associate Professor, Andrew contributes to the teaching of pharmacology and therapeutics within a range of medical and health degrees including the Doctor of Medicine, Bachelor of Paramedic Science, Bachelor of Medical Science and Master of Advanced Clinical Practice degrees.

Andrew has a highly active research profile, with a primary interest in translating pharmacokinetics into clinical practice through optimising drug dosing, specifically focusing on precision dosing of anticancer drugs. He has published more than 120 research articles and reviews in peer-reviewed international journals and has received numerous research awards including the prestigious Certara New Investigator Award from the Australasian Society of Clinical and Experimental Pharmacologists and Toxicologists and a Vice Chancellor's Award for Early Career Researchers.

Mary Bushell

Mary completed her Bachelor of Pharmacy (Honors) degree at Charles Sturt University and later worked in the Northern Territory, providing care as a practising pharmacist in some of the most remote communities in Australia. Mary's academic career began in 2011 at Charles Darwin University, where she advanced to a Senior Lecturer position coordinating and teaching pharmacology and pharmacy practice units. In 2016 Mary completed her PhD, which developed and validated a vaccination training program for pharmacy students.

Now a Clinical Assistant Professor in Pharmacy at the University of Canberra, Mary enjoys coordinating and teaching pharmacology and evidence-based medicine to a range of health courses including pharmacy, medicine, nursing, optometry, nutrition and health science. Mary takes great pride in the honour of fostering the next generation of health professionals.

DEDICATION

To the discipline of pharmacology, which provided the foundation of my academic career, and to those who enrich my life – my husband, John, and my family and friends.

Kathleen Knights

To my family and friends for their continuous encouragement and humour, to my colleagues for their support and guidance, and to my students for challenging and inspiring me.

Shaunagh Darroch

It is with gratitude and love that we dedicate this work to my wonderful wife, Angela, and amazing sons Aidan and Archer. Your kindness and love enrich every element of my life.

Andrew Rowland

To my greatest teachers – my parents, Penny and Tony. Thank you for inspiring my curiosity to learn science with nectarines, tennis balls and sheep's eyes. Forever grateful.

Mary Bushell

UNIT 1 Introduction to Pharmacology

CHAPTER 1
DRUGS AND MEDICINES

Mary Bushell

KEY ABBREVIATIONS

AMH	*Australian Medicines Handbook*
APF	*Australian Pharmaceutical Formulary and Handbook*
BP	British Pharmacopoeia
CFB	Clinical Focus Box
CMI	consumer medicine information
CTN	Clinical Trial Notification
DM	Drug Monograph
INN	International Non-proprietary Name
NZF	*New Zealand Formulary*
OTC	over-the-counter
RCCT	randomised controlled clinical trial
TGA	Therapeutic Goods Administration
WHO	World Health Organization

Chapter Focus

This chapter focuses on the origin, development and scope of pharmacology. It describes the physical and chemical characteristics of drugs, how drugs are named and classified and how drug information can be sourced. The stages of drug discovery and development, including the phases and important elements in clinical trials of investigational drugs, are outlined. Understanding basic pharmacology is integral for health professionals because it helps promote quality use of medicines, which subsequently improves health outcomes for their patients.

KEY TERMS

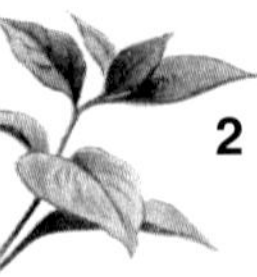

CRITICAL THINKING SCENARIO

Billy, a 28-year-old male, was recently diagnosed with depression and prescribed the antidepressant sertraline. Billy tells you, the health professional, that he does not like taking medicines. Up till now, Billy has only taken simple analgesia and the odd course of antibiotics.

Billy would like to learn more about the drug development stages and the phases of clinical trials that help promote safe and effective medicines.

1. Explain the stages of drug development.
2. Explain each of the phases of the clinical trial process.
3. Explain as a health professional how you would report a suspected adverse reaction to a medicine or vaccine.

Billy has looked at many online resources, blogs, tweets and relevant Facebook posts to search for information about the safety and effectiveness of sertraline. He tells you that a lot of information he has read is conflicting and, the more he reads, the more confused he gets. Billy read one online article that suggests that 'natural' medicines made from plants are safer than 'unnatural' synthetic medicines, like the one he has been prescribed.

4. Describe drug information sources that Billy can read to get evidence-based information about his new medicine.
5. Discuss if 'natural' drugs are safer than synthetic drugs.

Introduction

Pharmacology is the study of drugs, including their sources, nature, actions, effects in living systems and uses. The word '**drug**' is defined by the World Health Organization (WHO 2007) as 'any substance or product that is used or intended to be used to modify or explore physiological systems or pathological states for the benefit of the recipient'. The prefix 'pharmaco-' is derived from the Greek word *pharmakon*, meaning 'drug' or 'medicine'. Hence, we have related terms such as **pharmacy**, **pharmacodynamics**, **pharmacokinetics**, **pharmaceutics** and **pharmacopoeia** (Table 1.1).

Pharmacologists may study the origins, isolation, purification, chemical structure/synthesis, assay (measurement), actions/mechanisms, economics, genetic aspects and toxicity of drugs, as well as their fate in the body and medical uses. Pharmacologists work in hospitals, clinics, research institutions, drug companies, government departments of health, medical publishing and universities. In other words, wherever drugs are developed, studied and used.

Pharmacology deals with all drugs used in society – legal and illegal, prescription and '**over-the-counter**' (OTC) medications, endogenous substances (those produced within the body) and natural and synthetic products – with beneficial or potentially toxic effects. The pharmacological agents available today have controlled, prevented, cured, diagnosed and, in some instances, eradicated diseases, and have improved the quality of life of billions of people.

Medicines also have the potential to cause harm. (The ancient Greek word for 'drug' was also the word for 'poison'.) To administer a drug safely, one must know the appropriate **dose**, frequency, **route** of administration, **indications**, **contraindications**, significant adverse reactions, major drug interactions, dietary implications (if applicable) and appropriate monitoring techniques and interventions, and apply this knowledge to the particular patient and situation.

Drugs and medicines

Unfortunately, the word 'drug' has come to have connotations of illicit street drugs. However, it has a much simpler and wider meaning: a drug is a substance that usefully affects living tissues. The terms '**medication**', 'medicine' and '**pharmaceutical**' usually refer to drugs

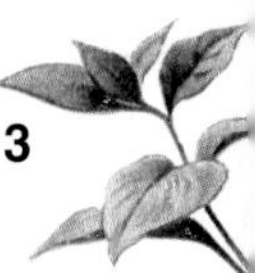

TABLE 1.1 Some common pharmacological terms[a]

TERM	DEFINITION
Adverse drug reaction	An unintended and undesirable response to a drug
Clinical pharmacology	Pharmacology applied to the treatment of human patients; the study of drugs 'at the bedside'
Dose	The quantity of a drug to be administered at one time, determined by experience as likely to be safe and effective in most people
Dose form/formulation	The form in which the drug is administered – for example, as a tablet, injection, eyedrops or ointment
Drug	A substance used to modify or explore the physiological system or pathological state for the benefit of the recipient
Indication	An illness or disorder for which a drug has a documented specific usefulness
Medicine	Drug(s) given for therapeutic purposes; possibly a mixture of drug(s) plus other substances to provide stability in the formulation; also, the branch of science devoted to the study, prevention and treatment of disease
Pharmaceutics	The science of the preparation and dispensing of drugs
Pharmacist[b]	A person licensed to store, prepare, dispense and provide drugs, and to make up prescriptions
Pharmacodynamics	What drugs do to the body and how they do it; refers to the interaction of drug molecules with their target receptors or cells, and their biochemical, physiological and possibly adverse effects
Pharmacokinetics	How the body affects a specific drug after administration; that is, how a drug is altered as it travels through the body (by absorption, distribution, metabolism and excretion)
Pharmacologist[b]	A person who studies drugs: their source, nature, actions/mechanisms, uses, fate in the body, medical uses and toxicity
Pharmacology	The study of drugs, including their actions and effects in living systems
Pharmacopoeia	A reference book listing standards for drugs approved in a particular country; may also include details of standard formulations and prescribing guidelines (a formulary)
Pharmacy	The branch of science dealing with preparing and dispensing drugs; also the place where a pharmacist carries out these roles
Receptor	Protein structure on or within a cell or membrane that is capable of binding to a specific substance (e.g. a transmitter, hormone or drug), initiating chemical signalling and causing altered function in the cell
Route	The pathway by which a drug is administered to the body; for example, in the oral route, the drug is taken by mouth and swallowed
Side effect	A drug's effect that is not necessarily the primary purpose for giving the drug in the particular condition; side effects may be desirable or undesirable. This term has been virtually superseded by the term 'adverse drug reaction', which is used throughout this book
Toxicology	The study of the nature, properties, identification, effects and treatment of poisons, including the study of adverse drug reactions

[a] See the Glossary (Appendix 2) for a more complete listing of pharmacological terms.
[b] The roles of these and many other health professionals are described in greater detail in Chapter 2.

mixed in a formulation with other ingredients to improve their stability, taste or physical form, in order to allow appropriate administration of the active drug.

Characteristics of drugs

Potency, selectivity and specificity

By our broad definition of a drug as a chemical having useful action on living tissue, many substances could be classed as drugs: even oxygen, sugar, salt and water usefully affect the body but can be toxic in overdose. However, useful drugs usually have other important attributes: potency, selectivity and specificity.

Potency relates to the amount of chemical required to produce an effect; it is an *inverse* relationship – the more potent the drug, the lower the dose required for a given effect (Fig 4.6, in Ch 4). One of the most potent chemicals known is the natural bacterial product botulinum toxin (commonly known as Botox), for which the estimated human median lethal dose (LD_{50}) is about $1–1.5 \times 10^{-7}$ g IV for a 70 kg adult. It is used to treat spasm of eye muscles and spasticity, and in neurological disorders and cosmetic surgery (DM 40.3).

Selectivity refers to the narrowness of a drug's range of actions on **receptors**, cellular processes or tissues. The antidepressant drugs known as selective serotonin reuptake inhibitors such as fluoxetine (Prozac – see DM 22.3) have fewer adverse effects than older antidepressants because of their more selective actions.

The term **specificity** may be used loosely like 'selectivity' – for example, cardiospecific or cardioselective β-blocking agents. Specificity may also refer to the relationship between the chemical structure of a drug and its pharmacological actions; for example, the effects of salbutamol and similar bronchodilators in asthma are due to their chemical similarity to the neurotransmitter noradrenaline (Fig 1.4, later), and hence their specificity for the β-adrenoceptor.

The ideal drug

In designing a new drug, a research pharmacologist might aim for it to be: easily administered (preferably orally) and fully absorbed from the gastrointestinal tract; not

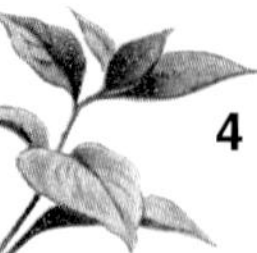

highly protein-bound in the blood plasma; potent; highly specific; selective, with rapid onset and useful duration of action; of high therapeutic index (no adverse drug reactions, no interference with body functions); unlikely to interact with any other drugs or foodstuffs; spontaneously eliminated; stable chemically and microbiologically; readily formulated into an easily taken form; and inexpensive.

Sadly, there is no *ideal drug*, whether natural product or synthetic. It has been said that any substance powerful enough to be useful is also powerful enough to do some harm. The decision to prescribe, administer or take a drug requires a risk–benefit analysis based on the best information available: Do the likely therapeutic benefits (efficacy) outweigh the possible harmful effects (toxicity)?

Physical aspects of drugs

In terms of their physical state, drugs may be solids, liquids or gases. Most are solids at room temperature, but some are liquids in the pure state, such as nicotine, halothane (a general anaesthetic) and ethanol, and some are gases, especially general anaesthetics such as nitrous oxide.

Chemical aspects of drugs

Inorganic/organic

Whether found naturally in plants, animals, minerals or microorganisms, or synthesised in a laboratory, all drugs are chemicals of one sort or another. They may be inorganic (do not contain carbon) molecules such as calcium salts used to prevent and treat osteoporosis, or iodine and iron used to prevent mineral deficiencies. Most drugs, however, are organic molecules; that is, they contain carbon in their structures. All the major classes of organic compounds, including hydrocarbons, proteins, lipids, carbohydrates, nucleic acids and steroids, are represented in pharmacopoeias (Fig 1.3, later). Many drug molecules are acids or bases, which is important not only for their taste and irritant effects but also for how the drugs move across membranes and are affected by metabolism and excretion (pharmacokinetics – see Ch 5).

Molecular size

The sizes of drug molecules can also vary enormously, ranging from tiny lithium, the third-lightest element with an atomic mass of about 7, used as a specific antimanic agent, through to proteins such as insulin (molecular mass 5808 daltons) and erythropoietin (molecular mass 34 kilodaltons). Most drugs are in a more intermediate size range, with molecular weights (relative molecular masses) of between 100 and 1000. For example, aspirin has a molecular weight of 180, testosterone (a steroid hormone) 288, digoxin (a cardiac glycoside) 781 and ciclosporin (an immunosuppressant with a cyclic polypeptide structure) 1203. The size and nature of the molecule have important implications: proteins taken orally would be digested in the gut, so they must be administered by injection; large molecules generally will not readily pass through cell membranes and may need to be administered directly to their site of action.

A brief history of pharmacology

Medicines in antiquity and pre-scientific eras

For many thousands of years and in all civilisations, people have searched for substances to prevent, treat and cure disease. Discovery of safe drugs presumably developed by trial and error, with many fatalities and adverse effects. Archaeological diggings show that Stone Age people used opium poppies (Ch 12) and Inca civilisations used cocaine (Ch 11). Artefacts discovered in the ruins of Pompeii indicate that first-century Romans used pills and potions, including plant materials (poppy, henbane, *Artemisia*, cannabis) and minerals. The timeline in Table 1.2 summarises the history of medicine and major drug discoveries, and Fig 1.1 shows portraits of four famous people from medical history.

TABLE 1.2 Timeline of medical history and major drug discoveries

TIME PERIOD	COMMENTS
3000–1500 BC	Sumerian civilisation: prescriptions inscribed on clay tablets; vegetable and mineral drugs prepared in milk, beer and wine; supernatural healing rituals carried out by healers and shamans. Egyptian period: diseases believed caused by evil spirits in the body; Imhotep, the god of medicine, and Isis and Horus, gods of pharmacy, worshipped. The Ebers Papyrus, from about 1500 BC, described formulations of more than 700 drugs from plant, mineral and animal sources. Chinese medicine dating back beyond 2000 BC included use of poisons and antidotes, acupuncture, diets and moxibustion (burning of incense herbs for heating skin); medicines included ephedra (ephedrine) for asthma and seaweeds (iodine) for goitre. Ancient Indian (Ayurvedic) medicine described many surgical practices and more than 1000 natural drugs, including wine (alcohol) and hemp (marijuana) for pain relief.
1100–146 BC	Ancient Greek civilisation: the god Asclepius considered the principal god of healing, with his wife Epione soothing pain, and daughters Hygeia helping prevent disease and Panacea representing treatment (hence the phrase 'a panacea for all ills'). Hippocrates, a Greek physician, is 'the father of medicine': emphasis on humours and doctrine of opposites.

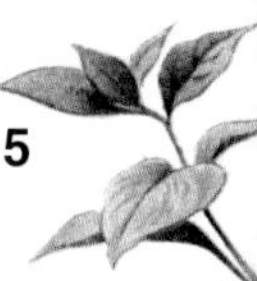

TABLE 1.2 Timeline of medical history and major drug discoveries—cont'd	
100 BC – AD 400	Roman Empire: medicine based on Greek traditions of herbal remedies and healing gods. Excellent public health measures introduced: safe water supplies and sanitation. Folk remedies included wound dressings of wine, vinegar, eggs, honey, worms and pig dung. Ephedra (ephedrine, a sympathomimetic agent) was used for asthma, cough and haemorrhage. Dioscorides' textbook *De Materia Medica* documented use of more than 600 medicinal plants and minerals including analgesics, antiseptics, emetics and laxatives; translated into Latin, Arabic and Persian. Indian surgeon wrote the *Sushruta Samhita*, the classic text of Ayurvedic medicine. Celsus described four cardinal signs of inflammation and stressed the importance of moderation, exercise, knowledge of anatomy and prevention of infection and haemorrhage.
2nd century	Galen, Greek physician/surgeon/druggist: pharmacy based on 'simples' and complex mixtures now called galenicals (see prescription A in Fig 2.4).
5th–11th centuries	Dark Ages in Europe: herbal medicine, folklore, magic, religion, bleeding, surgery and cosmology interwoven and practised in monasteries. Learning carried out in Latin; libraries held Greek, Roman and Arabic medical texts. In some countries, women allowed to practise medicine and midwifery. Meanwhile in Arabia, China and India, medicine and herbal pharmacy developed.
3rd–15th centuries	Golden Age of Islamic medicine: folk medicines included camphor, henna, syrup, aloes, amber and musk; first set of drug standards formulated. Classic Greek medical works translated into Arabic; an extensive library collected in Baghdad. Persian physician Avicenna now revered as 'the father of clinical pharmacology'. Great contribution of Islamic medicine: establishment of teaching hospitals and medical libraries such as in Baghdad, Cairo and Damascus; medical education has depended ever since on this style of training.
12th–14th centuries	Mediaeval period: in Europe, medical schools developed in Salerno, Bologna and Montpellier; pharmacy declared to be separate from medicine; apothecaries documented uses of herbs and spices; alchemists pursued the 'elixir of life'. The Black Death (plague) killed more than 25 million people in Europe. Victims of battle wounds usually succumbed to infection, haemorrhage and shock or pain. Hypnotic (sleep-inducing) and analgesic (pain-relieving) effects of the herbs poppy, henbane and mandrake known and valued.
14th–17th centuries	Renaissance in Europe: rebirth of interest in arts, sciences, politics, economics and medicine. Vesalius (anatomist), Gerard and Culpepper (herbalists) revolutionised medical knowledge. In the Ming dynasty in China, Li Shizhen documented Chinese medical knowledge in his compendium *Bencao Gangmu*, still the basis for traditional Chinese medicine. Paracelsus (1493–1541), Swiss alchemist and pharmacologist, denounced 'humoral pathology', substituted theory that diseases could be combated with specific remedies, and reduced prevalent overdosing. Infectious diseases, including measles and smallpox, spread from Europe to the 'New World'. Important pharmacological discoveries included: ♦ treating gout with colchicum (colchicine) and restriction of wine intake ♦ treating malaria with 'Jesuit's bark' (cinchona, containing quinine) ♦ preventing scurvy (vitamin C deficiency) with oranges and lemons ♦ using willow bark (salicylates) to treat fever, and foxglove (digitalis) to treat 'dropsy' (oedema) ♦ using extracts of opium, mandrake and hemlock in wine to relieve pain and to allow surgical procedures, and henbane (hyoscyamus, containing hyoscine) for inducing forgetfulness. Valerius Cordus (a German physician; 1515–1544) compiled the first pharmacopoeia (reference text with standard formulae and recipes); followed by the London Pharmacopoeia (1618), the French Codex (1818), and the pharmacopoeias of the United States (1820), Britain (1864) and Germany (1872).
18th–19th centuries	Rational medicine replacing trial-and-error empiricism. Deliberate clinical testing of drugs for their actions was carried out; studies of dose–response relationships led to safer use of drugs. Active constituents of plants isolated: first morphine (1804), followed by quinine, atropine and codeine; digitalis plant shown to be source of cardiac glycosides (digoxin, digitoxin); coca bark shown to contain a useful local anaesthetic, cocaine, purified and used in eye surgery; safer synthetic analogues soon developed. Anaesthetic gas nitrous oxide and volatile liquids ether and chloroform used in surgery, dentistry and obstetrics, providing first safe, painless surgery. Vaccinations developed for smallpox, diphtheria and rabies. Public health measures and quarantines imposed. Nursing developed as a profession. X-rays discovered. Advances in chemistry, especially coal-tar (organic) chemistry, allowed development of hypnotics and sedatives such as chloral hydrate, analgesics (including aspirin) and antiseptics such as carbolic acid.
20th century	Application of organic and synthetic chemistry, and biostatistics, to drug discovery; the first 'magic bullet': salvarsan against syphilis; receptor theories developed.
1920s	Insulin isolated (first protein to have chemical structure identified), the most important discovery for treatment of diabetes mellitus; penicillin discovered.
1930s–1940s	First safe oral antimicrobials: sulfonamides, penicillins and streptomycin developed. Use of muscle relaxants with general anaesthetics, making major surgery safer. Chemical warfare agents such as mustard gas led to 'nitrogen mustard' anticancer drugs. Cortisone, the hormone from the adrenal cortex, identified and synthetically prepared.
1940s–1950s	Autonomic pharmacology studies, structure–activity relationships on α- and β-receptors. DNA shown to be carrier of genetic information. First (modern) **randomised controlled clinical trial** (RCCT) (streptomycin against tuberculosis). World Health Organization (WHO) set up.
1950s	Chlorpromazine becomes the first effective antipsychotic drug to specifically treat schizophrenia. Structure of DNA determined, and understanding of molecular genetics expanded rapidly. Oral contraceptives developed – similar to natural estrogen and progesterone hormones, revolutionising family planning. Poliovirus vaccines eliminate deaths and paralysis from polio epidemics. First successful organ transplant.
1960s	Declaration of Helsinki prescribed ethical conduct of human medical research. Levodopa used to treat Parkinson's disease; immunosuppressants made organ transplantation feasible; treatment of hypertension with thiazide diuretics and β-blockers helped prevent strokes; cytotoxic agents (alkylating agents, antimetabolites and antibiotics) developed to treat cancers. Thalidomide disaster, with thousands of infants born with severe malformations, led to tightening of regulations for testing new drugs.

Continued

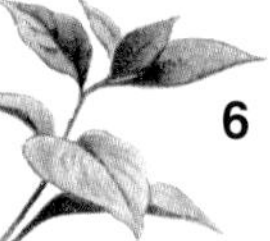

TABLE 1.2 Timeline of medical history and major drug discoveries—cont'd

1970s	Recombinant DNA technologies and monoclonal antibodies developed. Antivirals developed for prophylaxis and treatment of viral diseases. Childhood leukaemia treated successfully with cytotoxics and steroids. Ovulatory stimulants used in in-vitro fertilisation. Drug delivery methods and prodrug strategies improved.
1980s–1990s	HIV identified as the cause of AIDS. New drugs for thrombolysis, reduction of cholesterol levels, inhibition of synthesis of angiotensin or prostaglandins, antiretroviral therapy of AIDS, and treatment of impotence; new antineoplastic agents for chemotherapy of cancers, inhaled corticosteroids for asthma, atypical antipsychotics for schizophrenia; refinement of treatment protocols. Smallpox eradicated worldwide. The Human Genome Project successfully determined sequence of nucleotide base pairs in human DNA; all the genes of the human genome identified and mapped (2003).
2000–present	Stem cell therapy developed. Application of combinatorial chemistry and high-throughput screening allows rapid testing of millions of possible drug molecules. Recent innovations include chiral versions of optically active drugs (e.g. levobupivacaine, escitalopram), genetically engineered molecules (insulin glargine), prostaglandin analogues for glaucoma (latanoprost, travoprost), thiazolidinediones and incretin enhancers for type 2 diabetes; and tyrosine kinase inhibitors (imatinib, sorafenib), monoclonal antibodies (trastuzumab, ipilimumab) and BRAF inhibitors (vemurafenib) in cancer chemotherapy.

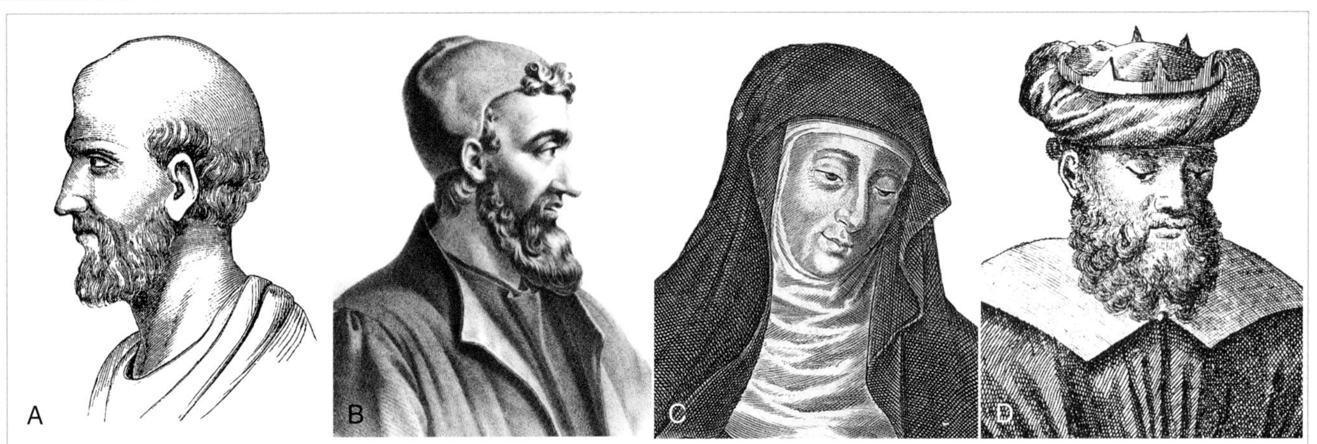

FIGURE 1.1 Famous people from medical history: **A** Hippocrates; **B** Galen; **C** Hildegard of Bingen; **D** Avicenna

A: Hippocrates (5th century BC, 'the father of medicine') taught that disease can be understood through careful diagnosis. He believed health was due to a balance of four 'humours' ebbing and flowing in the body (blood, phlegm, black bile and yellow bile); hence the related terms 'sanguine', 'phlegmatic', 'bilious', 'choleric' and 'melancholic'. His doctrine that opposites cure (cold treats fever, bleeding treats excess humours) was the basis of medicine for hundreds of years but eventually held up advances. Hippocrates still influences the practice of medicine, as in versions of the Hippocratic Oath proclaimed at many medical graduation ceremonies (CFB 2.9). **B:** Galen of Pergamon (2nd century) wrote voluminously on medical, scientific, philosophical, ethical and religious issues; he considered that bleeding (removal of large volumes of blood) was appropriate treatment for virtually all disorders. Galen was famous for his knowledge of drugs, both 'simples' (i.e. simple herbal or mineral remedies) and complex mixtures known as 'galenicals', including exotic herbs, amulets, excrement and antidotes. **C:** Hildegard of Bingen was a remarkable writer, composer, prophet, healer and abbess during the Middle Ages. Her books described the causes of many diseases and the medical and toxic properties of herbal, animal and mineral preparations. **D:** Avicenna (Abu-Ali Sina; Ibn Sina), the most famous ancient Persian physician, lived in central Asia and Persia around AD 980–1037. He was a 'man for all seasons' – physician, philosopher, astronomer, chemist, mathematician, poet, teacher. His most famous works, *The Book of Healing* and *The Canon of Medicine,* were standard medical textbooks for centuries, even in French medical schools. Avicenna is considered to be 'the father of clinical pharmacology', as he introduced systematic experimentation, quantification, randomised clinical trials and efficacy tests into the study of physiology and infectious diseases.

B Lithograph by Pierre Roche Vigneron, **C&D**: *Wellcome Library no. 4213i, CC BY 4.0.*

Into the 20th and 21st centuries: 'magic bullets'

Early in the 20th century, drugs commonly used in medicine were: morphine and codeine as analgesics; sodium bicarbonate and glycerine for gastrointestinal problems; sodium bromide as a sedative; sodium salicylate as an anti-inflammatory and antipyretic analgesic; and strychnine as a 'tonic'. During the 20th century, medicine made enormous advances, leading to therapeutic revolutions in all areas of medicine. Of 36 major events identified as the most significant in modern medicine from 1935 to 1999, at least half are directly due to developing effective drugs to treat previously life-threatening diseases (Le Fanu 2011).

As knowledge of chemistry, physiology, medicine and pharmacology developed, it was applied to the problem

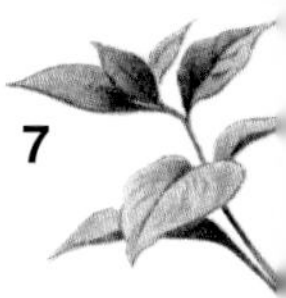

of finding drugs to treat specific conditions. The German chemist Paul Ehrlich, 'the father of chemotherapy', realised when working with synthetic dyes that the biological effect of a compound depends on its chemical composition. A major development was the production of safe, orally active synthetic antimicrobials (sulfonamides). In 1928, penicillin was discovered (by Alexander Fleming), and in the 1940s it was isolated and purified (by Howard Florey and Ernst Chain), revolutionising the treatment of microbial infections and leading to other antibiotics, such as streptomycin for tuberculosis.

These successes led to a search for the 'magic bullet' – the mythical goal of finding a specific drug to target a diseased tissue or cell while leaving all other tissues intact.

Advances in synthetic organic chemistry led to the establishment of large-scale chemical manufacturing plants to produce drugs. Structure–activity studies identified series of molecules with agonist or antagonist actions on many types of receptors. The importance of using a control group when testing drugs or other treatments was recognised, and the RCCT became the expected standard.

It is interesting to note that early in the 21st century most of the 'top 10 drugs' prescribed in developed countries are for lifestyle diseases, including statins for high cholesterol levels and calcium channel blockers and angiotensin-converting enzyme inhibitors for cardiovascular diseases (Tables 1.6 and 1.7, later).

The scientific revolution brought about by molecular biology techniques has enabled the identification and cloning of genes that code for therapeutically useful proteins, including monoclonal antibodies and receptors. Biochemical pathways in cell division are being elucidated, leading to new anticancer agents (Chs 32 and 33). Meta-analysis techniques have been developed (notably by Cochrane) to pool together and analyse results of clinical trials and medical research, and to evaluate scientific data in order to encourage implementation of evidence-based medicine.

KEY POINTS

Introduction to pharmacology

- Pharmacology is the study of drugs, which are substances used for their beneficial effects on living systems.
- People have searched for, been fascinated by, used and abused drugs throughout recorded history.
- Initially, useful natural compounds were discovered by trial and error; they were then studied for their medical actions and adverse effects.
- Drugs may be solids (most commonly), liquids or gases. Most are organic (carbon-containing) chemicals.

Drug discovery and development

The goal of the drug discovery and development process is to produce safe and effective therapeutic drugs. There are several ways in which potential therapeutic uses of chemicals – natural or synthetic – are determined, summarised as three steps: (1) understand the science, (2) unravel the story and (3) apply the technology. Drug discovery has been likened to the processes of evolution: a selection process with a high level of attrition and many influences affecting survival of the fittest. Recently, drug discovery has become more reliant on computational and artificial intelligence, accelerating the drug discovery process (Hinkson et al. 2020).

Where drugs come from

Drugs and biological products are derived from several main sources:

- microorganisms – for example, fungi used as sources of antibiotics (Fig 1.2A) and bacteria and yeasts genetically engineered to produce drugs such as human insulin
- plants – for example, *Atropa belladonna* (source of atropine), *Cannabis sativa* (marijuana), *Coffea arabica* (Fig 1.2B; coffee, caffeine), *Digitalis purpurea* (Fig 1.2C; digitalis), *Duboisia* species (hyoscine, nornicotine), *Eucalyptus* spp. (eucalyptus oil), *Papaver somniferum* (Fig 1.2D; opium, morphine[1])
- humans and other animals, from which drugs such as bovine insulin, human chorionic gonadotrophin and erythropoietin were or are obtained, sometimes by recombinant techniques
- minerals or mineral products – for example, iron, iodine and Epsom salts
- laboratories in which substances are synthesised, such as sulfonamides, β-blockers and antidepressants. Drugs may also be classed as semisynthetic when the starting material is a natural product, such as a plant steroid or microbial metabolite, which is then chemically altered to produce the desired drug molecule.

Development from natural or traditional remedies

For thousands of years, people have been trying natural products – animal, vegetable and mineral – to see if they are useful as foods or in treating disease (Table 1.3).

1 The isolation of the pure alkaloid morphine as the active pain-relieving constituent of opium poppies (in 1804) has been described as 'the single most important discovery in medicine', as it demonstrated that pharmacological activities of plants are due to the chemicals they contain.

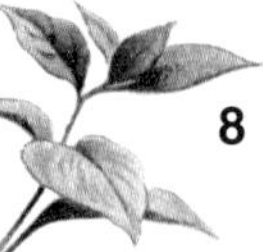

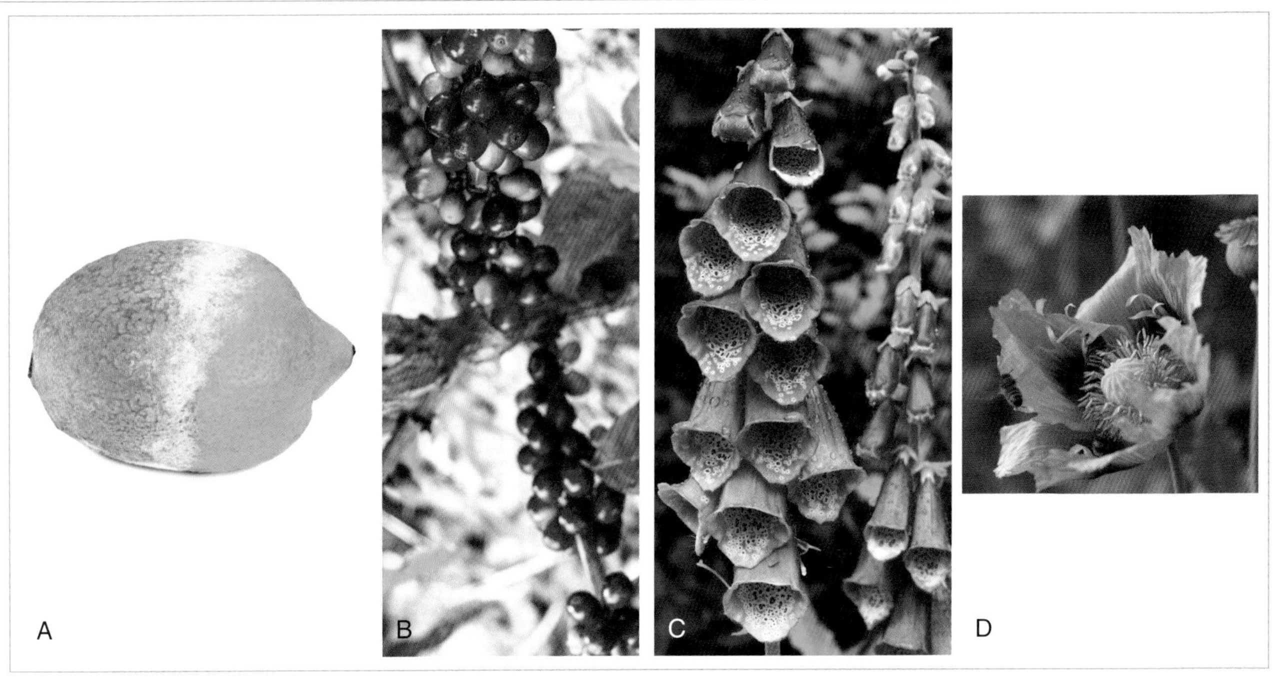

FIGURE 1.2 Natural sources of important drugs
A *Penicillium notatum* mould, source of penicillin; **B** *Coffea arabica*, source of caffeine (and coffee); **C** *Digitalis purpurea*, source of digoxin; **D** *Papaver somniferum*, source of morphine and codeine.
A–D: *iStockphoto/habari1; iStockphoto/kannika2013; iStockphoto/Petegar; iStockphoto/AtWaG*

TABLE 1.3 Some drugs from plants

DRUG	SOURCE	MAIN PHARMACOLOGICAL ACTIONS
Aromatic oils	For example, from eucalyptus, pine, mint	Decongestant, Rx common cold, mild antiseptics
Artemisinins	*Artemisia annua* (sagewort)	Antimalarial
Atropine	*Atropa belladonna* (deadly nightshade)	Antimuscarinic, premedication, Rx asthma
Bran	Indigestible vegetable fibre	Laxative, Rx constipation
Caffeine	*Coffea arabica* (coffee)	CNS stimulant, diuretic
Cocaine	*Erythroxylum coca*	CNS stimulant, local anaesthetic, addictive
Colchicine	*Colchicum autumnale* (crocus)	Anti-inflammatory, Rx gout
Coumarins	Sweet clover	Anticoagulants, prevent thrombosis
Digoxin	*Digitalis lanata* (woolly foxglove)	Cardiac glycoside, Rx heart failure
Ephedrine	*Ephedra sinica*	Sympathomimetic, Rx asthma
Ergot alkaloids (e.g. ergometrine)	Mould on *Claviceps* spp.	Oxytocic, Rx postpartum bleeding
Galantamine	*Galanthus nivalis* (snowdrop)	Anticholinesterase, used in neurological disorders and Alzheimer's disease
Hypericin	*Hypericum perforatum* (St John's wort)	Monoamine reuptake inhibitor, Rx depression
Ipecacuanha	Cephaelis root	Expectorant, emetic, Rx poisoning
Morphine	*Papaver somniferum* (opium poppy)	Analgesic, sedative, antidiarrhoeal, cough suppressant, addictive
Nicotine	*Nicotiana tabacum* (tobacco)	Vasoconstrictor, CNS stimulant, addictive
Paclitaxel	Yew tree bark	Antineoplastic, Rx cancer
Phytoestrogens	Clover, soybeans	Estrogenic, Rx menopausal symptoms
Pilocarpine	*Pilocarpus microphyllus*	Muscarinic agonist, Rx glaucoma
Quinine, quinidine	Cinchona bark	Antimalarial, Rx cardiac arrhythmias
Salicylates, including aspirin	*Salix* spp. (willow)	Anti-inflammatory, analgesic, antipyretic
Strychnine	*Strychnos nux-vomica*	CNS stimulant, convulsant
Vincristine	*Catharanthus roseus* (periwinkle plant)	Antineoplastic, Rx cancer

CNS = central nervous system; Rx = treatment of
Source: Evans (2009), Trease and Evans' Pharmacognosy, 16th edn [ch 6].

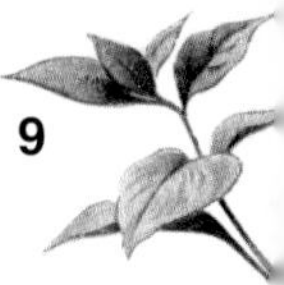

Natural products may be used as crude extracts, such as raw opium, tobacco leaves or herbal teas, or purified and/or synthesised and then formulated as pharmaceutical preparations, such as tablets, ointments and injections.

This is called the 'reefs and rainforests' route to new drugs, recognising that there are millions of natural chemicals in the environment to be identified and tested. As biodiversity is lost worldwide, we are losing the chance to discover novel drugs such as anticancer or antibiotic agents. (For example, the recent extinction of Australia's gastric-brooding frogs means we will now never know how the frog's eggs avoided digestion in the mother frog's stomach or being moved on into her small intestine – actions potentially useful in treating gastrointestinal tract disorders. Research into threatened bear species could elucidate their mechanisms for surviving months of hibernation without losing bone mass or dying of uraemia.) The Wellcome Trust in London has established the Millennium Seed Bank project at Kew Gardens to conserve and screen plants for possible future cures.[2]

Natural products not necessarily safer

There is a widely held belief that 'natural' products are safer than synthetic drugs, a belief encouraged by health-food and alternative therapy practitioners. A quick scan of naturally occurring substances such as arsenic, botulinum toxin, cantharidin, cocaine, cyanide, deadly nightshade, ipecacuanha, mercury, methanol, physostigmine, strychnine, thallium, tobacco and uranium shows that natural is not always good. It would be foolish to expect all natural products to be automatically safer than those synthesised in laboratories – or vice versa. Any drug's safety and quality must be tested and proved before it is approved for clinical use.

Active constituents of plant drugs

The leaves, roots, seeds and other parts of some plants may be dried, crushed, boiled and extracted or otherwise processed for use as medicine and, as such, are known as crude drugs or herbal remedies (Ch 3). Their therapeutic effects are produced by the chemical substances they contain. When the pharmacologically active constituents are separated, purified and quantified, the resulting substances usually have similar pharmacological actions to the crude drugs but are more potent (weight-for-weight), produce effects more reliably and are less likely to be affected by other constituents or contaminants in the crude preparations. Indeed, the herbal antidepressant St John's wort has been shown to have a similar mechanism of action – and hence similar therapeutic and adverse effects – as the synthetic selective serotonin reuptake inhibitors such as fluoxetine.

Some types of pharmacologically active molecules found in plants, grouped according to their chemical properties, are alkaloids, glycosides, steroids, hydrocarbons, alcohols/phenols, proteins, gums and oils (Table 1.4). Note that the groups are not mutually exclusive – there can be phenolic alkaloids, glycoproteins and phenolic glycosides. Fig 1.3 shows the chemical formulae of some drugs that are extracted from plant sources.

Serendipity (sheer good luck)

Although luck plays a part in some drug discoveries – such as Fleming's bacterial culture plate becoming contaminated with a growth of the fungus *Penicillium notatum*, which inhibited bacterial growth – it usually takes lateral thinking (e.g. questioning why bacteria were inhibited near the fungus), intelligence and years of hard work (extracting the natural antibacterial agent, determining its structure and developing methods of producing enough penicillin to treat people with bacterial infections) to exploit the lucky find.

Other examples of serendipity in pharmacological discovery are the findings that people treated with the first safe synthetic oral antibacterial agents, sulfonamides, had a lowering in their blood glucose levels, which led to sulfonylurea oral hypoglycaemic agents; and that hypertensive people treated with the vasodilator minoxidil tended to grow more hair. The drug is now used mainly as a hair restorer.

Chemical plus pharmacological studies

As chemical techniques developed in the 19th and 20th centuries, the structures of pharmacologically active substances could be determined and similar substances synthesised, then tested for activity. These **structure–activity studies** led to many drug groups:

- The second- and third-generation penicillins were modelled on the first penicillin.
- All the sympathomimetic amines were initially noradrenaline 'look-alikes': studies of *Ephedra sinica*, long known in traditional Chinese medicine to be useful in respiratory conditions (asthma), led to the purification of the active ingredient ephedrine, then to synthesis of the related β-receptor-activating antiasthma drugs isoprenaline and salbutamol (with fewer cardiovascular adverse reactions).
- β-blockers, such as propranolol and later atenolol, were designed to act as ligands at the receptor without activating it, and proved useful in cardiovascular diseases. (Chemical structures of β-receptor ligands are shown in Fig 1.4.)

2 There are many wonderful pharmaceutical gardens worth visiting, including the Jardin des Plantes de Montpellier in southern France, established in 1593, and the Chelsea Physic Garden (Garden of Medicinal Plants) in London, founded in 1673 as the Apothecaries' Garden.

TABLE 1.4 Pharmacologically active constituents of plant drugs

CHEMICAL CLASS AND STRUCTURE	CHARACTERISTICS	EXAMPLES
Alkaloids ♦ Organic nitrogen-containing compounds that are alkaline and usually bitter-tasting ♦ The nitrogen atom is usually in a heterocyclic ring of carbon atoms (Fig 1.3A)	♦ Many alkaloid drugs are amines, so their names often end in the suffix '-ine' ♦ Combined as salts to make them more soluble (e.g. morphine sulfate) ♦ Plants may have evolved the ability to synthesise bitter alkaloids as a defence against herbivorous animals	♦ Analgesics morphine (Fig 1.3A),* cocaine and codeine ♦ Antiasthma drugs ephedrine, theophylline and atropine ♦ Vinca alkaloids (anticancer) ♦ Alkaloids used in gout (colchicine), malaria (quinine) and obstetrics (ergot alkaloids) ♦ 'Social' drugs: nicotine and caffeine
Carbohydrates ♦ Organic compounds of carbon, hydrogen and oxygen	♦ Sugars are a source of energy ♦ Gums and mucilages are carbohydrate plant exudates; when water is added, some will swell and form a gelatinous mass, a useful laxative effect ♦ Gums are also used to soothe irritated skin and mucous membranes and may be a rich source of starch	♦ Sugars such as glucose ♦ Starches and fibres such as cellulose and inulin, a fructose–furanose polysaccharide (Fig 1.3B) used in kidney function tests (not to be confused with insulin, a protein from the pancreas) ♦ Gelling agents such as agar, and gums such as tragacanth and *Aloe vera* products (CFB 41.2)
Glycosides ♦ Particular type of carbohydrate that, on hydrolysis, yields a sugar plus one or more additional active substances	♦ The sugar part is believed to increase the solubility, absorption, permeability and cellular distribution of the glycoside	♦ Digoxin (Fig 1.3C), found in *Digitalis* (foxglove) plants; known as a cardiac glycoside because of its stimulant actions on the heart ♦ Glycosides present in oleanders and some other Australian plants are responsible for their poisonous nature ♦ Cane toads also contain cardioactive glycosides
Hydrocarbons ♦ Organic molecules consisting entirely of hydrogen and carbon ♦ May be straight-chain or aromatic (containing benzene rings)	♦ Derivatives such as organic alcohols and esters contribute the fragrances to many plants and perfumes ♦ Commonly used by drug companies and pharmacies when preparing topical formulations of drugs, especially creams and ointments	♦ Fats and waxes ♦ Oils such as castor, olive and coconut oil ♦ Fatty acids, prostaglandins and balsams
Oils ♦ A subgroup of hydrocarbons ♦ May be terpene-type compounds ♦ May contain many types of functional groups including ketones, phenols, alcohols, esters and aldehydes	♦ Viscous liquids high in hydrocarbon content ♦ Often flammable and immiscible with water and aqueous solvents ♦ Frequently used as flavouring agents, in perfumery, in chemical industries and as antiseptics ♦ A fixed oil dropped onto filter paper will leave a greasy stain, whereas a volatile oil (which evaporates) will not	♦ Eucalyptus, peppermint and clove oils are volatile oils used in medicine ♦ Castor oil (mainly composed of ricinoleic acid, Fig 1.3D) and olive oil are fixed oils ♦ Australian Myrtaceae family and *Melaleuca* genus plants contain many fragrant and useful oils, including eucalyptus and tea-tree oils
Phenols ♦ Phenols contain a benzene ring with a hydroxyl substituent	♦ Phenols are a specialised type of alcohol, a compound containing a hydroxyl group, –OH	♦ Salicylates, including aspirin-like compounds and flavouring agents (e.g. vanillin) ♦ Isoflavones, including phytoestrogens ♦ Coumarins, including the anticoagulant dicoumarol (Fig 1.3E) ♦ Cannabinols from marijuana ♦ Hypericin, from St John's wort, used in depression (Fig 1.3E)
Tannins ♦ A specialised type of phenol	♦ Astringent plant phenolics have the ability to tan hides (animal skins) by precipitating proteins ♦ Common plant constituents, especially in bark, accounting for some of the brown colour in swamps and rivers and in cups of tea	♦ In Australian native medicine, kino, the gum exuded from eucalyptus trees, was an important source of tannins, which were used to treat diarrhoea, haemorrhages and throat infections
Isoprenes, terpenes and steroids ♦ Terpenes are 10-carbon molecules built up from small 5-carbon building blocks called isoprenes ♦ Plant steroids are also synthesised naturally from isoprene sub-units	♦ Plant steroids, with their characteristic 4-ring structures, are used as the starting material for the production of many hormone drugs (Fig 28.2) ♦ The plant sterol diosgenin, from the *Dioscorea* species, has been used in the synthesis of estrogenic hormones	♦ Carotenoids such as β-carotene and vitamin A ♦ Salicylate analgesics including aspirin (acetylsalicylic acid) ♦ Pyrethrins (insecticides) ♦ Menthol (Fig 1.3F), camphor and thymol, aromatic compounds used in respiratory medicine ♦ Gossypol, a Chinese male contraceptive agent (Fig 1.3F)

* In Tasmania and Victoria, the opium poppy *Papaver somniferum* is grown and harvested for production of opium alkaloids, including morphine and codeine.

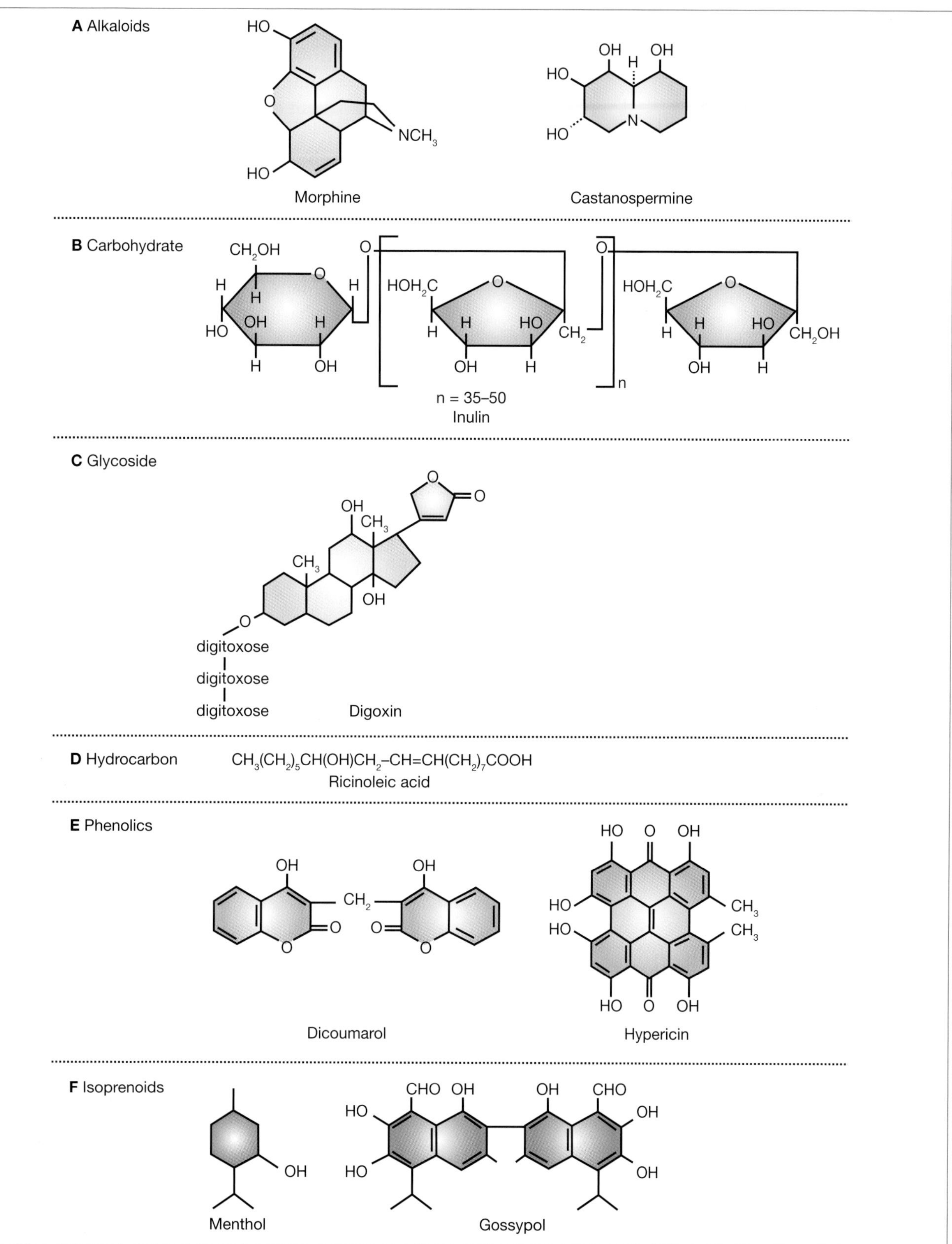

FIGURE 1.3 Chemical structures of some active drugs derived from plant sources

A Alkaloids: morphine and castanospermine. **B** A carbohydrate: inulin. **C** A glycoside: digoxin. **D** A hydrocarbon: ricinoleic acid. **E** Phenolics: dicoumarol and hypericin.* **F** Isoprenoids: menthol and gossypol.

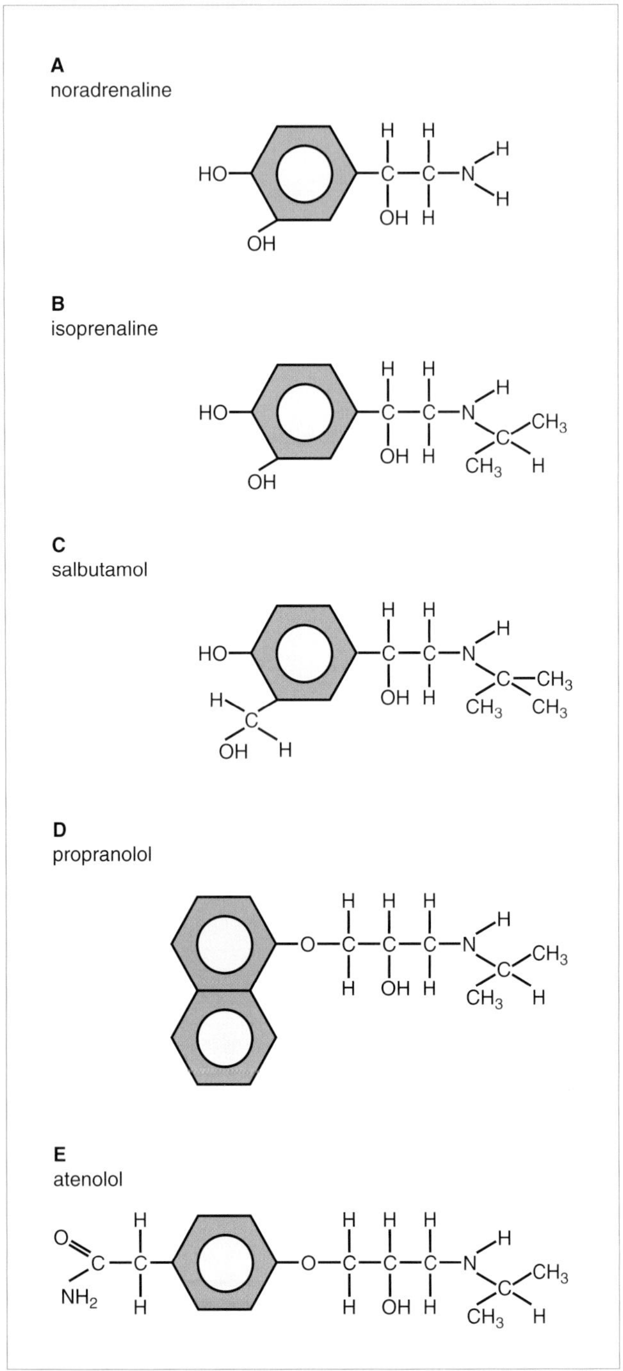

A
noradrenaline

B
isoprenaline

C
salbutamol

D
propranolol

E
atenolol

FIGURE 1.4 Structure–activity relationships for some drugs binding to adrenoceptors
A The sympathetic neurotransmitter noradrenaline.
B Isoprenaline, a non-selective β-adrenoceptor agonist.
C Salbutamol, a selective β_2-adrenoceptor agonist. **D** Propranolol, a non-selective β-adrenoceptor antagonist. **E** Atenolol, a selective β_1-adrenoceptor antagonist with less likelihood of causing asthma. Increasing the 'bulkiness' of the substituents at the catechol end (two adjacent –OH groups) or the amine end ($-NH_2$) may select for ligand-binding affinity or agonist/antagonist activity at specific receptors.

Research carried out by pharmacologists, biochemists and chemists in universities and research institutes may lead to the discovery of new drugs. The pharmaceutical industry monitors such research via the scientific literature, patent applications and scientific conferences.

Active metabolites of existing drugs

Sometimes drugs are found to be more active after metabolism in the body and so the metabolites are tested. Paracetamol is one of the metabolites of phenacetin, an early antipyretic analgesic agent, and is much safer than phenacetin. Many of the benzodiazepine antianxiety agents have pharmacologically active metabolites, some of which are drugs in their own right.

Rational molecular design

Structure–activity studies can predict the shape of the active site of a receptor and lead to the design of drugs that may be agonists or antagonists at that receptor. The early antihistamines were modelled on the histamine molecule. Subsequent brilliant pharmacology by Sir James Black[3] led to the discovery of histamine H_2-receptors and the development of specific H_2-antagonists, revolutionising the treatment of peptic ulcer (Fig 27.3).

Computer-aided design

Drug receptors, enzymes, ion channels and transporters are no longer simply 'black boxes' referred to by pharmacologists wishing to explain (or pretend that they understand) drug mechanisms; many are proteins with known amino acid sequences and tertiary structures (three-dimensional shapes), able to be cloned. Computer modelling of their active sites allows testing of chemicals for virtual binding affinity. Using such techniques, angiotensin-converting enzyme (ACE) inhibitors were designed for use in hypertension, dopa-decarboxylase inhibitors for administration with levodopa in Parkinson's disease, the anti-flu drug zanamivir to inactivate the flu virus and potential anticancer drugs to inhibit steps in the pathways of macromolecular synthesis.

Combinatorial chemistry ('combichem') techniques make it possible for millions of new molecules to be synthesised, either actually or virtually. This may involve systematic and repetitive use of commercially available chemical reagents to synthesise 'libraries' of new chemical compounds, preferably small molecules, which are then screened for activities on proteins, receptors, enzymes and transporters.

3 Black, a Scottish pharmacologist, was awarded the Nobel Prize in Medicine in 1988 for his work on 'important principles of drug treatment', discovering β-blockers and H_2-antagonists; when surprised to hear of his award, he quipped: 'I wish I had my beta-blockers handy!'

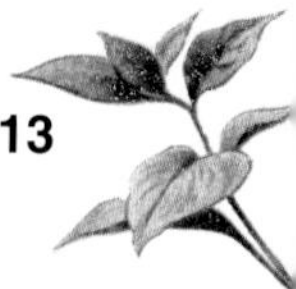

Standardisation of drugs

Formulations of drugs obtained from natural sources may fluctuate in strength, depending on how extracts are harvested and purified. Because accurate dosage and the reliability of drug effects depend on uniformity of strength and purity, **standardisation** (bringing the preparation to a specified concentration or quality, like the model) and publication of standards are necessary.

Drug standards in Australia and New Zealand

The main standards for drugs in Australia are those published in the *Martindale*, *British Pharmacopoeia*[4] and the *Australian Pharmaceutical Formulary* (APF; see later under 'Drug information sources'). The BP gives detailed, legally accepted standards for hundreds of drugs and herbal products, with chemical information and the approved formulations containing the substance. It lists criteria for purity; chemical methods for identification and assay (measurement); tests and maximum levels allowed for impurities; and storage conditions. Preparations meeting these standards are referred to as the BP preparation.

The APF is a reference book for **pharmacists** that helps promote quality use of medicines. It contains evidence-based information on medicine and pharmacy-specific topics – for example, dispensing, counselling and therapeutic management. It also contains key 'recipes' for commonly made formulations by pharmacists (i.e. extemporaneously prepared medicines). For example, Calamine Lotion APF is one 'recipe'. It lists the required quantity of individual ingredients (active and excipient), gives the method for preparation of the lotion and describes the use of the formulation. The New Zealand Formulary (NZF) is more like the Australian Medicines Handbook (AMH), with detailed information about drugs (see later under 'Drug information sources').

Assays

The technique, either chemical or biological, by which the strength and purity of a drug are measured is known as an **assay**; if available, a chemical method is used. For some drugs, either the **active ingredients** have not been completely identified or there are no available chemical methods. The pharmacological activity of such tissue extracts or pharmaceutical formulations may be standardised by biological methods, or **bioassay**.

4 The 'BP', as it is fondly known by generations of pharmacy students and pharmacists.

Bioassays

Bioassays are typically performed by determining the amount of a preparation required to produce a defined effect on a suitable living tissue (or animal, cell suspension, enzyme, microorganism, etc.) and then comparing the response to that produced by a standard preparation in the same bioassay system. Examples of early bioassays were for the potency of a sample of insulin measured by its ability to lower the blood glucose levels of rabbits, or for the strength of digoxin preparations assayed by their effects on contractions of isolated cardiac muscle tissue.

Bioassays are especially applicable to:

- substances that are poorly defined chemically
- mixtures containing chemically very similar substances (e.g. optical isomers, of which only one is active)
- highly active substances, especially endogenous mediators, present in very small amounts
- testing drugs in animals to predict effects in humans.

The bioassay method may be in vitro (in glass) – for example, using a suspension of an enzyme, cell or tissue culture, a microbiological culture, a standard preparation of an antibody or an isolated organ or tissue; or in vivo (in the living organism) – for example, testing the effect of a drug on blood pressure or behaviour.[5] Some drug actions are virtually impossible to test in animals either in vitro or in vivo, particularly the effects of CNS-active agents on mood, perception and thought processes. **Clinical trials** (see 'Clinical trials of drugs', later) are essentially bioassays in humans: the new drug (unknown) is tested against the best currently available therapy (standard drug or placebo) and compared for safety and efficacy.

The design of bioassays usually involves comparing two preparations and constructing log dose–response curves. If the substances act by similar mechanisms, the curves will be roughly parallel in their mid-sections and so the potency ratio can be determined, allowing the strength of the unknown to be calculated compared to the known standard (Fig 4.7). Because of biological variability, there may be variations in results quoting the absolute amount of biologically active material. Bioassays are not used as frequently as previously because techniques such as radioimmunoassay (itself a type of bioassay) and high-performance liquid chromatography have allowed very low levels of chemicals to be measured accurately without using animals.

5 There is currently a worldwide dearth of pharmacologists with the skills necessary to carry out many experimental methods in medical research or to train new generations of students in these techniques. This has come about largely because of the decrease in the number of practical classes held in pharmacology courses and the replacement of animal experiments with computer-modelled 'practicals'. In-vivo testing, however, is vital for the analysis of drug actions and development of new drugs–see discussion in Chapter 2 under 'Ethical aspects of pharmacotherapy'.

Bioassays in the BP

The *BP 2020* still gives several standard methods for bioassays, including for blood pressure–lowering substances, blood coagulation factors, anticoagulants, interferons, vaccines, antibiotics, endotoxins and pyrogens (substances that cause fever), plus tests for acute toxicity, microbiological sterility or contamination, including examination of herbal products.

Isolated organ experiments

In these pharmacological experiments, a small piece of animal tissue (e.g. a length of intestinal smooth muscle) or an entire organ (e.g. a heart) is 'isolated' from the animal's body and kept alive in warmed, oxygenated physiological saline solution in an organ bath, set up so that responses of the tissue (e.g. contractions of muscle, beats of the heart) can be monitored following administration of a drug solution into the organ bath. The classic experiment is the isolated guinea pig ileum preparation, in which a short strip of gastrointestinal tract smooth muscle responds (contracts) to stimulation by various neurotransmitters and other endogenous mediators; a great deal of classical pharmacology can be demonstrated and understood using this simple technique.

The use of isolated tissues for assaying responses reached a sophisticated level in the classic experiments of Sir John Vane at the Royal College of Surgeons in London in the 1960s. A set of five organ baths was set up in vertical series such that the physiological saline solution (or blood from an anaesthetised animal) from the top bath superfused (flowed down over) the next bath, and so on down the cascade. Small samples of gastrointestinal tract smooth muscle from four different species were set up in the baths, and the pattern of contraction or relaxation responses to seven endogenous mediators, including noradrenaline, bradykinin, prostaglandins and antidiuretic hormone, was studied. Vane discovered the mechanism of action of aspirin and other non-steroidal anti-inflammatory drugs, namely inhibition of the synthesis of prostaglandins; for this he was subsequently awarded the 1982 Nobel Prize for Medicine (and knighted by the Queen).

International units of activity

The strength of extracts of natural substances for which the purity is not 100% cannot be expressed in absolute terms such as grams or milligrams because the whole weight is not due to a single active ingredient. Such preparations are assayed biologically, and a unit of pharmacological activity is defined. A particular preparation – for example, of a hormone, enzyme, vitamin, vaccine, blood product or plant alkaloid – is designated by the WHO Expert Committee on Biological Standardization as the International Standard preparation, against which other national standard preparations are assayed. In Australia, for example, the Commonwealth Serum Laboratories (CSL) in Melbourne maintained the national standard for insulin, and all CSL insulin preparations were compared to it. The strengths of preparations are expressed in terms of International Units of Activity (IU)[6] measured in the particular bioassay (CFB 30.4), allowing comparison of preparations in terms of their biological efficacies.

Statistical methods in bioassays

It is well recognised that biological parameters, such as heights of adults, vary within a wide range, and the mean can be calculated as an average value. Consequently, biological experiments need to be repeated many times to get a mean result, and statistical tests can be applied to determine how likely this is to be the 'true value'. Values may be found to be normally distributed, and when plotted as a frequency distribution will assume a 'normal' bell-shaped curve.

Similarly, it can be expected that responses to a dose of a drug will also vary about a mean value. Variations may be due to many causes, especially errors in measurement and inherent biological variability both within and between individuals. In bioassays the same dose (or concentration) repeated several times may therefore give differing responses; likewise, the dose required to give the same response varies. Variability can be partly reduced by refining methods and using a very homogeneous population of animals or very similar subjects; however, this reduces the wide applicability of the results.

Statistical methods must then be applied to deal with random variations and to extrapolate from the sample mean to the population; such techniques are the province of biostatistics, rather than pharmacology. In the pharmacological context, statistical methods[7] are typically applied to bioassays studying dose–response relationships, cause–effect correlations, differences between groups of subjects treated differently and the results of clinical trials. Usually a 'null hypothesis' is defined (i.e. that there is no statistically significant difference between the groups being studied), and when results are analysed the null hypothesis is either accepted or rejected. The probability level (p) at which the results are accepted as being due to a real difference rather than occurring by chance is

6 The abbreviation IU may become confusing because the U may be misread as a V (IV: intravenous); some authorities recommend that the term 'unit' be written in full.

7 The first medical statistician credited with applying rigorous mathematical methods in the study of responses to drugs, and developing standard clinical trial methodologies, was Professor Austin Bradford Hill in the Medical Statistics Department of the London School of Hygiene and Tropical Medicine in the 1950s. Hill proved that two drugs together, streptomycin and para-aminosalicylic acid, given over a period of several months, markedly improved patients with tuberculosis and reduced development of microbial resistance to the antibiotic. And in an epidemiological study of lung cancer, by separating subjects into groups based on their smoking habits, Hill demonstrated conclusively that the more cigarettes people smoked, the greater their risk of lung cancer.

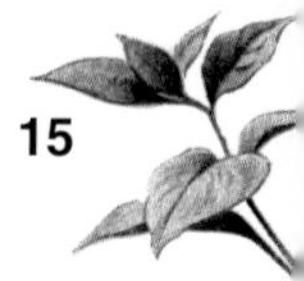

usually set at 0.05; that is, there is only a 5% likelihood (1 in 20 chance) that the results could have occurred by chance.

Typical statistical tests employed are either parametric (assuming a normal distribution of results), such as independent or paired *t*-test, analysis of variance; or non-parametric (when normal distribution cannot be assumed, i.e. the data is skewed) – for example, Mann–Whitney U test, or a chi-squared test.

Drug development

Development of new drugs is regulated by government legislation and administered by government authorities such as the Therapeutic Goods Administration (TGA) in Australia, the Ministry of Health and Medsafe in New Zealand and the Food and Drug Administration in the United States (Ch 2). Regulation protects consumers so that only safe and effective drugs are approved and protects sponsoring drug companies for their investment in terms of intellectual property and patents.

The pharmaceutical industry

The pharmaceutical industry is constantly searching for potential new drugs. The major markets are the United States, Europe, Japan, China and India; Australia accounts for only 1–2% of world sales of pharmaceuticals.

Stages of drug development

Drug development has traditionally been described as occurring in several clearly defined phases, involving multidisciplinary teams:

- the new idea or hypothesis – routes to drug discovery include selection of a target, new hypothesis for disease causation, ideas for new molecules, discovery of new natural products, optimisation of lead compounds, and research with new molecular biology, genetic engineering and formulation technologies
- design, purification or synthesis of the new molecule, from various sources (described above under 'Where drugs come from')
- screening new compounds for useful pharmacological activities or possible toxic effects – screening may be broad, to detect all actions, or specific, for affinity for a particular receptor, transporter or enzyme; high-throughput screening allows millions of compounds to be run through automated initial screens; these three stages may take between 2 and 5 years
- preclinical pharmacology – this includes in-vitro and in-vivo studies: pharmacodynamic actions and pharmacokinetic aspects (the fate of the molecule or compound in the body, including susceptibility to phases of metabolism) are studied usually in at least three mammalian species, including non-human primate species
- toxicology studies (adverse effects) – these include acute toxicity, long-term toxicity (chronic effects and effects on reproduction) and tests for mutagenicity and carcinogenicity; requirements depend on anticipated exposure and clinical use, whether acute or chronic
- pharmaceutical formulation and manufacturing – scale-up of the synthetic pathway, including stability tests and assay methods; these stages may take 1–2 years
- an application to drug-regulating authorities for approval to undertake a trial in humans, details of the molecule and its formulation, manufacturing information – all results of non-clinical studies, proposed clinical protocols, the sites for conduct of the study, names of personnel in the clinical trial team and approval from an ethics committee are submitted (note that in Australia many clinical trials are undertaken with approval from an ethics committee and notification to the TGA)
- clinical trials – if the drug appears to be safe, effective and worth testing, it will go to clinical trial while being closely monitored by the investigators and by the sponsor company or a clinical research organisation contracted by the sponsor (progress must be reported regularly to the national regulatory authority, which may sometimes undertake inspections; the first three phases of a clinical trial may take 5–7 years)
- registration – depending on the results of the full clinical trial program, the sponsors may apply for registration of the drug and approval to market it for clinical use
- ongoing post-marketing studies – these follow up the drug, monitoring its effects and interactions in the wider community for longer periods.

The costs in time, money and effort

The development of a drug takes a prodigious amount of money, effort and time, and it is a high-stakes, long-term, risky business. Drug development from idea to market typically takes 10–15 years. Once the idea, chemical or process is patented (to protect the developers from other companies stealing their ideas), the clock starts ticking! In most countries, the duration of a patent is 15–17 years, with a possible short extension. When the patent expires, other companies can manufacture and market the drug under their own trade names and as a 'generic' drug.[8]

8 Companies also try to extend their patent protection period when it is running out and maintain monopoly market share for blockbuster drugs by a process known as 'evergreening'–for example, by patenting an optical isomer of the drug, or a modified formulation.

It is estimated that every new drug costs around A$1 billion for basic and clinical studies and for the costs of application and promotion (a figure of US$2.6 billion has even been quoted), and that a drug company needs one to two new drugs every 3–4 years to remain financially viable. ('Me-too' drugs are significantly cheaper to develop because much of the expensive, time-consuming work has already been carried out for the original drug.) High costs are attributed to:

- the need for evidence of safety and cost-effectiveness
- increasing emphasis on 'lifestyle drugs', which require studies of long-term safety
- need for evidence about possible effects of concomitant medicines and the prevalence of polypharmacy, with inherent risks of drug interactions
- increasingly ageing populations, requiring drug testing in many chronic degenerative conditions
- the high attrition rate: drug development may be abandoned (or drugs withdrawn from use) at any stage because of problems with safety, efficacy, changes in fashion or a better competitor drug.

To achieve economies of scale, many drug company mergers have taken place, leaving only a few major research drug companies worldwide. Companies are trying to streamline testing procedures and get early information on toxicity or pharmacokinetic problems so as to waste as little time and money as possible.

Clinical trials of drugs

A clinical trial is a prospective study involving human participants that measures the effectiveness and safety of an intervention (e.g. diet, procedure, medical device) or treatment (e.g. drug, vaccine) (CFB 1.1). The intervention or treatment can be investigational (new and innovative) or established. Clinical trials report data on both safety (adverse reactions) and efficacy. The 'gold standard' of clinical trials is the **randomised controlled clinical trial** (RCCT), also known as the randomised controlled trial. In this type of study participants are randomly allocated to treatment groups; that is, they have an equal chance of being allocated to the new treatment (or the treatment undergoing investigation) or the control group. The control group will receive the current standard therapy (usually the best) treatment for the condition or a placebo treatment (if there is currently no available standard treatment). Placebo treatments contain no active ingredients. The outcomes of interest (e.g. reduction in blood pressure, blood glucose level or cholesterol) are measured in both groups and then compared. All clinical studies in humans must be approved by a local human research ethics committee.

Clinical trials are generally required for all new drugs and for new uses (new indications) or new formulations of old drugs; however, there are exceptions:

- Potentially toxic drugs (e.g. anticancer drugs) may go straight to phase II studies (see below) in a small number of people with the disease so volunteers without the disease are not subjected to adverse effects.
- The rules may be bent for orphan drugs (non-patentable, or for rare diseases; see Ch 2).
- There is public pressure for fast-tracking drugs potentially useful in otherwise fatal diseases such as cancers.

CLINICAL FOCUS BOX 1.1
The clinical trial process and the COVID-19 vaccines

In 2020 the world was waiting on a COVID-19 vaccine to mitigate the spread of the deadly SARS-CoV-2 virus. Once potential COVID-19 vaccines were developed, they had to undergo the rigorous clinical trial process to determine if the vaccines were safe and effective in humans before widespread use. Unfortunately, many vaccines did not progress through the clinical trial process. For example, the University of Queensland COVID-19 vaccine entered phase I human trials; however, after finding the vaccine induced false-positive HIV results, the vaccine did not progress to phase II.

The Pfizer/Biontech BNT162b2 mRNA vaccine (Ch 43) was one of several COVID-19 vaccines used in Australia and New Zealand. Prior to being approved, the vaccine went through a large (43,548 participants) randomised, observer-blind, placebo-controlled Phase II/III clinical trial. The trial was multicentre and multinational, with 152 sites worldwide. To ensure participants were 'blinded' to their treatment allocation, both groups received two injections, 21 days apart, delivered into the deltoid muscle.

The main outcome under examination in this RCCT was the efficacy of the COVID-19 vaccine against a COVID-19 diagnosis. The results showed eight cases of COVID-19 in the intervention and 162 in the placebo (control) group, equalling a vaccine efficacy of 95%. Results also showed the vaccine was safe. Although 27% of participants given the COVID-19 vaccine had local adverse reactions (indicative of an immune response), only four developed serious adverse effects, one of which was related to poor administration technique (Ch 43). The outcomes were then published in the *New England Journal of Medicine*. Following their own assessment, regulatory bodies across countries, including the TGA (Australia) and Pharmac (New Zealand), approved the vaccine for use. At the time of writing, this vaccine was still in phase IV of the clinical trial process (i.e. post-marketing surveillance). All health professionals play a role in reporting adverse drug reactions when they are available on the market – this is called pharmacovigilance.

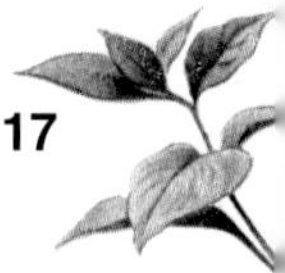

The objectives of RCCTs need to be realistic, valid and specific, yet allow for the results to be applied for the population at large (generalisation). Statisticians, researchers and clinicians are involved to optimise internal and external validity of the study. Clinical trials are a staged process, with few subjects in the early phases and stepwise decision making so that trials can be stopped if clear differences or toxicities become apparent; they are prolonged and expensive to run.

It is now customary for a Data Safety Monitoring Board to be appointed for a trial. Such a board is composed of a small number of independent experts who periodically review the emerging safety information from a trial.

Phase I: The first tests in humans using healthy volunteers

After extensive testing in vitro and in animals, the drug is administered initially in very low and increasing doses to small numbers of healthy volunteers, usually in a research centre or institution, under close medical and scientific supervision. The objectives are to determine in humans the pharmacological activities, pharmacokinetic parameters including bioavailability, tolerable dosage range and acute toxicity of the drug.

Phase II: The first administration to people with the condition the intervention or treatment is designed to treat

In phase II, the first studies on efficacy are conducted. To do this a small number of people with the condition that the intervention is designed to treat are given either the new investigational drug/intervention or the standard/placebo. There are approximately 50 subjects in each treatment group. The subjects are closely monitored, usually in major teaching hospitals. The tests may be 'single-blind'; that is, subjects do not know which treatment they are getting, but the investigators do, or 'double-blind'. Usually the investigators are specialists in the appropriate field, such as oncologists, psychiatrists or rheumatologists. Phase II studies indicate the pharmacokinetic and pharmacodynamic properties, therapeutic range of doses, maximum tolerated dose and common adverse reactions in those with the disease. They act as 'pilot studies' to optimise the protocol and determine dosing and sample sizes in the phase III trial.

Phase III: The full-scale randomised controlled clinical trial

This is 'the clinical trial', as commonly understood, in which the drug is administered to numerous (from several hundred to thousands) subjects under the guidance of experienced clinical investigators to ascertain whether, under defined conditions, the drug shows clinical benefit for the disease state, with an acceptably low rate of adverse drug reactions. The trial is usually 'multicentre', carried out simultaneously in different institutions or countries, to increase the number of subjects and investigators and achieve quicker results; many are partly carried out in Australia. A typical RCCT may cost up to AU$7 million, so it must be designed carefully to ensure statistically significant results can be extrapolated back to the target population. Important elements of the RCCT are as follows:

- Investigators must initially believe that the new treatment is at least as good as the old.
- Subjects must be randomised to ensure groups are initially similar in gender, age range, weight range and severity of disease.
- Participants must give informed consent. The 'informed consent' form for participants should contain detailed information about the study, potential benefits and adverse reactions and the option to withdraw at any stage.
- Double-blinding is usual, with coded packs of drugs so that neither investigators nor subjects know who received the new drug. After the trial has concluded, results are analysed and the code is revealed.
- The institution's ethics committee must have given approval to an application to run the trial (discussed in Ch 2).

Advance planning determines parameters such as: the study design (paired, crossover, parallel); criteria for those to be included or excluded (inclusions are generally wider than those in phase II trials); maximum length; outcome criteria (whether by changes in biomarkers or patient-improvement outcome); justification (who benefits?); information given to patients; protocols; sample sizes required for valid results; monitoring for adverse events; database management and statistical analysis methods; withdrawal procedures and follow-up schedules; regular auditing for safety; and quality control.

Usually the statistical basis for the trial is the null hypothesis – that there is in fact no difference between the two treatments; in other words, the new drug is just as good as the current therapy. If it becomes apparent that one group is benefiting statistically significantly more than the other, or suffering more adverse reactions, the trial is halted. Historically, results have been analysed for statistical equivalence and the null hypothesis is accepted or rejected. Increasingly, however, studies termed 'non-inferiority' studies are conducted. The study design allows that the new treatment may have a small degree of inferiority of efficacy. Prior to the study, an acceptable difference between the new treatment and

the comparator for the new treatment to be regarded as equivalent is decided by expert clinicians. Provided the new treatment does not exceed the acceptable difference, it may be judged as non-inferior. It is important that raw data from clinical trials be published (even negative results) so conclusions can be examined by outsiders not involved with the researchers, drug companies or funding bodies.

If the new drug is shown to be safe, efficacious and cost-effective, it may be approved for market by the government's regulatory body – the TGA in Australia and Medsafe in New Zealand. In both countries, advice is usually taken from the national advisory committee – the Advisory Committee on Medicines in Australia or the Medicines Assessment Advisory Committee in New Zealand.

Phase IV: Post-marketing studies

If the new drug is shown to be safe, efficacious and cost-effective, it may be approved for marketing. However, there are limitations in the testing and trialling processes: the number of people studied and the time allotted to the study have been limited (Fig 1.5); and certain types of subjects may have been excluded, such as children, pregnant women, the elderly and people with multiple disease states or taking other drugs.

Once marketed, the drug is used in many more people and for longer periods; extended monitoring of safety and efficacy (pharmacovigilance) is then possible. Inevitably, events will surface that were not seen during the trial such as rare adverse reactions, effects in subgroups of the population and drug interactions. Studies in older people are especially important because they may have comorbidities and require many drugs for prolonged periods.

Later, a meta-analysis may be conducted. A meta-analysis pools together all the results from similar clinical trials with the same or similar research question. Pooling the data increases the statistical power, making significant results more likely; however, meta-analyses suffer inevitably from 'publication bias' because negative results are less likely to be published than positive results. (Some regulating authorities and journals require authors to advise in advance when trials are to be carried out, and publish a study protocol, to ensure that results of all trials are published.) Sometimes, different trials will produce conflicting results; the choice to prescribe the drug is then based on clinical judgement.

As part of its post-market vigilance, the TGA encourages drug companies to share their large quantities of information about new drugs; it then rates companies' responses with a T-score for transparency. The TGA publishes detailed 'Australian Public Assessment Reports for new medicines and extended indications of prescription medicines' on its website. The *Australian Prescriber* publishes notes in a 'New Drugs' section of each issue. The TGA also carries out laboratory investigations of products on the market and ongoing monitoring to ensure compliance with legislation. The TGA publishes details about Australian reports of suspected adverse reactions in an online database called DAEN (Drug Adverse Event Notifications). Consumers are advised to discuss any concerns with a health professional. In New Zealand, Medsafe regulates clinical trials and carries out similar pharmacovigilance.

Pharmacovigilance: the 'blue card'

Through its Advisory Committee on Medicines, the TGA encourages and facilitates the reporting by consumers and health professionals of adverse events they suspect are related to medications and medical devices. Historically,

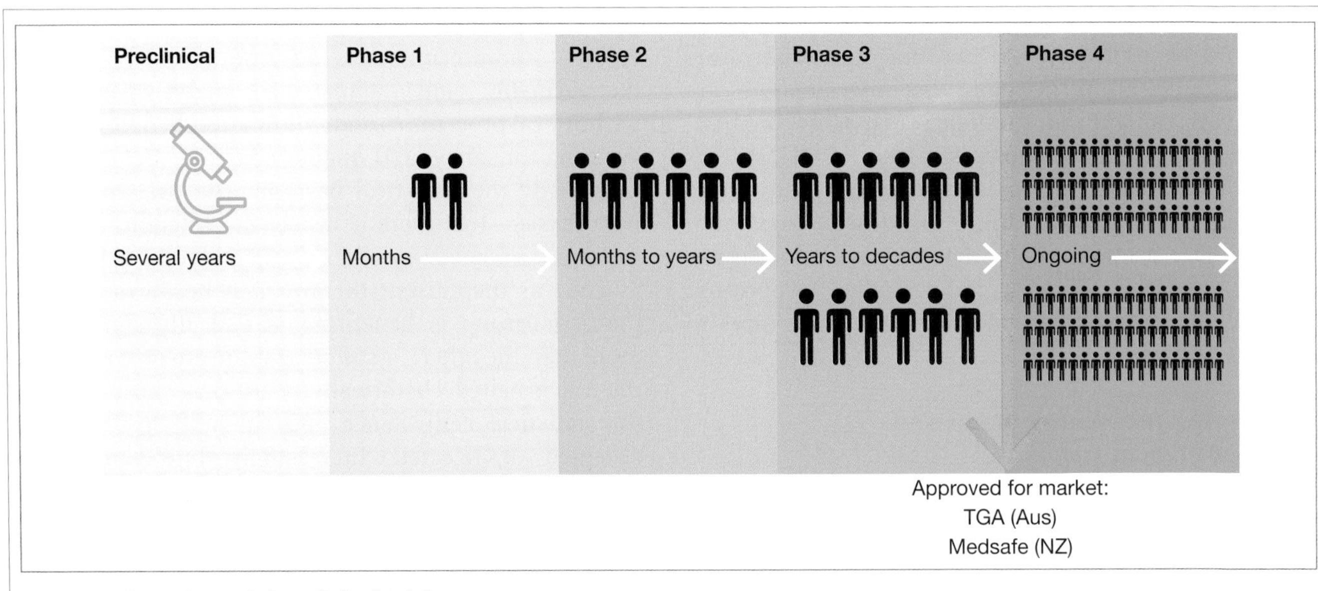

FIGURE 1.5 Overview of the clinical trial process

reporting has been by use of a one-page form (the 'blue card' – see Fig 1.6) that is readily available and can be completed. Online reporting is now also possible. Confidentiality is maintained. Consumers can also report their own adverse reactions via a 1300 telephone number designated as the Adverse Medicine Events Line (1300 134 237).

Reports of adverse reactions are reviewed, entered into DAEN and analysed for patterns. The Advisory Committee on Medicines informs health professionals about adverse events and can recommend actions ranging from no action required, to change of aspects of prescribing or dispensing, through to withdrawal of a drug from the

Australian Government
Department of Health
Therapeutic Goods Administration

TGA use only

Report of suspected adverse reaction to medicines or vaccines

See statement about the collection and use of personal information overleaf, and please attach any additional data to this form

Patient initials or medical record number:	Sex: M ☐ F ☐ / Weight (kg):	Date of birth or age:

Suspected medicine(s)/vaccine(s)

Medicine/vaccine (please use trade names; include batch number and AUST R or AUST L number if known)	**Dosage** (Dose number for vaccines eg 1st DTP)	Date begun	Date stopped	Reason for use

Other medicine(s)/vaccine(s) taken at the time of the reaction

Medicine/vaccine	**Dosage**	Date begun	Date stopped	Reason for use

Reaction(s): Date of onset of reaction (for vaccines time after administration): / /

Describe: (please provide as much detail as possible and include any results of relevant laboratory data and other investigations)

Seriousness: Life threatening ☐ Hospitalised ☐ Required a visit to doctor ☐

Treatment of reaction:

Outcome: Recovered ☐▸ Date: / / | Not yet recovered ☐ | Fatal ☐▸ Date: / / | Unknown ☐

Sequelae? No ☐ Yes ☐▸ Describe:

Reporting: Doctor ☐ Pharmacist ☐ Other ☐ | Contact details (email or phone)

Name:

Address:

Postcode: | Signature: Date: / /

Thank you for taking the time to complete this form PTO

FIGURE 1.6 The 'blue card', used by health professionals to report suspected adverse reactions to drugs and vaccines

Source: Adapted from Therapeutic Goods Administration <https://www.tga.gov.au/sites/default/files/blue-card-adverse-reaction-reporting-form.pdf>

Continued

Report of suspected reaction to medicines or vaccines ("Blue card")

Privacy statement
For general privacy information, go to <www.tga.gov.au/privacy>.
Information in this report is collected to assist in the post market monitoring of the safety of therapeutic goods under the *Therapeutic Goods Act 1989* (the Act). All reports are entered into the Therapeutic Goods Administration's (TGA's) Adverse Event Management System (AEMS). Further information about how the TGA uses adverse event information that is reported to it is available at <www.tga.gov.au/reporting-adverse-events>.

The TGA collects personal information in this report to:
- monitor the safety of medicines and vaccines under the Act
- contact the reporter of the adverse event if further information is required
- contact representatives of entities that supply therapeutic goods, to discuss reported adverse events
- check that the same information has not been received multiple times for the same adverse event.

At times, this information is collected from someone other than the individual to whom the personal information relates. This can occur when an adverse event is reported to a person or an entity other than the TGA (such as a health professional, a hospital or a sponsor), and that person or entity passes the information on to the TGA. In those cases, ordinarily the TGA will not collect the name and contact details of patients. However, the TGA may collect other information relating to patients, including the date of birth or age, gender, weight, initials and information about the relevant adverse event.

Personal information collected in this report may be disclosed as permitted under the Privacy Act 1988, including by consent or where the disclosure is required by, or authorised under, a law (for example, under section 61 of the Act). Where a report relates to vaccine events, personal information about the reporter or the patient may be disclosed to State and Territory health agencies under subsection 61(3) of the Act.

Fold here first (Please do not use staples on this form)

www.tga.gov.au/reporting-problems   Email: adr.reports@tga.gov.au   Fax: 02 6232 8392

What to report
You do not need to be certain, just suspicious!
Any information related to the reporter and patient identifiers is kept strictly confidential.
Adverse drug reaction reports should be submitted for prescription medicines, vaccines, over-the-counter medicines (medicines purchased without a prescription), and complementary medicines (herbal medicines, naturopathic and/or homoeopathic medicines, and nutritional supplements such as vitamins and minerals).
Please include timing of reactions relative to medicine administration where relevant.
The TGA particularly requests reports of:
- All suspected reactions to new medicines and vaccines
- All suspected drug interactions
- Unexpected reactions, that is not consistent with product information or labelling
- Serious reactions which are suspected of significantly affecting a patient's management, including reactions suspected of causing death, danger to life, admission to hospital, prolongation of hospitalisation, absence from productive activity, increased investigational or treatment costs, and birth defects.

Fold here second   D1073 June 2018

Delivery Address:
PO Box 100
WODEN ACT 2606

No stamp required
if posted in Australia

Medicines Safety Monitoring
Pharmacovigilance and Special Access Branch
Reply Paid 100
WODEN ACT 2606

FIGURE 1.6, cont'd

market. For example, the COX-2 inhibitor lumiracoxib was included in the Pharmaceutical Benefits Scheme in 2006 and became widely used; however, by late 2007 the TGA had received eight reports of serious liver damage (including two deaths), so the drug was deregistered. The TGA publishes (since 2010) Medicines Safety Updates. Sponsors of newly registered medicines must obtain TGA approval of a Medicines Risk Management Plan based on the European Medicines Agency's good-pharmacovigilance-practice (GVP) guideline.

Drug development in Australia

There is little basic research carried out by 'big pharma' drug companies in Australia or New Zealand, where most companies are offshoots of multinationals based overseas. Scientific work in Australian companies is mainly on formulations suitable for local conditions or preparation of submissions for the marketing of drugs developed overseas. Australia's share of global research and development is only about 1.3%, so Australia relies on the rest of the world to develop most advances in knowledge.

Australian medical schools and medical research institutes have an enviable reputation worldwide for medical and healthcare research; new compounds of interest may be discovered, and researchers collaborate with drug companies in developing drugs, after which commercial exploitation and 'value-adding' of the research usually happen overseas.

CSL (formerly Commonwealth Serum Laboratories) was established in Australia more than 100 years ago (1916) to develop 'immune sera' (vaccines). It is now a major international producer of blood products,

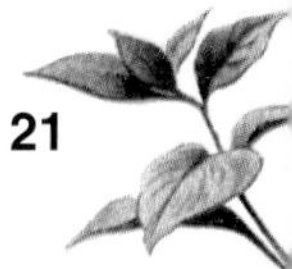

antivenoms and influenza and Q-fever vaccines, and markets many pharmaceutical drugs produced by other companies. CSL's subsidiary company Sequirus is the major manufacturer of the Oxford/AstraZeneca COVID-19 vaccine for Australia during the global pandemic. CSL employs more than 10,000 people in 27 countries.

Clinical trials in Australia and New Zealand

In Australia the TGA has overall control of therapeutic goods by regulating: pre-market evaluation and approval of products; clinical trials; roles of Human Research Ethics Committees (HRECs); trials involving gene therapy and related therapies; preventing or stopping a trial; indemnity and compensation; licensing of manufacturers; and post-market surveillance. Details of the relevant regulations and guidelines are covered in the TGA booklet *Australian Clinical Trial Handbook 2020* (see details in 'Online resources'). Use of a registered or listed product in a clinical trial beyond the conditions for which registration/listing has already been granted also requires approval. Overseas drug companies favour carrying out trials in Australia because our regulatory authority (the TGA) is respected, and data generated here is likely to be accepted in the United States and Europe. All clinical trials should be registered in advance at the Australian New Zealand Clinical Trials Registry, based at the National Health and Medical Research Council's Clinical Trials Centre in Sydney; thus, Australian and New Zealand researchers contribute to a worldwide initiative to make public the details of all clinical trials.

There are two main schemes under which drugs (and medical devices) may be trialled. The first is application for approval under the Clinical Trial Approval (CTA) scheme. An application to conduct a trial is submitted to the TGA, whose delegate reviews the data and may object to the trial or comment on the proposal. When any objections have been satisfactorily met and the local HREC has approved it, the trial may go ahead without further assessment from the TGA. Early phase I and II studies and trials of medical devices most commonly come under the CTA scheme. The scheme is complex, and few trials now come under these rules.

The second approach is notification under the Clinical Trial Notification (CTN) scheme, under which data are submitted to the local HREC, which reviews the data and the trial design and advises the institution if it approves the trial, or can refer the application to the CTA scheme. A CTN form must be submitted to notify the TGA of the trial. Phase III and IV trials and bioequivalence studies are best suited to the CTN scheme.

Principles of good clinical practice must be followed, such as those promulgated by the European Forum for Good Clinical Practice. These principles cover aspects such as: responsibilities of the investigators and the drug company; drug product handling, storage and accounting; reporting of adverse effects; and keeping and archiving of records. There are potential problems relating to lack of transparency about procedures, delaying or withholding of negative results, applying 'spin' to make drugs look better or participating doctors accepting funding or gifts from sponsoring drug companies.

In New Zealand, approval to trial a new drug not yet approved is submitted to the Standing Committee on Therapeutic Trials, a committee of the Health Research Council of New Zealand. Quite a few clinical trials are carried out in New Zealand because it is a small, closed, not too mixed population. Medsafe publishes *Guidelines on the Regulation of Therapeutic Products in New Zealand*; Part 11 concerns regulatory approval and good clinical practice requirements. Pharmaceutical companies conducting clinical research must comply with the principles contained in the guidelines; and participating doctors must be familiar with good clinical research practice requirements and assess the proposed research for compliance (see 'Online resources').

Future drug development

The new genetics

The discovery of the double-helical structure of DNA (published by Francis Crick and James Watson in 1953) and the determination of the sequence of nucleotide base pairs that make up the human genome[9] and mapping all its genes (declared complete in 2003) were arguably the most important scientific events of the 20th century. Although drugs are still being discovered by the old methods, there has been great interest in searching for new drugs using 'the new genetics' – application of molecular biology techniques to biochemistry and pathology. This has led to the discovery of genes associated with cancers, arthritis, cystic fibrosis, type 1 diabetes and various anaemias.

The human genome is estimated to encode from 20,000 to 25,000 gene products, of which many hundreds (especially proteins and receptors) are targets for existing drugs and thousands may be usefully exploited in the future (Oprea et al. 2018). The terms 'pharmacogenetics' and 'pharmacogenomics', and their relevance to expression of specific genes in diseases, related phenotypes, effects on drug responses and genetic differences in drug-metabolising enzymes or receptors, are discussed in more detail in Chapters 5 and 32.

Nanomedicines

The term 'nanotechnology' refers to the study of controlling matter at the nanometre (nm) level; a nanometre is one-billionth of a metre, or 10^{-9} m. Different

9 The suffix '-ome' has taken off. Originally used in 'genome' to imply a combination of gene and chromosome, it now seems to be added to almost any prefix to denote molecular biology technology applied to genetic information; thus, we now read about transcriptomics, proteomics, chemogenomics, metabolomics, glycomics, interactomics, even fluxomics. A paper given at the 2016 meeting of the Australasian Society of Clinical and Experimental Pharmacologists and Toxicologists in Melbourne included in its title the keyword 'Drugomics'!

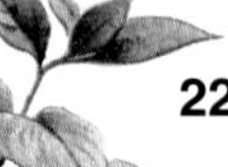

pharmacokinetic and toxicity issues can be expected from administering drugs in such tiny forms. Nanomedicines currently developed include polymeric particles, micelles, UV-blockers, particles of silver and gold, liposomes, magnetic particles enhancing selectivity of gene therapy delivery to cancer cells and multifunctional carriers.

KEY POINTS

How drugs are discovered and developed

- Drugs and biological products have been derived from several main sources:
  - microorganisms (e.g. antibiotics from fungi)
  - plants (e.g. morphine from the poppy *Papaver somniferum*; active plant constituents include alkaloids, carbohydrates, hydrocarbons, phenols and isoprenoid structures)
  - humans and other animals (e.g. human chorionic gonadotrophin)
  - minerals or mineral products (e.g. iron and iodine)
  - laboratories, in which substances such as β-blockers and antidepressants are synthesised chemically, or made by genetically engineered microorganisms (e.g. human insulin).

  New technologies, including those of combinatorial chemistry, high-throughput screening and genetic engineering are applied in the discovery of new drugs and diagnostic methods.
- Drug development takes place in various stages over many years:
  - design and synthesis of a new molecule
  - screening for useful and adverse biological activities
  - pharmaceutical formulation and manufacturing scale-up
  - clinical trials:
    - phase I: first in-human tests, for pharmacokinetics and safety
    - phase II: efficacy studies in a small cohort of people, for dose range
    - phase III: the randomised controlled clinical trial, double-blinded, statistically valid
    - if approved and marketed: ongoing post-marketing studies and pharmacovigilance.

  During the process of testing drugs, chemical and biological assays are carried out to determine their strength and purity. Bioassays may be of various types: in vitro, in vivo or in silico; drugs need to be tested in animals and humans before being approved as safe and effective.

  Legal requirements for drug regulation are implemented to remove unsafe or ineffective drugs.

Drug formulations

Drug formulations (pharmaceutics)

Depending on the route by which a drug is administered, different dosage forms are appropriate. **Pharmaceutics** is the science of formulating drugs – for example, into tablets, ointments, parenteral solutions, metered-dose inhalers or eyedrops; it is an important aspect of a pharmacist's work. The prescriber nominates the formulation best suited to the person and route of administration, according to whether the drug is intended to act locally or be absorbed.

A comprehensive listing of various forms of drug preparations is shown in Table 2.4; the routes of drug administration are discussed in Chapter 5. More details of formulations and routes of administration are given later for drugs administered locally to the respiratory system, eyes and ears and skin.

Formulations for oral administration

About three-quarters of all drugs prescribed are administered orally, in solid or liquid form. After swallowing, a solid **dose form** disintegrates into finer particles before dissolving into solution and becoming available for absorption.

Tablets

Of drugs taken orally, about 60% are in **tablet** form. Tablets are compressed mixtures of an active drug with other pharmacologically inert excipients: diluents (fillers), binders, adhesives, disintegrants, lubricants, flavours, colours, sweeteners or absorbents. (Supposedly inert excipients can cause adverse and hypersensitivity reactions.) Thus, the active drug may make up only a small fraction of the total tablet weight. The weight quoted for the tablet (e.g. aspirin 300 mg) refers to the average amount of *active drug* present. Tablets may appear as simple white discs or may be multilayered or coated with a film[10] to mask an unpleasant taste. Effervescent tablets fizz and dissolve in water for ease of swallowing.

The rate of release of active drug from a tablet – hence the rate of absorption and distribution to the active site – can be manipulated by pharmaceutical processing. Active

10 Brightly coloured film-coated tablets look dangerously like sweets such as 'Smarties' or 'M&Ms' and account for many cases of childhood poisoning annually–especially from iron tablets.

drug may be released slowly from a resin to delay absorption (**sustained-release** [SR] or controlled-release [CR] preparations) or a tablet may be coated to prevent nausea or to resist the digestive action of stomach contents (enteric coating, EC). SR, CR or EC tablets should not be cut.

Formulations for parenteral administration

Parenteral administration means administration of drugs by injection. The IV route, where the drug is injected directly into the circulation, avoids absorption delay. Other parenteral routes include intradermal (into the skin), intramuscular, intra-arterial and subcutaneous (into the fatty tissue under the skin); specialist techniques for local anaesthetics include the epidural (= extradural) and intrathecal routes (Ch 11).

Equipment and solutions

Because any injection is invasive with potential for irritation or infection, solutions for parenteral administration must be sterile, filtered, particle-free and preferably isotonic with body solutions (i.e. with 0.9% normal saline) and buffered to body pH. Injected solid particles can cause granulomas, ischaemia or phlebitis. If the drug to be administered parenterally is very insoluble in water, such as the general anaesthetic propofol, it can be formulated in an oily emulsion. Solutions for injection are usually presented in glass ampoules or bottles or plastic bags; typical equipment for delivery of a drug by IV infusion is shown in Figure 2.5.

Most institutions have guidelines for using IV sets, with lists of infusion solutions and possible compatible admixtures (agents added to IV fluids). The general rule is that, unless a combination is specifically approved by a hospital pharmacist or drug information centre, it should not be made. (As always, if in doubt, don't!)

Formulations for children

Formulations suitable for taking by children pose a special challenge to pharmacists and drug companies: very young children cannot swallow tablets or capsules; unpleasant tastes may need to be masked by sweeteners or flavours, but sugary mixtures encourage dental caries and impair management of diabetes. Unusual drug-delivery systems may not have been clinically trialled in children. One success story is the fentanyl 'lollipop', an applicator for self-administration of the opioid analgesic by rubbing on the inside cheek mucosa; these are manufactured in a wide range of strengths suitable for children with severe pain (DM 12.2).

Drug names and classifications

Drug names

As a drug passes through investigational stages (under a code number) before it is approved and marketed, it collects three different types of name: the **chemical name**, the approved (or generic or non-proprietary) name and the proprietary (or brand or trade) name or names. For example, the chemical name of amoxicillin, a commonly prescribed antibacterial antibiotic, is actually (2S,5R,6R)-6-{[(2R)-2-amino-2-(4-hydroxyphenyl)-acetyl]amino}-3,3-dimethyl- 7-oxo-4-thia-1-azabicyclo-[3.2.0] heptane-24-carboxylic acid, abbreviated to D(−)-α-**amino**-p-hydr**oxy**benzylpen**icillin**. Its approved (generic) name, amoxicillin, is clearly derived from parts of its chemical name. It is marketed under several proprietary names including Alphamox, Amoxil, Bgramin, Cilamox, Fisamox, GenRx Amoxycillin, Maxamox, Ranmoxy and Yomax; in various formulations such as injections, capsules, tablets, syrups, suspensions and paediatric drops, and in combinations with other antibacterials and proton-pump inhibitors.

It would be helpful if every drug had a name related to other drugs in the same class (Table 1.5); however, this tends to be true only of the more recent drug groups. Thus, we refer to 'the statins', 'gliptins' and 'the glitazones'. Names can be deceiving: names of most β-blockers end in '-olol', but stanozolol is an anabolic steroid, not a β-blocker; nystatin is an antifungal agent and somatostatin is a growth hormone release inhibitory factor – neither is a 'statin'; so we cannot assume that drugs whose names sound similar always have similar effects and uses. And Table 1.5 cannot be read backwards; that is, while the suffix '-vir' implies the drug is probably an antiviral, not all antiviral drugs end in -vir (think zidovudine and ribavirin).

Chemical names

The **chemical name** is a unique, precise description of the drug's chemical composition and molecular structure. It is particularly meaningful to medicinal chemists – who should be able to draw the chemical structure if given the chemical name – but may be unintelligible to others. Because chemical names are too complicated to remember, or fit on a prescription pad or bottle label, a drug likely to reach the market and to be used medically is allocated a name that is simpler and easier to spell.

Active ingredient names

The active ingredient name (sometimes referred to the approved or **generic name**) is usually suggested by the manufacturer and approved by a drug regulating authority; it becomes the official drug name. These should now be the same as the International Non-proprietary Name (INN; see below). It is shorter, often derived from the chemical name, and is the name listed in official compendia such as the AMH or the BP. The active ingredient name needs to be distinct in sound and spelling so it is not easily confused with other drugs. Names that are overly fanciful or optimistic about their beneficial effects, or that refer to medical conditions or body parts, are (supposed to be) rejected.

TABLE 1.5 Drug classes

PREFIX OR SUFFIX	DRUG GROUP	EXAMPLE GENERIC NAME
cefa/o-	Cefalosporins	Cefalexin
gli-	Sulfonylureas	Glibenclamide
-afil	Phosphodiesterase 5 inhibitors	Sildenafil
-a/oquine	Quinine antimalarials	Mefloquine
-artan	Angiotensin-II-receptor antagonists (sartans)	Candesartan
-a/ovir	Antivirals	Aciclovir
-azepam	Benzodiazepines	Diazepam
-azole	Azole antifungal agents	Fluconazole
-caine	Local anaesthetics	Lidocaine
-cillin	Penicillins	Ampicillin
-coxib	Cyclo-oxygenase-2 inhibitors (coxibs)	Celecoxib
-cycline	Tetracycline antibiotics	Doxycycline
-dipine	Calcium channel blockers (dihydropyridine-type)	Nifedipine
-dronate	Bisphosphonates	Alendronate
-eplase	Thrombolytics	Alteplase
-floxacin	Quinolone antibiotics	Ciprofloxacin
-glitazone	Thiazolidinediones (glitazones)	Pioglitazone
-i/ythromycin	Macrolide antibiotics	Azithromycin
-lutamide	Antiandrogens	Flutamide
-mab	Monoclonal antibodies	Rituximab
-olol (most)	β-blockers	Metoprolol
-onidine	Alpha$_2$-adrenoceptor agonists (α_2-agonists)	Clonidine
-oxifen(e)	Selective estrogen receptor modulators	Tamoxifen
-prazole	Proton-pump inhibitors	Omeprazole
-pril	ACE inhibitors	Captopril
-pristone	Progesterone receptor antagonists	Mifepristone
-prost	Prostaglandin analogues	Latanoprost
-rubicin	Anthracycline antineoplastic agents	Doxorubicin
-setron	5HT$_3$ antagonists	Ondansetron
-statin (some)	HMG-CoA reductase inhibitors (statins)	Simvastatin
-stim	Colony-stimulating factors	Filgrastim
-tidine	Histamine H$_2$-receptor antagonists (H$_2$-receptor antagonists)	Cimetidine
-tinib	Tyrosine kinase inhibitors	Imatinib
-triptan	5HT$_1$ agonists (triptans)	Sumatriptan
-zolamide	Carbonic anhydrase inhibitors	Acetazolamide

ACE = angiotensin-converting enzyme (converts angiotensin I to angiotensin II, which is a vasoconstrictor and hence raises blood pressure); HMG-CoA = 3-hydroxy-3-methylglutaryl coenzyme A (a coenzyme involved in the early stages of cholesterol synthesis); 5HT = 5-hydroxytryptamine or serotonin.
* For a full listing of the prefixes, suffixes and other stems approved for INN drug names, see the reference under 'International Non-proprietary Names', later.

Active ingredient (generic) prescribing and bioequivalence

Because numerous brand names may exist for the same drug, prescribers are mandated to use the active ingredient name (CFB 1.2). This helps to avoid confusion between drugs with similar brand names and reduces errors and costs. With some exceptions, most generic drug products sold (assuming same dose and type of formulation) are considered therapeutically equivalent (bioequivalent), and some 'generic' products are much less expensive than a particular brand name drug.

CLINICAL FOCUS BOX 1.2
Communicate the active ingredient name

In Australia, from February 2021, it became a legal requirement for all prescribers to write scripts using the name of a medicine's active ingredient. For example, instead of writing a script for *Lipitor 20 mg*, a brand (proprietary) name, the script should be written for *atorvastatin 20 mg* (the active ingredient). Prior to this, prescribers used a mix of brand and active ingredient names when prescribing, which was confusing for patients and led to medication errors.

It is not uncommon for there be many brand names for the one active ingredient. To continue using the atorvastatin example, there are many atorvastatin brands such as Atovachol, Torvastat and Trovas to name a few. In Australia and New Zealand, generic brands must show bioequivalence to the original brand before being available to the public. Bioequivalence is when two active ingredients result in similar blood concentration levels that lead to the same physiological effect.

Prior to the legislation, unless brand substitution was not permitted by the prescriber, a prescription written using a brand name could be substituted to another bioequivalent brand. For example, a script written for Torvastat 20 mg could be substituted to Atovachol 20 mg. In fact, because it would be impossible for hospital and community pharmacies to stock all the different brands of a medicine, it was routine for substitution to occur. It is hoped that active ingredient prescribing will reduce medication errors and simplify the language around medications. For example, Mr Smith will get used to calling his cholesterol-lowering medication 'atorvastatin' and looking for the active ingredient names on his medicines.

Another step you should take to improve medicines' safety is to use the active ingredient name when communicating with your patients and other health professionals. You will also note that this textbook does not often refer to brand names but to active ingredient names.

International Non-proprietary Names

WHO has a constitutional mandate to 'develop, establish and promote international standards with respect to biological, pharmaceutical and similar products' (WHO 2022). To this end, WHO collaborates with national nomenclature committees to select a single name of worldwide acceptability for each substance that is to be marketed as a drug. The name should be (as close as possible) the same in most countries and should aid harmonisation between jurisdictions and reduce prescribing errors.

Each INN is a unique name that is globally recognised and public property. The names of more than 8000 drugs are published in lists, each in eight languages, including a modernised version of Latin.[11] The general principles used by WHO in devising and approving INNs are given on its website (see 'Online resources'). They include:

- *ph* is replaced by *f* (dexamfetamine, not dexamphetamine)
- *th* is (sometimes) replaced by *t* (beclometasone, not beclomethasone)
- *y* is replaced by *i* (amoxicillin, not amoxycillin)
- *h* and *k* are avoided.

An exception to the Australian adoption of INNs is that we can keep referring to 'adrenaline' and 'noradrenaline', rather than adopting 'epinephrine' and 'norepinephrine'. However, the latter (US) terms must be included in parentheses whenever relevant – for example: 'Noradrenaline (norepinephrine) has a high affinity for ...'

American names

Sometimes, however, other approved names are used in the United States (USAN, the US Approved Name), Canada and countries that follow their lead. Australian and New Zealand students can become confused if they do not realise, for example, that a common drug with very different names is paracetamol, known as acetaminophen in the US/Canada.

Proprietary (trade or brand) names

When a drug company markets a particular drug product, it selects and copyrights a **proprietary, or trade, name** for its drug, thereby restricting use of the name to that individual drug company and to that formulation of the drug. To avoid confusion, which could jeopardise the safety of patients, trademark names should neither be derived from INNs nor contain common stems used in INNs. Drug companies carry out extensive advertising to encourage doctors to prescribe their particular version of the drug and to promote sales of trade name drugs; this expense is eventually borne by the consumer, or by government (i.e. taxpayers) if the drug is subsidised.

In this text, we will always use generic (approved) names for drugs but may sometimes add a trade name if it is sufficiently well known (e.g. Valium, Prozac, Viagra) to help readers identify a particular drug. (We do not imply thereby any preference for that particular brand of the drug.) Note that approved/generic names use lower-case letters, whereas a trade name always begins with an upper-case letter.

Drug classifications

Classification systems

Drug classification can be approached from many perspectives. Using the example of amoxicillin again, this could be classified by:

- source: where the drug comes from (semisynthetic antibiotic from *Penicillium* spp.)
- chemical formula or structure (β-lactam, penicillanic acid derivative)
- pharmacokinetic parameters: relating to how the drug is absorbed or metabolised in the body (acid-resistant, β-lactamase-sensitive)
- activity: relating to the effects of the drug in the body (wide-spectrum antibacterial agent)
- mechanism of action: explaining how the drug works (inhibitor of bacterial cell wall synthesis)
- clinical use: conditions for which the drug is prescribed (indicated for treatment of infections by sensitive Gram-positive and Gram-negative organisms)
- body systems affected by the drug (for infections of the respiratory system; ear, nose and throat; genitourinary tract, etc.)
- drug schedule: the group into which the drug is classified for legal purposes (S4 Prescription-Only medicine)
- pregnancy safety schedule: grouping drugs depending on their safety for use in pregnancy (A: considered safe)
- popularity (one of the most commonly prescribed drugs in the world)
- whether its use is allowed in sporting competitions (yes – approved by the World Anti-Doping Agency).

Not surprisingly, students are often confused by drug classification, particularly because sometimes the same drug may be classified into various groups depending on the clinical use. For example, aspirin-like drugs may be classified as analgesics, antipyretics, anti-inflammatory agents or antithrombotics. This book uses various

---

11 Classical scholars will be amused to hear that paracetamol becomes paracetamolum.

approaches where appropriate. For example, the title of Chapter 15, 'Psychotropic agents', refers to drug clinical effects. Antidepressants are grouped there as 'tricyclic antidepressants' (a chemical class), or by mechanism of action: 'monoamine oxidase inhibitors' or 'selective serotonin reuptake inhibitors'. Such drug classifications can simplify understanding about individual drugs.

Prototype drugs

Pharmacology is easier to understand and learn when **key, or prototype, drugs** are studied – that is, the most important drug in a class, to which other drugs in the class can be compared. In this text, many prototype drugs are described in detail in a consistent format called a Drug Monograph (DM); thus, insulin is the prototype antidiabetic agent (DM 30.2), and estradiol the prototype estrogenic hormone. When a new, similar drug becomes available, it can be associated with its prototype, and inferences made about its basic pharmacodynamic qualities before focusing on specific properties (usually pharmacokinetic) to differentiate it from the prototype and other similar drugs.

Prescription-Only or OTC drugs

A drug may be classified into schedules as a **Prescription-Only drug**, which means that it requires a legal prescription to obtain it, or it may be a non-prescription or **OTC drug**, which means that it may be purchased without a prescription, possibly in a pharmacy or supermarket. (Drug Schedules are considered in more detail in Ch 2.)

WHO Essential Medicines List

It is recognised that, with the enormous number of drugs available, few countries or health services can subsidise or provide the whole range of drugs, and no retail or hospital pharmacy could stock them all. To assist in deciding which drugs are the most important, WHO has derived a model Essential Medicines List, now comprising about 433 core drugs for adults and children in some 30 main categories that are 'deemed essential for addressing the most important public health needs globally' (see 'Online resources'). This is useful for all countries attempting to curtail rapidly increasing expenditure on drugs, particularly for developing countries, allowing them to allocate limited resources to essential drugs, defined as 'those that satisfy the priority health care needs of a population ... They are intended to be available in functioning health systems at all times, in appropriate dosage forms, of assured quality and prices individuals and health systems can afford' (WHO 2021).

The selection of drugs is determined by an Expert Committee on the Selection and Use of Essential Medicines and is updated regularly. These drugs first require market approval based on efficacy, safety, quality and value for money. Listing 'essential' drugs inevitably raises concerns, particularly from manufacturers of drugs not on the list, which may be seen as 'non-essential' (see 'Online resources').

Médecins Sans Frontières (MSF; Doctors Without Borders), the world's leading independent organisation for medical humanitarian aid, also publishes a list based on WHO's list. The MSF (2021) medical guidance is 'a practical manual intended for health professionals, physicians, pharmacists, nurses and health auxiliaries involved in curative care and drug management', especially in developing countries and those where MSF is involved in humanitarian care.

Australia's top 10 drugs

The Australian Commonwealth Department of Health regularly audits the usage of prescription drugs in Australia and publishes lists of the top 10 drugs, scored by numbers of defined daily doses, by prescription counts and by cost to the government (i.e. to taxpayers). The lists for drug use in the year 2019–20 are summarised in Table 1.6.[12] Note that only some subsidised drugs are audited here; it excludes those coming under 'co-payment' or 'closing-the-gap' schemes, bought OTC or provided under private prescriptions.

New Zealand's top 10 drugs

New Zealand's Pharmaceutical Management Agency (Pharmac) also publishes lists of the most prescribed medications, as a 'top 20'. Their top 10 (reported for 2019–20) were as follows: paracetamol, atorvastatin, omeprazole, aspirin (antithrombotic dosage), amoxicillin, ibuprofen, metoprolol, salbutamol, cilazapril, cholecalciferol (Table 1.7) – very similar to their 2015–16 list (Pharmac 2020a).

12 The three most expensive drugs (to government) in this list are new antivirals to treat hepatitis C.

TABLE 1.6 The top 10 drugs by prescription counts (in millions), Australia, 2019–20

ORDER	DRUG (MAIN INDICATION)	MILLIONS OF PRESCRIPTIONS
1	Rosuvastatin (lipid-lowering)	12.7
2	Atorvastatin (lipid-lowering)	11.0
3	Pantoprazole (oesophageal reflux)	8.0
4	Esomeprazole (oesophageal reflux)	8.0
5	Perindopril (hypertension)	6.6
6	Cefalexin (antibiotic)	5.3
7	Metformin (diabetes)	5.1
8	Escitalopram (depression)	4.9
9	Amoxicillin with clavulanic acid (antibiotic)	4.7
10	Sertraline (depression)	4.6

Source: Data from the Commonwealth Department of Health 2021

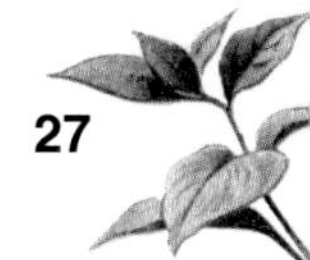

TABLE 1.7 The top 10 drugs by prescription counts (in millions), New Zealand, 2019–20		
ORDER	DRUG (MAIN INDICATION)	MILLIONS OF PRESCRIPTIONS
1	Paracetamol (analgesic)	2.88
2	Atorvastatin (lipid-lowering)	1.53
3	Omeprazole (oesophageal reflux)	1.48
4	Aspirin (anticoagulant)	1.14
5	Amoxicillin (antibiotic)	1.04
6	Ibuprofen (analgesic)	1.03
7	Metoprolol (cardiovascular)	0.95
8	Salbutamol (respiratory)	0.94
9	Cilazapril (hypertension)	0.84
10	Cholecalciferol (bone health)	0.46

Source: Data from the Commonwealth Department of Health 2021

The main cross-Tasman differences appear to be the slightly different statins and ACE inhibitors used in New Zealand (cilazapril is not available in Australia), the inclusion of amoxicillin and ibuprofen and the absence of an angiotensin-receptor antagonist (e.g. irbe- or candesartan), metformin (for diabetes) or pregabalin (for neuropathic pain/seizures) from the New Zealand list.

New Zealand's 10 most expensive drug groups (reported by Pharmac in 2020) were: immunosuppressants, antivirals (hepatitis C), vaccines, chemotherapeutic agents, antithrombotic agents, antidiabetic agents, long-acting β-adrenoceptor agonists, endocrine therapy, antipsychotics (Pharmac 2020b).

KEY POINTS

How drugs are named and classified

- A drug may have three main names:
  - its unique chemical name
  - an approved (generic) name, allocated by a regulating authority; in Australia and New Zealand, this now should be the official INN
  - a trade or brand name, given by the marketing company.
- Generic prescribing is encouraged, and dispensing of substituted products considered bioequivalent is sometimes permitted.
- Drugs are classified by any of a number of criteria – for example, by source, chemical group, pharmacokinetic parameters, pharmacological activity, mechanism of action, clinical use, body systems affected, legal drug schedule, pregnancy safety category, popularity, whether allowed in sporting competitions or whether considered 'essential'.
- Drug classifications help facilitate understanding of pharmacology by comparing the common characteristics of an example of a drug group or classification (the key, or prototype, drug) with those of other drugs in the same category.

Drug information

Important drug information

Our Drug Monographs summarise for selected prototype drugs the important basic information, including the drug's:

- group or category
- approved/generic name
- pharmacodynamic effects (what the drug does to the body)
- mechanisms of action
- indications for clinical use
- particular pharmacokinetic parameters (what the body does to this drug)
- common adverse effects (adverse drug reactions)
- **contraindications** (the medical conditions in which a drug should *not* be prescribed) and precautions
- significant drug interactions
- dosage and administration guidelines, optimum therapeutic plasma levels and monitoring techniques.

Information as to potential toxic effects and treatment of poisoning may also be relevant, as is safety of use in particular cohorts of people, such as infants or the elderly. The Australian Drug Evaluation Committee's Pregnancy Safety Category indicates the likely safety or risks with the use of a drug during pregnancy (see 'Online resources').

What patients want to know

There is a huge – often overwhelming – amount of information available on most drugs, especially on the internet, where its accuracy and bias cannot easily be judged. When it comes down to the basics, what patients most want to know is:

- What is the drug for?
- What will it do to me (risks and benefits)?
- How do I take it?
- What other treatment options are there?
- What might happen if I *don't* take it?

These are the questions that health professionals prescribing, recommending or administering drugs should be ready to answer.

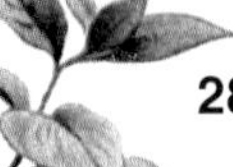

Drug information sources

Publication of data on new drugs and new information on old drugs is an ongoing process – in scientific journals, news releases, patient information brochures, reference books and textbooks. Much information (some of it of dubious quality) is found on the internet (Ioannidis et al. 2017). No single source will meet the varied and specialised needs of clinical practice today. It is always important to read critically, beware of bias or selectivity of information and consider what credibility can be given to the author and the publication, particularly with information found on the internet.

An excellent overview 'Where to find information about drugs' (Day & Snowden 2016) can be found via the *Australian Prescriber* website.

Official sources, pharmacopoeias and formularies

Official sources of drug information are published by government bodies such as departments of health and hospitals, and by pharmaceutical societies and medical colleges, containing legally or medically accepted standards for drugs. Pharmacopoeias are reference texts collecting together drug information relevant to a particular country, including descriptions, formulae, strengths, standards of purity and dosage forms.

Formularies are similar but may also include information on drug actions, adverse effects, general medical information, guidelines for pharmacists dispensing medicines and the 'recipes' for formulation or production of different medicines such as tablets, injections, ointments and eyedrops. A national **formulary** may also be used by government to limit the drugs available or subsidised, in order to encourage rational, cost-efficient prescribing and enhance the quality use of medicine (QUM; Ch 2).

The APF

The *Australian Pharmaceutical Formulary and Handbook: A Guide to Best Practice* is published by the Pharmaceutical Society of Australia. The APF now contains not just formulae ('recipes') for medicines but also principles of drug therapy, therapeutic management of common conditions (e.g. cough, head lice, tinea), monographs on complementary medicines, counselling guides, health information, physicochemical data on drugs, codes of ethics for pharmacists and Australian standards. It aims to underpin the expanding roles of pharmacists and encourage 'best practice' pharmacy (Pharmaceutical Society of Australia 2021).

New Zealand drug information sources

Medsafe is the New Zealand government's Medicines and Medical Devices Safety Authority. It is responsible for ensuring the regulation and safety of medicines and medical devices in New Zealand. The Medsafe website is a great source of independent information for health professionals and consumers (and students), with prescriber update articles, medicine data sheets, reporting of adverse reactions, 'patient info leaflets' and media releases, plus information about classification and regulation of medicines, medical devices, drug abuse, patient support groups, clinical trials and complementary medicines.

The New Zealand Ministry of Health and various organisations interested in medicines have developed a *New Zealand Formulary*, which provides point-of-care advice for health professionals and has a companion *New Zealand Formulary for Children*. It includes the New Zealand Universal List of Medicines, a list of all medicines prescribable in New Zealand. It is continuously updated and integrated with electronic prescribing and dispensing software packages. It provides four main components:

- preliminary general notes on use of drugs (medicines)
- practical notes on specific therapeutic categories
- datasheets (monographs) on individual drugs
- details of preparations available and relevant subsidy information.

The NZF therefore parallels much of the AMH, with the advantage that it is freely available and accessible online (in New Zealand), compared with the AMH, published annually at a cost to purchasers of approximately A$260.

Some other official sources

Other examples of official drug information sources are:

- *Martindale: The Complete Drug Reference*: monographs on drugs classified under therapeutic groups, such as analgesics, anthelmintics, vaccines; includes details of preparations, and lists of manufacturers and pharmaceutical terms (Buckingham 2020)
- *British Pharmacopoeia* (British Pharmacopoeia Commission): with official standards and monographs on thousands of drugs, formulated medicines, herbal drugs, blood products, radio-pharmaceuticals and surgical materials
- *United States Pharmacopeia* and the National Formulary (US Pharmacopeial Convention)
- *Handbook of Non-prescription Drugs: An Interactive Approach to Self-Care* (American Pharmaceutical Association): an authoritative source on 'non-prescription drug pharmacotherapy, nutritional supplements, medical foods, non-drug and preventive measures, and complementary therapies'.

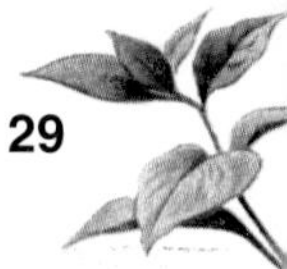

Semi-official sources

Semi-official sources of drug information may be published by government bodies or other groups, such as medical and pharmacology societies, and may include drug bulletins, reference books and updates, but no drug advertisements. While not official standards, they attempt to provide up-to-date, independent and unbiased information on drugs. Information such as lists of food additives, patient support organisations, poisons information centres and prescribing guidelines may be included.

Australian Medicines Handbook

In the years since the AMH was first published (1998), it has become virtually 'the bible' as a source of peer-reviewed, independent, authoritative information on therapeutic drugs and clinical practice in Australia. It is published by three national bodies concerned with drug therapy: ASCEPT (the Australasian Society of Clinical and Experimental Pharmacologists and Toxicologists), the PSA (Pharmaceutical Society of Australia) and the RACGP (Royal Australian College of General Practitioners). It aims to fulfil a need for 'an independent and up-to-date source of drug information to foster rational prescribing in Australia', much as the British National Formulary had done in the United Kingdom. It contains three main types of information:

- treatment considerations for common diseases, with comparisons between classes of drugs
- statements about classes of drugs, with comparisons between individual drugs in the class
- monographs on individual drugs, with some trade names and formulation types.

Preliminary sections provide general prescribing information, plus details on prescribing for patient groups. Appendices provide invaluable reference information, especially on significant drug interactions (see 'Online resources').

Therapeutic Guidelines series

Therapeutic Guidelines Limited is an independent not-for-profit organisation based in Melbourne, which started with a very small booklet called *Antibiotic Guidelines* published more than 20 years ago in a determined bid to encourage rational prescribing of antibiotics at the Royal Melbourne Hospital. Its aim was to reduce the risk of antibiotic resistance developing.

There is now (2021) a series of 19 guidelines, each dedicated to a branch of medicine or major drug therapy – for example, antibiotics, cardiovascular medicine and palliative care. The guidelines, each written by an 'Expert Group', are intended principally to provide prescribers with clear, practical, succinct and up-to-date therapeutic information, categorised according to diagnosis and updated every few years. They are published in print and electronic formats suitable for computers and mobile devices (see 'Online resources').

Cochrane

Cochrane is an international organisation that publishes systematic reviews and meta-analyses of the best evidence from research on healthcare interventions, with the aim of helping people to make well-informed decisions about health care. It aims to avoid duplication of studies, minimise bias and provide relevant, up-to-date, easily accessible information. There are Cochrane databases of reviews, clinical trials, methodologies and economic evaluations, among others (see 'Online resources').

Other semi-official sources

Other examples include:

- National Prescribing Service (NPS) MedicineWise: an independent, not-for-profit, evidence-based Australian organisation that works to improve the way health technologies, medicines and medical tests are prescribed and used; it provides newsletters, websites, fact sheets, apps and public campaigns to 'deliver meaningful information for health consumers, health professionals, government, research and other businesses to enable the best decisions about medicines and health technologies' (see 'Online resources')
- *Australian Prescriber*: a free bi-monthly independent review journal, published by the NPS, that provides critical commentary on drugs and therapeutics for health professionals, including Medicines Safety Updates; it has been freely available online since 1996, and articles are now included in the PubMed Central database
- reference books such as the *Australian Prescription Products Guide* ('PP Guide'), the *Merck Index*, *Drug Interactions: Analysis and Management* and journals such as *Current Therapeutics*, *Annals of Pharmacotherapy* and *Drugs* (references for current editions of these can best be found via a search engine).

Drug or poisons information centres and pharmacists

Drug information centres, usually located in the pharmacy departments of major teaching hospitals, are set up to disseminate information about drugs, adverse reactions, drug interactions, treatment of drug overdoses and other related information, to maximise safety, efficacy and economy in drug use (see AMH, Appendix, 'Drug

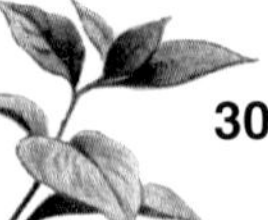

Information Centres'). They are excellent sources of information for both the public and health professionals. Community and hospital pharmacists, as medicines experts, are usually available and willing to provide drug information as part of their professional role.

Other drug information sources

- *Textbooks and drug guides:* An up-to-date pharmacology textbook is a valuable source of drug information for inclusion in the health professional's library! Various 'drug guides' also exist, acting as quick reference sources of summarised information on drugs. Most are now available online. Examples are the *MIMS Abbreviated* drug reference guides, published and updated four times per year. An app that is easily accessed on a smartphone, called 'Drug Names', provides concise information on a drug's class, mechanism of action, uses and dosage.
- *Reference books:* For example, *MIMS Annual* provides photographs to assist in identifying an unknown tablet or capsule. MIMS is now also published in various electronic formats (eMIMS) for android and Apple platforms, suitable for desktops, laptops, integratable to popular dispensing programs and as MIMSonline.
- *Drug companies' information:* Companies applying for registration of their products must supply to health authorities information on all aspects of the drug to prove its safety, efficacy and cost-effectiveness. A summary of this information is available in publications such as *MIMS Annual* and the PP Guide, and in consumer medicine information (see below) sheets, advertisements and promotions. Material supplied by drug companies is likely to be less objective than information in independent sources such as the AMH or *Australian Prescriber*. (Ethical aspects of drug advertising are discussed in Ch 2 of this text.)
- Consumer medicine information (CMI) pamphlets handed out to patients help improve people's understanding and usage of drugs they are prescribed. They are particularly important when a drug is first provided, the dose or formulation is changed or the information is revised. Previously, all products had to have CMI handouts/inclusions; however, many manufacturers now rely on consumers accessing information on their website.

The internet

With the proliferation of medical sites on the internet, many search engines (e.g. PubMed, Embase, eMedicine, Medline, Ovid, AusDI, Up-To-Date and the American Society of Health-System Pharmacists' drug information site) and directories are available to provide both general and specialised drug information for everyone – health professionals and consumers/patients. Some professional journals, databases, indexes and abstracting services also provide current drug information on the internet.

It is essential to read internet sites critically when seeking drug information because there is no screening system to determine the accuracy of internet information, and incorrect, commercial or biased information may be posted (Ioannidis et al 2017).[12]

KEY POINTS

Drug information sources

- Information about drugs is available from a wide variety of sources, ranging from official government publications through semi-official sources to drug company information and websites.
- Internet sources can be evaluated on the following criteria: accuracy, appearance, authority, currency and objectivity.

12 Students tempted to use Wikipedia as a quick source of drug information for assignments or revision purposes should beware. A comparison study looking at the accuracy and completeness of Wikipedia and Micromedex compared with FDA-approved production information found that Wikipedia was less complete and accurate. The authors concluded that Wikipedia should not be used by health professionals as a reference source (Reilly et al. 2017).

REVIEW EXERCISES

1. Mr MS is prescribed two new drugs, one for his blood pressure and one for his cholesterol. Mr MS does not like taking medicines and wants to know they are safe. He asks you, the health professional, to outline and describe the process from preclinical testing to post-marketing surveillance.
2. The doctor prescribes your patient an investigational drug that is new to you. Which drug information source would you select to find evidence-based information on this drug? What credibility could you give the information?
3. Compare the advantages and disadvantages of prescribing and using active ingredient (approved or generic) names rather than brand (or trade) names when communicating with patients.

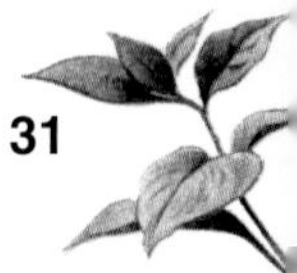

REFERENCES

Buckingham, R. (ed.). *Martindale: The Complete Drug Reference.* 40 ed, 2020, London, UK: Pharmaceutical Press.

Day, R.O., Snowden L., Where to find information about drugs. *Australian Prescriber*, 2016. **39**(3): p. 88.

Evans, WC (2009), Trease and Evans' Pharmacognosy, 16th edn, Edinburgh, 2009, Saunders. [ch 6].

Hinkson, I.V., Madej B., Stahlberg E.A., Accelerating therapeutics for opportunities in medicine: a paradigm shift in drug discovery. *Frontiers in Pharmacology*, 2020. **11**: p. 770.

Ioannidis, J.P., Stuart M., Brownless S., et al., How to survive the medical misinformation mess. *European Journal of Clinical Investigation*, 2017. **47**(11): pp. 795-802.

Le Fanu, J., *The rise and fall of modern medicine*. 2011: Hachette UK.

Médecins Sans Frontières (MSF) 2021. MSF medical guidelines. Online. https://medicalguidelines.msf.org/viewport/MG/en/guidelines-16681097.html

Oprea, T.I., Bologa C.G., Brunak S., et al., Unexplored therapeutic opportunities in the human genome. *Nature Reviews Drug Discovery*, 2018. **17**(5): p. 317–332.

Pharmac 2020a. *Year in Review: Top 20 community medicines by number of funded prescriptions dispensed*. Available from: https://pharmac.govt.nz/about/what-we-do/accountability-information/year-in-review/top-20-medicines-groups-by-prescription-volume/.

Pharmac 2020b. *Year in Review: Top 20 therapeutic groups by gross spend*. Available from: https://pharmac.govt.nz/about/what-we-do/accountability-information/year-in-review/top-20-therapeutic-groups-by-gross-spend/.

Pharmaceutical Society of Australia, *Australian pharmaceutical formulary and handbook*. 25 ed, ed. Sansom LN. 2021, Canberra: Pharmaceutical Society of Australia.

Reilly T, Jackson W, Berger V, et al. Accuracy and completeness of drug information in Wikipedia medication monographs. Journal of the American Pharmacists Association. 2017 Mar 1;57(2):193–6.

World Health Organization (WHO) 2007. A Model Quality Assurance System for Procurement Agencies: Recommendations for quality assurance systems focusing on prequalification of products and manufacturers, purchasing, storage and distribution of pharmaceutical products. WHO, Geneva.

World Health Organization (WHO) 2021. WHO model list of essential medicines – 22nd list, 2021. Online. https://www.who.int/publications/i/item/WHO-MHP-HPS-EML-2021.02

World Health Organization (WHO) 2022. International Nonproprietary Names Programme and Classification of Medical Products. Online. https://www.who.int/teams/health-product-and-policy-standards/inn

ACKNOWLEDGEMENTS

Evans WC: Trease and Evans' pharmacognosy, ed 16, Edinburgh, 2009, Saunders. [The definitive reference book on pharmacognosy (drugs from plants).]

ONLINE RESOURCES

Advisory Committee on the Safety of Medicines: https://www.tga.gov.au/ (follow links to Committees) (accessed 17 May 2021)

Australian Medicines Handbook: https://shop.amh.net.au (accessed 17 May 2021)

Australian Pharmaceutical Formulary: https://www.psa.org.au/apf (accessed 17 May 2021)

Australian Prescriber: https://www.nps.org.au/australian-prescriber/ (accessed 17 May 2021)

British Pharmacopoeia: https://www.pharmacopoeia.com (accessed 17 May 2021)

Centre for Adverse Reactions Monitoring (CARM) (New Zealand): https://www.medsafe.govt.nz/safety/report-a-problem.asp (accessed 17 May 2021)

Cochrane: https://www.cochrane.org/ (accessed 17 May 2021)

European Forum for Good Clinical Practice: https://efgcp.eu/ (accessed 17 May 2021)

General principles used by WHO in devising and approving INNs: www.who.int/medicines/services/inn/GeneralprinciplesEn.pdf?ua=1 (accessed 17 May 2021)

Martindale: The Complete Drug Reference: https://www.pharmpress.com/Martindale-The-Complete-Drug-Reference (accessed 17 May 2021)

Médecins Sans Frontières, essential drugs list: http://refbooks.msf.org/msf_docs/en/essential_drugs/ed_en.pdf (accessed 17 May 2021)

Medsafe (New Zealand): https://www.medsafe.govt.nz/ (accessed 17 May 2021)

MIMS Annual: https://www.mims.com.au/index.php/products/mims-annual (accessed 17 May 2021)

Prescribing Service (NPS) MedicineWise: https://www.nps.org.au/ (accessed 17 May 2021)

New Zealand Formulary (NZF): http://nzformulary.org (accessed 17 May 2021)

Pharmaceutical Management Agency, New Zealand (Pharmac): https://pharmac.govt.nz/

Pregnancy Safety Categories: https://www.tga.gov.au/prescribing-medicines-pregnancy-database (accessed 17 May 2021)

Therapeutic Goods Administration, adverse event notifications: https://www.tga.gov.au/reporting-adverse-events (accessed 17 May 2021)

Therapeutic Goods Administration, 'blue card': https://www.tga.gov.au/form/blue-card-adverse-reaction-reporting-form (accessed 17 May 2021)

Therapeutic Goods Administration, clinical trials guidelines: https://www.tga.gov.au/clinical-trials (accessed 17 May 2021)

Therapeutic Guidelines series: https://www.tg.org.au (accessed 17 May 2021)

United States Pharmacopeia (USP): https://www.uspnf.com/ (accessed 17 May 2021)

World Health Organization, Model List of Essential Medicines: https://www.who.int/publications/i/item/WHOMVPEMPIAU2019.06 (accessed 17 May 2021)

More weblinks at: http://evolve.elsevier.com/AU/Knights/pharmacology/.

CHAPTER 2

CLINICAL, ETHICAL AND LEGAL FOUNDATIONS OF PHARMACOTHERAPY

Mary Bushell

KEY ABBREVIATIONS

ADR	adverse drug reaction
Ahpra	Australian Health Practitioners Regulation Agency
Cth	Commonwealth
DUE	drug use evaluation
EBM/P	evidence-based medicine/ practice
FDA	US Food and Drug Administration
Medsafe	Medicines and Medical Devices Safety Authority (NZ)
NP	nurse practitioner
NPS	National Prescribing Service
OTC	over-the-counter
PBS	Pharmaceutical Benefits Scheme
PHARMAC	Pharmaceutical Management Agency (NZ)
QUM	Quality Use of Medicines
RCCT	randomised controlled clinical trial
SUSMP	*Standard for the Uniform Scheduling of Medicines and Poisons*
TGA	Therapeutic Goods Administration
UN	United Nations

Chapter Focus

'Pharmacotherapy' refers to the use of drugs for treating or preventing disease, as distinct from theoretical or experimental pharmacology, in which drugs may be studied to understand their mechanisms of action and effects. In this chapter, we focus first on the Australian laws relating to the regulation of prescription and over-the-counter (OTC) drugs, poisons, controlled substances, proscribed substances and investigational drugs, especially the *Therapeutic Goods Act 1989* (Cth); the drugs, poisons and controlled substances Acts and Regulations; and relevant customs, crimes and narcotic drugs Acts. The regulation and scheduling of drugs and controlled substances in Australia and New Zealand are compared.

Health professionals who prescribe, formulate, dispense or administer drugs are legally accountable for their actions related to drug therapy. This chapter reviews the roles of health professionals in relation to the use of medicines, and how quality use of medicines and drug use evaluations help optimise pharmacotherapy.

Many ethical principles also apply to drug use, based on human rights and bioethics; these should always underlie decisions related to pharmacology research and clinical practice. Controversy can arise as to how ethical principles are applied in clinical situations.

KEY TERMS

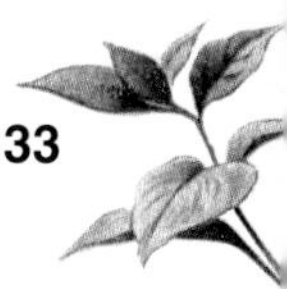

CRITICAL THINKING SCENARIO

Barbara, a 52-year-old female, recently experienced discomfort in her chest, arm, neck and jaw that lasted a couple of minutes. After an exercise tolerance test Barbara was diagnosed with stable angina. To relieve angina pain actively as it happens, her GP prescribed 400 microg glyceryl trinitrate spray to be administered sublingually. To prevent future episodes of angina Barbara was also prescribed aspirin 100 mg orally daily and atenolol 25 mg orally daily.

1. Discuss how we know the medicines that Barbara has been prescribed are safe and effective.
2. Discuss what the Poisons Standard (the SUSMP) is. Discuss the different levels of controls in access, supply/provision, labelling, storage, records and advertising for each of Barbara's prescribed drugs.

Barbara elects to have an electronic prescription, and her prescriber sends her a QR code via a text message to her phone. Barbara then forwards this QR code to her local pharmacy to be dispensed. The pharmacy has Barbara's Medicare and Commonwealth concession card details on file.

3. Outline what makes a legal prescription. Outline what makes a valid Pharmaceutical Benefits Scheme prescription.
4. Consistent with the National Health (Pharmaceutical Benefits) Amendment (Active Ingredient Prescribing) Regulations Barbara's GP used active ingredient prescribing. Discuss what active ingredient prescribing is and its benefits.
5. Discuss some of the benefits of electronic prescribing over paper-based prescribing.

Clinical aspects of pharmacotherapy

Introduction

To optimise use of drugs in a rational, clinically effective and cost-effective way, health professionals need to understand: the evidence on which clinical decisions are based; necessary decision-making processes before drugs are chosen, prescribed or advised; how prescriptions are written and dispensed; the types of formulations in which drugs are administered; and the factors that affect how people respond to drugs – in fact, basically the whole of clinical pharmacology!

Quality use of medicines

The foundation and chief purpose of pharmacotherapy is **Quality Use of Medicines** (QUM), described in Australia's *National Medicines Policy* (see 'Online resources') as the judicious, appropriate, safe and effective use of medicines. Specifically, QUM means:

- selecting management options wisely
- if a medicine is needed, selecting that medicine wisely – this means taking into consideration the person, the clinical condition, the benefits and harms of the medicine (based on the best evidence), the dosage and length of treatment, other medical conditions, other medicines the person may be taking, monitoring considerations and cost (to the individual, community and the healthcare system)
- using medicines safely and effectively – monitoring outcomes, minimising misuse, under- and overuse.

Some professional groups have incorporated a QUM policy within their own charter; for example, the Podiatry Board of Australia's Prescribing Information concludes with the necessity to have access to various reference texts and databases, plus 'access to Quality Use of Medicines principles' (see 'Online resources').

Evidence-based health care

Health professionals should practise **evidence-based medicine** (EBM)[1] – 'the conscientious, explicit and judicious use of current best evidence in making decisions about the medical care of individual patients' (Sackett et al. 1995).

1 Although the terms 'medicine' and 'medical' are sometimes used to imply health care provided by doctors, in the wider sense the term is defined as 'the branch of science devoted to the prevention of disease and the restoration of the sick to health' (The American Heritage Medical Dictionary 2007), so EBM is practised by a wide range of health professionals.

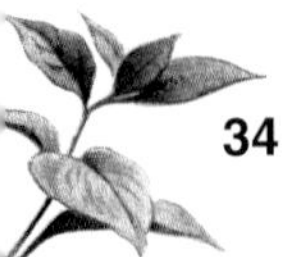

EBM (or EBP, evidence-based practice) applies to all therapy, whether with drugs or interventions such as physiotherapy techniques, lens prescriptions, dental care, nursing care or paramedic emergency aid.

Integrating evidence-based medicine improves patient outcomes and quality of life. It can also improve productivity and reduce healthcare costs. Despite this, studies show that as many as four in 10 adult patients receive care that is not based on current evidence, including ineffective, unnecessary and even harmful treatments (e.g. antibiotics for the common cold or otitis media).

Levels of evidence

Not all evidence or study types are considered equal. In research, there is a hierarchy of evidence. The strength of evidence on which EBM/EBP is based has been classified into levels of decreasing value:

- meta-analyses – evidence from a systematic review of all relevant randomised controlled clinical trials (RCCTs) such as Cochrane systematic reviews
- evidence from large, well-designed RCCTs
- evidence from small, randomised trials
- evidence from cohort or case-controlled studies
- evidence from case series or studies with no controls.

When using evidence to inform patient care, health professionals should critically appraise the evidence for its internal and external validity. Internal validity is the rigor in which the study was conducted. External validity is the applicability of the research findings to the real-life patient.

While clinical experience is an aspect of providing EBM, evidence based on clinical experience or expert opinion alone ('we've always done it this way') is considered the lowest form of evidence.

Drug information in objective databases such as PubMed, EMBASE (Excerpta Medica Database), the Cochrane Library and the Cumulative Index to Nursing and Allied Health Literature can be consulted. The *Australian Prescriber* website, **Medsafe**, the *Australian Medicines Handbook* (2021) and *Therapeutic Guidelines* are all based on the highest level of evidence available (see 'Online resources').

Targeting QUM

Australian medicines policies

In 1985 the World Health Organization held a conference on the rational use of drugs, calling on all governments to implement a national medicinal drug policy. In June 1996 the former Council of Australian Governments agreed on the central objectives of the *National Medicines Policy*:

- timely access to the medicines that Australians need, at a cost individuals and the community can afford
- medicines meeting appropriate standards of quality, safety and efficacy
- QUM
- maintaining a responsible and viable medicines industry (see 'Online resources': *National Medicines Policy*).

(The term 'medicine' includes prescription and non-prescription medicines, including complementary health products.)

QUM is implemented by health professionals, interested consumer groups, the **Therapeutic Goods Administration** (TGA), the Australian Government's Pharmaceutical Benefits Advisory Committee, agencies of government health departments and many other professional bodies. Examples of programs in QUM include: nominating a priority list of medicines commonly required for paediatric use; establishing guidelines for managing drugs in residential aged care facilities; setting up a system for recalling therapeutic goods; and programs for non-pharmacological aspects of health care such as diet, smoking cessation and exercise.

National Prescribing Service

The Australian **National Prescribing Service** (NPS) is an independent, not-for-profit organisation first established in 1998 to improve the way health technologies, medicines and medical tests are prescribed and used. Through its educational activities targeted to health practitioners, consumers and the pharmaceutical industry, the NPS has achieved some significant savings in drug costs.

NPS MedicineWise has programs for health professionals including Choosing Wisely Australia, MedicineInsight and Good Medicine Better Health. All programs aim to improve QUM

Medicines Australia

Medicines Australia 'leads the research-based medicines industry of Australia. Our members discover, develop and manufacture prescription pharmaceutical products, biotherapeutic products and vaccines that bring health, social and economic benefits to Australia. Our members invest in Australian medical research and take local discoveries and developments to the world' (Medicines Australia 2022). It is involved in developing health and industry policies, ensuring viable continuation of the industry, and administering the Code of Conduct for ethical marketing of prescription drugs. The industry body has QUM roles in developing medicines, providing evidence-based information and partnering with consumer organisations (see 'Online resources').

New Zealand medicines strategy

The New Zealand Ministry of Health / Manatū Hauora has several programs aimed at achieving QUM. (The roles of Pharmac [the Pharmaceutical Management Agency] and PTAC [the Pharmacology and Therapeutics Advisory

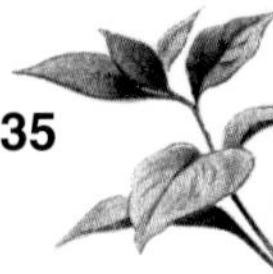

Committee] are described below, and those of SCOTT, Medsafe and the *New Zealand Formulary* were covered in Ch 1 in relation to clinical trials and drug information.)

The three main outcomes of the New Zealand medicines strategy include:

- access: New Zealanders have access to the medicines they need, regardless of ethnicity, location or wealth
- optimal use: medicines used to their best effect
- quality: medicines that are safe and effective.

The system includes several agencies with responsibilities for: QUM and **pharmacovigilance**, including Medsafe, District Health Boards and centres; programs for monitoring/implementing adverse drug reactions (ADRs), vaccines, best practice and quality improvement; primary health organisations; the *New Zealand Formulary*; and the *Universal List of Medicines*.

Drug use evaluation

The World Health Organization recommends that **drug use evaluation** (DUE; also known as drug utilisation review) be incorporated into QUM programs. DUE is a method of obtaining information related to drug use problems. Objectives may include: ensuring that drug therapy meets current standards of care; controlling drug costs; preventing or correcting problems related to medication; evaluating outcomes of drug therapy; identifying areas of practice that require further education of practitioners; and comparing activities between prescribers.

Some DUEs have been in the areas of:

- appropriate use of antibiotics in the primary care and hospital setting
- determining the list of drugs for acute care use in remote Indigenous Australian community health centres
- complementary medicines in public hospitals
- continuity of pharmacological care as patients are moved from hospital to the community
- reducing the prescribing of benzodiazepines in the community.

DUEs have been shown to save not only lives and time, but also money.

Modifying drug usage over time

Pharmacopoeias and formularies (and pharmacology textbooks) are in a constant state of change, and health professionals need to keep up to date. Some influences on evolving drug use are described below, with examples.

Why drugs appear

New technologies

Until the early 20th century, most drugs were from natural sources: plants (morphine, cocaine), minerals (iodine, iron) and animals (vaccines, tissue extracts). As chemical industries and pharmacological techniques developed, drugs such as antibiotics, oral contraceptives, antihypertensives, antipsychotic agents, human insulin and monoclonal antibodies became available (Table 1.2 in Ch 1).

New uses for old drugs

Drugs are sometimes found to have uses additional to original indications. Minoxidil, an antihypertensive agent, caused increased growth of hair and found new use as a hair-restorer. Methylphenidate, originally an appetite suppressant and stimulant, found new application in treating attention deficit hyperactivity disorder.

Better understanding of mechanisms

The discovery of the mechanism of action of aspirin (inhibiting synthesis of prostaglandins) and its antiplatelet actions led to its now widespread prophylactic use against thromboembolism, preventing myocardial infarction and strokes.

Better understanding of aetiology of disease

Studies of the causes of peptic ulcers first recommended sedatives to reduce stress, then antacids to neutralise gastric acid, then antimuscarinics, histamine H_2-receptor antagonists and proton-pump inhibitors to reduce the production of acid. Most recently, antibacterials to reduce infection with *Helicobacter pylori* were added (Ch 36). Similarly, rapid advances in understanding of the biochemical pathways involved in controlling cell division have led to many new anticancer drugs (Ch 33).

Changes in popularity of drugs

There is a recognised cycle in popularity of new drugs, just as for new gadgets, toys and mobile phones. As a drug is developed and marketed to prescribers and consumers, it rapidly surges in popularity. ADRs may become apparent, its expense is noted, and 'me-too' drugs compete, so its use wanes. Then, as the benefits and risks are evaluated rationally, the drug regains a medium but more stable position in usage.

Changes in availability of drugs

There may be a major change in the use of a drug as it is moved between poisons Schedules and becomes either more or less readily available or expensive. When new COX-2 inhibitors (celecoxib, rofecoxib) and statins (atorvastatin, simvastatin, etc.) were introduced, they were very expensive. Public (and drug company) pressure in Australia led to their being subsidised and listed on the PBS, and their use skyrocketed, at great expense to governments (i.e. taxpayers); statins are still the most frequently prescribed medicines in Australia. However, when patent protection for new drug molecules expires, other companies can legally manufacture and market the drug, so competition from 'generics' reduces the price.

Why drugs disappear

No longer optimal therapy

As better drugs are developed, many less effective and less safe drugs (such as bromide hypnotics and mercurial diuretics) have become obsolete. For centuries, syphilis was treated with toxic arsenic- or mercury-containing compounds, because the aetiology was unknown and no effective treatment was available until safe oral antibacterials were developed.

Medicine recalls

A medicine can be recalled when a deficiency is identified in its quality, safety or efficacy; or a disease may become less prevalent; or company mergers may bring competitor products into the same 'stable'. The manufacturer will notify wholesalers to cease distribution and pharmacists to return stock. Prescribers may then switch the patient to an alternative drug; however, a new drug may cause withdrawal reactions, recurrence of illness or new ADRs or interactions.

Adverse effects become apparent

ADRs appearing in post-marketing studies (phase IV trials; see Ch 1) may lead to withdrawal of the product. Thalidomide, for example, was marketed as a safe sedative and antinausea drug in pregnancy until thousands of congenital malformations became evident (CFB 2.1 and McBride[2]). Another example is the anti-inflammatory COX-2 inhibitor rofecoxib (Vioxx), which was introduced in Australia in 1999 and rapidly became popular. However, analyses of post-marketing use showed it caused about double the risk of heart attacks and strokes compared with a placebo (CFB 2.1).[3]

Drug combinations shown to be unjustified

From the times of the ancient Greeks into the mid-20th century, doctors often wrote prescriptions for complex mixtures 'for nerves' or as 'tonics' (see an example in Fig 2.3, later). More recently, combinations of antimicrobials, antiasthma drugs or antihypertensives may be formulated together. Adherence with therapy is enhanced when patients need only take one 'polypill'; however, it is usually better to prescribe drugs individually, as pharmacokinetic properties of components vary, and doses cannot be individually adjusted.

CLINICAL FOCUS BOX 2.1

The thalidomide disaster

Between 1958 and 1962, thousands of babies across Western countries, including Australia, were stillborn or born with congenital malformations, including short and absent limbs. The condition was termed phocomelia, meaning 'seal-like limbs', and had until that time been incredibly rare. Causes were proposed, including viral infections, radiation damage, nutritional deficiencies or environmental contaminants. In Germany alone, about 10,000 babies were affected. Dr Widukind Lenz, of Hamburg, asked mothers of affected babies to list all the drugs they had taken during pregnancy; Contergan, an apparently safe sedative, appeared in about 30% of the lists. Meanwhile, in Sydney, Dr William McBride had been consulted about several babies with phocomelia; all the mothers had taken Distaval, a mild sedative and antiemetic, during pregnancy. In 1961 Dr McBride wrote to the journal *The Lancet*, asking if similar cases had been reported. Lenz replied, and it became apparent that the same drug, thalidomide, was implicated in all cases.

More case reports flooded in, and the drug was withdrawn. However, cases kept appearing for many years because the drug was marketed under numerous trade names, warnings went unheeded, bottles of tablets lay around, the critical risk period was so short – between the 37th and 54th days of pregnancy – and effects not observed until many months later, and many mothers forgot having taken drugs in early pregnancy. (The drug had not been released in the United States because the Food and Drug Administration [FDA] had been concerned, not about its ability to cause congenital disabilities, but because it had adverse effects on the nervous system.)

Files published for the first time in 2013 revealed that many Australian women were used as 'human guinea pigs' by the Distillers Company in 1960, before tests in pregnant animals had been carried out, and that the German manufacturer suppressed warnings about fetal effects. Lawsuits and damages claims against the drug companies were still pursued in the courts decades later.

The thalidomide disaster led to tighter regulations of medicines and medical devices in Australia. It also saw the establishment of the Australian Drug Evaluation Committee. Today thalidomide is used as a non-cytotoxic antineoplastic to treat multiple myeloma. It is contraindicated in women of childbearing age who are not using contraception.

Source: McBride 1961.

2 A report by the Grattan Institute in Melbourne, dated 5 March 2017, claimed that 'Australians pay more than $500 million a year too much for their prescription drugs . . . Drug prices in Australia are . . . more than three times higher than in New Zealand.' The high prices not only hit the hip pocket - they mean that many Australians defer getting needed medicines due to the costs. The report was criticised by 'big pharma' drug companies and pharmacy bodies as being 'a simplistic response to a complex problem'.

3 Hundreds of patients in Australia joined legal class actions against the manufacturer of rofecoxib, claiming the manufacturer knew about increased risk of cardiovascular events long before the drug was withdrawn. It is reported that, in the year before its withdrawal, the manufacturer Merck reaped revenue of at least US$2.5 billion from sales of Vioxx.

When to use a new drug

Knowledge about a new drug, even after an RCCT, is still quite limited, and wider post-marketing use may show up unusual ADRs or efficacy in more subgroups of the population. The cautious approach suggests that doctors limit prescribing new drugs until pharmacovigilance in large populations.[4] In practice, despite the thousands of drugs in the pharmacopoeias, GPs prescribe mostly from a limited personal list of less than 100 tried-and-true preferred drugs – their 'P-list'.

There is often pressure from industry and consumers for particular drugs to be 'fast-tracked' through regulatory processes, with 'cutting of red tape' – for example, for new biologicals possibly effective in cancers. However, 'fast-tracked' drugs are more likely to be subsequently withdrawn than those subjected to the usual more careful vetting.

A pharmaceutical company may provide a 'product familiarisation program', to familiarise individual prescribers with a recently approved new drug while awaiting government subsidisation of it. This provides a small number of people with the new drug free of charge for a short period, thus saving the person and the government money, and increasing experience with the drug and the likelihood of adverse effects showing up. However, opponents of such programs 'argue that they are thinly disguised marketing exercises' that are aimed at increasing eventual usage of the drug, and thus making more profits for the company (Kyle 2017).

Pharmacoeconomics

Because of the blowout in demands for and costs of drugs, no country can provide all desirable drugs; hence, pharmacoeconomic rationalisation is essential, if possible without compromising good health care. Health economists need to evaluate and balance the costs of developing and providing drugs, the need for drugs by the increasing elderly population, the growing demands for 'lifestyle' drugs and indirect aspects such as savings from shorter hospital admissions, improved quality of life and surgery avoided. A statistic called the incremental cost-effectiveness ratio can be used to compare a new medicine with its comparator. Overall, policies such as generic substitution (dispensing the cheapest alternative among bioequivalent medicines), rationalisation of drug policies and QUM help to optimise access to essential drugs.

To be listed by the Australian Pharmaceutical Benefits Scheme (PBS) as a subsidised drug, it must be proved to be safe, effective and cost-effective. Listing as a 'restricted benefit' or as 'authority required to prescribe' helps limit use of an expensive drug to those in whom it will be most effective. (Such decisions have ethical implications, discussed later.)

Factors modifying responses to drugs

If the same dose of drug (on a mg drug dose per kg body weight basis) is given to similar people – or indeed to the same person on different occasions – the responses are likely to be different. Factors modifying drug responses need to be anticipated before prescribing and administering a drug, and afterwards when monitoring drug therapy. (Pharmaceutical factors affecting response, such as the form in which the drug is administered, are discussed later.)

Pharmacokinetic and pharmacodynamic factors

Factors that affect how a drug is absorbed from its site of administration, distributed around the body and eliminated by metabolism and excretion determine how much drug is available at any time to act. Pharmacokinetic principles are applied to dosage regimens and individual and life span aspects of drug therapy in Chapters 4–6.

'Pharmacodynamics' refers to what the drug does in the body, including useful therapeutic effects and ADRs, as well as studies of the drug's mechanism of action at the molecular level. These aspects are discussed in Chapters 3 and 7 and in subsequent chapters under drug groups and in Drug Monographs.

Adherence (compliance)

The primary determinant of drug response is whether or not the person takes the drug; as the old saying goes, 'the treatment can't work if the patient doesn't take it'.[5] **Adherence** is defined as 'the extent to which a person's behaviour . . . corresponds with agreed recommendations from a healthcare provider' (World Health Organization 2003); it therefore implies a more active role than the older term 'compliance'. In the context of pharmacotherapy, it implies administering the drug according to the six rights (Fig 2.1) and following all therapeutic advice, including lifestyle aspects such as diet modification, weight reduction, cessation of smoking and moderation in alcohol intake. This becomes a formidable challenge when multiple drugs are prescribed. Many studies have

4 The Public Citizen's Health Research Group, in the US, in fact recommended 'against the use of any new prescription drug, except for truly "breakthrough" drugs, for five years after approval by the FDA' (Wolfe 2012). This advice has been extended to a 7-year ban because 94% of drug safety withdrawals occurred within 7 years. However, this would be counterproductive because infrequent ADRs would be unlikely to show up; larger numbers require many doctors to prescribe, and many patients to take, the new drug. Someone somewhere has to start the ball rolling . . .

5 This has been recognised for thousands of years. The ancient Greek physician Hippocrates advised his medical students thus: 'Keep a watch also on the faults of patients, which often make them lie about the taking of things prescribed. For through not taking disagreeable drinks, purgative or other, they sometimes die. What they have done never results in a confession, but the blame is thrown upon the physician.' It seems that human nature has not changed much over thousands of years . . .

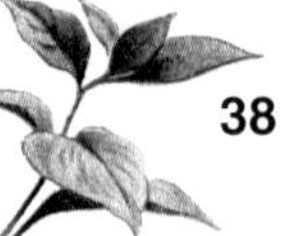

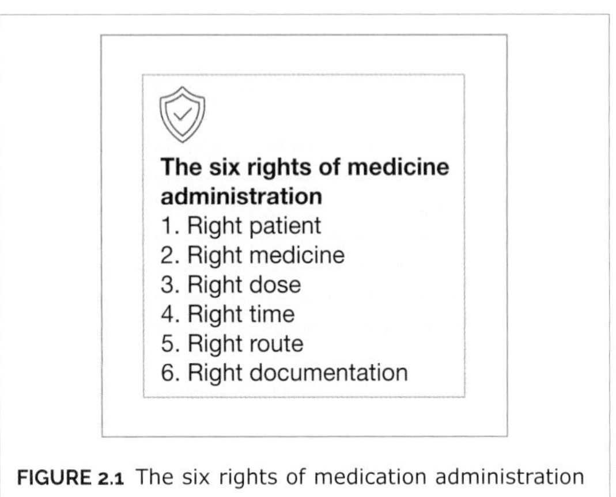

The six rights of medicine administration
1. Right patient
2. Right medicine
3. Right dose
4. Right time
5. Right route
6. Right documentation

FIGURE 2.1 The six rights of medication administration

shown that only approximately 50% of people with chronic conditions adhere to treatment recommendations (Usherwood 2017).

There are many causes of poor adherence, including intentional non-adherence, confusion over complicated drug regimens, bad taste or pain on administration, adverse effects occurring, not wanting to disturb or wake the person if sleeping, poor communication about the treatment, beliefs about the disease or treatment, lack of support or monitoring of therapy and cost or difficulty in obtaining medicines.

Poor adherence with long-term medication is common and, despite Hippocrates' warning, doctors are not good at predicting which patients are likely to adhere. The consequences of poor adherence, along with wasted drugs and time, include:

- reduced potential to benefit from treatment when drug levels in the body fall below the effective therapeutic range
- levels may rise and cause ADRs and toxicity
- the prescriber cannot properly monitor and adjust therapy and may waste effort revising the diagnosis, increasing doses or drugs or sending the person for more tests
- missed doses may have serious consequences such as with oral contraceptives (pregnancy), antiepileptic drugs (convulsions) or anticoagulant or antithrombotic drugs (strokes or heart attacks).

How to improve adherence

Ways of assessing adherence include careful counts of doses remaining after a specified period and measurements of drug levels in blood or urine samples (see 'Therapeutic drug monitoring' in Ch 5). Autonomy in medical care implies the patient's right to refuse to take drugs for good reasons. However, it is important that the prescriber be made aware if drugs are not being taken as directed so that doses can be adjusted or different drugs substituted.

Adherence can be improved if people understand and identify with their treatment, if it is the simplest possible regimen, if they know how to deal with **side effects** and if reminder packaging and administration aids are used. Studies have shown that young adults with asthma on preventer medications demonstrate significantly improved adherence when reminded by text messages, and that people with type 2 diabetes who receive their medications from only one pharmacy are more adherent than those who shop around for their drugs (Usherwood 2017).

Drug interactions

After a person has been stabilised on a drug, drug responses may be affected by interactions with any other drugs taken (prescribed, OTC or complementary) or with food and drinks. As more drugs are taken, the possibility of interactions rises exponentially, and drugs may be required to treat earlier adverse effects (the 'prescribing cascade'). Drug interactions may involve either pharmacokinetics (e.g. monoamine oxidase inhibitors inhibiting the metabolism of many other drugs) or pharmacodynamics (e.g. β-blockers taken for hypertension and β_2-agonists used for asthma having opposing effects).

Drug interactions are discussed in Chapter 8 and in Drug Interactions tables and individual Drug Monographs where clinically significant. There are exhaustive lists of common drug interactions in reference texts such as the *Australian Medicines Handbook* (2021) (Appendix B).

Placebo effect

The Latin word *placebo* literally means 'I will please.' In the pharmacological context, '**placebo**' refers to a harmless or inactive preparation prescribed to satisfy a person who does not require an active drug. In a clinical trial if there is no current best drug for comparison, the placebo is formulated to look identical to the active drug. This helps to maintain 'double-blinding' so neither subject nor clinician knows which drug is being taken.

Patients and subjects in trials frequently appear to respond to placebos with therapeutic or adverse effects. (See CFB 31.3 for placebo responses in trials of Viagra.) Factors inducing placebo response include the person's expectations, the relationship between the patient and health professional, the wish to be seen to comply, a response to increased care and attention and aspects such as the colour and taste of the dose form or pain from an injection.

Roles of health professionals in QUM

Traditionally the health professionals most involved with drugs were doctors who prescribed them, pharmacists who dispensed them and nurses who administered them. During the period that medicine was developing as a

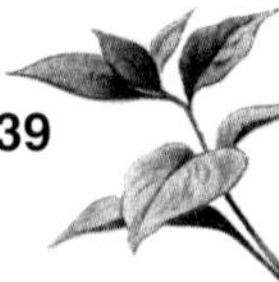

profession in England, physicians were allowed to prescribe 'physic' (medicine) compounded by apothecaries (pharmacists); now many more health professionals are involved with medicines or with people taking them and therefore need to know some pharmacological language and principles. The roles of many health professionals will be described briefly; specialised aspects, such as nursing roles in drug administration and pharmacists' roles in dispensing drugs, are beyond the scope of this text. National registration guidelines are being developed by many professional boards, under the auspices of the Australian Health Practitioner Regulation Agency (Ahpra).

In Australia, while the Commonwealth regulates therapeutic goods, each state has its own laws determining access to drugs. The Victorian Minister for Health has therefore approved prescriber lists for nurse practitioners (NPs), authorised optometrists, authorised podiatrists and authorised registered midwives. But whether the prescription is subsidised by the PBS is a Commonwealth decision; latest regulations should always be consulted.

Aboriginal and Torres Strait Islander health practitioners

Indigenous people throughout the world tend to be disadvantaged across a range of socioeconomic factors and suffer a greater burden of ill-health. As they move from traditional lifestyles, they may acquire diseases such as obesity, cardiovascular disease and type 2 diabetes. The average life expectancy of Indigenous Australians (Aboriginals and Torres Strait Islander peoples) is about 10 years less than that of non-Indigenous Australians, despite 'close-the-gap' policies.

About 25% of Indigenous Australians live in remote areas, where Indigenous health workers, with visiting doctors, nurses and pharmacists, provide knowledge about health, work in home medicine reviews and help with interviews and communication. The Aboriginal and Torres Strait Islander Health Practice Board of Australia comes under the auspices of Ahpra. The Certificate IV in Aboriginal and Torres Strait Islander Primary Health Care syllabus includes: units on safe use of medicines; assessment of needs of clients with alcohol and other drug issues; and strategies in sexual health and smoking cessation. Some drugs are listed on the PBS for prescribing specifically to Aboriginal and Torres Strait Islander peoples, to meet particular health needs (see 'Online resources').

Ambulance and mobile intensive care paramedics

The primary roles of a paramedic are rapid assessment, treatment and transport of individuals requiring medical care in the pre-hospital setting. Since 1 December 2018, paramedics must be registered with the Paramedicine Board of Australia to practise in Australia. Paramedics operate under written standing orders and are required to ensure compliance with legislation and standards associated with storage, documentation and administration of drugs. In Victoria, for example, paramedics can lawfully possess listed Schedule 4 and 8 poisons in accordance with health service permits held by Ambulance Victoria and/or St John Ambulance Australia (Vic).

Typical drugs used are: chewable aspirin for chest pain; intramuscular midazolam for seizures; methoxyflurane, morphine and ketamine as analgesics; glucose buccal gel for hypoglycaemic attacks; intramuscular naloxone for opioid overdoses; cardiovascular drugs; bronchodilators; and muscle relaxants.

Complementary and alternative medicine practitioners

Complementary and alternative medicine (CAM) practitioners use techniques including provision of herbal products, massage, acupuncture, naturopathy, homoeopathy and iridology. (Ch 44). The Boards for Chinese Medicine, Chiropractic and Osteopathy are regulated under Ahpra. There can be interactions between practices in Western medicine and CAM – for example, drug interactions between prescribed drugs and concurrent CAM preparations.

Dentists

Dentists are authorised to prescribe drugs related to their treatment, especially antibiotics, anti-inflammatories, analgesics, local anaesthetics, antiemetics, antianxiety agents and mouthwashes; those in the Australian PBS Dental Items List are subsidised (CFB 2.2). They frequently administer local anaesthetics and nitrous oxide during dental procedures to relieve pain. Amoxicillin is the antibiotic of first choice for severe superficial dental infections, with metronidazole added if necessary. Prophylactic antibiotic cover is advised for those with cardiac conditions that carry a risk of infective endocarditis, and those with recent joint surgery.

Doctors

Medical practitioners are responsible for advising on health issues, diagnosing disease and initiating and monitoring therapy, including prescribing drugs not available OTC (CFB 2.2). Doctors require extensive knowledge of pharmacology: actions and mechanisms of drugs (pharmacodynamics), drug handling by the body (pharmacokinetics) and clinical aspects, including ADRs, drug interactions, dosages, indications and contraindications for drug use, in all situations and patients.

The 'doctor's bag' of drugs

Traditionally, doctors visiting patients in the community carried a black bag holding drugs that the doctor could supply or administer as needed, particularly in emergencies

CLINICAL FOCUS BOX 2.2
Who can prescribe medicines in Australia?

An increasing number of health professionals can prescribe scheduled medicines, improving public access to medicines in a timely manner, consistent with the 1999 *National Medicines Policy*. To date (2021), medical doctors can prescribe, as can endorsed dentists, NPs, veterinary surgeons, midwives, optometrists and podiatrists. Physiotherapists and pharmacists cannot prescribe, but there is growing momentum for this to change (in countries such as New Zealand and the UK pharmacists can prescribe).

Medical and non-medical prescribing is regulated at the state and territory level (see relevant poisons legislation in Table 2.1). Therefore, there are slight variations between jurisdictions; however, the major aspects are somewhat uniform. In general, medical prescribers are less restricted when compared with non-medical prescribers.

There are two ways a non-medical prescriber can be endorsed to prescribe. One is where members of a profession are endorsed to prescribe from a restricted formulary. Endorsed dentists and optometrists, for example, can prescribe from a restricted formulary. In contrast, endorsed midwives and NPs, since 2019, do not prescribe from a restricted formulary; instead, they prescribe within their scope of practice. That is, they prescribe within their area of specialisation and specified circumstances. Subsequently, there is a wide variation between what one NP may prescribe when compared with another.

Prescribing may be restricted by indication, dose, route of administration and duration of therapy. For example, optometrists can prescribe atropine for ocular use (eyedrops) but not intravenous administration.

PBS prescribers

Not all prescribers can prescribe medicines that are subsidised under the PBS. To date (2021) they can only be prescribed by doctors, dentists, NPs, midwives and optometrists who are approved to prescribe PBS medicines under the *National Health Act 1953*. Podiatrists and veterinary surgeons can only prescribe non-PBS or private prescriptions. Pharmacists can dispense all legal prescriptions written by all the different 'types' of prescribers (even when the 'patient' is an animal).

or serious medical conditions in the surgery or person's home. The PBS still allows doctors to carry such drugs, most of them in parenteral (injectable) form – for example: adrenaline (epinephrine) for cardiac arrest and severe allergic reactions; haloperidol (for psychiatric emergencies); glucagon (for hypoglycaemia); morphine (to treat severe pain and pulmonary oedema); and oxytocin (for obstetric conditions). Non-injectable items include glyceryl trinitrate spray or patches (for angina or myocardial infarction), salbutamol aerosol (for asthma) and methoxyflurane inhalation (for painful procedures and trauma patients). It is suggested that doctors also carry supplies of normal saline and water for injection, a sharps container, disposable gloves and dressing packs. Logbooks of supplies need to be kept and a system for checking expiry dates implemented.

Midwives

Midwifery is the area of health care specialising in antenatal care, labour and childbirth in low-risk pregnancies. In Australia, registration is through the Nursing and Midwifery Board of Australia. Suitably qualified eligible midwives may be endorsed to supply and administer some Schedule 2, 3, 4 and 8 drugs only for 'women and their infants in the pre-natal, intra-partum and post-natal stages of pregnancy and birth' (Department of Health 2022). Appropriately trained and credentialled midwives may apply for a PBS prescriber number (see 'Online resources'). Only midwives with a PBS prescriber number can be recognised as an authorised prescriber. The medicines that midwives can prescribe is determined by state and territory legislation (Table 2.1), resulting in variations in what midwives can prescribe across the federation.

During antenatal care, midwives may recommend iron and folic acid to treat anaemias and prevent neural tube defects. During childbirth, nitrous oxide or oxygen may be administered and, in the absence of a doctor, midwives in some jurisdictions are allowed on phone order to administer oxytocin and/or ergometrine to stimulate uterine muscle contractions, and metoclopramide as an antiemetic. This must be followed up with a written doctor's prescription within 24 hours. Vitamin K is routinely administered to neonates to prevent haemorrhagic disease, and a single dose of hepatitis B vaccine at birth. A neonate may require oxygen, and they may need naloxone to reverse opiate-induced respiratory depression. 'Standing orders' from a medical team are required for prescription drugs.

In New Zealand, midwifery is an independent registration, so not all midwives are nurses. New Zealand midwives work as the lead maternity carer in low-risk pregnancies, during labour and up to 6 weeks postpartum. Midwives are Authorised Prescribers under the 1990

TABLE 2.1 Principal Australian and New Zealand legislation involved in the regulation of drugs

JURISDICTION	DRUG REGULATION LEGISLATION	ADDITIONAL DRUG OFFENCES ACTS
Australian Commonwealth (Cth)	*Therapeutic Goods Act 1989* (Cth) Therapeutic Goods Regulations 1990 (Cth) *National Health Act 1953* (Cth)	*Customs Act 1901* (Cth) *Crimes (Traffic in Narcotic Drugs and Psychotropic Substances) Act 1990* (Cth) *Narcotic Drugs Act 1967* (Cth) *Criminal Code Act 1995* (Cth)
Australian Capital Territory (ACT)	*Medicines, Poisons and Therapeutic Goods Act 2008* (ACT) *Drugs of Dependence Act 1989* (ACT) *Drugs in Sport Act 1999* (ACT) Drugs of Dependence Regulations 2009 (ACT)	Criminal Code 2002 (ACT)
New South Wales (NSW)	*Poisons and Therapeutic Goods Act 1966* (NSW) Poisons and Therapeutic Goods Regulations 2008 (NSW)	*Drug Misuse and Trafficking Act 1985* (NSW)
Northern Territory (NT)	*Medicines, Poisons and Therapeutic Goods Act 2012* (NT) Medicines, Poisons and Therapeutic Goods Regulations 2014 (NT)	*Misuse of Drugs Act 1990* (NT)
Queensland (Qld)	*Medicines and Poisons Act 2019* (Qld) Therapeutic Goods Regulation 2021 (Qld) Medicines and Poisons (Poisons and Prohibited Substances) Regulation 2021 (Qld)	*Drugs Misuse Act 1986* (Qld)
South Australia (SA)	*Controlled Substances Act 1984* (SA) Controlled Substances (Poisons) Regulations 2011 (SA) Controlled Substances (Controlled Drugs, Precursors and Plants) Regulations 2014 (SA)	*Criminal Law Consolidation Act 1935* (SA)
Tasmania (Tas)	*Poisons Act 1971* (Tas) Poisons Regulations 2018 (Tas) *Therapeutic Goods Act 2001* (Tas) Poisons (Declared Restricted Substances) Order 2017 (Tas)	*Misuse of Drugs Act 2001* (Tas) *Alcohol and Drug Dependency Act 1968* (Tas)
Victoria (Vic)	*Therapeutic Goods (Victoria) Act 2010* (Vic) *Drugs, Poisons and Controlled Substances Act 1981* (Vic) Drugs, Poisons and Controlled Substances Regulations 2006 (Vic)	*Crimes Act 1958* (Vic)
Western Australia (WA)	*Medicines and Poisons Act 2014* (WA) Medicines and Poisons Regulations 2016 (WA)	*Misuse of Drugs Act 1981* (WA)
New Zealand	*Medicines Act 1981* Medicines Regulations 1984 Medicines (Standing Order) Amendment Regulations 2016 Medicines (Designated Prescriber: Nurse Practitioners) Regulations 2016 Medicines (Designated Pharmacist Prescribers) Regulations 2013 Misuse of Drugs Regulations 1977	*Misuse of Drugs Act 1975*

amendments to the *Medicines Act* and Medicines Regulations (Table 2.1 and Midwifery Council of New Zealand under 'Online resources'). The New Zealand College of Midwives sets and reviews professional standards and provides continuing education (see 'Online resources'). Midwives are permitted to prescribe the controlled drugs pethidine, morphine and fentanyl for use only during childbirth.

Nurses

Traditionally, nurses have worked in hospitals, community health centres, specialist medical clinics, private practice, rural/district nursing services and in workplaces. In Australia, registration standards for nursing practice and continuing professional development are set by the Nursing and Midwifery Board of Australia. Nurses are involved, among other roles, in ensuring safe and reliable administration of drugs and in monitoring ADRs. In the hospital situation, this could include:

- assessing the person and taking a medication history
- noting the prescription, checking dosage and calculations and ensuring correct administration (the '**six rights**' – right patient, right medicine, right dose, right time, right route, right documentation)
- identifying problems relating to drug therapy and ensuring appropriate treatment
- ensuring adherence and signing the patient record after administering a dose
- ensuring safe storage of drugs on the ward
- following institutional procedures and maintaining documentation and records
- education about drug information, missed doses and continuation of therapy after discharge from hospital.

Nurses are not allowed to initiate or change prescribed drug therapy or alter labels on drug packs but may refuse to administer a prescribed drug if they think this is warranted. In an emergency, nurses may implement verbal directions from a doctor to administer a drug, but this must be confirmed by a written prescription.

Nurse practitioners

In a growing number of countries, legislation has been modified to allow nurses with special expertise and training (including in pharmacology and prescribing) to apply for endorsement as an NP. The Nursing and Midwifery Board of Australia and the Australian College of Nurse Practitioners have developed a set of National Competency Standards: 'A nurse practitioner (NP) is a registered nurse with the experience and expertise to diagnose and treat people of all ages with a variety of acute or chronic health conditions. NPs have completed additional university study at master's degree level and are the most senior clinical nurses in our health care system' (see 'Online resources').

The expanded role of the NP is defined by the context in which the individual is authorised to practise.

NP roles are to provide health care in areas where there are insufficient doctors, to improve QUM and access to treatment, to provide cost-effective care, to target at-risk populations, to provide outreach services and to provide mentorship and clinical expertise to other health professionals. NPs may specialise in areas such as rural health, diabetes management, geriatric medicine, palliative care or sexual health. NPs may apply for approval as PBS prescribers; the list of drugs permitted is wide (see listing for NPs under 'Pharmaceutical Benefits Scheme' in 'Online resources'), but for an individual NP the range may be determined by local state or territory legislation and be limited to their identified scope of practice.

Under the auspices of the *Health Professionals Competence Assurance Act 2003*, the Nursing Council of New Zealand approves the scope of practice, competency requirements and registration of NPs who are Authorised Prescribers working in collaborative teams to improve patient access to health care and medicines.

Optometrists and orthoptists

Optometrists specialise in primary eye care, including vision and ocular health assessment and prescribing spectacles (glasses) and contact lenses. The Optometry Board may endorse suitably qualified optometrists to prescribe a limited range of Schedule 4 drugs for optometric use: preparations (mainly eyedrops) of antimicrobials, local anaesthetics, anti-inflammatory drugs, antiallergy drugs, drugs to dilate the pupil (mydriatics) and drugs for treating glaucoma. The Optometry Board lists the scheduled medicines that an optometrist can prescribe. Endorsed optometrists can apply for approval as PBS prescribers.

Orthoptists traditionally worked with ophthalmologists (doctors specialising in eye disorders) to treat low vision and eye movement disorders such as strabismus (squint). Training of orthoptists has been extended to include prescribing of spectacles and lenses; currently, orthoptists in Victoria are allowed to 'possess and use' many drugs; prescribing drug rights and PBS accreditation may follow.

Pharmacists

Pharmacists are medicines experts and generally work in hospital or retail pharmacies. An increasing number of pharmacists are working in residential aged care facilities and general practice (medical) teams. Their major roles defined by the NPS are 'to prepare, and distribute for administration, medicines to those who are to use them. Dispensing includes: the assessment of the medicine prescribed in the context of the person's other medicines, medical history, and the results of relevant clinical investigations available to the pharmacist; the selection and supply of the correct medicine; appropriate labelling and recording; and counselling the person on the medicine and its use'. In New Zealand, suitably qualified, trained and experienced pharmacists may apply to be a Pharmacist Prescriber. To date, Australian pharmacists cannot prescribe.

Other roles of pharmacists include:

- detecting and preventing inappropriate doses, ADRs, drug interactions or misuse, and compounding of medicines – that is, the preparation from several ingredients of a product, such as an oral mixture, supplied for immediate use by a specific consumer
- monitoring sales of Schedule 2 and 3 medicines
- supervising staff, students and dispensary assistants
- ensuring the pharmacy is conducted according to the law and to standards of good pharmaceutical practice
- providing professional services such as administering vaccinations, blood pressure monitoring, weight management and cholesterol testing
- ordering, safe storage and disposal[6] of drug supplies
- maintaining all required equipment and reference materials
- collaborating with other health professionals to improve medicine safety
- participating in research and educational activities, business and professional competencies
- providing drug information services, therapeutic monitoring, pharmacovigilance and public health programs.

6 The National Return and Disposal of Unwanted Medicines program encourages people to return unwanted drugs to community pharmacies for safe disposal; this helps to minimise the risk of drugs ending up in waterways or with children or animals. A recent audit showed that the annual cost of wastage of PBS medicines was approximately A$2 million. The most commonly discarded drugs were salbutamol inhalers, insulin (most vials unused) and frusemide – a powerful diuretic. Doctors are encouraged not to prescribe too many repeats, and patients not to hoard drugs.

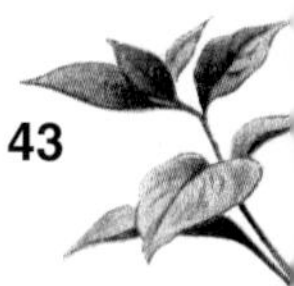

Accredited pharmacists (pharmacists who have completed additional certification) work collaboratively with GPs to optimise medication management services. They visit patients in their home or in residential aged care facilities, provide individualised counselling and medicines education and write a report to the GP about how to best improve QUM for that patient.

In hospitals, pharmacists carry out many roles such as: filling and maintaining ward stocks of drugs (imprest cabinets and drug trolleys); preparing sterile parenteral solutions, parenteral nutrition solutions and oncology drugs; participating in ward rounds, medication management plans, drug use evaluations and therapeutic drug monitoring; and providing advice on drug therapy and other drug information.

Physiotherapists

Physiotherapists (also known as physical therapists) deal with problems of movement, muscle coordination and posture. Because virtually all their patients are taking some drugs, physiotherapists need to be familiar with the principles of pharmacology and drugs used in obstetrics, neurological and cardiovascular conditions, asthma, inflammatory conditions and for pain control.

Podiatrists

Podiatrists specialise in disorders of the lower limbs, especially of the ankle and foot, and deal with biomechanical, medical, surgical and sports-related problems, especially in diabetes and rheumatology. Their patients are likely to be using cardiovascular drugs, hypoglycaemic agents, anti-inflammatories, analgesics and antimicrobials. Registered podiatrists administer local anaesthetics for pain relief in procedures involving the foot.

Those with extra training in pharmacology and microbiology and endorsed by the Podiatry Board of Australia and authorised under local legislation may prescribe a limited range of Schedule 4 drugs such as antimicrobials, anti-inflammatories, analgesics, anxiolytics and long-acting local anaesthetics. The board provides guidelines on approved courses of study, for writing private prescriptions and on supply and storage of permitted drugs. Currently (2021), podiatrists do not have access to PBS prescribing rights.

Other health practitioners working less closely with drugs

Most other health practitioners, while not actually prescribing, dispensing or administering drugs, are working with people who are likely to be taking drugs, whether for medical or social reasons. Understanding some of the language and principles of pharmacology is therefore helpful.

- Dietitians are involved with nutrition and food as they relate to health; there is overlap with pharmacology in parenteral nutrition, dietary supplements, vitamins and food–drug interactions.
- Health information managers deal with databases in epidemiology and clinical trials data, they code data from patient hospital records, they evaluate reports on accreditation and standards and they analyse 'casemix' information relevant to funding. They need to code accurately whether a condition is primary or a drug reaction and to understand why some conditions require expensive drugs and lengthy hospital stays.
- Occupational therapists work mainly with people who have disorders affecting activities of daily living; they facilitate and rehabilitate the person through activities, group therapy and adaptation of equipment and the environment.
- Prosthetists and orthotists specialise in prostheses (artificial body parts) and orthoses (devices to support limbs). Many of their clients have problems with motor control or poor circulation, so they need to know about neurological drugs and those used to improve circulation and treat diabetes or pain.
- Speech pathologists deal with people who have difficulties with verbal communication, language development and speech, hearing and swallowing. Their clients may be taking drugs for an underlying clinical problem such as strokes, other neurological impairments, cancer or psychiatric or behavioural disorders.

Drug prescriptions and formulations

Prescribing drugs

A **prescription** ('script') is a written direction for the preparation and administration of a specified amount of active drug for a specified person. In the ancient Babylonian civilisation, medical information on clay tablets recorded symptoms of illness, lists of pharmaceutical ingredients and directions for compounding, and invocations to the gods for healing. The prescription sign – sometimes shown in typeface as 'Rx' – may derive from the Egyptian character for the Eye of Horus, the symbol of good fortune and healing, or relate to the Roman god Jupiter, or be short for the Latin word '*recipe*', meaning the instruction 'take . . .', instructing the pharmacist to take the ingredients and compound them.

'Prescribing' is defined by the NPS as 'an iterative process involving information gathering, clinical decision making, communication and evaluation that results in the initiation, continuation, or cessation of a medicine'. It involves much more than simply writing the prescription.

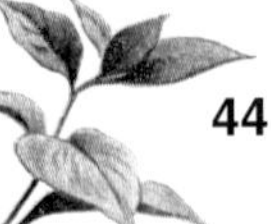

Decisions to be taken before prescribing

Any therapeutic intervention – whether administering a drug, implementing a physiotherapy program, carrying out a dental or podiatric surgical procedure, altering a person's diet or administering a complementary and/or alternative therapy such as acupuncture or herbal remedy – will interfere with the person's body systems. The first priority must follow the advice of Hippocrates: FIRST DO NO HARM. Then there are many questions that need to be answered, consciously or intuitively, before intervening. (A list presented in cartoon format in the textbook *Clinical Pharmacology: A Conceptual Approach* by Sweeney (1990) is reproduced here in Fig 2.2. See also Table 2.2 and sections on prescribing in the 'Preliminary information' pages in the current *Australian Medicines Handbook* (2021).)

Prescription orders

A prescription written by a licensed prescriber may present on a prescription form or an institutional order sheet (Figs 2.3B, 2.3C). Prescriptions must comply with legal formats – for example, as laid down in the Australian *Drugs, Poisons and Controlled Substances Act 1981* and Regulations. Prescriptions are then dispensed by a registered pharmacist. In some jurisdictions, appropriately qualified NPs, midwives, dentists, optometrists and podiatrists are licensed to prescribe a limited range of Prescription-Only drugs.

Prescriptions

A prescription must be clear, concise and correct. It requires the person's name and address (right patient); date written; active ingredient drug name (right drug); drug dose, strength, dosage form and quantity (right dose); route of administration (right route); dosage instructions or frequency of administration (right time); and must bear the signature, name, address and contact number of the prescriber (who has decided this is the right clinical situation). The number of times the prescription can be repeated should be specified, with clear instructions to the pharmacist and patient.

Prescriptions can be paper-based or electronic (with a QR code token). Potential benefits of electronic prescribing include:

- reduces prescribing and dispensing errors (electronic prescriptions are sent directly from the prescriber to the pharmacist supplying the medicine)
- improves prescribing and dispensing efficiency
- supports electronic medication charts in hospitals and residential aged care facilities
- reduces paper wastage and is environmentally friendly
- fewer lost prescriptions
- supports digital health services to optimise continuity of patient care and medicines safety
- reduces exposure to infectious diseases (e.g. COVID-19) by reducing the need to see health professionals face to face on multiple occasions
- supports patient privacy.

When typing or writing prescriptions, only accepted abbreviations should be used (Appendix 3). If any confusion or doubt exists, the prescriber is contacted for clarification.

Standing orders

Standing orders are in place in Australia and New Zealand to improve access to medicines. A standing order is 'a written instruction issued: by a medical practitioner . . . it authorises a specified person or class of people (e.g. registered nurses) who do not have prescribing rights to administer and/or supply specified medicines and some controlled drugs. The intention is for standing orders to be used to improve patients' timely access to medicines' (Taylor et al. 2017). Examples of standing orders include metoclopramide (antiemetic), paracetamol and ibuprofen.

Standing orders have no legal validity unless properly written, dated and signed. Repeating prescriptions without clinical review of the patient brings the risks of inappropriate drug use. Possession and use of prescription drugs by paramedics in ambulances may also be under 'standing orders'.

Hospital drug charts

Prescriptions in hospitals are usually written on a drug chart; this may be paper or electronic (Fig 2.3C). The chart has sections for general medications, intravenous (IV) drugs and fluids, nurse-initiated therapy (e.g. mild analgesics, laxatives, antacids), diabetes management and for admission drugs and a discharge prescription.

The Australian Commission on Safety and Quality in Health Care has developed 'PBS-friendly' proforma hospital medication charts and a National Residential Medication Chart (see 'Online resources').

Instructions and abbreviations in prescriptions

Many abbreviations and symbols are used in prescriptions; however, their use can lead to potentially serious errors in administration. The Australian Commission on Safety and Quality in Health Care has published a document, *Recommendations for Terminology, Abbreviations and symbols Used in Medicines Documentation*, which aims to establish consistent prescribing terminology, set recommended terms and abbreviations and list those that should be avoided as they frequently cause errors.

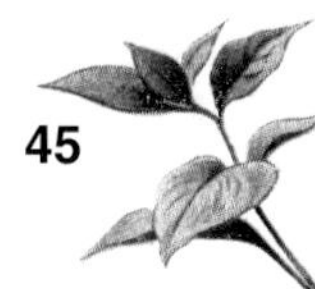

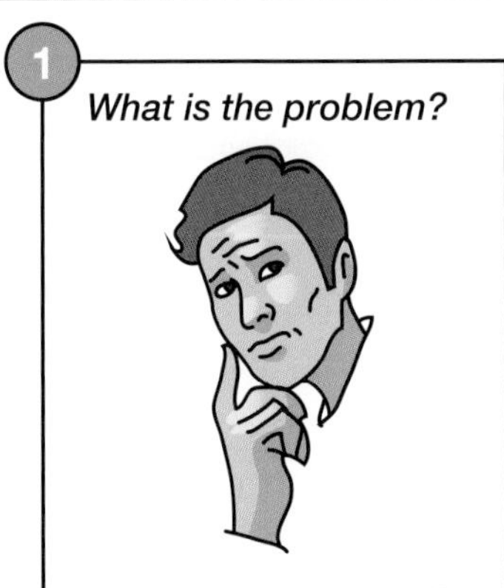
1
What is the problem?

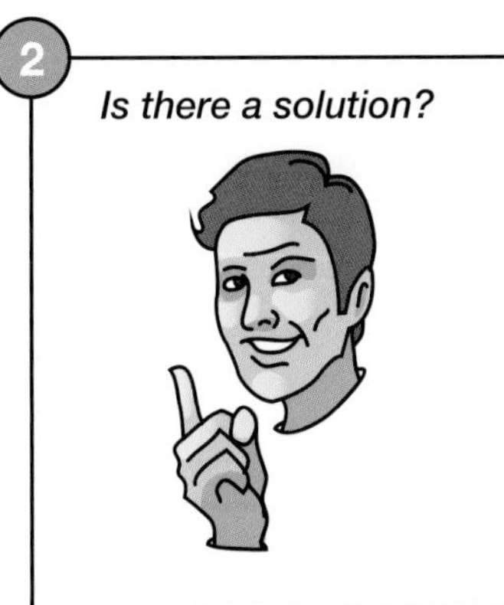
2
Is there a solution?

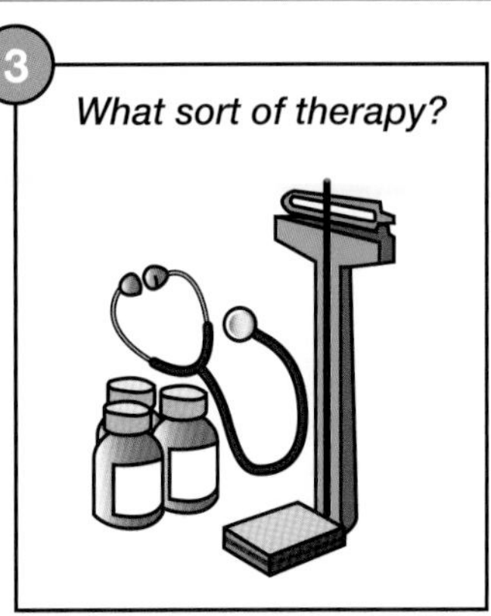
3
What sort of therapy?

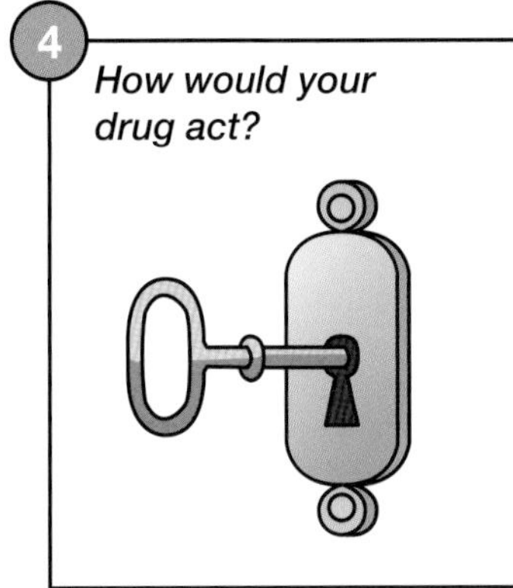

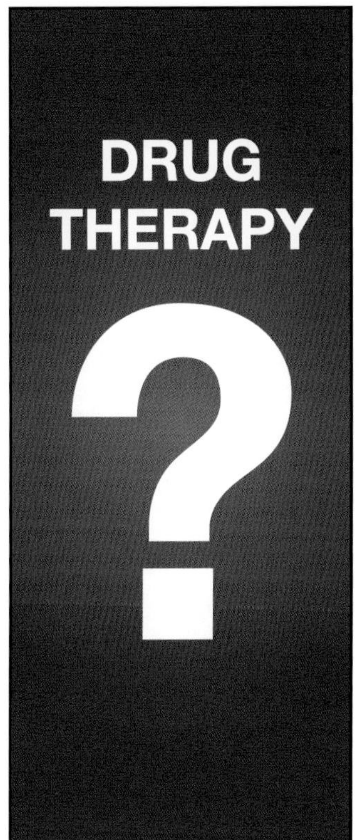

5
For how long will you treat?
CALENDAR
JANUARY

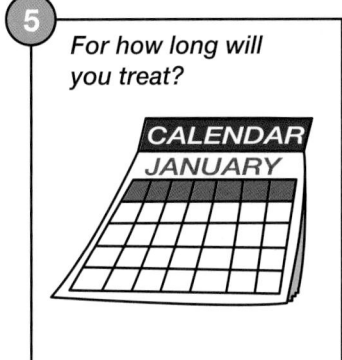

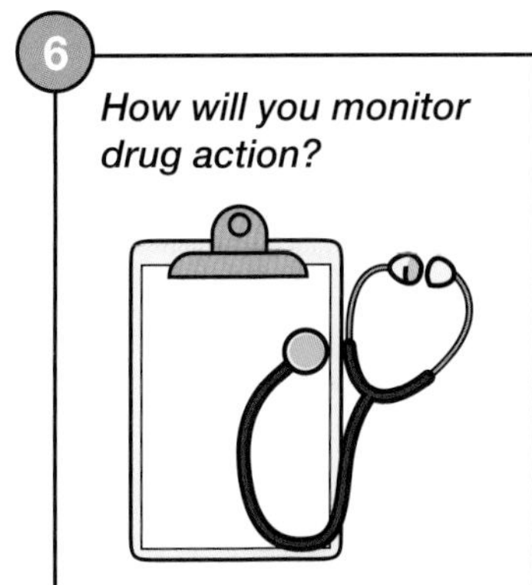

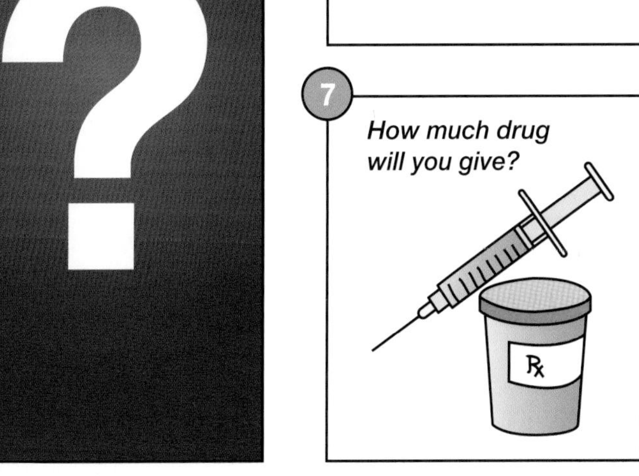

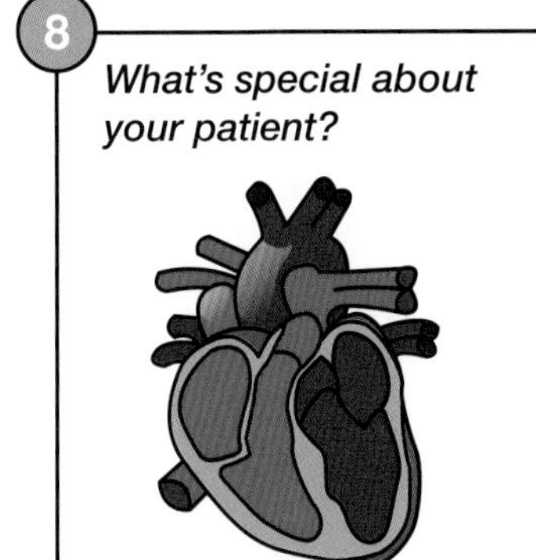

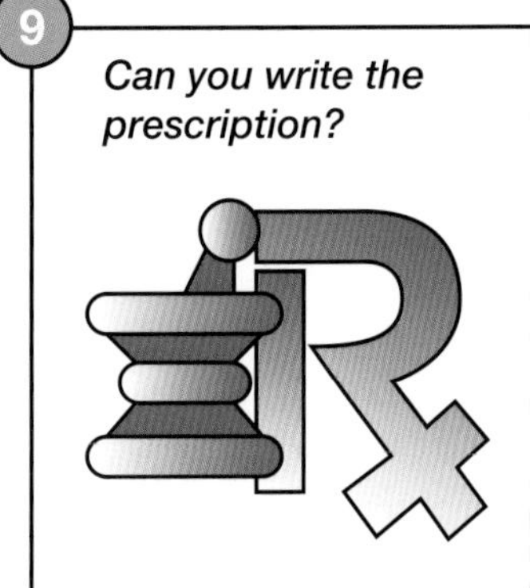

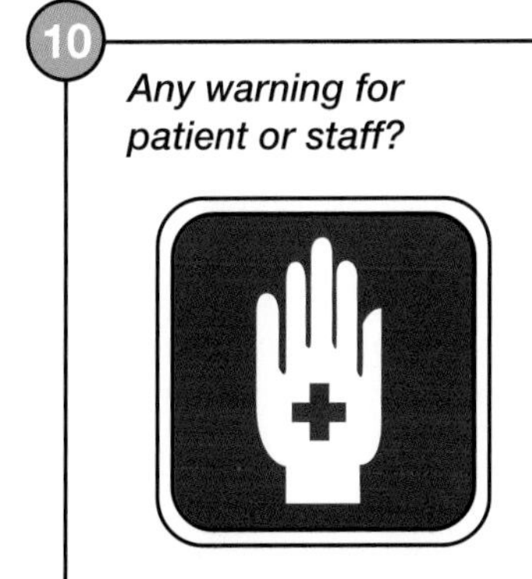

FIGURE 2.2 Questions to ask and answer when prescribing a drug

Source: Adapted from Sweeney 1990; used with permission.

TABLE 2.2 Questions to ask and answer when prescribing a drug

1. What is the problem?	2. Is there a (drug-based) solution?
The question is: 'What is going wrong here?' A full health history may take 30 minutes and should list all the person's current problems, relevant family history, past and current medications, allergies, ADRs and interactions, social drugs and all treatment modalities being used. The problems are specified in terms of pathophysiology or altered anatomy or psychology, not necessarily a diagnosis or 'label'.	Not all medical problems require drugs. Identify what changes need to be brought about in the person's functioning and whether drug treatment can improve the condition. Practitioners should keep an open mind and consider all modalities – surgery, nursing care, physiotherapy, podiatry, lifestyle changes (e.g. diet, exercise, stress, social drugs), psychotherapy and CAM methods, as well as drug treatment.
3. What sort of therapy?	4. How would your drug act? And what does it do?
Assuming there are suitable safe, effective drugs to treat the problem, there are many decisions: ♦ What class of drugs is appropriate? ♦ Are they all bioequivalent? Which particular drug should be selected? ♦ What do QUM guidelines recommend about this drug? What experience do we have with it? ♦ Is more than one drug required? ♦ Any cost factors to consider?	What is known about the pharmacodynamics of the drug? What is its mechanism and actions? Does it affect receptors, enzymes, ion channels, transport processes? How will it help the person's problems? What do we *not* know that could be important? What are the common ADRs and potential drug interactions? (Checking a data sheet for the drug is helpful here.)
5. For how long will you treat?	6. How will you monitor therapy?
What is the usual course of the condition and prognosis: will the person get better after short treatment, might there be ongoing relapses and remissions, or will the condition progress relentlessly? Are long-term effects of the drug different from immediate effects? When will you stop or change the therapy?	The person's progress must be monitored to evaluate the effects of the therapy – for example, by measuring: ♦ improvement in the problem ♦ adverse reactions to the drug ♦ plasma levels of the drug (e.g. for drugs with a low therapeutic index).
7. How much drug will you give?	8. What is special about this patient?
What dose is appropriate? Doses need to be individualised so, if necessary, look it up! Pharmacokinetic principles determine frequency of dosing and appropriate route. The therapeutic index of the drug will determine how critical the exact dose is. The route may determine the formulation, or there may be choices: if oral, will it be tablets, capsules, a mixture, a sustained-release form?	If the person is not an 'average' functioning adult, what are their age and weight? Are there concurrent conditions or susceptibility to adverse effects? Might a woman be pregnant or breastfeeding? How are liver and kidney functions? Is the drug contraindicated here? What might affect adherence or responses? What significant drug interactions are likely? What does the patient want from this prescribing?
9. Can you write (or dispense, or administer) the prescription?	10. Advice and warnings for the patient or staff?
Are the 'six rights' (patient, drug, dose, route, time, clinical situation) right? Does the prescription seem appropriate? Does it conform with legal and institutional requirements and QUM guidelines? Are the instructions to the patient adequate and correct?	Patients deserve as much medical information as they want about their condition, drugs being prescribed, how and when to take them, possible significant ADRs, drug and food (and alcohol) interactions and what to do if they miss a dose. Printed information should be included. Patients' carers, family and health professionals may need warnings.

Source: Prescribing guidelines predominantly adapted from the Australian Medicines Handbook (2021).

Some of the principles are:

- Use plain English; avoid jargon, Latin terms and Roman numerals.
- Avoid abbreviations wherever possible.
- Print all text, especially drug names.
- Use generic drug names; *never* abbreviate drug names.
- Express dose frequency unambiguously (e.g. three times a week, not three times weekly; 1/7 could mean for one day, or once daily, or for one week or once weekly).
- Avoid acronyms and abbreviations for medical terms and drug combinations.
- Avoid a trailing 0 after a decimal point (e.g. 1.0 mg may be read as 10 mg).
- Use 0 before a decimal point (e.g. 0.5 mL).
- Use commas in large numbers (e.g. 100,000 units).
- When a dose is to be taken only once per week, specify the day (e.g. 'on Tuesdays').[7]

Avoid error-prone and ambiguous abbreviations. These include μg (may be read as mg, resulting in a 1000× overdose; 'microgram' should be written in full), D/C (discharge or discontinue?), e/E (eye or ear?), HS/hs (half-strength or at bedtime [hora somni]?), IU (misread as IV), oc/c (eye ointment or eye-drops?), qd/QD (every day? or qid: 4 times a day), SSRI (selective serotonin

7 The importance of this labelling, and appropriate counselling, is highlighted by the many unintended dosing errors when methotrexate is prescribed to be taken once-weekly for arthritis, but patients inadvertently take it daily, leading to potentially life-threatening toxicity.

FOR LOSS OF APPETITE

Decoction of Aloes	2 fl. oz.
Decoction of Dandelion	1 fl. oz.
Infusion of Gentian	2 fl. oz.
Tincture of Cayenne	20 drops
Oil of Sassafras	10 drops
Rectified Spirit	1 dram
Borax	1 dram
Syrup	2.5 fl. oz.

Dose: 1 teaspoonful.
[fl. oz. = fluid ounce, approx. 28.4 mL;
fluid dram = approx. 3.7 mL; dram/drachm = approx. 3.9 g]

A

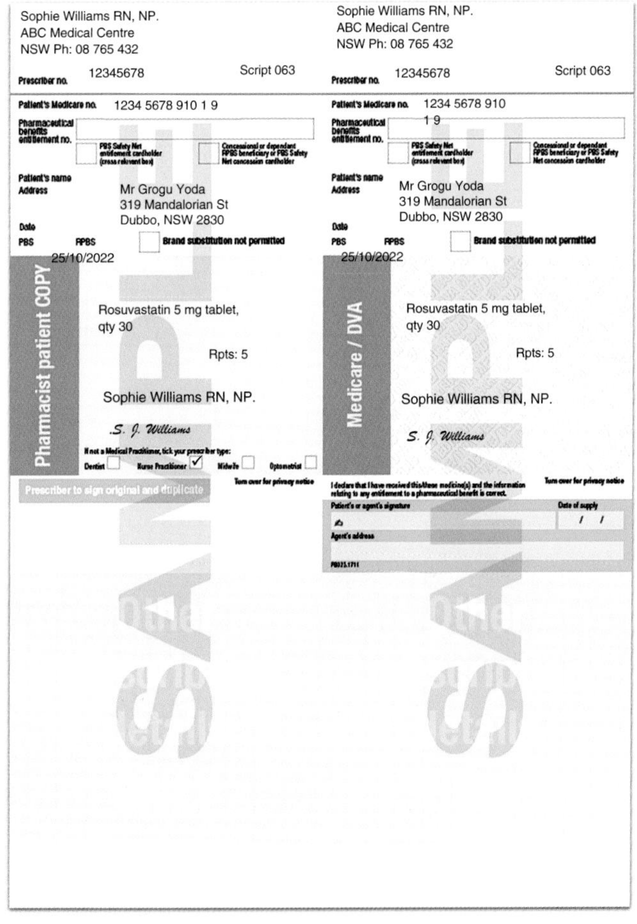
Sophie Williams RN, NP.
ABC Medical Centre
NSW Ph: 08 765 432
Prescriber no. 12345678 Script 063
Patient's Medicare no. 1234 5678 910 1 9
Pharmaceutical benefits entitlement no.
Patient's name
Address
Mr Grogu Yoda
319 Mandalorian St
Dubbo, NSW 2830
Date
PBS RPBS Brand substitution not permitted
25/10/2022
Pharmacist patient COPY
Rosuvastatin 5 mg tablet,
qty 30
Rpts: 5
Sophie Williams RN, NP.
S. J. Williams
Prescriber to sign original and duplicate

Sophie Williams RN, NP.
ABC Medical Centre
NSW Ph: 08 765 432
Prescriber no. 12345678 Script 063
Patient's Medicare no. 1234 5678 910
1 9
Pharmaceutical benefits entitlement no.
Patient's name
Address
Mr Grogu Yoda
319 Mandalorian St
Dubbo, NSW 2830
Date
PBS RPBS Brand substitution not permitted
25/10/2022
Medicare / DVA
Rosuvastatin 5 mg tablet,
qty 30
Rpts: 5
Sophie Williams RN, NP.
S. J. Williams
Patient's or agent's signature
Date of supply
Agent's address

B

FIGURE 2.3 Typical prescriptions
A Example of a prescription from the early 20th century, transcribed from a handwritten prescription in *Medical Prescriptions (for all diseases and ailments)*, Melbourne, c. 1929, Disabled Men's Association of Australia. This mixture would have contained extracts of at least 12 plants and an insect, plus four other chemicals including alcohol and water – truly a Galenical preparation (Ch 1)! **B** A typical current Pharmaceutical Benefits Scheme prescription; names and details have been changed.

Continued

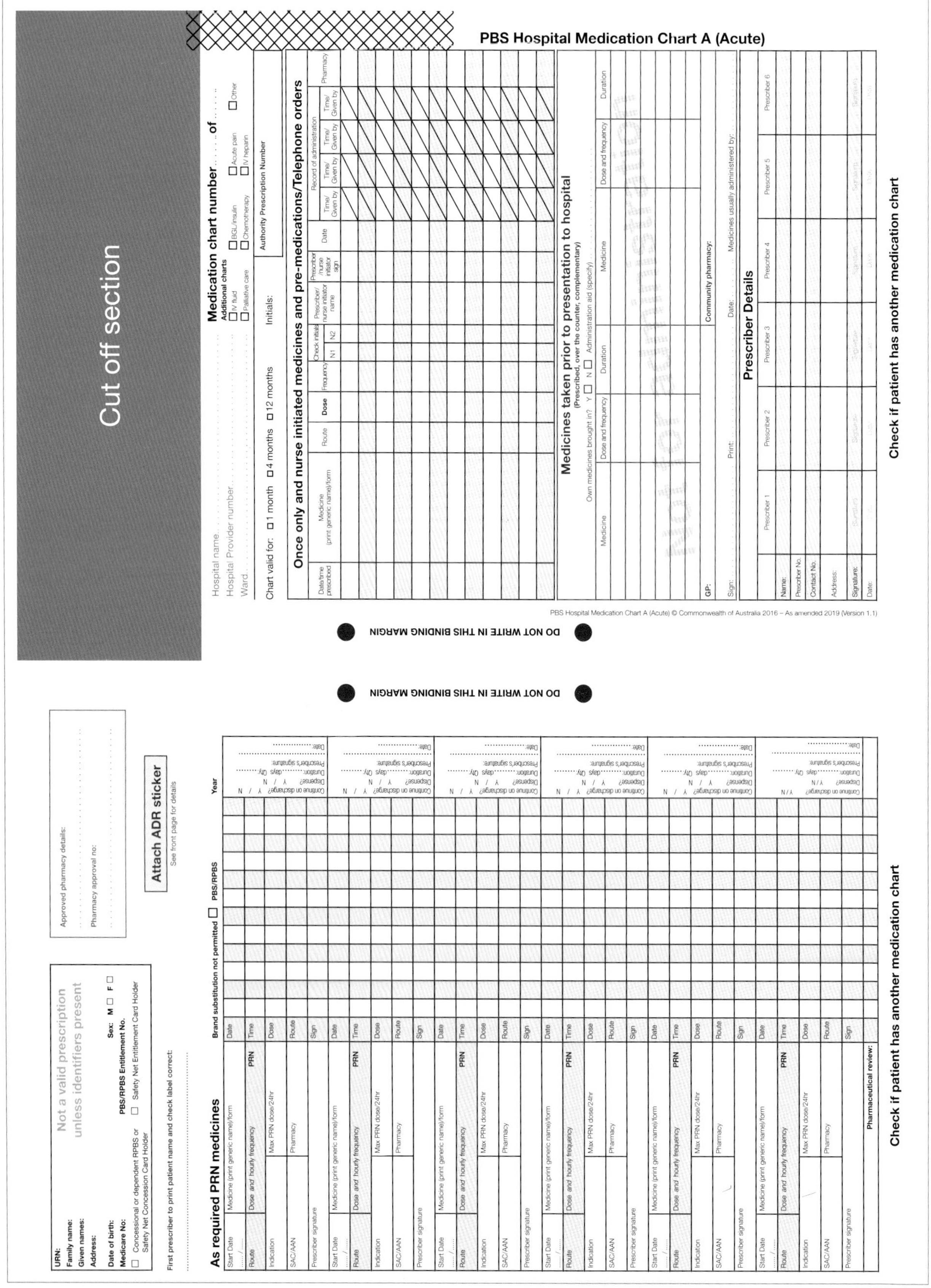

Cut off section

PBS Hospital Medication Chart A (Acute)

Medication chart number ...... of ......

Additional charts: ☐ IV fluid ☐ Palliative care ☐ BGL/insulin ☐ Chemotherapy ☐ Acute pain ☐ IV heparin ☐ Other

Hospital name ......

Hospital Provider number ......

Ward ......

Authority Prescription Number

Initials:

Chart valid for: ☐ 1 month ☐ 4 months ☐ 12 months

Once only and nurse initiated medicines and pre-medications/Telephone orders

Date/time prescribed	Medicine (print generic name)/form	Route	Dose	Frequency	Check initials N1	N2	Prescriber/nurse initiator name	Prescriber/nurse initiator sign	Date	Record of administration: Time/Given by	Time/Given by	Time/Given by	Time/Given by	Pharmacy

Medicines taken prior to presentation to hospital
(Prescribed, over the counter, complementary)

Own medicines brought in? Y ☐ N ☐ Administration aid (specify) ......

Medicine	Dose and frequency	Duration	Medicine	Dose and frequency	Duration

GP: Community pharmacy:

Sign: Print: Date: Medicines usually administered by:

Prescriber Details

	Prescriber 1	Prescriber 2	Prescriber 3	Prescriber 4	Prescriber 5	Prescriber 6
Name:						
Prescriber No.						
Contact No.						
Address:						
Signature:						
Date:						

Check if patient has another medication chart

PBS Hospital Medication Chart A (Acute) © Commonwealth of Australia 2016 – As amended 2019 (Version 1.1)

DO NOT WRITE IN THIS BINDING MARGIN

DO NOT WRITE IN THIS BINDING MARGIN

URN:
Family name:
Given names:
Address:
Date of birth: Sex: M ☐ F ☐
Medicare No: PBS/RPBS Entitlement No.
☐ Concessional or dependent RPBS or Safety Net Concession Card Holder ☐ Safety Net Entitlement Card Holder

Not a valid prescription unless identifiers present

First prescriber to print patient name and check label correct: ......

Approved pharmacy details: ......

Pharmacy approval no: ......

Attach ADR sticker
See front page for details

As required PRN medicines

Brand substitution not permitted ☐ PBS/RPBS Year

Start Date	Medicine (print generic name)/form		PRN	Date	Time	Dose	Route	Sign
Route	Dose and hourly frequency							
Indication		Max PRN dose/24hr						
SAC/AAN		Pharmacy						
Prescriber signature								

Continue on discharge? Y / N
Dispense? Y / N
Duration: ......days Qty ......
Prescriber's signature:
Date: ......

(The PRN medicine block above is repeated six times on the chart.)

Pharmaceutical review:

Check if patient has another medication chart

FIGURE 2.3, cont'd C A typical medication therapy chart from a patient's hospital record (also known as the patient's drug chart).
Source: Services Australia 2021; reproduced with permission.

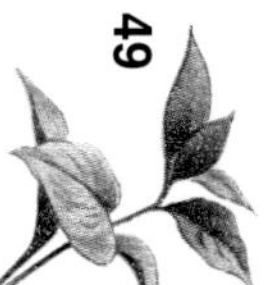

Cut off section

Attach ADR sticker

Allergies and adverse drug reactions (ADR)

☐ Nil known ☐ Unknown (tick appropriate box or complete details below)

Medicine (or other)	Reaction / type / date	Initials

Sign .... Print .... Date ....

Affix patient identification label here and overleaf

URN:
Family name:
Given names:
Address:

Not a valid prescription unless identifiers present

Date of birth: Sex: M ☐ F ☐
Medicare No: PBS/RPBS Entitlement No.
☐ Concessional or dependent RPBS or Safety Net Concession Card Holder ☐ Safety Net Entitlement Card Holder

First prescriber to print patient name and check label correct:
....

Weight (kg): .... Height (cm): ....

Regular Medicines

Brand substitution not permitted ☐ PBS/RPBS Year

Variable dose medicine — Date and month →

Start Date ...... / ...... | Medicine (print generic name)/form | Drug level | Time level taken | Dose | Prescriber | Time to be given | Nurse initial
Route | Frequency – Prescriber to enter dose times and individual dose
Indication | Pharmacy
Prescriber signature | SAC/AAN

Continue on discharge? Y / N
Dispense? Y / N
Duration: ......days Qty: ......
Prescriber's signature: ......
Date: ......

VTE risk assessed: Yes ☐ Prophylaxis not required ☐ Contraindicated ☐ Signature: Date:

Start Date ...... / ...... | Medicine (print generic name)/form
Route | Dose and Frequency – and now enter times →
Indication: VTE prophylaxis | Pharmacy
Prescriber | SAC/AAN
Mechanical prophylaxis | AM check
Signature / NI signature | Print name | PM check

Continue on discharge? Y / N
Dispense? Y / N
Duration: ......days Qty: ......
Prescriber's signature: ......
Date: ......

Start Date ...... / ...... | Warfarin | Marevan / Coumadin – Circle brand | INR Result
Route | Prescriber to enter individual doses | Target INR Range | Dose (mg mg mg mg mg mg mg mg mg mg)
Indication | Pharmacy | Prescriber
Prescriber signature | Initial 1 (18:00) | Initial 2

Continue on discharge? Y / N
Dispense? Y / N
Duration: ......days Qty: ......
Prescriber's signature: ......
Date: ......

Prescriber to enter administration times ↓

Start Date ...... / ...... | Medicine (print generic name)/form | Tick if slow release
Route | Dose and Frequency – and now enter times →
Indication | Pharmacy
Prescriber signature | SAC/AAN

Continue on discharge? Y / N
Dispense? Y / N
Duration: ......days Qty: ......
Prescriber's signature: ......
Date: ......

Start Date ...... / ...... | Medicine (print generic name)/form | Tick if slow release
Route | Dose and Frequency – and now enter times →
Indication | Pharmacy
Prescriber signature | SAC/AAN

Continue on discharge? Y / N
Dispense? Y / N
Duration: ......days Qty: ......
Prescriber's signature: ......
Date: ......

Pharmaceutical review:

Check if patient has another medication chart

Recommended administration times
Guidelines only

Morning	Mane	0800				
Night	Nocte			1800 or 2000		
Twice a day	BD	0800		2000		
Three times a day	TDS	0800	1400	2000		
Regular 6 hourly	6 hrly	0600	1200	1800	2400	
Regular 8 hourly	8 hrly	0600	1400	2200		
Four times a day	QID	0600	1200	1800	2200	

Tick if slow release

SR = Sustained, modified or controlled release formulation.
If scored tablet, then half can be given.
Dose must be swallowed without crushing.

Anticoagulant education record
Medicine: ....
Education
Provided ☐ Declined ☐
Not appropriate ☐
Written information
Provided ☐ Declined ☐
Written information provided:
CMI ☐ Other: ☐ ....
Signature: ....
Designation: .... Date: ......

Reason for not administering
Codes MUST be circled

Absent	(A)
Fasting	(F)
On leave	(L)
Not available – obtain supply or contact prescriber	(N)
Refused – notify prescriber	(R)
Self administered	(S)
Vomiting	(V)
Withheld – enter reason in clinical record	(W)

SAC: Streamline Authority Code
AAN: Authority Approval Number

Regular Medicines

Brand substitution not permitted ☐ PBS/RPBS Year

Date and month →
Prescriber to enter administration times ↓

Start Date ...... / ...... | Medicine (print generic name)/form | Tick if slow release
Route | Dose and Frequency – and now enter times →
Indication | Pharmacy
Prescriber signature | SAC/AAN

Continue on discharge? Y / N
Dispense? Y / N
Duration: ......days Qty: ......
Prescriber's signature: ......
Date: ......

Start Date ...... / ...... | Medicine (print generic name)/form | Tick if slow release
Route | Dose and Frequency – and now enter times →
Indication | Pharmacy
Prescriber signature | SAC/AAN

Continue on discharge? Y / N
Dispense? Y / N
Duration: ......days Qty: ......
Prescriber's signature: ......
Date: ......

Start Date ...... / ...... | Medicine (print generic name)/form | Tick if slow release
Route | Dose and Frequency – and now enter times →
Indication | Pharmacy
Prescriber signature | SAC/AAN

Continue on discharge? Y / N
Dispense? Y / N
Duration: ......days Qty: ......
Prescriber's signature: ......
Date: ......

Start Date ...... / ...... | Medicine (print generic name)/form | Tick if slow release
Route | Dose and Frequency – and now enter times →
Indication | Pharmacy
Prescriber signature | SAC/AAN

Continue on discharge? Y / N
Dispense? Y / N
Duration: ......days Qty: ......
Prescriber's signature: ......
Date: ......

Start Date ...... / ...... | Medicine (print generic name)/form | Tick if slow release
Route | Dose and Frequency – and now enter times →
Indication | Pharmacy
Prescriber signature | SAC/AAN

Continue on discharge? Y / N
Dispense? Y / N
Duration: ......days Qty: ......
Prescriber's signature: ......
Date: ......

Start Date ...... / ...... | Medicine (print generic name)/form | Tick if slow release
Route | Dose and Frequency – and now enter times →
Indication | Pharmacy
Prescriber signature | SAC/AAN

Continue on discharge? Y / N
Dispense? Y / N
Duration: ......days Qty: ......
Prescriber's signature: ......
Date: ......

Pharmaceutical review:

Check if patient has another medication chart

FIGURE 2.3, cont'd

reuptake inhibitor or sliding scale regular insulin), ung (not understood as ointment), tid (may be misread as bd), 6/24 (may be read as every 6 hours or six times per day), cc (could mean cubic centimetre or with meals), SC and SL are sometimes confused.

Some common abbreviations are shown in Appendix 3; only those shown asterisked are recommended in the *Australian Medicines Handbook*. If there is any possibility of confusion, words should be written in full: 'If in doubt, write it out!'

Substitution of drug brands: active ingredient prescribing

In February 2021 it became mandatory for Australian prescribers to include the active ingredient on prescriptions. If a prescriber would like to include a specific brand name, it must appear after its active ingredient.

Although there is a cost saving associated with supplying the generic over the brand, there are clinical and practical reasons why a person should stay with a specific brand – for example, avoiding patient confusion.

Prescribing for special groups

Most published dosage regimens are suitable for 'average' adults. However, average doses are often inappropriate. For example, dosages may vary in the following cases:

- Children: weight, skin texture, body surface area, hormone levels and likely adherence vary depending on age; suitable formulations and administration techniques may be required.
- The elderly: pharmacokinetics and pharmacodynamics of drugs may vary depending on renal and cardiovascular functions; homeostatic mechanisms and adherence may be impaired; multiple diagnoses and polypharmacy are issues; administration aids may assist dosing and enhance adherence.
- Pregnant women: risks of drugs to the fetus must always be considered.
- Breastfeeding mothers: effects of drugs on the infant or on lactation will determine need for drug or timing of doses relative to feeds (Ch 30).
- People with renal impairment: may require dose reductions for renally-cleared drugs.
- People with obesity: drug distribution, clearance and half-lives may be altered.
- Family and friends: it is generally considered unethical and inappropriate for practitioners to prescribe for family and friends, except in exceptional circumstances.

(More details are given in Ch 6, 'Pharmacokinetics and dosing regimens'; in the 'Preliminary information' pages of the *Australian Medicines Handbook*; and in the *AMH Children's Dosing Companion*.)

Off-label prescribing

When a drug is prescribed for an indication, a patient group or by a route that is not included in the approved Product Information for that drug, the prescribing is 'off-label'. The term does not apply to prescribing for a condition for which the drug is approved but not subsidised by government.

The drugs most commonly used 'off-label' are psychotherapeutics: antidepressants, antipsychotics and anxiolytics/sedatives. Off-label prescribing is not illegal but may be unethical; it may be risky for patient and doctor, and costly to the patient if not subsidised. The onus is on the prescriber to act in the patient's best interest and be able to defend the prescribing on high-level evidence. The patient should be allowed to give informed consent and be warned that their situation may not be listed in the consumer medicine information sheet for the drug.

Inappropriate prescribing

Prescribing errors occur frequently, particularly when busy prescribers ignore some 'questions to answer' before prescribing, and when people 'doctor shop' or move between health professionals. Most common is underprescribing, where drugs are not prescribed despite guidelines recommending them, or doses are sub-therapeutic. Elderly people are often not treated optimally, for fear of polypharmacy (Rankin et al. 2018).

Overprescribing (e.g. various anti-inflammatories for different conditions in one patient) and irrational prescribing (e.g. antibiotics for viral infections, or cough suppressants in productive cough) also contribute to unsuccessful prescribing.

Polypharmacy

Polypharmacy is the concurrent use of multiple medications, usually five or more drugs including all prescribed, OTC and CAM medicines. (Using 10 or more concurrent drugs has been described as 'hyperpolypharmacy'.) It has connotations of unnecessary drugs or use at frequencies greater than essential. Polypharmacy leads to multiple ADRs and drug interactions, and drugs may be needed to treat side effects of earlier-prescribed drugs – the 'prescribing cascade'.[9] Older people are particularly at risk: nearly two-thirds of Australians aged 75 or older regularly take more than four medications, with a high risk of adverse consequences.

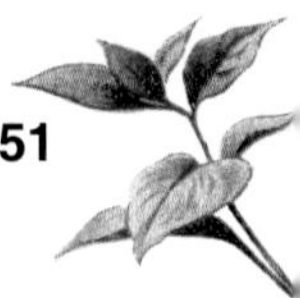

Interventions recommended for managing polypharmacy are:

- prevention – avoid using drugs for minor complaints
- regular medication review – assess the need for therapy, and dosage; check for ADRs, drug interactions and adherence
- non-pharmacological approaches – use lifestyle measures whenever possible
- communication – with the patient, about expectations and difficulties with adherence, and with other health professionals about changes in drug regimens
- simplification – reduce regimens to essential drugs, at the lowest effective doses and frequencies.

Such interventions successfully reduce inappropriate prescribing (Rankin et al. 2018).

Deprescribing – that is, cessation of long-term therapy, or stopping medicines when no further benefits will be achieved compared with potential harms – should be initiated carefully by weaning off slowly.

Teaching prescribing

Medical students (in retrospect) often say that insufficient time is devoted to teaching **clinical pharmacology** and prescribing in medical courses, resulting in anxiety as interns when suddenly being required to write prescriptions. The Australian NPS recognises that many (suitably qualified) health professionals now require prescribing competencies. NPS has produced a National Prescribing Curriculum, a series of interactive case-based modules that encourage confident and rational prescribing. The modules follow a stepwise approach as outlined in the World Health Organization's *Guide to Good Prescribing*.

Drug formulations (pharmaceutics)

Drugs are available in many different formulations (see Table 2.3). The science of formulating drugs is known as pharmaceutics.

KEY POINTS

Clinical aspects of pharmacotherapy

- National drug policies in Australia and New Zealand encourage evidence-based practice and QUM; this is enhanced by educational bodies disseminating objective information about drugs and by studies of drug use in hospitals.
- Many pharmacodynamic and pharmacokinetic factors may affect how a person responds to drugs; in the clinical situation, adherence, drug interactions and placebo effects are particularly important.
- Many health professionals are involved with pharmacotherapy, whether prescribing, dispensing, administering or monitoring drugs; responsibilities and challenges vary accordingly.
- The range of drugs available for prescribing (or recommending) is very wide; individual practitioners usually prescribe from a limited list of preferred drugs.
- The drugs allowable for subsidised prescribing on the Australian PBS depend on the profession and authorisation status of the prescriber.
- Before a drug is prescribed or advised, factors relating to the person, the drug and the clinical situation must be considered.
- Prescriptions are legally regulated documents, with specific requirements for format; abbreviations in prescriptions should be used only cautiously.
- Drugs may be formulated in many dose forms to maximise safe administration and clinical effect; formulations for oral and **parenteral administration** are common in general practice and hospital use, respectively.

TABLE 2.3 Various drug formulations

PREPARATIONS FOR ORAL USE	PREPARATIONS FOR TOPICAL USE
Liquid ◆ Aqueous solution (substances dissolved in water) ◆ Aqueous suspension (solid particles suspended in water; must be shaken well before measuring out) ◆ Draught (oral liquid in single-dose volume, e.g. 50 mL) ◆ Elixir (aromatic, sweetened alcohol/water solution) ◆ Emulsion (two-phase system of two immiscible liquids, fine droplets of one phase dispersed in the other by action of an emulsifying agent) ◆ Extract (syrup or dried form of natural product) ◆ Mixture (liquid preparation of drugs) ◆ Spirit or essence (alcoholic solution of volatile substances) ◆ Syrup or linctus (aqueous solution containing high concentration of sugars) ◆ Tincture (alcohol extract of plant or vegetable substance)	◆ Aerosol (fine mist of powder or solution; may contain propellant) ◆ Cream (semi-solid emulsion that contains drug, usually oil-in-water) ◆ Dusting powder (dry substances in fine powder form) ◆ Gel or jelly (semi-solid preparation in aqueous base) ◆ Liniment (liquid preparation for lubricating or soothing, applied by rubbing) ◆ Lotion (liquid preparation applied to skin) ◆ Ointment (semi-solid preparation usually in an oily base for local or systemic effects) ◆ Paste (thick ointment primarily used for skin protection) ◆ Plaster (solid preparation spread on fabric) ◆ Transdermal patch (adhesive patch impregnated with drug that is absorbed continuously through the skin and acts systemically)

Continued

TABLE 2.3 Various drug formulations—cont'd

Solid ♦ Capsule (soluble case, usually of gelatine, containing liquid or dry drug; convenient for drugs with unpleasant taste) ♦ Lozenge (flavoured tablet, dissolves slowly in mouth) ♦ Pill (spherical or ovoid rolled mass containing a single dose of drug mixed with excipients) ♦ Powder/granule (loose fine/moulded drug substance in dry form) ♦ Tablet (compressed, powdered drug(s) in small disc for single-dose administration)	Preparations for use on mucous membranes ♦ Aqueous solutions of drugs, usually for topical action but may be for systemic effects, including enemas, douches, mouthwashes, nasal and throat sprays and gargles ♦ Sublingual tablet (dissolves in mouth for systemic absorption across buccal membranes) ♦ Aerosol sprays, nebulisers and inhalers (deliver drug in fine droplet form or finely dispersed powder to target membrane, e.g. bronchodilators to airways) ♦ Drops (aqueous solutions, with or without gelling agent to prolong retention time; used for eyes, ears or nose) ♦ Foam (powders or solutions of medication in volatile liquids with a propellant, e.g. vaginal foams for contraception) ♦ Lamella (small gelatine disc impregnated with drug for use in the eye, e.g. to treat glaucoma) ♦ Suppository (small bullet-shaped solid form containing drug mixed in firm but dissolvable base such as cocoa butter, to facilitate insertion into the rectum; may be for local or systemic effect) ♦ Pessary (a vaginal suppository) Miscellaneous drug delivery systems ♦ Intradermal implant (sterile pellet or rod containing small deposit of drug for insertion into dermal pocket, allowing the drug to leach slowly into tissue; usually for administration of hormones such as testosterone or estradiol) ♦ Micropump system (a small external pump, attached by belt or implanted, that delivers medication via a needle in a continuous steady dose, e.g. for insulin, anticancer chemotherapy or opioid analgesic) ♦ Targeted drug-carrier system, e.g. liposomes, protein drug carriers (designed to deliver a specific drug to a particular capillary bed, cell or receptor)
Preparations for parenteral use (injections) ♦ Ampoule (sealed glass container for sterile injectable liquid) ♦ Cartridge (unit of parenteral medication to be used with specific injecting device) ♦ Injection (sterile solution or suspension for parenteral administration) ♦ Vial (glass container with rubber stopper for liquid or powdered medication)	
Intravenous infusions (for continuous injection via indwelling cannula) ♦ Glass bottles, flexible collapsible plastic bags, or semi-rigid plastic containers in sizes from 100 to 1000 mL containing fluid replacement with or without drug; solution may flow in via gravity or be delivered by pump ♦ Heparin lock or Angiocath (a port site for direct administration of intermittent IV medications without the need for primary IV solution) ♦ Intermittent IV infusions (usually small secondary IV set to which drug is added; it runs as a 'piggyback' to the primary IV infusion; see Fig 2.4)	

Ethical aspects of pharmacotherapy

Introduction

The practice of formulating, prescribing, administering and monitoring drugs needs to be not only clinically and legally appropriate but also carried out in an ethical manner. Ethics is defined as the science of morals in human conduct, or moral principles. The consideration of ethical principles is to answer the question, '*What should I do in this situation?*'

Human rights, the basis for bioethics

The basic human rights, acknowledged by the United Nations (UN) and accepted by most countries, are the rights to life, security, health, dignity, privacy, autonomy, marriage and procreation, and freedom of thought and religion. Codes of bioethics are based on these human rights and date back as far as the Hippocratic Oath (5th century BC). The ancient vow poses several modern problems, not least those relating to abortion, euthanasia, treating family members, risks of litigation and swearing to ancient Greek gods! More recently, bioethics, and indeed the policy of the Australian Medical Association, are based on the Nuremberg Code (1947), Declaration of Geneva (1948), the *International Code of Medical Ethics* (1949) agreed to by the UN after World War II, the Declaration of Helsinki (1964), and their subsequent amendments. Modern versions of the Hippocratic Oath have been devised.

Medical ethics

Medical ethics are the principles and values that guide the decisions of medical practitioners and, by extension, apply to all health practitioners. They are usually listed as:

- *non-maleficence* (not doing harm)
- *beneficence* (doing good); together these first two principles underlie the duty of care owed to patients and clients and imply the importance of risk–benefit analysis
- *justice*, whereby all persons have equal access to health care
- *veracity*, that the truth will be told to all persons about their condition and treatment
- *confidentiality* of personal and health records – principles set out in Australian privacy legislation relate to collection, use and correction of information; data quality and security; openness of policies, assignment of identifiers to individuals, and data flow across borders
- *autonomy* of the patient – the person always retains the right to choose or refuse treatment or participation, and the right to have sufficient information to give 'informed consent'.

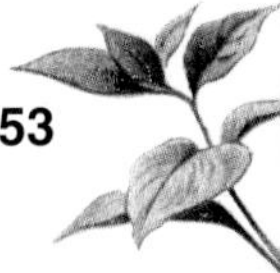

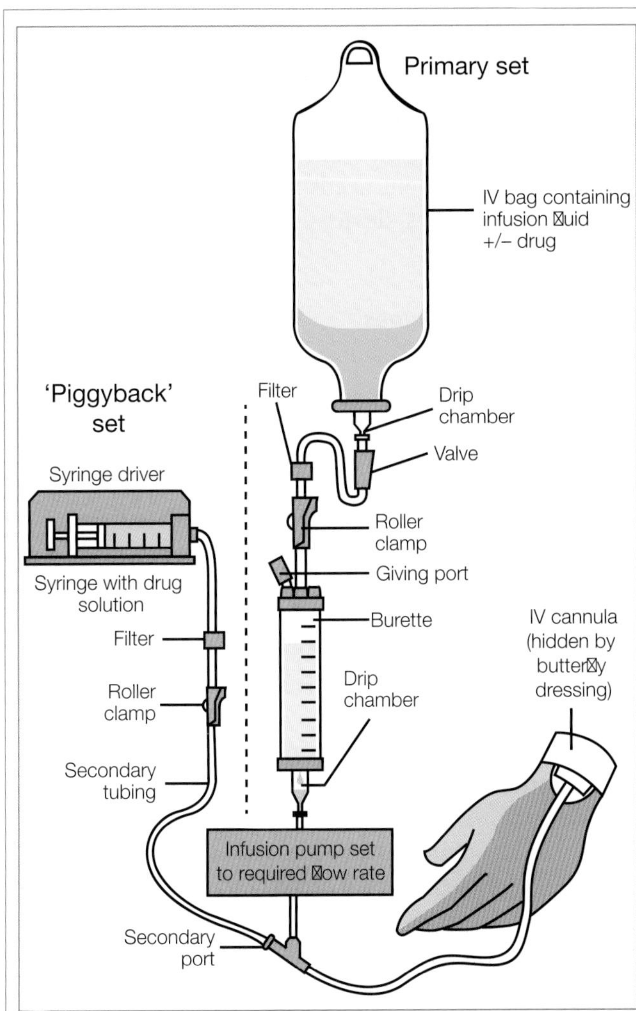

FIGURE 2.4 Diagram of a typical intravenous infusion set-up, showing a bag with IV infusion fluid and primary drug, flexible tubing, valves, filters, a giving port (for addition of another drug) with burette, infusion pump, plus a secondary 'piggyback' set with a reservoir of secondary drug in a pump-driven syringe; all leading to an IV cannula indwelling in the person's vein.

Responsibilities of health practitioners

All health practitioners have responsibilities to practise ethically: to use all appropriate resources in the best interests of their patients, to remain competent and up to date in their practice and to accord their patients all basic human rights. What constitutes unethical conduct may be hard to determine; in the healthcare context, it can mean serious misconduct compared with what would reasonably be expected by a general body of colleagues.

Ethical dilemmas: current issues in bioethics

Medical ethics issues arise frequently, and are often hard to resolve. Typically, they involve professional secrecy, consent to treatment and procedures with legal implications (sterilisation, abortion, assisted pregnancies, euthanasia and experimentation). This section cannot attempt to cover all ethical dilemmas relevant to pharmacology, but aspects of some current issues are summarised below.

Warnings of risks

If every possible adverse effect or drug interaction is explained in detail, a patient might never consent to any treatment, therefore putting their health further at risk; however, this does not justify withholding information. The High Court of Australia has said that the patient must be informed about 'material' (i.e. significant) risks.[8] Health professionals have an ethical obligation not to recommend inappropriately risky treatments.

Animal rights

It is generally recognised that in the testing of drugs, medical devices or procedures, animals should be used only when absolutely necessary. Although results from animal tests cannot automatically be extrapolated to humans, such tests do protect humans. The Australian and New Zealand Council for the Care of Animals in Research and Teaching works diligently to protect animal rights and promote 'the three Rs': **R**eplacement of animals wherever possible, **R**eduction in the numbers of animals used and **R**efinement of techniques to minimise harm.

Information technology and 'telemedicine'

The advent of the internet has raised many new issues. Should medical information and consultations be widely available – for example, on the web? Should pharmacists be allowed to supply drugs by mail? Does this erode the professional's role or the clinical relationship, or is it the patient's right to know about and obtain drugs anywhere? Is prescription- or drug-shopping from countries with the most lax drug regulations allowable?

Equal access to drugs and medical care

In 2000 the UN launched the Millennium Development Goals – eight goals to be achieved by 2015 to address underlying inequalities in health including: reduce child mortality; improve maternal health; and combat HIV/AIDS, malaria and other diseases. However, increasing costs of medical technologies and new drugs, demands of ageing populations, patients' expectations, doctors' fear of litigation, commercial demands of the pharmaceutical industry and governments' need for tight budget controls all make the rationing of health care a difficult ethical

8 Hundreds of Australians have been awarded compensation by the drug company Pfizer after court battles claiming that they were not warned adequately about possible adverse effects of the drug cabergoline, a dopamine agonist prescribed to treat Parkinson's disease and restless legs syndrome. Many patients developed pathological gambling and shopping habits, losing hundreds of thousands of dollars. The *Australian Medicines Handbook* now warns that adverse effects include 'impulse control disorders'.

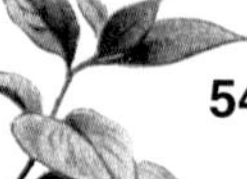

issue. (See the earlier discussion on pharmacoeconomics.) Principles of equity and fairness need to be applied or high-quality care will only be available to the wealthy, those in cities or those in manufacturer-subsidised trials.

The TGA's Pharmaceutical Benefits Advisory Committee has to weigh demands from the public for subsidised access to all (safe) drugs and demands from drug companies wanting subsidies for their products against demands from other interests competing for scarce government health funds. The decision by the PBS to fund a new class of drugs to treat people with hepatitis C cost over a billion dollars, effectively curing many people but leading to opportunity cost against wider public health programs. Although drugs on the PBS have been approved as being cost-effective, it is still true that more lives might be saved by 'employing more nurses, or even . . . building bicycle paths' (Moulds 2012). At the least, decisions as to subsidising drugs onto the PBS should be justifiable and transparent.

Examples of inequitable access to health care include:

- Some groups are excluded from participation in clinical trials – for example, children, pregnant women, elderly people or people with concurrent conditions; results of trials will not necessarily be applicable to them.
- Clinical trials that would not be approved in countries with strong regulations may be carried out in underdeveloped countries,[9] putting participants at risk.
- Children have been described as 'therapeutic orphans' because they can be denied access to new medications, and drugs may not be marketed in dose forms suitable for children; some authorities now require that drugs likely to be used in children are trialled in children.
- Australian Aboriginal and Torres Strait Islander people have greater morbidity and mortality than other Australians but lower access to health care, including drugs under the PBS.
- People in developing countries are often denied drugs due to prohibitive costs and lack of government subsidies; allowing production of generic drugs can be life-saving and reduce much suffering.
- Thirty 'neglected diseases': a UNESCO report shows significant reduction in funding for developing-world diseases such as trachoma, leprosy, Buruli ulcer and diarrhoeal diseases. The G-FINDER (Global Funding of Innovation for Neglected Diseases) report by the Policy Cures Research project, funded by the Bill & Melinda Gates Foundation, showed that more than 11 million people die from these diseases each year, and there are urgent needs for investment in related drugs, diagnostics, devices, vaccines and vector-control products.

Promotion of medicines

The World Health Organization has a code of 'ethical criteria for medical drug promotion'. Drug companies obviously consider that advertising of drugs to doctors is effective, otherwise it would not be carried out; however, advertising adds to the cost of new drugs. In Australia, 'detailing' of drugs to doctors is regulated by TGA legislation, guidelines and the Code of Conduct of Medicines Australia, and by complaints from consumers and 'watchdogs'. Breaches of the Code can require withdrawal of promotional material and heavy fines, plus exposure in professional journals (e.g. annually in the *Australian Prescriber*).[10]

Advertising of prescription medicines to the public is not permitted in Australia, but advertising of OTC drugs is allowed. 'Direct-to-consumer' prescription drug advertising is legal in New Zealand and the US and is effective in increasing demand for medicines. Drug companies can boost demand for their products by defining common mild problems (e.g. dyspepsia, headache or baldness) as diseases requiring drug treatment, adding to the heavy costs of drugs to governments (i.e. taxpayers).

Advertisements often emphasise the benefits of a drug rather than the risks and mention adverse reactions only in the finest print. They should be monitored for superficial or misleading information, shock tactics, insidious comparisons and stereotyping (pictures of middle-aged male doctors treating anxious housewives, blond blue-eyed children, confused elderly women or stressed hypertensive male executives).

Relationships between health practitioners and the pharmaceutical industry

Prescribers are often 'wooed' by drug company representatives to increase their prescribing of a particular drug; incentives may range from 'starter packs' of drugs, equipment for the desk and lunches after seminars, to subsidisation of trips to overseas conferences or funding for research. Accepting even a small gift puts the prescriber

9 This was described graphically in the book by John le Carré (and later a movie), *The Constant Gardener*. Interestingly, in 2009 the drug company Pfizer signed a US$75 million agreement with Nigeria in settlement of charges that Pfizer had illegally tested an antibiotic on Nigerian children during a meningitis epidemic in 1996. Pfizer denied wrongdoing but settled, paid legal costs and agreed to set up a fund to support patients who took part in the trial.

10 In 2017–18, several drug companies were sanctioned by Medicines Australia with fines up to $100,000 for breaches of the Code of Conduct with respect to inappropriate promotional material, media releases and misleading claims, and were forced to withdraw the offending material. The fact that this happens every year implies that, for the companies concerned, the fine is minimal compared with the marketing benefits gained (Medicines Australia Code of Conduct 2018).

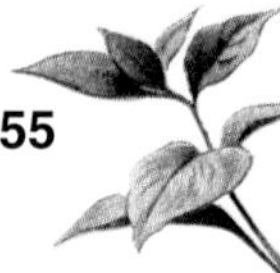

in a conflict-of-interest position. Although doctors generally maintain that they can resist such pressures, studies have shown that even subconsciously their prescribing patterns are affected by donations from drug company 'reps'. There is a range of positions that prescribers can adopt, from refusing all gifts, so as to avoid any compromise, through to acceptance of generous gifts while hoping to maintain independence.

The chief concerns about these practices are that commercial objectives override properly prioritised health care, education and research, and that there may be distortions in scientific evaluations and publications. Most biomedical journals now require that authors declare all conflicts of interest. Institutions and learned colleges expect there will be minimal acceptance of gifts or support, that research and publication will be guided by scientific and ethical values and that Australian clinicians and researchers will be required to make full public disclosure of all financial and other ties with commercial interests.

Ethical aspects of clinical trials

The Declaration of Helsinki, declared in 1964 and recognised internationally, outlines the ethical considerations related to medical research involving human subjects:

> *Every biomedical research project involving human subjects should be preceded by careful assessment of predictable risks in comparison with foreseeable benefits to the subject or to others. Concern for the interests of the subject must always prevail over the interests of science and society (World Health Organization – see 'Online resources').*

Many of the general issues in medical ethics discussed above also apply to the situation of a clinical trial. Particularly relevant are:

- personal autonomy and the subject's right to withdraw at any stage (individual rights versus welfare rights)
- the doctor being in a position of potential conflict (the healer versus the investigator)
- randomisation into groups, denying the control group access to the test drug, and the test group access to the current best treatment
- the extent to which subjects should be paid or compensated for expenses
- appropriate makeup of ethics committees
- special guidelines necessary for testing of reproductive technologies or for people who cannot give consent (e.g. minors, or those who have dementia, are aggressive or unconscious)
- trials being subsidised by the manufacturer company, and participating doctors having conflicts of interest if accepting emoluments.

Through the efforts of the International Conference on Harmonisation, standards of conduct for clinical trials have been determined that are now essentially uniform for all the major regulatory agencies worldwide, including Australia's TGA.

KEY POINTS

Ethical aspects of pharmacotherapy

- The ethical principles on which clinical practice is based are underpinned by basic human rights and international Declarations.
- Application of medical ethics principles can be controversial in many situations; it is important for health professionals to consider and discuss issues.
- During drug development, drugs need to be tested in animals and humans before being approved as safe and effective; many ethical issues become relevant.

Legal aspects of pharmacotherapy

Introduction

Before the 20th century there were few controls on the use of drugs, most of which were natural products with low efficacy. Official books of standards for medicinal products (pharmacopoeias) date back as far as the *Salerno Medical Edict* issued by Frederick II of Sicily (1240), who ordered apothecaries to prepare remedies always in the same way. In England in 1540 the manufacture of medicinal concoctions was subjected to supervision under the Apothecaries Wares, Drugs and Stuffs Act, which established the appointment of inspectors to police the Act. There was little information available about drugs compared with what we expect today. As chemical industries developed, more potent and efficacious drugs were synthesised (see again Table 1.2) and as trade in drugs of dependence (addictive drugs) increased in the early 20th century, it was recognised that controls on drugs were required.

International drug controls

Controls on narcotic drugs

The control of drugs in international law began in 1912 when the first Opium Conference was held at The Hague, Netherlands. International treaties were drawn up, calling on governments to:

- limit the manufacturing of and trade in medicinal opium to medical and scientific needs
- control the production and distribution of raw opium
- establish a system of governmental licensing to control the manufacture of and trade in drugs covered by the treaties.

In 1961, government representatives formulated the *United Nations Single Convention on Narcotic Drugs*, which became effective in 1964. The Convention needs to be ratified and signed by a country before it is binding, then appropriate legislation must be enacted. The Convention consolidated all existing treaties into one document for the control of all **narcotic** substances,[11] except for medical treatment and research, by:

- outlawing the production, manufacture, trade and use of narcotic substances for non-medicinal purposes
- limiting possession to authorised persons
- providing for international control of all opium transactions and production by the national monopolies in countries designated to produce opium, such as Australia and Turkey
- requiring import certificates and export authorisations.

The Convention, which comes under the auspices of the UN Office on Drugs and Crime (UNODC), lists drugs in schedules depending on their liability for abuse and production of adverse effects.

Australia has signed the following international treaties about drugs:

- *Single Convention on Narcotic Drugs 1961 (described above)*
- *Convention on Psychotropic Substances 1971*
- *UN Convention Against Illicit Traffic in Narcotic Drugs and Psychotropic Substances 1988.*

The International Narcotics Control Board was established to enforce the *Single Convention on Narcotic Drugs* and monitor implementation of the UN's drug control conventions. The Board has representatives from governments and the World Health Organization and monitors compliance with conventions regarding the manufacture, traffic and trade in drugs and government control over chemicals used in illicit manufacture.

Because enforcement is an immense task, it is impossible to prevent illicit trafficking. The UN's 2020 *World Drug Report* noted that 269 million people globally used illicit drugs. Treaties and international attempts to control illicit drugs are only as strong as the determination of member countries to introduce, update and enforce local laws. However, fines are less than the gains to be made by illicit trafficking. New means of distribution, such as 'internet pharmacies', pose new problems (CFB 2.2 and Hensey & Gwee 2016[10]). Acknowledging that many countries face high rates of crime related to drug trafficking, the UNODC has recently responded with a two-pronged approach: to integrate programs to reduce illicit drug supply and demand; and to focus on prevention, treatment, alternative development and protection of fundamental human rights (see UNODC in 'Online resources', and Ch 25).

Controls on therapeutic drugs

Drugs used therapeutically also need to be controlled because most people assume but cannot assess their safety and efficacy. When 'patent medicines' first flooded markets in developed countries early in the 20th century, there were few controls. Many tragic situations occurred, notably the 1937 fatal poisoning of more than 100 children in the United States by the Massengill Company's preparation of the new antimicrobial drug sulfanilamide, leading to demands for legislation to control marketing of all medicinal substances. The birth of thousands of deformed babies in the 1960s after use of thalidomide led to more rigorous testing and controls of drugs (CFB 2.1 and McBride[3]). More recently, post-marketing studies and meta-analyses of risks/benefits have led to worldwide recalls of drugs such as rofecoxib and aprotinin.

Most governments take a risk assessment role and require that drugs available in their country be assessed for safety, efficacy, quality of manufacture and cost-effectiveness. This provides protection not only for the public but also for drug manufacturers (and governments). The principles generally adopted are that:

- most people are not sufficiently knowledgeable about drugs to self-medicate safely
- all drugs should be assessed for potential risks and benefits
- a licence to market a drug is granted for a specified period subject to review
- government guidelines with respect to Good Laboratory Practice, Good Manufacturing Practice and Good Clinical Practice should be observed.

As world trade and health practices become ever more globally based, requirements for drug registration and licensing should become uniform in all developed countries.

Regulation of drugs in Australia

The regulation of medicinal drugs in Australia via the Therapeutic Goods Act has three primary aims: to control the supply of drugs prone to abuse; to regulate the availability of substances for therapeutic use (to ensure safety and quality); and to include certain products on government-sponsored assistance schemes.

11 The term 'narcotic' literally means 'causing numbness, sleep or unconsciousness', and so could apply to all central nervous system (CNS) depressants. It was originally used to refer to the 'narcotic analgesics', such as opium and derivatives such as morphine, to distinguish them from 'non-narcotic analgesics' such as aspirin. The term came to be extended to all drugs likely to cause addiction, and therefore to include drugs such as cocaine and amphetamines – certainly not CNS depressants – and even LSD and marijuana. It is now used more or less interchangeably with the terms 'illicit' or 'proscribed' to refer to all drugs for which there are international controls on trade and importation; these drug groups are discussed in detail in Chapter 19.

Australian laws related to drug regulation can be broadly divided into two types: laws that regulate drugs used for medicinal purposes in humans (discussed in this section); and laws that prohibit the possession, production and supply of **proscribed drugs** (i.e. prohibited drugs; discussed under 'Australian Drug Offences'). Legal non-medicinal drugs such as alcohol and tobacco are also subject to regulation (Ch 25). Drug availability can also be controlled at state and local levels – for example, by a hospital's drug committee.

Underpinning all healthcare-related laws are the fundamental principles of human rights and ethics (discussed later). Some aspects of common laws (developed by judicial precedence and interpretation) are also relevant: health professionals are considered to have a 'duty of care' and are expected to carry out their roles with their patients' best interests as the first priority.

Commonwealth and state laws

In Australia, drugs are controlled by extensive complex and overlapping pieces of Commonwealth, state and territory legislation (Table 2.1). Commonwealth legislation cannot apply in all situations, for constitutional reasons, and recent attempts to harmonise the criminal laws of states and territories have not yet succeeded. The Model Criminal Code, developed in 2009, is a set of criminal laws promulgated to facilitate the development of national criminal laws by all states and territories – that is, 'harmonisation' between jurisdictions. The Commonwealth, Australian Capital Territory and Northern Territory have enacted parts of the code, but other jurisdictions have made little progress.

Broadly, state and territory laws control 'poisons', and Commonwealth legislation controls 'therapeutic goods'; the role of the Commonwealth is increasing steadily. (Note that the term 'poison' is used broadly to cover drugs used clinically, as well as veterinary, agricultural and domestic chemicals.) Offences related to international drug trafficking are set out in Commonwealth legislation, while the state and territory criminal laws cover the production, possession, use and distribution of proscribed drugs within those jurisdictions. Additional legislation in most states covers drug use related to road safety. A substance may be subject to both Commonwealth and state regulation. For example, states and territories have their own guidelines on prescribing and dispensing of methadone and buprenorphine in treatment of opioid dependence; the scheduling and policing of these addictive drugs remain a Commonwealth responsibility.

Therapeutic Goods Administration

The Therapeutic Goods Act regulates 'therapeutic goods' for use in humans for preventing, treating or diagnosing a disease or pregnancy – for example, drugs, medical devices, diagnostic devices and biological entities, excluding foods and cosmetics. Before a therapeutic good can be marketed in Australia it must be approved and registered by the TGA, a division of the Commonwealth Department of Health, which evaluates the product pre-marketing for quality, safety, efficacy and cost-effectiveness, and access for the public (Fig 2.1).

In the case of a new drug, the sponsor, usually a drug company, submits material to the TGA, including chemical and manufacturing data and results from pharmacological testing in vitro, in vivo and in clinical trials (Therapeutic Goods Administration 2021). Experienced evaluators in the relevant advisory committee examine the material closely over months. The TGA makes the final decision on registering the drug for therapeutic use in Australia and decides into which schedule it should be classified. The process also applies to non-prescription drugs and some complementary and alternative remedies, to traditional medicines and to medical devices such as breast implants, diagnostic test kits, prostheses, dental materials, contact lenses and tampons. The TGA also regulates therapeutic goods post-marketing, enforces standards of practice, licenses manufacturers and verifies compliance.

Drugs that are legal but unregistered may be accessed via various schemes (see Donovan 2017):

- the Special Access Scheme, which allows the importation or supply of an unapproved drug for a single patient on a case-by-case basis, subject to TGA approval
- the Authorised Prescriber Scheme
- importation for personal use
- investigational drugs in notified and approved clinical trials.

Classification into schedules: Standard for the Uniform Scheduling of Medicines and Poisons

Historically, regulation of drug availability in Australia was a state responsibility, which led to anomalies such as a drug being available over the counter in one state – for example, in Albury, NSW – whereas a prescription might be required in Albury's sister town, Wodonga, on the opposite bank of the Murray River in Victoria (or vice versa). In the late 20th century, a review strongly supported a uniform regulatory scheme across states and territories, noting the benefits in terms of QUM and a balance between the many vested interests involved: drug companies want drugs to be as widely bought as possible, governments want to minimise costs and protect the public, while health professionals wish to perform and protect their roles in the supply of drugs.

The Australian Advisory Committee on Medicines Scheduling recommends classification of most drugs and many chemicals into schedules, in the *Standard for the Uniform Scheduling of Medicines and Poisons* (SUSMP). The Standard is published by the Australian Government under Commonwealth law and is registered on the Federal Register of Legislation as the *Poisons Standard* (see, for example, the *Poisons Standard,* in 'Online resources'). The SUSMP is updated at least annually; it is important to refer to the most recent version. Decisions in relation to the Standard have no force in Commonwealth law; but most states and territories have adopted the Standard in their legislation and regulations determining how consumers access a particular drug, and how it is to be packaged and labelled. More information on state/territory scheduling, including contact details for drugs and poisons units, is available on the TGA website (see 'Online resources').

Trans-Tasman harmonisation

The SUSMP also attempts to unify scheduling and control of drugs and poisons between Australia and New Zealand. This trans-Tasman scheduling harmonisation has been largely effective, with a few minor discrepancies (see below under 'Regulation of Drugs in New Zealand').

The drug schedules

The *Poisons Standard* contains 10 schedules of 'poisons' (i.e. drugs and other chemicals) that are subject to varying levels of controls on labels, containers, storage, disposal, record keeping, sale, supply, possession and use and advertising of the scheduled substances. First aid instructions, warning statements and labelling requirements are given in appendices. Drugs are labelled with the 'signal words' of the classification – for example, 'Pharmacy-Only' medicine. This change was made to counteract the false perception in the community that higher S numbers necessarily meant higher toxicity. In fact, the schedules listed in order of greatest to least restrictions are 9, 10, 8, 4, 7, 3, 2, 6, 5.

The decision to classify a substance into a particular schedule depends not only on the potential toxicity of the drug but also on the purposes for which it is used, the dose in the particular preparation, its potential for abuse, other ingredients present, the formulation (e.g. oral tablet, parenteral injection or topical ointment) and the need for access to the drug.

Most drugs for therapeutic use are in Schedule 2, 3, 4 or 8. A drug may appear in more than one schedule; for example, aspirin appears in various schedules (2, 4, 5 and 6) depending on the strength and type of the formulation, the route of administration, the quantity of doses in the package, whether other drugs are present and whether it is intended for human or veterinary use. Where a preparation contains two or more substances, the preparation is in the schedule that is the most restrictive. A few human medicines are included in Schedule 5 and 6 such as head lice preparations and some essential oils.

There may be varying provisions within a schedule; for example, isotretinoin is a S4 Prescription-Only medicine used to treat severe acne (tretinoin cream; DM 41.2) but is teratogenic (causes congenital malformations), so there are strict requirements relating to prescribing and labelling it for women of childbearing age. Drugs may be moved around between schedules as clinical experience and drug usage patterns change. In general, there is a trend to down-schedule medicines, improving access to the public in line with one of the central objectives of the *National Medicines Policy*. The most recent version of the SUSMP should always be consulted to answer the question, 'What schedule is this drug in?' Some examples are given in the lists below.

Unscheduled substances

If a substance does not appear in a schedule or appendix of the SUSMP (i.e. is unscheduled) it is not a poison by definition and can be supplied to the public (unless it is subject to other legislative controls).

Includes: laxatives, contact lens products, infant formulae, vitamins, sunscreens, many topical antiseptics, herbal remedies and small packs of some drugs with high safety margins – for example, non-sedating antihistamines for short-term treatment of hay fever.

Pharmaceutical substances

Schedule 2 Pharmacy Medicine

Available to the public only from pharmacies, where a pharmacist's advice is available if required; or, where a pharmacy service is unavailable, from persons licensed to sell Schedule 2 poisons.

Includes: some cough and cold preparations, oral antihistamines in larger packs or in combination preparations, mild analgesics, worm tablets, anti-inflammatory agents, topical antifungal preparations, histamine H_2-receptor antagonists (in small packs, for relief of heartburn), topical local anaesthetics (not eyedrops), corticosteroids in some topical formulations, decongestant eyedrops and some herbal preparations.

Schedule 3 Pharmacist-Only Medicine

Available to the public only from a pharmacist or from medical, dental or veterinary practitioners but without need for a prescription. Safe use of these substances requires professional advice; storage must not be accessible to the public.

Includes: some metered-dose bronchodilator asthma aerosols, topical corticosteroids (some low-strength preparations in small packs), glucagon, antivirals for cold sores, adrenaline (epinephrine) injections for anaphylaxis,

serotonin receptor agonists for migraine treatment and hormones for emergency contraception.

Schedule 4 Prescription-Only Medicine or Prescription Animal Remedy

May be used or supplied only under prescription from an Authorised Prescriber. Must be stored in a dispensary. In some Australian states, specially qualified nurses, optometrists and podiatrists may prescribe from a limited range of S4 Prescription-Only drugs.

Includes: most drugs – for example, antibiotics, antidepressants, hormones including insulins and hormonal contraceptives (except for emergency contraception), most cardiovascular and central nervous system drugs, antineoplastic agents and most injections.

Agricultural, domestic and industrial substances

Schedule 5 Caution

Substances with a low potential for causing harm, supplied with simple warnings and safety directions on the label. For sale by a pharmacist, Poisons Licence holder or general dealer. Must not be stored or supplied in a drink or food container.

Includes: some veterinary medicines, household poisons, ether, naphthalene, petrol; some head lice lotions.

Schedule 6 Poison

More dangerous chemicals than those in Schedule 5, with moderate potential for harm. Extra storage and packaging controls and strong warning labels required.

Includes: many household and garden pesticides and solvents; some iodine tinctures.

Schedule 7 Dangerous Poison

Substances with a high potential for causing harm at low exposure, which require special precautions. A permit is required to buy these chemicals, the purchaser must be over 18 years of age. Special regulations may restrict their availability, possession, storage or use.

Includes: varying strengths of chemicals such as arsenic, azo dyes, strychnine, cyanide and commercial pesticides.

Controlled drugs and prohibited substances

Schedule 8 Controlled Drug

Controlled drugs are substances that may produce addiction or dependence. Possession without authority is illegal. Tight controls are applied to reduce abuse and dependence. Drugs must be stored in a locked cabinet and records kept for 2 years in most states, 5 years in WA.

Includes: opioids such as morphine, methadone, fentanyl and high-dose codeine alone; CNS stimulants such as dexamfetamine; cocaine, ketamine and some cannabis extracts.

Schedule 9 Prohibited Substances

Substances of which the manufacture, possession, sale or use is prohibited except in special circumstances. Drugs that may be abused or drugs possibly required for teaching, research or analytical purposes, but which are too toxic for therapeutic use.

Includes: heroin and most recreational drugs such as amphetamine derivatives, LSD and muscimol (except alcohol and tobacco).

Schedule 10: Substances of such danger to health as to warrant prohibition of sale, supply and use

Substances (other than those in Schedule 9) so dangerous that sale, supply and use are prohibited; included are many poisonous plants, herbs and chemicals, poisons such as amygdalin, cinchophen and aristolochia derivatives and many dyes.

Other regulation by the TGA

Drugs are subject to strict regulation in all Australian states and territories from the moment of their manufacture through selling, purchasing, using, storing, prescribing and dispensing until their administration. The Therapeutic Goods Act also contains provisions covering:

- licences for manufacturers of therapeutic goods for use in humans (most registered health professionals and some alternative practitioners are already covered in the practice of their profession)
- supply: wholesaling and retailing:
  - it is an offence to supply by wholesale any therapeutic goods that are not on the register
  - access, labelling and record keeping, etc. depend on the schedule of the drug
  - drug companies and the TGA endeavour to maintain regular supplies
- possession:
  - certain persons are authorised to possess Schedule 4 and 8 drugs for legitimate commercial, professional or emergency purposes
  - unauthorised possession of Schedule 8 or 9 poisons is a criminal offence
- advertising:
  - various state Acts prohibit advertising Schedule 4, 8 and 9 poisons to the public
  - advertisements are allowed in bona fide professional publications or journals (e.g. *Australian Pharmacist*)
  - unscheduled substances and some in Schedules 2 and 3 can be advertised directly to the public within SUSMP guidelines

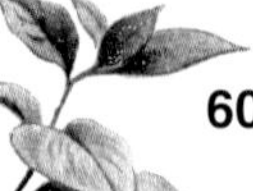

- prescriptions:
  - generally, Schedule 4 or 8 drugs can be prescribed by medical practitioners, dentists and veterinary surgeons in the lawful practice of their respective professions
  - some optometrists, podiatrists and NPs with specialised training have limited prescribing rights
- dispensing:
  - legal prescriptions for Schedule 4 and 8 drugs can be filled by pharmacists (or by a 'dispensing doctor' for their own patients, in areas without adequate pharmacy coverage)
  - in most states and territories a pharmacist can, at a doctor's request, dispense a small supply of Schedule 4 drugs without a prescription in an emergency; a valid written prescription must be provided as soon as practicable
- packaging and labelling:
  - labelling and packaging of drugs are governed by orders and regulations; it is an offence to fail to comply with these standards
  - pharmacists must ensure that medicines are labelled correctly to ensure safe storage and administration, as determined by the drug's schedule
  - labels may be advisory, explanatory or reminders, such as: 'this medicine may cause drowsiness'; 'discard contents after dd/mm/yyyy'; 'this prescription may be repeated . . . times'; 'take immediately before food'
- administration:
  - as a general rule, administration of Schedule 4 and 8 poisons to a person requires written or verbal authorisation by the prescriber, except in emergencies
- storage and destruction:
  - storage and destruction of Schedule 4 and 8 poisons by manufacturers, wholesalers and pharmacists, and in hospitals, are strictly regulated
  - on hospital wards an 'imprest' system of lockable cupboards, trolleys and bedside drawers provides access; strict security procedures must be maintained
  - storage requirements imposed on doctors, dentists and veterinary surgeons are less stringent, as they are less likely to store large quantities of drugs
- record keeping:
  - Schedule 4 and 8 drugs must be accounted for at every stage of manufacture, supply, storage and dispensing
  - hospital drug charts (Fig 2.3C, earlier) show how each drug was prescribed and administered
- testing of drugs:
  - provisions in the Therapeutic Goods Act and regulations govern the use of experimental drugs and testing in animals and humans
- counterfeiting (CFB 2.3), recall procedures and reporting of adverse effects are also covered.

Orphan drugs

An **orphan drug** is designated by the TGA as an agent that is intended to treat, prevent or diagnose a rare disease, or that is not commercially viable to supply to treat, prevent or diagnose another disease or condition (see Therapeutic Goods Administration, in 'Online resources'). This designation recognises that people with rare conditions have as much right as all others to safe, effective drugs.

The TGA's Orphan Drug Program encourages sponsors (drug companies) by reducing the costs and controls associated with drug development, evaluation and approval. Drugs already rejected on safety grounds, or already registered or considered essential drugs, are not considered. Some hundred formulations are designated as orphan drugs by the TGA. Examples include the drug

> **CLINICAL FOCUS BOX 2.3**
>
> **Fake pharmaceuticals and pharmacies**
>
> In Australia, thanks to drug regulation and customs surveillance, the prevalence of fake or substandard medicines is estimated (by the World Health Organization) to be very low: less than 1% of market value. However, the increasing number of drugs purchased online from illegal pharmacies poses a risk. There are at least 36,000 active internet pharmacies globally, of which fewer than 5% are legitimate (i.e. staffed by qualified pharmacists and selling drugs according to regulations). Illegal online pharmacies pose a risk to public safety because they often sell counterfeit and contaminated drugs (with unknown safety profiles) and illicit substances. In some cases, drugs have been ineffective (leading to travellers contracting malaria) or toxic (causing death due to contamination with diethylene glycol). Illegal online pharmacies encourage people to self-diagnose and remove the opportunity for patient monitoring and the provision of pharmaceutical care.
>
> Health professionals play a vital role in improving medicines safety by educating individuals and the public about the harms of purchasing medicines from illegal internet pharmacies.
>
> *Source: Hensey & Gwee 2016.*

patisiran for the treatment of hereditary transthyretin mediated amyloidosis in individuals who have neuropathy and tafasitamab for the treatment of diffuse large B-cell lymphoma, an aggressive type of non-Hodgkin lymphoma.

In New Zealand there is a comparable program facilitated through Pharmac funding medicines for rare disorders.

Legal aspects of special concern to pharmacists

As the supplier of many OTC and all Pharmacy- (S2), Pharmacist- (S3) and Prescription-Only (S4) drugs, the final responsibility for safe supply rests with the pharmacist. State and territory Acts, Regulations and Pharmacy Board guidelines cover aspects such as: training, examination and registration of pharmacists; good pharmaceutical practice, including control of the dispensary, dispensing, labelling, counselling and record keeping; possession, storage and supply of drugs; and services to residential care facilities.

Typical day-to-day issues of legal concern for pharmacists involve:

- clients who appear to be 'doctor shopping' for excessive prescriptions
- concern about possible forgery of prescriptions
- loss or theft of drugs
- suspected self-prescribing by professionals with prescribing rights
- ensuring that requests for Schedule 3 (Pharmacist-Only) drugs are warranted by an appropriate condition being diagnosed
- administration of the methadone maintenance program (Ch 25).

Other issues relate to accreditation programs for pharmacists and pharmacies, unprofessional conduct and disciplinary processes, extemporaneous preparation of medicines not subject to control by the TGA, mandatory notification obligations, ethical aspects (described later), drug regulation and advertising, and workplace health and safety matters.

Pharmaceutical Benefits Scheme

The PBS began as a limited scheme in 1948, as a list of 139 'life-saving and disease preventing' medicines provided free of charge for Australians. By June 2020, 902 different drugs (and 5371 brands) deemed to be essential to the community but too expensive for individual purchase were partially subsidised by the government. Most PBS-listed medicines are dispensed by pharmacists and used by patients at home. Some (e.g. chemotherapy drugs and potent hormones) need medical supervision or can only be prescribed by authorised doctors (the S100 items).

There is a separate section, the Repatriation Pharmaceutical Benefits Scheme, subsidising a wider range of medications and dressings to armed forces veterans and eligible dependants.

Costs of the PBS

In the financial year 2019–20, total PBS government expenditure was over A$12.6 billion, an increase of almost 6.7% on the previous year. The number of PBS prescriptions was 208.5 million. Growth was mainly driven by listing of expensive biological therapies ('biologicals'), new antivirals and small-molecule anticancer drugs. The average dispensed price per prescription of PBS medicines increased to $67.34. The costs increase every year, causing blow-outs in the health budget (see Table 1.8 for the most prescribed drugs).

The Pharmaceutical Benefits Advisory Committee evaluates the efficacy, safety and cost-effectiveness of a drug compared with current therapies, then may recommend the drug for subsidy and a price is negotiated. When a drug is listed on the PBS it makes it more affordable for the individual (because part of the cost is subsidised by the government),[12] and so members of the committee, government and doctors are under pressure from drug companies to ensure PBS listing.

In Australia, only doctors, dentists, midwives, optometrists and NPs who are approved to prescribe PBS medicines under the National Health Act can prescribe PBS drugs. The number and type of drugs that a prescriber can prescribe under the PBS is related to that prescriber's scope of practice. Podiatrists who are endorsed to prescribe scheduled drugs may prescribe from a list of drugs, but these are not yet subsidised by the PBS.

Access to drugs outside the PBS

Drugs not subsidised by the PBS may be obtained by other means: via private prescriptions (where the patient pays the full price), or available over the counter in pharmacies, health shops and supermarkets (Ch 3). Life-saving drugs for very rare diseases may be funded under the Orphan Drug Program.

Medicines in pregnancy

The TGA, through its Advisory Committee on Prescription Medicines, maintains an 'Australian categorisation of risk of drug use in pregnancy' (Ch 30). Categories range from A (drugs taken by a large number of pregnant women without harmful effects on the fetus) to X (drugs with a high risk of permanent fetal damage that should not be

12 For example, in 2020 atezolizumab, a new treatment for liver cancer, cost approximately A$10,000 per prescription prior to its PBS listing, and only the normal PBS drug fee (then approximately A$41 per prescription) afterwards; taxpayers subsidise the difference. Patients prescribed atezolizumab needs multiple prescriptions while undergoing treatment.

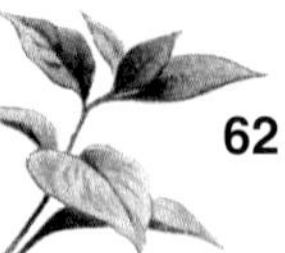

used in pregnancy). The classification is a warning to users and prescribers, rather than a legally enforceable regulation.

Drugs in sport

The use of drugs by athletes and during sporting competitions is regulated not so much by the government (although there is some Commonwealth and state legislation – for example, SUSMP Appendix D and the *Australian Sports Anti-Doping Authority Act 2006*) as by the International Olympic Movement and its Anti-Doping Rules, and the World Anti-Doping Agency, implemented in Australia by the Australian Sports Anti-Doping Authority. Drugs are classified into groups depending on whether they are allowed under certain circumstances, prohibited or prohibited in some sports.

Australian drug offences

Historical aspects

The enactment of drug legislation in Australia has followed the social trends and scientific knowledge of the time, dating from the 1890s in relation to opium and the early 1900s for other drugs. Historically in Australia the selective enactment of drug laws has been influenced by racism, powerful international pressures and the vested interests of bureaucrats, politicians and the medical profession. For example, in 19th-century Australia, opium was freely available and used, and the line dividing medical 'use' from non-medical 'abuse' was not yet apparent. By the late 1880s opium was seen as a 'pollutant, moral as well as physical' and was associated with Chinese 'opium dens'. Soon after, its non-medical use was criminalised.

Two pieces of Commonwealth legislation that relate to certain dealings in drugs, both within and outside Australia, the *Crimes (Traffic in Narcotic Drugs and Psychotropic Substances) Act 1990* (Cth) and the *Narcotic Goods Act 1967* (Cth), were introduced pursuant to UN Conventions.

Legislation

Drug offences (i.e. breaches of the local laws relating to the manufacture, production, sale, supply, possession, handling or use of certain poisons, drugs and other substances) and responsibility for the policing of drug laws are set out in Commonwealth, state and territory legislation. Generally, for offences for which possession of the drug is necessary, it will be a defence to show that professional possession was authorised under the relevant state law.

Which drugs are proscribed (illegal)?

The drugs that are proscribed in the states, territories and the Commonwealth are very similar; they are set out in authoritative lists, usually based on the SUSMP (see above).

Commonwealth offences

The principal piece of Commonwealth legislation containing drug offences is the *Criminal Code Act 1995* (Cth), supplemented by the *Customs Act 1901* (Cth), the *Narcotic Goods Act 1967* (Cth) and the *Narcotic Drugs Amendment Act 2016* (Cth). Part 9.1 of the Criminal Code addresses the trafficking, illegal manufacture, supply and possession of controlled drugs and plants. Prohibited conduct under the Criminal Code includes: the cultivation of certain plants (e.g. opium poppy) to produce narcotic drugs; making narcotic drugs or psychotropic substances; and the sale, supply or possession of a narcotic drug or psychotropic substance, including dealings on board an Australian aircraft in flight or an Australian ship at sea, and outside Australia in various circumstances.

The Customs Act also details offences relating to importing or exporting narcotic goods. The Narcotic Goods Act forbids the manufacture of a drug without a licence, and contains other restrictions on manufacture, labelling and destruction. The Australian Government can now update and expand the list of prohibited substances by regulation rather than by changing the Criminal Code to respond rapidly to new 'designer drugs'.

State and territory offences

In most Australian states and territories it is an offence, unless authorised, to produce, manufacture, use, possess, consume, self-administer, deal in, distribute, traffic in, sell or supply or possess equipment related to a proscribed drug. A range of related offences exists in certain jurisdictions, such as the theft of proscribed drugs, 'spiking' of food and drinks, the possession of property derived from drug dealing, possessing instructions or equipment for producing proscribed drugs and offences related to prescriptions for proscribed drugs

The practices of health professionals are usually governed by relevant Acts of Parliament (e.g. the *Health Practitioner Regulation National Law Act 2009*) and by the regulations of the appropriate professional board (e.g. the Podiatry Board of Australia). These boards are specific to the profession concerned.

Regulation of drugs in New Zealand

In New Zealand, legislation relevant to drugs is contained in the *Medicines Act 1981* and regulations (1984), plus in the *Medicines Amendment Act 2013*, and various subsequent notices and regulations relating to medical devices, approved laboratories, hazardous substances, and to Designated Prescribers, including now some NPs, midwives, pharmacists and optometrists (see 'Online resources: New Zealand Drug Regulatory Information'). The four key elements of the regulatory framework (administered by Medsafe, the Medicines and Medical Devices Safety Authority) are: availability, quality, access and information. Medsafe's mission is 'to enhance the health of New Zealanders by regulating medicines and medical devices to maximise safety and benefit' (see 'Online resources').

Scheduling and prescribing of drugs

In New Zealand, 'Scheduled Medicines' are classified into three main categories, unless the Minister of Health has gazetted departures from the SUSMP listings:

- prescription medicine (similar to S4 of the SUSMP)
- restricted medicine (also known as pharmacist-only medicine – S3 of the SUSMP)
- pharmacy-only medicine (S2 of the SUSMP).

These are listed in the First Schedule to the Medicines Regulations 1984 and Amendments.

For a shift from 'prescription' to 'non-prescription' status, a medicine should have been marketed and in wide use for 3 or more years, have a low risk of serious reactions and be suitable for non-prescription sale based on criteria including convenience, toxicity, potency, precautions, abuse potential and availability of similar products.

All other products (other than controlled drugs, see below) are deemed unclassified and are 'general sale medicines'. There are no registration numbers assigned to show that products have been approved for sale, as there are in Australia. New Zealand allows direct-to-consumer advertising of drugs, which is prohibited in Australia for prescription drugs. New Zealand follows Australian guidelines and categories for safety of drugs in pregnancy.

Trans-Tasman harmonisation

The general principles of scheduling harmonisation (between New Zealand and Australia) state that there should be: equivalent scheduling and general exemptions; common definitions, criteria, guidelines and drug classes; common nomenclature, using international non-proprietary names; and harmonisation of labelling, packaging, warnings, etc. Despite efforts at simplification and harmonisation, there are still some differences in scheduling of drugs and terminology. It is recognised that differences should be re-assessed, preferably harmonising to the less restrictive schedule.

Pharmac

Pharmac is a Crown body with the responsibility for managing the pharmaceutical budget and funding of medicines, vaccines and some medical devices. It tenders for subsidised drugs, and its committees set access criteria. Pharmac publishes its Pharmaceutical Schedule (not to be confused with the SUSMP Schedules) under two sections: Section B: Community Pharmaceuticals and Section H: Hospital Pharmaceuticals, showing the drugs (and brands) that are subsidised by the government.

The *New Zealand Universal List of Medicines* is provided under the auspices of the Ministry of Health, with input from Medsafe, Pharmac and the Pharmacy Guild. It is a 'dictionary of trusted, standardised information about medicines covering medicines approved for supply in New Zealand as well as products listed in Pharmac's Pharmaceutical Schedule . . .' (see 'Online resources').

Pharmacology and Therapeutics Advisory Committee

The Pharmacology and Therapeutics Advisory Committee is Pharmac's primary clinical advisory committee. It considers and makes recommendations on applications for funding medicines, management of and amendments to the Pharmaceutical Schedule and the need for reviews of drugs. The committee is made up of senior health practitioners from a range of specialties, who review evidence before recommending and negotiating subsidies. Generally, New Zealanders pay much lower co-payment prices for drugs than do Australians (unless on a special scheme). Many more drugs within a class are subsidised in Australia, whereas New Zealand limits the number of bio-equivalent 'me-too' drugs subsidised: a comparative study showed that of the five most popular drug classes, 81 different drug products were subsidised in New Zealand, whereas over 650 were subsidised by the PBS.

Controlled drugs (drugs of dependence) in New Zealand

The New Zealand *Dangerous Drugs Act 1927* dealt with the controls required by the League of Nations for opium and non-opiate drugs. Before this, opium was readily available; the main drugs causing problems (then as now) were alcohol and tobacco.

After World War II, cannabis and amphetamines began to appear as problem drugs, and in the 'hippy' days of the 1960s and 1970s, people also experimented with *Datura* (containing the plant alkaloids atropine and hyoscine), amphetamines, hallucinogens and solvent sniffing. The *Narcotics Act 1965* included controls on mescaline, cocaine and LSD, as well as opiates. The *United Nations Single Convention on Narcotic Drugs* (1961, 1972) imposed wider controls on drugs, including marijuana. Countries signatory to this Convention are constrained to abide by its agreements. In New Zealand, the *Misuse of Drugs Act 1975* and subsequent regulations (1977) classified controlled drugs into schedules to allow penalties depending on the severity of the abuse, and contain the requirements for the manufacture, sale, supply, prescribing and labelling of controlled drugs. Alcohol and tobacco are excluded from the Acts; alcohol is subject to the *Sale of Liquor Act 1989* and amendments. There is some debate in New Zealand about including marijuana along with more damaging drugs such as heroin and cocaine.

KEY POINTS

Legal aspects of pharmacotherapy

- Drugs are controlled at many levels: international, national and state; local institutions also regulate access to medicines.
- Laws apply to the classification and control of chemicals, poisons, drugs and other therapeutic goods. Some chemicals are proscribed, and criminal law relates to offences under relevant Acts.
- Drugs are classified into various *Poisons Schedules* to control access, supply and provision, labelling, storage, records and advertising.
- Special arrangements exist for 'orphan drugs' to treat very rare diseases, for classifying drugs for safe use in pregnancy, and with respect to drug use in sport.
- The trans-Tasman harmonisation policy attempts to maintain similar regulations between New Zealand and Australia.
- Governments determine which drugs will be subsidised for consumers; local institutions may determine which can be prescribed.

REVIEW EXERCISES

1. In Australia and New Zealand, there are a number of different types of prescribers. As a health professional it is important you know who can prescribe what. Discuss the different types of prescribers and what they can prescribe in the country in which you (will) practise. Discuss where you would find the legislation outlining the different types of prescribers and which prescribers can prescribe medicines that are subsidised via the Pharmaceutical Benefits Scheme.
2. Ms JC, a 38-year-old family lawyer, presents to her local pharmacy and requests something to alleviate the signs and symptoms of her common cold. The pharmacist asks if she is taking any other medicines, including those purchased over the counter and complementary therapies. Ms JC states that she takes rosuvastatin 10 mg (a medicine to reduce cholesterol) daily. The pharmacist recommends paracetamol 500 mg two tablets every 4–6 hours for her fever and pseudoephedrine 60 mg once daily for short term use to relieve her nasal congestion. Ms JC selects a box of 100 paracetamol tablets and presents her driver's licence as a requirement to purchase the box of pseudoephedrine. Why does the pharmacist ask if Ms JC is taking any other medicines? List the poisons schedule that paracetamol, pseudoephedrine and rosuvastatin are in. Are the drugs subsidised by your government (i.e. via the PBS in Australia or the New Zealand Pharmaceutical Schedule)? Why did Ms JC have to show her driver's licence?
3. As a health professional you are wanting to determine if a new drug is safe and effective for your patients. To do this you want to read the related peer reviewed research. Discuss what databases you might search to obtain relevant primary and secondary studies. You find a relevant well-designed RCCT, a meta-analysis, a case-control study and a case report. Discuss the hierarchy of evidence and which study holds the greatest weight when informing evidence-based care.

REFERENCES

Australian Medicines Handbook 2021, ***Australian medicines handbook 2021***, Adelaide, AMH.

Department of Health 2022. Authorised midwives – legislative requirements. Victorian Government, Melbourne. Online: https://www.health.vic.gov.au/drugs-and-poisons/authorised-midwives-legislative-requirements

Donovan, P., Access to unregistered drugs in Australia. Australian Prescriber, 2017. 40(5): 194–196.

Hensey, C.C., Gwee A., Counterfeit drugs: an Australian perspective. Medical Journal of Australia, 2016. 204(9): 344.

Kyle, G., Product familiarisation programs. Australian Prescriber, 2017. 40(6): 206–207.

McBride, W.G., Thalidomide and congenital abnormalities The Lancet, 1961. 278(7216): 1358.

Medicines Australia 2022. Who we are. Online: https://www.medicinesaustralia.com.au/about-us/who-we-are/

Medicines Australia Code of Conduct: breaches 2017–18. Australian Prescriber, 2018. 41(6): 195–195.

Moulds R. Deferring PBAC decisions: rationing as a reality. Australian Prescriber 2012; 35(1): 2–3

Rankin, A., Cadogan C.A., Patterson S.M. et al., Interventions to improve the appropriate use of polypharmacy for older people. Cochrane Database Systemic Review, 2018. 9(9): Cd008165.

Sackett, D.L., Rosenberg W.M., Gray J.A. et al., Evidence based medicine: what it is and what it isn't. 1996, British Medical Journal Publishing Group.

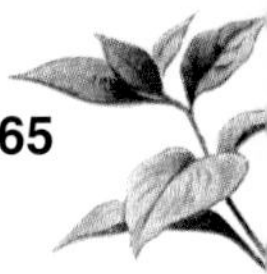

Services Australia 2021. Stationery for medical practitioners. Australian Government, Canberra. Online: https://www.servicesaustralia.gov.au/pbs-and-rpbs-stationery-for-medical-practitioners?context=22851

Sweeney, G.D., Clinical Pharmacology: A Conceptual Approach. 1990: New York: Churchill Livingstone.

Taylor, R., McKinlay E., Morris C. Standing order use in general practice: the views of medicine, nursing and pharmacy stakeholder organisations. Journal of Primary Health Care, 2017. 9(1): 47–55.

The American Heritage Medical Dictionary 2007. Definition: Medicine. Houghton Mifflin Company.

Therapeutic Goods Administration, The Australian clinical trial handbook, Department of Health, Editor. 2021, Australian Government: Canberra.

Usherwood, T., Encouraging adherence to long-term medication. Australian Prescriber, 2017. 40(4): 147–150.

Wolfe, SM. The seven-year rule for safer prescribing. Australian Prescriber 2012;35:138–9.

World Health Organization 2003, Adherence to long-term therapies. Evidence for action. World Health Organization, Geneva.

ONLINE RESOURCES

AMH Children's Dosing Companion 2017: https://shop.amh.net.au/cdcbook (accessed 2 November 2021)

Australian categorisation system for prescribing drugs in pregnancy: https://www.tga.gov.au/prescribing-medicines-pregnancy-database (accessed 2 November 2021)

Australian College of Nurse Practitioners: https://acnp.org.au (accessed 2 November 2021)

Australian Commission on Safety and Quality in Health Care: https://www.safetyandquality.gov.au/our-work/medication-safety/medication-charts/national-standard-medication-charts/pbs-hospital-medication-chart (accessed 2 November 2021)

Australian Health Practitioner Regulation Agency (Ahpra): https://www.ahpra.gov.au/ (accessed 2 November 2021)

Australian Pharmaceutical Formulary: https://www.psa.org.au/apf (accessed 2 November 2021)

Australian Prescriber: https://www.nps.org.au/australian-prescriber/ (accessed 2 November 2021)

Declaration of Geneva (1948): https://www.wma.net/what-we-do/medical-ethics/declaration-of-geneva/ (accessed 2 November 2021)

Declaration of Helsinki: https://www.wma.net/policies-post/wma-declaration-of-helsinki-ethical-principles-for-medical-research-involving-human-subjects/ (accessed 2 November 2021)

International Code of Medical Ethics (1949): https://www.wma.net/policies-post/wma-international-code-of-medical-ethics/ (accessed 2 November 2021)

Medicines Australia: http:// https://medicinesaustralia.com.au (accessed 2 November 2021)

Medsafe NZ: https://www.medsafe.govt.nz/index.asp (accessed 2 November 2021)

Midwifery Council of New Zealand: https://www.midwiferycouncil.health.nz (accessed 2 November 2021)

National Medicines Policy (Australia): https://www.health.gov.au/nationalmedicinespolicy/ (accessed 2 November 2021)

National Prescribing Service (NPS): https://www.nps.org.au/ (accessed 2 November 2021)

New Zealand College of Midwives: https://www.midwife.org.nz/ (accessed 2 November 2021)

New Zealand Drug Regulatory Information: https://www.medsafe.govt.nz/regulatory/Guideline/GRTPNZ/overview-of-therapeutic-product-regulation.pdf (accessed 2 November 2021)

New Zealand Formulary: https://www.nzformulary.org/ (accessed 2 November 2021)

New Zealand Ministry of Health / Manatu– Hauora: https://www.health.govt.nz/ (accessed 2 November 2021)

New Zealand Ministry of Health: https://www.health.govt.nz/our-work/primary-health-care/about-primary-health-organisations/ (accessed 2 November 2021)

New Zealand *Universal List of Medicines*: https://www.nzulm.org.nz/ (accessed 2 November 2021)

Pharmac (NZ): https://www.pharmac.govt.nz/ (accessed 2 November 2021)

Pharmaceutical Benefits Scheme: https://www.pbs.gov.au/pbs/home (accessed 2 November 2021)

Therapeutic Goods Administration (TGA): https://www.tga.gov.au/ (accessed 2 November 2021)

More weblinks at: http://evolve.elsevier.com/AU/Knights/pharmacology/.

CHAPTER 3

MOLECULAR DRUG TARGETS AND PHARMACODYNAMICS

Andrew Rowland

KEY ABBREVIATIONS

ATP	adenosine triphosphate
cAMP	cyclic adenosine monophosphate
cGMP	cyclic guanosine monophosphate
GDP	guanosine diphosphate
GPCR	G-protein-coupled receptors
GTP	guanosine triphosphate
HMG-CoA	3-hydroxy-3-methylglutaryl coenzyme A

KEY TERMS

Chapter Focus

Drugs have been a mainstay in the treatment of disease for centuries. Belief in their 'magical' powers has now been replaced by scientific understanding of the basis of drug action. This knowledge has enabled health professionals to use drugs more effectively and safely, and pharmaceutical companies and scientists to develop new drugs that produce more targeted therapeutic effects with diminished adverse effects. An understanding of the molecular targets for drug action and the relationship between exposure to a drug and the pharmacological response it produces underpins many aspects of the use of drugs.

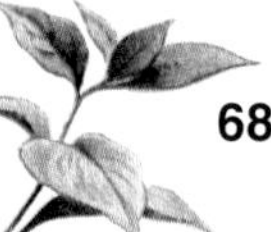

CRITICAL THINKING SCENARIO

Sam is a 65-year-old male with a history of asthma and chronic obstructive pulmonary disease. Since he was young, he has had two puffers at home: a blue one that contains salbutamol (a β-adrenoceptor agonist) and a white one that contains ipratropium (a muscarinic acetylcholine receptor antagonist). While these two drugs have opposing effects (one is an agonist and the other is an antagonist) and act at different targets, there is a lot of overlap in how and why they are used. How can this be the case?

Introduction

Drugs don't confer new functions on a tissue or organ; instead, they modify existing physiological, biochemical or biophysical processes in order to change existing functions of a tissue or organ to achieve a therapeutic outcome. For example, when a hypoglycaemic drug is prescribed for a person with diabetes, the health professional can monitor the effectiveness of the drug by repeated measurements of the person's blood glucose concentration. Drugs can act by interacting with endogenous small molecules (e.g. antacids neutralise gastric acid), altering the activity of a cell membrane (e.g. local anaesthetics) or interaction with protein (e.g. adrenaline (epinephrine) increases the heart rate by interacting with receptors in the heart). The site at which a drug binds is called the 'molecular target' or 'site of action'. In the vast majority of cases the molecular target is a protein, but there are exceptions such as antimicrobials and cytotoxic chemotherapy drugs that bind to deoxyribonucleic acid (DNA), which is not a protein.

Drug specificity, selectivity and affinity

The **specificity** of a drug describes the number of effects the drug produces, while **selectivity** describes the number of molecular targets the drug interacts with. An ideal drug would interact with a single molecular target, at a single site, and cause only one effect. Such a drug would be described as having complete specificity; unfortunately, no drugs can lay claim to that title. Most drugs show some degree of selectivity – that is, a preference for a molecular target – but may lack specificity either because they act on more than one molecular target or because they act on a molecular target that is located in multiple organs or tissues throughout the body. For example, isoprenaline is non-selective because it interacts with β_1 adrenoceptors in the heart, causing an increase in heart rate and force of contraction, and with β_2 adrenoceptors in the lungs, causing bronchodilation. In contrast, salbutamol is selective for β_2 adrenoceptors, and greater site (in this case, tissue) selectivity is achieved when the drug is inhaled. At higher doses, salbutamol causes muscle tremor by interacting with β_2 adrenoceptors in skeletal muscle. Although selectivity for β_2 adrenoceptors is retained at higher doses, tissue selectivity is lost, leading to a loss of specificity and multiple effects.

To understand how drugs act, we need to understand the site on the molecular target at which they bind, the molecular mechanisms by which an extracellular signal alters an intracellular pathway and causes a functional change in a cell and why under some circumstances the response to drugs decreases with time. The binding of a drug to its molecular target can occur via multiple interactions, including simple hydrogen bonding, ionic or hydrophobic interactions, van der Waals forces (these are the forces between molecules of non-polar compounds) and covalent interactions. The last may increase the duration of drug action – for example, the effects of aspirin on platelets or of acetylcholinesterase inhibitors. The strength of the interaction between a drug and its molecular target – that is, the avidity with which a drug binds – is defined as the **affinity** of a drug for its molecular target. A drug's selectivity and affinity for a target can be determined in a laboratory by spraying the drug over a surface coated with the target of interest and measuring the scattering of light caused as the drug binds to the target and changes the structure of the surface. The selectivity and affinity of a drug depend on its chemical structure, molecular size and electrical charge. Changes in any of these parameters can dramatically increase or decrease the binding of a drug to its molecular target, altering its therapeutic efficacy and/or toxicity.

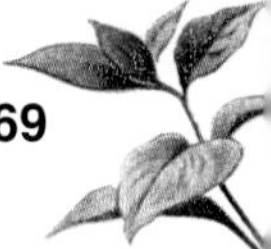

KEY POINTS

Drug specificity, selectivity and affinity

- With the exception of drugs that target cancer and infection by acting on nucleic acids, most drugs act by binding to proteins, which are referred to as molecular targets.
- An ideal drug would interact with only one molecular target, at one site and have only one effect; that is, it would be specific. Most drugs show selectivity; that is, they display a preference for a molecular target.

Molecular drug targets

Most drugs cause their effect by acting on one of four main types of protein targets. These are called regulatory proteins because they mediate the actions of hormones, neurotransmitters and other chemical messengers. The four types of regulatory proteins are:

- transporters
- ion channels
- enzymes
- receptors.

Transporters

The integrity of the cell membrane is essential for maintaining homeostasis. Many small molecules and ions are too polar to passively diffuse across membranes and so must be transported. In some cases, transport across a cell membrane can be passive (e.g. carrier-mediated diffusion), but more commonly it is an active process. In many cases, active transport requires the hydrolysis of adenosine triphosphate (ATP) as an energy source to actively pump a substance across the membrane against an electrochemical gradient. Transporters that facilitate this type of passage across a membrane contain a distinct ATP binding site and are called ABC (ATP-binding cassette) transporters. In other cases, transport of an organic molecule is coupled to transport of an ion such as sodium through a process of secondary active transport. If the movement of both molecules across the membrane is in the same direction, the transporter is called a symporter (e.g. the transport of sodium/potassium/chloride in the Loop of Henle). If the molecules are moved across the membrane in opposite directions, the transporter is called an antiporter (e.g. the exchange of sodium and potassium in the proximal convoluted tubule). Other important transporters that function this way include those involved in the uptake of neurotransmitters such as noradrenaline (norepinephrine), serotonin and glutamate. These specific transporters are often targets for drugs. Venlafaxine and cocaine are examples of drugs that inhibit transporter-mediated uptake of noradrenaline, an important transmitter in the sympathetic nervous system. The role of transporters in the uptake and efflux of drugs and in drug–drug interactions is becoming increasingly recognised as important in the clinical use of drugs.

Ion channels

Ion channels are proteins embedded within the cell membrane that control this flow of ions into and out of the cell, thereby maintaining an electrochemical gradient between the interior and exterior of the cell. Ion channels are present in the membranes of all cells and represent one of the two classes of ion transporting proteins, the other being ion transporters. Ion channels have two distinct features that differentiate them from other transporters:

- The rate of flow through the channel is very high (millions of ions can flow through a channel every second).
- Ions can only pass through an ion channel down their electrochemical gradient from a compartment containing a higher concentration of ions to a compartment containing a lower concentration.

A variety of drugs target ion channels. These include the diuretic amiloride, which blocks entry of sodium into renal tubular cells, and various calcium channel-blocking drugs such as verapamil, nifedipine and diltiazem.

Enzymes

Enzymes are biological catalysts that control biochemical reactions within the cell. Although it is possible for a drug to either activate or inhibit an enzyme, in clinical practice almost every drug that acts on an enzyme works by inhibiting the enzyme. For example, the anticoagulant drug warfarin inhibits the enzyme vitamin K epoxide reductase, preventing activation of vitamin K1 and blocking production of vitamin K1–dependent clotting factors. This drug is used to reduce the risk of future events in patients who have previously experienced a blood clot. Drugs that interact with enzymes are usually able to do so by virtue of their structural resemblance to **substrate** molecules of the enzyme – that is, the substances acted on by an enzyme. A drug may resemble the substrate of an enzyme so closely that the enzyme combines with the drug instead of the substrate. An example is the lipid-lowering drug atorvastatin. This drug closely resembles the endogenous substrate 3-hydroxy-3-methylglutaryl coenzyme A (HMG-CoA), which is normally metabolised to the cholesterol precursor mevalonate by the enzyme HMG-CoA reductase. Atorvastatin is an HMG-CoA

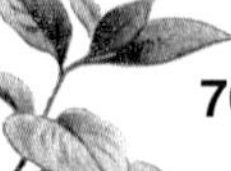

reductase inhibitor. Drugs resembling enzyme substrates are often termed 'antimetabolites' and can either block normal enzymatic action or result in the production of other substances with different biochemical properties. An example of an antimetabolite is the anticancer drug methotrexate. Common drugs that act on enzymes are listed in Table 3.1, which also identifies the chapters in which the individual drugs are discussed.

Receptors

Receptors are signalling proteins that recognise and respond to chemical messengers, including hormones, neurotransmitters and other mediators, to change function within a cell. Receptors are the largest and most diverse type of molecular drug target.

Families of receptors

Receptors respond to a variety of signals and control many different functions within a cell. In some cases, such as synaptic transmission, receptor-mediated effects occur very rapidly – usually over a millisecond time scale. In other cases, such as steroid hormone signalling, the effects occur much more slowly – over hours to days. Differences in time scale of effect are due to the different coupling (signal transduction) mechanisms that link the occupation of the receptor by a ligand (drug or endogenous chemical) to the ensuing response. Receptors are divided into four types (superfamilies) based on differences in their structure and coupling mechanisms:

- *Type 1:* Ligand-gated ion channels are membrane-bound channels that are activated when a ligand binds to a specific site (orthosteric site) on the protein. Examples of type 1 receptors include the nicotinic acetylcholine receptor and type A γ-aminobutyric acid (GABAA) receptor. Type 1 receptors are responsible for functions such as central and peripheral synaptic transmission mediated by excitatory neurotransmitters (e.g. acetylcholine and glutamate) and inhibitory neurotransmitters (e.g. glycine and GABA). The response time of ligand-gated ion channels is very rapid, usually in the order of milliseconds.
- *Type 2:* G-protein-coupled receptors (GPCRs) are discussed in the following section. GPCRs have a slightly slower response than the type 1 receptors, usually in the order of seconds because of the associated signal transduction mechanisms.
- *Type 3:* Kinase receptors are similar in structure to GPCRs but with different signal transduction mechanisms. Response is typically measured in hours because these receptors are linked to processes that alter gene transcription and therefore protein synthesis, which does not occur rapidly. Receptors of this type include tyrosine kinase receptors acted on by epidermal growth factor, atrial natriuretic peptide, vascular endothelial growth factor, nerve growth factor and many more trophic hormones. Drugs that inhibit kinase receptors are increasingly used to treat neoplastic disorders.
- *Type 4:* Nuclear receptors regulate gene transcription and include the peroxisome proliferator activated receptor that binds some hypolipidaemic drugs, the retinoic and retinoid X receptors and the steroid hormone receptors. Although called 'nuclear', they are often located in the cytosol and require binding of various other molecules before translocating to the nucleus where they interact with specific response elements located on genes – for example, steroid hormone receptors. Response time for nuclear receptor activation is similar to the type 3 receptors, usually occurring hours later because of the time taken to alter cell processes such as gene transcription. A notable example, the pregnane X receptor (PXR), does not have an endogenous ligand; instead, PXR detects the presence of foreign toxic substances and upregulates the expression of proteins involved in detoxification.

Type 1, 2 and 3 receptors are all located in the cell membrane and have an orthosteric site (ligand binding site) that faces outwards to respond to extracellular

TABLE 3.1 Common enzyme-inhibiting drugs

ENZYME	DRUGS	EXAMPLE USE(S)
5α-reductase	Finasteride	Hair loss Benign prostatic hyperplasia
Acetylcholinesterase	Neostigmine	Myasthenia gravis
Angiotensin-converting enzyme (ACE)	Captopril Lisinopril	Hypertension Heart failure
Cyclo-oxygenase	Aspirin Celecoxib Ibuprofen	Inflammation Osteoarthritis Rheumatoid arthritis
Dihydrofolate reductase	Methotrexate Trimethoprim	Autoimmune diseases Bacterial infection Cancer Ectopic pregnancy
HMG-CoA reductase	Atorvastatin Simvastatin	Hypercholesterolaemia
Phosphodiesterase • PDE3 • PDE5	Milrinone Sildenafil	Heart failure (milrinone) Erectile dysfunction (sildenafil)
Thymidine kinase	Aciclovir	Herpes simplex virus
Topoisomerase IV	Ciprofloxacin	Bacterial infection
Vitamin K epoxide reductase	Warfarin	Deep vein thrombosis Pulmonary embolism Stroke prevention
Xanthine oxidase	Allopurinol	Gout Kidney stones

messengers. Type 4 receptors affect gene transcription (e.g. the glucocorticoid receptor) and are located in the cytosol, migrating into the cell nucleus when activated.

G-protein-coupled receptors

Comprising at least 800 unique receptors, GPCRs are the largest family of plasma membrane receptors. GPCRs mediate responses to the majority of our hormones and neurotransmitters, as well as our sense of smell, taste and sight. These receptors are often more familiar to health professionals as muscarinic acetylcholine receptors, the receptors for adrenaline and noradrenaline (adrenoceptors), dopamine receptors, adenosine receptors, histamine receptors, dopamine receptors and opioid and opioid-like receptors. GPCRs are important targets exploited in pharmacotherapy.

GPCRs consist of an extracellular (amino) terminus that projects above the membrane, seven membrane-spanning helices (designated I–VII) separated by loops of varying sizes and an intracellular (carboxyl) terminus (Fig 3.1). When a ligand (e.g. a drug such as salbutamol or an endogenous transmitter such as acetylcholine) binds to a cleft within the membrane-spanning regions or a ligand-binding domain located in the extracellular amino terminus of a GPCR, the ligand-receptor complex that is formed then associates with a G-protein. It is important to appreciate that G-proteins comprise three sub-units (α, β and γ), which are essential for normal function. The guanine nucleotides bind to the α sub-unit, while the β and γ sub-units remain together as a complex. When an agonist binds (e.g. morphine to the opiate receptor), the bound guanosine diphosphate (GDP) dissociates from the α sub-unit in exchange for guanosine triphosphate (GTP). This leads to a change from the inactive state of a GDP-bound G-protein to an active GTP-bound G-protein. The α-GTP complex dissociates from both the receptor and the $\beta\gamma$ complex and interacts with the effector protein – for example, an ion channel or

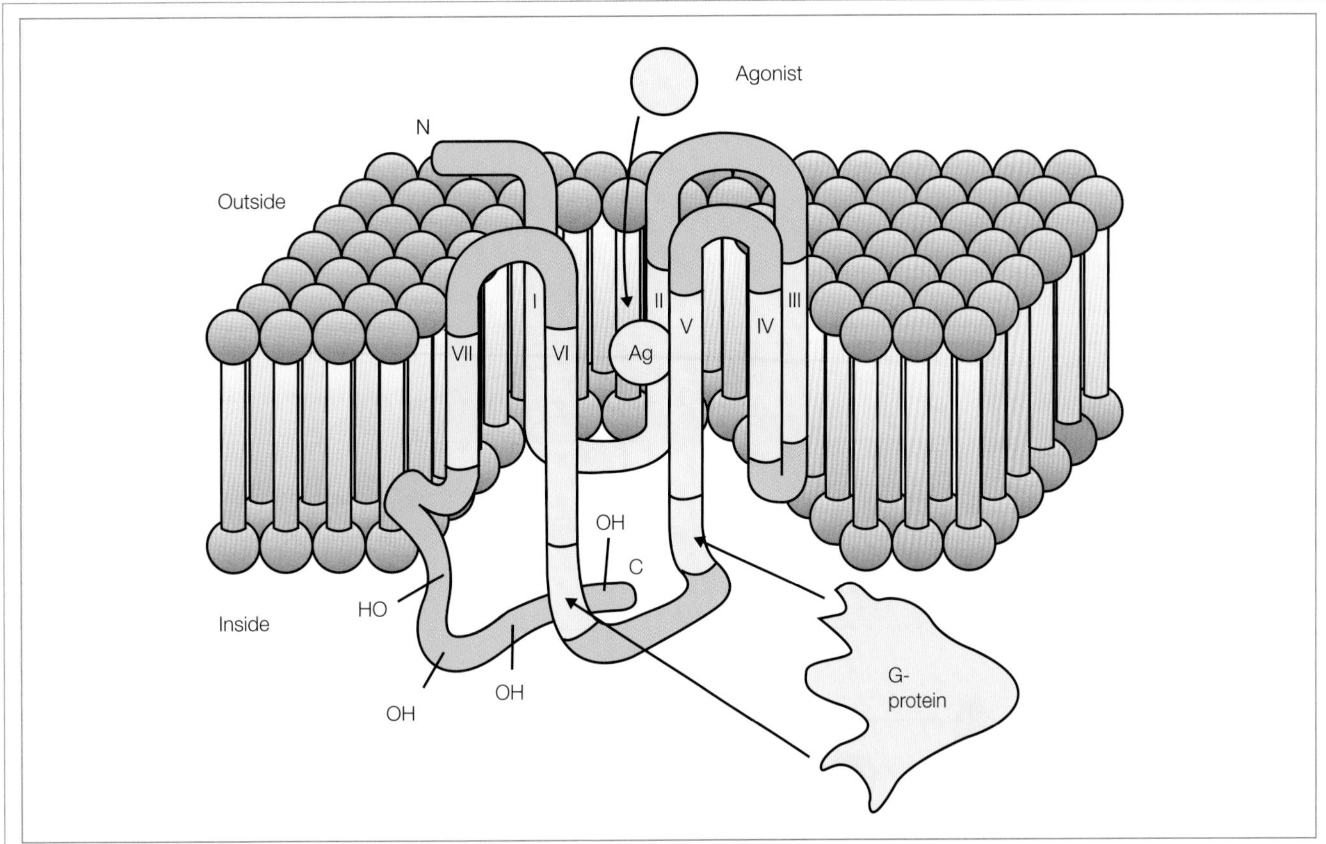

FIGURE 3.1 Transmembrane topology of a typical 'serpentine' GPCR

The amino (N) terminus of the receptor is extracellular (above the plane of the membrane) and the carboxyl (C) terminus is intracellular. The termini are connected by a polypeptide chain that traverses the plane of the membrane seven times. The hydrophobic transmembrane segments (light colour) are designated by Roman numerals I–VII. The agonist (Ag) approaches the receptor from the extracellular fluid and binds to a site surrounded by the transmembrane regions of the receptor protein. G-proteins (G) interact with cytoplasmic regions of the receptor, especially with portions of the third cytoplasmic loop between transmembrane regions V and VI. The cytoplasmic terminal tail of the receptor contains numerous serine and threonine residues whose hydroxyl (–OH) groups can be phosphorylated. This phosphorylation may be associated with diminished receptor-G-protein interaction.

Source: Katzung et al. 2012, Figure 2-11; reproduced with permission of The McGraw-Hill Companies.

adenylyl cyclase. The βγ complex can also interact with a second effector protein. The G-protein remains active until GTP is hydrolysed, by the intrinsic GTPase activity of the G-protein, to GDP, and the G-protein returns to its inactive GDP-bound state (Fig 3.2). Cells may express more than 20 GPCRs and each has a specific function. There are many different types of G-proteins and, through a series of reactions, the activated G-protein changes the activity of a second messenger specific to the type of G-protein. A simplified schema is shown in Figure 3.3.

Second messengers

For a cell to respond to an external stimulus (e.g. binding of a drug or hormone to a receptor), the signal has to be communicated from the exterior of the cell to the respective response elements within the cell. This mechanism of communication often involves a second messenger system, which initiates signalling within the cell through a specific biochemical pathway. The signal and the response are highly coordinated within the cell and this often involves multiple highly integrated pathways.

cAMP and cGMP

One of the most studied second messengers is cyclic adenosine monophosphate (cAMP), which is synthesised by membrane-bound adenylyl cyclase under the control of a number of GPCRs. cAMP mediates effects such as the breakdown of fat, conservation of water by the kidney and the rate and force of contraction of the heart. It exerts most of its effects through a series of protein kinases that control cell function by phosphorylating proteins (adding phosphate groups to the protein) (Fig 3.3). The breakdown of cAMP by phosphodiesterase enzymes terminates its action. Inhibition of phosphodiesterase, which results in an increase in the intracellular concentration of cAMP and hence calcium, is one of the mechanisms by which caffeine and theophylline are thought to produce cardiac effects. The cAMP second messenger system is linked to the action of β-adrenoceptors and many other receptors.

Another important second messenger is cyclic guanosine monophosphate (cGMP), which is involved in controlling the function of smooth muscle and nerve cells and monocytes and platelets. cGMP is formed by two distinct forms of guanylyl cyclase; the soluble form is activated to cGMP by nitric oxide. Nitric oxide is important in cardiovascular health and plays a role in both the autonomic and the central nervous systems. The second form of guanylyl cyclase is membrane-bound and is activated by natriuretic peptides. Similar to cAMP, the effects of cGMP are terminated by the phosphodiesterase enzymes. Sildenafil, a drug used to treat erectile dysfunction, inhibits phosphodiesterase 5 (PDE5), which results in an increased concentration of nitric oxide that enhances the action of it on penile vascular smooth muscle.

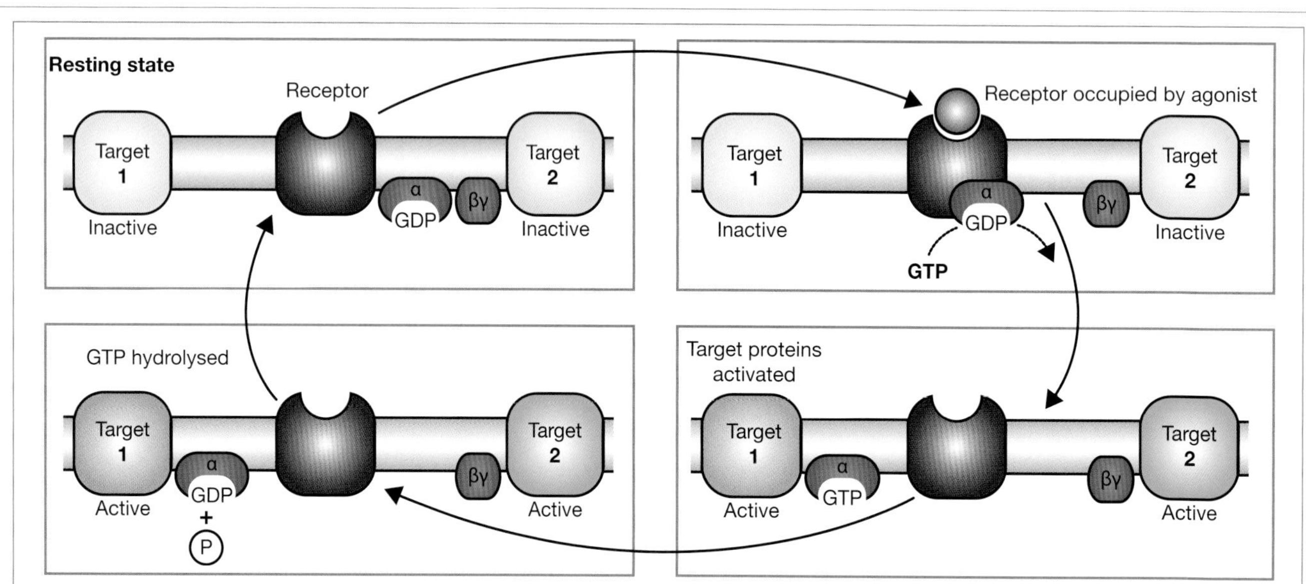

FIGURE 3.2 The function of the G-protein
The G-protein consists of three sub-units (α, β,γ) which are anchored to the membrane through attached lipid residues. Coupling of the α sub-unit to an agonist-occupied receptor causes the bound GDP to exchange with intracellular GTP; the α-GTP complex then dissociates from the receptor and from the βγ complex, and interacts with a target protein (target 1, which may be an enzyme such as adenylyl cyclase, or an ion channel). The βγ complex may also activate a target protein (target 2). The GTPase activity of the α sub-unit is increased when the target protein is bound, leading to hydrolysis of the bound GTP to GDP, whereupon the α sub-unit reunites with βγ.
Source: Rang HP, Dale MM, Ritter JM, et al: Pharmacology, Edinburgh, 2012, Elsevier.

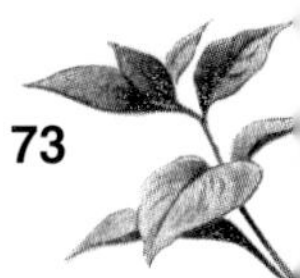

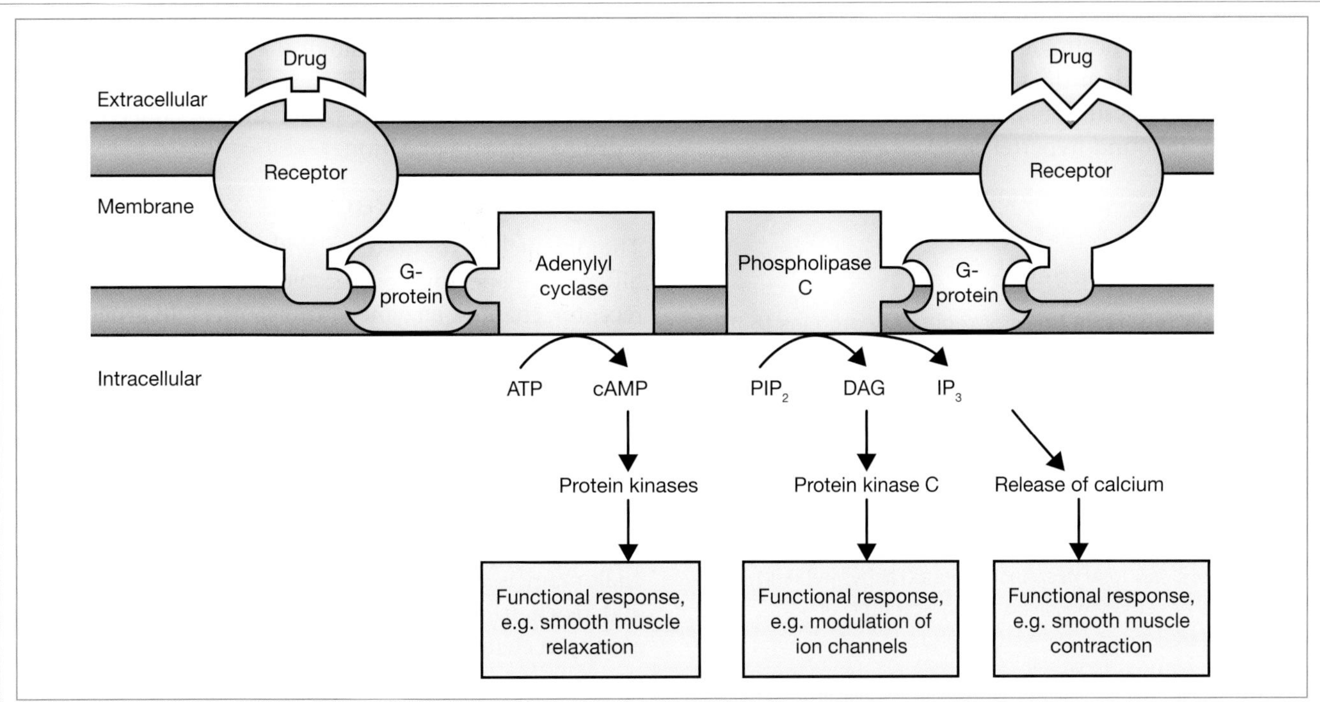

FIGURE 3.3 Schematic representation of activation of G-protein-coupled receptors by drugs
The second messenger systems involved include: (1) cAMP, which activates various protein kinases linked to cellular functions (e.g. smooth muscle relaxation); and (2) activation of phospholipase C, which cleaves phosphatidylinositol-4,5-bisphosphate (PIP_2) to form diacylglycerol (DAG), which activates protein kinase C, and inositol triphosphate (IP_3), which releases intracellular calcium. ATP = adenosine triphosphate.

Phosphoinositides and calcium

Another well-studied second messenger system involves hydrolysis of a minor component of cell membranes, splitting it into two second messengers, diacylglycerol and inositol triphosphate (Fig 3.3). The diacylglycerol is confined to the cell membrane where it activates protein kinase C, which causes changes in the activity of other enzymes that ultimately produce the functional response (e.g. increased glandular secretions). The inositol triphosphate diffuses through the cytoplasm and causes the release of calcium from storage sites. The increased intracellular calcium then regulates the activity of other enzymes, producing a response such as increased contractility. These particular second messengers are important for producing the effects mediated by α-adrenoceptors and muscarinic receptors.

Desensitisation and receptor turnover

Receptor populations are not static and receptors may undergo several changes, including loss of responsiveness at the individual receptor level or a change in the number of receptors. The term used clinically to describe diminished responsiveness after repeated exposure to the same concentration of the drug that stimulates the receptor is 'tachyphylaxis'. It is rapid in onset and the person's initial response to the drug cannot be reproduced, even with larger doses of the drug. Transdermal glyceryl trinitrate used to treat angina is an example of a drug that requires intermittent dosing (12 hours on, 12 hours off) to limit the problem of tachyphylaxis (Ch 21).

Desensitisation (also referred to as adaptation or refractoriness) refers more specifically to a decrease in the response of the receptor–second messenger system and is a common feature of many receptors. The mechanisms underlying receptor desensitisation are complex and include: (i) an uncoupling of the receptor from its second messenger system, (ii) altered binding of the drug to the receptor or (iii) a decrease in the total number of receptors. Phosphorylation and dephosphorylation of proteins (adding or removing phosphate groups, respectively) is an important mechanism for controlling protein function. With the GPCRs, uncoupling occurs when phosphorylation of the agonist-bound GPCR complex facilitates recruitment of arrestin which, in turn, uncouples the G-protein from the receptor. This can be thought of as 'arresting' or halting the function of the receptor. Further details on desensitisation will be provided in later chapters where relevant to specific drugs – for example, glyceryl trinitrate.

The total number of receptors in the cell membrane at any one time can also change. A decrease in receptor number is called downregulation and can contribute to desensitisation and loss of response. An increase in receptor number is referred to as upregulation and can cause receptor hypersensitivity. For example, upregulation of receptors often occurs after chronic use of drugs that block receptors; when the drug is abruptly removed, the person may experience increased responsiveness to stimuli (e.g. rebound hypertension).

KEY POINTS

Molecular drug targets

- There are four main types of regulatory proteins that drugs act on: transporters, enzymes, ion channels and receptors.
- A large group of proteins that are targets for drugs are receptors, which are cellular macromolecules directly concerned with chemical signalling that initiates a change in cell function.
- Receptors can lose responsiveness (tachyphylaxis), become desensitised or be downregulated or upregulated.

Pharmacodynamics

Pharmacodynamics is the study of the interaction between a drug and its molecular target and of the pharmacological response: what the drug does to the body (Fig 3.4). The magnitude of a pharmacological effect of a drug depends on the nature of the interaction with the target, the affinity of the drug for the target and the concentration of a drug at the site of action.

Drug target interactions

The interaction of a drug with its target is classified differently depending on the type of molecular target (i.e. receptor, channel, enzyme or transporter). In general terms, the binding of a drug with its target will either make something happen ('switch the target on') or stop something from happening ('switch the target off'). Clinically used drugs that act on enzymes, transporters and channels elicit their effect by switching the target off; these drugs are called 'inhibitors' when they act on an enzyme (e.g. atorvastatin is an HMG-CoA reductase inhibitor) or transporter (e.g. citalopram is a serotonin reuptake transporter inhibitor), and 'blockers' when they act on a channel (e.g. verapamil is a calcium channel blocker). Drugs that act on receptors can either 'switch on' or 'switch off' the target and are classified according to what they do, and how they do it.

Receptor agonists

Binding of a drug to a receptor causes a functional response, which is governed initially by the affinity of the

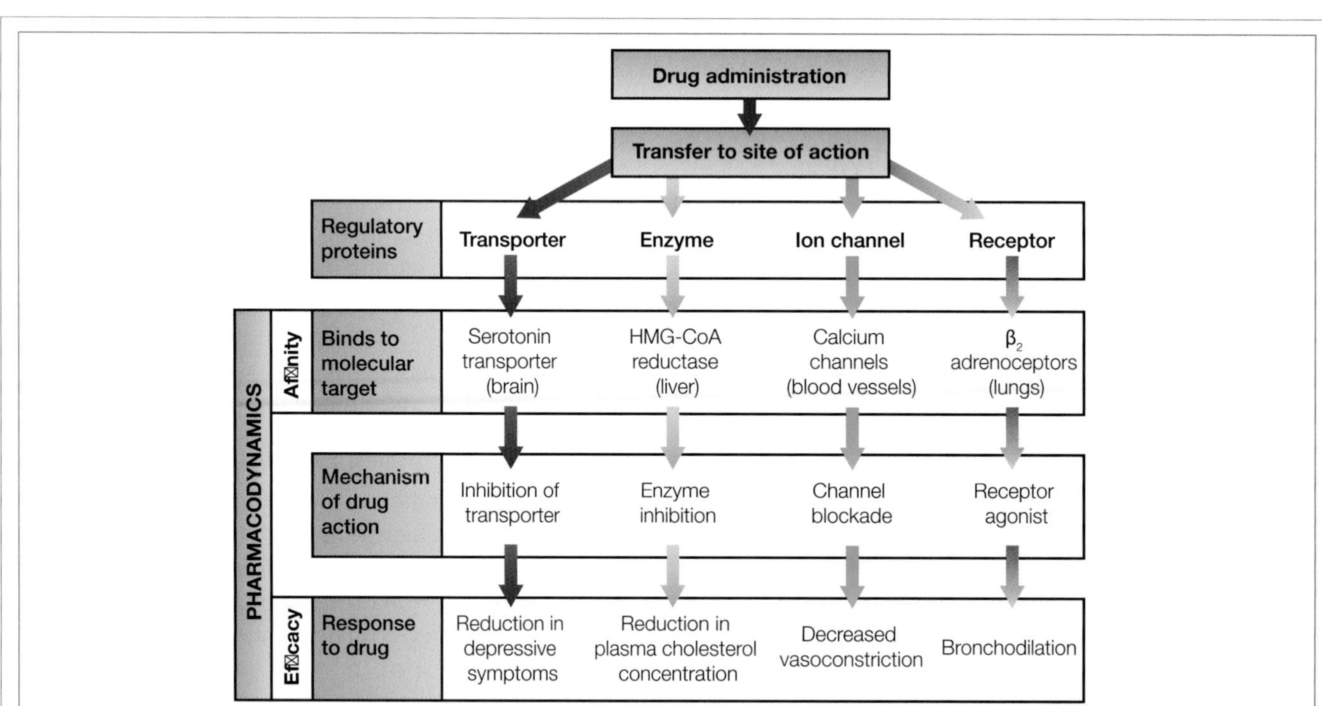

FIGURE 3.4 Principles of pharmacodynamics

The figure shows the four main types of regulatory proteins and illustrates the concept of pharmacodynamics by using an example of each type of protein. Note the interrelationships between the affinity of a drug and drug efficacy (response). This illustration does not take into account the effects of absorption, distribution, metabolism and excretion, which all affect the concentration of drug reaching the molecular target.

drug for the receptor as determined by the chemical forces that cause the drug to bind. Once bound, the ability to activate the receptor (i.e. to produce an effect or response) is determined by the **efficacy** of the drug. Defining the response caused by a drug binding to a receptor can be complex. For example, an **agonist** may be a full agonist or a partial agonist, depending on the capacity to cause a response; and it may be a direct agonist or an allosteric agonist, depending on which part of the receptor it binds to. At the least complex level, drugs that bind to a receptor are simply termed agonists or **antagonists**. A drug that functions as an agonist binds to the orthosteric site and activates the receptor producing the same response as the endogenous (natural) ligand (Fig 3.5). Examples of endogenous ligands include hormones (e.g. estrogen), neurotransmitters (e.g. dopamine) and catecholamines (e.g. adrenaline).

Partial agonists

Partial agonists bind to and activate a receptor but cannot elicit the same maximal response as the endogenous ligand for that receptor, even when all receptors are

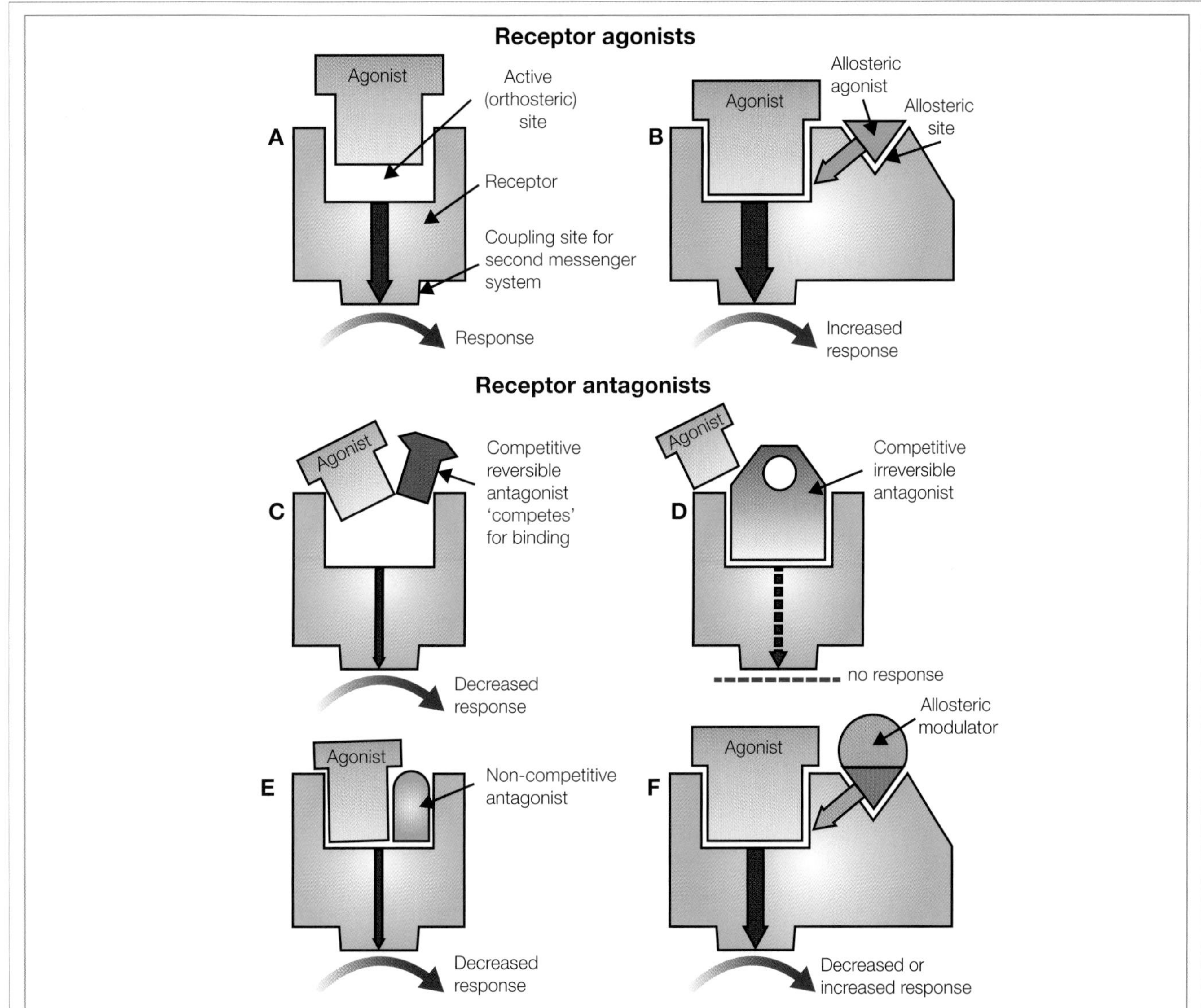

FIGURE 3.5 Illustration of drug–receptor interactions
A An agonist drug binds to the active site of the receptor and produces a response; **B** An allosteric agonist binds at a site distinct to the active site and in this case increases the response elicited by the agonist; **C** A competitive inhibitor 'competes' with the agonist for binding, ultimately causing a decreased response; **D** A competitive irreversible antagonist binds to the receptor, irreversibly preventing agonist binding – hence, no response; **E** A non-competitive antagonist binds independently, blocking the response to the agonist at some point within the receptor-coupling cascade and causes a decreased response; **F** An allosteric modulator binds to the allosteric site producing a change in the protein, either causing reduced affinity of the primary agonist (antagonism) and hence reducing the response or potentiating (facilitating) the effect of the primary agonist and hence increasing the response.

occupied. An example of this type of drug is the non-selective β-adrenoceptor antagonist pindolol, which is an antagonist but also possesses slight intrinsic agonist (sympathomimetic) activity that lessens the negative cardiovascular effects of β-blockade.

Antagonists

Receptor antagonists bind to the orthosteric site of the receptor (they retain affinity for the receptor) without eliciting a response (they have no efficacy). In doing so, the antagonist prevents the binding of an agonist to the receptor and so prevents activation of the receptor (Fig 3.5). An example of a receptor antagonist is naloxone; this drug is a μ-opioid receptor antagonist that is used to reverse the harmful effects caused by the administration of excess opioid agonist (e.g. morphine, heroin). Antagonists are classified based on how and where they bind to the receptor. The two defining characteristics that are of greatest clinical importance are reversibility and competitiveness.

Reversible competitive antagonists

Reversible competitive antagonists interfere with the binding of the endogenous agonist to the orthosteric site: that is, they 'compete' for binding to the receptor. Their action can be overcome by increasing the concentration of the agonist. In essence, the agonist, when there is a higher concentration of molecules, out-competes the antagonist and the responsiveness of the tissue returns with agonist occupancy of the vacant receptors. For example, higher concentrations of adrenaline are used to overcome the competitive blockade of β-adrenoceptors by propranolol. Competitive antagonists reduce the potency of the receptor agonist, but they do not alter the efficacy of the agonist; that is, they shift the agonist concentration response curve to the right but do not alter the slope or maxima.

Irreversible competitive antagonists

Irreversible competitive antagonists have limited therapeutic usefulness because they make the target receptor permanently unavailable for binding of the endogenous agonist. This is explained by the competitive antagonist having a high affinity for the receptor and dissociating from the receptor so slowly it is in essence an 'irreversible' antagonist. Used experimentally to investigate receptor function, their action is usually prolonged and it is not terminated until the receptors 'die' and are replaced by new receptors. Examples of chemicals in this class include some inhibitors of acetylcholinesterase and chemicals such as nerve gases (Ch 9). Therapeutically used drugs of this class include aspirin, which irreversibly inhibits a platelet enzyme, and omeprazole, which irreversibly inhibits the gastric proton pump (Ch 23). As these drugs permanently occupy the receptor and effectively remove them from the system, they reduce both the potency and the efficacy of the receptor agonist; that is, they cause the agonist concentration response curve to shift to the right and reduce the slope and maxima.

Non-competitive antagonists

Non-competitive antagonists block the response to an agonist at some point within the cascade of intracellular events. Both the antagonist and the agonist bind independently of each other, and the antagonist drug may dissociate so slowly from the receptor that its action is very prolonged. In general, non-competitive antagonists reduce both the maximal response and the slope of the agonist concentration–response curve. An example of a drug in this category is buprenorphine, which is a partial agonist at μ-opioid receptor but that acts as a non-competitive antagonist in the presence of an opioid receptor agonist because it occupies and dissociates slowly from the receptor.

Allosteric effects

Allosteric modulators indirectly alter the function of a receptor in either a positive (allosteric agonist) or a negative (allosteric antagonist) way. These drugs bind to a distinct (allosteric) site on the receptor that is separate from the orthosteric site (Fig 3.5). Allosteric modulators can alter the function of receptors and produce a pharmacological response by:

- activating the receptor, causing a different biological response to the agonist
- altering the binding affinity of the receptor agonist
- changing the efficacy of receptor activation by the agonist.

The most prominent example of allosteric modulators is a class of drugs called benzodiazepines (Ch 20). Binding of benzodiazepines to an allosteric site on the GABAA receptor increases the affinity of the receptor for the endogenous inhibitory neurotransmitter GABA, thus inhibiting neurotransmission and leading to a range of sedative effects.

Concentration–response relationship

When making decisions about the use of a drug, it is important to know how big an effect the drug will have and how much drug is required to have an effect. These considerations are addressed by the concentration–response relationship, which is commonly depicted as a drug concentration–response curve.

How does knowledge of the concentration–response relationship for a drug serve a useful purpose? When an agonist drug is administered, the response usually increases in proportion to the dose until the receptors are saturated. Increasing the dose further at this stage does not produce any further increase in response. The sigmoidal shape of the concentration–response curve on a logarithmic plot includes a linear portion that occurs between 20% and 80% of the maximal response. This section 'most often applies to drugs at therapeutic concentrations and increasing drug concentration above 80% maximal response achieves very little in terms of extra therapeutic effects, but increases the risk of adverse effects' (Birkett 1995) (Fig 3.6). This relationship is described by the equation:

$$E = \frac{E_{max} \times C}{C + EC_{50}}$$

where E is the effect observed at a given drug concentration of C, E_{max} is the maximal response that the drug can produce and EC_{50} is the concentration at which the drug produces 50% of its maximal response.

Potency

Drugs are often referred to as being 'potent' or 'very potent', but what does this mean and how is it calculated? If we think about the concentration–response relationship, **potency** is the measure of how much drug is required to have an effect. For example, fentanyl and oxycodone are two opioid analgesics that relieve pain by activating μ-opioid receptors. As a highly potent drug, fentanyl is able to elicit a response at a very low concentration; oxycodone, which is a less potent drug, is able to elicit the same response but requires a much higher concentration to do so. The functional consequence is that the more potent a drug, the lower the dose that is required (i.e. a lower dose of fentanyl compared with oxycodone to achieve the same analgesic effect). Potency is measured as the EC_{50}, which can reflect either the concentration that causes half the maximal effect (graded relationship) or the concentration that causes an effect in half the population (quantal relationship). Plotting the concentration–response data for several drugs using a semi-logarithmic scale allows us easily to visualise the relative potencies of the drugs (Fig 3.7).

Efficacy

Another term that is also commonly used to describe drugs is their maximal efficacy. Often simply called efficacy, this is a measure of 'how big an effect the drug will have' when all targets are occupied. Again, the concentration–response curves allow us to visualise the efficacy of a drug – that is, the maximum response a drug can produce (E_{max}). Several drugs may have the same potency but differ in their efficacy (Fig 3.8). Conversely, as shown in Figure 3.7, drugs may differ in potency but have the same efficacy. This is important clinically, because the maximal effectiveness of a drug depends on its efficacy and not on its potency. To illustrate this point, let us assume that the three drugs in Figure 3.8 are used as bronchodilators to treat asthma. The question could be asked: Does it matter which drug is used if each is equipotent as a bronchodilator? Knowing the concentration–response curves for the various drugs

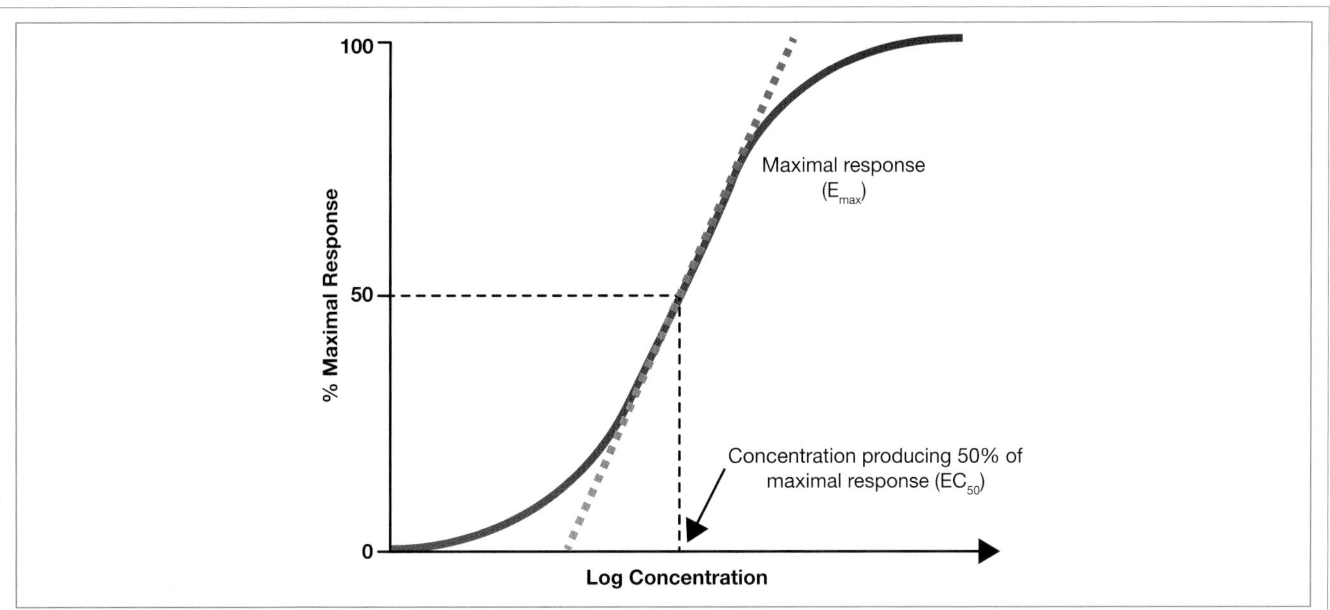

FIGURE 3.6 A drug concentration–response curve plotted on a logarithmic scale

The EC_{50} is the drug concentration at which 50% of the maximal response is observed. E_{max} is the maximal response when all the receptors are occupied.

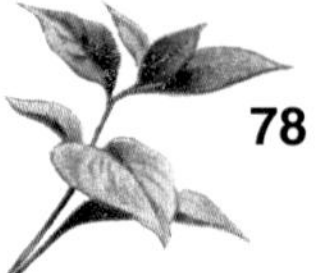

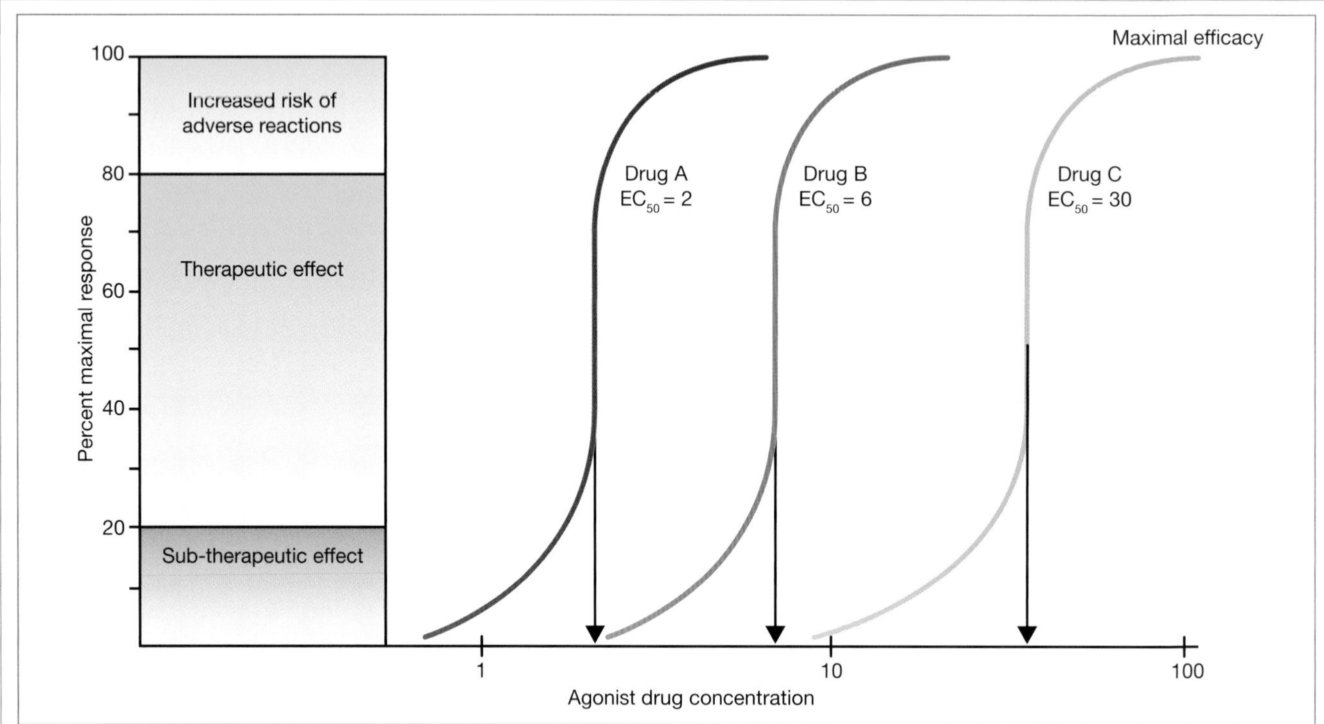

FIGURE 3.7 Theoretical concentration–response curves on a logarithmic scale for drugs A, B and C
The drugs are all agonists acting on the same receptor and eliciting the same response. Drug A (EC_{50} = 2) is three times more potent than drug B (EC_{50} = 6), which is five times more potent than drug C (EC_{50} = 30). Drugs A, B and C all differ in their potency but have the same maximal efficacy.

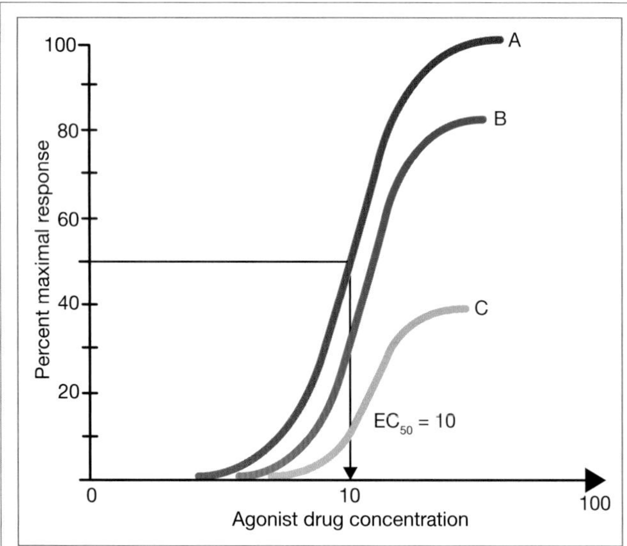

FIGURE 3.8 Concentration–response curves for three drugs A, B and C, all with the same potency (EC_{50} = 10) but different maximal efficacies
In this example, drugs B and C are classed as partial agonists as they produce less than the maximal effect achieved with the full agonist drug A.

would provide the answer. Drugs A and B would provide a greater clinical response (bronchodilation) than drug C because they have greater efficacy.

Let us now consider the effect on the concentration–response curve of an agonist in the presence of a competitive antagonist. The curve is shifted to the right. How far it is shifted to the right depends on the concentration of the competitive antagonist in displacing the agonist and the affinity of the antagonist for the receptor. This indicates that a much higher concentration of agonist is needed to produce 50% of the maximal response (EC_{50}), but in this situation maximal efficacy of the agonist is unchanged (Fig 3.9).

For health professionals, understanding drug efficacy is clinically very important. For example, consider two drugs that have the same affinity for β_2 adrenoceptors, which mediate bronchodilation in the lung. Drug A is an agonist and drug B is an antagonist. If you administer drug A to an asthmatic, it will produce bronchodilation; if you administer drug B, it will result in bronchoconstriction. This is a prime example of how two drugs can have the same affinity but differ widely in clinical efficacy – you might say the difference can be between life and death.

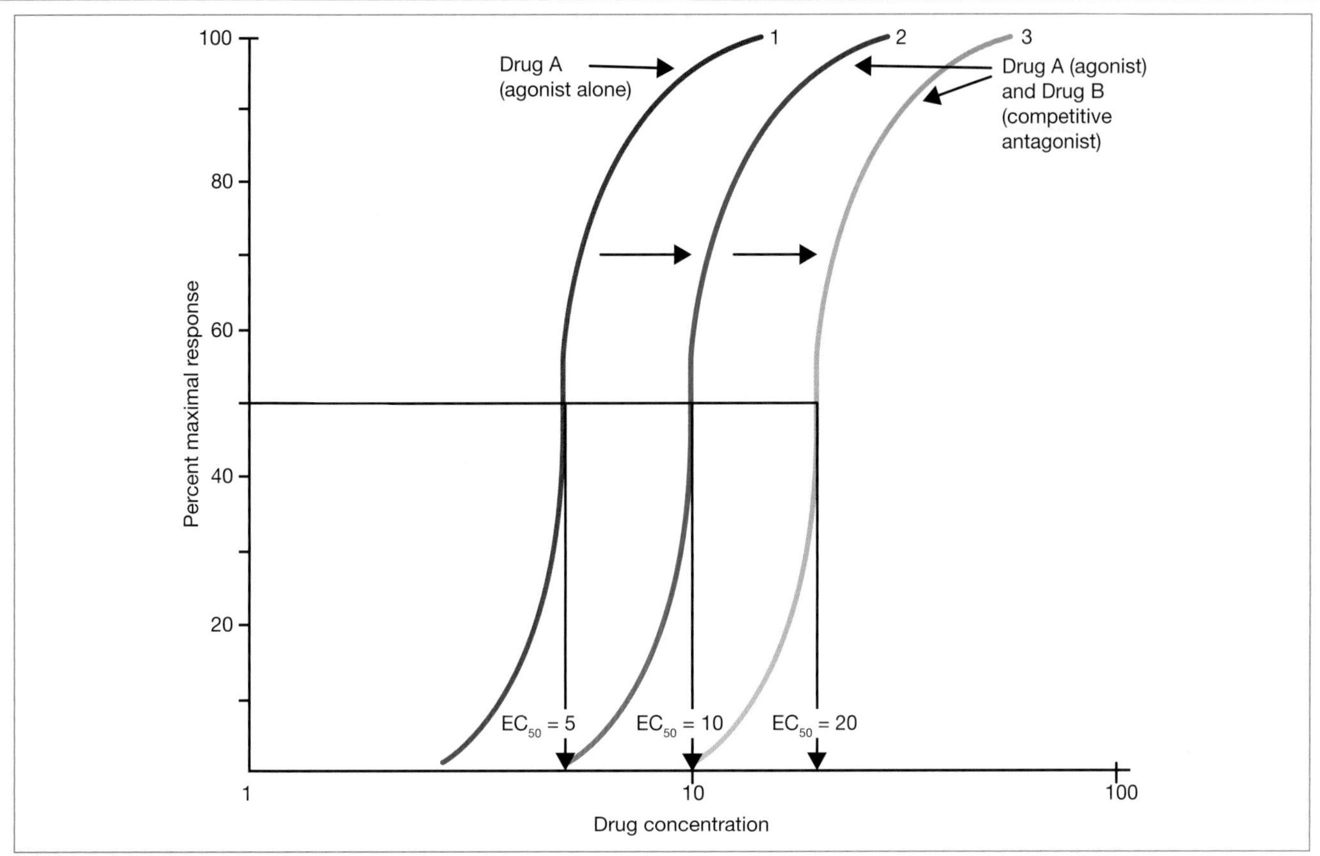

FIGURE 3.9 Competitive antagonism of the response produced by drug A (curve **1**) by increasing concentrations (curves **2** and **3**) of the competitive antagonist drug B

Note the shift of the concentration–response curve to the right without a change in the maximal efficacy of drug A.

KEY POINTS

Pharmacodynamics

- An agonist binds to the orthosteric site of the receptor (governed by affinity) and activates the receptor (governed by efficacy) to produce the same response as the endogenous ligand.
- Partial agonists produce less than the maximal effect caused by the endogenous ligand, even when all receptors are occupied.
- An antagonist binds to a receptor and blocks access of the endogenous ligand, diminishing the normal response.
- When a drug is administered, the response usually increases in proportion to the dose until the receptors are saturated. Increasing the dose further does not produce any further increase in response.
- Potency is measured as the EC_{50}, which is the concentration at which a drug produces 50% of its maximal response.
- 'Efficacy' refers to the ability of a drug to elicit a response once it is bound to the molecular target. The maximal efficacy of a drug is the maximum response a drug can produce.
- The clinical effectiveness of a drug depends on its efficacy, not on its potency.

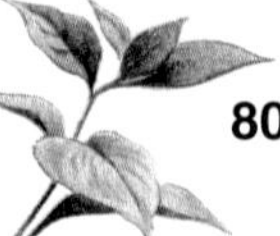

REVIEW EXERCISES

1. Mr TP presents to his GP having experienced shortness of breath while playing basketball. He is diagnosed with exercise-induced asthma and prescribed salbutamol, a short acting beta-adrenoceptor agonist, to manage his symptoms. Exacerbations of asthma may also be treated with ipratropium, an acetylcholine receptor antagonist. Considering the pathways that these two drugs work on, explain how a receptor agonist or a receptor antagonist could both be used to treat the same disease state.
2. Ms SM is being treated in hospital for an exacerbation of congestive heart failure (CHF). At home Ms SM manages her CHF with a diuretic called hydrochlorothiazide, but in hospital she is treated with a different diuretic called frusemide, which has 1/10th the potency, but double the efficacy of hydrochlorothiazide. Using this comparison of drugs from the same broad therapeutic class to support your answer, discuss the clinical value of knowledge of the concentration–response relationship of different drugs.
3. Mr TS presents to the emergency department of a local hospital with a broken ankle and you need to manage his pain. There are many drug options that are available to you for managing pain. As a health professional, discuss the practical importance of maximal drug efficacy.

REFERENCES

Birkett D. Pharmacokinetics made easy 10 Pharmacodynamics - the concentration-effect relationship. Aust Prescr 1995;18:102–4.

Katzung BG, Masters SB, Trevor AJ: Basic and Clinical Pharmacology, 2012, Figure 2-11; reproduced with permission of The McGraw-Hill Companies.

Rang HP, Dale MM, Ritter JM, et al: Pharmacology, Edinburgh, 2012, Elsevier.

CHAPTER 4

DRUG ABSORPTION, DISTRIBUTION, METABOLISM AND EXCRETION

Andrew Rowland

KEY ABBREVIATIONS

ABC	ATP binding cassette
ATP	adenosine triphosphate
CYP	cytochrome P450
GIT	gastrointestinal tract
MRP	multidrug resistance protein
SLC	solute carrier
UGT	UDP-glucuronosyltransferase

KEY TERMS

Chapter Focus

The duration and extent of exposure by an individual to a drug is a key determinant of its therapeutic efficacy and tolerability; inadequate exposure results in a lack of efficacy ('therapeutic failure'), while excessive exposure increases the risk of toxicity and reduces tolerability. Drug exposure is determined by the processes of absorption, distribution, metabolism and excretion. Understanding these processes provides a theoretical framework for inter-individual variability in exposure and the design of drug dosing regimens.

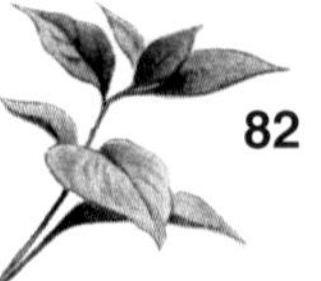

CRITICAL THINKING SCENARIO

Michelle is a 43-year-old female who has been in hospital following surgery to repair a torn ACL. While in hospital she was receiving 10 mg of intravenous morphine twice daily. As part of her hospital discharge, she is given a prescription for oral morphine. The prescription is for 10 × 30 mg morphine tablets and the instructions say to take one tablet every 12 hours for the next 5 days.

1. Is this a medication error?
2. If not, what is the reason for Michelle now being given an oral dose of morphine that is three times greater than the intravenous dose she was taking while in hospital?

Introduction

For a drug to produce an effect, it must interact with a molecular target. The concentration of drug that interacts with the target is influenced by how the drug passes through the body via the processes of **absorption**, **distribution**, **metabolism** and **excretion**. The relationship between these processes is shown in Figure 4.1. The study of the passage of a drug through the body via these processes is collectively described by the term **pharmacokinetics**, or simply 'what the body does to the drug'.

Drug absorption

Absorption is an important factor for all routes of drug administration with the exception of the intravenous route, where the drug is administered directly into the systemic circulation and does not require absorption from the site of administration.

Before a drug can be distributed to its site of action, it must be absorbed from the point of application into the systemic circulation. An oral drug may be in a solid form (tablet, capsule or powder) or in liquid form (solution or suspension). Disintegration of solid dosage forms must occur before dissolution, a process by which a drug goes into solution and becomes available for absorption (Fig 4.2). The drug formulation is important because the faster the rate of dissolution, the more rapidly the drug can be absorbed. For orally administered drugs, absorption is fastest for liquids, elixirs and syrups > suspensions > powders > capsules > tablets > coated tablets > enteric-coated tablets and sustained (or controlled or 'slow' release) formulations.

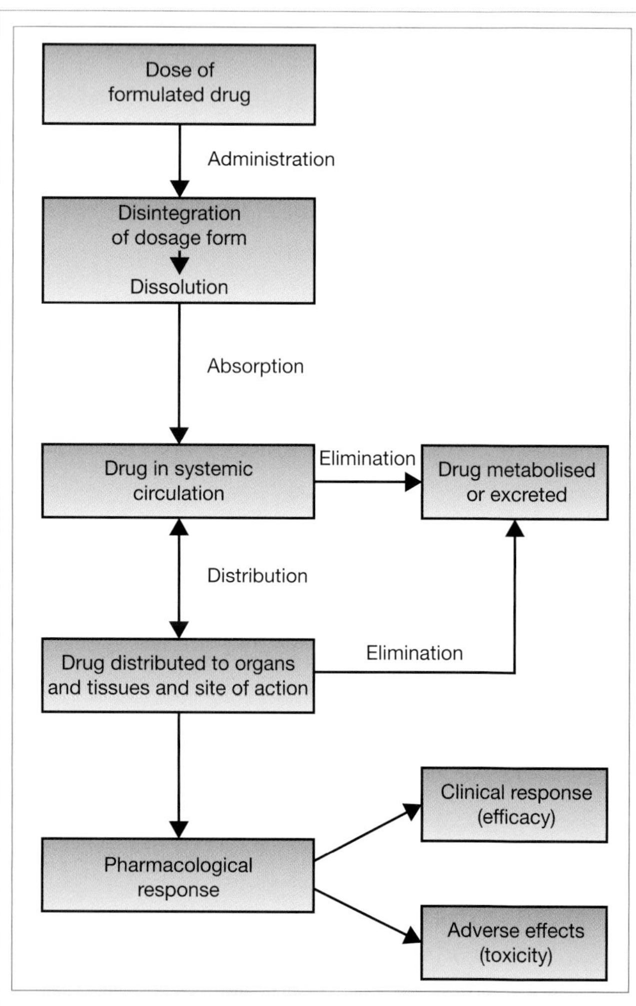

FIGURE 4.1 Interrelationship between drug absorption, distribution, metabolism and elimination
Note: For some drugs the site of action is the vascular system.

Absorption across biological membranes

For absorption to occur, it is necessary for a drug to cross a membrane and enter the blood vessels on the other

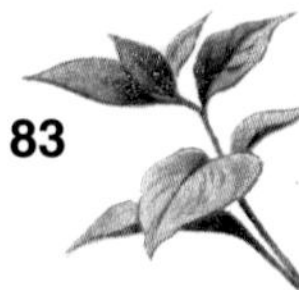

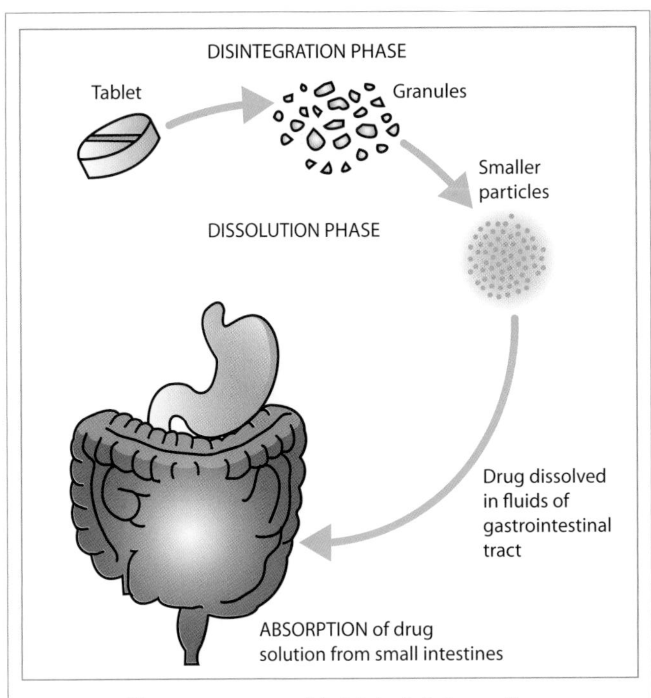

FIGURE 4.2 The processes of tablet disintegration, dissolution and drug absorption

Source: Salerno 1999, Figure 4-2; used with permission.

side. The membrane typically consists of a lipid bilayer that contains protein molecules irregularly dispersed throughout it. These proteins, which provide the membrane with structural order, may themselves act as carriers (transporters), enzymes, receptors, ion channels or antigenic sites. Lipid-soluble drugs readily pass through the lipid membrane, while ionised (charged) drugs have difficulty crossing cell membranes. The membrane also contains narrow-diameter aqueous channels called aquaporins, which permit the passage of small uncharged water-soluble substances such as urea as well as water itself, but not the passage of drugs given their larger size (Fig 4.3).

When free to move to their sites of action, drug molecules are transferred from one body compartment to another by way of the blood; however, free movement can be limited because membranes also enclose these various sites. Whether the barrier to drug transfer consists of a single layer of cells, such as the intestinal epithelium, or several layers of cells, such as skin, in order for a drug to gain access to the interior of a cell or a body compartment it has to penetrate cell membranes. All of the physiological processes mediating absorption, distribution, metabolism and excretion are predicated on two main processes: passive diffusion and **carrier-mediated transport**.

Passive diffusion

Most drugs cross membranes by a process of passive diffusion, which is the transfer of the drug across the membrane from a region of higher concentration to a region of lower concentration until equilibrium is established on either side of the membrane (Fig 4.3). Passive diffusion is influenced by the surface area of the membrane exposed to the drug, the concentration gradient of the drug and its lipid–water partition coefficient. For acidic and basic drugs, diffusion is also influenced by the ionisation state.

Carrier-mediated transport

In contrast to passive diffusion, carrier-mediated transport requires the involvement of a membrane protein for the

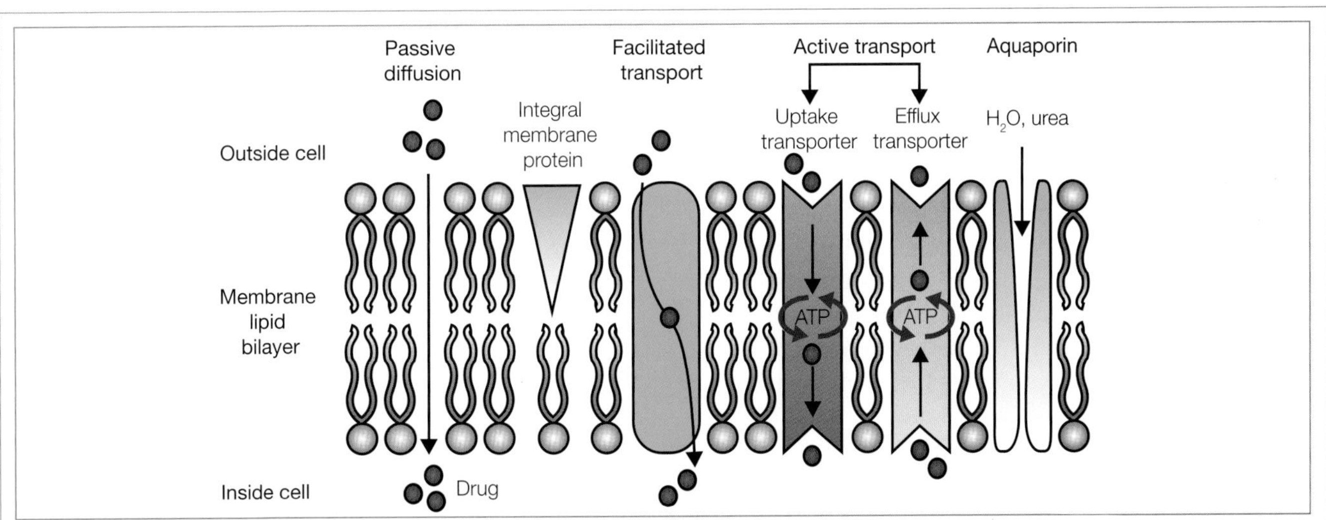

FIGURE 4.3 Movement of drugs across biological membranes by passive diffusion, facilitated transport and active transport

Aquaporins allow passage of water and urea, but not drugs.

movement of a compound across a biological membrane. Carrier-mediated transport may be active (requiring energy) or facilitated (not requiring energy – Fig 4.3). Active transport processes permit the movement of a compound against a concentration gradient (from an area of low concentration to an area of high concentration) or, in the case of ions, against the electrochemical gradient (e.g. the sodium–potassium 'pump'). In addition to its role in the transport of amino acids, glucose, some vitamins, neurotransmitters and ions, carrier-mediated transport also contributes to drug absorption, distribution and elimination. Membrane transporters are classified in two 'superfamilies': the ATP binding cassette (ABC) and solute carrier (SLC) transporters. The ABC transporters require the hydrolysis of ATP to provide the energy to 'pump' substrates across membranes. Within the ABC family there are seven subclasses of transporters, within the SLC superfamily there are 43 families and currently there are in excess of 300 known transporters. The role of transporters in drug disposition is complex, and this is an ongoing area of research. It is now clear, however, that both the ABC and the SLC family transporters play important roles in drug disposition. Carrier-mediated transport of drugs is particularly important in the kidney, gastrointestinal tract (GIT), liver and the blood–brain barrier.

The best characterised member of the ABC family is the efflux transporter P-glycoprotein (P-gp; also known as MDR1, which stands for 'multi-drug resistance'), which was first discovered in tumour cells. It is associated with the multidrug resistance phenomenon observed in patients treated with cancer chemotherapeutic drugs for extended periods. Drug resistance can result from the over-expression of P-gp, which leads to an increased efflux of the cytotoxic drug from the cancer cell, thus lowering the intracellular concentration of drugs such as paclitaxel, vincristine and doxorubicin. P-gp is found in the intestine, kidney, liver, blood–brain barrier, placenta and testes. Another transporter called breast cancer resistance protein (BCRP or ABCG2) that transports several anticancer drugs has also been implicated in resistance. Other efflux transporters include the multidrug resistance proteins (MRPs) and the multidrug and toxin extrusion proteins (MATEs). BCRP, MRPs and MATEs are variably expressed in a number of tissues, including the intestine, liver and kidneys, and they tend to differ in terms of the classes of compounds they transport.

The major uptake transporters are the organic anion transporting polypeptides (OATPs), organic anion transporters (OATs) and organic cation transporters (OCTs), which are all members of the SLC family of transporters. OATP1B1, OATP1B3 and OATP2B1 are expressed in the liver where they play a major role in the hepatic uptake of a diverse range of compounds that include bile acids, sulfate and glucuronide conjugates, and drugs such as fexofenadine, rifampicin, telmisartan and 'statin' HMG-CoA reductase inhibitors (atorvastatin, pravastatin and rosuvastatin). OATs and OCTs transport organic anions (negatively charged drugs such as furosemide [frusemide]) and cations (positively charged drugs such as metformin and ranitidine), respectively. These transporters variably contribute to the uptake of drugs in the kidney and liver.

Variables that affect drug absorption

The rate and extent to which a drug is absorbed are influenced by the following variables.

Nature of the cell membrane that the drug must traverse

The surface area of the absorbing site is an important determinant of drug absorption. Larger absorbing surfaces ease greater drug absorption and the more rapid effects. Gaseous anaesthetics are absorbed immediately from the pulmonary epithelium because of the large surface area of the lung. The small intestine, which also offers a large surface area, is another site from which drugs are efficiently absorbed.

Blood flow

Blood circulation to the site of administration is a significant determinant of the rate and extent of drug absorption. A rich blood supply (e.g. the sublingual route) enhances absorption, whereas a poor vascular site (e.g. the subcutaneous route) delays it. This is because removal of the drug in blood following absorption maintains the concentration gradient necessary for passive diffusion. An individual in shock, for example, may not respond to intramuscularly administered drugs because of poor peripheral circulation. Drugs injected intravenously, on the other hand, are placed directly into the systemic circulation and are immediately available to exert an effect. Food increases splanchnic blood flow and can enhance absorption of orally administered drugs.

Solubility

To be absorbed, a drug must be in solution; the more soluble the drug, the more rapidly it will be presented for absorption. Because cell membranes are composed of a lipid bilayer, lipid solubility is an essential attribute of drugs absorbed from certain areas (e.g. the GIT). Chemicals and minerals that form insoluble precipitates in the GIT, such as barium salts, drugs that are resins (e.g. the bile acid-binding resin cholestyramine) and drugs that are not soluble in water or lipids are not absorbed.

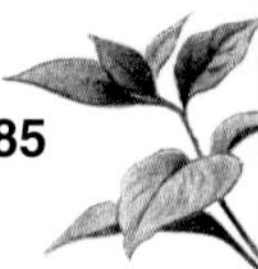

Ionisation

Many drugs are weak acids or weak bases that are present in body fluids as either ionised or un-ionised forms. The ionised (charged polar) form is usually water-soluble (lipid-insoluble) and does not diffuse readily through the cell membranes of the body. In contrast, the un-ionised (neutral, non-polar) form of a drug is more lipid-soluble (less water-soluble) and is more capable of crossing cell membranes. In general, an acidic drug is relatively un-ionised in an acid environment such as the stomach, but a basic drug tends to ionise in the same acid environment. In contrast, a basic drug is less ionised in a less acidic site such as the small intestine, while the acidic drug tends to be more ionised. Despite the varying states of ionisation, negligible drug absorption occurs in the stomach (because of the small surface area, the thick lining of mucus and tight intracellular junctions), whereas most drugs are absorbed in the small intestine (duodenum, jejunum and ileum).

The extent of ionisation is determined by the pH of the environment. To illustrate how a change in pH affects ionisation, consider the following example. Drug X is a weak acid with a pKa of 5. In an acidic environment of pH 2, pH – pKa = –3 and drug X will be ~0.1% ionised. In this situation the majority of drug X is un-ionised and hence available to diffuse across cell membranes. However, in a more basic environment (pH 8), pH – pKa = 3 and drug X will be ~99.9% ionised. Conversely, if a drug is a weak base (pKa ~8), in an acidic environment of pH 3, pH – pKa = –5 and hence a basic drug will be over 99.9% ionised and only the 0.1% of the drug that is un-ionised will diffuse across cell membranes.

Formulation

Drug formulations can be manipulated to achieve desirable absorption characteristics. A drug can be coated with a resin or contained in a matrix from which it is slowly released. Sustained (or controlled) release formulations are useful for drugs that have a short elimination half-life (Ch 5). Drugs may also be prepared with a coating that offers relative resistance to the acidic environment of the stomach (e.g. enteric coating). Enteric coatings on drugs are used to:

- prevent decomposition of chemically sensitive drugs by gastric acid (e.g. penicillin G and erythromycin are unstable at an acidic pH), thus improving bioavailability
- prevent dilution of the drug before it reaches the intestine
- prevent nausea and vomiting induced by the effect of the drug in the stomach
- provide delayed release of the drug.

Routes of drug administration

The route of drug administration can affect both the rate of onset of action and the magnitude of the therapeutic response that results. When a drug is given for a systemic effect, absorption is an essential first step before the drug enters the systemic circulation and is distributed to a location distant from the site of administration.

A drug may enter the circulation either by being injected there directly (intravenously) or by absorption from other extravascular sites. The traditional or standard routes of drug administration fall into the following major categories:

- oral (also called enteral)
- parenteral – includes subcutaneous, intramuscular, intravenous, intrathecal or epidermal
- inhalation
- topical
- rectal.

However, new technologies continue to emerge, with drugs delivered by drug-eluting stents in the field of cardiology, the application of nanoparticles targeting brain tumours, administration of antibody–drug conjugates in cancer chemotherapy, the use of nanocarriers for transdermal vaccine administration and miniature micro-electromechanical devices for passive and active drug delivery.

Oral route

Oral, or enteral, ingestion is the most common route for drug administration. It is a safe, convenient and economical route of administration. However, the frequent changes in the GIT environment produced by food, emotion, physical activity and other medications may at times make absorption of drugs unreliable and slow. Drugs may be absorbed from several sites along the GIT and they may also be metabolised by enzymes in the gastrointestinal mucosa before they are absorbed and enter the systemic circulation.

Absorption from the oral cavity

Although the oral cavity possesses a thin lining, a rich blood supply and a slightly acidic pH, little absorption occurs in the mouth. However, despite its small surface area, the oral mucosa is capable of absorbing certain drugs as long as they dissolve rapidly in the salivary secretions (i.e. drugs given by sublingual or buccal routes). In sublingual administration the drug is placed under the tongue to permit tablet dissolution in salivary secretions. Fentanyl, an analgesic medicine, can be administered in this manner, and the person is advised to refrain as long as possible from swallowing saliva containing the tablet form of the drug. Drugs absorbed sublingually enter the systemic circulation directly without entering the portal system, thus bypassing the liver and escaping first-pass metabolism. Accordingly, absorption is rapid and the effects of the drug may become apparent within 2 minutes. With buccal administration the drug (tablet) is placed between the teeth and the mucous membrane of the cheek. Some hormones and enzyme preparations are administered by this route and are rapidly absorbed.

Absorption from the stomach

Although the stomach has a rich blood supply, it has a thick layer of mucus, tight intracellular junctions and a relatively small surface area; hence, it is not a major site of drug absorption (despite the common misconception that significant drug absorption occurs in the stomach). However, the length of time a drug remains in the stomach is a significant variable in determining the rate of gastrointestinal absorption. Generally, a slow gastric emptying rate decreases the rate of drug absorption in the small intestine. This is why many drugs are administered on an empty stomach, with sufficient water to ensure dissolution of the drug and rapid passage into the small intestine. (Drugs that cause gastric irritation are usually given with food.) After solid-dose drug administration the recipient should be encouraged to sit upright for at least 30 minutes to shorten gastric emptying time (the time required for the drug to reach the small intestine) and also to reduce the potential for tablets or capsules to lodge in the oesophageal area.

Absorption from the small intestine

The small intestine is highly vascularised and, with its many villi, presents a significantly larger and more permeable absorption surface compared with the stomach. It is the major site for absorbing orally administered drugs that pass from the stomach into this region, and drugs are absorbed primarily in the upper part of the small intestine. The pH of the intestinal fluid, which is close to neutral (ranging from 5.5 to 7 in the duodenum to 7.5 in the ileum), influences the extent of ionisation of a drug within the lumen of the GIT. It should be noted, however, that ionisation of a weak acid or a weak base does not prevent absorption from the small intestine.

Weak acids and weak bases exist in biological fluids in a dynamic equilibrium between the more lipid-soluble un-ionised form and the more water-soluble ionised forms (Fig 4.4). The un-ionised (lipid-soluble) form of the drug is readily absorbed across the small intestinal membrane. Because of the dynamic nature of the equilibrium, more ionised drug is then converted to the un-ionised form to compensate for the amount absorbed, and the un-ionised drug then in turn becomes available for absorption. As a consequence of this process, most weak acids and weak bases are well absorbed after oral administration. By contrast, strongly acidic (e.g. the H_1 receptor antagonist proxicromil) and basic drugs (e.g. gentamicin) are not absorbed when given orally because essentially all drug present in the small intestine will be ionised.

Although passive diffusion is the dominant process involved in the absorption of most drugs, a number of uptake transporters, including OATP1A2, OCT3 and PEPT1, have been identified on the apical (luminal) membrane of enterocytes. It is therefore possible that these transporters contribute to the absorption of drugs. It is also important to recognise that the efflux transporters P-gp, BCRP and MRP2 are also expressed on the apical membrane of enterocytes. It is well established that P-gp limits the absorption of some drugs since, following oral absorption, the drug may be actively transported back into the lumen of the small intestine.

Absorption from the rectum

The surface area of the rectum is not very large, but drug absorption does occur because of extensive vascularity. The veins of the rectum include the superior, middle and inferior veins. Only the superior rectal veins unite to form the inferior mesenteric vein, which is a tributary of the portal vein. Drug absorbed via the superior rectal veins flows to the liver via the portal vein and is metabolised, while the remainder of the drug that is absorbed (approximately 50%) escapes first-pass metabolism as it bypasses the liver. Rectal drug administration may be used for both local and systemic effects. This route is often used in unconscious individuals, in fasting patients, in those unable to swallow or when severe vomiting is present. Disadvantages to rectal drug administration include erratic absorption because of rectal contents, interruption of drug absorption resulting from defecation, local drug irritation with some medications, uncertainty of drug retention and patient acceptability.

Parenteral route

'Parenteral administration' commonly refers to the administration of drugs by injection. Intravenous administration is the most rapid route of drug administration, with high concentrations being achieved quickly in the systemic circulation. The **bioavailability** of a drug administered intravenously is 100% because the entire dose is delivered directly into the systemic circulation. Absorption from subcutaneous or intramuscular injection sites is faster than via the oral route but is less reliable because local blood flow and diffusion through the tissue influences the pattern of absorption.

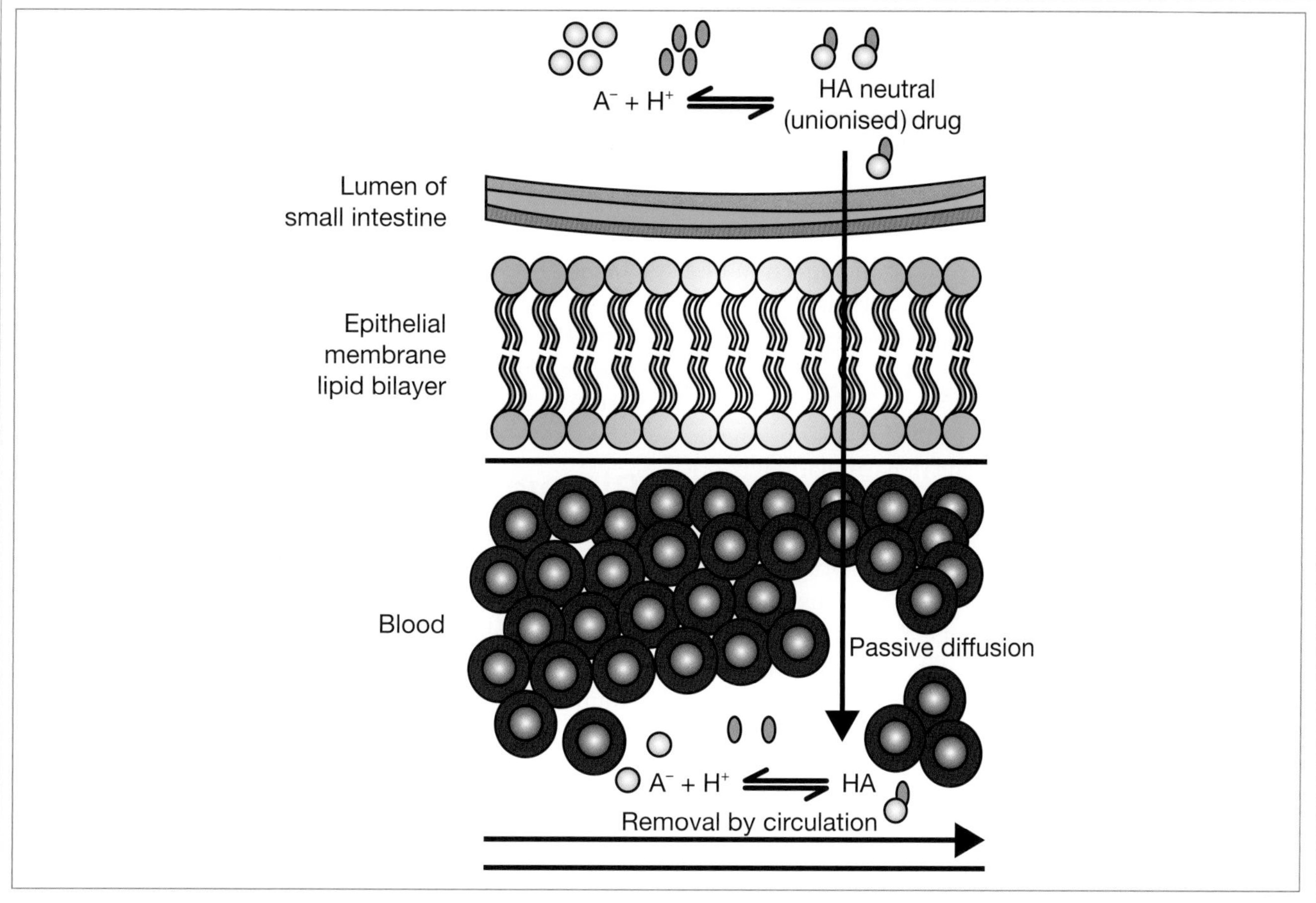

FIGURE 4.4 Weak acids and weak bases exist in biological fluids in a dynamic equilibrium between the more lipid-soluble un-ionised form (HA) and the more water-soluble ionised form ($A^- + H^+$)

The un-ionised form of the drug (HA) is readily absorbed across the small intestinal membrane into the bloodstream where it dissociates, re-establishing the dynamic equilibrium between HA and $A^- + H^+$. In the lumen of the small intestine, because of the dynamic nature of the equilibrium, more ionised drug is then converted to the un-ionised form to compensate for the amount absorbed; the un-ionised drug then in turn becomes available for absorption.

Subcutaneous

A subcutaneous injection of a drug is given beneath the skin into the connective tissue or fat immediately underlying the dermis. This site can be used only for drugs that are not irritating to the tissue, otherwise severe pain, necrosis and sloughing of tissue may occur. The rate of absorption is slow and can provide a sustained effect.

Intramuscular

'Intramuscular administration' refers to the injection of a drug solution into muscle. Most often the drug is fully soluble in an aqueous solution and absorption occurs more rapidly than with subcutaneous injection because of greater tissue blood flow. However, not all drugs are formulated as aqueous solutions. Procaine penicillin is poorly soluble and is injected as an aqueous suspension that is slowly absorbed and hence has a prolonged duration of action. Some steroid hormones are synthesised as chemical esters, which increases their solubility in oil and slows the rate of absorption. Drug absorption via this route may not be 'normal' in obese or emaciated people because of differences in subcutaneous fat distribution.

Intravenous

This route of drug administration has both advantages and disadvantages. The intravenous route produces an immediate pharmacological response because the desired amount of drug is injected directly into the bloodstream, thereby circumventing the absorption process. However, adverse effects may occur as a result of the rapid attainment of a high plasma concentration. Intravenous drugs may be given as a small bolus dose or by constant infusion, which should generally be administered slowly to prevent adverse effects.

Intrathecal

Intrathecal drug administration means the drug is injected directly into the spinal subarachnoid space, bypassing the

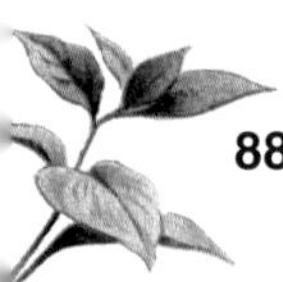

blood–brain barrier. Many compounds cannot enter the cerebrospinal fluid or are absorbed in this region only very slowly. When rapid central nervous system effects of drugs are desired – for example, with spinal anaesthesia or in treatment of acute infection of the central nervous system – this route may be used.

Epidural

'Epidural drug administration' refers to the injection of a drug within the spinal canal on or outside the dura mater that surrounds the spinal column.

Inhalation

The lungs provide a large surface area for absorption and the alveolar membrane is thin. The rich capillary network adjacent to the alveolar membrane promotes ready entry of drugs into the bloodstream. Drug delivery via the lungs avoids first-pass extraction by the liver. Drugs such as bronchodilators are administered by various metered-dose inhalation devices (nebulisers, 'puffers') that deliver the drug during inhalation into the airway, producing primarily a local effect with reduced systemic adverse effects compared with oral administration.

Topical route

Depending on the site of application, absorption of drugs applied topically to the skin and mucous membranes is generally rapid. Examples include cutaneous application, nasal sprays and eyedrops.

Skin

Drugs applied to the skin are used to produce either a local or a systemic effect through the use of ointments or transdermal patches. Passage across the stratum corneum, the outer hard layer of skin, is rate-limiting in the dermal absorption of drugs. However, following passage through the stratum corneum, lipophilic drugs diffuse freely through the remainder of the epidermis and dermis. The dermis is perfused by capillaries, which aids dermal drug absorption by maintaining a concentration gradient. Absorption occurs more readily through abraded or burnt skin, and factors that enhance cutaneous blood flow or hydrate the skin also increase absorption – for example, massaging, warming the skin or covering with an occlusive dressing.

Eyes

Topical administration of ophthalmic drugs produces a local effect on the conjunctiva or anterior chamber. Systemic absorption can occur through drainage from the naso-lacrimal canal and, as this route bypasses the liver (no first-pass metabolism), adverse systemic effects may occur (e.g. unwanted effects due to the use of corticosteroids as eyedrops). Suspensions and ointments are also used and eye/lid movements may promote the distribution of drug over the surface of the eye.

Ears

Otic administration of drops into the auditory canal may be chosen to treat local infection or inflammatory conditions or to help remove wax in the external ear.

Nose

Nasal drops or sprays containing medications may be applied or sprayed directly onto the nasal mucosa. This route is commonly used for treatment of sinus conditions resulting from viral infection or hay fever.

Bioavailability

After a drug crosses the membranes of the GIT, it enters the portal vein. The portal vein then carries the blood containing the drug to the liver, which is the main site of drug metabolism. The drug may pass through the liver and enter the systemic circulation as intact parent drug (unmetabolised) or may undergo metabolism in the liver. The extent to which a drug is metabolised (extracted) by the liver is highly variable.

The two factors that determine the amount of intact drug reaching the systemic circulation are:

- The fraction of the drug dose absorbed from the GIT; designated as f_g. When $f_g = 1$, the drug is completely absorbed; when $f_g = 0$, none of the drug is absorbed.
- The fraction of absorbed drug that escapes first-pass metabolism by the liver; designated as f_H. The fraction of drug not extracted by the liver can be calculated as 1 minus the hepatic extraction ratio $(1 - E_H)$ (Fig 4.5).

First-pass metabolism

Orally administered drugs that are absorbed travel first through the portal system and the liver before entering the systemic circulation. Depending on whether the drug is metabolised or not, a variable amount of drug can be extracted (E_H) by the liver before the drug ever reaches the systemic circulation. In the example shown in Figure 4.5, 80 mg of the drug reaches the liver and 60 mg is extracted in the first pass through the liver. Consequently, the bioavailability of that drug is 20% and hence only 20 mg (a small fraction of the original 100 mg dose) is available for distribution and to produce a pharmacological effect. For such medications the oral drug dose is calculated to compensate for **first-pass effect**. For example, morphine undergoes significant first-pass metabolism – 30 mg oral morphine is equivalent to 10 mg morphine administered intramuscularly, intravenously or subcutaneously.

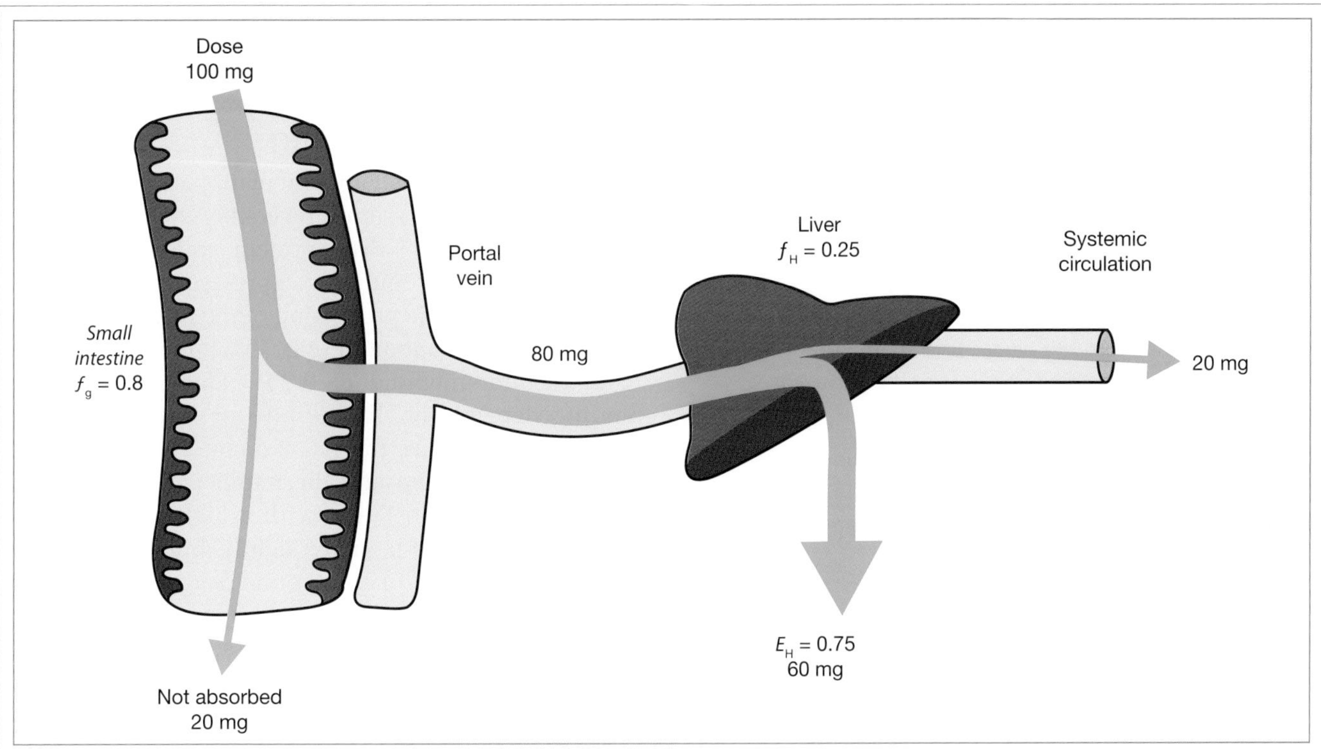

FIGURE 4.5 Factors affecting bioavailability

In this example, 80 mg of the original 100 mg dose is absorbed intact into the portal circulation. (The fraction absorbed is 0.8.) The hepatic extraction ratio is 0.75; that is, 60 mg is extracted in the first pass through the liver, and 20 mg escapes extraction and is available for distribution via the systemic circulation. The bioavailability is $F = f_g \times f_H$, which is $0.8 \times 0.25 = 0.2$ (20%).

Source: Birkett 2010, Figure 5.1; reproduced with permission from McGraw-Hill.

Bioequivalence

The term bioequivalence is used when referring to two formulations of the same drug containing an identical concentration of the active ingredient in the same dosage form and administered by the same route. Once the patent expires on a drug, other pharmaceutical companies can produce a generic equivalent of the original patented drug under a new proprietary name. The generic product must be tested against the original product to determine its relative exposure. The two products are considered to be bioequivalent if parameters describing the exposure to the new product are within 20% of the original product (i.e. within the range 0.85 to 1.2) and if there are no clinically important differences between their therapeutic or adverse effects. When granting a licence for a generic product, regulatory authorities place particular importance on evidence of bioequivalence.

Biosimilars

Most drugs are relatively low molecular-weight organic chemicals and, once the patent has expired, the synthesis of a generic version is relatively easy. However, more recently, biopharmaceutical drugs (or 'biologics') have been introduced into clinical medicine. These drugs are most commonly proteins or 'humanised' monoclonal antibodies produced using biotechnology methods – for example, the expression of recombinant proteins in cell culture and mouse hybridoma technology. Examples of engineered, recombinant proteins include human growth hormone and insulin, while cetuximab and bevacizumab are examples of humanised monoclonal antibodies. Often the biologic is produced using microbial cells, and during the production process any small change (e.g. in post-translational modification) can cause a major impact on the biological activity of the protein drug. Once the patent expires, a biosimilar can be produced.

According to European Medicines Agency guidelines, a biosimilar is not considered a generic medicinal product because it is often impossible to determine the bioequivalence of a protein. This is understandable when you consider that biologics are often manufactured from unique cell lines, and it is virtually impossible to produce an 'identical' copy of the original patented protein. For example, glycosylation of the proteins (which is important for biological activity), ligand recognition and pharmacokinetics were found to differ between the original patented epoetin and a number of biosimilar epoetins. These differences are thought to account for the altered clinical profiles of the biosimilars. Similarly, differences in clinical activity and adverse effects have been reported for interferon-alpha-2a and enoxaparin biosimilars.

KEY POINTS

Absorption

- Absorption is defined as the process by which unchanged drug proceeds from the site of administration into the blood. It is an important factor for all routes of administration with the exception of intravenous administration.
- Variables that affect drug absorption include the nature of the absorbing membrane, blood flow, the solubility of the drug, the degree of ionisation and formulation characteristics.
- Bioavailability of a drug is defined as the proportion of the administered dose that reaches the systemic circulation intact.
- Two factors determining bioavailability are the amount of drug absorbed from the GIT and the amount of drug escaping hepatic extraction.

Distribution

After a drug reaches the systemic circulation, it can be distributed to various interstitial and intracellular compartments within the body, including blood, bone, fat, total body water and extracellular water. Distribution is defined as the process of reversible transfer of a drug between one location and another (one of which is usually blood) in the body (Fig 4.1). Some drugs remain almost exclusively in blood; these include penicillin and warfarin. Other drugs are distributed to organs that are well perfused (e.g. heart, liver and kidneys), and the local drug concentration in these organs may be high initially. Drugs are also distributed more slowly to organs with poor blood supply, which include skeletal muscles and fat. Drugs that are widely distributed in the body include amiodarone, digoxin and morphine.

The rate and extent to which a drug enters the different compartments of the body depends on the permeability of the capillaries, the partitioning of the drug between the vascular and tissue compartment, perfusion and the presence of drug transporters (e.g. the blood–brain barrier). As already discussed, lipid-soluble (un-ionised) drugs can readily cross capillary membranes to enter most tissues and fluid compartments, whereas ionised (lipid-insoluble) drugs do not diffuse readily across membranes.

Plasma protein binding

On entry into the systemic circulation, a proportion of free drug molecules bind reversibly to proteins and lipoproteins to form drug–protein complexes. Plasma protein binding is commonly expressed as a percentage, which represents the proportion of the total drug bound, or as the fraction unbound (e.g. 75% bound corresponds to a fraction unbound of 0.25). The extent of drug binding depends on the affinity or attraction of the drug for the protein, the relative concentrations of the drug and the protein and the number of drug binding sites on the protein. Drugs with a high affinity for the binding protein will be more 'tightly' but still reversibly bound and the fraction of unbound drug will be low (i.e. the percentage bound is higher). Although plasma protein binding is a saturable process, the concentrations of most drugs in blood following therapeutic doses are generally lower than that required to saturate the binding sites on these proteins. However, there are exceptions. For example, the high plasma concentrations of salicylate achieved with anti-inflammatory doses as used in the treatment of rheumatoid arthritis can result in non-linear binding to albumin. Non-linear binding occurs when the concentration of the drug saturates the protein binding sites and adding more drug increases disproportionately the unbound concentration of the drug in plasma. Protein binding is a reversible and dynamic process, with bound and unbound drug in equilibrium:

$$\text{Free drug} + \text{protein} \leftrightarrow \text{drug} - \text{protein complex}$$

As free drug is removed from the circulation (e.g. by distribution, metabolism, excretion), the drug–protein complex dissociates very rapidly so more 'free' drug is released to replace what is 'lost'. This is very important, as it is only the free or unbound drug that exerts a pharmacological effect. This is illustrated below. In this example, the initial plasma drug concentration is 100 mg/L, the fraction of drug that is bound to plasma proteins is 0.8 (80%) and the unbound fraction is 0.2 (20%).

Historically, the convention is that acidic drugs (e.g. ibuprofen) bind mainly to plasma albumin, while basic drugs (e.g. quinine) bind to α_1-acid glycoprotein; however, many newer drugs, such as small-molecule kinase inhibitors, do not follow this convention. In this case, these drugs, which are weak bases, bind primarily to albumin. Among the highly protein-bound drugs is warfarin, which is about 99% protein-bound. This means that at any given time, 99% is bound to plasma proteins and only 1% of free drug is available for distribution (the drug–protein molecule is too large to diffuse through the blood vessel membrane) and to exert a pharmacological effect. Other examples of highly protein-bound drugs include kinase inhibitors over 99%, nonsteroidal anti-inflammatory drugs over 95%, alfentanil 92%, atorvastatin ~98% and candesartan 99.8%. Drugs with low protein binding include cefalexin 14%, codeine 7%, fluconazole 11% and paracetamol 10%. Because albumin and (to a lesser extent) other plasma proteins provide a number of binding sites, two drugs can compete with one another for the same site and displace each other.

Hypoalbuminaemia

Hypoalbuminaemia, or low levels of albumin in the blood, may be caused by hepatic dysfunction such as cirrhosis or by failure of the liver to synthesise sufficient plasma proteins. The decrease in albumin concentration results in an increase in the amount of free drug available for distribution to tissue sites. When a person is given the usual dosage of a drug in the presence of decreased plasma protein binding, more of the free (unbound) drug is available to exert a pharmacological effect. This may result in toxicity, and the drug dosage should be reduced. This is illustrated using the anticonvulsant drug phenytoin.

Tissue binding

Adipose tissue

Lipid-soluble drugs have a high affinity for adipose tissue, which is where these drugs are stored. Moreover, the relatively low blood flow in adipose tissue makes it a stable reservoir for a limited number of drugs. For example, the lipid-soluble barbiturate anaesthetic thiopental sodium is initially rapidly distributed to the brain, producing anaesthesia, but then redistributes to and accumulates in fatty tissue at concentrations 6–12 times those in the plasma. Continued administration of thiopental sodium causes a progressively longer period of anaesthesia as the drug accumulates in the body. This is one of the reasons why thiopental sodium is used for the induction of anaesthesia and not for surgical anaesthesia. Accumulation in adipose tissue is one reason for a drug having a prolonged half-life (Ch 5).

Bone

Some drugs have an unusual affinity for bone; for example, the tetracycline antibiotics accumulate in bone after being absorbed onto the bone-crystal surface. This serves as a storage site for tetracycline antibiotics, which can depress bone growth in premature infants. Distribution of tetracycline to the teeth in a young child results in discolouration, which is thought to be due to formation of a tetracycline–calcium–orthophosphate complex. Brownish pigmentation of permanent teeth may also result if this drug is given during the prenatal period or early childhood.

Tissue-specific barriers to drug distribution

A number of tissues and organs where it is particularly important to minimise drug or toxin exposure are 'protected' by barriers, which typically involve specific characteristics of the capillary membranes (e.g. tighter junctions between cells and thicker basement membrane), reinforcement by secondary cell types (e.g. astrocytes in the brain) and high levels of expression of efflux transporters (e.g. P-gp). Examples of organ-specific barriers include the blood–brain, blood–retina and placental barriers.

Blood–brain barrier

The blood–brain barrier comprises the endothelial cells of brain capillaries, which are joined to each other by tight junctions. The capillary structure is further reinforced by astrocytic end-feet that project from astrocytes to form a near continuous layer over the thick basement membrane that underlies the endothelial cells. Although the barrier does allow penetration of lipid-soluble drugs into the brain and cerebrospinal fluid, further protection of the brain is provided by transporters. On the luminal membrane of brain capillary endothelial cells a number of drug transporters are expressed, including the efflux transporters P-gp and BCRP. In some circumstances, such as meningitis, the blood–brain barrier can become 'leaky', and this allows access of drugs that would not normally be able to penetrate the brain. Using penicillin systemically to treat bacterial meningitis is an example of taking advantage of the inflammatory disruption of the blood–brain barrier.

Placental barrier

The placenta separates the blood vessels of the mother and the fetus and constitutes for some compounds a protective barrier. In addition, placental enzymes such as sulfotransferase can metabolise catecholamines, inactivating them as they travel from the maternal circulation to the embryo. Despite the thickness of the placenta, it does not afford complete protection to the fetus. Like the blood–brain barrier, lipophilic drugs readily diffuse across the placenta while the passage of more polar compounds is generally impeded. Consequently, many drugs intended to produce a therapeutic response in the mother may also cross the placental barrier and exert harmful effects on the fetus.

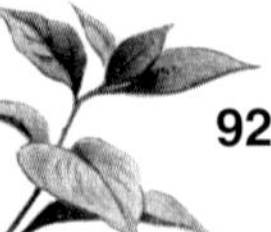

KEY POINTS

Distribution

- Distribution is defined as the process of reversible transfer of a drug between one location and another (one of which is usually blood) in the body.
- On entry into the systemic circulation, free drug molecules bind reversibly to proteins to form drug–protein complexes. Protein binding decreases the free drug concentration and limits tissue distribution. As free drug is removed from the circulation, the protein–drug complex dissociates so more free drug is released.
- Only free or unbound drug exerts a pharmacological effect.

Drug metabolism

Drug metabolism is the process of chemical modification of a drug and is almost invariably carried out by enzymes. The liver is the primary site of drug metabolism but, with certain drugs, other organs (e.g. kidneys, lungs and intestine) may also be involved to a limited degree. Most drugs (around 70%) undergo metabolism to some extent, and in most (but not all) cases, the products of metabolism have less biological activity than the parent drug. An exception to this is the use of prodrugs, which are drugs that require activation (often in the liver) in order to elicit a therapeutic action. Examples of prodrugs are the anti-rheumatic drug leflunomide, the analgesic codeine and the antiplatelet clopidogrel. For most therapeutic drugs, metabolism results in the formation of a more water-soluble compound or metabolite, which can be more readily excreted. Metabolism clears the parent compound from the systemic circulation and promotes urinary excretion.

Classification of drug metabolism reactions

The vast majority of drugs are metabolised in the liver by either functionalisation and/or conjugation reactions. It is important to recognise that a drug may:

- be excreted as unchanged parent drug (e.g. gentamicin)
- undergo functionalisation and be directly excreted (e.g. caffeine)
- undergo conjugation and be directly excreted (e.g. paracetamol)
- undergo functionalisation then conjugation prior to excretion (e.g. phenytoin).

These reactions are not necessarily sequential and can occur simultaneously (e.g. the metabolism of codeine by oxidation to morphine and by glucuronidation to codeine-6-glucuronide).

Functionalisation reactions

These reactions generally involve introducing or unmasking a polar functional group into the molecule, thereby producing more water-soluble metabolite. Common functionalisation reactions include dealkylation (de-ethylation or demethylation), hydrolysis, hydroxylation and oxidation. In some cases, metabolites are more pharmacologically active than the parent compound and, uncommonly, may be more toxic. (For example, N-acetyl-p-benzoquinone imine [NAPQI] is the toxic metabolite of paracetamol responsible for the severe liver damage associated with overdose of this drug.) Cytochrome P450 is the major family of enzymes associated with these reactions. Other functionalisation enzymes include esterases, alcohol dehydrogenase, flavin-containing mono-oxygenases and xanthine oxidase.

Cytochrome P450

The enzymes of greatest importance in functionalisation reactions are the superfamily of cytochrome P450 (CYP) enzymes. CYP are found in the smooth endoplasmic reticulum of cells and are particularly abundant in hepatocytes. CYP are involved not only in drug metabolism but also in the metabolism of environmental pollutants and dietary chemicals, and in the synthesis and metabolism of bile acids, steroids, hormones and fatty acids. There are more than 50 individual human CYP, which are classified based on amino-acid sequence identity into families and sub-families; of these, approximately 18 enzymes in families 1, 2 and 3 can metabolise drugs. In naming them, the suffix 'CYP' is followed by a number designating the family, which is followed by a letter denoting the sub-family and then another number in order of their discovery. For example, CYP3A4 is the fourth member of CYP family 3, sub-family A. The human CYPs of greatest importance in hepatic drug metabolism are CYP1A2, CYP2C8, CYP2C9, CYP2C19, CYP2D6, CYP2E1 and CYP3A4. Table 4.1 lists some common therapeutic drugs that are substrates for these CYPs.

Conjugation reactions

These involve joining a suitable functional group present in the drug molecule with the polar group of an endogenous substance in the body (e.g. glucuronic acid, sulfate, acetyl-coenzyme A or glutathione). The conjugated drug molecule is generally more polar or more water-soluble, which enhances urinary excretion.

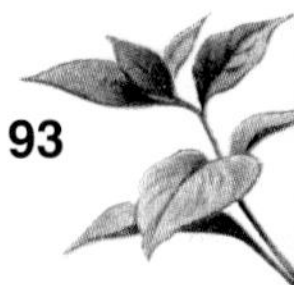

TABLE 4.1 Representative drugs metabolised by CYP enzymes

CYP	DRUGS METABOLISED
CYP1A2	Amitriptyline, caffeine, clozapine, haloperidol, lidocaine (lignocaine), olanzapine, ondansetron, tamoxifen
CYP2C8	Chloroquine, montelukast, paclitaxel
CYP2C9	Celecoxib, diclofenac, gliclazide, ibuprofen, irbesartan, losartan, naproxen, phenytoin, sildenafil, sulfonylurea, S-warfarin
CYP2C19	Citalopram, clopidogrel, diazepam, esomeprazole, omeprazole, pantoprazole, sertraline
CYP2D6	Amitriptyline, codeine, dexamfetamine, dextromethorphan, fluoxetine, fluvoxamine, haloperidol, metoprolol, mirtazapine, perhexiline, quetiapine, risperidone, timolol, venlafaxine
CYP2E1	Ethanol, halothane, methoxyflurane
CYP3A4	Amiodarone, aprepitant, atorvastatin, carbamazepine, ciclosporin, erythromycin, felodipine, hydrocortisone, HIV protease inhibitors (e.g. saquinavir), simvastatin, tacrolimus, tyrosine kinase inhibitors (e.g. axitinib), verapamil, zolpidem

The relationship between drug metabolism and renal excretion is illustrated in Figure 4.6. The various types of conjugation reactions are identified in Table 4.2 along with the enzymes and co-factors that are involved in their catalysis.

UDP-glucuronosyltransferases

UDP-glucuronosyltransferase (UGT) are a superfamily of enzymes that catalyse the conjugation of glucuronic acid, which is derived from the co-factor UDP-glucuronic acid (UDPGA), to a substrate (drug) that contains a suitable functional group. To date, 21 UGTs have been identified; these are grouped into the 1A, 2B, 3A and 8A families. Of these, UGT 1A1, 1A4, 1A6, 1A9, 2B7 and 2B15 are of greatest importance in drug metabolism. UGT enzymes also metabolise many endogenous chemicals of physiological significance. For example, bilirubin is glucuronidated by UGT1A1, and people who are deficient in this enzyme become jaundiced.

Variability in drug metabolism

Differences can occur between individuals in both the extent and the rate of metabolism of many drugs. Metabolism therefore becomes very important in

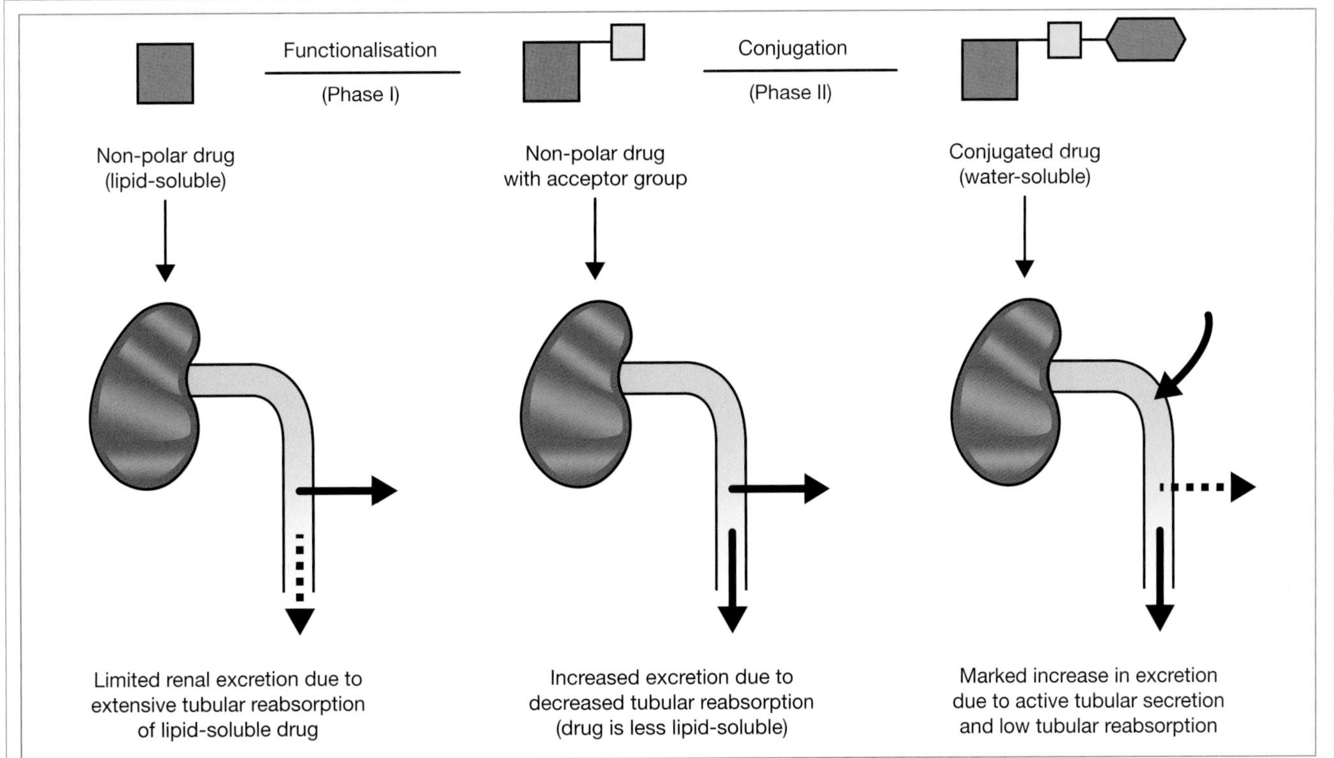

FIGURE 4.6 Relationship between drug metabolism and renal excretion
Metabolism via functionalisation and conjugation reactions results in decreasing lipid solubility, increasing water solubility and progressive enhancement of urinary excretion.
Source: Birkett et al. 1979, Figure 2; reproduced with permission.

TABLE 4.2 Conjugation reactions

ENZYME	COFACTOR	REACTION	SUBSTRATE / METABOLITE
UDP-glucuronosyltransferases	UDP-glucuronic acid	Glucuronidation	Morphine/morphine-3-glucuronide Codeine/codeine-6-glucuronide
Sulfotransferases	Sulfate	Sulfation	Salbutamol/salbutamol sulfate Paracetamol/paracetamol sulfate
N-acetyltransferases	Acetyl-CoA	Acetylation	Isoniazid/acetylisoniazid Clonazepam/7-acetamido-clonazepam
Glutathione-S-transferases	Glutathione	Glutathione conjugation	Paracetamol/paracetamol–glutathione conjugate

determining the therapeutic and toxic effects of many drugs. This variability can be due to a range of factors including:

- genetics
- environmental factors – for example, co-administered drugs, diet, alcohol, smoking
- age and gender
- disease states – for example, hepatic, cardiovascular
- hormonal changes – for example, pregnancy.

Drug interactions

Metabolic drug interactions can occur when two or more chemicals (drugs, herbs or environmental chemicals) are present in the body at the same time. In this situation, one chemical (the interaction perpetrator) alters the activity of the enzyme involved in eliminating the other chemical (the interaction victim). Metabolic drug interactions are typically caused by the co-administration of two drugs (drug–drug interactions) but may also occur when a chemical present in a herbal preparation (herb–drug interaction) or food item (diet–drug interaction) alters the metabolism of a drug. Such reactions result from either induction or inhibition of enzyme activity. Induction of drug metabolism usually arises from increased synthesis of more of the enzyme protein via an effect on the genes that encode the specific drug-metabolising enzyme. The clinical impact of enzyme induction depends on the extent to which the plasma drug concentration is decreased (suboptimal) over the course of treatment with normal dosing. For example, cigarette smoke induces expression of CYP1A2 and therefore increases the metabolism of clozapine and olanzapine; this can result in a substantially higher dose requirement for some patients.

Inhibition of drug metabolism typically occurs when two drugs compete for metabolism by the same enzyme. This invariably results in a decrease in metabolism of one or both of the drugs. The clinical consequences of inhibition of drug metabolism include a decreased rate of elimination from the body, resulting in an increased plasma concentration and risk of toxicity. Examples include:

- inhibition of warfarin metabolism by amiodarone or fluconazole, increasing the risk of bleeding
- inhibition of azathioprine metabolism by allopurinol, increasing the risk of severe bone marrow toxicity and death
- inhibition of ciclosporin and tacrolimus metabolism by erythromycin, increasing the risk of nephrotoxicity and neurotoxicity
- inhibition of diazepam metabolism by cimetidine, prolonging central nervous system depression.

Disease states

In people with cardiac failure, liver perfusion and oxygenation may be decreased, and this can reduce the activity of drug-metabolising enzymes. In liver disease the effects are harder to predict because they depend on the disease type and severity, both of which can influence drug metabolism. In general, in severe cirrhosis and viral hepatitis the clearance of drugs metabolised by CYP is decreased.

Hormonal factors

Although gender-related differences have been observed for drug-metabolising enzymes in animal species, differences in humans are often minor and clinically insignificant. However, hormonal factors during pregnancy can have an important effect on drug metabolism, particularly during the third trimester when increased activity of many CYP and UGT enzymes occurs. For example, it is well established that doses of the anticonvulsant drugs carbamazepine (metabolised by CYP3A4) and phenytoin (metabolised by CYP2C9) must be increased during pregnancy to maintain plasma concentrations in the therapeutic range. Following birth, doses decline to pre-pregnancy requirements. CYP2D6 activity is also induced during pregnancy. In contrast, there is evidence suggesting that the metabolism of caffeine (a CYP1A2 substrate) declines during pregnancy. Thus, although induction occurs most commonly, effects of pregnancy on drug metabolism are not always predictable.

KEY POINTS

Metabolism

- Drug metabolism, or biotransformation, is the process of chemical modification of a drug and is almost invariably carried out by enzymes.
- The vast majority of drugs are metabolised in the liver by functionalisation and/or conjugation reactions. The major drug-metabolising enzyme superfamilies are the cytochrome P450 (CYP) and UDP-glucuronosyltransferase (UGT) enzymes.
- Large differences may occur between individuals in the rate of metabolism of drugs. This variability may be due to genetic, environmental, age or disease-related factors.

Excretion of drugs and drug metabolites

In pharmacokinetic terms, elimination refers to the irreversible loss of drug from the site of measurement and occurs by the processes of metabolism and excretion. For example, after administration, a drug may be metabolised by the liver but its metabolites may remain in the body. In this case, the parent drug is considered to have been eliminated. The terms 'elimination' and 'excretion' are often used interchangeably, but excretion applies solely to the loss of (chemically) unchanged drug or metabolites in, for example, urine or bile. The term 'unchanged' in this context may appear confusing, but it refers to the immediate chemical species that is being excreted, which can be either a parent molecule or a metabolite. In this regard, the liver, being the major site of drug metabolism, is the main organ of elimination, while the kidneys are the main organs of excretion.

Hepatic uptake and biliary excretion

Although lipophilic drugs freely diffuse across the membrane of hepatocytes, the presence of uptake transporters of the OCT, OATP, OAT and sodium/taurocholate co-transporting polypeptide (NTCP) families facilitate the uptake of drugs that are organic anions and cations as well as other polar compounds. Once in the hepatocyte, the drug becomes available for metabolism by enzymes such as CYP and UGT or for excretion into bile by the efflux transporters (P-gp, BCRP, MATE1 and MRP2) located on the canalicular membrane. Thus, drugs such as small-molecule kinase inhibitors, which are substrates for uptake transporters (OATP), drug-metabolising enzymes (CYP) and efflux transporters (P-gp and BCRP), are eliminated by both metabolism and biliary excretion. Metabolites formed within the hepatocyte may (1) diffuse, or (2) be transported (by MRP) across the apical membrane back into blood for subsequent excretion in urine, or (3) be transported into the bile (by the transporters present on the canalicular membrane), passed into the duodenum and excreted in faeces.

Drugs and drug metabolites that are excreted into bile become available for reabsorption once the bile is released into the small intestine. In the small intestine the drug may be reabsorbed and returned to the liver via the portal vein, a process referred to as enterohepatic recycling. Since many drugs (e.g. atorvastatin, digoxin, ethinylestradiol, indometacin, morphine, rifampicin, kinase inhibitors and many antimicrobials) are excreted in bile to some extent, they are likely to undergo enterohepatic cycling to some degree. Glucuronide metabolites excreted into the bile can be hydrolysed by bacterial enzymes in the GIT to re-form the parent drug, which can subsequently undergo enterohepatic recycling.

Renal excretion

Renal excretion of drugs and drug metabolites is influenced by the processes of glomerular filtration, tubular secretion and reabsorption (Fig 4.7). Glomerular

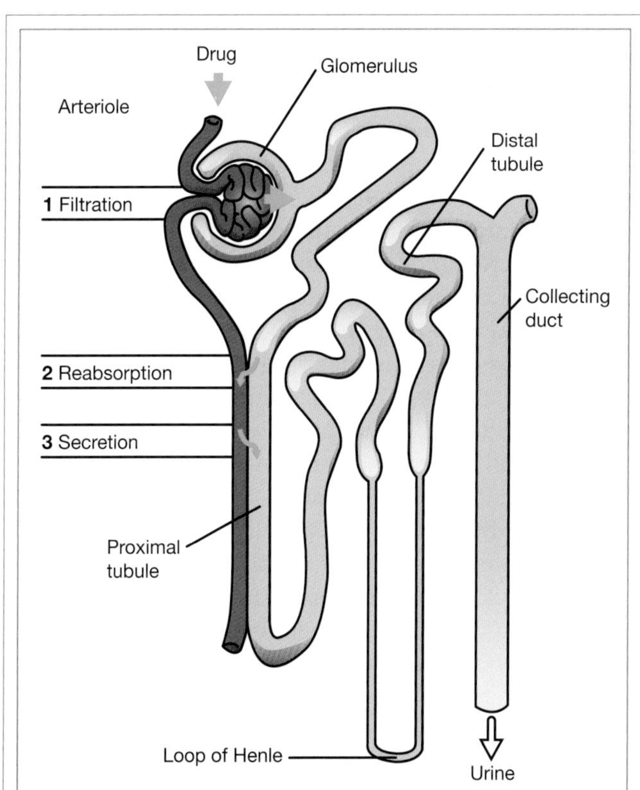

FIGURE 4.7 The drug excretion process, illustrating: **1** glomerular filtration, **2** tubular reabsorption and **3** secretion

Source: Salerno 1999, Figure 4-6; used with permission.

filtration and tubular secretion facilitate the transfer of drugs and metabolites from blood into urine, while reabsorption counters these processes. Free unbound drugs and water-soluble metabolites are filtered by the glomeruli (the glomerular filtration rate [GFR] is around 120 mL/min), whereas protein-bound substances are not filtered. Since there are no drugs that circulate in blood completely bound to protein or erythrocytes, all drugs and metabolites will undergo glomerular filtration to some extent. Drug transporters in the proximal tubule transfer those drugs and metabolites that are organic acids and bases from the interstitial fluid into the tubule cell. However, once in the urine, lipophilic drugs can transfer back into the tubule cell and interstitial fluid (reabsorption). Most of the 120 mL of water from the plasma filtered at the glomerulus is reabsorbed during its passage through the renal tubule, and only about 1–2 mL finally appears as urine. As the water is reabsorbed, a concentration gradient is established between the drug in the tubular fluid and the unbound drug in the blood. (That is, the drug in the urine is concentrated relative to that in the blood.) If the drug is lipid-soluble enough to pass through the membranes, it will be reabsorbed from the tubular fluid back into the systemic circulation. If the urine flow rate is high, there is less of a concentration gradient and less drug is reabsorbed. Conversely, if the urine is more concentrated due to a low urine flow rate, there is more of a concentration gradient and more drug is reabsorbed. In contrast to lipophilic drugs, polar, water-soluble compounds such as acids, bases and polar drug metabolites (e.g. glucuronides) are not reabsorbed and are excreted in the urine (Fig 4.6).

The proximal tubule is the main site of transporter-mediated secretion of drugs and/or their metabolites into the lumen of the nephron. Initially, both acidic and basic drugs are taken up from the interstitial fluid into tubular cells via the basolateral uptake 'acid' and 'base' transporters. These include OAT 1, 2 and 3 and OCT 2 and 3. The apical membrane of proximal tubular cells additionally expresses efflux transporters, including P-gp, OAT4, MATE 1 and 2 and MRP 2 and 4, which serve to export compounds from the tubular cell into urine. Another family of transporters found in the kidney, the so-called novel organic cation transporters (OCTNs) that are localised on the apical membrane, also appear to contribute to the transfer of organic cations into the tubular lumen. From a clinical perspective, at times it may be useful to reduce the excretion of a drug. One way of doing this is to competitively inhibit tubular secretion. For example, probenecid, which is used to treat gout, reduces the renal excretion of penicillin. It does this by inhibiting the efflux of penicillin via OATs from the tubular cell into the lumen of the nephron and hence reduces excretion of penicillin in urine. Clinically, this prolongs the effect of the antibiotic by maintaining a therapeutic plasma concentration for a longer period.

Pulmonary excretion

Gases and volatile drugs (e.g. general anaesthetics such as halothane) are inhaled and excreted (exhaled) via the lungs. On inspiration, these agents enter the bloodstream and, after crossing the alveolar membrane, access the systemic circulation. Excretion from the lungs depends on the rate of respiration. Volatile chemicals, such as ethanol, which are highly soluble in blood, may be excreted in limited amounts by the lungs. Approximately one part in 2000 of the ethanol in blood is in the gaseous state, and pulmonary excretion is the basis of the alcohol breath test.

Excretion in sweat and saliva

Drug excretion through sweat and saliva is relatively unimportant because this process is slow relative to other forms of excretion and represents only a minor proportion of total excretion.

KEY POINTS

Excretion

- The major organs for the excretion of unchanged drugs and drug metabolites are the kidneys.
- The process of renal excretion of drugs is influenced by glomerular filtration, tubular secretion and reabsorption.

Pharmacokinetics during pregnancy and early life

Many physiological changes that occur during pregnancy affect the pharmacokinetics of drugs. In addition to these changes that affect the mother's exposure to a drug during pregnancy and after birth while the mother is breastfeeding, it is also important to consider the potential drug exposure of the developing fetus and child.

Pharmacokinetic changes during pregnancy

Absorption

Although pregnancy does not directly affect drug absorption from the GIT, it does delay gastric emptying and decreases motility, which can increase or decrease drug absorption. For example, drugs that require an acidic environment for absorption may have a delayed absorption pattern because of the typical decrease in production of hydrochloric acid in the stomach during pregnancy. In addition, frequent vomiting may not only prevent normal oral drug administration but may also alter the plasma concentration of a drug because of unpredictable absorption.

Distribution

In addition to the substantial physiological change of essentially rapidly developing an additional organ (the placenta), more subtle changes in the woman's body mass and fluid distribution may also change the volume of distribution of a drug. During pregnancy, there is an increase in maternal plasma volume (30–50%) and a 25% increase in body fat. The latter may affect the distribution of drugs that are deposited in fatty tissues and can result in a fall in their plasma concentrations. Albumin concentration decreases from the second trimester through to the time of birth by approximately 20%. This affects the protein binding of drugs such as phenytoin and valproate where dosage adjustment is difficult because the development of fetal abnormalities is dose-dependent with both these drugs.

The placenta maintains separation of the blood supply of the mother and fetus while at the same time it is perfused by blood from both the maternal and the fetal circulations. It is crucial for delivery of oxygen and nutrients and as an endocrine organ, but the placenta also functions as a 'barrier' to protect the fetus from infectious and toxic agents. Exposure to drugs during pregnancy may result in fetal exposure if the drug ingested crosses the placenta. The fetus is then at risk of both the pharmacological and the teratogenic effects of the drug. However, for the first 10 weeks of embryonic development the maternal circulation does not perfuse the placenta and the fetal–placental–maternal circulation is not fully developed. Hence, drugs that produce dysmorphogenesis during this period reach the fetus via diffusion through extracellular fluid. After 10 weeks gestation the transfer of a drug across the placenta depends on the physicochemical properties of the drug, polarity, protein binding, lipid solubility and duration of exposure to the drug. The main process involved in transplacental transfer of nutrients and drugs is passive diffusion, with facilitated diffusion and active transport having lesser roles.

The amount of free drug crossing the placenta at any given time depends on the maternal plasma drug concentration. Eventually the concentration of drug on either side of the placenta will equalise; that is, the fetal plasma drug concentrations will equal the maternal drug concentration. In pregnancy, low-molecular-mass drugs (250–500 Da) freely cross the placenta, while drugs of molecular mass over 1000 Da (e.g. heparin) cross very poorly. Additionally, lipid-soluble drugs easily cross the placenta while diffusion of hydrophilic drugs is poor. In late gestation, the enhanced utero–placental blood flow and the thinner membranes that separate maternal blood flow and placental capillaries result in an increased placental transfer of un-ionised, lipophilic unbound drugs. Facilitated diffusion requires the presence of a carrier but does not require the input of energy. Again, the end result is equal concentrations of drug in the maternal and fetal circulations. Drug transporters are found in the maternal-facing apical membrane and in the fetal-facing basolateral membrane. An example of a placental transporter that transports drugs from the maternal circulation to the fetus is the organic cation transporter (OCTN2) that transports methamphetamine and verapamil. Many more transporters have been identified that have the potential to transport drugs from the fetus to the maternal circulation. These include P-gp, which is thought to have evolved to protect the fetus by effluxing potentially toxic environmental chemicals and drugs from the fetal compartment. Transporters of the MRP family have also been identified in the human placenta and again it has been suggested that they function to protect the fetus by transporting metabolites from the fetus to the maternal circulation.

Metabolism

Maternal hepatic drug-metabolising enzyme activity can either increase or decrease during pregnancy depending on the CYP or UGT enzyme(s) involved (Table 4.3). For

TABLE 4.3 Pregnancy-induced changes in hepatic drug-metabolising enzyme activity

ENZYME	EFFECT ON CLEARANCE	TRIMESTER	EXAMPLES OF DRUGS AFFECTED
CYP1A2	Decrease	1st, 2nd and 3rd	Caffeine
CYP2A6	Increase	2nd and 3rd	Nicotine
CYP2C9	Increase	3rd	Phenytoin
CYP2C19	Decrease	2nd and 3rd	Proguanil
CYP2D6	Increase	3rd	Dextromethorphan, metoprolol, fluoxetine, nortriptyline
CYP3A4	Increase	3rd	Nifedipine, saquinavir, ritonavir, lopinavir
UGT1A4	Increase	1st, 2nd and 3rd	Lamotrigine
UGT2B7	Increase	3rd	Morphine, zidovudine, oxazepam

example, in pregnant women metabolism of caffeine is decreased, but the metabolism of the antiepileptic drug phenytoin is increased, often necessitating adjustments in drug dosage during pregnancy. For the majority of drugs, effects on hepatic clearance occur most commonly in the third trimester. Paracetamol is metabolised predominantly by UGT1A6 with a contribution from UGT1A1 and UGT1A9 (Miners et al. 2011). Increased paracetamol clearance via glucuronidation increases in the third trimester, but it is unclear whether this affects a single UGT enzyme (e.g. UGT1A6) or a variable combination of all three enzymes. The effects of these changes on drug therapies are difficult to predict because the alterations can vary enormously between individual pregnant women.

Drug metabolism in the placenta

Our knowledge of drug metabolism in human placenta is limited, and it appears in general to play a minor role in limiting the exposure of the fetus to drugs. However, it is well established that the activity of placental drug-metabolising enzymes is altered in pregnant women who either abuse drugs, smoke or consume alcohol. Drug-metabolising enzymes identified to date include CYP1A1, which is present in placenta throughout pregnancy, while CYP1A2 is present in the first trimester. The activity of CYP1A1 is increased by smoking, and the extent of induction depends on the stage of pregnancy. Importantly, CYP1A1 activates polycyclic aromatic hydrocarbons found in tobacco, which can lead to detrimental effects on the fetus. CYP2E1, which metabolises ethanol, is present in the placenta from the first trimester, but the levels of this enzyme vary enormously, possibly reflecting variable alcohol consumption in pregnant women. UGT1A and UGT2B enzymes are present in the placenta throughout pregnancy but, like the CYP enzymes, UGT enzyme activity is highly variable. It is thought that placental UGT enzymes play a role in placental metabolism through formation of polar metabolites that are then more easily eliminated from the fetal compartment.

Drug metabolism in the fetus

Drugs that cross the placenta enter the fetal circulation via the umbilical vein; 40–60% of umbilical venous blood enters the liver, with the remainder entering directly into the fetal circulation. Drug effects in the fetus can be more significant and prolonged than in the mother because the fetus in general has immature liver drug-metabolising enzymes and thus metabolises drugs differently from adults. Increased exposure of the fetus to a drug or its metabolites can occur if the metabolite produced by the fetus is toxic and binds to fetal plasma proteins, or if metabolism by the fetal liver results in the formation of a water-soluble metabolite that does not readily cross the placenta. Under these circumstances, drugs and metabolites accumulate in amniotic fluid, resulting in increased fetal exposure.

Renal excretion

During pregnancy renal blood flow and GFR increase 50–80%, causing an increase in the elimination rate of drugs excreted predominantly unchanged by the kidney, which may lead to the need for dosage adjustment. This increase in renal function starts shortly after conception and persists until the last few weeks of pregnancy when a reduction in GFR may be observed. To date there is very little information on whether pregnancy has any effect on drugs that are secreted or reabsorbed in the renal tubule. Drugs shown to have increased renal clearance include the antibiotics, ampicillin, cefuroxime, ceftazidime and piperacillin. Other drugs include lithium, sotalol, dalteparin and enoxaparin sodium (Anderson 2005). If drugs are absolutely necessary during pregnancy, they should be carefully selected and titrated to the desired clinical response.

Pharmacokinetic development during early life

Neonates

Although drug use in infants/children requires advanced knowledge and skills, neonates require special consideration because they lack many of the protective mechanisms of older children and adults. Their skin is thin and permeable, their stomachs lack acid and their lungs lack much of the mucous barrier. Neonates regulate body temperature poorly and become dehydrated easily. After the transition from in utero to life, neonates are solely dependent on their own drug-metabolising enzymes to metabolise drugs and chemicals. Delayed maturation of hepatic drug functionalisation and conjugation enzymes may account for the toxicity of some drugs in the newborn. Expression of CYPs changes markedly during development; CYP2E1 activity surges within hours of birth, as does that of CYP2D6. During the first week of life, activity of CYP2C9 and CYP2C19 becomes evident, while activity of CYP1A2 appears at 1–3 months of age. This immaturity of metabolic capacity results in slower drug clearance and prolonged elimination. For example, phenobarbital (phenobarbitone) plasma half-life is 70–500 hours in neonates (younger than 7 days), 20–70 hours in those younger than 1 month, 20–80 hours in children 1–15 years of age and 60–180 hours in young adults. UGTs also have unique maturation profiles. For example, glucuronidation of paracetamol is decreased

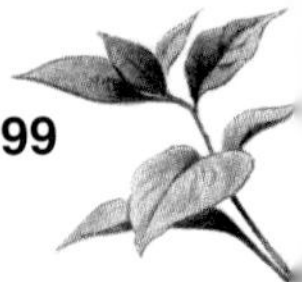

in newborns and young children in comparison to adolescents and adults, which reflects the delayed development of UGT1A6 and UGT1A9.

Infants/children

When an infant is 1 year old, drug absorption, distribution and excretion are in general similar to those of an adult. The exception is hepatic metabolism, where there is evidence of an age-dependent increase in hepatic clearance in comparison to adults. This increased drug clearance in children under the age of 10 years often necessitates a higher weight-based drug dosage. This concept is illustrated with the example of phenobarbital (phenobarbitone). The child reaches adult parameters at puberty, so drugs primarily eliminated by hepatic metabolism may require dosage adjustment and this must be individually determined and carefully monitored.

In infants, GFR reaches adult capacity between 8 and 12 months, while tubular function does not mature until the infant is around 12 months old. For drugs excreted primarily by the kidneys, the plasma half-life will be prolonged during the first week of life. (The lower the renal drug clearance, the longer the drug half-life in the body.) These developmental changes can alter dramatically the clearance of drugs that are renally excreted. Tobramycin is eliminated principally by glomerular filtration. Dosing for neonates (1 week of age or less) is up to 4 mg/kg per day. This may be administered in two equal doses every 12 hours.

Many drugs that are safe and effective for adults may not have been tested for use with children, nor have doses been established because of the complex medico–legal issues associated with the conduct of clinical trials involving children. Often a standard paediatric medication dosage is non-existent and doses are usually calculated according to the weight or body surface area of the child. Calculation formulae based either on the child's weight and age related to the adult or on the adult dose are inaccurate and should not be used. Children are not small adults and their pharmacodynamic and pharmacokinetic differences will definitely affect the dose of drug needed to produce a therapeutic effect. An infant's body composition is about 75% water (adults have 50–60%), and an infant has less fat content than the adult; therefore, water-soluble drugs are generally administered in larger doses to infants and children in proportion to body weight than to adults. A good example of this is the water-soluble drug gentamicin, an intravenous antibiotic. Recommended dosages (normal renal function) (intramuscular/intravenous) from the *Australian Medicines Handbook* are as follows.

For adults:

- systemic infection, severe UTI: 3 mg/kg/day in three divided doses (> 60 kg: usually 80 mg/dose, less than or equal to 60 kg: usually 60 mg/dose)
- life-threatening infection: initially 5 mg/kg/day in 3–4 divided doses, then 3 mg/kg/day when clinically indicated
- therapy duration usually 7–10 days.

For children aged 0–12 years:

- administer in 2–3 divided doses
- uncomplicated UTI: 3 mg/kg/day
- systemic infection: initially 4.5–6 mg/kg/day
- life-threatening infection: initially 5–7.5 mg/kg/day
- dose by age.

Drug exposure from breast milk

Many drugs or their metabolites cross the epithelium of the mammary glands and are excreted in breast milk. The risk to the infant of exposure to these drugs during breastfeeding depends on the maternal plasma drug concentration and the amount of milk ingested by the infant. Breast milk is acidic (pH 6.5); therefore, basic compounds with low plasma protein binding and high lipid solubility such as narcotics (e.g. morphine and codeine) achieve high concentrations in this fluid. A major concern arises over the transfer of such drugs from mothers to their breastfed babies, which can result in adverse effects such as sedation and failure to thrive.

KEY POINTS

Pregnancy and early life

- Physiological changes that occur during pregnancy can affect the absorption, distribution, metabolism and excretion of drugs.
- During pregnancy, increases in renal blood flow and GFR cause an increase in the elimination rate of drugs excreted predominantly unchanged by the kidney. This may lead to the need for dosage adjustment.
- The amount of drug diffusing at any given time depends on the maternal plasma drug concentration. Eventually, the fetal plasma drug concentration will equal the maternal drug concentration.
- Activities of placental drug-metabolising enzymes are altered in pregnant women who either abuse drugs, smoke or consume alcohol.
- The disposition of drugs in infants and children differs from that in adults because of factors such as growth, maturation of drug-metabolising enzymes, plasma and tissue binding, and physiological maturation of organ systems.

REVIEW EXERCISES

1. Following oral administration of a 100 mg dose of drug A to Mr MS, 60 mg is recovered in the urine as either unchanged drug or metabolites, and the remaining 40 mg is recovered as unchanged drug in the faeces. The hepatic clearance of drug A is 13.5 L/hr. Showing all calculations and stating all assumptions, determine the oral bioavailability of drug A.
2. Mr MS develops difficulty swallowing but still requires drug A (from review exercise 1), which must now be administered intravenously. Providing a short justification, estimate the intravenous dose of drug A that would be equivalent to a 100 mg oral dose of this drug.
3. Ms D has been prescribed the antiepileptic drug carbamazepine, but her seizures are not well controlled. Discuss the range of factors that could be contributing to her variability in response to the drug.
4. Mr G has presented to the emergency department of his local hospital with an aspirin overdose. A number of management measures were instituted, including administration of sodium bicarbonate. Explain why he has been administered sodium bicarbonate.

REFERENCES

Anderson GD: Pregnancy-induced changes in pharmacokinetics: a mechanistic-based approach, *Clinical Pharmacokinetics* 44:989–1008, 2005. [Seminal paper describing the changes in drug exposure that occur during pregnancy.]

Birkett DJ 2010, *Pharmacokinetics Made Easy: Pocket Guide* (2nd Edition), McGraw Hill, Sydney.

Birkett DJ, Grygiel JJ, Meffin PJ, et al: Fundamentals of clinical pharmacology; 4 Drug biotransformation, *Current Therapeutics* 6:129–138, 1979.

Miners JO, Bowalgaha K, Elliot DJ, et al: Characterization of niflumic acid as a selective inhibitor of human liver microsomal UDP-glucuronosyltransferase 1A9: application to the reaction phenotyping of acetaminophen glucuronidation, *Drug Metabolism and Disposition* 39:644–652, 2011.

Salerno E: *Pharmacology for health professionals*, St Louis, 1999, Mosby.

CHAPTER 5

PHARMACOKINETICS AND DOSING REGIMENS

Andrew Rowland

KEY ABBREVIATIONS

AUC	area under the plasma concentration versus time curve
CL	clearance
CL_S	systemic clearance
C_{SS}	steady-state plasma drug concentration
E_H	hepatic extraction ratio
F	bioavailability
$t_{1/2}$	half-life
V_D	volume of distribution

KEY TERMS

Chapter Focus

The choice of a drug for a patient is influenced by many factors, and using the right dose is essential both for achieving the desired effect and for limiting adverse effects. An understanding of pharmacokinetic principles allows selection of the right dose and the prediction of the effects of disease states, drug interactions and environmental factors on dosing regimens. The importance of the key pharmacokinetic concepts of clearance, volume of distribution and half-life are illustrated in this chapter using clinically relevant examples.

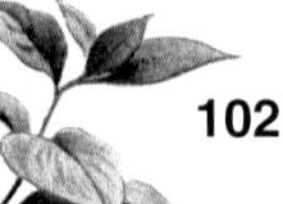

CRITICAL THINKING SCENARIO

Bernadette is a 43-year-old female with a history of epilepsy and has recently started taking 600 mg of carbamazepine (an antiseizure medication) twice daily to help control her seizures.

She has been admitted to hospital with suspected carbamazepine toxicity and a blood sample reveals that her carbamazepine blood concentration is 40 microg/mL. The reference target blood concentration range for carbamazepine is 4–12 microg/mL and the half-life of this drug is approximately 18 hours. It's important that Bernadette starts taking carbamazepine again (at a lower dose) as soon as possible to avoid a risk of having a seizure, but you need to wait long enough for it to be safe. Approximately how long (in terms of hours or doses) should staff wait before giving another dose of carbamazepine?

Introduction

The rational use of drugs is based on an assumption that a particular concentration of a drug will have the desired therapeutic effect and that adverse effects will be negligible. For many drugs, there is a sufficient relationship between plasma drug concentration and clinical response for dosing regimens to be designed to maintain the concentration within a therapeutic range. Because therapeutic ranges are generally derived from population-level data rather than from individuals, they are considered to reflect the range of drug concentrations having a high probability of producing the desired therapeutic effect and a low probability of producing adverse effects. For a limited number of drugs it is possible, and in some cases necessary, to adjust the dosing regimen to achieve the desired plasma concentration for an individual by considering their characteristics (e.g. age, health status, liver and kidney function) and the pharmacokinetics of the drug. This process, which has had many titles, is increasingly known as precision dosing.

Plasma concentration–time profile of a drug

Measuring the plasma concentration–time profile of a drug allows the relationship between the plasma drug concentration and the therapeutic response or toxicity to be visualised. For example, the theoretical drug in Figure 5.1 has been administered as a single oral dose. It

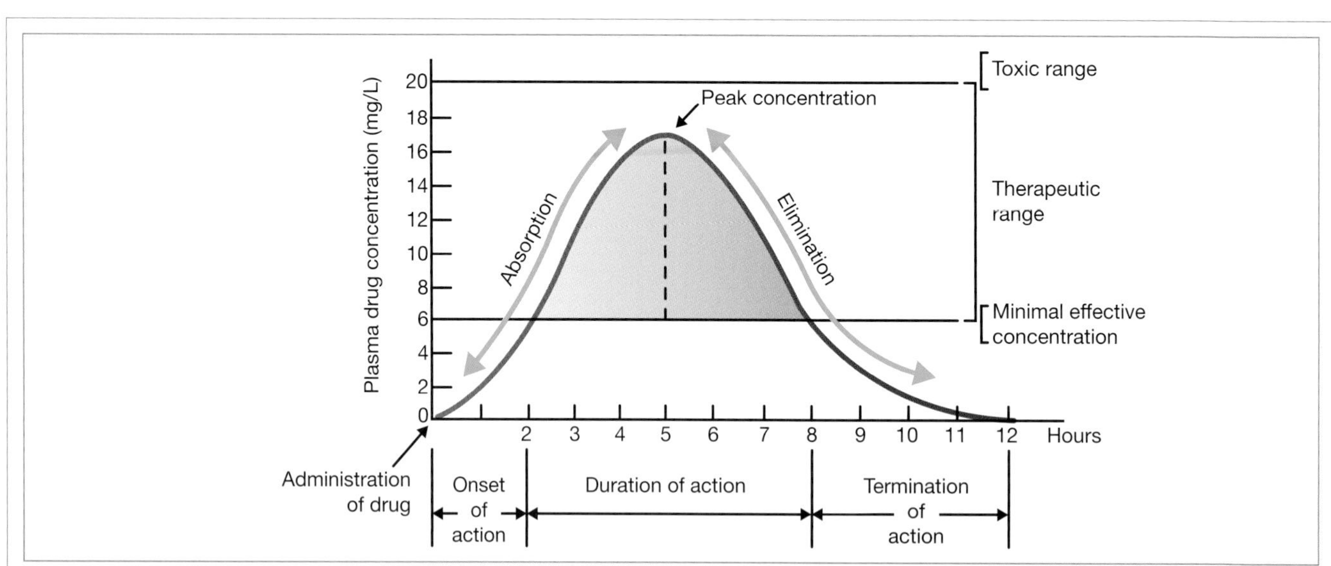

FIGURE 5.1 Plasma concentration–time profile for a theoretical drug administered as a single oral dose

Source: Adapted from Salerno 1999, Figure 4-7; used with permission.

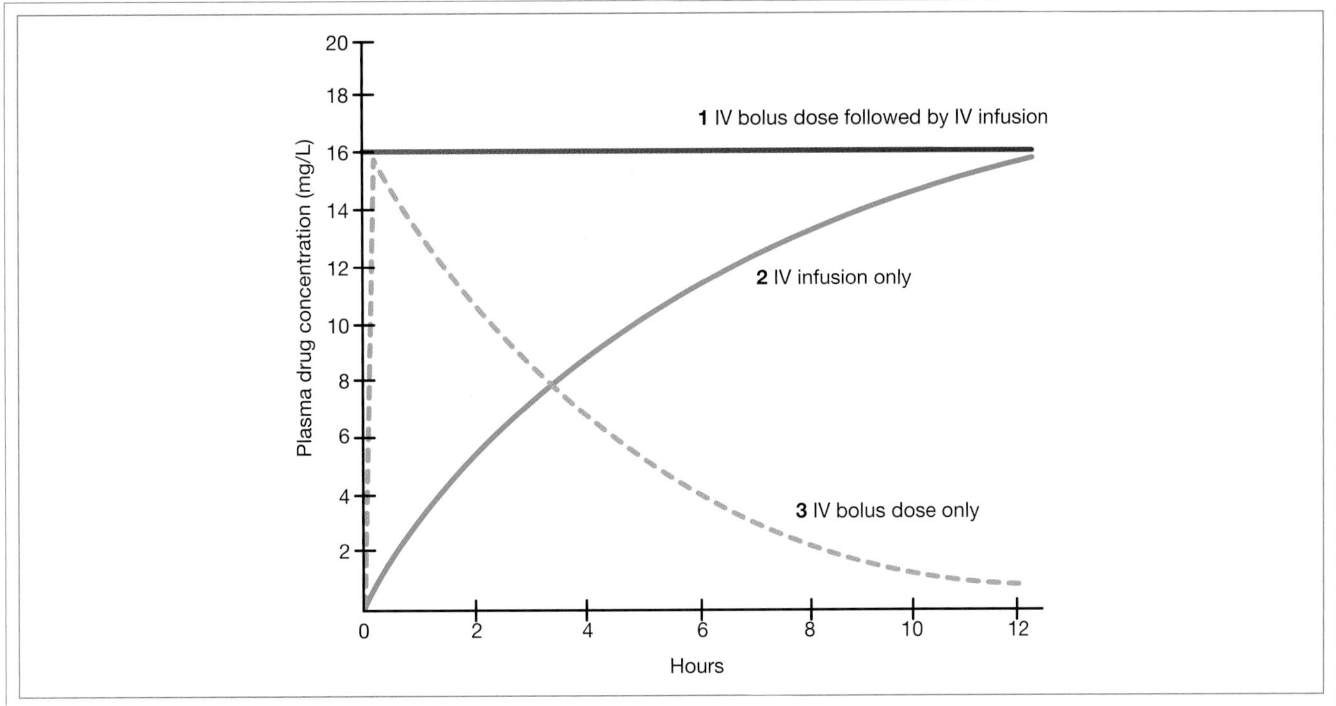

FIGURE 5.2 Plasma concentration–time profiles for a drug administered as (1) a single IV bolus dose followed by an IV infusion, (2) an IV infusion only and (3) a single IV bolus dose

has an onset of action of approximately 2 hours, a peak plasma concentration at 5 hours and a 6-hour duration of action (the length of time the plasma drug concentration remains within the therapeutic range). In this case, the processes of absorption, distribution and elimination (i.e. metabolism and excretion) influence the plasma concentration–time profile of the drug.

Intravenous (IV) administration of a drug as a single bolus dose followed by an infusion, or as a single bolus dose alone, or as an infusion alone, all give different plasma concentration–time profiles that are influenced by distribution and elimination but not by absorption (Fig 5.2).

How does this knowledge help you to design an appropriate dosing regimen? Buried within these plasma drug concentration–time profiles are the key pharmacokinetic parameters of **clearance**, **volume of distribution** and **half-life**. The clearance of a drug and its volume of distribution are determined by the characteristics of both the patient and the drug, whereas the plasma half-life of the drug is a composite parameter that is related directly to the volume of distribution of the drug and inversely to the clearance of the drug.

Area under the plasma concentration versus time curve

The **area under the plasma concentration versus time curve** (AUC) is exactly what the title suggests: the total area under the curve that describes the concentration of the drug in the systemic circulation as a function of time post-dose (normally zero until infinity). It can be used to calculate both the clearance of a drug after IV administration and its **bioavailability**. The latter is calculated by comparing the respective AUC values after IV and oral administration of the same dose of the same drug.

The AUC is most commonly determined by the 'trapezoid method', whereby the curve is divided into equal-sized strips, the areas of which are calculated and added together to give the final value. This process is illustrated in Figure 5.3.

Key pharmacokinetic concept: clearance

Clearance (CL) describes the ability of either an individual organ or the body to eliminate a drug. Clearances by each organ are additive and, hence, total clearance from the systemic circulation – that is, systemic clearance (CL_S) – reflects the total sum of all the clearance processes relevant to the particular drug (Fig 5.4):

$$CL_{Systemic} = CL_{Renal} + CL_{Hepatic} + CL_{Other}$$

In general, for most drugs unless indicated otherwise, clearance by other organs (e.g. the lungs) is negligible. For a particular drug and a specific person, providing they remain physiologically stable, clearance is constant. For example, if you measured the clearance of paracetamol

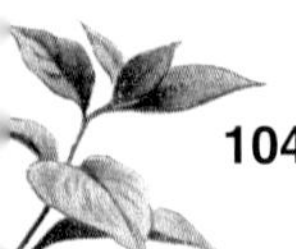

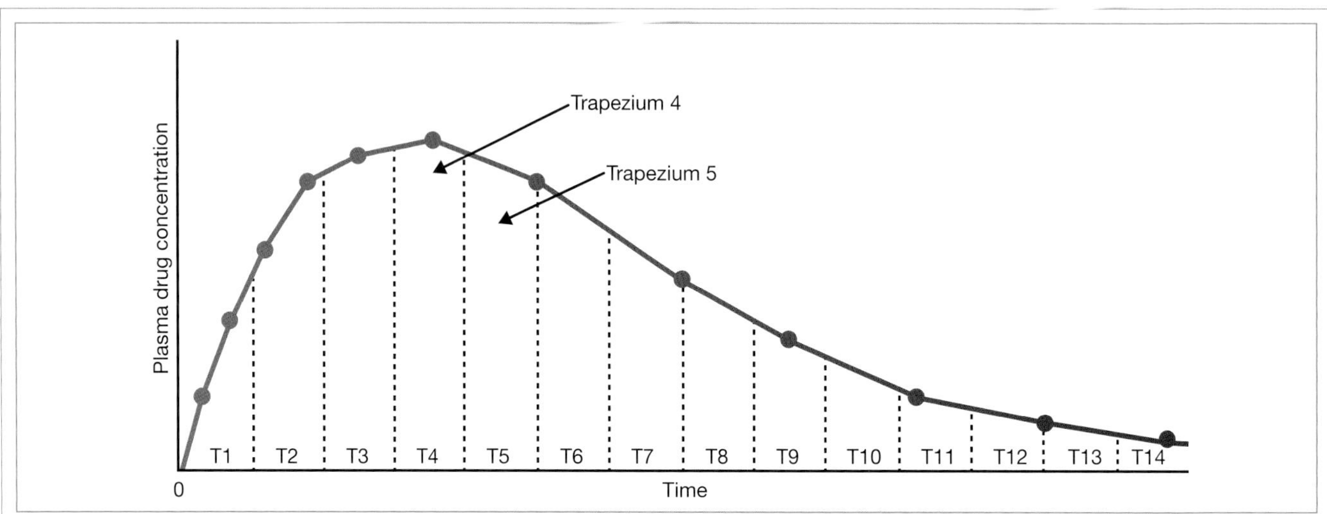

FIGURE 5.3 Plasma drug concentration versus time curve after an oral dose of a drug
The AUC is determined by calculating the area of each trapezium and summing the values. AUC = Area T1 + Area T2 + Area T3 + Area T4 ... + Area Tn.

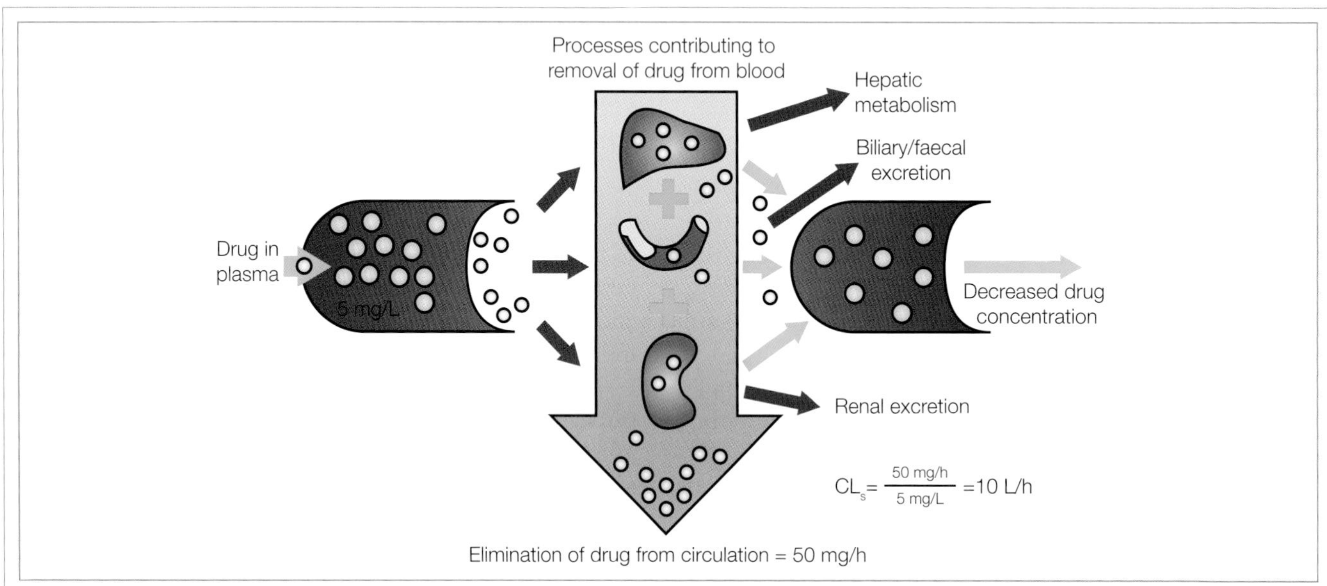

FIGURE 5.4 Concept of systemic (total body) clearance of a drug from plasma
Only some drug molecules are extracted from plasma on each pass of blood through the kidneys, liver or other sites contributing to drug elimination. In this example, the plasma drug concentration is 5 mg/L and the elimination rate is 50 mg/h; hence, systemic clearance is 10 L/h.

in yourself it should not change very much from day to day, provided the activity of your liver enzymes that metabolise paracetamol did not change. However, paracetamol clearance in a population will broadly reflect the inter-individual variability in the activity of drug-metabolising enzymes in that population.

Hepatic clearance

A drug will enter the liver in the blood delivered via the portal vein, which comes from the gastrointestinal tract, and via the hepatic artery, which comes from the systemic circulation. The rate of drug entering the liver is determined by multiplying liver blood flow (which is abbreviated as Q_H and assumed to be equal to 90 L/hr) by the concentration of drug in blood entering the liver (which is abbreviated as C_{in}). A drug will leave the liver in the blood via the hepatic vein and be returned to the systemic circulation. The rate of drug leaving the liver is determined by multiplying liver blood flow Q_H by the concentration of drug in the blood leaving the liver (which is abbreviated as C_{out}). By definition, we can say that the difference between the concentration of drug entering the liver and the concentration of drug exiting the liver (i.e. the amount that is extracted) divided by the concentration of drug entering the liver is equal to the hepatic extraction ratio (E_H), which defines the proportion of drug that is extracted. Hepatic clearance (CL_H) is simply calculated as this extraction ratio multiplied by the volume of blood passing through the liver per unit of time using the equation:

$$CL_H = E_H \times Q_H$$

Drugs cleared by the liver are classified, according to the relationship between CL_H and Q_H, as having either a low, intermediate or high hepatic clearance based on the following criteria:

- low hepatic clearance: $CL_H < 20$ L/h or $E_H < 0.2$
- intermediate hepatic clearance: CL_H between 20 and 60 L/h, or E_H between 0.2 and 0.67
- high hepatic clearance: $CL_H \geq 60$ L/h or $E_H \geq 0.67$.

Low hepatic clearance drugs are considered to be 'capacity limited'; that is, the capacity of the enzymes in the liver to clear the drug is the limiting factor in determining extraction, whereas high hepatic clearance drugs are considered to be availability limited; that is, the delivery of the drug (in the blood) to the liver is the limiting factor determining extraction. Examples of drugs in these categories are shown in Table 5.1. Low hepatic clearance does not mean that the drug is then cleared by the kidneys; it indicates that the capacity of the hepatic enzyme or enzymes to metabolise the drug is low and therefore the drug will simply be cleared more slowly.

TABLE 5.1 Examples of drugs with either a low, intermediate or high hepatic clearance

LOW CLEARANCE	INTERMEDIATE CLEARANCE	HIGH CLEARANCE
Carbamazepine	Caffeine	Lidocaine (lignocaine)
Diazepam	Fluoxetine	Morphine
Ibuprofen	Midazolam	Propofol
Phenytoin	Omeprazole	Propranolol
Warfarin	Paracetamol	Zidovudine

Effects of enzyme induction and inhibition on hepatic clearance

For an orally administered drug, induction of drug metabolism will typically result in a decrease in drug exposure, and inhibition will typically result in an increase in drug exposure; however, the way this happens differs between high- and low-CL_H drugs. Recalling that the liver can play a role in determining both bioavailability and clearance, the impact of altered enzyme activity will depend on how significant the induction or inhibition is in proportion to the role of the liver in the given context. For example, for a low hepatic clearance drug, the effect of first-pass metabolism on oral bioavailability will always be low (as by definition $E_H < 0.2$ for a low-CL_H drug, f_H for a low-CL_H drug will be greater than 0.8), meaning that most of the drug escapes first-pass metabolism. Because the overall effect of first-pass metabolism on bioavailability for a low-CL_H drug is inherently minor, the impact of any change in first-pass metabolism will also be negligible. However, as by definition clearance is 'capacity limited' for a low-CL_H drug, any changes in this capacity limited clearance process are likely to be important. The different impacts of induction and inhibition of hepatic drug metabolising enzyme activity on bioavailability and clearance (and drug exposure) for low- and high-CL_H drugs is summarised in Table 5.2.

Renal clearance

Renal drug clearance is the net effect of glomerular filtration, active secretion and passive reabsorption. Because only unbound drug (f_u = fraction of drug unbound in plasma) is filtered at the glomerulus, clearance by glomerular filtration (CL_{GF}) can be calculated as:

$$CL_{GF} = f_u \times GFR$$

where GFR is the glomerular filtration rate (assumed to be 7.2 L/hr for a healthy adult).

As all drugs must be partially unbound in plasma, they must be filtered to some extent. We can therefore assume that renal clearance always has a component of $f_u \times$ GFR. Hence, for any drug where renal clearance is greater than $f_u \times$ GFR, there must be a significant component of the

TABLE 5.2 Impact of changing enzyme activity on clearance and bioavailability for low- and high-CL_H drugs

EFFECT ON ENZYME ACTIVITY	LOW-CL_H DRUG		HIGH-CL_H DRUG	
	CLEARANCE (CL_H)	BIOAVAILABILITY (F)	CLEARANCE (CL_H)	BIOAVAILABILITY (F)
Induction	Increased *(decreased drug exposure)*	Negligible *(drug exposure essentially unchanged)*	Negligible *(drug exposure essentially unchanged)*	Decreased *(decreased drug exposure)*
Inhibition	Decreased *(increased drug exposure)*	Negligible *(drug exposure essentially unchanged)*	Negligible *(drug exposure essentially unchanged)*	Increased *(increased drug exposure)*

drug secreted into the renal tubule. There may also be some reabsorption of the drug, but it would always be minor in comparison to secretion. Conversely, if renal clearance is less than $f_u \times$ GFR the drug must be significantly reabsorbed and secretion would then be the minor component. For most drugs, changes in renal function do not always necessitate an adjustment in drug dosage. However, when renal function is reduced to less than half and the drug is more than 50% cleared by the kidneys, dosage adjustment is necessary. Digoxin and gentamicin are examples of drugs cleared by the kidneys for which the dosing regimen needs to be changed in those with renal impairment.

The importance of clearance

Continued drug administration eventually leads to a situation where the rate of drug going in equals the rate of drug going out and the plasma drug concentration remains constant. Clearance determines the maintenance dose rate (DR) required to achieve a target plasma concentration at **steady state** (C_{ss}).

$$\text{Maintenance dose rate (DR)} = CL_s \times \text{target steady-state plasma drug concentration } (C_{ss})$$

A sample calculation for a theoretical drug is shown below.

Maintenance dose calculation

Let us consider drug A, for which the target plasma concentration at steady state is 12.5 mg/L. Because the person to be given the drug has an acute condition, it is decided to administer drug A initially as an IV infusion. The clearance of drug A is 8 L/h and the volume of distribution is 40 L. With IV administration, the bioavailability is 1 (100%).

$$\begin{aligned} DR &= CL_s \times C_{ss} \\ &= 8 \text{ L/hr} \times 12.5 \text{ mg/L} \\ &= 100 \text{ mg/hr} \end{aligned}$$

Thus the infusion rate should be 100 mg/h.

Because the person's condition improves, it is decided to switch to an oral dosing regimen, but it is essential to maintain the plasma drug concentration. The oral formulation has a bioavailability (F) of 0.8 (80%) and the recommended dosing interval is 8-hourly. Thus, the oral maintenance dose can be calculated.

$$\begin{aligned} \text{Maintenance dose} &= DR \div F \times \text{dosing interval} \\ &= 100 \text{ mg/hr} \div 0.8 \times 8 \text{ hr} \\ &= 1000 \text{ mg} \end{aligned}$$

A formulation close to the ideal dose would then be prescribed. In this case, drug A is available as a 500 mg capsule, so two capsules would be administered 8-hourly.

KEY POINTS

Clearance

- Clearance determines the maintenance dose rate required to achieve the target plasma concentration at steady state.
- The impact of induction and inhibition of drug metabolising enzyme activity on bioavailability and clearance differs between high- and low-CL_H drugs.

Key pharmacokinetic concept: volume of distribution

It is important to understand that the term 'volume of distribution' (V_D) of a drug is an abstract term and that it is not referring to a 'real' volume.

For example, if a drug is tightly bound to plasma proteins, most of it will remain within the circulatory system and it will have a volume of distribution similar to that of the blood volume. If, however, it is distributed out of the circulatory system and binds to tissue components (e.g. protein, fats), less remains in the blood and the drug will appear to be distributed in a larger volume. The larger the volume, the more widespread (tissue-bound) the drug is within the body. This is illustrated in Figure 5.5 using a bucket filled to its maximum capacity of 5 L, which is its actual or real volume. When the drug remains in the 'blood', volume of distribution remains at 5 L. However, when the drug distributes out of the 'blood', even though it is still a 5 L bucket, volume of distribution becomes 50 L.

If the volume of distribution is 'not a real volume', of what use is it clinically? First, it provides an indication of accumulation of drugs in extravascular (tissue) compartments (e.g. fat, muscle).

Second, it is a major determinant of the half-life of a drug. Third, on occasion it is necessary to achieve a high plasma concentration quickly to produce the desired therapeutic response. To do this, a loading dose is administered to 'fill up' the volume of distribution. The size of the loading dose is calculated by knowing the volume of distribution of the drug:

$$\text{Loading dose} = V_D \times \text{target plasma concentration (C)}$$

If we now consider drug A used in the maintenance dose calculation, the volume of distribution of drug A was known to be 40 L and the target plasma drug concentration was 12.5 mg/L.

$$\begin{aligned} \text{Loading dose} &= V_D \times C \\ &= 40 \text{ L} \times 12.5 \text{ mg/L} \\ &= 500 \text{ mg} \end{aligned}$$

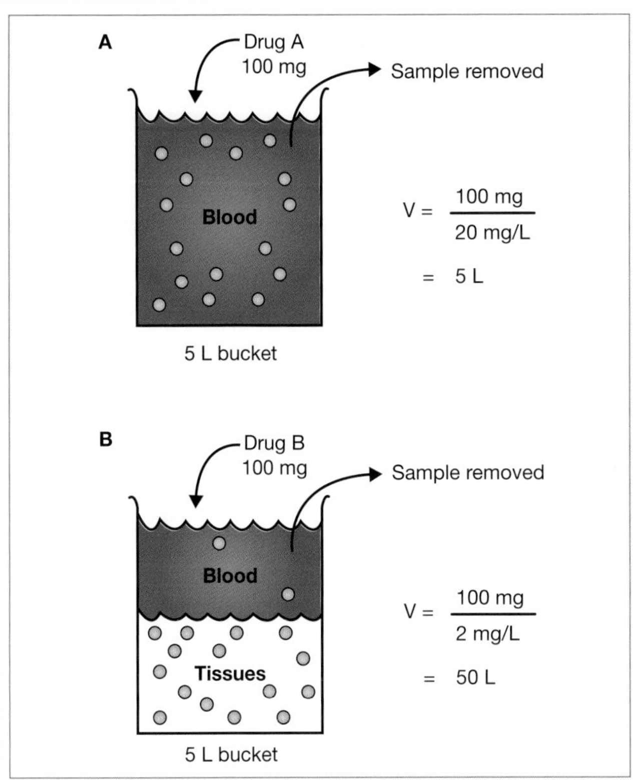

FIGURE 5.5 In this example, the volume of the full bucket is 5 L and the amount of drug placed in each bucket is 100 mg

After the drug has distributed, a 'blood' sample is removed from each bucket and the concentration of the drug is measured. **A** Bucket A is filled with 'blood' to represent the circulatory system. Drug A binds tightly to plasma proteins and remains within the circulation. The concentration of drug measured in the 'blood' sample is 20 mg/L and the calculated volume of distribution of drug A is 5 L, the same as the volume of the bucket. **B** Bucket B is filled with a mixture of 'blood' and 'tissues' to represent the intravascular and extravascular compartments. Drug B moves from the 'blood' and is distributed to the 'tissues', where it binds strongly to tissue proteins. The concentration of drug measured in the 'blood' sample is 2 mg/L, and the calculated volume of distribution of drug B is 50 L, 10 times greater than the volume of the bucket!

Thus, the loading dose would be 500 mg. Because rapid intravenous administration is often undesirable because of the high plasma concentrations achieved before the distribution phase, loading doses may be given over a period of minutes or even hours. In the example described above with drug A, the medical condition was acute and a loading dose (provided it was not contraindicated) could have been administered to produce a rapid pharmacological effect. Figure 5.2 shows that with the infusion alone it would take around 8 hours to achieve the desired plasma drug concentration (curve 2). In contrast, an IV bolus dose would raise the plasma drug concentration to the desired level almost immediately (Fig 5.2, curve 3).

The volume of distribution changes with age, body composition and disease states, and differs between males and females. For example, in infants under 1 year of age, volume of distribution is approximately 75–80% of body weight; in adult males, it is approximately 60% of body weight; and in adult females, it is 55% of body weight. As we age, there is also a progressive reduction in total body water and lean body mass with a relative increase in body fat.

> **KEY POINTS**
>
> **Volume of distribution**
>
> - The volume of distribution of a drug is defined as the volume in which the amount of drug in the body would need to be uniformly distributed in order to produce the observed concentration in blood.
> - The loading dose is the initial amount of drug required to fill the volume of distribution.

Key pharmacokinetic concept: half-life

Half-life ($t_{1/2}$) is a useful and commonly used parameter when describing a person's exposure to a drug. Indeed, half-life is the major determinant of:

- The duration of action of a drug after a single dose. If a drug is administered as a single dose, the longer the drug's half-life the longer the plasma drug concentration will remain within the therapeutic range (Clinical Focus Box 5.1).
- The time taken to reach steady state with chronic dosing. In general, it takes three to five half-lives to reach the desired steady-state plasma drug concentration (Fig 5.6).
- The dosing frequency required to avoid massive fluctuations in plasma drug concentration during the dosing interval. Once steady state has been reached, the half-life and the dosing interval determine the extent to which the plasma drug concentration fluctuates. If a drug is given orally every half-life, then the concentration will fall by one-half between doses and the plasma drug concentration will remain within the therapeutic range between doses (Fig 5.6).

Determinants of half-life

The two processes that influence half-life are distribution and clearance. Changes in either of these processes will alter the half-life of a drug. It can be seen from Figure 5.7 that, if two drugs have the same clearance but different

CLINICAL FOCUS BOX 5.1

The dilemma of the missed dose

Often the question is raised, 'What do I do if I forget to take my medication?' Inevitably, on one or more occasions, a person will miss a dose of their drug. The simple issue of what to do if this occurs is rarely explained to patients, and an unintentionally missed dose is construed too readily as noncompliance. For some drugs (e.g. a lipid-lowering drug), a missed dose is of little consequence, but for others a missed dose can result in a decrease in the therapeutic plasma concentration and subsequent clinical manifestations (e.g. epilepsy). Pregnancy as a result of missing a dose of the oral contraceptive pill is well recognised.

Knowledge of the drug's half-life is useful for making a recommendation if a dose is missed. In general, when the clinical effect of a drug is related to its half-life, a single missed dose is less of a problem for a drug with a long half-life than for a drug with a short half-life, for which the therapeutic effect will be lost rapidly. For some drugs (e.g. the oral contraceptive pill), specific recommendations exist for when a single dose is missed. A double dose should usually not be taken to make up for the dose missed because with many drugs (e.g. warfarin) this can cause adverse effects. The normal dosing regimen should be resumed and the next prescribed dose taken at the normal time.

Source: Gilbert et al. 2002.

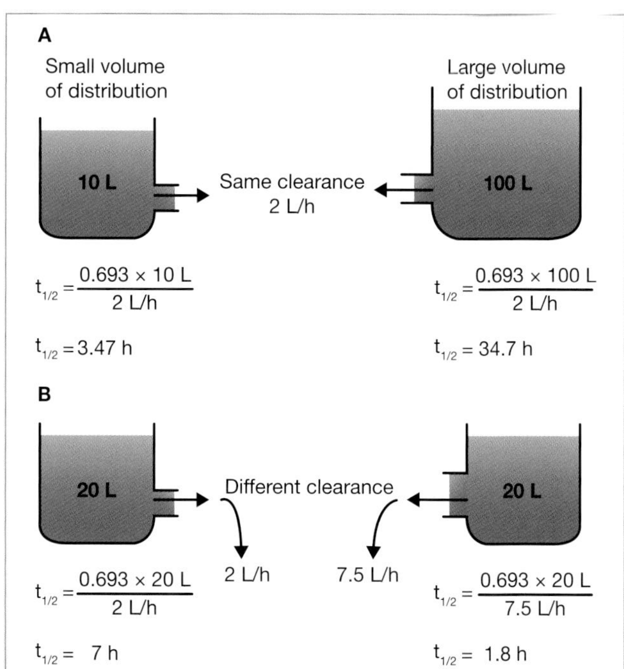

FIGURE 5.7 Effects of volume of distribution and clearance on half-life

In A the drugs have the same clearance but differing volumes of distribution, and the half-lives differ by about 10-fold. In B the drugs have the same volume of distribution but clearances differ about fourfold. In both examples the half-life alters in relation to the change in volume of distribution or the change in clearance.

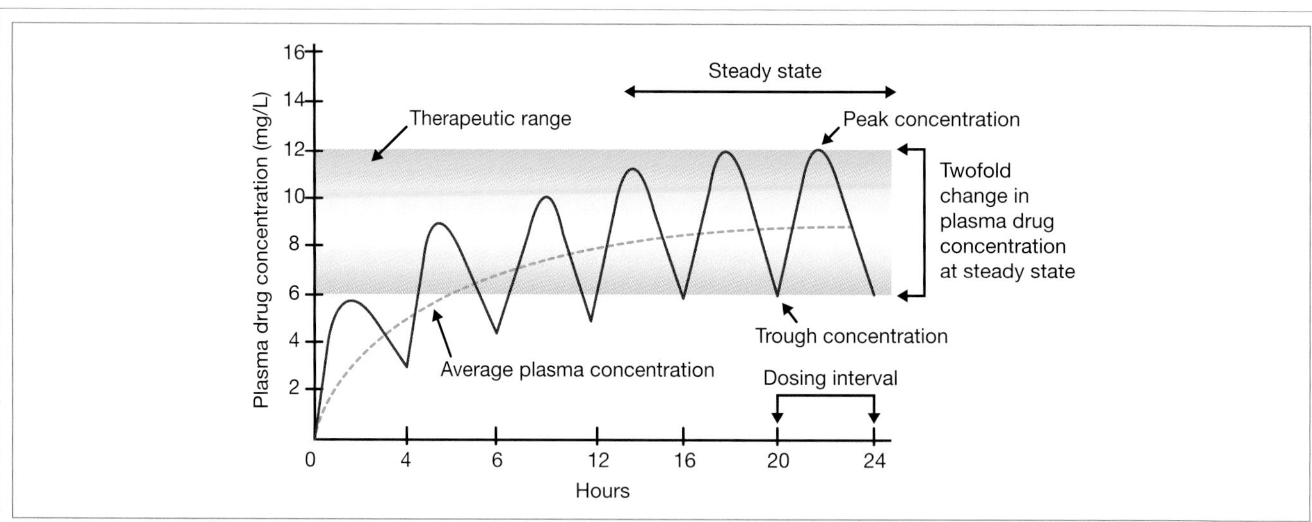

FIGURE 5.6 In this example, the drug has a half-life of 4 hours and is given orally every 4 hours

After one half-life the average plasma concentration is 50% of the eventual steady-state concentration, which is reached after three to five half-lives. Once steady state is reached, the plasma drug concentration will fluctuate twofold between doses if dosing continues on the half-life.

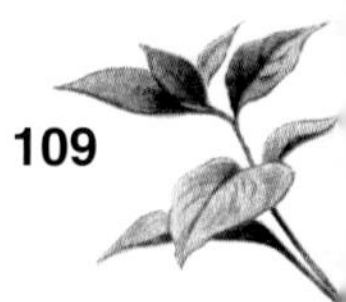

volumes of distribution, the half-life will be shorter for the drug with the smaller volume of distribution. Similarly, if the two drugs have the same volume of distribution but different clearances, the half-life will be shorter for the drug with the higher clearance. This simple relationship explains why the half-life of a drug can change in people with heart failure because of decreased volume of distribution and decreased liver blood flow, and in those with liver or kidney disease because of changes in clearance. Changes in half-life may necessitate changes in the dosing regimen.

KEY POINTS

Half-life

- Half-life is the major determinant of the duration of action of a drug after a single dose, the time taken to reach steady state with chronic dosing and the dosing frequency to minimise fluctuations in plasma drug concentration.
- The processes influencing half-life are volume of distribution and clearance.

Saturable metabolism

The last situation to consider is saturable metabolism, which is particularly relevant to some hepatically cleared drugs. Anyone who has consumed alcohol to excess will have experienced the consequences of saturable hepatic metabolism. How often the comment is made that 'It was the last drink that made me drunk', and how true that is!

Our previous discussion of half-life assumed first-order kinetics; that is, a constant proportion of the drug is eliminated per unit of time. In that situation, clearance and half-life are constant for a particular drug and the person. As the blood concentration of the drug increases, the rate of elimination also increases. This process is illustrated in panel A of Figure 5.8.

However, when saturable metabolism occurs, the maximum capacity and the rate of metabolism cannot increase further as the dose increases. This is called zero-order kinetics, and in this situation the rate of elimination does not increase in proportion to the dose and concentration. At this stage, metabolism is said to be 'saturated' and clearance and half-life are no longer constant. Clearance continually decreases, and half-life continually increases, as the dose and blood concentration increase. In this situation, a small change in dose can cause a large increase in the plasma drug concentration

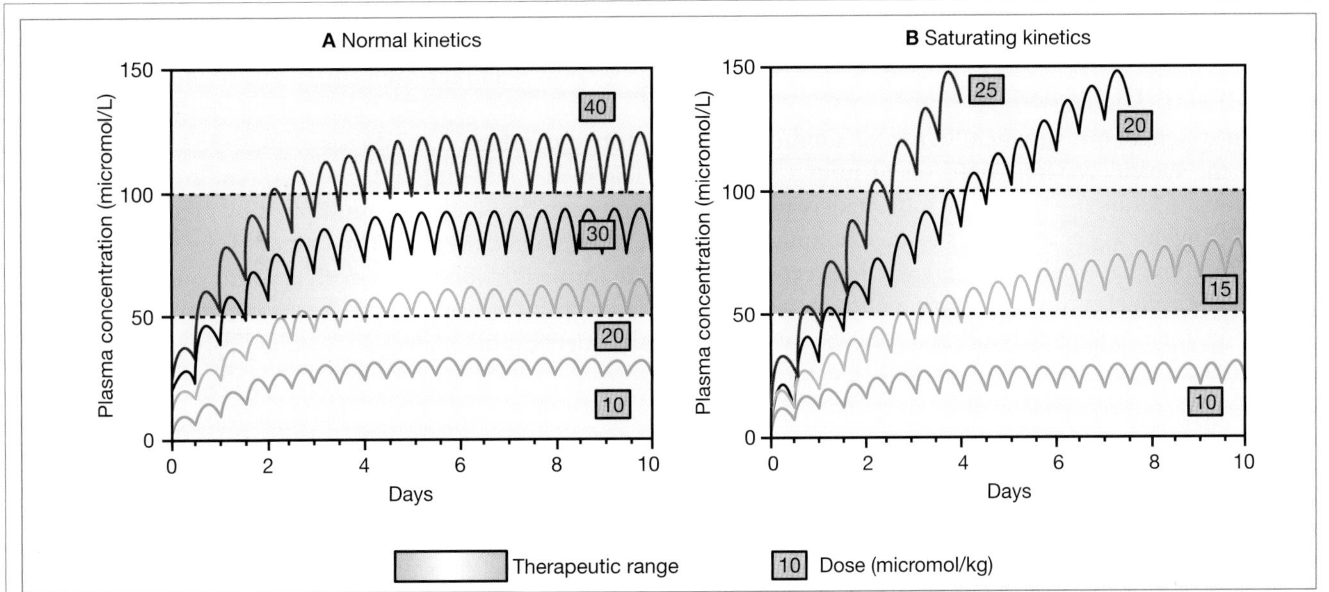

FIGURE 5.8 Comparison of non-saturating and saturating kinetics for drugs given orally every 12 hours
A The curves show an imaginary drug, similar to the antiepileptic drug phenytoin at the lowest dose, but with linear kinetics. The steady-state plasma concentration is reached within a few days, and is directly proportional to dose. **B** Curves for saturating kinetics calculated from the known pharmacokinetic parameters of phenytoin. Note that no steady state is reached with higher doses of phenytoin and that a small increment in dose results after a time in a disproportionately large effect on the plasma concentration. (Curves were calculated with the Sympak pharmacokinetic modelling program written by Dr JG Blackman, University of Otago.)
Source: Rang et al. 2012, Figure 10.9; reproduced with permission from Elsevier.

TABLE 5.3 Summary of key pharmacokinetic concepts

CONCEPT	SYMBOL	EQUATION	PARAMETERS AND COMMON UNITS
Bioavailability	F	$F = f_g \times f_H$	f_g = fraction of oral dose absorbed f_H = fraction of drug escaping hepatic extraction
Systemic clearance	CL_S	$CL_H + CL_R + CL_{Other}$	CL_S = L/h
Hepatic clearance	CL_H	$CL_H = E_H \times Q_H$	CL_H = L/h or mL/min Q_H = liver blood flow = 90 L/h
Hepatic extraction ratio	E_H	$E_H = CL_H \div Q_H$	Ratio
Renal clearance by glomerular filtration	CL_{GF}	$CL_{GF} = f_u \times GFR$	f_u = fraction of drug unbound in plasma GFR = glomerular filtration rate
Maintenance dose rate (IV dose)	DR	$DR = CL \times C_{SS}$	DR = mg/h C_{SS} = mg/L
Concentration at steady state (IV dose)	C_{SS}	$C_{SS} = DR \div CL$	CL = L/h or mL/min
Concentration at steady state (oral dose)	C_{SS}	$C_{SS} = F \times DR \div CL$	F = bioavailability = 0–1
Loading dose	LD	$LD = V_D \times C$	V_D = volume of distribution (L) C = target plasma concentration (mg/L)
Half-life	$t_{1/2}$	$t_{1/2} = 0.693 \times V_D \div CL$	$t_{1/2}$ units can be minutes or hours or days or weeks, etc.

because clearance is decreased. This is illustrated in panel B of Figure 5.8 for the antiepileptic drug phenytoin. As a consequence of the zero-order kinetics, it is necessary to increase the phenytoin dose in small increments. Other drugs that exhibit saturable metabolism include salicylic acid and, of course, ethanol.

Key pharmacokinetic concepts are summarised in Table 5.3.

Dosage measurements and calculations

Measurement systems

The main system of measurement in use for administering drugs is the metric system, based on SI units (Système International d'Unités) – this is the most widely used and the most convenient because units change in multiples of 10. Useful conversion tables to convert between metric measures and imperial ones, such as inches or pints, are included in some reference books, or conversions can be done online.

Metric system

The metric system has several basic units of measure including:

- length, the metre (m)
- time, the second (s)
- mass, the kilogram (kg)
- amount of substance, the mole (mol).

Derived units

Other useful derived units are: for volume, the cubic metre (m^3); for area, the square metre (m^2); for temperature, degrees Celsius (°C); and for mass, the gram (g). Other accepted units are the minute (min), the litre (L; 1 L = 1000 cm^3) and, for mass of atoms or molecules, the atomic mass unit (u), approximately equal to the mass of a hydrogen atom (also sometimes referred to as the dalton, Da).

The mole is the amount of any substance that contains Avogadro's number (about $6.022 \times 10_{23}$) of atoms or molecules of the substance, and is equivalent to the molecular weight expressed in grams. The mole is therefore a different weight depending on the substance; for example, 1 mole of sodium chloride (molecular weight 58.5) is present in 58.5 g pure NaCl and 1 mole of water in 18 g pure H_2O. This unit is used mainly in laboratories and research situations, not for dosing drugs.

Metric prefixes

The metric system is a decimal system in which the basic units can be divided or multiplied by 10, 100 or 1000 to form a secondary unit. The names of the secondary units are formed by joining a Greek or Latin prefix to the name of the primary unit (Table 5.4); for example, the gram is the metric unit of weight commonly used in weighing

TABLE 5.4 Metric prefixes, meanings and relations

PREFIX	MEANING	POWER OF 10
giga (G)	billions (thousand millions)	10^9, 1 000 000 000
mega (M)	millions	10^6, 1 000 000
kilo (k)	thousands	10^3, 1 000
hecto (h)	hundreds	10^2, 100
deca, deka (da)	tens	10^1, 10
deci (d)	tenths	10^{-1}, 1/10, 0.1
centi (c)	hundredths	10^{-2}, 1/100, 0.01
milli (m)	thousandths	10^{-3}, 1/1000, 0.001
micro	millionths	10^{-6}, 0.000 001
nano (n)	billionths	10^{-9}

chemicals and various pharmaceutical preparations. A gram is 1/1000 of a kilogram, and 1000 times greater than a milligram. Hence to change milligrams to grams, divide by 1000, and to change metres to centimetres, multiply by 100. When performing dose calculations the unit micro (µ) should be written out or micro used if there is a possibility of confusion with 'm'. (A mistake, such as dosing a patient with 250 mg digoxin instead of 250 microg, could be fatal.)

Conventional notations

The following is the style of notation as recommended for the International System of Units:

- Units are not capitalised (gram, not Gram).
- No full stop should be used with unit abbreviations (mL, not m.L. or mL.).
- Only decimal notation should be used, not fractions (0.25 kg, not 1/4 kg).
- Quantities less than 1 should have a zero placed to the left of the decimal point (0.75 mg, not .75 mg) to avoid mistakes.
- Abbreviations should not be made plural (10 kg, not kgs).
- There is a space between the numerical value and the unit symbol (100 g, not 100g).

There are some situations in medicine in which SI units are not used. These include:

- Percentage solutions, where the strength of a solution may be expressed as a percentage (e.g. 2% solution) rather than in mol/L or g/L. By convention, in this context '%' means grams of solute per 100 mL solution.
- Drip rates for infusion sets. Commonly, a standard set delivers 20 drops of aqueous liquid per mL (15 drops for blood), whereas a microdrip set delivers 60 drops per mL.
- Electrolyte solutions, which may be expressed in milliequivalents (mEq). For example: 1 L of a 1 mM solution of calcium chloride ($CaCl_2$) contains 1 mEq calcium ions and 2 mEq chloride ions.

Dosage calculations

When in doubt, it is advisable to double-check all calculations with another health professional, especially with a pharmacist who will be highly trained in dose and concentration calculations. The examples of dose calculations in Appendix 4 are the types of problems that may be encountered. Each problem is solved in a step-wise manner, in some cases showing alternative possible methods. Where appropriate, helpful hints are included.

Body surface area for paediatric drug dosing

Nomograms for the estimation of body surface area from weight and height can be found in common drug guides. When specific dosage information is not available, specialist information should be sought from the drug information services in major hospitals.

Although rules have been devised for converting adult dosage schedules to those for infants and children, it must be emphasised that no rules or charts are adequate to guarantee safety of dosage at any age, particularly in the neonate. Always take care to check whether the drug doses are expressed either as a mg/kg/dose or on a mg/kg/24 hours basis. No method takes into account all variables, particularly inter-individual differences. The calculated dose is a guide for initiating therapy, but the severity of the primary disorder, the presence of co-existing conditions, clinical response and therapeutic drug monitoring all contribute to ascertaining the optimal dose.

Rounding off

As dosage calculations underpin a physical activity, there are some logistical limitations associated with this activity that need to be accounted for. For example:

- the capacity to administer a fraction of a drop in an infusion (round off to whole number)
- the capacity to administer a small fraction of a mL in a syringe (round off to 1 decimal place).

REVIEW EXERCISES

1. Mr DE is taking propranolol (a high-hepatic clearance drug) and is administered a second drug that is known to inhibit the metabolism of propranolol. Should his dose of propranolol be adjusted? If the current dose is maintained, what are the possible clinical consequences?
2. Mrs WS is to be changed from her IV drug infusion to an oral formulation and it is important that the plasma drug concentration is maintained: the current dose rate is 50 mg/h, the dosing interval for the oral formulation is 6-hourly and the bioavailability of the oral drug is 0.75. Calculate the dose required every 6 hours.
3. Mr CK is commenced on a low dose of the antiepileptic drug phenytoin and his dose increased in small increments to achieve a desirable effect. Explain why it is important that increases in doses of phenytoin are made in small increments.

REFERENCES

Gilbert A, Roughead L, Sansom L: I've missed a dose; what should I do? Australian Prescriber 25:16–18, 2002.

Rang HP, Dale MM, Ritter JM, et al: Rang and Dale's pharmacology, ed 7, Edinburgh, 2012, Churchill Livingstone.

Salerno E: Pharmacology for health professionals, St Louis, 1999, Mosby.

CHAPTER 6
PRECISION MEDICINE
Andrew Rowland

KEY ABBREVIATIONS

CYP	cytochrome P450
DNA	deoxyribonucleic acid
EM	extensive metaboliser
HLA	human leucocyte antigen
PM	poor metaboliser
RNA	ribonucleic acid
SNP	single nucleotide polymorphism
TDM	therapeutic drug monitoring
TPMT	thiopurine methyltransferase
URM	ultra-rapid metaboliser

KEY TERMS

allele 114
genetic polymorphism 115
pharmacogenetics 114
phenotype 115
precision medicine 114
single nucleotide polymorphism 115
therapeutic drug monitoring 121

Chapter Focus

Two unfortunate features associated with the use of drugs are therapeutic failure and adverse reactions. It is not surprising that substantial effort is expended in trying to match the right dose of the right drug with the right patient. For some drugs it is useful to measure the concentration in the blood, while for others biological markers in the blood can assist in individualising the drug therapy to optimise response or avoid toxicity. If factors such as age, gender and disease are taken into consideration, the one remaining variable that can influence either efficacy or toxicity of a drug is the genetic makeup of the person. The Human Genome Project provided enormous advances in our ability to elucidate the genetic basis of inter-individual variability in drug response. Polymorphisms have been identified in drug-metabolising enzymes, drug transporters and multiple drug targets including receptors, ion channels and enzymes. This chapter provides an overview of the contemporary approaches used to individualise drug therapies and describes examples where these approaches have had an impact on patient care.

KEY DRUG GROUPS

Anticoagulants
Antiepileptics
Antineoplastics
Antiretrovirals
Immunosuppressants

CRITICAL THINKING SCENARIO

William, a 72-year-old male, started taking warfarin (an anticoagulant medicine) 6 months ago after experiencing a heart attack. Warfarin is a narrow therapeutic drug that is cleared by CYP2C9, an enzyme that has generic variants that are known to reduce warfarin clearance. We can predict a person's warfarin dose requirement based on their CYP2C9 genotype, or measure their warfarin blood concentration, but instead, when a person starts taking warfarin, we measure their INR (a marker of coagulation and response to warfarin). Considering the hierarchy of things we care about when giving someone a drug, why does this make sense?

Introduction

Wide variability in drug response between individuals is a feature of many drugs, and this has led in more recent times to the concept of **precision medicine**. If we start from the basic premise of choosing the *right drug* for the *right patient* at the *right dose* and *time*, hence maximising efficacy and minimising toxicity, how then do we explain dramatically different responses to an optimised dosage regimen in different patients?

Variability in response can result from pharmacodynamic and/or pharmacokinetic factors. The latter include altered absorption (of orally administered drugs), distribution, metabolism and excretion. Factors known to influence renal drug clearance include age (neonatal period and elderly), renal dysfunction and cardiac failure, and these are often taken into account when determining drug dosage. However, accounting for variability in hepatic drug metabolism is more complex. Hepatic clearance can be affected by age, diet, hormonal factors, disease states, interactions (drug–drug, drug–herb) and environmental chemicals. However, of the plethora of factors that can influence hepatic drug clearance, it is now recognised that the largest inter-individual variability in drug response/toxicity often arises from inherited (genetic) differences that alter drug metabolism and/or the molecular targets of drugs, including transduction mechanisms downstream of the receptor.

Pharmacogenetics

The term '**pharmacogenetics**' was first proposed by Vogel in 1959 as the 'study of the role of genetics in drug response' (Müller & Rizhanovsky 2020). Simply stated, pharmacogenetics relates to the inheritance of genes that define a person's variability in drug exposure and response. Studies conducted more than 40 years ago demonstrated that identical twins resembled each other in terms of how they metabolised a drug, whereas fraternal twins (developed from separate eggs) showed variations similar to the general population. This was consistent with fraternal twins having different patterns of inheritance. Early examples of adverse outcomes led to research that focused primarily on identifying people with 'genetic differences' that placed them at risk of drug toxicity or adverse drug reactions. However, it is now evident that genetic factors can also predispose people to therapeutic failure.

DNA and protein synthesis

Deoxyribonucleic acid (DNA) has long been considered as the building block of life. The importance of DNA lies in the fact that it contains the information that codes for the synthesis of the proteins that ultimately determine the physical and chemical characteristics of the human body. Genes are arranged along chromosomes; human somatic cells have 46 chromosomes or 23 homologous pairs, one chromosome in each pair inherited from your father and one from your mother. Each chromosome consists of an uninterrupted length of DNA that represents multiple genes that may exist in alternative forms (**alleles**). Genetic information is stored in DNA (as well as in RNA, ribonucleic acid) as a set of three nucleotides called a triplet comprising a combination of adenine, cytosine, guanine or thymine (Fig 6.1). Each triplet is transcribed (copied) as a complementary sequence of three RNA nucleotides called a codon. Each codon specifies one amino acid, and a sequence of amino acids forms a protein molecule.

Variations in proteins not only occur between different species but also between people of the same species. This genetic variation between humans arises through mutations in genes that may occur in either our own cells or occurred in the genes we have inherited from our ancestors. Spontaneous mutations are a common occurrence in all species and occur as a result of either

Amino acid	Codon
Lysine (Lys)	AAA AAG
Glutamine (Gln)	CAA CAG
Aspartic acid (Asp)	GAC GAU
Histidine (His)	CAC CAU
Glycine (Gly)	CGA GGC GGG GGU

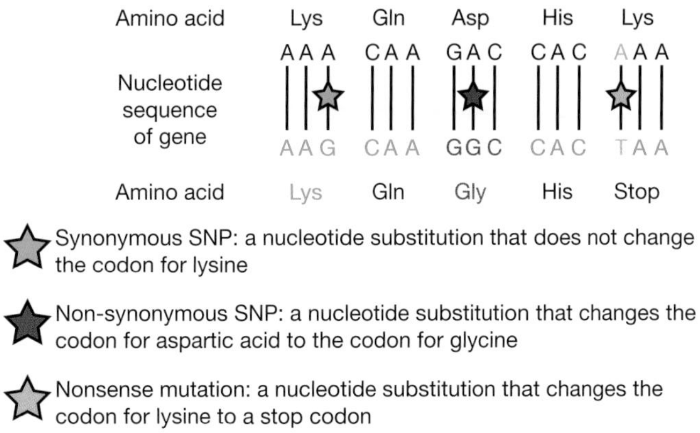

Amino acid	Lys	Gln	Asp	His	Lys
Nucleotide sequence of gene	AAA	CAA	GAC	CAC	AAA
	AAG	CAA	GGC	CAC	TAA
Amino acid	Lys	Gln	Gly	His	Stop

☆ Synonymous SNP: a nucleotide substitution that does not change the codon for lysine

★ Non-synonymous SNP: a nucleotide substitution that changes the codon for aspartic acid to the codon for glycine

☆ Nonsense mutation: a nucleotide substitution that changes the codon for lysine to a stop codon

FIGURE 6.1 Examples of single nucleotide polymorphisms (SNPs)
Most amino acids are represented by more than one codon, which is composed of three successive nucleotides. The codon specifies the amino acid, and the sequence of codons in the gene controls how the cell orders the assembly of amino acids into a specific protein. The Asp–Gly substitution illustrated is the molecular basis of the deficiency in butyrylcholinesterase activity.

normal cell function or random interactions with the environment. These mutations account for evolution. However, in some instances the mutation has consequences for our health; for example, a genetic disease may arise from a change in a single amino acid in a protein, or a mutation that arises from an environmental exposure (e.g. radiation exposure) may result in cancer.

Genetic polymorphism

It is well recognised that there is greater variability in drug response within a population than there is in an individual administered a drug on different occasions or between identical twins. Pharmacogenetic variability results from **genetic polymorphism** – that is, the presence of different allelic forms of a gene. Genetic polymorphism refers to a change in DNA sequence that occurs at an allele frequency of at least 1% in a population. DNA variations or mutations arise from changes in the components of DNA (i.e. the bases adenine, cytosine, guanine or thymine), which then results in a change in the nucleotide sequence. A change in the nucleotide sequence gives rise to a variant allele compared with the reference or 'wild-type' allele.

Polymorphisms that arise from substitution of one nucleotide for another are called **single nucleotide polymorphisms** (SNPs) (Fig 6.1). If an SNP that occurs in the coding region of a gene is a non-synonymous (missense) SNP it results in a change in an amino acid in the encoded protein, potentially altering the structure, stability, activity and ligand-binding properties of the protein. Synonymous (silent) SNPs do not incorporate a change in an amino acid but may alter a functional activity such as transcription efficiency. A nucleotide substitution that leads to a stop codon is called a nonsense mutation. Nucleotide insertions/deletions and frameshift mutations involving single or multiple nucleotides can also occur, and these may alter gene expression and/or protein structure and function. Additionally, genes may either be duplicated, resulting in enhanced protein synthesis, or completely deleted, with a consequential reduction in protein synthesis. All of these mechanisms have the potential to cause a 'genetic difference' in a person and hence to alter drug response.

Examples of drug-metabolising enzymes that exhibit genetic polymorphisms that influence drug response include:

- cytochrome P450 (CYP) (CYP1A2, CYP2A6, CYP2B6, CYP2C8, CYP2C9, CYP2C19, CYP2D6, CYP3A5)
- N-acetyltransferase (NAT2)
- thiopurine methyltransferase (TPMT)
- UDP-glucuronosyltransferases (UGT1A1, UGT1A4, UGT1A9, UGT2B15, UGT2B17).

Pharmacogenetic phenotypes

In general, if a mutation occurs in a single gene it gives rise to a monogenic trait that is evident from the phenotype. The **phenotype** refers to the clinical manifestation – for example, a person described as a 'slow acetylator' or 'fast acetylator' of isoniazid. For drug-metabolising enzymes, the genotype–phenotype associations for a monogenic trait are shown in Table 6.1 for people with wild-type (allele denoted as *1) and/or variant or 'mutant' (allele denoted as *2, *3, etc.) alleles. People who are homozygous for the wild-type allele are generally referred to as 'extensive metabolisers', and those who are homozygous for the recessive allele are referred to as 'poor metabolisers'. 'Intermediate metabolisers' carry

TABLE 6.1 Genotype–phenotype relationship

DRUG METABOLISING ENZYME PHENOTYPE	RELATIVE ENZYME ACTIVITY	GENOTYPE
Ultra-rapid metaboliser	High	*1/*1/*1 (>2 copies of gene)
Extensive metaboliser	Normal	*1/*1 (homozygous wild-type)
Intermediate metaboliser	Intermediate	*1/*2 (heterozygote)
Poor metaboliser	Low or absent	*2/*2 (homozygous variant)

one copy of the wild-type allele and one copy of the recessive allele. An 'ultra-rapid' metaboliser phenotype results in people who carry more than two copies of a gene. For example, CYP2D6 ultra-rapid metabolisers inherit between three and 13 copies of the CYP2D6 gene. Whereas people who are poor metabolisers eliminate drugs more slowly than extensive metabolisers, ultra-rapid metabolisers have high rates of metabolism. Plasma drug concentration–time profiles for all metabolisers of a hypothetical intermediate hepatic clearance drug are shown in Figure 6.2.

Ethnic and race-specific polymorphisms

The frequency of genetic polymorphisms differs between ethnic groups and between different races. For example, the homozygous silent variant of butyrylcholinesterase occurs at a frequency of one in 100,000 in European and American populations. In contrast, in ethnic groups such as the Vysya of India and the Alaskan Inuit, the frequency of the homozygous silent butyrylcholinesterase is one in 50 people.

Regarding CYP, the frequency of the CYP2D6 PM phenotype is 7–10% in Caucasians but only 1–2% in North Asian populations (Japanese, Chinese and Koreans). The frequency of the CYP2D6 URM phenotype is 2–3% in Caucasians, but as high as 25% in Northeast African populations (e.g. Ethiopians and Somalis). The CYP2D6 phenotype is of considerable clinical significance because CYP2D6 metabolises many clinically used drugs, some of which have narrow therapeutic indices. Examples include:

- antianginals – perhexiline
- antidysrhythmic – flecainide, propafenone
- β-adrenoceptor antagonists – metoprolol, timolol
- antidepressants – clomipramine, doxepin, fluoxetine, nortriptyline, paroxetine, venlafaxine
- antipsychotics – haloperidol, risperidone
- opioids – codeine, dextromethorphan, tramadol.

It is evident from these and other examples that genetic polymorphisms frequently differ between different races and ethnic groups. Clearly, in multicultural societies

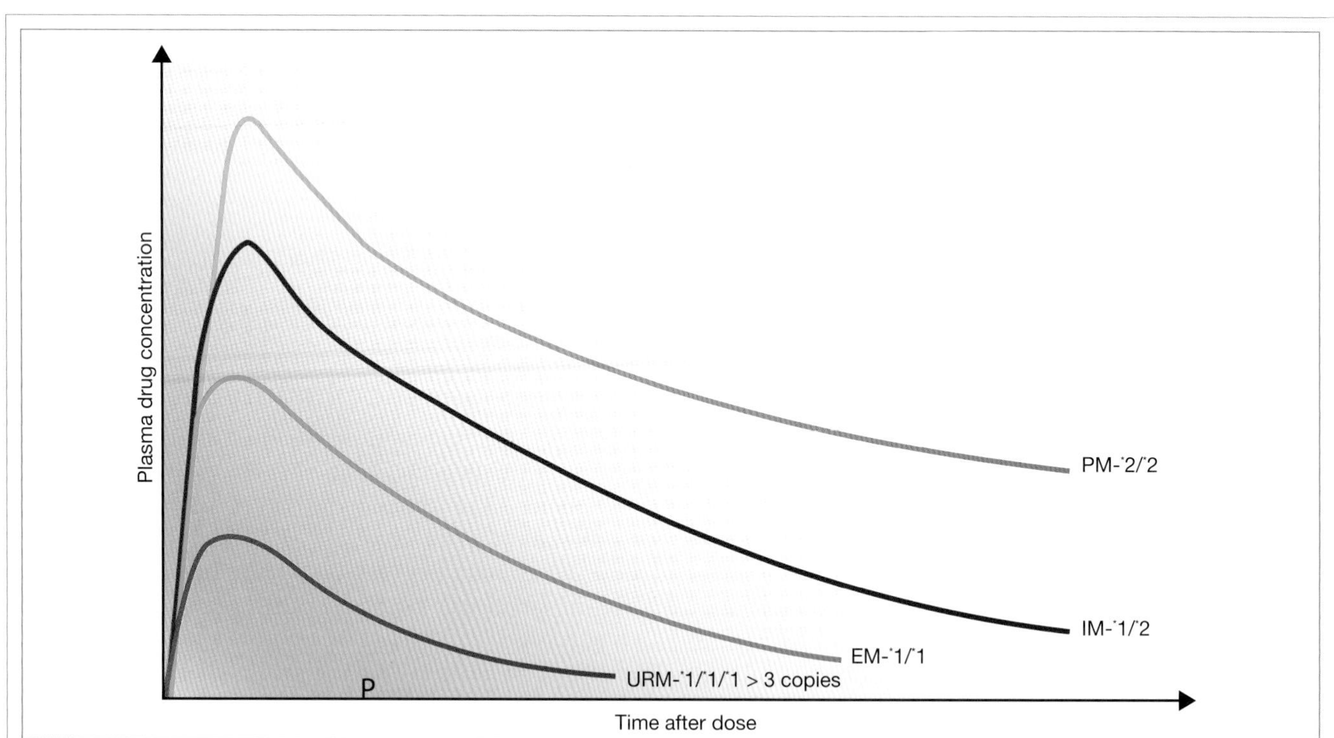

FIGURE 6.2 Impact of genotype and phenotype on drug clearance
Plasma drug concentration–time profiles for an ultra-rapid metaboliser (URM), extensive metaboliser (EM), intermediate metaboliser (IM) and poor metaboliser (PM) of a hypothetical intermediate/high hepatic clearance drug.

this creates a further layer of complexity when attempting to 'individualise drug therapy'.

KEY POINTS

Principles of pharmacogenetics

- Pharmacogenetic variability results from genetic polymorphism – that is, the presence of different allelic forms of a gene.
- A change in the nucleotide sequence gives rise to a variant or 'mutant' allele compared with the reference or 'wild-type' allele.
- Polymorphisms that arise from substitution of one nucleotide for another are called single nucleotide polymorphisms (SNPs).
- If a change occurs in a single gene, it gives rise to a monogenic trait that is evident from the phenotype. The phenotype refers to the clinical manifestation – for example, a person described as a 'poor metaboliser', 'extensive metaboliser' or 'ultra-rapid metaboliser'.

Pharmacogenetics in clinical practice

Arguably the greatest advances in the clinical use of pharmacogenetic testing in recent years have been in response to the rapid development of targeted anticancer medicines. In many cases, these drugs are specifically designed to target mutated proteins that promote tumour growth and metastatic invasion. The benefit derived from the use of targeted anticancer drugs may be influenced by the genotype of either the drug target or downstream proteins involved in the associated signalling cascade (Clinical Focus Box 6.1). When testing is performed to optimise drug dosing, it is generally based on phenotype using either measurement of a metabolic ratio (i.e. the metabolite-to-drug ratio in blood or urine) or direct measurement of the enzyme activity. The potential consequences of polymorphic drug-metabolising enzymes include:

- increased plasma drug concentration and duration of action
- decreased plasma drug concentration and therapeutic failure
- adverse drug reactions/toxicity
- failure to activate a prodrug
- drug metabolism via alternative pathways
- exacerbation of drug interactions.

The following sections describe some examples of clinically relevant pharmacogenetic polymorphisms.

CLINICAL FOCUS BOX 6.1
Predictive and prognostic genotypes in the treatment of colorectal cancer

An important example of the use of pharmacogenetic testing to influence treatment decisions is testing for mutations in the BRAF and RAS viral oncogenes in people with metastatic colorectal cancer (mCRC). mCRC can be treated with either an anti-EGFR mAb such as cetuximab and panitumumab or an anti-vascular endothelial grow factor mAb such as bevacizumab. People with an mCRC tumour bearing a mutation in one of the RAS oncogenes do not benefit from treatment with an anti-EGFR mAb and hence should be treated with bevacizumab. In this case, the RAS mutation status is predictive of treatment effect and can be used to directly guide the selection of one medicine over another. In subtle contrast to this, people with an mCRC tumour bearing a mutation in the BRAF oncogene have a more aggressive cancer and poorer prognosis, although the proportional size of the treatment benefit they derive from using an anti-EGFR mAb is not affected. In this case, the BRAF mutation status is prognostic of disease progression, but not predictive of treatment effect. As such, BRAF mutation status is not used to directly guide the selection of one medicine over another, but can be used by clinicians, along with other patient and tumour characteristics, in a more general manner to guide treatment.

Source: Sorich et al. 2016.

HER2

Trastuzumab targets the extracellular domain of the human epidermal growth factor receptor 2 (HER2). HER2 is encoded by the HER2/neu gene and plays a significant role in the proliferation of certain tumour cells. Clinically, the level of HER2 expression is important in guiding treatment decisions for those with breast cancer because it determines response to trastuzumab. HER2 expression is determined by the number of copies of the HER2/neu gene. This type of genotypic effect is known as copy number variation.

EGFR

Small-molecule kinase inhibitors inhibit the intracellular kinase domain of mutated kinase receptors in cancer cells and the therapeutic outcome is therefore dependent on the presence of specific mutations in the target kinase(s). Genotype can confer both sensitivity and resistance to these drugs. For example, activating mutations in exons 19 or 21 of the epidermal growth factor receptor (EGFR) confer sensitivity to small-molecule EGFR inhibitors such as erlotinib and gefitinib, while mutation of exon 20 (primarily T790M) of EGFR confers resistance to these drugs. Interestingly, second- and third-generation small-molecule EGFR inhibitors such as osimertinib have been developed specifically to overcome resistance caused by this T790M mutation.

BRAF

Mutations resulting in substitution of the valine residue at position 600 of the BRAF protein are observed in approximately 50% of people with advanced melanoma. The most common of these mutations, accounting for 90% of BRAF V600 mutations, is designated V600E. This mutation results in substitution of the valine residue at position 600 with a glutamic acid residue. BRAF is involved in the signalling pathway of growth factors (e.g. EGRF) required for normal cell proliferation and survival. BRAF V600E is 10 times more active as a protein kinase compared with wild-type BRAF and its presence leads to uncontrolled cell growth. Dabrafenib and vemurafenib are kinase inhibitors used in the treatment of metastatic melanoma that specifically target BRAF V600 mutations, inhibiting the mutated protein.

CYP2D6

Tamoxifen

Tamoxifen is commonly used to treat estrogen-responsive breast cancer. CYP2D6 metabolises tamoxifen to 4-hydroxytamoxifen, which is the precursor to endoxifen. Endoxifen is 100-fold more potent than tamoxifen as a selective estrogen receptor modulator (antagonist), and variability in the plasma concentration of endoxifen has been linked to CYP2D6 genotype and phenotype. If a person was a CYP2D6 PM, a lower plasma concentration of endoxifen would be predicted in comparison with a person who was an extensive metaboliser. While several retrospective studies have demonstrated an association between the CYP2D6 PM phenotype and a worse outcome on tamoxifen, other studies have been inconclusive. Prospective studies are required to confirm the benefit of CYP2D6 genotype-guided tamoxifen therapy.

Opioid analgesics

The analgesic effect of codeine arises largely from its conversion to morphine; about 10% of the codeine dose is converted to morphine by CYP2D6. Decreases in the plasma morphine concentration and analgesic response are observed in CYP2D6 PMs treated with codeine. By contrast, there is increased conversion of codeine to morphine in CYP2D6 URM and this may result in severe adverse effects, including respiratory depression (Clinical Focus Box 6.2). High plasma morphine concentrations and opioid toxicity, which may be fatal, have been observed in the breastfed infants of mothers taking codeine who are CYP2D6 URMs. Like codeine, tramadol is also converted to an active metabolite by CYP2D6. The active metabolite, O-desmethyltramadol, exhibits 200-fold higher affinity for the μ-opioid receptor than tramadol itself and thus the metabolite is a potent analgesic. Compared with CYP2D6 EMs, the efficacy of tramadol in poor metabolisers appears to be lower.

> **CLINICAL FOCUS BOX 6.2**
> **Codeine use in children**
>
> The US Food and Drug Administration (FDA) issued a safety warning in 2012 (updated in 2013) regarding the use of codeine as an analgesic in children after tonsillectomy and/or adenoidectomy. The FDA identified 13 cases of paediatric death in children receiving therapeutic doses of codeine, mostly in the setting of either adeno-tonsillectomy for obstructive sleep apnoea (eight cases) or respiratory tract infection (three cases). CYP2D6 metaboliser status was available for seven of the children who died: three were classified as CYP2D6 ultra-rapid metabolisers, three were extensive metabolisers and one was a likely ultra-rapid metaboliser. The enhanced conversion of codeine to morphine, particularly in the children who were CYP2D6 ultra-rapid metabolisers, can lead to high plasma concentrations of morphine and respiratory depression, even at therapeutic doses of codeine. Children with sleep apnoea and respiratory disorders may be more vulnerable as their breathing is already compromised. The contraindication to codeine and codeine-containing medications applies to all children undergoing tonsillectomy and/or adenoidectomy, irrespective of whether they have sleep apnoea. The FDA further advised that codeine should only be used for the treatment of other types of pain in children if the benefits outweigh the risk.
>
> *Source: Food and Drug Administration – see 'Online resources'.*

Perhexiline

Perhexiline is prescribed in Australia and New Zealand for the management of refractory angina. It has a narrow therapeutic index (plasma drug concentration range 0.15–0.6 mg/L) and exhibits dose-dependent kinetics. High plasma concentrations are linked to peripheral neuropathy and potentially fatal hepatotoxicity. The normal dose range for perhexiline to maintain a therapeutic plasma concentration varies markedly, from 50–100 mg/week in poor metabolisers to 50–400 mg/day in extensive and ultra-rapid metaboliser patients. Perhexiline is metabolised by CYP2D6, and this variability in dose requirement is explained by the presence of defective CYP2D6 alleles. There is good concordance between the ratio of plasma hydroxy-perhexiline (the principal metabolite of perhexiline) and plasma perhexiline concentration and CYP2D6 genotype.

CYP2C9

Warfarin

Warfarin is an anticoagulant drug that is administered as a racemic mixture (R- and S- enantiomers). S-warfarin is

TABLE 6.2 Warfarin maintenance doses based on CYP2C9 and VKORC1 genotypes

VKORC1	CYP2C9					
	*1/*1	*1/*2	*1/*3	*2/*2	*2/*3	*3/*3
GG	5–7 mg	5–7 mg	3–4 mg	3–4 mg	3–4 mg	0.5–2 mg
AG	5–7 mg	3–4 mg	3–4 mg	3–4 mg	0.5–2 mg	0.5–2 mg
AA	3–4 mg	3–4 mg	0.5–2 mg	0.5–2 mg	0.5–2 mg	0.5–2 mg

three to five times more potent as an anticoagulant than R-warfarin. S-warfarin is metabolised primarily by CYP2C9. In Caucasians the most common variants of CYP2C9 are CYP2C9*2 and CYP2C9*3, which occur at frequencies of 11% and 7%, respectively. The CYP2C9*2 variant causes a 40% reduction in the rate of S-warfarin metabolism, while CYP2C9*3 causes almost a complete loss of capacity to metabolise S-warfarin. In both cases, significantly lower daily dosage of warfarin is required to maintain a therapeutic international normalised ratio. In addition to this pharmacogenetic variability in the enzyme responsible for removing warfarin from the body, the use of warfarin is further complicated by genetic variability in the target for this drug. VKORC1 is the gene that encodes vitamin K epoxide reductase, which is the molecular target that is inhibited by warfarin. Warfarin dosing guidance on the basis of CYP2C9 and VKCOR1 genotypes have been proposed (Table 6.2) and illustrate the complexity of accounting for genetic variability in both the drug clearance and drug target.

CYP2C19

Clopidogrel

Clopidogrel is a prodrug that is converted in a two-step process to an active thiol metabolite by CYP enzymes, including CYP2C19. The thiol metabolite binds irreversibly to a cysteine residue in the P2Y12 receptor, which blocks ADP-induced platelet aggregation (Ch 13). Clopidogrel is used widely to prevent vascular ischaemic events, especially in dual antiplatelet therapy with aspirin to prevent atherothrombotic events in acute coronary syndromes managed with percutaneous coronary intervention (PCI). Two loss-of-function alleles, CYP2C19*2 and CYP2C19*3 (which occur only in Asian populations), primarily account for the CYP2C19 PM; the frequencies of the poor metaboliser phenotypes in Caucasians and Asians are approximately 3% and 20%, respectively. Given the important role of CYP2C19 in clopidogrel metabolic activation, numerous studies have investigated the impact of CYP2C19 genetic polymorphism on cardiovascular outcomes during clopidogrel therapy.

UGT1A1

Irinotecan

Irinotecan is a prodrug used in the treatment of colorectal cancer. It is metabolised to the active metabolite SN-38, which functions as a topoisomerase I inhibitor. SN-38 is metabolised via glucuronidation, principally by UGT1A1 with a minor contribution by UGT1A9. Currently, there are more than 60 known polymorphisms in the UGT1A1 gene and some of these have functional consequences. The UGT1A1*28 polymorphism arises from the insertion of an extra thymine–adenine repeat, making a total of seven instead of the normal six repeats, in the promoter region of the gene. People who are homozygous for UGT1A1*28 have reduced UGT1A1 gene expression and the UGT1A1*28 allele is thought to contribute about 40% of the variability in enzyme activity of UGT1A1.

TPMT

Cytotoxic immunosuppressants

Mutant TPMT alleles (TPMT*2, TPMT*3A, TPMT*3B, TPMT*3C) are a classic example of the syntheses of defective drug-metabolising enzymes that increase the risk of adverse drug reactions. TPMT metabolises the cytotoxic immunosuppressant drugs azathioprine (the prodrug of mercaptopurine) and mercaptopurine. Normally, mercaptopurine is 'detoxified' by TPMT, and reduced TPMT activity is associated with a high frequency of myelosuppression (Fig 6.3). People who do not carry wild-type TPMT alleles have extremely low TPMT activity and almost always develop neutropenia. Indeed, people with the wild-type alleles (TPMT*1/*1) tolerate therapy for around 20 times longer than people heterozygous for mutant TPMT alleles (39 versus 2 weeks). Mercaptopurine and azathioprine both have a narrow therapeutic index and phenotyping provides a useful way of identifying those potentially at risk of developing myelosuppression. As erythrocyte TPMT activity mirrors that of the liver, which metabolises azathioprine and mercaptopurine, phenotyping is determined by measuring erythrocyte TPMT activity prior to treatment. The dose of azathioprine or mercaptopurine is then adjusted and people with a poor metaboliser phenotype receive about 10% of the dose of those with the extensive metaboliser phenotype.

Drug transporters

Polymorphisms of membrane transporters that are involved in drug transport have also been reported. The most widely studied is P-glycoprotein (P-gp, also called MDR1), which is encoded by the gene ABCB1. However, results from studies investigating the activity of polymorphic variants of P-gp and responses to anticancer drugs, antihistamines, anticonvulsants, antiviral drugs, cardiac glycosides and

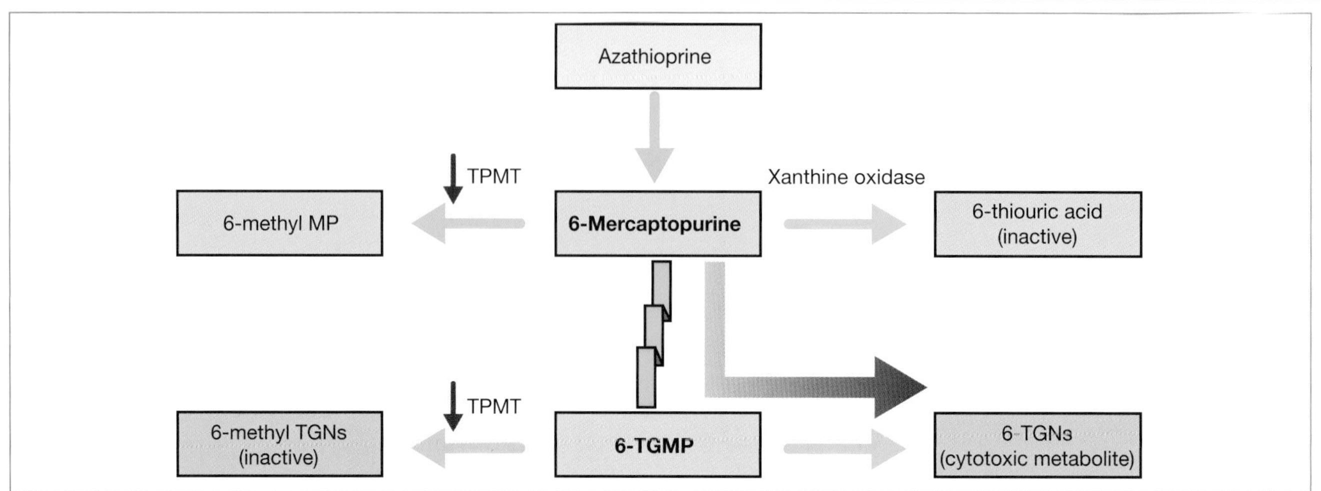

FIGURE 6.3 Metabolism of azathioprine and mercaptopurine
Mercaptopurine is either metabolised by TPMT (to 6-methyl MP) and xanthine oxidase (to 6-thiouric acid) or converted via hypoxanthine-guanine phosphoribosyltransferase to 6-thioguanine monophosphate (6-TGMP), which serves as the precursor to the pharmacologically active cytotoxic metabolites, 6-thioguanine nucleotides (TGNs). 6-TGMP is also metabolised via TPMT to the inactive 6-methyl-TGMP. In the presence of low TPMT activity (indicated by the downward arrows) metabolism occurs predominantly via 6-TGMP, resulting in increased formation of 6-TGNs (indicated by the large solid arrow) and severe myelosuppression.

immunosuppressants have been controversial. The transporter OATP1B1 facilitates the hepatic uptake of several drugs, including HMG-CoA reductase inhibitors ('statins'). Inhibition of OATP1B1 – for example, by ciclosporin – increases plasma concentrations of simvastatin and the risk of myopathy. There is also evidence indicating that a mutation in OATP1B1 (which results in substitution of the amino acid valine for arginine at position 174) also affects the pharmacokinetics of simvastatin, and perhaps other statins, more than doubling the risk of myopathy. However, myopathy can still occur in the absence of this polymorphism.

Human leucocyte antigen

Abacavir

Abacavir is a nucleoside reverse transcriptase inhibitor used in the treatment of HIV. Five to eight per cent of Caucasian people treated with abacavir develop hypersensitivity reactions characterised by acute respiratory symptoms, rash, fever, malaise and gastrointestinal symptoms. With continued treatment the symptoms worsen and, in people with abacavir hypersensitivity, recommencing therapy may result in life-threatening hypotension. There is a strong association between potentially fatal abacavir hypersensitivity and the human leucocyte antigen (HLA) allele HLA-B*57:01. HLA complexes have a vital role in the immune system where they bind peptides derived from 'self' cells or from exogenous ('non-self') proteins for presentation to T-cells, thereby initiating antigen-specific responses. Genetic testing (genotyping) is now routinely performed before starting abacavir therapy.

Allopurinol

Polymorphic HLA alleles are also associated with the hypersensitivity reactions that occur in some people receiving allopurinol. Allopurinol hypersensitivity, which may result in severe cutaneous adverse reactions such as Stevens-Johnson syndrome and toxic epidermal necrolysis, shows an association with the variant HLA-B*58:01 allele. The frequency of the HLA-B*58:01 allele ranges from 5% to 10% in East and Southeast Asian populations but is less common in Caucasians (< 1%) and rare in Indigenous Australians. Despite the potential seriousness of allopurinol hypersensitivity, testing for HLA-B*58:01 in those commencing allopurinol appears not to be warranted since a hypersensitivity response does not occur in all carriers of this allele. Rather, people taking allopurinol should be monitored for severe cutaneous adverse reactions.

Pharmacogenetics and adverse drug reactions

The role of genetics in predisposing people to adverse drug reactions has been known since the late 1950s through the discovery of deficiencies of enzymes such as pseudocholinesterase and the link to succinylcholine suxamethonium apnoea. This easily recognised and diagnosed enzyme deficiency led many to conclude that we would be able to identify using genetic tests those that were more likely to develop adverse reactions to some drugs. This concept, although attractive, has been replaced by the realisation that pharmacogenetic testing

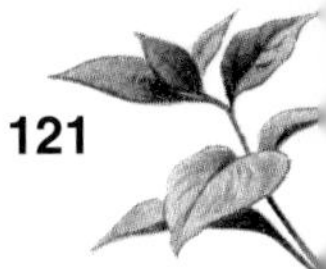

will aid in the prediction and prevention of only a limited number of adverse reactions, and as such the uptake of this testing has been rather variable and limited.

Individualising drug dosing

In addition to the selection of an appropriate medicine, tailoring of drug therapy can also often involve the individualisation of drug dosing. There are various strategies that can be applied to guide dose selection on the basis of exposure, response or toxicity. These strategies may be used to guide:

- initial dose selection based on a predicted capacity to eliminate the drug (genotyping or phenotyping)
- dose adaptation in order to tailor the drug effect or respond to a change in circumstance.

Exposure-guided dosing

Therapeutic drug monitoring (TDM) is a commonly used approach to guide dosing decisions on the basis of drug exposure. TDM typically involves measuring the drug concentration in the blood in order to adjust the dosage rationally. There are multiple reasons a clinician may use TDM for a drug including to:

- individualise therapy
- monitor medication adherence
- detect sub-therapeutic treatment
- minimise risk of toxicity
- detect drug interactions
- monitor the impact of changing physiology
- guide withdrawal of a therapy.

The general characteristics of a treatment that are consistent with a benefit from the use of TDM are:

- established relationship between plasma concentration and effect
- well-defined therapeutic and toxic levels
- substantial variability in drug exposure between people or within a person over time
- narrow therapeutic index
- no readily measured response marker.

When undertaking TDM, the measured drug concentration is compared with a therapeutic range (published values of the concentration of the drug in plasma at steady state during effective therapy). Therapeutic ranges are valid for about 80% of the population and are a guide to expected plasma concentration of the drug. Trough levels (the lowest level likely to be in blood, measured by taking a blood sample immediately before the next dose) are usually evaluated. In some situations – for example, to avoid toxic levels – peak levels are evaluated at the time of maximum plasma concentration.

Response-guided dosing

Drug therapy can be monitored by measuring various effects of drugs. Examples include measuring blood pressure in a person receiving an antihypertensive agent, blood clotting times for anticoagulant therapy and blood glucose levels for hypoglycaemic agents. Response-guided dosing may also be crudely applied in acute situations where a drug is repeatedly administered (titrated) in order to achieve a desired effect, such as the management of severe pain with opioid analgesics.

Toxicity-guided dosing

Particularly in the case of drugs with a narrow therapeutic index, adverse reactions may limit the level to which the dose can be increased. In people with cancer, cytotoxic therapy is frequently monitored by checking the person's white blood cell count; if this falls too much, the person is at risk of overwhelming infection. Only when the white blood cell count has recovered sufficiently is another course of chemotherapy instituted. The aminoglycoside antibiotics can cause severe damage to the kidneys and to hearing, so people who require these drugs may have their hearing and renal function monitored. A common adverse reaction to the non-steroidal anti-inflammatory drugs is dyspepsia and exacerbation of peptic ulcers. The prescriber might monitor this by advising the person: 'Stop taking the drug if you start to feel sick, and let me know.'

Future challenges to precision medicine

While gaining increasing acceptance in certain therapeutic domains (primarily oncology), the broader translation of pharmacogenetics and precision medicine into clinical practice remains challenging. Assigning causation of genetic variants to a diagnostic association is technically onerous and time-consuming, necessitating rigorous analytic validation and quality assurance/control to ensure meaningful translation to clinical practice. Additionally, the conduct of trials to establish that clinical outcomes are improved when drug therapy is individualised is difficult because of ethical issues surrounding privacy/confidentiality and record retention, potential misuse of a person's genetic information and health/life insurability, the problem of non-genomic confounding effects (e.g. diet, smoking, drug interactions) and the enormous expense of such trials.

KEY POINTS

Individualised drug dosing

- Drug dosing may be guided on the basis of exposure, therapeutic response or toxicity.
- Dose individualising strategies may be used to select the optimal initial dose or to guide dose adaptation.

REVIEW EXERCISES

1 You observe that two residents at the local aged care facility are receiving quite different doses of warfarin. (Mrs AC's dose is much lower than the normal dosage.) After enquiring, you are advised that Mrs AC has a 'genetic deficiency'. Discuss what 'genetic' deficiencies can account for the requirement for a lower dose of warfarin in Mrs AC.

2 Mr GB has been diagnosed recently with HIV and is due to start treatment with abacavir. Discuss why Mr GB has been advised that he must be genotyped for HLA-B*57:01 before drug therapy can begin. In the absence of genotyping, what are the risks to Mr GB from abacavir therapy?

3 Mr ST has been diagnosed with metastatic colorectal cancer. Genetic screening reveals that his tumour harbours a mutation in codon 12 of the KRAS gene. Citing relevant evidence, discuss how this information should be incorporated into the person's treatment plan.

REFERENCES

Müller DJ, Rizhanovsky Z. From the origins of pharmacogenetics to first applications in psychiatry. Pharmacopsychiatry. 2020 Jul;53(4):155–161. doi: 10.1055/a-0979-2322.

Sorich MJ, Wiese MD, Rowland A, et al: Extended RAS mutations and anti-EGFR monoclonal antibody survival benefit in metastatic colorectal cancer: a meta-analysis of randomized controlled trials, Annals of Oncology 26: 13–21, 2016.

CHAPTER 7

ADVERSE DRUG REACTIONS AND DRUG INTERACTIONS

Andrew Rowland

KEY ABBREVIATIONS

ADR adverse drug reaction
CAM complementary and alternative medicine
DDI drug–drug interaction

KEY TERMS

adverse drug event 124
adverse drug reaction 124
complementary and alternative medicine 125
drug–drug interaction 125
pseudoallergic reaction 126

Chapter Focus

With the increasing use of multiple concurrent medications (polypharmacy), drug interactions are increasingly a cause for concern because they may result in loss of efficacy (decreased benefit) or the development of toxicity (unwanted effects). Additionally, with the widespread use of complementary and alternative medicines (CAMs) (e.g. vitamin, herbal, aromatherapy and homoeopathic products), drug–CAM interactions are adding to the burden. Many studies have confirmed that adverse drug reactions and drug interactions are major clinical problems, accounting for a significant number of hospital admissions, extended hospital stays and substantial costs to the healthcare system. It is important that health professionals are aware of the adverse reaction and drug interaction profiles of drugs and CAMs and be ever vigilant for the occurrence of adverse outcomes.

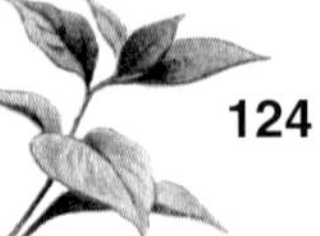

CRITICAL THINKING SCENARIO

Terry, a 61-year-old male, was diagnosed with renal cell cancer 2 years ago and has been taking 50 mg of sunitinib (a cancer medicine) daily without any complications ever since. Last week Terry contracted COVID-19. Fearing that he is quite frail, Terry's doctor prescribed a 5-day course of Paxlovid (nirmatrelvir/ritonavir) to help minimise his symptoms. What, if any, impact is Paxlovid likely to have on Terry's cancer medicine and how might this be addressed?

Introduction

The Ancient Greeks first described the concept of a medicine and a poison in scientific terms. Throughout the centuries, the use of medicinal products has gone hand in hand with reports of **adverse drug reactions** (ADRs). Public concern about ADRs arose in the late 19th century because of the number of sudden deaths associated with the use of chloroform. This led to the development of regulatory bodies, such as the Food and Drug Administration in the United States, which establish the safety of new drugs. Despite regulatory frameworks, there have been many notable incidences of ADRs that have resulted in withdrawal of the offending drug (Table 7.1). Public interest in the safety of drugs has increased as a result of better communication between consumers and health professionals.

Adverse drug reactions

The World Health Organization defines an ADR as 'any response to a drug which is noxious, unintended, and which occurs at doses normally (and appropriately) used in man for the prophylaxis, diagnosis, or therapy of disease' (World Health Organization 1984). The general wording of this definition has been in use for the last 34 years and at various times has been modified slightly because the word 'noxious' is perhaps not correct in the context of the definition. Clinical responses to an ADR include modifying the dose, discontinuing the drug, hospitalising the person or providing supportive measures. This definition does not encompass the situations of drug overdose, drug withdrawal, drug abuse or error in administration. The last is included within the definition of an **adverse drug event**.

Risk factors for developing an adverse drug reaction

Risk factors for ADRs are specific to both the person and the drug. Factors relating to the person can include:

- age – the elderly and neonates
- gender – women appear to be more susceptible

TABLE 7.1 Notable adverse drug reactions necessitating withdrawal of the drug

YEAR	DRUG	USE	ADVERSE DRUG REACTION
1961	Thalidomide	Sedative	Congenital malformations
1982	Benoxaprofen	Anti-inflammatory	Liver/kidney damage
1983	Zomepirac	Anti-inflammatory	Anaphylaxis
1992	Temafloxacin	Antibiotic	Blood dyscrasias
1997	Dexfenfluramine	Anorectic	Pulmonary hypertension and cardiac valve disorders
1998	Terfenadine	Antihistamine	Ventricular dysrhythmia
2000	Troglitazone	Hypoglycaemic	Liver damage
2001	Cerivastatin	Lipid lowering	Deaths from severe rhabdomyolysis
2004	Rofecoxib	Anti-inflammatory	Cardiovascular events
2007	Aprotinin	Antifibrinolytic	Increased mortality
2007	Lumiracoxib	Anti-inflammatory	Hepatotoxicity
2008	Rimonabant	Antiobesity	Severe depression and suicide
2009	Efalizumab	Immunosuppressant	Progressive multifocal leucoencephalopathy
2010	Sibutramine	Antiobesity	Increased risk of cardiovascular events
2011	Sitaxentan	Treatment of pulmonary hypertension	Fatal idiosyncratic hepatic failure

- kidney or liver disease
- genetic factors
- history of prior drug reactions
- polypharmacy (five drugs or more).

Factors specific to the drug can include:

- chemical characteristics – for example, large molecules such as heparin can themselves be immunogenic
- class of drug – for example, anticoagulants
- route of drug administration – topical and oral routes generally involve a lower incidence of drug allergy
- dose – many ADRs are dose-related
- duration and frequency – prolonged and frequent use can increase the risk of an ADR.

Incidence of adverse drug reactions

In developed countries, many elderly individuals take on average four to five prescription drugs and two over-the-counter drugs at any time. Taking multiple types of drugs contributes to the incidence of ADRs. In addition to prescribed medications and those bought over the counter, Australians have embraced the use of **complementary and alternative medicines** (CAMs). The trend has been strongest among women and includes the use of herbal medicines and aromatherapy oils. ADRs occur in people of all ages and are twice as common in women. They are a major cause of morbidity and mortality, especially in the elderly. Many studies have evaluated polypharmacy in the elderly in recent years, typically finding that 25–30% of elderly people were taking 6–10 medications, and 10–15% take more than 10 types each day. The drugs most commonly implicated were antihypertensives, anticoagulants, cardiovascular drugs, cytotoxics and non-steroidal anti-inflammatory drugs (Held et al. 2017).

Classification of adverse drug reactions

The current classification system is not ideal, and not every ADR may fit perfectly into one of the categories. It is generally accepted that there are two main categories of ADR, type A (augmented) and type B (bizarre), and two subordinate categories, type C (chronic) and type D (delayed). A further two classes include end-of-use or withdrawal effects (type E) and unexpected failure of therapy (type F).

Type A (augmented, dose-related) ADRs

Type A ADRs are characterised by:

- predictable reaction based on the pharmacology of the drug (often an exaggeration of effect)
- relationship to dose
- common occurrence (about 80% of ADRs)
- usually mild
- high morbidity and low mortality
- reproducibility in animal models.

Factors predisposing to type A reactions include the dose, pharmaceutical variation in drug formulation, pharmacokinetic variation (e.g. renal failure), pharmacodynamic variation (e.g. altered fluid and electrolyte balance) and **drug–drug interactions** (DDIs) (e.g. inhibition of metabolism of one drug by another concomitantly administered drug). Examples include:

- sedation with the use of antihistamines
- bleeding with anticoagulants
- hypoglycaemia from the use of insulin
- hypokalaemia with the use of diuretics.

Type B (bizarre, non-dose-related) ADRs

Type B ADRs are characterised by:

- unpredictability
- no relationship to dose
- uncommon occurrence (about 20% of ADRs)
- increased severity
- high morbidity and high mortality
- lack of reproducibility in animal models.

These reactions are less common but often cause death. Factors contributing to type B reactions include pharmaceutical variation, receptor abnormalities, unmasking of a biological deficiency (e.g. glucose-6-phosphate dehydrogenase deficiency), abnormalities in drug metabolism (e.g. slow acetylators of the antituberculosis drug isoniazid), drug allergy and DDIs (e.g. rare incidence of hepatitis). Examples include interstitial nephritis with the use of non-steroidal anti-inflammatory drugs and eosinophilia with the use of anticonvulsants such as carbamazepine and phenytoin.

Type C (chronic, dose-related and time-related) ADRs

Type C ADRs are characterised by occurrence as a consequence of long-term use. Examples include:

- adaptive changes (e.g. development of drug tolerance and physical dependence)
- appearance of tardive dyskinesia in those treated long term with neuroleptic drugs for schizophrenia
- rebound phenomena (e.g. rebound tachycardia after the abrupt discontinuation of β-blockers and acute adrenal insufficiency after abrupt withdrawal of corticosteroids).

Type D (delayed, time-related) ADRs

Type D ADRs are characterised by the appearance of delayed effects. These may be acceptable if the benefit of

drug therapy outweighs the risk, as in the case of irreversible infertility in young people receiving cytotoxic drugs for malignancies. In general, however, they are considered unacceptable. Examples include carcinogenesis (e.g. the association of lymphoma with immunosuppressive drugs) and teratogenesis.

Type E (end-of-use, withdrawal) ADRs

Type E ADRs are uncommon and are related to withdrawal of a drug. They include opiate withdrawal syndrome and myocardial ischemia after abrupt cessation of β-blockers.

Type F (failure, unexpected failure of therapy) ADRs

Type F ADRs are increasingly common and are often caused by a drug interaction (e.g. inadequate dose of the oral contraceptive when a drug that induces the metabolism of estrogen is administered concomitantly).

Drug allergy

A drug allergy, or hypersensitivity, is a type B ADR. Drug allergies are characterised by:

- occurrence in a small number of people
- the requirement for previous exposure to either the same or a chemically related drug
- the rapid development of an allergic reaction after re-exposure
- production of clinical manifestations of an allergic reaction.

The diagnosis of a drug allergy is often difficult to establish because there are no reliable laboratory tests that can identify the relevant drug, and in some cases the symptoms can imitate infectious disease symptoms. The situation may be easier if the drug administered is commonly suspected of causing an allergic reaction (e.g. penicillin), but it is difficult if the drug used is seldom reported to produce an allergic reaction.

Some drugs can produce a pseudoallergic reaction that resembles an allergic reaction but has no immunological basis. Usually, these reactions occur as a result of mast cell degranulation and subsequent release of histamine. Clinically, they resemble the type I hypersensitivity reaction, but they do not involve drug-specific immunoglobulin E. An example of a pseudoallergic reaction is the release of histamine that occurs with opiates (e.g. morphine), vancomycin and radiological contrast media. Allergic reactions to drugs generally follow the type I–IV classification. Table 7.2 lists the types of reactions, the main clinical manifestations and examples of drugs commonly implicated.

Immune modulating drugs and adverse drug reactions

Drugs that modulate the immune system are commonly used to treat diseases such as cancer, rheumatoid arthritis, multiple sclerosis, inflammatory bowel disease and lupus. Although beneficial in many clinical settings the use of immune-modulating drugs is also associated with a significant number of ADRs (Table 7.3). Suppression of

TABLE 7.2 Allergic drug reactions

(TYPE)/REACTION	CLINICAL MANIFESTATIONS	EXAMPLES OF DRUGS
(I) Immediate hypersensitivity	Urticaria, anaphylaxis, angio-oedema, bronchospasm	Penicillins, local anaesthetics, neuromuscular blocking drugs, radiological contrast media
(II) Antibody-dependent cytotoxic	Cytopenia, vasculitis, haemolytic anaemia	Quinine, rifampicin, metronidazole
(III) Complex-mediated	Serum sickness, vasculitis, interstitial nephritis	Anticonvulsants, antibiotics, hydralazine, diuretics
(IV) Cell-mediated or delayed hypersensitivity	Contact sensitivity	Local anaesthetic creams

TABLE 7.3 Commonly used immune-modulating drugs and associated ADRs

DRUG GROUP	THERAPEUTIC EFFECT	ADVERSE DRUG REACTIONS
Corticosteroids	Immune suppression; decreased expression of nitric oxide synthase; decreased expression of intracellular adhesion molecules	Increased risk of infections such as *Pneumocystis carinii* and systemic fungal infections
Cytotoxic drugs	Inhibition of cell proliferation	Increased risk of infections (e.g. herpes zoster, cytomegalovirus) and life-threatening infections; increased risk of malignancies
Calcineurin inhibitors	Immune suppression	Increased risk of lymphomas and non-melanoma skin cancers
Biological agents	Immune-modulating	Formation of autoantibodies; increased risk of infection and malignancies such as lymphomas (infliximab); progressive multifocal leucoencephalopathy (rituximab)
Sphingosine agonists	Immune suppression	Increased risk of infections

the immune response increases the risk of infection and cancer and, paradoxically, some of these drugs can also induce hypersensitivity (type B reactions) and/or autoimmune syndromes.

KEY POINTS

Adverse drug reactions

- An ADR is defined as any response to a drug that is noxious and unintended, and that occurs at doses normally used for the prophylaxis, diagnosis or therapy of disease.
- ADRs occur in people of all ages and are twice as common in women. They are a major cause of morbidity and mortality, especially in the elderly.
- There are two main categories of ADR, type A (predictable) and type B (unpredictable), and subordinate categories, type C (chronic use), type D (delayed reactions), type E (end-of-use or withdrawal effects) and type F (unexpected failure of therapy).
- The diagnosis of a drug allergy can often be difficult to establish because there are no reliable laboratory tests that can identify the relevant drug, and the symptoms can sometimes imitate infectious disease symptoms (e.g. fever).
- Risk factors for developing an ADR include, but are not limited to, age, gender, presence of concurrent disease, multiple chronic medical problems, drug class, polypharmacy, renal/hepatic impairment, genetics, history of prior drug reaction, the drug dose and the duration and frequency of drug use.
- Practical points for decreasing inappropriate drug use in the elderly include frequent medication review, simplified drug regimens, use of low doses and providing simple written and verbal instructions.

Drug–drug interactions

A DDI occurs when a drug's pharmacological effect is altered by another drug: that is, there is an increased therapeutic and/or adverse effect or a decreased therapeutic and/or adverse effect. DDIs are often unanticipated and go unrecognised, and the clinical and economic importance is frequently underestimated.

Frequency of drug interactions

The exact frequency of drug interactions is unknown, although anecdotal evidence suggests that they are relatively common and result in a significant number of hospital admissions. The possibility of a drug interaction exists whenever two or more medications are prescribed to an individual, and the likelihood of an interaction will increase as the number of medications used increases (polypharmacy). For a person taking two drugs the estimated incidence of a DDI is 5.6%, while a person taking six drugs has an estimated incidence of a DDI of 56%. One of the problems in identifying a DDI is that the physiological/biochemical changes resulting from a DDI may be masked by, or confused with, the clinical signs and symptoms of the illness or other comorbidities. Additionally, it may be difficult to identify which 'drugs' are involved in a DDI, especially if the prescriber is unaware of other medicines the person is taking – for example, over-the-counter drugs, CAMs and/or dietary/nutritional supplements. Those at greatest risk of a drug interaction are:

- the severely ill, who typically receive multiple drugs
- those receiving chronic therapy, often comprising a cocktail of drugs (e.g. in the treatment of either HIV infection or cancer)
- older adults, who tend to have multiple pathologies and often receive multiple drugs concurrently.

Drug interactions are of greatest concern with drugs that have a narrow therapeutic index. Even a small change in the concentration of the drug available at the target site (e.g. receptor, enzyme) can lead to a major alteration in response. For example:

- enhanced anticoagulation (bleeding) with warfarin resulting from concomitant use of the antidysrhythmic drug amiodarone, which inhibits the metabolism of warfarin
- bradycardia with digoxin resulting from concomitant administration of the antidysrhythmic drug amiodarone, which decreases renal or biliary excretion of digoxin.

Interactions involving drugs with a wide therapeutic index (e.g. penicillin antibiotics, β-adrenoceptor antagonists) cause fewer problems. Knowledge of the mechanisms of drug interactions is essential to enable health professionals to prevent interactions occurring (wherever possible) and to systematically analyse potentially new drug interactions. Indeed, analysis of known and potential interactions is critical in the planning of a therapeutic regimen.

Classification of drug interactions

Drug interactions are broadly classified, according to their pharmacological mechanism, into either pharmacodynamic or pharmacokinetic interactions.

Pharmacodynamic drug interactions

Pharmacodynamic drug interactions may be 'direct' or 'indirect'. Direct pharmacodynamic interactions involve additive effects at a common target (and possibly potentiation) or antagonism due to actions at different sites in an organ. An example of antagonism at a common receptor site is the concurrent use of a β_2-adrenoceptor agonist (used to treat asthma, e.g. salbutamol) and a non-selective β-adrenoceptor antagonist (used to treat hypertension, e.g. propranolol). Both drugs have opposing effects at the same receptor (i.e. the β_2-adrenoceptor). Unintentional drug interactions of this type should not occur because they are so obvious from the known pharmacology of the drugs.

Examples of direct pharmacodynamic interactions involving drugs with different mechanisms of action include the following:

- Monoamine oxidase (MAO) inhibitors, which are used in the treatment of depression and which increase the amount of noradrenaline (norepinephrine) stored in nerve terminals, interact dangerously (to cause marked hypertension) with 'sympathomimetic' drugs such as ephedrine that cause the release of stored noradrenaline. Tyramine, which is present in foods such as cheese, yeast extracts and Chianti-type wines, produces a similar response in people treated with MAO inhibitors because it is an indirect-acting sympathomimetic, which displaces noradrenaline from the nerve terminals.
- Warfarin is an anticoagulant that inhibits vitamin K–mediated synthesis of clotting factors. The risk of bleeding is increased by co-administration of aspirin, which decreases platelet aggregation by inhibiting the synthesis of thromboxane A_2.

An indirect pharmacodynamic interaction occurs when the pharmacological effect of one drug alters the response to another drug, even though the two effects are not themselves directly related. Common examples include certain diuretics (e.g. furosemide [frusemide] or hydrochlorothiazide), which lower the blood potassium concentration. This will enhance the toxic effects of the cardiac glycoside digoxin, which is used to treat atrial fibrillation and cardiac failure, and of type III antidysrhythmic drugs (e.g. amiodarone) that prolong the cardiac action potential.

Pharmacokinetic drug interactions

The plasma concentration of a drug may be altered by interactions occurring during absorption, distribution, metabolism and excretion.

Absorption

Absorption interactions involve a change in either the rate or the extent of absorption. Drugs that change the rate of gastric emptying (i.e. the time it takes for the contents of the stomach to empty into the small bowel) will alter the rate of absorption of co-administered drugs. Muscarinic receptor antagonists (e.g. hyoscine) delay gastric emptying and gastrointestinal motility. This combination of effects delays drug absorption from the gastrointestinal tract. Many drugs, including tricyclic antidepressants and histamine-1-receptor antagonists that possess antimuscarinic properties, delay the absorption of co-administered drugs. Gastric emptying rate is slowed by opioid drugs, including morphine and pethidine, and hence the time to reach the peak plasma concentration is generally increased for a drug co-administered with an opioid.

Co-administered drugs may also decrease the extent of drug absorption. Whereas changes in the rate of absorption generally affect only the time to onset of action, changes in extent of absorption can alter response. For example, colestyramine is a bile acid-binding resin used to treat hypercholesterolaemia. Unfortunately, colestyramine also binds other drugs, reducing the amount of drug that is absorbed. Because colestyramine reduces the absorption of corticosteroids, digoxin, thyroxine and warfarin (and probably other drugs), these drugs should be administered either several hours before or after the colestyramine dose.

Distribution

Because many drugs circulate in the blood bound (at least in part) to the proteins albumin and α_1-acid glycoprotein, they may compete for the same binding sites. Displacement from plasma protein of one drug by another is common, and this leads to an increase in the unbound, pharmacologically active, concentration of the drug in the blood. Although it is still widely believed that the increase in unbound concentration arising from 'displacement interactions' may precipitate drug toxicity, this is rarely the case. Following a drug displacement interaction, the concentration of unbound drug in blood does indeed increase. However, the unbound drug is available for distribution into tissues, leading to an increase in the volume of distribution, hepatic clearance and renal excretion. There is, however, a decrease in total drug concentration (i.e. bound plus unbound drug) because of the higher clearance.

Metabolism

Administration of some drugs can lead to decreased (inhibited) or increased (induced) activity of drug-metabolising enzymes such as cytochrome P450 (CYP). Many important drug interactions arise from altered metabolism, and the clinical importance of the interaction will depend on the change in clearance and the therapeutic index of the altered drug. A 10% change in clearance is unlikely to be important, but a 30% change in the clearance of a narrow-therapeutic-index drug such as warfarin can have serious implications. Importantly, just as there is considerable inter-individual variability in the clearance of metabolised drugs, there is significant variability in the magnitude of the change in clearance associated with any metabolic drug interaction. Drugs known to cause induction are generally non-selective in their effects on CYP enzymes. Examples include:

- the antituberculosis drug rifampicin, which appears to induce all CYP and UDP-glucuronosyltransferase (UGT) isoforms, therefore potentially decreasing the blood concentration of all co-administered drugs that are metabolised by these enzymes
- the anticonvulsant drugs phenobarbital (phenobarbitone), phenytoin and carbamazepine induce CYP2C9 and CYP3A4, and possibly other enzymes of CYP and UGT families. People with epilepsy receiving these drugs are prone to drug interactions and their consequences (e.g. unwanted pregnancy due to enhanced metabolism of oral contraceptive steroids)
- chronic consumption of ethanol (alcohol), which induces CYP2E1, although there are relatively few clinically used drugs that are metabolised by this enzyme.

Inhibitory drug interactions are relatively common, and inhibition of metabolism increases the steady-state blood concentration and the likelihood of drug toxicity. Some drugs, notably the H_2 antagonist cimetidine, inhibit the activity of most CYP enzymes (although UGT is unaffected). Conversely, probenecid inhibits most UGT enzymes (without affecting CYP). Most inhibitory interactions are relatively selective for one or a limited number of drug-metabolising enzymes because they most commonly arise from competition for metabolism at the enzyme active site. It is generally not correct to refer to a drug as 'an inhibitor of drug metabolism'. Rather, a drug will normally selectively inhibit the metabolism of other drugs for a limited number of enzymes, and this specificity of interaction is used to predict and interpret metabolic drug interactions. Some selective inhibitors of CYP enzymes are shown in Table 7.4. As an example, fluoxetine causes interactions with many drugs metabolised by CYP2D6 (e.g. other antidepressants and perhexiline), which generally requires a reduction of the dose. The clearances of drugs metabolised by CYP3A4 are similarly decreased by the commonly used antibiotic erythromycin, again generally requiring a dose reduction. The following are examples of CYP metabolic drug interactions:

- Amiodarone and its active metabolite desethylamiodarone inhibit CYP2C9, which metabolises S-warfarin. This DDI increases the risk of major bleeding.
- Paroxetine, a CYP2D6 inhibitor, reduces the plasma concentration of endoxifen, an active metabolite of tamoxifen used in breast cancer treatment.
- Many azole antifungals inhibit CYP3A, decreasing clearance of some statins, which increases the risk of statin-induced myopathy.

Metabolic drug interactions also occur with other drug-metabolising enzymes. Probenecid is a 'universal' inhibitor of drug glucuronidation, and there is evidence to suggest that rifampicin, phenobarbital (phenobarbitone), phenytoin and carbamazepine may induce numerous UGT enzymes. For example, fluconazole appears to inhibit only UGT2B7 (which metabolises morphine and zidovudine). In the case of the fluconazole–morphine drug interaction, a rise in the plasma concentration of morphine may result in respiratory depression.

A potentially fatal interaction occurs when azathioprine and allopurinol are co-administered. Allopurinol is an inhibitor of the enzyme xanthine oxidase, and is used to treat gout and gouty arthritis (Ch 34). Azathioprine (used mainly in cancer treatment) is converted to an active metabolite, 6-mercaptopurine, which is metabolised by xanthine oxidase. Co-administration of azathioprine and allopurinol leads to accumulation of 6-mercaptopurine, resulting in potentially life-threatening bone marrow suppression.

TABLE 7.4 Examples of clinically significant inhibitors of CYP enzymes

ENZYME	INHIBITORS
CYP1A2	Ciprofloxacin, fluvoxamine
CYP2C8	Gemfibrozil, trimethoprim
CYP2C9	Fluconazole
CYP2C19	Fluconazole, fluvoxamine, moclobemide, ticlopidine
CYP2D6	Cinacalcet, doxepin, fluoxetine, paroxetine, perhexiline, quinine
CYP3A4	Clarithromycin, diltiazem, erythromycin, itraconazole, ritonavir, saquinavir, verapamil

Excretion

Interactions may occur between drugs that are substrates for secretory and efflux transporters in the kidney. The mechanism of such interactions is simply 'competition' for the same transporter. For example, the plasma concentrations of penicillin, ciprofloxacin, furosemide (frusemide) and tenofovir are increased as a result of co-administration of probenecid, which inhibits an organic anion secretory transporter (OAT1/3) in the basolateral membrane of the proximal tubule, thereby reducing active secretion of the drugs into the renal tubule.

Drug interactions with nutrients and CAMs

Although there is wide appreciation of drug interactions, interactions between nutrients and/or food components and CAMs are often not considered and, in fact, may be discounted. Chemicals present in food may alter the activity of drug-metabolising enzymes. Notable in this regard are chemicals present in grapefruit juice that inhibit the activity of CYP3A4 present in the gastrointestinal tract. (CYP3A4 is localised in both the liver and the small bowel.) The enzyme present in the small bowel appears to contribute significantly to the first-pass metabolism of numerous CYP3A4 substrates. Thus, the bioavailability of a number of drugs, such as ciclosporin, felodipine, midazolam, triazolam and verapamil, increases significantly when they are taken with grapefruit juice, which enhances the potential for toxicity.

There is also interest in the effects of herbal medicines on drug metabolism and the consequences of herb–drug interactions, which are based on the same pharmacokinetic and pharmacodynamic mechanisms as DDIs. Herbal medicines are used widely, particularly by women, given the perception that 'natural' products are a safe and effective alternative to pharmaceuticals. As plant products, herbal medicines typically contain hundreds of different chemicals; it is not surprising that some of these will alter the activity of drug-metabolising enzymes. In the United States, the seven top-selling herbal medicines in descending order are: ginkgo, St John's wort, ginseng, kava, saw palmetto, garlic and echinacea. Interestingly, the top 10 herbal/botanical supplements reported to have the most interactions with individual drugs are (in descending order): St John's wort, ginkgo, kava, digitalis, willow, Asian ginseng, astragalus, licorice, saw palmetto and garlic; and the drugs involved in the most interactions were warfarin, insulin, aspirin and digoxin.

Important in terms of drug interaction is St John's wort, which is taken to treat the symptoms of depression. St John's wort contains chemicals called hyperforins, which mimic the effects of rifampicin as an inducer of CYP enzymes. Consumption for 2 weeks significantly induces the activity of both hepatic and intestinal CYP3A4 and the intestinal transporter P-glycoprotein. Thus the clearances of amitriptyline, carbamazepine, ciclosporin, HIV protease inhibitors, warfarin and several other drugs have been shown to be increased in subjects taking St John's wort, with risk of therapeutic failure. Similarly, the plasma concentrations of alprazolam and midazolam have been shown to be reduced in healthy volunteers taking St John's wort. Furthermore, oral contraceptives contain ethinylestradiol, which is metabolised by CYP3A4. Concomitant administration of St John's wort increases the metabolism of ethinylestradiol, and unplanned pregnancy has been reported as an issue in women who use oral contraceptive steroids and St John's wort. Not surprisingly given its use in depression, interactions with 'synthetic' antidepressants have been reported. The combination of St John's wort and the serotonin reuptake inhibitors (sertraline, paroxetine and venlafaxine) may result in headaches, changes in mental state, tremors, autonomic instability, gastrointestinal upset, myalgias and motor restlessness (symptoms similar to central serotonin excess). These symptoms may be explained by inhibition of serotonin reuptake in the brain by St John's wort.

There is evidence to suggest that multiple complementary medicines interact (pharmacodynamically or pharmacokinetically) with 'pharmaceutical' drugs, and studies investigating the mechanisms involved and quantifying the magnitudes of any interactions are ongoing. Interactions between herbal medicines and conventional drugs are increasingly observed, and it is likely that their incidence is more common than anticipated initially. It is essential that information on the use of complementary medicines is obtained from any individual, including pregnant women, prior to prescribing any drug, as it is essential to determine if concomitant use of complementary medicines may exacerbate the potential for drug interactions.

KEY POINTS

Drug interactions

- Drug interactions are broadly classified according to their pharmacological mechanisms – that is, pharmacodynamic or pharmacokinetic.
- Pharmacodynamic drug interactions may be 'direct' or 'indirect'.
- Direct pharmacodynamic interactions involve additive effects at a common target (and possibly potentiation) or antagonism due to actions at different sites in an organ.
- An indirect pharmacodynamic interaction occurs when the pharmacological effects of one drug alter the response to another drug, even though the two types of effects are not themselves directly related.
- A pharmacokinetic drug interaction can alter the concentration of drug in the systemic circulation through interactions occurring at any stage – that is, during absorption, distribution, metabolism or excretion.
- Multiple CAMs (including St John's wort, ginkgo and kava) are known to interact either pharmacodynamically or pharmacokinetically with prescription drugs.
- Strategies for reducing the incidence of ADRs and drug interactions include careful history-taking, considering non-drug treatment, correct and appropriate dosing, frequent review of therapeutic goals and drug regimens, avoiding polypharmacy and careful communication with the person or carer.

REVIEW EXERCISES

1. Mr CF presents with a rash that occurs coincidentally with having been prescribed an antibiotic. Which class of antibiotics is most frequently implicated in causing a rash? Potentially what type of adverse drug reaction is this, and what will be your advice to Mr CF in terms of future administration of antibiotics?
2. Mrs ED has atrial fibrillation and is prescribed warfarin. You are aware that there are several drug interactions with warfarin. Discuss the clinical implications for Mrs ED of an inhibitory drug interaction involving warfarin.
3. Mr AR has just received a kidney transplant and has heard from a friend that St John's wort can help his new kidney work a bit better because it helps to get rid of some of the extra fluid. Why is it important to counsel transplant patients against the consumption of St John's wort?

REFERENCES

Held F, Le Couteur DG, Blyth FM, et al: Polypharmacy in older adults: Association Rule and Frequent-Set Analysis to evaluate concomitant medication use, Pharmacological Research 116:39–44, 2017.

World Health Organization: Collaborating centres for international drug monitoring, Geneva, 1984, WHO. (WHO publication DEM/NC/84:153 (E)).

CHAPTER 8

DRUGS AFFECTING CHOLINERGIC TRANSMISSION

Shaunagh Darroch

KEY ABBREVIATIONS

ACh	acetylcholine
AChE	acetylcholinesterase
ANS	autonomic nervous system
CNS	central nervous system
mAChRs	muscarinic acetylcholine receptors
nAChRs	nicotinic acetylcholine receptors
NMJ	neuromuscular junction
PNS	peripheral nervous system

KEY TERMS

Chapter Focus

The peripheral nervous system is subdivided functionally and anatomically into two divisions: the autonomic and the somatic nervous systems. The autonomic nervous system comprises the parasympathetic and sympathetic divisions and is responsible for regulating the internal viscera such as the heart, blood vessels, digestive organs, kidneys and reproductive organs. The somatic nervous system is the division of the peripheral nervous system that coordinates consciously controlled functions such as movement, posture and respiration; a single motor neuron connects the central nervous system to the skeletal muscles, which are the effector organs.

The parasympathetic and somatic components of the peripheral nervous system use acetylcholine as the principal neurotransmitter. The action of acetylcholine on muscarinic receptors leads to responses primarily in the gastrointestinal and respiratory tracts, bladder, heart, eye and glands. The action of acetylcholine on nicotinic receptors in the autonomic ganglia and skeletal muscle leads to autonomic post-ganglionic neurotransmission and skeletal muscle contraction, respectively.

This chapter provides a general overview of autonomic and somatic nervous system function and reviews clinically relevant drugs that mimic, intensify or block the action of acetylcholine on muscarinic receptors in the parasympathetic system, on the ganglion-type nicotinic receptors of the autonomic nervous system and on the muscle-type nicotinic receptors at the skeletal neuromuscular junction.

KEY DRUG GROUPS

ACETYLCHOLINESTERASE:

- Acetylcholinesterase reactivator: pralidoxime
- Anticholinesterase agents: **donepezil**, **galantamine**, **neostigmine** (Drug Monograph 8.3), **rivastigmine**

PARASYMPATHETIC NERVOUS SYSTEM:

- Muscarinic receptor agonists: **bethanechol** (Drug Monograph 8.1)
- Muscarinic receptor antagonists: **atropine** (Drug Monograph 8.2), **glycopyrronium bromide** (**glycopyrrolate**), **ipratropium bromide**

SOMATIC NERVOUS SYSTEM:

- Depolarising neuromuscular blocking drugs: **suxamethonium** (Drug Monograph 8.4)
- Non-depolarising neuromuscular blocking drugs: **atracurium**, cisatracurium, pancuronium, **rocuronium** (Drug Monograph 8.4)

CRITICAL THINKING SCENARIO

In the early afternoon, 26-year-old horticulturist Jonah was brought by ambulance to the emergency department. The treating paramedics noted that he was working in the orchard when he initially complained to his supervisor of blurred vision and watery eyes. Within the hour he had become agitated, disoriented and had difficulty breathing. It had been noted by his supervisor that the apple trees had been sprayed with pesticide early in the morning. Organophosphate poisoning was suspected to be the cause.

1. What is the cause of each of his symptoms?
2. What is the mechanism of action of this agent?
3. What would be the initial treatment of Jonah and, if poisoning, what would be the antidote?
4. Discuss the mechanism of action of any antidotes. Should the paramedics and staff at the orchard also be taking precautions against poisoning?

Introduction: General overview of the autonomic and somatic nervous systems

The two principal divisions of the nervous system are the central nervous system (CNS) and the peripheral nervous system (PNS). The PNS is divided further, on a functional and anatomical basis, into two subdivisions: the autonomic and the somatic nervous systems. The **autonomic nervous system** (ANS) primarily maintains the internal environment of the body at an optimal level (**homeostasis**) and cannot function independently of the CNS. The activities regulated by the ANS are not under direct conscious control and include the contraction and relaxation of smooth muscle, regulation of heartbeat and glandular secretions. The ANS is organised into two subdivisions (Fig 8.1):

- **parasympathetic nervous system** (Fig 8.2)
- sympathetic nervous system (Fig 8.2 and Ch 9).

There are also interactions with the enteric nervous system (Ch 16).

The afferent (incoming) fibres of both systems carry sensory information to the CNS, which is integrated at various levels within the brain. The information that flows out from the CNS is conducted along efferent (outgoing) motor neurons of either the autonomic efferent system or the somatic efferent system (see 'Homeostatic Actions' below). These systems innervate various organs and tissues (commonly called effectors) that produce a physiological response when stimulated

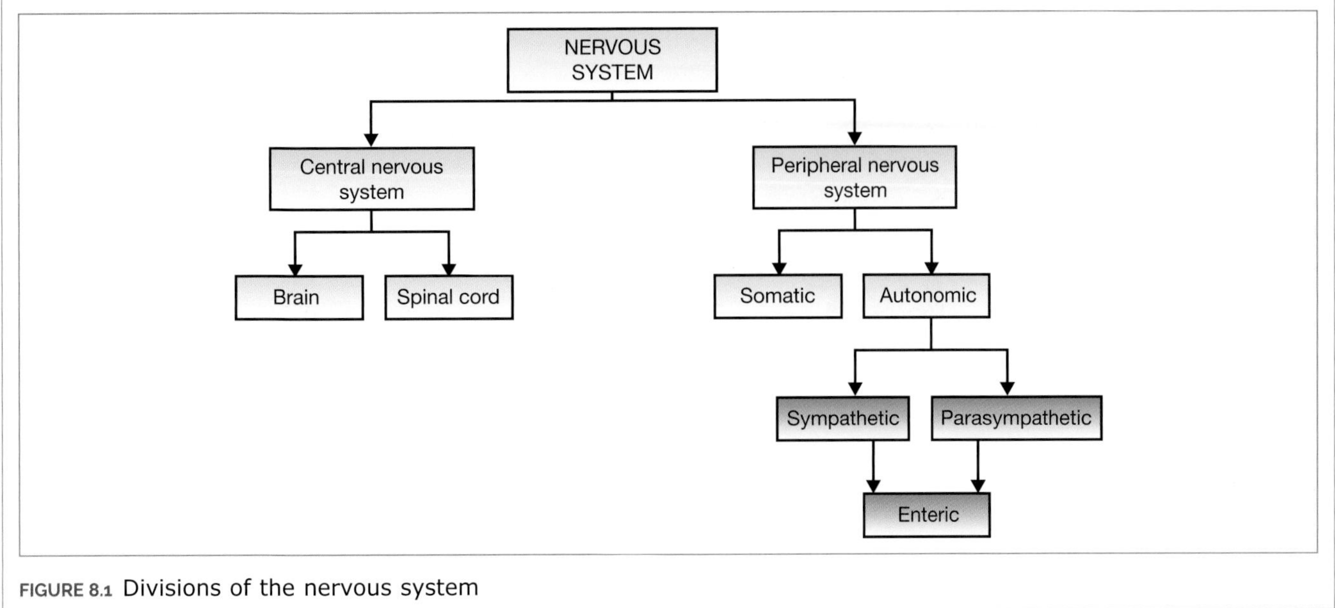

FIGURE 8.1 Divisions of the nervous system

by the appropriate nerves (Figs 8.2 and 8.3). Innervation of skeletal muscle is principally coordinated by the somatic nervous system.

Homeostatic actions

The simplest means by which homeostasis is maintained is via autonomic (visceral) reflexes. The first component of the reflex arc is the receptor, which detects changes such as a rise or fall in temperature or in pressure in blood vessels or distension in the viscera. Information from the receptor is then transmitted via a sensory (afferent) neuron to the CNS, the site of integration. The preganglionic, autonomic efferent (motor) neuron then conveys nerve impulses from the CNS to ganglia and onwards to the effector, which produces the appropriate alteration of activity of muscles and glands. The information carried to the CNS (sensory or input) and instructions sent from the CNS (motor output) constitute a feedback control mechanism. Nerve impulses may vary in frequency and pattern according to the degree of activity required of the effector. The control of visceral function is involuntary, so the feedback mechanism must include all the components of a control system essential to performing the reflex act, the sole purpose of which is to prevent extreme changes in function that may create a disturbance in the internal environment.

Most organs receive dual innervation from the parasympathetic and sympathetic systems. In general, the opposing actions of the two systems balance one another; for example, a rise in parasympathetic activity is accompanied by a fall in sympathetic input (Fig 8.2 and Table 8.1). In many instances, therefore, the systems produce opposite effects, but they may also produce the same effect; for example, in salivary glands stimulation from both systems produces secretion. The noticeable exceptions are the lacrimal (tear) glands of the eye, which receive only parasympathetic fibres. In contrast, the arrector pili muscles attached to hair follicles in the skin, adipocytes (fat cells), kidneys and blood vessels are innervated solely by sympathetic fibres. Regarding the human airway, the situation is even more complex. The dominant neural control is exerted through parasympathetic cholinergic nerves that mediate bronchoconstriction. In contrast, sympathetic innervation of the airways is sparse, and few noradrenergic fibres have been demonstrated in human airways. However, both α- and β-adrenoceptors are present in airways, and these are activated by circulating catecholamines, predominantly adrenaline[1] (Chs 9 and 15).

Physiological differences between the subdivisions of the ANS

The parasympathetic nervous system functions mainly to conserve energy and restore body resources and is often referred to as initiating 'resting and digesting'. This includes reducing heart rate, increasing gastrointestinal activity and secretion of digestive enzymes associated with increased digestion and absorption. In contrast, the sympathetic nervous system dominates the body during

1 Reminder: In the American literature, noradrenaline and adrenaline are known as norepinephrine and epinephrine, respectively, from an old name for the adrenal gland, the epinephric gland. From April 2016, medicines containing adrenaline and noradrenaline include the international names 'epinephrine' and 'norepinephrine' on labels and information leaflets. Refer to Ch 9.

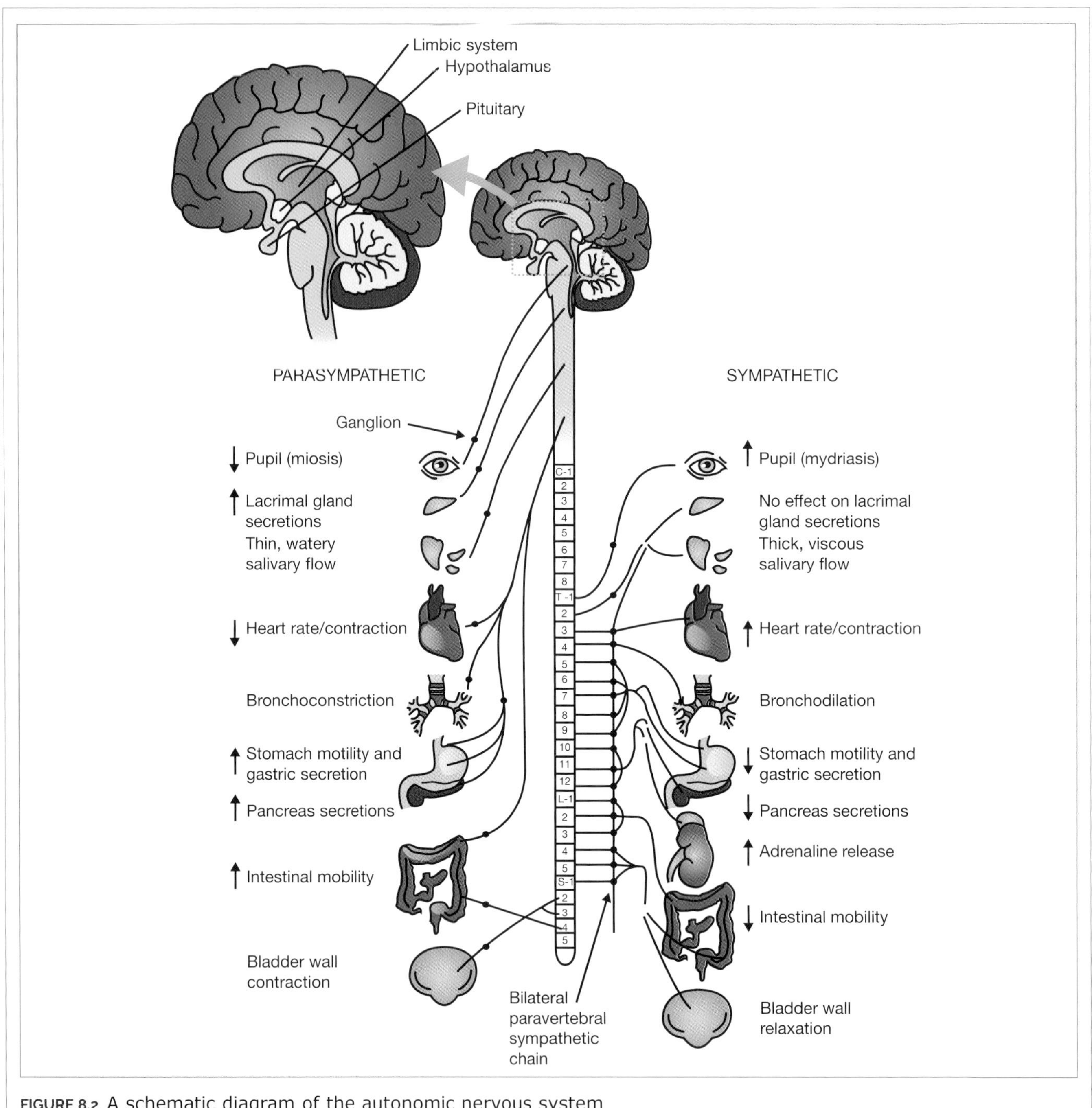

FIGURE 8.2 A schematic diagram of the autonomic nervous system
Source: Adapted from Salerno 1999, Figure 14.3; used with permission.

emergency and stress situations and is often called the 'fight-or-flight' system. The sympathetic response to physical or emotional stress involves expenditure of energy and includes an increase in the blood glucose concentration, heart activity and blood pressure (Table 8.1). The concept of these two extreme situations (rest and flight) in humans is outdated. In everyday life the ANS functions continually, and the balance of sympathetic and parasympathetic control depends on the needs of a particular organ at any given time.

Anatomical differences between the subdivisions of the ANS

The parasympathetic and sympathetic efferent pathways consist of two **neurons** (nerve cells) and an **autonomic ganglion**, which is a collection of neuronal cell bodies. The first neuron is known as the preganglionic neuron and extends from the cell body in the CNS to the autonomic ganglion. The second neuron is called the postganglionic neuron and extends from the autonomic

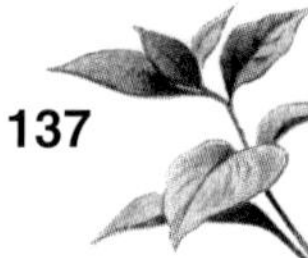

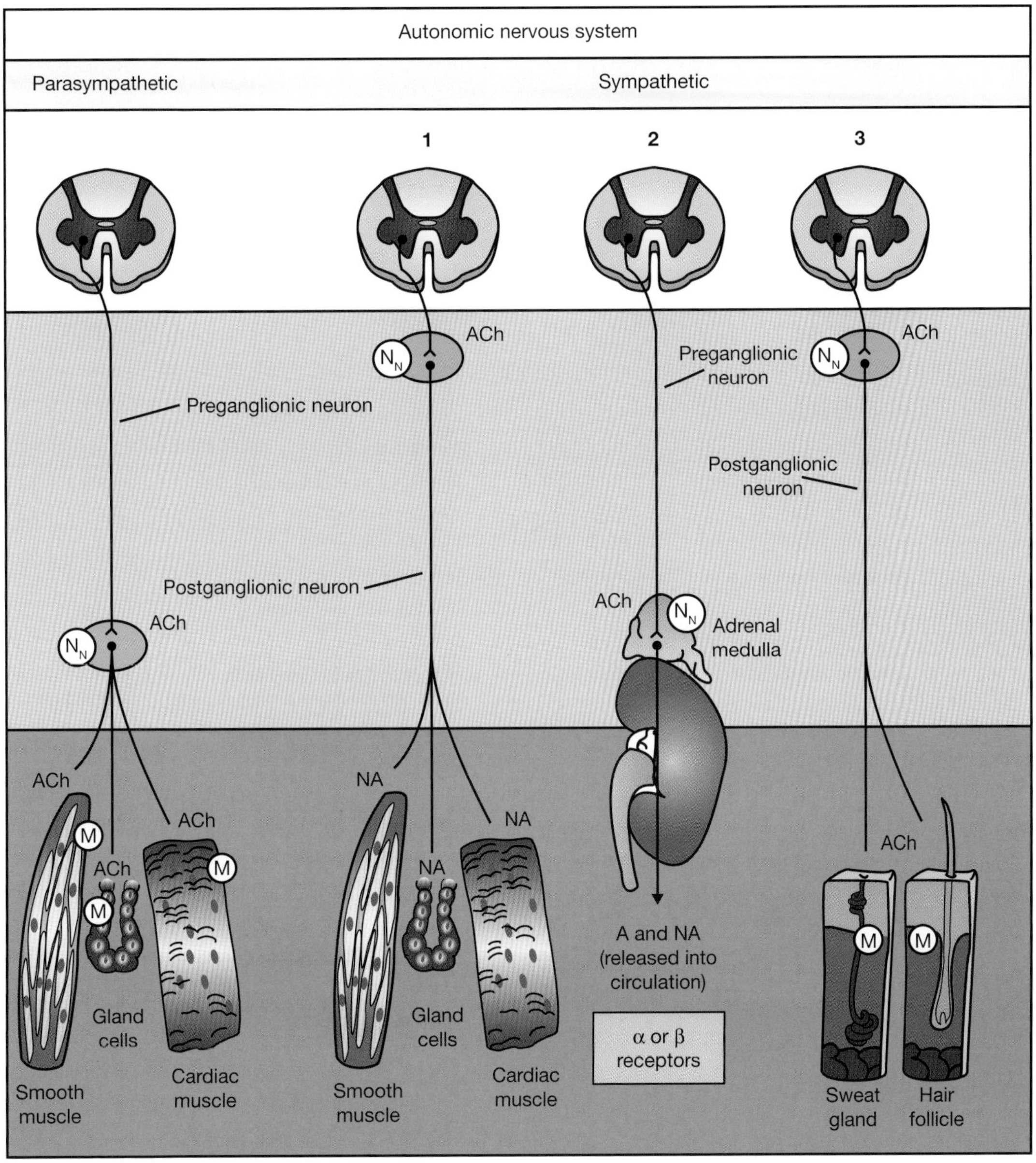

FIGURE 8.3 Chemical neurotransmitters and receptor sites in the autonomic nervous system
A = adrenaline; ACh = acetylcholine; NA = noradrenaline; NN = neuronal nicotinic receptor; M = muscarinic receptor.
Source: Adapted from Salerno 1999, Figure 14.2; used with permission.

ganglion to the effector organ, gland or cell. The parasympathetic preganglionic fibres emerge with the cranial nerves (III, VII, IX and X) and at the sacral spinal levels from about S2 through S4 (Fig 8.2). The tenth cranial nerve (X), or vagus nerve, has extensive branches that supply fibres to the heart, lungs and almost all the abdominal organs. The parasympathetic ganglia are located close to the effectors that produce the physiological response, and consequently the preganglionic axon tends to be long.

The sympathetic system is also called the thoracolumbar system because its preganglionic fibres originate in the spinal cord from thoracic segment T1 to the lumbar segment at L2 level (Fig 8.2). The sympathetic ganglia lie on either side of the vertebral column in two chains, called the paravertebral sympathetic chains; hence the sympathetic preganglionic axons tend to be short. The only exception to the two-neuron arrangement is the adrenal medulla, which is supplied directly by a preganglionic neuron.

The enteric nervous system consists of the neurons whose cell bodies lie in the intramural plexuses of the gastrointestinal tract and incoming nerves from both the sympathetic and the parasympathetic systems that

TABLE 8.1 Responses to autonomic nerve impulses and relevant receptors

	PARASYMPATHETIC		SYMPATHETIC	
EFFECTOR ORGANS	RESPONSE	RECEPTOR	RESPONSE	RECEPTOR
Heart				
Sinoatrial node	↓ Heart rate	$M_2{>}{>}M_3$	↑ Heart rate	$\beta_1{>}\beta_2$
Atrioventricular node	↓ Conduction velocity	$M_2{>}{>}M_3$	↑ Automaticity ↑ Conduction velocity	$\beta_1{>}\beta_2$
Atria	↓ Force ↓ AP duration	$M_2{>}{>}M_3$	↑ Force ↑ Conduction velocity	$\beta_1{>}\beta_2$
Ventricles	↓ Contractility (slight)	$M_2{>}{>}M_3$	↑ Force of contraction ↑ Conduction velocity ↑ Automaticity	$\beta_1{>}\beta_2$
Arterioles (smooth muscle)				
Coronary	No innervation	M_3[a]	Constriction (+), dilation (++)	α_1, α_2, β_2
Skin and mucosa	No innervation	M_3[a]	Constriction	α_1, α_2
Skeletal muscle	Dilation (no innervation)	M_2[b] (indirect)	Constriction and dilation	α_1, β_2
Cerebral	No innervation	M_3[a]	Slight constriction	α_1
Mesenteric	No innervation	M_3[a]	Constriction and dilation	α_1, β_2
Renal	No innervation	M_3[a]	Constriction and dilation	α_1, α_2, β_1, β_2
Veins (systemic)	No innervation	–	Constriction and dilation	α_1, α_2, β_2
Lung				
Bronchial muscle	Bronchoconstriction	$M_3 > M_2$	Bronchodilation (no direct sympathetic innervation)	β_2 (dilated by circulating adrenaline)
Bronchial glands	Secretion	M_2, M_3	↓ Secretion ↑ Secretion	α_1 β_2
Gastrointestinal tract				
Motility	↑ Motility	$M_2 = M_3$	↓ Motility	α_1, α_2, β_1, β_2
Sphincters	Relaxation (open)	M_2, M_3	Contraction (closed)	α_1
Exocrine glands	↑ Secretion Gastric acid secretion	M_3 M_1	Inhibition	α_2
Salivary glands	Copious watery secretion	M_2, M_3	Thick, viscous secretion	α_1
Gallbladder and ducts	Contraction	M_2, M_3	Relaxation	β_2
Kidney (renin secretion)	No innervation	–	Decrease; increase	α_1; β_1
Urinary bladder				
Detrusor muscle	Contraction	$M_3{>}M_2$	Relaxation	β_2
Trigone and sphincter	Relaxation	$M_3{>}M_2$	Contraction	α_1
Eye				
Radial muscle, iris	–	–	Contraction (mydriasis)	α_1
Sphincter muscle, iris	Contraction (miosis)	M_2, M_3		
Ciliary muscle	Contraction for near vision	M_2, M_3	Relaxation for far vision (slight)	β_2
Aqueous humour			Formation, outflow	β_1, β_2
Skin				
Sweat glands	No effect	–	↑ Sweating	α_1, mainly cholinergic
Arrector pili muscle	No innervation	–	Piloerection (gooseflesh)	α_1
Lacrimal glands	↑ Secretion	M_2, M_3	Secretion	α_1
Nasopharyngeal glands	↑ Secretion	M_2, M_3	No innervation	–
Male sex organs	Erection	M_3	Ejaculation	α_1

α = alpha receptor, β = beta receptor, M = muscarinic receptor

[a] Stimulation of muscarinic receptors on blood vessel endothelial cells causes the release of nitric oxide, which is a vasodilator. These muscarinic receptors are not directly innervated but respond only to circulating muscarinic agonists.

[b] In skeletal muscle blood vessels acetylcholine binding to presynaptic M_2 receptors on postganglionic sympathetic neurons inhibits the release of noradrenaline. Inhibition of noradrenaline-induced vasoconstriction results in vasodilation.

Source: Brunton L.L., & Hilal-Dandan R, & Knollmann B.C.(Eds.), (2017). Goodman & Gilman's: The Pharmacological Basis of Therapeutics, 13e. McGraw Hill.

terminate on enteric neurons in the wall of the intestine. The enteric nervous system, however, is pharmacologically more complex than the sympathetic or parasympathetic systems, involving many neuropeptides and other transmitters (e.g. 5-hydroxytryptamine and nitric oxide) (Ch 16).

KEY POINTS

The autonomic nervous system

- The principal divisions of the nervous system are the central nervous system (CNS) and the peripheral nervous system (PNS), which has three subdivisions – the autonomic nervous system (ANS), the somatic nervous system (SNS) and the enteric nervous system.
- The ANS regulates the function of smooth muscle, cardiac muscle and glandular secretions, which are not under direct conscious control.
- The ANS is organised into two subdivisions: the parasympathetic and sympathetic systems.
- The principal neurotransmitters in the ANS are acetylcholine and noradrenaline.
- Autonomic reflexes play a key role in maintaining homeostasis.
- The parasympathetic system functions to conserve energy (the resting and digesting response), while activity of the sympathetic system increases in response to demand and is best known for mediation of the fight or flight response.
- There are physiological and anatomical differences between the subdivisions of the ANS.

Neurochemical transmission

The passage of a nerve impulse from one neuron to another neuron (e.g. at autonomic ganglia) or from a neuron to an effector via a chemical signal is called **neurochemical transmission**. When the action potential reaches the presynaptic nerve terminal, the electrical signal is converted to a chemical signal by release of a **neurotransmitter**, which acts as a chemical messenger enabling nerve cells to communicate signals to the structures they innervate. The site at which communication between neurons occurs is called a **synapse**. Communication between a neuron and an effector occurs at a **neuroeffector junction**. In the parasympathetic and sympathetic nervous systems, synapses occur at ganglia, which are the sites of synapses between the preganglionic and postganglionic neurons and between the postganglionic neuron and the effector tissue or organ. The presence of a specific chemical at these synapses determines the type of information a neuron can receive and the range of responses it can yield in return. Receptors on the postsynaptic membrane bind the transmitter, which initiates a postsynaptic response that can be either excitatory or inhibitory. There are more than 100 specific neurotransmitters, and these are discussed in the context of the relevant pharmacology in the appropriate chapters.

Acetylcholine and cholinergic transmission

There are multiple neurotransmitters in the ANS, but the two transmitters we have the most extensive knowledge of are **acetylcholine** (ACh) and noradrenaline. Nerves that release ACh are called **cholinergic neurons** and are involved in cholinergic transmission (Fig 8.3). ACh is the neurotransmitter released from:

- preganglionic neurons in both the parasympathetic and the sympathetic systems
- postganglionic parasympathetic nerve fibres
- postganglionic sympathetic neurons that innervate sweat glands and the base of hair follicles
- somatic neurons.

For correct transmission across synapses to occur the neurotransmitter must first be synthesised, stored and then released, so it can bind to and activate receptors and finally be inactivated. Many autonomic and somatic drugs affect one of these individual events, so it is essential to understand the basic mechanisms involved in neurotransmission.

The process involves several steps:

1. ACh is synthesised in the cytoplasm of the nerve terminal from free choline and acetyl coenzyme A via the action of the enzyme choline acetyltransferase.
2. Once synthesised, ACh is transported by the vesicular ACh transporter into synaptic vesicles or granules, which are located in the nerve terminal (Fig 8.4).
3. The arrival of an action potential at the nerve ending facilitates the entry of calcium, which induces the synaptic vesicles containing ACh to attach to specific docking sites on the synaptic membrane. This process of vesicle–membrane fusion is driven by the vesicle protein synaptobrevin and the two membrane proteins SNAP-25 and syntaxin 1.

   The release of the neurotransmitter molecules from the vesicle into the synaptic cleft occurs via a process called exocytosis, which is driven by the synaptotagmin family of proteins. The whole process of vesicle docking, cycling and exocytosis is under the control of these various trafficking proteins.

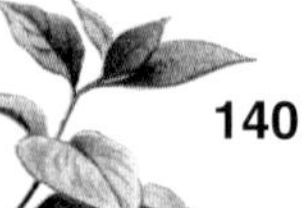

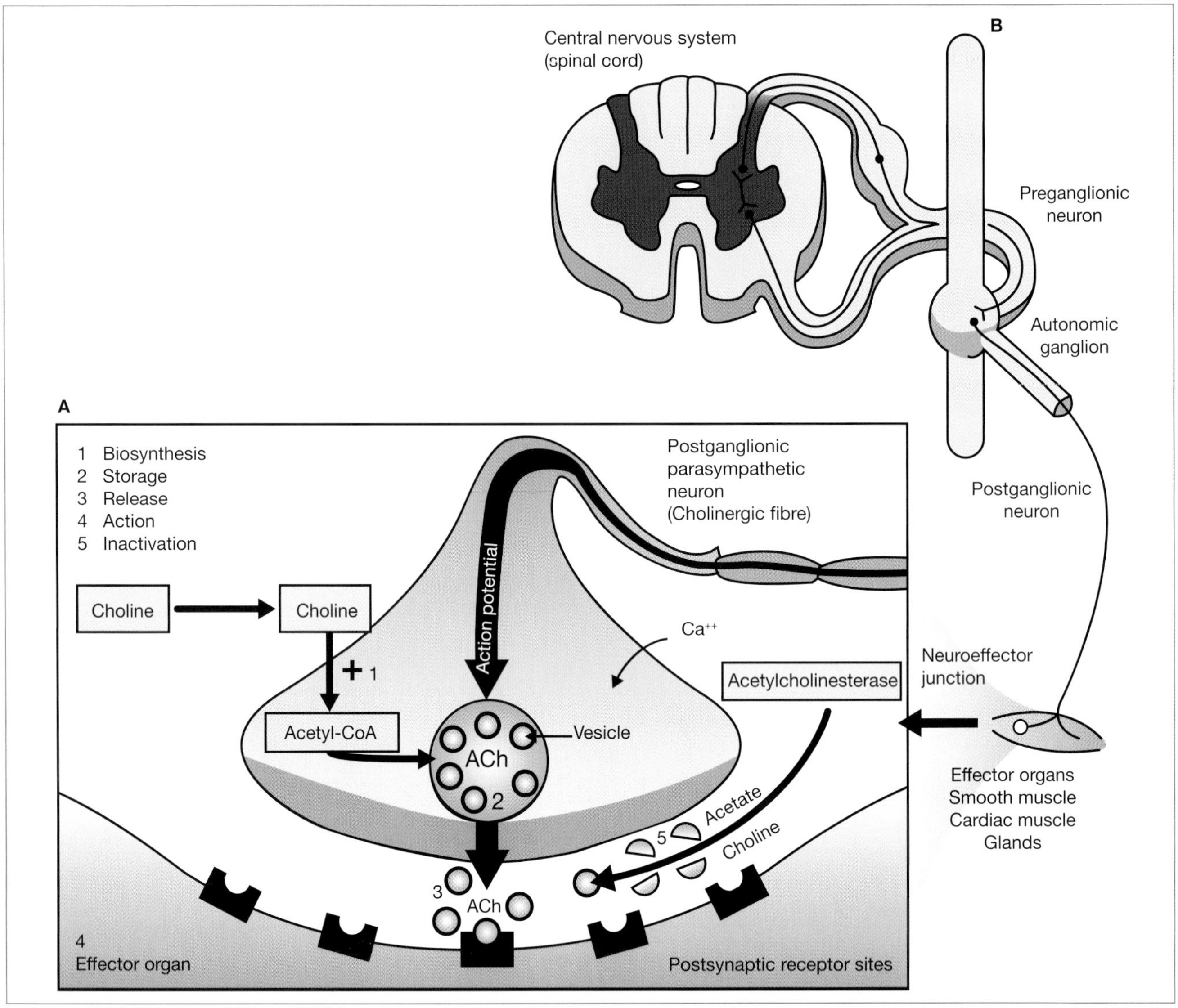

FIGURE 8.4 **A** Cholinergic transmission at a neuroeffector junction; **B** Schematic representation of the relation between a neuron in the CNS, a preganglionic neuron and an effector organ innervated by a postganglionic parasympathetic neuron. **1** *Biosynthesis of ACh:* choline is taken up by the axon terminal and ACh is synthesised from choline and acetyl coenzyme A. **2** *Storage:* after synthesis, ACh is stored in the vesicle until the arrival of a nerve impulse. **3** *Release:* an action potential arriving at the nerve terminal causes the vesicle to attach itself to the membrane and release ACh, which then diffuses across the synaptic cleft and combines with the receptors on the effector cell. **4** *Action:* the interaction of ACh with the receptors results in a response. **5** *Inactivation of ACh:* at the synaptic cleft, ACh is hydrolysed by the enzyme acetylcholinesterase.
Source: Adapted from Salerno 1999, Figure 14.4; used with permission.

4 Once ACh has been released from the synaptic vesicles it diffuses across the synaptic cleft and attaches to specialised postsynaptic receptors on the membrane of the next neuron or effector site (e.g. glands, skeletal muscles).

   The binding of ACh to the nicotinic receptor increases the permeability of the postsynaptic membrane of the **neuromuscular junction** (NMJ) to sodium and potassium ions, via nicotinic receptor activation, which results in excitation or inhibition of skeletal muscle activity, or activation of specific muscarinic G-protein-coupled receptors regulating glandular or smooth and cardiac muscle activity at the neuroeffector junction (Figs 8.3 and 8.4).

5 Inactivation of ACh ensues.

Cholinergic receptors

Sir Henry Dale, investigating the pharmacological properties of ACh in 1914, distinguished two actions that are reproduced by the alkaloids[2] muscarine (obtained from the toadstool *Amanita muscaria*) and nicotine, which

2 In general, alkaloids are a broad group of compounds containing nitrogen that are found predominantly in various plants and fungi.

is an alkaloid from the nightshade family of plants (e.g. tobacco plant *Nicotiana tabacum*). As the effects of muscarine mimic the parasympathetic nervous system, he termed the receptors 'muscarinic', while those in autonomic ganglia and at the skeletal NMJ were termed 'nicotinic receptors' because the effects of nicotine mimic actions of the somatic and autonomic nervous systems. Five distinct subtypes of muscarinic acetylcholine receptors (mAChRs) have been identified, of which three are relevant clinically. These subtypes are classified broadly as the neural type (M_1), the cardiac and presynaptic type (M_2) and the glandular or smooth muscle type (M_3) (Table 8.1). In the periphery mAChRs, which are all G-protein-coupled receptors (Ch 3), are located in smooth muscle, cardiac muscle and glands, while, in the CNS, mAChRs are involved in functions such as motor control, memory and cardiovascular and temperature regulation.

Nicotinic receptors (nAChRs) are classed as peripheral or central neuronal (CNS) types, and the skeletal muscle type (N_M). The peripheral neuronal nicotinic receptors (N_N) are found in the adrenal medulla and in the ganglia of both the parasympathetic and the sympathetic systems (Fig 8.3). The CNS types of nAChRs are widespread throughout the brain.

Cholinergic activity

As above, ACh has two major actions via the relevant receptors:

- stimulant effects on the ganglia, adrenal medulla and skeletal muscle (nicotinic receptors)
- stimulant effects at postganglionic nerve endings in cardiac muscle, smooth muscle and glands (muscarinic receptors).

KEY POINTS

Acetylcholine and cholinergic transmission

- Neurons communicate with each other or with effectors via generation of an electrical signal or action potential.
- Information transfer (signal transmission) at synapses is facilitated by neurotransmitters.
- Neurotransmitters are stored in presynaptic vesicles, released by exocytosis and have their actions terminated by metabolism, reuptake into nerve terminals and diffusion.
- Parasympathetic and sympathetic efferent (motor) pathways consist of preganglionic neurons that extend from cell bodies in the CNS to the autonomic ganglia, and postganglionic neurons that extend from the ganglia to various effector organs.
- ACh is the transmitter between pre- and postganglionic neurons in both the parasympathetic and the sympathetic systems, and between postganglionic parasympathetic nerves and effector organs.
- The cholinergic receptors stimulated by ACh are either nicotinic or muscarinic receptors.
- Nicotinic receptors exist in the ganglia of the parasympathetic and sympathetic systems, adrenal medulla and skeletal muscle (somatic motor system) and CNS.
- Five distinct subtypes of mAChRs have been identified. The three that are relevant pharmacologically are classified broadly as the neural type (M_1), the cardiac and presynaptic type (M_2) and the glandular or smooth muscle type (M_3).
- Muscarinic receptors are located mainly at postganglionic parasympathetic sites in smooth muscle, cardiac muscle and glands. Sympathetic cholinergic neurons activate muscarinic receptors on sweat glands and arrector pili muscles on hair follicles.

Drugs acting at muscarinic receptors

Although ACh is important physiologically, it has no therapeutic value because it lacks selectivity, binding to both nicotinic and muscarinic receptors, and its duration of action is exceedingly brief (< 1 millisecond) due to rapid hydrolysis by anticholinesterase. The lack of tissue selectivity, which is due to the widespread distribution of muscarinic receptors, is common to many of the drugs discussed in this chapter.

Muscarinic receptor agonists

Muscarinic receptor agonists, also referred to as **parasympathomimetics** or **cholinomimetics** (e.g. bethanechol), bind to **muscarinic receptors** and mimic the action of ACh from the parasympathetic nervous system. These drugs are divided into two groups:

- **choline esters**, which are chemically similar to the neurotransmitter ACh and include carbachol, methacholine and bethanechol. Bethanechol is used systemically for urinary retention, increasing the tone of the bladder detrusor muscle (Drug Monograph 8.1)
- **cholinomimetic alkaloids** and synthetic analogues, which include muscarine, pilocarpine and oxotremorine. Pilocarpine is used to treat glaucoma, inducing miosis, contracting the ciliary muscle and allowing the outflow of aqueous humour (Ch 40). Refer to Fig 8.5 for the pharmacological effects of muscarinic receptor agonists.

Drug Monograph 8.1
Bethanechol

Bethanechol acts on muscarinic receptors (possibly M_3 receptors, although it is not certain) on the detrusor muscle of the urinary bladder and smooth muscle of the gastrointestinal tract. In the bladder, the resulting contraction of the smooth muscle is sufficiently strong to initiate micturition and empty the bladder. In the gastrointestinal tract, the drug stimulates gastric motility, increases gastric tone and often restores impaired peristaltic activity of the oesophagus, stomach and intestine. It also promotes defecation. Its actions are similar to, although longer acting than, those of the physiological mediator ACh, and its effect is blocked by atropine. Therapeutic doses in normal human subjects have little effect on heart rate, blood pressure or the peripheral circulation.

Indications

More effective drugs have generally replaced bethanechol; it is available for treating postoperative and postpartum non-obstructive urinary retention (although not recommended because the effect is inconsistent) and for neurogenic atony of the urinary bladder associated with retention.

Pharmacokinetics

Bethanechol is a polar (charged) quaternary ammonium compound. Despite being poorly absorbed from the gastrointestinal tract, bethanechol chloride is effective orally. It does not penetrate the blood–brain barrier in therapeutic doses, but it is distributed to areas of low blood flow. Unlike ACh, bethanechol, because it has a different chemical structure, is not degraded by AChE, and its effects therefore are more prolonged than those of ACh. Onset of action is between 30 and 90 minutes of oral administration, peak effect occurs within 90 minutes and duration of action is up to 6 hours, depending on the dose administered. When the drug is administered subcutaneously, the onset of action is between 5 and 15 minutes, peak effect occurs between 15 and 30 minutes and the duration of action is about 2 hours. Routes of metabolism and excretion are unknown.

Drug interactions

The following effects can occur when bethanechol is given with the drugs listed:

- Other muscarinic agonists or anticholinesterase drugs: enhanced cholinergic effects and perhaps toxicity; monitor closely for adverse effects or, if possible, avoid this combination of medications.
- Muscarinic receptor antagonists or drugs with anticholinergic effects: may decrease clinical effectiveness.

Adverse reactions

Adverse reactions are presented in Table 8.2. The adverse effects of this drug, which include bradycardia, hypotension, sweating, salivation, vomiting, diarrhoea and intestinal cramps, are a consequence of parasympathetic stimulation.

Warnings and contraindications

Use is contraindicated in people with known bethanechol hypersensitivity, Parkinson's disease (will worsen symptoms), asthma (will cause bronchoconstriction), epilepsy, hypotension, severe bradycardia (will decrease heart rate further), coronary artery disease, gastrointestinal obstruction, hyperthyroidism (may precipitate atrial fibrillation) and peptic ulcer (will stimulate gastric acid secretion). No data are available regarding excretion in breast milk. Bethanechol should be avoided during pregnancy because of excitatory effects on bladder smooth muscle.

Muscarinic receptor antagonists

Muscarinic receptor antagonists are often referred to as **parasympatholytics** or **anticholinergics** (e.g. atropine) because they competitively block the action of ACh at muscarinic receptors (e.g. they block the effects of stimulation of the parasympathetic nervous system). (See Fig 8.3 and Table 8.1 for muscarinic receptor sites.) These drugs are categorised as:

- naturally occurring alkaloids (e.g. atropine and hyoscine) that are lipid-soluble, absorbed from the gastrointestinal tract and the conjunctiva and penetrate the blood–brain barrier
- semisynthetic derivatives (e.g. homatropine)
- synthetic drugs that exhibit some degree of muscarinic receptor selectivity – for example, the quaternary ammonium compounds ipratropium (acts on M_2 presynaptic autoreceptors and M_3 postsynaptic receptors) and tiotropium (acts on M_1 and M_3 receptors) used to treat asthma (Ch 15); the M_3 receptor antagonists oxybutynin (Ch 17) and propantheline used for urinary dysfunction; tropicamide used for eye disorders (Ch 40); and the M_1 selective antagonist pirenzepine (not available in Australia and New Zealand), which inhibits gastric acid secretion but has little effect elsewhere in the body.

The best-known muscarinic antagonists are atropine and hyoscine. *Atropa belladonna* (deadly nightshade)

Pupil constriction (miosis), lacrimation
Decreased intraocular pressure (treatment of glaucoma)
Increased cognition and arousal
Increased salivation
Bronchoconstriction, increased airways mucus secretion
Increased sweating (sympathetic cholinergic effect)
Bradycardia–decreased heart rate and force of contraction
Nausea and vomiting
Increased stomach motility
Increased gastrointestinal secretions
Increased peristalsis (contraction of GI tract)–diarrhoea
Treatment of atony (paralytic ileus)
Micturition (urinary incontinence)
Increased blood flow to skeletal muscles

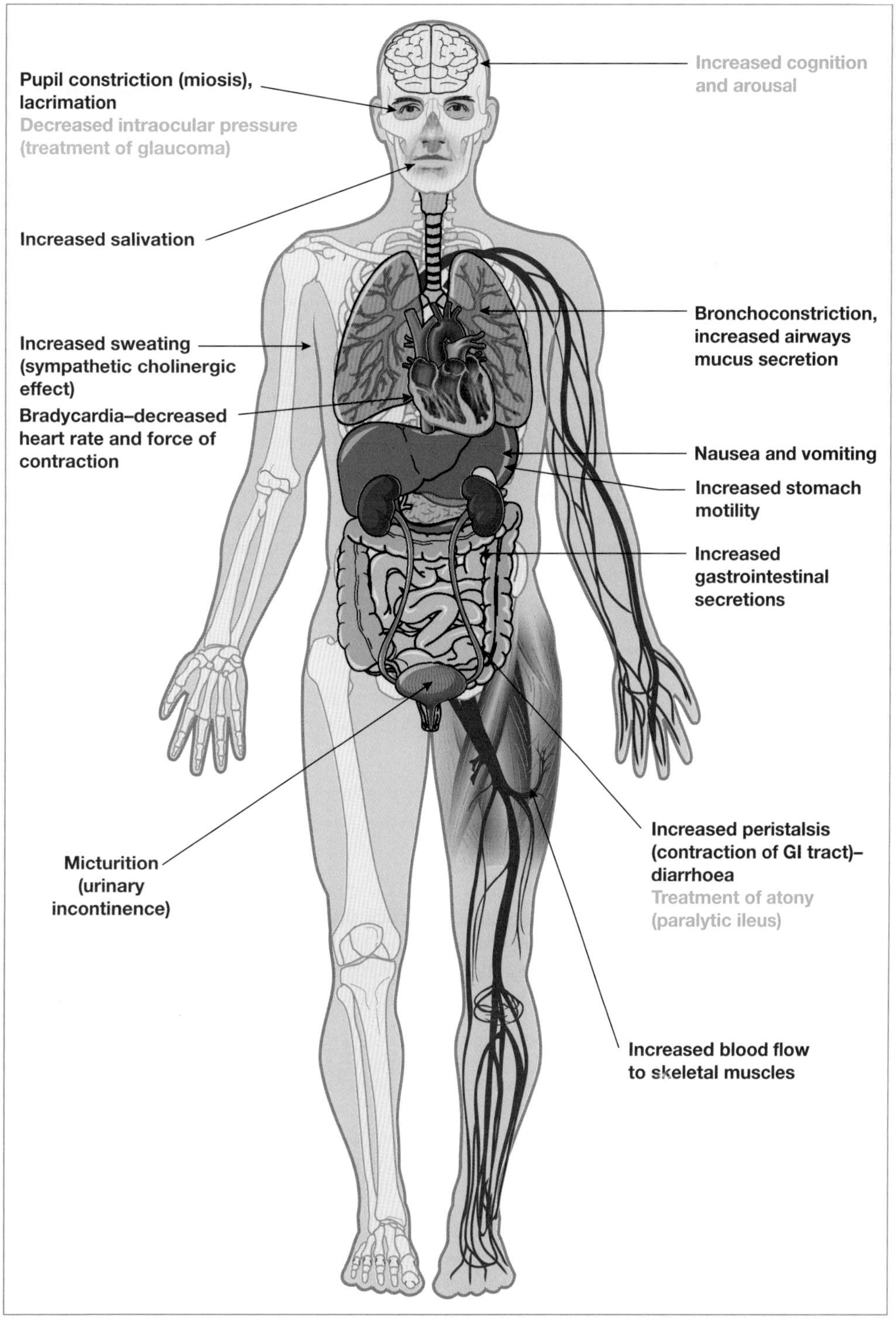

FIGURE 8.5 Pharmacological effects of muscarinic receptor agonists

contains mainly atropine, whereas *Hyoscyamus niger* (henbane) and *Datura stramonium* (jimsonweed) contain hyoscine. Atropine (Drug Monograph 8.2) is the prototype muscarinic antagonist and its use for more than half a century is testimony to its therapeutic effectiveness. With the exception of some degree of selectivity for the heart and gastrointestinal tract (M_2 and M_3 receptor subtypes, respectively), all the muscarinic receptor antagonists produce peripheral effects similar to those observed with atropine. To avoid the widespread unwanted effects of muscarinic receptor antagonism, more selective drugs have been developed. Synthetic anticholinergic drugs

with fewer central adverse effects than atropine are used to treat Parkinson's disease. These include benzatropine and trihexyphenidyl. Their usefulness is limited by peripheral anticholinergic (atropinic) adverse reactions and their tendency to be less effective with continued use. They are also used to control extrapyramidal reactions, such as rigidity, akinesia (difficulty in or lack of ability to initiate muscle movement), tremor and akathisia, induced by antipsychotic drugs (Ch 22). Muscarinic receptor antagonists and their main uses are shown in Table 8.3. Refer to Fig 8.6 for the pharmacological effects of muscarinic receptor antagonists.

Drug Monograph 8.2
Atropine

Atropine is a non-selective muscarinic receptor antagonist that has very little effect on the actions of ACh at nicotinic receptors. It produces a wide range of pharmacological effects because of the widespread distribution of muscarinic receptors in the body. The main effects are summarised below.

Eyes

The pupil is dilated (mydriasis) and relaxation of the ciliary muscle causes failure of accommodation (cycloplegia), impairing near vision. Pupil dilation may reduce outflow of aqueous humour, causing a rise in intraocular pressure, a hazardous situation for people with narrow-angle glaucoma. These effects in the eye occur with local and systemic administration of atropine, although the usual single therapeutic dose of atropine given orally or parenterally has little effect on the eye. Following pupil dilation photophobia occurs, and the usual reflexes to light and accommodation disappear.

Skin and mucous membranes

Low doses of atropine inhibit secretion from lacrimal, bronchial, salivary and sweat glands. This produces the characteristic drying of the mucous membranes of the mouth, nose, pharynx and bronchi, and causes the skin to become hot and dry.

Respiratory system

Atropine relaxes the smooth muscle of the bronchial tract but is less effective than adrenaline as a bronchodilator and is not used for asthma.

Cardiovascular system

When very low doses of atropine are administered, the heart rate is temporarily slowed because of a central action that augments vagal activity (paradoxical bradycardia). Larger doses block the effect of vagal stimulation on the sinoatrial node and atrioventricular junction, which leads to an increased heart rate. In therapeutic doses, atropine has little or no effect on blood pressure because most vascular beds lack significant cholinergic innervation.

Gastrointestinal tract

The effect of atropine on the secretions of the pancreas and intestinal glands is not therapeutically significant, but atropine (in larger doses) incompletely inhibits gastrointestinal motility. Gastric acid secretion is reduced slightly.

Urinary tract

Atropine slightly relaxes smooth muscle of the urinary tract, and therapeutic doses decrease the tone of the fundus of the urinary bladder. It also causes constriction of the internal sphincter, which can produce urinary retention, particularly in elderly men with prostatic enlargement.

Central nervous system

As atropine penetrates the blood–brain barrier it has prominent effects on the CNS and in large doses causes excitement, agitation, irritability, hallucinations, delirium and, finally, stupor and coma. These effects are due to blockade of central muscarinic receptors. A rise in temperature is sometimes seen, especially in infants and young children, probably as a result of suppression of sweating. Because they reduce cholinergic transmission, muscarinic receptor antagonists are used to treat the extrapyramidal effects (tremor, involuntary movements and rigidity) associated with both Parkinson's disease and antipsychotic drug use.

Pharmacokinetics

Atropine is a racemic tertiary ammonium compound that due to its lipid solubility is readily absorbed after oral and parenteral administration; it is also absorbed from mucous membranes. After intramuscular administration, peak plasma concentration is reached within 30 minutes. The duration of action is 4–6 hours, but ocular effects can last longer. Approximately 50% of the drug is bound to plasma proteins and unbound drug readily crosses the placental barrier and the blood–brain barrier. Atropine is metabolised primarily in the liver (~45%) to noratropine, atropine-*N*-oxide, tropine and tropic acid, and approximately 55% is excreted as unchanged drug in the urine.

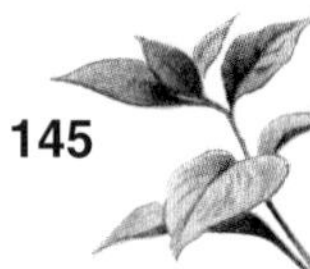

Drug interactions and adverse reactions

The anticholinergic effect of drugs such as tricyclic antidepressants (e.g. amitriptyline, nortriptyline, clomipramine, dosulepin [dothiepin]), some antihistamines (e.g. promethazine) and the phenothiazines (e.g. chlorpromazine) may be additive with atropine, increasing the therapeutic and adverse effects, including central delirium. Avoid a combination of drugs with anticholinergic effects and muscarinic receptor antagonists if possible. The reduction in gastric motility caused by atropine can also impair the absorption of other drugs. For adverse reactions, see Table 8.2.

Warnings and contraindications

Avoid use in people with atropine hypersensitivity or known hypersensitivity to other muscarinic antagonists. Atropine is contraindicated in myasthenia gravis, severe cardiac disease, gastrointestinal obstructive disease, narrow-angle glaucoma, acute haemorrhage, prostatic hypertrophy, urinary retention, pyloric obstruction, ulcerative colitis, toxaemia of pregnancy and febrile conditions and in debilitated patients with intestinal atony or paralytic ileus. Caution should be exercised in any situation where there is a higher likelihood of adverse effects – for example, Down syndrome, the elderly, people with autonomic neuropathy and hepatic and renal disease.

Dosage and administration

Atropine is used in a variety of circumstances including as a premedication prior to anaesthesia, to treat bradycardia during resuscitation and to treat poisoning with organophosphates. Current drug information sources or, if applicable, a Poisons Information Centre should be consulted before administration. As a premedication to prevent excessive salivation and respiratory tract secretions in adults during anaesthesia, 0.3–0.6 mg may be given intramuscularly about 1 hour before anaesthesia or intravenously immediately before induction.

TABLE 8.2 Drugs affecting the parasympathetic nervous system: adverse reactions

DRUG	ADVERSE REACTIONS
Muscarinic agonists	
Bethanechol Pilocarpine	Abdominal pains or upset, increased salivation and sweating, nausea or vomiting; flushed skin; blurred or disturbed vision; unsteadiness; headache and diarrhoea Nausea, blurred vision and visual impairment and reduced visual acuity, dizziness
Muscarinic antagonists	
Atropine and hyoscine	Inhibition of sweating; constipation; dry mouth, throat and skin; blurred vision; urinary retention; headache; photophobia; drowsiness; weakness; nausea or vomiting; urticaria; dermatitis and eye pain from raised intraocular pressure. In addition, euphoria, amnesia and insomnia are reported more often with hyoscine
Glycopyrronium bromide (glycopyrrolate) (synthetic antispasmodic)	Abdominal distension; headache; dizziness; constipation; nausea; vomiting; sedation; dry mouth, nose, throat and skin; blurred or disturbed vision; dysuria; weakness; hypotension and decreased sexual ability

Hyoscine hydrobromide

Similar to atropine, hyoscine is a non-selective muscarinic receptor antagonist. The peripheral effects of hyoscine are similar to those of atropine but, due to greater permeation of the blood–brain barrier, it has marked effects on the CNS. At therapeutic doses, it depresses the CNS and causes drowsiness, euphoria, memory loss, relaxation and sleep. It does not increase blood pressure or respiration.

Because of its depressant action on vestibular function, it is used for motion sickness, to prevent nausea and vomiting and as an adjunct medication with general anaesthesia to reduce respiratory tract secretions. The pharmacokinetic properties of hyoscine are similar to those of atropine. For adverse reactions, refer to Table 8.2.

The elderly are more sensitive to this drug at the usual adult dosage; sensitivity can manifest as confusion, blurred vision and ataxia.

Synthetic and semisynthetic derivatives of atropine

The usefulness of atropine is limited by the fact that it is a complex drug and because it produces effects in a range of organs or tissues simultaneously, owing to the widespread distribution of muscarinic receptors. When it is administered for its antispasmodic effects, it also produces prolonged effects in the eye, causing dilated pupils and blurred vision. It also causes dry mouth and possibly tachycardia. Atropine does have some desirable effects, and a large number of drugs have been synthesised in an effort to take advantage of the antispasmodic effect of atropine without its other effects (Table 8.3).

Many products are marketed as antispasmodic and anticholinergic drugs, and their formulations are either modifications of a belladonna alkaloid or include one or more of the natural alkaloids as their active ingredients. The pharmacological properties are therefore similar to

TABLE 8.3 Muscarinic receptor antagonists: clinical use and route of administration

DRUG	CLINICAL USE	ROUTE OF ADMINISTRATION
Atropine	Mydriatic, cycloplegic, antisecretory, organophosphate poisoning	IV, IM, SC, topical (eye-drops)
Trihexyphenidyl (benzhexol) (Ch 24)	Parkinson's disease, drug-induced extrapyramidal disorders	Oral
Benzatropine mesilate (Ch 24)	Parkinson's disease, drug-induced extrapyramidal disorders, acute dystonic reaction	Oral, IV, IM
Glycopyrronium bromide (glycopyrrolate)	Antisecretory	Inhaled (powder)
Hyoscine butylbromide	Antispasmodic, sedative, antisecretory	Oral, IV, IM
Hyoscine hydrobromide (Ch 16)	Motion sickness, sedative, antisecretory	Oral, IV, IM, SC, transdermal
Ipratropium bromide (Ch 15)	Bronchodilator	Inhalational, nasal spray
Oxybutynin[a] (Ch 17)	Bladder dysfunction	Oral, topical (patch)
Propantheline bromide	Bladder dysfunction	Oral
Solifenacin succinate	Bladder dysfunction	Oral
Tiotropium (Ch 15)	Bronchodilator	Inhalational
Tropicamide (Ch 40)	Mydriatic, cycloplegic	Topical (eyedrops)

[a] Has calcium channel-blocking and local anaesthetic activity at high doses.
IM = intramuscular; IM = intravenous; SC = subcutaneous

atropine. One of the more commonly used systemic agents is glycopyrronium bromide (glycopyrrolate).

Glycopyrronium bromide (glycopyrrolate)

Glycopyrronium bromide (glycopyrrolate) is a synthetic non-selective muscarinic receptor antagonist with effects similar to those of atropine. Unlike atropine, it is unable to easily cross lipid membranes (e.g. the blood–brain barrier) and hence has minimal CNS effects. It is also less likely to produce pupillary or ocular effects. Glycopyrronium bromide (glycopyrrolate) is indicated as an antimuscarinic drug to reduce salivary, tracheobronchial and pharyngeal secretions preoperatively, to prevent bradycardia induced during anaesthesia and to prevent or reduce the peripheral effects of AChE inhibitors (neostigmine or pyridostigmine).

Following an IV dose, the onset of action occurs within about 1 minute, and following an IM dose, about 15–30 minutes. Vagal blocking action lasts 2–3 hours and the antisialogogue effect (inhibition of the flow of saliva) can last up to 7 hours. Glycopyrronium bromide (glycopyrrolate) is predominantly excreted by the kidneys as unchanged drug.

KEY POINTS

Muscarinic receptor agonists and antagonists

- Muscarinic agonists are also referred to as parasympathomimetic drugs (e.g. bethanechol). They mimic the action of ACh on muscarinic receptors.
- Muscarinic antagonists are also referred to as parasympatholytic or anticholinergic drugs (e.g. atropine). They block the action of ACh and, hence, the effect that would result from parasympathetic nervous system stimulation.
- Muscarinic agonists such as bethanechol are used systemically for non-obstructive urinary retention and for atony of the urinary bladder associated with retention. Pilocarpine is used to treat glaucoma (as a miotic).
- Adverse reactions to bethanechol include abdominal pain or upset, increased salivation and sweating, nausea or vomiting, flushed skin, blurred or disturbed vision, unsteadiness, headache and diarrhoea.
- Muscarinic antagonists such as atropine and synthetic derivatives are used clinically as mydriatics, cycloplegics and in treating bladder dysfunction and Parkinson's disease. They are also used as preanaesthetic (premedication) drugs to decrease secretions.
- Adverse reactions to atropine include: constipation; dry mouth, throat and skin; blurred vision; urinary retention; and headache (Table 8.2).

Acetylcholinesterase

The action of released ACh is brief (< 1 millisecond); after ACh has bound to the post-synaptic receptors it dissociates quickly from the receptors and is inactivated rapidly by the enzyme **acetylcholinesterase** (AChE) (Fig 8.4).

The enzyme hydrolyses (breaks down) about 600,000 molecules of ACh per minute, making it one of the most efficient enzymes. Hydrolysis of the neurotransmitter

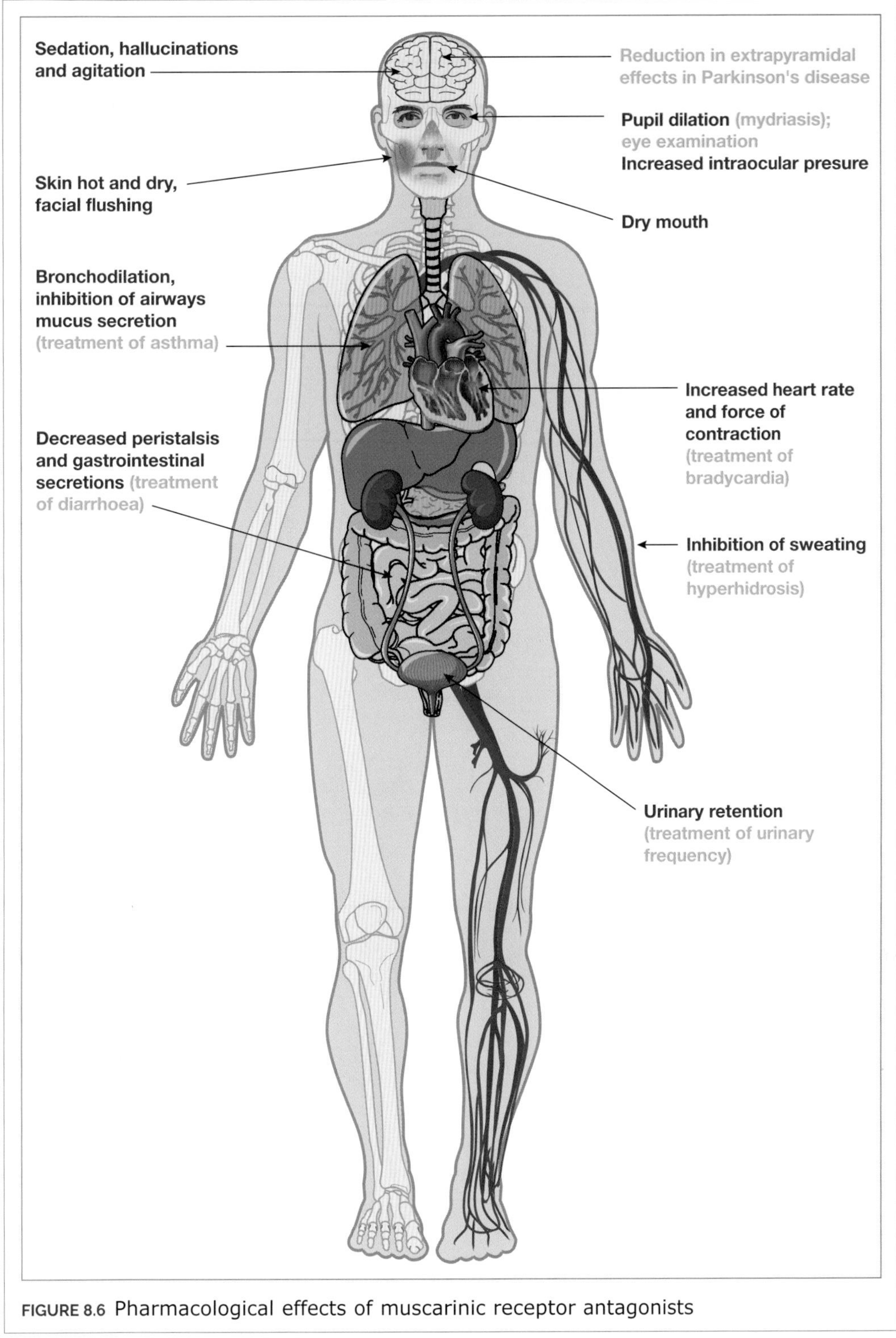

FIGURE 8.6 Pharmacological effects of muscarinic receptor antagonists

ACh forms choline and acetate (Fig 8.4, earlier) and thus the action of ACh is terminated. Choline has no transmitter action and is recycled for synthesis of ACh after reuptake into the presynaptic nerve terminal by the choline transporter CHT1.

The enzyme is found in high concentrations between the presynaptic nerve terminal and the postsynaptic membrane – that is, in the synaptic cleft where ACh is present. It is bound to the postsynaptic membrane and the active site, which resembles a deep gorge, and contains within its structure two distinct sites that are determined by the presence of crucial amino acids: a serine plus a histidine, which form the esteratic (catalytic) site; and a glutamate residue that binds the choline moiety of ACh

Increased cognition and arousal (treatment of Alzheimer's disease)
Headache, insomnia, dizziness
Pupil constriction (miosis), lacrimation
Bradycardia
Skeletal muscle cramps; tremor and paralysis, myalgia, diaphragmatic paralysis
Bronchoconstriction, increased airways secretions (bronchorrhoea)
Nausea, vomiting
Micturition; Urinary incontinence
Increased peristalsis–diarrhoea

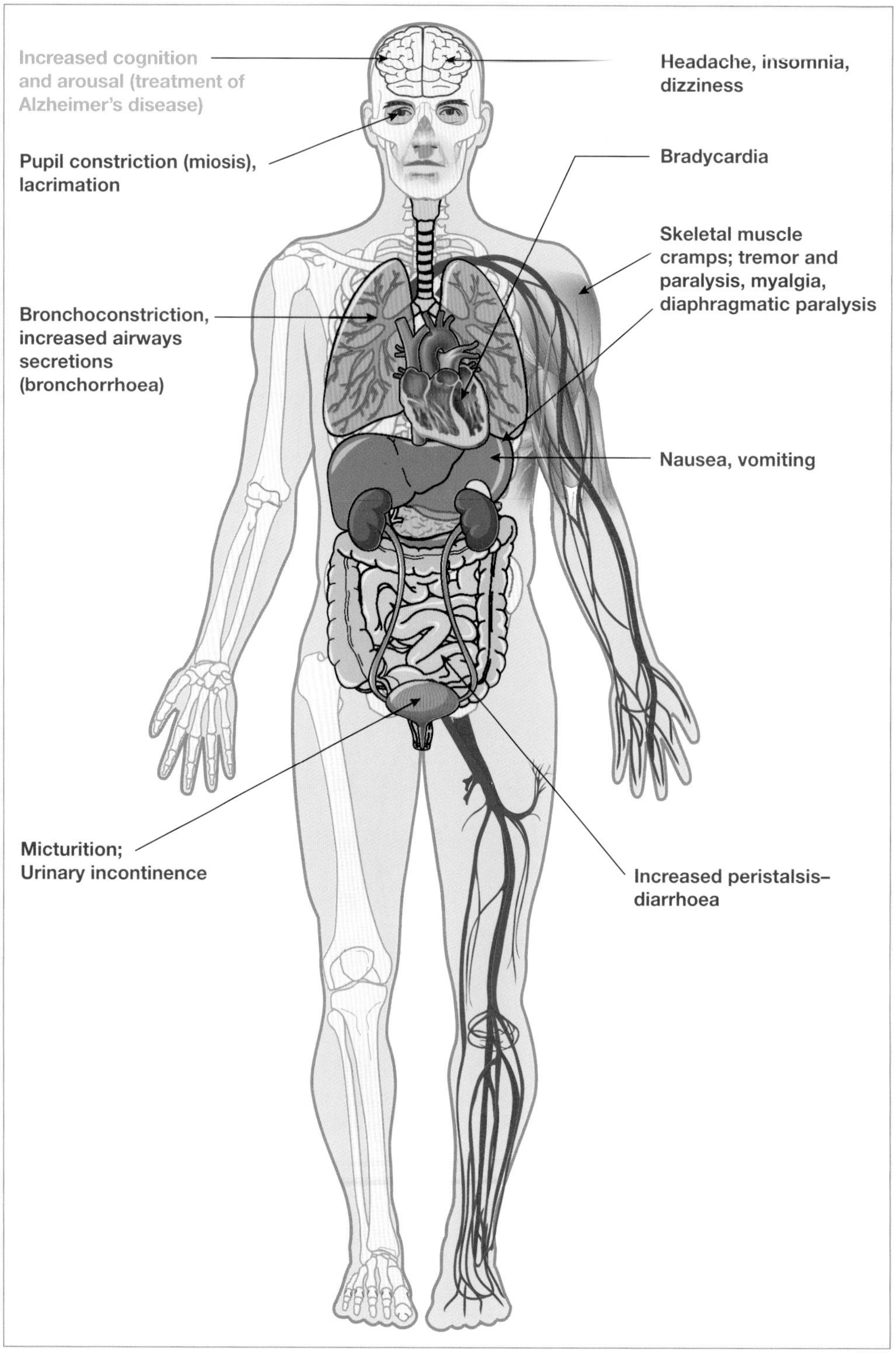

FIGURE 8.7 Pharmacological effects of anticholinesterases

(Fig 8.8) found in the anionic site. Together, these three amino acids are crucial for hydrolysis of ACh and are the targets for the reversible and irreversible AChE inhibitors.

Although ACh was discovered in 1914, at that time 'esteratic' activity (i.e. enzyme activity that breaks down [hydrolyses] the ester bonds in ACh) was only observed in serum. It wasn't until 1937 that AChE was found to exist in high concentrations at the NMJ. AChE can exist in multiple forms, as a single enzyme and as complexes of two or three enzyme molecules, and it exists as both a

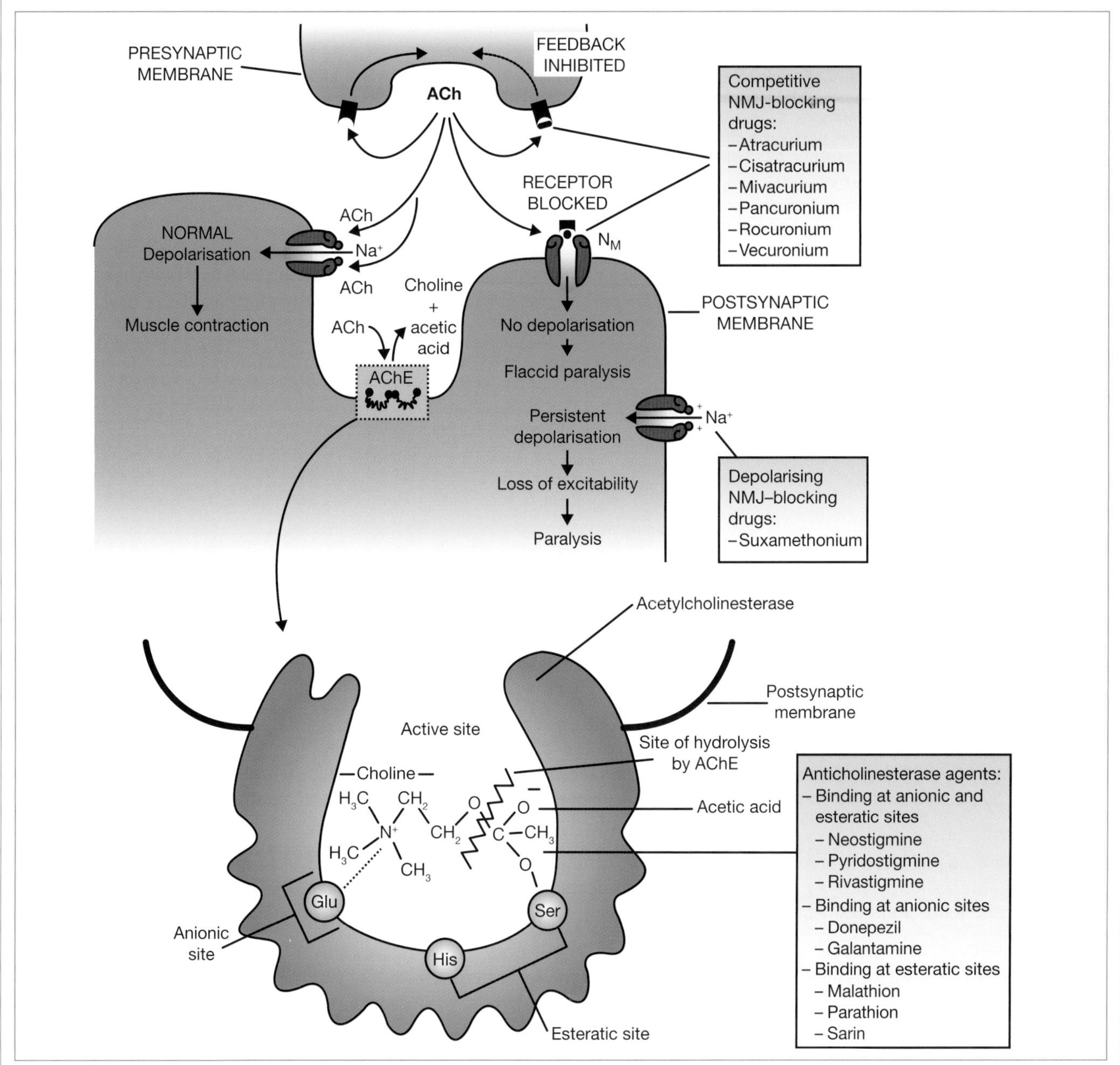

FIGURE 8.8 Sites of action of neuromuscular blocking drugs and anticholinesterase agents

Schematic representation of the postsynaptic membrane of the motor end-plate showing nicotinic receptors and acetylcholinesterase (AChE). The enlargement shows acetylcholine (ACh) within the active site of acetylcholinesterase. The critical amino acids forming the catalytic site are indicated: Glu = glutamate, His = histidine, Ser = serine. The zigzag line indicates the site of hydrolysis of acetylcholine, yielding choline and acetic acid. NMJ = neuromuscular junction.

membrane-bound and a secretable form. It is expressed in multiple tissues in the body, including central and peripheral neurons, endocrine and exocrine glands, skeletal muscle, smooth muscle and cardiac muscle cells. In humans it is also found in erythrocytes and lymphocytes. This enzyme, which is also bound to the synaptic basal lamina of skeletal muscle, is a target for drugs, insecticides and nerve gases.

Anticholinesterase agents

The main pharmacological and toxicological effects of all the **anticholinesterase agents** (Fig 8.7) are explained by enhanced levels of ACh (Table 8.4). They are used for conditions such as Alzheimer's disease and myasthenia gravis, and to reverse neuromuscular blockade after anaesthesia. In addition, AChE is the biological target of

TABLE 8.4 Therapeutic and toxicological effects of anticholinesterase agents

SITE	EFFECT
NMJ	Inhibition of AChE leads to an increased synaptic concentration of ACh, which antagonises the action of the competitive non-depolarising NMJ blockers. This results in reversal of blockade. Toxicological effects include fasciculations, weakness, muscular paralysis. In myasthenia gravis, which is characterised by muscle weakness and profound fatigue, inhibition of AChE results in an increase in synaptic ACh, which increases the likelihood of postsynaptic action potential at the NMJ.
Postganglionic, parasympathetic synapses	Increased ACh leads to increased stimulation of muscarinic ACh receptors causing salivation, lacrimation (tears), increased gastrointestinal tract and bronchial secretions, bronchospasm, bradycardia, hypotension, constricted pupils, vomiting, diarrhoea and urination.
CNS	Overstimulation of both central nicotinic and muscarinic receptors causes confusion, headache, anxiety, irritability, ataxia, fatigue, amnesia, hypothermia, lethargy, unconsciousness, convulsions, coma, central respiratory depression.
Cardiovascular system	Actions on the cardiovascular system are complex, reflecting both ganglionic and postganglionic effects resulting from accumulation of ACh. This initially causes excitation at the ganglia but, with increasing concentration of ACh, ganglionic blockade occurs through persistent depolarisation. Augmentation of vagal action results in bradycardia, shortening of the effective refractory period of the atria and increases in the refractory period and conduction time at the SA and AV nodes. Overstimulation of sympathetic ganglionic nicotinic receptors results in tachycardia and hypertension.

Drug Monograph 8.3
Neostigmine

Neostigmine is a reversible inhibitor of AChE, forming a carbamylated enzyme complex at the active site.

Indications

Neostigmine is most commonly used for the reversal of neuromuscular blockade induced by non-depolarising blockers such as rocuronium. In addition to its use as an adjunct to anaesthesia, it is used to treat myasthenia gravis.

Pharmacokinetics

Neostigmine is a quaternary ammonium compound, poorly absorbed from the gastrointestinal tract and does not cross the blood–brain barrier. The plasma half-life is in the order of 0.5–1.5 hours and it is hydrolysed slowly by AChE over the following 3–4 hours. It is predominantly excreted in the faeces (> 50%) and urine (about 30%). It is metabolised principally by plasma cholinesterases, and the pharmacokinetics of the drug are unlikely to be affected by liver disease.

Drug interactions

Many of the drug interactions are more relevant to the situation where the drug is used to treat myasthenia gravis as any drugs with anticholinergic activity may antagonise the effects of neostigmine; for example, the effect of drugs used in urinary incontinence and Parkinson's disease will be substantially diminished by administering an anticholinesterase drug.

Adverse reactions

These often relate to the overdose situation and resemble a cholinergic crisis, with many of the symptoms listed in Table 8.4.

Warnings and contraindications

The drug should be used with care in people with a history of asthma, cardiac disease, hypotension or peptic ulceration. Safety of neostigmine in pregnancy has not been established.

Dosage and administration

For reversal of neuromuscular blockade in adults, 0.04–0.07 mg/kg to a maximum of 5 mg is administered IV over 1 minute simultaneously with atropine (0.6–1.2 mg).

pesticides and chemical warfare agents. Poisoning can be a result of the additional use of these organophosphate anticholinesterases.

Three broad categories of AChE agents exist:

- Short-acting drugs – for example, edrophonium (used in the diagnosis of myasthenia gravis), donepezil and galantamine (used for Alzheimer's disease). These drugs bind reversibly to the anionic site of the enzyme and, due to rapid hydrolysis, the duration of action is short.
- Medium-acting drugs – for example, neostigmine (used for myasthenia gravis and reversal of NMJ blockade; see Drug Monograph 8.3), pyridostigmine (for myasthenia gravis; see Ch 24) and rivastigmine (used for Alzheimer's disease; see Ch 24). These drugs bind to both the anionic and the esteratic sites of the enzyme and are hydrolysed more slowly, increasing their duration of action.
- Irreversible drugs – for example, pesticides and chemical warfare agents ('nerve gases'), bind to the esteratic site and inactivate the enzyme.

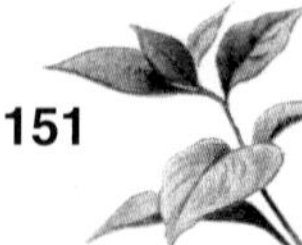

Donepezil, galantamine and rivastigmine

These three anticholinesterase drugs and the *N*-methyl-D-aspartate (NMDA) antagonist memantine are approved to treat Alzheimer's disease but not for other types of dementia (Ch 24). The use of donepezil, galantamine and rivastigmine increases the level of ACh in the brain and provides marginal improvements in cognition and global assessment of dementia.

Donepezil is a synthetic reversible inhibitor of AChE that exhibits a relatively high degree of selectivity for neuronal AChE with little effect on intestinal or cardiac AChE. Galantamine is also a reversible inhibitor of AChE, while rivastigmine is classed as a reversible carbamylating AChE inhibitor, which has high lipid solubility and readily crosses the blood–brain barrier. It is important to appreciate that the AChE drugs are classified on the basis of their duration of inhibition of AChE, which differs from the pharmacokinetics of the drug. For example, donepezil forms a stable complex with AChE but is hydrolysed within minutes, while its plasma half-life is 70 hours. Table 8.5 provides a comparison of the pharmacokinetics of these three drugs.

Donepezil and galantamine are subject to drug interactions with agents that are substrates, inducers or inhibitors of the liver enzymes CYP3A4 and CYP2D6. For example, increased plasma concentrations of donepezil and galantamine are likely to occur with co-administration of the CYP3A4 inhibitor erythromycin. In contrast, as rivastigmine is hydrolysed by cholinesterase, interaction with other drugs metabolised by the CYP family is unlikely. As would be anticipated, combination with drugs with anticholinergic activity may antagonise the effect of anticholinesterases and worsen the dementia. Classes of drugs that may antagonise the effects of AChE inhibitors include drugs for bladder dysfunction (Ch 17), antihistamines and some antipsychotics and antidepressants.

Adverse effects of the anticholinesterases are commonly cholinergic effects such as nausea, vomiting, diarrhoea, anorexia, headache, insomnia, dizziness, tremor and urinary incontinence. Infrequently, bradycardia occurs and combination with drugs that also cause bradycardias may increase the risk of bradycardia and hypotension.

Irreversible anticholinesterase agents

With the exception of echothiopate, which was formerly used to treat glaucoma, most irreversible inhibitors of AChE are pesticides of the organophosphate class or chemical warfare agents such as the nerve gases sarin, tabun and soman. The organophosphate pesticides (e.g. chlorpyrifos, diazinon, parathion and malathion) are widely used in agriculture, horticulture and urban gardening, and are a common cause of poisoning in humans. It is estimated that in rural regions of the world around 200,000 people die every year from intentional self-poisoning with organophosphorus pesticides. The organophosphate pesticides inhibit AChE by forming a very stable complex principally with the esteratic site (see Fig 8.8, earlier). This phosphorylated form of the enzyme is not functional, ACh is not degraded and return of AChE activity depends on synthesis of a new enzyme. In addition, some of these agents also inhibit plasma butyrylcholinesterase that hydrolyses many different choline-based esters. (Plasma butyrylcholinesterase is also known as pseudocholinesterase or plasma cholinesterase.)

As above, nerve gases are also irreversible organophosphate anticholinesterase agents. A great deal of interest has been rekindled since the use of chemical nerve agents in various wars since the 1980s and in terrorist attacks – for example, in Japan in a subway attack in 1995 and in the Gulf War and more recently in March 2018 in the town of Salisbury in the United Kingdom (Clinical Focus Box 8.1). These agents are highly volatile and pose a significant health problem. Toxicity or cholinergic crisis occurs as a result of irreversible inactivation of AChE leading to an accumulation of ACh. Persistent stimulation by ACh at presynaptic and postsynaptic receptors occurs initially, followed finally by paralysis of cholinergic

TABLE 8.5 Pharmacokinetics of anticholinesterase drugs used to treat Alzheimer's disease

VARIABLE	DONEPEZIL	GALANTAMINE	RIVASTIGMINE
Inhibition of AChE	Short	Short	Intermediate
Bioavailability	~100%	~88.5%	Dose-dependent
Metabolism	CYP2D6, CYP3A4	CYP2D6, CYP3A4	Hydrolysis by cholinesterase
Renal excretion[a]	17%	~18–20%	Negligible
Half-life (h)	~70	~8	~1

[a] Unchanged drug.
Source: Brunton et al, Goodman and Gilman's The Pharmacological Basis of Therapeutics (2011); Jann (1998); Zarotsky et al (2003). Brown JH, Laiken N. Muscarinic receptor agonists and antagonists. In: Brunton LL, Chabner B, Knollman B (eds). Goodman & Gilman's The Pharmacological Basis of Therapeutics. 12th edn. New York: McGraw-Hill, 2011 Zarotsky V, Sramek JJ, Cutler NR. Galantamine hydrobromide; an agent for Alzheimer's disease. American Journal of Health-System Pharmacy; 60: 446–452. 2003

CLINICAL FOCUS BOX 8.1

Organophosphate and chemical warfare agents poisoning and treatment

Chemicals (chlorine and phosgene) hazardous to humans were first used as 'weapons of mass destruction' during World War I. Since that time, refinement of chemical processes has resulted in the continued production of chemical weapons. Organophosphate nerve agents such as tabun, sarin, cyclosarin and soman were manufactured during World War II, and sarin and soman have been stockpiled in several countries, including the United States. Another class of nerve gases is the V class, which are organophosphate esters of various 2-aminoethanethiols of which VX is the most lethal.

These agents are inhibitors of AChE; the antidote carried by military personnel is atropine, which antagonises the persistent stimulation of muscarinic receptors. However, it is ineffective in antagonising the nicotinic effects of ACh and hence muscle weakness and paralysis does not improve.

neurotransmission. This ultimately affects the somatic, autonomic and central nervous systems (Table 8.4; Drug Monograph 8.3).

The signs and symptoms of poisoning from pesticides and nerve gases can be categorised according to whether excessive stimulation occurs at muscarinic or nicotinic receptors. The mnemonic 'DUMBELS' describes the muscarinic symptoms: **D**iarrhoea; **U**rination; **M**iosis; **B**ronchorrhoea, bronchoconstriction and bradycardia; **E**mesis; **L**acrimation; **S**alivation (Geoghegan & Tong 2006). Nicotinic effects would occur more from stimulation of the somatic nervous system (e.g. skeletal muscle twitching, weakness and flaccid paralysis, paralysis of the diaphragm) and from the release of catecholamines from the adrenal medulla (Table 8.4 and Fig 8.7, earlier).

Treatment of organophosphate poisoning

This is a complex area and requires considerable expertise to recognise the effects of common chemical warfare agents and interpret the severity of nerve poisoning based on clinical symptoms. Drugs that are used include atropine, which antagonises the muscarinic effects of excess ACh but is ineffective in antagonising the nicotinic effects of ACh (Clinical Focus Box 8.1). Pralidoxime is an AChE-reactivating oxime that exerts a nucleophilic attack on the phosphorylated esteratic site (disrupts the covalent bond between the nerve agent and AChE), resulting in formation of a phosphoryloxime, which 'regenerates' the enzyme. This reverses nicotinic receptor dysfunction and reduces the paralysis. Early administration (usually IV) is necessary because, as the phosphorylated enzyme 'ages' (within hours), it becomes resistant to reactivation. Pralidoxime is excreted unchanged by the kidney and a continuous infusion is usually administered for 24 hours after symptoms resolve (Geoghegan & Tong 2006). As this drug has anticholinesterase activity, adverse effects include cholinergic symptoms such as nausea and blurred vision. The treatment of organophosphate poisoning due to pesticides is similar and involves use of atropine, pralidoxime and diazepam; the last is used to treat agitation and to provide adequate sedation (Eddleston et al. 2008).

KEY POINTS

Acetylcholinesterase and anticholinesterase agents

- The enzyme AChE is responsible for the highly efficient breakdown and termination of the action of ACh.
- AChE is the biological target for anticholinesterase drugs, pesticides and chemical warfare agents such as nerve gases.
- Blockers of the enzyme cholinesterase inhibit ACh breakdown and increase levels of the transmitter at the ganglia of the ANS and postjunctional sites.
- The anticholinesterase drug neostigmine is commonly used to reverse neuromuscular blockade produced by non-depolarising neuromuscular blockers; it is also used as an adjunct to anaesthesia.
- Donepezil, galantamine and rivastigmine are approved for the treatment of Alzheimer's disease but not for other types of dementia. They increase the level of ACh in the brain and provide marginal improvements in cognition and global assessment of dementia.
- Irreversible anticholinesterase agents are, in general, organophosphates. They are used as pesticides (e.g. parathion and malathion) and chemical warfare agents (e.g. sarin, tabun and soman).
- Toxicity of anticholinesterase agents occurs as a result of accumulation of ACh and excessive stimulation of the somatic, autonomic and central nervous systems.
- Drugs that are used to treat nerve agent poisoning include atropine (Drug Monograph 8.2), which antagonises the muscarinic effects of excess ACh, and pralidoxime, which 'regenerates' AChE.

Drugs acting at nicotinic receptors

Nicotinic receptors

Nicotinic acetylcholine receptors are members of the Cys-loop super family of transmitter-gated ion channels

TABLE 8.6 Nicotinic receptor subtypes

	MUSCLE TYPE (N_M)	GANGLION TYPE (N_N)	CNS TYPE (N_N)
Molecular form	$(\alpha1)^2\beta1\delta\epsilon$ (adult form)	$(\alpha3)^2(\beta4)^3$	$(\alpha4)^2(\beta4)^3$
Location	Skeletal NMJ	Autonomic ganglia	Many brain regions pre- and postsynaptic
Membrane response	Excitatory. Increased cation permeability (mainly Na^+ and K^+)	Excitatory. Increased cation permeability (mainly Na^+ and K^+)	Pre- and postsynaptic excitation Increased cation permeability (Na^+, K^+ and Ca^{2+})

Source: Adapted from Rang et al. 2016; Brunton et al. 2017

(ionotropic receptors). This family includes the $GABA_A$ and $5\text{-}HT_3$ receptors. All nicotinic receptors are pentamers in which each of the five sub-units contains four α-helical transmembrane domains. The sub-units are designated using a Greek letter: Genes encoding a total of 17 sub-units (α1–10, β1–4, γ, δ and ϵ) have been identified (Table 8.6). The sub-units combine to form many different nicotinic receptor subtypes. Subtypes include muscle (N_M), ganglion and CNS types (N_N) (Gotti et al. 2019).

Nicotinic receptor agonists

There are few clinical uses for nicotinic receptor agonists due to their lack of specificity. Nicotinic agonists include ACh and nicotine and the depolarising neuromuscular blocking drug suxamethonium (or succinylcholine; see Drug Monograph 8.4) (Hoskin et al. 2019).

Nicotinic receptor antagonists are known as ganglion blocking agents (acting at the ANS) or non-depolarising neuromuscular blocking drugs (acting as somatic agents – see next section).

Ganglion-blocking drugs

The major neurotransmitter at all autonomic ganglia is ACh. Ganglion-blocking drugs, such as hexamethonium and mecamylamine, block the action of ACh at autonomic ganglia by competing with ACh at the synapse. This results in reduced impulse transmission from preganglionic to postganglionic neurons in both the sympathetic and the parasympathetic systems. Because of the profound physiological effects (hypotension, loss of cardiovascular reflexes) elicited by ganglion-blocking drugs, they are now clinically obsolete, used in research only. The first

Drug Monograph 8.4
Suxamethonium

Mechanism of action

Suxamethonium, an analogue of ACh, was introduced into clinical practice in 1951 and is still widely used. It is an agonist at muscle endplate nicotinic receptors and maintains the depolarised state. In addition, suxamethonium stimulates nicotinic receptors in ganglia of both sympathetic and parasympathetic nerves and also muscarinic receptors in the heart. It is the only truly short-acting muscle relaxant, and reversal by an anticholinesterase drug is unnecessary because of the short duration of action of suxamethonium but also because use of an anticholinesterase agent will prolong the depolarisation blockade.

Indications

It is used when brief muscle relaxation is required (e.g. for electroconvulsive therapy, tracheal intubation, short surgical procedures and orthopaedic manipulations).

Pharmacokinetics

The onset of action of suxamethonium is rapid and the estimated half-life is in the order of 2–4 minutes. Blockade persists for about 10 minutes and the drug is rapidly hydrolysed by plasma butyrylcholinesterase (also known as pseudocholinesterase or plasma cholinesterase) to choline and succinylmonocholine; the latter is then hydrolysed to choline and succinic acid. In some individuals with an inherited genetic deficiency, which manifests as a diminished activity of plasma butyrylcholinesterase, blockade can persist for an extended period of time. This is often referred to as 'scoline apnoea'.

Drug interactions

Many drugs enhance the neuromuscular blocking activity of suxamethonium (e.g. lidocaine [lignocaine]), non-penicillin antibiotics, β-blockers, metoclopramide, lithium carbonate, high-dose corticosteroids and some cancer chemotherapy drugs). Current sources should be consulted for a more extensive list.

Adverse reactions

Suxamethonium can cause profound and complex effects on the cardiovascular system, including bradycardia (most likely due to stimulation of vagal ganglia causing enhanced vagal nerve activity), tachycardia (due to stimulation of nicotinic receptors in sympathetic ganglia), dysrhythmias, hypertension and cardiac arrest. Because of loss of potassium from the motor endplate, an increase in plasma potassium concentration can occur and this is important in situations of extensive burns and massive trauma and in people with muscular disorders; release of potassium can cause ventricular tachyarrhythmias. In rare situations, suxamethonium can precipitate malignant hyperthermia, an often fatal condition characterised by intense muscle spasm and a rapid rise in body temperature. Although the action of suxamethonium is short, in some people prolonged apnoea occurs as a result of either a butyrylcholinesterase deficiency, the use of anticholinesterase drugs that inhibit the action of butyrylcholinesterase or the presence of liver disease, which can result in a low plasma butyrylcholinesterase concentration.

Warnings and contraindications

Care should be taken with the use of suxamethonium in people with electrolyte disturbances, low butyrylcholinesterase activity, renal disease and concomitant digitalis therapy. The drug is contraindicated in people with a known or suspected familial history of malignant hyperthermia and in cases of extensive burns or multiple traumas.

Dosage and administration

Dosage is individualised depending on the circumstances of use and the degree of relaxation required. The drug is usually administered IV, but the IM route may be used when a suitable vein is not accessible. Under no circumstances should suxamethonium be administered to a conscious person.

effective antihypertensive agent was hexamethonium and in 1954 Paton described 'Hexamethonium Man'; a gentleman who was exhibiting the theoretical side effects of this drug (see Evolve website and Paton 1954). Although this drug is not in clinical use, this description illustrates that blockade of the ANS activity produces diverse actions.

KEY POINTS

Drugs acting at nicotinic receptors

- Nicotinic acetylcholine receptors are members of the superfamily of transmitter-gated ion channels.
- There are skeletal muscle, ganglion and CNS types of receptors.
- There are few clinical uses for agonists such as nicotine due to their lack of specificity.
- Nicotinic receptor antagonists include ganglion-blocking drugs such as hexamethonium and non-depolarising neuromuscular blocking drugs such as rocuronium (see later).

Somatic nervous system

As noted previously, the first major division of the PNS is the ANS, comprised of parasympathetic and sympathetic divisions. The second major division of the PNS is the **somatic nervous system** (Fig 8.1, earlier), which coordinates consciously controlled functions, including movement, posture and respiration. In this system, a single motor neuron connects the CNS to the skeletal muscles, which are the effector organs of the somatic nervous system. Often called the voluntary nervous system, this system allows conscious control of skeletal muscles and hence movement. Initiating and controlling both gross movements (e.g. jumping or walking) and precise movements (e.g. those done with the hands) involves the motor cortex, which initiates and controls movement, the basal ganglia, which integrate and establish our muscle tone, and the cerebellum, which ensures that movements are smooth and coordinated. Integration of these systems aids in the maintenance of normal posture and balance.

Once the primary motor area of the cerebral cortex initiates a voluntary movement, nerve impulses propagate from the motor cortex through upper motor neurons that cross over in the medulla oblongata to the other side; thus, muscles on the right side of the body are controlled by the left motor cortex, and the right side of the brain controls the muscles on the left side of the body. The upper motor neurons terminate in the anterior grey horn of the spinal cord at each spinal segment. In many instances, the upper motor neurons synapse first with interneurons, which act as the connection with the lower motor neurons; they in turn innervate skeletal muscles of the trunk and limbs (Fig 8.9). The lower motor neurons are the final common pathway that connects the CNS to the skeletal muscles.

The neuromuscular junction and nicotinic receptors

The synapse between the lower motor (somatic) neuron and the skeletal muscle is called the **neuromuscular junction** (NMJ). At the NMJ, the motor neuron divides, forming a cluster of synaptic end bulbs that contain

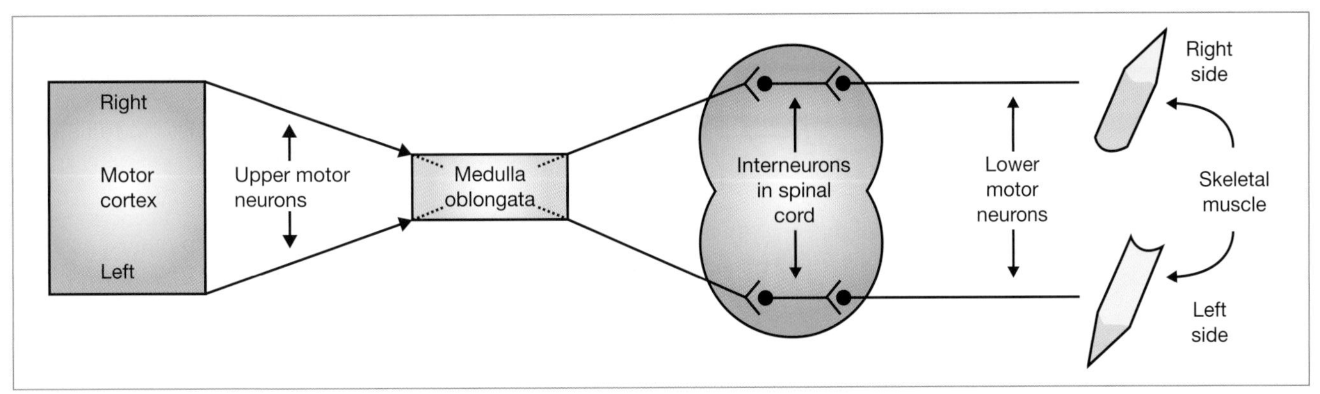

FIGURE 8.9 Diagrammatic representation of motor pathways from the right and left sides of the motor cortex innervating skeletal muscles on the opposite sides of the body

vesicles carrying ACh. Following arrival of a nerve action potential (Fig 8.10, later), ACh is released from the vesicles and diffuses across the synaptic cleft to act on postsynaptic nicotinic receptors on the motor endplate of the muscle fibre. As muscle fibres tend to be long, the NMJ is usually near the centre of the fibre. This allows the impulse to spread evenly towards the ends of the muscle fibre and ensures that contraction occurs simultaneously throughout the length of the muscle. Each nerve impulse produces only one muscle contraction. The release and metabolism of ACh occur by the same mechanisms as those described for the parasympathetic nervous system. The difference is that, in the somatic nervous system, ACh acts on postsynaptic nicotinic ACh receptors (nAChRs) of the skeletal muscle-type (N_M) on the motor endplate (Fig 8.10, later), whereas the postsynaptic receptors in the parasympathetic system are muscarinic receptors.

Muscle-type nicotinic receptors

Skeletal muscle-type nicotinic receptors (N_M) are members of a superfamily of ligand-gated ion channels that mediate the effect of ACh on skeletal muscles (Table 8.6 earlier); they are the main biological targets of the tobacco alkaloid nicotine. The N_M receptor is composed of five sub-units arranged in a circular manner with the ion channel in the centre. To date, 10 types of the α sub-unit, four types of β sub-units and one each of the remaining sub-units have been identified. The bulk of the receptor faces the extracellular surface. The density of the receptors is very high on the motor endplate. When two molecules of ACh bind (one molecule to each of the α sub-units), the channel opens immediately and sodium ions flow through, causing depolarisation of the motor endplate. This triggers the muscle action potential, causing muscle contraction (Fig 8.10). Contraction occurs because of a sliding filament mechanism involving actin and myosin.

There are many sites at which drugs and toxins can interrupt neuromuscular transmission. These include blockade of action potential generation in the motor neuron, inhibition of release of ACh (botulinum toxin causing generalised muscle weakness: see Evolve), inhibition of the breakdown of ACh and blockade of postsynaptic receptors. The pharmacological agents of clinical relevance anticholinesterase agents (see earlier), botulinum toxin (uses include blepharospasm, upper limb spasticity and cosmetic correction) and drugs blocking postsynaptic receptors commonly referred to as neuromuscular blocking drugs.

KEY POINTS

Somatic nervous system pharmacology

- The somatic nervous system coordinates consciously controlled functions such as posture, movement and respiration.
- The synapse between the lower motor (somatic) neuron and the skeletal muscle is called the NMJ.
- The transmitter at the NMJ is ACh, which acts on both nicotinic and muscarinic presynaptic autoreceptors and postsynaptic nicotinic receptors.
- Skeletal muscle-type nicotinic receptors (N_M) are members of a superfamily of ligand-gated ion channels that mediate the effect of ACh on skeletal muscles (at the motor endplate).

Neuromuscular blocking drugs

Neuromuscular blocking drugs produce relaxation of skeletal muscles including the diaphragm, which is particularly valuable for facilitating endotracheal intubation and, hence, control of the airway in both acute situations and during general anaesthesia for surgical purposes (Ch 18). During general anaesthesia, neuromuscular blockade facilitates mechanical ventilation, prevents reflex muscle contractions and

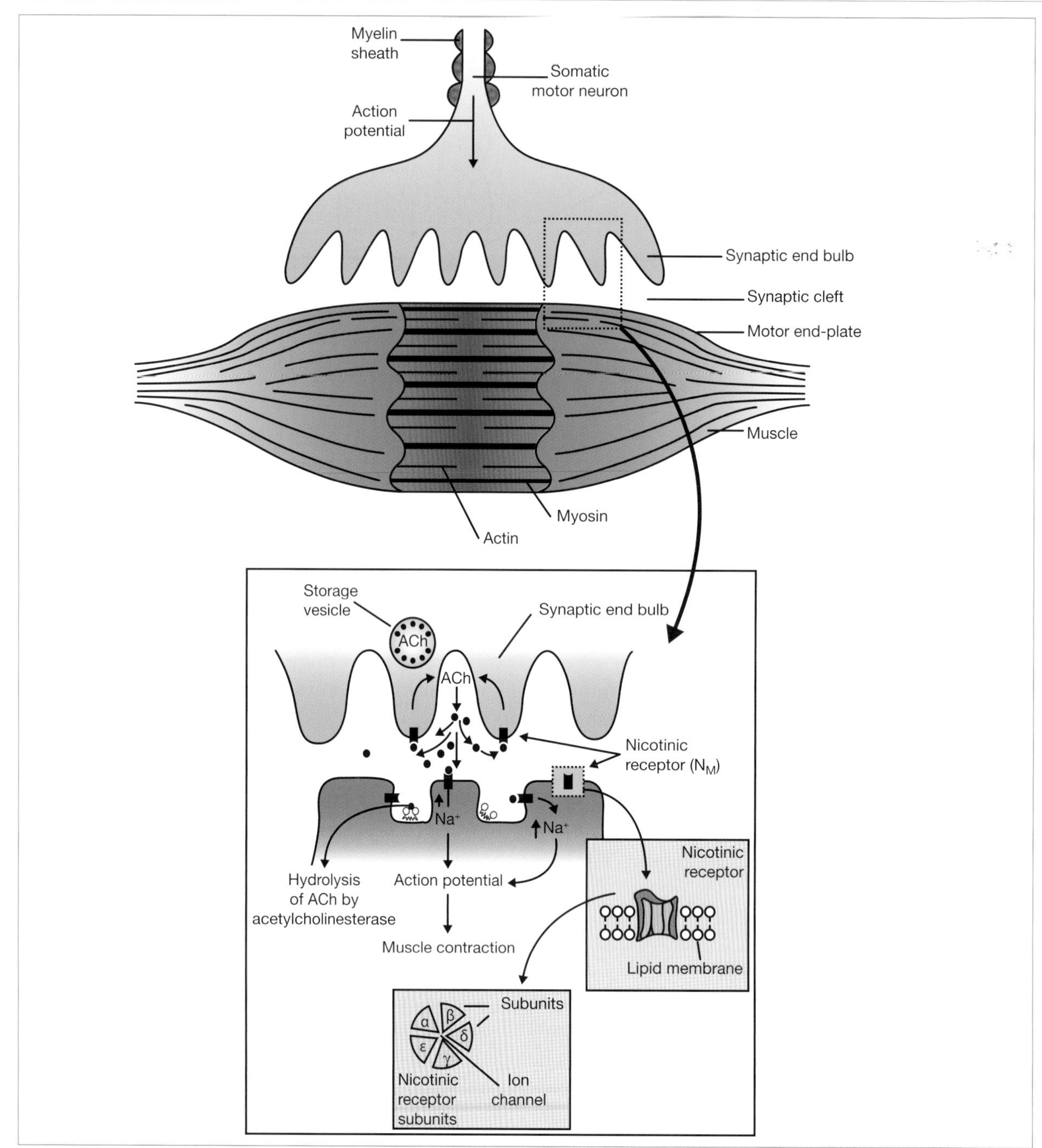

FIGURE 8.10 The neuromuscular junction, showing release of acetylcholine (ACh), which acts on both postsynaptic nicotinic receptors and presynaptic nicotinic autoreceptors
The insets show enlargements of the relevant structures.

improves access to the surgical field. The neuromuscular blocking drugs are principally of two types:

- Competitive drugs, or **non-depolarising neuromuscular blocking drugs**, competitively block the action of ACh at postsynaptic nicotinic receptors and also the presynaptic nicotinic autoreceptors, blocking the normal feedback loop that increases ACh release under conditions of enhanced stimulation. The action of the non-depolarising drugs, which include rocuronium, can be reversed by anticholinesterase drugs (Fig 8.8, earlier).
- Nicotinic receptor agonists which are **depolarising neuromuscular blocking drugs** maintain the depolarised state of the motor endplate, thus preventing transmission of another action potential. The only agent that is used clinically is suxamethonium (Figs 8.8 and 8.11 later and Drug Monograph 8.4).

Depolarising neuromuscular blocking drug

Currently, the only depolarising neuromuscular blocking drug in clinical use is suxamethonium (also known as succinylcholine, see Drug Monograph 8.5). In contrast to tubocurarine, which blocks nicotinic receptors and produces flaccid muscle paralysis, suxamethonium acts as an agonist at the nicotinic receptors on the motor endplate and produces spastic paralysis. Binding to the receptor results in persistent stimulation and maintains the depolarised state of the motor endplate.

Loss of electrical excitability ensues because the sodium channels remain open and the motor endplate can no longer respond to an electrical stimulus. Suxamethonium causes excessive salivation due to muscarinic-like actions, which can be prevented by the use of atropine. In addition, initial muscle fasciculations (twitching) occur because, as each endplate is depolarised, it produces a localised action potential in the muscle fibre. As each fibre has only one motor endplate, when they are depolarised individually it is not sufficient to produce complete muscle contraction. These fasciculations subside quickly and neuromuscular blockade follows. Suxamethonium causes histamine release from mast cells and severe anaphylactoid reactions are more frequent in women.

KEY POINTS

Neuromuscular blocking drugs

- The neuromuscular blocking drugs are principally of two types: competitive non-depolarising neuromuscular blocking drugs (which are nicotinic receptor antagonists) and depolarising neuromuscular blocking drugs (which are nicotinic receptor agonists).
- Non-depolarising drugs such as rocuronium competitively block the action of ACh. They produce rapid blockade at the motor endplate, which is characterised by initial motor weakness that progresses to flaccid paralysis.
- Non-depolarising drugs characteristically cause a release of histamine that may manifest as a rash or, in more severe cases, as hypotension and bronchoconstriction.
- The only depolarising drug in clinical use is suxamethonium, an agonist at nicotinic receptors on the motor endplate causing sustained depolarisation.
- Adverse effects of suxamethonium include bradycardia, tachycardia, dysrhythmias, hypertension and cardiac arrest. In rare situations, suxamethonium can precipitate malignant hyperthermia, an often fatal condition characterised by intense muscle spasm and a rapid rise in body temperature.

Non-depolarising neuromuscular blocking drugs

Curare is synonymous with the South American arrow-tip poisons that were used by indigenous people along the Amazon and Orinoco Rivers for killing animals. The pharmacologist Claude Bernard investigated the muscle paralysing effect of curare in 1856. He showed that the drug prevents the response of skeletal muscle to nerve stimulation but does not inhibit contraction from a direct stimulus, nor does it block nerve conduction. These elegant experiments established the concept of nerve–muscle conduction, and in 1942 curare was introduced for promoting muscle relaxation during general anaesthesia. This development heralded the search for other curare-like drugs. Although tubocurarine (the active constituent of curare) is no longer in clinical use, various synthetic drugs have been produced. These include atracurium, cisatracurium, mivacurium, pancuronium, rocuronium and vecuronium. As these drugs are quaternary ammonium compounds, they are poorly absorbed and do not readily cross the blood–brain barrier or placenta; the latter is an advantage when operating on pregnant women.

Effects on skeletal muscle

In general, the **non-depolarising drugs** produce rapid blockade characterised by motor weakness that progresses to total flaccid paralysis. Small muscles (e.g. those of the eyelid) are affected first, proceeding through to the limbs, neck, trunk and, finally, the diaphragm and intercostal muscles. With paralysis of the respiratory muscles, respiration ceases and mechanical ventilatory support is required. Return to normal muscle function varies markedly between people and between individual muscle groups. Normally, function returns first to the respiratory system, the diaphragm and intercostal muscles; pharyngeal and facial muscles recover more slowly.

Effects on mast cells

Typically, the non-depolarising drugs atracurium and mivacurium cause histamine release from mast cells. This often manifests as harmless cutaneous reactions (flushing and rash), but more severe symptoms can occur, including hypotension and bronchospasm. The effect is not related to an action at nicotinic receptors but is more likely due to the highly basic nature of these drugs.

Drug Monograph 8.5 describes rocuronium. The main characteristics of the other non-depolarising drugs are summarised in Table 8.7.

Drug Monograph 8.5
Rocuronium

Mechanism of action

Rocuronium is a potent competitive antagonist of acetylcholine at nicotinic receptors on the skeletal muscle motor end-plate and at presynaptic nicotinic autoreceptors, blocking the normal feedback loop that increases ACh release under conditions of enhanced stimulation. Interruption of neuromuscular transmission requires occupancy of more than 70% of the nicotinic receptors, while blockade requires more than 95% occupancy. Blockade of muscarinic receptors leads to its mild vagolytic properties.

Indications

To aid control of the airway by facilitating endotracheal intubation, as an adjunct to general anaesthesia to provide muscle relaxation during surgery and in intensive care.

Pharmacokinetics

Rocuronium is widely distributed following intravenous administration. It has very limited lipid solubility. The time of onset is 75 seconds, and clinical duration of action is over 30 minutes. The parent compound is largely excreted in bile with 30% renal excretion.

In the presence of preexisting renal disease, clearance can be reduced and the half-life prolonged.

Drug interactions

Potentiation of effect can occur with inhalation anaesthetics (e.g. sevoflurane, isoflurane), suxamethonium, antibiotics such as the aminoglycosides (which inhibit both ACh release and non-competitively block nicotinic receptors), diazepam, calcium channel blockers (the mechanism is unclear, but may involve a reduction in calcium-dependent release of ACh), lithium, propranolol and magnesium salts. A decrease in effect can occur with adrenaline, carbamazepine and anticholinesterase agents such as neostigmine, high-dose corticosteroids and the chloride salts of calcium, and potassium.

Adverse reactions

These are uncommon; there is no effect on heart rate, cardiac output and blood pressure. A life-threatening anaphylactoid reaction can occur, with the incidence reported to the around 1 in 2500 patients.

Warnings and contraindications

Care should be exercised with using rocuronium in people with impaired hepatic or renal function and cardiovascular disease. The drug is contraindicated in people with known hypersensitivity to rocuronium.

Dosage and administration

Rocuronium is administered intravenously and the dosage should be individualised. The initial dose range for intubation is 0.6–1.2 mg/kg in adults and in children older than 1 month of age, depending on the surgical procedure. The maintenance dose range is 0.15 mg/kg, and in long-term inhalational anaesthesia it should be reduced to 0.075–1 mg/kg body weight.

TABLE 8.7 Comparative information on non-depolarising neuromuscular blocking drugs

DRUG	ONSET OF BLOCKADE (MIN)	DURATION OF BLOCKADE (MIN)	COMMENTS
Atracurium	2–6	30–60	Transient hypotension. Histamine release at higher clinical doses. Metabolised by plasma esterases to inactive metabolites. Also undergoes spontaneous non-enzymatic chemical degradation, which is pH-dependent. It is stable at acidic pH, but its duration of action is much shorter due to greater degradation under conditions producing alkalosis, e.g. hyperventilation.
Cisatracurium	2–7	10–35	Low incidence of flushing, hypotension and bronchospasm due to histamine release. Cisatracurium is an isomer of atracurium and is more potent. It also undergoes spontaneous non-enzymatic degradation.
Pancuronium	4–6	60–120	Pancuronium produces little histamine release, but blockade of muscarinic receptors decreases vagal activity resulting in tachycardia.
Rocuronium	1–3	30–40	Limited adverse effects. Potential for anaphylactic reactions. No significant tachycardia or hypotension.
Vecuronium	2–4	20–40	Limited adverse effects. Potential for anaphylactic reactions. Allergic cross-sensitivity with pancuronium.

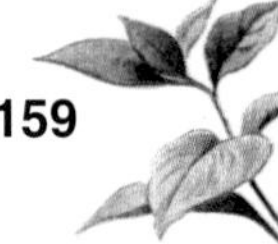

Reversal of neuromuscular blockade

Sugammadex is a modified gamma cyclodextrin approved for use in Australia to selectively reverse the effects of the neuromuscular blockers rocuronium and vecuronium, thus accelerating recovery from drug-induced muscle relaxation for surgical purposes (i.e. neuromuscular blockade). It works by forming a complex with the neuromuscular blockers (Fig 8.11), reducing their availability to bind to nicotinic receptors in the NMJ. Sugammadex is currently registered for use in Australia and New Zealand.

Impaired accommodation, dry eyes, impaired eyelid closure
Skeletal muscle relaxation and paralysis:
• Flaccid paralysis– non depolarising blockers
• Spastic paralysis – depolarising blockers
Diaphragmatic paralysis for rapid sequence intubation
Anaphylaxis: mast cell histamine release- bronchoconstriction and vasodilation (non-depolarising)
Decreased blood pressure (non-depolarising)

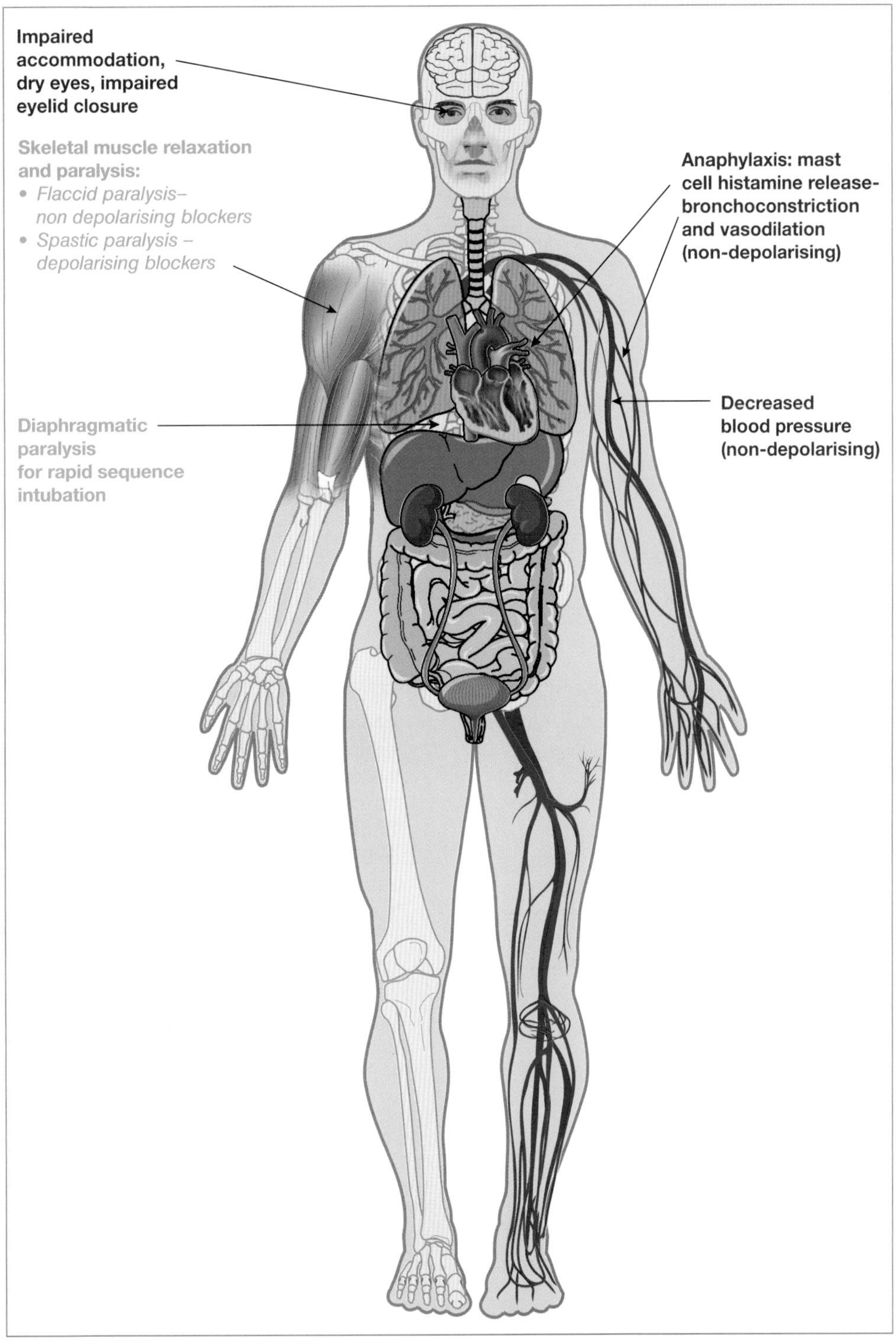

FIGURE 8.11 Pharmacological effects of neuromuscular blockers: depolarising and non-depolarising

DRUGS AT A GLANCE
Drugs affecting cholinergic transmission

PHARMACOLOGICAL GROUP AND EFFECT	KEY EXAMPLES	CLINICAL USE
Parasympathomimetics/cholinomimetics (muscarinic receptor agonists) Stimulate muscarinic receptors on smooth muscle, cardiac muscle and glandular tissue	Bethanecol, pilocarpine	Urinary retention Glaucoma
Parasympatholytic/anticholinergics/antimuscarinics (muscarinic receptor antagonists) Block muscarinic receptors on smooth muscle, cardiac muscle and glandular tissue preventing activation by the parasympathetic nervous system	Atropine	Bradycardia Reversal of anticholinesterase poisoning
	hyoscine	Motion sickness
	ipratropium bromide	Asthma reliever
	glycopyrrolate	Antisialogogue
	tropicamide	Mydriasis (pupil dilation) and cycloplegia (paralysis of accommodation) for eye examinations
Drugs that inhibit cholinesterases (anticholinesterases) Bind to and block the active site of cholinesterase enzyme inhibiting the breakdown of ACh	Neostigmine	Myasthenia gravis (reversal of muscle weakness)
	Donepezil, galantamine, rivastigmine	Alzheimer's disease (CNS)
Neuromuscular-blocking drugs (nicotinic receptor agonists) Maintain the depolarised state of the motor endplate, thus preventing transmission of another action potential	Suxamethonium	Rapid sequence intubation/endotracheal intubation
Neuromuscular-blocking drugs (nicotinic receptor antagonists) Blockade of somatic nervous system activation of neuronal nicotinic receptors on motor endplate producing flaccid paralysis	Rocuronium	Neuromuscular blockade during general anaesthesia Endotracheal intubation

REVIEW EXERCISES

1. Mrs QR has presented with early symptoms of the extrapyramidal effects (tremor, involuntary movements and rigidity) associated with Parkinson's disease. Explain why her doctor has prescribed her trihexyphenidyl (benzhexol). What advice should be given regarding the adverse effects of the drug?
2. Mrs AB has Alzheimer's disease and has just been commenced on 5 mg donepezil daily. You notice that she has developed diarrhoea, urinary incontinence and is sweating. Mrs AB is also complaining of fatigue and a headache. Explain why she has developed these adverse effects.
3. Mr BB has just been brought into the emergency department with severe asthma accompanied by an altered level of consciousness and rising PCO_2 levels. As his condition deteriorated, the decision was made to intubate. Explain why rocuronium was administered, and discuss its classification, the mechanism of action and duration of action. What drug would be used to reverse its effects? The paramedics, in their handover, state that as part of the initial treatment he was given a dose of ipratropium bromide. Discuss the mechanism of action of this drug as it relates to the clinical management of his asthma.

REFERENCES

Appiah Ankam, J and Hunter J. Pharmacology of Neuromuscular Blocking drugs. Continuing Education in Anaesthesia, Critical Care & Pain | Volume 4 Number 1 2004

Brunton L.L., Hilal-Dandan R. & Knollmann B.C. (Eds.), Goodman & Gilman's The Pharmacological Basis of Therapeutics, ed 13, New York, 2017, McGraw-Hill.

Eddleston M, Buckley NA, Eyer P, et al: Management of acute organophosphorus pesticide poisoning, Lancet 371:597–607, 2008.

Geoghegan J, Tong JL: Chemical warfare agents, Continuing Education in Anaesthesia, Critical Care & Pain 6:230–234, 2006.

Gotti C, Marks MJ, Millar NS, Wonnacott S. Nicotinic acetylcholine receptors (nACh) (version 2019.4) in the IUPHAR/BPS Guide to Pharmacology Database. IUPHAR/BPS Guide to Pharmacology CITE. 2019; 2019(4). Available from: https://doi.org/10.2218/gtopdb/F76/2019.4.

Hoskin JL, Al-Hasan Y, Sabbagh MN. Nicotinic Acetylcholine Receptor Agonists for the Treatment of Alzheimer's

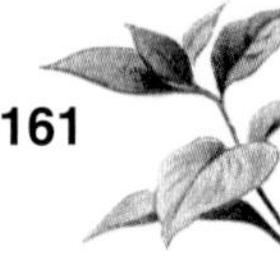

Dementia: An Update. Nicotine & Tobacco Research. 2019; Feb 18;21(3):370–376. doi: 10.1093/ntr/nty116. PMID: 30137524; PMCID: PMC6379052.

Jain A, Wermuth HR, Dua A, et al. Rocuronium. [Updated 2022 May 5]. In: StatPearls [Internet]. Treasure Island (FL): StatPearls Publishing; 2022 Jan-. Available from: https://www.ncbi.nlm.nih.gov/books/NBK539888/

Moore E.W., Hunter, J.M. The new neuromuscular blocking agents: do they offer any advantages?, BJA: British Journal of Anaesthesia, Volume 87, Issue 6, 1 December 2001, Pages 912–925, https://doi.org/10.1093/bja/87.6.912

MIMS Australia. (2022). Rocuronium In MIMS Online. http://www.mimsonline.com.au

Paton W.D.M. The Hexamethonium Man. Pharmacological Reviews. 1954; 6, 59.

Rang HP, Dale MM, Ritter JM, et al: Rang and Dale's Pharmacology, ed 8, Edinburgh, 2016, Elsevier Churchill Livingstone.

Salerno E: Pharmacology for health professionals, St Louis, 1999, Mosby.

ONLINE RESOURCES

IUPHAR database of receptors and ion channels: https://www.guidetopharmacology.org/ (accessed 6 October 2021)

More weblinks at: http://evolve.elsevier.com/AU/Knights/pharmacology/.

CHAPTER 9

DRUGS AFFECTING NORADRENERGIC TRANSMISSION

Shaunagh Darroch

KEY ABBREVIATIONS

COMT catechol-*O*-methyltransferase
DOPA dihydroxyphenylalanine
ENT extraneuronal transporter
ISA intrinsic sympathomimetic activity
MAO monoamine oxidase
NET noradrenaline (norepinephrine) uptake transporter
VMA vanillylmandelic acid
VMAT2 vesicular monoamine transporter 2

KEY TERMS

Chapter Focus

The sympathetic (adrenergic) nervous system is the second major subdivision of the autonomic nervous system. This system acts in concert with the parasympathetic nervous system to regulate the heart, secretory glands and vascular and non-vascular smooth muscle. Drugs that stimulate or block α- and β-adrenoceptors are common in clinical practice today. Understanding the physiological responses mediated by adrenergic receptors aids in rationalising the pharmacological and adverse effects of drugs affecting noradrenergic transmission.

KEY DRUG GROUPS

Direct-acting α- and/or β-adrenoceptor agonists:

- **adrenaline (epinephrine)** (Drug Monograph 9.1), **dopamine**, **isoprenaline**, **noradrenaline (norepinephrine)**

Mixed-acting α- and β-adrenoceptor agonists:

- **ephedrine**, **metaraminol**, **pseudoephedrine**

Non-selective α_1 and α_2 adrenoceptor antagonists:

- **phenoxybenzamine**, phentolamine

Selective α_1-adrenoceptor antagonists:

- **prazosin** (Drug Monograph 9.2)

Non-selective α_1, β_1 and β_2 adrenoceptor antagonists:

- **carvedilol** (Drug Monograph 9.3), labetalol, **propranolol**, sotalol

Selective β_1 adrenoceptor antagonists:

- atenolol, bisoprolol, metoprolol, **nebivolol**

Non-selective β_1 and β_2 adrenoceptor antagonists:

- pindolol

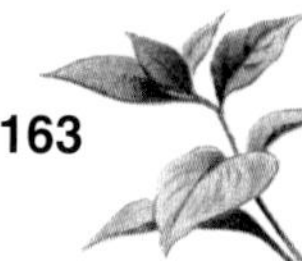

CRITICAL THINKING SCENARIO

Samuel, who suffers from asthma and hypertension, visits his local doctor complaining of shortness of breath. He states that despite using a reliever (salbutamol) and preventer (beclomethasone) his asthma seems to be worsening. The doctor notes that he is also taking propranolol for his hypertension. What are the mechanisms of action of his reliever and of propranolol? Discuss the possibility of drug interactions. What are the adverse effects of β-adrenoceptor agonists?

Introduction

This chapter reviews the anatomy and physiology of the sympathetic nervous system as a basis for discussing the pharmacology of sympathetic agonists and antagonists. A knowledge of the fundamentals of sympathetic nervous system pharmacology is important in treating peripheral disorders including cardiovascular, gastrointestinal and respiratory conditions.

The sympathetic nervous system

In the sympathetic nervous system, the preganglionic fibres originate in the spinal cord from thoracic segment T1 to the lumbar segment L2 (Fig 8.2, in Ch 8). The sympathetic ganglia lie on either side of the vertebral column in two chains, called the paravertebral sympathetic chains; hence the sympathetic preganglionic axons tend to be short, whereas the postganglionic axons are long. The only exception to the two-neuron arrangement is the adrenal medulla, which is supplied directly by a preganglionic neuron. Sympathetic activity increases in periods of stress ('fight-or-flight' reactions; Fig 9.1), although under normal conditions it exerts control over specific organ systems. See Chapter 8 for a discussion of the actions of sympathetic cholinergic neurons.

There are three endogenous **catecholamines** in the body: **dopamine**, **noradrenaline** and **adrenaline**. Dopamine is the precursor for the synthesis of noradrenaline and adrenaline, and has a major role as a neurotransmitter in certain areas of the central nervous system (CNS). (For more information on CNS transmission, refer

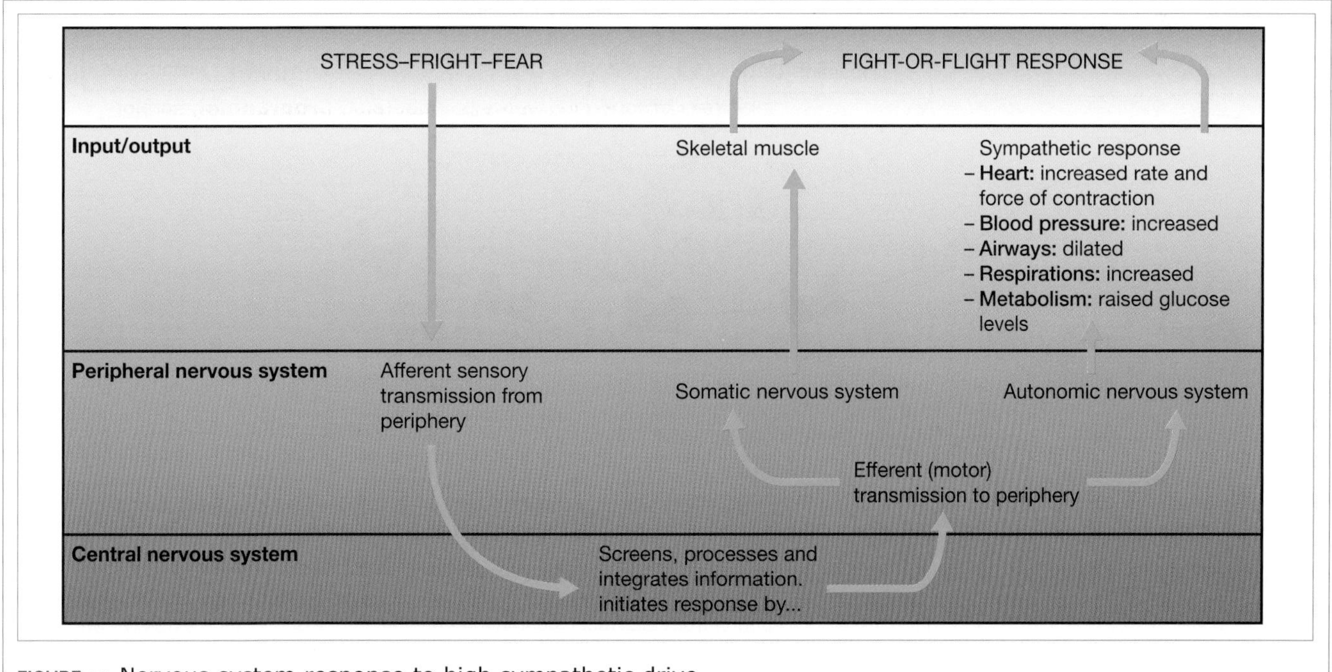

FIGURE 9.1 Nervous system response to high sympathetic drive

to various chapters in Unit 8.) Noradrenaline acts as the neurotransmitter between sympathetic postganglionic nerves and the organs they innervate (Figs 9.2 and 9.3), a process known as adrenergic transmission. Both noradrenaline and the major circulating catecholamine, adrenaline, are released by chromaffin cells of the adrenal medulla; sympathetic nervous system stimulation of these specialised cells leads to secretion of both noradrenaline (20%) and adrenaline (80%). The synthesis of noradrenaline is mediated by different enzymes located in the postganglionic sympathetic nerve terminals (Fig 9.2). Clinically, an abnormally high secretion of adrenaline and noradrenaline, which causes palpitations, excessive sweating, hypertension, headaches and skin pallor, occurs in phaeochromocytoma, a rare chromaffin cell tumour.

The following steps are involved in synthesising noradrenaline, mediated by different enzymes located in the postganglionic sympathetic nerve terminals:

1. The amino acid tyrosine is obtained from dietary proteins.

   Tyrosine is taken up by adrenergic neurons and enzymatically converted by the cytosolic enzyme tyrosine hydroxylase into dihydroxyphenylalanine (DOPA). Tyrosine hydroxylase is specific to catecholamine-containing cells. Because it is solely responsible for converting tyrosine to DOPA, it is considered the rate-limiting (controlling) step in the synthesis of noradrenaline.

   DOPA, in turn, is metabolised (decarboxylated) to dopamine by the cytosolic enzyme DOPA decarboxylase.

2. Dopamine is then taken up into neuronal storage vesicles, or granules, where it is metabolised into the neurotransmitter noradrenaline by the enzyme dopamine β-hydroxylase, which is located in the storage vesicles.

   Unlike adrenergic neurons, in the adrenal medulla the enzyme phenylethanolamine *N*-methyltransferase converts noradrenaline to adrenaline. On stimulation, both adrenaline and noradrenaline are released from the adrenal medulla and carried by the systemic circulation to all parts of the body.

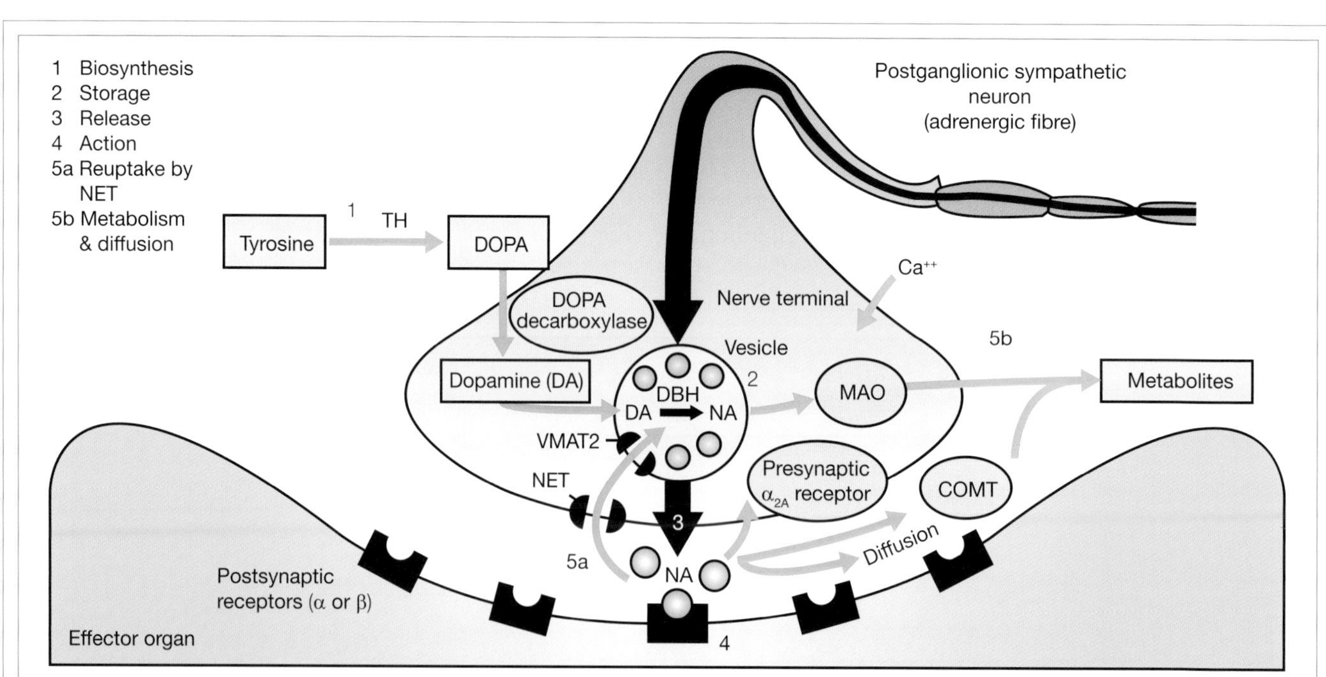

FIGURE 9.2 Adrenergic transmission at a neuroeffector junction
1 Biosynthesis and storage of noradrenaline: tyrosine is taken up by adrenergic neurons and metabolised to DOPA by the cytosolic enzyme tyrosine hydroxylase. DOPA is metabolised to dopamine by the cytosolic enzyme DOPA decarboxylase.
2. Dopamine is taken up into storage vesicles where it is metabolised by the vesicular enzyme dopamine β-hydroxylase to noradrenaline.
3 Release: an action potential arriving at the nerve terminal causes the vesicle to attach itself to the membrane and release noradrenaline, which then diffuses across the synaptic cleft and combines with post-junctional receptors on the effector cell and with presynaptic α_{2A} receptors.
4 Action: the interaction of noradrenaline with the receptors results in a response.
5 The action of noradrenaline is terminated predominantly by reuptake of noradrenaline into the nerve terminal by NET (5a) and sequestration back into vesicles by VMAT2, and with a lesser contribution from enzymatic degradation by MAO and COMT and by diffusion away from the receptors (5b).
Source: Adapted from Salerno 1999, Figure 14-5; used with permission.

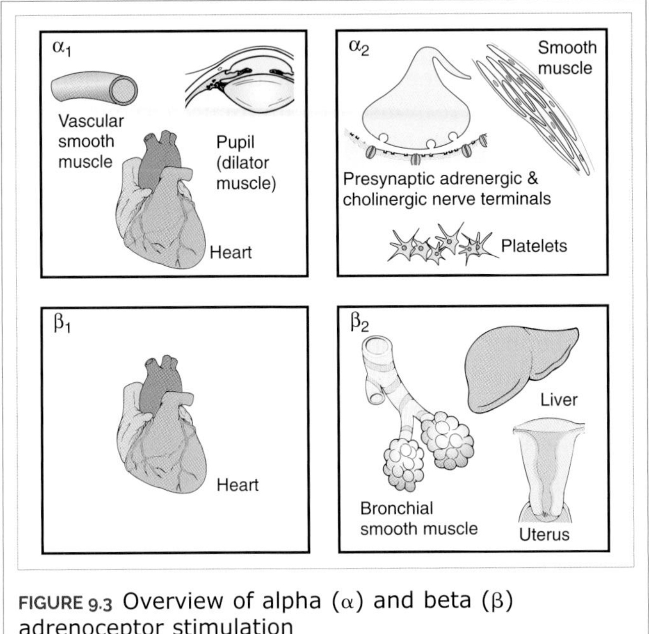

FIGURE 9.3 Overview of alpha (α) and beta (β) adrenoceptor stimulation

3. In manner similar to that of cholinergic transmission, the arrival of an action potential at the nerve terminal of the postganglionic neuron causes an influx of calcium ions, fusion of vesicles with the cell membrane and release of stored noradrenaline into the junctional cleft.
4. Noradrenaline then diffuses across the cleft to the receptor sites on the postjunctional membrane of neuroeffector cells (smooth muscle, cardiac muscle or glands). Negative feedback occurs via the prejunctional α_{2A}-adrenoceptor: when stimulated inhibits the release of noradrenaline (Fig 9.4).

   The uptake and degradation of catecholamines differs substantially from that of acetylcholine. Once noradrenaline has bound to an adrenoceptor, its action must be rapidly terminated to prevent prolongation of its effects, which could lead to a loss of regulatory control of visceral function. The termination of action of noradrenaline occurs by the following mechanisms, as indicated in Figure 9.2:

5a. Reuptake of the noradrenaline into nerve terminals by the noradrenaline uptake transporter (NET), which is located on the presynaptic membrane. (This process was previously referred to as uptake 1.) A proportion of the intraneuronal noradrenaline is then sequestered back into vesicles aided by vesicular monoamine transporter 2 (VMAT2) and the remainder is metabolised.

5b. Uptake into extraneuronal cells by the extraneuronal transporter (ENT) (this process, previously called uptake 2, also transports adrenaline and isoprenaline) and subsequent metabolism.

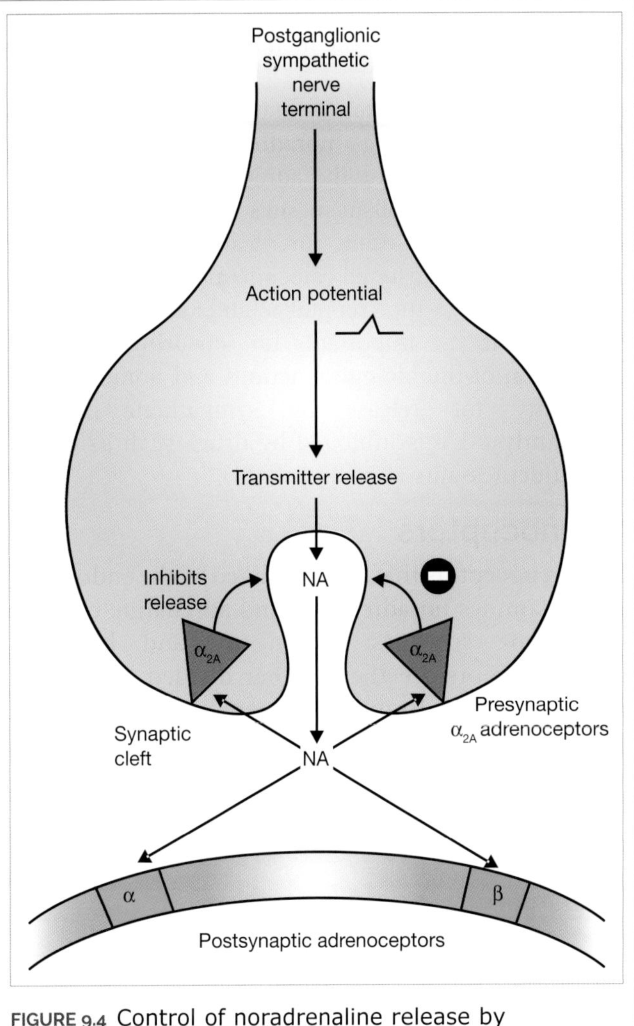

FIGURE 9.4 Control of noradrenaline release by presynaptic α_{2A}-adrenoceptors

The dominant process for terminating the action of noradrenaline released from sympathetic neurons is reuptake by NET, with a lesser contribution from metabolism by monoamine oxidase (MAO) and catechol-*O*-methyltransferase (COMT).

Diffusion into the bloodstream and metabolism at non-neuronal sites.

Catecholamines are metabolised by the enzymes MAO and COMT. Two types of MAO have been identified, MAO-A and MAO-B. These enzymes, and drugs that inhibit them, are discussed in Chapter 22 in the context of the antidepressants.

Free noradrenaline in the cytoplasm of the nerve terminal is metabolised by MAO, which is bound to the surface membrane of intraneuronal mitochondria. COMT is widely distributed throughout the body, with the highest concentration found in the liver, followed by the kidney and gastrointestinal tract (GIT). It is a membrane-bound enzyme in chromaffin cells and a cytosolic enzyme in non-neuronal tissue. It metabolises both noradrenaline and the metabolites produced by the action of MAO.

Non-neuronal uptake, facilitated by ENT, is a minor pathway for clearing noradrenaline produced in sympathetic neurons or the adrenal medulla. However, non-neuronal metabolism in sites such as the liver and kidney is very important for clearing circulating and exogenously administered catecholamines.

In summary, the reuptake and sequestration of noradrenaline is important for ensuring both the termination of the biological actions and noradrenaline's availability for release by sympathetic neurons. Importantly, NET is inhibited by drugs such as cocaine and antidepressants (Chs 22 and 23).

Adrenoceptors

The adrenoceptors that are stimulated by the endogenous catecholamines noradrenaline and adrenaline comprise two major subtypes: alpha (α) and beta (β). α-adrenoceptors are then further divided into α_1 and α_2 subtypes; the former has been further subdivided into α_{1A}, α_{1B} and α_{1D} subtypes and the latter into α_{2A}, α_{2B} and α_{2C} subtypes. A summary of the subtypes (α and β adrenoceptors), their tissue localisation and their dominant response to autonomic nervous system stimulation is shown in Table 8.1 (Ch 8), Table 9.1 and Figure 9.3.

The **α-adrenoceptors** are differentiated primarily by their location. α_1-adrenoceptors are located postjunctionally on, for example, vascular smooth muscle cells. They are generally located close to the nerve terminal on the postjunctional membrane so that the action of released noradrenaline is rapid. α_2-adrenoceptors are found on presynaptic nerve terminals and on sites remote from the nerve terminals, such as platelets. The inhibitory presynaptic α_{2A} autoreceptors are pharmacologically distinct from the postjunctional α_1-adrenoceptors and control the amount of noradrenaline released through a negative feedback mechanism. When the concentration of noradrenaline in the synaptic cleft reaches a high level, it stimulates the α_{2A}-adrenoceptors, which prevent the further release of noradrenaline (Figs 9.2 and 9.4). This feedback prevents excessive and prolonged stimulation

TABLE 9.1 α- and β-adrenoceptor subtypes, examples of tissue localisation and dominant physiological response

LOCALISATION	α_{1A}	α_{1B}	α_{1D}	α_{2A}	α_{2B}	α_{2C}	β_1	β_2	β_3
Aorta			✓						
Brain	✓	✓	✓	✓		✓	✓	✓	
Blood vessels	✓	✓			✓			✓	
Coronary vessels			✓	✓					
Heart	✓						✓	✓	✓
Kidney		✓			✓		✓	✓	
Liver	✓				✓			✓	
Lung	✓	✓						✓	
Platelets			✓	✓	✓				
Prostate	✓		✓						
Smooth muscle (e.g. bladder, airways, uterus)	✓							✓	✓
Sympathetic neurons (prejunctional receptors)				✓					
Skeletal muscle							✓	✓	✓

Dominant physiological response
α_{1A}Arterial vasoconstriction
Vascular smooth muscle contraction
Promotes cardiac hypertrophy
α_{1B}Promotes cardiac hypertrophy
α_{1D}Arterial vasoconstriction
α_{2A}Reduces sympathetic neurotransmission (including central sympathetic outflow)
Arterial vasoconstriction
α_{2B}Vasoconstriction
α_{2C}Modulates dopamine neurotransmission
Inhibits hormone release from adrenal medulla
β_1 Heart (SA and AV nodes and His-Purkinje systems) increased automaticity, conduction velocity and contractility
β_2 Dilation of vasculature: arterioles and arteries
Relaxation of bronchial smooth muscle
Relaxation of pregnant uterine smooth muscle
β_3 Relaxation of bladder detrusor muscle

Source: Brunton et al. 2017.

of postjunctional α_1-adrenoceptors on effector organs such as the eye, arterioles, veins, male sex organs and bladder neck.

Important responses mediated by α-adrenoceptor stimulation in humans include:

- vasoconstriction of arterioles in the skin and splanchnic area and increased peripheral resistance, which results in a rise in blood pressure
- pupil dilation (mydriasis)
- relaxation of gastrointestinal smooth muscle, contraction of gastrointestinal sphincters
- increase in smooth muscle tone of bladder neck.

β-adrenoceptors show wide tissue distribution (Table 8.1 in Ch 8; Table 9.1 and Fig 9.3) and are divided into three types:

- β_1-adrenoceptors, which are primarily located on the heart
- β_2-adrenoceptors, which mediate the actions of catecholamines on smooth muscle, especially the smooth muscle of bronchioles, arteries and arterioles of skeletal muscle
- β_3-adrenoceptors, which are located on the plasma membrane of adipocytes and mediate lipolysis (Schena & Caplan 2019). They are present on skeletal muscle and are also expressed in human brain, heart, gallbladder, GIT, prostate and urinary bladder detrusor muscle. A β_3-adrenoceptor agonist, mirabegron, is used to treat overactive bladder (Schena & Caplan 2019).

Important responses mediated by β-adrenoceptor stimulation include:

- increase in heart rate and contractility
- vasodilation of arterioles supplying skeletal muscles
- bronchial relaxation
- uterine relaxation
- aqueous humour formation.

Most arteries and veins contain both α- and β-adrenoceptors. A change in blood pressure will depend on the degree of vasoconstriction in the skin and splanchnic area, and the extent of vasodilation in skeletal muscle blood vessels, along with changes in heart rate. Refer to Table 8.1 in Chapter 8 and Table 9.1.

KEY POINTS

The sympathetic nervous system

- The sympathetic nervous system is responsible for major physiological changes in the body in response to high demand or stressful situations (e.g. 'fight-or-flight' reactions).
- The catecholamine noradrenaline acts as the neurotransmitter between sympathetic postganglionic nerves and effector organs.
- Adrenaline is a catecholamine released from modified postganglionic neurons in the adrenal medulla into the bloodstream (hormone) and from certain neurons.
- There are two major subtypes of adrenoceptors – alpha (α) and beta (β) – and they are stimulated by noradrenaline and adrenaline.
- The subtypes of adrenoceptors are alpha (α_{1A}, α_{1B}, α_{1D}, α_{2A}, α_{2B}, α_{2C}) and beta (β_1, β_2, β_3).

Drugs acting at adrenergic receptors

Specific drugs that stimulate or block α- and β-adrenoceptors are available, and many of these drugs are discussed in other chapters in the context of the relevant pharmacology (see, for example, short- and long-acting β-adrenoceptor agonists in the context of asthma in Ch 15). Except for agonists at central α_2-adrenoceptors, which are discussed in the context of schizophrenia in Chapter 22, these agents all act at peripheral autonomic sites. The extent of sympathetic innervation or the presence of adrenoceptors on various organs will determine the magnitude of response to an individual adrenergic drug.

Drugs affecting noradrenergic activity in the body include:

- direct-acting adrenoceptor agonists (**sympathomimetic drugs**) that mimic the effects of either noradrenaline released from sympathetic nerve terminals or adrenaline released from the adrenal medulla acting on α- and β-adrenoceptors
- mixed-acting adrenoceptor agonists that release noradrenaline indirectly and also directly activate the adrenoceptors
- indirect-acting adrenoceptor agonists that either facilitate the release of noradrenaline from, or block the uptake of noradrenaline into, nerve terminals or inhibit metabolism by MAO or COMT (e.g. methamphetamine)
- adrenoceptor antagonists (blockers), also referred to as **sympatholytic drugs**, which block the action of the sympathetic nervous system.

Direct-acting adrenoceptor agonists

During circulatory shock due to, for example, cardiogenic factors or distributive factors (e.g. anaphylaxis), the autonomic nervous system plays an essential compensatory role in an attempt to restore normal haemodynamics; therefore, many drugs that target the sympathetic nervous system are used to manage this condition. The direct-acting adrenoceptor agonists directly stimulate α- and **β-adrenoceptors**, mimicking the effects of sympathetic stimulation, such as increasing cardiac output, vasoconstriction of arterioles and veins, regulation of body temperature, bronchodilation and a variety of other effects. (For more information on the effects of the sympathetic nervous system, see Ch 8, Table 8.1.) Although there are other agents, five drugs are widely used for circulatory shock:

- catecholamines: adrenaline (epinephrine), noradrenaline (norepinephrine)[1] and dopamine
- synthetic catecholamines: dobutamine and isoprenaline.

1 A reminder that in the American literature, noradrenaline and adrenaline are known as norepinephrine and epinephrine, respectively, from an old name for the adrenal gland, the epinephric gland. From April 2016, in Australia and New Zealand medicines containing adrenaline and noradrenaline have started to include the international names 'epinephrine' and 'norepinephrine' on labels and information leaflets (Therapeutic Goods Administration 2021). In this chapter we use 'noradrenaline' and 'adrenaline'.

Refer to Drug Monograph 9.1 for a description of the pharmacology of adrenaline.

Adrenaline is an important drug that stimulates α- and β-adrenoceptors. It is commonly used in the treatment of bronchospasm and croup, emergency treatment of anaphylactic reactions and cardiac arrest, as a haemostatic agent and during ocular surgery.

The use of isoprenaline in shock is limited by β_2-adrenoceptor-mediated vasodilation that may worsen hypotension (Table 9.2).

Noradrenaline acts principally on α_1-, β_1- and β_3-adrenoceptors, with less selectivity for β_2-adrenoceptors. In contrast, adrenaline acts on all α- and β-adrenoceptor subtypes, with significantly greater effects on α-adrenoceptors at higher doses. Isoprenaline, a synthetic catecholamine, acts only on β-adrenoceptors.

Drug Monograph 9.1
Adrenaline (epinephrine)

Mechanisms of action

Adrenaline stimulates α- and β-adrenoceptors. The primary action of adrenaline is on the β-adrenoceptors of the heart, smooth muscle of the bronchi and blood vessels. At low doses, adrenaline has predominantly β-adrenoceptor actions, but with increasing doses an increase in α-adrenoceptor activity is observed.

Cardiac effects

Adrenaline produces a significant increase in myocardial contraction (positive **inotropic effect**) as a result of activating β_1-adrenoceptors and increased influx of calcium into cardiac fibres. The strong myocardial contractions result in more complete emptying of the ventricles and an increase in cardiac work, oxygen consumption and cardiac output. This positive inotropic effect provides the rationale for using adrenaline in cardiac arrest.

Adrenaline cannot be used repeatedly to improve the function of a failing heart (congestive heart failure) because it increases oxygen consumption by cardiac muscle.

A significant increase in cardiac rate (positive **chronotropic effect**) occurs as a result of the increased rate of membrane depolarisation in the pacemaker cells in the sinus node during diastole. Action potential threshold is reached sooner, pacemaker cells fire more often and heart rate increases. Adrenaline may also produce spontaneous firing of Purkinje fibres, which may cause them to exhibit pacemaker activity. This effect can cause ventricular extrasystoles and increase the susceptibility of ventricular muscle to fibrillation. An improvement in atrioventricular conduction (positive **dromotropic effect**) may also occur in conduction abnormalities.

Vascular effects

Vascular effects of adrenaline depend on the dose and the vascular bed affected. Low doses of adrenaline decrease total peripheral vascular resistance and lower blood pressure. At low doses, adrenaline acts via β_2-adrenergic receptors causing vasodilation through L-type calcium channels. In large doses, adrenaline activates α-receptors in the peripheral vascular system, which results in an increase in peripheral resistance and in blood pressure. The dominant net response is often, however, vasodilation; for example, during situations of high sympathetic demand, the release of adrenaline from the adrenal medulla constricts blood vessels in the skin and splanchnic areas but dilates those of skeletal muscles, thus shunting blood to the areas needed for 'fight-or-flight'-type responses.

Renal artery constriction and increased resistance occurs with adrenaline, and renal blood flow may be substantially reduced. Direct action on β_1-adrenoceptors on juxtaglomerular cells increases the secretion of renin.

Central nervous system effects

Adrenaline in therapeutic doses is not a CNS stimulant. Signs of restlessness, tremors and anxiety may be secondary to the effects of adrenaline on skeletal muscle, the cardiovascular system and changes in metabolism. Beneficial cerebral

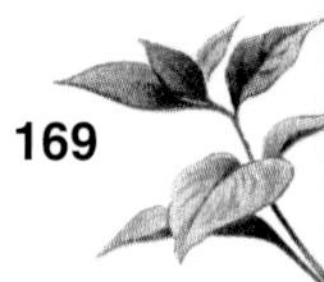

effects from adrenaline in people with hypotension are thought to be the result of increased systemic pressure with a resultant improvement in cerebral blood flow.

Smooth muscle effects

Generally, adrenaline relaxes smooth muscle of the GIT. The stomach is relaxed and the amplitude and tone of intestinal peristalsis are reduced. In theory, this may retard gastrointestinal emptying and propulsion of food; however, this effect is rare in humans with therapeutic doses of catecholamines. In the urinary bladder, adrenaline causes trigone and sphincter constriction via α-adrenoceptor stimulation and detrusor relaxation (β-adrenoceptor agonist activity), which may cause a delay in the desire to void and hence urine retention. Adrenaline inhibits uterine contraction during the last months of pregnancy, and the β_2-adrenoceptor agonists such as salbutamol are used to prevent premature labour.

Respiratory effects

Adrenaline is a powerful bronchodilator and relieves respiratory distress due to allergens such as bee venom. In asthma, it is likely that beneficial effects also occur through the effect of adrenaline on mast cells and on bronchial mucosa (Ch 15).

Metabolic effects

Adrenaline inhibits insulin secretion and decreases the uptake of glucose by peripheral tissues, thus raising blood glucose levels. It stimulates lipolysis in adipose tissue, which results in an increase in free fatty acids in blood. Therefore, in response to high sympathetic drive, there is an abundant supply of fuel and energy. Adrenaline also has a calorigenic effect, primarily as a result of increased metabolism, which increases oxygen consumption.

Indications

Adrenaline is used:

- for the emergency treatment of anaphylactic reactions and severe acute reactions to drugs, animal serums, insect stings and other allergens; in severe/life-threatening asthma, to relieve bronchospasm, croup with life-threatening airway compromise, angio-oedema and swelling of the mucosa and upper airway obstruction (e.g. laryngeal oedema). Pulmonary congestion is also alleviated by constriction of mucosal blood vessels
- as an adjunct to local anaesthetics. Concurrent administration of adrenaline with local anaesthetics reduces circulation to the site, which results in a slowing of vascular absorption (this promotes the local effect of the anaesthetic and prolongs its duration of action)
- as a haemostatic agent to control superficial bleeding from arterioles and capillaries in the skin, mucous membranes or other tissues
- in ocular surgery to control bleeding, induce mydriasis and conjunctival decongestion, and to lower intraocular pressure
- to provide inotropic support in acute exacerbations of chronic heart failure and in situations of acute heart failure, cardiogenic shock and septic shock
- to treat cardiac arrest.

Pharmacokinetics

Adrenaline is not given orally because of rapid metabolism in the mucosa of the GIT and liver by COMT and MAO. Following parenteral administration, adrenaline is rapidly metabolised by COMT, taken up into extraneuronal tissue (e.g. liver) by ENT and further metabolised to vanillylmandelic acid (VMA). VMA is the major urinary metabolite excreted by the kidneys in humans and is used as a diagnostic marker for catecholamine-secreting tumours. The plasma half-life of adrenaline is in the order of 2 minutes.

Drug interactions

If indicated, adrenaline is not withheld because of concerns of drug interactions. The following effects can occur when adrenaline is given with the drugs listed:

- α-adrenoceptor antagonists (α-blockers): β-adrenoceptor-mediated effects predominate, producing hypotension.
- β-adrenoceptor antagonists (β-blockers): α-adrenoceptor-mediated vasoconstriction predominates, resulting in hypertension, severe bradycardia and possibly heart block. Effects are less marked with atenolol, bisoprolol and metoprolol. If using non-selective β-blockers (e.g. propranolol), reduce adrenaline dose. In all cases, monitor blood pressure and heart rate.
- Entacapone: Entacapone inhibits COMT and hence the metabolism of adrenaline, increasing the risk of dysrhythmias. Reduce the dose of adrenaline and monitor closely.
- Digitalis glycosides: Digitalis sensitises the myocardium to the effects of adrenaline; the additive effect of the adrenaline increases the risk of dysrhythmias.
- Halogenated anaesthetics (e.g. isoflurane): May sensitise the heart, increasing the risk of severe dysrhythmias. Monitor closely – a reduction in dose of adrenaline is usually necessary.
- Oxytocics: Concurrent use may produce severe hypertension.
- Tricyclic antidepressants, MAO inhibitor antidepressants, cocaine: Potentiate the effect of adrenaline. Concurrent use may result in dysrhythmias, tachycardia and hypertension or hyperpyrexia. Avoid, or a serious drug interaction may occur.

Adverse reactions

Adverse reactions include increased nervousness, restlessness, insomnia, tachycardia, tremors, sweating, hypertension, nausea, vomiting, pallor and weakness. With inhalation devices, adverse reactions include bronchial irritation and coughing

(with high doses), dry mouth and throat, headaches and flushing of the face and skin. High doses may cause ventricular dysrhythmias.

Warnings and contraindications

Adrenaline is used with caution in persons with diabetes mellitus, closed-angle glaucoma, hypertension, ischaemic heart disease, heart failure, arrhythmias, hyperthyroidism, phaeochromocytoma and Parkinson's disease. When used in end-artery areas, such as the fingers, toes or penis, the reduced blood supply to the area may result in ischaemia and gangrene. Avoid use in people with known hypersensitivity to adrenaline (or sympathomimetics), organic brain damage, coronary insufficiency or shock.

Dosage and administration

Intravenous (IV) administration (e.g. infusion or slow IV injection) should only be done by highly experienced health professionals (e.g. emergency medicine practitioners, Advanced Life Support [ALS]-credentialled personnel) because of the risk of systemic adverse effects. When administering via the IV route, continuous monitoring of the ECG, use of pulse oximetry and recording of blood pressure should be instigated. Absorption after intramuscular (IM) injection into the mid-anterolateral thigh can be slow because of local vasoconstriction, but it is the preferred route of administration at the first sign of an anaphylactic reaction. Administration via an endotracheal tube has been de-emphasised and subcutaneous administration is not recommended because of erratic absorption. Nebulised adrenaline is used for upper airway obstruction and for treating croup, and has a rapid onset of action of 1–5 minutes. The adrenaline autoinjectors EpiPen, and the junior version EpiPen Jr, are approved for use in Australia and New Zealand and contain a single fixed dose of adrenaline. Health professionals should familiarise themselves with the appropriate procedures.

Adrenaline is available in ampoules as: 1:1000, which is 1 mg adrenaline in 1 mL; and 1:10,000, which is 0.1 mg in 1 mL or 1 mg in 10 mL. When giving adrenaline IV, the more dilute formulation (1:10,000) is used. Adrenaline is also available as the fixed-dose autoinjectors; EpiPen is 300 microgram/0.3 mL and the equivalent junior versions are 150 microgram/0.3 mL. In severe anaphylaxis or cardiac arrest, doses of adrenaline may need to be repeated; this will depend on the initial dosage used and the clinical response. For specific clinical situations, consult guidelines such as those of the Australasian Society of Clinical Immunology and Allergy and the Australian Resuscitation Council (see 'Online resources').

Noradrenaline

At α-adrenoceptors:

- Noradrenaline has a high affinity for α-adrenoceptors and, because the blood vessels of the skin, visceral organs and kidneys (both arteriolar and venous beds) and mucous membrane contain α-adrenoceptors, it produces vasoconstriction in these tissues. As a consequence, noradrenaline causes reduced blood flow in the kidneys and other visceral organs.

  At β-adrenoceptors:

- Although noradrenaline activates β_1-adrenoceptors on the heart, effecting changes in diastolic and systolic pressure, peripheral vascular resistance coupled with compensatory vagal reflexes results in no change in heart rate and cardiac output.

Stimulation of α- and β_1-adrenoceptors with noradrenaline is dose-related. At low doses (< 0.002 mg/min infusion), β_1-adrenoceptors are stimulated; at doses higher than 0.004 mg/min, stimulation of α-adrenoceptors increases total peripheral resistance. Titration of the dose in steps of 0.002–0.004 mg/min is based on haemodynamic response.

Clinical uses

Noradrenaline is selectively used for restoring blood pressure in acute hypotensive states such as sympathectomy,

TABLE 9.2 Comparative information on adrenoceptor agonists

	ADRENOCEPTOR AND EFFECTS[a]			ORGAN RESPONSE[b]		
DRUG	β_1	β_2	α_1	KIDNEYS	CARDIAC	BP
Adrenaline (high dose)	++	0	+++	D	I	I/D
Dobutamine	+++	+	0/+	0	I	0/I
Dopamine (high dose)	++	0	+++	I		0/I
Isoprenaline	+++	+++	0	I/D	I	#
Noradrenaline	+	+	+++	D	0/D	I

+ = minimal effect; ++ = moderate effect; +++ = greatest effect; 0 = no effect; I = increased; D = decreased; # = usual doses maintain or raise systolic pressure.
[a] Adrenoceptor and effects: α_1 = vasoconstriction; β_1 = inotropic effect; β_2 = vasodilation
[b] Organ response: kidneys = renal perfusion; cardiac = cardiac output; BP = blood pressure

myocardial infarction, phaeochromocytomectomy and blood transfusion reactions. It is also used as adjunct therapy in cardiac arrest.

The main therapeutic effect of noradrenaline results from peripheral arteriolar vasoconstriction in all vascular beds. Both systolic and diastolic pressures are elevated, causing a rise in mean arterial pressure. Of importance during shock is constriction of the venous capacitance vessels, which reduces splanchnic and renal blood flow. This is brought about by severe restriction of tissue perfusion in these regions. In persistent hypotension after blood volume deficit has been corrected, noradrenaline helps to raise the blood pressure to an optimal level and establishes a more adequate circulation.

Pharmacokinetic considerations

Oral noradrenaline is rapidly metabolised by COMT and MAO in the mucosa of the GIT, liver and other tissues. Noradrenaline has limited therapeutic value and is administered IV, preferably via a central venous access device to minimise the risk of extravasation and subsequent tissue necrosis. Onset of action is rapid by the IV route and distribution is mainly to the heart, spleen and glandular tissues. The half-life is short and ranges from approximately 30 seconds to 3 minutes. Following parenteral administration, the most significant clearance occurs by uptake into sympathetic nerves by NET and, to a lesser extent, by uptake into extraneuronal tissues by ENT. Most of the dose is excreted in urine as VMA. Subcutaneous noradrenaline is poorly absorbed owing to local vasoconstriction at the site of injection.

Adverse drug reactions and drug interactions

Drug interactions with noradrenaline are similar to those of adrenaline and include interactions with halogenated inhalational anaesthetics, β-blocking agents, digitalis glycosides, tricyclic antidepressants, MAO inhibitors, cocaine and oxytocics. Adverse reactions include anxiety, dizziness, pallor, tremor, insomnia, headache, palpitations and, infrequently, hypertension and bradycardia.

Warnings and contraindications

Noradrenaline should be used with caution in people living with atherosclerosis, mesenteric and peripheral vascular thrombosis or other occlusive vascular diseases, metabolic acidosis, hypoxia or hyperthyroidism. It should also be avoided in those with hypertension, hypersensitivity to sodium metabisulfite (the preservative in the solution), hypovolaemia, myocardial infarction and ventricular dysrhythmias. Importantly, noradrenaline solution should be protected from light and not used if a brown colouration is present.

Isoprenaline

Isoprenaline, a synthetic catecholamine, is a non-selective β-adrenoceptor agonist – it stimulates both β_1- and β_2-adrenoceptors (Fig 9.5). The β_1-adrenoceptor activity produces an increase in the force of myocardial contraction and heart rate. The β_2-adrenoceptor response of the smooth muscle of the bronchi, skeletal muscle blood vessels, GIT and blood vessels of the splanchnic bed is relaxation. This drug also stimulates insulin secretion through β-adrenoceptor activation of beta cells of the pancreatic islets, and causes the release of free fatty acids from adipocytes.

Isoprenaline is used to increase automaticity and atrioventricular (AV) nodal conduction in Stokes-Adams syndrome and serious episodes of heart block. It may also be used as adjunctive therapy in treatment of hypovolaemic states, septic shock, congestive heart failure and cardiogenic shock.

Haemodynamically, activation of β_1-adrenoceptors by isoprenaline on the heart increases cardiac output and venous return to the heart. However, peripheral vascular resistance is reduced, and in normal individuals this may cause a significant drop in blood pressure with excessive dosage.

Pharmacokinetic considerations

Absorption of orally administered isoprenaline is erratic and this route is no longer recommended. Following IV administration, the plasma concentration of isoprenaline declines in a biphasic manner. The initial phase corresponds to rapid uptake into smooth muscle and cardiac tissue (around 5 minutes), while the second phase, which reflects widespread metabolism, lasts for more than 2.5 hours. Isoprenaline is metabolised by COMT in the GIT, liver and lungs and is excreted in the urine, predominantly as unchanged drug (~60%).

Adverse drug reactions and drug interactions

Drug interactions with isoprenaline include β-adrenoceptor antagonists, which antagonise the therapeutic effect of isoprenaline (may precipitate asthma). Also, avoid concurrent administration of isoprenaline with other sympathomimetic amines because additive effects may occur and cardiotoxicity may result. The range of adverse reactions for isoprenaline is similar to that for adrenaline.

Warnings and contraindications

Use isoprenaline with caution in the elderly and in people living with diabetes mellitus, hyperthyroidism or ischaemic heart disease. Isoprenaline is contraindicated in the presence of tachycardia, ventricular dysrhythmias and myocardial infarction, and in those with known hypersensitivity to isoprenaline.

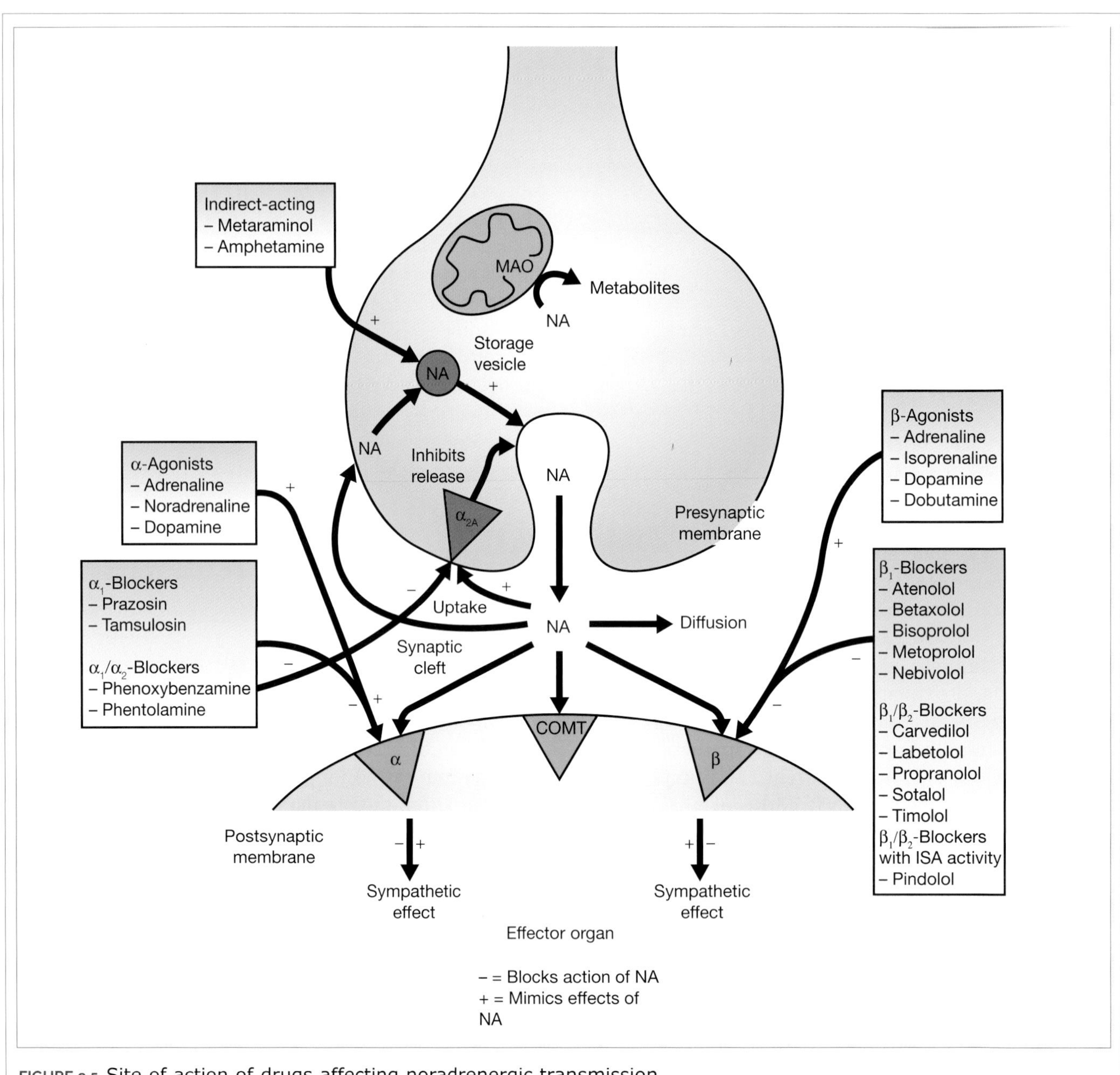

FIGURE 9.5 Site of action of drugs affecting noradrenergic transmission

Dopamine

Dopamine is a catecholamine and is the immediate precursor of noradrenaline (Fig 9.2). It acts directly on both adrenergic and dopaminergic receptors. Dopamine stimulates dopaminergic receptors (see Ch 18 for subtypes of dopamine receptors in the CNS), β_1-adrenoceptors and, in high doses, α_1- and α_2-adrenoceptors. Its actions are dose-dependent and very complex.

Low doses

Unlike noradrenaline, in low doses (0.5–2 microgram/kg/min), dopamine acts mainly on dopaminergic (D_1) receptors to cause vasodilation of the renal and mesenteric arteries. Renal vasodilation increases renal blood flow, usually accompanied by greater urine and sodium excretion.

Low to moderate doses

In low to moderate doses (usually 2–10 microgram/kg/min), DA acts directly on the β_1-adrenoceptors on the myocardium and indirectly by releasing noradrenaline from myocardial presynaptic sympathetic storage sites. These actions increase myocardial contractility and stroke volume, thereby increasing cardiac output. Systolic blood pressure and pulse pressure may rise, with either no effect or a slight elevation in diastolic blood pressure. Nevertheless, total peripheral resistance is usually unchanged. Coronary blood flow and myocardial oxygen consumption increase, while heart rate increases only slightly at low doses.

Higher doses

With higher doses of dopamine (10 microgram/kg/min or more), α-adrenoceptors are stimulated, increasing peripheral resistance. As a consequence, higher doses may reduce urinary output, eliminating the benefit of D_1 receptor-mediated renal vasodilation.

Clinical uses

Unlike noradrenaline, dopamine aids perfusion of vital splanchnic organs. The combination of cardiac and vascular effects has led to successful use of dopamine in the treatment of circulatory shock and refractory heart failure. Dopamine is used to correct haemodynamic imbalances associated with shock syndrome caused by myocardial infarction, trauma, endotoxin septicaemia, open heart surgery, renal failure and chronic cardiac decompensation (as in congestive heart failure).

Pharmacokinetic considerations

Dopamine is administered by IV infusion. The drug has a rapid onset of action (2–5 minutes) and a short duration of action (5–10 minutes). It is widely distributed throughout the body and is actively taken up into sympathetic nerves but does not cross the blood–brain barrier and therefore does not act on central dopaminergic receptors. Dopamine is rapidly metabolised by COMT and MAO in peripheral tissues to the major metabolite homovanillic acid, which is excreted in urine at twice the rate of VMA.

Adverse reactions

Adverse reactions include headache, nausea, vomiting, angina, respiratory difficulties, decreased blood pressure and, less frequently, hypertension, irregular or ectopic heart beats, tachycardia and palpitations. For drug interactions, warnings and contraindications, see the discussion of noradrenaline.

Dobutamine

Dobutamine is a synthetic catecholamine directly stimulating cardiac β_1-adrenoceptors to increase the force of myocardial contraction. At the same time, dobutamine produces comparatively little increase in heart rate or peripheral vascular resistance.

Clinical uses

Dobutamine is used primarily in the short-term management of people requiring inotropic support, as in those with congestive heart failure, cardiogenic shock due to myocardial infarction or after cardiac surgery. Its beneficial effects include a progressive increase in cardiac output and a decrease in pulmonary capillary wedge pressure, thereby improving ventricular contraction. By enhancing stroke volume, this agent is an effective positive inotropic drug. Because of its minimal influence on heart rate and blood pressure (both major determinants of myocardial oxygen demand), it is valuable for use in people with low cardiac output. Dobutamine does not have any effect on dopamine receptors and does not cause vasodilation in the kidney.

Pharmacokinetic considerations

Dobutamine is administered IV during short-term management of people requiring inotropic support. The onset of action of dobutamine is within 1–2 minutes, and it has a duration of action of approximately 10 minutes. Its plasma half-life is less than 3 minutes because it is rapidly metabolised by hepatic COMT to methyldobutamine, which is conjugated with glucuronic acid and excreted in the urine. The glucuronide metabolite has no significant cardiovascular activity.

Adverse reactions and drug interactions

Drug interactions are similar to those of adrenaline with regard to α- and β-blockers, general anaesthetics and oxytocin. Additive vasodilatory effects also occur with the co-administration of sodium nitroprusside and additive chronotropic effects with other drugs producing the same effect. Adverse reactions include nausea, headache, respiratory distress, angina, palpitations, tachycardia, hypertension and, commonly, ventricular ectopic beats. Hence, dobutamine is contraindicated in people with atrial fibrillation, ventricular dysrhythmias and phaeochromocytoma.

Other direct-acting adrenoceptor agonists

Table 9.2, earlier, provides comparative information on the endogenous and synthetic catecholamines. In addition to the catecholamines, other direct-acting **α-adrenoceptor agonists** include the topical ocular drugs naphazoline, tetryzoline (tetrahydrozoline), phenylephrine and oxymetazoline (α_1-adrenoceptor agonist), which are used to treat ocular congestion and are freely available as over-the-counter products (Ch 40). Oxymetazoline is also used for nasal decongestion. Brimonidine and apraclonidine are α_2 receptor agonists used to reduce intraocular pressure in glaucoma (Ch 40).

Mixed-acting adrenoceptor agonists

The prototypical mixed-acting adrenoceptor agonist is ephedrine, a racemic drug isolated from the plant Ephedra, with pseudoephedrine being the stereoisomer of ephedrine (*L*-ephedrine) and with a similar pharmacological profile.

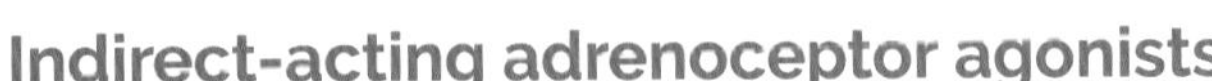

Indirect-acting adrenoceptor agonists

Indirect-acting adrenoceptor agonists can trigger the release of noradrenaline and adrenaline from their storage sites (see mechanism of action of ephedrine, above) in the adrenal medulla and sympathetic neurons; these neurotransmitters are then free to stimulate α- and β-adrenoceptors (e.g. amphetamine [Ch 23] and tyramine). Others block the uptake of noradrenaline into sympathetic neurons by NET (e.g. cocaine) or inhibit MAO/COMT (e.g. entacapone [Ch 24]).

Centrally acting adrenoceptor agonists

Clonidine is an α_2 adrenergic agonist used to treat hypertension and severe cancer pain and to treat withdrawal symptoms from opioids. It acts at the prejunctional α_2 receptor to decrease noradrenergic outflow.

KEY POINTS

Adrenergic nervous system drugs; agonists

- Drugs that affect this system are either:

  adrenoceptor agonists (sympathomimetic) drugs (i.e. they mimic the effects of sympathetic nerve stimulation), or

  adrenoceptor antagonists (sympatholytic) drugs (i.e. drugs that compete at receptor sites to inhibit adrenergic sympathetic stimulation).
- These agents may be direct-acting, mixed-acting or indirect-acting drugs and affect α- and/or β-adrenoceptors.
- Adrenaline is an important drug (a direct-acting catecholamine) that stimulates α- and β-adrenoceptors. It is commonly used in the treatment of bronchospasm and croup, emergency treatment of anaphylactic reactions and cardiac arrest, as a haemostatic agent and during ocular surgery.
- Noradrenaline has a high affinity for α-adrenoceptors and is therefore a potent peripheral arteriolar vasoconstrictor. It raises both systolic and diastolic pressure.
- Isoprenaline is a non-selective **β-adrenoceptor agonist** that increases myocardial contraction and heart rate and produces bronchodilation.
- Dopamine, the immediate precursor of noradrenaline, in low doses stimulates dopaminergic receptors, in low to moderate doses β_1-adrenoceptors and, in higher doses, α_1- and α_2-adrenoceptors.
- Dobutamine is used for people with low cardiac output because it directly stimulates the β_1-adrenoceptors of the heart.
- Both dopamine and dobutamine have been used to treat circulatory shock.
- The mixed-acting sympathomimetics include ephedrine and pseudoephedrine.

Adrenoceptor antagonists

α-adrenoceptor antagonists

α-adrenoceptor antagonists compete with catecholamines for binding at α-adrenoceptors and inhibit sympathetic stimulation (Figs 9.5 and 9.6). The main groups of drugs are:

- α_1-adrenoceptor selective antagonists such as alfuzosin, prazosin and silodosin and tamsulosin. These drugs have largely replaced the non-selective antagonists phenoxybenzamine and phentolamine
- non-selective α_1- and α_2-adrenoceptor antagonists such as phenoxybenzamine and phentolamine
- non-selective α_1- and β-adrenoceptor antagonists such as labetalol and carvedilol
- ergot alkaloids, which usually act as partial α-adrenoceptor antagonists. These have many actions, but the α-blocking effect is not used therapeutically. Ergot alkaloids have previously been used to treat migraine (Ch 24).

α_1-adrenoceptor antagonists

The principal use of prazosin (Drug Monograph 9.2) is in the treatment of hypertension and benign prostatic hyperplasia, while alfuzosin and tamsulosin are only indicated for symptomatic relief of urinary obstruction in benign prostatic hypertrophy (Ch 31). Selective blockade of postsynaptic α_1-adrenoceptors results in a decrease in peripheral vascular resistance because of inhibition of catecholamine-induced vasoconstriction. Only a minor increase in heart rate occurs in comparison to the non-selective antagonists because this drug has negligible α_2-adrenoceptor antagonist activity and does not cause an increase in noradrenaline release from nerve terminals.

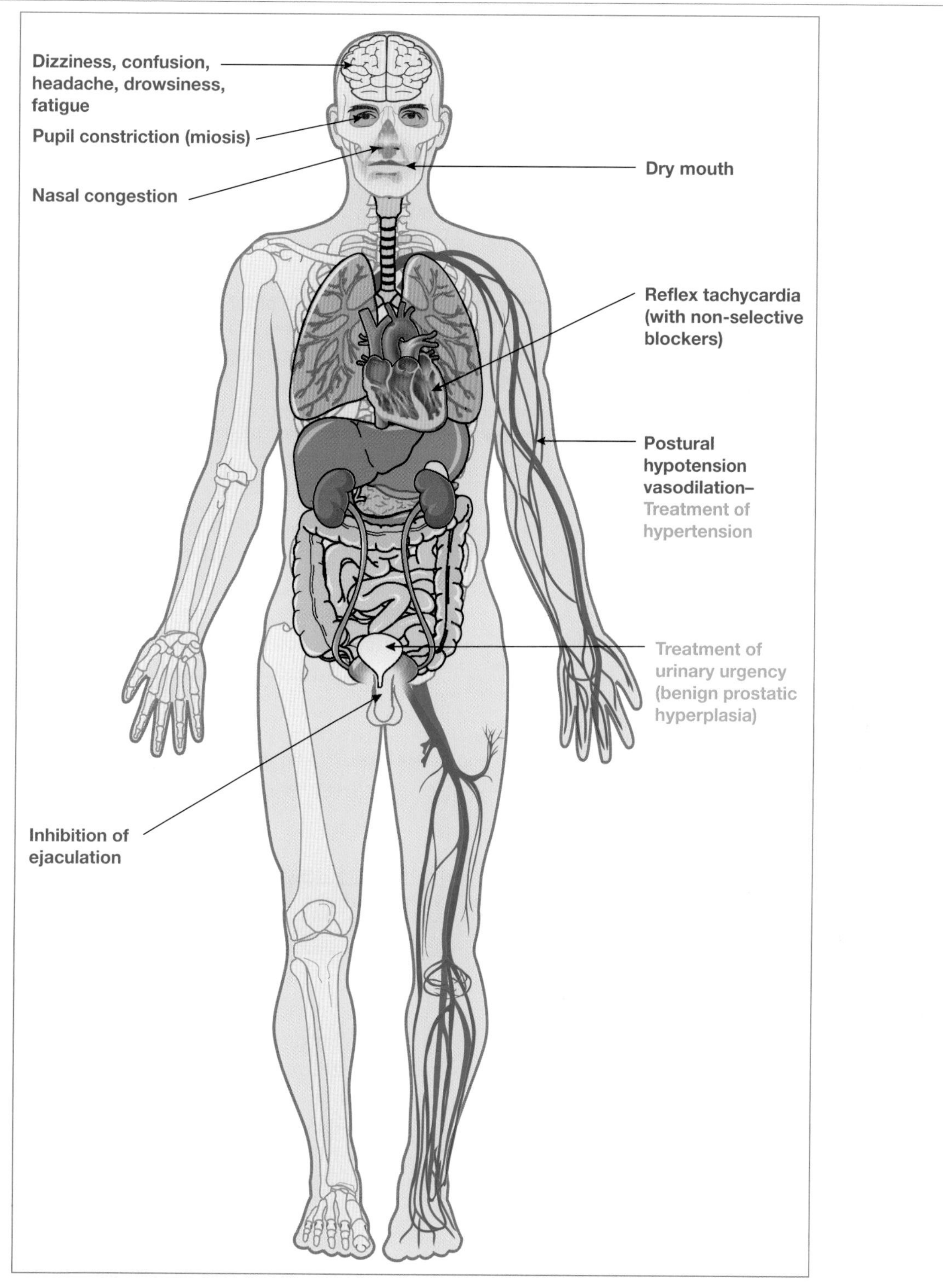

FIGURE 9.6 Pharmacological effects of α-adrenoceptor antagonists

Drug Monograph 9.2
Prazosin

Mechanism of action
Prazosin, developed in the 1970s, was the first of the α_1-adrenoceptor selective antagonists. It has high affinity for the α_{1A}, α_{1B} and α_{1D} subtypes of adrenoceptors and little affinity for α_2 receptors. Blockade of α_1-adrenoceptors in arterioles and veins leads to a decrease in peripheral vascular resistance, reducing venous return to the heart. Unlike other vasodilator drugs, prazosin does not produce a reflex tachycardia.

Pharmacokinetics
Prazosin is well absorbed after oral administration, with bioavailability in the order of 50–80%. Peak concentration occurs about 1–2 hours after an oral dose. Prazosin is highly bound (~95%) in plasma to albumin and α_1-acid glycoprotein. The plasma half-life ranges from 2.5 to 3.5 hours. More than 90% of the drug is metabolised in the liver to O-demethylated metabolites that are excreted in bile.

An increase in plasma half-life (about 7 hours) and bioavailability (2–3-fold) occurs in people with congestive cardiac failure. Some of the metabolites of prazosin also have weak antihypertensive activity, which may contribute to the effect of the drug.

Drug interactions
The first dose of prazosin may cause hypotension. Syncope may occur within 30–90 minutes of the initial dose of drug. The risk of this first-dose phenomenon may be increased by β-blockers, diuretics and calcium channel blockers and those on phosphodiesterase inhibitors.

Adverse reactions
Common adverse reactions include postural hypotension, dizziness, headaches, drowsiness, fatigue, nasal congestion and urinary urgency.

Warnings and contraindications
Care should be exercised in people with preexisting renal disease (which may exacerbate the first-dose effect), liver disease (which may necessitate a dosage reduction) and in the elderly (who are often more likely to suffer orthostatic hypotension). Prazosin is contraindicated in heart failure associated with mechanical obstruction such as aortic stenosis and in those with known sensitivity to prazosin.

Dosage and administration
For the treatment of hypertension, the dosage initially is 0.5 mg twice daily for 3–7 days, increasing to 1 mg 2–3 times daily. The maintenance dose range is 3–20 mg daily in 2–3 divided doses, and the optimal response may take up to 6 weeks to occur.

Non-selective α_1- and α_2-adrenoceptor antagonists

These agents include phenoxybenzamine and phentolamine (not registered for use in Australia or New Zealand)

Phenoxybenzamine is a long-acting, irreversible α_1- and α_2-adrenoceptor antagonist that abolishes or decreases the receptiveness of α-adrenoceptors to adrenergic stimuli. At higher doses, it also antagonises the actions of acetylcholine, histamine and 5-hydroxytryptamine (5-HT, serotonin) because it covalently binds to the various receptors. This covalent interaction with α-adrenoceptors results in a long duration of action and a progressive decrease in peripheral vascular resistance.

Phenoxybenzamine elicits a reflex increase in heart rate that may be exacerbated by blockade of presynaptic α_2-adrenoceptors. The α_2-adrenoceptor is located on vascular prejunctional nerve terminals where its stimulation inhibits the release of noradrenaline in a form of negative feedback. Blockade of this receptor results in the release of noradrenaline, which in turn causes tachycardia (see Fig 9.4, earlier). Phenoxybenzamine is used in the management of phaeochromocytoma and in the preparation of people with this condition for surgery.

The drug has variable oral absorption, and the onset of action is 1–2 hours. Its clinical effect can persist for 3–4 days, and this most probably relates to turnover time of the receptor. The half-life is in the order of 24 hours, with metabolism in the liver and excretion via urine and faeces.

Warnings and contraindications
Avoid concurrent use of phenoxybenzamine with sympathomimetics, such as adrenaline, as unopposed stimulation of β_2-adrenoceptors will exacerbate the hypotension and reflex tachycardia.

The drug is contraindicated when hypotension is undesirable – for example, after cerebrovascular accident and myocardial infarction.

Adverse reactions

Adverse reactions include dizziness (postural hypotension), miosis, tachycardia, nasal congestion, confusion, dry mouth, headache and inhibition of ejaculation. Use with caution in people with heart failure, coronary artery disease, respiratory infections or renal impairment.

Phentolamine competitively blocks α_2- (presynaptic) and α_1- (postsynaptic) adrenoceptors equally. The action occurs at both arterial and venous vessels. This causes direct relaxation of vascular smooth muscle and lowers total peripheral resistance, inducing a marked reflex tachycardia. The drug is used to prevent or control hypertensive episodes in the individual with phaeochromocytoma, especially preoperatively and during surgery. It is not registered for use in Australia or New Zealand.

Pharmacokinetics

It is administered IM and IV. Its half-life is approximately 19 minutes after IV administration, but the haemodynamic response may persist for up to 12 hours. About 13% of the drug is excreted in urine unchanged.

Drug interactions, adverse effects and warnings and contraindications are similar to those of phenoxybenzamine.

Non-selective α_1- and β-adrenoceptor antagonists

See Drug Monograph 9.3 for information on carvedilol.

Labetalol acts on both α_1- and β-adrenoceptors and competitively antagonises the action of catecholamines. It is a complex drug that selectively blocks α_1-, β_1- and β_2-adrenoceptors but also partially stimulates β_2-adrenoceptors and inhibits the neuronal uptake of noradrenaline (similar to the action of cocaine). Blockade of α_1-adrenoceptors leads to a fall in peripheral vascular resistance, while blockade of β_1-adrenoceptors prevents the reflex sympathetic stimulation of the heart. The drug is indicated for treating hypertension.

Pharmacokinetics

Rapid absorption occurs after oral administration, and peak plasma concentration occurs within 20–90 minutes. Bioavailability is highly variable (11–86%), due primarily to extensive presystemic metabolism. Labetalol is extensively metabolised to glucuronide conjugates that are excreted in urine (55–60%) and faeces (12–27%).

Drug interactions, adverse effects, warnings, contraindications, dosage and administration are discussed in the following section in the context of the predominant β-blocking activity of labetalol.

Drug Monograph 9.3
Carvedilol

Multiple clinical trials (including COMET, COPERNICUS and CAPRICORN) have shown that carvedilol reduces mortality and morbidity in people with mild-to-severe congestive heart failure. Additionally, in combination with standard drug therapy, carvedilol reduces mortality in the setting of myocardial infarction.

Mechanism of action

Carvedilol is a unique cardiovascular drug with a wide range of therapeutic benefits. Its predominant haemodynamic effects are derived from blockade of β_1-, β_2- and α_1-adrenoceptors. A racemic drug, both the R (+) and S (−) enantiomers possess similar α_1-blocking activity, but only S (−) carvedilol exhibits non-selective β-blocking activity while the drug has little or no affinity for α_2-adrenoceptors nor intrinsic sympathomimetic activity.

Carvedilol is a potent antihypertensive and the reduction in blood pressure primarily due to blockade of β_1-, β_2- and α_1-adrenoceptors is not associated with a reflex tachycardia. Total peripheral resistance decreases due to blockade of α_1-adrenoceptors; this vasodilatory effect reduces afterload and offsets the negative inotropic effect of cardiac β-blockade. Consequently, cardiac output and stroke volume are maintained.

Carvedilol and some of its metabolites possess antioxidant properties protecting the vascular system from reactive oxygen species. In addition, this drug has antiproliferative and antiatherogenic actions, as well as anti-ischaemic, antihypertrophic and antidysrhythmic actions. A further additional benefit arises from improved insulin sensitivity.

Pharmacokinetics

- Carvedilol is rapidly and completely absorbed after oral administration and undergoes extensive first-pass metabolism, which accounts for its bioavailability of 20–25%. Peak plasma concentration occurs within 1–2 hours.
- More than 95% of the drug is bound to plasma proteins (predominantly albumin) and the volume of distribution is 100–140 L.
- Carvedilol is metabolised in the liver by the enzymes CYP2D6 (R (+) enantiomer) and the S(-) enantiomer by CYP2C9 with a half-life of 4–7 hours.

- The predominant route of excretion is biliary with less than 2% of the dose excreted as unchanged drug in urine. No dosage adjustment is necessary in people with renal disease; however, in those with hepatic disease, bioavailability is increased.

Drug interactions and adverse reactions

See the text for general information on drug interactions and adverse reactions with β-blockers. Inhibitors or inducers of CYP2D6 and CYP2C9 enzymes may affect plasma concentrations of carvedilol. A combination of carvedilol and rifampicin (rifampin) may result in decreased plasma concentration of carvedilol due to induction of metabolism (CYP2C9) by rifampicin. An increase in the dose of carvedilol may be necessary; alternatively, consider use of a renally cleared β-blocker.

Warnings and contraindications

β-blockers are in general contraindicated in shock and people living with asthma, diabetes, hyperthyroidism, phaeochromocytoma, myasthenia gravis or bradycardia (45–50 beats/minute).

Dosage and administration

For the treatment of hypertension, the usual adult dose is 12.5 mg daily for 2 days and then 25 mg once daily increased at intervals greater than 2 weeks up to a maximum once-daily dose of 50 mg or in two divided doses. For people living with heart failure, the dose must be individualised and closely monitored. The commencing dose is half the usual daily adult dose, increasing at intervals greater than 2 weeks to a maximum of 25 mg twice daily. Refer to expert texts for specific information.

β-adrenoceptor antagonists

β-adrenoceptor antagonists, commonly referred to as β-blockers, competitively block the actions of catecholamines (Table 9.3, Figs 9.5 and 9.7). The main group is the β_1-selective blockers that are frequently referred to as cardioselective blockers because these agents block β_1-adrenoceptors on the heart. At high doses, however, β_1-adrenoceptor selectivity diminishes, and the adverse effects of β_2-adrenoceptor blockade then need to be considered. Drugs that block both types of adrenoceptors, β_1- and β_2-, are referred to as non-selective β-adrenoceptor antagonists. The use of all of these drugs is contraindicated in people with asthma because of inhibition of bronchodilation mediated by β_2-adrenoceptors. The exception is the newer drug nebivolol, which is the most highly selective drug of the β_1-adrenoceptor antagonists with a more than 300-fold higher affinity for β_1-adrenoceptors than β_2-adrenoceptors. In addition, nebivolol is unique in that it causes vasodilation mediated through the release of nitric oxide in endothelial cells.

TABLE 9.3 Classification of β-adrenoceptor antagonists

TYPE	DRUGS
Selective β_1-adrenoceptor antagonists	Atenolol, betaxolol,[a] bisoprolol, metoprolol, nebivolol[b]
Non-selective β_1- and β_2-adrenoceptor antagonists	Carvedilol,[c] labetalol, propranolol, sotalol, timolol[a]
Non-selective β_1- and β_2-adrenoceptor antagonist with ISA activity	Pindolol[d]

[a] Available as eyedrops only.
[b] Highly selective antagonist at β_1-adrenoceptors, and also causes vasodilation through release of nitric oxide.
[c] Also an α_1 antagonist.
[d] Not marketed in Australia or New Zealand.

A further differentiation of β-blockers relates to **intrinsic sympathomimetic activity** (ISA). ISA was initially believed to be advantageous when compared with agents that exhibit β-blocking effects only. It was suggested that fewer serious adverse effects would occur with such agents but, clinically, the significance of this property has not been proven. ISA causes partial stimulation of the β-adrenoceptor, although this effect is less than that of a pure agonist. For example, if a person has a slow heart rate at rest, the partial agonists may help to increase the heart rate; however, if the person has a rapid heart rate or tachycardia from exercise, these agents may help to slow the heart rate, primarily due to the predominant β-blocking effect.

Table 9.3 notes the classification of adrenergic blocking drugs by receptor activity. The prototype of the β-adrenoceptor antagonists is propranolol, the drug against which all others are compared.

Mechanism of action

β-adrenoceptor antagonists competitively block β-adrenoceptor sites located on the heart, smooth muscle of the bronchi and blood vessels, kidney, pancreas, uterus, brain and liver. Cardiac muscle contains principally β_1-adrenoceptors, while smooth muscle sites contain primarily β_2-adrenoceptors (Table 8.1 [Ch 8] and Table 9.3).

Cardiovascular effects

Pharmacologically, blockade of β_1-adrenoceptors on the heart decreases rate, conduction velocity, myocardial contractility and cardiac output.

The antianginal effects produced by β-blockers are primarily a result of the reduction in myocardial oxygen requirements because of the diminished heart rate and myocardial contractility (see Fig 9.7).

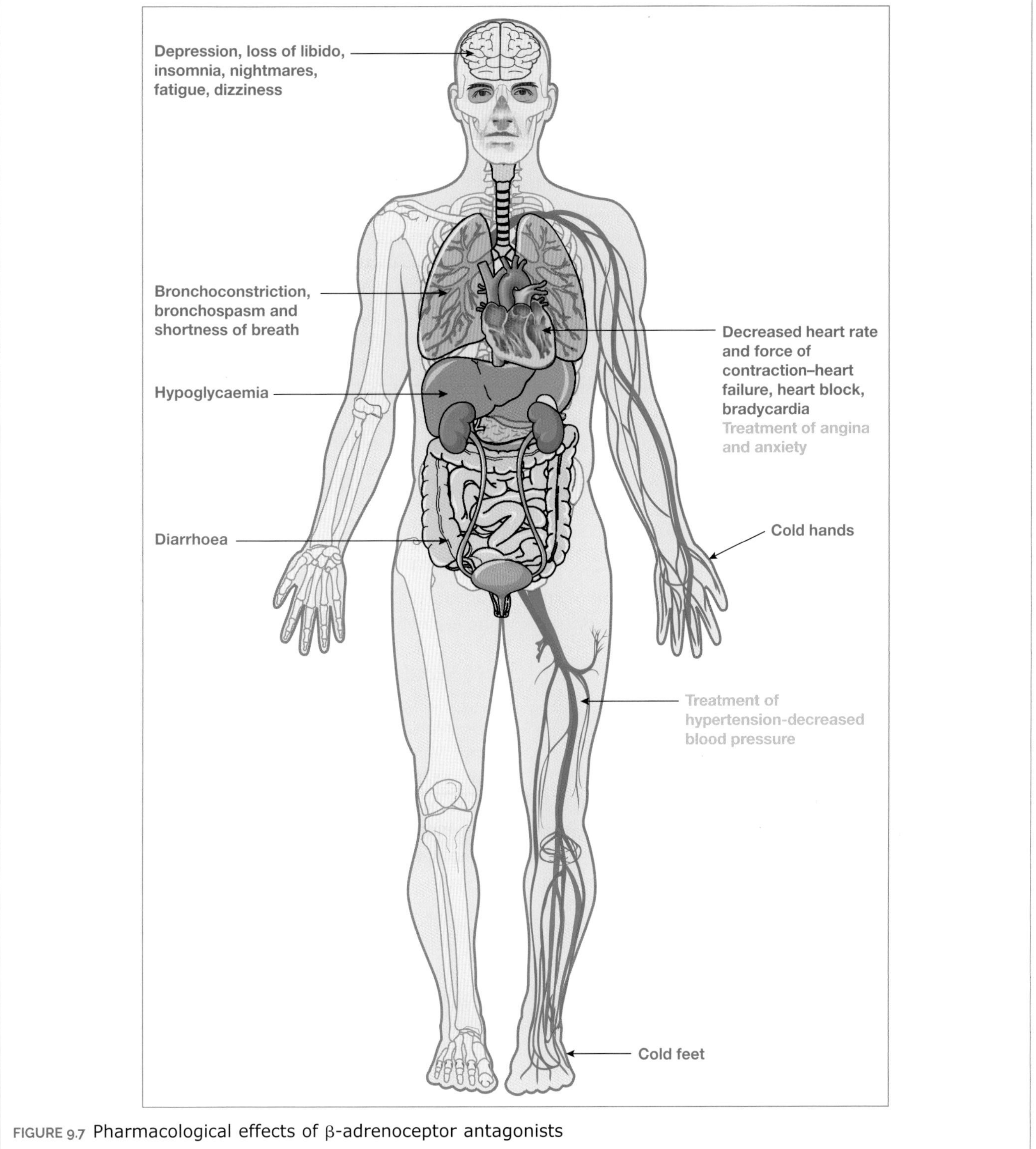

FIGURE 9.7 Pharmacological effects of β-adrenoceptor antagonists

Their antihypertensive actions result from decreased cardiac output (without a reflex increase in peripheral vascular resistance), diminished sympathetic outflow from the vasomotor centre in the brain to the peripheral blood vessels and reduced renin release by the kidney.

Antidysrhythmic activity is associated with depression of sinus node function, slowing of conduction in the atria and the atrioventricular node and an increased refractory period of the AV node.

Central nervous system effects

Adverse effects of β-blockers include fatigue, insomnia, nightmares and depression. Although many studies have investigated an association between lipophilicity and CNS effects, no clear correlation has been established. Studies have also identified that β-blockers decrease melatonin release via inhibition of central β_1-adrenoceptors. Lower nocturnal melatonin concentration may contribute to the sleep disturbances.

Metabolic effects

Catecholamines are involved in the regulation of lipid and carbohydrate metabolism and, in response to hypoglycaemia, promote glycogen breakdown and mobilisation of glucose. Hence, blockade of β-adrenoceptors prevents an adequate response to hypoglycaemia in people with insulin-dependent diabetes and may also mask the symptoms.

Non-selective β-blockers raise plasma triglyceride concentration and lower high-density lipoprotein concentration, raising concerns that this may be undesirable in people with hypertension.

Indications

β-blocking drugs are used to treat angina pectoris, hypertension, Fallot's tetralogy, tremors and tachycardia associated with anxiety and hyperthyroidism; to prevent or treat cardiac dysrhythmias, myocardial infarction (acute and in the long term), vascular headaches, phaeochromocytoma and glaucoma (topical eyedrops); and as an adjunct to conventional therapy for heart failure. (The only approved drugs in this setting are bisoprolol, carvedilol, metoprolol and nebivolol.)

Pharmacokinetics

For the pharmacokinetics and usual adult dose range of β-blockers, see Table 9.4. These drugs are either metabolised in the liver or excreted as unchanged drug by the kidneys. This allows the use of different agents in preexisting conditions of hepatic or renal impairment; for example, a drug such as metoprolol is metabolised by the liver, which is more suitable for use in those with renal impairment, whereas atenolol is more suitable in a person with hepatic disease because it is predominantly cleared by the kidneys.

Drug interactions and adverse reactions

See Drug Interactions 9.1 for the drug interactions of β-blockers. Common adverse effects of β-blockers include insomnia, nightmares, depression, nausea, diarrhoea, dizziness, fatigue, hypotension, heart failure, heart block, bradycardia, cold hands and feet, bronchospasm and shortness of breath. Use β-blockers with caution in people living with liver or renal function impairment, heart failure, diabetes, hyperlipidaemia, peripheral vascular disease, hyperthyroidism, myasthenia gravis or phaeochromocytoma. β-blockers are contraindicated in people with drug hypersensitivity, cardiogenic shock, heart block, bradycardia, severe hypotension and asthma and chronic obstructive airways disease.

Withdrawal of a β-blocking drug

Abrupt cessation of β-blockers can cause a rebound phenomenon that exacerbates hypertension, angina or ventricular dysrhythmias, and may precipitate a myocardial infarction. It is recommended that the dose of a β-blocking drug be halved every 2–3 days, reducing the dose over 8–14 days. The person should be advised to avoid vigorous physical exercise or activity during this time to decrease the risk of a myocardial infarction or cardiac dysrhythmia. If withdrawal signs occur (angina or chest pain, sweating, rebound hypertension, dysrhythmias, tremors, tachycardia or respiratory distress), these may be controlled by temporary reinstitution of the drug.

TABLE 9.4 Pharmacokinetics and adult dose range of β-adrenoceptor antagonists[a]

DRUG	ORAL BIOAVAILABILITY (%)	HALF-LIFE (H)	ELIMINATION	ADULT DOSE RANGE
Atenolol	~50	7–9	Renal (85–100%)	25–100 mg/day
Betaxolol	Ophthalmic preparation	14–22	Hepatic/renal (> 80%)	Eyedrops (5 mg/mL)
Bisoprolol	~88	10–12	Hepatic (50%) / renal (50%)	1.25–10 mg/day
Carvedilol	~30	6–10	Hepatic (> 75%)	6.25–50 mg/day
Labetalol	~33	6–8	Hepatic (95%)	200–800 mg/day
Metoprolol	~50	3–5	Hepatic (90%)	50–300 mg/day
Nebivolol	13% (EM)[b] and ~100% (PM)[b]	10 (EM)[b] and 35 (PM)[b]	Hepatic (99%)	1.25–10 mg/day
Propranolol	~25	3–6	Hepatic (> 99%)	40–320 mg/day
Sotalol	~100	7–18	Renal (90%)	80–320 mg/day
Timolol	Ophthalmic preparation	5–6	Hepatic (85%)	Eyedrops

[a] Consult approved product information for individual drugs and doses for specific indications – for example, heart failure.
[b] CYP2D6 extensive metaboliser (EM) and poor metaboliser (PM) phenotypes

DRUG INTERACTIONS 9.1
β-adrenoceptor antagonists

DRUG	POSSIBLE EFFECTS AND MANAGEMENT
Adrenaline	Severe hypertension and bradycardia may occur with the use of non-selective beta antagonists. Use with extreme caution and monitor closely.
Antidiabetic agents, oral hypoglycaemic agents, insulin	May mask symptoms of hypoglycaemia such as increased heart rate and lowered blood pressure, and may prolong hypoglycaemic episodes, making monitoring difficult. Monitoring of blood glucose levels and dosage adjustments of the hypoglycaemic agent may be necessary.
Digoxin	May have an additive effect, increasing atrioventricular conduction time. Monitor heart rate and use with caution.
Calcium channel blockers (diltiazem and verapamil)	Enhanced cardiac-depressant effects, further decreasing rate, contractility and conduction.
Clonidine	Combination may produce severe adverse reactions. Each drug is associated with withdrawal symptoms such as rebound hypertension. Avoid combination.
MAO inhibitors	Combination may result in hypotension and bradycardia. Use with caution and monitor closely.
Nonsteroidal anti-inflammatory drugs	Antihypertensive effect of β-blockers may be reduced. Monitor blood pressure and avoid concurrent use.

KEY POINTS

Adrenoceptor antagonists

- The adrenoceptor antagonists (sympatholytics) are classified by their receptor activity – that is, α- and/or β-adrenoceptor antagonist effects.
- The main groups of α-adrenoceptor antagonists are the α_1-selective antagonists such as alfuzosin, prazosin and tamsulosin; the non-selective α_1- and α_2-adrenoceptor antagonists such as phenoxybenzamine; and the mixed α_1- and β-adrenoceptor antagonists, which include carvedilol and labetalol.
- The classification of β-blocking drugs includes the selective β_1 (cardioselective) agents such as atenolol, bisoprolol, metoprolol and nebivolol; the non-selective β-blocking agents such as propranolol; and the non-selective β-blocking agents with ISA activity such as pindolol.
- Abrupt cessation of β-blockers can cause a rebound phenomenon. When stopping treatment reduce dose gradually.

DRUGS AT A GLANCE
Drugs affecting noradrenergic neurotransmission

PHARMACOLOGICAL GROUP AND EFFECT	KEY EXAMPLES	CLINICAL USE
Sympathomimetics Adrenergic receptor (adrenoceptor) agonists α_1-receptor agonists • Stimulate α_1 receptors on smooth muscle of vasculature to induce vasoconstriction	Adrenaline (epinephrine) noradrenaline (norepinephrine)	Anaphylaxis
α_2-receptor agonists	Dopamine	Low doses enhance renal blood flow; high doses enhance peripheral resistance
• CNS: Stimulate prejunctional α_2 receptors on adrenergic to reduce adrenergic outflow	Clonidine	Hypertension, severe cancer pain, drug withdrawal
β_1-receptor agonists • Stimulate β receptors on cardiac muscle and AV and SA nodes to induce positive inotropic and chronotropic effects	Adrenaline	Cardiogenic shock Anaphylactic shock
	Dobutamine	Inotropic support in congestive heart failure, cardiogenic shock
	Isoprenaline	Bradycardia, heart block
β_2-receptor agonists • Stimulate β receptors on smooth muscle of the bronchi to induce relaxation and bronchodilation	Short-acting • Salbutamol • Terbutaline	Asthma Premature labour (salbutamol)

α-receptor antagonists Selective α_1-receptor antagonists • Blockade of α_1 receptors on smooth muscle of blood vessels leading to vasodilation Non-selective α-receptor antagonists (As above)	Prazosin Phenoxybenzamine	Hypertension Symptomatic relief in benign prostatic hyperplasia Phaeochromocytoma Symptomatic relief in benign prostatic hyperplasia
β-receptor antagonists Non-selective β_1-receptor antagonists (As above) Selective β_1-receptor antagonists Blockade of β_1 receptors on cardiac muscle and AV and SA nodes to induce negative inotropic and chronotropic effects	Propranolol Atenolol, bisoprolol, metoprolol, nebivolol	Hypertension Angina Tachyarrhythmias Acute coronary syndromes Cardiac failure

REVIEW EXERCISES

1 Ms FG, a 14-year-old, presents to the emergency department after an allergic reaction after eating peanuts at a party. She first experienced breathing difficulties and swelling of her lips and hands. As she is being triaged, she collapses. She is administered adrenaline 1:1000 IM injection into her thigh. Explain the effect of adrenaline on the cardiovascular and respiratory systems. Explain why this drug is useful in treating anaphylactic shock.

2 Ms MC has recently been diagnosed with moderate heart failure. She has been prescribed an ACE inhibitor to reduce fluid load and now her cardiologist has prescribed the beta-blocker nebivolol. She has now titrated her dose from 1.25 mg to a 5 mg dose. She returns to the clinic in 2 weeks complaining of tiredness, insomnia and vivid dreams. What is your explanation as to why these symptoms have occurred? Should she stop taking nebivolol immediately?

REFERENCES

Brunton LL, Chabner BA, Knollmann BC, editors: Goodman & Gilman's the pharmacological basis of therapeutics, ed 13, New York, 2017, McGraw-Hill.

Salerno E: Pharmacology for health professionals, St Louis, 1999, Mosby.

Schena G, Caplan MJ. Everything You Always Wanted to Know about β3-AR * (* But Were Afraid to Ask). Cells. 2019 Apr 16;8(4):357. doi: 10.3390/cells8040357. PMID: 30995798; PMCID: PMC6523418.

Therapeutic Goods Administration 2021. Changes to adrenaline and noradrenaline labels [online] Available at: <https://www.tga.gov.au/changes-adrenaline-and-noradrenaline-labels [Accessed 9 Oct 2021].

ONLINE RESOURCES

Australasian Society of Clinical Immunology and Allergy: https://www.allergy.org.au/ (accessed 24 February 2022)

Australian Resuscitation Council: https://www.resus.org.au/ (accessed 24 February 2022)

More weblinks at: http://evolve.elsevier.com/AU/Knights/pharmacology/.

CHAPTER 10

DRUGS AFFECTING CARDIAC FUNCTION

Kathleen Knights

KEY ABBREVIATIONS

ANP	atrial natriuretic peptide
ATP	adenosine triphosphate
AV	atrioventricular
BNP	B-type natriuretic peptide
CNP	C-type natriuretic peptide
CO	cardiac output
HR	heart rate
mV	millivolts
NA	noradrenaline
SA	sinoatrial
SV	stroke volume

KEY TERMS

Chapter Focus

Knowledge of the anatomy and physiology of the heart and vascular system is essential for understanding the action and use of drugs in the treatment of hypertension, cardiac failure, angina and thromboembolic disorders. Numerous drugs affect the heart both directly and indirectly and include the autonomic transmitter adrenaline (epinephrine) and related drugs, antidysrhythmic drugs, the cardiac glycoside digoxin and the calcium channel blockers (Ch 11). The drugs used to treat dysrhythmias are very potent, with the potential to cause sudden cardiac death. Careful drug selection, along with close monitoring of a person's clinical condition, is crucial to achieving the goal of safe and effective antidysrhythmic therapy.

KEY DRUG GROUPS

Antidysrhythmic drugs:

- **adenosine** (DM 10.4), **amiodarone** (DM 10.3), digoxin (a cardiac glycoside), **disopyramide** (DM 10.1), esmolol, **flecainide** (DM 10.2), lidocaine (lignocaine) (see Ch 11), **sotalol**

Drugs for heart failure:

- **milrinone**, **sacubitril/**valsartan

Antianginal drug:

- **ivabradine**

CRITICAL THINKING SCENARIO

Mavis, a 72-year-old woman, has presented to the emergency department with gastrointestinal disturbances (nausea, vomiting and diarrhoea) and is complaining that her 'eyes have gone funny'. You ascertain that she is currently prescribed digoxin for atrial fibrillation 62.5 micrograms once daily. What explanations can you think of that may explain her symptoms? A digoxin plasma drug concentration is measured and you are advised that the result is 2.9 microgram/L. Discuss what further laboratory tests would be undertaken to help explain why her plasma digoxin concentration is high.

Introduction: The heart

The heart, which lies in the mediastinum slightly to the left of the midline of the thoracic cavity, consists of four chambers – the upper right and left atria and the lower right and left ventricles (Fig 10.1A). The heart wall consists of the external smooth epicardium, the middle layer of myocardium (or muscle tissue) and the inner endocardium, which lines the chambers of the heart and the valves. The pumping action of the heart depends on the ability of the cardiac muscle to contract. Contractility of the heart is energy-dependent, and the heart derives most of its energy from oxidative metabolism of fatty acids and lactate, which occurs in mitochondria and cardiac muscle cells.

The myocardium is composed of interconnected branching muscle fibres, or cells, that form the walls of the atria and the ventricles. The thickness of the myocardium of the atria and ventricles varies. The atrial walls tend to be thinner because the atria act more as delivery containers, whereas the ventricular walls tend to be thicker because the ventricles forcibly contract and pump blood against a resistance. The resistance of the pulmonary bed is low, so the wall of the right ventricle is not as thick as that of the left ventricle, which has to pump blood to all parts of the body against total systemic vascular resistance.

Coronary vascular supply of the heart

Blood supply to the myocardium is provided by the right and left coronary arteries, which arise from the base of the aorta (Fig 10.1B). The right atrium and ventricle are supplied with blood from the right coronary artery. The left coronary artery divides into the anterior (descending) branch and the circumflex branch and supplies blood to the left atrium and ventricle. These main coronary vessels continue to divide, forming numerous branches, resulting in a profuse network of coronary vessels. The major arterial vessels supplying the heart are located on the external surface of the ventricles. Branches penetrate the myocardium towards the endocardial (inner) surface. Venous coronary blood drains via the coronary sinus into the right atrium. Coronary perfusion occurs as a result of the high pressure of blood in the aorta and occurs primarily when the ventricles have relaxed and the coronary vessels are no longer compressed. Ventricular contraction compresses the coronary vascular bed but increases coronary outflow. Increased oxygen delivery to the myocardium is supported almost exclusively by the increased coronary blood flow.

When the demand for oxygen and nutrients by body tissues increases, cardiac output (CO) must increase. At the same time, the heart muscle itself must be supplied with enough oxygen and nutrients to replace the energy it expends. In other words, a balance must be maintained between energy expenditure and energy restoration. The increase in heart rate (HR) increases the metabolic needs of the heart and, normally, coronary dilation occurs in an attempt to meet the higher metabolic demand and to overcome restricted blood inflow. Whenever the delivery of oxygen to the myocardium is inadequate to meet the increased oxygen consumption by the heart, myocardial ischaemia occurs. Atheroma formation is one of the main causes of ischaemia, which manifests in the signs and symptoms of angina (Ch 11), while rupture of a plaque may cause a myocardial infarction.

Control by the autonomic nervous system

The cardiac conduction system possesses the inherent ability for spontaneous rhythmic initiation of the cardiac impulse, but the autonomic nervous system has an important role in regulating the rate, rhythm and force of myocardial contraction of the heart. Postganglionic fibres of the sympathetic nervous system, which release noradrenaline (NA), innervate the sinoatrial (SA) node, atria and ventricles. Action of NA on β_1 receptors located in both nodes and atrial/ventricular muscles increases HR, automaticity, conduction velocity and force of contraction. Circulating adrenaline from the adrenal medulla also elicits cardiac responses – for example, tachycardia. Clinically, high doses of administered adrenaline (epinephrine) may exert a direct effect on the electrophysiological properties of cardiac tissue, causing cardiac dysrhythmias.

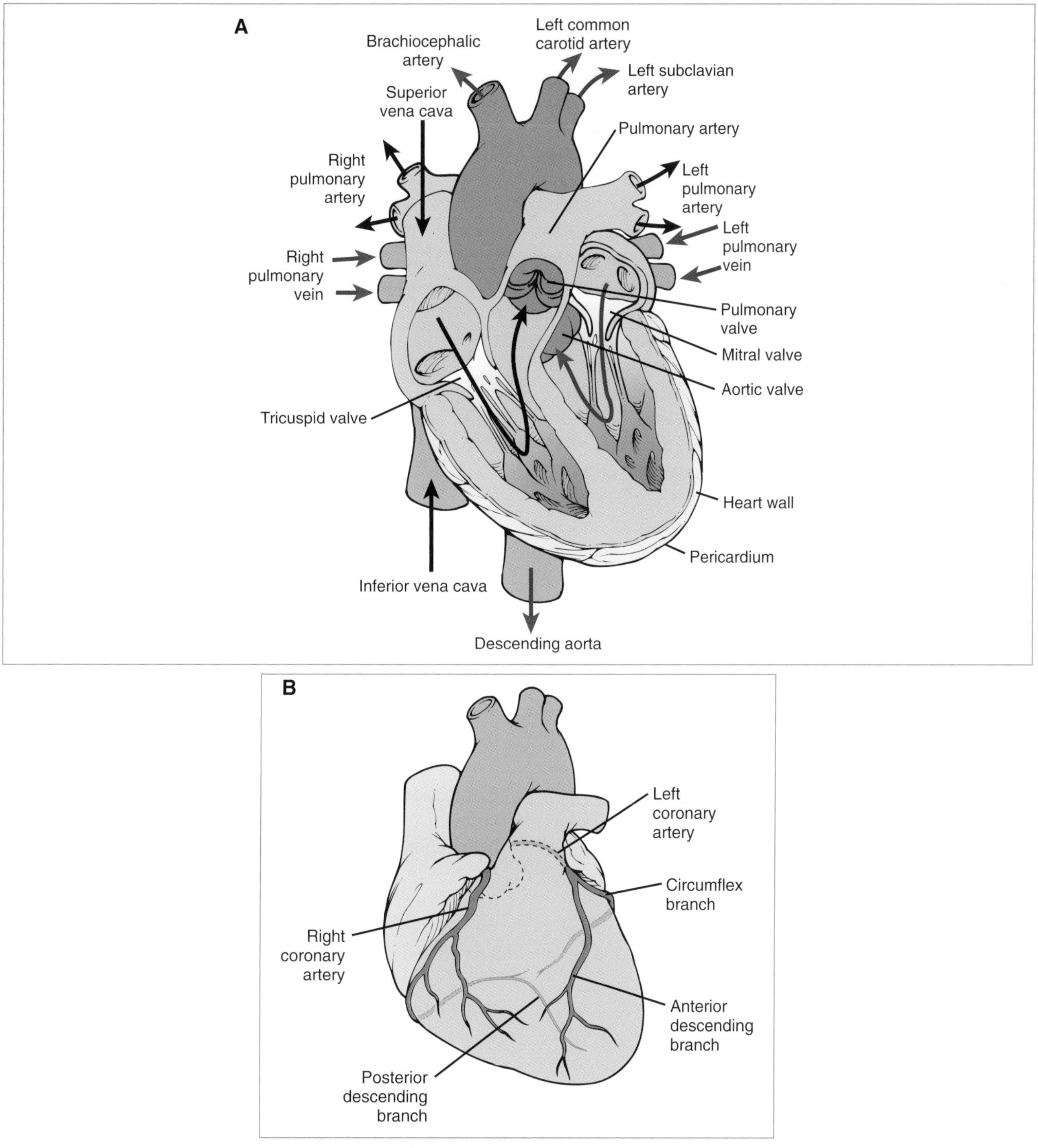

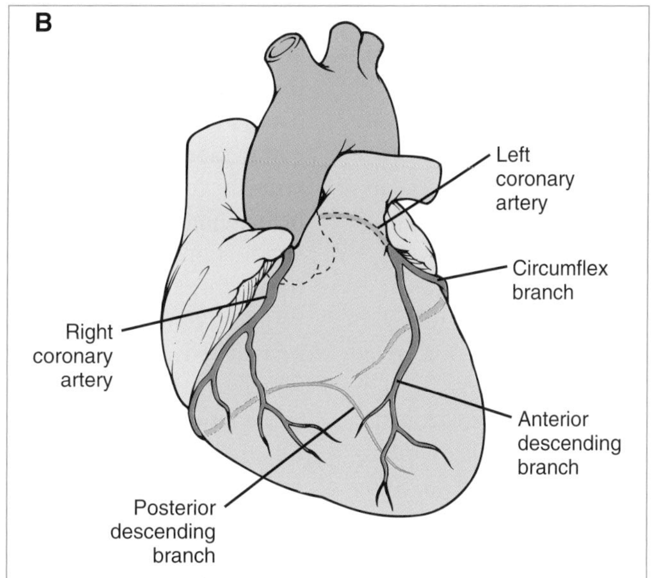

FIGURE 10.1 A schematic diagram of the heart, blood flow and valves

A Schematic diagram of the heart, valves, major blood vessels and blood flow. Black arrows indicate the direction of flow of deoxygenated blood, and blue arrows the flow of oxygenated blood. **B** Coronary blood supply to the heart. Dark-shaded vessels are those located on the external surface of the ventricles; light-shaded vessels show penetration of arterial branches towards the endocardial surface.

Vagal nerve fibres of the parasympathetic branch, which release acetylcholine, are found primarily in the SA and atrioventricular (AV) nodes and atrial muscle. Acetylcholine acts on muscarinic (M_2) receptors of the SA node to decrease HR, on the AV node to decrease conduction velocity and, to a limited extent, on the M_2 receptors on cardiac myocytes to reduce cardiac contractility. Control by the vagus nerve ensures the HR is slowed to approximately 75 beats/minute. In the absence of input from the parasympathetic nervous system the heart would contract at about 90–100 beats/minute, which is the normal automatic firing rate of the SA node. Normally, the HR is under the continuous influence of

both parasympathetic and sympathetic nervous systems; the resting HR is the result of their opposing influences and at rest the firing rate of the sympathetic cardiac nerves is less than that of the vagus nerve.

Cardiac natriuretic peptides

The natriuretic peptides include atrial natriuretic peptide (ANP), brain or B-type natriuretic peptide (BNP) and C-type natriuretic peptide (CNP). CNP has antithrombotic and antifibrotic properties. The beneficial effects of ANP and BNP arise from their actions as direct vasodilators, promoting natriuresis and diuresis by increasing the glomerular filtration rate and reducing renin release from renal juxtaglomerular cells, which reduces plasma angiotensin II concentration and, consequently, aldosterone secretion. These actions result in a decrease in arterial pressure, systemic vascular resistance, ventricular preload and total body sodium and fluid load. ANP is located in secretory granules of atrial myocytes and is released by stretching of the atria. In contrast, BNP and CNP are located in the ventricles and vascular smooth muscle, respectively. Stretching of the ventricles results in the release of BNP, and the circulating concentration of BNP correlates with the severity of heart failure (Bozkurt et al. 2021). In this situation, the rise in BNP is ineffective in combating fluid overload.

ANP and BNP are metabolised by the membrane-bound endopeptidase neprilysin, which is found principally in the kidney. In addition, neprilysin contributes to the metabolism of the potent vasoconstrictor angiotensin II. Not surprisingly, inhibitors of neprilysin have been developed with the aim of providing effective drugs for the management of heart failure (see later section on sacubitril with valsartan).

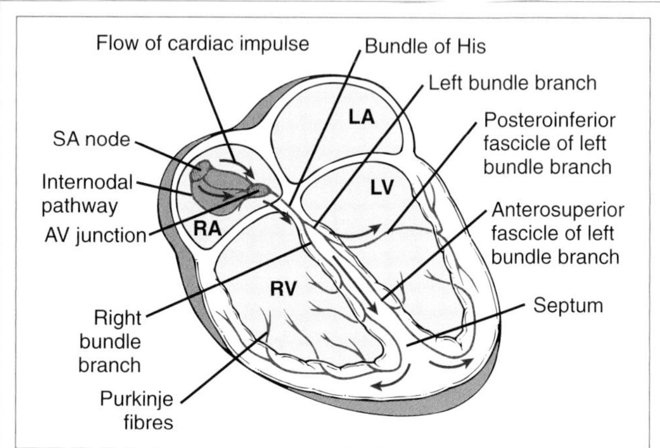

FIGURE 10.2 Cardiac conduction system
Cardiac impulses are initiated at the SA node and transmitted through the internodal pathways to the two atria, resulting in atrial contraction. At the AV node, the electrical impulse is delayed. Conduction then speeds up at the bundle of His, with the impulse travelling through the right bundle branch and the left bundle branch and continuing through the posteroinferior fascicle and anterosuperior fascicle of the latter bundle branch. Finally, the arrival of impulses at the Purkinje fibres results in their distribution to all parts of both ventricles where, on excitation, ventricular contraction is produced. RA = right atrium; RV = right ventricle; LA = left atrium; LV = left ventricle; SA = sinoatrial
Source: Adapted from Salerno 1999, Figure 18.3; used with permission.

The cardiac conduction system

Contraction of the heart depends on the regularity of events occurring in the cardiac cycle. Each cycle consists of a period of relaxation, **diastole**, followed by a period of contraction, **systole**. The rhythm and rate of the cardiac cycle are regulated by the conduction system, specialised cardiac cells that have the ability to initiate and transmit the electrical impulses needed to stimulate contraction of the cardiac muscle.

The conduction system (Fig 10.2) comprises:

- the SA node
- internodal pathways
- the AV node
- the bundle of His
- right and left bundle branches
- Purkinje fibres.

Normally, the SA node, located in the right atrium, is the primary site of electrical activity in the human heart and initiates the heartbeat. The impulses generated are conducted through the interatrial and internodal pathways to both atria, producing atrial contraction. Having travelled through the atria the impulses arrive at the AV node, which links the conducting pathways of the atria to the ventricles. Electrical conduction is delayed at the AV node, allowing time for the atria to contract fully and the ventricles to finish filling before ventricular contraction. At the bundle of His, conduction speeds up and the impulses travel through the right and left bundle branches, then through the posteroinferior and anterosuperior fascicles of the left bundle branch. The transmission of impulses at the Purkinje fibres, which consist of tiny fibrils that spread around the ventricles and connect directly with the myocardial cells, is very rapid. Finally, the synchronised depolarisation of both ventricles produces ventricular contraction, resulting in the ejection of blood through both the pulmonary artery and the aorta by the ventricles. The coordinated pumping action of the heart is initiated and regulated by the specialised fibres of the conduction system that possess three basic electrophysiological properties: automaticity, conductivity and refractoriness.

Automaticity

The cells that possess this property of **automaticity** (ability to spontaneously initiate an electrical impulse) are called pacemaker cells. They are found in the SA and AV nodes and the His–Purkinje system.

Normally, impulses are spontaneously and regularly initiated at the SA node. During the resting phase the membrane of the cell depolarises spontaneously and gradually, until it reaches the threshold and generates an action potential (see later section, 'Electrical Excitation'). The slow depolarisation of the membrane in the resting state is called spontaneous diastolic depolarisation, or phase 4 depolarisation, and defines automaticity. In the SA and AV nodes, this property is attributed to changes in potassium and calcium currents and the pacemaker current. The resting potential of automatic pacemaker cells differs from that of contractile myocardial cells. After full repolarisation, the membrane of myocardial cells maintains a steady resting potential until an external stimulus causes it to depolarise. Automaticity is thus a property of fibres of the conduction system that normally controls heart rhythm – it is not a feature of 'working' muscle (atria and ventricles). However, in some circumstances (e.g. cardiac disease, use of certain drugs), myocardial cells have the potential to exhibit spontaneous depolarisation. This is often referred to as an 'early after-depolarisation', which occurs because of a shift closer to the threshold for an action potential resulting from an abnormal interaction of the calcium current and the repolarising potassium current. If an early after-depolarisation is sufficiently large, it may trigger an extrasystole, often referred to as a premature ventricular contraction. If a run of extrasystoles occurs, this may result in ventricular tachycardia (120–150 beats/minute), which has the potential to degenerate into ventricular fibrillation.

The spontaneous excitation of pacemaker cells establishes the normal rhythm of the heart. The regularity of such pacemaking activity is termed rhythmicity. Under normal circumstances, only one functional pacemaker, the SA node, predominates because it has the highest frequency of depolarisation. The normal rate of impulse formation is about 72 beats/minute. If the SA node substantially slows its rate of impulse formation, then the AV node becomes the primary pacemaker of the heart and will drive the heart at approximately 40 beats/minute.

Conductivity

'Conductivity' refers to the ability of a cell to transmit an action potential along its plasma membrane. The property of conductivity therefore exists not only in the cells of the conduction system but also in the cardiac musculature. The speed with which electrical activity is spread within the SA node is quite slow – about 0.05 m/s. The impulse then spreads out rapidly over the atrial musculature at a rate of about 1 m/s. When the impulse reaches the AV node, there is a delay of about 0.01 second, then atrial systole occurs, allowing the atria to contract fully and the ventricles to fill. The impulse then spreads rapidly at about 2–4 m/s, along the right and left bundle branches and Purkinje fibres. This rapid activation of contractile elements evokes a synchronous contraction of the ventricles. The conduction velocity is determined by the threshold size of the resting potential of the cell membrane and by membrane responsiveness.

Refractoriness

Cardiac tissue is non-responsive to stimulation during the initial phase of systole (contraction). This is known as **refractoriness**, and it determines how closely together two action potentials can occur. Throughout most of the repolarisation phase, the cell cannot respond to a stimulus. The effective refractory period represents that period in the cardiac cycle during which a stimulus, no matter how strong, fails to produce an action potential. After the effective refractory period and as repolarisation nears completion, a relative refractory period occurs. This is defined as that period during which a propagated action potential can be elicited, provided that the stimulus is stronger than normally required in diastole. When this happens, the fibre is stimulated to contract prematurely, giving rise to an ectopic (extra) beat. Drugs such as digoxin, caffeine and nicotine can trigger ectopic activity.

Myocardial contraction

Cardiac cells are electrically coupled to each other through gap junctions that allow the action potential to propagate from cell to cell. Cardiac muscle contraction begins with a rapid change in the resting membrane potential of the cell. This electrical current spreads to the interior of the cell, where it causes the release of calcium ions from the sarcoplasmic reticulum. The calcium ions then initiate the chemical events of contraction. The overall process for controlling cardiac muscle contraction, called excitation–contraction coupling, involves electrical excitation, mechanical activation and contractile mechanisms.

Electrical excitation

Cardiac muscle contraction begins with an action potential initiated by the SA node. The action potential occurs in the membrane of the myocardial cell. The resting state of a muscle cell in the ventricle is created by the difference in electrical charge across the sarcolemma. In this case, the inside of the cell is negative with respect to the outside, which is positively charged. Because the sarcolemma separates these opposite charges, the membrane is in effect polarised. At rest, the extracellular environment is rich in sodium ions (Na^+) and the intracellular environment in potassium ions (K^+), with a rich calcium ion (Ca^{2+}) concentration in the region of the sarcolemma and where it invaginates on the sarcotubule (Fig 10.4, later).

The cardiac action potential is divided into two stages, depolarisation and repolarisation. These stages are further subdivided into five phases, 0–4. The resting potential of a myocardial cell is called phase 4; in this phase, the membrane is polarised with a charge of around −90 millivolts (mV). At this voltage, the interior of the cell is negative with respect to the exterior and the membrane is relatively impermeable to ions. Any stimulus that changes the resting membrane potential to a critical value, called the threshold, can generate an action potential. See Fig. 10.3A for the stages of an action potential.

- Phase 0 begins when the critical threshold for depolarisation (around −60 mV) is reached as a result of normal pacemaker activity or of propagation of an electrical impulse from a nearby cell, which opens voltage-dependent sodium channels. The fast inward current of sodium ions (fast channel) results in a membrane that is positively charged to 20 mV. This difference in membrane potential results in depolarisation and is designated as phase 0 (the upstroke) of the action potential. Within a few milliseconds, the sodium channels close and are unavailable for initiation of another action potential until repolarisation has occurred. Soon after, repolarisation occurs in three phases.
- In phase 1 a partial repolarisation occurs due to inactivation of the sodium current.
- Phase 2 is the plateau phase that is prominent in ventricular muscle and results from a slow inward current of calcium ions via L-type voltage-sensitive calcium channels and a small outward flow of potassium ions. Calcium ion entry into the cell is essential for the excitation–contraction coupling mechanism.
- Phase 3 results from rapid potassium ion efflux from the cell via voltage-gated potassium channels. As more potassium leaves the cell and less calcium enters during this phase, the membrane potential reverts to −90 mV.
- After repolarisation phase 4, a resting period ensues during which the cell membrane actively transports sodium ions out and potassium ions in, against their concentration gradients. These cation exchanges during recovery require an adenosine triphosphate (ATP)-dependent transport mechanism, the Na^+–K^+ pump located in the sarcolemma. Binding to the sarcolemma, Na^+–K^+-ATPase contributes to the pharmacological effects of digoxin on myocardial contraction.

In the cells of the SA and AV nodes, the action potential consists of only phases 0, 3 and 4 (Fig 10.3B). The principal distinguishing feature of the pacemaker fibre resides in phase 4 or the pacemaker potential. A slow spontaneous depolarisation occurs that requires no external stimulus and is termed diastolic depolarisation. This is responsible for automaticity.

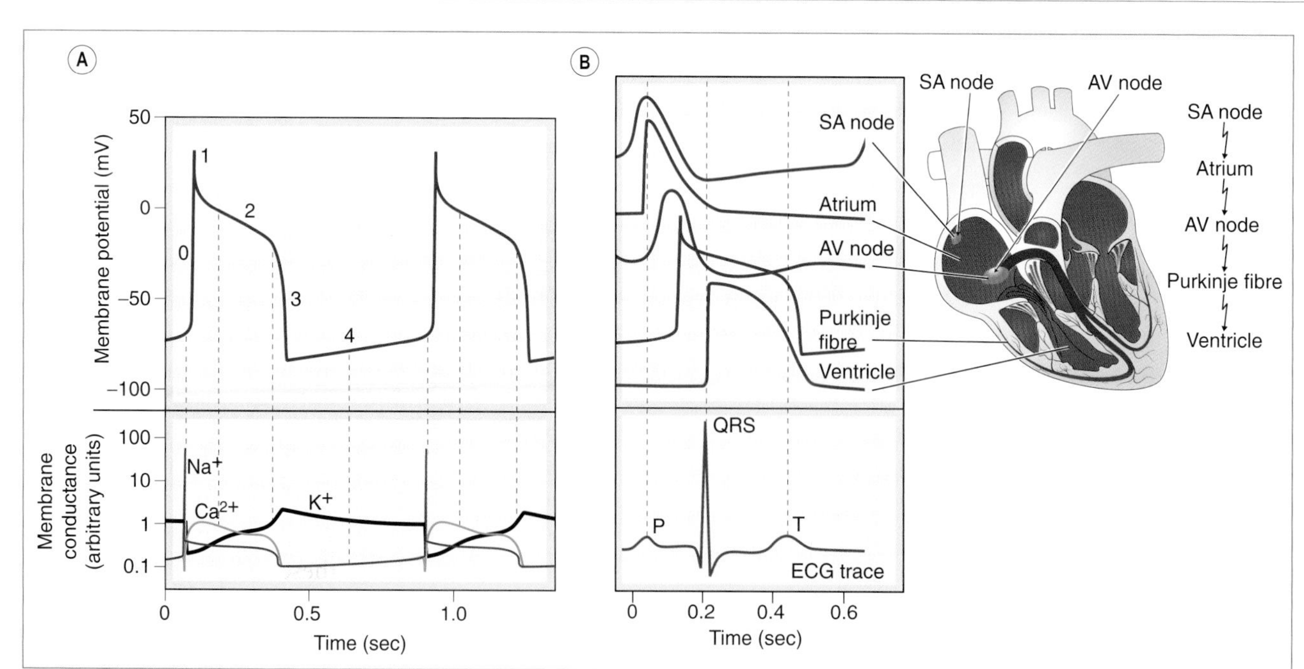

FIGURE 10.3 The cardiac action potential

A Phases of the action potential: 0, rapid depolarisation; 1, partial repolarisation; 2, plateau; 3, repolarisation; 4, pacemaker depolarisation. The lower panel shows the accompanying changes in membrane conductance for Na^+, K^+ and Ca^{2+}. **B** Conduction of the impulse through the heart, with the corresponding ECG trace. Note that the longest delay occurs at the AV node, where the action potential has a characteristically slow waveform. SA = sinoatrial

Source: Adapted from Noble 1975; reproduced with permission from Rang 2012, Figure 21.1.

In 1979, the I_f or 'funny' current was identified and explains more fully the changes that occur during diastolic depolarisation of the SA and AV nodes. The I_f channels are known as hyperpolarisation-activated cyclic nucleotide-gated (HCN) channels and are found mainly in the membrane of the SA and AV node pacemaker cells. The HCN channels open at the end of the action potential, allowing the 'funny' current to flow, which drives the membrane voltage towards the threshold of the next action potential, thus determining the slope of phase 4 (Fig. 10.3B). The slope of phase 4 determines the frequency of the action potentials and, hence, HR. Unlike the fast sodium channels of the myocardium, depolarisation (or phase 0) is achieved predominantly by the slower current carried by calcium ions (to a minor extent by sodium ions) through the slow calcium channels of nodal cells. Thus, phase 0 results in a slower conduction velocity in nodal cells than in myocardial cells. Calcium channel blockers inhibit these slow channels. Repolarisation is more gradual and involves only phase 3. The membrane then finally returns to phase 4.

An electrocardiogram (ECG) is a graphic representation of electrical currents produced by the heart and is typified by three distinct waves on the ECG (P, QRS and T, which always precede mechanical contraction). The P wave represents atrial depolarisation and follows the firing of the SA node. After the P wave, a short pause or interval (P–R interval) occurs while the electrical activity is transmitted to the AV node, conduction tissue and ventricles. The second wave, the QRS complex, represents ventricular depolarisation and the ventricles contract shortly after it begins. Repolarisation, or recovery, of the ventricles is indicated by the third and smaller T wave. Rarely, a U wave may be seen, which is thought to represent repolarisation of papillary muscle. Atrial recovery or repolarisation does not show on the ECG because it is hidden in the QRS complex (Fig 10.3B).

Mechanical activation

Each individual cardiac muscle cell contains a nucleus in the middle and a plasma membrane (cell membrane), the sarcolemma (Fig 10.4A). By joining end to end, the cells form a long fibre, with each cell contacting its neighbour through a thickening of the sarcolemma called the intercalated disc. These discs contain desmosomes, which hold the fibres together, and gap junctions, which provide sites of low electrical resistance, permitting the spread of muscle action potentials throughout the cardiac muscle.

Each individual muscle fibre (cell) comprises a group of multiple parallel myofibrils, the end unit of which is the myofilament. The myofibrils are arranged end-to-end in a series of repeating units called sarcomeres (Fig 10.4B, C). At the point of separation of the sarcomeres, known as the Z line, the sarcolemma of the muscle fibre interlocks (invaginates) at its end with the sarcomere to form the transverse sarcotubule, or T system, which penetrates deeply into the cell. An extensive network of internal membranes, the sarcoplasmic reticulum, encircles groups of myofibrils and makes contact with the sarcotubules.

The sarcomere, which is the basic unit of contraction in the heart, lies between two successive Z lines and consists of two contractile proteins, actin and myosin, which combine to help effect cardiac contraction (Fig 10.4D). Contraction is initiated when the impulse reaches the myocardial cell and travels along the sarcolemma of the muscle fibre. As the depolarisation wave spreads along the sarcotubules, calcium enters through 'L-type' (long-lasting and large) voltage-sensitive calcium channels, causing a secondary release of calcium from the sarcoplasmic reticulum. Hence the plateau, which is phase 2 of the action potential, is maintained through this slow inward calcium current. Calcium ion movement is the chief component that couples electrical excitation of the sarcolemma with muscle activation of the myofilaments in the sarcomere. Normally, interaction between actin and myosin is prevented by tropomyosin, which is bound to the actin filament. Binding of calcium ions to troponin C, a component of the troponin complex, results in a conformational change that moves tropomyosin out of the way and allows binding of the myosin cross-bridges to the actin filaments. These changes initiate the contractile mechanism.

The contractile mechanism

Activation of the actin filaments by calcium ions allows formation of the myosin cross-bridges. This interaction pulls the actin along the immobile myosin filaments towards the centre, shortening the sarcomere and producing muscle contraction (Fig 10.4E). In this process, the lengths of individual filaments remain unchanged. The greater the quantity of calcium ions delivered to troponin, the greater the rate and numbers of interactions between actin and myosin. As a result of this response, the development of tension and contractility is increased.

When magnesium is present, ATP is cleaved by myosin ATPase. This reaction provides the energy necessary for the actin filaments to move along the myosin and produce muscle contraction. Muscle relaxation depends on removing calcium ions from the sarcomere, thereby allowing the actin–myosin filaments of the sarcomere to return to their resting positions. This is achieved by a calcium ATPase (located in the walls of the sarcoplasmic reticulum), which actively returns some calcium ions to the sarcoplasmic reticulum while the remainder are removed from the cell by a Na^+–Ca^{2+} exchange protein that exchanges three sodium ions for every calcium ion.

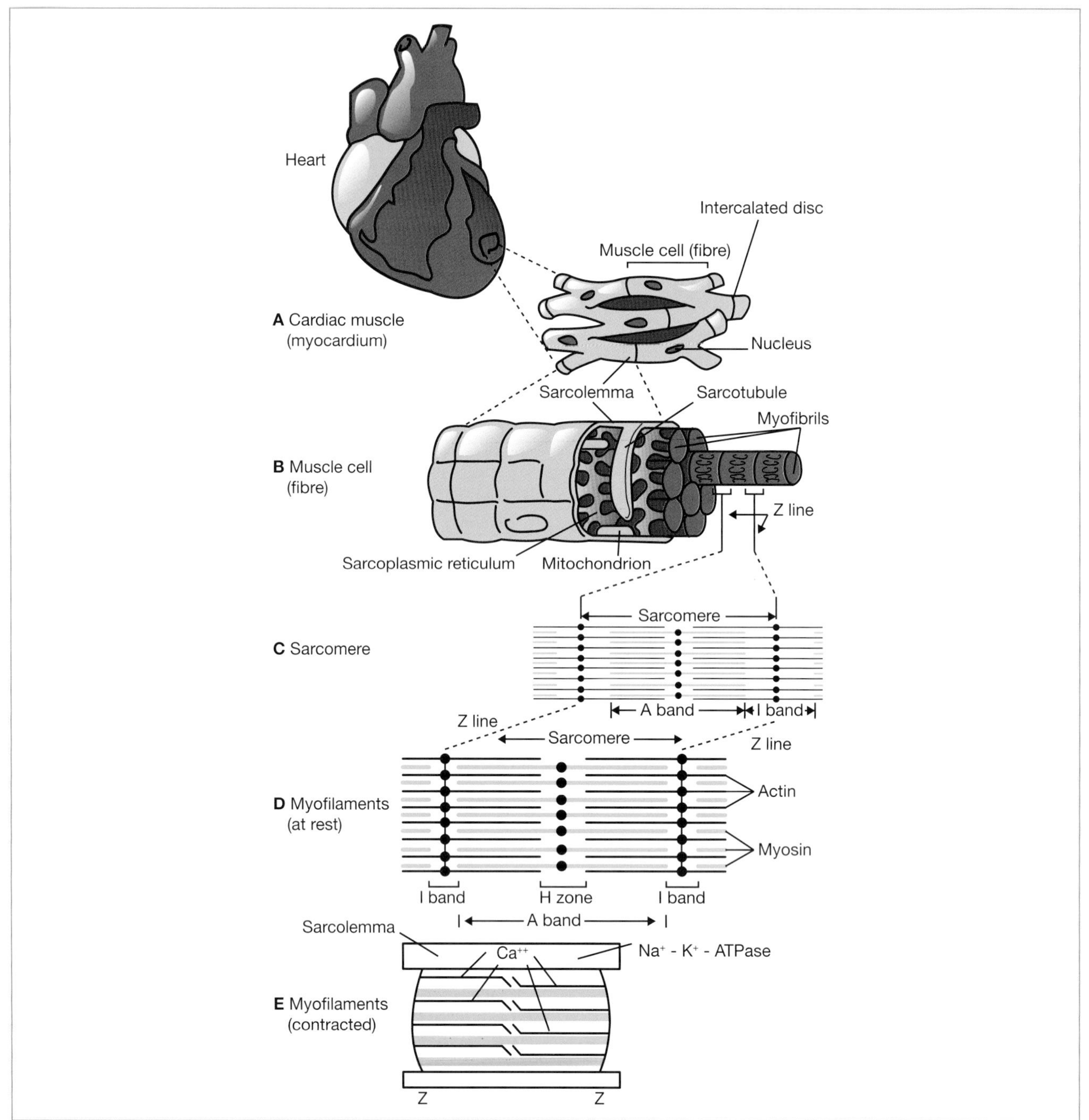

FIGURE 10.4 Structure of heart and cardiac muscle cell fibres

The enlargement of the square illustrates a portion of the cardiac muscle (myocardium) **(A)**, which is composed of myocardial cells. Each cell contains a centrally located nucleus and a limiting plasma membrane (sarcolemma), which forms the intercalated disc at the termination of each cell. An individual muscle cell (fibre) **(B)** consists of multiple parallel myofibrils. Each myofibril is arranged longitudinally in a series of light and dark repeating units. Each unit is called a sarcomere. At the Z line, the sarcolemma invaginates to form the transverse sarcotubules, or T system. An extensive network, called the sarcoplasmic reticulum, encircles groups of myofibrils and makes contact with the sarcotubules. The sarcoplasmic reticulum contains a high concentration of calcium ions. The mitochondria appear in long chains between the myofibrils. The sarcomere **(C)** is the unit of muscle contraction. It is composed of two types of bands, the A band and the I band. The Z line divides the latter. Myofilaments **(D)** of the sarcomere include the thin filament, actin, and the thick filament, myosin. The dark appearance of the A band is caused by the myosin and the lighter appearance of the I band by the actin. When contracted **(E)**, the sarcomere shortens so that the thick filaments approach the Z line and the width of the H zone between the thin filaments narrows. Calcium ions are required for contraction.

Source: Adapted from Salerno 1999; used with permission.

Cardiac output

The primary function of the heart is the supply of oxygenated blood to the rest of the body, both during periods of rest and during increased physical activity. When the body's requirement for oxygen increases, HR and CO increase to meet the demand. CO is a function of both the **stroke volume** (SV) and HR; that is:

$$CO = SV \times HR$$

SV of the heart depends on the volume of blood remaining in the heart at the end of diastole and the volume that remains after ventricular contraction. For example, in a healthy resting adult, if SV was about 70 mL and HR 72 beats/minute, CO would equal 5040 mL/min.

The factors that regulate SV include the degree of stretch of heart fibres before contraction (**preload**), the force of contraction of the ventricles and the pressure that must be overcome before the ventricles can eject the blood (**afterload**). The greater the preload, the greater is the stretch and the greater the contraction. This relation means that the longer the muscle fibres are at the end of diastole, the more forceful the contraction will be during systole. This mechanism applies only when the muscle fibre is lengthened within physiological limits and is known as the Frank-Starling relation (or the Frank-Starling law of the heart). This relation ensures that outputs from the right and left ventricles are the same.

If a diseased heart is dilated and the fibres are stretched to a critical point beyond their limit of extensibility, the forces of contraction and CO are both diminished and ineffective. If the right ventricle fails, blood pools in systemic vessels, causing peripheral oedema, while failure of the left ventricle results in pulmonary oedema because of the backing up of blood in the lungs. Thus the functional significance of the Frank-Starling relation is that effective CO can be brought about only by adequate relaxation and refilling of cardiac chambers after each myocardial contraction.

KEY POINTS

The heart

- The heart comprises four chambers, two upper atria and two lower ventricles, which are supplied with blood and nutrients by the right and left coronary arteries.
- The myocardium or cardiac muscle tissue is comprised of sarcomeres, the basic contractile unit of the heart.
- Postganglionic fibres of the sympathetic nervous system release NA and innervate the SA node, atria and ventricles. Action of NA on β_1 receptors located in both nodes and in atrial and ventricular muscles increases HR, automaticity, conduction velocity and force of contraction.
- Vagal nerve fibres of the parasympathetic nervous system, which release acetylcholine, are found primarily in the SA and AV nodes and atrial muscle. Acetylcholine acts on M_2 receptors of the SA node to decrease HR, on the AV node to decrease conduction velocity and, to a limited extent, on the M_2 receptors on cardiac myocytes to reduce cardiac contractility.
- The natriuretic peptides include ANP, BNP and CNP. These endogenous neurohormones increase sodium and water excretion by the kidney and, with the exception of the efferent arterioles of the kidney, they relax vascular smooth muscle.
- Stretching of the ventricles results in the release of BNP, and the circulating concentration of BNP correlates with the severity of heart failure.
- The cardiac conduction system comprises the SA and AV nodes, internodal pathways, the bundle of His, right and left bundle branches and the Purkinje fibres.
- The cardiac conduction system exhibits automaticity, conductivity and refractoriness, attributes required for the initiation and transmission of electrical impulses necessary for myocardial contraction.
- The overall process of cardiac muscle contraction involves electrical excitation, mechanical activation and contractile mechanisms.
- The cardiac action potential is divided into two stages, depolarisation and repolarisation, which are further subdivided into five phases (0–4) on the basis of ion movement.
- Cardiac output is a function of stroke volume and heart rate: $CO = SV \times HR$.
- Factors regulating stroke volume include the degree of stretch of heart fibres before contraction (preload), the force of contraction of the ventricles and the pressure that must be overcome before the ventricles can eject the blood (afterload).
- The Frank-Starling law of the heart defines the relationship between the force of ejection and the length of cardiac muscle fibres.

Drugs affecting cardiac function

Numerous drugs affect the heart and vascular system and provide the mainstay for treating diseases such as **heart failure**, which is characterised by reduced CO and the consequential failure to provide adequate perfusion to meet the metabolic requirements of the body (Fig 10.5 and Clinical Focus Box 10.1), dysrhythmias, hypertension, ischaemic heart disease (angina), peripheral vascular disease and shock and hypotension.[1] Many of these drugs exert a direct effect on the heart or vasculature, while others indirectly affect cardiac function as a consequence of actions on vascular tissue.

Drugs acting directly on the heart include:

- the sympathomimetics adrenaline (epinephrine), noradrenaline (norepinephrine) and the related drugs discussed in Chapters 8 and 9
- the antianginal drug ivabradine
- milrinone and sacubitril/valsartan used to treat heart failure
- antidysrhythmic drugs – for example, adenosine, amiodarone, atropine (Ch 8), digoxin, disopyramide, esmolol, flecainide, lidocaine (Ch 18) and sotalol
- the antihypertensive calcium channel blockers, which also act on vascular smooth muscle (Ch 11).

Drugs with a positive **inotropic effect** increase the force of myocardial contraction (e.g. digoxin, dobutamine, adrenaline and isoprenaline), whereas drugs with a negative inotropic effect decrease the force of myocardial contraction (e.g. propranolol).

Drugs with a positive **chronotropic effect** accelerate the HR by increasing the rate of impulse formation in the SA node (e.g. adrenaline). A drug with a negative chronotropic effect has the opposite effect and slows the HR by decreasing impulse formation (e.g. digoxin, ivabradine).

A drug with a positive **dromotropic effect** increases conduction velocity through specialised conducting tissues (e.g. phenytoin), while a drug with a negative dromotropic effect delays conduction (e.g. verapamil, see Ch 11).

1 The authors acknowledge that the prefix 'a' means 'without', and the only arrhythmia is asystole. The correct term is 'dysrhythmia', the prefix 'dys' meaning 'difficulty with'. Although the terms 'arrhythmia' and 'anti-arrhythmic drugs' occur frequently in the literature, we have chosen to use 'dysrhythmia' and 'antidysrhythmic drugs'.

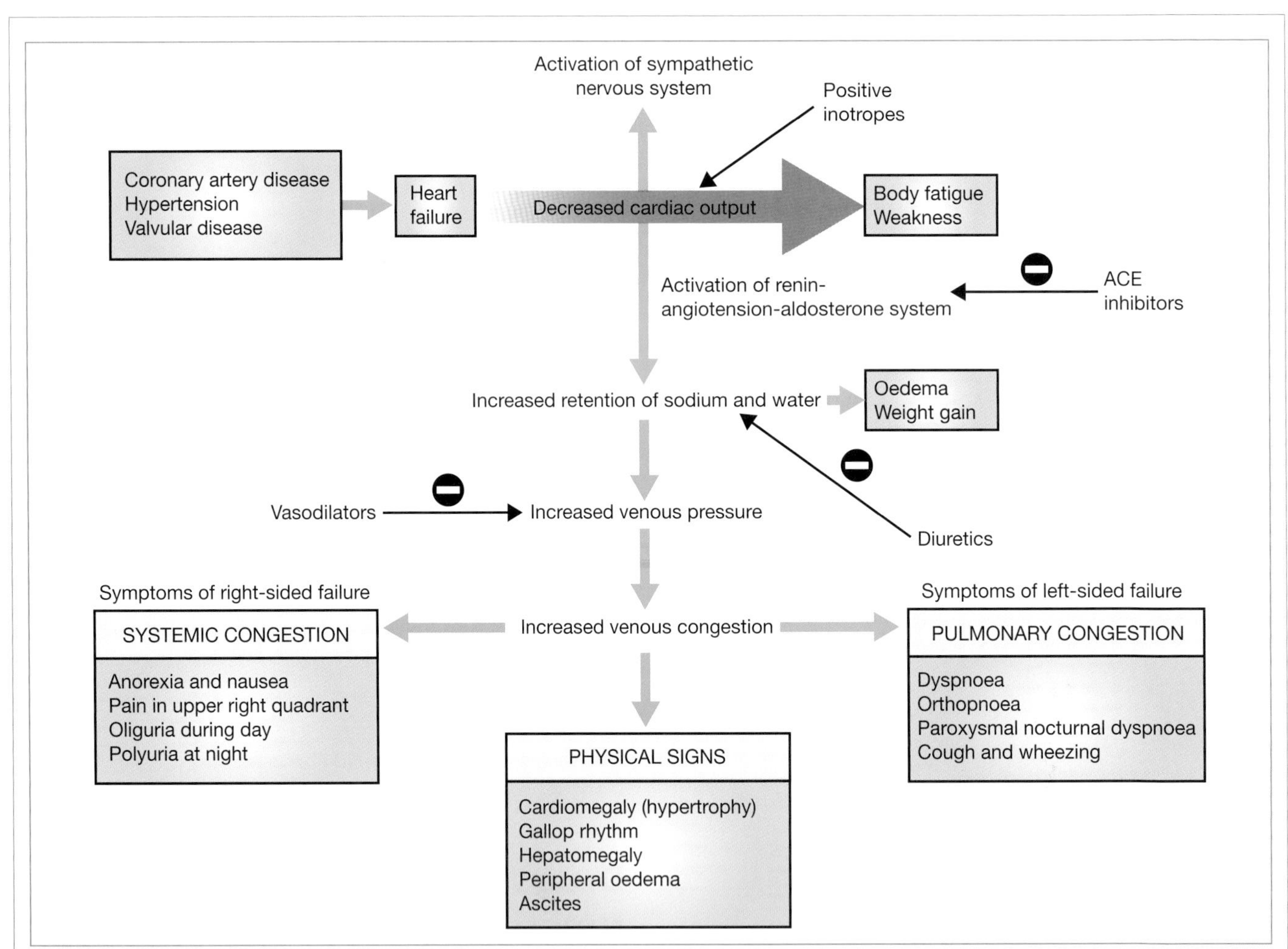

FIGURE 10.5 Signs and symptoms of heart failure and site of action of commonly used drugs
– = inhibitory effect
Source: Adapted from Salerno 1999, Figure 19.1; used with permission.

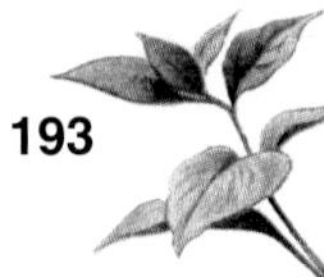

CLINICAL FOCUS BOX 10.1
Management of heart failure

In general, the prevalence of heart failure increases from about 10% in people aged 70 years to over 50% in those 85 years and older. Risk factors predisposing to heart failure include coronary artery disease (the cause in ~66% of people with systolic heart failure), hypertension and diabetes. Heart failure is a complex clinical syndrome, and the symptoms (fatigue, shortness of breath and congestion) are related to inadequate CO (and, hence, inadequate tissue perfusion) during exertion and to the retention of fluid.

The short-term goals of therapy are to relieve symptoms and improve the quality of life. Long-term management is aimed at slowing disease progression and prolonging survival. Non-pharmacological approaches include modifying risk factors (diet, smoking and alcohol intake), encouraging exercise, often through rehabilitation programs, and providing home support.

Pharmacological therapy includes the angiotensin-converting enzyme (ACE) inhibitors (e.g. enalapril, lisinopril), diuretics (e.g. loop and thiazide), β-blockers (e.g. bisoprolol, carvedilol, metoprolol or nebivolol), aldosterone antagonists (e.g. eplerenone, spironolactone), angiotensin receptor blockers (ARBs) (e.g. candesartan, valsartan), the neprilysin/ARB combination sacubitril/valsartan and the I_f channel inhibitor ivabradine. Studies have shown that β-blockers may have favourable effects in some cases of heart failure; however, because of adverse effects on left ventricular function, these drugs are started in low doses and titrated upwards. Digoxin still provides valuable therapy in people with chronic heart failure accompanied by AF.

Source: National Heart Foundation of Australia and Cardiac Society of Australia and New Zealand 2018.

Ivabradine, a selective sinus node I_f channel inhibitor

Ivabradine was developed originally to treat myocardial ischaemia and supraventricular dysrhythmias and is the first selective inhibitor of the I_f channel in the SA node (Flarakos et al. 2016). It is indicated for treating stable angina in patients with normal sinus rhythm and as an adjunct to standard treatment of stable chronic heart failure in patients with normal sinus rhythm and with an HR over 77 beats/minute.

Mechanism of action

Ivabradine selectively blocks the I_f channel, decreasing the slope of the spontaneous diastolic depolarisation of the SA node, hence lowering HR at rest and during exercise. It does not affect myocardial contractility or AV conduction, and the beneficial effect in angina occurs from the reduction in cardiac work and myocardial oxygen demand.

Pharmacokinetics

Ivabradine is hepatically metabolised by CYP3A4 forming either active or inactive metabolites while 4% of the parent drug is cleared renally. N-desmethylation leads to formation of the major active metabolite S18982 that is also a substrate for CYP3A4. Bioavailability has been reported as 40–53% due to first-pass metabolism in both the gut and the liver; maximal plasma concentration was observed between 1 and 1.5 hours after oral dosing. The half-life of ivabradine is in the order of 11 hours. Concomitant administration of inhibitors of CYP3A4 (e.g. diltiazem, itraconazole and clarithromycin) is contraindicated because of the risk of adverse effects due to reduced hepatic clearance. Additionally, carbamazepine and St John's wort, known inducers of CYP3A4 activity, reduce the bioavailability of ivabradine.

Adverse reactions

Not surprisingly, bradycardia is a predictable dose-related adverse effect giving rise to dizziness and hypotension. Ivabradine also causes luminous effects (enhanced brightness in part of the visual field) because it interacts with a retinal current that normally attenuates the retinal response to bright light stimuli. The interaction results from the fact that the retinal current is very similar to the cardiac I_f current.

Milrinone, a phosphodiesterase inhibitor

Milrinone is indicated for short-term treatment (about 48 hours) of severe heart failure refractory to other drugs, and for low-cardiac-output states (e.g. following cardiac surgery). It is principally used in coronary and intensive care units, and prolonged use is associated with increased mortality.

Mechanism of action

Phosphodiesterases (PDE) are a family of enzymes comprising 11 subtypes. Milrinone is a selective inhibitor of phosphodiesterase 3 (PDE3), which is expressed in heart and metabolises cAMP in cardiac and vascular tissue (Fig 10.6). Inhibition of the breakdown of cAMP results in elevated levels of cAMP within those tissues. This then results in increased calcium influx and uptake by the sarcoplasmic reticulum, causing improvement in myocardial contractility and vasodilation without increasing myocardial oxygen consumption and HR. Milrinone is a positive inotrope and, as a result of a balanced vasodilation of both resistance and capacitance vessels, systemic and pulmonary vascular resistance and right and left heart-filling pressures decrease.

Pharmacokinetics

Administered intravenously, milrinone has a half-life of 2.5 hours and duration of action of 3–6 hours. It is

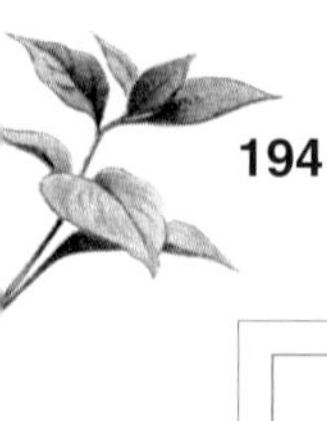

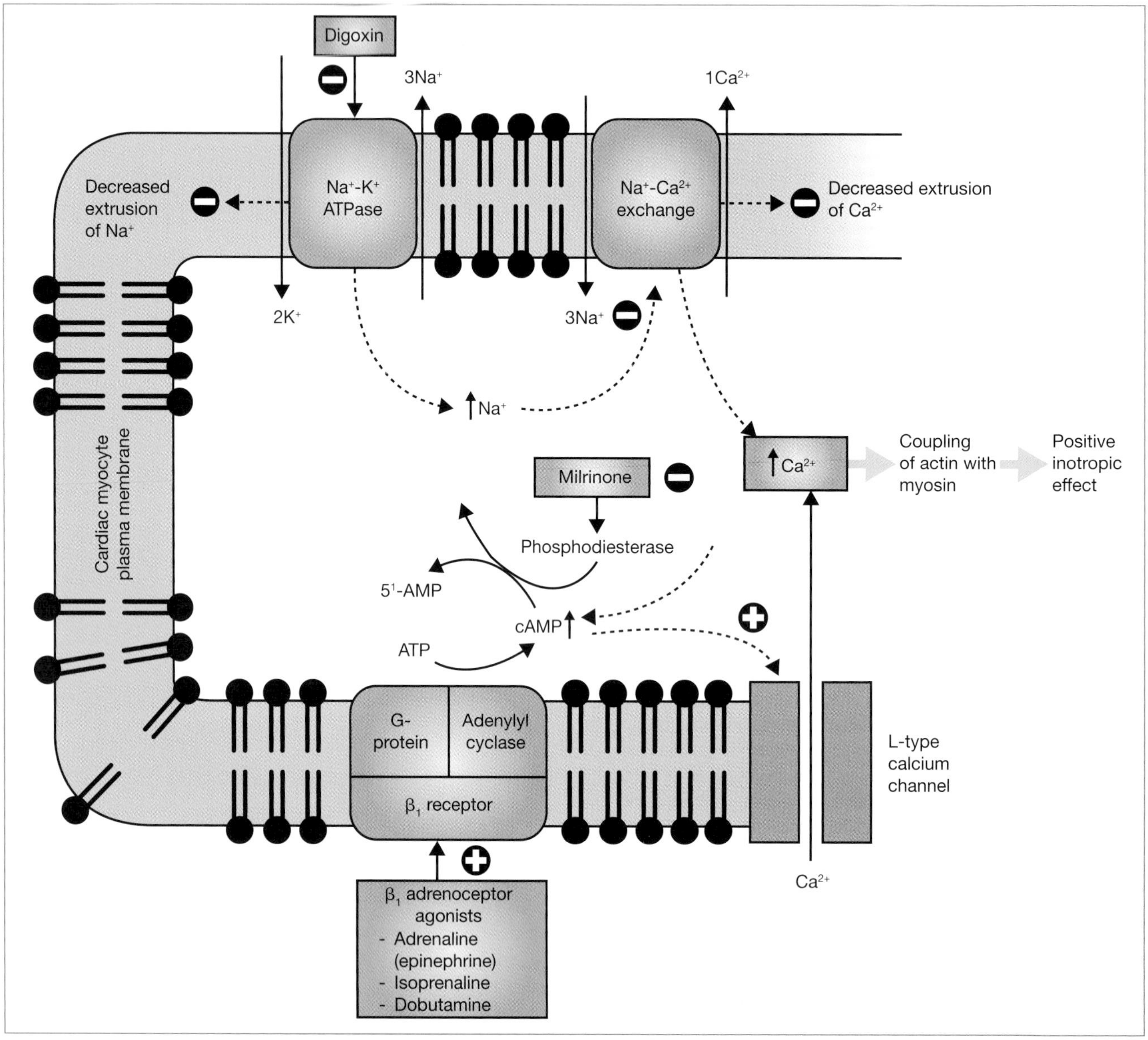

FIGURE 10.6 Schematic representation of cardiac myocyte indicating sites of action of digoxin, milrinone and β-adrenoceptor agonists − = inhibitory effect; + = positive effect

excreted by the kidneys, and a reduction in dose is necessary in people with severe renal impairment. This drug should not be administered with other PDE3 inhibitors (e.g. anagrelide).

Adverse reactions

Common adverse reactions include ventricular dysrhythmias, angina, hypotension, nausea and headache.

Sacubitril/valsartan, a neprilysin/angiotensin (AT_1) receptor inhibitor

Sacubitril/valsartan is a drug combination indicated for treating NYHA class II–IV heart failure with reduced ejection fraction (Vardeny et al. 2014). Current clinical data support a role for this drug combination in the treatment of heart failure. However, large trials in different heart failure patient populations are ongoing.

Mechanism of action

Sacubitril, which is a prodrug, is metabolised to the active neprilysin inhibitor LBQ657 within 3.5 hours following oral dosing. The pharmacological effect of neprilysin inhibition results in an increased concentration of natriuretic peptides, which then produce an array of advantageous cardiovascular effects (see previous section 'Cardiac Natriuretic Peptides'). The combination with valsartan (Ch 11) is used to negate the deleterious effects of angiotensin II that may accumulate due to neprilysin

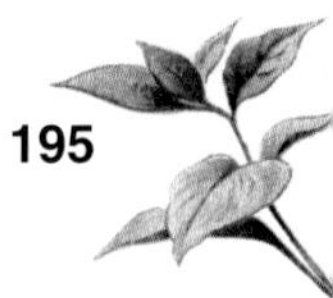

inhibition. In addition, this drug combination produces vasodilation, reduces sympathetic tone, increases glomerular filtration rate and reduces aldosterone release.

Pharmacokinetics

Once administered, the drug combination dissociates into sacubitril and valsartan. The maximum plasma concentration of sacubitril is achieved within 1.5–2 hours and for valsartan within 0.5–1 hour. Although the majority (~85%) of LBQ657 is excreted via urine and faeces, there is limited knowledge of the metabolism of both sacubitril and LBQ657.

Adverse reactions

Common adverse reactions include hypotension, dizziness, fainting, hyperkalaemia and renal impairment.

KEY POINTS

Drugs affecting cardiac function

- Numerous drugs that affect the heart and vascular system are used to treat heart failure, dysrhythmias, hypertension and ischaemic heart disease.
- Many drugs exert a direct effect on the heart or vasculature; others indirectly affect cardiac function as a consequence of actions on vascular tissue.
- Drugs acting directly on the heart include the catecholamines (Ch 9), ivabradine, milrinone, cardiac glycosides (typified by digoxin) and antidysrhythmic drugs.
- Ivabradine is the first selective inhibitor of the I_f channel in the SA node. It decreases the slope of the spontaneous diastolic depolarisation of the SA node, hence lowering HR at rest and during exercise. It does not affect myocardial contractility or AV conduction, and the beneficial effect in angina occurs from the reduction in cardiac work and myocardial oxygen demand.
- Milrinone, a selective inhibitor of phosphodiesterase 3 (PDE3), improves myocardial contractility and vasodilation without increasing myocardial oxygen consumption and HR. It is indicated for short-term treatment (~48 hours) of severe heart failure refractory to other drugs, and for low-cardiac-output states.
- Sacubitril/valsartan is a neprilysin/angiotensin (AT_1) receptor inhibitor used to treat heart failure. The active metabolite of sacubitril increases natriuretic peptides, which then produce an array of advantageous cardiovascular effects. The combination with valsartan negates the adverse effects of angiotensin II accumulation.

Dysrhythmias and antidysrhythmic drugs

Dysrhythmias

A cardiac **dysrhythmia** is defined as any deviation from the normal rhythm of the heartbeat (Table 10.1). Disorders of cardiac rhythm arise because of abnormality in spontaneous initiation of an impulse (i.e. in automaticity) or abnormality in impulse conduction (i.e. in conductivity). In some circumstances, a combination of both processes occurs.

Abnormality in automaticity

A disturbance in automaticity can alter the heart's rate, rhythm or site of origin of impulse formation. When the rate of pacemaker activity is affected, a decrease in automaticity of the SA node produces sinus bradycardia (an abnormal condition in which the heart contracts steadily but at < 60 beats/minute). An increase in automaticity of the SA node results in sinus tachycardia (an abnormal condition in which the heart contracts regularly but at > 100 beats/minute). A shift in the site of origin of impulse formation can generate an abnormal pacemaker or an ectopic focus, resulting in activation of a part of the heart other than the SA node. This is called an ectopic pacemaker, and it may discharge at either a regular or an irregular rhythm. It occurs because the cardiac fibres depolarise more frequently than the SA node. Abnormal automaticity can develop in cells that usually do not initiate impulses (e.g. atrial or ventricular cells). Clinical disorders such as hypoxia or ischaemia can cause impulse disturbances in automaticity and in conductivity, and both manifestations are responsible for ectopic beats. Ectopic beats are classified as escape beats, premature beats or extrasystoles, and ectopic tachydysrhythmia.

Abnormality in conductivity

Altered conduction of cardiac impulses probably accounts for more dysrhythmias than changes in automaticity. A disturbance in conductivity may be caused by a delay or block of impulse conduction or by the re-entry phenomenon. In abnormal circumstances, conduction of an atrial impulse to the ventricles can be delayed or blocked in the AV node or in conduction pathways beyond this region. In first-degree AV block, the impulses from the SA node pass through to the ventricles very slowly; this is shown by a prolonged P–R interval on the ECG. In second-degree block, some atrial beats fail to pass into the ventricles through the AV node. In third-degree block, or complete heart block, no impulses reach the ventricle, in which case the Purkinje fibres initiate their own spontaneous depolarisation at a very slow rate. This results in independent ventricular and atrial rhythms referred to as ventricular 'escape'.

TABLE 10.1 Examples of dysrhythmias

TYPE	DESCRIPTION	POSSIBLE CAUSES
Bradydysrhythmias		
Atrioventricular block	Intermittent or absent conduction between atria and ventricles. Commonly occurs at AV node or within bundle branch system.	Drug induced (e.g. β-blockers, digoxin, diltiazem, verapamil), infection, myocardial infarction
Sick sinus syndrome	Associated with SA node dysfunction, usually SA block or inadequate SA node conduction. Characterised by severe sinus bradycardia and symptoms of weakness, dizziness, lethargy and syncope. Treatment usually requires a pacemaker.	Various cardiomyopathies, inflammatory myocardial disease, myocardial ischaemia, digoxin toxicity
Tachydysrhythmias		
Atrial tachydysrhythmias		
Atrial fibrillation	Common sustained dysrhythmia characterised by disordered electrical activity in atria resulting in a fast, irregular ventricular response. High risk of stroke and heart failure.	Acute myocardial infarction, can be idiopathic, cardiac surgery, mitral stenosis, rheumatic disease, advanced age (> 65 years)
Atrial flutter	Atrial tachycardia characterised by contraction rate 230–380/minute with ventricular contractions in 1:2, 1:3, 1:4 or variable ratio.	Cause often unknown, heart disease, AV node dysfunction, chronic hypertension, overactive thyroid
Supraventricular tachycardia	Atrial tachycardia and dysrhythmias arising from AV junction.	Hypoxia, electrolyte and acid–base abnormalities, enlarged atria, digoxin toxicity
Ventricular tachydysrhythmias		
Premature ventricular ectopics	Ectopics	Alcohol, caffeine, stress
Ventricular tachycardia	> 100 beats/minute	Acute myocardial infarction
Torsades de pointes	Characterised by a prolonged ventricular action potential (prolonged QT interval). Can be congenital (mutations in the cardiac sodium or potassium channels) or acquired.	Acquired: electrolyte disturbances or from a number of drugs and drug classes, such as antidysrhythmic drugs (e.g. amiodarone, disopyramide, sotalol), antipsychotics, antimicrobial drugs, methadone, tacrolimus, tricyclic antidepressants

Re-entry phenomenon

The re-entry phenomenon is the mechanism responsible for initiating ectopic beats. For example, when an impulse travels down the Purkinje fibre, it normally spreads along two branches, and when it enters the connecting branch impulses are extinguished at the point of collision in the centre (Fig 10.7A). At the same time, other impulses that begin laterally from the Purkinje fibres activate ventricular muscle tissue. In an abnormal situation, the impulse descending from the central Purkinje fibre travels down one branch normally but encounters a block in the other branch due to ischaemia or injury (Fig 10.7B). This is a unidirectional block because the impulse can pass in one direction only. In the injured branch, where the impulse is blocked in the forward direction at the site of injury, a retrograde (reverse) impulse from the ventricular tissue re-enters the depressed region from the other direction, provided the pathway proximal to the block is no longer refractory. When the effective refractory period of the blocked area is over, re-entry of the impulse from the ventricular muscle into this site causes the impulse to circulate or recycle repetitively through the loop, resulting in a circus-type movement that produces dysrhythmia.

Drugs that decrease or slow conduction velocity can convert a unidirectional block to a two-way or bidirectional block (Fig 10.7C). As the impulses travelling in the antegrade (forward) direction and those moving in a retrograde (reverse) direction are blocked at the injured site, the re-entry pathway is interrupted, abolishing the ectopic beats. In Fig 10.7D, the conditions required for preventing re-entry by another mechanism are illustrated.

Antidysrhythmic drugs

The rationale for use of antidysrhythmic drugs includes restoration of haemodynamic stability, prevention of life-threatening dysrhythmias, prevention of sudden cardiac death, controlling ventricular rate and preventing thromboembolism in AF. Despite their use for the treatment of dysrhythmias, these drugs all possess **prodysrhythmogenic** potential and can worsen the dysrhythmia and cause sudden death. Use of these drugs requires careful consideration of other treatment options and, following institution of therapy, careful monitoring of the person's clinical condition.

Antidysrhythmic drugs were classified based on their fundamental effects on cardiac electrophysiology by Vaughan Williams in 1970. This classification is of value in predicting the drug's therapeutic efficacy, although not all drugs belonging to a particular class necessarily possess identical actions. The pharmacokinetics and classification of currently available antidysrhythmic drugs are shown in Table 10.2 and Fig 10.8, but there are several drugs not classified in the Vaughan Williams system.

Classification of antidysrhythmic drugs

Antidysrhythmic drugs are classified into classes I–IV.

Class I

Class I drugs block voltage-sensitive sodium channels interfering with sodium influx during phase 0 of the

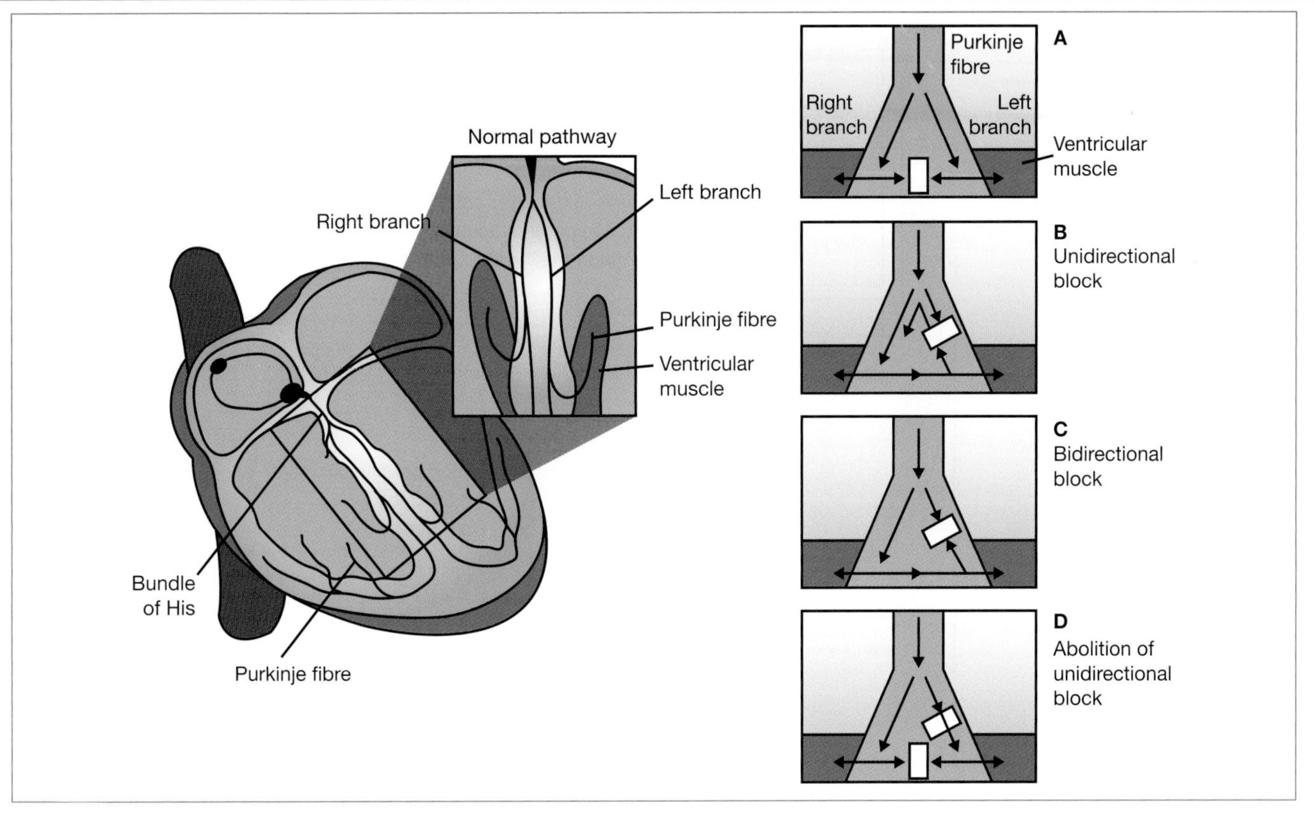

FIGURE 10.7 Re-entry phenomenon
Illustration of a branched Purkinje fibre that activates ventricular muscle.
Source: Adapted from Salerno 1999, Figure 20.1; used with permission.

TABLE 10.2 Pharmacokinetics of selected antidysrhythmic drugs

DRUG	ONSET OF ACTION (h)	HALF-LIFE (h)	THERAPEUTIC RANGE[a]
Class Ia drug			
Disopyramide	0.5–3	4–10	2–4 mg/L (6–12 micromol/L)
Class Ib drugs			
Lidocaine	IV: 1 min	1.6	–
	IM: 3–15 min		
Class Ic drug			
Flecainide	1–6	Varies (12–27)	0.2–0.9 mg/L
Class II drugs – β-adrenoceptor antagonists (Ch 9)			
Class III drugs			
Amiodarone	3–7	14–59 days (metabolite 60–90 days)	1–2.5 mg/L (1.6–4 micromol/L)
Sotalol	2–3	12–14	
Class IV drugs – calcium channel blockers (Ch 11)			

[a] Local or regional laboratories should be consulted.
Sources: Australian Medicines Handbook. Adelaide: Australian Medicines Handbook Pty Ltd; 2021; Thummel KE, Shen DD, Isoherranen N. Design and optimization of dosage regimens: Pharmacokinetic data. In: Brunton LL, Hilal-Dandan R, Knollmann BC, editors. Goodman & Gilman's The Pharmacological Basis of Therapeutics. 13th ed. New York: McGraw Hill; 2018, p1325-1378.

action potential. In general, class I drugs bind to the sodium channel when it is in the open or refractory state and less so during the resting state. Thus, the more frequently the channel is activated the greater the degree of block by the class I drugs. Although they all share the same basic mechanism, there are differences between the drugs based on their binding to either the resting, open or refractory states of the sodium channel. These minor differences give rise to the subclasses:

- **Class Ia** drugs (e.g. disopyramide, Drug Monograph 10.1) are the oldest antidysrhythmics and previously included quinidine and procainamide. Quinidine is not registered for use in Australia and New Zealand because of evidence of increased mortality with chronic use. Disopyramide binding properties lie between the Ib and Ic drugs, but in addition it prolongs the repolarisation phase but not to the same extent as the class III drugs.
- The **class Ib** drug lidocaine (Ch 18) differs from class Ia drugs because, in general, it does not affect conduction velocity. Lidocaine binds to the open sodium channels during phase 0 such that many of the channels are blocked when the action potential peaks. The drug dissociates from the channel rapidly, leaving it available for the next action potential if cardiac rhythm is normal. However, conduction of premature beats is blocked while the channel remains occupied. Additionally, lidocaine binds to refractory channels and is particularly effective in ischaemic myocardium when the cells are depolarised. Lidocaine is useful for acute

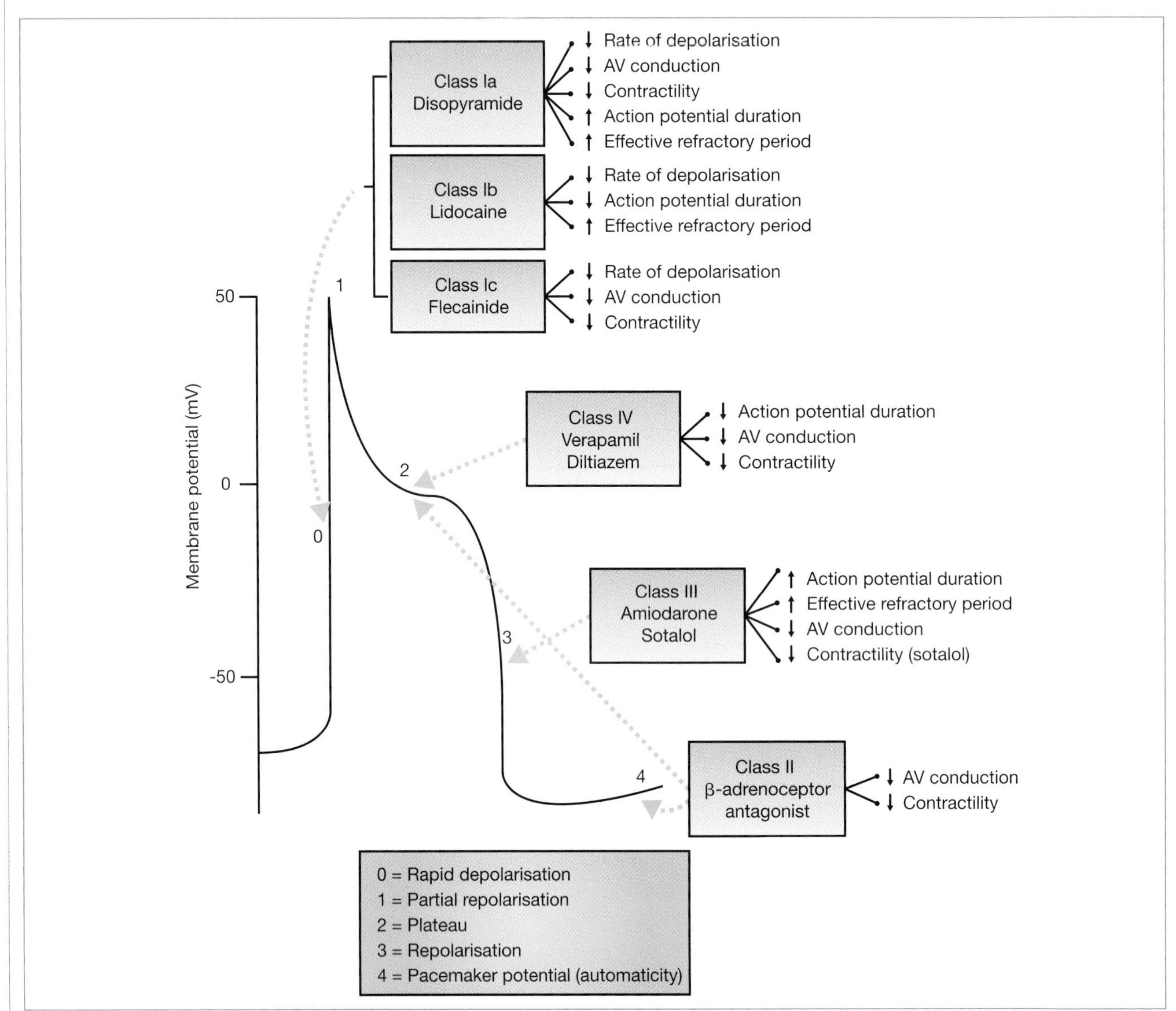

FIGURE 10.8 Phases of the cardiac action potential and the effects produced by the various classes of antidysrhythmic drugs

ventricular dysrhythmias. Like the class Ia drugs, lidocaine can worsen dysrhythmias, and a high incidence of adverse effects has limited its usefulness.

- The **class Ic** drug flecainide (Drug Monograph 10.2) is used to treat AF and flutter and serious ventricular dysrhythmias. It binds to and dissociates from the sodium channels slowly, effectively maintaining the block throughout the cardiac cycle. As binding to refractory channels is marginal, this drug does not have greater efficacy in ischaemic/damaged myocardium. It also inhibits conduction in the His–Purkinje system. The potential for prodysrhythmic effect is of special concern, especially in people with poor left ventricular function or sustained ventricular dysrhythmias. The class Ic drugs can also aggravate congestive heart failure.

Class II

Class II drugs include atenolol, esmolol and metoprolol. (These drugs are discussed extensively in Ch 9.) All three drugs are β-adrenoceptor antagonists used to control cardiac dysrhythmias caused by excessive sympathetic activity. They reduce the rate of the SA node, slow conduction in the atria and AV node and increase the functional refractory period. These drugs are the only

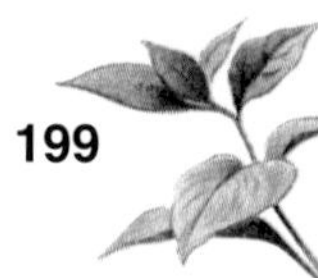

DRUG MONOGRAPH 10.1
Disopyramide

Mechanism of action

Disopyramide prevents the movement of sodium and potassium across cell membranes. The inhibition of cation exchange results in a decrease in the rate of diastolic depolarisation from the resting potential during phase 4 and an increase in the threshold potential (the voltage shifts towards 0 mV) causing decreased impulse conduction and delayed repolarisation in the atria, ventricles and Purkinje fibres. The delay repolarisation probably exerts an important antidysrhythmic action. The tissue remains refractory for a period after full restoration of the resting membrane potential. This property is believed to influence the conversion of unidirectional block to bidirectional block, thereby abolishing the re-entry type of dysrhythmia (Fig 10.7C). Additionally, by decreasing impulse generation at ectopic sites, disopyramide suppresses or abolishes dysrhythmias. Abnormal or ectopic pacemaker tissue appears to be more sensitive to disopyramide than the SA node, thus permitting the SA node to re-establish control over impulse formation in the heart.

Disopyramide also exerts an anticholinergic effect, resulting in inhibition of vagal action on the SA node and AV junction. This effect permits the sinus node to accelerate and can often provoke a dangerous sinus tachycardia. The latter is the reason why a drug that slows AV conduction may be administered with disopyramide when it is used in the treatment of atrial flutter or AF.

Pharmacokinetics

Disopyramide is well absorbed and is metabolised by the liver to the weakly active metabolite (mono-N-dealkylated disopyramide), which has both antidysrhythmic and anticholinergic effects. The half-life of disopyramide is about 4 hours, and about 50% is excreted as unchanged drug in urine. The therapeutic plasma concentration range for disopyramide is 2–4 mg/L (Table 10.2).

Drug interactions

The following drug interactions may occur with disopyramide:

- Azole antifungals: Increase disopyramide plasma concentration. Avoid combined use.
- Erythromycin: Increases disopyramide plasma concentration. Avoid combined use.
- Other antidysrhythmic agents, such as diltiazem, flecainide, lidocaine, verapamil and β-adrenergic blocking agents: Require close monitoring for evidence of negative chronotropic (bradydysrhythmia) and inotropic effects (heart failure). β-adrenergic blocking agents may exacerbate heart failure, especially in individuals with compromised ventricular function. Avoid combined use, or potentially serious drug interactions may occur.
- Phenytoin: Promotes induction of hepatic drug-metabolising enzymes, which reduces disopyramide plasma concentration. Monitor plasma concentration and increase dose if required.
- Tricyclic antidepressants: Should not be co-administered. Avoid combined use, as prolongation of the Q–T interval increases the risk of prodysrhythmic effect.

Adverse reactions

Common adverse reactions include:

- blurred vision, constipation, urinary retention and dry mouth (due to anticholinergic effects)
- hypersensitivity reactions
- severe disturbances of cardiac rhythm and exacerbation of heart failure.

Warnings and contraindications

Disopyramide should be used with caution in people with diabetes mellitus, glaucoma (closed-angle), hypokalaemia, myasthenia gravis, enlarged prostate or renal impairment. Avoid use in people with disopyramide hypersensitivity, AV block, cardiogenic shock, cardiac conduction abnormality, cardiomyopathy or heart failure.

Dosage and administration

Dosage and oral administration are individualised according to response and tolerance, and the dose is reduced in people with impaired renal function.

class of antidysrhythmics to show a reduction in mortality post-myocardial infarction.

Drugs such as atenolol are used to treat atrial tachydysrhythmias and ventricular dysrhythmias, whereas esmolol is indicated for short-term treatment of SVT induced by AF or atrial flutter.

Class III

Class III drugs include amiodarone (Drug Monograph 10.3) and sotalol. The electrophysiological properties of amiodarone and sotalol differ markedly from those of the other classes. Drugs in this group prolong the effective refractory period by prolonging the action potential duration.

DRUG MONOGRAPH 10.2
Flecainide

Mechanism of action

Flecainide is a sodium channel-blocking agent used to treat ventricular dysrhythmias; it has minimal effects on repolarisation and no anticholinergic properties. It suppresses premature ventricular contractions, and in high doses can exacerbate dysrhythmias in people with a pre-existing ventricular tachydysrhythmia or with a previous myocardial infarction.

Pharmacokinetics

Flecainide is well absorbed after oral administration. It is hepatically metabolised by CYP2D6 to inactive metabolites and about 45% is renally excreted as unchanged drug. The therapeutic range for flecainide is 0.2–0.9 mg/L (Table 10.2).

Drug interactions

The administration of flecainide with other antidysrhythmic drugs (digoxin, β-blockers, verapamil) can result in enhanced adverse cardiac effects. In people with diuretic-induced hypokalaemia, there is an increased risk of dysrhythmias.

Adverse reactions

Adverse reactions include:

- blurred vision, dizziness, headaches
- constipation, nausea
- chest pain, irregular heartbeats and dysrhythmias.

Warnings and contraindications

Use flecainide with caution in people with heart failure, hypokalaemia or hyperkalaemia, and renal impairment. Flecainide is contraindicated in post-myocardial infarction, in people with heart block or in situations of cardiogenic shock.

Dosage and administration

Flecainide is available as both an oral and an IV formulation. Dosage is adjusted based on clinical response and drug concentration monitoring.

Sotalol is a β-adrenoceptor antagonist that also blocks cardiac potassium channels, prolonging the action potential duration and increasing the effective refractory period in atrial and ventricular tissue and at the AV node. It is indicated for treatment and prevention of atrial and serious ventricular dysrhythmias. Sotalol is predominantly cleared renally (around 90%) and therefore accumulates in people with renal impairment (Table 10.2). Additive depressant effects occur with other antidysrhythmic drugs, including verapamil and diltiazem, producing bradydysrhythmia, AV block and an increased risk of heart failure. Increased risk of dysrhythmias also occurs in the presence of diuretic-induced hypokalaemia.

Common adverse effects include hypotension, dyspnoea, fatigue, dizziness, impotence, nausea, vomiting and diarrhoea. Similar to the other classes of antidysrhythmic drugs, sotalol is prodysrhythmogenic, potentially producing new or worsening dysrhythmias. Care should be exercised in people with heart failure, airways disease, diabetes or peripheral vascular disease. Sotalol is contraindicated in the presence of heart block, sinus bradycardia, severe heart failure and hypotensive states. Sotalol is available as both an IV and an oral formulation.

Class IV

Class IV drugs are the calcium channel blockers (e.g. verapamil, see Ch 11). Drugs in this class are used to treat SVT and for controlling ventricular rate in AF and atrial flutter.

Clinical Uses of Antidysrhythmic Drugs

Class Ia e.g. disopyramide
- Ventricular tachydysrhythmias

Class Ib e.g. lidocaine
- Serious ventricular dysrhythmias

Class Ic e.g flecainide
- Paroxysmal AF or atrial flutter
- Serious ventricular dysrhythmias

Class II e.g. esmolol
- Control of dysrhythmias provoked by increased sympathetic activity
- Non-compensatory sinus tachycardia

Class III e.g. amiodarone
- Serious tachydysrhythmias e.g. VT, AF and SVT

Class IV e.g. verapamil
- SVT, AF or atrial flutter

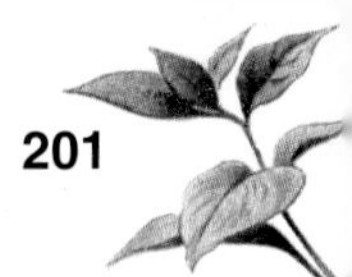

DRUG MONOGRAPH 10.3
Amiodarone

Mechanism of action

Amiodarone increases the refractory period in all cardiac tissues through a direct effect on the tissues. It decreases automaticity, prolongs AV conduction and decreases the automaticity of fibres in the Purkinje system. It can block potassium, sodium (class I effect) and calcium channels (class IV effect) and β receptors (class II effect). It has the potential to cause a variety of complex effects in the heart and has serious adverse effects. Its main active metabolite, desethylamiodarone (DEA), produces increasing depression of the rate of depolarisation during phase 0, and hence the changing electrophysiological effects observed with chronic dosing may reflect accumulation of both amiodarone and DEA.

Indications

Amiodarone is used to prevent and treat serious atrial and ventricular dysrhythmias, and for managing acute tachydysrhythmias.

Pharmacokinetics

The pharmacokinetics of amiodarone are subject to large inter-individual variability in bioavailability, plasma concentration and elimination half-life. Additionally, there are pharmacokinetic differences between single dose and chronic administration. Amiodarone is a structural analogue of thyroid hormone and is highly lipophilic. It is poorly absorbed, and its bioavailability ranges from 20% to 86%. It is highly protein bound (> 99%), widely distributed in the body (e.g. in adipose tissues, liver and lung) and reaches steady-state plasma concentration after several weeks. Its onset of action varies from several days to weeks, even if loading doses are administered. It has a biphasic elimination half-life: the initial half-life is 2.5–10 days, and the terminal half-life is 26–107 days. It has one active metabolite, DEA, which has a terminal half-life of about 60 days (Table 10.2).

Drug interactions

Amiodarone inhibits CYP1A2, CYP2C9, CYP2D6 and CYP3A4 and is subject to multiple drug interactions. Examples include:

- Digoxin: Amiodarone increases the plasma concentration of digoxin, causing toxicity. Monitor plasma digoxin concentration and reduce dose of digoxin as necessary. Can also see additive effects of both drugs on the SA node and AV junction.
- Other antidysrhythmic agents: Can increase cardiac effects and the risk of inducing tachydysrhythmias. It also increases the plasma concentration of flecainide by inhibiting its metabolism. If amiodarone must be given with class I antidysrhythmic agents, reduce the dose of the class I drug by 30–50% several days after starting amiodarone.
- Phenytoin: Can result in increased plasma concentration of phenytoin, possibly resulting in toxicity. Monitor plasma concentration of phenytoin and decrease dosage if necessary.
- Warfarin: Can increase anticoagulant effect by inhibiting metabolism of warfarin. Decrease warfarin dose as necessary and monitor the international normalised ratio.

Adverse reactions

These include:

- dizziness, ataxia, bitter taste, headache, blurred vision
- flushing, nausea, vomiting, constipation, weight loss
- tremors, paraesthesiae of fingers and toes
- photosensitivity, blue–grey skin discolouration
- thyroid dysfunction (hypo-, hyperthyroidism)
- pulmonary fibrosis or pneumonitis, cough, fever
- allergic reactions.

Warnings and contraindications

Use amiodarone with caution in people with heart failure and liver or thyroid function impairment.

Avoid use in people with amiodarone hypersensitivity, second- or third-degree AV block and bradycardia.

Dosage and administration

Local protocols for treatment of dysrhythmias should be consulted for oral and IV dosing. Because a variety of IV doses are used in emergencies, local protocols/guidelines/specialist personnel should be consulted before use (e.g. Advanced Life Support [ALS] Guidelines, Australian Resuscitation Council).

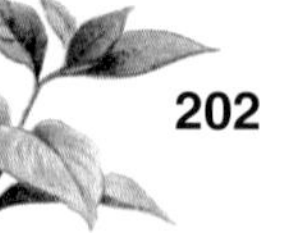

Unclassified antidysrhythmic drugs

Drugs not classified under this scheme include adenosine (Drug Monograph 10.4), atropine (Ch 8), adrenaline (epinephrine) (Ch 9), digoxin and magnesium sulfate heptahydrate.

Digoxin

The digitalis glycosides – that is, those glycosides derived from the *Digitalis* species (e.g. digoxin and digitoxin) – are among the oldest drugs known to affect both cardiac

DRUG MONOGRAPH 10.4
Adenosine

Mechanism of action

Adenosine is a naturally occurring biologically active endogenous molecule in humans that arises following the breakdown of ATP. Adenosine binds to adenosine receptor types A_1, A_{2A}, A_{2B} and A_3, which are G-protein coupled receptors that transduce intracellular signals that modulate different cell responses. Adenosine receptors are widespread throughout the central nervous system but are also found in peripheral tissues including the heart, liver, kidney, adipose tissue, gastrointestinal tract, lung and blood vessels. Examples of actions and physiological responses mediated by adenosine receptor subtypes in the cardiovascular system and kidney are shown below

ADENOSINE RECEPTOR SUBTYPE	ACTION/PHYSIOLOGICAL RESPONSE
A_1	In cardiac tissue, binding to A_1 receptors opens potassium channels, which results in hyperpolarisation of myocytes and a decrease in cyclic adenosine monophosphate (cAMP); this inhibits L-type calcium channels and calcium entry into the cell. In the SA node, adenosine inhibits pacemaker activity, which decreases the slope of phase 4 of the action potential (Fig 10.8), decreasing the spontaneous firing rate and causing a negative chronotropic effect. Inhibition of L-type calcium channels at the AV node causes a negative dromotropic effect because of a reduction in conduction velocity.
	In the kidney, A_1 receptor activation results in vasoconstriction, decreased glomerular filtration rate and inhibition of renin secretion.
A_{2A}	Activation of A_{2A} receptors on coronary smooth muscle cells results in stimulation of adenylyl cyclase, which increases cAMP and ultimately results in smooth muscle relaxation. Increased cAMP also causes smooth muscle relaxation by inhibiting myosin light chain kinase, which leads to decreased myosin phosphorylation and a decrease in contractile force. Upregulation of A_{2A} receptors has been reported in patients with end-stage chronic heart failure.
A_{2B}	A_{2B} receptors found in vascular endothelium and smooth muscle cells of the heart and kidney are thought to regulate vascular tone by exerting vasodilatory effects. Activation of A_{2B} receptors is also thought to prevent cardiac remodelling after myocardial infarction.

Indications

Adenosine is used for:

- acute treatment of supraventricular tachycardia
- cardiac diagnostic procedures.

Pharmacokinetics

Adenosine has a rapid onset of action of less than 2 minutes, and action persists only for the duration of administration. It is rapidly transported into vascular cells and red blood cells (within 10 seconds) where it is phosphorylated by adenosine kinase to form AMP and also metabolised to inosine by adenosine deaminase. Inosine is rapidly (within minutes) metabolised by nucleoside phosphorylase to hypoxanthine, which is detectable in blood. Hypoxanthine is then metabolised by xanthine oxidase to xanthine, which is further metabolised by xanthine oxidase to uric acid. Hypoxanthine, xanthine and uric acid are excreted in urine by the kidneys.

Drug interactions

As caffeine and theophylline are methylxanthines and theophylline acts at adenosine receptors, it is not unexpected that both drugs would antagonise the effects of adenosine. Both caffeine and theophylline should be avoided for 24 hours before any cardiac imaging procedure. A clinically relevant interaction occurs with the antiplatelet drug dipyridamole, which inhibits the cellular uptake of adenosine thereby increasing the risk of bradycardia. If possible, dipyridamole should be ceased 24 hours before any planned use of adenosine or, alternatively, adenosine should be used at a significantly reduced dose.

Adverse reactions

Adverse effects are dose-related and resolve rapidly once drug administration is ceased. The most commonly reported adverse effects include:

- flushing of the head, face and body with a sensation of heat

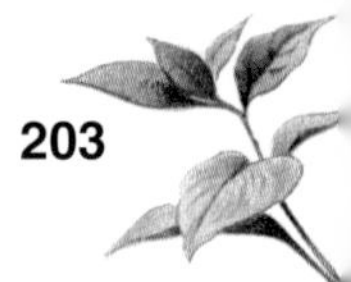

- headache, nausea and dizziness
- chest discomfort, dyspnoea.

With higher doses, first-, second- and third-degree AV block have been reported. Hypotension has also been reported in patients with ischaemic heart disease.

Warnings and contraindications

- Adenosine is contraindicated in patients without a pacemaker who have second- or third-degree heart block or sick sinus syndrome.
- Patients with cardiac dysrhythmias (e.g. AF or atrial flutter) may experience an acceleration in ventricular rate.
- In severe reactive airways disease, adenosine may cause significant bronchoconstriction and hence should be used with extreme caution.

Dosage and administration

For acute treatment of SVT or for diagnostic techniques, hospital or other approved protocols should be consulted before use. Adenosine is administered as an IV bolus followed by a further dose if unsuccessful within 1–2 minutes. For cardiac perfusion imaging, adenosine is administered as an IV infusion.

contractility and rhythm. They increase the force of contraction (positive inotropism) and alter the electrophysiological properties of the heart by slowing the HR (negative chronotropism) and slowing conduction velocity (negative dromotropism).

Digitalis was originally a herbal remedy that was used for hundreds of years by 'common' people (farmers and housewives) for dropsy (fluid accumulation). In the mid-1700s, a female patient shared an old family recipe for curing dropsy with Dr William Withering, who then used it with his dropsy patients. After studying digitalis for 10 years, he published his conclusions in *An Account of the Foxglove*. This remarkable publication stressed instructions that are still valid today – for example, the necessity of individualising dosage according to response. Digitalis was listed in the *London Pharmacopoeia* in 1722.

Indications

Digoxin is the only cardiac glycoside used clinically and was previously a first-line drug for treating heart failure. Its use in that setting has declined in the face of more effective drugs. It is used to treat cardiac dysrhythmias, especially AF, atrial flutter, paroxysmal atrial tachycardia and heart failure. During AF, several hundred impulses originate from the atria, but only a few of them are transmitted through the AV junction. Digoxin slows the ventricular rate because it increases the refractory period of the AV junction and slows conduction at this site, thereby reducing the possibility of ventricular tachycardia.

Mechanism of action

The mechanisms of action of the cardiac glycosides (digoxin, digitoxin and ouabain) are fundamentally the same, with minor differences occurring among the pharmacokinetic parameters of the individual agents. Digoxin inhibits the active transport of sodium and potassium across the myocardial cell membrane by inhibiting the action of the membrane-bound enzyme Na^+–K^+-ATPase. Normally, this enzyme hydrolyses ATP to provide the energy for the Na^+–K^+ pump that expels intracellular sodium and transports potassium into the cardiac cell during repolarisation. Digoxin binds specifically to the α sub-unit of the Na^+–K^+-ATPase and inhibits its action (Fig. 10.6). Intracellular sodium accumulates, which inhibits the extrusion of calcium ions, and hence more intracellular calcium is available to be taken up by the sarcoplasmic reticulum. Free calcium ions are essential for linking the electrical excitation of the cell membrane to the mechanical contraction of the myocardial cell, a mechanism known as excitation–contraction coupling. The increased availability of calcium ions released from the sarcoplasmic reticulum increases the coupling of actin and myosin, which results in more forceful myocardial contraction with a concomitant increase in CO. Inhibition of Na^+–K^+-ATPase activity is proposed to be the mechanism by which the cardiac glycosides increase myocardial contraction without causing increased oxygen consumption.

Digoxin decreases HR and slows conduction velocity by altering the electrophysiological properties of cardiac tissues. At a therapeutic plasma concentration, digoxin decreases automaticity and increases the effective refractory period of atrial tissue and the AV node. These actions are partly direct and partly occur as a result of augmentation of vagal activity (slowing of HR) by a direct effect on the central vagal nuclei, which modifies the excitability of efferent vagal fibres, and by a decrease in the sensitivity of the SA and AV nodes to catecholamines and sympathetic impulses.

With increasing plasma concentration of digoxin, prolongation of the refractory period and depressed conduction in the AV conduction system leads to severe bradycardia and complete heart block. In addition, at toxic plasma concentrations digoxin can increase sympathetic nervous system activity and directly increase automaticity. This increases the rate of spontaneous depolarisation and is one of the mechanisms responsible

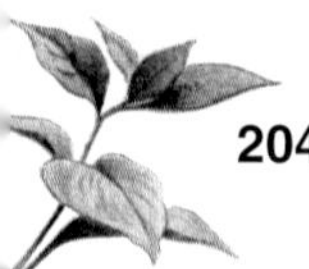

for digitalis-induced ectopic pacemakers. Toxic doses of digitalis can significantly increase impulse formation in latent or potential pacemaker tissue, causing dysrhythmias.

Pharmacokinetics

The absorption of digoxin is influenced by both the oral formulation and the activity of the intestinal efflux transporter P-gp, which reduces absorption. Digoxin is 60–80% absorbed from tablets and 70–85% from the oral liquid. Digoxin is not hepatically metabolised; about 20% of the dose is eliminated by biliary excretion and the remainder is renally excreted as unchanged drug (about 70–80%) in urine. Digoxin is both filtered and secreted, and renal elimination of digoxin is impaired (~16% reduction) by co-administered drugs that inhibit digoxin efflux via the renal P-gp transporter (Fenner et al. 2009). In the presence of normal renal function, the plasma half-life of digoxin is 36–50 hours, thus permitting once-daily dosing, and steady-state plasma concentration is achieved after about 5–7 days. In situations of impaired renal function, the half-life can increase to 3–5 days necessitating dosage adjustment. Use of a loading dose is not usually required for heart failure but is used to treat dysrhythmias. Digoxin is widely distributed to all body tissues, and the concentration of digoxin in tissues such as the heart, liver and skeletal muscle tends to be higher than that in plasma.

Drug interactions

There are multiple drug interactions with digoxin, and relevant drug information sources should always be consulted. Drug Interactions 10.1 lists examples of interactions that decrease absorption and increase or decrease digoxin plasma concentration.

Adverse reactions

Adverse reactions include anorexia and gastrointestinal disturbances such as nausea, vomiting and diarrhoea. Central nervous system effects, such as visual disturbances, confusion, nightmares, agitation and drowsiness, are less frequent, as are dysrhythmias. The dysrhythmias seen with digitalis toxicity are premature ventricular beats, paroxysmal atrial tachycardia with AV block, progressing AV block and ventricular dysrhythmias such as ventricular tachycardia or fibrillation. Loss of appetite, nausea, vomiting and abdominal distress may indicate digoxin toxicity.

Digoxin toxicity

Digoxin has a narrow therapeutic range and people can display toxic effects when the plasma drug concentration is within the therapeutic range (Clinical Focus Box 10.2). Dosage should be individualised depending on the underlying condition (i.e. heart failure or AF) and on assessment of renal function, clinical response and plasma drug concentration monitoring. Elderly people may have

DRUG INTERACTIONS 10.1
Digoxin

DRUG	POSSIBLE EFFECTS	MANAGEMENT
Amiodarone	Marked increase in plasma concentration of digoxin, with increased risk of toxicity; additive effect on slowing cardiac conduction	Reduce dosage of digoxin and monitor plasma digoxin concentration and clinical status, especially bradydysrhythmias
Colestyramine	Decreased absorption of digoxin and reduced efficacy	Separate administration of these drugs; consult relevant sources for further information
Calcium channel-blocking drugs (verapamil and diltiazem)	Increased plasma digoxin concentration, enhanced negative effect on AV conduction and HR	Monitor plasma digoxin concentration and anticipate need to reduce dose
Quinine	Possibly an increase in plasma concentration of digoxin	Monitor plasma concentration and clinical response closely; dosage reduction may be necessary
Spironolactone	Increased plasma digoxin concentration	Monitor plasma digoxin concentration and anticipate need to reduce dose
St John's wort	Possibly decreases plasma digoxin concentration and clinical effect	Avoid combination
Suxamethonium	Risk of dangerous dysrhythmias (e.g. bradydysrhythmia)	Avoid, or potentially serious drug interaction may occur
Ticagrelor	Possibly an increase in plasma concentration of digoxin	Monitor plasma digoxin concentration; observe for adverse effects; anticipate need to reduce dose

Note: This is not an exhaustive list and appropriate drug information resources should be consulted for further drug interactions with digoxin.

Source: Australian Medicines Handbook 2021.

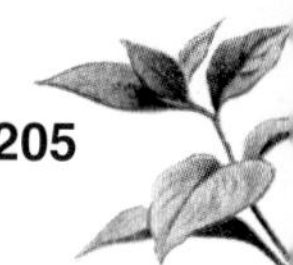

CLINICAL FOCUS BOX 10.2
Therapeutic drug monitoring of plasma digoxin concentration

Digoxin has a narrow therapeutic range of 0.5–2 microgram/L (0.6–2.6 nanomol/L). In situations of chronic heart failure, studies suggest that a plasma concentration of 0.5–0.8 microgram/L (0.6–1.0 nanomol/L) should be the target range. Although adverse effects are in general related to plasma digoxin concentration, often the plasma concentration does not clearly delineate patients with toxic concentrations from those with non-toxic concentrations. Plasma digoxin concentration should be used as a guide in conjunction with clinical observations.

Criteria for determining plasma digoxin concentration include:

- suspected toxicity
- the person's adherence to drug therapy being questionable or unreliable
- failure to respond appropriately to therapy
- presence of impaired renal function
- use of drugs with documented interactions (e.g. quinine, calcium channel blocking drugs)
- confirmation of unusual or abnormal plasma digoxin concentration.

The time that a blood sample is drawn for determination of plasma digoxin concentration is critical. Blood should be taken at least 6 hours after the last oral dose or immediately before the next dose (trough concentration).

age-related renal or hepatic impairment and a decreased volume of distribution for digoxin; thus, lower doses are necessary to avoid toxicity.

Almost every type of dysrhythmia can be produced by digoxin, and the type of dysrhythmia produced varies with age and other factors. Premature ventricular contractions and bigeminal rhythm (two beats and a pause) are common signs of digoxin toxicity in adults, whereas children tend to develop ectopic nodal or atrial beats. Other digoxin-induced dysrhythmias result from depression of the SA and AV nodes, which results in various conduction disturbances (first- or second-degree heart block or complete heart block). Digoxin can also cause increased myocardial automaticity, producing extrasystoles or tachycardia.

Health professionals need to be aware of the predisposing factors for digoxin toxicity. The presence of any of these factors indicates the need for close observation for signs and symptoms of toxicity:

- Hypokalaemia – low potassium concentration can increase digoxin cardiotoxicity. Potassium competes with digoxin for binding to the Na^+–K^+-ATPase pump; a depletion of potassium increases cardiac excitability. Low extracellular potassium increases digoxin binding and enhances ectopic pacemaker activity. Potassium loss can occur as a result of vomiting, diarrhoea or gastric suctioning. Poor dietary intake or severe dietary restrictions that decrease electrolyte intake can also alter potassium levels. The use of corticosteroids and various diuretic agents (e.g. furosemide and thiazide preparations) can induce potassium loss. Corticosteroids cause potassium loss and sodium retention.
- Hypercalcaemia – excess calcium in the presence of digoxin may cause sinus bradycardia, AV conduction block and ectopic dysrhythmia.
- Hypomagnesaemia – low magnesium concentration increases the risk of digoxin toxicity.
- Co-existing conditions – approximately 70% of digoxin is excreted by the kidneys and, in cases of diminished renal function, the plasma half-life of digoxin increases, necessitating dosage reduction. If the patient should develop digoxin toxicity, management becomes an issue because the plasma half-life of digoxin may be in the order of 5 days.

Treatment of digoxin poisoning

The antidote for life-threatening digoxin poisoning is an ovine digoxin-specific antibody fragment (fab). These fragments, which are derived from anti-digoxin antibodies, bind the digoxin molecules, preventing them from binding to the site of action. The digoxin–fragment complex accumulates in blood and is excreted by the kidneys. As more tissue digoxin is released into the blood to maintain equilibrium, it is bound by the antibody fragments and removed, which results in a lower concentration of digoxin in tissues, thereby reversing its effects.

After IV administration the onset of action is rapid and initial signs of improvement in digoxin toxicity may be seen within 15–30 minutes. The half-life of digoxin immune fab appears to be in the order of 15–20 hours, but data on use in humans are limited.

Close monitoring is necessary, as withdrawal of digoxin can result in a decrease in CO, congestive heart failure and hypokalaemia. An increase in ventricular rate may be seen in people with AF. Safety of digoxin immune fab has not been completely defined because of its limited use. There are no known contraindications to use, but caution should be exercised in people with kidney function impairment, a history of allergies (particularly to sheep proteins) and in those previously treated with digoxin immune fab.

The adult dose varies according to the amount of digoxin that is required to be complexed. One vial of antibody binds approximately 0.5 mg digoxin. The dose required can be calculated from the number of tablets ingested or from the plasma digoxin concentration. The full product information should be consulted for calculation of the dosage of digoxin antibodies, and the shelf expiration date of the product checked before use.

Magnesium sulfate heptahydrate

Magnesium sulfate heptahydrate blocks calcium entry by inhibiting L-type calcium channels during phase 3 of the action potential, an effect that potentially could shorten the QT interval. It also blocks the outward movement of potassium via potassium channels, which could potentially prolong the QT interval. These counterbalancing cellular actions may terminate torsade de pointes independently of the QT interval. Magnesium sulfate heptahydrate also decreases early after-depolarisations, contributing to an antidysrhythmic effect.

It is cleared renally, and hypermagnesaemia is an issue in situations of renal impairment. Adverse effects relate to hypermagnesaemia and include loss of deep tendon reflexes and respiratory depression resulting from neuromuscular blockade. The latter is potentiated in combination with aminoglycosides, and the combination should be used with extreme caution and with monitoring of respiratory function.

KEY POINTS

Dysrhythmias and antidysrhythmic drugs

- Antidysrhythmic drugs are used to prevent and treat cardiac rhythm disorders.
- Cardiac dysrhythmias are usually the result of an abnormality in the electrophysiology of the cells in the cardiac conduction system or cardiac muscle cells.
- The antidysrhythmic drugs are subdivided into four classes (I–IV) according to their mechanism of action.
- Class Ia, Ib and Ic drugs suppress automaticity. Class Ia includes disopyramide, which decreases conduction velocity and prolongs the action potential.
- Class Ib drugs (e.g. lidocaine) may increase or have no effect on conduction velocity.
- The class Ic drug flecainide is indicated for treating or preventing supraventricular tachydysrhythmias.
- Class II drugs have β-adrenergic-blocking action and are discussed in Chapter 9.
- The class III drugs are amiodarone and sotalol.
- The class IV drugs have calcium channel blocking activity and are discussed in Chapter 11.
- Unclassified antidysrhythmic agents include adenosine, digoxin and magnesium sulfate heptahydrate.
- Digoxin decreases HR and slows conduction. It is used to treat cardiac dysrhythmias, especially atrial flutter and fibrillation, and heart failure.
- Digoxin has a narrow therapeutic index, can exacerbate or worsen dysrhythmias and is subject to many serious drug interactions.
- Several factors, such as hypokalaemia, hypercalcaemia and hypomagnesaemia, may predispose to digoxin toxicity.
- Ovine digoxin-specific antibody fragment is used to treat digoxin poisoning.
- All antidysrhythmic drugs are potent medications that require careful selection and close monitoring to avoid drug-induced adverse effects.

DRUGS AT A GLANCE

Drugs affecting cardiac function

PHARMACOLOGICAL GROUP AND EFFECT	KEY EXAMPLES	CLINICAL USE
Antidysrhythmic drugs[a] • ↓ AV conduction • ↓ contractility • ↑ or ↓ action potential duration • ↑ effective refractory period • ↓ rate of depolarisation	Adenosine	• Acute treatment of SVT • Aid in myocardial perfusion imaging
	Amiodarone	• Serious tachydysrhythmias
	Disopyramide	• Life-threatening ventricular tachydysrhythmias
	Flecainide	• Serious ventricular dysrhythmias • SVT • Paroxysmal AF or atrial flutter
	Lidocaine (lignocaine)	• Serious ventricular dysrhythmias

	Propafenone[b]	• Supraventricular extrasystoles • Supraventricular tachycardia • Wolff-Parkinson-White syndrome • Serious ventricular tachydysrhythmias
	Sotalol	• Treatment and prevention of dysrhythmias
Antianginal drug • I_f channel inhibitor • Interferes with depolarisations of SA node • ↓ HR	Ivabradine	• Angina with HR > 70 beats/minute
Cardiac glycoside • ↑ myocardial contraction • ↓ HR and AV nodal conduction • ↑ vagal tone	Digoxin	• AF and atrial flutter • Heart failure
Drugs for heart failure • PDE3 inhibitor • ↑ calcium influx into sarcoplasmic reticulum • ↑ force of myocardial contraction	Milrinone	• Severe heart failure • Low CO states
• Neprilysin inhibitor • ↓ degradation of natriuretic peptides • Blocks angiotensin II • Vasodilator • ↓ sympathetic tone	Sacubitril with valsartan	• Heart failure

[a] Not all antidysrhythmic drugs have all properties
[b] New Zealand only
AF = atrial fibrillation; SVT = supraventricular tachycardia

REVIEW EXERCISES

1 Mr BC is a 65-year-old male with a history of atrial fibrillation. He has been feeling unwell for several weeks and was recently admitted for observation. The admitting doctor has taken some blood to determine Mr BC's plasma digoxin concentration. The student nurse asks you to explain why digoxin is beneficial for AF and why the blood was taken before Mr BC's next digoxin dose.

2 Edith, a nurse practitioner, has been explaining to you the classification of antidysrhythmic drugs. She asks you to explain the pharmacological effects of amiodarone and why it is contraindicated for use in people with second- or third-degree heart block.

REFERENCES

Australian Medicines Handbook. Adelaide: Australian Medicines Handbook Pty Ltd; 2021

Bozkurt B, Coats AJS, Tsutsui H, et al. Universal definition and classification of heart failure: A report of the Heart Failure Society of America, Heart Failure Association of the European Society of Cardiology, Japanese Heart Failure Society and Writing Committee of the Universal Definition of Heart Failure. European Journal of Heart Failure 2021;23:352-80.

Fenner KS, Troutmen MD, Kempshall S, et al. Drug–drug interactions mediated through P-glycoprotein: clinical relevance and in vitro-in vivo correlation using digoxin as a probe drug. Clinical Pharmacology & Therapeutics 2009;85:173–81.

Flarakos J, Du Y, Bedman T, et al. Disposition and metabolism of [^{14}C] Sacubitril/Valsartan (formerly LCZ696) an angiotensin receptor neprilysin inhibitor, in healthy subjects. Xenobiotica 2016;46:986-1000.

National Heart Foundation of Australia and Cardiac Society of Australia and New Zealand: Guidelines for the Prevention, Detection, and Management of Heart Failure in Australia 2018. Heart, Lung and Circulation 2018; 27:1123–208.

Noble D: The initiation of the heartbeat, Oxford, 1975, Oxford University Press.

Rang HP: Rang and Dale's pharmacology, ed 7, 2012, Elsevier.

Salerno E: Pharmacology for health professionals, St Louis, 1999, Mosby.

Thummel KE, Shen DD, Isoherranen N. Design and optimization of dosage regimens: Pharmacokinetic data. In: Brunton LL, Hilal-Dandan R, Knollmann BC, editors. Goodman & Gilman's The pharmacological basis of therapeutics. 13th ed. New York: McGraw Hill; 2018, p1325–1378.

Vardeny O, Miller R, Solomon SD. Combined neprilysin and renin-angiotensin system inhibition for the treatment of heart failure, JACC: Heart Failure 2014;2:663–70.

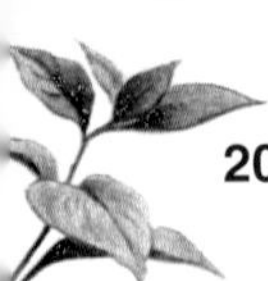

ONLINE RESOURCES

American Heart Association: https://www.heart.org/ (accessed 28 February 2022)
Cardiac Society of Australia and New Zealand: https://www.csanz.edu.au/ (accessed 28 February 2022)
European Society of Cardiology: https://www.escardio.org/ (accessed 28 February 2022)
Heart Foundation: https://www.heartfoundation.org.au/ (accessed 28 February 2022)

More weblinks at: http://evolve.elsevier.com/AU/Knights/pharmacology/.

CHAPTER 11

DRUGS AFFECTING VASCULAR SMOOTH MUSCLE

Kathleen Knights

KEY ABBREVIATIONS

ACE	angiotensin-converting enzyme
ARB	angiotensin receptor blocker
CYP	cytochromes P450
eNOS	endothelium nitric oxide synthase
GTN	glyceryl trinitrate
NO	nitric oxide
RAAS	renin–angiotensin–aldosterone system

KEY TERMS

Chapter Focus

The focus of this chapter is drugs that produce vasodilation by relaxing vascular smooth muscle by either a direct or an indirect action. Some drugs act primarily on veins or arterioles, while others dilate both types of blood vessels. The principal uses of these drugs, which include the organic nitrates, calcium channel blockers, potassium channel activators, angiotensin-converting enzyme inhibitors and angiotensin receptor antagonists, are in the treatment of angina, hypertension and heart failure. These drugs are frequently prescribed, either alone or in combination therapy.

KEY DRUG GROUPS

Drugs for angina:

- Nitrates: **glyceryl trinitrate** (Drug Monograph 11.1)
- Potassium channel activator: **nicorandil**

Drugs for hypertension:

- Aldosterone receptor antagonists: **eplerenone** (Drug Monograph 11.4), **spironolactone**
- Angiotensin-converting enzyme (ACE) inhibitors: **captopril**, **enalapril**, **fosinopril**, **lisinopril**, **perindopril** (Drug Monograph 11.2), **quinapril**, **ramipril**, **trandolapril**
- Angiotensin-receptor (AT_1) antagonists (also called angiotensin-receptor blockers [ARBs]): **candesartan**, **eprosartan**, **irbesartan**, **losartan**, **olmesartan**, **telmisartan**, **valsartan** (Drug Monograph 11.3)
- Calcium channel blockers: **amlodipine**, **clevidipine**, **diltiazem**, **felodipine**, **lercanidipine**, **nifedipine**, **nimodipine**, **verapamil**
- Centrally acting adrenergic inhibitors: **clonidine**, **methyldopa**, **moxonidine**
- Potassium channel activators: **diazoxide**, **minoxidil**

Drugs for peripheral vascular disease:

- Pentoxifylline (oxpentifylline), oxerutins (hydroxyethylrutosides)

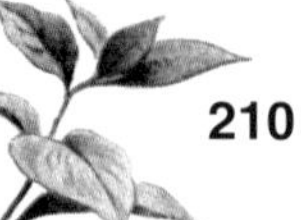

CRITICAL THINKING SCENARIO

For acute angina, glyceryl trinitrate sublingual spray (400 micrograms/dose) was prescribed for Andrea, with instructions to use 1–2 sprays and repeat after 5 minutes if necessary but to not exceed 2 sprays in total. Discuss the physiological/pharmacological reasons why glyceryl trinitrate is preferentially administered sublingually rather than via the oral route.

Introduction: The vascular system

The vascular system comprises arteries and arterioles, and venules and veins, that carry blood away from and back to the heart, respectively. Arterioles and capillaries are the main resistance vessels and regulate afterload, while the venules and veins are capacitance vessels, contributing to preload of the ventricles. The arterial wall consists of three layers: the inner (*tunica intima*), the middle (*tunica media*) and the outer (*tunica adventitia*). The middle (thickest) layer is composed of elastic and smooth muscle fibres, and the outer of elastic and collagen fibres. Actin and myosin are present in smooth muscle, but the striations are not visible (unlike skeletal and cardiac muscle) and the relationship between actin and myosin is less highly organised.

The smooth muscle is arranged in a circular layer, and stimulation by the sympathetic nervous system causes contraction of the smooth muscle, which narrows the lumen of the vessel (vasoconstriction). In contrast, a diminution in sympathetic stimulation results in relaxation of the smooth muscle (vasodilation). The elastic properties of the arteries enable distension when the ventricles eject a volume of blood, and the elastic recoil aids in the forward propulsion of the blood.

Arteries branch to form arterioles and capillaries, the main resistance vessels, which play a key role in blood pressure regulation. Capillaries are the smallest of the arterial vessels and connect the arterioles to the venules. The combined resistance of the systemic blood vessels, but principally the arterioles, capillaries and venules, is referred to as systemic vascular resistance (SVR) or total peripheral resistance.

Venules are the conduits through which blood flows from the capillaries to the veins. Veins consist of the same three layers as arteries, but these differ in terms of their relative thickness, with the *tunica adventitia* forming the thickest layer. Unlike arteries, veins have a system of valves that ensure blood flows in a forward direction towards the heart. About 60% of the blood volume is contained within the systemic veins and venules; hence, they are referred to as capacitance vessels.

The vascular endothelium

The luminal surface of the *tunica intima* is lined with a single layer of nucleated endothelial cells that are linked together laterally by tight junctions. Endothelial cells act as a barrier (which may be ruptured, see Ch 12), control contraction of vascular smooth muscle and play an active role in haemostasis and thrombosis (Ch 13). In addition, these cells are a source of multiple endogenous mediators that influence vascular function through either vasodilation or vasoconstriction (Fig 11.1). An important mediator is nitric oxide (NO), which is synthesised from L-arginine, present in endothelial cells, by the action of an isoform of NO synthase called endothelium nitric oxide synthase (eNOS) or NOS-III. Endothelium-dependent agonists such as acetylcholine and substance P bind to receptors on the surface of the endothelial cell and increase the intracellular concentration of calcium ions that, in a complex with calmodulin, activate eNOS. The NO formed acts locally on the adjacent vascular smooth muscle cell where it activates guanylyl cyclase, which converts guanosine triphosphate (GTP) into cyclic guanosine monophosphate (cGMP). The increase in cGMP inactivates myosin light-chain kinase and the accompanying decrease in intracellular calcium results in vascular relaxation (Fig 11.1). Other important endothelium-derived mediators include PGI_2 (prostacyclin) (Ch 34), angiotensin (discussed later in this chapter) and endothelin-1, which causes vasoconstriction (Fig 11.1).

Smooth muscle action potentials

Vascular smooth muscle depends primarily on the presence of calcium ions to initiate and sustain contraction. It is believed that the onset of depolarisation (phase 0) in smooth muscle is caused mainly by calcium ions rather than by sodium ions. There are three mechanisms that can lead to an increase in calcium ions, which then triggers smooth muscle contraction: (1) calcium entry through voltage-gated L-type calcium channels; (2) calcium release from the smooth endoplasmic reticulum of the smooth muscle cell; and (3) calcium entry through either ligand-gated channels or channels activated by

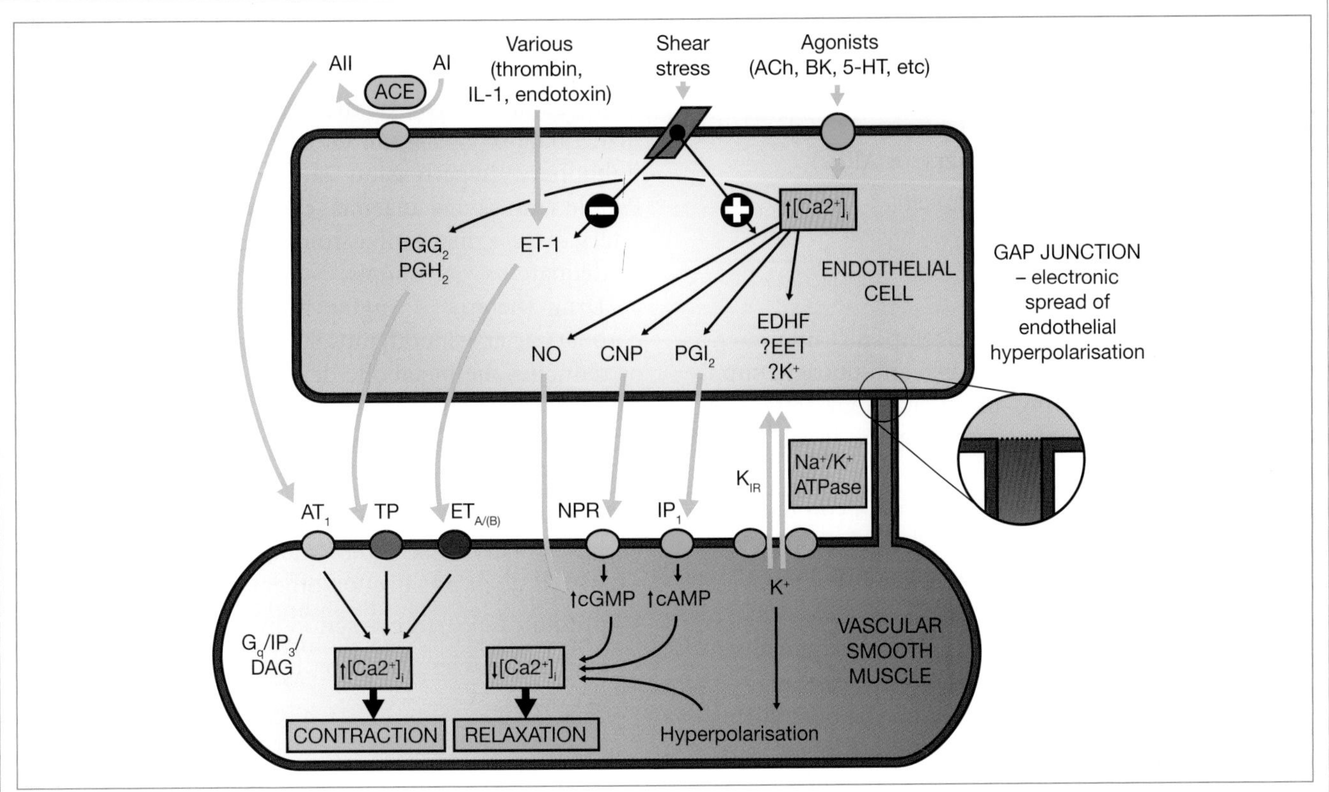

FIGURE 11.1 Endothelium-derived mediators The schematic shows some of the more important endothelium-derived contracting and relaxing mediators; many (if not all) of the vasoconstrictors also cause smooth muscle mitogenesis, while vasodilators commonly inhibit mitogenesis. 5-HT = 5-hydroxytryptamine; A = angiotensin; ACE = angiotensin-converting enzyme; ACh = acetylcholine; AT_1 = angiotensin AT_1 receptor; BK = bradykinin; CNP = C-natriuretic peptide; DAG = diacylglycerol; EDHF = endothelium-derived hyperpolarising factor; EET = epoxyeicosatetraenoic acid; ET-1 = endothelin-1; $ET_{A/(B)}$ = endothelium A (and B) receptors; G_q = G-protein; IL-1 = interleukin-1; IP_1 = prostanoid receptor; IP_3 = inosinol 1,4,5-trisphosphate; K_{IR} = inward rectifying potassium channel; Na^+/K^+ ATPase electrogenic pump; NPR = natriuretic peptide receptor; PG = prostaglandin; TP = T prostanoid receptor.

Source: Adapted from Rang et al. 2012, Figure 22.1; used with permission.

G-protein-coupled receptors. In smooth muscle the action potential generally has a slower upstroke and longer duration than that observed in skeletal muscle action potentials. The upstroke or depolarising phase reflects the opening of voltage-gated L-type calcium channels and influx of calcium ions that causes more voltage-gated calcium channels to open. The slow rise of the action potential is due to the slowness of opening of the calcium channels in contrast to the more rapid opening of sodium channels in skeletal and cardiac muscle. The repolarisation phase is also relatively slow because of a combination of the slow inactivation of L-type calcium channels and the slow activation of voltage-gated potassium channels and calcium-activated potassium channels.

The rise in free calcium ion concentration is considered to be the primary event in triggering smooth muscle contraction via the calcium–calmodulin complex that activates myosin light chain kinase (Ch 10), increasing smooth muscle tone and causing vasoconstriction (Fig 11.1). Activation of smooth muscle can reduce the calibre of small vessels markedly, as is apparent from the 'spasm' that may occur in coronary vessels. Calcium channel-blocking drugs are capable of blocking the slow calcium ion influx in smooth muscle of blood vessels, thereby producing relaxation. Modulation of calcium concentration forms the basis for the actions of a range of drugs that affect the vascular system. Drugs causing vasoconstriction by acting on α-adrenoceptors (e.g. α-adrenoceptor agonists such as adrenaline (epinephrine)) and vasodilation (α_1-adrenoceptor antagonists such as prazosin) are discussed in Chapter 9.

This chapter describes drugs that directly and indirectly affect vascular smooth muscle contraction. Emphasis is on **vasodilator drugs** used for to treat a variety of disorders including hypertension, angina, shock, cardiac failure and peripheral vascular conditions. The main groups of drugs to be discussed are:

1 Direct-acting vasodilators:
   - nitrates
   - calcium channel blockers
   - potassium channel activators.

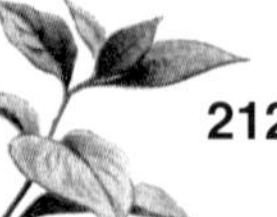

2 Indirect-acting vasodilators:
- centrally acting adrenergic inhibitors
- angiotensin-converting enzyme (ACE) inhibitors
- angiotensin (AT_1) receptor antagonists (also called angiotensin receptor blockers, or ARBs)
- aldosterone receptor antagonists.

Angina

The term **angina pectoris** refers to temporary interference with blood flow that reduces oxygen and nutrient supply to heart muscle, resulting in intermittent myocardial ischaemia, typically characterised by pain. It can be of a number of types:

- *Stable angina* is usually associated with coronary arteriosclerosis, and the pain predictably occurs with exertion or stress (e.g. cold, fear, emotion) and after eating.
- *Unstable angina* is a progressive form of angina in which pain occurs more frequently and becomes more severe with time. The pain may appear during rest and may last longer, with less relief by antianginal drugs. People with this condition eventually show signs and symptoms of impending MI or coronary failure.
- *Variant angina* (Prinzmetal's angina) is uncommon and is caused by focal spasm of coronary arteries. In about 75% of people, the spasm occurs near an area of atherosclerosis. The pain often occurs during rest or without any cause.

When coronary blood flow is inadequate, hypoxia causes an accumulation of pain-producing substances such as lactic acid (an anaerobic metabolite) and other chemicals such as potassium ions, kinins and adenosine. Stimulation of cardiac sensory nerve endings, which transmit impulses to the central nervous system (CNS), results in the typical anginal pain. Coronary atherosclerosis or vasomotor spasm of the coronary vessels may cause inadequate oxygenation. Other causes of angina may be pulmonary hypertension and valvular heart disease. People with severe anaemia, even with minimal coronary artery disease, may suffer from anginal attacks because of inadequate oxygen supply.

Drug therapy of angina is aimed at either relaxing coronary artery smooth muscle, thus improving perfusion, or reducing the metabolic demand of the heart, or both. An ideal antianginal drug:

- establishes a balance between coronary blood flow and the metabolic demands of the heart
- has a local rather than a systemic effect, acting directly on coronary vessels to promote coronary vasodilation with little or no effect on other organ systems
- promotes oxygen extraction by the heart
- is effective when taken orally and has a sustained action
- is devoid of tolerance.

Currently, no one drug meets all these criteria and the drugs now available provide only temporary relief (Clinical Focus Box 11.1).

KEY POINTS

The vascular system

- Arterioles and capillaries are the main resistance vessels and regulate afterload. Venules and veins are capacitance vessels contributing to preload.

CLINICAL FOCUS BOX 11.1

Management of acute coronary syndrome

Guidelines for the management of acute coronary syndromes (ACS) were published jointly by the National Heart Foundation of Australia and the Cardiac Society of Australia and New Zealand in 2016 (Chew et al. 2016). The key evidence-based recommendations include:

- initial assessment of ACS should involve a 12-lead ECG with clinical interpretation within 10 minutes of first presentation
- care is guided by a Suspected ACS Assessment Protocol
- cardiac-specific troponin concentration is measured on presentation and at clearly defined periods thereafter.

Recommendations for long-term management include, where appropriate:

- dual antiplatelet therapy with aspirin (100–150 mg/daily) and either clopidogrel or ticagrelor for up to 12 months irrespective of whether coronary revascularisation was performed
- the highest tolerated dose of a statin should be initiated and continued indefinitely.

Not surprisingly, lifestyle education, cardiac rehabilitation programs and chest pain action plans now form part of the long-term management strategy. Check regularly for updates and amendments on the Heart Foundation website (see 'Online resources').

- Endothelial cells control vascular smooth muscle tone and play an active role in haemostasis and thrombosis.
- Endothelial mediators include NO, prostacyclin (PGI_2), angiotensin II and endothelin-1.
- A rise in free calcium ion concentration is considered the primary event in increasing smooth muscle tone and causing vasoconstriction.
- 'Angina' refers to temporary interference with coronary blood flow that reduces oxygen and nutrient supply to heart muscle. Intermittent myocardial ischaemia is typically characterised by pain.

Direct-acting vasodilator drugs

Organic nitrates

The nitrates – glyceryl trinitrate, isosorbide dinitrate and isosorbide mononitrate – are very effective drugs for treating angina pectoris because of their dilating effects on veins and arteries (Drug Monograph 11.1). The resulting pooling of blood in the veins (capacitance blood vessels) decreases the amount of blood returned to the heart (preload), which reduces left ventricular end-diastolic volume. This decrease in venous return helps reduce myocardial oxygen demand. (Chest pain caused by angina pectoris largely results from an inadequate supply of oxygen to the heart.)

DRUG MONOGRAPH 11.1
Glyceryl trinitrate

Glyceryl trinitrate (GTN) is the key drug in the organic nitrate category. It is available as a spray, transdermal patch or injection (IV infusion). The other drugs in this category include isosorbide dinitrate, which is available as a sublingual tablet, and isosorbide mononitrate, available as a controlled-release formulation.

Mechanism of action

Chemically, GTN is a polyol ester of nitric acid, which is metabolised initially by mitochondrial aldehyde dehydrogenase (ALDH-2) to nitrite prior to the release of the biologically active gaseous NO. The release of NO activates soluble guanylyl cyclase in vascular smooth muscle, thereby increasing formation of cGMP. This in turn leads to changes in the degree of phosphorylation of smooth muscle proteins. Ultimately, dephosphorylation of the myosin light chain leads to relaxation (Fig 11.1).

GTN at low doses causes venodilation, with little effect on arterial resistance vessels. This reduces preload and stroke volume. With higher doses, dilation of arteries occurs, resulting in a reduction in arterial pressure which, coupled with venous pooling when standing, often results in postural hypotension and dizziness. The reduction in both cardiac output and arterial pressure reduces the oxygen demand by the myocardium. Nitrates also dilate normal coronary and coronary collateral vessels. The resultant increased coronary perfusion, and hence oxygen delivery, ensures more efficient distribution of blood to ischaemic areas of the myocardium. The organic nitrates do not significantly change contractility or heart rate.

Indications

GTN is used to:
- prevent or treat stable angina
- treat unstable angina and heart failure associated with acute MI.

Pharmacokinetics

GTN is rapidly metabolised by the liver to dinitrates that have about 10% of the biological activity of the parent drug (Table 11.1).

Drug interactions

The concurrent use of nitrates with alcohol, antihypertensives, other drugs causing hypotension and vasodilators (including sildenafil, tadalafil and vardenafil) may result in enhanced orthostatic hypotensive effects.

Adverse reactions

These primarily result from vasodilation and include:
- headache, dizziness, orthostatic hypotension, palpitations
- nausea or vomiting
- agitation, facial flushing, dry mouth, rash and blurred vision.

Warnings and contraindications

Nitrates are contraindicated in people with:

- cardiomyopathy, hypotension, hypovolaemia
- aortic or mitral stenosis
- severe anaemia
- raised intracranial pressure and glaucoma
- concurrent use of sildenafil.

Dosage and administration

See Table 11.1. Sublingual tablets and the sublingual spray are used during an acute attack or during an episode of angina. The sublingual tablet is placed under the tongue or in the buccal pouch allowing it to dissolve fully, or the aerosol is sprayed under the tongue. The person should not swallow, eat, drink or smoke while the tablet is in the mouth. After use of sublingual preparations, a transient headache lasting 15–20 minutes and flushing may occur.

The sublingual tablets should be stored in a tightly closed container and dated when first opened. The container should not be left opened, exposed to heat or moisture and should be stored below 30 degrees Celsius.

The sublingual spray should not be inhaled, and the mouth should be closed immediately after delivering the dose. If using a pump delivery system, the pump may need to be primed to ensure an even spray.

Oral controlled-release tablets should not be crushed or chewed but swallowed whole with a full glass of water.

Transdermal GTN is a patch system that contains a drug reservoir from which the drug is slowly released (passive diffusion). The drug is absorbed through the skin and transported by blood to the site of action to produce its beneficial effects. This system is applied daily to a hairless skin area, usually on the chest (preferred site), shoulder or inside upper arm. The site should be changed to avoid skin irritation but avoid applying the patch to extremities, especially below the knee or elbow.

Transdermal systems with different release rates are available (releasing ~0.2–0.6 mg/h), and each has a different mechanism for drug delivery. The systems should not be considered interchangeable. (Figure 11.2 provides an illustration of transdermal systems.) As tolerance develops to GTN, it is recommended that the patch be applied for 12–14 hours and removed for 10–12 hours each day. This drug-free interval helps to maintain the efficacy of the product.

TABLE 11.1 Pharmacokinetics and dosages of nitrates

DRUG	ONSET OF ACTION	DURATION OF ACTION (h)	METABOLISM	EXCRETION	USUAL ADULT DOSE
Glyceryl trinitrate			Liver	Kidneys	
Sublingual spray	2–4 minutes	< 1			Acute angina: 400–800 micrograms (1 or 2 sprays) after 5 minutes 1 further spray (maximum of 3 sprays)
Transdermal patch	30–60 minutes	Depends on duration of application			Prevention of chronic angina: use 5 mg/24 hours patch once daily for ~12–14 hours/day
IV infusion	Immediate	Variable[a]			Unstable angina: 5–10 micrograms/minute increased by 5 micrograms/minute every 3–5 minutes until desired response
Isosorbide dinitrate			Liver	Kidneys	
Sublingual tablet	2–5 minutes	1–2			Acute angina: 5–10 mg
Isosorbide mononitrate			Liver/kidneys	Kidneys	
Controlled-release tablet	1–2 hours	~24			Prevention of angina: 30–60 mg once daily to a maximum of 120 mg daily

[a] Depends on duration of infusion.

Source: Dosage information: Australian Medicines Handbook 2021, pp. 243–245. Verify adult dose range using up-to-date drug/product information sources.

Calcium Channel Blockers

Mechanism of action

The **calcium channel blockers**, while having diverse chemical structures, all block the inward movement of calcium through the slow channels of the cell membranes of cardiac and smooth muscle cells. This activity, however, varies according to the tissue/cells: cardiac muscle, or myocardium; the cardiac conduction system (SA and AV nodes); and vascular smooth muscle. These drugs are used to treat angina, supraventricular tachydysrhythmias (verapamil), hypertension and cerebral vasospasm after subarachnoid haemorrhage (nimodipine).

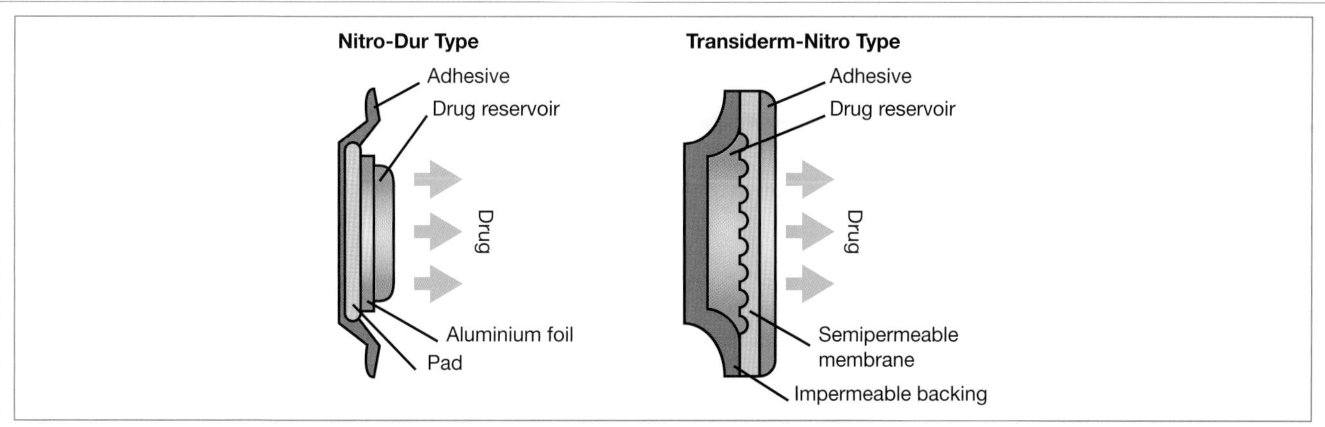

FIGURE 11.2 Transdermal systems Nitro-Dur is a gel-like matrix surrounded by fluid. Transiderm-Nitro contains a semipermeable membrane between the drug reservoir and the skin that controls the drug delivery.

Effects on myocardium

Calcium channel blockers decrease the force of myocardial contraction by blocking the inward flow of calcium ions through the slow channels of the cell membrane during phase 2 (plateau phase) of the action potential (Fig 10.3 in Ch 10). The diminished entry of calcium ions fails to trigger the release of large amounts of calcium from the sarcoplasmic reticulum within the cell. This free calcium is needed for excitation–contraction coupling, an event that activates contraction by allowing cross-bridges to form between the actin and myosin filaments of muscle. The force of contraction by the heart is determined by the number of actin–myosin cross-bridges formed within the sarcomere. Decreasing the amount of calcium ions released from the sarcoplasmic reticulum results in fewer actin–myosin cross-bridges being formed, thus decreasing the force of contraction and resulting in a negative inotropic effect.

Effects on SA node and AV junction

In these tissues, calcium channel blockers decrease automaticity in the SA node and decrease conduction in the AV junction. Depolarisation (phase 0) of the action potential is normally generated by the inward calcium ion current through the slow channels. These drugs block the inward calcium ion current across the cell membrane of the SA node, decreasing the rate of depolarisation and depressing automaticity. The result is a decrease in heart rate (negative chronotropic effect). Similarly, decreasing calcium ion influx across the cell membrane of the AV junction slows AV conduction (negative dromotropic effect) and prolongs AV refractory time. When AV conduction is prolonged, fewer atrial impulses reach the ventricles, thus slowing the rate of ventricular contractions.

Effects on vascular smooth muscle

The effect of calcium channel blockers on smooth muscle of the coronary and peripheral vessels has a significant influence on cardiovascular haemodynamics. Coronary artery dilation occurs, which lowers coronary resistance and improves blood flow through collateral vessels, as well as improving oxygen delivery to ischaemic areas of the heart.

These agents also inhibit the contraction of smooth muscle of the peripheral arterioles. This results in widespread reduction in resistance to blood flow through the body (determined by the tone of the vascular musculature and the diameter of the blood vessels) and blood pressure. The haemodynamic change reduces afterload, which also decreases oxygen demand of the heart.

The calcium channel blockers include the:

- phenylalkylamine type (verapamil)
- benzothiazepine type (diltiazem)
- dihydropyridine type (amlodipine, clevidipine, felodipine, nifedipine, nimodipine and lercanidipine).

Verapamil was the first calcium channel blocker released. It has greater effects on the heart, reducing AV conduction and blocking the SA node, resulting in a decrease in heart rate and contractility. It is considered a moderate peripheral vasodilator. Diltiazem has similar pharmacological effects on vascular tissue but has less effect on the heart than verapamil. These agents dilate coronary arteries and arterioles, inhibit coronary artery spasm and dilate peripheral arterioles, reducing total peripheral resistance (afterload), thus lowering arterial blood pressure at rest and during exercise.

The dihydropyridine drugs, exemplified by nifedipine, have minimal effect on cardiac tissue at therapeutic doses. They act principally on vascular smooth muscle, reducing peripheral vascular resistance. In some circumstances, the reflex sympathetic response to vasodilation results in tachycardia, which may be deleterious. Table 11.2 provides a comparison of the cardiovascular effects of different types of calcium channel blockers. Clevidipine is an

TABLE 11.2 Comparison of cardiovascular effects of calcium channel-blocking drugs

EFFECTS	AMLODIPINE	DILTIAZEM	FELODIPINE	NIFEDIPINE	VERAPAMIL
Contractility	↑	↓	↑	0/↓	↓↓
Vasodilation					
Coronary	↑	↑↑↑	↑	↑↑	↑↑
Peripheral	↑↑↑	↑	↑↑	↑↑↑	↑
Heart rate	+/−	0/↓	↑	↑	↑↓
Cardiac output	↑	0/↑	↑	↑	↑↓

↑ = slight increase; ↓ = slight decrease; ↑↑ = intermediate increase; ↓↓ = intermediate decrease; ↑↑↑ = significant increase; ↓↓↓ = significant decrease; +/− = minimal effect; 0 = no effect.

TABLE 11.3 Pharmacokinetics and dosages of oral calcium channel-blocking drugs

DRUG/INDICATION	TIME TO PEAK CONCENTRATION (h)	DURATION OF ACTION (h)	METABOLISM	USUAL ADULT ORAL DAILY DOSE
Amlodipine/A, H	6–8	~24	Hepatic	2.5–5 mg daily, max 10 mg/daily
Diltiazem/A, H	2–3	4–8	Hepatic	For angina, atrial flutter and AF 30 mg 3–4 times daily; increase gradually as required to a max of 360 mg/day
Controlled-release	6–11	12	Hepatic	180 mg once daily to a max of 360 mg once daily
Felodipine/H (controlled-release)	2.5–5	24	Hepatic	Maintenance dose; 5–10 mg once daily to a max of 20 mg once daily
Lercanidipine/H	1.5–3	24	Hepatic	10 mg once daily increasing to 20 mg (max) once daily. Use 10 mg dose for at least 2 weeks before increasing dose
*Nifedipine/A, H	0.5–1	4–8	Hepatic	❖10–20 mg twice daily to a max of 20–40 mg twice daily
Controlled-release			Hepatic	Hypertension: initially 30 mg/day; may titrate over 7–14 days to max 120 mg/day according to response Chronic stable angina: initially 30 mg/day; may increase to max 90 mg/day
+Nimodipine	1–1.5	No data	Hepatic	Consult local protocols. 60 mg 6 times daily
#Verapamil/A, H	1–2	8–10	Hepatic	For angina, 80 mg 2–3 times daily to a max of 160 mg 2–3 times daily
Controlled-release		24		180–240 mg daily to a max of 240 mg twice daily

A = angina: H = hypertension
*Also used for preterm labour
Conventional tablets: + Used following aneurysmal subarachnoid haemorrhage; # also used for SVT, AF, atrial flutter and cluster headache.
Source: Dosage information: Australian Medicines Handbook 2021, pp. 264–268. Verify adult dose range using up-to-date drug/product information sources.

arterial vasodilator administered IV and is used short term mainly for perioperative hypertension when oral dosing is not appropriate. It is unique in that its onset and termination of action are both rapid, the latter due to rapid hydrolysis by blood and tissue esterases. Nimodipine, a dihydropyridine, was developed specifically to dilate cerebral blood vessels. It is indicated to treat cerebral ischaemia after subarachnoid haemorrhage.

Pharmacokinetics

See Table 11.3 for pharmacokinetics of the calcium channel-blocking agents. Most of these drugs are metabolised to some degree by CYP3A4. Diltiazem is metabolised to a major metabolite, desacetyldiltiazem, which may be responsible for up to 50% of its coronary vasodilation. Norverapamil, the active metabolite of verapamil, accounts for about 20% of the antihypertensive effect of verapamil. Nifedipine has no known active metabolite, while the other agents have metabolites that have varying therapeutic effects. Nimodipine is highly lipophilic and crosses the blood–brain barrier, having a greater effect on cerebral arteries than other arteries in the body.

Drug interactions

With the exception of clevidipine, the common involvement of CYP3A4 leads to extensive drug interactions that vary for each of the other calcium channel-blocking drugs. Relevant drug information sources should always be consulted. Examples include:

- *β-adrenoceptor antagonists:* An increased risk of bradycardia occurs with co-administration with diltiazem, and monitoring of cardiac function is necessary. The combination with verapamil is not recommended because of the risk of heart block.

- *Carbamazepine and ciclosporin:* Diltiazem and verapamil increase plasma concentrations of carbamazepine and ciclosporin. Monitor such combinations closely, as dosage adjustments may be necessary.
- *Digoxin:* Increased plasma concentration of digoxin has been reported with co-administration of verapamil or diltiazem. Monitor digoxin plasma concentration closely whenever a calcium channel-blocking agent is started or discontinued or when dosage is changed. Monitor for prolonged AV conduction, bradycardia or AV blocks, especially during the initial week of therapy, as digoxin dose may need to be changed.
- *Inhibitors of CYP3A4* (e.g. erythromycin, itraconazole, grapefruit juice): May decrease metabolism of the calcium channel blockers, increasing the potential for adverse effects. Monitor and adjust dose if necessary.

Adverse reactions

Common adverse reactions are shown in Figure 11.3. Gingival hyperplasia is a rare adverse effect reported with amlodipine, diltiazem, felodipine, verapamil and, most often, nifedipine. It starts as an inflammation of the gums, usually in the first 9 months of therapy. When the drug is discontinued, this effect usually improves within 1–4 weeks. Good dental hygiene, along with professional teeth cleaning, is necessary to reduce the potential for this adverse effect.

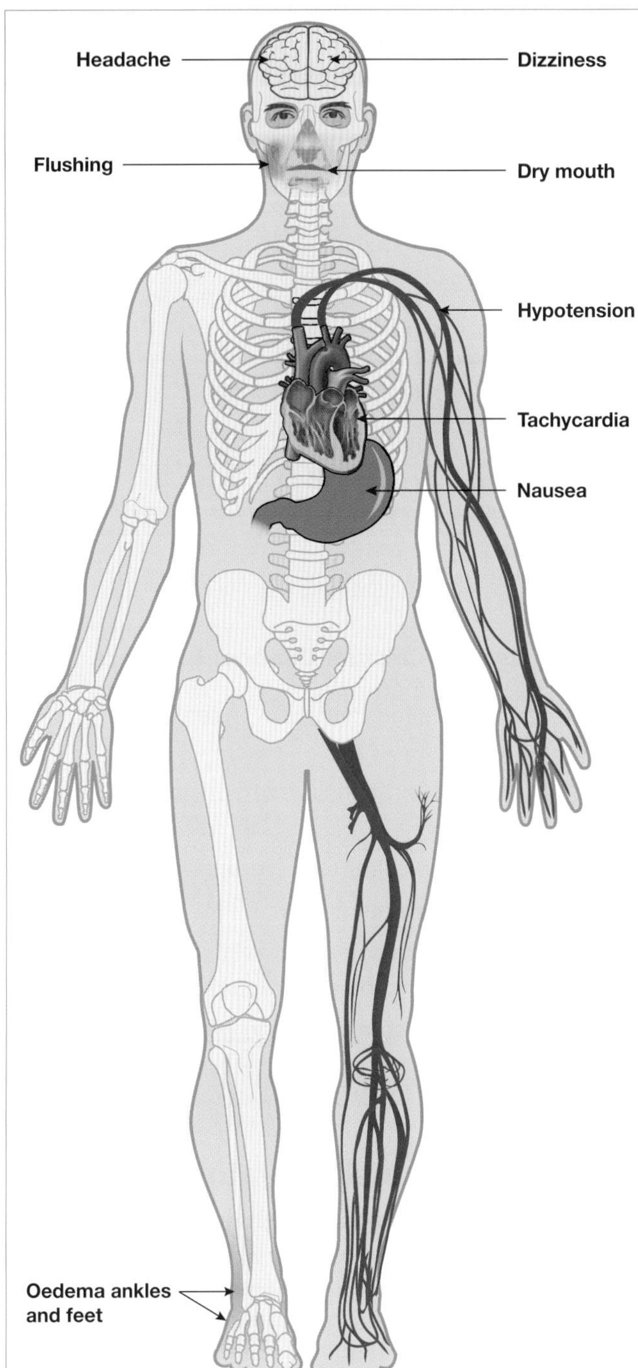

FIGURE 11.3 Common adverse effects of calcium channel blockers Adverse effects vary between the drugs depending on the degree of vasodilation, which is greatest with the dihydropyridines such as nifedipine.

Warnings and contraindications

Calcium channel blockers should be used with caution in people with severe bradycardia, congestive heart failure (caution with felodipine, nifedipine and nimodipine, as they have a slight negative inotropic effect), hypotension, acute MI, or liver or kidney impairment. Avoid use in people with hypersensitivity to calcium channel blockers, cardiac shock, severe bradycardia or congestive heart failure. (Use extreme caution with diltiazem and verapamil.) The use of clevidipine is contraindicated in severe aortic stenosis.

The elderly are more susceptible to these drugs and the adverse effects of increased weakness, dizziness, fainting episodes and falls. In the presence of hepatic impairment, treatment should be started at a lower dose for amlodipine and felodipine because reduced hepatic metabolism may result in increased plasma drug concentration. Plasma half-life increases in the elderly with amlodipine, diltiazem, felodipine and verapamil. These agents should not be discontinued abruptly, as severe rebound angina attacks may result. (Gradual drug withdrawal is recommended.)

The antianginal drugs discussed in preceding sections (nitrates and calcium channel blockers) provide symptomatic relief in people with angina. These drugs may be used alone or in combination because they improve the balance between myocardial oxygen supply and demand. A comparison of the effects of these drugs on cardiovascular parameters is shown in Table 11.4.

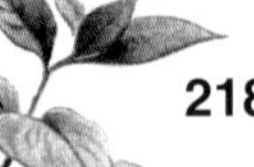

TABLE 11.4 Comparison of cardiovascular effects of nitrates, β-blockers and calcium channel blockers

EFFECT	NITRATES	β-BLOCKERS	CALCIUM CHANNEL BLOCKERS
Systolic blood pressure	(−)	(−)	(−)
Ventricular volume	(−)	(+)	(−) or (0)
Heart rate	(+)	(−)	(−), (+) or (0)
Myocardial contractility	(0)	(−)	(−)
Coronary blood flow	(+)	(+) or (0)	(+)
Coronary vessel resistance	(−)	(+) or (0)	(−)
Coronary spasm	(−)	(+) or (0)	(−)
Collateral blood flow	(+)	(0)	(−)

(−) = decreased; (+) = increased; (0) = no change.

Clinical Uses of Calcium Channel Blockers

- Angina (amlodipine, diltiazem, nifedipine, verapamil)
- Aneurysmal subarachnoid haemorrhage (nimodipine)
- Atrial fibrillation (diltiazem, verapamil)
- Atrial flutter (verapamil)
- Hypertension (amlodipine, clevidipine, diltiazem, felodipine, lercanidipine, verapamil)
- Prevention of cluster headache (verapamil)
- SVT (verapamil)

Potassium channel activators

Potassium channel activators include nicorandil, which may be used as an alternative to long-acting nitrates to reduce the frequency of anginal attacks, and diazoxide and minoxidil, which have limited use in treating hypertension. These drugs relax smooth muscle by acting on ATP-sensitive potassium channels. Normally, intracellular ATP closes the channel, causing the smooth muscle cells to depolarise. Drugs that activate the potassium channel antagonise the action of ATP, preventing closure of the channel. This results in hyperpolarisation and relaxation of the vascular smooth muscle.

Nicorandil

In addition to its action as an activator of potassium channels, which leads to arterial vasodilation and a reduction in afterload, nicorandil relaxes the venous vascular system. This is due to an increase in cGMP brought about by the nitrate moiety of the drug (a similar effect to that of GTN). Nicorandil is used in chronic stable angina because of evidence that it exerts a direct effect on normal and stenotic coronary arteries.

After oral administration, nicorandil is absorbed rapidly, with bioavailability in the order of 75%, indicating no extensive first-pass metabolism. Maximal plasma concentration is reached in 30–60 minutes and the drug has a rapid elimination phase, with a half-life of about 60 minutes. Nicorandil is metabolised by denitration, with the metabolites excreted in the urine within 24 hours.

Common adverse reactions include nausea, flushing, headache, dizziness, palpitations and myalgia. At high doses, hypotension may be problematic. Caution should be exercised in people with severe hepatic impairment, as lower doses may be required. Nicorandil is contraindicated in people with hypotension or left ventricular failure.

Diazoxide

The antihypertensive action of diazoxide results from potassium channel activation and hence relaxation of smooth muscles in the peripheral arterioles, which causes a decrease in peripheral resistance. As blood pressure falls, a reflex increase in heart rate and cardiac output occurs, with resultant maintenance of coronary and cerebral blood flow. This cardiovascular reflex mechanism also inhibits the development of orthostatic hypotension. Concurrent use with other antihypertensives or peripheral vasodilators may result in additive effects.

Diazoxide is administered intravenously to rapidly reduce blood pressure in hypertensive emergencies such as malignant hypertension and hypertensive crisis. Intravenous diazoxide is ineffective in reducing elevated blood pressure in people with monoamine oxidase (MAO)-induced hypertension or phaeochromocytoma. Because of its adverse effects, the drug is not normally used orally to treat chronic hypertension. Administered intravenously (intermittently or by infusion) the onset of action is 1 minute, the peak effect occurs within 2–5 minutes, the half-life is about 28 hours and the duration of effect is 2–12 hours. Diazoxide is metabolised by the liver forming oxidative metabolites and sulfate conjugates. Both metabolites and unchanged drug are excreted by the kidneys.

Adverse reactions include hyperglycaemia, tachycardia, anorexia, headache, flushing, dizziness, constipation, abdominal cramps, changes in taste perception and oedema (sodium and water retention). Relevant hospital or other protocols should be consulted prior to use. With rapid IV injection, severe adverse reactions that may occur including angina, bradycardia, hypotension, cerebral ischaemia and confusion. Use diazoxide with caution in people with gout, diabetes and heart failure. Avoid use in people with diazoxide hypersensitivity, coronary or cerebral insufficiency or aortic dissection.

Diazoxide also opens potassium channels in the plasma membrane of pancreatic β-cells. The subsequent hyperpolarisation of the membrane inhibits insulin release from the pancreas. Hence, it can be used to treat intractable hypoglycaemia. Capsules and oral liquid diazoxide are available through the Special Access Scheme. The oral route is not normally used to treat hypertension because of poor tolerance of oral diazoxide.

Minoxidil

Minoxidil is an orally effective direct-acting peripheral vasodilator. It reduces blood pressure by decreasing peripheral vascular resistance in the arteriolar vessels, with little effect on veins. It does not cause orthostatic hypotension. It is a potent vasodilator and also causes a reflex increase in cardiac output, induces sodium retention, promotes development of oedema and increases plasma renin activity. Minoxidil is reserved for severe hypertension unresponsive to traditional agents – that is, severe hypertension associated with chronic renal failure. Concomitant administration of a β-blocking drug such as propranolol is necessary to prevent severe reflex tachycardia. Administration of a diuretic agent is also essential to counteract sodium and water retention. The more commonly recognised topical use is for male-pattern baldness in both men and women.

The onset of action of minoxidil is 30 minutes, with the peak effect occurring in 2–3 hours (after a single dose). Although the plasma half-life is about 4 hours, the duration of its hypotensive action may exceed 24 hours. With daily administration, steady-state plasma concentration is achieved after 3–7 days. It is metabolised (~90%) in the liver, principally forming an *N*-glucuronide, and the metabolites are excreted by the kidneys.

Adverse reactions occur with oral dosing and include nausea, vomiting, tachycardia, anorexia, headache, excessive hair growth (hypertrichosis; usually on face, arms and back), red flushing of skin, oedema, angina and pericarditis. Use with caution in people with heart failure, angina, phaeochromocytoma, cerebrovascular disease and post MI. Avoid use in people with minoxidil hypersensitivity or pulmonary hypertension secondary to mitral stenosis, and in pregnant or lactating women.

Miscellaneous vasodilators

The drugs discussed below include hydralazine and sodium nitroprusside. Both agents are used during hypertensive emergencies because they are rapid direct-acting vasodilators that produce an immediate fall in arterial pressure.

Hydralazine

Hydralazine hydrochloride produces its hypotensive effects by direct relaxation of vascular smooth muscle, particularly the arterioles, with a lesser effect on veins, leading to reduction in peripheral resistance. Consequently, renal blood flow is increased, providing an advantage in situations of renal failure. Hydralazine also maintains cerebral blood flow, but it causes sodium and water retention. The resulting hypotension is thought to stimulate the baroreceptor reflex, causing an increase in heart rate and cardiac output. Unfortunately, this response offsets the antihypertensive effects of the drug. Tolerance to the antihypertensive action may be counteracted by combination with other antihypertensive drugs. Hydralazine also increases plasma renin activity. It is used to treat hypertensive emergencies and in combination with a β-blocker and a diuretic in patients with hypertension refractory to other drugs.

An oral dose of hydralazine has an onset of action of 45 minutes; with IV administration the onset is within 10–20 minutes. The peak effect is within 1 hour (orally) or 15–30 minutes (IV). The plasma half-life is 3–7 hours and duration of action is 3–8 hours. It is metabolised principally by acetylation in the liver, with the metabolites excreted by the kidneys. Identification of a 'slow-acetylator' phenotype (Ch 5) in both Caucasians (about 50%) and Asians (about 20%), which results in significant increases in the plasma concentration of the drug and hence the risk of toxicity, has limited the usefulness of this drug. Concurrent drug administration with MAO inhibitors or other antihypertensives may result in severe hypotension.

Adverse reactions include diarrhoea, nausea, vomiting, tachycardia, anorexia, headache, facial flushing, stuffy nose, oedema, angina, rash, peripheral neuritis and a systemic lupus erythematosus (SLE)-like syndrome. The SLE-like syndrome may include myalgia, arthralgia, arthritis, weakness, fever and skin changes. Use with caution in people with angina, cerebral artery disease and renal and hepatic impairment. The drug is contraindicated in people with hydralazine hypersensitivity, aortic dissection, severe tachycardia and heart failure and SLE.

Sodium nitroprusside

Sodium nitroprusside (nitroferricyanide) is a potent and rapid direct-acting arterial and venous vasodilator that greatly reduces arterial blood pressure. It is indicated for rapid reduction of blood pressure in hypertensive

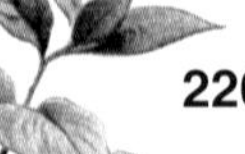

emergencies and for controlled hypotension during surgery.

It contains five cyanide groups and when the drug is administered IV, one molecule of nitroprusside reacts with one molecule of haemoglobin to form one molecule of cyanmethaemoglobin, four cyanide ions and NO, the active substance. NO then activates the enzyme guanylyl cyclase to produce cGMP and vasodilation. The decrease in systemic resistance causes a reduction in preload and afterload, improving cardiac output.

Its onset of action and peak effect occur almost immediately (within minutes) after administration by IV infusion. The duration of effect is 1–10 minutes after discontinuation of the infusion and the half-life of nitroprusside is 2 minutes. The free cyanide ions react with thiosulfates, catalysed by the mitochondrial enzyme rhodanase, forming the final metabolite thiocyanate, which is excreted by the kidneys. Processing of cyanide ions from sodium nitroprusside to thiocyanate can proceed normally at a rate of about 2 micrograms/kg/minute. Infusion rates greater than this can lead to accumulation of cyanide ions. In people with normal renal function the half-life of thiocyanate is 3 days, but this may double or triple in people with renal failure.

The hypotensive effect of sodium nitroprusside is exacerbated by other antihypertensive drugs, volatile anaesthetics and other negative inotropes. Adverse reactions include dizziness, excessive sweating, headache, anxiety, abdominal cramps, tachycardia, hypothyroidism, flushing, rash and muscle twitching. Thiocyanate toxicity is characterised by ataxia, blurred vision, headache, nausea, vomiting, tinnitus, shortness of breath, delirium and unconsciousness. In contrast cyanide toxicity manifests as hypotension, metabolic acidosis, pink colouration of skin and mucous membranes, very shallow breathing, decreased reflexes, coma and widely dilated pupils.

Use with caution in people with hypothyroidism, hypothermia or lung disease. Avoid use in patients with nitroprusside hypersensitivity, cerebrovascular or coronary artery disease, liver disease, kidney disease or metabolic-induced vitamin B12 deficiency.

For a hypertensive emergency, the solution should be freshly prepared using 5% glucose intravenous infusion (no other solution should be used) and protected from light by wrapping the container in the supplied opaque sleeve, aluminium foil or other opaque material. The prepared solution should be discarded within 24-hours. A freshly prepared solution has a faint brown tinge; discard if it is highly coloured (e.g. blue, green or dark red).

KEY POINTS

Direct-acting vasodilator drugs

- Vasodilator drugs are used to treat a range of disorders, including hypertension, angina, shock, cardiac failure and peripheral vascular conditions.
- Vasodilator drugs relax vascular smooth muscle in either veins or arterioles, while others dilate both types of blood vessels.
- The main groups of direct-acting vasodilator drugs are the organic nitrates, calcium channel blockers and potassium channel activators.
- Metabolism of organic nitrates results in the release of NO, which increases cGMP levels leading to vasodilation.
- At low doses, GTN causes venodilation, reducing preload and stroke volume. Higher doses dilate arteries, and the overall effect is a reduction in myocardial work and oxygen demand, hence their beneficial effect in angina.
- Calcium channel-blocking drugs block the inward movement of calcium ions through the slow channels of cardiac and vascular smooth muscle cell membranes.
- These drugs decrease the force of myocardial contraction (negative inotropic effect), decrease automaticity in the SA node and decrease conduction in the AV junction (negative chronotropic and negative dromotropic effects, respectively) and inhibit calcium ion influx in smooth muscle cells (reduction in peripheral vascular resistance).
- These drugs are very effective for treating angina, hypertension and cardiac dysrhythmias, but not all calcium channel blockers have equivalent therapeutic effects.
- Drugs such as diazoxide, nicorandil and minoxidil relax smooth muscle by activating ATP-dependent potassium channels. They activate the potassium channel, antagonising the action of ATP and preventing closure of the channel. This results in hyperpolarisation and relaxation of the vascular smooth muscle.
- Diazoxide and minoxidil have limited use in the treatment of hypertension, while nicorandil is used to treat angina.
- Hydralazine and sodium nitroprusside are rapid direct-acting vasodilators used during hypertensive emergencies to produce an immediate fall in arterial pressure.

Indirect-acting vasodilator drugs

The main groups of drugs in this category, which are primarily used to treat hypertension (Clinical Focus Box 11.2) include:

- centrally acting drugs that inhibit vasoconstriction mediated by the sympathetic nervous system
- inhibitors of the **renin–angiotensin–aldosterone system** (RAAS).

CLINICAL FOCUS BOX 11.2
Hypertension

Hypertension is defined as an elevated systolic blood pressure, diastolic blood pressure, or both. In clinical practice, elevated systolic blood pressure is a greater predictor of cardiovascular risk than elevated diastolic pressure. Worldwide definitions of hypertension vary, and a suggested classification has been developed following a review of systems in the United States and Europe (Gabb et al. 2016).

CATEGORY	SYSTOLIC BP (mmHg)	DIASTOLIC BP (mmHg)
Optimal	< 120	< 80
Normal	120–129	80–84
High–normal	130–139	85–89
Grade 1 (mild hypertension)	140–159	90–99
Grade 2 (moderate hypertension)	160–179	100–109
Grade 3 (severe hypertension)	≥ 180	≥ 110
Isolated systolic hypertension	≥ 140	< 90

This classification also stratified individuals based on blood pressure, the presence of risk factors and the degree of target-organ damage secondary to hypertension. The major risk factors in hypertensive patients include cigarette smoking, diabetes mellitus, raised total or LDL cholesterol or reduced HDL cholesterol, age (> 55 years male, > 65 years female), family history of heart disease, male gender (increased risk at any age compared with females), obesity, excessive alcohol intake and a sedentary lifestyle. Psychosocial risk factors include depression, social isolation and lack of quality support. Those populations most at risk include people of Aboriginal, Torres Strait Islander, Māori or Pacific Islander origin and those in lower socioeconomic groups. The target-organ damage or cardiovascular disease in hypertensive people includes stroke or transient ischaemic attacks, kidney disease, retinopathy and various cardiac diseases such as angina, heart failure, left ventricular hypertrophy and prior MI.

Source: Adapted with permission from the National Heart Foundation of Australia. Guideline for the diagnosis and management of hypertension in adults 2016. © 2016 National Heart Foundation of Australia.

Drug therapy for hypertension

Non-pharmacological measures are the first step for managing hypertension and include weight and alcohol reduction, smoking cessation, limiting dietary sodium intake and embarking on a program of regular physical activity of at least 30 minutes of moderate-intensity exercise daily on most days of the week. In addition, it is important to ascertain if an individual is taking any over-the-counter drugs or complementary or alternative medicines (Clinical Focus Box 11.3).

CLINICAL FOCUS BOX 11.3
Drugs, medications and hypertension

Many people take drugs (prescribed) and medications purchased at pharmacies, health-food stores or online. Some of these products may elevate blood pressure and should be excluded as a contributing factor when taking an individual's history. The following list of examples is by no means an exhaustive one:

- alcohol (excessive consumption)
- amphetamine
- bupropion
- bromocriptine (rebound hypertension with abrupt withdrawal)
- caffeine pills and caffeine-containing products
- clonidine (rebound hypertension with abrupt withdrawal)
- clozapine
- cocaine
- corticosteroids
- energy drinks
- ginseng
- guarana
- haemopoietic drugs (darbepoetin, epoetin alpha, epoetin beta, methoxy pegepoetin beta)
- hormone replacement therapy
- methamphetamine
- modafinil
- MAO inhibitors (moclobemide, phenelzine, tranylcypromine)
- natural licorice
- non-steroidal anti-inflammatory drugs (NSAIDs)
- oral estrogen contraceptives
- serotonin-noradrenaline reuptake inhibitors (SNRI, e.g. venlafaxine)
- sympathomimetics such as decongestants
- St John's wort (may decrease efficacy of some CV drugs).

Source: Adapted with permission from the National Heart Foundation of Australia. Guideline for the diagnosis and management of hypertension in adults 2016. © 2016 National Heart Foundation of Australia.

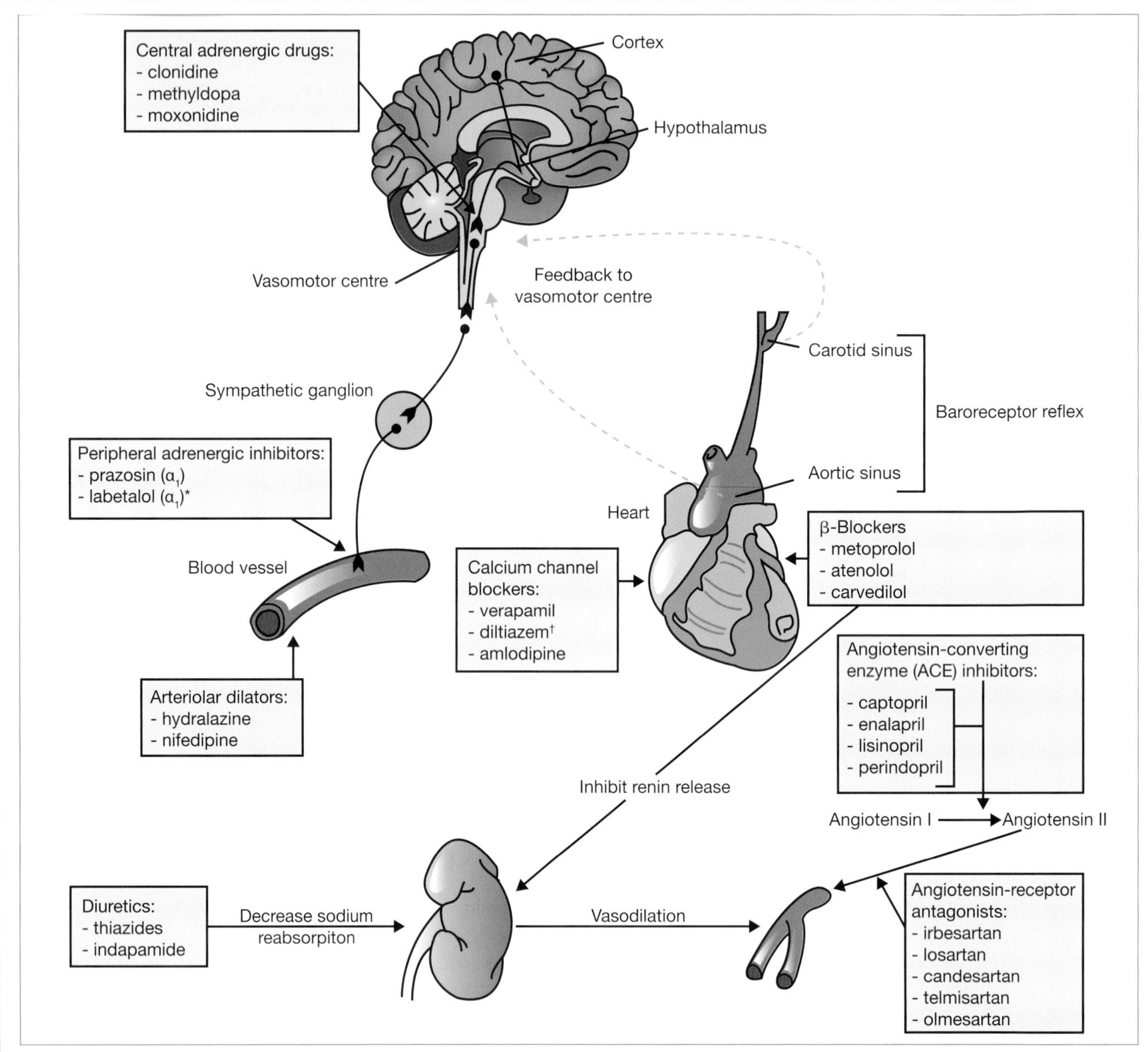

FIGURE 11.4 Physiological control of blood pressure and sites of action of some currently used oral antihypertensive drugs * Labetalol acts on both α_1- and β_1-adrenoceptors. † Diltiazem acts on both the heart and arteriolar vascular smooth muscle.

When instituting drug therapy, the lowest dose of the chosen drug is used, adding a second drug from a different drug class if necessary. The overriding goal of drug therapy is to lower the blood pressure, with minimal adverse effects. Long-acting drugs that allow once-daily dosing are preferable because they aid adherence. Figure 11.4 summarises the physiological factors controlling blood pressure (the sympathetic nervous system and the RAAS) and indicates the sites of action of currently used oral antihypertensive drugs.

Effective first-line monotherapy regimens include:

- **angiotensin-converting enzyme (ACE) inhibitors**
- **angiotensin receptor antagonists (ARBs)**
- dihydropyridine calcium channel blockers
- thiazide diuretics (for people 65 years or older).

Effective drug combinations include:

- an ACE inhibitor or ARB plus a calcium channel blocker
- an ACE inhibitor or ARB plus a thiazide diuretic
- an ACE inhibitor or ARB plus a β-blocker
- a β-blocker plus a dihydropyridine calcium channel blocker (amlodipine, felodipine, lercanidipine or nifedipine)
- a thiazide diuretic plus a β-blocker
- a thiazide diuretic plus a calcium channel blocker.

Centrally acting adrenergic inhibitors

The **centrally acting adrenergic inhibitors** clonidine, methyldopa and moxonidine are effective antihypertensive drugs, but are not considered first-line drugs because of their adverse effects profiles and lack of clinical evidence of significant cardiovascular benefit.

Clonidine

Clonidine is a centrally acting α_2 adrenergic agonist. It reduces systolic and diastolic blood pressure by stimulating central α_2 receptors, which decreases sympathetic outflow from the brain to the blood vessels and heart. Blood pressure is lowered as a result of decreased cardiac output, heart rate and peripheral vascular resistance. The effect on cardiac output is the result of a reduction in both heart rate and stroke volume, which can lead to bradycardia.

The decreased sympathetic outflow to the kidneys reduces renal vascular resistance, preserving renal blood flow. In some people, renin activity may be suppressed. With continued clonidine use, a diuretic is used to correct fluid retention.

Clonidine is marketed to treat hypertension and menopausal flushing, but is also used for the diagnosis of phaeochromocytoma. At a low dose, clonidine is also used for migraine or recurrent vascular headache prophylaxis in adults unresponsive to other drug therapies.

Clonidine is well absorbed after oral administration, with bioavailability approaching 100%. Oral clonidine has an onset of action within 0.5–1 hour, a peak effect in 2–4 hours and a duration of action of up to 8 hours. Clonidine is excreted predominantly as unchanged drug in urine (60%), with the remainder excreted as hydroxylated metabolites.

Clonidine is subject to a number of drug interactions, including:

- *β-adrenoceptor antagonists:* Concurrent administration with clonidine may lead to loss of blood pressure control. Bradycardia may be exacerbated. Monitor pulse rate closely. If discontinuing both drugs, the β-blocker should be stopped first. Discontinuing clonidine first may increase the risk of inducing a withdrawal hypertensive crisis.
- *Tricyclic antidepressants:* The antihypertensive effectiveness of clonidine may be reduced. This usually occurs in the first or second week of therapy. Monitor closely, as dosage adjustments and/or an alternative drug may need to be considered.

Adverse reactions are numerous and include dry mouth, headache, constipation, weakness, postural hypotension, impotency or decreased sexual drive, insomnia, anxiety, anorexia, nausea, vomiting and pruritus.

Clonidine is used with caution in the elderly and in people with impaired AV node or sinus node function, coronary insufficiency, depression or a history of depression, Raynaud's syndrome or a recent MI. Clonidine is contraindicated in sick sinus syndrome and heart block.

Methyldopa

Methyldopa is often used to treat hypertension in pregnant women, but in non-gestational hypertension its usefulness is limited by CNS and hepatic adverse effects. Although the exact hypotensive mechanism of methyldopa is unknown, the theory is that a metabolite of methyldopa (α-methylnoradrenaline) stimulates the central α_2 adrenergic receptors, which results in a reduction in sympathetic outflow to the heart, kidneys and peripheral vasculature.

The peak effect of methyldopa occurs 4–6 hours after a single dose or 48–72 hours with multiple dosing. The duration of action is 12–24 hours (after a single oral dose), 1–2 days (after multiple oral doses) or 10–16 hours (after IV administration). Methyldopa is metabolised to α-methylnoradrenaline within adrenergic nerve endings and in the liver to a sulfate conjugate (30–60%). Excretion is primarily by the kidneys. Methyldopa is subject to a number of drug interactions, including:

- *Iron:* Ferrous sulfate or gluconate may reduce bioavailability, interfering with blood pressure control.
- *Tricyclic antidepressants:* May reduce the antihypertensive effect of methyldopa, and an alternative antihypertensive should be considered.

Adverse reactions include drowsiness, dry mouth, headache, oedema of the feet and legs, fever, postural hypotension, impotency, insomnia, depression, anxiety and nightmares. Use with caution in people with depression (may be worsened) or renal dysfunction. Avoid use of methyldopa in people with methyldopa hypersensitivity, hepatitis, cirrhosis, haemolytic anaemia or phaeochromocytoma.

Moxonidine

Unlike clonidine and methyldopa, moxonidine has minimal actions on α_2 adrenoceptors. Moxonidine acts on central imidazoline I_1 receptors present in the rostral ventral medulla, decreasing sympathetic tone. Adrenaline, noradrenaline and renin concentrations fall, resulting in a decrease in blood pressure and systemic vascular resistance. Heart rate, cardiac output and stroke volume are unaffected. The drug is well absorbed and bioavailability is about 90%. Moxonidine is largely excreted as unchanged drug (~60%) and the half-life is about 2.5 hours. Renal dysfunction decreases clearance and increases half-life. Moxonidine is contraindicated in heart failure and may exacerbate symptoms of coronary heart disease. Adverse effects are fewer in comparison with clonidine and include somnolence, weakness, dizziness, hypotension and bradycardia. This drug should be withdrawn gradually over several days.

The renin–angiotensin–aldosterone system

The kidneys are by far the most important organs in the body for long-term regulation of blood pressure and, normally, excessive fluid retention is controlled by negative feedback mechanisms that operate to restore normal fluid and electrolyte balance. The RAAS regulates blood pressure by increasing or decreasing blood volume through modulation of renal function (Fig 11.5). Abnormal activation of the RAAS plays a key role in the development and pathophysiology of hypertension and cardiovascular disease and correlates directly with the incidence and extent of end-organ damage. The major effector molecules of the RAAS are renin, angiotensin II and the mineralocorticoid **aldosterone**. Additionally, it is now recognised that aldosterone is a proinflammatory molecule that plays a major role in the progression of ischaemic heart disease and that a raised aldosterone-to-renin ratio is common in people with hypertension.

A reduction in blood flow through the kidneys decreases renal arterial pressure, which causes the release of renin into the circulation. Renin is secreted from the juxtaglomerular cells located in the afferent arteriolar walls of the nephron and catalyses the cleavage of angiotensinogen, a plasma globulin, to form angiotensin I, a weak vasoconstrictor. Subsequently, in endothelial cells, primarily in the lung, angiotensin I is converted by angiotensin-converting enzyme to angiotensin II.

Angiotensin II, acting via AT_1 receptors, is one of the most potent vasoconstrictors known. It effectively constricts arterioles, which increases peripheral resistance and raises blood pressure. In addition, angiotensin II acts on the adrenal cortex to stimulate the secretion of aldosterone, which promotes reabsorption of sodium by the kidneys and the excretion of potassium. The increased sodium elevates the osmotic pressure of plasma, causing a release of antidiuretic hormone from the hypothalamus, leading to increased reabsorption of water from the renal tubules, which adds further to the rise in blood pressure. Angiotensin II itself also acts on the kidney tubules to promote reabsorption of water. Furthermore, activation of

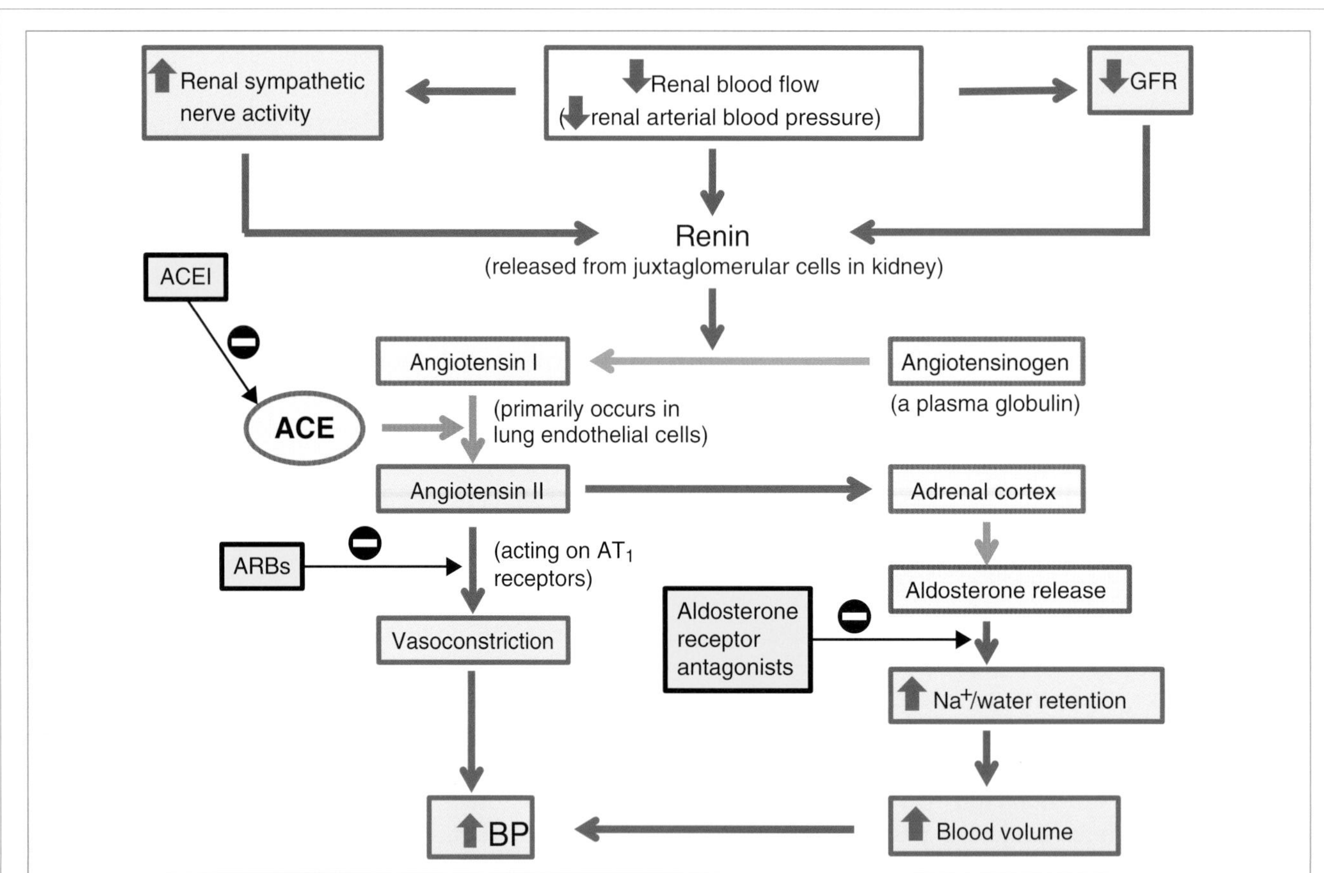

FIGURE 11.5 Interrelationship between renal perfusion, the renin–angiotensin–aldosterone system, hypertension and the sites of action of drugs targeting RAAS ACE = angiotensin-converting enzyme; ACEI = angiotensin-converting enzyme inhibitors; ARBs = angiotensin receptor (AT_1) antagonists; - = inhibitory effect

AT_1 receptors produces adverse effects on the cardiovascular system, including the promotion of vascular and cardiac hypertrophy, inflammation and fibrosis.

In addition to vascular effects, angiotensin II reduces insulin sensitivity and impairs insulin secretion. Not surprisingly, there is a close association between the metabolic syndrome, the risk of type 2 diabetes and the RAAS system, as blockade of the RAAS results in an antidiabetogenic effect improving measures of diabetic nephropathy.

Inhibition of the RAAS is now a common therapeutic strategy used to intervene in the pathogenesis of cardiovascular and renal dysfunction. A large clinical trial found that ARBs in a fixed dose combination with a calcium channel blocker were as effective as ACE inhibitors in reducing the risk of major cardiovascular events and hospitalisations for congestive heart failure (Hsiao et al. 2015).

The key drug groups used are those that:

- inhibit the conversion of angiotensin I to angiotensin II – ACE inhibitors
- block the action of angiotensin II on AT_1 (angiotensin II type I) receptors – the ARBs
- block aldosterone receptors – aldosterone-receptor antagonists.

Angiotensin-converting enzyme inhibitors

ACE inhibitors competitively block the angiotensin-converting enzyme necessary for the conversion of angiotensin I to angiotensin II. Angiotensin II is a powerful vasoconstrictor that raises blood pressure and also causes aldosterone release, resulting in sodium and water retention (Fig 11.4). Inhibition of ACE results in:

- a decrease in vascular tone, thereby directly lowering blood pressure
- inhibition of aldosterone release, reducing sodium and water reabsorption; the resultant excretion of fluid is thought to cause only a secondary reduction in blood pressure (decrease in aldosterone secretion does lead to a slight elevation in serum potassium)
- an increase in plasma renin activity, caused by a loss of negative feedback on renin release.

Large clinical studies have now established that ACE inhibitors reduce cardiovascular mortality and morbidity in subjects with coronary artery disease and reduce the incidence of stroke and the need for revascularisation procedures compared with placebo. Further studies have demonstrated the beneficial effects of ACE inhibitors in delaying progression of renal impairment in people with early diabetic nephropathy and showed a reduction in cardiovascular mortality and morbidity in people with congestive heart failure.

Captopril is the prototype drug of this class, which now also includes enalapril, fosinopril, lisinopril, perindopril (Drug Monograph 11.2), quinapril, ramipril and trandolapril.

Clinical Uses of ACE Inhibitors

- Hypertension
- Chronic heart failure
- Diabetic nephropathy (type 1 diabetes)
- Left ventricular dysfunction post MI
- Reduction of risk of MI or cardiac arrest in people with coronary artery disease

Drug interactions

A consequence of ACE inhibition is potassium retention, which may lead to hyperkalaemia. Combination of ACE inhibitors with other drugs that cause potassium retention should be avoided and the plasma potassium concentration should be monitored closely. Other drug interactions include:

- *Loop diuretics:* Concurrent administration with an ACE inhibitor may result in first-dose hypotension. Withhold diuretic for 24 hours before initiating ACE inhibitor therapy. Combination may increase the risk of ACE inhibitor-induced renal dysfunction. Monitor renal function and decrease dose or cease drug administration if indicated.
- *Lithium:* Reduced excretion of lithium, with increased risk of toxicity. Monitor plasma lithium concentration and renal function.
- *NSAIDs, including COX-2 inhibitors:* Increased risk of hyperkalaemia and reduced hypotensive effect of ACE inhibitor. Avoid combined use.
- *Potassium-sparing diuretics, potassium supplements:* Closely monitor plasma electrolytes, especially potassium, because of the high risk of hyperkalaemia.

Adverse reactions

These include headache, diarrhoea, loss of taste, weakness, nausea, dizziness, hypotension, rash, fever and joint pain. The cough associated with ACE inhibitor use occurs in a significant number of people and is thought to be due to the inhibition by the ACE inhibitor of the enzyme that degrades bradykinin (Clinical Focus Box 11.4). Although rare, ACE inhibitors can cause angio-oedema, which may be fatal. This is of particular concern if there is a previous history of hereditary or idiopathic angio-oedema or a previous reaction of this type to an ACE inhibitor.

Warnings and contraindications

Avoid use in people with ACE inhibitor hypersensitivity, history of angio-oedema or hyperkalaemia and in renal

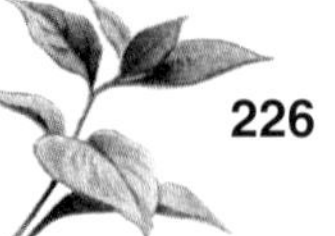

DRUG MONOGRAPH 11.2
Perindopril

Perindopril is a competitive inhibitor of angiotensin-converting enzyme, which converts angiotensin I into angiotensin II, a potent vasoconstrictor. It is indicated to treat hypertension and heart failure, and to reduce the risk of a cardiovascular event in people with stable coronary artery disease.

Pharmacokinetics

Perindopril is rapidly absorbed following oral administration with peak plasma concentration occurring within about 1 hour. It is extensively metabolised with less than 10% of the dose recovered in urine as parent drug. Perindopril is a prodrug and there are six metabolites. The two main metabolites are the pharmacologically active diadic metabolite perindoprilat (formed from perindopril by the action of carboxylesterases) and perindoprilat glucuronide. The half-life of perindopril is 1–1.5 hours, while that of perindoprilat ranges from 30 to 120 hours because of the slow dissociation of perindoprilat from ACE. The latter accumulates in renal failure, augmenting the pharmacodynamics effect of ACE inhibition.

Drug interactions

Concomitant use of the drugs listed below with perindopril can cause (1) hyperkalaemia, and/or (2) increase the risk of hypotension, and/or (3) cause renal impairment:

- ARBs (sartans) avoid combination (1, 2, 3)
- loop diuretics (2, 3)
- NSAIDs (1, 3, and reduce antihypertensive effect of ACEI) – avoid combination in the elderly
- thiazide diuretics (2, 3)
- ciclosporin (1).

Warnings and contraindications

These drugs should be used with caution in people with:

- a history of angio-oedema (e.g. previous ACEI use)
- volume or sodium depletion
- **peripheral vascular disease** (PVD) or other conditions with increased likelihood of renal artery stenosis, and are contraindicated in women planning to conceive or who are pregnant. (Use in the second or third trimester may cause fetal abnormalities.)

Adverse reactions

These include:

- hypotension, headache, dizziness
- hyperkalaemia, renal impairment
- fatigue, nausea
- cough (Clinical Focus Box 11.4).

Dosage and administration

Perindopril is administered orally (Table 11.5), and is also available as a fixed-dose combination with either amlodipine or indapamide.

With the exception of captopril and lisinopril, the other ACE inhibitors are ester prodrugs that, following cleavage by esterases, form the active metabolite (listed in Table 11.5). With the exception of captopril, most of these drugs maintain an antihypertensive effect for up to 24 hours, allowing once-daily dosing. Some of these drugs are also available in combination with either the diuretic hydrochlorothiazide (enalapril, fosinopril, quinapril) or indapamide (perindopril arginine, perindopril erbumine) or with a calcium channel blocker (enalapril, perindopril arginine, ramipril).

TABLE 11.5 Pharmacokinetics and adult dosing of ACE inhibitors in hypertension

DRUG	ONSET OF ACTION (h)	DURATION OF EFFECT (h)	ACTIVE METABOLITE	ADULT DOSE RANGE (mg/day)[a]
Captopril	0.25–1	6–12	–	50–100
Enalapril	1	24	Enalaprilat	10–20
Fosinopril	≤ 1	24	Fosinoprilat	10–40
Lisinopril	1	24	–	5–40
Perindopril (erbumine)	3–6	24	Perindoprilat	4–8
Perindopril (arginine)	3–4	24	Perindoprilat	5–10
Quinapril	≤ 1	≤24	Quinaprilat	5–40
Ramipril	1–2	24	Ramiprilat	1.25–10
Trandolapril	0.5	48	Trandolaprilat	1–4

[a] Oral doses titrated as needed and tolerated.

Source: Dosage information: Australian Medicines Handbook 2021, pp. 254–259. Verify adult dose range using up-to-date drug/product information sources.

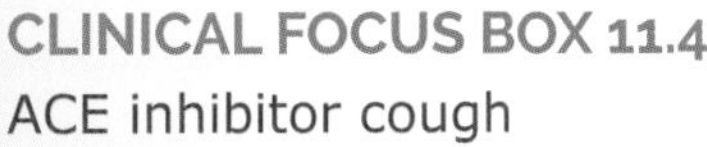

CLINICAL FOCUS BOX 11.4

ACE inhibitor cough

A well-known adverse effect of ACE inhibitors is a dry persistent cough that has been reported to occur in 5–35% of people prescribed ACE inhibitors. The cough:

- occurs more often in women, non-smokers and Chinese patients
- is not dose-dependent
- can occur within hours of the first dose
- may take weeks to months to develop
- normally resolves within 1–4 weeks of cessation of therapy
- may persist for 3 months after stopping the ACE inhibitor.

It is thought that the cough occurs as a consequence of inhibition of ACE, which is normally responsible for the metabolism of bradykinin (a vasodilator peptide) to inactive fragments. Inhibition of ACE results in accumulation of bradykinin and substance P, protussive mediators that sensitise airway nerves that produce a cough as a result of a tickling or scratching sensation in the throat (Dicpinigaitis 2006).

artery stenosis or renal impairment. ACE inhibitors should be avoided in pregnancy because of their potential to produce a range of abnormalities. Further precautions are advisable for a number of select situations (e.g. primary hyperaldosteronism, treatment with mTOR inhibitors), and specialist drug information resources should be consulted.

Angiotensin receptor (AT_1) antagonists

Although ACE inhibition clearly has beneficial effects in people with hypertension, ischaemic heart disease and congestive heart failure, approximately 10% of people have adverse effects that limit the usefulness of ACE inhibitors. This led to an investigation of the potential of drugs to inhibit angiotensin II. After the discovery of two subtypes of angiotensin II receptors, it was found that stimulation of the type 1 receptor (AT_1) mediated all the actions of angiotensin II. This meant a more precise target was available for blocking the vasoconstrictor effects of angiotensin II, rather than the broader effects (and possibly adverse effects) resulting from inhibition of ACE.

The AT_1 receptor quickly became the target for the development of a new group of antihypertensive drugs, the non-peptide angiotensin receptor (AT_1) antagonists (blockers, or ARBs). These agents, commonly called 'sartans', include candesartan, eprosartan, irbesartan, losartan, olmesartan, valsartan (Drug Monograph 11.3) and telmisartan (Table 11.6). They block the AT_1 receptor, thus inhibiting angiotensin II-mediated vasoconstriction and aldosterone release. They have little effect on plasma potassium concentration but may cause hyperkalaemia in people with renal disease or in those taking a potassium-sparing diuretic or a potassium supplement. In addition, they do not inhibit the breakdown of the cough-producing bradykinin. Losartan was the first AT_1 receptor antagonist synthesised and, with the exception of losartan, the ARBs are available as combination products with hydrochlorothiazide while valsartan is also available as a combination product with amlodipine.

Indications

ARBs are indicated to treat hypertension and/or heart failure in people unable to tolerate ACE inhibitors. These drugs reverse endothelial dysfunction and atherosclerosis and reduce the risk of cardiovascular events. Additionally, ARBs reduce end-organ damage of the kidney, brain and heart and decrease mortality of patients with congestive heart failure.

Pharmacokinetics

(Refer to Table 11.6.) Some of the ARBs are metabolised to varying degrees by cytochromes P450 and UDP-glucuronosyltransferases and the resulting metabolites in general (with the exception of losartan and the prodrug candesartan cilexetil) have a lower affinity for the AT_1 receptor. Valsartan and candesartan are minimally metabolised and are excreted primarily as unchanged drug. In contrast, irbesartan is extensively metabolised with less than 2% excreted in urine as unchanged drug. The ratio of hepatic to renal clearance varies for each individual sartan; for example, 35–50% of olmesartan is excreted as unchanged drug in urine. In general, the sartans are well absorbed and bioavailability varies from 13% (eprosartan) to 60–80% (irbesartan).

Drug interactions

Similar to the ACE inhibitors, drug interactions with the sartans include those drugs that cause potassium retention, and the combination should be avoided or the plasma potassium concentration monitored closely. Additional interactions occur with loop diuretics, NSAIDs and lithium (refer to the information on ACE inhibitors).

Adverse reactions

As expected, adverse reactions include hyperkalaemia, dizziness and headache (Drug Monograph 11.3).

Warnings and contraindications

Caution should be exercised if prescribing an ARB to people with peripheral vascular disease, renal dysfunction or volume or sodium depletion. Sartans are contraindicated in pregnancy, although there are limited data.

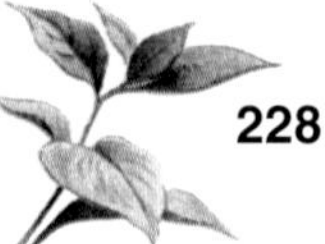

DRUG MONOGRAPH 11.3
Valsartan

Valsartan is a commonly used potent orally active non-peptide ARB with 20,000-fold greater selectivity for AT_1 receptors than AT_2 receptors. In 2015 it was approved in combination with the neprilysin inhibitor sacubitril (Ch 10) to treat heart failure. Multiple clinical trials have attested to the efficacy of valsartan in treating hypertension and heart failure.

Pharmacokinetics

Valsartan is rapidly absorbed following oral administration, achieving maximal plasma drug concentration within 1–4 hours. Bioavailability is about 25% (range 10–35%). Valsartan is extensively bound to plasma proteins (95%) and the elimination half-life ranges from 7 to 10 hours depending on the route of administration and the formulation. Most of the drug is excreted unchanged in faeces (83%) and urine (13%). Minor hepatic metabolism to valeryl 4-hydroxy valsartan is catalysed by CYP2C9.

Drug interactions

Concomitant use of the drugs listed below with valsartan can cause hyperkalaemia:
- ACE inhibitors
- ciclosporin
- heparin
- NSAIDs
- potassium-sparing diuretics, potassium supplements.

Adverse reactions

These include:
- hyperkalaemia (common in the presence of renal disease)
- headache and migraine
- malaise, back or muscle pain
- dose-related orthostatic hypotension, dizziness.

Warnings and contraindications

The sartans in general are:
- used with caution in people with evidence of volume or sodium depletion, as severe hypotension may result
- avoided in people with bilateral renal artery stenosis, as there is an increased risk of renal failure
- contraindicated in women planning to conceive or who are pregnant. (Use in the second or third trimester may cause fetal abnormalities.)

Dosage and administration

Valsartan is administered orally (Table 11.6) and is also available as a fixed-dose combination with either amlodipine or hydrochlorothiazide or as a combination with both.

TABLE 11.6 Pharmacokinetics and adult dosing of angiotensin receptor (AT_1) antagonists in hypertension

DRUG	BIOAVAILABILITY	TIME TO PEAK EFFECT (h)	HALF-LIFE (h)	ADULT DOSE RANGE (mg/day)[a]
Candesartan	15%	6–8	5–10	4–32
Eprosartan	13%	1–2	5–9	400–600
Irbesartan	60–80%	3–6	11–15	75–300
Losartan	14%	6	1.5–2 (parent)	50–100
			4–9 (metabolite)	
Olmesartan	26%	1.4–2.8	12–18	20–40
Telmisartan	40%	0.5–1	24	40–80
Valsartan	23%	2	6–9	80–320

[a] Once-daily dosing. Verify adult dose range using up-to-date drug information sources.

Sources: Australian Medicines Handbook 2021, pp. 259–263; Kirch et al. 2001; Schwocho & Masonson 2001.

Aldosterone-receptor antagonists

In addition to a role in sodium and water homeostasis, aldosterone increases magnesium and potassium excretion, impairs endothelial and baroreceptor function, reduces vascular compliance and promotes myocardial fibrosis, thus contributing to cardiovascular and renal disease. Aldosterone binds to mineralocorticoid receptors (Ch 29) that increase the absorption of sodium ions and water through epithelial sodium channels and promote potassium excretion by epithelial cells in the distal nephron.

Spironolactone, the prototypical aldosterone-receptor antagonist, was launched in 1960 to treat primary hyperaldosteronism, oedematous conditions and resistant hypertension.

Structurally, spironolactone is similar to progesterone and non-selectively binds to mineralocorticoid receptors and to progesterone and androgen receptors. Use of spironolactone for extended periods of time results in profound hyperkalaemia (resulting from antagonism of aldosterone) and major endocrine effects, including loss of libido, menstrual irregularities, gynaecomastia and impotence. This non-selectivity limits the use of spironolactone. However, in recognising the deleterious actions of aldosterone on the cardiovascular system, this led to a trial in 1999 of spironolactone in subjects with severe heart failure, RALES (Randomised Aldactone Evaluation Study). Subjects randomised to receive spironolactone had a 35% reduction in hospitalisation and a 30% reduction in mortality. However, hyperkalaemia and progestogenic and antiandrogenic adverse effects limits its usefulness in this setting.

Further investigations led to the development of eplerenone, which is a competitive aldosterone receptor antagonist with greater mineralocorticoid receptor selectivity and reduced progestogenic and antiandrogenic actions. In 2005 the Eplerenone Post-Acute Myocardial Infarction Heart Failure Efficacy and Survival Study (EPHESUS) showed that eplerenone reduced all-cause mortality by 15% in subjects post MI and with clinical signs of heart failure, which is now its indication for use (Drug Monograph 11.4).

DRUG MONOGRAPH 11.4
Eplerenone

Eplerenone is approved to treat heart failure and left ventricular impairment post MI. It blocks the action of aldosterone at mineralocorticoid receptors preventing aldosterone-induced sodium and water reabsorption and potassium excretion by epithelial cells in the distal nephron. Due to its mineralocorticoid receptor selectivity, eplerenone provides clinical advantages in comparison to spironolactone.

Pharmacokinetics

The absolute oral bioavailability of eplerenone is unknown, but absorption is not affected by food. Peak plasma concentration occurs within 1.5 hours post dose. Eplerenone is extensively metabolised by CYP3A4 to the major metabolites 6β-hydroxy eplerenone (32%), 6β, 21-hydroxy eplerenone (21%) and 21-hydroxy eplerenone (8%). Approximately 67% of the dose is excreted, predominantly as metabolites (< 2.5% is excreted as unchanged drug, in urine and 32% in faeces). The plasma half-life is about 3 hours.

Drug interactions

- The aldosterone antagonists cause hyperkalaemia, particularly in the presence of renal impairment or when co-administered with other drugs that cause potassium retention or with potassium supplements.
- CYP3A4 inhibitors amiodarone, diltiazem, erythromycin, fluconazole, itraconazole, saquinavir or verapamil increase the plasma concentration of eplerenone and the risk of hyperkalaemia.
- Aldosterone antagonists in combination with NSAIDs increase the risk of hyperkalaemia and worsening of renal function.

Adverse reactions

Common adverse effects include:

- hyperkalaemia, renal dysfunction
- hypotension, dizziness.

Warnings and contraindications

Eplerenone is contraindicated in the following existing situations:

- hyperkalaemia (potassium > 5.5 mmol/L). Plasma potassium concentration should be checked regularly and the eplerenone dose reduced or ceased if hyperkalaemia occurs. Current drug information sources should be consulted for further advice

- diabetes and/or proteinuria
- severe hepatic impairment.

Dosage and administration

The initial dose is 25 mg once daily, increasing over a period of a month to a maintenance dose of 50 mg daily if potassium concentration is less than 5.5 mmol/L. If potassium concentration is 5.5 mmol/L or greater, consult appropriate drug information sources for further dosing advice.

KEY POINTS

Centrally acting adrenergic inhibitors and RAAS inhibitors

- Five drug classes are used to treat hypertension. These include ACE inhibitors, angiotensin receptor (AT_1) antagonists, calcium channel blockers, diuretics (Ch 17) and β-blockers (Ch 9).
- Depending on a patient's response to therapy, combination drug therapies are often required for good control of hypertension. Such combinations are based on an understanding of the physiological control of blood pressure and the sites of action of the drugs used.
- The main indirect-acting vasodilator drugs are the centrally acting drugs that inhibit sympathetic outflow and inhibitors of the RAAS.
- The centrally acting agents, clonidine and methyldopa, are effective antihypertensives, especially when combined with a diuretic, but are not first-line drugs and are used in limited circumstances. When given as a sole agent, clonidine and methyldopa cause sodium and water retention.
- ACE inhibitors such as captopril competitively block the angiotensin-converting enzyme necessary for the conversion of angiotensin I to angiotensin II. Angiotensin II is a powerful vasoconstrictor that raises blood pressure and causes aldosterone release, resulting in sodium and water retention.
- ACE inhibitors are indicated to treat hypertension, heart failure, diabetic nephropathy, left ventricular dysfunction and after MI. All drugs of this class demonstrate similar antihypertensive efficacy, and adverse reactions do not differ significantly among the individual ACE inhibitors.
- Angiotensin receptor (AT_1) antagonists inhibit the action of angiotensin II, thereby preventing vasoconstriction, and are indicated to treat hypertension.
- In addition to a role in sodium and water homeostasis, aldosterone contributes to the progression of cardiovascular and renal disease. Spironolactone and eplerenone are aldosterone receptor antagonists.
- Spironolactone is used to treat primary hyperaldosteronism, oedematous conditions, resistant hypertension and female hirsutism. Although beneficial in a setting of heart failure, hyperkalaemia and progestogenic and antiandrogenic adverse effects limit the usefulness of spironolactone.
- Eplerenone is a competitive aldosterone antagonist with greater mineralocorticoid receptor selectivity and reduced progestogenic and antiandrogenic actions. It is primarily used to reduce the risk of cardiovascular death in a setting of heart failure and left ventricular dysfunction.

Peripheral vascular disease

PVD, which results in coolness or numbness of the extremities, intermittent claudication and leg ulcers, is a common problem in the elderly. The primary risk factors include hyperlipidaemia, diabetes, obesity, hypertension and smoking. The use of various direct-acting vasodilators for peripheral occlusive arterial disease has generally been very disappointing. Pentoxifylline (oxpentifylline), a xanthine derivative, and the oxerutins (hydroxyethylrutosides) are used for symptomatic relief, but there is a lack of convincing evidence for efficacy of these drugs. If no benefit is seen after a short trial of use, the drugs should be stopped.

KEY POINTS

Drugs for peripheral vascular disease

- PVD commonly afflicts the elderly, and drugs such as pentoxifylline and the oxerutins are used.
- Pentoxifylline is a xanthine derivative that improves haemorrhagic disorders in the microcirculation, which involves the flow of blood through the fine vessels (arterioles, capillaries and venules).
- The oxerutins (hydroxyethylrutosides) are flavanoids that reduce microvascular permeability, capillary leakage and oedema.
- Improvement with these drugs is marginally better than with a supervised exercise program.

DRUGS AT A GLANCE

Drugs affecting vascular smooth muscle

PHARMACOLOGICAL GROUP AND EFFECT	KEY EXAMPLES	CLINICAL USE
Antianginal drugs *Nitrates* • Metabolism results in release of NO, a vasodilator • Primarily venodilator • ↓ preload • ↓ oxygen demand of myocardium	Glyceryl trinitrate Isosorbide dinitrate	• Prevention/treatment of stable angina • Heart failure
	Isosorbide mononitrate	• Prevention of angina
Potassium channel activator (see below) Antihypertensives	Nicorandil	• Prevention/treatment of stable angina
Calcium channel blockers • Block inward movement of calcium through cell membranes of cardiac and smooth muscle cells • ↓ force of myocardial contraction • Dilate coronary arteries, which improves oxygen delivery to myocardium • Dihydropyridines are arteriolar vasodilators, which results in reduction in peripheral vascular resistance and blood pressure	Amlodipine	• Hypertension
	Clevidipine	• Hypertension (absence of oral treatment)
	Diltiazem	• Angina • Hypertension (controlled release)
	Felodipine	• Hypertension
	Lercanidipine[AUS]	• Hypertension
	Nifedipine	• Angina • Hypertension
	Nimodipine	• Prevention/treatment of neurological issues following aneurysmal subarachnoid haemorrhage
	Verapamil	• Angina • Atrial fibrillation/flutter • Hypertension • Supraventricular tachycardia (SVT)
Potassium channel activators • Relax vascular smooth muscle by acting on ATP-sensitive potassium channels • Antagonise action of ATP, which prevents closure of potassium channels • Cause hyperpolarisation and relaxation of vascular smooth muscle	Diazoxide	• Hypertensive emergency
	Minoxidil	• Severe refractory hypertension
Vasodilators • Direct arteriolar vasodilator (hydralazine) • Direct arteriolar/venous vasodilator (sodium nitroprusside)	Hydralazine	• Hypertensive emergency
	Sodium nitroprusside	• Hypertensive emergency • Controlled hypotension during surgery • Acute heart failure
Centrally acting antihypertensives • α_2 adrenoceptor agonist • ↓ sympathetic tone • ↓ blood pressure	Clonidine	• Hypertension
	Methyldopa	• Hypertension

ACE inhibitors
• Inhibit angiotensin converting enzyme which:
  • blocks conversion of angiotensin I to angiotensin II
  • reduces vasoconstricting effects of angiotensin II
	Captopril	• Hypertension
		• Chronic heart failure with reduced ejection fraction
		• Diabetic nephropathy (type 1 diabetes)

	Cilazapril[NZ]	• Hypertension • Chronic heart failure adjunct to digoxin/diuretic
	Enalapril	• Hypertension • Chronic heart failure with reduced ejection fraction
	Fosinopril[AUS]	• Hypertension • Chronic heart failure with reduced ejection fraction
	Lisinopril	• Hypertension • Chronic heart failure with reduced ejection fraction • Post MI (acute treatment)

	Perindopril	• Hypertension • Chronic heart failure with reduced ejection fraction • Reducing risk of myocardial infarction (MI) in patients with coronary artery disease (CAD)
	Quinapril	• Hypertension • Chronic heart failure with reduced ejection fraction
	Ramipril	• Hypertension • Post MI in presence of heart failure • Prevention of progressive renal failure (presence of persistent proteinuria)
	Trandolapril	• Hypertension • Post MI

Angiotensin receptor (AT_1) antagonists
• Inhibit binding of angiotensin II to AT_1 receptors which:
  • ↓ vasoconstricting effects of angiotensin II
  • ↓ sodium reabsorption
  • inhibits aldosterone release
	Candesartan	• Hypertension
		• Chronic heart failure with reduced ejection fraction

	Eprosartan	• Hypertension
	Irbesartan	• Hypertension • Reduction of renal disease progression in type 2 diabetes
	Losartan	• Hypertension • Reduction of renal disease progression in type 2 diabetes
	Olmesartan[AUS]	• Hypertension
	Telmisartan[AUS]	• Hypertension • Prevention of cardiovascular morbidity/mortality in patients with CAD, peripheral artery disease (PAD), diabetes or stroke
	Valsartan	• Hypertension • Chronic heart failure with reduced ejection fraction • Post MI

Drugs for heart failure
Aldosterone-receptor antagonists
• Antagonise action of aldosterone which:
  • ↑ sodium and water excretion
  • ↓ potassium excretion
	Eplerenone	• Heart failure to reduce risk of cardiovascular death
		• Mild heart failure

	Spironolactone	• Resistant hypertension • Primary hyperaldosteronism • Refractory oedema • Hirsutism in females
Drugs for peripheral vascular disease *Vasodilator* • Vasodilator	Pentoxifylline	• Relief of claudication in PAD

[AUS] *Australia only*
[NZ] *NZ only*

REVIEW EXERCISES

1 Mr ED has recently been prescribed olmesartan (40 mg) in combination with amlodipine (5 mg) and hydrochlorothiazide (25 mg) to treat hypertension. When last out shopping, he fainted in the street and was found to be hypotensive. Discuss the physiological/pharmacological factors that could have contributed to his hypotensive episode.

2 You are assisting the anaesthetist when he requests that you prepare an IV solution of sodium nitroprusside. He advises that the solution must be protected from light and that you are to closely monitor the patient's heart rate and blood pressure. Explain the basis for his directions to you.

3 Ms VG, a 71-year-old female, has been taking an ACE inhibitor and a thiazide diuretic to treat hypertension. This morning she twisted her ankle and decided to take some ibuprofen to reduce the swelling. Discuss the impact of ibuprofen on her renal haemodynamics considering her use of an ACE inhibitor and a diuretic.

REFERENCES

Australian Medicines Handbook. Adelaide: Australian Medicines Handbook Pty Ltd 2021.

Chew DP, Scott IA, Cullen L, et al. National Heart Foundation of Australia and Cardiac Society of Australia and New Zealand: Australian clinical guidelines for the management of acute coronary syndromes 2016. Medical Journal of Australia 2016; 205:128–33.

Dicpinigaitis PV: Angiotensin-converting enzyme inhibitor-induced cough. Chest 2006;129(Suppl 1):169S–173S.

Gabb GM, Mangoni A, Anderson CS, et al. Guideline for the diagnosis and management of hypertension in adults 2016. Medical Journal of Australia 2016: 205;85–9.

Hsiao F-C, Tung Y-C, Chou S-H, et al. Fixed-dose combination of renin-angiotensin system inhibitors and calcium channel blockers in the treatment of hypertension. Medicine 2015; 94:1–10.

Kirch W, Horn B, Schweizer J. Comparison of angiotensin II receptor antagonists, European Journal of Clinical Investigation 2001; 31:698–706.

Rang HP, Dale MM, Ritter JM, et al: Rang and Dale's pharmacology, ed 7, 2012, Elsevier.

Schwocho LR, Masonson HN. Pharmacokinetics of CS-866, a new angiotensin II receptor blocker, in healthy subjects. Journal of Clinical Pharmacology 2001;41:515–27.

ONLINE RESOURCES

National Heart Foundation of Australia – Guideline for the diagnosis and management of hypertension in adults 2016: https://www.heartfoundation.org.au (accessed 20 January 2022)

More weblinks at: http://evolve.elsevier.com/AU/Knights/pharmacology/.

CHAPTER 12
LIPID-LOWERING DRUGS
Kathleen Knights

KEY ABBREVIATIONS

CAD	coronary artery disease
HDL	high-density lipoproteins
HMG-CoA	3-hydroxy-3-methylglutaryl coenzyme A
IDL	intermediate-density lipoproteins
LDL	low-density lipoproteins
LPL	lipoprotein lipase
PCSK	proprotein convertase subtilisin/kexin
PPAR	peroxisome proliferator activated receptor
VLDL	very-low-density lipoproteins

KEY TERMS

apolipoproteins 235
atherosclerosis 235
high-density lipoproteins 235
HMG-CoA reductase 238
lipoprotein lipase 235
low-density lipoproteins 235
proprotein convertase subtilisin/kexin type 9 236
very-low-density lipoproteins 235

Chapter Focus

Dyslipidaemia, or increased plasma concentrations of cholesterol and triglycerides, is clinically associated with atherosclerosis. Atherosclerosis is characterised by cholesterol deposits in the lining of arteries, which eventually produce degenerative changes and obstruct blood flow. Atherosclerosis can result in angina, heart failure, myocardial infarction, cerebral artery disease and renal artery insufficiency. It is also a factor in hypertension. The treatment guidelines for managing dyslipidaemia include dietary and lifestyle modifications and drug treatment.

KEY DRUG GROUPS

- Bile acid-binding resin: **colestyramine**
- Fibrates: **fenofibrate**, **gemfibrozil**
- HMG-CoA reductase inhibitors (commonly known as statins): **atorvastatin** (Drug Monograph 12.1), **fluvastatin**, **pravastatin**, **rosuvastatin**, **simvastatin**
- PCSK9 inhibitors: **alirocumab**, **evolocumab** (Drug Monograph 12.2)
- Additional drugs: **ezetimibe**, **nicotinic acid**

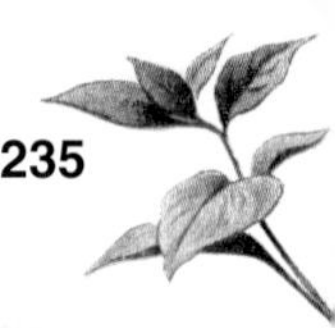

CRITICAL THINKING SCENARIO

Rita, a 63-year-old female, has been prescribed atorvastatin (10 mg/daily) for hypercholesterolaemia. As the prescribing health professional, explain to Rita how atorvastatin works, and discuss the beneficial effects you expect to see in her plasma lipid profile after 4 weeks. She returns regularly for her monthly check up and over a further 2 months her dose is gradually increased to 40 mg daily. On her current visit Rita complains of extensive muscle discomfort, which she indicates started when she resumed her daily glass of grapefruit juice at breakfast time. You immediately advise her to cease the grapefruit juice and you take a blood sample to measure creatinine kinase. Explain the relationship between her atorvastatin dose, her myalgia, her consumption of grapefruit juice and the measurement of creatine kinase.

Introduction

Dyslipidaemia is a metabolic disorder characterised by increased concentrations of lipids and lipoproteins. Lipid-lowering drugs are used along with dietary modifications and exercise to treat dyslipidaemia. Clinical and experimental studies have provided evidence of an important relationship between high levels of circulating triglycerides and cholesterol and atherosclerosis. **Atherosclerosis**, a disorder that involves large- and medium-sized arteries, is characterised by cholesterol deposits in the arterial wall, which eventually produce degenerative changes and obstruct blood flow.

Atherosclerosis is a causative factor in coronary artery disease (CAD), which can result in angina, heart failure and myocardial infarction (MI); cerebral arterial disease that results in senility or cerebrovascular accidents; peripheral arterial occlusive disease, which can cause gangrene and loss of limb; and renal arterial insufficiency. It is also a factor in hypertension.

Lipids do not circulate freely in the bloodstream. Instead, they are transported as complexes called lipoproteins, which are assembled from a mixture of lipids and proteins. They are generally spherical in shape and comprise an interior core, consisting of cholesteryl esters and triglycerides, which are covered by a layer of phospholipids, free cholesterol and apolipoproteins, which are located near the surface. Hyperlipoproteinaemias are always associated with an increased concentration of one or more lipoproteins.

Apolipoproteins

Apolipoproteins have a variety of functions: they serve as ligands for cell receptors, activate enzymes involved in lipoprotein metabolism and provide structure for the lipoprotein. If apolipoprotein metabolism is impaired, an increased risk of atherosclerosis exists; thus, plasma concentrations of apolipoproteins are important in evaluating lipid disorders. The apolipoproteins include apoA-I, apoA-II, apoA-IV, apoA-V, apoB-100, apoB-48, apoC-I, apoC-II, apoC-III, apoE and apo(a). The last is associated with Lp(a), a lipoprotein (structurally related to plasminogen) that promotes thrombosis. Apolipoprotein A-I is thought to confer the beneficial effect of **high-density lipoproteins** (HDL); HDL particles that have both A-I and A-II appear not to be as atheroprotective. In contrast, a deficiency of the C-II apolipoprotein in **very-low-density lipoprotein** (VLDL) particles results in impaired triglyceride metabolism and hypertriglyceridaemia.

Classification of lipoproteins

Chylomicrons are the largest plasma lipoproteins and transport dietary cholesterol and triglycerides absorbed from the gastrointestinal tract (GIT) to the liver. This is known as the exogenous pathway, whereas the lipoproteins transporting cholesterol between the liver and peripheral cells are part of the endogenous pathway. Chylomicrons consist mainly of triglycerides (85–95%) and are produced in the small intestine during absorption of a fatty meal. They are cleared from the bloodstream by **lipoprotein lipase** (LPL) after 12–14 hours. The chylomicron that remains following the removal of the triglyceride content is cleared rapidly by the liver and is not converted into **low-density lipoprotein** (LDLs). The three primary lipoproteins found in the blood of fasting patients are VLDLs, LDLs and HDLs. The intermediate-density lipoproteins (IDLs) have short half-lives (from minutes to a few hours) and their concentrations in plasma tend to be very low.

Very-low-density lipoproteins

VLDLs, which carry lipid from the liver to the peripheral cells, contain a large amount of triglyceride (50–65%) and 20–30% cholesterol, and are formed in the liver from endogenously synthesised triglycerides, cholesterol and phospholipid. These lipoproteins contain 15–20% of the total blood cholesterol and most of the triglyceride found in the body. The apolipoproteins apoB-100, apoE and apoC-I-III are synthesised in the liver and, once incorporated, result in the final assembly of VLDL. After VLDL particles are secreted from the liver into the circulation, their triglyceride content is released as a result of the action of the enzyme LPL, which is located in the endothelium of adipose, muscle and cardiac tissue capillaries. As the triglycerides are hydrolysed by LPL, the resulting free fatty acids are taken up by adjacent tissues. Drugs that enhance the action of LPL (e.g. the fibrates) will lower plasma triglyceride concentrations.

Low-density lipoproteins

When triglyceride hydrolysis is almost complete, the remnant VLDL (termed IDL) is released from the capillary endothelium and re-enters the circulation. Approximately 40–50% of the IDL is cleared from plasma by the liver via LDL receptors, which recognise the apoB-100 and apoE components of the remnants. The remainder of the IDL is converted to the cholesterol-rich lipoprotein LDL, which contains 60–70% of total blood cholesterol; its relationship with the development of atherosclerosis has resulted in its label of 'bad' cholesterol. LDL particles have a half-life of 1–2 days, which accounts for their high concentration in plasma in comparison to VLDL and IDL. The quantity and density of systemic LDL particles correlate with the risk of atherosclerosis, and elevated LDL levels indicate that an individual has a greater risk of developing atherosclerosis. LDL (~75%) is cleared from plasma mainly via hepatic LDL receptors, and defects in the LDL receptor gene are associated with high plasma concentrations of LDL and familial hypercholesterolaemia.

High-density lipoproteins

The function of HDL is to carry about 25% of plasma cholesterol from the periphery back to the liver, where it is processed into bile acids. As the cholesterol HDL carries is ultimately for excretion, it is known as 'good' cholesterol. HDLs are the smallest and most dense lipoproteins and can be separated based on density into HDL2 (larger and more cholesterol-rich) and HDL3 particles (smaller, less cholesterol-rich). Their function is to transfer cholesterol from peripheral cells to the liver, either directly or by exchanging cholesteryl esters for triglycerides from LDL and VLDL. This exchange is mediated by cholesteryl ester transfer protein and accounts for approximately 66% of the removal of cholesterol from HDL. The LDL particles are then cleared from plasma by LDL receptors principally in the liver, and the level of hepatic LDL receptors generally controls the level of circulating LDL in humans. High levels of HDL are considered beneficial and decrease the risk of coronary heart disease. This transport mechanism prevents the accumulation of cholesterol in the arterial walls, thereby providing protection against the development of atherosclerosis.

Synthesis and degradation of LDL receptors

Plasma lipoproteins are usually in a state of dynamic equilibrium. When the liver and tissues outside the liver need cholesterol, they increase the synthesis of LDL receptors on their respective cell surfaces (Fig 12.1). These receptors are necessary for the binding of LDL, thus enabling the release of free fatty acids. When the cellular need for cholesterol is met, the synthesis of LDL receptors decreases, and this controls the plasma level of LDL. The enzyme that 'up' or 'down' regulates the LDL receptor in response to the cell cholesterol concentration is PCSK9 (**proprotein convertase subtilisin/kexin type 9**), which belongs to a family of proprotein convertases that help maintain homeostasis of cell surface receptors such as the LDL receptor. Simply, when PCSK9 attaches to an LDL receptor it is internalised, making the receptor susceptible to lysosomal degradation and thus decreasing the number of LDL receptors. If PCSK9 is not bound to the LDL receptor when it is internalised, it is not degraded in the lysosome and instead is recycled to the cell surface where it continues to clear LDL (see Fig 12.3, later, on PCSK9 inhibitors). Modulation of the number of hepatic LDL receptors is an integral part of the therapeutic approach to the management of hypercholesterolaemia. Figure 12.1 illustrates cholesterol transport in tissues and indicates the sites of action of the lipid-lowering drugs discussed in the following sections.

Hyperlipoproteinaemias

Dyslipidaemias can be classed as primary or secondary. The primary, or genetically determined, hyperlipoproteinaemia forms are classified into six phenotypes, depending on the lipoprotein particle elevated (Table 12.1). Phenotypes IIa and IIb carry the highest risk of atherosclerosis, while phenotypes II and IV have a moderately elevated risk. Factors such as diabetes mellitus, obesity, hypothyroidism, nephrotic syndrome, excess alcohol consumption and drug treatment (e.g. corticosteroids, thiazide diuretics) constitute the secondary causes of dyslipidaemia. In these cases, investigation of underlying disease pathology or current drug treatment is necessary before instituting lipid-lowering drug therapy.

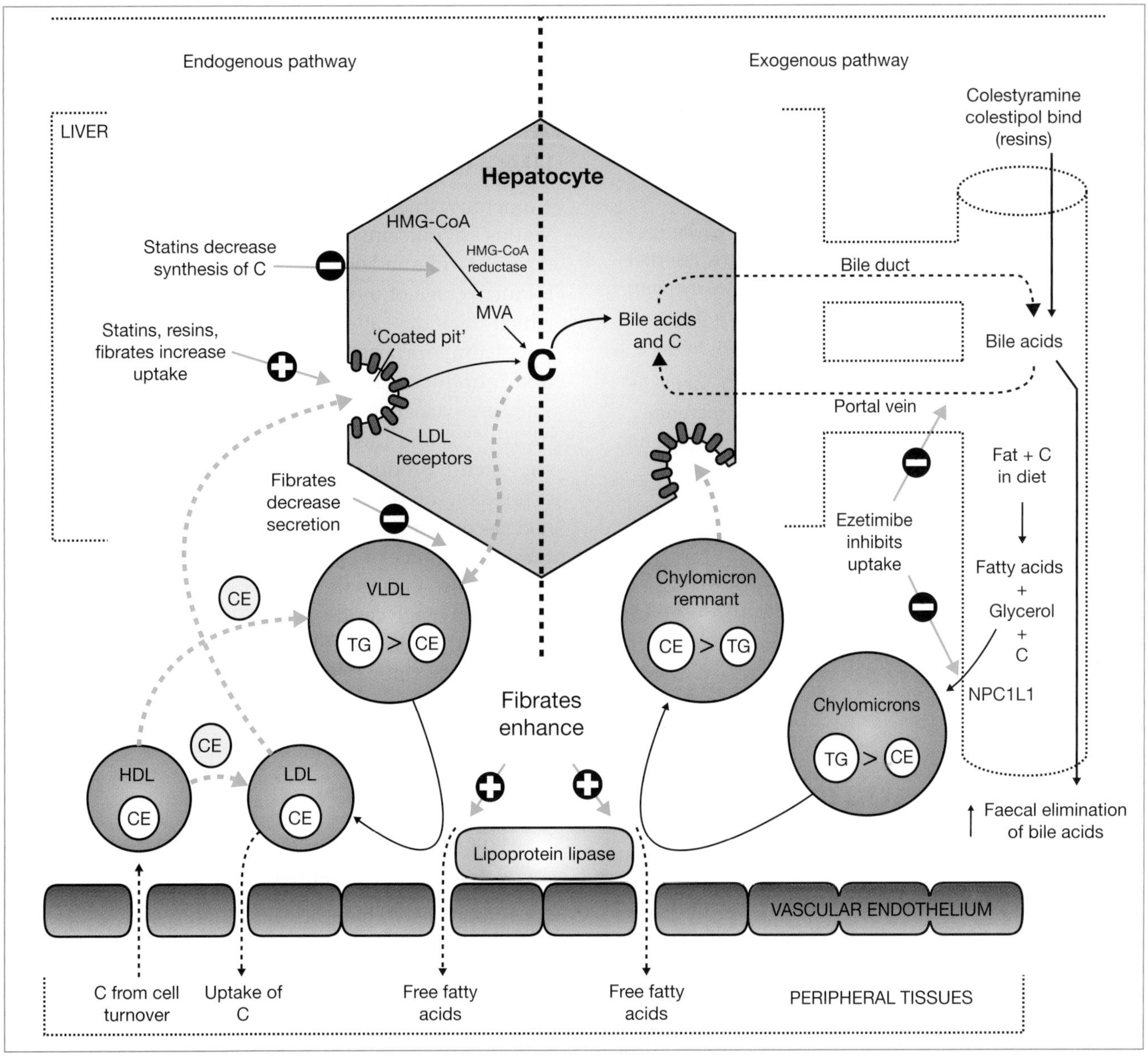

FIGURE 12.1 Schematic diagram of cholesterol transport in the tissues, with sites of action of the main drugs affecting lipoprotein metabolism C = cholesterol; CETP = cholesteryl ester transport protein; HDL = high-density lipoprotein; HMG-CoA reductase = 3-hydroxy-3-methyl-glutaryl-CoA reductase; LDL = low-density lipoprotein; MVA = mevalonate; NPC1L1 = a cholesterol transporter in the brush border of enterocytes; VLDL = very-low-density lipoprotein.

Source: Adapted from Rang et al. 2012, Figure 23.1; used with permission.

TABLE 12.1 Frederickson / World Health Organization classification of hyperlipoproteinaemia

PHENOTYPE	DISORDER	LIPOPROTEIN ELEVATED	LIPIDS ELEVATED
I	Familial lipoprotein lipase deficiency	Chylomicrons	Triglycerides
IIa	Familial hypercholesterolaemia	LDL	Cholesterol
IIb	Familial combined hyperlipidaemia	LDL + VLDL	Cholesterol > triglycerides
III	Familial dysbetalipoproteinaemia	Chylomicron remnants + IDL	Triglycerides + cholesterol
IV	Familial hypertriglyceridaemia	VLDL	Triglycerides
V	Severe hypertriglyceridaemia	Chylomicron remnants + VLDL	Triglycerides > cholesterol

KEY POINTS

Dyslipidaemia

- Dyslipidaemia is a metabolic disorder characterised by increased concentrations of plasma cholesterol and triglycerides and can be classified as primary or secondary.
- High circulating levels of cholesterol and triglycerides have been associated with atherosclerosis, a disorder in which lipids are deposited in the linings of medium- and large-sized arteries, eventually producing degenerative changes and obstructing blood flow.
- Atherosclerosis is a causative factor in CAD, which in turn can result in angina, heart failure, MI, cerebral artery disease, peripheral artery occlusive disease and renal arterial insufficiency.
- The primary lipoproteins found in the blood of fasting patients are VLDL, LDL ('bad') and HDL ('good').
- In non-pathological conditions, lipoproteins, cholesterol and LDL receptors are usually in a state of dynamic equilibrium.

Management strategies for dyslipidaemia

Dietary modification and identification and management of modifiable risk factors (e.g. smoking, alcohol intake, physical activity, weight) are important in the treatment of a high LDL-cholesterol (LDL-C) concentration. Identification of higher risk patients can be aided by a number of tools that can be found online at the Heart Foundation website (see 'Online resurces').

In the absence of a satisfactory reduction of high plasma lipid concentrations through exercise, diet and lifestyle modification, lipid-lowering drugs offer health professionals a management strategy for treating dyslipidaemia. This is of proven benefit in patients with high cardiovascular risk factors (Gurgle & Blumenthal 2018).

The main classes of lipid-lowering drugs are:

- inhibitors of 3-hydroxy-3-methylglutaryl coenzyme A (HMG-CoA) reductase (commonly referred to as statins)
- PCSK9 inhibitors
- bile acid-binding resins
- fibrates
- additional agents, including nicotinic acid, ezetimibe and fish oil.

The choice of drug depends on the patient's plasma lipid profile and whether the aim is to reduce the concentration of LDL-C (hypercholesterolaemia) or triglycerides (hypertriglyceridaemia), or both LDL-C and triglycerides (hyperlipidaemia).

HMG-CoA reductase inhibitors

Numerous studies over 30 years have established that 'statins' significantly reduce the risk of coronary heart disease, stroke and death in patients undergoing treatment for an average of more than 5 years. This group of drugs, which includes atorvastatin (Drug Monograph 12.1), fluvastatin, pravastatin, rosuvastatin and simvastatin, was first introduced into clinical practice in the late 1980s. They are particularly effective, lowering total cholesterol by 10–45% and raising HDL by 2–13%. The decrease in cholesterol production in the liver leads to increased expression of the LDL receptor gene with subsequent increased synthesis of LDL receptors, resulting in a greater clearance of LDL-C from the circulation. A modest increase also occurs in HDL, as well as a slight reduction in plasma triglycerides. The widespread use of these drugs worldwide is attributable to their proven efficacy in randomised clinical trials in reducing CAD, angina, strokes and the need for angioplasty and coronary artery bypass grafts.

Clinical Uses of Statins

- Hypercholesterolaemia
- Patients with a high risk of coronary heart disease
- Hypertensive patients with high risk of CAD
- Post MI

Mechanism of action

Statins are reversible competitive inhibitors of **HMG-CoA reductase**, the rate-limiting enzyme necessary for cholesterol biosynthesis. HMG-CoA reductase catalyses the conversion of HMG-CoA to mevalonate, which is an essential precursor in the synthesis of cholesterol (Fig 12.2). Simvastatin and pravastatin are chemically modified derivatives of the original fungal metabolite lovastatin, whereas atorvastatin, fluvastatin and rosuvastatin are synthetic compounds. In addition to beneficial effects on lipid profiles, the statins have a number of other 'antiatherosclerotic' or pleiotropic effects (Corsini et al. 1999). Clearly, these actions may contribute to the overall beneficial effects observed with statin therapy (Ruscica et al. 2018). These include:

- beneficial effects on endothelial function
- reduced vascular inflammatory response
- reduced platelet aggregability

Drug Monograph 12.1
Atorvastatin

Atorvastatin is a second-generation synthetic drug that resembles the natural substrate HMG-CoA; hence, it is a reversible inhibitor of HMG-CoA reductase. Unlike simvastatin, atorvastatin is administered as the active hydroxy acid form.

Indications

Atorvastatin is indicated for the treatment of hypercholesterolaemia and mixed hyperlipidaemia.

Pharmacokinetics

Atorvastatin is well absorbed, and maximum plasma concentrations occur within 1–2 hours. Bioavailability is low (~12%), which may be accounted for by high hepatic first-pass metabolism and presystemic (gut wall) metabolism. Two active metabolites have been detected in plasma, 2-hydroxy-atorvastatin and 4-hydroxy-atorvastatin, both of which are in equilibrium with their respective inactive lactone forms. CYP3A4 is the main enzyme responsible for formation of the two active metabolites, which are then glucuronidated by UGT1A1 and UGT1A3. The biliary route is the main route of elimination of atorvastatin and its metabolites with less than 2% excreted as unchanged drug in urine; hence, changes in renal function have no significant effect on the pharmacokinetics of atorvastatin. The half-life of atorvastatin is about 20 hours, which may be increased in patients with hepatic disease.

Drug interactions

See Drug Interactions 12.1.

Warnings and contraindications

Use of atorvastatin is contraindicated in the following instances:
- where there is a condition of pre-existing liver disease
- in women of childbearing age unless adequate contraceptive cover is assured
- in people with severe intercurrent illness (infection, trauma).

Adverse reactions

Common adverse reactions include:
- GIT discomfort, headaches, insomnia and dizziness
- an elevation of hepatic transaminase levels within the first few weeks of treatment (dose-related, start at lower end of the dosage range)
- development of myopathy, which can progress to rhabdomyolysis and renal failure. The latter is more likely when the statins are combined with inhibitors of CYP3A4, but an increased incidence has also been observed in combination with the fibrate class of lipid-lowering drugs and nicotinic acid.

Dosage and administration

The initial dose is 10 mg, increasing to a maximum of 80 mg daily. Effectiveness of the dose is determined by monitoring plasma lipids. Atorvastatin is also available in combination with amlodipine for patients stabilised on at least 5 mg of amlodipine daily and in combination with ezetimibe to increase reduction in LDL-C.

- modification of thrombus formation
- stabilisation of atherosclerotic plaques
- decreased smooth muscle cell migration and proliferation
- increased fibrinolytic activity
- decrease in C-reactive protein, a marker of inflammation and coronary heart disease risk.

Pharmacokinetics

At the pharmacokinetic level the statins currently available have some important differences, which are summarised in Table 12.2. Atorvastatin, fluvastatin, pravastatin and rosuvastatin are administered as the active β-hydroxy acid form, whereas simvastatin is administered as an inactive lactone (a prodrug) that requires metabolic activation by the liver to the active hydroxy acid form. Although rosuvastatin is the most hydrophilic statin and simvastatin is more lipophilic, all statins are absorbed rapidly following oral administration, reaching peak concentrations within 5 hours. Food variably affects absorption: there is no apparent effect on the absorption of simvastatin and rosuvastatin, while bioavailability of fluvastatin, pravastatin and atorvastatin is decreased. However, the overall lipid-lowering efficacy of statins is not affected by whether the statin is taken with an evening meal or at bedtime.

All of the statins have low systemic bioavailability, indicating extensive first-pass metabolism. With the exception of pravastatin, which is metabolised by cytosolic

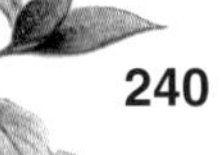

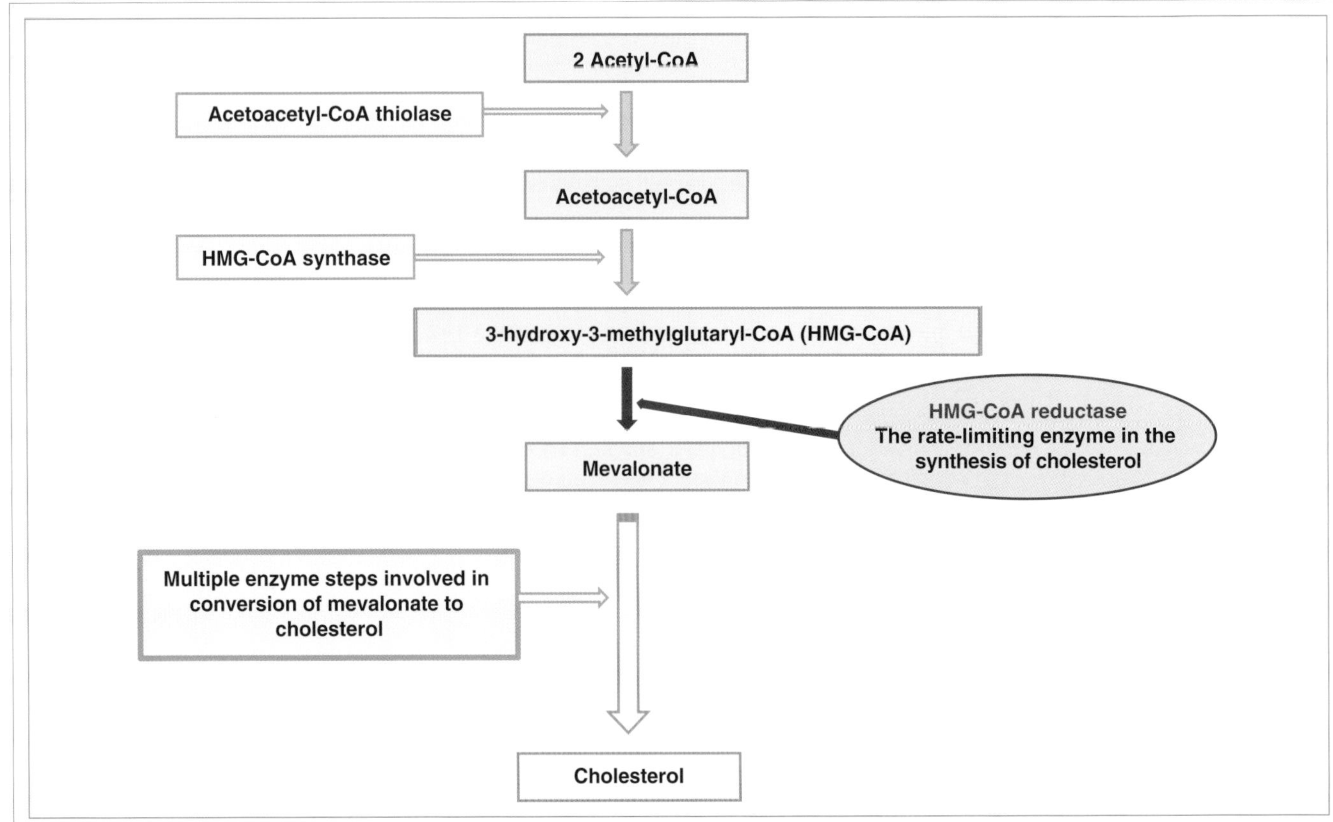

FIGURE 12.2 Synthesis of cholesterol from acetyl-CoA This pathway involves at least 30 enzyme reactions. HMG-CoA reductase catalyses the rate-limiting step in cholesterol synthesis and inhibition of this step reduces formation of cholesterol.

TABLE 12.2 Comparative pharmacokinetics of the statins and reduction in LDL-C*

PARAMETER	ATORVASTATIN	FLUVASTATIN	PRAVASTATIN	ROSUVASTATIN	SIMVASTATIN
Bioavailability (%)	12	19–29	18	17–23	5
T_{max}[a] (h)	2–3	0.5–1	0.9–1.6	3–5	1.3–2.4
Protein binding (%)	80–90	> 99	43–55	88	94–98
Metabolism	CYP3A4	CYP2C9	SULT	CYP2C9, CYP2C19 (minor)	CYP3A4
Metabolites	Active	Inactive	Inactive	Active (minor)	Active
Hepatic extraction (%)	> 70	> 68	46–66	70	78–87
Systemic clearance (L/h/kg)	0.25	0.97	0.81	0.63	0.45
$t_{1/2}$[b] (h)	15–30	0.5–2.3	1.3–2.8	14–26	2–3
OATP transporters	1B1	1B1, 1B3, 2B1	1B1, 1B3, 2B1	1B1, 1B3, 2B1	1B1
Urinary excretion (%)	2	6	20	10	13
Faecal excretion (%)	70	90	71	90	58
Reduction in LDL-C (%)	~50	~28	~30	~52	~38

*Information based on a 40 mg oral dose.
[a]T_{max} = time to reach peak concentration.
[b]$t_{1/2}$ = terminal elimination half-life.
Sources: Bellosta et al. 2004; Corsini et al. 1999; Noe et al. 2007.

sulfotransferases (SULT), all statins are substrates for cytochrome P450 (CYP). Fluvastatin exhibits saturable first-pass metabolism and is metabolised by CYP2C9 and, to a lesser extent, by CYP3A4; atorvastatin and simvastatin are metabolised by CYP3A4; while rosuvastatin is metabolised to a minimal extent by CYP2C9 and CYP2C19.

Interaction with various drug transporters is complex. Atorvastatin is both a substrate and an inhibitor of the efflux transporter P-glycoprotein and a substrate and an inhibitor of the sinusoidal uptake organic anion transporter OATP1B1. Pravastatin is a substrate of OATP1B1, OATP2B1 and OATP1B3 (all expressed on the basolateral membrane on human hepatocytes), which contributes to the efficient hepatic uptake of pravastatin. Hepatic uptake by the various transporters enhances the pharmacological effect of the statins by delivering the drugs directly to the liver as the target organ. Together, hepatic uptake and extensive first-pass metabolism minimise the 'escape' of the drug into the systemic circulation, hence limiting the adverse effects in muscle tissue.

The predominant route of excretion of the statins is via the faeces, with renal excretion accounting for less than 2% with atorvastatin, 6% with fluvastatin, 20% with pravastatin and 30% with rosuvastatin. An initial response is seen within 1–2 weeks and the maximum therapeutic response occurs within 4–6 weeks of chronic drug administration. Bile acid-binding resins can impede absorption, so statins should be administered either 1 hour before or 4 hours after administration of the resin.

Drug interactions

Potential drug interactions with the statins should always be considered, especially because these drugs are often one of multiple medications taken by people with cardiovascular disease. Interactions occur with drugs that can either inhibit or induce CYP enzymes and with other drugs that may be substrates for transporters. Fluvastatin and rosuvastatin are metabolised by CYP2C9 and pravastatin by SULT and hence they are less subject to interactions than the other statins (Drug Interactions 12.1).

Warnings and contraindications

These drugs are used cautiously and at the lowest dose in patients with hepatic or renal impairment because the risk of myopathy and rhabdomyolysis is related to the dose of statin administered and the plasma drug concentration. Hence, reduction in the metabolism of statins (e.g. impaired hepatic function) or the excretion of statins and their active metabolites (e.g. impaired renal function) will increase the likelihood of these adverse effects.

They are avoided in people with hypersensitivity to any HMG-CoA reductase inhibitor, organ transplant recipients receiving immunosuppressant drugs and people with any disease state or condition that may predispose them to renal failure. They are also avoided in women planning pregnancy or with inadequate contraception.

Adverse drug reactions

Although these drugs are well tolerated, adverse drug reactions include:

- stomach cramps or pain, constipation or diarrhoea, nausea
- headache, sleep disturbances (e.g. insomnia, nightmares)
- muscle toxicity (Clinical Focus Box 12.1). This ranges from myalgia (common) through to myopathy, myositis and rhabdomyolysis (rare). Currently, there is no consensus on the exact definition of statin-induced myopathy and the underlying mechanisms are poorly understood (Joy & Hegele 2009). Predisposing factors include older age, female, excessive alcohol intake and concomitant administration of fibrates, ciclosporin, protease inhibitors, macrolide antibiotics or amiodarone. Statin treatment should be ceased if persistent unexplained muscle pain occurs, and the creatine kinase concentration is elevated. In the absence of any identified cause of the myopathy (e.g. hypothyroidism, neuromuscular diseases), statin therapy may be recommenced after a month if the creatine kinase concentration is within the normal range.
- diabetes – data from clinical trials and meta-analyses have indicated that, despite the beneficial effects on cardiovascular health, statins increase the risk

DRUG INTERACTIONS 12.1
Atorvastatin and simvastatin

DRUG*	POSSIBLE EFFECTS AND MANAGEMENT
Clarithromycin, diltiazem, HIV protease inhibitors, antifungal drugs (itraconazole and fluconazole)	Increased plasma concentration of atorvastatin and simvastatin. Increased risk of myopathy or rhabdomyolysis. Stop statin for duration of treatment or use an alternative (e.g. pravastatin). Some combinations contraindicated by manufacturer.
Grapefruit juice	Should be avoided if taking atorvastatin or simvastatin because grapefruit juice inhibits presystemic metabolism of both of these drugs by CYP3A4. Inhibition of presystemic metabolism leads to increased bioavailability and hence an increased plasma drug concentration and the likelihood of adverse effects – in particular, myalgia and myopathy.
St John's wort	Induction of CYP3A4 activity may decrease plasma concentration of both atorvastatin and simvastatin, decreasing clinical effect. Avoid combination with St John's wort.

*This is not an exhaustive list and multiple interactions involving all of the statins with other drugs have been reported. Consult relevant drug information sources before administering atorvastatin or simvastatin.

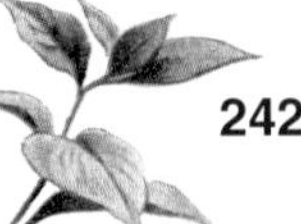

CLINICAL FOCUS BOX 12.1
Overview of the symptoms and progression of statin-induced muscle toxicity

PROGRESSIVE SYMPTOMS	CHARACTERISTICS
Myalgia – diffuse muscle discomfort involving predominantly proximal muscles	♦ Common adverse drug reaction ♦ Dose-related ♦ Reversible ♦ Creatine kinase level normal or slightly elevated
Myopathy – muscle pain with creatine kinase level >10 × upper limit of normal	♦ Dose-related ♦ Affects predominantly upper limb proximal muscles ♦ Muscle fibre necrosis and electromyography changes
Myositis – characterised by muscle weakness with or without elevated creatine kinase levels	♦ Dose-related ♦ Characterised by variation in muscle fibre size and inflammatory cell infiltrate
Rhabdomyolysis – characterised by muscle destruction, presence of myoglobin in urine, muscle pain and swelling, and elevated creatine kinase	♦ Rare (< 1 in 100,000) ♦ Acute renal failure may occur ♦ Can be fatal (< 1 in 1,000,000)

Source: Adapted from Evans 2004.

of incident type 2 diabetes. The risk appears to be greater with higher doses than with lower doses. The mechanism by which statins induce diabetes is unknown but has been suggested to involve perturbation of glucose transport and possible insulin resistance. A further analysis of the JUPITER trial has confirmed the beneficial effect of statins in reducing cardiovascular events in the trial participants irrespective of whether they did or did not have diabetic risk factors. Further, in subjects with a higher risk of developing diabetes (e.g. metabolic syndrome, impaired fasting glucose, body mass index greater than 30 kg/m^2, raised glycated haemoglobin A_{1c}), the benefits of statins therapy still exceeded the diabetes hazard. The data further showed that the risk of developing diabetes was limited to those subjects who already had biochemical evidence of impaired glucose metabolism. However, in comparison to placebo, the average time to diagnosis of diabetes was earlier in the participants receiving statin therapy (Ridker et al. 2012).

Statin dosages

Hepatic cholesterol synthesis is maximal in the early hours of the morning (midnight to 2 am) and statins with short half-lives (fluvastatin, pravastatin and simvastatin) are taken in the evening to maximise efficacy. The recommended adult doses are: atorvastatin range 10–80 mg once daily; fluvastatin 80 mg once daily (controlled release tablet); pravastatin, 10–80 mg daily (in 1 or 2 doses); rosuvastatin, 5–10 mg once daily (range 5–20 mg once daily) to a maximum of 40 mg once daily under specialist supervision; simvastatin, 10–80 mg once daily.

PCSK9 inhibitors

The PCSK9 inhibitors are a newer class of lipid-lowering drug (Dullaart 2017, Page & Watts 2016, Schmidli 2016). They include alirocumab, which is not subsidised by the Pharmaceutical Benefits Scheme, and evolocumab (Drug Monograph 12.2), which is subject to a range of clinical criteria to meet Pharmaceutical Benefits Scheme subsidy requirements. Both drugs are human monoclonal antibodies that bind to circulating PCSK9, preventing it from binding to the hepatocyte LDL receptor and thus promoting continued clearance of cholesterol (Fig 12.3 and previous section on synthesis and degradation of LDL receptors).

Both drugs are administered subcutaneously either fortnightly or once a month. Following administration, maximal inhibition of PCSK9 occurs in 4–8 hours, the plasma drug concentration peaks in 3–4 days, and both drugs have a half-life in the range of 11–20 days. As these drugs are proteins, the most likely metabolism will occur via proteolytic pathways; interactions with CYP enzymes or drug transporters are not anticipated.

The adverse effect profile for both drugs is not fully known, but to date reports of injection site reaction, influenza-like symptoms, upper respiratory tract infections and GIT disturbances (e.g. nausea, diarrhoea) have been documented.

Bile acid-binding resin

Colestyramine is a non-absorbable anion-exchange resin, also called bile acid sequestrant. This drug is no longer a first-line lipid-lowering therapy because of the high incidence of adverse effects and drug interactions and is now principally used as adjunct therapy to the statins. Cholesterol is the major precursor of bile acids, which are secreted from the gallbladder into the small intestine. Bile acids perform two functions in the small intestine: they emulsify fat from food to facilitate chemical digestion; and they are required for absorption of lipids (including the fat-soluble vitamins, A, D, E and K). Bile acids are returned to the liver via enterohepatic recirculation.

Colestyramine binds bile acids in the intestine, thereby decreasing absorption of exogenous cholesterol. To compensate for the loss of bile acids removed by the resins and excreted in the faeces, the liver increases the rate of endogenous metabolism of cholesterol into bile acids and increases the expression of hepatic LDL receptors, and hence the uptake of LDL-C from plasma. Long-term increased faecal loss of bile acids causes a reduction in plasma cholesterol concentration that is blunted by the

Drug Monograph 12.2
Evolocumab

With the discovery of PCSK9 in 2003 and recognition of its role in modulating LDL-C concentration, the development of drugs to target PCSK9 quickly ensued. Evolocumab is a human monoclonal immunoglobulin (IgG2) that binds human PCSK9 (Fig 12.3). It is indicated for treating homozygous familial hypercholesterolaemia, heterozygous familial hypercholesterolaemia in the presence of statin intolerance or suboptimal therapeutic response to a statin, and primary hypercholesterolaemia with preexisting CAD and suboptimal response/intolerance to a statin.

Pharmacokinetics

Following administration, evolocumab has an estimated absolute bioavailability of about 72%. The maximal plasma drug concentration occurs in 3–4 days, and the half-life is in the range of 11–17 days, while steady state is not achieved for 12 weeks (Henry et al. 2016). As expected, the drug has a small volume of distribution (~3.3 L). Evolocumab is primarily a protein; thus, it is unlikely to be metabolised by the liver or kidney. It is anticipated that the drug will be degraded to small peptides and amino acids via normal immunoglobulin clearance pathways. When administered as either monotherapy or a combination therapy, the reduction in LDL-C is in the range of 53–75%.

Adverse reactions

From current clinical trial data, evolocumab appears to be well tolerated, with high participant completion rates (> 90%) in several trials to date. Adverse reactions documented so far include:

- injection site reactions (e.g. redness, pain, bruising)
- nasopharyngitis
- myalgia, back pain, fatigue
- neurocognitive effects (e.g. memory impairment, confusion, delirium).

Warnings and contraindications

To date, human data are limited, and up-to-date drug information sources should be consulted. The manufacturer does not recommend continued breastfeeding if taking evolocumab.

Dosage and administration

Administered subcutaneously, the dosage depends on the type of dyslipidaemia. The usual dosage is either 140 mg once every 2 weeks or 420 mg once a month. If administering the large dose, three injection sites should be used.

increased synthesis of cholesterol by the liver. An increase in plasma triglycerides limits the use of a bile acid-binding resin in people with hypertriglyceridaemia.

Colestyramine is used to treat hypercholesterolaemia and mixed hyperlipidaemia. Plasma cholesterol concentration usually decreases within 1–2 weeks, but in some patients, it may increase or exceed previous concentration with continued therapy. With colestyramine, plasma cholesterol concentration may continue to fall for up to 1 year. However, after withdrawal of colestyramine, the plasma cholesterol concentration tends to rise in 2–4 weeks. Colestyramine is also used to treat pruritus induced by bile acid deposits in dermal tissues (from partial biliary obstruction) and for diarrhoea following ileal resection. Pruritus will return in about 1–2 weeks after discontinuation of the drug. Close monitoring for effectiveness is necessary.

Colestyramine is not absorbed from the GIT and hence there are no major systemic effects. It binds bile acids in the intestine and is excreted via the faeces. See Drug Interactions 12.2 for drug interactions with colestyramine and possible outcomes.

Adverse reactions include:

- constipation, indigestion, abdominal pain, nausea, vomiting, flatulence
- dizziness, headache
- rarely, gallstones, pancreatitis, bleeding ulcers and malabsorption syndrome.

Colestyramine is used with caution in people with gallstones, hypothyroidism, haemorrhoids, kidney disease or bleeding disorders. Avoid use in people with colestyramine hypersensitivity, biliary obstruction or constipation. Colestyramine is contraindicated in the presence of phenylketonuria because of the presence of aspartame in the product. (Aspartame is metabolised to phenylalanine.) Safety in pregnancy has not been established.

Fibrates

Although several fibric acid derivatives are available overseas, only fenofibrate and gemfibrozil are available in Australia. Gemfibrozil and fenofibrate are more effective in reducing VLDL that is rich in triglycerides than in lowering LDL-C that is high in cholesterol. These drugs have not been shown to reduce the overall incidence of cardiovascular mortality, fatal MI or stroke. The mechanism of action is not completely understood, but recent studies indicate that fibrates interact with peroxisome proliferator activated receptors (PPARs), which regulate gene transcription. Specifically, an interaction with a PPAR may provide an explanation for the reduction of triglycerides via stimulation of fatty acid oxidation, increased LPL activity and the reduction in apoC-III synthesis. These drugs are indicated principally to treat severe hypertriglyceridaemia and mixed hyperlipidaemia, and as second-line treatment for hypercholesterolaemia.

Additional drugs

Several additional drugs are discussed below, and a comparison of their lipid-lowering effects is given in Table 12.3.

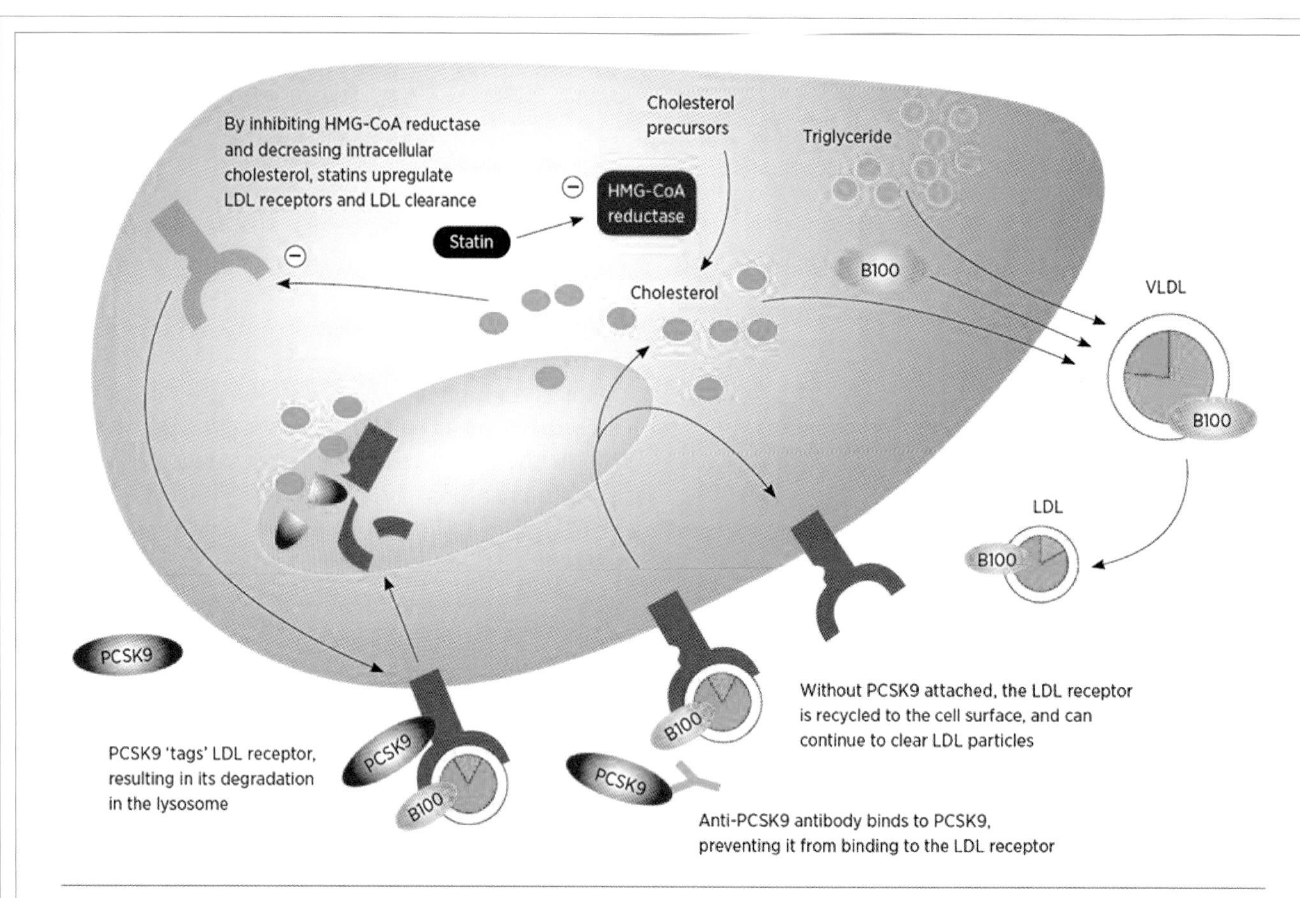

FIGURE 12.3 Mechanism of action of statins and anti-PCSK9 monoclonal antibodies VLDL is secreted by the liver and converted to LDL, which delivers cholesterol to peripheral tissues and is atherogenic. LDL particles are taken up via LDL receptors, primarily on hepatocytes, and degraded. The production of LDL receptors is decreased by intracellular cholesterol, so lowering intracellular cholesterol with statins results in increased LDL receptors and LDL uptake. LDL-receptor degradation is enhanced by PCSK9, so inhibiting PCSK9 with antibodies increases LDL-receptor recycling and LDL uptake.

Source: Page & Watts 2016; reproduced with permission.

DRUG INTERACTIONS 12.2

Bile acid-binding resin[a]

DRUG	POSSIBLE EFFECTS AND MANAGEMENT
Warfarin	Concurrent use significantly decreases absorption of warfarin; thus the anticoagulant effect might be reduced. It is suggested that warfarin be given 1 hour before, or 4–6 hours after, colestyramine. Also, monitor the international normalised ratio and adjust warfarin dose as necessary.
Digoxin	Reduced absorption occurs with a bile acid-binding resin. It is recommended that drugs be administered at least 1 hour before, or 4–6 hours after, administration of resin. Monitor plasma digoxin concentration.
Thyroxine	Decreased absorption of thyroxine. Separate doses of thyroxine and colestyramine by at least 4 hours and monitor clinical response to thyroxine.

[a]Multiple interactions with other drugs affecting either absorption and/or enterohepatic recycling have been reported. Consult relevant drug information sources before administering a bile acid-binding resin.

TABLE 12.3 Comparison of lipid-lowering effects

	EFFECT ON LIPIDS[a]		EFFECT ON LIPOPROTEINS			
DRUG	CHOLESTEROL	TRIGLYCERIDES	VLDL	LDL	HDL	TYPICAL RESPONSE
Colestyramine	↓	0 or slight ↑	0 or ↑	↓	0 or ↑	Decreases cholesterol 20–40%
Evolocumab	↓↓	0	↓	↓	↑	Decreases cholesterol 50–60%
Ezetimibe	↓	↓	–	↓	0 or ↑	Decreases cholesterol 10–18%
Fenofibrate	↓	↓	↓	↓ or ↑	↑	Significantly lowers triglycerides 20–50%
Gemfibrozil	↓	↓	↓	↓ or ↑	↑	Decreases triglycerides; only slight decrease in cholesterol
Nicotinic acid	↓	↓	↓	↓	↑	Decreases triglycerides (40–80%) and cholesterol 10–20%
Simvastatin	↓	↓	↓	↓	↑	Decreases cholesterol 30–50%

[a]↑ = increase; ↓ = decrease; 0 = no change.

Nicotinic acid

The lipid-lowering effect of nicotinic acid (niacin) has been known since 1955. Nicotinic acid is a water-soluble vitamin that inhibits mobilisation of free fatty acids from peripheral tissue via an inhibition of hormone-sensitive lipase activity. This results in a reduction in the transport of free fatty acids to the liver and, hence, reduced hepatic synthesis of triglycerides and the secretion of VLDL. Nicotinic acid also increases the plasma HDL concentration markedly (20–30%) via a reduction in clearance of apoA-I. It is used principally as an adjunct to other therapies, such as the fibrates and colestyramine, to treat severe and mixed hypertriglyceridaemia. It is also used to treat niacin (vitamin B3) deficiency and, because it increases blood flow through skin and muscle, it is used to treat peripheral vascular disease.

Nicotinic acid is well absorbed orally and has a plasma half-life of about 45 minutes. Extensive metabolism occurs in the liver where nicotinic acid is conjugated with glycine-forming nicotinuric acid, which is excreted in urine. Approximately 35% of the dose is excreted as unchanged drug in urine. Reduction in plasma triglyceride concentration occurs within several hours of the start of dosing.

Combination with HMG-CoA reductase inhibitors can result in myopathy and rhabdomyolysis. Potentiation of the effect of antihypertensive drugs has also been reported. Adverse reactions include increased feelings of warmth and flushing of the face and neck. Flushing can be very intense and can be reduced in severity by taking aspirin 30–60 minutes before each dose of nicotinic acid. Other common adverse effects include hypotension, nasal stuffiness, diarrhoea, vomiting and dyspepsia. Less frequently encountered are pruritus, skin rash, dry skin or eyes, hyperglycaemia, hyperuricaemia and jaundice. Liver toxicity has been reported with doses of 2 g per day and higher doses. Use with caution in people with gout, diabetes mellitus, peptic ulcer, liver disease and CAD. A reduction in dose may be necessary in situations of renal impairment. Nicotinic acid is contraindicated in people with a recent MI or symptomatic hypotension.

Ezetimibe

Ezetimibe is a novel lipid-lowering drug that inhibits intestinal absorption of both cholesterol and phytosterols. It is effective in inhibiting both intestinal absorption of dietary cholesterol and reabsorption of cholesterol excreted in bile (Fig 12.1). The exact mechanism of action is unknown, but ezetimibe localises at the brush border of the small intestine and is thought to inhibit absorption of cholesterol by binding to a specific transport protein (NPC1L1) in the small intestine wall. Ezetimibe inhibits intestinal absorption of plant sterols but does not alter absorption of fat-soluble vitamins and nutrients. The average reduction in LDL-C with ezetimibe is about 18% and it has minimal effect on HDL-C and triglycerides. It is primarily used as an adjunct to diet for the treatment of hypercholesterolaemia and homozygous phytosterolaemia.

Ezetimibe is conjugated in the intestine, forming an active glucuronide, which accounts for approximately 90% of the drug in plasma after 30 minutes. Ezetimibe and ezetimibe glucuronide are then transported to the liver and subsequently secreted in bile back into the intestine (enterohepatic recycling). The half-life of both is approximately 22 hours, and about 80% of the administered dose is excreted in faeces and about 11% in urine. As ezetimibe is not metabolised to any major extent in the liver, significant interactions with most drugs used to treat dyslipidaemia are not a major issue. However, coadministration with colestyramine reduces bioavailability, and hence these drugs should be administered several hours apart.

Ezetimibe is administered once daily as a 10 mg dose. Commonly, ezetimibe causes headache and diarrhoea and, as with the statins, muscle disorders (e.g. myalgia, muscle cramps, weakness and pain) have been reported. Combinations of ezetimibe (10 mg) and simvastatin (10–80 mg) or atorvastatin (10–80 mg) or rosuvastatin

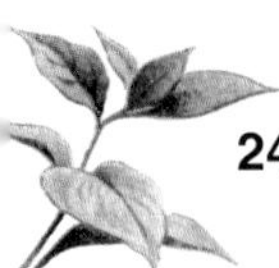

(5–40 mg) increases the lipid-lowering effect of the statin by up to 20% and is a valuable combination for patients who cannot tolerate a higher dose of a statin.

Fish oils

In general, the consumption of omega-3 fatty acids by humans has decreased as a result of marked changes in dietary habits. One of the active components of fish oil is docosahexaenoic acid (DHA), which is present in oily fish such as mackerel, salmon and tuna. Consumption of a fish-rich diet is thought to account for the lower incidence of coronary heart disease in the Japanese and in Greenland Inuit. Omega-3 fatty acids are thought to exert their beneficial effects through reducing VLDL formation and accelerating VLDL metabolism to LDL particles. This ultimately reduces triglyceride levels, but also potentially increases LDL-C levels. Similar to the fibrates, omega-3 fatty acids have a high affinity for PPARα and may upregulate the metabolism of fatty acids in the liver.

Although fish oil supplements appear to be relatively safe, high doses may increase bleeding time. Current information from the Heart Foundation suggests eating a healthy diet rich in fruit and vegetables and consuming two or three serves (150 g serve) of oily fish per week (see 'Online resources').

KEY POINTS

Lipid-lowering drugs

- In the absence of a satisfactory reduction of high plasma lipid concentrations through exercise, diet and lifestyle modification, lipid-lowering drugs are used to treat dyslipidaemia.
- Effectiveness of lipid-lowering drugs varies depending on the specific type of dyslipidaemia.
- The main classes of lipid-lowering drugs are the HMG-CoA reductase inhibitors ('statins'), PCSK9 inhibitors, bile acid-binding resin and fibrates.
- Statins (HMG-CoA reductase inhibitors) significantly reduce the risk of coronary heart disease, stroke and death in patients undergoing treatment for more than 5 years.
- The newer PCSK9 inhibitors substantially reduce LDL-C, and long-term trials are ongoing to determine their safety, efficacy and impact on cardiovascular disease outcomes.
- Colestyramine is a non-absorbable anion-exchange resin, also called bile acid sequestrant.
- The HMG-CoA reductase inhibitors and colestyramine are subject to numerous drug interactions.
- Gemfibrozil and fenofibrate are more effective in reducing VLDL that is rich in triglycerides than in lowering LDL that is high in cholesterol.
- Ezetimibe is a novel lipid-lowering drug that inhibits intestinal absorption of both cholesterol and phytosterols. It is effective in inhibiting both intestinal absorption of dietary cholesterol and reabsorption of cholesterol excreted in bile.
- An additional agent used to treat dyslipidaemia is nicotinic acid.

DRUGS AT A GLANCE
Lipid-lowering drugs

PHARMACOLOGICAL GROUP AND EFFECT	KEY EXAMPLES	CLINICAL USE
Lipid-lowering drugs *Statins - HMG-CoA reductase inhibitors* • ↓ cholesterol synthesis • ↑ LDL receptors • ↓ triglycerides *Line up with Alirocumab* • Bind to PCSK9 which inhibits its binding to LDL receptors • ↑ LDL clearance *Line up with Colestyramine* • Bind bile acids in small intestine • ↓ absorption of cholesterol • ↑ expression LDL receptors	Atorvastatin	• Hypercholesterolaemia • Hypertensive patients at risk of cardiovascular disease
	Fluvastatin	• Hypercholesterolaemia • CAD after PCI
	Pravastatin	• Hypercholesterolaemia • After MI • Unstable angina
	Rosuvastatin	• Hypercholesterolaemia • High risk of cardiovascular disease
	Simvastatin	• Hypercholesterolaemia • High risk of cardiovascular disease
	Alirocumab	• Hypercholesterolaemia after inadequate response to statins
	Evolocumab	• Homozygous familial hypercholesterolaemia • Inadequate response to statins

<table>
<tr><td rowspan="8">Line up with Bezafibrate
• Interact with PPARs to regulate gene transcription
• ↓ triglycerides
• ↑ HDL
Line up with Ezetimibe
• Inhibits absorption of exogenous cholesterol
• Inhibits lipase activity
• ↓ mobilisation of free fatty acids from periphery
• ↓ synthesis of triglycerides
• ↑ HDL</td><td>Colestyramine</td><td>• Hypercholesterolaemia
• Bile acid induced pruritus
• Diarrhoea following ileal resection</td></tr>
<tr><td>Colestipol[NZ]</td><td>• Hypercholesterolaemia</td></tr>
<tr><td>Bezafibrate[NZ]</td><td>• Primary hyperlipidaemia types IIa, IIb, III, IV and V
• Severe hypertriglyceridaemia</td></tr>
<tr><td>Fenofibrate[AUS]</td><td>• Severe hypertriglyceridaemia
• Dyslipidaemia associated with type 2 diabetes</td></tr>
<tr><td>Gemfibrozil</td><td>• Severe hypertriglyceridaemia with risk of pancreatitis
• Dyslipidaemia associated with diabetes</td></tr>
<tr><td>Ezetimibe[AUS]</td><td>• Hypercholesterolaemia
• Homozygous sitosterolaemia</td></tr>
<tr><td>Nicotinic acid</td><td>• Hypercholesterolaemia
• Mixed hyperlipidaemia
• Severe triglyceridaemia</td></tr>
</table>

[AUS]Australia only
[NZ]NZ only

REVIEW EXERCISES

1 Mr BG, a 59-year-old male, has been diagnosed previously with hypercholesterolaemia. His HDL-C was less than 1 mmol/L, his total cholesterol was 8.1 mmol/L and his triglycerides were normal. After a period of time Mr BG found he was unable to tolerate the higher dose of atorvastatin (80 mg daily) and he has now been commenced on a fixed-dose combination of ezetimibe (10 mg) and atorvastatin (20 mg). Discuss the pharmacological effect of the combination drug and indicate what you expect/hope to see when he has his next lipid profile done.

2 Mrs BK has a history of gall stones and has previously been treated with colestyramine to relieve the itching, which was caused by the deposition of bile acids in her dermal tissue. Explain why colestyramine, which is generally prescribed for hypercholesterolaemia, is effective under these circumstances.

3 Mr DE has been diagnosed with severe hypertriglyceridaemia. With regard to the lipid-lowering drugs groups available to you, make a table listing the pros and cons of each drug group in terms of the impact on the lipid profile. Which drug groups are indicated for hypertriglyceridaemia?

REFERENCES

Bellosta S, Paoletti R, Corsini A. Safety of statins: focus on clinical pharmacokinetics and drug interactions. Circulation 2004;109:III-50–III-57.

Corsini A, Bellosta S, Baetta R, et al. New insights into the pharmacodynamic and pharmacokinetic properties of statins. Pharmacology & Therapeutics 1999;84:413–428.

Dullaart RPF. PCSK9 inhibition to reduce cardiovascular events. The New England Journal of Medicine 2017;376(18): 1790–91.

Evans M. Statin safety in perspective – maximising the risk:benefit. British Journal of Cardiology 2004;11:449–454.

Gurgle HE, Blumenthal DK: Drug therapy for dyslipidemia. In: Brunton LL, Hilal-Dandan R, Knollman BC, editors: Goodman & Gilman's The pharmacological basis of therapeutics. New York: McGraw-Hill; 2018, 13 edn, pp. 605–618.

Henry CA, Lyon RA, Ling H. Clinical efficacy and safety of evolocumab for low-density lipoprotein cholesterol reduction. Vascular Health and Risk Management 2016;12:163–69.

Joy TR, Hegele R.: Narrative review: statin-related myopathy. Annals of Internal Medicine 2009;150:858–868.

Noe J, Portmann R, Brun ME, Funk C. Substrate-dependent drug–drug interactions between gemfibrozil, fluvastatin and other organic anion-transporting peptide (OATP) substrates on OATP1B1, OATP2B1 and OATP1B3. Drug Metabolism and Disposition 2007;35:1308–14.

Page MM, Watts GF. PCSK9 inhibitors– mechanisms of action. Australian Prescriber 2016; 39:164–67.

Rang HP, Dale MM, Ritter JM, et al: Rang and Dale's pharmacology, ed 7, 2012, Elsevier.

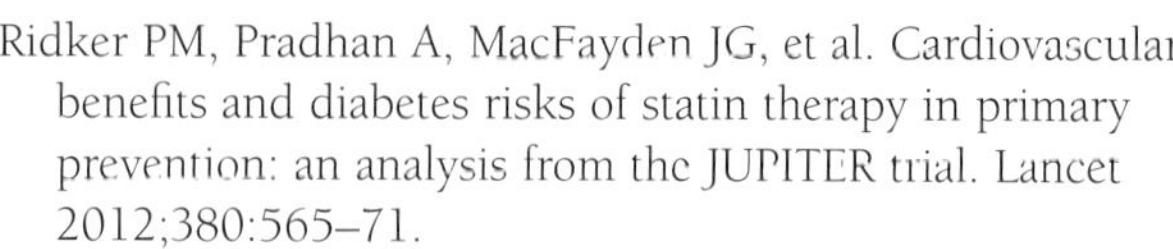

Ridker PM, Pradhan A, MacFayden JG, et al. Cardiovascular benefits and diabetes risks of statin therapy in primary prevention: an analysis from the JUPITER trial. Lancet 2012;380:565–71.

Ruscica M, Ferri N, Macchi C, et al. Lipid-lowering drugs and inflammatory changes: an impact on cardiovascular outcomes? Annals of Medicine 2018;50:461–484.

Schmidli R. PCSK9 inhibitors – clinical applications. Australian Prescriber 2016; 39:168–701.

ONLINE RESOURCES

Australian Heart Foundation. You're probably not eating enough fish – here's what you should do: https//www.heartfoundation.org.au/blog/not-eating-enough-fish (accessed 31 May 2021)

More weblinks at: http://evolve.elsevier.com/AU/Knights/pharmacology/.

CHAPTER 13

DRUGS AFFECTING THROMBOSIS AND HAEMOSTASIS

Kathleen Knights

KEY ABBREVIATIONS

ADP	adenosine diphosphate
aPTT	activated partial thromboplastin time
INR	international normalised ratio
LMWHs	low-molecular-weight heparins
NOACs	new oral anticoagulants
PT	prothrombin time

KEY TERMS

anticoagulant drugs 252
antifibrinolytic drugs 263
antiplatelet drugs 260
embolus 250
haemostasis 250
haemostatic drugs 263
low-molecular-weight heparins 252
thrombolytic (fibrinolytic) drugs 262
thrombus 250

Chapter Focus

Globally, tens of thousands of people die each year from coronary heart disease and stroke, and many more are diagnosed with deep vein thrombosis, pulmonary embolus, transient cerebral ischaemic attacks and other non-fatal thrombotic events. The formation of thrombi or acute thromboembolic disorders requires the use of anticoagulant, thrombolytic and antiplatelet agents. In contrast, in some instances excessive bleeding needs to be reversed by the use of specific haemostatic and antifibrinolytic drugs that hasten clot formation and reduce bleeding. All of these drugs are potent, effective medications requiring a thorough knowledge of their pharmacology for safe administration and usage.

KEY DRUG GROUPS

Anticoagulants:

- Antithrombin III-dependent: **fondaparinux**
- Direct factor Xa inhibitors: **apixaban**, **rivaroxaban**
- Direct thrombin inhibitors: **bivalirudin**, **dabigatran etexilate**
- Heparins: dalteparin, **enoxaparin** (Drug Monograph 13.1), **heparin**, nadroparin
- Vitamin K antagonists: **warfarin** (Drug Monograph 13.2)

Antiplatelet drugs:

- **Aspirin**, **dipyridamole**
- Glycoprotein IIb/IIIa receptor inhibitors: **eptifibatide**, **tirofiban**
- $P2Y_{12}$ inhibitors: **clopidogrel**, **prasugrel**, **ticagrelor**

Haemostatic and antifibrinolytic drugs:

- Factor VIII, factor IX, **idarucizumab**, **protamine**, **tranexamic acid**, **vitamin K**

Thrombolytics:

- **Alteplase**, **tenecteplase**, urokinase

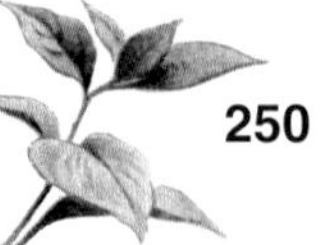

CRITICAL THINKING SCENARIO

Jennifer, a 69-year-old woman, has been admitted to her local hospital for an elective knee replacement. Following surgery, she returns to the ward at 4 pm. At 10 pm she is started on fondaparinux 2.5 mg subcutaneously once daily, which is continued for the next 5 days while she remains in hospital. The orthopaedic surgeon advises Jennifer that the drug will be continued until she is fully mobile.

1. Discuss the mechanism of action of fondaparinux.
2. Explain why Jennifer was commenced on this drug 6 hours postoperatively and should remain on the drug until fully mobile.

Introduction

This chapter reviews anticoagulant, antiplatelet, thrombolytic, haemostatic and antifibrinolytic drugs. Although blood clotting normally provides protection against excessive haemorrhage, the development of a **thrombus** (an aggregation of platelets, fibrin, clotting factors and the cellular elements of blood) that becomes attached to the inner wall of a blood vessel can obstruct blood flow and cause ischaemia. An **embolus**, a mass of undissolved matter that breaks off from the thrombus, can travel in the vascular system and lodge, causing ischaemia, infarction and death. In contrast, a defect in the blood coagulation cascade can lead to excessive bleeding or haemorrhage, even after a minor injury.

Basically, inappropriate activation of coagulation mechanisms is responsible for forming two types of thrombi: arterial thrombi and venous thrombi. Both are associated with significant morbidity and mortality, and the risk of thrombosis increases with age. Thousands of people die each year from coronary heart disease and stroke, and many more are diagnosed with deep vein thrombosis, pulmonary embolus, transient cerebral ischaemic attacks and other non-fatal thrombotic events. Local trauma, vascular stasis and systemic alterations in blood coagulation are considered the main factors in the initiation of a thrombosis in an unbroken vessel. The pathogenesis of arterial thrombosis is complex and involves genetic and environmental factors. Arterial thrombi are most frequently associated with ruptured atherosclerotic plaques, high blood pressure and turbulent blood flow, which damage the endothelial lining of the blood vessel causing platelets to aggregate and stick in the arterial system.

Venous thrombosis is also a multifactorial problem that occurs in areas where blood flow is reduced or stasis occurs, which initiates clotting and produces a thrombus in the venous system. Risk factors for venous thrombosis include inherited thrombophilia disorders (e.g. antithrombin deficiency), prolonged immobilisation (e.g. long-haul flights, major trauma), operative procedures (e.g. orthopaedic surgery), certain types of cancer (e.g. myeloproliferative disorders), pregnancy, use of the oral contraceptive pill and hormone replacement therapy.

Drugs affecting thrombosis and haemostasis include:

- anticoagulants
- antiplatelet drugs
- thrombolytics
- haemostatic and antifibrinolytic drugs.

The haemostatic mechanism

Haemostasis is a process that spontaneously stops bleeding from damaged blood vessels and is achieved by three sequential steps:

Step 1. Vasoconstriction

This response instantly slows the flow of blood from and through the ruptured vessel.

Step 2. Platelet plug formation

After injury to a blood vessel, interruption of the continuity of the endothelial lining exposes collagen (a fibrous protein) in the underlying connective tissue. Platelets become activated, changing their shape (Ch 14) and becoming spherical with long dendritic extensions that facilitate adhesion to the exposed collagen; a dense aggregate is formed, in a process known as platelet adhesion. This attachment triggers the release of adenosine diphosphate (ADP) and thromboxane A_2 from the dense granules in the platelet cytoplasm. Liberation of these factors causes further activation of nearby platelets and vasoconstriction through the action of thromboxane A_2, which further limits blood flow through the damaged vessel. Platelet membrane glycoprotein receptors mediate adhesion to the subendothelial tissue, and the outer surfaces of the platelets become extremely sticky. The surface protein glycoprotein IIb/IIIa undergoes a conformational change during platelet activation, expressing receptor function for fibrinogen. Binding of fibrinogen to glycoprotein IIb/IIIa mediates platelet aggregation, and eventually the mass forms the haemostatic plug (Fig 13.4, later). Because this plug is relatively unstable, it can stop the bleeding quickly as long as the damage to the vessel is minute. However, for long-term effectiveness the platelet plug must be reinforced with fibrin. This involves a series of chemical coagulation or clotting reactions. Blood coagulation ultimately results in the formation of a stable fibrin clot, which comprises a meshwork of fibrin threads that entraps platelets, blood cells and plasma. Thus, the physical formation of a blood clot or thrombus plays a key role in haemostasis by permanently closing the hole in the injured vessel, preventing further bleeding.

Step 3. Blood coagulation

The chemical events in blood coagulation involve two distinct pathways: the intrinsic pathway and the extrinsic pathway.

Intrinsic pathway

Because all the chemical substances involved in coagulation are normally found in circulating blood, this pathway is referred to as the intrinsic pathway of coagulation. In this complex pathway, activation by proteolysis of the first inactive blood coagulation factor causes activation of the next factor, and this cascading process continues through the whole pathway. See Figure 13.1 for a summary of the main steps in the intrinsic pathway.

The process occurs over several minutes and is initiated by injury to the endothelial lining of the blood vessel wall. Briefly:

1. When blood contacts the exposed underlying collagen, factor XII (Hageman factor) is activated by proteolysis to the active 'a' form (factor XIIa). The simultaneous damage of platelets also causes the release of platelet phospholipid (platelet factor III), which is required later in the coagulation process.
2. Factor XIIa then activates factor XI, converting it to factor XIa.
3. In the presence of calcium ions, factor XIa then reacts with factor IX to form activated factor IXa.
4. Factor IXa, in the presence of calcium ions and platelet phospholipid, interacts with factor VIII and thrombin to form a complex. This combination then speeds up the activation of factor X, forming factor Xa.

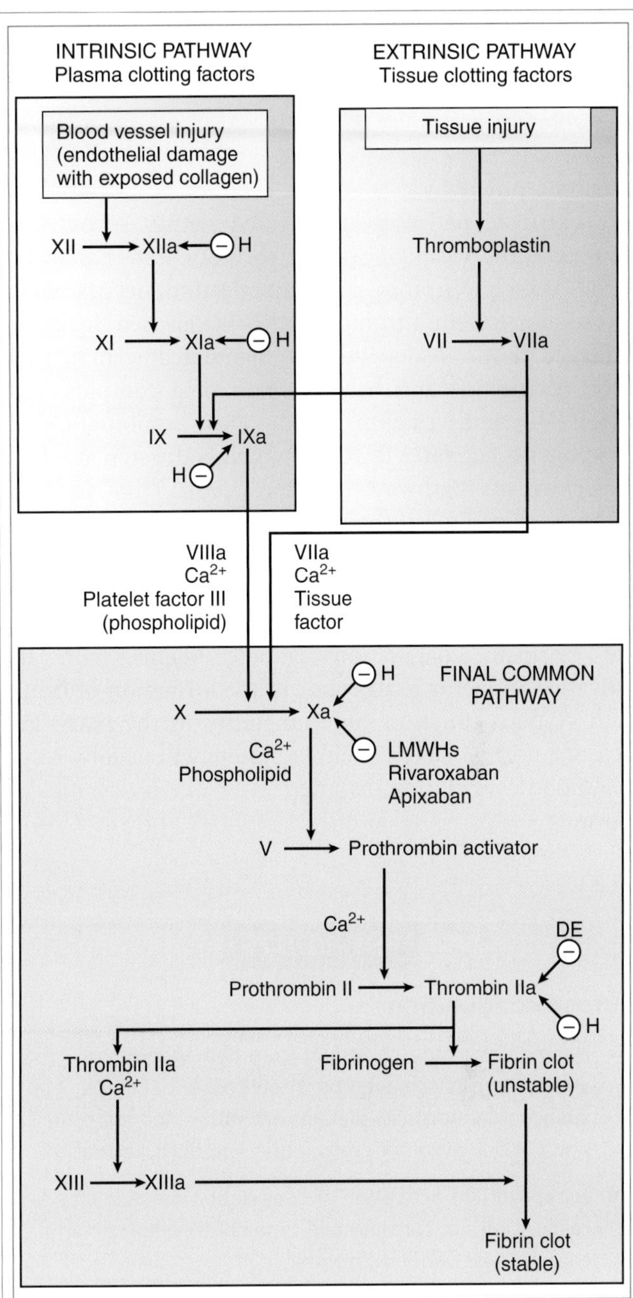

FIGURE 13.1 **Coagulation cascade for the intrinsic and extrinsic pathways** Final pathway (activation of factor X) is common to both the intrinsic and the extrinsic pathways. Sites of action of anticoagulant drugs denoted; H = heparin; LMWHs = low-molecular-weight heparins; DE = dabigatran etexilate; ⊖ = inhibition

5. Factor Xa combines with factor V, calcium ions and platelet phospholipid to form a complex known as the prothrombin activator (factor IIa).
6. Factor IIa initiates the cleavage of prothrombin to form thrombin, which then converts fibrinogen into fibrin, forming an unstable clot.

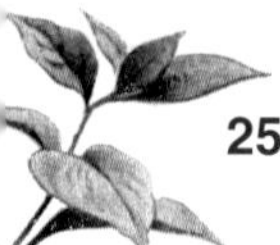

7 The final step involves the action of factor XIII (a fibrin-stabilising factor), thrombin and calcium ions, which catalyse the formation of a stronger, stable fibrin clot.

Extrinsic pathway

The extrinsic pathway is activated within seconds by trauma to the vascular wall or to tissue external to the blood vessels. In this pathway, clotting occurs when the tissue protein thromboplastin is released from the damaged tissue, leaks into the bloodstream (hence the name 'extrinsic') and becomes part of a complex with factor VII and calcium ions. This combination of components activates factor X, which is the step at which the extrinsic pathway converges with the intrinsic pathway; coagulation then continues through a common route with the resultant formation of a stable clot (see Fig 13.1 for the extrinsic pathway).

The final pathway common to both the intrinsic and the extrinsic coagulation cascade begins with the activation of factor X and ends in the formation of fibrin. Both systems function simultaneously in the body, and lack of a normal factor in either system will usually result in a blood coagulation disorder.

KEY POINTS

Blood coagulation

- Haemostasis stops bleeding from damaged blood vessels and is achieved by three sequential steps: (1) vasoconstriction; (2) platelet activation and adhesion; and (3) activation of coagulation and fibrin formation.
- Inappropriate activation of coagulation mechanisms is responsible for forming two types of thrombi: arterial thrombi and venous thrombi.
- Both types of thrombi are associated with significant morbidity and mortality, and the risk of thrombosis increases with age.
- Arterial thrombi are most frequently associated with ruptured atherosclerotic plaques, high blood pressure and turbulent blood flow, which damage the endothelial lining of the blood vessel, causing platelets to aggregate and adhere in the arterial system.
- Venous thrombosis occurs in areas where blood flow is reduced or stasis occurs.
- Blood coagulation involves two distinct pathways: the intrinsic pathway and the extrinsic pathway.

Anticoagulant drugs

Anticoagulant drug therapy (Fig 13.2) is primarily prophylactic because these agents act by preventing fibrin deposits, extension of a thrombus and thromboembolic complications. Although long-term anticoagulant therapy remains controversial, there is evidence that anticoagulant therapy reduces the incidence of thrombosis and therefore prolongs life. These drugs have no direct effect on a blood clot that has already formed or on ischaemic tissue injured by an inadequate blood supply because of the clot.

The main groups of **anticoagulant drugs** include:

- heparin and the **low-molecular-weight heparins** (LMWHs) dalteparin, enoxaparin (Drug Monograph 13.1) and nadroparin, and the LMW heparinoid danaparoid
- the vitamin K antagonist warfarin (Drug Monograph 13.2, later)
- the antithrombin III-dependent anticoagulant fondaparinux
- the direct thrombin inhibitors bivalirudin and dabigatran etexilate
- the direct factor Xa inhibitors apixaban and rivaroxaban.

Heparin and the LMWHs are the drugs of first choice if a rapid anticoagulant effect is required because their onset is immediate if administered intravenously.

Low-molecular-weight heparins

Currently, there are three LMWHs on the market – dalteparin, enoxaparin and nadroparin – and one heparinoid, danaparoid. The LMWHs are fragments approximately one-third the size of standard heparin and are prepared by enzymatic or chemical cleavage of unfractionated heparin. This difference in molecular weight produces an anticoagulant with properties considerably different from those of heparin. The LMWHs are administered subcutaneously and are considered to be safer and require less monitoring than standard heparin.

Mechanism of action

Both types of heparin can inactivate factor Xa. Unfractionated heparin also inactivates thrombin (IIa) by binding, at the same time, to both antithrombin III and thrombin. In contrast, LMWHs increase the action of antithrombin III on factor Xa but, because of their small size, LMWHs cannot bind antithrombin III and thrombin at the same time. Hence, they have both an enhanced capacity to inhibit factor Xa, which contributes to their improved antithrombotic effect, and a relatively minor effect on aPTT (Clinical Focus Box 13.1). Danaparoid is a more selective inhibitor of factor Xa than the LMWHs. See Table 13.1 for a comparison of unfractionated heparin and LMWHs.

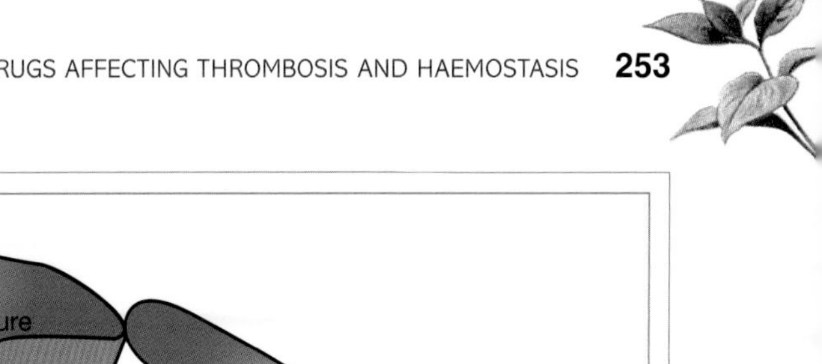

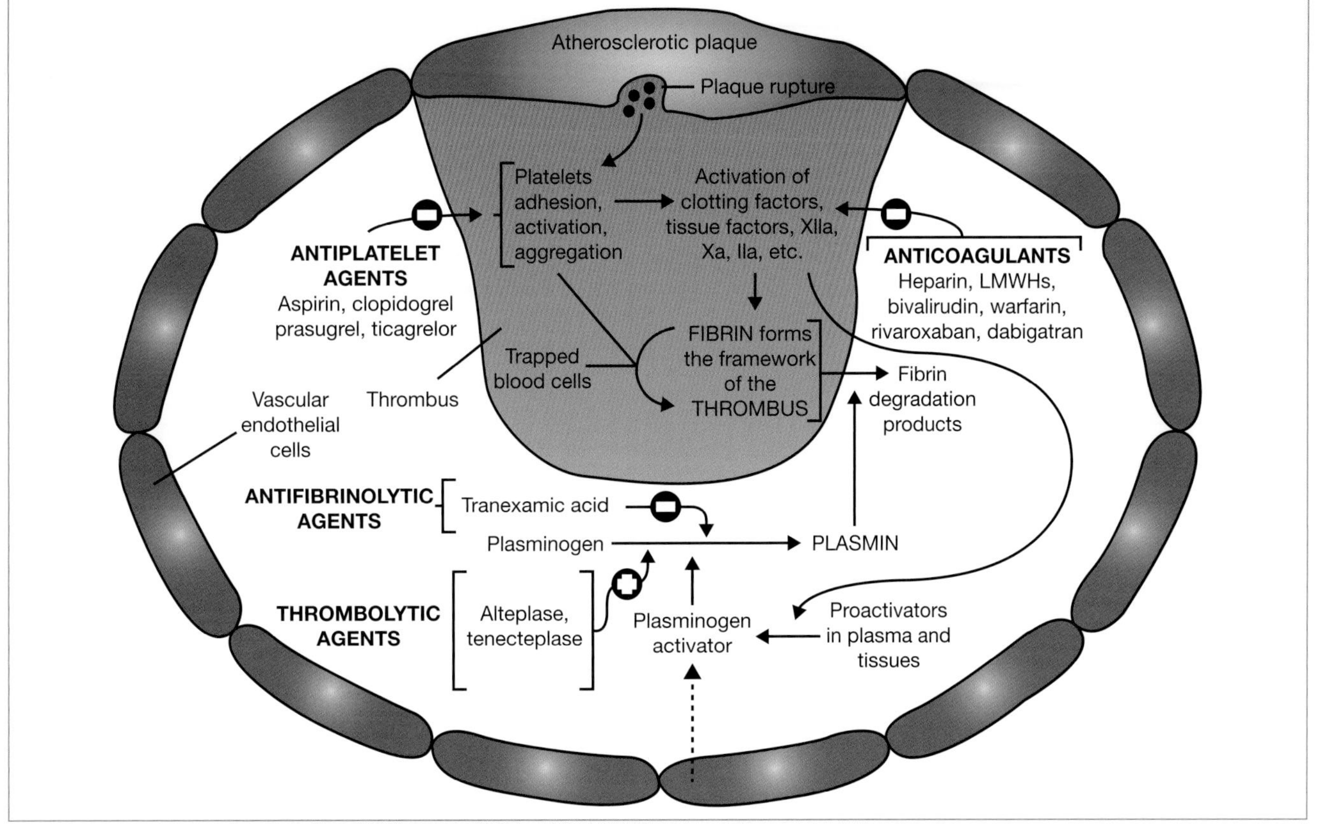

FIGURE 13.2 Sites of action of drugs interacting with the coagulation cascade and the fibrinolytic and platelet activation pathways

Source: Adapted from Rang et al 2012, Figure 24.10; reproduced with permission.

Drug Monograph 13.1
Enoxaparin

Enoxaparin is an LMWH produced by partial depolymerisation of unfractionated heparin. It is indicated for preventing and treating venous thromboembolism (VTE) (e.g. in surgical patients and in bedridden people with an acute illness). Additionally, enoxaparin is used to treat acute myocardial infarction.

Mechanism of action

The LMWHs, including enoxaparin, bind to and accelerate the action of antithrombin III (Fig 13.1). Binding potentiates inactivation of factor Xa and factor IIa (thrombin), ultimately resulting in decreased thrombin formation and hence preventing fibrin clot formation. Enoxaparin has a four-fold greater effect on factor Xa than on factor IIa.

Pharmacokinetics

Following subcutaneous administration, the bioavailability of enoxaparin is 91% and the volume of distribution is small (5–9 L) due to confinement to the vascular space. Enoxaparin undergoes desulfation and depolymerisation in the liver, producing smaller fragments with decreased biological activity. Both the parent drug (~10%) and the smaller inactive fragments (~40%) are renally excreted. The elimination half-life is in the range of 3–5 hours.

Drug interactions

Drug interactions with the LMWHs include any drugs that potentially affect the clotting process, and current drug information sources should be consulted. In addition, the heparins can cause hyperkalaemia, and combinations that increase this risk should be avoided or the plasma potassium concentration should be monitored.

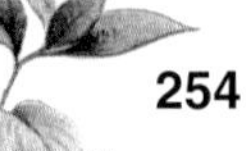

Adverse reactions

Adverse reactions commonly include:

- bleeding, bruising
- injection site reactions – for example, pain (rarely skin necrosis)
- hyperkalaemia.

Warnings and contraindications

Refer to the section on heparins in the text.

Dosage and administration

Enoxaparin is administered subcutaneously, and the dosage varies depending on the situation; for example, in surgical patients 20 mg is administered once daily for 7–14 days (maximum) or until mobile. Alternatively, in immobilised medical patients, the dosage is 40 mg once daily for 6–14 days or until ambulatory.

CLINICAL FOCUS BOX 13.1
Coagulation tests

Activated partial thromboplastin time

The activated partial thromboplastin time (aPTT) test measures the overall activity of the intrinsic coagulation pathway (Winter et al. 2020). It is performed by warming a thromboplastin reagent containing an activator with an aliquot of the person's plasma and then recalcifying this mixture after a set incubation period.

The length of time taken for the mixture to clot is called the aPTT and the normal range is usually about 26–39 seconds, depending on the analyser and the brand of reagent used.

A prolonged test can indicate:

- a deficiency of one or more coagulation factors in the intrinsic coagulation pathway (Fig 13.1)
- the presence of a 'lupus'-type coagulation inhibitor
- the presence of heparin.

The test is used to monitor heparin administration to a person. The therapeutic range for the aPTT in someone on heparin is about 50–90 seconds. The aPTT test cannot be used to monitor the effect of LMWH.

Prothrombin time

The prothrombin time (PT) test measures the overall activity of the extrinsic coagulation pathway (Fig 13.1). It is performed by adding thromboplastin to an aliquot of the person's plasma and measuring the time it takes for the mixture to clot.

This clotting time is used to determine the INR (international normalised ratio). The same test is performed using normal control plasma, and the prothrombin ratio is then derived by dividing the patient's clotting time by the mean normal control clotting time.

Finally, the INR is calculated using the 'international sensitivity index' of the thromboplastin reagent, so that the ratio obtained is independent of the reagent brand or testing laboratory. The normal range for the INR is about 1.0–1.3.

A prolonged test can indicate:

- a deficiency of a coagulation factor in the extrinsic pathway
- the presence of a 'lupus'-type coagulation inhibitor
- the presence of warfarin.

The test is used to monitor warfarin administration. The range for the INR in a person on warfarin is 2.0–4.0.

TABLE 13.1 Comparison of regular heparin and low-molecular-weight heparins

PROPERTY	REGULAR HEPARIN	LOW-MOLECULAR-WEIGHT HEPARIN
Molecular weight range	3000–30,000	1000–10,000
Average molecular weight	12,000–15,000	4000–6000
Mechanism of action	Inactivates factor Xa and IIa (thrombin)	Inactivates factor Xa
aPTT monitoring required	Yes	No
Inhibition of platelet function	++++ (high)	++ (medium)
Route of administration	IV, SC	SC
Protein binding	++++ (high)	+ (low)
Vascular permeability increased	Yes	No
Treatment of bleeding	Protamine	Protamine (partially effective)

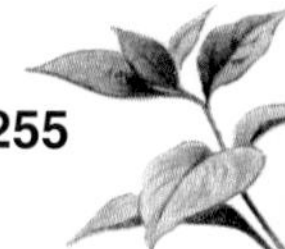

Clinical Uses of Low-Molecular-Weight Heparins

- Prevention of VTE in surgical and high-risk medical patients
- Prevention of VTE in surgical patients (sole indication for danaparoid)
- Prevention of clotting during haemodialysis
- Treatment of DVT
- Treatment of acute STEMI, non-STEMI and unstable angina (enoxaparin)

Pharmacokinetics

In comparison with standard heparin, LMWHs have a lower affinity for endothelial cells, macrophages and plasma proteins; an increased bioavailability; and a more predictable clearance that is independent of dose. Hepatic clearance plays a minor role and elimination is principally via the kidneys, hence their biological half-life is prolonged in people with renal failure. For LMWHs, consider dose reduction in severe renal impairment and avoid completely in end-stage renal disease. LMWHs have a longer half-life than heparin (2–4 times greater) when given subcutaneously and their anticoagulant effect also lasts longer. The elimination half-life for dalteparin is 3–5 hours, enoxaparin 3–6 hours and nadroparin 3–11 hours.

Drug interactions and adverse reactions

Drug interactions with the heparins include any drugs that potentially affect the clotting process, and current drug information sources should be consulted. In addition, the heparins can cause hyperkalaemia, and combinations that increase this risk should be avoided or the plasma potassium concentration should be monitored.

Bleeding is a well-known complication of heparin therapy, and the LMWHs have a similar risk. Common adverse reactions include local irritation effects such as erythema, haematomas, urticaria and pain at the injection site. The incidence of thrombocytopenia is less (around 0.6%) and data on osteoporosis also indicate a decreased incidence. Danaparoid may be used as an alternative to heparin or LMWH in people with heparin-induced thrombocytopenia, as cross-reactivity occurs in fewer than 10% of patients.

Warnings and contraindications

Use LMWH with caution in people undergoing any medical/surgical procedure that increases the potential of bleeding. Avoid use in people with LMWH or heparin hypersensitivity, bleeding disorders, severe hypertension, stroke, thrombocytopenia, severe liver or kidney disease, endocarditis or retinopathy. In people with renal impairment, the risk of bleeding with LMWHs is greater because they are eliminated by renal excretion. See the section 'Haemostatic and Antifibrinolytic Drugs', later in the chapter, for the role of protamine in reversing heparin-induced bleeding.

Vitamin K antagonists

These drugs were discovered following an outbreak of a haemorrhagic disorder in cattle eating spoiled sweet clover in 1929, when the active constituent was identified as bis-hydroxycoumarin. Synthesised analogues, including warfarin (the name comes from the **W**isconsin **A**lumni **R**esearch **F**oundation, and **arin** from coumarin), were originally thought to be too toxic and were used as rodenticides. Following survival of a man in 1951 after repeated suicide attempts using high doses of the rat poison, warfarin was introduced as an anticoagulant for humans in 1959 (Drug Monograph 13.2). Table 13.2 provides a comparison of heparin and warfarin. Figure 13.3 illustrates the site of action of warfarin and the importance of the role of vitamin K (see later section, 'Haemostatic and Antifibrinolytic Drugs').

Antithrombin-III-dependent anticoagulant

A synthetic antithrombin-III-dependent anticoagulant is fondaparinux, which binds AT III potentiating the neutralisation of factor Xa by antithrombin, inhibiting both thrombin formation and thrombus development. It does not inhibit thrombin (activated factor IIa) and has no antiplatelet activity. It is as effective and as safe as the LMWHs. It is used to prevent VTE in high-risk surgery such as hip fracture or replacement, or knee replacement. Administered subcutaneously, the long half-life of 17 hours permits once-daily administration. As with the heparins, this drug is contraindicated in co-existing bleeding disorders and in cases of renal impairment. The latter is important because fondaparinux is excreted unchanged in urine. At present, there are limited data in pregnancy and breastfeeding.

Direct thrombin inhibitors

The use of medicinal leeches (*Hirudo medicinalis*) has its origins more than 2500 years ago. In 1884 it was discovered that blood in the leech gut did not coagulate. This led to the isolation in pure crystalline form of the anticoagulant hirudin from leech pharyngeal glands by Markwardt in 1957. Hirudin is a direct irreversible non-covalent inhibitor of thrombin, but the extent of anticoagulation is unpredictable.

Bivalirudin is a 20-amino-acid synthetic polypeptide analogue of hirudin, which binds directly and reversibly

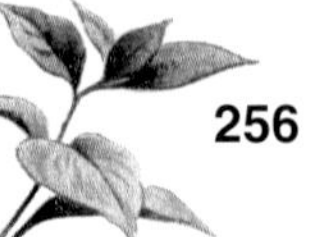

Drug Monograph 13.2
Warfarin

Warfarin interferes with hepatic synthesis of the vitamin K–dependent clotting factors through inhibition of the vitamin K epoxide reductase complex 1 (VKORC1). As a consequence, interference in the γ-carboxylation of the glutamic acid residues on factors II, VII, IX and X, and on various anticoagulant proteins by γ-glutamyl carboxylase, leads to the production of non-functional coagulation factors (Fig 13.3). Factor VII is depleted quickly; the sequential depletion of factors IX, X and II follows. Warfarin does not affect established clots but prevents further extension of formed clots, thereby diminishing the potential for secondary thromboembolic complications. The main advantage of warfarin is that it is effective orally and can be given once daily after the maintenance dose has been established.

Indications

Warfarin is indicated for the prophylaxis and treatment of DVT and pulmonary thromboembolism. It is also used for the prophylaxis of thromboembolism associated with chronic atrial fibrillation, myocardial infarction or in people with prosthetic heart valves.

Pharmacokinetics

Warfarin is a racemic drug comprising equal concentrations of S- and R-warfarin. It is well absorbed from the gastrointestinal tract and has a systemic bioavailability of more than 95%. Peak plasma concentration occurs in 3–9 hours and its duration of action is 2–5 days. Warfarin is highly protein-bound (99%), and the plasma half-life varies from 25 to 60 hours, with an average of 40 hours. Warfarin crosses the placenta, and fetal plasma attains a similar plasma concentration to that of the maternal circulation.

S-warfarin is metabolised in the liver by CYP2C9 with a minor contribution from CYP2C8, CYP2C18 and CYP2C19. The predominant role of CYP2C9 (which exhibits significant pharmacogenetic variation, refer to Ch 6) in S-warfarin metabolism accounts for the large variability observed in warfarin dose requirements. Some people with certain CYP2C9 variant alleles have reduced metabolism of S-warfarin and thus increased warfarin plasma concentration. This is more prevalent in European, African and Asian populations. There is limited evidence to support that genotyping improves anticoagulation control or reduces the risk of haemorrhage. In contrast, R-warfarin is metabolised by CYP1A2 and CYP3A4 and, to a minor extent, by CYP1A1, CYP2C8, CYP2C18, CYP2C19 and CYP3A5.

Drug interactions

Numerous drugs, including antimicrobials, cardiovascular drugs, analgesics, anti-inflammatory drugs, immunomodulators, gastrointestinal drugs, antineoplastics and central nervous system drugs and St John's wort interact with warfarin, and current drug information resources should always be consulted. The INR should be monitored frequently when instituting, ceasing or altering other drug therapy.

Adverse reactions

Adverse reactions include:

- bleeding (common)
- rarely, alopecia, anorexia, abdominal cramps or distress, leucopenia, nausea, vomiting, diarrhoea, purple toes syndrome and kidney damage.

Warnings and contraindications

- Avoid use in the elderly. Risk factors for bleeding include age older than 70 years, previous history of stroke and falls, liver disease, chronic renal failure, drug interactions and evidence of gastrointestinal bleeding in the previous 18 months.
- Contraindicated in alcoholics.
- Avoid use in pregnancy (except for women with prosthetic heart valves). Risk of abortion and teratogenicity is high, and fetal abnormalities and facial anomalies have been reported if warfarin is administered during the first trimester. Administration during the second and third trimesters is associated with central nervous system abnormalities.
- Avoid use in people with known anticoagulant drug hypersensitivity, any medical or surgical condition associated with bleeding (aneurysm, cerebrovascular bleeding, surgery and severe trauma), blood disorders, severe uncontrolled hypertension, pericarditis, severe diabetes, ulcers, visceral cancer, vitamin C or vitamin K deficiencies, endocarditis or severe liver or kidney impairment.
- Brands of warfarin should not be interchanged due to a lack of bioequivalence data.

Dosage and administration

Warfarin should be taken at the same time each day, and the usual dose is 5 mg daily for 2 days and then adjusted according to the INR. The maintenance dose is in the range 1–10 mg daily. The INR range varies with specific indications, and local guidelines should be consulted. A number of algorithms are available to aid health professionals with warfarin dosing and these can be accessed at the International Warfarin Pharmacogenetics Consortium website (https://www.pharmgkb.org/page/iwpc) and www.warfarindosing.org.

TABLE 13.2 Anticoagulant drugs: comparison of heparin and warfarin

	HEPARIN	WARFARIN
Onset of action	Immediate	Slow (24–48 hours)
Route of administration	Parenteral	Oral
Duration of action	Short (< 4 hours)	Long (2–5 days)
Laboratory test for dosage control	Activated partial thromboplastin time (aPTT)	Prothrombin time (PT)
Antidote	Severe bleeding, protamine	Vitamin K, whole blood or plasma
Pregnancy	Heparin and LMWH used. LMWH not recommended in pregnant women with prosthetic heart valves due to evidence of inadequate anticoagulation	Contraindicated (mental retardation, blindness and other central nervous system abnormalities have been reported in association with second and third trimester exposure)
Lactation	Safe to use	Safe to use

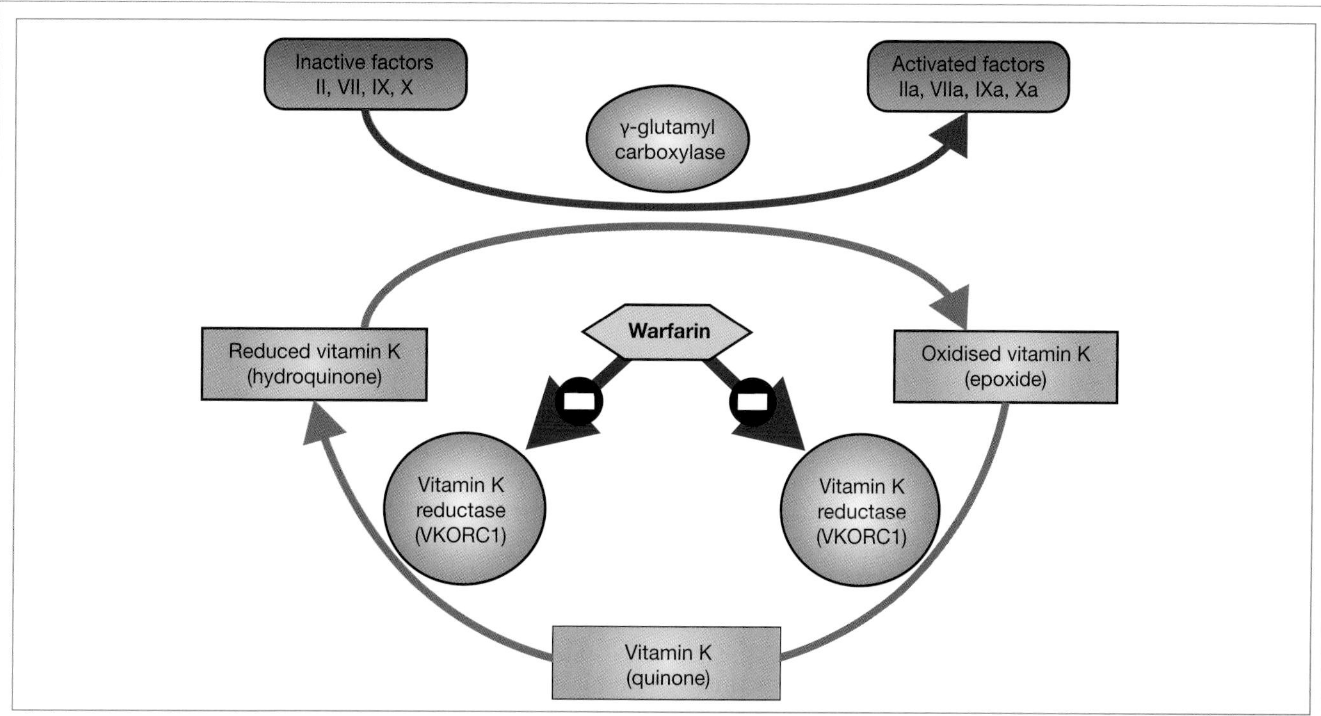

FIGURE 13.3 Site of action of warfarin and the role of vitamin K The oxidation of the reduced form of vitamin K (the hydroxyquinone) forming oxidised vitamin K (the epoxide) is coupled to the carboxylation of the inactive factors II, VII, IX and X. The vitamin K reductase complex 1 (VKORC1) then regenerates the reduced form of vitamin K via initial formation of vitamin K quinone. Warfarin inhibits VKORC1 and, hence, both the regeneration of reduced vitamin K and the formation of the activated clotting factors.

to thrombin independently of AT III and hence blocks the thrombogenic activity of thrombin. Relatively quick dissociation of the drug from thrombin leaves a small amount of active thrombin free for the control of haemostasis. Bivalirudin has a plasma half-life of 25 minutes and is administered as an intravenous bolus and by intravenous infusion. Bleeding disorders and significant reduction in renal function are factors for consideration prior to use of bivalirudin. Severe bleeding is common with bivalirudin and, rarely, anaphylaxis has been reported.

Dabigatran etexilate is an oral direct thrombin inhibitor. Dabigatran itself has low bioavailability (~7%), and dabigatran etexilate, the prodrug of dabigatran, was developed to aid gastrointestinal absorption. Following hydrolysis of dabigatran etexilate by hepatic carboxylesterases, the active moiety dabigatran specifically and competitively inhibits both free and clot-bound thrombin by binding to the active site of the thrombin molecule. It is indicated for the prevention of thromboemboli after major lower limb surgery (e.g. knee replacement) and total hip replacement and in the prevention of stroke and systemic embolism in people with non-valvular atrial fibrillation at high risk of stroke.

Pharmacokinetics

Maximal plasma concentration occurs in ~1.5 hours, and the plasma half-life is in the order of 8–10 hours following single-dose administration and 14–17 hours after multiple doses. Approximately 80% of the drug is excreted unchanged in urine (Chan et al. 2020). The remainder is excreted as dabigatran glucuronides in the bile. Moderate renal impairment (CrCl 30–50 mL/min) results in decreased renal excretion and an increased plasma concentration of dabigatran.

Drug interactions

In the absence of extensive metabolism by the liver, dabigatran is not subject to major drug–drug interactions. However, dabigatran is a substrate of the efflux transporter P-glycoprotein and drug interactions involving the P-glycoprotein inhibitors quinine and verapamil have been reported. Inhibition of P-glycoprotein results in an increase in the plasma concentration of dabigatran and an increased risk of bleeding. Verapamil is contraindicated in people already on dabigatran and who have had major orthopaedic surgery.

Warnings and contraindications

Dabigatran doubles the aPTT and the PT and current data indicate a tendency for increased bleeding, in comparison to warfarin, in those aged older than 75 years and taking a standard dose of 150 mg twice daily for VTE. A reduced dose of 110 mg twice daily is recommended in those with reduced renal function or who are over 75 years of age. Routine monitoring of the INR is not undertaken as the results are highly variable and unpredictable. Bleeding is a significant clinical problem (see the later section 'Haemostatic and Antifibrinolytic Drugs' for the role of idarucizumab in reversing dabigatran-induced bleeding).

Unfractionated heparins, heparin derivatives, LMWHs, fondaparinux, thrombolytic drugs, GPIIb/IIIa receptor antagonists, clopidogrel, dextran and vitamin K antagonists should not be administered concomitantly with dabigatran etexilate. Close observation should be carried out when there is an increased haemorrhagic risk – for example, major trauma or recent biopsy, active gastrointestinal ulcers or recent gastrointestinal bleeding, intracranial haemorrhage or spinal, ophthalmic or brain surgery.

Direct factor Xa inhibitors

Rivaroxaban was the second of the new oral anticoagulants (NOAC) (after dabigatran etexilate) to become available since the introduction of warfarin. It is a direct reversible dose-dependent competitive inhibitor that binds directly to the active site of factor Xa generated in both the intrinsic and the extrinsic pathways, thereby attenuating thrombin generation and preventing conversion of fibrinogen to fibrin. The drug prolongs both PT and aPTT, and prolongation of PT correlates with the plasma drug concentration.

Rivaroxaban is absorbed rapidly and bioavailability ranges from 60% to 80%. Approximately 30% of the dose is excreted unchanged in urine, while the remainder is metabolised by CYP3A4, CYP2C8 and CYP-independent mechanisms. There are limited data on drug interactions, but the incidence appears low. As rivaroxaban is a substrate for P-gp and CYP3A4, concomitant administration of strong inhibitors of P-gp and CYP3A4 (e.g. itraconazole, posaconazole, voriconazole and ritonavir) is contraindicated because of increased risk of bleeding.

Clinical evidence supports efficacy of rivaroxaban for VTE prevention after hip or knee replacement surgery. Recommended duration of therapy is 14 days after knee replacement and 35 days after hip replacement. Monitoring is not undertaken, as there is no way to relate prothrombin time to either therapeutic or adverse effects, and the effect of rivaroxaban cannot be monitored by using the INR.

Apixaban is the newest NOAC and, like rivaroxaban, is a direct inhibitor of factor Xa. It is indicated to treat VTE following elective knee or hip replacement.

The drug is rapidly absorbed with a bioavailability of ~50%. Similar to rivaroxaban, it is a substrate for P-gp, and it is metabolised by demethylation and hydroxylation by CYP3A4/5 with minor roles for CYP1A2, 2C8, 2C9, 2C19 and CYP2J2. Apixaban has multiple routes of elimination: ~25% is excreted as unchanged drug in urine, ~25% is excreted as metabolites the majority of which occur in faeces, and there is also evidence of direct biliary excretion. Again, similar to rivaroxaban, strong inhibitors of CYP3A4 and P-gp are contraindicated. Inducers of CYP3A4 and P-gp (e.g. carbamazepine, rifampicin, phenytoin, phenobarbital (phenobarbitone) and St John's wort) have been shown to reduce the plasma drug concentration of apixaban, reducing clinical efficacy. For the same reasons as stated above, monitoring of the anticoagulant effect is not undertaken and hence there is no method to guide dosage adjustment. However, limited clinical data indicate an increase in the plasma drug concentration in severe renal failure (CrCl 15–29 mL/min) and dosage adjustment is recommended.

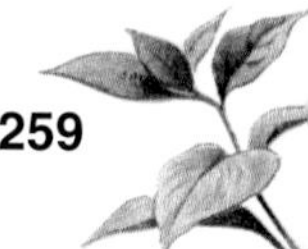

CLINICAL FOCUS BOX 13.2

Andexanet: reversing anticoagulation of apixaban and rivaroxaban

Andexanet alpha is a 'decoy' drug. It is a recombinant modified human factor Xa that is catalytically inactive (Connolly et al. 2019; Heo et al. 2018). When in the vascular space (volume of distribution is 5L) it has high binding affinity and sequesters apixaban and rivaroxaban. This results in a reduction in the circulating drug concentration reversing the anticoagulant effect and a restoring the endogenous activity of factor Xa. Reversal is achieved in 2–5 minutes. In 2018 the US Food and Drug Administration approved the use of andexanet alfa as a reversing agent and the European Medicines Agency granted conditional approval in 2019. Approval has not yet been granted in Australasia.

Bleeding is a common adverse effect of both rivaroxaban and apixaban and reversing the effect of the drugs is now possible (Clinical Focus Box 13.2).

KEY POINTS

Anticoagulants

- Heparin produces its anticoagulant effect by combining with antithrombin III to form a complex that acts at multiple sites in the normal coagulation system, inactivating factors IXa, Xa, XIa and XIIa. Inactivation of factor Xa of the intrinsic and extrinsic pathways prevents the conversion of prothrombin to thrombin, thereby inhibiting the formation of fibrin from fibrinogen.
- The LMWHs are fragments of standard heparin prepared by enzymatic or chemical cleavage. They inactivate factor Xa more potently than factor IIa and hence have a relatively minor effect on aPTT.
- LMWHs are considered safer, easier to administer and require less monitoring than standard heparin. Bleeding is a well-known complication of heparin therapy, and the LMWHs have a similar risk.
- Warfarin is an orally administered anticoagulant and is indicated for the prophylaxis and treatment of DVT and pulmonary thromboembolism.
- Many drugs interact with warfarin, and the INR should be monitored frequently when instituting, ceasing or altering other drug therapy.
- The synthetic antithrombin-III-dependent anticoagulant is fondaparinux, which binds to AT III, potentiating the neutralisation of factor Xa by antithrombin and inhibiting both thrombin formation and thrombus development.
- The direct thrombin inhibitors include bivalirudin and dabigatran etexilate.
- Bivalirudin binds directly and reversibly to thrombin independently of AT III and hence blocks the thrombogenic activity of thrombin.
- Dabigatran specifically and competitively inhibits both free and clot-bound thrombin by binding to the active site of the thrombin molecule.
- Rivaroxaban and apixaban are direct reversible dose-dependent competitive inhibitors of factor Xa. They bind directly to the active site, thereby attenuating thrombin generation and preventing conversion of fibrinogen to fibrin.

Antiplatelet agents

Platelets play a critical role in thrombosis following vascular damage. Platelets adhere to a thrombogenic surface and are activated by mediators such as platelet activating factor, thromboxane A_2 (which binds to Tx receptors), ADP (which binds to $P2Y_{12}$ and $P2Y_1$ receptors) and thrombin, resulting in platelet aggregation. The last occurs because the platelets stick to one another via fibrinogen bridges that link between the specific glycoprotein receptors, expressed on the surfaces of the platelets. ADP binding to the $P2Y_{12}$ receptor stimulates the activation of the glycoprotein IIb/IIIa receptor.

Glycoprotein IIb/IIIa is the most abundant surface protein (~8000 molecules/platelet) and during platelet activation it undergoes a conformational change to express receptor function, which results in the binding of fibrinogen that mediates prolonged platelet aggregation. This is an autocatalytic process, as exposure of certain lipids on the surface of the platelets promotes further thrombin formation, platelet aggregation and fibrin formation. Although this process is desirable when forming a haemostatic plug, it is undesirable when triggered intravascularly.

Our knowledge of the role of platelets in thromboembolic disease and our understanding of the pharmacology of aspirin has led to considerable development of drugs with 'antiplatelet activity'.

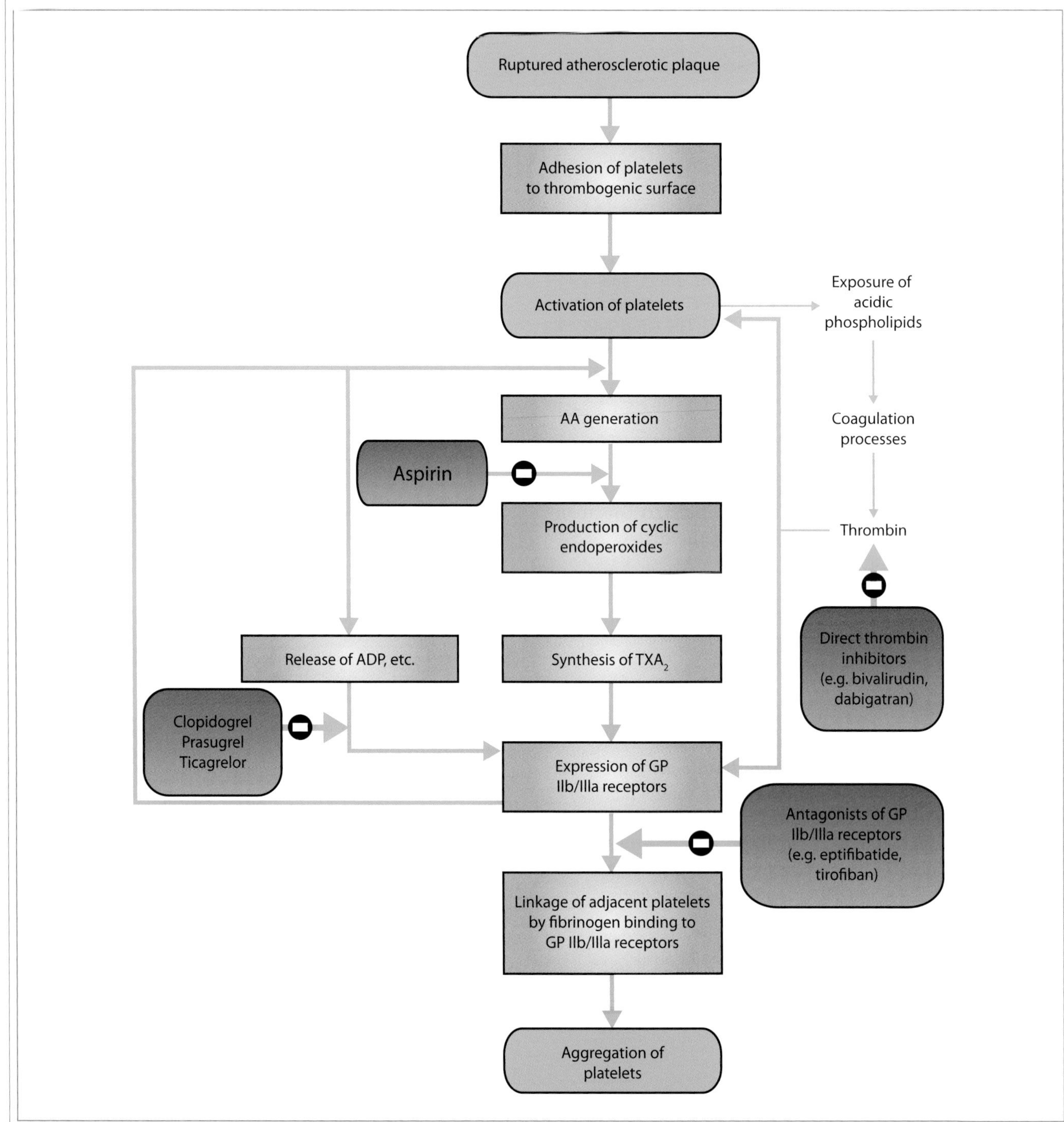

FIGURE 13.4 Platelet activation Events involved in platelet adhesion and aggregation are shown, with the sites of action of various drugs. AA = arachidonic acid; ADP = adenosine diphosphate; GP = glycoprotein; TXA_2 = thromboxane A_2

Source: Adapted from Rang et al 2012, Figure 24.7; reproduced with permission.

Antiplatelet drugs are used to treat arterial thrombosis and include:

- aspirin and dipyridamole
- the $P2Y_{12}$ inhibitors clopidogrel, prasugrel and ticagrelor
- the glycoprotein IIb/IIIa receptor inhibitors eptifibatide and tirofiban (Fig 13.4).

(The role of aspirin as an analgesic is discussed in Ch 19, and as an anti-inflammatory agent in Ch 34.)

Aspirin

Mechanism of action

Aspirin causes a long-lasting functional deficit in platelets by irreversibly inhibiting the cyclooxygenase enzyme

COX-1 that is necessary for thromboxane A_2 synthesis. Thromboxane A_2 promotes platelet aggregation and vasoconstriction, and thus aspirin suppresses these actions. Platelets lack the metabolic capacity to synthesise new COX-1, and the deficit induced by aspirin lasts 8–10 days until new platelets are synthesised. This effect on platelet function explains both the effectiveness of aspirin as an antiplatelet agent and why it prolongs bleeding time.

Numerous studies have established the effectiveness of aspirin therapy in people with acute myocardial infarction and demonstrated conclusively a significant reduction in mortality. Aspirin is standard treatment (both primary and secondary prevention) in both cardiovascular and cerebrovascular diseases. The antiplatelet effect of aspirin is achieved at a dose of 75–300 mg daily, and no additional benefit has been observed at higher doses. Low-dose aspirin (75–150 mg/day) does not cause changes in bleeding time. Aspirin is also available as a fixed-dose combination with clopidogrel (clopidogrel 75 mg/aspirin 100 mg) and with dipyridamole (dipyridamole 200 mg [controlled release]/aspirin 25 mg).

In some people on chronic low-dose aspirin, the risk of a thrombotic event remains due to incomplete inhibition of platelet aggregation; this is called 'aspirin resistance'. Strategies to address the problem include avoidance of drugs that interfere with the action of aspirin (e.g. non-steroidal anti-inflammatory drugs [NSAIDs]) and twice-daily dosing.

Dipyridamole

The mechanism of action of dipyridamole is unclear but is thought to include inhibition of thromboxane A_2 formation; inhibition of phosphodiesterase activity, which results in an increase in platelet cAMP; and inhibition of red blood cell uptake of adenosine, a platelet aggregation inhibitor. Oral dipyridamole is used in combination with aspirin (dipyridamole 200 mg, aspirin 25 mg controlled release) for the secondary prevention of ischaemic stroke and transient ischaemic attacks, and is administered intravenously for cardiac stress testing.

After an oral dose, dipyridamole is rapidly absorbed and reaches peak plasma concentrations within 45–75 minutes. Bioavailability ranges from 40% to 70% and is limited by hepatic first-pass metabolism. It is highly protein-bound, metabolised in the liver and excreted principally as glucuronides in bile. Drug interactions include:

- *Adenosine:* cellular uptake of adenosine is inhibited and a reduction in dose of adenosine might be necessary.
- *Thrombolytic agents:* concurrent use increases risk of severe bleeding and haemorrhage.

Adverse reactions include headache, dizziness, abdominal upset, rash, allergic reaction, angina pectoris, blood pressure lability (hypertension, hypotension) and tachycardia. Use dipyridamole cautiously in people with unstable angina or recent myocardial infarction and in the presence of aortic stenosis.

$P2Y_{12}$ inhibitors

Mechanism of action

The $P2Y_{12}$ inhibitors inhibit ADP-induced platelet aggregation by either irreversibly (clopidogrel and prasugrel) or reversibly (ticagrelor) binding to the $P2Y_{12}$ platelet receptor. This prevents ADP-mediated activation of the glycoprotein IIb/IIIa complex and hence platelet aggregation. The $P2Y_{12}$ receptors lose their ability to bind ADP for the life of the platelet. On cessation of treatment, platelet function returns within about a week.

Pharmacokinetics

Clopidogrel, a second-generation thienopyridine derivative, is a prodrug that is predominantly metabolised (85%) to an inactive carboxylic acid metabolite. The remaining 15% is metabolised to an active metabolite in a two-step process involving CYP2C19, CYP1A2 and CYP2B6 in the first step and CYP2C9, CYP2C19, CYP2B6 and CYP3A in the second step. Maximum concentration of the active metabolite is reached about 1 hour after dosing. Unlike aspirin, the active thiol metabolite has no effect on prostaglandin synthesis. Variability in clopidogrel response has been observed in multiple studies, and current evidence suggests a combination of genetic (e.g. CYP2C19 polymorphism that leads to a loss of function and reduced platelet inhibition) and clinical causes (e.g. poor adherence to therapy). This variability in response has led to the development of more potent third-generation $P2Y_{12}$ inhibitors (e.g. prasugrel and ticagrelor).

Prasugrel is also a prodrug that is rapidly absorbed. In the intestine prasugrel is hydrolysed, initially forming an intermediate (R-95913) that is then subsequently metabolised in the liver to the active metabolite R-138727 by CYP3A4, 2B6, 2C9 and 2C19. R-138727 is then further metabolised to two inactive metabolites that are excreted in the urine. Peak concentration of the drug occurs within 30 minutes and the onset of action is more rapid, more potent and more consistent than that of clopidogrel. Although the plasma half-life of the active metabolite is about 4 hours because prasugrel binding to the $P2Y_{12}$ receptor is irreversible its action is prolonged even after discontinuation of the drug.

Ticagrelor, unlike clopidogrel and prasugrel, is not a prodrug and it reversibly binds to the $P2Y_{12}$ receptor. The drug is rapidly absorbed after oral administration, reaching peak plasma concentration at 1.5–3 hours.

Ticagrelor is metabolised by CYP3A4 predominantly to the active metabolite AR-C124910XX, which constitutes about 40% of the overall plasma drug concentration. Inhibition of platelet aggregation is greater and more consistent than that of clopidogrel. Co-administration of strong CYP3A4 inhibitors and inducers is not recommended, and digoxin concentration should be monitored as ticagrelor is an inhibitor of P-gp.

Clinical Uses of $P2Y_{12}$ Inhibitors

- Acute coronary syndrome (with aspirin)
- Stent implantation (prasugrel with aspirin)
- Prevention of thromboembolism in people with ACS (clopidogrel)

Adverse reactions, warnings and contraindications

Bleeding is a common adverse reaction and may be quite severe. To lessen the risk of bleeding these drugs are contraindicated in patients with severe active bleeding and in those with a history of stroke or transient ischaemic attack or bleeding disorders or severe hepatic disease. Prasugrel is not recommended in those over 75 years of age. With ticagrelor precaution should be exercised in persons presenting with cardiac dysrhythmias – in particular, bradycardia, second- to third-degree atrioventricular block and sick sinus syndrome. In addition, ticagrelor may worsen asthma/chronic obstructive pulmonary disease and exacerbate hyperuricaemia.

Glycoprotein IIb/IIIa receptor inhibitors

Mechanism of action

As was seen in Figure 13.4, inhibition of glycoprotein IIb/IIIa receptors will inhibit the final pathway of platelet aggregation by preventing binding of fibrinogen.

The inhibitors eptifibatide and tirofiban are peptides based on a common sequence that occurs in glycoprotein IIb/IIIa receptors. These drugs are administered parenterally and are used in combination with heparin or aspirin (low-dose) to prevent ischaemic cardiac complications in people undergoing percutaneous transluminal coronary angioplasty or intracoronary stenting. To date, development of oral formulations has not been successful.

Drug interactions include:

- *Oral anticoagulants:* administration within 1 week of the oral anticoagulants is not recommended because of the increased risk of bleeding.
- *Antiplatelet drugs (dipyridamole):* monitor closely if administered concurrently, as the risk of bleeding is increased.
- *Dextran/LMWHs/NSAIDs:* concurrent usage results in increased risk of bleeding and haemorrhage.
- *Thrombolytic drugs:* combined use can result in increased risk of bleeding. Monitor closely if combination or sequential drug therapy is used.

Adverse reactions include bleeding (minor and major), thrombocytopenia, visual changes, confusion, nausea, vomiting and hypotension. Monitor PT, aPTT, creatinine clearance, platelet count, haemoglobin and haematocrit before and during treatment.

KEY POINTS

Antiplatelet drugs

- Platelets play a critical role in thrombosis following vascular damage.
- Platelets adhere to a thrombogenic surface and are activated by mediators such as platelet activating factor, thromboxane A_2 (which binds to Tx receptors), ADP (which binds to $P2Y_{12}$ and $P2Y_1$ receptors) and thrombin, resulting in platelet aggregation.
- Antiplatelet drugs inhibit platelet aggregation and reduce the risk of arterial thrombosis.
- The sites of action of antiplatelet drugs include the enzyme COX-1, the platelet receptors $P2Y_{12}$ and glycoprotein IIb/IIIa receptors.
- The antiplatelet drugs include:

  aspirin, which binds irreversibly to platelet COX-1

  dipyridamole, which is thought to inhibit thromboxane A_2 formation, phosphodiesterase activity (which results in an increase in platelet cAMP) and red blood cell uptake of adenosine, a platelet aggregation inhibitor

  the $P2Y_{12}$ inhibitors clopidogrel, prasugrel and ticagrelor

  the glycoprotein IIb/IIIa receptor inhibitors eptifibatide and tirofiban.

Thrombolytic drugs

Thrombolytic (fibrinolytic) drugs have similar biochemical mechanisms of action on the fibrinolytic system, converting blood plasminogen to plasmin. Plasmin, a fibrinolytic enzyme, digests or dissolves fibrin clots wherever they can be reached by plasmin (Fig 13.2).

These drugs, which are used to treat acute thromboembolic disorders, alter haemostatic capability more profoundly than does anticoagulant therapy. Consequently, when bleeding occurs, it is more severe and very difficult to control. The main drugs in this class include alteplase (also known as recombinant tissue plasminogen activator, rt-PA), tenecteplase and urokinase. Alteplase and tenecteplase are produced using recombinant DNA technology, and urokinase is a product isolated from human urine.

Alteplase and tenecteplase are indicated for ST-segment-elevation myocardial infarction (STEMI); additional uses include in pulmonary embolism, acute-ischaemic stroke (alteplase), peripheral arterial embolism and thrombosed cannulae (e.g. intravenous cannulae, central venous cannulae, haemodialysis shunts). Urokinase is not marketed in Australia but may be available via the Special Access Scheme (SAS).

These agents are administered intravenously. Alteplase and urokinase have elimination half-lives of 35 minutes and up to 20 minutes, respectively. The time to peak effect after intravenous injection is from 20 minutes to 2 hours. Duration of the thrombolytic effect is about 4 hours for alteplase and urokinase. Tenecteplase shows biphasic elimination kinetics, with an initial half-life of about 25 minutes and a terminal half-life of 130 minutes. The exact mechanisms of elimination for many of these drugs are not fully established.

Drug interactions include:

- *Anticoagulants (oral) or heparin:* concurrent use increases haemorrhage risk, but the combination of heparin and thrombolytic therapy is often prescribed for treatment of an acute coronary artery occlusion. Monitor closely if concurrent therapies are administered.
- *Antiplatelet drugs:* concurrent use can increase the risk of bleeding episodes. Combination is not recommended, with the exception of aspirin when indicated for an acute myocardial infarction.

The commonest adverse reaction is bleeding, including intracerebral haemorrhage. Others occurring less often include fever, headache, nausea, vomiting, hypotension, dysrhythmias, allergic reaction, facial flushing, arthralgia and bronchospasm. With urokinase, adverse reactions include stomach pain or swelling, backache, bloody urine and stools, constipation, severe headaches, dizziness, arthralgia, tachycardia, bradycardia and fever.

In an acute coronary artery thrombosis evolving into a transmural myocardial infarction, thrombolytic therapy is most effective when started as early as possible or within 6–12 hours of the onset of symptoms. In general, bolus administration followed by an intravenous infusion is used. The drug regimens for acute myocardial infarction, pulmonary embolism, DVT and arterial thromboembolism vary, and local institutional or manufacturer's guidelines should be consulted.

KEY POINTS

Thrombolytic drugs

- Thrombolytic (fibrinolytic) drugs are used to dissolve already formed clots and to treat acute thromboembolic disorders.
- These drugs convert blood plasminogen to plasmin, a fibrinolytic enzyme that digests or dissolves fibrin clots wherever they can be reached by plasmin.
- The main drugs in this class include alteplase (also known as recombinant tissue plasminogen activator, rt-PA), tenecteplase and urokinase.

Haemostatic and antifibrinolytic drugs

Haemophilia is a hereditary disorder caused by a deficiency of one or more plasma protein clotting factors. This condition usually leads to persistent and uncontrollable haemorrhage after even minor injury. The symptoms include excessive bleeding from wounds and haemorrhage into joints, the urinary tract and, on occasion, the central nervous system. There are two types of haemophilia: haemophilia A, the classic type in which factor VIII activity is deficient; and haemophilia B, or Christmas disease, in which factor IX complex activity is deficient. In recent years, a correct diagnosis of the coagulation disorder has led to specific factor replacement therapy, and this medical advance has resulted in effective management of people at home.

Haemostatic and **antifibrinolytic drugs** are compounds used to control and prevent bleeding in the treatment of both haemophilia and drug-induced over-anticoagulation. This group of drugs includes factor VIII, factor IX and tranexamic acid. Idarucizumab, protamine and vitamin K are commonly used to reverse the effects of anticoagulants. All of these agents are used to control rapid loss of blood.

Factor VIII

Factor VIII, or the antihaemophilic factor, is a glycoprotein necessary for haemostasis and blood clotting. In the intrinsic pathway the antihaemophilic factor is required for the transformation of prothrombin to thrombin. In the treatment or prevention of haemophilia A, factor VIII administration is based on replacing the missing plasma clotting factor to control and prevent bleeding.

When administered intravenously, factor VIII has a distribution half-life of 2.4–8 hours and an elimination half-life of 8.4–19.3 hours. The time to peak effect is 1–2 hours after intravenous administration. No significant drug interactions have been reported with factor VIII, but anticoagulants and antiplatelet drugs should not be administered to haemophiliacs.

Mild to severe allergic reactions have been reported, such as bronchospasm, elevated temperature, chills or rash. Other adverse reactions, which might be related to the rate of infusion, include headache, increased heart rate, tingling of fingers, fainting, lethargy, sedation, hypotension, back pain, nausea or vomiting, visual disturbances and chest constriction.

Use factor VIII with caution in people with sensitivity to mouse, hamster or bovine proteins. Avoid use in people with antihaemophilic factor hypersensitivity. People who develop antibodies to factor VIII might not respond to factor VIII therapy.

Factor IX complex

Factor IX complex is a purified plasma fraction prepared from pooled units of plasma. It contains factors II, VII, IX and X, which are known as the vitamin K coagulation factors. This agent is used for therapy in people with a deficiency of these factors during haemorrhage or before surgery. It is also indicated for people with haemophilia B in whom factor IX is deficient (Christmas disease). Factor IX complex is used to prevent or control bleeding in people with factor IX deficiency. It is also used to treat people with bleeding problems who have antibodies to factor VIII, and it will reverse haemorrhage induced by warfarin.

Factor IX has an elimination half-life of 18–32 hours, and the time to peak effect after intravenous administration is 10–30 minutes. Interactions with other drugs have not been established.

Adverse reactions include chills and fever, especially when large doses are given. Also, if the intravenous infusion is given too rapidly, headache, flushing, rash, nausea, vomiting, sedation, lethargy, elevated temperature and tingling have been reported. The infusion should be stopped and, in most people, it can be resumed at a much slower rate.

Thrombosis and disseminated intravascular coagulation have occurred as a result of the administration of factor IX. Myocardial infarction, pulmonary embolism and anaphylaxis have also been reported. It should not be used in people undergoing elective surgery because they are at a greater risk of thrombosis.

Use factor IX with caution in people with trauma injuries and severe liver impairment, and in those who have recently had surgery. Avoid use in people with factor IX, hamster protein or mouse protein hypersensitivity, disseminated intravascular coagulation and those with a history of thromboembolism. Factor IX should be administered slowly by intravenous injection or by intravenous infusion. The dosage is individualised according to the person's haematology results. Check current references for specific dosing recommendations.

Tranexamic acid

Tranexamic acid, an antifibrinolytic drug, is a competitive inhibitor of plasminogen activation; at high doses, it is a non-competitive inhibitor of plasmin. It is indicated for use in a number of situations, including heavy menstrual bleeding, to prevent haemorrhage in people with mild-to-moderate coagulopathies undergoing minor surgical procedures (e.g. cervical conisation, dental surgery) and to prevent hereditary angio-oedema. No significant drug interactions have been reported.

Adverse reactions include nausea, vomiting, diarrhoea, visual disturbances, thrombosis, hypotension, thrombo-embolism and menstrual discomfort.

Use with caution in women who are breastfeeding. Avoid use in people with tranexamic acid hypersensitivity, colour vision defects, haematuria, subarachnoid haemorrhage, a history of thrombosis or renal impairment.

Drugs reversing anticoagulation

Idarucizumab (reverses dabigatran)

Idarucizumab is a humanised monoclonal antibody fragment that binds free dabigatran, thrombin-bound dabigatran and the acyl glucuronide metabolites of dabigatran. It has a 350-fold greater affinity for dabigatran than dabigatran's affinity for thrombin, and it does not reverse the effects of other anticoagulants or antithrombotic agents. Idarucizumab itself has no antithrombotic or prothrombotic properties.

Following intravenous administration, peak plasma concentration is achieved immediately at the end of the infusion and reversal of the anticoagulant effect of dabigatran is immediate. The anticoagulant effect of dabigatran may re-emerge up to 24 hours after the infusion and a further intravenous infusion may be necessary. The drug has a small volume of distribution as it is confined to the plasma compartment. Idarucizumab is biodegraded to small peptides and amino acids, and renal excretion is the main route of elimination with 32% of the dose appearing in urine within 6 hours.

Idarucizumab is indicated for rapid reversal of dabigatran in situations of emergency surgery/procedures or for life-threatening uncontrolled bleeding. The main adverse reactions include headache and local infusion site reactions (e.g. mild erythema, swelling, pain) (Reilly et al. 2016).

Protamine (reverses heparins)

Protamine, a protein-like substance derived from the sperm and mature testes of salmon and other fish, is a heparin antagonist and is used in over-anticoagulation. Protamine is a very weak anticoagulant alone, but when the sulfate form is given in conjunction with heparin, a complex is formed that dissociates the heparin–AT III complex, thus reducing the anticoagulant action of heparin. Protamine is a basic protein (containing many free amino groups) and combines with heparin to form an inactive complex.

Protamine is indicated to treat an overdose of LMWH or standard heparin that has resulted in haemorrhaging. Blood transfusions may be necessary. It is also used to neutralise the effects of heparin administered during either dialysis or cardiac or arterial surgery. It is administered intravenously and has an onset of action within 1 minute. Its duration of action is approximately 2 hours.

Adverse reactions include back pain, a feeling of warmth or tiredness, flushing, nausea and vomiting. Less often reported are bradycardia, sudden hypotension, shock and dyspnoea (all related to the too-rapid administration of protamine), bleeding (caused by protamine overdose or a rebound of heparin activity), hypertension and anaphylaxis.

Use protamine with caution in people who have been exposed to either protamine or protamine insulin in the past. Antibodies to protamine may have developed, which increases the risk of an allergic reaction. Avoid use in people with protamine hypersensitivity.

Protamine is administered by slow intravenous injection over 10 minutes. One milligram of protamine is necessary to neutralise around 100 units of standard heparin, if injected within 15 minutes of heparin administration. As heparin is cleared quite rapidly, a reduction in the dose of protamine is necessary if it is administered more than 15 minutes after the heparin dose. Seek specialist advice before administering protamine. Close monitoring with blood coagulation tests is required.

Vitamin K (reverses warfarin)

Vitamin K (phytomenadione) is essential to the hepatic synthesis of prothrombin (factor II) and factors VII, IX and X. It acts as a co-factor for the carboxylase enzyme, which is necessary for the formation of prothrombin. Vitamin K may be given as an antidote for excessive anticoagulation with warfarin if simple cessation of warfarin therapy is not sufficient (Fig 13.3). Local guidelines should be followed when administered to reverse the anticoagulant effect of warfarin (Tran et al. 2013). When vitamin K is given concurrently with warfarin, the anticoagulant effect is reduced.

A deficiency of vitamin K leads to hypoprothrombinaemia and haemorrhage; vitamin K is also used to prevent and treat hypoprothrombinaemia. Prothrombin deficiency can occur because of inadequate absorption of vitamin K from the intestine (usually caused by biliary disease in which bile fails to enter the intestine) or because of destruction of intestinal organisms, which might occur with antibiotic therapy. It is also seen in the newborn because of a lack of establishment of intestinal organisms. Vitamin K is routinely administered to newborns to help prevent haemorrhage. Although prothrombin levels may be normal at birth, they decline until about day 6–8, when the liver is then able to form prothrombin.

Vitamin K is also indicated in the preoperative preparation of patients with deficient prothrombin, particularly those with obstructive jaundice.

The onset of action for oral phytomenadione is 6–12 hours, and for the injectable form it is 1–2 hours. Vitamin K is metabolised in the liver and excreted via the kidneys and in the bile. Hence it is used with caution in people with biliary atresia, pancreatic insufficiency or fat malabsorption syndromes. Adverse reactions include facial flushing, taste alterations and redness or pain at the injection site.

KEY POINTS

Haemostatic and antifibrinolytic drugs

- The haemostatic and antifibrinolytic agents are used to control and prevent bleeding and reduce blood loss.
- This group of drugs includes eptacog alfa (factor VII), factor VIII, factor IX and tranexamic acid and idarucizumab, protamine and vitamin K.
- Idarucizumab is used to reverse the anticoagulant effects of dabigatran.
- Protamine reverses the anticoagulant effects of the heparins.
- Vitamin K reverses the action of warfarin.

DRUGS AT A GLANCE
Drugs affecting thrombosis and haemostasis

PHARMACOLOGICAL GROUP AND EFFECT	KEY EXAMPLES	CLINICAL USE
Anticoagulants *Heparins* • Inactivate factor IIa (thrombin) and factor Xa by binding to antithrombin III • ↑ action of antithrombin III on factor Xa (LMWHs) • ↓ binding to thrombin (LMWHs)	Dalteparin (LMWH)	• Prevention of VTE in surgical patients • Prevention of thrombosis during dialysis
	Danaparoid[AUS] (heparinoid)	• Prevention of VTE in surgical patients
	Enoxaparin (LMWH)	• Prevention of VTE in high-risk surgical/medical patients • Prevention of thrombosis during dialysis • Treatment of venous thrombosis • Treatment of unstable angina/acute STEMI/non-STEMI
	Heparin	• Prevention of VTE in high-risk surgical/medical patients • Prevention of arterial thrombosis (coronary angioplasty) • Prevention of extracorporeal thrombosis during haemodialysis/cardiopulmonary bypass • Treatment of ACS and VTE
	Nadroparin (LMWH)	• Prevention of DVT during surgery • Treatment of DVT • Prevention of thrombosis during dialysis • Prevention of VTE (high-risk medical patients)
Vitamin K antagonist • Inhibits VKORC1, which inhibits synthesis vitamin K–dependent clotting factors (II, VII, IX and X)	Warfarin	• Prevention/treatment of VTE • Prevention of thromboembolism (prosthetic heart valves) • Prevention of stroke in high-risk patients • In patients with AF and high-risk of stroke/systemic embolism
Direct thrombin inhibitors • Reversibly bind to thrombin which, • Prevents conversion of fibrinogen to fibrin • Prevents thrombus formation	Bivalirudin	• Unstable angina (moderate-to-high-risk) • Non-STEMI undergoing PCI
	Dabigatran etexilate	• Prevention of VTE (hip/knee replacement) • Treatment of acute VTE • Patients with AF and high-risk of stroke/systemic embolism
Antithrombin-III-dependent anticoagulant • Binds ATIII potentiating neutralisation of factor Xa by antithrombin • Inhibits thrombin formation and thrombus development	Fondaparinux	• Prevention of VTE (hip/knee replacement/abdominal surgery) • Treatment of VTE • Treatment of unstable angina/non-STEMI • Treatment of STEMI

Antifibrinolytics
• Competitive inhibitor of plasminogen activation
	Tranexamic acid	• Reduction of bleeding in:
		  • minor surgery
		  • major surgery
		  • heavy menses
		  • knee/hip arthroplasty

Direct factor Xa inhibitors • Competitive inhibitor binds to factor Xa • Attenuates thrombin generation and prevents conversion of fibrinogen to fibrin	Apixaban	• Prevention of VTE (hip/knee replacement) • Treatment of acute VTE • Patients with AF and high-risk of stroke/systemic embolism
	Rivaroxaban	• Same as apixaban
Antiplatelet drugs *Glycoprotein IIb/IIIa receptor inhibitors* • Occupy receptors and prevent binding of fibrinogen	Eptifibatide	• Unstable angina • Non-STEMI • Elective PCI with stenting
	Tirofiban	• Unstable angina • Non-STEMI
$P2Y_{12}$ inhibitors • Bind $P2Y_{12}$ platelet receptors and inhibit platelet aggregation	Clopidogrel	• Symptomatic atherosclerosis • ACS (with aspirin)
	Prasugrel	• ACS (with aspirin)
	Ticagrelor	• ACS (with aspirin)

Other antiplatelet drugs • Inhibitor of COX-1 • ↓ thromboxane A_2 synthesis and platelet aggregation	Aspirin	• Symptomatic atherosclerosis • ACS
• Inhibits phosphodiesterase activity • ↑ platelet cAMP	Dipyridamole	• Cardiac stress testing (IV) • Ischaemic stroke and transient ischaemic attack (with aspirin)
Haemostatics *Dabigatran antagonist* • A monoclonal antibody fragment • Binds free dabigatran, thrombin-bound dabigatran and metabolites of dabigatran	Idarucizumab	• Reversal of dabigatran anticoagulation (life-threatening or uncontrolled bleeding/emergency surgery)
Heparin antagonist • Forms complex with heparin • Dissociates the heparin-AT III complex reducing the anticoagulant effect of heparin	Protamine	• Overdose with either heparin, dalteparin or enoxaparin • Risk of severe haemorrhage
Thrombolytics • Convert plasminogen to plasmin • Plasmin digests or dissolves fibrin clots	Alteplase	• Acute STEMI • Acute ischaemic stroke • Pulmonary embolism (massive)
	Tenecteplase	• Acute STEMI

AUS = Australia only
ACS = acute coronary syndrome; AF = atrial fibrillation; DVT = deep vein thrombosis; LMWH = low-molecular-weight heparins; PCI = percutaneous coronary intervention; STEMI = ST-elevation myocardial infarction; VTE = venous thromboembolism

REVIEW EXERCISES

1 Ms B, a 26-year-old female, has a prosthetic heart valve and is on warfarin therapy. She has been advised that if she becomes pregnant her warfarin will need to be stopped and she will change to heparin therapy. She asks you to explain why she will need to cease warfarin and change to heparin. Make a list of the key points you would discuss with her to answer her query.

2 Mrs TG, a 69-year-old woman, is taking warfarin and on admission to hospital her INR was 5.0. She was administered oral vitamin K to counter the excessive anticoagulation. Explain how vitamin K counteracts excessive anticoagulation due to warfarin.

3 Mr D presented with an acute coronary event and, following insertion of two coronary stents, he was commenced on aspirin and clopidogrel. A junior member of staff asks you to explain to them how each drug works and why Mr D has been commenced on a combination. What are your explanations?

REFERENCES

Chan N, Sobieraj-Teague M, Eikelboom JW. Direct oral anticoagulants: evidence and unresolved issues. Lancet 2020;396:1767–76.

Connolly SJ, Crowther M, Eikelboom JW, et al. Full study report of andexanet alfa for bleeding associated with Factor Xa inhibitors. The New England Journal of Medicine. 2019;380:1326–35.

Heo Y-A. Andexanet alfa: First global approval. Drugs 2018;78:1049–55.

Rang HP, Dale JM, Ritter JM, et al., Rang and Dale's Pharmacology, 7th ed. Elsevier Ltd; 2012.

Reilly PA, van Ryn J, Grotthe O, et al. Idarucizumab, a specific reversal agent for dabigatran: mode of action, pharmacokinetics and pharmacodynamics, and safety and efficacy in Phase 1 subjects. American Journal of Emergency Medicine 2016;129:S64–S72.

Tran HA, Chunilal SD, Harper PL, et al. An update of consensus guidelines for warfarin reversal. Medical Journal of Australia 2013;198(4):198–99.

Winter WE, Greene DN, Beal SG, et al. Clotting factors: Clinical biochemistry and their roles as plasma enzymes. Advances in Clinical Chemistry 2020;94:31–84.

ONLINE RESOURCE

International Warfarin Pharmacogenetics Consortium: https://www.pharmgkb.org/page/iwpc (accessed 8 June 2021)

More weblinks at: http://evolve.elsevier.com/AU/Knights/pharmacology/.

CHAPTER 14
DRUGS AFFECTING THE HAEMOPOIETIC SYSTEM

Kathleen Knights

KEY ABBREVIATIONS

CSF	colony-stimulating factor
EPO	erythropoietin
G-CSF	granulocyte colony-stimulating factor
RBCs	red blood cells
WBCs	white blood cells

KEY TERMS

anaemia 271
colony-stimulating factors 269
erythropoietin 269
ferritin 272
granulocyte colony-stimulating factor 274
haematinics 271
haemosiderin 272
thrombocytopenia 271

Chapter Focus

The haemopoietic system comprises principally blood and bone marrow and the accessory organs: the liver, spleen and kidneys. Blood is crucial for the maintenance of homeostasis, and perturbations of the haemopoietic system may manifest in illnesses such as anaemia, haemophilia, thromboembolic disease and leukaemia. This chapter reviews the haematinic agents and erythropoietin agonists used in the treatment of anaemia and the haemopoietic colony-stimulating factors often used as adjuncts to chemotherapy.

KEY DRUG GROUPS

Colony-stimulating factors:

- **Filgrastim, lipegfilgrastim, pegfilgrastim**

Erythropoietin agonists:

- **Darbepoetin alfa, epoetin alfa, epoetin beta, methoxy polyethylene glycol-epoetin beta**

Haematinic agents:

- **Folic acid, iron, vitamin B12**

CRITICAL THINKING SCENARIO

Ari, a 48-year-old male, was diagnosed 3 months ago with cancer and has been undergoing regular chemotherapy cycles. Immediately after his last round of treatment the oncologist ordered filgrastim subcutaneously (10 micrograms/kg) daily, with a further full blood count to be repeated in 3 days. The filgrastim was administered 24 hours after his last chemotherapy cycle was completed. With reference to the pharmacology of filgrastim explain why the drug has been prescribed for Ari and what beneficial effects the oncologist is anticipating. Explain why the administration of filgrastim has been delayed for 24 hours and what the purpose is of a full blood count in 3 days.

Introduction

The haemopoietic system comprises primarily the blood and bone marrow, complemented by the liver (storage of vitamin B12 for erythrocyte production), spleen (removal of expired blood cells and storage of platelets) and kidneys (erythropoietin production). Blood is the major transport medium, carrying drugs and nutrients absorbed from the gastrointestinal tract, oxygen from the lungs and hormones, electrolytes and so on to cells throughout the entire body. In addition, it transports metabolic products from cells to the liver, kidneys and lungs for excretion. Blood further helps to regulate body temperature in concert with changes in the vascular system that varies blood flow through the skin. Buffering is also an important function of blood; the pH of human blood ranges from 7.35 to 7.45. In addition to its transportation and regulatory roles, blood is integral to the process of coagulation (Ch 13) and aids in immunity by producing antibodies.

Blood composition

Blood is composed of two components: cells and plasma. The blood volume of an average-sized adult is approximately 5 L, of which approximately 3 L is usually plasma. There are principally three types of blood cells: red blood cells (RBC), or erythrocytes, which transport oxygen and carbon dioxide; white blood cells (WBCs), or leucocytes, which aid in the defence of the body against bacteria and infections; and platelets, or thrombocytes, which are necessary for blood coagulation. Plasma is about 92% water and 8% plasma proteins (e.g. albumin, globulins and fibrinogen). Plasma proteins (e.g. albumin, α_1 acid glycoprotein, fatty acid binding proteins) play an important role in maintaining the osmotic pressure of blood, which is important for fluid exchange through capillary walls. Albumin is important for transporting some steroid hormones and in binding numerous drugs (Ch 4). Fatty-acid-binding proteins that transport fatty acids also bind some drugs. The globulins include the immunoglobulins, also called antibodies, which are important in the body's defence against viruses and bacteria. Fibrinogen is essential for blood clotting and is converted to fibrin by thrombin in the presence of calcium ions. In addition to the proteins, plasma may contain thousands of other substances such as glucose, electrolytes, vitamins, hormones and products of metabolism.

Blood cell production

Haemopoiesis, or blood cell production, occurs within certain parts of bone, principally the red bone marrow. During fetal development, many tissues (e.g. the liver, spleen and thymus gland) participate in blood cell production; however, after birth, haemopoiesis occurs only in the red bone marrow and, after 20 years of age, principally in the bone marrow of the vertebrae, sternum, ribs and ilia. Differentiation and proliferation of precursor cells into the various types of blood cells is regulated by haemopoietic growth factors such as **erythropoietin** (EPO), thrombopoietin and the cytokines, which include **colony-stimulating factors** (CSFs) and interleukins (Ch 34).

Secretion by the kidneys of EPO, a hormone that regulates the production of RBCs by the bone marrow, is stimulated by hypoxia and/or blood loss. With maximal bone marrow stimulation, RBC production can be increased seven-fold. Thrombopoietin, another hormone, is produced by the liver and substantially increases platelet production, while CSFs and interleukins stimulate formation of leucocytes. A simplified diagram of blood cell differentiation is shown in Figure 14.1.

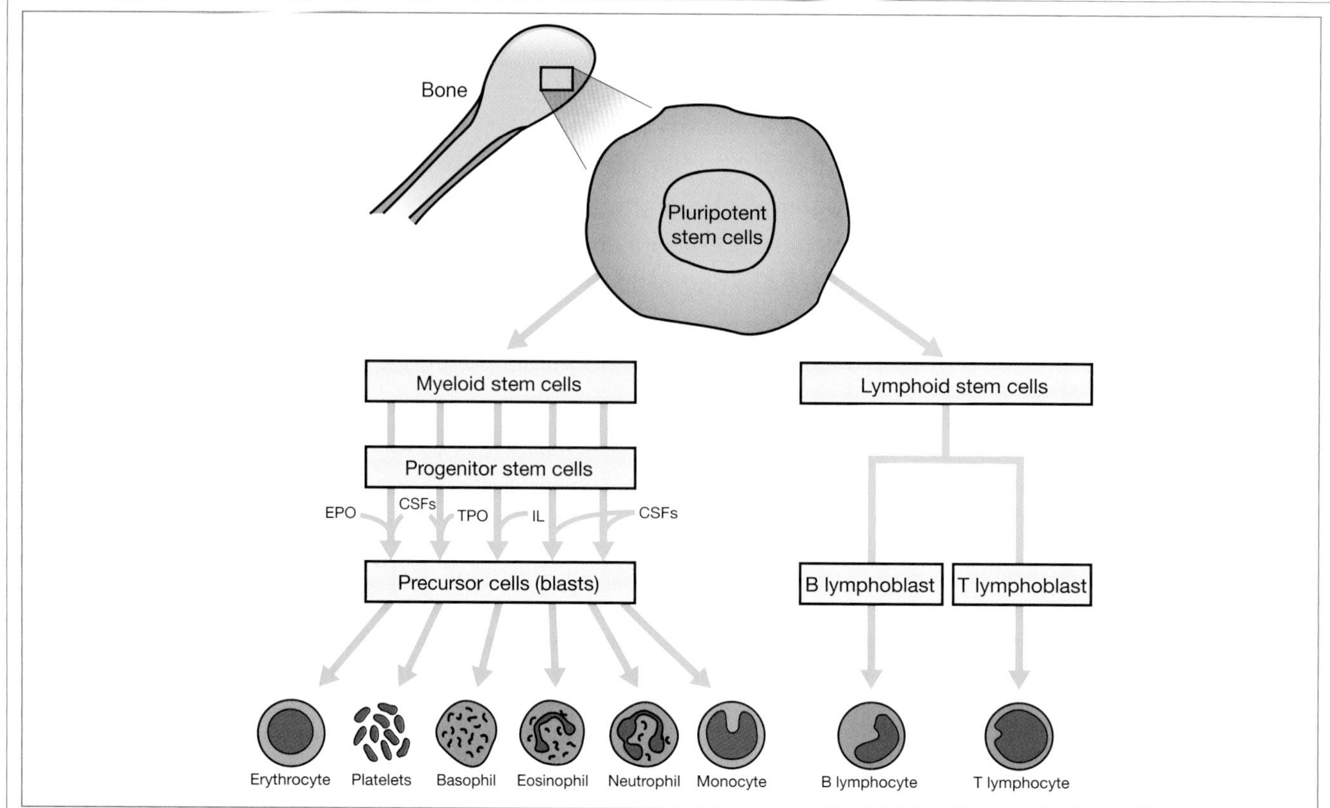

FIGURE 14.1 A simplified diagram of blood cell production (haemopoiesis) and the involvement of growth factors
Cells originating from myeloid stem cells are produced in the bone marrow. Lymphoid stem cells arise in bone marrow, but development of lymphocytes is completed in lymphatic tissue. CSFs = colony-stimulating factors; EPO = erythropoietin; IL = interleukin; TPO = thrombopoietin.

Red blood cells (erythrocytes)

RBCs, or erythrocytes, are small, non-nucleated, biconcave disc-shaped cells present in large quantities in the bloodstream. Without a nucleus, RBCs have negligible synthetic capacity and hence their life span is short (about 120 days). Expired cells are removed from the circulation and destroyed by phagocytes resident in the liver and spleen. A healthy adult female has 3.8–5.8 $\times 10^{12}$ cells/L of blood. It is estimated that more than 100 million RBCs are produced/minute during adulthood, and production (erythropoiesis) and destruction of these cells is balanced to maintain a relatively constant level of RBCs.

Within the cytosol of RBCs are haemoglobin molecules, the main function of which is the transport of oxygen. Each haemoglobin molecule consists of a protein called globin, composed of four polypeptide chains, four non-protein haem pigment molecules and four iron atoms. Each polypeptide chain is associated with one haem and one iron ion (Fe^{2+}); thus, one haemoglobin molecule combines in total with four oxygen molecules. Oxygen is transported from the lungs to the tissues, where it is released from the haemoglobin and diffuses through the interstitial fluid into the cells. Haemoglobin can also combine with carbon dioxide that is carried from the cells to the lungs for excretion. Haemoglobin has also been reported to be involved in blood pressure regulation by transporting the vasodilator nitric oxide, produced by endothelial cells that line blood vessels.

White blood cells (leucocytes)

There are five types of nucleated leucocytes found in the blood. They are produced primarily in the bone marrow and are classified according to the presence or absence of granules in the cell cytoplasm (Fig 14.1). The three types of granular leucocytes are neutrophils, eosinophils and basophils. Aged cells that have different-shaped nuclear lobes and an increased number of nuclei (> 2, > 3 or > 5) are referred to as polymorphonuclear leucocytes, or polymorphs. The other two types of leucocytes are lymphocytes and monocytes, which are produced mainly in lymph tissues and the spleen, thymus, tonsils and various other lymphoid tissues, in the bone marrow, gastrointestinal tract and elsewhere. Neutrophils, basophils, monocytes and lymphocytes are very mobile; they leave the capillaries and migrate to sites of infection. The neutrophils and monocytes ingest and destroy the pathogens, a process known as phagocytosis, while the

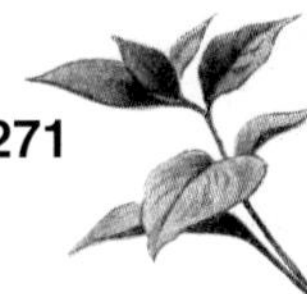

lymphocytes defend the body against bacteria, fungi and viruses. (See Ch 34 for an overview of the immune system.) In contrast, eosinophils play a dominant role during allergic reactions and parasitic infections.

The life span of granulocytes is estimated to be 4–8 hours in the bloodstream and 3–5 days in body tissues. If involved in phagocytosis of pathogens, this life span can be reduced to a few hours because granulocytes can also be destroyed. Monocytes also have a short life span in the blood, but in body tissues they can increase in size and differentiate to become tissue macrophages (the main phagocytic cells of the immune system that ingest foreign antigens and cell debris), providing a first line of defence against tissue infections. The agranular T and B lymphocytes may live for several years.

Platelets

Unlike RBCs and WBCs, platelets, or thrombocytes, are small, disc-shaped, non-nucleated colourless cell fragments that split off from the megakaryocytes produced by the bone marrow (Fig 14.1). They have a short life span of about 5–8 days. Time-expired platelets are engulfed by resident macrophages in the spleen and liver. Platelets are essential for coagulation (Ch 13). People with a low concentration of platelets have **thrombocytopenia**. Such people tend to bleed, and their skin usually displays small purple spots (hence the name thrombocytopenia purpura). Thrombocytopenia is often induced by irradiation injury to the bone marrow, or results from aplasia of the bone marrow induced by specific drugs.

KEY POINTS

Haemopoietic system

- The haemopoietic system comprises primarily the blood and bone marrow, complemented by the liver (which stores vitamin B12 for erythrocyte production), the spleen (which removes expired blood cells and stores platelets) and the kidneys (which produce EPO).
- Blood transports drugs and nutrients absorbed from the gastrointestinal tract, oxygen from the lungs and hormones and electrolytes and other substances to cells throughout the entire body.
- Blood is composed principally of plasma and three types of blood cells: red blood cells, or erythrocytes (which transport oxygen and carbon dioxide); white blood cells, or leucocytes (which defend the body against bacteria and infections); and platelets, or thrombocytes (which are necessary for blood coagulation).

Haematinics

A condition in which there is a reduced oxygen-carrying capacity of the blood is referred to as **anaemia**, and often manifests as fatigue. The different types of anaemia are classified on the basis of the size and number of functional RBCs and haemoglobin concentration. A combination of measuring serum ferritin, iron, vitamin B12 and folic acid, and microscopic examination of a blood smear and a bone marrow smear, allows a precise diagnosis of the type of anaemia.

Agents used to treat anaemias include the **haematinics**: iron, folic acid and vitamin B12 and the EPO agonists.

Iron and iron deficiency anaemia

Iron deficiency anaemia is characterised by small RBCs with reduced haemoglobin, and other causes of iron deficiency should be excluded prior to treatment. These include, but are not limited to, blood loss (e.g. chronic non-steroidal anti-inflammatory drug use and gastrointestinal ulceration), blood donation, pregnancy and lactation (increased iron requirement), malabsorption (e.g. after gastric surgery), inadequate diet (e.g. due to

CLINICAL FOCUS BOX 14.1
Blood and bone smears

A blood smear provides evidence of:

- hypochromic, microcytic anaemia, commonly caused by iron deficiency due to either inadequate intake or absorption or excessive loss of iron giving rise to small RBCs with a low haemoglobin content
- macrocytic anaemia, characterised by large RBCs that are few in number
- normochromic normocytic anaemia, evident from a reduced number of normal RBCs with normal haemoglobin content
- a mixed blood picture.

A bone marrow smear increases diagnostic precision by providing evidence of:

- anaemia due to nutritional deficiency (e.g. deficiency in absorption of vitamin B12 from the small intestine caused by a lack of intrinsic factor, inadequate or no intake of red meat, iron deficiency or folic acid deficiency)
- haemolytic anaemia due to excessive destruction of RBCs (e.g. adverse reaction to drugs or inappropriate immune reaction [transfusion incompatibility])
- anaemia resulting from bone marrow suppression (e.g. caused by radiation therapy or cancer chemotherapeutic agents).

socioeconomic status, low consumption of meat or a vegetarian/vegan lifestyle) and previous history of iron deficiency. Iron deficiency not only causes anaemia: iron is also an essential component of myoglobin, enzymes with a haem moiety (e.g. cytochromes and peroxidases) and metallo flavoproteins such as xanthine oxidase, which is involved in purine metabolism. (See the section on hyperuricaemia and gout in Ch 34.)

Iron is a transition metal. The majority of iron (~65%) circulates as haemoglobin, which contains four haem moieties, each having one iron atom to which one oxygen molecule binds reversibly. In general, iron is obtained through a meat-containing diet, creating a problem for cultures reliant on grain as a major food source. Iron is absorbed from the duodenum and upper jejunum and carried in plasma bound to transferrin. Iron that leaves the plasma is used for synthesis of haemoglobin by red cell precursors that bind the transferrin molecules, releasing them after the uptake of the iron. Iron as **ferritin** is stored in all cells and, on average, plasma contains approximately 4 mg iron; the daily turnover is about 30 mg (Fig 14.2). The majority of the iron is stored in erythrocytes, with the next highest concentrations occurring in liver and bone marrow (stored as ferritin and haemosiderin) and in muscle, with small amounts in the spleen and bound in enzymes. **Haemosiderin** is a degraded form of ferritin. Iron concentration is tightly controlled by the absorptive process, as the body has virtually no mechanism for excreting iron.

Once iron deficiency anaemia has been diagnosed, iron is administered orally but can also be given parenterally if required. Iron dosage is expressed in terms of elemental iron:

- 1 mg elemental iron = ~3 mg ferrous sulfate (dried)
- 1 mg elemental iron = ~5 mg ferrous sulfate (as liquid)
- 1 mg elemental iron = ~3 mg ferrous fumarate.

Iron is also available in combination with folic acid for preventing and treating iron and folate deficiency during pregnancy. To prevent an excessive intake of iron, the oral and parenteral formulations of iron should not be used together. In addition, although a rare occurrence, there is a risk of an anaphylactoid reaction with parenteral iron preparations.

Adverse reactions with iron are gastrointestinal disturbances (e.g. abdominal pain, nausea, vomiting, diarrhoea and black-coloured faeces). As acute iron toxicity can be serious or even fatal in small children, iron formulations should be kept well out of reach and preferably

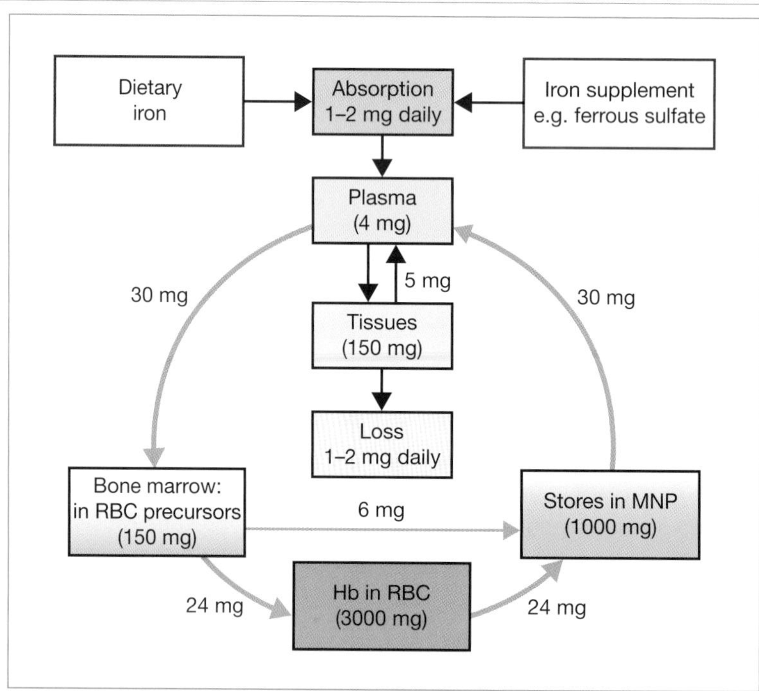

FIGURE 14.2 Distribution and turnover of iron in the body
The quantities by the arrows indicate the usual amounts transferred each day. The transfer of 6 mg from red cell precursors to phagocytes represents aborted cells that fail to develop into functional red blood cells. Hb, haemoglobin; MNP, mononuclear phagocytes (mainly in liver, spleen and bone marrow); RBC, red blood cells.
Source: Rang et al. 2016, Chapter 25, Figure 25.1; used with permission.

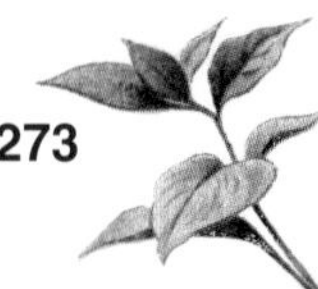

locked away. In cases of chronic iron overload, the iron chelators deferasirox, deferiprone or desferrioxamine are administered. These drugs form complexes with the iron, which are then excreted in faeces or urine.

Folic acid and vitamin B12

In general, folic acid deficiency occurs through poor diet, while vitamin B12 deficiency arises from absorptive problems in the terminal ileum (e.g. in Crohn's disease). Folic acid and vitamin B12 are both obtained through the diet, and both are interrelated in the synthesis of DNA. Folic acid is essential for DNA synthesis, and dietary folic acid is reduced to tetrahydrofolate (FH_4). Vitamin B12 is required for conversion of methyl-FH_4 to FH_4; hence, a deficiency of either results in defective DNA synthesis.

Always exclude vitamin B12 deficiency before prescribing folic acid to treat megaloblastic anaemia. In addition, check medications, as some drugs (e.g. anti-epileptics and dihydrofolate reductase inhibitors such as methotrexate and trimethoprim) cause folic acid deficiency. Except in special circumstances, folic acid is administered orally. Adverse reactions with folic acid are rare.

Vitamin B12 (available as hydroxocobalamin and cyanocobalamin) is used principally to treat vitamin B12 deficiency and optic neuropathies. (The vitamin is essential to nerve development.) Confirm diagnosis before use, as vitamin B12 may mask the clinical signs of folic acid deficiency. Hydroxocobalamin is administered intramuscularly, while cyanocobalamin is available as both an oral and an injectable (IM) formulation. In cases of malabsorption syndrome, oral formulations are inappropriate and vitamin B12 injections will be required. As with folic acid, adverse reactions are rare.

Clinical Uses of Iron, Folic Acid and Vitamin B12

Iron

- Prevention/treatment of iron deficiency anaemia

Folic acid

- Folate deficiency anaemia
- Prevention of neural tube defect in fetuses
- Prevention of chronic haemo/renal dialysis induced folate deficiency
- Prevention/treatment of methotrexate-induced toxicity

Vitamin B12

- Prevention/treatment of vitamin B12 deficiency
- Treatment of optic neuropathies

KEY POINTS

Haematinics

- A reduced oxygen-carrying capacity of the blood is referred to as anaemia.
- Different types of anaemia exist and are classified on the basis of the size and number of functional RBCs and the haemoglobin concentration.
- Iron concentration is tightly controlled by the absorptive process, as the body has virtually no mechanism for excreting iron.
- The haematinics commonly used to treat anaemia include iron, folic acid and vitamin B12.
- Iron is absorbed from the duodenum and upper jejunum carried in plasma bound to transferrin and stored in cells as ferritin.
- Folic acid is used to treat folate-deficiency anaemia, to prevent neural tube defects in the growing fetus and to treat or prevent toxicity from methotrexate.
- Vitamin B12 (available as hydroxocobalamin and cyanocobalamin) is used principally to treat pernicious anaemia and optic neuropathies.

Haemopoietics

The continuous replacement of RBCs is called haemopoiesis and is regulated by growth factors such as EPO, thrombopoietin and the cytokines, which include the CSFs. EPO is not the sole haemopoietic growth factor, but it is important, and in its absence severe anaemia is invariably observed. EPO stimulates the division and differentiation of erythroid progenitors in the bone marrow. When the haemoglobin concentration decreases or tissue oxygenation is low, plasma EPO concentration rises and within 3–4 days circulating RBCs begin to rise. It is produced in the kidney, and production is impaired in chronic renal failure.

Erythropoietin agonists

Recombinant human EPOs (epoetin alfa and epoetin beta) are almost identical to the human hormone, while darbepoetin alfa, also a recombinant hormone, is a slightly larger version of EPO (due to glycosylation) but nevertheless has the same actions. Methoxy polyethylene glycol-epoetin beta is a complex of recombinant epoetin beta with methoxy-polyethylene glycol – that is, pegylated epoetin beta. Epoetin alfa (Drug Monograph 14.1) and darbepoetin alfa act specifically through the EPO receptor on the surface of erythroid progenitor cells, stimulating erythropoiesis, increasing reticulocyte count and increasing haematocrit and haemoglobin concentration. The EPO receptor is also expressed on mast cells and in gastric mucosa and brain neurons.

The duration of action of darbepoetin alfa and methoxy polyethylene glycol-epoetin beta is longer, allowing once-weekly and once-monthly dosing, respectively, while epoetin alfa is administered three times weekly. These drugs are used to treat anaemia associated with chronic renal failure; surgery with expected blood loss; in cancer chemotherapy; and to stimulate RBC production prior to autologous blood collection in people with anaemia who are undergoing elective surgery.

Adverse reactions are common and include hypertension (due to a rapid rise in haemoglobin), flu-like symptoms (e.g. headache, bone pain, myalgia and fever) and rash, peripheral oedema, dyspnoea and gastrointestinal disturbances (e.g. nausea, vomiting and diarrhoea). Administered SC/IV, pain at the injection site is more common with darbepoetin alfa, while the development of epoetin antibodies (which may limit usefulness) has been reported.

Colony-stimulating factors

Colony-stimulating factors are cytokines that regulate cell proliferation, differentiation and growth through an action on progenitor cells. Currently available drugs include the **granulocyte colony-stimulating factors** (G-CSFs) filgrastim, pegfilgrastim and lipegfilgrastim. G-CSF is primarily regarded as a haemopoietic growth factor of the granulocyte lineage controlling the development of neutrophils.

The G-CSFs are indicated for preventing and treating chemotherapy/drug-induced neutropenia and severe chronic neutropenia, and for mobilising stem cells in donors for use in allogenic transplantation. The G-CSFs shorten the period of severe neutropenia after high-dose chemotherapy and improve outcomes in terms of reduced hospitalisation rates for opportunistic bacterial and fungal infections and decreased frequency of interruptions to chemotherapy protocols through hospitalisation for febrile neutropenia.

Rare adverse effects include cardiovascular toxicity, pulmonary oedema, pericardial effusion, splenic rupture and toxic epidermal necrolysis. Of concern is the suggestion of a link with secondary malignancies, although a causal relationship has not been established.

Granulocyte colony-stimulating factors

Filgrastim is a recombinant non-glycosylated form of human G-CSF produced in culture using *Escherichia coli*, pegfilgrastim is filgrastim complexed with a polyethylene glycol moiety at the *N*-terminus of the recombinant protein, while lipegfilgrastim is a more complex molecule comprising filgrastim covalently linked to a single polyethylene glycol molecule via a glycine/sialic acid/*N*-acetylgalactosamine moiety.

Pegylation of filgrastim reduces its clearance by glomerular filtration, increases its half-life and thus prolongs its action and allows less frequent dosing. Lipegfilgrastim is predominantly cleared by a neutrophil-mediated pathway that becomes saturated at higher doses. Filgrastim may be administered SC/IV, while pegfilgrastim and lipegfilgrastim are administered subcutaneously. Specialist protocols should be consulted for information on dosage, route of administration and precautions prior to administration.

Adverse effects are common and include headache, bone pain, fever, injection site reactions and splenomegaly.

KEY POINTS

Haemopoietics

- Haemopoiesis, or blood cell production, occurs principally in the bone marrow.
- Differentiation and proliferation of precursor cells into the various types of blood cells is regulated by haemopoietic growth factors such as EPO, thrombopoietin and the cytokines, which include CSFs and interleukins.
- Erythropoietin agonists include recombinant human erythropoietin (epoetin alfa and epoetin beta), which are almost identical to the human hormone, while darbepoetin alfa and methoxy polyethylene glycol-epoetin beta are recombinant hormones that are a slightly larger version of EPO but nevertheless have the same actions.
- CSFs are cytokines that regulate cell proliferation, differentiation and growth through an action on progenitor cells.
- G-CSF is primarily regarded as a haemopoietic growth factor of the granulocyte lineage controlling the development of neutrophils.
- Currently available drugs include the G-CSFs, filgrastim, pegfilgrastim and lipegfilgrastim.

DRUGS AT A GLANCE
Drugs affecting the haemopoietic system

PHARMACOLOGICAL GROUP AND EFFECT	KEY EXAMPLES	CLINICAL USE
Haematinics • Agents used to treat anaemias	Iron	• Prevention/treatment of iron deficiency anaemia
	Folic acid	• Folate deficiency anaemia • Prevention of neural tube defect in fetus • Prevention of chronic haemo/renal dialysis induced folate deficiency • Treat/prevent methotrexate induced toxicity
	Vitamin B12	• Prevention/treatment of vitamin B12 deficiency • Treatment of optic neuropathies
Haemopoietics Erythropoietin agonists • Stimulate erythropoiesis by binding to erythropoietin receptor on surface of erythroid progenitor cells	Darbepoetin alfa	• Treat anaemia of chronic renal failure • Chemotherapy-induced anaemia (non-myeloid deficiency)
	Epoetin alfa	• Treat anaemia of chronic renal failure • Chemotherapy-induced anaemia (non-myeloid deficiency) • Surgery with expected blood loss • In people with anaemia before autologous blood collection before surgery
	Epoetin beta	• Treat anaemia of chronic renal failure • Chemotherapy-induced anaemia (non-myeloid deficiency) • Increase yield of autologous blood collection • Preventing anaemia of prematurity
	Methoxy polyethylene glycol-epoetin beta[AUS]	• Treat anaemia of chronic renal failure
Granulocyte colony-stimulating factors • Haemopoietic growth factor controlling development of neutrophils from progenitor cells	Filgrastim	• Prevention/treatment of neutropenia • Stem cell mobilisation (autologous infusion/allogenic transplantation) • Severe chronic neutropenia
	Lipegfilgrastim	• Prevention/treatment of neutropenia • Stem cell mobilisation (autologous infusion/allogenic transplantation) • Severe chronic neutropenia
	Pegfilgrastim	• Prevention/treatment of neutropenia • Stem cell mobilisation (autologous infusion/allogenic transplantation) • Severe chronic neutropenia

AUS = Australia only

REVIEW EXERCISES

1 Ms GH, a 28-year-old, has been diagnosed with iron deficiency anaemia and has been treated with iron 100 mg daily. However, her most recent haemoglobin 3 weeks after commencing iron therapy was unchanged from her previous test. Make a list of possible explanations.

2 Mr CD is a 22-year-old elite cyclist who casually asks you if you know anything about EPO. What are the purported physiological advantages of EPO administration in elite cyclists? What are the risks to Mr CD's health from doping with EPO?

REFERENCE

Rang HP, Dale MM, Ritter JM et al. Rang & Dale's Pharmacology, 8th edition, Churchill Livingstone, London; 2016

ONLINE RESOURCES

American Society of Hematology: https://www.hematology.org/ (accessed 28 February 2022)

European Hematology Association: https://ehaweb.org/ (accessed 28 February 2022)

Haematology Society of Australia and New Zealand: https://www.hsanz.org.au/ (accessed 28 February 2022)

More weblinks at: http://evolve.elsevier.com/AU/Knights/pharmacology/.

CHAPTER 15

DRUGS USED IN RESPIRATORY DISORDERS

Shaunagh Darroch

KEY ABBREVIATIONS

cAMP	cyclic 3,5-adenosine monophosphate
CF	cystic fibrosis
COPD	chronic obstructive pulmonary disease
DPI	dry powder inhaler
GMP	guanosine monophosphate
ICS	inhaled corticosteroids
IgE	immunoglobulin E
LABAs	long-acting β_2-agonists
LAMAs	long-acting muscarinic antagonists
MDI	metered-dose inhaler
$PaCO_2$	partial pressure of carbon dioxide in arterial blood
PaO_2	partial pressure of oxygen in arterial blood
PGs	prostaglandins
pMDI	pressurised metered-dose inhaler
SABAs	short-acting β_2-agonists
SAMAs	short-acting muscarinic antagonists

Chapter Focus

The respiratory system maintains the exchange of oxygen and carbon dioxide between the lungs and cells, and regulates the pH of body fluids. This chapter briefly reviews relevant respiratory system anatomy and physiology, and describes how drugs are administered by inhalation. Drugs used for effects in the respiratory tract are discussed: medical gases (oxygen and carbon dioxide), respiratory stimulants, drugs affecting mucus and surfactant secretions, antiasthma medications (bronchodilators, symptom controllers and anti-inflammatory agents) and drugs used in the management of chronic obstructive pulmonary disease, respiratory tract infections and conditions affecting the nose. The effects of respiratory depressants are discussed. Olfaction, the sense of smell (or, rather, impairment of it), is discussed in the context of respiratory and other conditions and various drug groups that may impair this sense.

Australia and New Zealand have high prevalences of respiratory tract diseases; respiratory-related conditions including acute and chronic illness. One in nine Australians (11%) reported having asthma in 2020-2021, and 1.5% of Australians reported having chronic obstructive pulmonary disease. An underpinning knowledge of the structure, function and pathophysiology of the respiratory tract is fundamental to understanding the drug groups used to treat the various disorders.

KEY TERMS

β_2-adrenoceptor agonists 296
aerosol 281
allergic rhinitis 292
analeptics 287
anticholinergics 301
asthma 294
bronchoconstriction 290
bronchodilator 295
carbonic anhydrase 280
controller 298
corticosteroids 301
cough suppressant 308
cromones 303
decongestants 309
expectorants 288
hypercapnia 280
hypoxia (hypoxaemia) 285
immunomodulating drugs 294
leukotriene-receptor antagonists 303
long-acting β_2-agonists 298
long-acting muscarinic antagonists 301
mast-cell stabilisers 303
mucociliary transport 281
mucolytics 288
muscarinic receptors 309
nebuliser 283
oxygen free radicals 285
pressurised metered-dose inhaler 283
preventer 301
puffer 283
reliever 298
respiration 279
rhinitis 292
short-acting β_2-agonists 298
short-acting muscarinic antagonists 301
spacer 283
surfactant 281
xanthine derivatives 299

KEY DRUG GROUPS

Bronchodilator drugs:

- Anticholinergics (muscarinic antagonists):
  - Long-acting (LAMAs): **tiotropium**, **aclidinium**, **umeclidinium**, **glycopyrronium bromide (glycopyrrolate)**; Short-acting (SAMAs): **ipratropium bromide**
- β_2-adrenoceptor agonists
  - Long-acting (LABAs; controllers): **formoterol (eformoterol)**, **salmeterol**, **indacaterol**
  - Short-acting (SABAs): **salbutamol**, **terbutaline** (Drug Monograph 15.2)
- Methylxanthines: **aminophylline**, **theophylline** (Drug Monograph 15.3)

Drugs for respiratory tract infections:

- Antivirals: **amantadine**, neuraminidase inhibitors: **zanamivir**, oseltamivir
- Cough suppressants: **codeine**, **pholcodine** (Drug Monograph 15.5)
- Decongestants: **xylometazoline** (Drug Monograph 15.1)
- Drugs for influenza and (SARS-CoV-2): **vaccines**

Drugs for rhinitis:

- Antihistamines: levocabastine; nasal corticosteroids: beclometasone; sympathomimetics: phenylephrine, xylometazoline, oxymetazoline

Expectorants:

- Irritant expectorants: guaifenesin; diluents: **normal saline**, **water**

Medical gases:

- **Carbon dioxide**, nitric oxide, nitrous oxide, **oxygen**

Mucolytics:

- **Dornase alfa**, **bromhexine**, **acetylcysteine**

Prophylactic antiasthma drugs (preventers):

- Cromones (cromolyns): **sodium cromoglycate**, **nedocromil**
- Inhaled (gluco)corticosteroids: **beclometasone** (Drug Monograph 15.4), **budesonide**, fluticasone, ciclesonide
- **Other drug groups:**
  - Leukotriene-receptor antagonists (LTRAs): **montelukast**
  - Monoclonal antibodies: **omalizumab**, **mepolizumab**

Pulmonary surfactants:

- **Beractant**, **poractant alfa**

CRITICAL THINKING SCENARIO

Acute asthma in a child

Pablo calls an ambulance for his 12-year-old son, Josh, who has a runny nose, dry cough and rapid-onset breathing difficulties. The boy was diagnosed with chronic persistent asthma earlier that year and prescribed an asthma preventer puffer of low-dose inhaled fluticasone propionate, 50 micrograms pMDI via spacer, one puff taken twice daily. The paramedics note that the boy has moderate work of breathing, tight wheeze on stethoscope auscultation of the chest, and tachycardia. He can speak in

sentences. He is given six puffs of salbutamol 100 micrograms via spacer over 5 minutes, with some improvement in his symptoms. This dose is repeated during transit to the local hospital.

1. Why was Josh originally prescribed low dose fluticasone propionate and administered salbutamol by the paramedics?
2. What classes of drugs are these and what are their mechanisms of action?
3. Explain the roles of the pMDI and spacer.

Source: Acknowledgment to Dr Philippa Shilson, paediatrician.

Introduction: The respiratory system, respiratory disease and its treatment

This chapter reviews the anatomy and physiology of the respiratory system as a basis for a discussion of pathophysiology and the pharmacological treatment of respiratory conditions. An understanding of basic respiratory anatomy and physiology is important for a deeper understanding of the treatment of respiratory conditions. The respiratory system includes all structures involved in the movement and exchange of oxygen and carbon dioxide: the nose and nasal cavities, airway passages, lungs, pharynx, larynx, trachea, bronchi, bronchioles, pulmonary lobules with their alveoli, the diaphragm and all muscles concerned with respiration itself (Figs 15.1 and 15.2). Oxygen is supplied to the body through the process of **respiration**, a term loosely used to describe three distinct but interrelated processes: pulmonary ventilation (inspiration and expiration), gas transport and cellular respiration.

The respiratory system also participates in warming, filtering and moistening inspired air and in the senses of smell and taste, producing sounds (speech) and assisting in the control of pH, in removal of foreign bodies and mucus, in immune system defence mechanisms, in

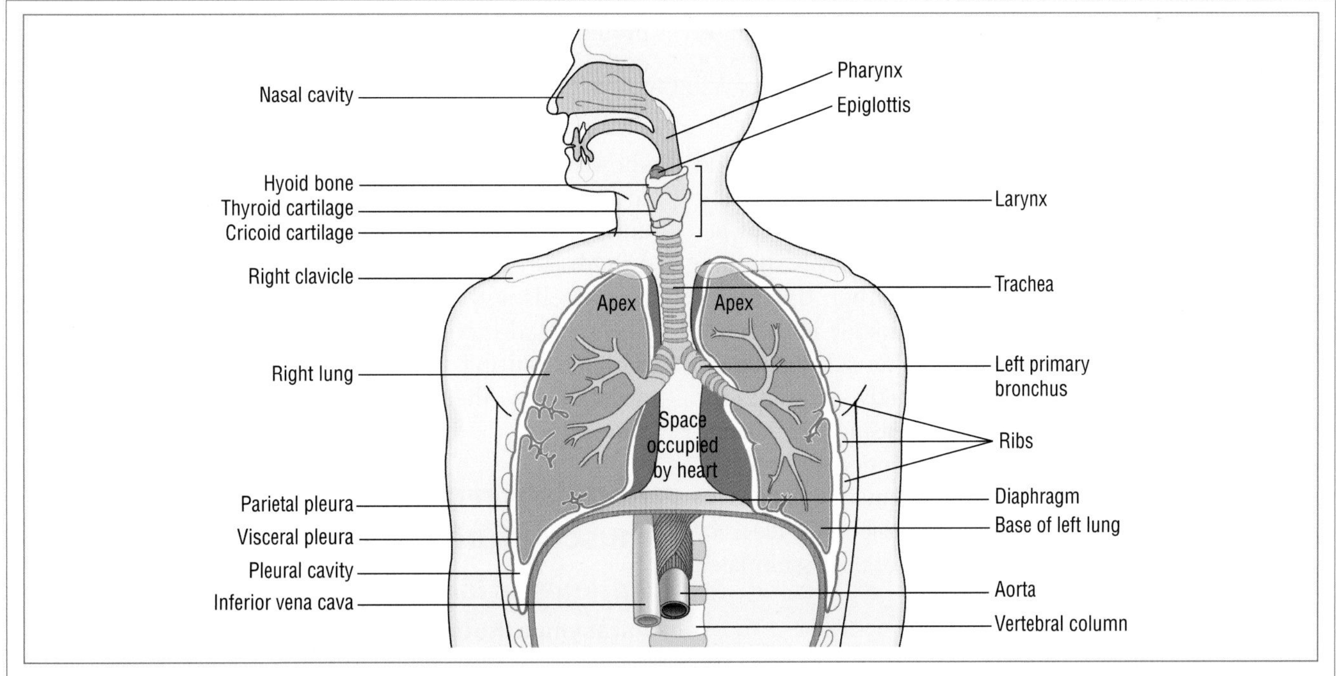

FIGURE 15.1 Structures associated with the respiratory system

Source: ©2022 Medtronic. All rights reserved. Used with the permission of Medtronic

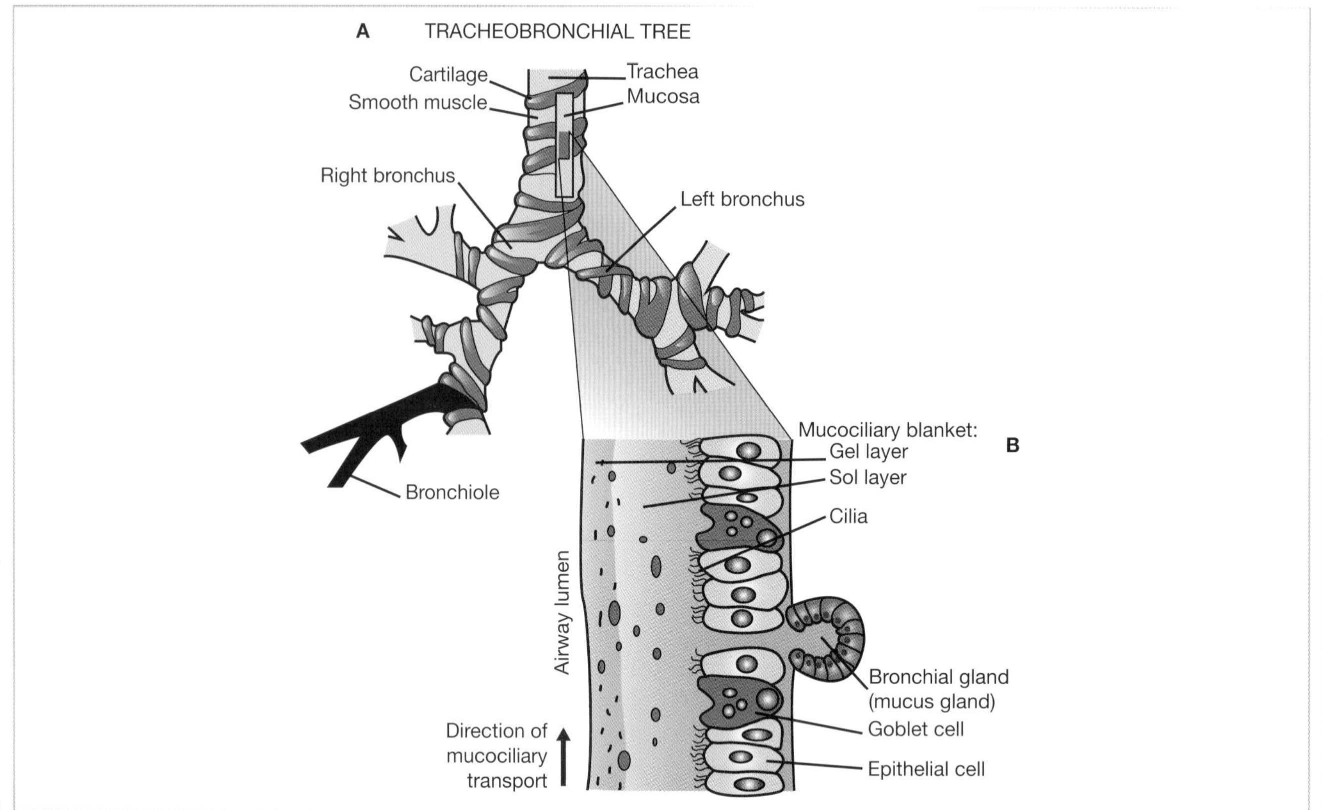

FIGURE 15.2 Tracheobronchial tree and bronchial smooth muscle
A Diagram of tracheobronchial tree. **B** Longitudinal section of the inner lining of an airway, magnified approximately ×200.
Source: Salerno 1999; used with permission.

inactivation of many biogenic amines and autacoids, and in temperature regulation.

Control of respiration

Respiration is normally under involuntary central and autonomic control. The basic rhythm for respiration is maintained via the medulla oblongata at 12–18 breaths per minute in adults. Regulation is achieved primarily through changes in concentrations of oxygen, carbon dioxide or hydrogen ions in body fluids; carbon dioxide is the chief respiratory stimulant. An increase in the carbon dioxide tension of the blood (**hypercapnia**) directly stimulates the inspiratory and expiratory centres, increasing the rate and depth of breathing. If arterial oxygen concentration falls below about 60% of normal (hypoxaemia), such as in chronic obstructive pulmonary disease (COPD) or exposure to high altitude, chemoreceptors are stimulated to increase alveolar ventilation.

Control of pH

Respiration regulates the pH of blood by controlling the carbon dioxide tension; bicarbonate ions (HCO_3^-) and proteins in the blood function as buffer systems, according to the equation

$$CO_2 + H_2O \rightleftharpoons H_2CO_3 \rightleftharpoons HCO_3^- + H^+$$

showing the combination of carbon dioxide with water to form carbonic acid, which dissociates to bicarbonate and hydrogen ions. This reaction is catalysed by **carbonic anhydrase** enzymes, widely distributed especially in red blood cells and epithelia. High carbon dioxide content of the blood increases formation of carbonic acid in the blood, resulting in respiratory acidosis. Conversely, a decrease in the carbon dioxide content results in alkalosis.

Regulation of the glands and musculature of the respiratory tract

Autonomic innervation

Parasympathetic

The predominant innervation of human airways is by the cholinergic nerves which, via the vagus nerve, synapse in ganglia located in the wall of the bronchi. Parasympathetic postganglionic nerve stimulation leads to activation of M_3 muscarinic receptors on the smooth muscle and also the glandular tissue, leading to contraction, and thus bronchoconstriction, and secretion, respectively (Ch 8).

Sympathetic

There are no sympathetic nerves innervating the airways; however, there is a preponderance of B_2 receptors, activation of which by circulating catecholamines, predominantly adrenaline (epinephrine), leads to bronchial smooth muscle relaxation (Ch 9).

Respiratory tract secretions

Mucus

Mucus secreted by the goblet cells and bronchial glands located in the submucosa of the tracheobronchial tree moistens and lubricates the branching tubular airways, as shown in Figure 15.2B. As above, the mucus glands are under vagal (parasympathetic) control; mucus secreted into the lumen of the airways is an extracellular gel containing water and mucins, heavily glycosylated proteins. It is moved up the tracheobronchial tree towards the larynx by **mucociliary transport** (or mucokinesis). Excessive mucus or impaired clearance contributes to the pathophysiology of all the common airway diseases.

Pulmonary surfactant

Pulmonary **surfactant** (i.e. *surf*ace-*act*ive *a*ge*nt*) is a phosphatidylcholine–apoprotein lipoprotein mixture secreted from alveolar epithelial type II cells and present in the secretions in the alveoli. Surfactant reduces surface tension in the lung, stabilises the alveoli and improves lung mechanics. Synthesis and secretion of surfactant is low in the fetus until immediately before birth, when a surge in maternal glucocorticoids triggers surfactant release. Natural or synthetic surfactant is administered to premature babies with respiratory distress syndrome (see later).

KEY POINTS

The respiratory system

- The respiratory system comprises structures involved in the movement of gases from the nose via conducting airways (trachea, bronchi, bronchioles) to the respiratory bronchioles and alveoli in the lungs.
- The primary function of the lungs is gas transport and exchange between air and blood in pulmonary capillaries. The processes involved are pulmonary ventilation, gas transport across membranes and cellular respiration.
- Other functions are regulation of blood pH, immunological defence, participation in speech, taste and smell and metabolic functions.
- The main buffering capacity of the blood is provided by the bicarbonate–carbonic acid–carbon dioxide equilibrium, catalysed by carbonic anhydrase enzymes.
- Bronchial smooth muscle is innervated by the parasympathetic nervous system. The parasympathetic nervous system mediates bronchoconstriction via activation of M_3 muscarinic receptors leading to smooth muscle contraction.
- Although there is no functional evidence for direct sympathetic innervation of airway smooth muscle, β_2-adrenoceptors are activated by circulating adrenaline. Relaxation of smooth muscle ensues, leading to bronchodilation.
- Respiratory tract secretions, produced by goblet cells and bronchial glands (M_3 receptors), form a protective mucociliary blanket and epithelial type II cells in the alveoli provide surfactant functions.

Considerations for drug delivery to the airways: drugs by inhalation

Aerosols

An **aerosol** is a suspension of fine liquid or solid particles dispersed in a gas or in solution. Aerosol drugs are most commonly inhaled, and can also be administered to the skin (as topical sprays) or to body cavities (ear, nose). After inhalation, some particles are deposited in the respiratory tract; the remainder tends to be swallowed, depending on droplet size. Inhalation may be via steam, from a nasal spray or with devices such as metered-dose inhalers (MDI – Fig 15.3A), spacers (Fig 15.3B), dry powder inhalers (DPI – Fig 15.3C, D), face masks and nebulisers (Fig 15.3F). Liquid or solid particles range in size from about 0.005 to 50 micrometres in diameter.

Aerosol therapy has many advantages:

- Drug administration is convenient.
- There is minimal irritation, contamination or systemic adverse effects.
- Lower doses can be given than by systemic administration.
- The drug is delivered rapidly to the desired site of action.

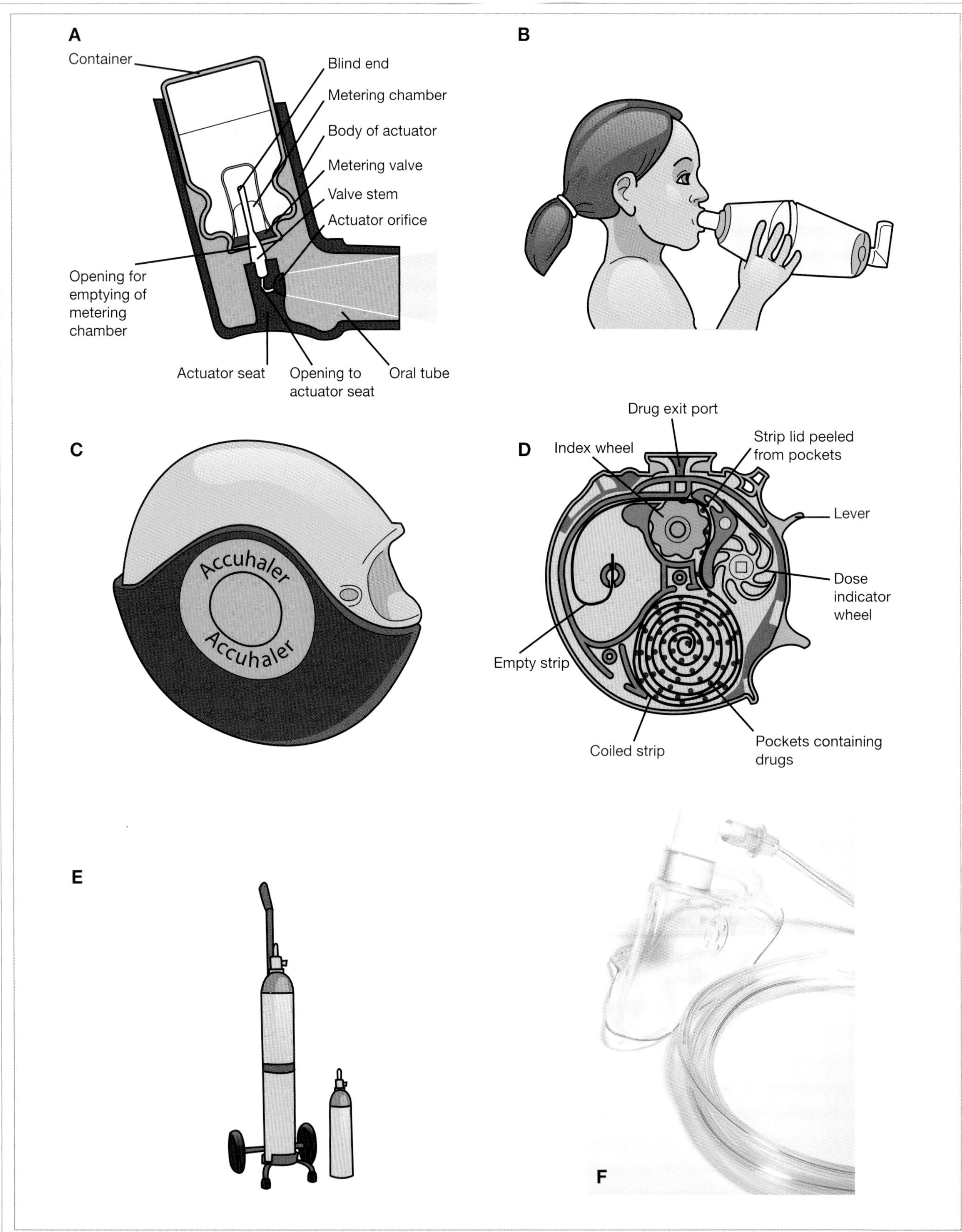

FIGURE 15.3 Devices for drug administration by inhalation

A Pressurised metered-dose inhaler (pMDI, or 'puffer') shown in cross-section. **B** pMDI in combination with a large-volume spacer. **C** Accuhaler™. **D** Accuhaler; cross-section. **E** Gas cylinder on trolley. **F** Adult nebuliser bowl, tubing and mask.

Sources: ***A**, **C** and **D**: courtesy GlaxoSmithKline, Australia; used with permission; **E**: Dreamstime/Podius; **F**: istock/Hulldude30*

- Inhaled aerosols can promote bronchodilation, pulmonary decongestion, loosening of secretions, topical application of corticosteroids and other drugs and moistening of inspired air.

A disadvantage of aerosol therapy is that if the person has poor control of inhalers, there is poor asthma control. Most inhalers are used incorrectly, and it is important that health professionals assist the client with correct usage of the devices (see 'Online resources' – inhaler techniques).

Pressurised metered-dose inhalers

Pressurised metered-dose inhalers (pMDIs), invented more than 50 years ago, are small hand-held 'puffers' containing multiple doses of the active drug, mixed with a dispersing agent and a propellant, in a canister (Fig 15.3A). The canister is shaken and then the top is depressed (while inhaling) to deliver an accurate dose of the aerosol along with the inert propellant gas, usually a hydrofluoroalkane. (Previously, chlorofluorocarbons were used; while biologically inert, these were infamous for their deleterious effects on the Earth's ozone layer.)

Effective use of pMDIs requires good hand–breath coordination, which may be difficult for young children; breath-activated MDIs, spacers (Fig 15.3B) and face masks help improve drug administration (Clinical Focus Box 15.1). Breath activated MDIs release a mist of medicine when inhalation occurs.

Dry powder inhalers

DPIs are similar to breath-activated MDIs, except that the drug is delivered as finely divided particles rather than in aerosol solution. Examples are the 'Accuhaler', a compact device with a foil strip inside containing doses of finely powdered drug (Fig 15.3C, D). Seretide Accuhaler™ (fluticasone with salmeterol) 100/50 recommends use in children from the age of 4 years.

The 'Turbuhaler', in which the drug is loaded as a capsule that is broken open when the base is rotated, releases the active drug. They should not be prescribed for use by children younger than 8 years, although Symbicort (budesonide and formoterol) turbuhalers are recommended for use in children older than age 6. Mouthpieces of inhalers may need regular cleaning; manufacturers' instructions for specific devices should be followed.

Nebulisers

Nebulisers ('pumps'; Fig 15.3F) use compressed air or oxygen, or ultrasonic energy, to produce a fine mist of drug in aerosol form from a solution. They are useful for delivering large doses inhaled by mouth over long periods, especially in severe asthma attacks. The aerosol drug or solution may irritate facial skin and may contribute to the spread of bacteria. They may also be costly to purchase.

CLINICAL FOCUS BOX 15.1
Puffers and spacers

Correct use of inhaler devices maximises drug delivery to the airways, so users need to be shown and reminded of the best way to use inhalers, how to know when they are nearly empty and how to clean them. With pMDI **puffers**, the technique is as follows:

1. Take the cap off the puffer's mouthpiece.
2. Hold the puffer upright and shake it well.
3. Breathe out slowly and gently without emptying the lungs.
4. Put the mouthpiece between the teeth and close the lips around it without biting.
5. Tilt the head back slightly and, while breathing in slowly, press down on the top of the aerosol canister and continue to breathe in deeply.
6. Take the puffer away from the mouth and hold the breath for as long as possible, then breathe out gently.
7. Click the cap back onto the puffer.
8. If the inhaler contained a corticosteroid drug, rinse the mouth with water and spit out.

The technique for handling different styles of inhalers varies, but the inhaling drug–breath holding–exhaling method is similar. Cleaning techniques for devices should be checked from information supplied with the inhaler. The simplest way to determine when a puffer is running out of drug is to count and keep a record of the number of times it has been used.

Children and people with poor hand–breath coordination sometimes find it easier to use a puffer with a **spacer** (Fig 15.3B), which reduces the amount of drug deposited in the mouth and throat. With children under 5 years of age, a small-volume spacer or nebuliser and face mask may be useful. Spacers should be washed monthly (with dishwashing detergent) and allowed to air-dry.

Droplet size

Effectiveness of aerosol therapy depends on the number and size of droplets that can be suspended in an inhaled aerosol. Large droplets (>40 micrometres in diameter) will be deposited primarily in the upper airway (mouth, pharynx, trachea and main bronchi), useful for keeping large airways (nose and trachea) moist and for loosening secretions. Medium-sized droplets (8–15 micrometres in diameter) will be deposited primarily in the bronchioles and bronchi. Smaller droplets (2–4 micrometres in diameter) are more likely to reach alveolar ducts and sacs. Droplets smaller than about 0.6 micrometres are unlikely to be deposited, and will be exhaled.

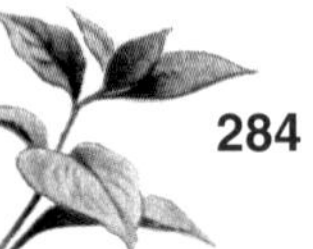

Inhaled drugs

Drugs administered by inhalation are generally intended for local effects only. However, the lung is an absorptive organ (think: oxygen), so it is a route for drugs to enter the systemic circulation. As an example, inhaled bronchodilator β_2-agonist aerosols do produce systemic effects after absorption: the drug stimulates β_3-and β_1-adrenoceptors, causing tremor and tachycardia, respectively. Absorption of drugs is generally rapid because of the highly vascular pulmonary capillary system, and depends on the lipid solubility of the inhaled drug, the aerosol particle size and pulmonary function. (For inhaled general anaesthetic gases, refer to Ch 18, Table 18.2.)

Potential problems from aerosol administration include oral fungal infections after corticosteroid inhalation, or ocular effects if the aerosol mist reaches the eyes (e.g. in the case of ipratropium administration). A considerable proportion of an inhaled drug dose is swallowed, so it may produce systemic effects or be digested or metabolised rapidly.

When two or more inhalers are prescribed together, such as when a corticosteroid or mast-cell stabiliser puffer is prescribed along with a bronchodilator puffer, it is important that the *bronchodilator* is administered 5 minutes *before* the other drug to promote bronchodilation and maximise inhalation of the second aerosol.

KEY POINTS

Drug delivery to airways

- An aerosol is a suspension of fine particles, liquid or solid dispersed in gas to body cavities.
- Aerosol therapy is convenient and rapid, provides minimal systemic effects, allows for lower doses of drugs, promotes bronchodilation and decongestion and enables topical administration of drugs such as corticosteroids to airways.
- Devices for drug administration by inhalation include nasal sprays, pMDIs, DPIs and nebulisers.
- Effectiveness of inhaled drugs depends on the number and size of droplets.
- Systemic effects can occur with inhaled drugs.
- Users need to be taught proper techniques for use and cleaning of a pMDI or other inhalation devices. Spacer units are often suggested, especially for young children. Home use of peak-flow meters is recommended for early detection of airflow obstruction.

Medical gases

Medical gases are supplied in a range of container sizes, from small portable aluminium cylinders (about 170 L capacity) to steel cylinders of compressed gases (capacity of several thousand litres), through to systems of tanks (capacity > 115,000 L) and plumbed-in gas lines servicing hospitals and research institutions. The colour coding adopted in Australia for medical gases is shown in Table 15.1. Equipment used to handle and administer gases includes regulators and flow meters, carry bags, trolleys, oxygen concentrators and conserving devices, pressure gauges, masks, cylinder backpacks, suction units, cannulae, tubing and connectors (Fig 15.3 E, F) (BOC Limited 2011).

Oxygen

Oxygen is colourless, odourless and tasteless. Inspired air normally contains 20.9% oxygen, which at atmospheric pressure of 760 mmHg exerts a partial pressure (PO_2) of 159 mmHg. Haemoglobin in the pulmonary vein is normally 97% saturated with oxygen, and the partial

TABLE 15.1 Examples of medical gases

GAS	COLOURS	USES
Air, compressed	White cylinder, black and white shoulder	Breathing apparatus; carrier gas for anaesthesia; driving surgical air tools
Carbogen (usually 5% CO_2 in oxygen)	White cylinder, green-grey and white shoulder	Respiratory stimulant; oxygenation of isolated tissues in physiological and pharmacological research
Carbon dioxide	White cylinder, grey-green shoulder	Respiratory stimulant; in anaesthesia; in cryosurgery; to facilitate vasodilation
Helium	White cylinder, brown shoulder	Vehicle gas; gaining access to obstructed airways; in magnetic resonance imaging machines; in balloons
Nitrous oxide	White cylinder, ultramarine blue shoulder	Analgesia and anaesthesia (with oxygen); vehicle gas in anaesthesia; in cryosurgery
Heliox (oxygen with helium)	White cylinder, brown and white shoulder	Severe COPD, bronchiolitis, bronchiectasis, decompression sickness
Entonox (50% oxygen, 50% nitrous oxide)	White cylinder, ultramarine blue and white shoulder quadrants	Self-administered anaesthetic in obstetrics, first aid, dentistry, doctors' surgeries, ambulances, etc.
Oxygen, compressed	White cylinder, white shoulder	Respiratory therapy; carrier gas in anaesthesia; resuscitation; high-altitude and underwater breathing; hyperbaric chambers

Note: The New Zealand manufacturer refers to green/grey as 'French grey', and to ultramarine blue as 'royal blue'.

Source: BOC Limited 2011.

pressure of oxygen in arterial blood (PaO_2) is normally greater than 80 mmHg.

If oxygen is not continuously supplied to cells, they suffer **hypoxia** (inadequate cellular oxygen). The brain is most susceptible: an acute reduction of PaO_2 level to 50 mmHg decreases mental functioning, emotional stability and fine muscular coordination; further reduction impairs judgement and muscular coordination, decreases pain perception and eventually causes unconsciousness and irreversible damage. When circulation is impaired, blood flow to the brain, kidneys and heart tends to be preserved at the expense of other less vital organs.

Indications for oxygen therapy

While essential for life, oxygen is also potentially toxic (see 'Adverse Effects of Oxygen', below). Oxygen is used chiefly to treat hypoxia and **hypoxaemia** (oxygen deficiency in arterial blood). The most common form of hypoxia necessitating oxygen treatment is hypoxic hypoxia, produced in airway obstruction (asthma, COPD), hypoventilation or at high altitude. Oxygen should be administered in appropriate dosage regimens (% concentration, flow rate and duration) with monitoring of blood gas concentrations. It is also used as a carrier gas in general anaesthetic techniques.

Oxygen is further used in the treatment of severe influenza, cyanosis, chest wounds, shock, severe haemorrhage, cardiac or respiratory arrest, collapsed or punctured lung, coronary artery occlusion (heart attack, angina) and in neonatal resuscitation. It is frequently administered by paramedics in prehospital situations.

Oxygenation of the blood can be measured using pulse oximeters; British Thoracic Society guidelines recommend aiming for normal to near-normal oxygen saturation (94–98%) for all acutely ill people except for those at risk of hypercapnic respiratory failure (88–92%).

The effectiveness of oxygen administration depends on the carbon dioxide content of blood, as a high CO_2 level is the main stimulant to respiration. such as in pulmonary embolism or oedema, myocardial infarction or status asthmaticus (acute severe asthma). People with COPD, however, are subject to hypercapnia (high $PaCO_2$) with low PaO_2. Their medullary centres are relatively insensitive to stimulation by carbon dioxide; rather, low PaO_2 stimulates respiration. Oxygen concentration (25%) and flow rates (1–2 L/min) are therefore kept low for these people; however, the guiding principle is that hypoxaemia is more dangerous than hypercapnia, so adequate oxygen levels must always be maintained.

Administration

Oxygen is administered by inhalation via catheters, nasal cannulae (prongs) or masks. Regulators and fittings on gas cylinders are non-interchangeable, to minimise risk of inadvertent administration of the wrong gas (Table 15.1, above). The gas is under pressure and potentially explosive, so tanks must be handled carefully. Most of the oxygen administered in hospitals is provided from a central source, where it is stored as a gas or liquid oxygen. Oxygen cylinders may also be carried in a backpack or supplied to homes (domiciliary oxygen therapy) of people with severe persistent hypoxaemia – for example, due to chronic bronchitis, emphysema, pulmonary hypertension or cancer affecting the lungs. Oxygen-rich air may be provided from an oxygen concentrator, a small mobile floor-standing electrically powered machine that removes nitrogen from room air.

Hyperbaric oxygen

Hyperbaric oxygen is used in circulatory disturbances such as air or gas embolism, decompression sickness, wounds and infections (e.g. with *Clostridium welchii* [gas gangrene]), carbon monoxide or cyanide poisoning, acute traumatic ischaemia, crush injury and compartment syndrome, and in compromised (ischaemic) skin grafts and flaps, and radiation necrosis.

Adverse effects of oxygen

While oxygen is essential for life, it has also been described as a toxic mutagenic gas; aerobic organisms including humans survive because they have evolved antioxidant defences against oxygen. Exposure to 80–100% oxygen for a prolonged period can cause an inflammatory response and destruction of the alveoli–capillary membrane of the respiratory tract. Toxicity symptoms are substernal distress (ache or burning sensation behind the sternum), respiratory distress with decreased vital capacity, nausea, vomiting, restlessness, tremors, twitching, paraesthesias, convulsions and a dry, hacking cough. Excessive oxygen supplied to preterm infants to treat respiratory distress syndrome can cause blindness (Clinical Focus Box 15.2).

Oxygen free radicals

Free radicals are chemical species containing one or more unpaired electrons that readily participate in oxidation–reduction reactions. **Oxygen free radicals** (reactive oxygen species, ROS) include the superoxide radical ($O_2^{\bullet -}$) and hydroxyl radical ($^{\bullet}OH$), formed in many biochemical reactions in the body by peroxidases, xanthine oxidase and nitric oxide synthase, and in the electron transport chain.

Oxygen free radicals are implicated in many pathological processes – for example, post-ischaemic reperfusion injury, processes of ageing and carcinogenesis, radiation-induced damage, atherosclerosis, inflammatory bowel disease and some types of adverse drug reactions. It causes oxidative stress when there is imbalance between ROS and levels of antioxidant defences, leading either to

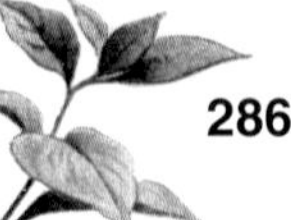

CLINICAL FOCUS BOX 15.2
Oxygen administration in premature infants

Health professionals caring for premature infants must be aware of the danger of retinopathy of prematurity (ROP; retrolental fibroplasia). This is a vascular proliferative disorder of the retina that occurs in some premature infants and is the leading cause of childhood blindness worldwide. Infants are administered high concentrations of oxygen after birth to treat respiratory distress of the newborn. The use of supplemental oxygen, oxygen concentration, duration and prolonged mechanical ventilation were among the most frequently identified risk factors for severe and treatment-requiring ROP. Oxygen constricts the developing retinal vessels in the eye, suppressing normal vascularisation. On return to normal oxygen levels, the tissue becomes relatively hypoxic, blood vessels proliferate, endothelial cells become disorganised and there can be destruction of the immature retina, resulting in blindness.

Historically, in 1951 Dr Kate Campbell, a Melbourne paediatrician, was the first person to demonstrate the link between oxygen levels in humidicribs and ROP. She showed that incidence was highest in premature babies nursed in neonatal units equipped with 'oxygen-cots' that could provide high levels of oxygen, thus associating the blindness with oxygen toxicity. Other purported causes are maternal factors such as hypertensive disorders of pregnancy, age, smoking and maternal medication use such as β-blockers and antihistamines later in pregnancy. Caffeine use associated with apnoea of prematurity has been associated with decreased incidence of ROP.

Careful monitoring of arterial blood gases is essential, and the oxygen concentration of inspired air should be kept between 30% and 40%. Oxygen saturation should be targeted within the range of 91–95% in preterm neonates. Some incubators are equipped with a safety valve that automatically releases any excess oxygen outside the chamber. More recent advances in treatment include cryotherapy, laser photocoagulation and surgical vitrectomies (Kim et al. 2018).

adaptation or to cell injury and cell death. To protect against ROS toxicity, mitochondria in bacteria and humans have evolved defence mechanisms, including the enzymes superoxide dismutase and catalase.

A diet high in antioxidants may protect against disorders of old age; the antioxidant vitamins E (tocopherols) and C (ascorbic acid) and α-lipoic acid are protective, and a diet rich in fruit, vegetables, nuts, beans and lentils is encouraged.

Carbon dioxide

Carbon dioxide is a colourless, odourless gas that is heavier than air; normal air contains only 0.04% CO_2. Inhalation of 3–5% CO_2 for a short period increases both rate and depth of respiration unless the respiratory centre is depressed by drugs or disease.

Excess carbon dioxide in inhaled air (> 7%) may cause acidosis and unresponsiveness of the respiratory centre to carbon dioxide; impaired nerve conduction and transmission; depression of activity of the cerebral cortex, myocardium and smooth muscle of peripheral blood vessels; and, at high doses, carbon dioxide narcosis (sleepiness and confusion, and anaesthetic and convulsant effects).

Indications

Indications for clinical use of carbon dioxide are:

- carbon monoxide poisoning – 5–7% CO_2 in oxygen is sometimes used to increase the rate of separation of carbon monoxide from carboxyhaemoglobin
- respiratory depression – when carbon dioxide is used as a respiratory stimulant, close monitoring by pulse oximetry and PaO_2 is important
- general anaesthesia and postoperative uses – mixtures of oxygen and carbon dioxide may be used during anaesthesia; carbon dioxide initially hastens anaesthesia by increasing pulmonary ventilation and reducing struggling; in the recovery period, it hastens elimination of inhaled anaesthetics
- facilitation of vasodilation and increased cerebral blood flow, to promote venous return to the heart and therefore to improve the rate and force of myocardial contraction
- for insufflation into body cavities in gynaecological investigations and keyhole surgery.

Other uses

- Solid carbon dioxide ('dry ice', at –78°C) destroys tissues; in cryotherapy, it is applied directly to warts and other skin lesions.
- Carbon dioxide has been used to treat intractable hiccups.
- Carbon dioxide in solution (as carbonated 'fizzy' drinks) stimulates absorption of liquids by mucous membranes and rapidly relieves thirst (and hastens absorption of alcohol).
- A mixture of carbon dioxide (usually 5%) in oxygen, known as Carbogen, is used in many pharmacological and physiological experiments to oxygenate isolated tissues (Table 15.1, above).

Administration and toxicity

A 5–10% concentration of carbon dioxide in oxygen delivered through a tight-fitting face mask is inhaled by the person until depth of respiration is increased in conditions where there is absent or reduced breathing. A simpler way of administering carbon dioxide is to allow the person to hyperventilate with a paper bag held over the face; re-inhaling expired air causes the CO_2 content to be continually increased. Administration should be stopped as soon as the desired effects have been obtained.

Signs of carbon dioxide over-dosage are dyspnoea, breath-holding, markedly increased chest and abdominal movements, nausea and raised systolic blood pressure. Prolonged administration of 5% CO_2 may produce severe central nervous system (CNS) depression; a 10% concentration can lead to loss of consciousness within 10 minutes.

Other gases

Other gases used medically include nitrous oxide (as an analgesic/anaesthetic, see Ch 18), nitric oxide (as a vasodilator) and helium (to assist oxygen flow) – see Table 15.1. Entonox, a mixture of 50% nitrous oxide and 50% oxygen, is used for acute, short-term pain relief. Heliox, a mixture of 79% helium and 21% oxygen, is used in obstructive airways disease.

Nitric oxide

A use for the gas nitric oxide (NO) is to improve tissue oxygenation in neonates suffering hypoxic respiratory failure resulting from meconium aspiration or pulmonary hypertension. Nitric oxide is a mediator generated locally in tissues, with many physiological actions including vasodilation. When administered as a gas (provided at 800 ppm in nitrogen), NO dilates blood vessels in the lungs, enhances oxygenation and helps overcome hypoxia. While administration of NO over a period of 4 days reduces the need for extracorporeal membrane oxygenation in babies, there are many adverse effects (including formation of methaemoglobin, hypotension and haematuria), and overall survival of very premature babies is not markedly increased. It is only approved for use in neonates of over 34 weeks' gestation, but is also used in adults in intensive care units.

KEY POINTS

Medical gases

- Oxygen, as a therapeutic gas, is used in many clinical situations to treat hypoxia. Oxygen toxicity is a potential problem.
- Carbon dioxide in low concentrations is used as a respiratory stimulant.
- Other medical gases include nitrous oxide, helium and nitric oxide.

Respiratory stimulants and depressants

Respiratory stimulants: analeptics

Direct respiratory stimulants are referred to as **analeptics** and are a subgroup of CNS stimulants (Ch 23). They act directly on respiratory and vasomotor centres in the medulla to increase respiratory rate and tidal exchange, and also raise blood pressure. In large doses, they may cause convulsions, CNS depression and respiratory paralysis. The only drug routinely used as a respiratory stimulant is caffeine (Drug Monograph 23.2), indicated in respiratory distress and apnoea in preterm infants.

Reflex respiratory stimulants

Reflex stimulation of the medullary centre occurs through peripheral irritation of sensory nerve receptors in the pharynx, oesophagus and stomach. The rate and depth of respiration (and blood pressure) are then increased. Aromatic ammonia spirit (commonly called sal volatile) and the natural compounds camphor, menthol and thujone (a constituent of absinthe) have been given by inhalation for their actions as reflex respiratory stimulants.[1]

Respiratory depressants

Respiratory depression is seldom desirable but is sometimes unavoidable. The most important drugs causing respiratory depression as an adverse reaction are the opioid analgesics. They depress the sensitivity of the respiratory centre to carbon dioxide, thereby making breathing slower and more shallow. Pholcodine is used as an antitussive (cough suppressant) for painful or harmful cough (Drug Monograph 15.5, later); however, codeine, dihydrocodeine and dextromethorphan are used as alternatives to pholcodine. Many other CNS-depressant drugs, including benzodiazepines, barbiturates, antihistamines and alcohol, also cause respiratory depression.

Drugs affecting secretions and mucociliary transport

Pulmonary surfactant use in respiratory distress syndrome

Infants born preterm at less than 32 weeks' gestation are at risk of respiratory distress syndrome due to immature mechanisms for producing surfactant, and are likely to suffer rapid shallow breathing, hypoxaemia and acidosis unless treated with synthetic surfactant. Surfactant can be purified from animal lung sources or

1 In cases of fainting, they were administered by inhaling the vapours as 'smelling salts'.

produced by genetic engineering techniques in bacterial cell cultures. Two forms used in Australia are beractant (a modified bovine product) and poractant alfa (derived from pigs' lungs). They are supplied as solutions for intratracheal administration, normally used only in neonatal intensive care units for premature infants suffering or at risk of respiratory distress syndrome. Surfactant reduces dependence on a ventilator, reduces risk of pneumothorax, increases oxygenation and has improved survival rates of premature babies from 30% in the 1970s to 90% today. Concomitant nasal positive airways pressure enhances survival. If premature birth is anticipated, glucocorticoids given prophylactically to the mother can enhance fetal lung maturation and synthesis of surfactant.

Mucoactive agents

Mucoactive agents are drugs that aid in the clearance of mucus from the upper and lower airways and include expectorants, diluents, mucolytics and mucoregulators.

Expectorants

Sputum (phlegm) is an abnormal viscous secretion of the lower respiratory tree, consisting mainly of mucus, a mucopolysaccharide–glycoprotein material; the characteristic thickness and yellow colour are due to leucocytes, bacteria and DNA derived from the breakdown of mucosal cells. **Expectorants** are drugs that aid in the removal (swallowing or spitting out) of sputum from the bronchial passages.

In respiratory disorders such as chronic bronchitis the mucus clearance process is impaired, causing mucus plugging of airways and alveoli (Fig 15.4) and pathogenic colonisation by microorganisms, leading to overproduction of thick, tenacious sputum. Expectorants, diluents and mucolytic drugs alter the consistency of the sputum, either by diluting thickened secretions (diluents, irritants) or by chemically breaking down mucus (mucolytics), enhancing eventual expectoration, or spitting out, of these secretions.

Irritant expectorants

The action of irritant expectorants on the mucous membranes increases secretion of mucus from bronchial secretory cells, facilitates ciliary action and productive coughing and lubricates dry tissues. Irritant expectorants include the natural compounds *Hedera helix*, ipecacuanha, squill, guaifenesin, iodides, senega, ammonia and volatile oils (lemon, eucalyptus, menthol and ti-tree). While these contribute much to the colour, flavour, smell and placebo effect of many old-fashioned over-the-counter cough mixtures (see later section), there is little objective evidence of any pharmacological efficacy. In higher doses, these compounds also have direct and irritant emetic actions.

Diluents

Water and saline solutions

Water is most commonly used to dilute respiratory secretions, administered by ultrasonic nebuliser or, more traditionally, by inhaling steam over a basin of boiling water. Water deposited on the gel layer of the respiratory tree reduces the adhesive characteristics and general viscosity of the gelatinous substances. (For those receiving restricted fluid intake, water absorbed through the inhalation route must be added to the intake record.) Normal saline (0.9% sodium chloride) administered by nebulisation is well tolerated, resulting in hydration of respiratory secretions. Inhalation of hypotonic solution (e.g. 0.45% sodium chloride) may provide deeper penetration into the more distal airways, whereas inhalation of hypertonic solution, 1.8% sodium chloride, stimulates a productive cough.

Mucolytic drugs

Mucolytics help disintegrate mucus by breaking down the structure of mucus, facilitating removal of mucus or other exudates from the lung, bronchi or trachea by postural drainage, coughing, spitting or swallowing.

Mucolytics in cystic fibrosis

The disease cystic fibrosis (CF), an inherited autosomal-recessive condition, involves abnormally thick mucus secretions in many organs (including lungs, sweat glands, pancreas and liver) due to abnormal chloride transport, sodium hyperabsorption, deregulation of calcium homeostasis and an enhanced inflammatory response (Masel 2012; Villanueva et al. 2017). Life expectancy used to be very short, but is now more than 35 years.

Most people suffer from severe respiratory infections due to impaired mucociliary transport. Standard treatment involves use of antibiotics for bacterial infections, enzymes and mucolytics to reduce mucus viscosity (dornase alfa, mannitol [see later] or saline), chest physiotherapy and exercise to clear mucopurulent secretions, bronchodilators, oxygen, anti-inflammatory agents and nutritional support. Nebulised antibiotics are administered for control of *Pseudomonas aeruginosa* infections.

Dornase alfa

Dornase alfa is a prescribed respiratory inhalant product with proven mucolytic efficacy, administered to increase expectoration in CF. It is recombinant human deoxyribonuclease, a DNA-degrading enzyme that digests extracellular DNA released from degenerating neutrophils and cellular debris in purulent sputum, thus improving pulmonary function and reducing the risk of respiratory tract infections. Its use has decreased hospitalisations and medical costs, but it is expensive.

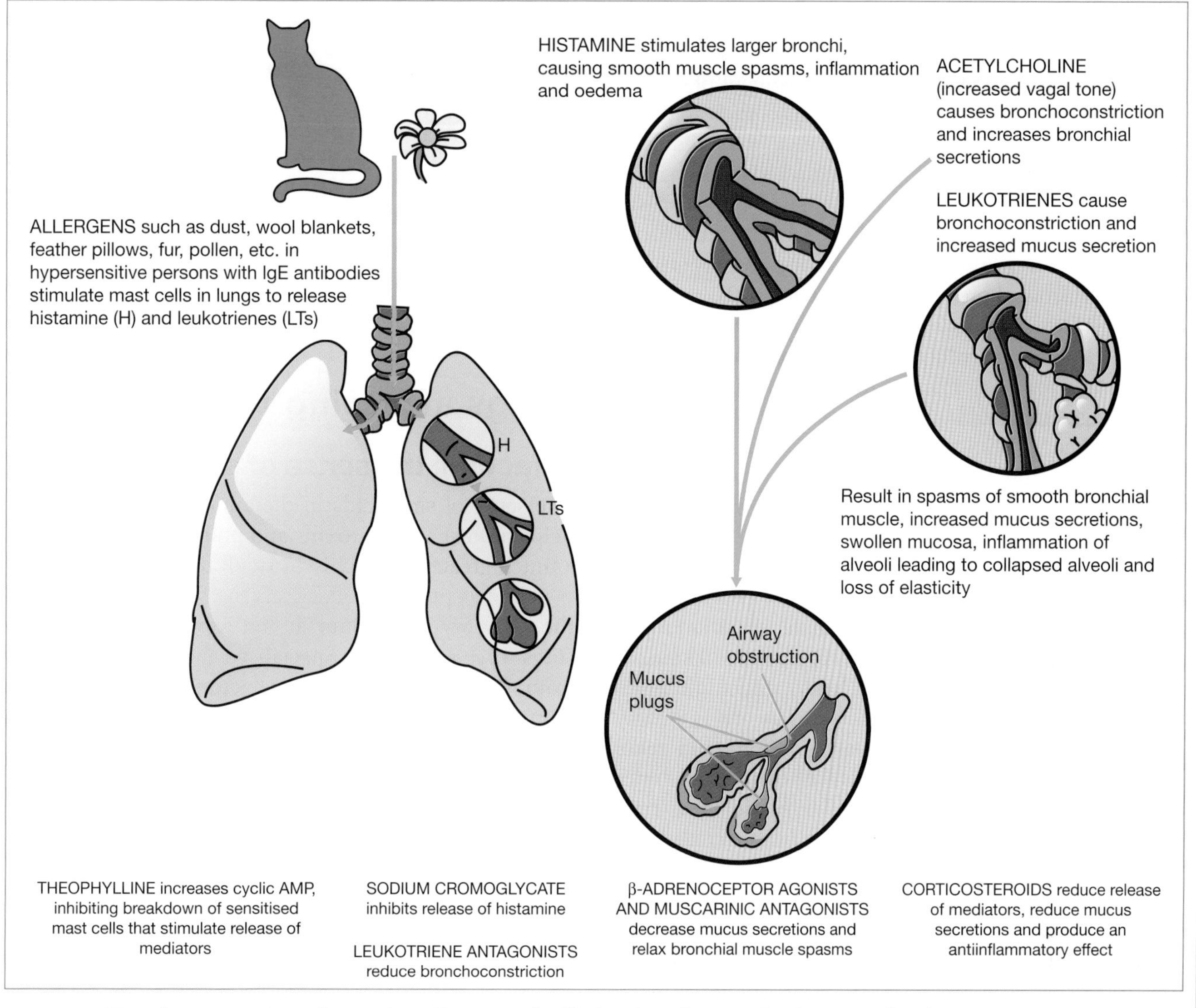

FIGURE 15.4 The airways and mediators in asthma, and effects of various antiasthma medications H = histamine; LTs = leukotrienes.

Source: Adapted from Rang et al. 2003; used with permission.

The solution is inhaled via a nebuliser – usually one 2.5 mg ampoule/day regularly for 6–12 months. Inhaled enzyme acts locally in the respiratory tract and is not absorbed. Significant improvement in pulmonary function may be seen within 3–7 days and a decrease in respiratory infections within weeks. Multi-action antibiotics are also used to treat chronic biofilm infections.

Gene therapy in cystic fibrosis

The gene for CF was identified in 1989 and its product, the CF transmembrane conductance regulator (CFTR), has been studied intensively; this membrane protein in epithelial cells is defective in people with CF. The aim of gene therapy is to transfer the gene into cells of the airways of people with CF, so that they can express the CFTR protein and so improve chloride and sodium conductance. Other methods include drugs aimed at suppressing premature termination of the synthesis of the protein, stabilising the protein structure, activating the protein or enhancing normal chloride channel functions. Drugs currently available include tezacaftor, lumacaftor and ivacaftor in various combinations. Tezacaftor and lumacaftor increase the amount and function of CFTR protein on the cell surface, while ivacaftor increases channel opening of the CFTR protein to facilitate chloride transport across cell membranes.

Other mucolytics

Mannitol, a sugar that is an impermeable solute, increases osmotic pressure and acts to draw water out of cells. When the powder is inhaled via a DPI in the treatment of CF, the osmotic pressure in the airways secretions is increased and water is moved into the airway's lumen, thus reducing viscosity of the mucus. Cough, throat pain and vomiting and diarrhoea are common adverse effects, and bronchospasm may worsen asthma. Mannitol is also administered systemically for its osmotic effect in treating acute glaucoma or raised intracranial pressure (Nevitt et al. 2020).

Older mucolytics are acetylcysteine, which splits disulfide bonds in mucoproteins, and bromhexine, thought to improve mucus flow by enhancing the hydrolysing activity of lysosomal enzymes. There is little hard evidence of clinical efficacy for either compound, except in reducing exacerbations in people with COPD. Acetylcysteine may be used in tracheostomy care.

Mucoregulators

The M_3 muscarinic receptors, present on bronchial smooth muscle cells and gland cells, mediate stimulation of bronchial secretions (Fig 15.4) and contraction of smooth muscle (**bronchoconstriction**); and anticholinergics (muscarinic receptor antagonists, antimuscarinic drugs) such as atropine inhibit bronchial secretions and relax smooth muscle (Drug Monograph 8.2). Anticholinergics ipratropium and tiotropium are used in bronchial asthma as bronchodilators (see later), but potential adverse effects include inhibition of bronchial secretion and mucociliary transport, and accumulation of thickened secretions; however, as there is often excessive mucus production in asthma, the effects tend to cancel out. Tiotropium and glycopyrronium bromide (glycopyrrolate) are indicated in COPD to improve exercise capacity and reduce morbidity and mortality (see later).

KEY POINTS

Stimulants, depressants, expectorants and mucolytics

- Analeptics, such as caffeine, act directly to stimulate respiration via the vasomotor and respiratory centres in the medulla.
- Respiratory depression is a seldom desirable side effect of drugs such as opioids.
- Drugs affecting secretions and mucociliary transport include:
    - pulmonary surfactants, used in respiratory distress syndrome in premature infants
    - expectorants to aid removal of sputum
    - diluents, which are used to dilute respiratory secretions
    - mucolytics such as dornase alfa, which break down and reduce the viscosity of sputum in people with abnormal or excessive respiratory tract secretions
    - anticholinergics to inhibit bronchial secretions and promote relaxation of bronchial smooth muscle (mucoregulators).

Drugs affecting the nose

Olfaction: the sense of smell

The sense of smell aids in the appreciation of foods and helps protect against toxins and pollutants. Humans have a much greater sensitivity to smell than to taste.

The receptors for olfaction (the sense of smell) are in the olfactory epithelium at the top of the nasal cavity (Figs 15.1 and 15.5). Specialised cilia projecting down from the dendrites of the olfactory receptor cells are stimulated by chemicals in the inhaled air and initiate an action potential in the olfactory neurons. These synapse within the olfactory bulb and form the olfactory tract of the first cranial nerve, passing eventually to the lateral olfactory area of the temporal lobe of the cortex and to other regions of the limbic system and the hypothalamus.

The sensation of smell may be impaired in many situations – for example, by ageing, radiation, dental treatment, poor oral hygiene, psychiatric and neurological disorders, tumours, trauma, epilepsy, migraine, infections/inflammation, renal failure and deficiencies of vitamin B or zinc. Dysfunctions are more common in the elderly and can significantly reduce the quality of life. Anosmia (lack of sense of smell) can occur as a genetic trait. Hyposmia, a mild general defect in olfaction, is a common symptom of colds and rhinitis and is due to inflammation and obstruction of the nasal passages. Drugs are used to decongest airways and so improve the sense of smell. That food often becomes tasteless during these conditions indicates that components of the flavour can no longer be smelled.

Hyperosmia (heightened sense of smell) occurs in CF, adrenal insufficiency and states of hysteria. In schizophrenia and epilepsy, olfactory hallucinations may occur. There are few specific medical treatments for these olfactory dysfunctions; zinc supplements may be useful, as may be nasal decongestants.

Drugs impairing the sense of smell

A great variety of drugs have been noted to cause alterations in smell as an adverse effect; these are summarised in Table 15.2. For example, antimigraine

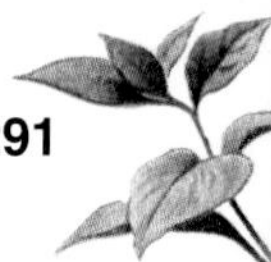

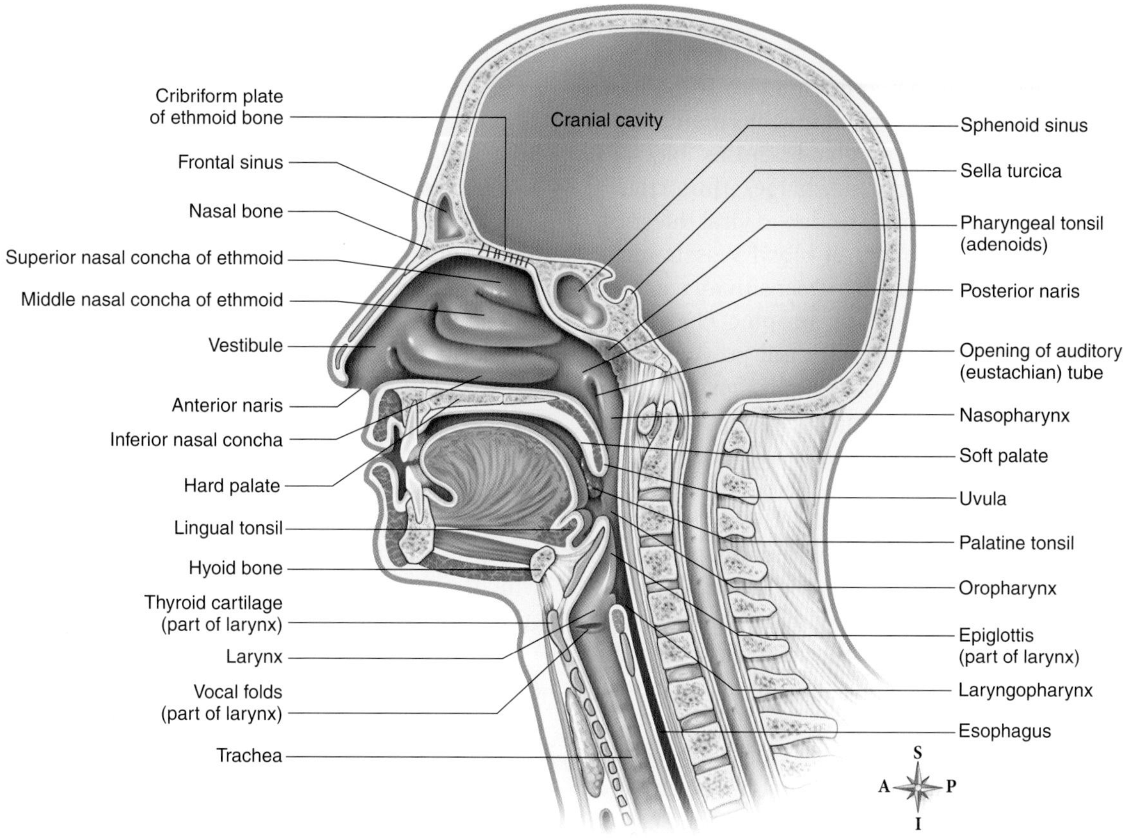

Cribriform plate of ethmoid bone
Frontal sinus
Nasal bone
Superior nasal concha of ethmoid
Middle nasal concha of ethmoid
Vestibule
Anterior naris
Inferior nasal concha
Hard palate
Lingual tonsil
Hyoid bone
Thyroid cartilage (part of larynx)
Larynx
Vocal folds (part of larynx)
Trachea
Cranial cavity
Sphenoid sinus
Sella turcica
Pharyngeal tonsil (adenoids)
Posterior naris
Opening of auditory (eustachian) tube
Nasopharynx
Soft palate
Uvula
Palatine tonsil
Oropharynx
Epiglottis (part of larynx)
Laryngopharynx
Esophagus
S
A
P
I

FIGURE 15.5 Sagittal section of the head and neck showing the locations of the respiratory structures
Source: Netter Images; used with permission.

TABLE 15.2 Drug effects on smell

DRUG GROUP: EXAMPLE	EFFECT ON SMELL	PROPOSED MECHANISM
Calcium channel blockers: nifedipine, diltiazem	×	Inhibit receptor events
Diuretics: acetazolamide, hydrochlorothiazide, spironolactone	×	
Fluoroquinolones: o/ciprofloxacin	×	Inhibit cytochrome P450
Others: minocycline, griseofulvin, metronidazole	×	
H_2-antagonists: cimetidine	⇓	Inhibit receptor events
Corticosteroids: prednisolone	⇓	Inhibit receptor membrane activity
Antithyroid: carbimazole	⇓	Hypothyroidism, Zn interactions
Antimigraine: triptans	×	Inhibit receptor events
Antiparkinsonian drugs: levodopa/carbidopa	×	Enhanced DA activity
Anticonvulsants: carbamazepine, phenytoin	×	
α-agonists: phenylephrine	⇓	Inhibit receptor events

Sensory effects: ⇓ = decreased sense; × = impaired sense; – = no effect or not known.
DA = dopamine; Zn = zinc. Only drug groups for which the adverse effects are well documented have been included. Many groups and individual drugs have been omitted.
(For details, see Bromley 2000; Doty et al. 2008; Henkin 1994.)

drugs may impair – or corticosteroids may decrease – the sense of smell. The mechanisms may vary for the specific drugs. Chronic exposure to chemicals, especially metals, plastics, solvents and tobacco smoke, also adversely affects olfaction.

In most cases, the mechanism by which the chemical sense is altered is poorly understood, and the doses at which the effects occur are very variable. The impaired sensation takes some days or weeks of chronic dosing to develop, and the impairment may persist for weeks or months. People who notice that 'things are starting to smell different' may need reassurance that this is an acknowledged adverse effect of a particular drug, which is usually reversible after stopping treatment.

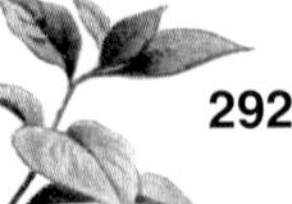

Rhinitis and nasal obstruction

Obstruction to free airflow in the nose occurs very commonly as a feature of the common cold. It is due to **rhinitis**, or inflammation of the nasal mucous membranes, in which overactivity of mucus glands causes excessive mucus production and watery discharge (rhinorrhoea, 'runny nose'). The condition may be due to viral infection, impaired nervous system control of blood vessels in the membrane (vasomotor rhinitis), hypersensitivity reactions (allergic rhinitis), hypertrophic or atrophic changes or drug adverse effects. Nasal polyps (nasal polyposis) are benign growths of the nasal passages, and they may grow and cause chronic nasal congestion.

Allergic rhinitis

Allergic rhinitis, or 'hay fever', is an atopic disorder (type 1 hypersensitivity reaction) mediated by immunoglobulin E (IgE) antibodies. Sensitised mast cells and basophils release autacoids, including histamine, serotonin, prostaglandins and leukotrienes, which mediate inflammatory and immune responses. Prevalence of allergic rhinitis is highest in children and young adults (20%). There is a strong association in children with asthma and with eczema (atopic dermatitis). Inhaled allergens such as grass or flower pollens and moulds cause seasonal symptoms (e.g. 'spring fever'), whereas other allergens (house dust mites, animal fur and foods) cause chronic or perennial rhinitis. Specific allergens can be identified by skin testing or in-vitro testing. Common symptoms include sneezing, nasal congestion and hypersecretion, blocked ears, irritated pharynx and itchy nose, palate and eyes.

Management programs include attempts to identify and reduce exposure to specific allergens or environments, immunotherapy against antigens and symptomatic drug treatment.

Nasal corticosteroids

First-line treatment for rhinitis and nasal polyposis is now topical corticosteroids, administered intranasally by nasal spray or drops. Nasal formulations are available for beclometasone, budesonide, ciclesonide, fluticasone and mometasone (see later under 'Drugs Used in Asthma' and Ch 29 for a discussion of corticosteroids); they can be used as needed or regularly. Nasal administration reduces inflammation, mucus production and risk of systemic adverse effects of corticosteroids. The main adverse effects are local: stinging, nose-bleeding, itching and sore throat.

H_1-receptor antagonists (antihistamines)

The other common drugs used to treat allergic rhinitis are the antihistamines (oral and intranasal H_1-receptor antagonists), An example is levocabastine as an intranasal preparation. They are also useful for their antiemetic, sedative, dual anticholinergic activity (mucoregulatory) effects and may be present in cough suppressant preparations (Chs 8, 16 and 20). The many actions of histamine as an autacoid are discussed in Chapter 34, and clinical uses of H_2-receptor antagonists in peptic ulcer are described in Chapter 16.

Mechanism of action

In allergic rhinitis, H_1-receptor antagonists are useful for blocking of histamine-induced vasodilation, thus decreasing capillary permeability, erythema and oedema. While released histamine normally contracts bronchial smooth muscle (bronchoconstriction, Fig 15.4), H_1-antihistamines are not useful bronchodilators and are not effective in allergic asthma and anaphylaxis, in which more powerful mediators are implicated. These include the historically known slow-reacting substance of anaphylaxis (SRS-A), which consists of three bioactive cysteinyl leukotrienes (CysLTs): leukotriene B_4 (LTB_4), LTC_4 and LTD_4.

Adverse effects

The older H_1-antihistamines such as promethazine and diphenhydramine have powerful sedative effects;[2] hence the common warning on packets of tablets: 'Do not drive or operate machinery after taking this drug'. They may be useful at night for hay-fever sufferers, but should not be given to infants younger than 2 years because there is increased risk of sudden infant death syndrome. The sedative effect common to older antihistamines is additive with that of other CNS depressants, including alcohol.

Second and third-generation H_1-antihistamines such as loratadine and fexofenadine were developed to minimise this effect; they are called 'non-sedating'. Cetirizine, however, does not claim to be non-sedating and may still cross the blood–brain barrier and have some CNS-depressant effects.

Other intranasal drugs for allergic rhinitis

Many drugs are formulated as nasal sprays or drops for topical use in rhinitis. They include:

- normal saline solutions such as nasal drops or sprays
- sympathomimetic **decongestants** including xylometazoline nasal spray or drops (Drug Monograph 15.1); also formulations of ephedrine, oxymetazoline, tramazoline and phenylephrine (see Ch 9 for a discussion of sympathomimetic agents)

2 This sedative effect may be appreciated by the parents of children given an antihistamine as an antiemetic to prevent travel sickness during long car or plane journeys. However, children sometimes react paradoxically to CNS-active drugs, and may instead be hyper-stimulated – not a good outcome!

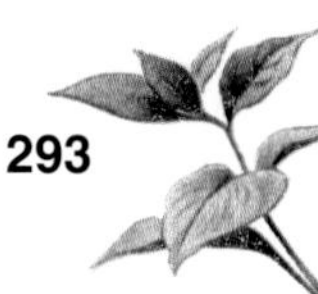

Drug Monograph 15.1

Xylometazoline nasal spray

Sympathomimetic amines such as xylometazoline, oxymetazoline and tramazoline are administered for decongestant effects as nasal sprays and phenylephrine as spray, drops, tablets and cough syrups.

Mechanism of action

These agonists have α-receptor-mediated vasoconstrictor actions.

Tolerance can occur rapidly to these actions.

Indications

Xylometazoline nasal spray is indicated for symptomatic relief of congestion (inflammation and excess secretions) and red eyes associated with acute rhinitis, common cold and sinusitis. Intranasal administration also assists intranasal examination.

Pharmacokinetics

Topically applied (in the eyes or nose), vasoconstrictors act rapidly. After intranasal administration, plasma levels of xylometazoline are below the limits of detection, so pharmacokinetic parameters cannot be determined.

Adverse effects

Transient stinging and throat dryness may be felt. Systemic sympathomimetic effects can occur, such as headache and insomnia, so decongestants should not be taken by people with hypertension.

Warnings and contraindications

Prolonged use (4–5 days) of nasal vasoconstrictor sprays can cause rebound nasal congestion, known as rhinitis medicamentosa, and the drug may become less effective due to tolerance.

Sympathomimetics should not be used by people taking antidepressants because of potentiation of effects, or in children under 6 years.

Dosage and administration

The nose should be blown gently first before administration of the drops or spray, as directed. Xylometazoline is formulated as nasal spray or drops, 0.05% or 0.1%.

- nasal formulations of cromones used prophylactically
- nasal anticholinergics, which dry up nasal secretions and reduce rhinorrhoea (ipratropium)
- volatile oil decongestants, often administered as inhalation or chest rub: may include menthol or camphor, or volatile oils such as wintergreen (methyl salicylate).

Sinusitis

Sinusitis, or inflammation of the mucous membranes lining the bone cavities of the face (Fig 15.5, earlier), usually results from infection. Clinical features include feeling of fullness or pain in the forehead or cheeks, fever and nasal congestion. Bacterial infection causes purulent discharge. Specific antibiotics are prescribed if the infecting organism is bacterial: for example, amoxicillin, doxycycline hyclate, cefuroxime and cefaclor are usually suitable. Treatment with antipyretic analgesics (e.g. paracetamol), nasal corticosteroids, saline irrigations and decongestants helps to relieve symptoms. Chronic sinusitis, persisting for more than 12 weeks, may require oral corticosteroids, and possibly surgery to remove polyps.

KEY POINTS

Drugs affecting the nose and olfaction

- Drugs can be administered via the nose for local and/or systemic effects.
- Drugs can have varying effects on olfaction.
- Sinusitis usually results from infection. Treatment includes antibiotics, antipyretic analgesics (e.g. paracetamol), nasal corticosteroids, saline irrigations and sympathomimetic decongestants. If the cause is bacterial, specific antibiotics are prescribed.
- Chronic sinusitis may require oral corticosteroids.
- Allergic rhinitis, or 'hay fever', is an atopic disorder (type 1 hypersensitivity reaction) and is treated with:
  - nasal corticosteroids or antihistamines (oral and intranasal H_1-receptor antagonists)
  - immunotherapy
  - sympathomimetic decongestants, nasal saline and volatile oil decongestants.

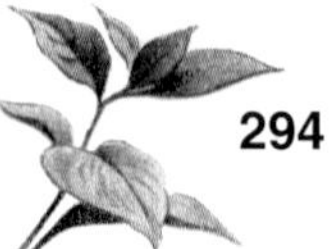

Drug treatment of asthma

Asthma is a chronic inflammatory disease of the airways in which the passage of air into and out of the lungs is obstructed. It has been described since ancient civilisations; the word comes from the Greek word for 'panting'. By the early 20th century, asthma was being treated with adrenaline (epinephrine) injections, anticholinergics and coffee (containing methylxanthines); other β-agonists and corticosteroids were introduced in the 1950s, and long-acting β-agonists (LABAs) in the 1980s. Later treatments include long-acting muscarinic antagonists (LAMAs) and **immunomodulating drugs** (Global Initiative for Asthma 2022; Trivedi et al. 2014) (Asthma Australia – see 'Online resources').

Pathophysiology of asthma

The hallmarks of asthma are reversible bronchoconstriction, chronic inflammation of the epithelium of the airways and increased mucus secretion; there is airway hypersensitivity to a variety of stimuli, leading to episodes of wheezing, breathlessness and coughing. Asthma affects more than 300 million people worldwide, including 11% of Australians and 12% of adult New Zealanders reported taking current asthma medication.

The prevalence of asthma varies by socioeconomic area, in Australia being highest for those living in the lowest socioeconomic areas compared with those living in the highest areas (males: 13% and 10%, respectively; females: 16% and 10%, respectively).

Effective asthma management requires accurate diagnosis, achieving and maintaining good control and regular monitoring and review. The rationales for use of drugs in asthma are to relieve and control symptoms, prevent acute asthma and deaths and maintain best lung function and quality of life (Australian Medicines Handbook 2020; Ministry of Health 2018; NAC 2018; National Asthma Council Australia 2022).

Airways inflammation and remodelling

Asthma is not only a disease of impaired autonomic control of the airways lumen diameter; it is now recognised that many physiological mediators are involved in the pathogenesis of an asthma attack, including leukotrienes, interleukins, histamine,[3] prostaglandins (PGs) and other cytokines and nitric oxide, as well as autonomic neurotransmitters (Page et al. 2017). In fact, the term asthma has been more recently understood to be an umbrella diagnosis for several diseases with distinct pathways (endotypes) and variable clinical presentations (phenotypes) (Kuruvilla et al. 2019; Page et al. 2017).

The early phase of an acute attack involves vasodilation and increased capillary permeability, with infiltration of bronchial mucosa by white blood cells. Numerous immune cell types are involved, particularly mast cells, eosinophils, macrophages and Th2 and $CD4^+$ lymphocytes. Activation of these cells leads to release of dozens of pro-inflammatory mediators and cytokines, notably nuclear factor κB, interleukin-2, -4, -5 and -13 and tumour necrosis factor-α, as well as immunoglobulin E (IgE).

The inflammatory process involves vascular leakage, contraction of bronchial smooth muscle (bronchoconstriction), inflammatory cell infiltration, increased oedema and mucus production, impaired mucociliary function and, eventually, thickening of airway walls, airway hyper-reactivity and irreversible airways obstruction (Fig 15.4). The late-phase (chronic) response involves inflammation, proliferation of fibroblasts and fibrosis, oedema of the airway mucosa, necrosis of bronchial epithelial cells and airway wall remodelling, with increased collagen deposition. Expiration is particularly impaired, leading to air trapping, hypoxaemia and raised PCO_2. The principal signs and symptoms are wheezing and cough, tachypnoea or dyspnoea (rapid or difficult breathing), chest tightness, tachycardia, fatigue, sweating, difficulty speaking sentences and anxiety. If bronchoconstriction is not reversed, status asthmaticus occurs, with respiratory acidosis and possibly life-threatening respiratory failure.

Allergic asthma

In most people with asthma there is an allergic component mediated by IgEs. Extrinsic (atopic, allergic) asthma is triggered by allergens such as pollens, house dust mites, animal fur, moulds or proteins in foods such as eggs; some drugs, including penicillins and aspirin, can also precipitate allergic asthma. 'Westernisation' of environments (reduced infant infections, reduced exposure to some allergens and increased use of antibiotics) may be associated with increased risk of childhood asthma. Other common triggers are drugs that cause bronchoconstriction, including β-blockers (see review questions), chemicals such as sulfites used as preservatives, exercise (breathing cold air), emotional stress, respiratory infections and environmental pollutants including cigarette smoke. All people with asthma are hypersensitive to bronchoconstrictor agents, including acetylcholine and PGD_2.

Non-allergic asthma

In non-allergic or 'intrinsic asthma', there is no identified causative agent: however it is proposed that it may involve viral and bacterial superantigens, tobacco smoke, small particulate matter and volatile organic compounds.

3 However, antihistamine drugs are not clinically useful in asthma treatment, suggesting that histamine plays only a minor role in the pathophysiology.

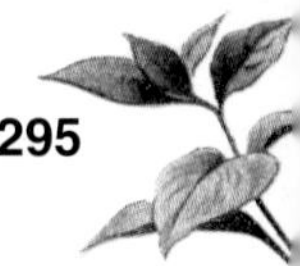

KEY POINTS

The pathophysiology of asthma

- Asthma is a condition that involves impaired autonomic control as well as inflammatory processes.
- The principal signs and symptoms of asthma include wheezing and cough, tachypnoea or dyspnoea (rapid or difficult breathing), chest tightness, tachycardia, fatigue, sweating, difficulty speaking sentences and anxiety.
- The early phase of an acute attack involves vasodilation and increased capillary permeability, infiltration of immune cell types and the release of dozens of pro-inflammatory mediators and cytokines. Constriction of the airways can be produced by neuropeptides and cytokine mediators released during inflammatory responses.
- The late-phase (chronic) response involves inflammatory processes, proliferation of fibroblasts and fibrosis, oedema of the airway mucosa, necrosis of bronchial epithelial cells and airway wall remodelling, with increased collagen deposition.

Drugs used in asthma

Not surprisingly, many types of drugs are used to inhibit the pathological effects of the various mediators. The main groups are:

- bronchodilators (β_2-receptor agonists, theophyllines and anticholinergics)
- controller or preventer medications (long-acting β_2-receptor agonists (controllers), inhaled corticosteroids (ICS), leukotriene-receptor antagonists, 5-lipoxygenase inhibitors, cromones and antibodies).

Figure 15.6 gives an overview of the mechanisms of action of asthma medications on inflammation and bronchial smooth muscle contraction. Aspects of their clinical use are summarised in Table 15.3.

There is a large degree of variability in the response of asthmatics to bronchodilators, ICS and leukotriene modifiers. Some variability is attributed to genetic variation, with many variants of single nucleotide polymorphisms identified that alter airways' responsiveness and lead to exacerbations. Choice of drugs depends on client factors, aetiological factors, drug factors such as adverse drug reactions and classified severity and frequency of asthma attacks. Triggering factors should be avoided if possible.

The stepwise pharmacological treatment is discussed later in this chapter (Fig 15.7). Older classifications referred to asthma as mild, moderate or severe:

- Mild – intermittent attacks (fewer than 1–2 per week), or nocturnal asthma twice or less monthly. Peak expiratory flow (PEF) over 80% predicted (i.e. > 80% of the expected level); normal after bronchodilator use; PEF variability under 20%.
- Moderate – attacks more than twice weekly, nocturnal asthma symptoms more than twice per month, and use of a bronchodilator β-agonist inhaler required nearly daily. PEF 60–80% predicted; normal after bronchodilator use; PEF variability 20–30%.
- Severe – frequent and continuous asthmatic symptoms, including nocturnal asthma and having been hospitalised for asthma in the previous year.

Currently, the severity of asthma is assessed retrospectively, reviewing the level of treatment that has been required to control the symptoms and exacerbations. This is once the client has been on a controller for several months and, if possible, step-down treatment has been undertaken to determine the minimum effective level of treatment.

According to the *Australian Asthma Handbook* (2021), good asthma control is having, in the previous 4 weeks:

- daytime symptoms fewer than 2 days a week
- need for short-acting reliever fewer than 2 days a week (not including doses for preventing exercise-induced bronchoconstriction)
- no limitation of activity
- no symptoms during the night or on waking.

Further classification includes partial control or poor control.

The overall management of asthma is summarised after discussion of the groups of drugs commonly used in treatment.

Bronchodilator drugs

β-adrenoceptor agonists

Bronchodilator drugs are used to treat pulmonary diseases such as asthma, chronic bronchitis and emphysema. The classification of anticholinergic and adrenoceptors agonists and the effects of agents that stimulate or block specific receptors are discussed in Chapters 8 and 9; reviewing these chapters will help in understanding the mechanisms and actions of bronchodilators.

Bronchodilators have been used in respiratory medicine for more than 5000 years: ephedrine, an alkaloid from the plant *Ephedra sinica*, was introduced from traditional Chinese medicine into Western medicine in 1923. Ephedrine is a sympathomimetic amine related structurally to adrenaline (a hormone from the adrenal medulla); it has a predominantly indirect action via release of noradrenaline from adrenergic nerve terminals; thus, it has effects on both α- and β-adrenoceptors.

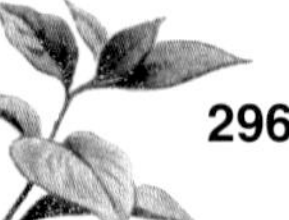

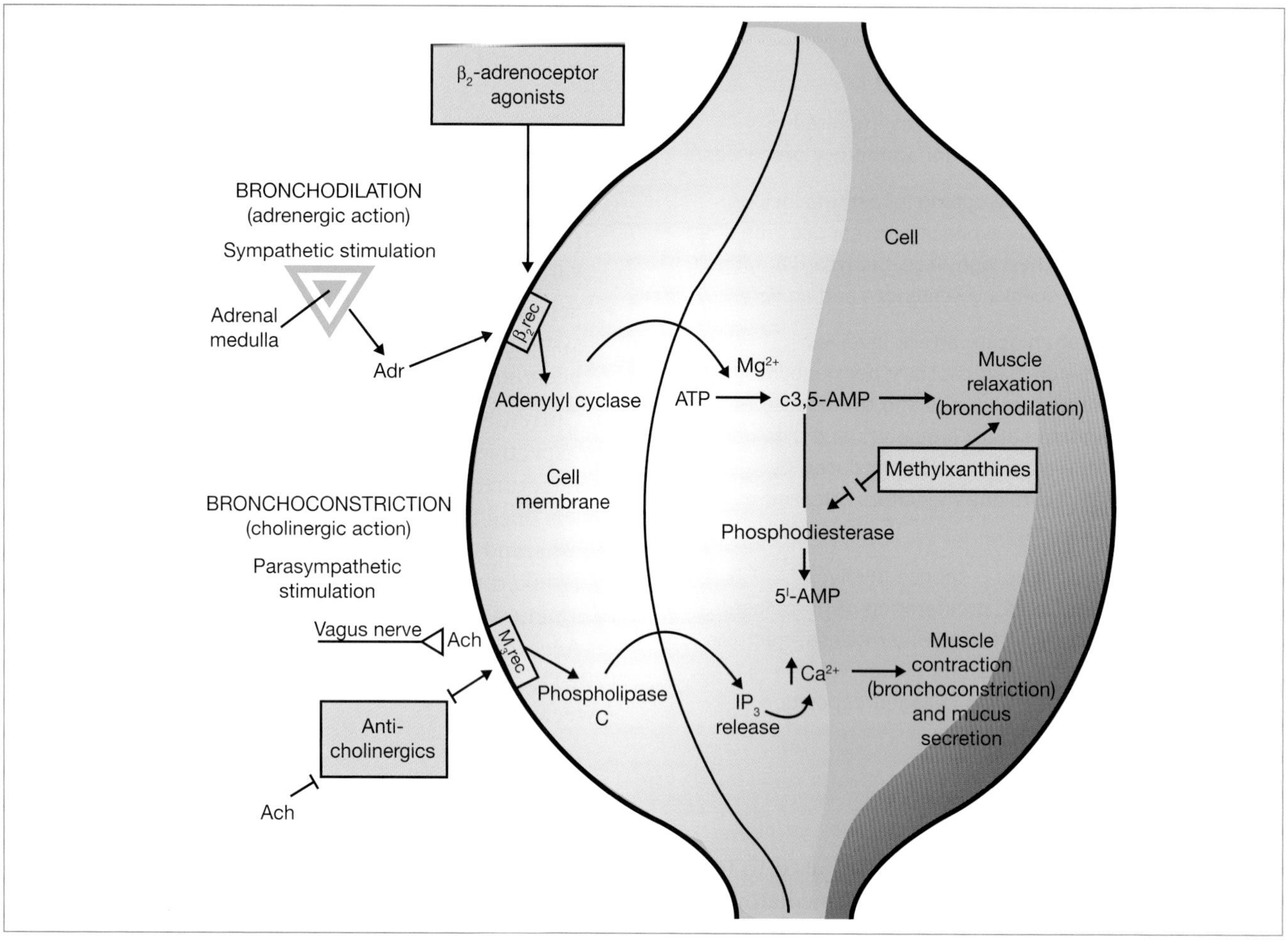

FIGURE 15.6 Typical mechanisms of action of drugs on bronchial smooth muscle **A** Bronchodilation pathway. **B** Bronchoconstriction pathway. Note that tachykinins also cause bronchoconstriction, and nitric oxide and VIP bronchodilation; however, there are as yet no common antiasthma drugs acting via these mediators. ACh = acetylcholine; Adr = adrenaline; $\beta_2$rec = β_2-adrenoceptor; c3,5-AMP = cyclic 3,5 adenosine monophosphate; IP = inositol phosphate; M_3rec = M_3 muscarinic receptor

Adrenaline, also a non-selective α- and β-adrenoceptor agonist, is still used clinically for asthma (and for anaphylactic reactions and cardiovascular effects) but has a short duration of action (Drug Monograph 9.1). Effects mediated by α-adrenoceptors (especially vasoconstriction and hypertension) and β_1-adrenoceptors (cardiac stimulation) count as adverse reactions in the context of asthma therapy, so much research effort has gone into the development of specific β_2-agonist bronchodilators (Matera et al. 2020b).

Mechanism of action

Activation of β_2-adrenoceptors in bronchial smooth muscle leads to increased formation of cyclic 3,5-adenosine monophosphate (cAMP), enhancement of calcium extrusion from the cell and binding of intracellular calcium, which lowers the concentration of intracellular calcium and strongly relaxes bronchial smooth muscle (Fig 15.6). **β_2-adrenoceptor agonists** are the most effective bronchodilators, acting as functional antagonists of airway smooth muscle contraction. (Agonist actions on β_2-adrenoceptors in a pregnant uterus can cause relaxation of uterine smooth muscle, so the drugs are also used to delay threatened miscarriage; see Ch 30.)

Administration

The optimal route of administration of β_2-agonists is by inhalation; 'puffers' and 'pumps' deliver low doses of drug directly to the airway smooth muscle and have rapid and relatively specific effects. Some inhaled drug is inevitably deposited in the oropharynx and swallowed; it may be absorbed into the systemic circulation and cause adverse reactions. In rare cases, propellants may induce cardiac dysrhythmias or allergic reactions. In emergencies, systemic administration may be required: adrenaline, salbutamol and terbutaline can be administered by

TABLE 15.3 Summary of drugs used in asthma

DRUG GROUP	EXAMPLE	FORMULATION/ROUTE	ONSET (min)	DURATION (h) OR FREQUENCY (/d)	USAGE
Relievers					
SABAs	Salbutamol	DPI, pMDI, neb, PO, IV (IM, SC)	5–15	3–6 h; neb: 3–4/d	Reliever + ex-ind
	Terbutaline	DPI, SC	5–15	3–6 h	Reliever + ex-ind
LABAs (rapid)	Formoterol (eformoterol)	DPI	Fast 1–3	>12 h; admin 2/d	Reliever + controller in people on inhaled CSs
Anticholinergics (SAMAs)	Ipratropium	pMDI, neb	Short	6 h; admin 3–4/d	COPD; adjunct in acute severe asthma
Anticholinergics (LAMAs)	Tiotropium	DPI	30	Long-acting up to 24 h	Long-term COPD
	Aclidinium	DPI	10	Long-acting up to 24 h twice daily	Long-term COPD
	Glycopyrronium bromide (glycopyrrolate)	DPI		Long-acting up to 24 h	Long-term COPD
	Umeclidinium	DPI	5-15	Long-acting up to 24 h	
Theophyllines	Aminophylline	Slow IV injection or infusion			Long-term COPD
	Theophylline	CR tablets, syrup	1–2 hrs	CR admin 2/d; syrup 4/d	Adjunct in severe persistent asthma
Controllers					
LABAs	Indacaterol	DPI	< 5	Up to 24; 1/d	Controller combined with inhaled CSs in COPD
	Salmeterol	DPI, pMDI	10–20	>12	Controller combined with inhaled CSs
Preventers					
Corticosteroids (ICS)	Beclometasone	pMDI		Admin 2/d	Maintenance in persistent asthma
	Budesonide	DPI, neb		Admin 2/d	Maintenance in persistent asthma
	Ciclesonide	pMDI		Admin 1/d	Maintenance in persistent asthma
	Fluticasone	DPI, pMDI, neb		Admin 2/d	Maintenance in persistent asthma
Cromones (cromolyns)	Sodium cromoglycate	DPI, pMDI, neb		Admin 2–4 times/daily	Alternative to inhaled CSs in persistent asthma; ex-ind
	Nedocromil	pMDI		Admin 2–4/d	Alternative to inhaled CSs in persistent asthma; ex-ind
Leukotriene receptor antagonist	Montelukast	PO		1/d	Alternative to inhaled CSs in persistent asthma; ex-ind
Anti-IgE antibody	Omalizumab	SC		Every 2–4 weeks	Allergic asthma in people on inhaled CSs

Notes:

1. Combination inhalers available include the following:
   - LABA + LAMA – formoterol + aclidinium (DPI)
   - ICS + LABA budesonide + formoterol (DPI), and fluticasone + salmeterol (DPI, pMDI)
   - ICS + LABA + LAMA (mometasone + indacaterol + glycopyrronium; DPI).
2. Most drugs used in asthma are also indicated for treatment of acute exacerbations of COPD; COPD is the only accepted indication for indacaterol and tiotropium.

Admin = administer; COPD = chronic obstructive pulmonary disease; CR = controlled-release; CSs = corticosteroids; d = day; DPI = dry powder inhaler; ex-ind = prevention of exercise-induced asthma; ICS = inhaled corticosteroids; IV = intravenous; LABA= long-acting β_2-agonist; LAMA = long-acting muscarinic antagonist; neb = nebuliser; PO = oral; pMDI = pressurised metered-dose inhaler; SAMA = short-acting muscarinic antagonist; SABA= short-acting β_2-agonist; SC = subcutaneous

Sources: Based on information in Australian Medicines Handbook 2021; Respiratory Expert Group 2020.

injection. Salbutamol is also available in a syrup form, useful for children.

Adverse effects

While agonists with relatively specific actions on β_2-adrenoceptors are available, they may in high doses also stimulate α- and β_1-receptors, so adverse effects in the cardiovascular system (vasoconstriction, vasodilation and reflex tachycardia, pulmonary vasodilation), skeletal muscle (fine tremor), metabolism[4] (ketoacidosis, mobilisation of triglycerides) and CNS (headaches, nausea and anxiety) may occur. The reverse is also true: β_1-adrenoceptor antagonists used in cardiovascular disease may have potentially life-threatening bronchoconstrictor (β_2 antagonism) effects in people with asthma.

4 Hence they may be abused in sport for their anabolic effects.

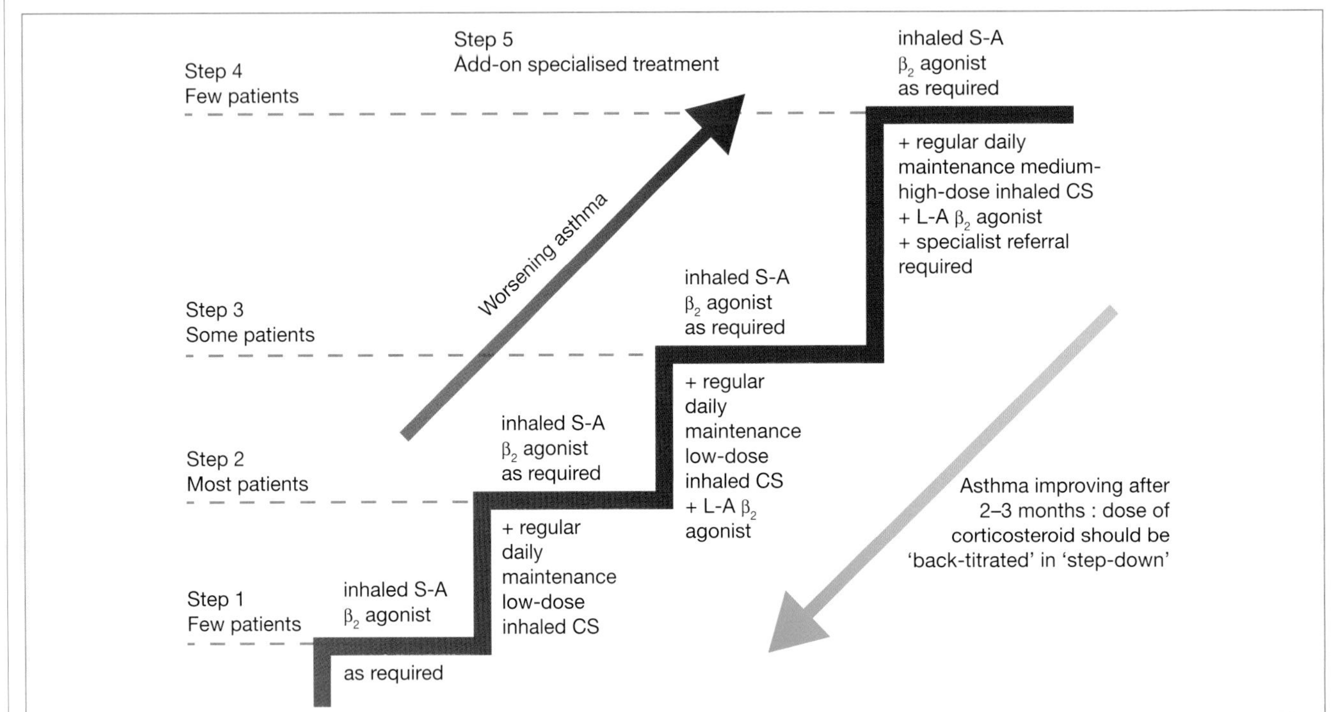

FIGURE 15.7 Stepwise maintenance of asthma in adults CS = corticosteroid; L-A = long-acting; S-A = short-acting. Persistent: > 3–4 attacks/week; moderate: asthma not controlled by low-dose inhaled CS + β_2-agonist

Source: National Asthma Council Australia 2022.

'Epidemics' of deaths from asthma occurred in the 1960s in Britain (attributed to over-the-counter preparations of high-dose isoprenaline) and in the 1980s in New Zealand (attributed to high doses of the LABA fenoterol). Non-selective β-agonists may downregulate receptors, leading to tolerance to the bronchodilator effects of these agents, which encourages overuse and exacerbates adverse effects arising from cardiac and vascular actions. In addition, people with particular polymorphisms of the β_2-adrenoceptor appear to experience reduced lung function and increased asthma exacerbations.

Short-acting β_2-agonists (relievers)

Short-acting β_2-agonists (SABAs) are fast-acting bronchodilators, used as **relievers** in first-line treatment for acute relief of asthma symptoms; salbutamol (also known as albuterol, and by its first trade-name Ventolin) and terbutaline are described in Drug Monograph 15.2. SABAs-only treatment is no longer recommended. They are also used for symptom relief in COPD and during allergic reactions, and to prevent exercise-induced asthma. Over-dependence on β_2-agonists (high dose use on more than 3 days per week) may indicate that other aspects of asthma management, including preventive use of anti-inflammatory drugs and monitoring of FEV_1 (forced expiratory volume in 1 second), are not optimal.

Long-acting β_2-agonists (controllers)

Long-acting β_2-agonists (LABAs) commonly used include salmeterol and formoterol (eformoterol), and indacaterol. They are used for asthma and COPD (Crisafulli et al. 2017). Due to their allosteric actions at the β_2 receptors and greater lipid solubilities they have prolonged actions, with half-lives in the range of 6–12 hours (indacaterol up to 24 hours), and are administered once or twice daily by MDI or DPI. They are useful against night-time symptoms and are symptom **controllers**, used in conjunction with ICS (preventers) or long-acting muscarinic antagonists (see below) in maintenance treatment of asthma or COPD. Formoterol (eformoterol) has a rapid onset of action (Table 15.3) and can also be used for quick relief. Indacaterol is currently indicated for long-term once-daily maintenance treatment of COPD. Other newer ultra-long-acting LABAs include olodaterol and vilanterol, used in combination with tiotropium, and umeclidinium and/or fluticasone respectively (for COPD and emphysema).

There is some controversy about the safety of LABAs: their use may increase tolerance to SABAs and increase exacerbations of asthma, especially if LABAs are used alone (i.e. without ICS). There may be a genetic component to this increased susceptibility. They are not recommended for use in children under 6 years.

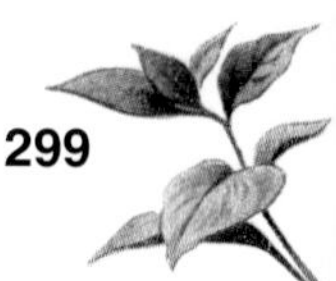

Drug Monograph 15.2
Salbutamol and terbutaline

Mechanism of action
These are SABA bronchodilators.

Indications
For the symptomatic relief of acute asthma and protection against exercise-induced asthma, and for symptomatic relief of bronchospasm in COPD, for allergic reactions and after smoke inhalation.

Pharmacokinetics
Onset of action by inhalation is rapid, within 5–15 minutes, with peak effect within 1–2 hours and duration of action of 3–6 hours.

Salbutamol is metabolised in the liver and excreted in the kidneys.

Terbutaline is excreted largely unchanged. Small amounts of either drug swallowed are rapidly metabolised.

Drug interactions
Concomitant therapy with other sympathomimetic amines will cause excessive sympathetic stimulation (tremor, tachycardia). β-blockers, including those for hypertension and in eyedrops for glaucoma, antagonise the effects of β_2-agonists and may precipitate asthma, so they are contraindicated. Hypokalaemia resulting from β_2-agonist therapy may be potentiated by xanthine derivatives, steroids or diuretics; potassium levels should be monitored. Antidepressant drugs may potentiate cardiovascular effects.

Adverse effects
These include tremor, palpitations, anxiety, restlessness, headaches, muscle cramps, hyperglycaemia and tachycardia, an unusual taste in the mouth and hyperactivity in children. Symptoms of overdose are those of excessive α- or β_1-adrenoceptor stimulation – for example, hypertension or palpitations.

Precautions
Precautions are needed in people with cardiovascular disease, diabetes or hyperthyroidism. Excessive use of bronchodilator aerosols, or lack of response, may indicate worsening asthma control. Both drugs are safe in pregnancy and when breastfeeding although, as a Category A drug, care should be taken with use of terbutaline in the first 3 months of pregnancy. No data is available for use of terbutaline in the elderly. Treatment of asthma or COPD should be in accordance with current national treatment guidelines.

Dosage and administration
The adult bronchodilator dose for both is 1–2 inhalations (100 micrograms of salbutamol, 500 micrograms of terbutaline), with the second inhalation at least 1 minute after the first, then again every 4–6 hours. Both drugs can be administered by nebuliser, orally or parenterally in acute severe attacks, and are commonly administered by paramedics.

Methylxanthines
The xanthine group of drugs includes the methylxanthines: caffeine, theophylline and theobromine. Beverages from the extracts of plants containing these alkaloids have been used by humans since ancient times, and strong coffee was used as a remedy for asthma. (CNS stimulation by xanthines is discussed in Ch 23, and social use as drinks is discussed in Ch 25.)

Xanthine derivatives relax smooth muscle (particularly bronchial muscle); stimulate cardiac muscle, diaphragm contractility and the CNS (hence their social use); and produce diuresis, through increased renal perfusion and increased sodium and chloride excretion. The main medical use of these natural products and their synthetic analogues is as bronchodilators.

The most active xanthine bronchodilator is theophylline (Drug Monograph 15.3), sometimes used as its derivative aminophylline (a more soluble but highly alkaline ethylene-diamine-theophylline derivative, given IV). It has a narrow therapeutic index and many drug interactions (Drug Interactions 15.1). Although a weak bronchodilator, theophylline has useful anti-inflammatory effects and may increase responsiveness to corticosteroids in those resistant to steroids.

Mechanisms of action
Despite their long history and wide social and medical usage, the mechanism of action of xanthines is not well understood. One explanation for their bronchodilator effect is inhibition of phosphodiesterase (the enzyme that metabolises cAMP), leading to increased intracellular levels of cAMP, smooth muscle relaxation and bronchodilation (Fig 15.6); however, the concentrations of theophylline required to inhibit the enzyme in vitro are much greater

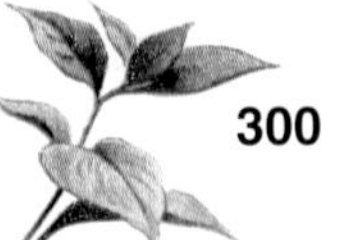

Drug Monograph 15.3
Theophylline

Theophylline is the prototype xanthine bronchodilator. It is most commonly prescribed as controlled-release tablets for maintenance treatment of poorly controlled moderate-to-severe asthma and COPD.

Mechanism of action

Theophylline is a phosphodiesterase inhibitor, the concominant cyclic AMP and cyclic GMP activation leads to bronchiolar smooth muscle relaxation. It is also an adenosine receptor antagonist thus reversing adenosine-induced bronchoconstriction.

Pharmacokinetics

- Absorption is little altered by food. Sustained-release (SR) tablets are formulated to optimise absorption. Although enteric-coated tablets and sustained-release dosage forms have delayed and unreliable absorption patterns, most provide a bioavailability of 100%.
- Peak level of theophylline is reached in 1–2 hours with the oral solution, and in 4–13 hours for sustained-release products.
- Protein binding is moderate (50–70%), and theophylline distributes across the placenta (Pregnancy Category A) and into breast milk.
- Liver metabolism produces various uric acid and xanthine derivatives (some with low activity), which are excreted via the kidneys.
- The half-life of theophylline varies with age and with concurrent illness: in premature newborns the half-life is around 30 hours; it is 3.5 hours for children 1–9 years of age, and 3–12 hours for adult non-smokers with uncomplicated asthma. In an adult smoker it is only 3–4 hours, and in the elderly 10 hours. Theophylline has a narrow therapeutic window: trough plasma levels are between 10 and 20 mg/L; however, therapeutic responses are variable and close supervision is necessary.
- Excretion is by the kidney and about 10% of the dose is excreted unchanged in the urine.

Drug interactions

There are many drug interactions with theophylline (DI 15.1); reference databases should be consulted for specific drugs and therapy monitored closely.

Adverse effects

These are dose-dependent and are related to the other main actions of xanthines (CNS and cardiac stimulation and diuresis), and include nausea, headache, insomnia, increased anxiety, vomiting, gastro-oesophageal reflux and increased urination. Tachycardia and convulsions may appear at high plasma levels (> 30 mg/L); toxicity may occur even at therapeutic levels. Older adults have an increased risk of toxicity due to reduced clearance.

Precautions

Use with caution in people with fever, gastrointestinal or cardiovascular disorders, thyroid or liver dysfunction, and in the elderly. Monitoring plasma levels is strongly recommended.

Dosage and administration

The dosage of theophylline preparations should be adjusted to maintain a serum concentration of 10–20 microgram/mL (see previous comments on serum levels). Doses are increased gradually over several days while monitoring for adverse effects, and plasma concentration should be measured.

DRUG INTERACTIONS 15.1
Theophylline

DRUG	POSSIBLE EFFECTS AND MANAGEMENT
Aciclovir, alcohol, allopurinol, cimetidine, cipro- and norfloxacin, disulfiram, fluvoxamine, interferon alpha, macrolide antibiotics, oral contraceptives, propranolol	Theophylline concentration may be increased; its dose may need to be reduced
Phenobarbital (Phenobarbitone), phenytoin, rifampicin, ritonavir, sucralfate	Theophylline concentration may be decreased; its dose may need to be increased
β_2-agonists or diuretics	Theophylline can potentiate hypokalaemia caused by these drugs
Lithium, macrolides, pancuronium, phenytoin	Theophylline may decrease concentration of or response to these drugs, so dose of the other drug may need to be increased

than therapeutic levels. Other mechanisms proposed include inhibition of cyclic GMP-specific phosphodiesterase; competitive antagonism of adenosine at adenosine receptors (adenosine activates adenylate cyclase, and has cardiac-depressant, bronchoconstrictor, anti-inflammatory and platelet-aggregation-suppressant effects); increased histone deacetylase 2 activity, which may help reverse corticosteroid resistance; and selective inhibition of phosphoinositide 3-kinase, a regulator of inflammation. In treatment of asthma, theophylline derivatives act as bronchodilators, inhibit the late (inflammatory) phase of asthma and directly stimulate the medullary respiratory centre.

Anticholinergics

Plants from the *Atropa* or *Datura* genera have been smoked or inhaled for relief of respiratory symptoms for hundreds of years. These plants contain the alkaloids atropine or stramonium, competitive antagonists at muscarinic receptors. **Anticholinergics** produce bronchodilation by blocking vagal tone and parasympathetic reflexes mediating bronchoconstriction (Ch 8 and Fig 15.6); they may also decrease secretions and make them hard to expectorate. Typical 'atropinic side effects' are dry mouth and throat, urinary retention and constipation; anticholinergics can exacerbate glaucoma or prostatic hypertrophy. Anticholinergics include the short- and long-acting muscarinic antagonists (Matera et al. 2020a).

Short-acting muscarinic antagonist: ipratropium

The **short-acting muscarinic antagonist** (SAMA) ipratropium has useful bronchodilator actions after inhalation; and can be used as maintenance treatment in severe asthma and COPD (Table 15.3 and later discussion). Ipratropium is a quaternary (charged) ammonium compound, unlikely to cross the blood–brain barrier after administration, so has fewer adverse effects than does atropine.

Ipratropium is available as an MDI or nebuliser and may be used 3–4 times daily (commonly administered by paramedics in emergency situations).

Long-acting muscarinic antagonists

Long-acting muscarinic antagonists (LAMAs) include tiotropium, glycopyrronium bromide (glycopyrrolate), aclidinium and umeclidinium. LAMAs cause bronchodilation, have a duration of action of over 24 hours and are used once daily. Aclidinium is used twice daily. Tiotropium is more selective for M_3 receptors: it is inhaled via a DPI once daily and is longer acting than ipratropium. A newer product for tiotropium, Spiriva respimat, is a solution for inhalation.

The muscarinic antagonists should not be used prophylactically or for relief of symptoms, except in severe asthma, or COPD (e.g. ipratropium bromide (Atrovent)); instead, they are used as adjunctive controller therapy with corticosteroids (ICS). They can be used in combination with LABAs. Interactions with other drugs with anticholinergic effects are common, and combinations should be avoided.

They have a wide therapeutic margin when administered by inhalation, as there is little systemic absorption. However, if the aerosol mist or powder reaches the eyes, it can cause mydriasis, blurred vision and risk of glaucoma (see 'Mydriatics' and 'Cycloplegics' in Ch 40).

Novel classes of bronchodilators

As there is no single best drug to treat asthma, research is ongoing to find better therapies. Novel classes of bronchodilators being studied include:

- biological therapies, with targets that include IgE, IL-5, the IL-5 receptor and the IL-4/IL-13 receptor-α subunit
- e-type prostanoid receptor 4 agonists
- bitter-taste receptor agonists
- gene-2 relaxin hormone.

Preventers: prophylactic antiasthma drugs

These drugs are collectively known as **preventers**; they include the corticosteroids, cromones and newer drugs that prevent inflammatory responses.

Corticosteroids

Corticosteroids are used in chronic asthma to decrease airway obstruction. The adrenal cortex hormones are discussed in detail in Chapter 29; the anti-inflammatory and immunosuppressant actions of glucocorticoids such as cortisone and prednisolone are useful in asthma. Prophylactic use of ICS, preventing the late-phase inflammatory response and decreasing bronchial hyper-reactivity, has revolutionised the management of asthma. The products available now as DPI, pMDI or nebuliser forms (ICS) are beclometasone (Drug Monograph 15.4), budesonide, ciclesonide and fluticasone (furoate and propionate forms) – see Table 15.3, and Figure 15.7 (earlier) for stepwise adjustment of dosage in asthma management according to level of symptom control. A spacer should be used with a pMDI to enhance drug delivery to the airways including in children.

Mechanism of action

Corticosteroids enter the cytoplasm of cells, bind to specific glucocorticoid receptors, then translocate into the nucleus where they bind to response elements in target genes and bring about induction or repression of gene transcription. They also inhibit the enzyme phospholipase A_2, thereby inhibiting the production of COX enzymes and subsequently the production of PGE_2

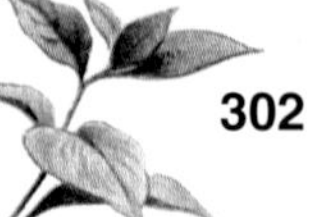

Drug Monograph 15.4
Beclometasone inhaled

Mechanism of action
As a glucocorticoid beclometasone inhibits both inflammatory cells and release of inflammatory mediators associated with the pathophysiology of asthma.

Indications
ICS are indicated for maintenance treatment and prophylaxis in persistent asthma.

Pharmacokinetics
A considerable proportion (up to 80%) of an inhaled dose of beclometasone is likely to be swallowed, then absorbed from the intestinal tract. Qvar breath activated formulations automatically release the metered dose through the mouthpiece and overcome the need for clients to coordinate actuation with inspiration. There is increased lung deposition and reduced oropharyngeal deposition compared with are these still around in order to make comparison with?

Peak plasma concentrations are reached 3–5 hours after administration; the drug is subject to metabolism in the liver and excretion in faeces and urine.

Adverse effects
Local adverse effects include dysphonia (changed voice), oropharyngeal candidiasis (oral thrush) and allergic reactions; systemic effects are rare.

Drug interactions
None are clinically significant; other antiasthma medications may be continued.

Warnings and precautions
- Oral deposition of drug (and hence oral infections and systemic absorption) can be reduced by use of a spacer and by rinsing the mouth and throat after each dose.
- The drug is not useful for acute asthma attacks because it is not a bronchodilator.
- If prescribed with an inhaled bronchodilator, the β_2-agonist or anticholinergic should be inhaled (to open the airways) before the corticosteroid.
- Dosage should not be reduced or stopped unless advised.
- Qvar is Category B3 and there is inadequate clinical evidence on safety. The therapeutic benefits of Qvar should be weighed against the potential hazards to the mother and baby.

Contraindications
Hypersensitivity to any ingredient.

Dosage and administration
Dosage starts at levels likely to be effective, and is reduced to the minimum dose that controls symptoms and then is 'stepped down' by 25% every 3 months if possible. Dosage may be doubled if asthma worsens or respiratory tract infection occurs.

and PGI_2. Their exact mechanism in asthma is still poorly understood but involves:

- decreased activation of lymphoid cells and eosinophils
- decreased production and action of many cytokines, including interleukins involved in chemotaxis and bronchospasm
- decreased generation of vasodilator PGs and the immunoglobulins IgE and IgG
- decreased histamine release from basophils and (long-term) decreased production of mast cells.

Overall, corticosteroids reduce both the early and the late (proliferative) stages of the inflammatory response. They are indicated prophylactically in maintenance treatment of severe asthma and COPD (e.g. LABA + long-acting anticholinergic + ICS), and in acute asthma and croup. The maximum improvement in pulmonary function may take 1–4 weeks.

Systemic administration and adverse effects
Regular systemic (oral) administration of corticosteroids can cause significant adverse 'cushingoid' effects, including adrenal suppression and growth suppression; altered deposition of muscle, fat, skin, hair and bone; ocular changes, infections, mineralocorticoid effects and psychological disturbances (Ch 29). This has led to the use of the alternate-day schedules of treatment. Systemic

corticosteroids are still used (e.g. short courses of prednisolone orally) when inhaled medications (corticosteroids, β_2-agonists, anticholinergics) and oral theophylline cannot adequately control asthma. In emergencies, corticosteroids may be administered parenterally (e.g. IV hydrocortisone, dexamethasone).

- Chemical modifications of the steroid molecule produced compounds such as beclometasone with enhanced absorption after inhalation and reduced risk of systemic adverse effects.
- Local effects of inhaled steroids include hoarse voice and oral or oesophageal candida infections. To prevent fungal infections, individuals are advised to rinse their mouth out with water after use of a corticosteroid inhaler.
- Frequent use of ICS may lead to a dose-related decrease in bone mineral density and increased risk of osteoporosis, so postmenopausal women taking inhaled steroids are advised to have their bone mineral density monitored every 2 years.

Glucocorticoid resistance

Resistance to steroid therapy can develop, and increase asthma severity without impairing the metabolic effects of steroids. There may be multiple endotypes represented by different immunological and inflammatory phenotypes.

Many mechanisms for steroid resistance have been proposed, including increased expression of a variant steroid receptor, over-expression of many cytokines (Th2, TNF-α and TGF-β), increased production of inflammatory mediators in macrophages, a reduction in histone deacetylase-2 activity and increased oxidative stress.

Cromones (mast-cell stabilisers)

Sodium cromoglycate (Clinical Focus Box 15.3) and nedocromil are examples of **cromones** (also known as cromolyns, or **mast-cell stabilisers**); these drugs are anti-inflammatory agents that inhibit the release of histamine, leukotrienes and other mediators of inflammation from mast cells and macrophages. They are inhaled 2–4 times daily, or 15 minutes before exercise, to reduce the risk of asthma attacks (in addition to maintenance doses). The puffers must be cleaned every day.

Mechanism of action

The mechanism is not clear: they are said to stabilise mast cells (Fig 15.4, earlier), but may also act by blocking chloride channels, suppressing activation of sensory nerves, desensitising neuronal reflexes and inhibiting release of cytokines, or acting through ion channels. Inhaled before an attack, the overall effect is to inhibit bronchoconstriction and reduce bronchial hyper-reactivity. Neither drug has any bronchodilator effect, nor do they have any effect on any inflammatory mediators already released in the body.

Other drug groups

Leukotriene-receptor antagonists (LTRAs)

The only **leukotriene-receptor antagonist** (Fig 15.4) currently used is montelukast. The mechanism of action of this drug group is blockade of receptors for the cysteinyl leukotrienes (LTC_4, LTD_4 and LTE_4), which are components of the 'slow-reacting substance of anaphylaxis (SRS-A)' as it is historically known; it is thought to be a mediator of inflammation in both early and late phases of asthma. They also inhibit other pro-inflammatory

CLINICAL FOCUS BOX 15.3
Sodium cromoglycate: a most unusual drug

Sodium cromoglycate, also known as cromolyn sodium and as [di]sodium cromoglycate, has many unusual properties:

- It was developed as an analogue of a plant compound khellin, a smooth muscle relaxant; however, it has no bronchodilator activity.
- It can reduce antigen-mediated bronchoconstriction.
- It is so highly water-soluble (with 11 oxygen atoms per molecule) that it is not absorbed to any useful extent from the gastrointestinal tract; thus, it is always administered topically, by DPI or MDI, or as eyedrops or nasal spray.

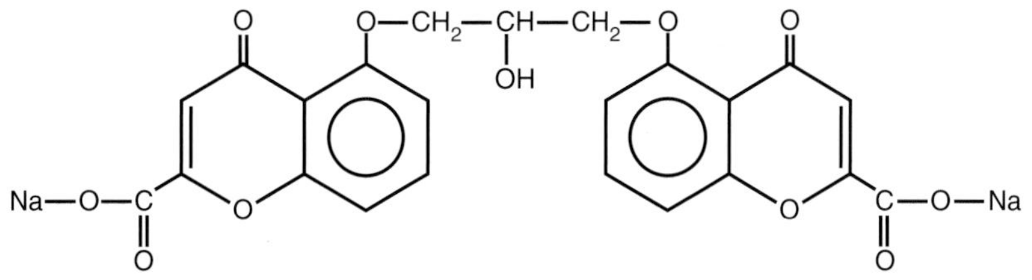

O—CH$_2$—CH—CH$_2$—O
OH
Na—O—C
C—O—Na

Sodium cromoglycate

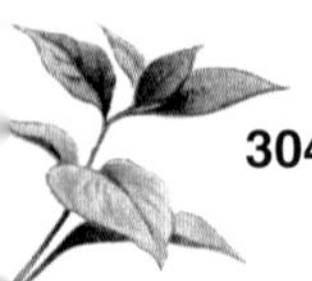

cytokines, so they reduce the inflammation, mucus secretion and bronchoconstriction associated with asthma.

Montelukast is not indicated for reversal of bronchospasm in acute asthma attacks, but has additive effects to β_2-agonists and is useful adjunctive therapy for those inadequately controlled with ICS, as it may allow a reduction in corticosteroid dosage. Improvement in asthma symptoms should be noted within a few days. In children older than 2 years, it may be used for mild persistent or frequent intermittent asthma.

Administered orally, montelukast is rapidly absorbed and has a rapid onset of action. Adverse effects include headache, nausea and abdominal upset or pain. Adverse neuropsychiatric events, including suicidal ideation, depression, aggressive behaviour and hallucinations, may occur; patients (and caregivers of young patients) are warned to seek medical advice. There appears to be limited evidence for congenital defects due to use in pregnancy and it is safe in breastfeeding women.

5-lipoxygenase inhibitors

This group of drugs act by inhibition of the enzyme 5-lipoxygenase, thus preventing synthesis of leukotrienes from arachidonic acid. Zileuton, no longer used in Australia, was the first of these drugs; approved in the United States, it reduces mucus plugs and constriction of bronchial airways. The late inflammatory response is also impaired; similar drugs are being tested in models of cancer and inflammatory disorders.

Monoclonal antibodies

Monoclonal antibodies used for reactive airways diseases include mepolizumab and omalizumab. Mast-cell activation is reduced by omalizumab, a recombinant humanised monoclonal antibody that complexes with free IgE antigens to prevent their binding to mast cells and the subsequent cascade of inflammation. The drug has a slow onset and long duration of action after subcutaneous injection; it effectively reduces IgE concentrations and asthma symptoms in people with allergic asthma, allowing reduction or cessation of steroid dosage. Interestingly, the drug itself can cause an anaphylactic reaction, and injection site reactions and bleeding. Its clinical use has been associated with an increased rate of malignancies, presumably because of reduced immune responsiveness.

Mepolizumab is a humanised monoclonal antibody (IgG1, kappa) that is indicated as an add-on treatment for severe refractory eosinophilic asthma in people aged 12 years or older.

The drug targets human interleukin-5 (IL-5) with high affinity and specificity. IL-5 is the major cytokine for the growth and differentiation, recruitment, activation and survival of eosinophils.

New drugs for asthma

New drugs are constantly being developed and tested for use in asthma, particularly as the pathogenesis is better understood. It has been reported that 5–10% of people have various subtypes of inadequately controlled and difficult-to-treat asthma. Newer, 'add on' therapies include biological therapies including monoclonal antibodies and drugs that target innate cytokines. In future, for severe asthma, therapies will target different phenotypes and endotypes (Pelaia et al. 2021).

Responses to antiasthma drugs can vary greatly, suggesting pharmacogenetic differences in the metabolising enzymes or receptors involved. Studies on variant polymorphisms of genes for β_2 receptors, M_2 or M_3 receptors, glucocorticoid receptors or cys-leukotriene receptors may assist understanding of variable responses and enhance personalised, targeted therapies.

KEY POINTS

Drugs used in the treatment of asthma

Asthma relievers/bronchodilators

- Bronchodilators include β_2-receptor agonists, methylxanthines and anticholinergics.
  - β_2-receptor agonists relax smooth muscle in airways by activation of β_2-adrenoceptors.
  - β_2-receptor agonists include the non-selective agonist adrenaline, SABAs including salbutamol and terbutaline and the LABAs or symptom controllers formoterol (eformoterol), salmeterol and indacaterol. LABAs may be combined with corticosteroids or anticholinergics.
  - The methylxanthines caffeine and theophylline can induce bronchial smooth muscle relaxation by the proposed inhibition of phosphodiesterase. Also proposed is the antagonism of adenosine at adenosine receptors.
  - Anticholinergics block the M_3 muscarinic receptors on bronchial smooth muscle leading to smooth muscle relaxation. They may also decrease airways' glandular secretions.
- SAMAs include ipratropium. The LAMAs include tiotropium, glycopyrronium bromide (glycopyrrolate), aclidinium and umeclidinium.

Preventers/controllers

- (Gluco)corticosteroids:
  - include beclometasone, budesonide, fluticasone and ciclesonide

- enter the cytoplasm, bind to specific glucocorticoid receptors, then translocate into the nucleus and bring about induction or repression of gene transcription. They also inhibit the enzyme phospholipase A_2. 'Cushingoid' effects, including adrenal suppression and growth suppression, are side effects of corticosteroids.

- Cromones (cromolyns):
  - are also known as mast-cell stabilisers and include sodium cromoglycate and nedocromil
  - inhibit the release of histamine, leukotrienes and other mediators of inflammation from mast cells and macrophages.
- Leukotriene antagonists:
  - block receptors for the cysteinyl leukotrienes
  - also inhibit other pro-inflammatory cytokines.
- 5-lipoxygenase inhibitors act by inhibition of the enzyme 5-lipoxygenase, preventing synthesis of leukotrienes from arachidonic acid.
- Monoclonal antibodies:
  - Omalizumab, a recombinant humanised monoclonal antibody, complexes with free IgE antigens to prevent their binding to mast cells.
  - Mepolizumab targets human interleukin-5 (IL-5) with high affinity and specificity.

Overview of asthma management

Combination therapy

Combined inhalers containing both a long-acting symptom controller and a corticosteroid preventer are now considered the 'gold standard' for asthma management; an example is formoterol (eformoterol) plus budesonide (ICS), thus reducing the risk of severe exacerbations compared with regimens with a single reliever. A combination is indicated for regular treatment of asthma when use of both drugs is appropriate. A budesonide (ICS)–formoterol (eformoterol; LABA) inhaler can be used as a reliever therapy as required, with the same inhaler used twice daily as maintenance therapy (Global Initiative for Asthma 2022; National Asthma Council Australia 2022).

The pharmacokinetic parameters of each drug appear to be unaffected by co-administration, and adverse reactions, precautions and interactions are as for each component drug. The advantages are: convenience of using only one inhaler, cost reduction, better control of asthma, regular use of a low-dose steroid and likely better compliance with therapy.

Suboptimal therapy

Despite the availability of several groups of drugs for the treatment of asthma, many of which date back thousands of years, asthma therapy is frequently not optimal, and there is still an unacceptably high level of mortality and morbidity. In particular, studies in children with asthma show that only 40% are well controlled. Possible reasons for unsuccessful therapy include:

- overreliance on short-acting bronchodilator relievers
- under-use of controller medications or inhaled corticosteroid preventers
- poor control over MDIs
- poor inhaler technique and poor compliance (Harris et al. 2016)
- low parental expectations of asthma control in children
- lack of understanding that asthma is a chronic condition
- lack of objective measurements of severity of asthma
- inadequate monitoring of therapy and compliance
- pharmacogenetic differences.

Stepwise management

Guidelines have been published by groups of specialist doctors to encourage appropriate evidence-based treatment. The emphasis in guidelines is on stepwise management, with treatment stepped up to stronger drugs to achieve good control of symptoms, and cautious stepping down after improvement and review of therapy. Asthma is classified and treated according to symptoms and severity. It is also important to assess future risk of adverse outcomes. Severity is determined retrospectively, after 2–3 months of treatment of specific symptoms. An example of the stepwise approach for management of adult asthma is shown in Figure 15.7 (earlier) (Global Initiative for Asthma 2020; National Asthma Council Australia 2020).

Chronic asthma

Before treatment of chronic asthma begins, severity needs to be assessed with spirometry/peak flow meters testing and trigger factors identified and managed. Treatment is tailored to suit the person and the severity. ICS are started at a dose sufficient to be effective, as monitored by peak-flow meter readings, then reduced to the minimum required to maintain control. Antibacterials are reserved for specific infections, antihistamines are rarely useful and sedatives are contraindicated because of agitation from dyspnoea.

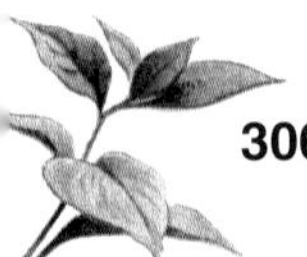

Acute asthma

Acute asthma is a life-threatening situation and may require systemic corticosteroids, adrenaline, aminophylline, oxygen and nebulised bronchodilators, and close monitoring of lung function, blood gases and CNS function. Adrenaline is one of the drugs commonly carried and used in ambulance vehicles; paramedics can administer it by nebuliser in severe asthma and croup, and also by intramuscular injection. (See also Drug Monograph 9.1 for its use in cardiac and anaphylactic conditions.) Drugs also administered include ipratropium bromide and salbutamol.

Asthma action plans

Each client should have an individualised written action plan, including education and self-management aspects, so clients can recognise their own symptoms, start and step-up treatment and promptly reach medical attention. Action plans need to consider factors such as closeness to hospital help, as people in rural areas face added risk factors (isolation, lack of support networks and seasonal high levels of environmental allergens).

Proposed by Australian and New Zealand groups through the National Asthma Council are various action plans that advise patients and carers to:

- ensure they know when and where to get medical care including in emergencies, who wrote the plan and its date
- achieve best lung function (regularly monitor FEV_1)
- assess the severity of the condition and symptom control
- identify and avoid trigger factors
- optimise a client's medication programs (minimise the number of drugs, doses and adverse effects)
- ensure they know their usual asthma and allergy medications and have clear instruction on how to change medications (example: when asthma is getting worse or substantially worse or when peak flow falls below an agreed rate)
- follow action plans
- educate the client, and review responses, lung function, compliance and inhaler technique regularly.

Specific stepwise plans are developed for exercise-induced asthma; asthma in athletes, children and infants, pregnant women, the elderly and travellers; occupational asthma, home management of acute asthma; and asthma in accident and emergency departments (see the Asthma Foundation Handbook and National Asthma Council: action plans – 'Online resources').

The Australian 'GP Asthma Initiative' promotes the 'Asthma Cycle of Care' plan as the best practice model for managing asthma. It involves at least two asthma-related consultations within 12 months for a person with moderate to severe asthma, with at least one of these visits (the review visit) planned (see Department of Health [Australian Government] and National Asthma Council in 'Online resources').

Asthma in pregnancy

Pregnant women tend to overestimate the risks of taking asthma medications; however, during pregnancy optimal asthma control is the priority, to maintain the health of the mother and fetus. Inhaled SABAs are safe throughout, and LABAs in the second and third trimesters if needed. Inhaled or oral corticosteroids appear to pose no risk to mother or child; budesonide may be preferred. Inhaled antiasthma drugs are safe for lactating women and their babies; however, spacing dose and breastfeeding times may be necessary when using oral corticosteroids. General advice is to take the dose immediately after feeding the baby.

Athletes with asthma

The World Anti-Doping Agency has responsibility for controlling the use of drugs by athletes, to keep sport drug-free. The main drugs prohibited during competitions include β_2-agonists, systemic adrenaline and corticosteroids. This poses problems for athletes with asthma. Most β_2-agonists are prohibited because they have anabolic actions: they can increase lean (muscle) mass and reduce body fat. While there is no evidence that they enhance sporting performance, they are often abused by athletes. The ban is relaxed for four β_2-agonists (salbutamol, salmeterol, formoterol [eformoterol] and vilanterol), which can be used via inhalation at recommended doses by athletes who have previously registered with their sporting authority as being asthmatic and been granted a Therapeutic Use Exemption.

KEY POINTS

Overview of asthma management

- Combined inhalers containing both a long-acting symptom controller and a corticosteroid preventer are now considered the 'gold standard' for asthma management.
- Despite the availability of several groups of drugs for the treatment of asthma, asthma therapy is frequently not optimal, and there is still an unacceptably high level of mortality and morbidity.
- Management plans for asthma involve educating the person, regular monitoring of lung function and compliance, avoiding trigger factors and evidence-based stepwise management with antiasthma drugs and individualised written asthma action plans.

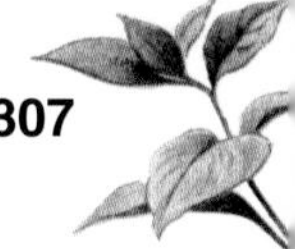

Drug treatment of chronic obstructive pulmonary disease

COPD, also known as chronic obstructive airways disease or as chronic airways limitation, is a disorder characterised by airflow obstruction that is not fully reversible. COPD is often associated with cough, emphysema, airways damage, excessive mucus and sputum production, and recurrent respiratory infections, so drugs used in respiratory tract infections may be indicated.

COPD includes three important disorders: chronic bronchitis, emphysema and chronic asthma with fixed airflow obstruction. Asthma (characterised by *reversible* airways narrowing) can occur with COPD. COPD typically affects middle-aged and older people. Cigarette smoking is the main aetiological factor, and stopping smoking is the only measure that slows progression. Inherited conditions such as deficiency of the α_1-antitrypsin enzyme predispose people to alveolar collapse and exacerbate smoking problems. Dyspnoea (difficult, laboured breathing) develops insidiously over many years and the FEV_1 is typically reduced to less than 70% of forced vital capacity. Cardiac disease and disordered breathing during sleep (sleep apnoea) are also common with COPD and need to be effectively treated. Management involves cessation of smoking, oxygen for hypoxaemia, regular immunisations, pulmonary rehabilitation (exercises, education and behavioural modification) and possible lung-reduction surgery for those with emphysema, plus drug therapy.

Drug therapy for COPD

Pathological changes of COPD cannot be reversed, but drugs may relieve symptoms, prevent or treat exacerbations, slow the decline and improve quality of life. The drugs used in COPD and in acute exacerbations are all considered in other sections of this chapter (Table 15.3), similar to those used in the treatment of asthma; a brief summary of their use in COPD follows.

Bronchodilators

Bronchodilators may be administered by puffer with a spacer or by nebuliser, starting with an inhaled SABA. Long-acting drugs such as salmeterol and indacaterol and tiotropium (and similar combinations) are effective at reducing symptoms and increasing exercise capacity. Tiotropium and glycopyrronium bromide (glycopyrrolate) may improve quality of life and reduce COPD mortality.

Inhaled corticosteroids

ICS (budesonide or fluticasone) can slow the decline in respiratory function and reduce mortality; however, there is increased risk of pneumonia. Oral corticosteroid for less than 14 days may reduce severity of exacerbations and hasten recovery.

Combination therapy

This can include a SABA or ipratropium bromide. Add or switch to LABA or LAMA for persistent symptoms. If still symptomatic use a LABA-LAMA combination and add an ICS if symptoms worsen (LABA + long-acting anticholinergic + ICS).

Oxygen

'Domiciliary oxygen' – that is, long-term continuous oxygen therapy in the home – for at least 15 hours per day reduces mortality in people with severe hypoxia (Table 15.1). There is less evidence of benefit from intermittent ambulatory oxygen therapy.

Other treatments

Other drugs used in COPD include theophylline, mucoactive agents (saline or acetylcysteine via nebuliser) and antibiotics specific to the current pathogen. Clients are recommended to have pneumococcal vaccination, severe acute respiratory syndrome coronavirus 2 (SARS-CoV-2; COVID-19) and annual influenza vaccination. Respiratory rehabilitation, exercise programs, weight reduction and antianxiety or antidepressant drugs are also effective and improve quality of life. Support networks with a multidisciplinary team of health professionals and self-management plans are important. Severe disease unresponsive to treatment may require lung volume reduction surgery or lung transplantation; in the terminal situation, palliative care should be considered.

Cessation of smoking

The most important measure to improve COPD is to quit smoking. Smoking is the largest single preventable cause of death and disability in Australia, causing respiratory disease including lung cancer, and increasing risk of cardiovascular, cerebrovascular and peripheral vascular disease. The pharmacological effects of nicotine are discussed in Chapter 8, and the social use and abuse of nicotine in Chapter 25.

Bronchiectasis

Bronchiectasis – chronic necrotising infection of the bronchi and bronchioles, with purulent sputum and airways damage – is usually due to CF but can occur in pneumonia and other respiratory diseases. Drugs useful in CF include expectorants and mucolytics along with antibiotics, bronchodilators, ICS, vaccinations (pneumococcal, influenza, COVID-19) and chest physiotherapy, as noted earlier.

Drugs used in respiratory tract infections

Treatment of viral infections

Most upper respiratory tract infections (URTIs), including acute bronchitis, are caused by viruses for which there are no safe, specific antiviral agents available. The recommended treatment is therefore symptomatic, as for the common cold. Refer to Chapter 43 for a discussion on vaccines and Chapter 37 for antivirals, in prophylaxis and treatment.

Viral infections are notorious for lowering the body's immune defences and predisposing the person to secondary bacterial infections, possibly dangerous in those with chronic conditions such as asthma, COPD or rheumatic heart disease. Antibiotics appropriate for the specific infecting bacteria may be prescribed, following current therapeutic guidelines (see Antibiotic Expert Group 2021). For example: for exacerbations of COPD with *Streptococcus pneumoniae,* use amoxicillin and doxycycline.

Common cold (coryza)

The viruses most commonly responsible for the common cold are RNA rhinoviruses, spread by contact and by droplets, often via the conjunctiva. The virus multiplies mainly in cells lining the nostrils, causing inflammation of the nose and throat, hence the common symptoms of redness and watery secretions of the nose, eyes and throat.

Development of vaccines against the common cold has been largely unsuccessful due to the different and variable antigenic types of rhinoviruses.

Treatment of the common cold is mainly symptomatic, with decongestants, antiseptics, expectorants, aspirin-like antipyretic analgesics and rest. Antihistamines, whisky or brandy, and 'hot toddies' have no proven efficacy in colds, other than as sedatives or placebos.

'Cough mixtures'

Cough is a protective reflex by which a sudden blast of compressed air from the bronchial tubes expels irritating, infective or obstructive material. 'Cough receptors' are sensory nerves (vagal afferents with terminals in airway walls) activated by various stimuli including inhaled foreign bodies, chemical irritants, inflammatory mediators, intraluminal material and mechanical stimulation to airway epithelium. Common causes of cough are URTIs, pollutants including cigarette smoke, asthma, COPD, gastro-oesophageal reflux and adverse reactions to drugs such as β-blockers and angiotensin-converting enzyme (ACE) inhibitor drugs (Ch 11).

Cough may also occur in more serious disorders such as CF, tuberculosis, bronchiectasis, lung cancer or heart failure. Such underlying disorders should be treated, rather than simply using a cough suppressant (antitussive agent).

As well as a cough suppressant (see opioids below), 'cough mixtures' may include (with varying degrees of efficacy):

- anticholinergics, expectorants and mucolytics (see earlier in this chapter)
- antihistamines
- antipyretic analgesics (commonly, paracetamol)
- sympathomimetic decongestants
- demulcent (soothing) liquids, flavouring and sweetening agents and alcohol.

The combination of a cough suppressant and an expectorant (cough stimulant) in a cough mixture is illogical and should be avoided. If there is bronchial hyper reactivity with the cough, an inhaled cromone or corticosteroid (e.g. beclometasone) may be effective. There is little evidence for efficacy other than demulcent (soothing) or placebo effect for over-the-counter cough mixtures in children with acute cough.[5] Cough and cold remedies for children under 2 years of age have been rescheduled to Prescription-Only (S4) due to reports of adverse events, accidental overdoses and lack of efficacy. Parents are advised to use simple remedies for their coughing children, such as rest, hydration and demulcents.

Opioid cough suppressants

Cough suppressants are reserved for a non-productive (dry, hacking) cough that is inadequately controlled by over-the-counter medications; the objective is to decrease the intensity and frequency of the cough, yet permit adequate elimination of tracheobronchial secretions and exudates. The underlying disorder should be treated first with the relevant agents; for example, cough secondary to gastro-oesophageal reflux may be relieved with histamine H_2-receptor antagonists and proton pump inhibitors (Ch 16).

Opioids such as morphine potently suppress the cough reflex by direct depression of the medullary cough centre, a mechanism unrelated to their analgesic or respiratory depressant actions. Codeine, pholcodine (Drug Monograph 15.5), dextromethorphan and dihydrocodeine exhibit less pronounced cough suppressant effects than morphine, with fewer adverse effects. They are widely used, and many products containing them are available over the counter (see also Chs 19 and 25). Pentoxyverine, an opioid-type cough suppressant that is an agonist at sigma-opioid receptors, is in some proprietary cough syrups used for dry cough.

Adverse effects

Opioids' clinical usefulness as cough suppressants is limited by adverse effects: they inhibit the ciliary activity of the respiratory mucous membrane, may cause bronchoconstriction in people with allergies or asthma and cause drowsiness, drug dependence and constipation.

5 It has been suggested that sugar and flavourings in cough syrups act by causing release of endogenous opioids – a possible explanation for Mary Poppins' tuneful observation that 'A spoonful of sugar helps the medicine go down'.

Drug Monograph 15.5
Codeine and pholcodine

Mechanism of action
Opioids produce antitussive effect by direct action on the cough centre of the medulla in the CNS.

Indications
Opioid cough suppressants such as codeine and pholcodine are indicated in non-productive cough for their depressant actions on the medullary cough centre. They are generally formulated as oral liquids known as linctuses or 'cough mixtures'.

Pharmacokinetics
Onset of action is rapid, with duration 6–8 hours. Codeine is normally metabolised to morphine and norcodeine, and metabolites are excreted by the kidneys. Pholcodine undergoes two-compartment distribution and extensive liver metabolism and has a very long elimination half-life, with metabolites and parent drug excreted in urine.

Drug interactions
Opioids have additive effects with other CNS depressants, including antihistamines and alcohol, and concurrent use should be avoided. Pholcodine has been linked to an increased risk of anaphylaxis with neuromuscular blocking drugs (Crilly & Rose 2014).

Adverse effects
These include drowsiness, respiratory depression, nausea, vomiting and constipation. Adverse effects in the CNS, including dependence and withdrawal, are more likely with codeine. Excessive constipation tends to limit use of codeine.

Warnings and contraindications
People should be warned of drowsiness and should not drive or operate machinery if affected. Avoid use in respiratory failure or asthma, in children or if the person has a productive cough.

Dosage and administration
The cough suppressant dosage of codeine for adults is 15–30 mg, 3–4 times daily, and for pholcodine 10–15 mg, 3–4 times daily. (For comparison, the analgesic oral dose of codeine, 200 mg, is equivalent in analgesia to 10 mg IM/SC morphine.)
Dosage should be reduced in renal or hepatic impairment and in the elderly.

Decongestants
Vasoconstriction in mucous membranes, leading to decongestion, may be achieved by the topical application of sympathomimetic amine **decongestants** such as xylometazoline (Drug Monograph 15.1), oxymetazoline, phenylephrine and pseudoephedrine, which stimulate α_1-adrenoceptors on vasculature leading to vasoconstriction. If administered systemically, these drugs cause generalised sympathetic effects including vasoconstriction, hypertension and cardiac stimulation.

Decongestion may also be achieved by blocking **muscarinic receptors**, which mediate increased respiratory secretions, with atropinic drugs such as ipratropium. The preferred treatment for 'blocked nose', especially in infants and children, is simply isotonic (0.9%) saline solution, as nasal drops or spray.

Influenza and coronavirus
Influenza is a common viral respiratory infection occurring during most winters, sporadically or in epidemics. Systemic symptoms of headache, myalgia, fever and chills occur 1–2 days before the respiratory symptoms (sore throat, cough, nasal obstruction).

Coronavirus disease (COVID-19) was first reported in Wuhan, China in late December 2019 and the World Health Organization declared a pandemic in early March 2020.

Vaccines currently in use include Vaxzevria (AstraZeneca) and the mRNA vaccines, Comirnaty (Pfizer) and Spikevax (Moderna). Refer to Chapter 43 for information on vaccine usage.

Vaccination
As with rhinoviruses causing the common cold, the influenza virus, for example, shows great antigenic variation with frequent mutations. Influenza vaccine (Drug Monograph 15.6) for active immunisation must be prepared regularly against strains currently in circulation. Vaccines are manufactured to conform to annual requirements of the Australian or New Zealand ministries of health; recommendations as to who should receive vaccination vary. Vaccination is strongly recommended for pregnant women, parents and guardians of young infants, health workers and community care workers, Indigenous Australians, people with underlying chronic conditions and those who are severely obese.

Approved indications for vaccines should be followed accurately, especially in children, with children being closely monitored after vaccination. Refer to Chapter 43 for further information.

Treatment of influenza
Otherwise healthy people with influenza infections are advised to treat symptoms with rest, increased fluid intake and paracetamol for fever; those at high risk of complications may be prescribed anti-flu drugs to minimise complications.

Zanamivir is a neuraminidase inhibitor for treating infections due to influenza viruses. Viral replication is inhibited by blocking the viral surface enzyme neuraminidase, preventing release of new virus from cells. This drug and oseltamivir have been reported to

Drug Monograph 15.6
Influenza vaccine

Influenza vaccines are prepared from viral cultures that have been inactivated, purified and preserved.

Indications

Administration of the current vaccine before winter induces antibodies against viral surface antigens and proteins, and provides protection against infection. Australian National Health and Medical Research Council recommendations are that the following groups be vaccinated annually:

- people over 65 years of age
- Aboriginal and Torres Strait Islander people over 50 years (and free annual influenza vaccine be made available for all Indigenous people (i.e. all aged 6 months and older))
- adults and children over age 6 months with chronic debilitating diseases, including severe asthma and diabetes mellitus
- children with congenital heart disease or CF
- adults and children on immunosuppressant therapy
- residents of chronic care facilities.

Adverse effects

Mild localised reactions, fever and malaise have been reported; very rarely, neurological reactions occur.

Warnings and contraindications

The vaccine is contraindicated during acute febrile illnesses, in people with allergies to neomycin, polymyxin or gentamicin and in those with allergies to egg proteins (because the virus vaccine is prepared in hen eggs).

Dosage and administration

One or two doses are administered intramuscularly or by deep subcutaneous injection; volume depends on age and brand/formulation. Several formulations are manufactured; not all are suitable for children, as those under 5 years are more likely to suffer febrile reactions.

have limited beneficial effect in the treatment of influenza, at best shortening the duration of symptoms by about half a day. Peramivir is a new drug in this class.

Amantadine is an antiviral drug that specifically inhibits replication of the A2 (Asian) flu strain; however, many strains have become resistant. Interestingly, amantadine is also used as an antiparkinsonian agent, as it has indirect dopamine-receptor agonist actions and blocks receptors for acetylcholine and NMDA.

An example of a new drug for the treatment of influenza (flu) as part of an international work-sharing initiative is Baloxavir marboxil (Xofluza). It is indicated for the treatment of uncomplicated influenza in people 12 years of age and older who have been symptomatic for no more than 48 hours and who are otherwise healthy, or at high risk of developing influenza complications.

Treatment of coronavirus

The treatment of coronavirus includes monoclonal antibodies and antivirals and well as symptomatic management. Monoclonal antibodies include Sotovimab (XEVUDY) and Asirivimab + imdevimab (RONAPREVE), an example of a new combination monoclonal antibody treatment, provisionally approved and included in the Australian Register of Therapeutic Goods for the treatment of COVID-19 in adults and adolescents aged 12 years. Other drugs provisionally approved include the antiviral remdesivir (VEKLURY) used to treat the severely unwell, requiring oxygen or high-level support to breathe, and in hospital care and nirmatrelvir + ritonavir (PAXLOVID) (see Therapeutic Goods Administration in 'Online resources').

Other respiratory tract infections

Antimicrobial agents are considered in detail in Chapter 36.

Pneumonia

Pneumonia involves inflammation of the lower respiratory passages (bronchioles) and alveoli arising from infections, irritation or toxic material. Clinical features include fever and chills, shortness of breath and tachypnoea, coughing of green or blood-stained sputum, tachycardia and use of accessory muscles in breathing. It is most common at the extremes of life and is frequently the specified cause of death in frail elderly people ('the old man's friend'). Significant predisposing factors include underlying cardiorespiratory disorders, influenza and immunodeficiency states.

Various pathogenic organisms may be involved; community-acquired pneumonia is most commonly caused by *Streptococcus pneumoniae* and there is often occupational exposure – for example, *Mycoplasma pneumoniae* in healthcare institutions and *Legionella pneumophila* from air-conditioning systems.

The spectrum of pathogens causing hospital-acquired pneumonia differs, and ill people are often immunocompromised, so recommendations for antibiotic therapy vary. Pneumococcal vaccines are recommended for elderly people and those who are immunocompromised or at particular risk.

Antibiotic therapy

Selection of appropriate antibiotics depends on identifying the pathogenic organisms (usually bacteria) and their levels of resistance; current local prescribing guidelines must be followed rigorously.

Tuberculosis

Globally, tuberculosis (TB; infection with *Mycobacterium tuberculosis*) is a leading cause of death from infection, second only to AIDS; it is estimated that one-third of the world's population has latent TB. People who are immunocompromised (e.g. HIV-AIDS) are at risk of becoming ill. In 2020 a total of 1.5 million people died from TB and there were an estimated 10 million new cases. 1.7 billion people were infected with tuberculosis. It is a notifiable disease in Australia, which has a very low prevalence (5.8 per 100,000 population in 2018). Incidence is highest in immigrants, especially those from South Asia and sub-Saharan Africa.

Many strains of *Mycobacterium tuberculosis* have developed resistance to previously effective antibiotics, so multidrug regimens are necessary in all cases for several months. Multidrug-resistant bacteria do not respond to isoniazid and rifampicin, and second-line drugs such as the aminoglycosides must be used.

Standard **d**irectly **o**bserved **t**reatment **s**hort-course therapy (DOTS, adopted by the World Health Organization in 1993) consists of combination chemotherapy, with rifampicin, isoniazid, pyrazinamide and ethambutol. Regimens with daily, twice-weekly or thrice-weekly doses for 2–6 months have been devised; taking the dose must be directly observed to ensure compliance This strategy leads to cure in about 95% of cases; recommendations for antimycobacterial drugs and regimens depend on local resistance patterns.

Croup

Croup (acute laryngotracheobronchitis) is an acute syndrome of hoarse voice, barking cough and noisy breathing usually occurring at night, with fever, runny nose and sore throat. Inflammation produces the classic high-pitched respiratory stridor. It is a common respiratory tract infection of childhood, usually occurring in autumn in children from 3 months to 3 years. Most cases have a viral aetiology: parainfluenza, respiratory syncytial virus or adenoviruses; no vaccine is available. Corticosteroids, either systemic or inhaled, are effective in reducing symptoms of airway obstruction and respiratory distress, and reduce time spent in hospital. Severe croup requires hospitalisation and nebulised adrenaline 0.1% with oxygen plus corticosteroids.

Whooping cough

Pertussis (whooping cough) is a highly contagious respiratory infection caused by the bacterium *Bordetella pertussis*. While infants (who have not been vaccinated) are most at risk of life-threatening disease, peak incidence now occurs in people aged over 15 years. Antibiotics, especially macrolides such as erythromycin, may reduce the infectious period, but have little effect on the duration or severity of the disease. Antibiotics effectively eliminate *Bordetella pertussis* from the nasopharynx. Antibiotic prophylaxis for household contacts reduces the risk of spread among infants. Azithromycin or clarithromycin or trimethoprim plus sulfamethoxazole are used. Booster vaccinations are recommended for adolescents and adults, at about 10-year intervals.

Nasal Infection

The nose can become a carrier site for infections, notably of *Staphylococcus aureus* in staff of hospitals, where methicillin-resistant *Staphylococcus aureus* can pose serious risks to immunocompromised people. An ointment containing the antibiotic mupirocin (2%) is formulated for administration to the nasal passages to treat nasal staph carriage.

KEY POINTS

Drugs used in COPD and respiratory tract infections

- COPD is best prevented by cessation of smoking; bronchodilators, ICS and oxygen are used.
- Cough suppressants such as opioids are used to reduce non-productive cough.
- Viral respiratory tract infections (e.g. cold, influenza, croup) are treated largely symptomatically, with antipyretic analgesics and decongestants.
- Bacterial infections (e.g. pneumonia, TB) are treated with antibiotics specific to the pathogenic organism.
- Complementary and alternative medicine treatments (CAMs) for respiratory disorders are discussed in Clinical Focus Box 15.4.

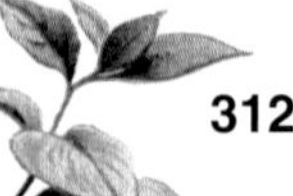

CLINICAL FOCUS BOX 15.4
CAMS for respiratory disorders

There are good pharmacological rationales for many traditional, complementary and alternative medicine treatments for respiratory disorders:

- Garlic and horseradish contain several antiallergy and moistening sulfur compounds.
- Coffee and tea contain xanthine bronchodilators.
- Saltpetre (potassium nitrate) is a smooth-muscle relaxant.
- The herb *Ephedra sinica* (ma huang), from traditional Chinese medicine, contains the bronchodilator ephedrine.
- New Zealand green-lipped mussels have anti-inflammatory actions.
- Echinacea extracts may stimulate phagocyte activity in the non-specific immune system.
- Fijian plants traditionally used are dilo (*Calophyllum inophyllum*) for TB, weleti (*Carica papaya*, pawpaw) for asthma, kalakalabucidamu (*Acalypha wilkesiana*) for pleurisy and uci flowers (*Euodia hortensis*) for chest colds.
- Various other Chinese, Japanese, Indian and Native American herbs are used, some of which may have steroidal components with anti-inflammatory activities.

Also tried are dietary methods (avoidance of allergenic foods; supplementation with fish oils, vitamin C, magnesium, selenium or zinc) and mind–body techniques, including meditation and biofeedback.

Volatile scented oils, discussed previously under 'Expectorants', are present in many cough and cold 'cures'. They may be inhaled in mists or sprays or vaporised over a candle. One popular over-the-counter ointment, Vicks Vaporub, formulated to be applied topically or inhaled via steam, contains oils of camphor, menthol, thymol, eucalyptus, turpentine, nutmeg and cedarleaf.

Indigenous Australians use native plants to treat cough and respiratory tract congestion, either by inhalation or drinking a decoction (tea) containing plant oils and cineoles with mucolytic and decongestant properties. These are present in eucalypt species, the liniment tree (*Melaleuca symphocarpa*), lemon grasses (Cymbopogon) and river mint (*Mentha australis*).

Sources: Adapted from Braun & Cohen 2015; Cambie & Ash 1994.

DRUGS AT A GLANCE
Drugs affecting the respiratory system

PHARMACOLOGICAL GROUP AND EFFECT	KEY EXAMPLES	CLINICAL USE
Medical gases	Oxygen Carbon dioxide Nitrous oxide Nitric oxide	Hypoxia Carbon monoxide poisoning Anaesthesia Respiratory stimulant in neonates
Analeptics	Caffeine	Respiratory stimulant
Drugs Affecting Secretions and Mucociliary Transport		
Pulmonary surfactants	Beractant Poractant	Respiratory distress in premature infants
Mucoactive agents Expectorants • Irritants • Diluents Mucolytics • Recombinant human deoxyribonuclease, a DNA-degrading enzyme that digests extracellular DNA released from degenerating neutrophils and cellular debris in purulent sputum Other • Increases osmotic pressure and acts to draw water out of cells, reducing viscosity of the mucus enhancing the hydrolysing activity of lysosomal enzymes Mucoregulators • Block muscarinic receptors on glands to reduce secretions	Guaifenesin Normal saline Dornase alfa Mannitol Bromhexine Ipratropium bromide	Respiratory tract infection Cystic fibrosis Respiratory tract infection

Drugs for allergic rhinitis Nasal corticosteroids • Inhibit gene transcription and the enzyme phospholipase A_2, inhibiting the production of inflammatory mediators H_1 receptor antagonists • Block histamine-induced vasodilation, thus decreasing capillary permeability, erythema and oedema, also antimuscarinic effects Sympathomimetic decongestants • Stimulate α-adrenergic receptors on vasculature and induce vasoconstriction Cromones • Prevent release of histamines from mast cells Anticholinergics • Block muscarinic receptors on glands to reduce secretions	Budesonide, fluticasone and mometasone Levocabastine Xylometazoline Sodium cromoglycate Ipratropium bromide	Allergic rhinitis
Drugs to treat asthma and COPD		
Relievers Bronchodilators Short-acting β_2-receptor agonists (SABAs) • Stimulate β_2-adrenoceptors in bronchial smooth muscle leads to relaxation of bronchial smooth muscle Methylxanthines • Proposed inhibition of phosphodiesterase (the enzyme that metabolises cAMP), leading to increased intracellular levels of cAMP, smooth muscle relaxation and bronchodilation • Inhibit cyclic GMP (guanosine monophosphate) specific phosphodiesterase • Competitive antagonism of adenosine at adenosine receptors Short-acting muscarinic antagonists (SAMAs) • Block muscarinic M_3 receptors on glands and smooth muscles to reduce secretions and relax smooth muscles of airways Long-acting muscarinic antagonists (LAMAs) • Block muscarinic M_3 receptors on glands and smooth muscles to reduce secretions and relax smooth muscles of airways (duration of action of over 24 hours)	Salbutamol and terbutaline Theophylline, aminophylline Ipratropium bromide Tiotropium, glycopyrronium bromide (glycopyrrolate), aclidinium and umeclidinium	Acute relief of asthma and COPD symptoms Acute relief of asthma and COPD symptoms (rarely used) Symptomatic treatment of asthma and COPD Maintenance treatment of asthma and COPD (with adjuncts; ICS, LAMA, LABA combinations)
Controller medications Long-acting β_2-receptor agonists (LABAs) • Allosteric binding of agonists at the β_2 receptors leads to prolonged relaxation of bronchial smooth muscle	Salmeterol Formoterol (eformoterol) Indacaterol	Maintenance treatment of asthma and COPD (with inhaled corticosteroids)
Preventer medications Corticosteroids • Inhibit gene transcription and the enzyme phospholipase A_2, inhibiting the production inflammatory mediators Monoclonal antibodies • Recombinant humanised monoclonal antibody, complexes with free IgE antigens to prevent their binding to mast cells • Target human interleukin-5 (IL-5) (inflammatory mediator) with high affinity and specificity Leukotriene-receptor antagonists (LTRAs) • Block receptors for the cysteinyl leukotrienes (LTC_4, LTD_4 and LTE_4), mediators of inflammation in both early and late phases of asthma; also inhibit other pro-inflammatory cytokines Oxygen • Reduces mortality in people with severe hypoxia	Fluticasone, budesonide, beclometasone Omalizumab Mepolizumab Montelukast	Maintenance treatment of asthma and COPD Maintenance treatment of moderate-to-severe allergic asthma in people treated with inhaled corticosteroids and with raised serum IgE levels Severe refractory eosinophilic asthma in those aged 12 years or older Maintenance treatment of asthma COPD Acute severe asthma
Drugs used in respiratory tract infections Cough suppressants (antitussives) • Suppress the cough reflex by direct depression of the medullary cough centre, acting at opioid receptors Decongestants • Sympathomimetic amine decongestants • Stimulate α_1-adrenoceptors on vasculature leading to vasoconstriction Muscarinic receptor antagonists • Block muscarinic M_3 receptors on glands in airways to reduce secretions	Dextromethorphan, codeine Xylometazoline, oxymetazoline, phenylephrine Ipratropium bromide	Productive cough Respiratory tract infection Allergic rhinitis Rhinorrhoea associated with allergic and non-allergic rhinitis, and common cold

Anti-influenza agents Vaccine • Prepared from viral cultures that have been inactivated, purified and preserved, stimulate immune response to antigen Neuraminidase inhibitors • Viral replication is inhibited by blocking the viral surface enzyme neuraminidase, preventing release of new virus from cells	Zanamivir Oseltamivir	Prevention of influenza infection

REVIEW EXERCISES

1. Mr BB attends his local pharmacy for salbutamol as he has been suffering from wheezing and chest tightness lately. He tells the pharmacist that his friend mentioned that he should try Ventolin spray. Two months later Mr BB attends his GP for a repeat prescription for his blood pressure medication; he is on metoprolol for hypertension. He mentions that he has been wheezing a lot lately. When questioned further, Mr BB admitted he had had asthma when a teenager, but no exacerbation since then. Explain to Mr BB why his asthma recurred, and suggest a change in prescription that might help prevent further episodes.
2. JS, a 12-year-old boy, is transported to the emergency department in acute respiratory distress with tachycardia, tachypnoea, moderately severe increased work of breathing with oxygen saturations 87% in room air and widespread wheeze; he is speaking in two- to three-word phrases. After medical assessment, 2.5 mg of nebulised salbutamol and supplemental oxygen 8 L/minute are delivered via face mask, then nebulised ipratropium bromide 250 micrograms. The salbutamol/ipratropium nebules are repeated at 20-minute intervals for a further two doses, with only temporary improvement in his breathing difficulties. IV access is obtained, and full cardiac monitoring is commenced. Hydrocortisone 4 mg/kg is administered IV stat. He is then loaded with IV aminophylline 10 mg/kg over 1 hour, and ambulance transfer is arranged to the nearest tertiary paediatric hospital for further care. Over the following 12 hours, the boy's air entry, respiratory effort and oxygen requirements begin to improve. What are the mechanisms of action of ipratropium bromide, hydrocortisone and aminophylline? Should the boy's daily inhaled corticosteroid preventer be continued while he is in hospital receiving methylprednisolone?
3. Ms RK is a 20-year-old student who suffers from allergic rhinitis, triggered by the dust and cat fur in her share house. She has been taking over-the-counter levocabastine spray for the past 3 months and, because this did not work sufficiently, she has been taking xylometazoline nasal spray three times daily for the past 2 months. She is finding that she is unable to breathe through her nose and the symptoms are not resolving. Discuss the clinical use of nasal decongestants and antihistamines. What could be the cause of her worsening symptoms?

REFERENCES

Antibiotic [published 2022 Feb]. In: Therapeutic Guidelines [digital]. Melbourne: Therapeutic Guidelines Limited; 2022 Feb. https://www.tg.org.au

Australian Medicines Handbook 2021: Australian medicines handbook 2020, Adelaide, AMH.

BOC Limited 2011. Medical gas cylinder data chart. Available from: https://www.boc-healthcare.com.au/en/quality-safety/safety-technical-data/medical-gas-cylinder-chart.html

Braun L, Cohen M: Herbs and natural supplements: an evidence-based guide, ed 4, Sydney, 2015, Elsevier.

Bromley SM: Smell and taste disorders: a primary care approach. American Family Physician. 2000; 61(2):427–436, 438.

Cambie RC, Ash J: Fijian medicinal plants, Australia, 1994, CSIRO.

Crilly H, Rose M: Anaphylaxis and anaesthesia: can treating a cough kill? Australian Prescriber 2014; 37(3):74–76.

Crisafulli E, Frizzelli A, Fantin A, et al: Next generation beta adrenoreceptor agonists for the treatment of asthma. Expert Opinion in Pharmacotherapy. 2017; 18(14):1499–1505.

Doty RL, Shah M, Bromley SM: Drug-induced taste disorders. Drug Safety 2008; 31(3):199–215.

Global Initiative for Asthma. Global Strategy for Asthma Management and Prevention, 2022. Available at: http://www.ginasthma.org.

Harris K, Mosler G, Williams S, et al: Suboptimal asthma control and asthma medication adherence in UK secondary school children. American Journal of Respiratory and Critical Care Medicine. 2020; 193: A2162.

Henkin RI: Drug-induced taste and smell disorders: incidence, mechanisms and management related primarily to treatment of sensory receptor dysfunction. Drug Safety 1994; (5): 318–377.

Kim SJ, Port AD, Swan R, et al. Retinopathy of prematurity: a review of risk factors and their clinical significance. Survey of Ophthalmology. 2018; 63(5):618–637. doi:10.1016/j.survophthal.2018.04.002

Kuruvilla ME, Lee FE, Lee GB. Understanding Asthma Phenotypes, Endotypes, and Mechanisms of Disease. Clinical Reviews in Allergy and Immunology. 2019; 56(2):219–233. doi:10.1007/s12016-018-8712-1

Masel P: Management of cystic fibrosis in adults. Australian Prescriber 2012; 35(4):118–121.

Matera MG, Belardo C, Rinaldi M, et al. 2020a. Emerging muscarinic receptor antagonists for the treatment of asthma. Expert Opinion in Emergency Drugs. 2020; 25:2, 123–130, DOI: 10.1080/14728214.2020.1758059

Matera MG, Page CP, Calzetta L, et al. 2020b. Pharmacology and Therapeutics of Bronchodilators Revisited. Pharmacological Reviews 72(1):218–252. doi: 10.1124/pr.119.018150. PMID: 31848208.

Ministry of Health. 2018. Annual Data Explorer 2018/19: New Zealand Health Survey. Wellington: Ministry of Health. URL: https://minhealthnz.shinyapps.io/nz-health-survey-2018-19-annual-data-explorer.

NAC (National Asthma Council Australia) 2018. National Asthma Strategy 2018. Melbourne: National Asthma Council Australia. AIHW

National Asthma Council Australia. Australian Asthma Handbook. Version 2.2. Melbourne: National Asthma Council Australia; 2022. http://www.asthmahandbook.org.au [cited 2022 Sep 13]

Nevitt SJ, Thornton J, Murray CS, et al. Inhaled mannitol for cystic fibrosis. Cochrane Library. 2020; 5(5), CD008649. https://doi.org/10.1002/14651858.CD008649.pub4

Page C, O'Shaughnessy B, Barnes P: Pathogenesis of COPD and asthma. Handbook of Experimental Pharmacology 2017; 237:1–21.

Pain and Analgesia [published 2021 Mar]. In: Therapeutic Guidelines [digital]. Melbourne: Therapeutic Guidelines Limited; 2021 Mar. https://www.tg.org.au

Pelaia C, Pelaia G, Crimi C, et al. Biologics in severe asthma. Minerva Medica 2021; Feb 8. doi: 10.23736/S0026-4806.21.07296-7.

Rang HP, Dale MM, Ritter JM, et al: Pharmacology, ed 5, Edinburgh, 2003, Churchill Livingstone.

Respiratory Expert Group: Therapeutic guidelines: respiratory, edn 6, Melbourne, 2020, Therapeutic Guidelines Limited.

Salerno E: Pharmacology for health professionals, St Louis, 1999, Mosby.

Trivedi R, Richard N, Mehta R, et al: Umeclidinium in patients with COPD: a randomised, placebo-controlled study. European Respiratory Journal. 2014; 43:72–81.

Villanueva G, Marceniuk G, Murphy M S, et al. Diagnosis and management of cystic fibrosis: summary of NICE guidance. The BMJ. 2017; 359: j4574 doi:10.1136/bmj.j4574

Waugh A, Grant A: Ross & Wilson Anatomy & Physiology in Health and Illness, ed 12, London, 2014, Churchill Livingstone.

ONLINE RESOURCES

Asthma and Respiratory Foundation (New Zealand): http://www.asthmafoundation.org.nz/ (accessed 20 January 2022)

Asthma Australia: https://www.asthmaaustralia.org.au (accessed 20 January 2022)

Australian Government Department of Health (search keyword 'asthma'): http://www.health.gov.au/ (accessed 20 January 2022)

BOC Limited: http://www.boc.com.au/ (accessed 20 January 2022)

Cystic fibrosis: https://www.cysticfibrosis.org.au/ (accessed 20 January 2022)

Global Initiative for Asthma: http://www.ginasthma.org/ (accessed 20 January 2022)

Global Initiative for Chronic Obstructive Lung Disease (GOLD): global strategy for the diagnosis, management and prevention of COPD: http://www.goldcopd.org/ (accessed 20 January 2022)

Medsafe (for specific New Zealand drugs): http://www.medsafe.govt.nz/ (accessed 20 January 2022)

National Asthma Council – Australian asthma handbook: https://www.nationalasthma.org.au/health-professionals/australian-asthma-handbook (accessed 20 January 2022)

National Asthma Council Australia – Action plans: https://www.nationalasthma.org.au/health-professionals/asthma-action-plans/asthma-action-plan-library (accessed 20 January 2022)

National Asthma Council Australia – Asthma cycle of care: https://www.nationalasthma.org.au/living-with-asthma/resources/health-professionals/reports-and-statistics/asthma-cycle-of-care (accessed 20 January 2022)

National Asthma Council Australia – Asthma mortality statistics: https://www.nationalasthma.org.au/living-with-asthma/resources/health-professionals/reports-and-statistics/asthma-mortality-statistics (accessed 20 January 2022)

National Asthma Council Australia – Inhaler technique: https://www.nationalasthma.org.au/living-with-asthma/resources/health-professionals/information-paper/hp-inhaler-technique-for-people-with-asthma-or-copd (accessed 20 January 2022)

Therapeutic Goods Administration – COVID-19 treatments provisional determinations: https://www.tga.gov.au/covid-19-treatments-provisional-determinations (accessed 20 January 2022)

World Anti-Doping Agency: http://www.wada-ama.org/en/ (accessed 20 January 2022)

World Health Organization: http://www.who.int/tb/en/ (accessed 20 January 2022)

More weblinks at: http://evolve.elsevier.com/AU/Knights/pharmacology/.

CHAPTER 16

DRUGS AFFECTING THE UPPER AND LOWER GASTROINTESTINAL TRACT

Shaunagh Darroch

KEY ABBREVIATIONS

CTZ	chemoreceptor trigger zone
GIT	gastrointestinal tract
GORD	gastro-oesophageal reflux disease
IBS	irritable bowel syndrome
KGF	keratinocyte growth factor
NERD	non-erosive reflux disease
NSAIDs	non-steroidal anti-inflammatory drugs
PEG	polyethylene glycol
PPI	proton pump inhibitor

KEY TERMS

antidiarrhoeal 343
antiemetics 335
constipation 339
Crohn's disease 344
cytoprotective agents 329
diarrhoea 339
gastrin 325
gastritis 325
gastrointestinal tract 318
gustation 322
H_2-receptor antagonists 330
Helicobacter pylori 325
histamine 325
histamine (H_2) receptors 330
inflammatory bowel disease 344
irritable bowel syndrome 344
laxatives 340
parietal cells 325
pepsin 325
peristalsis 319
ulcerative colitis 344

Chapter Focus

This chapter reviews the various topical and systemic medications used to treat illnesses or disorders affecting the upper and lower gastrointestinal tract. Many gastrointestinal disorders – such as peptic ulcers, nausea and vomiting, constipation, diarrhoea, inflammatory bowel disease and irritable bowel syndrome – negatively impact affected individuals, and knowledge of the drugs used can improve the quality of a person's life. Drugs discussed include dentifrices, mouthwashes and gargles, antacids and proton pump inhibitors, antiemetics, laxatives, antidiarrhoeal drugs and drugs used to treat inflammatory bowel disease.

KEY DRUG GROUPS

Antiemetics:

- Dopamine antagonists: **domperidone**, **metoclopramide** (Drug Monograph 16.3), **prochlorperazine**
- Miscellaneous: dexamethasone, lorazepam
- Muscarinic receptor antagonists: **hyoscine hydrobromide**
- NK_1-receptor antagonists: **aprepitant**, **fosaprepitant**
- 5-HT_3-receptor antagonists: **granisetron**, **ondansetron** (Drug Monograph 16.4), **palonosetron**, **tropisetron**

Drugs affecting the mouth:

- Dentrifices
- Drugs used to treat mouth blistering
- Drugs used to treat oral candidiasis: **nystatin** (Drug Monograph 16.1)
- Drugs used to treat oral mucositis: **palifermin**
- Mouthwashes and gargles
- Saliva substitutes

Drugs that neutralise or inhibit gastric acid secretion:

- Antacids: magnesium–aluminium combinations
- Cytoprotective agents: **misoprostol**, **sucralfate**
- H_2-receptor antagonists: **famotidine**, **nizatidine**, **ranitidine**
- Proton pump inhibitors: **esomeprazole**, lansoprazole, **omeprazole** (Drug Monograph 16.2), pantoprazole, rabeprazole
- ***Helicobacter pylori*** **treatment regimens:** e.g. proton pump inhibitor, clarithromycin, amoxicillin

KEY DRUG GROUPS—cont'd

Antidiarrhoeal drugs:

- **Diphenoxylate**, **loperamide**

Drugs that affect the lower gastrointestinal tract:

- laxatives
- antidiarrhoeals

Drug therapy for inflammatory bowel disorders:

- Corticosteroids

5-aminosalicylates (5-ASA)

- **Balsalazide**, **mesalazine** (Drug Monograph 16.6), **olsalazine**, **sulfasalazine**
- Immunosuppressants
- TNF-a [alpha symbol] antagonists

Laxatives:

- Bulk forming: psyllium
- Faecal softening: **docusate**
- Stimulant: **bisacodyl**, **senna**
- Osmotic: **lactulose** (Drug Monograph 16.5)

CRITICAL THINKING SCENARIO

A 21-year-old man, Patrick, was admitted to the emergency department of a hospital complaining of nausea/vomiting and cramping periumbilical pain. The initial diagnosis was bacterial gastroenteritis. He was admitted to the short stay ward and treated with intravenous fluids and antibiotics. He subsequently improved and was discharged.

Two weeks later, Patrick presented again with complaints of recurrent abdominal pain, new-onset diarrhoea and rectal bleeding. He complained that he was losing weight. A CT scan of the abdomen/pelvis revealed ileal thickening and a small bowel obstruction. Colonoscopy revealed ulcerations of the ileum and colon consistent with ulcerative colitis. Patrick was prescribed mesalazine and prednisolone.

1. Describe the mechanism of action of mesalazine.
2. If Patrick continues to vomit, what are the options for dosages of mesalazine?
3. What are the precautions associated with this drug?
4. Why was he also prescribed prednisolone?

Introduction: The gastrointestinal system, gastrointestinal disease and drugs affecting the gastrointestinal system

Disorders of the upper **gastrointestinal tract** (GIT), such as indigestion, gastritis and peptic ulcers, are common problems reported by a large proportion of the population. Disorders affecting the entire lower GIT are diarrhoea and constipation, while others affecting the large intestine include diverticular disease, inflammatory bowel disease, irritable bowel syndrome and carcinoma. The causes of many gastrointestinal diseases remain unclear. Various medications are used to treat illnesses or disorders affecting the upper and lower GIT, although drug treatment is often focused on relieving symptoms rather

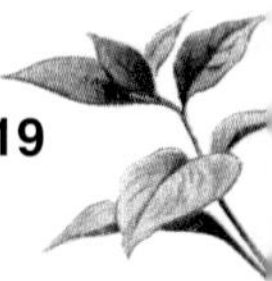

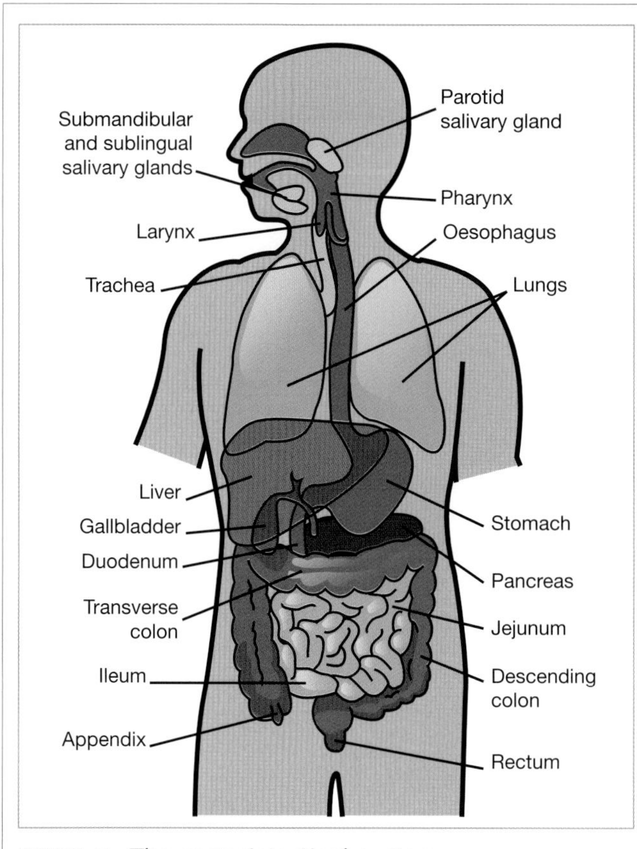

FIGURE 16.1 The gastrointestinal system

Source: Salerno 1999, Figure 34.1.

than on control or cure. A fundamental understanding of the anatomy and physiology of the gastrointestinal system is important to understand its associated pathophysiology and pharmacology.

The digestive system has four main activities – motility, secretion, digestion and absorption – and is made up of the GIT, also called the alimentary canal, and the accessory organs of digestion such as the teeth, tongue, biliary system (liver and gall bladder) and pancreas (Fig 16.1). Mechanical digestion involves processes such as chewing and churning, while chemical digestion relies on secretion of digestive enzymes such as those in the mouth (salivary amylase), stomach (pepsin) and small intestine (pancreatic amylase). Movements by the smooth muscle fibres surrounding the GIT mix the contents by segmental contractions and propel the material through the tract by **peristalsis**.

The secretory and muscular activities of the GIT are regulated by both intrinsic and extrinsic neural mechanisms.

Neuronal control of the gastrointestinal system

Intrinsic neuronal control of the GIT is via the enteric nervous system, an interconnecting network of neurons that innervates, for example, the in smooth muscle and secretory cells of the GIT and relays information via the autonomic nervous system and local reflexes. This intrinsic system is self-regulating and is capable of controlling exocrine gland secretions and muscular contractions independently of the central nervous system (CNS). Neurotransmitters in the enteric nervous system include acetylcholine, nitric oxide, 5-hydroxytryptamine (5-HT, serotonin) and substance P. The extrinsic innervation of the GIT is supplied by the divisions of the autonomic nervous system (Chs 8 and 9). These divisions coordinate activities among different regions of the GIT; plus, there is communication between the GIT and the CNS. The parasympathetic division relays nerve impulses via two branches of the vagus nerve and exerts mostly an excitatory action, which increases digestive secretions and muscular activity. The splanchnic nerves of the sympathetic division are primarily inhibitory nerves and decrease digestive secretions and muscular activity. Under normal conditions, the two divisions of the autonomic nervous system and the enteric nervous system maintain a delicate balance of control over the functions of the GIT.

KEY POINTS

The gastrointestinal system

- There are four main activities of the digestive system: motility, secretion, digestion and absorption.
- The primary functions of the gastrointestinal system are digestion and absorption. These processes are facilitated by the motile and secretory properties of the GIT and associated organs.
- The secretory and muscular activities of the GIT are regulated by both intrinsic and extrinsic neural mechanisms.

The upper gastrointestinal tract

The upper GIT consists of the mouth (buccal cavity) and pharynx, oesophagus, stomach and the accessory organs – the pancreas, liver and gall bladder. Drugs are used to maintain oral hygiene and to treat the various disorders affecting the function of the upper GIT.

The mouth (buccal cavity) and pharynx

The mouth, or buccal cavity, functions as the starting point of the digestive process. Ingested food is chewed and mixed with saliva that contains the enzymes amylase, which initiates the breakdown of disaccharide sugars and starches (polysaccharides), and lingual lipase, which initiates digestion of dietary triglycerides (fats).

Three pairs of salivary glands secrete saliva via ducts into the mouth – the sublingual and submandibular salivary glands and the parotid glands. When food has been chewed and is reduced to a soft spongy mass in the mouth, it is swallowed. Swallowing (deglutition) is a complex process that begins as a voluntary movement but is continued as an involuntary muscular reflex as the bolus of food is propelled through the pharynx into the oesophagus.

Systemic diseases, nutritional deficiencies and mechanical trauma can cause irritation or inflammation of buccal structures. Dental disorders (e.g. caries and gingivitis) and bacterial, viral or fungal infections (e.g. candidiasis or herpes simplex) can affect the structures of the oral cavity, causing symptoms such as mouth blistering or other lesions, swelling, pain and inflammation. The pharynx (throat), which connects the mouth and the oesophagus, is important in swallowing. When food and fluid pass through the pharynx into the oesophagus, the trachea is closed to prevent aspiration into the lungs and respiration is inhibited. The oral and pharyngeal phases of swallowing last less than one second. Like the mouth, the pharynx can be affected by viral infections and become irritated and inflamed (e.g. due to sinusitis or the common cold; see Ch 15). Neurological lesions and cerebrovascular accidents involving the medulla and the swallowing centre can result in difficulties in the pharyngeal phase of swallowing. (See the discussion of the skeletal motor system in Ch 8.)

Drugs affecting the mouth

Good oral hygiene – which includes brushing the teeth properly after meals and at bedtime, flossing and gum stimulation – has a major influence on the health of the tissues of the mouth. Many mouth and throat preparations containing anti-inflammatory agents, anaesthetics and antiseptics are available for various disorders of the oral cavity, including chapped lips, sun and fever blisters, inflammatory lesions, ulcerative lesions secondary to trauma, gingival lesions, teething pain, toothache, irritation caused by orthodontic appliances or dentures, and oral cavity abrasions. Most topical agents that affect the mouth may be purchased over the counter. In addition, some medications may cause dry mouth as an adverse effect (e.g. muscarinic receptor antagonists such as atropine and the anticholinergic drugs used to treat Parkinson's disease), and prolonged loss of secretions may contribute to poor oral health (Deutsch & Jay 2021).

Mouthwashes and gargles

Mouthwashes and gargles are dilute aromatic solutions that often contain a sweetener and an artificial colouring agent. They may also contain an antiseptic (e.g. alcohol, cetylpyridinium chloride or chlorhexidine gluconate), an anaesthetic (e.g. benzocaine, lignocaine hydrochloride), an analgesic (e.g. choline salicylate) or an anticaries agent (sodium fluoride). Using mouthwashes with high alcohol content may be problematic in some groups of the general population (e.g. children and people with cultural or religious objections to alcohol use). The leading mouthwashes usually contain 7–30% alcohol and the use of a mouthwash in young children is not recommended, as children often swallow the mouthwash rather than expectorating it. Products that inhibit plaque formation are available, and clinical trials have demonstrated some success with volatile oils and the antiseptics cetylpyridinium chloride and chlorhexidine.

Mouthwashes are often used for halitosis, or 'bad breath'. They can improve mouth odour briefly; however, if such a problem persists, the underlying cause (e.g. poor dental hygiene or various gum diseases) needs to be identified and treated. Mouthwashes containing anaesthetics and antibacterials are also used as gargles to treat colds or sore throats. They are generally not considered effective for such problems. Sore throats are usually caused by infection, most often viral rather than bacterial. Gargling might not reach the site of infection, which is often deep in the throat tissues. In addition to commercial preparations (e.g. Betadine Sore Throat Gargle), sodium chloride solution (half a teaspoon of salt in an average-sized glass of warm water) has been commonly used as a gargle and mouthwash. Non-alcoholic chlorhexidine mouthwash can inhibit plaque formation and may be used in moderate-to-severe gingivitis, as an adjunct to improved oral hygiene and teeth scaling by dentist. In more severe cases antibacterial treatment may be required.

Several fluoride-containing preparations, including mouthwash, toothpaste, tablets and solutions, are available for use as anticaries agents. The exact mechanism of action of fluoride in preventing caries is not fully understood; however, fluoride ions appear to exchange for hydroxyl or citrate (anion) ions and then settle in the anionic space in the surface of the enamel. This results in a harder outer layer of tooth enamel (a fluoridated hydroxyapatite) that is more resistant to demineralisation. Fluoridated mouthwashes have been used in communities with both limited fluoridated and unfluoridated water supplies, and their use has been associated with a significant decrease in tooth decay.

Fluoridated mouthwashes are generally rinsed for a minute and expectorated, preferably after brushing and flossing. Eating and drinking should be avoided for about 30 minutes after use.

Dentifrices

A dentifrice is a substance used to aid in cleaning teeth and is also available for treating hypersensitive teeth. Ordinary dentifrice contains one or more mild abrasives, a foaming agent and flavouring materials made into a powder or paste (toothpaste) to be used as an aid in the mechanical cleansing of accessible parts of the teeth. Fluoride dentifrices are effective anticaries agents. Dentists often suggest desensitising dentifrices that contain potassium nitrate, such as Sensodyne toothpaste.

Saliva substitutes

Saliva substitutes such as Biotene moisturising mouth spray and Biotene Oralbalance gel are used to relieve dry mouth caused by factors such as salivary gland dysfunction or occurring as a result of drug administration (e.g. anticholinergics and tricyclic antidepressants). Available as solutions and as pump sprays and gels, saliva substitutes contain electrolytes (potassium, magnesium, calcium and sodium chloride), potassium phosphate, saccharin, sorbitol solution and carboxymethylcellulose as the base.

Drugs used to treat mouth blistering

Acute viral diseases such as herpes simplex, herpes zoster and varicella are treated symptomatically with antipyretic analgesics such as paracetamol and aspirin. In worsening cases and in recurrent herpetic infection, treatment with the antiviral drug aciclovir should be considered. Aciclovir acts to reduce viral shedding, time to crusting, duration of local pain and severity of symptoms. In addition to viral infections, mouth lesions can be caused by local irritation, medications, radiation, dental manipulations or systemic disease. Instituting proper treatment involves initial identification of the causative factor.

Drugs used to treat oral candidiasis

The term 'candidiasis' ('thrush') is used commonly to refer to a superficial fungal infection; in the case of the mouth, rarely are fungi other than *Candida* involved. Local factors predisposing to an outbreak of visible oral fungal lesions include smoking, the wearing of dentures, decreased salivation and the use of inhaled corticosteroids. In some people, however, the precipitating factor may be associated with systemic antibiotic or corticosteroid use or cancer chemotherapeutic treatment regimens. Although there are various antifungal agents, amphotericin (lozenge), miconazole (oral gel) and nystatin (oral tablets, capsules and oral suspension) are the most commonly used drugs for oral candidiasis. In contrast, in severely immunocompromised people, the oral antifungal drug fluconazole is preferred. Only nystatin will be reviewed in this section (Drug Monograph 16.1), as the azole antifungal agents are discussed in Chapter 37.

Drugs used to treat oral mucositis

Inflammation of or injury to the mucous membrane of the mouth and throat may result from several factors, including infections, use of chemotherapeutic agents (e.g. high-dose methotrexate) and irradiation. In some cases, mucositis is associated with an increased risk of severe or life-threatening infections. Treatments vary depending on the cause and include basic oral care (e.g. brushing, flossing) and use of mouthwashes, topical antifungal drugs, topical and systemic analgesics and the recombinant human keratinocyte growth factor palifermin.

Palifermin is a recombinant truncated version of endogenous keratinocyte growth factor and has similar biological activity to the native protein, but with increased stability. Keratinocyte growth factor (KGF) is a member of the family of fibroblast growth factors and binds to KGF receptors, which are located on epithelial cells of the tongue, buccal mucosa, salivary glands, oesophagus, stomach and various other tissues of the GIT. Activation of KGF receptors leads to proliferation, differentiation and migration of epithelial cells.

Palifermin treatment results in an increase in the thickness of oral epithelium, decreased ulcer formation and a reduction in atrophy of the oral mucosa. It is only available in Australia under the Special Access Scheme.

KEY POINTS

The mouth and pharynx

- The mouth, or buccal cavity, functions as the starting point of the digestive process.
- Drugs affecting the mouth and pharynx include a variety of medications and formulations:
  - Dentrifices are used to clean teeth and to treat sensitive teeth, and include toothpastes (also for sensitive teeth).
  - Saliva substitutes are used in syndromes where there is underproduction of saliva or where medications have suppressed the secretion of saliva (e.g. anticholinergics).
  - Mouthwashes, gargles and dentifrices are used for maintaining oral hygiene. Mouthwashes and gargles are used for halitosis and to treat sore throats (e.g. contain antiseptics and local anaesthetics).

- Topical antivirals are used to treat viral diseases with associated mouth blistering.
- Antifungals such as nystatin are one of the most commonly used drugs to treat oral candidiasis. Nystatin is administered as tablets, capsules and oral suspension and miconazole (oral gel). The term 'candidiasis' ('thrush') is used commonly to refer to a superficial fungal infection; in the case of the mouth, rarely are fungi other than *Candida* involved.
- Palifermin, a keratinocyte growth factor used to stimulate the growth of mucosa, is used to treat oral mucositis.

Gustation: The sense of taste

Gustation (the sense of taste) is a chemical sense closely linked to smell, but it is much less sensitive. The sense of taste aids in the appreciation and normal digestion of foods and helps protect against toxins and pollutants. Molecules dissolved in saliva in the mouth are sensed by gustatory receptors on taste buds (specialised epithelial cells) located mainly on the back of the tongue and elsewhere in the mouth, throat and oesophagus. The chemical contacts a gustatory 'hair' passing through a pore on the surface of the cell, stimulating receptors on the membrane and inducing action potentials in the primary afferent sensory neurons that make contact with the receptor cells. The chemical information is transduced into cellular signals via stimulation of G-protein-coupled membrane receptors, second messengers, enzymes and ion channels. Subsequent neurons in the taste pathway run via the pons and medulla to the thalamus, then to the taste centre in the parietal lobe of the cerebral cortex, where the taste is perceived. Trace metals, especially zinc and copper, are involved at the active site of taste receptors, and zinc or copper deficiencies may cause loss or distortion of taste. Other common causes of taste

Drug Monograph 16.1
Nystatin

Nystatin is a polyene antifungal product of *Streptomyces noursei* and was one of the first antifungal drugs to be discovered and used clinically. It exhibits fungicidal activity against a broad spectrum of fungal pathogens (e.g. *Candida albicans*, *Candida krusei* and *Candida tropicalis*). It is used to treat cutaneous, intestinal, oropharyngeal and vulvovaginal candidiasis.

Mechanism of action

It is thought to exert its effect by interacting with the sterol moiety of ergosterols primarily in the cell membrane (Ch 37). This interaction leads to the formation of pores or channels that result in leakage of essential intracellular components such as ions, amino acids and sugars.

Pharmacokinetics

Nystatin is not absorbed from mucous membranes of the mouth, GIT and vagina, or from the skin, and most passes unchanged in the stools. Due to systemic toxicity, as occurs when low amounts may be absorbed due to tissue inflammation, its use is limited to treat mucocutaneous and intestinal candidiasis.

Drug interactions

Nystatin is not metabolised, and no drug interactions have been documented.

Adverse reactions

The most common adverse reactions of nausea, vomiting and diarrhoea occur more frequently with higher doses. Oral irritation or sensitisation may occur.

Warnings and contraindications

Nystatin is contraindicated in people with a previous history of hypersensitivity to the drug. As gastrointestinal absorption is negligible, use in pregnancy is considered safe.

Dosage and administration

The oral dose ranges from 100,000 IU four times daily to 500,000–1,000,000 IU three times daily and is taken as a suspension, tablet or capsule. It may also be used in vaginal pessaries and creams. In general, the preparation should be held within the mouth for as long as possible to increase contact time with the mucosa. The oral liquid should be swallowed, as expectorating the drug may lead to failure to treat infections of the mucosa of the posterior pharynx or oesophagus.

disturbance are oral infections and appliances, dental procedures and exposure to toxic chemicals.

The gustatory receptors are sensitive to four main classes of taste: sour (acids), sweet (sugars, some alcohols, amino acids and lead salts), bitter (many alkaloids and acids) and salty (metal ions, especially sodium). A taste more recently described is called umami (Japanese for 'delicious'), the taste elicited by glutamate in some meats and cheeses. The threshold for bitter tastes is the lowest: brucine, a compound from the plant nux vomica and closely related to strychnine, is detectable at the level of about 0.4 parts per million. This sensitivity to bitter tastes may have developed as a protective function, as many potentially poisonous natural substances (including drugs such as quinine, strychnine, nicotine and cocaine) are very bitter.

The sensation of taste, as with smell (Ch 15), may be impaired in many situations – for example, by ageing, radiation, dental treatment, poor oral hygiene, psychiatric and neurological disorders, tumours, trauma, epilepsy, migraine, hypothyroidism, infections and inflammation, renal failure and deficiencies of vitamin B or zinc. Dysfunctions of these senses are more common in the elderly and can significantly reduce the quality of life. A great variety of drugs have been noted to cause alterations in taste as an adverse effect; these are summarised in Table 16.1.

TABLE 16.1 Drug effects on taste

DRUG GROUP: EXAMPLE	SENSORY EFFECT	PROPOSED MECHANISM
Cardiovascular drugs		
ACE inhibitors: captopril, enalapril	⇓, ×	Zn chelation
Calcium channel blockers: nifedipine, diltiazem	⇓, ×	Inhibit receptor events
β-blockers: propranolol, betaxolol	⇓, ×	Antagonise adrenoceptors
Diuretics: acetazolamide, hydrochlorothiazide, spironolactone	×	
Antimicrobials		
Penicillins: ampicillin	⇓	Inhibit receptor turnover
Quinolones: o/ciprofloxacin	×	Inhibit cytochrome P450
Others: minocycline, griseofulvin, metronidazole	×	
Antivirals: zidovudine	⇓, ×	Inhibit receptor events
Drugs acting on the GI tract		
H_2 antagonists: cimetidine	⇓, ×	Inhibit receptor events
Anti-inflammatory agents		
NSAIDs: aspirin	⇓, ×	Inhibit PGs; deplete Zn
Corticosteroids: prednisolone	⇓	Inhibit receptor membrane activity
Antirheumatics: penicillamine	⇓	Zn, Cu interactions
Endocrine drugs		
Antithyroid: carbimazole	⇓	Hypothyroidism, Zn interactions
Hypoglycaemics: insulin	⇓	Inhibit receptor events
Hypoglycaemics: sulfonylureas	×	Inhibit receptor events
Drugs affecting the CNS		
Antimigraine: triptans	×	Inhibit receptor events
Antidepressants: im/desipramine, ami/nortriptyline	⇓, ×	Altered NA effects, dry mouth
Antidepressants: sertraline	⇓, ×	Altered 5-HT effects
Anorectics: amphetamines	×	Altered NA effects
Antiparkinsonian drugs: levodopa/carbidopa	⇓, ×	Enhanced DA activity
Anticonvulsants: carbamazepine, phenytoin	×	
Autonomic drugs		
Nicotine	×	Binds to ACh receptor
Antineoplastic drugs		
Antimetabolites: fluorouracil	×	Inhibit receptor turnover
Antimetabolites: methotrexate	⇓	Inhibit receptor turnover, stomatitis
Antibiotics: bleomycin, doxorubicin	⇓	Inhibit receptor turnover, stomatitis

Sensory effects: ⇓ = decreased sense; × = impaired sense; – = no effect or not known.
ACE = angiotensin-converting enzyme; ACh = acetylcholine; CNS = central nervous system; Cu = copper; DA = dopamine; H_2 = histamine H_2 receptor; 5-HT = 5-hydroxytryptamine (serotonin); NA = noradrenaline; NSAID = non-steroidal anti-inflammatory drug; PG = prostaglandin; Zn = zinc
Only drug groups for which the adverse effects are well documented have been included. Many groups and individual drugs have been omitted. (For details, see Audo & Warchol 2012; Bromley 2000; Doty et al. 2008; Henkin 1994.)

Drugs affecting taste

Loss or decrease of taste sensation (ageusia, hypogeusia) may occur as a result of neuronal damage or as an adverse effect of drugs. In some conditions, the sense of taste is distorted (dysgeusia), giving unexpected tastes sensed as metallic, bitter, burned or rotten. Although these conditions cannot readily be treated medically, zinc supplements have been shown to be effective in some trials. Some drugs implicated in reducing or impairing the sense of taste are listed in Table 16.1; those most commonly implicated are antihypertensives, antimicrobials and antidepressants.

In most cases the mechanism by which the chemical sense is altered is poorly understood, and the doses at which the effects occur are very variable. The impaired sensation takes some days or weeks of chronic dosing to develop, and the impairment may persist for weeks or months.

Sweeteners

Sugars

Chemicals from many different classes may taste sweet – even salts of beryllium and lead. However, the most important sweet-tasting compounds are sugars, synthetic sweet-tasting compounds such as aspartame and saccharin, and amino acids. The sweetest known sugar is β-d-fructose, but its sweetness decreases with increasing concentration and at higher temperatures. In decreasing order of sweetness, other sugars rank as follows: sucrose ('sugar'), glucose, galactose = mannose = lactose, maltose, raffinose. There are many other naturally occurring sweet substances, including honey and plant extracts.

Sucrose solutions are safe and effective orally for analgesia in newborns and infants up to 12 months undergoing painful procedures such as heel-pricks or taking blood (Ch 19).

Artificial sweeteners

Aspartame, the methyl ester of the aspartic acid/phenylalanine dipeptide, is an artificial sweetener that is about 180 times sweeter than sucrose and is included in many pharmaceutical preparations. It is contraindicated in people with phenylketonuria. Earlier sweeteners (saccharin and cyclamates) have been superseded due to a suspected risk of cancers. Other sugar substitutes include acesulfame potassium (Ace-K), sucralose and sugar alcohols such as xylitol and mannitol.

Stevia is a natural sweet compound from the South American plant *Stevia rebaudiana*; glycosides in the extract stevioside impart the sweet taste. Because it is 300 times sweeter than sugar and provides no kilojoules, stevia is overtaking aspartame as a sugar substitute in drinks and as a 'tabletop sweetener'. The market for stevia is growing rapidly and there are plans to develop an Australian industry in stevia crops.

However, there is some debate about the usefulness of such substitutes: by providing a sweet taste without kilojoules (or calories), they should lower the energy intake of foods and drinks. However, some studies show that people using such sweeteners actually eat more due to an increased appetite for sweet foods, and that highly refined starch products added to replace the bulk of sugar also actually increase the kilojoules.

The oesophagus and stomach

Anatomy and physiology

An understanding of the anatomy and physiology of the oesophagus and stomach is essential in understanding the mechanisms of actions of drugs affecting upper GIT disorders.

The oesophagus is a collapsible muscular structure about 25 cm in length that extends from the pharynx to the upper region (cardia) of the stomach at the upper oesophageal sphincter.

The stomach is a J-shaped, pouch-like structure lying below the diaphragm and has four divisions: the cardia, the fundus, the body and the pylorus. The stomach wall is composed of the mucosa, which contains the gastric glands responsible for the secretion of pepsinogen, gastric lipase, hydrochloric acid and intrinsic factor, and the submucosa, which connects the mucosa to the underlying muscularis mucosae.

The muscularis has three layers of smooth muscle – longitudinal, circular and oblique layers – which allow the stomach to churn and mix the contents.

In general, vagal stimulation (parasympathetic) increases the force and frequency of contractions, while input from the sympathetic nervous system decreases both activities. The enteric nervous system plays an important part in digestive processes.

The stomach functions as a temporary storage site for food as it is being digested and is capable of holding 1500–2000 mL. When a bolus of food arrives, the proximal region of the stomach relaxes to accommodate the ingested meal. Gentle peristaltic movements pass over the stomach and the food is mixed with the gastric secretions to form a liquid called chyme. More vigorous mixing movements occur in the body of the stomach, and the velocity and force of contractions increase as the chyme is moved towards the pylorus. The contractions, which last 2–20 seconds and occur at a rate of 3–5 per minute, are responsible primarily for the mixing of the chyme with the digestive juices, but they also assist the propulsion of the chyme into the duodenum. Negligible nutrient and drug absorption takes place in the stomach.

As the peristaltic contraction approaches the pylorus, a small volume of the chyme is forced into the duodenum; however, the majority is forced back into the body of the stomach, where further mechanical and chemical digestion occurs. The pyloric sphincter controls communication between the stomach and the duodenum.

The time required for digestion in the stomach depends on the amount and type of food eaten. Normal gastric emptying time is 2–6 hours, but certain drugs, physical activity of the individual and body position during digestion may affect this. Liquids empty more rapidly, whereas solids must be reduced in size to particles less than 2 mm^3 in volume before emptying occurs. Neural and hormonal reflexes control the balance between the gastric emptying rate and the processing capacity of the small intestine.

Gastric secretions

The major stimulant to gastric acid secretion is protein. Gastric juice is comprised of **pepsin**, hydrochloric acid, mucus and intrinsic factor. The secretion of hydrochloric acid by **parietal cells** kills bacteria in food, denatures protein and converts inactive pepsinogen into active pepsin, which aids further in protein degradation. Mucus and bicarbonate ions secreted by superficial mucosal cells form a gel-like layer that serves to protect the stomach from the acid environment and provides lubrication between the superficial cells and bulky undigested material. The parietal cells also secrete intrinsic factor, a protein essential for the binding of vitamin B12 before its absorption in the ileum. The stimuli for gastric secretion and the cells involved are illustrated in Figure 16.2.

The hormone **gastrin**, the neurotransmitter acetylcholine and the local hormone **histamine** all directly stimulate acid secretion by parietal cells. In contrast, prostaglandins E_2 and I_2 inhibit acid secretion. The process of gastric acid production and secretion is illustrated in Figure 16.3. Binding of prostaglandins of the E (PGE_2) and I (PGI_2) series (Ch 34) to EP_3 prostaglandin receptors on parietal cells decreases gastric acid secretion. Additionally, PGE_2 increases gastric cytoprotective mucus and bicarbonate secretion, and increases mucosal blood flow.

Parietal cells secrete 1000–2000 mL hydrochloric acid per day, so maintenance of the gastric mucosal barrier is essential to prevent ulceration. Changes in mucosal blood flow, decreased secretion of protective mucus, bacterial infection and damage by agents such as alcohol and aspirin may all lead to weakening of the mucosal barrier and ulceration.

Disorders affecting the oesophagus

Oesophageal disorders include such conditions as gastro-oesophageal reflux disease (GORD) (Clinical Focus Box 16.1) and non-erosive reflux disease (NERD) and are characterised by retrosternal pain (heartburn) and difficulty in swallowing (dysphagia) (Woo et al. 2020). The sources of the pain are numerous; potential causes include diffuse oesophageal spasm, achalasia (failure of lower oesophageal sphincter to relax), pyloric or duodenal ulcers, postural changes (bending forward) and excessive alcohol ingestion. Heartburn commonly results from reflux oesophagitis (backflow of gastric contents into the oesophagus) or from hiatal hernia (protrusion of a part of the stomach through the diaphragm). Dysphagia can be a symptom, for example, of oesophageal obstruction, mechanical interference with or paralysis of the muscles, or anxiety states. Inflammation of the oesophagus can have many causes (e.g. reflux oesophagitis associated with hiatal hernia, irritant ingestion, infection, peptic ulceration or prolonged gastric intubation).

Disorders affecting the stomach

Acute **gastritis** is an inflammatory response of the stomach lining to ingestion of irritants, such as ethanol (alcohol) or non-steroidal anti-inflammatory drugs (NSAIDs), including aspirin. The NSAIDs inhibit prostaglandin synthesis, which reduces the effectiveness of the protective mechanisms and can result in gastric ulcer formation. Symptoms include epigastric discomfort, nausea, abdominal tenderness and gastrointestinal haemorrhage.

Chronic gastritis is a long-term inflammation of the stomach lining, generally with degeneration of the gastric mucosa. It is thought that causative factors may include autoimmune reactions, the bacteria *Helicobacter pylori* (*H. pylori*) and NSAIDs. Infection with *H. pylori* causes chronic active gastritis and is associated with the development of gastric and duodenal ulcers, and gastric carcinoma.

Chronic gastritis is more common in women, and the incidence increases with age, excessive smoking and ethanol use. Symptoms are non-specific but may include flatulence, epigastric fullness after meals, diarrhoea and bleeding. Iron deficiency anaemia and pernicious anaemia may result from chronic gastritis. Treatment of symptoms and elimination of possible causative or aggravating factors (e.g. aspirin use) comprise the usual therapeutic regimen. Treatment of chronic and acute gastritis includes lifestyle modifications, antacids, PPIs and H_2-receptor antagonists (see below).

Peptic ulcer disease is a broad term encompassing both gastric and duodenal ulcers. Understanding the role of the various hormones, neurotransmitters and prostaglandins in regulating acid secretion provides the basis for the pharmacological management of peptic ulcer disease.

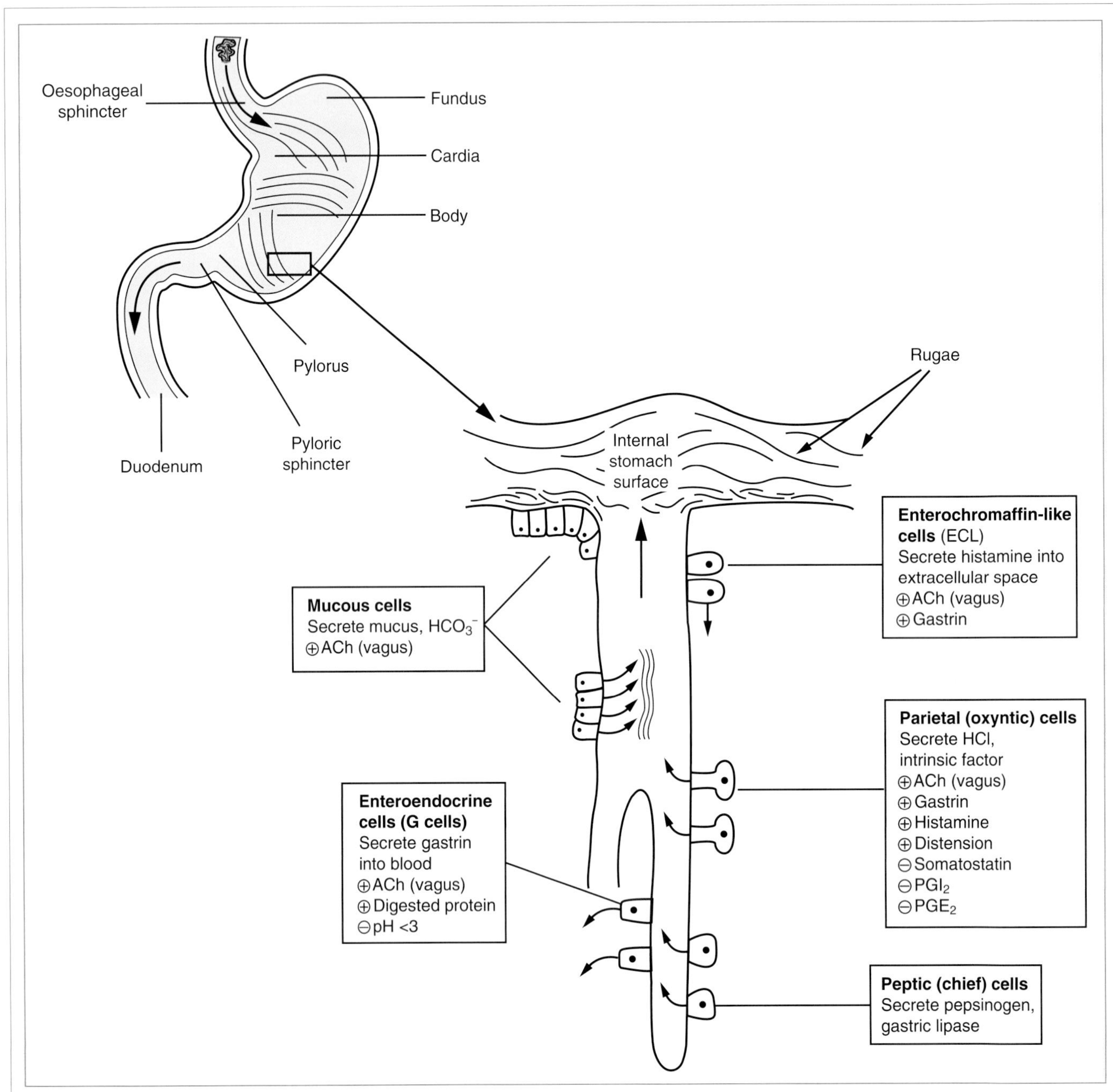

FIGURE 16.2 Schematic diagram of stomach, gastric glands and secretory cells
Note: + = stimulatory factors; − = inhibitory factors.

Although both types of ulcers produce a break in the gastric mucosa, the causes differ. With gastric ulcers, the ability of the gastric mucosa to protect and repair itself seems to be defective; in duodenal ulcers, hypersecretion of acid and pepsin is responsible for the erosion of the duodenal mucosa. Gastric colonisation with *H. pylori*, a common Gram-negative bacillus, has been identified as a major causative agent in individuals with peptic ulcer disease not caused by NSAIDs (see Clinical Focus Box 16.2 and later). Treatment with various drug combinations results in healing and a low peptic ulcer recurrence rate.

Duodenal ulcers are more common than gastric ulcers, accounting for nearly 80% of all peptic ulcers, and usually occur more frequently in younger people. Overall, the reported incidence of peptic ulcers is much lower in females. In addition to various drug treatment regimens, diet and lifestyle modifications are equally important. Hereditary factors, use of some drugs (e.g.

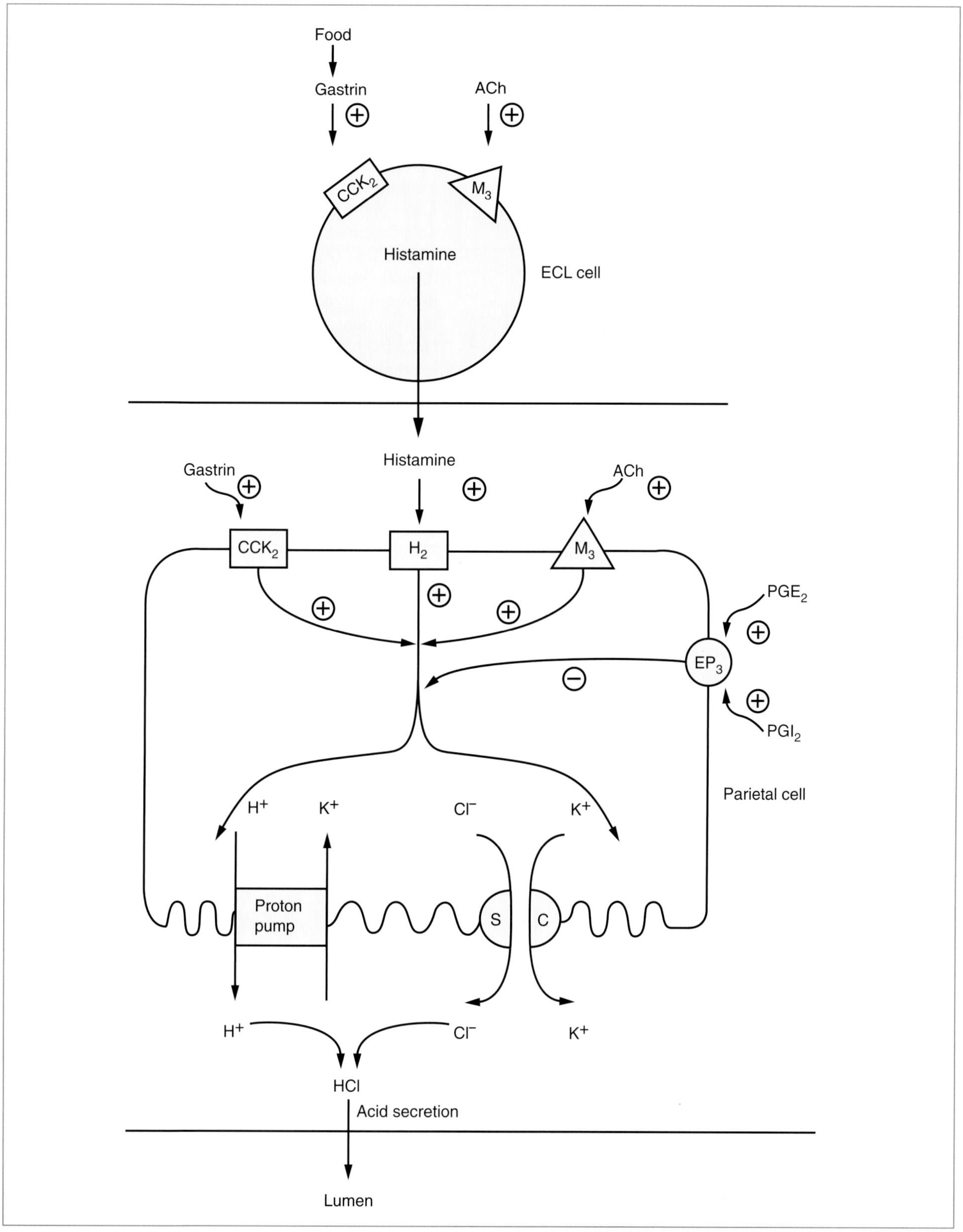

FIGURE 16.3 Schematic diagram of gastric acid secretion, etc.

Source: Adapted from Rang et al. 2012, Figure 29.2; used with permission.

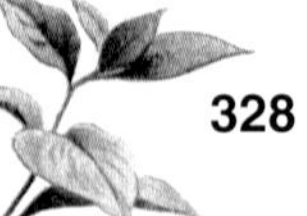

CLINICAL FOCUS BOX 16.1

Gastro-oesophageal reflux disease and non-erosive reflux disease

GORD, characterised by reflux of acidic gastric contents into the oesophagus, is extremely common, and as much as 25% of the population experience symptoms. Considered a disease with a high relapse rate, the prevention of recurrences of symptoms, mucosal lesions and complications is the main aim of therapy. The pathogenesis of GORD is multifactorial and includes impaired function of the lower oesophageal sphincter and delayed gastric emptying. Approximately 30% of people with GORD have erosive oesophagitis, while the remaining 70% have NERD. Use of proton pump inhibitors (PPIs) results in successful symptom control of GORD, enabling healing of the oesophagus and decreasing risk of complications; there is a reduction in night-time heartburn and improving sleep-related disturbances. Lifestyle and changing causative medications are recommended. NERD is a more heterogeneous disorder overlapping with functional dyspepsia, and evidence indicates that the response to PPIs is less consistent than in people with clearly established erosive disease.

GORD can also occur in infants due to oesophageal sphincter immaturity and a predominantly fluid dietary intake. Pharmacological management is reserved for infants presenting with symptoms of irritability, disrupted sleep patterns, anorexia, frequent vomiting, respiratory problems or poor weight gain. Acid-suppressing medication such as PPIs, H_2 antagonists and, to a lesser extent, antacids are used as first-line therapy. GORD resolves in most infants by 2–3 years of age.

CLINICAL FOCUS BOX 16.2

Helicobacter pylori

H. pylori is a Gram-negative bacterium that commonly infects around 30–40% of Australian-born adults. It is more common in people older than 40 years (< 10% incidence in children) and in people of Middle Eastern, Asian and Eastern European origin. There appears to be no difference between males and females in the frequency of infection (Australian Gastroenterology Institute – see 'Online resources'). It is a spiral (helical)-shaped organism that has evolved to inhabit the highly acidic environment of the stomach, particularly the pylorus. Once the bacterium adheres to the gastric epithelial cells, it breaks down endogenous urea, creating a protective cloud of ammonia and bicarbonate that enables it to protect itself against the effects of gastric acid. The ability of the bacterium to degrade urea and release carbon dioxide forms the basis of the *H. pylori* breath test, which is used to detect infestation and also to monitor the effectiveness of drug-mediated eradication (see the section '*Helicobacter pylori* treatment regimens'). *H. pylori* has been established as a causal agent in developing chronic gastritis, duodenal and gastric ulcers and gastric cancer.

aspirin and corticosteroids), psychological factors, stress and diet have also been implicated in developing peptic ulcer disease.

Conditions of the oesophagus and stomach requiring drug therapy include hyperacidity, GORD, gastritis, ulcer disease, and also nausea, vomiting and hypermotility. Drugs used include antacids, anticholinergics, antidepressants, anxiolytics, H_2-receptor antagonists, PPIs and cytoprotective agents (substances that protect cells from damage) such as sucralfate and the prostaglandin analogue misoprostol.

Drugs that neutralise or inhibit gastric acid secretion

The following sections are limited to those drugs not covered elsewhere in this book and which neutralise or inhibit gastric acid secretion: antacids, cytoprotective agents, PPIs and H_2-receptor antagonists. Anticholinergic use has been superseded by H_2-receptor antagonists.

Antacids

Antacids are chemical compounds that buffer or neutralise hydrochloric acid in the stomach and thereby raise the gastric pH. They have been used for centuries, often in the form of 'baking soda' (sodium bicarbonate), and are indicated for the relief of symptoms associated with peptic ulcer disease, gastritis, GORD (Clinical Focus Box 16.1) and dyspepsia. The main ingredients in antacids include aluminium hydroxide, calcium carbonate, magnesium salts and sodium bicarbonate, alone or in combination. Heartburn, indigestion and stomach upset are common, and most antacids may be purchased over the counter.

Although there are many antacid preparations on the market, the magnesium–aluminium combinations (e.g. Mylanta, Gaviscon) are among the most common antacids selected by individuals and health professionals. Combination antacids have been formulated to reduce the risk of diarrhoea or constipation as an adverse effect. In some formulations, alginic acid or simethicone may also be included. Gaviscon contains sodium alginate, which forms a viscous cohesive foam; this is thought to be beneficial in reflux oesophagitis by increasing adherence of mucus to the lower oesophageal mucosa.

Simethicone, a defoaming agent, relieves flatulence by dispersing and preventing the formation of mucus-surrounded gas pockets in the GIT.

Dosage and administration

The amount of antacid needed to neutralise hydrochloric acid depends on the person, the condition being treated and the buffering capability of the preparation used. The acid-neutralising property of antacids varies and is defined as the quantity (milliequivalents [mEq]) of hydrochloric acid brought to a pH of 3.5 in 15 minutes (Table 16.2). The maximum dosages listed on antacid packages should be followed; however, many people exceed the recommendations, thus increasing the potential for producing many of the adverse reactions (Table 16.3).

Antacids are considered either rapid-acting (e.g. sodium bicarbonate) or less rapid-acting (e.g. aluminium hydroxide). When administered in a fasting state, the antacid effect lasts 20–40 minutes. If administered 1 hour after meals, the effects may be extended for up to 3 hours. Liquid and powder dosage forms have been found to be more effective antacids than the tablet dosage form. Most tablets require chewing before swallowing to ensure complete dissolution of the antacid in the stomach. Absorption of antacids varies, and those that contain aluminium, calcium or magnesium are absorbed to a lesser extent than those containing sodium bicarbonate. Most of the unreacted insoluble antacids are excreted in the faeces.

Adverse reactions

As sodium bicarbonate is also absorbed in the intestine, prolonged use of this antacid should be avoided, particularly in people with heart failure or hypertension and other conditions where a sodium-restricted diet is recommended. Additionally, antacids should be avoided in the presence of co-existing conditions such as constipation (worsened by aluminium) or diarrhoea (aggravated by magnesium). Antacids are generally considered safe for use in pregnancy if prolonged use or high doses are avoided.

In people with normal renal function, absorption of cations (e.g. Al^{3+}, Mg^{2+}, Ca^{2+}) causes little in the way of systemic problems; however, in the presence of renal insufficiency, absorption of, for example, Ca^{2+} may cause hypercalcaemia, or Mg^{2+} may cause hypermagnesaemia (Wu & Carter 2007).

Milk-alkali syndrome

The characteristic features of the syndrome arising from prolonged and excessive intake of milk and antacids are irritability, distaste for milk, occasional nausea and vomiting, headache, mental confusion, anorexia, muscle ache, weakness and malaise. Impairment of renal function ensues, with elevated plasma calcium, phosphorus and bicarbonate. Calcium and phosphate precipitate in the kidney tubules, contributing to the renal damage. The syndrome has a reported mortality of around 5%.

Adverse reactions

A concise list of adverse reactions and contraindications to antacids is given in Table 16.3.

Drug interactions

Antacid–drug interactions depend on the composition of the antacid used. In general, antacids have been reported most frequently to reduce or delay the absorption of many drugs. In some instances, however, the reverse occurs and, in particular, antacids containing magnesium hydroxide can increase the absorption of some hypoglycaemic drugs, thus potentially placing the person at risk of hypoglycaemia.

There are multiple drug interactions, including the following:

- *Bisphosphonates:* antacids significantly reduce absorption.
- *Tetracyclines (oral):* antacids may combine with tetracyclines, decreasing their absorption in the GIT. Advise patients to take antacids at least 3–4 hours before or after tetracycline antibiotics.

Health professionals should be aware of the need for careful scheduling of antacids, as most medications need to be separated by at least 2 hours from an antacid. Refer to individual drug interactions.

Cytoprotective agents

Protection of the gastric and duodenal mucosa is aided by secretion of bicarbonate ions into a mucus layer that protects the underlying epithelial cells against erosion from gastric acid. **Cytoprotective agents** enhance the

TABLE 16.2 Antacids: acid-neutralising capacity

ANTACID	PRIMARY INGREDIENTS	ACID-NEUTRALISING CAPACITY
Liquid preparations		(mEq / 5 mL)
Gastrogel	Aluminium hydroxide, magnesium hydroxide, magnesium trisilicate	8.22
Tablet preparations		(mEq/tablet)
Mylanta 2go Original	Aluminium hydroxide, magnesium hydroxide, simethicone	11.5
Mylanta Double Strength	Aluminium hydroxide, magnesium hydroxide, simethicone	23

TABLE 16.3 Adverse reactions associated with antacids

CONSTITUENT OF ANTACID	ADVERSE REACTIONS[a]	CONTRAINDICATIONS/CO-EXISTING CONDITIONS
Aluminium hydroxide	Common: constipation, chalky taste. Infrequent: phosphate depletion, faecal impaction, intestinal obstruction, encephalopathy	Chronic renal failure because of increased risk of aluminium toxicity
Calcium carbonate	Belching, flatulence, constipation, abdominal distension, hypercalcaemia, alkalosis, phosphate depletion, renal calculi, milk–alkali syndrome	Hypercalcaemia, hyperparathyroidism, renal impairment (increased risk of hypercalcaemia)
Sodium bicarbonate	Belching, abdominal distension, metabolic alkalosis (high doses), hyperventilation, hypokalaemia, hyperirritability, tetany, volume overload, pulmonary oedema	Metabolic or respiratory alkalosis, chloride depletion, hypoventilation, oedema associated with heart failure, renal failure or cirrhosis, renal impairment (increased risk of sodium retention)
Magnesium salts	Diarrhoea, chalky taste, belching, elevated plasma magnesium	Diarrhoea (may be aggravated), renal impairment (increased risk of raised plasma magnesium)

[a]Adverse reactions are listed in order of most common through to rare.

protection afforded by the mucus layer or provide a physical barrier over the ulcerated surface. The two main agents are sucralfate and the prostaglandin analogue misoprostol.

Sucralfate is composed of sulfated sucrose and aluminium hydroxide. It is a non-absorbable drug that in the presence of acid undergoes a chemical reaction that results in formation of a sticky, yellow–white gel that forms a protective, acid-resistant shield in the ulcer crater. This barrier hastens the healing of the ulcer by protecting the mucosa for up to 6 hours. The binding to the ulcer crater is thought to be the main therapeutic effect, but sucralfate also stimulates angiogenesis, production of mucus and protective prostaglandins. It is administered orally with minimal systemic absorption (up to 5%). This product is indicated for short-term (up to 8 weeks) peptic ulcer treatment and for preventing stress-induced ulcers.

Drug interactions

Drug interactions include:

- *Antacids:* concurrent use can interfere with sucralfate binding, thus reducing its effect.
- *Ciprofloxacin, norfloxacin, tetracycline antibiotics:* decreased absorption and bioavailability of these antibiotics.
- *Digoxin, warfarin and theophylline:* decreased absorption and bioavailability.

Adverse reactions

The most common adverse reaction is constipation, which occurs in 1–15% of people. Infrequently, there are reports of nausea, vomiting, dry mouth, dizziness, back pain, rash and headache.

Misoprostol, a synthetic analogue of prostaglandin E_1, is indicated for the treatment of peptic ulcers and the prevention of gastric ulcers associated with the use of NSAIDs. Similar to prostaglandins of the E and I series, misoprostol protects the stomach by decreasing gastric acid secretion via an action at EP_3 prostaglandin receptors on parietal cells and increasing gastric cytoprotective mucus and bicarbonate. Misoprostol is rapidly absorbed after oral administration and undergoes rapid first-pass metabolism to an active metabolite, misoprostol acid, which is then further metabolised to inactive metabolites.

Drug interactions and adverse reactions

No significant drug interactions have been reported. Infrequent adverse reactions reported include constipation, gas, headache, nausea and vomiting. In about 30% of people, diarrhoea limits its usefulness.

As misoprostol can cause hypotension in people with cerebrovascular or coronary artery disease, it should be used with caution in these groups. Importantly, as misoprostol can induce premature labour and may be teratogenic in large doses, it should not be used to treat peptic ulcers in pregnant women or in those contemplating pregnancy. However, for further information on its obstetric indications, refer to Chapter 30.

H_2-receptor antagonists

Histamine is produced in enterochromaffin-like cells of the oxyntic mucosa by decarboxylation of l-histidine by histidine decarboxylase. Released histamine then acts on **histamine (H_2) receptors** to increase gastric acid secretion (Fig 16.3, earlier). The **H_2-receptor antagonists** include famotidine, nizatidine and ranitidine, which competitively block histamine from stimulating the H_2 receptors located on the gastric parietal cells, thus reducing (~70%) gastric acid secretion.

These drugs are indicated for treating peptic ulcer disease, GORD and dyspepsia, and for stress ulcer

TABLE 16.4 H_2-Receptor Antagonists Pharmacokinetics (Oral Administration)

DRUG	ORAL BIOAVAILABILITY	TIME TO PEAK PLASMA CONCENTRATION (h)	HALF-LIFE (h)	DURATION OF ACTION (h)	% METABOLISM/EXCRETION
Famotidine	40–45%	1–4	2.5–4	10–12 basal and nocturnal	Liver (5%)/renal
Nizatidine	> 70%	0.5–3	1–2	Up to 8 basal, up to 12 nocturnal	Liver (about 35%)/renal
Ranitidine	50%	1–3	2–3	Up to 4 basal, up to 13 nocturnal	Liver (about 25%)/renal

prophylaxis. They have similar structural and pharmacokinetic characteristics, which are summarised in Table 16.4. All of these drugs are well absorbed, achieving maximal plasma concentration in around 1–3 hours.

Drug interactions and adverse reactions

All H_2-receptor antagonists reduce the bioavailability of drugs that require an acidic environment for absorption. In general, these drugs are well tolerated. Common adverse reactions include diarrhoea, constipation, headache, dizziness, rash and confusion in the elderly.

Dosages vary, depending on the condition being treated (peptic ulcer disease, GORD, dyspepsia, stress ulcer prophylaxis). Consult the relevant drug information sources for dosing recommendations.

Proton pump inhibitors

PPIs suppress gastric acid secretion by inhibiting the proton pump (H^+, K^+ ATPase enzyme system) at the secretory surface of the gastric parietal cells (Fig 16.3, earlier, for the location of the proton pump, and Drug Monograph 16.2 for an example; omeprazole). These drugs consist of a benzimidazole and a pyridine ring and are weak bases. Following administration, the drugs accumulate in the highly acidic environment (pH ~0.8) of the secretory canaliculi of the parietal cells, where they are converted to a thiophilic sulfenamide (a permanent cation), which interacts covalently with H^+, K^+ ATPase involved in hydrogen ion transport. When sufficient drug molecules bind to the proton pump, the final step of acid production is inhibited, thus suppressing both basal and stimulated gastric acid secretion.

The covalent (irreversible) interaction with H^+, K^+ ATPase explains why the duration of action of PPIs exceeds their plasma half-life. PPIs are the most potent inhibitors of gastric acid secretion available, and dosing once daily inhibits maximal acid output by about 85%. When administration of a PPI is ceased, acid secretion is restored following synthesis of new H^+, K^+ ATPase.

The first of these drugs to be developed was omeprazole (Drug Monograph 16.2), which binds irreversibly to the proton pump; others now available include lansoprazole, pantoprazole, rabeprazole and esomeprazole (the *S*-isomer of omeprazole).

Helicobacter pylori treatment regimens

It is now well established that infection with *H. pylori* causes chronic active gastritis, is associated with the development of gastric and duodenal ulcers and is a recognised risk factor in the development of gastric carcinoma (Clinical Focus Box 16.2). Eradicating *H. pylori* is considered first-line treatment because it vastly improves the odds of non-recurrence of the ulcer. Early therapies involved using a single drug such as an antibiotic, a PPI or bismuth; however, monotherapy was found to be effective in less than 30% of people, so combinations were developed.

The recommended therapy is triple therapy – three drugs administered twice a day for 14 days.

Current triple therapy regimens include:

- PPI, clarithromycin and amoxicillin (> 90% eradication) – duration of treatment 14 days, preferred regimen.
- PPI, clarithromycin and metronidazole (> 80% eradication) – duration of treatment 14 days, used if amoxicillin is unsuitable.
- PPI, amoxicillin and metronidazole (> 80% eradication) – duration of treatment 14 days, used if clarithromycin is unsuitable.

Combining the individual agents in a single packet helps simplify a complicated drug schedule, and omeprazole/esomeprazole, clarithromycin and amoxicillin are available as a 'single script' combination pack (Nexium Hp7).

The success of *H. pylori* eradication hinges on adherence to therapy and susceptibility of the bacterium to the antibiotics. Bacterial resistance is an ever-increasing problem, and resistance of strains to clarithromycin hinders success in about 10% of the population in the United States, southwestern Europe and Japan, and in about 20% of the Australian population. The World Health Organization prioritises research into clarithromycin resistance as high priority due to the relationship between *H. pylori* and stomach cancers. If two courses that include clarithromycin and metronidazole fail to eradicate *H. pylori*, patients are likely to have at least single resistance and more frequently double resistance (Mitchell & Katelaris 2016).

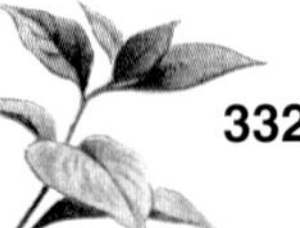

Drug Monograph 16.2

Omeprazole

Omeprazole, the prototype drug, is a racemate comprising R-omeprazole and S-omeprazole. (S-omeprazole is marketed as esomeprazole.) It is indicated for the treatment of peptic ulcer disease, treatment and prevention of NSAID-induced peptic ulceration, severe erosive oesophagitis that occurs with GORD and long-term treatment of hypersecretory gastric conditions such as Zollinger–Ellison syndrome.

Mechanism of action

See the description of the mechanism of action of PPIs in the text.

Pharmacokinetics

After a single oral dose, the onset of action of omeprazole as indicated by decreased gastric acid secretion is within 1 hour; its peak effect is in 2 hours and its duration of action is 3–5 days (the time needed for return of secretory activity).

Bioavailability is in the range of 30–40%, and the plasma half-life is around 0.5 hours. It is extensively metabolised in the liver by CYP2C19 to the major metabolite hydroxyomeprazole (with a minor contribution by CYP3A4) and to a lesser extent to omeprazole sulfone by CYP3A4 (with a minor contribution by CYP2C19).

Drug interactions

In view of its metabolism by CYP2C19 and CYP3A4, interactions with other drugs should be expected. Concurrent administration of omeprazole with diazepam or phenytoin can lead to increased plasma concentrations of diazepam and phenytoin, and dosage reduction might be necessary. Similarly, co-administration with warfarin can lead to increased anticoagulation, and monitoring of the international normalised ratio should be considered.

Additionally, PPIs can decrease the bioavailability of drugs that rely on an acidic environment for absorption (e.g. atazanavir [HIV-protease inhibitor] and digoxin).

Adverse reactions

Omeprazole is generally well tolerated. Minor adverse effects include abdominal pain, dizziness, headache, nausea, vomiting, diarrhoea, flatulence and skin rash. Decreased absorption of vitamin B_{12} has also been observed with chronic treatment.

Warnings and contraindications

Avoid use in people with omeprazole hypersensitivity. Care should be exercised in people with impaired hepatic function because of the risk of accumulation of the drug when high doses are used. Avoid concomitant use with clopidogrel.

Dosage and administration

The adult oral dose for symptomatic GORD is 10–20 mg daily for 4 weeks. For erosive oesophagitis use 20 mg once daily for 4 weeks. Maintenance therapy is 10 mg daily if needed and up to 20 mg. For gastric hypersecretory conditions, the maintenance dose is 20–120 mg daily, adjusting as necessary. The capsule formulation should not be opened, crushed or chewed, as the drug will degrade in the acidic environment of the stomach. For peptic ulcer disease with *H. pylori* 40 mg once daily or 20 mg twice daily in association with a combination of antibacterials.

Alternative drug regimens are required in those where the standard triple therapy is ineffective due to suspected antibiotic-resistant *H. pylori* strains (O'Connor et al. 2020). Continued maintenance of acid suppression may also be necessary in people where eradication treatment either fails or is contraindicated, in those with gastric ulcers, or ulcers bigger than 1 cm in diameter, or if peptic ulcers recur in the absence of reinfection.

KEY POINTS

Oesophageal and stomach disorders and their treatment

- The oesophagus extends from the pharynx to the upper region (cardia) of the stomach and passes through the diaphragm at the oesophageal hiatus into the abdominal cavity.
- Oesophageal disorders are characterised by retrosternal pain (heartburn) and difficulty in swallowing (dysphagia).
- In the stomach, gastric acid secretion is regulated by neural (parasympathetic) and hormonal (gastrin, histamine) mechanisms.
- Drugs that neutralise or inhibit gastric acid secretion include antacids, H_2-receptor antagonists, PPIs and cytoprotective agents and previously anticholinergics.
- Antacids are chemical compounds that buffer or neutralise hydrochloric acid in the stomach and thereby raise the gastric pH.

- Antacid–drug interactions depend on the composition of the antacid used; in general, antacids have been reported most frequently to reduce or delay the absorption of many drugs.
- The drugs used to treat peptic ulcer include cytoprotective agents, H_2-receptor antagonists and the PPIs.
- Cytoprotective agents enhance the protection afforded by the mucus layer or provide a physical barrier over the ulcerated surface. The two main agents are sucralfate and the prostaglandin analogue misoprostol.
- Histamine is produced in enterochromaffin-like cells of the oxyntic mucosa. Released histamine then acts on H_2-receptors to increase gastric acid secretion. The H_2-receptor antagonists block the action of histamine at the receptors. They include cimetidine, famotidine, nizatidine and ranitidine, and uses include peptic ulcer disease and GORD.
- PPIs reduce gastric acid secretion by irreversibly inhibiting the hydrogen–potassium ATPase enzyme system at the secretory surface of the gastric parietal cells.
- It is now well established that infection with *H. pylori* causes chronic active gastritis, is associated with the development of gastric and duodenal ulcers and is implicated in the development of gastric carcinoma.
- Use of *H. pylori* eradication regimens improves the odds of non-recurrence of peptic ulcers. Success hinges on adherence to therapy and susceptibility of the bacterium to the antibiotics. The most successful therapy is triple therapy.

The vomiting reflex

The induction of vomiting involves a complex coordinated response between two areas: an area of sensory nerve cells called the chemoreceptor trigger zone (CTZ), located in the floor of the fourth ventricle of the brain, and the vomiting centre, or emetic centre, located in the medulla. The emetic centre receives inputs from:

- the CTZ
- the vestibular apparatus
- higher brain centres relaying sensory inputs such as pain, smell and sight
- organs such as the heart, and parts of the GIT.

In the absence of the blood–brain barrier, the CTZ (Fig 16.4) is activated by both cerebrospinal fluid-borne and blood-borne emetics, such as chemical toxins and drugs, and by the neurotransmitter 5-HT, released from afferent nerve pathways from the stomach and small intestine. The CTZ itself is not able to induce vomiting, but is stimulated by smells, strong emotion, severe pain, raised intracranial pressure, labyrinthine disturbances (motion sickness), endocrine disturbances, toxic reactions to drugs, gastrointestinal disease, radiation treatments and chemotherapy. The CTZ then relays messages to the emetic centre through actions of the neurotransmitters acetylcholine, 5-HT, histamine and dopamine. Discharge from both the sympathetic and the parasympathetic nervous systems often leads to the accompanying symptoms of salivation, sweating, rapid breathing and cardiac dysrhythmias.

Vomiting is characterised by forceful expulsion of the contents of the stomach (and sometimes that of the duodenum) through the mouth. This occurs as a result of impulses sent via efferent nerves from the emetic centre to the upper GIT, diaphragm and abdominal muscles. Strong contraction of the abdominal muscles then forces the contents past the oesophageal sphincter and into the mouth. Relaxation of the abdominal muscles allows any material remaining in the oesophagus to empty back into the stomach. This cycle may be repeated many times. Although vomiting in many instances is a protective mechanism to rid the body of toxic substances, it may in severe cases lead to fluid and electrolyte disturbances.

Drugs for nausea and vomiting

Vomiting is a complex process involving multiple nerve pathways and neurotransmitters (e.g. ACh acting on muscarinic receptors, histamine on H_1 receptors, dopamine on D_2 receptors, substance P acting on neurokinin-1 [NK_1] receptors and 5-hydroxytryptamine acting on 5-HT_3 receptors).

There are numerous causes of nausea and vomiting, and treatment differs for acute situations such as pregnancy (Clinical Focus Box 16.3) and gastroenteritis, for chronic situations such as gastric or metabolic diseases and for psychogenic vomiting such as that occurring with bulimia. The cerebral cortex is also involved in anticipatory nausea and vomiting, a conditioned response caused by a stimulus connected with a previous unpleasant experience. Control of vomiting is important and at times it can be very difficult, which can be distressing to the individual concerned.

Cancer chemotherapy-induced vomiting

Vomiting caused by cancer chemotherapy and radiotherapy can be severe enough that treatment can be delayed, and many clients vehemently refuse further treatment. Often when cancer chemotherapeutic agents are used in combination, the emetogenic potentials of the agents are additive. Typically, vomiting starts within 4 hours of treatment, peaks towards 10 hours and subsides

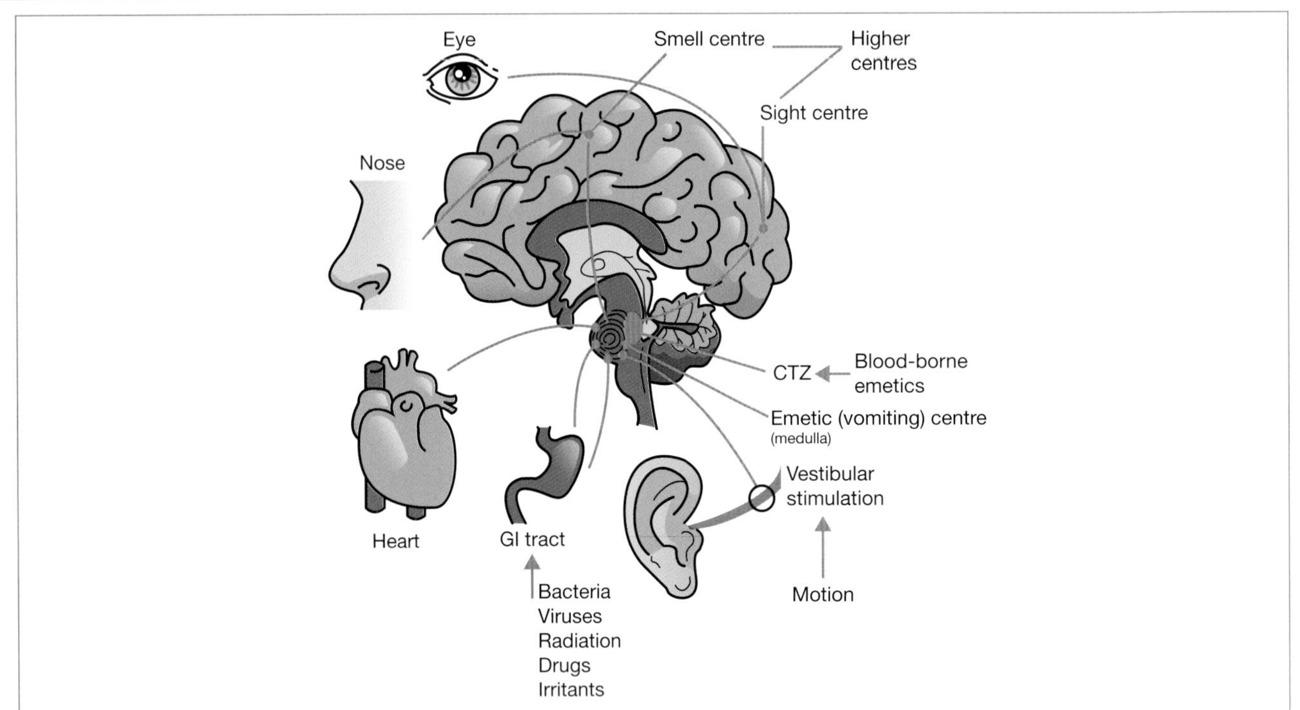

FIGURE 16.4 The chemoreceptor trigger zone (CTZ) and the sites activating the emetic centre

Source: Adapted from Salerno 1999, Figure 35.1.

CLINICAL FOCUS BOX 16.3

Nausea and vomiting in pregnancy

Nausea, often described as 'morning sickness', affects up to 80% of pregnant women and as many as 50% experience vomiting. Its onset is in the early stages of pregnancy. In severe cases of 'hyperemesis gravidarum' (1–2%), women are hospitalised for correction of dehydration and electrolyte imbalance. This phase of nausea and vomiting tends to last 7–12 weeks, beginning around week 6 and resolving around week 12. In many cases, dietary changes are sufficient to relieve symptoms (low-fat, high-carbohydrate, small meals) and pharmacological intervention is not necessary. Where possible, avoid drug therapy and ensure adequate hydration.

In the wake of the thalidomide disaster of the early 1960s, most antiemetics are contraindicated in pregnancy. If drug therapy is considered because of impaired quality of life, health professionals should refer to the category of risk for an individual drug. Drugs used include ondansetron, metoclopramide, pyridoxine (vitamin B6), doxylamine prochlorperazine, promethazine and vitamin B12. For hyperemesis gravidarum, intravenous rehydration is the cornerstone of management; however, if symptoms are prolonged and intractable, drugs such as domperidone, metoclopramide, prochlorperazine or ondansetron may be used. Caution with combined doxylamine/pyridoxine, which is not teratogenic and may be effective in treating nausea and vomiting in pregnancy. Ondansetron is commonly used to treat hyperemesis gravidarum, but studies are urgently needed to determine whether it is safer and more effective than using first-line antiemetics. Thiamine (vitamin B1) should be introduced following protocols to prevent refeeding syndrome and Wernicke encephalopathy. Data from the National Birth Defects Prevention Study has identified an increased risk of cleft palate in infants when mothers were treated for nausea and vomiting during the first trimester with ondansetron, and of hypospadias if mothers were treated with steroids. The authors acknowledged that the results may be 'chance findings' but were of the view that the relationships should be further investigated (Anderka et al. 2012).

over the following 12–24 hours. Delayed vomiting can occur with high-dose cisplatin and can last 3–5 days. It is not surprising that anticipation of therapy and the sight and smell of the hospital can trigger nausea and vomiting in as many as 25% of people. Because antiemetics are usually more effective in preventing vomiting (e.g. ondansetron) than they are in treating it, they should be administered (often in high doses) prophylactically before cytotoxic therapy. Chemotherapy-induced vomiting may also require several antiemetic agents with different sites of action for effectiveness (e.g. metoclopramide and lorazepam, metoclopramide and dexamethasone or prochlorperazine and dexamethasone; see below). In addition to drug therapy, behavioural and psychological support should be provided.

Antiemetics

Antiemetics act principally by blocking the neurotransmitters in the vomiting centre, the cerebral cortex, the CTZ or the vestibular apparatus. A variety of miscellaneous drugs are also used to control vomiting caused by various factors; these include corticosteroids (dexamethasone and methylprednisolone) via, for example, their anti-inflammatory effect and direct central action at the glucocorticoid receptors in the nucleus of the solitary tract; benzodiazepines used primarily for their sedative and anxiety-relieving actions (e.g. lorazepam used for anticipatory nausea and vomiting associated with chemotherapy); and the common spice, ginger (*Zingiber officinale*). The potential role of the endocannabinoid system to treat nausea and vomiting is an emerging field of research. According to the TGA, 'At this time, the use of medicinal cannabis for the treatment of nausea and vomiting in managing the adult patient's symptoms should be considered only where conventional treatments have been appropriately tried and proven unsuccessful' (Therapeutic Goods Administration 2017).

The drugs used to control and prevent nausea and vomiting and associated neurotransmitters are summarised in Table 16.5.

Dopamine antagonists

Drugs within this class include prochlorperazine, domperidone, droperidol, haloperidol and metoclopramide (Drug Monograph 16.3). Prochlorperazine is a phenothiazine derivative and first-generation antipsychotic with antiemetic effects, probably by an inhibitory action on the CTZ and vomiting centre. Phenothiazines are thought to act mainly as D_2-receptor antagonists, but they also have antihistamine and antimuscarinic properties. Only their actions relevant to nausea and vomiting are discussed here; other information on phenothiazines and their use as antipsychotic drugs can be found in Chapter 22.

Prochlorperazine is indicated for the treatment of nausea and vomiting due to causes such as migraine and vertigo, as in Ménière's disease. It is more effective than antihistamines in severe vomiting, especially in vertigo and migraine, and is available as tablets, injections and suppositories (Ch 24). It is carried by ambulances and commonly administered by paramedics as treatment or prophylaxis of nausea and vomiting in motion sickness, for planned aeromedical evacuation and when there is allergy or contraindication to administration of metoclopramide as an antiemetic.

Use is contraindicated where there is evidence of previous hypersensitivity to phenothiazines and in situations of CNS depression. Adverse reactions are common and include constipation, dry mouth, sleepiness, dizziness, blurred vision and extrapyramidal effects (parkinsonism in the elderly and dystonia in younger people). Less common reactions include skin rash, hypotension and peripheral oedema. (For additional information, including phenothiazine warnings and contraindications, see Chapter 22.)

Muscarinic receptor antagonists (anticholinergics)

Hyoscine hydrobromide is a competitive antagonist of the actions of ACh at muscarinic receptors and is used to prevent motion-induced (sea, air, car, train) nausea and vomiting by depressing conduction in the labyrinth of the inner ear. Overstimulation in this area is responsible for the nausea and vomiting of motion sickness. The adverse effects of hyoscine are related to its anticholinergic effects; these include dry mouth, tachycardia, blurring of vision and, less commonly, constipation, mental confusion, fatigue and restlessness and irritability. Administration is

TABLE 16.5 Drugs for controlling nausea and vomiting, and the associated neurotransmitters

NEUROTRANSMITTER AND RECEPTOR	DRUG CLASS	ANTIEMETIC AGENT
Dopamine acting via (D_2) receptors located in the stomach and CTZ	Dopamine antagonists	Domperidone, droperidol, haloperidol, metoclopramide, prochlorperazine
Acetylcholine acting on muscarinic receptors in the vestibular and vomiting centres*	Muscarinic receptor antagonists (anticholinergics)	Hyoscine hydrobromide
Histamine (H_1) receptors in vestibular and vomiting centres	H_1-receptor antagonists (antihistamines)	Dimenhydrinate, promethazine
5-hydroxytryptamine (5-HT_3) receptors in the GIT, CTZ and vomiting centres	5-HT_3-receptor antagonists	Granisetron, ondansetron, tropisetron, palonosetron
Substance P acting via neurokinin-1 (NK_1) receptors located in the CNS	NK_1-receptor antagonists	Aprepitant, fosaprepitant

*Overstimulation of the labyrinth (inner ear) results in the nausea and vomiting of motion sickness

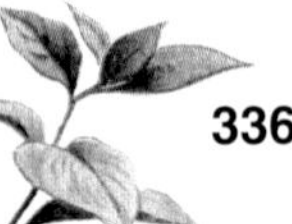

Drug Monograph 16.3
Metoclopramide

Metoclopramide is used for diabetic gastroparesis, GORD and, parenterally, for preventing nausea and vomiting secondary to emetogenic cancer chemotherapeutic agents, radiation and opioid medications. It is also used as an adjunct for gastrointestinal radiological examinations because it hastens the transit of barium through the upper GIT by its stimulation of gastric emptying and acceleration of intestinal transit. Parenteral metoclopramide may be used to facilitate small-intestinal intubation.

Mechanism of action

Metoclopramide has both central and peripheral actions in preventing or relieving nausea and vomiting. Centrally it blocks dopamine (D_2) receptors in the CTZ (in high doses, 5-HT_3 antagonism may be observed), while peripherally it accelerates gastric emptying (sensitising tissues to the action of ACh), reduces reflux from the duodenum and stomach into the oesophagus (via an action on D_2 receptors) and enhances motility of the upper GIT. The enhanced motility effect may be mediated through an action on muscarinic cholinergic systems within the GIT.

Pharmacokinetics

It is almost completely absorbed following oral dosing, and peak plasma concentrations occur 30–180 minutes after oral administration, 10–15 minutes after an intramuscular dose and within 5–20 minutes of an intravenous dose. The half-life in plasma is 2.5–5 hours. Metoclopramide is metabolised predominantly by hepatic CYP2D6 with a minor contribution by CYP1A2. In addition, metoclopramide is also an inhibitor of CYP2D6. Approximately 20–30% of the drug is excreted unchanged in urine, with the remainder excreted as metabolites.

Drug interactions

As many CNS antidepressant drugs are metabolised by CYP2D6, additive CNS-depressant effects are observed in combination with metoclopramide. A potentially serious drug interaction could occur with this combination, which should be avoided. In surgical patients, metoclopramide can reduce inactivation of suxamethonium and hence prolong neuromuscular blockade. The effects of metoclopramide are antagonised by anticholinergic drugs and narcotic analgesics.

Adverse reactions

These include diarrhoea, sleepiness, restlessness, dizziness, headache, extrapyramidal (parkinsonian) effects, hypotension, tachycardia and, rarely, agranulocytosis and tardive dyskinesia. Onset reported within first 5 days of treatment. In 2009 the Food and Drug Administration in the United States implemented a Black Box Warning advising health professionals of the risk of tardive dyskinesias following long-term or high-dose use.

Warnings and contraindications

Metoclopramide is contraindicated where a previous reaction to dopamine antagonists has been reported, and in phaeochromocytoma because of a risk of a hypertensive crisis. The drug should be used with caution in Parkinson's disease and depression, as it can worsen the symptoms. Dosage reduction (25–50%) should be considered in situations of severe renal impairment and low doses used in children because of an increased risk of extrapyramidal adverse effects.

Dosage and administration

To treat nausea or vomiting in an adult weighing over 60 kg, the oral dose of metoclopramide is 10 mg three times daily. Decreasing doses are used in people weighing under 60 kg. Nausea and vomiting in children (< 10 kg) is treated with a dose of 0.1 mg/kg (maximum 1 mg) twice daily. The maximum dose is 0.5 mg/kg/day for all age groups (except children below 1 year of age) to a maximum of 30 mg/day.

Source: Australian Medicines Handbook 2021.

recommended 30 minutes prior to travel. Travacalm Original contains dimenhydrinate, hyoscine hydrobromide and caffeine.

5-HT_3-receptor antagonists

Ondansetron (Drug Monograph 16.4), granisetron, palonosetron and tropisetron are selective 5-hydroxytryptamine (5-HT, serotonin) antagonists. 5-HT_3 receptors are located peripherally on the vagus nerve terminal and centrally in the CTZ. One theory is that cancer chemotherapeutic agents cause the release of stored 5-HT from the enterochromaffin cells of the GIT, which stimulates 5-HT_3 receptors located in the vagus nerve in the GIT. Stimulation of vagal afferents via 5-HT_3 receptors results in the CTZ initiating the vomiting reflex. When ondansetron is administered before antineoplastic therapy, 5-HT_3 receptors in the brainstem and GIT are blocked. As a result, 5-HT released in response to the administration of antineoplastic agents cannot bind to 5-HT_3 receptors and thus vomiting is prevented.

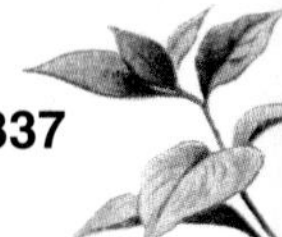

Drug Monograph 16.4
Ondansetron

Ondansetron was the first of the 5-HT-receptor (5-HT_3) antagonists approved for the prevention of nausea and vomiting associated with the use of cytotoxic agents and radiotherapy.

Pharmacokinetics

Oral absorption of ondansetron is maximal after 1–1.5 hours, oral bioavailability is about 60% and its plasma half-life is 3–4 hours. It is extensively metabolised (via hydroxylation) in the liver (~90%) by CYP1A2, CYP2D6 (minor role) and CYP3A4, and less than 10% is excreted as unchanged drug in urine.

Drug interactions

There is no evidence that ondansetron either induces or inhibits metabolism of other drugs currently. The combination of apomorphine and ondansetron should be avoided because of the risk of severe hypotension and bradycardia. Data from small studies have shown loss of consciousness. The combination with tramadol can decrease the analgesic effect of tramadol.

Adverse reactions

Common adverse reactions include constipation, headache, anxiety and dizziness. Chest pain, hypotension and rash are infrequent and, rarely, anaphylaxis, extrapyramidal effects and seizures have been reported.

Warnings and contraindications

Ondansetron should be used with caution in people with impaired liver function, as plasma clearance can be reduced and dosage adjustment may be necessary.

Dosage and administration

To prevent cancer chemotherapy-induced nausea and vomiting in children older than 1 year, ondansetron is administered at a dosage of 5 mg/m^2 (maximum 8 mg) intravenously immediately before the start of chemotherapy. The oral adult dose is 16–24 mg 1–2 hours before the start of cancer chemotherapy. The intravenous dose is 8–12 mg, with a maximum of 8 mg in people aged older than 75 years.

Source: Australian Medicines Handbook 2021.

Palonosetron, a second-generation drug, is given intravenously 30 minutes before chemotherapy. It has a long half-life (~40 hours), and it has yet to be established if further doses are required for chemotherapy regimens of more than 1 day.

Aprepitant and fosaprepitant

Substance P, a neurotransmitter that acts on neurokinin-1 (NK_1) receptors, is widely distributed in the CNS. It is thought to be involved in pain transmission and emetic pathways. Aprepitant and fosaprepitant (the prodrug of aprepitant) are oral NK_1-receptor antagonists that act centrally to control, in particular, chemotherapy-induced vomiting. They are most effective when used in combination with a 5-HT_3-receptor antagonist and the corticosteroid dexamethasone. As a consequence of aprepitant metabolism by CYP3A4, potential drug interactions are likely with agents such as dexamethasone (a substrate for CYP3A4). When aprepitant is used concomitantly with oral dexamethasone, the dose of dexamethasone is halved. At present there are no data for its use in severe hepatic impairment, in children or in pregnancy and lactation. Common adverse effects include diarrhoea, fatigue, headache, hiccups and, rarely, angio-oedema and urticaria.

Corticosteroids

Corticosteroids have been reported to be effective for chemotherapy-induced nausea and vomiting, either alone or when used in combination with other antiemetics. The mechanism of action is unknown, but it has been proposed that these drugs may inhibit prostaglandin synthesis and decrease 5-HT turnover in the CNS, which might be involved in cancer chemotherapy-induced vomiting. Research has indicated that certain prostaglandins (especially the E series) can induce nausea and vomiting. A full discussion of the pharmacology of corticosteroids can be found in Chapters 29 and 33.

KEY POINTS

Vomiting and the antiemetics

- The induction of vomiting involves a complex coordinated response between the CTZ, located in the floor of the fourth ventricle of the brain, and the vomiting or emetic centre, located in the medulla. The process involves multiple nerve pathways and

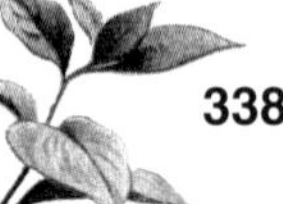

neurotransmitters (e.g. acetylcholine, histamine, dopamine, substance P and 5-hydroxytryptamine).

- Antiemetics, which include dopamine, muscarinic, 5-HT_3- and NK_1-receptor antagonists, are given for the relief of nausea and vomiting, including that associated with cancer chemotherapy.
  - Dopamine antagonists include prochlorperazine, domperidone, droperidol, haloperidol and metoclopramide (Drug Monograph 16.3). Prochlorperazine is a phenothiazine derivative with antiemetic effects, probably by an inhibitory action on the CTZ and vomiting centre.
  - Muscarinic receptor antagonists include hyoscine hydrobromide, a competitive antagonist of the actions of ACh at muscarinic receptors. It is used to prevent motion-induced (sea, air, car, train) nausea and vomiting by depressing conduction in the labyrinth of the inner ear.
  - Ondansetron, granisetron, palonosetron and tropisetron are selective 5-HT_3 antagonists. They act at $5HT_3$ receptors on vagal nerve terminals and centrally in the CTZ.
  - Aprepitant and fosaprepitant (the prodrug of aprepitant) are oral NK_1-receptor antagonists that act centrally to control chemotherapy-induced vomiting.

The pancreas

Continued digestion and absorption of food in the small intestine relies on secretions from the accessory organs – the pancreas, liver and gall bladder. The pancreas (see also Ch 30) secretes about 1500 mL liquid daily, comprising water, sodium bicarbonate and enzymes such as pancreatic amylase, trypsin and chymotrypsin. The acidic duodenal chyme is neutralised by the aqueous component of the pancreatic secretions, which brings the pH within range for further digestion of nutrients by the pancreatic enzymes. Regulation of pancreatic secretion is complex; for example, to prevent erosion of the duodenal mucosa, the rate of delivery of acidic chyme into the duodenum is equalled by the rate of secretion of bicarbonate ions, which neutralise the chyme.

With the exception of diabetes mellitus (Ch 28), many pancreatic diseases have symptoms that are not readily diagnosed. Inflammation of the pancreas may be acute or chronic. Among the many causes are blockage of the pancreatic ducts, trauma to the pancreas, excessive alcohol consumption, drug use and tumours, cysts or abscesses. Symptoms are non-specific, but ultimately include severe pain. Carcinoma of the pancreas is as difficult to diagnose as other pancreatic disorders.

Pancreatic enzyme supplements

The pancreas releases digestive enzymes and bicarbonate into the duodenum to help in the digestion of fats, carbohydrates and proteins. Bicarbonate neutralises acid and thus helps to protect the enzymes from both acid and pepsin. When acid chyme enters the duodenum, vagal stimulation regulates pancreatic secretion, and enzyme replacement therapy may be necessary for people who have had the vagal fibres surgically severed or who have had surgical procedures that cause food to bypass the duodenum. In addition, replacement therapy is usually necessary in exocrine pancreatic enzyme deficiency states, chronic pancreatitis, cystic fibrosis, pancreatic tumours and pancreatic obstruction.

The supplements are all of porcine origin and contain principally lipase with protease and amylase. The supplements are in capsule form containing mini microspheres. If possible, use enteric-coated products because the microsphere formulation resists gastric inactivation, so the enzymes reach the duodenum to hydrolyse fats into glycerol and fatty acids, proteins into peptides and starch into dextrins and sugars.

The most common adverse reactions include nausea, vomiting and abdominal pain. Hyperuricaemia and intestinal obstruction occur rarely. Dosage should be adjusted as necessary to suit the individual and is guided by the quality and quantity of stools. Use of these products should be avoided in people with hypersensitivity to pork proteins.

The gall bladder

Hepatocytes secrete into the bile canaliculi 800–1000 mL of bile per day, which flows into the gall bladder, a pear-shaped organ lying on the under surface of the liver. Bile, a yellowish-green liquid (pH 7.6–8.6), contains water, bile acids, bile salts, cholesterol, phospholipids and bile pigments such as bilirubin. The gall bladder stores and concentrates the bile and, after a meal, contracts rhythmically, expelling bile into the duodenum. The bile salts aid in the emulsification and absorption of lipids in the small intestine.

Cholecystitis (i.e. inflammation of the gall bladder) is often associated with the presence of gallstones. The stones lodge in the gall bladder neck or ducts, causing congestion and oedema as bile builds up. This may be an acute or a chronic condition. Malignant tumours of the gall bladder are infrequent.

Drugs that affect the biliary system

Ursodeoxycholic acid is a minor constituent of human bile. Its administration results in a change in bile acid composition and an increase in bile acid output and bile flow. It is indicated for the treatment of chronic cholestatic liver disease and cholestasis related to cystic fibrosis. There are limited data on its use in children and pregnant women. Drugs such as colestyramine, colestipol, charcoal and antacids can bind ursodeoxycholic acid, resulting in reduced absorption of the drugs. Diarrhoea is a common adverse reaction.

The lower gastrointestinal tract

The small and large intestine

The small intestine, comprising the duodenum, jejunum and ileum, begins at the pyloric sphincter, coils through the abdominal cavity and connects with the large intestine at the ileocaecal sphincter. The small intestine is actually about 6–7 m long; however, under normal conditions, muscle tone keeps it to about 3 m in length. Chyme remains in the small intestine for 3–5 hours, during which time more than 90% of the nutrients and water are absorbed. Any undigested material passes to the large intestine.

The caecum, colon and rectum make up the large intestine, which is about 1.5 m in length. The distal 2.5 cm of the rectum is known as the anal canal. The final stages of digestion in the large intestine occur through bacterial action, including fermentation of carbohydrate, with the release of carbon dioxide, hydrogen and methane gas. These bacteria also synthesise vitamin K, which is absorbed by simple diffusion in the colon. Around 400–800 mL water is also reabsorbed in the large intestine. Decomposition of bilirubin contributes to the brown colour of faeces. Secretion of mucus by the lining of the large intestine protects the bowel from the rough undigested faecal matter. Peristaltic movements push the faeces to the rectum, where they are expelled through the reflex action known as defecation.

Distension of the rectum by faeces stimulates stretch receptors. This sends sensory information to the CNS via the sacral segment of the spinal cord. Parasympathetic motor impulses to the colon, rectum and anus result in contraction of rectal muscles. This increases pressure in the rectum which, coupled with contraction of the diaphragm and abdominal muscles, relaxation of the internal sphincter and voluntary relaxation of the external sphincter, results in expulsion of faeces through the anus.

Disorders of the small and large intestine

Two disorders affecting the entire lower GIT are constipation and diarrhoea. Others affecting the large intestine include diverticular disease, which has no specific therapy; inflammatory bowel disease, which is the collective term used to describe ulcerative colitis and Crohn's disease, irritable bowel syndrome (see later); and carcinoma. Haemorrhoids (varicosities of the external or internal haemorrhoidal veins) are also common.

Everyone has regular bowel movements that range from three per day to three per week. Changes to bowel habits should be investigated thoroughly and causative factors eliminated before instituting drug therapy. Bowel function is often a major concern, particularly constipation in the elderly and diarrhoea in children and immunosuppressed people.

Constipation

Constipation is defined as difficult faecal evacuation as a result of hardness and dryness of faeces and perhaps infrequent movements. Causes of constipation include disordered bowel habits, various disease states, lack of dietary fibre, inadequate fluid intake or certain drugs such as codeine and morphine (Ch 19). Approximately 16–17% of the adult population in Europe and the US suffer with constipation and the condition is more than two times more common in women than men (International Longevity Centre–UK and Norgine – see 'Online resources').

Chronic constipation is sometimes simply caused by a lack of dietary fibre and reduced fluid intake. Often, however, the underlying cause is organic disease such as tumours; bowel obstruction; diseases of the liver, gall bladder or muscles; neurological abnormalities such as multiple sclerosis and Parkinson's disease; or pregnancy. Other factors that contribute to constipation include a failure to respond to defecation impulses, a sedentary lifestyle characterised by insufficient exercise and impaired physical mobility.

Constipation is often an adverse reaction of many commonly used drugs, and simply changing or stopping drug therapy may be all that is required to restore normal bowel habit. Drugs causing constipation include aluminium antacids, anticholinergics, tricyclic antidepressants, opioids and the calcium channel blockers verapamil and amlodipine and antipsychotics such as clozapine. (See Ch 22 for a description of clozapine-induced constipation.) The elderly appear to have a higher incidence of constipation, often because of multiple illnesses that require a variety of medications. The ageing process itself is associated with a decline in both physiological function and physical activity, and people who suffer from disorders of the GIT frequently complain of constipation (Clinical Focus Box 16.4). On the other hand, a person may complain of constipation when no organic disease or lesion can be found.

Diarrhoea

Diarrhoea is characterised by defecation of liquid faeces occurring as a result of decreased absorption by the small and large intestine, accumulation of non-reabsorbable

CLINICAL FOCUS BOX 16.4
Alternatives to laxative therapy

The elderly often use or misuse laxatives because of the view that regularity implies a daily bowel movement. Long-term-care residents are susceptible to constipation and medications may contribute. As lifestyle factors may predispose to constipation, health professionals should obtain from the person a dietary and laxative history, including use of herbal preparations. Encouragement to simply increase fluid intake and undertake a regular exercise routine, such as a daily walk or active and passive exercise for bedridden clients, may prove beneficial.

Individuals who regularly consume a low-fibre diet or foods that tend to harden stools (e.g. cheese, hard-boiled eggs, liver, cottage cheese, foods high in sugar content and rice) should be encouraged to increase their intake of dietary fibre. A high-fibre diet with adequate fluid intake helps reduce constipation by stimulating bowel activity. High-fibre foods include orange juice with pulp or fresh citrus fruits, bran or whole-grain cereals and breads, and leafy vegetables. Other fruits high in dietary fibre are prunes, bananas, figs and dates. Prunes (*Prunus domestica*) contain a laxative substance in addition to being high in dietary fibre. Daily consumption of prunes or a small glass of prune juice is therefore often suggested for constipation. Avoid fibre supplements in non-ambulatory people or those who are on restricted or limited fluid intake.

solutes (osmotic diarrhoea) or excessive secretion in the small intestine and colon (secretory diarrhoea). The term 'diarrhoea' generally describes the increased passage of semi-liquid or liquid stools. Causes of diarrhoea range from gastroenteritis caused by a virus or bacteria, parasitic infections, food poisoning and food intolerances to carcinomas.

Drugs can cause diarrhoea; these include NSAIDs, antibiotics, cytotoxic agents, magnesium-containing antacids and laxatives.

Diarrhoea may be acute, with a sudden onset in a previously healthy individual, lasting about 3 days to 1–2 weeks; this is usually self-limiting and resolves without sequelae. Chronic diarrhoea can last for 3–4 weeks or more, with recurring passage of liquid stools, and may be accompanied by fever, anorexia, nausea, vomiting, weight reduction and chronic weakness. In many instances, chronic diarrhoea in adults signifies an underlying disease that necessitates definitive treatment directed to the organic cause. Persistent diarrhoea in any age group, but particularly in infants, can lead to significant fluid and electrolyte disturbances and circulatory collapse.

Drugs that affect the lower gastrointestinal tract

Laxatives

Laxatives are drugs given to enhance transit of food through the intestine. The duration of treatment with laxatives should be as short as possible, and the desirability of limiting reliance on laxatives should be discussed with the person. Figure 16.5 summarises the types of laxatives and describes alternatives to pharmacological treatment. Clinical Focus Box 16.5 describes some traditional medicines from Australian plants.

Bulk-forming laxatives

Bulk laxatives absorb water and increase the volume, bulk and moisture of non-absorbable intestinal contents, thereby distending the bowel and initiating reflex bowel activity. The laxatives constituting this group are natural plant gums such as psyllium (ispaghula), bran and *Sterculia*, and semisynthetic cellulose derivatives such as methylcellulose. These agents are polysaccharide polymers that are not broken down by normal digestive processes. They stimulate peristalsis by increasing the bulk of the stool through absorption of water in the colon. This mechanism of laxative action is a normal stimulus and is one of the least harmful. These drugs do not interfere with absorption of food, but need to be administered with sufficient fluids to ensure an adequate effect.

The effect of these laxatives may not be apparent for 12–24 hours, and their full effect may not be achieved until the second or third day after administration. Some health professionals maintain that bran and dried fruits (e.g. prunes, prune juice and figs) exert the same effect, and they prefer to suggest these foods rather than the bulk-forming laxatives. Although bulk-forming laxatives are indicated for constipation, they have also been found to improve stool consistency in diarrhoea and for colostomy and ileostomy patients. Adverse reactions are minimal, the most commonly reported being flatulence and bulky stools.

Faecal softening agents

Faecal softening agents act as dispersing wetting agents, facilitating mixture of water and fatty substances within the faecal mass, producing soft faeces. The faecal softening agents include docusate, liquid paraffin and poloxamer. They are commonly used to treat acute constipation and to prevent straining (e.g. after bowel surgery).

Docusate acts like a detergent, permitting water and fatty substances to penetrate and to become well mixed with the faecal material. It may also inhibit water absorption from the bowel and stimulate water secretion into the GIT. Softened stools are usually excreted in 1–3 days after oral administration and about 15 minutes after rectal administration. These agents may be used for people with rectal impaction, haemorrhoids, postpartum

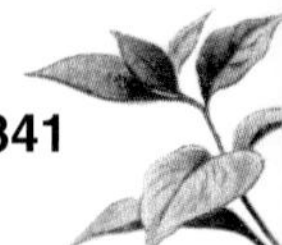

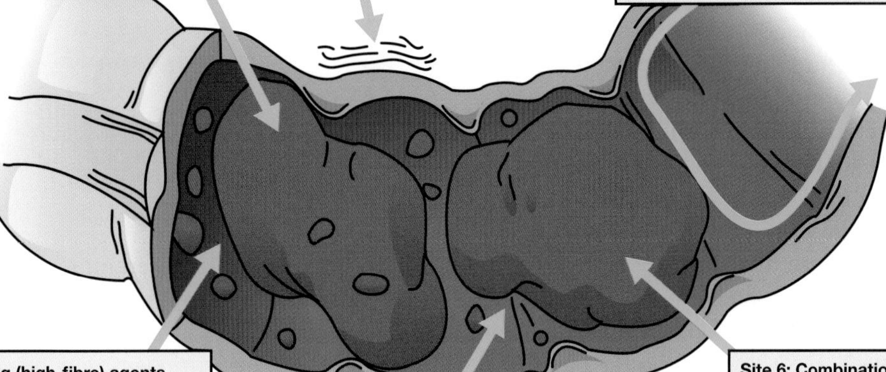

Site 1: Faecal softeners
Example: docusate
Mechanism: wetting agent used to soften faecal matter
Onset of action: 1–3 days
Comments: Liquid dosage form may cause throat irritation; dilute in fruit juice or milk before administering

Site 3: Stimulants
Example: senna
Mechanism: increases peristalsis via nerve stimulation in the colon
Onset of action: 6–12 hours
Comments: May cause discolouration of faeces and urine (alkaline urine from pink, red to brown; acid urine from yellow to brown)

Site 5: Lubricants/faecal softeners
Example: liquid paraffin
Mechanism: coats surface of faeces and eases passage of stool; also softens faecal mass
Onset of action: 6–8 hours
Precaution: Avoid administering within 2 hours of meals, as it may impair absorption of vitamins A, D, E and K. Avoid use in dysphagic and bedridden persons as aspiration of liquid parafin may result in lipid pneumonitis

Site 2: Bulk forming (high-fibre) agents
Example: psyllium hydrophilic
Mechanism: absorbs water to increase bulk, distending bowel to initiate reflex bowel activity
Onset of action: 12 hours to 3 days
Comments: Contraindicated in persons with dysphagia, as oesophageal obstruction may result. Avoid in dehydrated persons or individuals with limited or restricted fluid intake

Site 4: Osmotics
Example: lactulose
Mechanism: increases volume of fluid in lumen, resulting in distension, peristalsis and evacuation
Onset of action: 1–3 hours
Comments: Avoid use in colostomy and ileostomy, and in persons with impared renal function or dehydration

Site 6: Combination of stool softener and stimulant
Example: docusate and senna
Mechanism: stool softener and stimulant
Onset of action: 6–12 hours
Precaution: As noted for individual laxatives

FIGURE 16.5 Classification of laxatives according to site of action

Source: Adapted from Salerno 1999, Figure 3.1.

CLINICAL FOCUS BOX 16.5

Australian medicinal plants for gastrointestinal disorders

Indigenous Australians have long used plant-derived astringents such as mucilage or tannins for symptomatic treatment of GIT disorders.

Astringents obtained from exudates, barks and roots of several plants, most commonly eucalypt and wattle species, can be used to treat diarrhoea and dysentery. Exudates, commonly known as kinos, provide a rich source of the astringent tannins. Kinotannic acid is thought to be the active ingredient. Exudates of the river red gum (*Eucalyptus camaldulensis*) are dissolved in water and drunk, as are those of the coastal sheoak (*Casuarina equisetifolia*) and sassafras (*Cinnamonium oliveri*). Indigenous Queenslanders use the inner roots, leaves and boiled fruits (named jelly boys) of the dysentery bush (*Grewia retusifolia*) for relief of gastric upsets. The fruits form a jelly-like substance, which is ingested. Similarly, the roots and stems of some species of orchid (*Cymbidium albuciflorum*) provide a rich source of mucilage or pseudostarch.

Stomach upsets of unspecified cause are treated with infusions of either the bark of black wattle (*Acacia mearnsii*) or the leaves of wild or native raspberry (*Rubus moluccanus*). Small balls of white clay, perhaps similar to kaolin, may be chewed, sometimes with pieces of termite mounds. The termite mound pieces might also provide nutritional benefit, as they are a rich source of iron, with levels as high as 2%.

Natural purgatives or laxatives include the mildly active ingredient mannitol, found in the sugary exudate of manna gum (*Eucalyptus viminalis*). The leaves and pods of the native senna (*Cassia pleurocarpa* or *Cassia australis*) also provide a laxative effect. Although the active constituents are not known, the leaves do contain triterpenes.

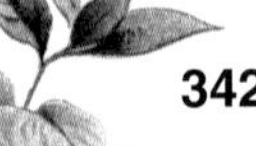

constipation and painful conditions of the rectum and anus, and for people who should avoid straining during defecation (e.g. after rectal or eye surgery). Docusate may be useful for immobile patients, especially children. Adverse reactions are infrequent, and oral formulations should be given with plenty of fluid.

Liquid paraffin, a mixture of liquid hydrocarbons obtained from petroleum, is not digested and absorption is minimal. Liquid paraffin penetrates and coats the faecal mass and prevents excessive absorption of water. Liquid paraffin is especially useful when it is desirable to keep faeces soft and when straining must be avoided.

Liquid paraffin can impair the absorption of fat-soluble vitamins A, D, E and K. If liquid paraffin is taken with meals, gastric emptying time may be delayed. An objection to its use is that in large doses it tends to leak or seep from the rectum, which can cause anal pruritus and interfere with healing of postoperative wounds in the region of the anus and perineum. This leakage is often an embarrassment to the person. Although absorption of liquid paraffin is limited, after prolonged use it may cause a chronic inflammatory reaction in tissues where it is found.

Poloxamer is a surfactant that increases penetration of fluid into faeces, thereby softening the faecal mass. It is a component of Coloxyl and is primarily used in infants and children. Care should be exercised, as continued or high use may lead to abdominal discomfort and excessive fluid and electrolyte loss, particularly of potassium.

Stimulant laxatives

Stimulant laxatives promote accumulation of water and increase peristalsis in the colon by irritating intramural sensory nerve plexi endings in the mucosa. The principal stimulant laxatives are bisacodyl, sodium picosulfate and preparations of senna. These agents promote accumulation of water and electrolytes in the lumen and stimulate nerve endings to increase intestinal motility. The stimulant laxatives usually act in 6–12 hours. Their primary effect is on the small and large intestines, which explains their tendency to produce cramping. Stimulant laxatives are used in preparation for diagnostic and surgical bowel procedures. Adverse effects of stimulant laxatives include abdominal cramping and fluid and electrolyte imbalance. Except for spinal patients, these agents are not recommended for regular use. Table 16.6 compares the stimulant laxatives in use today.

Bisacodyl is a relatively non-toxic laxative agent that stimulates peristalsis on contact with the mucosa of the colon. It is the chemical triphenylmethane, related to the pH indicator phenolphthalein. The enteric coating is formulated to dissolve in intestinal fluids and, when released, produces its stimulating effects on the colon. It should not be chewed, crushed or taken with milk or antacids because it can irritate the stomach, manifesting as severe abdominal cramps. The tablets produce evacuation of the bowel in 6–12 hours, and suppositories and enemas act within 15–60 and 5–15 minutes, respectively. The suppositories may cause a burning sensation and proctitis.

TABLE 16.6 Stimulant laxatives

NAME	ONSET OF ACTION (h)	REMARKS
Bisacodyl	6–12 (oral)	To prevent premature dissolving of enteric coating and GIT irritation, bisacodyl should not be taken with, or within 1 hour of ingestion of, milk or antacids
Sodium picosulfate	6–12 (oral)	Often used in preparation for surgery
Senna	6–12 (oral)	Crude senna may cause urine discolouration, contraindicated in intestinal obstruction

Senna is obtained from the dried leaves of the *Cassia* plant. It produces a thorough bowel evacuation in 6–12 hours, and this may be accompanied by abdominal pain or griping. It is found in proprietary remedies such as Laxettes and Senokot.

Osmotic and saline laxatives

The osmotic laxatives include Macrogols or polyethylene glycols (PEGs), glycerol, lactulose (Drug Monograph 16.5) and sorbitol. These are not absorbed. By exerting an osmotic effect, they increase the volume of fluid in the lumen. This increased volume accelerates the transfer of the gut contents and leads to increased defecation. Glycerol suppositories are available in adult, child and infant sizes. These suppositories act as osmotic agents by absorbing water, but they also lubricate and increase stool bulk. Local irritation of the mucous membrane of the rectum may promote peristalsis, and evacuation occurs 5–30 minutes after insertion.

Saline laxatives retain and increase the water content of faeces by virtue of an osmotic effect and stimulate peristalsis. Saline laxatives are soluble salts (e.g. magnesium salts, sodium salts and PEG Macrogol electrolyte solutions) that are only slightly absorbed from the alimentary canal. Because of their osmotic effect, they retain and increase the water content of faeces. The water in the intestinal lumen produces fluid accumulation and distension, leading to peristalsis and eventual evacuation of bowel contents. The result is a faecal mass of liquid or semi-liquid stools. The laxative dose promotes laxation in 6–8 hours, whereas a cathartic dose works in less than 3 hours.

The intestinal membrane is not entirely impermeable to the passage of saline laxatives, and as much as 20% of

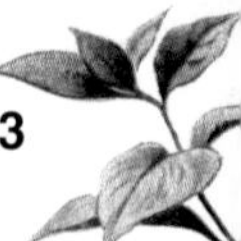

Drug Monograph 16.5
Lactulose

Lactulose is a semisynthetic disaccharide of galactose and fructose.

Mechanism of action

In the GIT the normal colonic bacteria (*Lactobacillus* and *Bacteroides*, *Escherichia coli* and *Streptococcus faecalis*) metabolise lactulose to organic acids, primarily lactic, acetic and formic acids. These acids produce an osmotic effect, an increase in fluid accumulation, distension, peristalsis and bowel movement within 24–72 hours.

Indications

Lactulose is indicated for constipation and is used to decrease blood ammonia levels in people with hepatic encephalopathy secondary to chronic liver disease. The latter effect is thought to result from the trapping by the lactulose of intestinal ammonia (as NH_4^+) and hence the excretion of excess ammonia in the faeces.

Pharmacokinetics

Absorption is minimal ($< 1\%$) after oral administration; this exceedingly small dose is excreted via the kidneys.

Drug interactions

The effectiveness of lactulose can be reduced if it is used concomitantly with an antibiotic that destroys the normal colonic bacteria. Conflicting reports exist regarding the concomitant use of neomycin and lactulose. Closer monitoring of patients should occur with concomitant oral antibiotic therapy.

Adverse reactions

These include flatulence, intestinal cramps, increased thirst and belching. Excessive doses might produce some diarrhoea and nausea (caused by the sweet taste).

Contraindications

Avoid use in people with intestinal obstruction or galactose or lactose intolerance.

Dosage and administration

The adult dose for constipation is 15–45 mL daily to a maximum of 45 mL. If the sweet taste is a problem, suggest mixing with water, milk, fruit juice or a citrus-flavoured beverage.

the salt may be absorbed. Electrolyte disturbances have been reported with their long-term daily use, and sodium salts should be avoided in people with congestive cardiac failure. Renal impairment can lead to the accumulation of magnesium and sodium ions, and hence significant electrolyte disturbances. A common formulation of magnesium sulfate is Epsom salts.

Isosmotic solutions containing PEG and electrolytes are marketed as gastrointestinal solutions specifically for bowel evacuation before surgery or gastrointestinal diagnostic procedures. These powders (ColonLYTELY, Moviprep and Glycoprep-C) consist of a mixture of PEG (a non-absorbable osmotic substance) with sodium salts (sulfate, bicarbonate and chloride) and potassium chloride that is isosmotic with body fluids. The large volume of non-absorbable fluid, commonly 2–4 L, leads to copious watery diarrhoea. Because it is isosmotic, dehydration does not occur. These products can cause failure of regular medication (e.g. the oral contraceptive pill). All saline laxatives can cause nausea, vomiting, bloating and electrolyte disturbances, and are used with caution in people with intestinal obstruction or suspected perforation.

Antidiarrhoeal drugs

In some circumstances, specific anti-infective drug treatment is indicated but, in the main, the rationale for using **antidiarrhoeal** drugs relates to relief of symptoms and the prevention of fluid and electrolyte loss. These drugs should not be used in infants and children with acute diarrhoea because of potential delay in expulsion of organisms and because they do not cause a reduction in fluid and electrolyte loss (Australian Medicines Handbook 2021). Many over-the-counter antidiarrhoeal drugs contain limited amounts of opioids (loperamide and diphenoxylate), aluminium hydroxide, attapulgite, kaolin, pectin and belladonna alkaloids (hyoscyamine, hyoscine and atropine).

Opioid antidiarrhoeals

Loperamide and diphenoxylate are over-the-counter opioids that activate μ-opioid receptors on intestinal smooth muscles, resulting in a reduction in secretions and inhibition of propulsive movements in the gut. This slows the passage of intestinal contents and allows reabsorption of water and electrolytes, reducing stool frequency.

These agents are indicated for short-term treatment of diarrhoea and for reducing the frequency and fluidity of motions in people with an intestinal stoma. Adverse reactions are usually minimal.

Diphenoxylate is chemically related to pethidine and also inhibits intestinal propulsive motility by acting directly on μ-opioid receptors on intestinal smooth muscles. The addition of atropine to diphenoxylate formulations has no therapeutic benefit but it is included in the formulation to discourage abuse; the combination can produce dizziness, dry mouth and blurred vision as a result of the muscarinic antagonist properties of atropine.

Common adverse reactions include abdominal pain, nausea, vomiting and constipation. Rash, dizziness and paralytic ileus occur rarely. Accidental or deliberate overdosage can produce additional symptoms of flushing, hyperthermia, tachycardia, dry mouth, agitation, pinpoint pupils, lethargy, respiratory depression and coma.

Concurrent use with alcohol can lead to increased CNS effect. With anticholinergics or other drugs with anticholinergic effects (e.g. tricyclic antidepressants), there is an increase in anticholinergic effects. Concurrent use with monoamine oxidase (MAO) inhibitors can result in a hypertensive crisis. Caution should be exercised where there is evidence of co-existing inflammatory bowel disease and severe hepatic impairment.

Inflammatory bowel disease

Inflammatory bowel disease includes Crohn's disease and ulcerative colitis. Although initially recognised in developed countries, inflammatory bowel disease is a global problem without geographical boundaries. Genetic and environmental factors are thought to play a role in both conditions, and smoking is a risk factor. Management includes not only drug therapy but also consideration of dietary and lifestyle factors. Excellent information can be obtained from Crohn's and Colitis Australia. Management is primarily aimed at inducing and maintaining remission of the disease state and preventing complications such as fistulae and abscesses. This, in turn, improves quality of life and ensures adequate nutrition and growth in children.

Crohn's disease is a chronic recurring inflammatory disease characterised by episodes of active flare-up and periods of remission when people are relatively free of symptoms such as abdominal pain, bowel obstruction or diarrhoea, nausea and tiredness. It can occur in any segment of the GIT but commonly small and large bowel. Treatment involves the use of various drugs, with the main aim of inducing and maintaining remission. In about 60% of cases, surgery may be required to remove affected portions of the bowel.

Ulcerative colitis is also a chronic inflammatory bowel disorder; however, unlike Crohn's disease, it affects the colonic mucosa starting in the colon and extending to the rectum. It is more common than Crohn's disease and is characterised by diffuse mucosal inflammation. Clinical symptoms include bloody diarrhoea, abdominal pain and rectal urgency. Similar to Crohn's disease, people experience acute flare-ups of the disease and long periods of remission. In a proportion of people, the disease is so severe a colectomy will be required. Aggressive pharmacotherapy limits progression and maintains remission in patients (Adams & Bornemann 2013). The aim is to increase steroid-free remission periods, reduce hospitalisations, enhance mucosal healing and improve quality of life for all affected people (Feuerstein et al. 2019).

Drug therapy for inflammatory bowel disease

Current therapy (summarised in Table 16.7) for these conditions includes corticosteroids (e.g. prednisolone and budesonide), which are discussed in detail in Chapter 29; the 5-aminosalicylates (5-ASA), which include balsalazide, mesalazine, olsalazine and sulfasalazine; and the immunosuppressants, such as azathioprine, mercaptopurine and methotrexate (discussed in Ch 34). Currently, Crohn's disease is an indication for the use of the TNF-α antagonists adalimumab and infliximab.

5-aminosalicylates (5-ASA)

Sulfasalazine consists of the sulfonamide antibiotic sulfapyridine, linked to the anti-inflammatory drug 5-aminosalicyclic acid, also called mesalazine. Sulfasalazine is poorly absorbed and, in the colon, it is split by bacteria into sulfapyridine and mesalazine, which is the active component effective in the treatment of bowel disease (Drug Monograph 16.6). Olsalazine (a dimer of two molecules of 5-ASA) and balsalazide (5-ASA linked to 4-aminobenzoyl-β-alanine, an inert carrier) are azo-bonded prodrugs that following azo reduction by anaerobic bacteria in the colon release the active drug mesalazine directly to the colon. Variability in efficacy and tolerability may be related to the different formulations.

Irritable bowel syndrome

The cause of **irritable bowel syndrome** (IBS) is unknown. The condition is common and affects up to 20% of adults in the industrialised world. Although IBS is often thought of as a predominantly female condition, symptoms are found equally in men and women. The female tag to the syndrome probably arose because women more frequently seek medical advice. Symptoms of IBS include long-term recurrent abdominal pain, change in bowel habits, anorexia, nausea, bloating and flatulence. The condition is often precipitated by stress and anxiety, and may occur after severe intestinal infection.

Management of IBS varies enormously and no real consensus on treatment exists. Dietary manipulation – for example, exclusion-type diets and low-wheat, low-lactose and low-fructose diets – is a popular approach, as is psychotherapy. Although beneficial in multiple settings,

TABLE 16.7 Drugs used to treat ulcerative colitis and Crohn's disease

	ULCERATIVE COLITIS	CROHN'S DISEASE
Mild-to-moderate disease	Initial therapy for active proctitis or distal colitis: Mesalazine + 5-ASA (add budesonide or corticosteroids if ineffective) Extensive disease: 5-ASA +/− prednisolone or budesonide	1 Prednisolone 2 Budesonide (controlled ileal release formulation)
Acute, severe disease or frequently relapsing	1 Acute severe (medical emergency): Methylprednisolone sodium succinate or hydrocortisone 2 If unresponsive to steroids, salvage therapy is continued with ciclosporin or infliximab	1 Induction therapy for severe disease: Hydrocortisone[a] or Methylprednisolone sodium succinate 2 If intolerant or refractory to above: azathioprine or mercaptopurine or methotrexate plus folic acid 3 If no response after 3 months of therapy: Infliximab or adalimumab or vedolizumab
Chronic active disease – moderate to severe	Severe chronically active frequently relapsing: 1 Azathioprine or mercaptopurine 2 If adverse effects are intolerable, methotrexate + folic acid 3 If unresponsive or intolerant of 5-ASA +/− corticosteroid, infliximab or vedolizumab	1 Azathioprine or mercaptopurine or methotrexate + folic acid
Maintenance therapy	1 5-ASA 2 If frequent relapses, azathioprine or mercaptopurine or methotrexate + folic acid 3 If refractory to above, use infliximab or vedolizumab	Severe chronically active frequently relapsing: 1 Azathioprine or mercaptopurine 2 If adverse effects are intolerable, methotrexate + folic acid 3 If unresponsive or intolerant of 5-ASA +/− corticosteroid, infliximab or vedolizumab

[a] Corticosteroids are used for acute attacks but should not be used for maintenance therapy because of evidence of limited efficacy and serious adverse effects with high-dose, long-term use. Refer to expert texts for full details.

Source: Adapted from Therapeutic Guidelines Limited 2021.

Drug Monograph 16.6
Mesalazine

Mechanism of action
The exact mechanism of action of mesalazine (5-ASA) is unknown, but it is thought to exert an anti-inflammatory effect in ulcerative colitis and Crohn's disease by inhibiting the production of (1) inflammatory mediators of the lipoxygenase pathways, (2) platelet-activating factor, (3) interleukin-1 and TNF-α, and (4) inhibition of the transcription factor NFκB, which is involved in production of inflammatory mediators. It also inhibits activation of B cells and the production of oxygen radicals. It activates PPAR-γ receptors, which counteract nuclear activation of intestinal inflammatory responses

Pharmacokinetics
Disintegration of the enteric-coated formulation (Pentasa) takes place in the small bowel about 5 hours after administration, and about 80% of the drug is available to exert its action on the intestinal mucosa. In addition to oral formulations, mesalazine can be delivered directly into the rectum or left colon by using enemas (Salofalk, Pentasa), foam preparations (Salofalk) and suppositories (Pentasa). Mesalazine is metabolised by acetylation forming N-acetyl-5-ASA, and 20–40% of the dose is excreted in faeces and 30–50% in urine. The plasma half-life is 0.5–1 hour.

Adverse reactions
These are more common with higher doses and include headache, nausea, rash, abdominal discomfort and diarrhoea.

Warnings and contraindications
Mesalazine is contraindicated in people with known hypersensitivity to salicylates or sulfasalazine, and in the presence of impaired renal function.

Dosage and administration
A dose of 500 mg (as Mesasal tablet) three times daily is recommended for acute exacerbations of ulcerative colitis and Crohn's disease, and 250 mg three times daily as a maintenance regimen. Mesalazine is also available as a 1200 mg prolonged-release tablet for once-daily administration. It is also available as modified release granules, enema and suppositories.

increase in dietary fibre may worsen symptoms, especially in those most affected by constipation, and may lead to bloating and flatulence.

The use of drug therapy is still debated and includes antispasmodic agents (e.g. hyoscine, hyoscyamine), loperamide if diarrhoea predominates and short-term use of laxatives if constipation predominates. It has been shown that IBS sufferers improve significantly when treated with Chinese herbal medicines. Among the many herbal medicines that have calming properties, peppermint oil has found its way into mainstream medicine. Although conflicting studies have been published, the current balance of data tends to support a role for peppermint oil to treat IBS (Dimidi et al. 2017; Ford et al. 2020). Mintec capsules contain 0.2 mL peppermint oil; the dosage is 1–2 capsules three times daily 30 minutes before food (Australian Medicines Handbook 2021).

KEY POINTS

Drugs affecting the lower gastrointestinal tract

- Drugs affecting the lower GIT include laxatives and antidiarrhoeal medications, and specific drugs used to treat inflammatory bowel disease (e.g. mesalazine) and IBS (e.g. peppermint oil).
- Laxatives are drugs given to enhance transit of food through the intestine.
- Bulk laxatives (e.g. psyllium, bran and methylcellulose) absorb water and increase the volume, bulk and moisture of non-absorbable intestinal contents, thereby distending the bowel and initiating reflex bowel activity.
- Faecal softening agents act as dispersing wetting agents, facilitating mixture of water and fatty substances within the faecal mass, producing soft faeces. The faecal softening agents include docusate, liquid paraffin and poloxamer.
- Stimulant laxatives promote accumulation of water and increase peristalsis in the colon by irritating intramural sensory nerve plexi endings in the mucosa. The principal stimulant laxatives are bisacodyl, sodium picosulfate and preparations of senna.
- Osmotic laxatives are not absorbed and, because they exert an osmotic effect, they increase the volume of fluid in the lumen. The osmotic laxatives glycerol, lactulose and sorbitol are not absorbed.
- Loperamide, diphenoxylate and codeine are opioid antidiarrhoeal drugs that activate μ-opioid receptors in the gut wall, resulting in a reduction in secretions and inhibition of propulsive movements in the gut.
- Current therapy for ulcerative colitis and Crohn's disease includes:
  - corticosteroids (e.g. prednisolone and budesonide)
  - 5-ASA, which include balsalazide, mesalazine, olsalazine and sulfasalazine
  - immunosuppressants such as azathioprine, mercaptopurine and methotrexate.
- Treatment for IBS includes antispasmodic agents (e.g. hyoscine, hyoscyamine), loperamide if diarrhoea predominates and short-term use of laxatives if constipation predominates. Complementary therapies such as peppermint oil may also be used.

DRUGS AT A GLANCE
Drugs affecting the upper and lower gastrointestinal tracts

PHARMACOLOGICAL GROUP AND EFFECT	KEY EXAMPLES	CLINICAL USE
Antifungals	**Nystatin**	**Oral candidiasis**
Drugs for acid-related disorders		
Antacids • Buffer or neutralise hydrochloric acid in the stomach and thereby raise the gastric pH	Magnesium aluminium combinations	Heartburn GORD NERD
Cytoprotective agents • Sulfated sucrose and aluminium hydroxide provide a protective barrier over mucosa • Synthetic analogue of prostaglandin E_1 decreasing gastric acid secretion via an action at EP_3 prostaglandin receptors on parietal cells and increasing gastric cytoprotective mucus and bicarbonate	Sucralfate Misoprostol	Gastritis GORD Gastric and duodenal ulcers (also preventative)
H_2 receptor antagonists • Block receptors involved in gastric acid secretion	Famotidine, ranitidine, nazitidine	Gastritis GORD Gastric and duodenal ulcers
Proton pump inhibitors • suppress gastric acid secretion by inhibiting the proton pump (H_1, K_1 ATPase enzyme system) at parietal cells	Esomeprazole, lansoprazole, omeprazole	Gastritis GORD Gastric and duodenal ulcers

Antiemetics		
Dopamine antagonists • Block DA receptors in vomiting centre of the CNS	Metoclopramide, prochlorperazine, domperidone	Include chemotherapy induced vomiting, migraine, gastroenteritis
5-HT_3 antagonists • Block receptors in vomiting centre of the CNS and on vagus nerve in the GIT	Ondansetron, granisetron, palonosetron, tropisetron	Include chemotherapy, induced vomiting, migraine, gastroenteritis
NK_1-receptor antagonists (substance P receptor antagonists) • Block receptors in vomiting centre of the CNS	Aprepitant Fosaprepipant	Include chemotherapy, induced vomiting
H_1 receptor antagonists and muscarinic antagonists • Block receptors in vestibular apparatus and vomiting centres	Promethazine (H_1) Hyoscine (M_1)	Motion sickness (preventative/ prophylaxis)
Laxatives		
Bulk forming	Natural plant gums and cellulose derivatives	Constipation
Faecal softening agents • Wetting agents, facilitating mixture of water and fatty substances within the faecal mass, producing soft faeces	Docusate, liquid paraffin	Constipation
Stimulant laxatives • Increase peristalsis in the colon by irritating intramural sensory nerve plexi endings in the mucosa	Bisacodyl, sodium picosulfate	Constipation
Osmotic laxatives • Exert an osmotic effect, increase the volume of fluid in the lumen and induce peristalsis	Glycerol, lactulose	Constipation
Antidiarrhoeals		
Opioid antidiarrhoeals • Activate μ-opioid receptors on intestinal smooth muscles, resulting in a reduction in secretions and inhibition of propulsive movements in the gut	Codeine, loperamide, diphenoxylate (with atropine)	Diarrhoea
Drugs to treat inflammatory bowel disorders		
Corticosteroids • Inhibit the production of inflammatory mediators		Crohn's disease, ulcerative colitis
5-aminosalicylates (5-ASA) • Inhibit the production of (1) inflammatory mediators of the lipoxygenase pathways, (2) platelet-activating factor, (3) interleukin-1 and TNF-α, and (4) inhibition of the transcription factor NFκB	Balsalazide[AUS], mesalazine, olsalazine, sulfasalazine	Crohn's disease, ulcerative colitis
Immunosuppressants • Inhibit inflammatory mediators	Azathioprine, mercaptopurine, methotrexate	Crohn's disease, ulcerative colitis
TNF-α antagonists • Inhibit inflammatory mediators	Adalimumab, infliximab	Crohn's disease

GORD = gastro-oesophageal reflux disease; NERD = non-erosive reflux disease
AUS = Australia

REVIEW EXERCISES

1. Mrs XP is a 55-year-old woman who was referred to the gastroenterology clinic by her GP due to consistent discomfort and significant weight loss. For the past 6 months she has had burning pain in the epigastric region and chest that worsens after eating meals and drinking coffee and alcohol. She takes antacids to relieve the pain. She undergoes a breath test and gastroscopy and is diagnosed with *H. pylori* infection. She is recommended to undertake 'triple therapy'. Describe the classes of drugs that are in this type of therapy. If the bacteria is resistant to the therapy, what are the other options for Mrs XP?
2. Mrs CJ, an 80 year old, lives in an aged care facility. She has been prescribed oxybutynin for her urinary incontinence and Panadol Forte (paracetamol and codeine) for pain associated with a recent fall. Mrs CJ complains of constipation and associated abdominal pain. Could any of her medications have caused the constipation? Briefly,

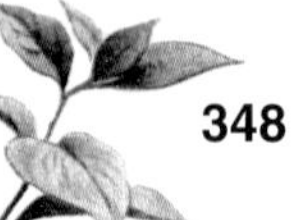

what are the mechanisms of action of her medications and could they contribute to any adverse effects?

3. Mr AJ, while on holiday in a tropical location, developed acute diarrhoea causing significant dehydration. He was prescribed codeine but mistakenly took triple the recommended dose in an attempt to alleviate the symptoms. Explain why he has presented to the local hospital with diverse adverse reactions affecting the gastrointestinal, respiratory and central nervous systems.

REFERENCES

Adams SM, Bornemann PH: Ulcerative colitis. American Family Physician 87(10):699–705, 2013.

Anderka M, Mitchell AA, Louik C, et al: Medications used to treat nausea and vomiting of pregnancy and the risk of selected birth defects. Birth Defects Research. Part A, Clinical and Molecular Teratology 94:22–30, 2012.

Audo I, Warchol ME: Retinal and cochlear toxicity of drugs: new insights into mechanisms and detection. Current Opinion in Neurology 25(1):76–85, 2012.

Australian Medicines Handbook P/L: Australian medicines handbook 2021, Adelaide, 2021, AMH.

Bromley SM: Smell and taste disorders: a primary care approach. American Family Physician 61(2):427–436, 438, 2000.

Deutsch A, Jay E. Optimising oral health in frail older people. Australian Prescriber [Internet]. 2021 Oct [cited 2021 Nov 2];44(5):153–60. Available from: https://search.ebscohost.com/login.aspx?direct=true&AuthType=shib&db=afh&AN=152787358&site=eds-live

Dimidi E, Rossi M, Whelan K: Irritable bowel syndrome and diet: where are we in 2018? Current Opinion in Clinical Nutrition and Metabolic Care 20(6):456–463, 2017.

Doty RL, Shah M, Bromley SM: Drug-induced taste disorders. Drug Safety 31(3):199–215, 2008.

Feuerstein JD, Moss AC, Farraye FA. Ulcerative colitis. Mayo Clinic Proceedings. 2019 Jul;94(7):1357–1373. doi: 10.1016/j.mayocp.2019.01.018. Erratum in: Mayo Clinic Proceedings. 2019 Oct;94(10):2149. PMID: 31272578.

Ford AC, Sperber AD, Corsetti M, et al. Irritable bowel syndrome. Lancet. 2020 Nov 21;396(10263):1675–1688. doi: 10.1016/S0140-6736(20)31548-8. Epub 2020 Oct 10. PMID: 33049223.

Henkin RI: Drug-induced taste and smell disorders: incidence, mechanisms and management related primarily to treatment of sensory receptor dysfunction. Drug Safety 11(5):318–377, 1994.

Mitchell H, Katelaris P: Epidemiology, clinical impacts and current clinical management of Helicobacter pylori infection. Medical Journal of Australia 204(10):376–380, 2016.

O'Connor A, Furuta T, Gisbert JP, et al. Review – Treatment of *Helicobacter pylori* infection 2020. Helicobacter. 2020 Sep;25 Suppl 1:e12743. doi: 10.1111/hel.12743. PMID: 32918350.

Rang HP, Dale JM, Ritter JM, et al: Rang and Dale's pharmacology, ed 7, 2012, Elsevier Inc.

Salerno E: Pharmacology for health professionals, St Louis, MO, 1999, Mosby.

Therapeutic Goods Administration 2017. Guidance for the use of medicinal cannabis for the prevention or management of nausea and vomiting in Australia. Version 1. Available from: https://www.tga.gov.au/publication/guidance-use-medicinal-cannabis-prevention-or-management-nausea-and-vomiting-australia

Therapeutic Guidelines Limited 2021. Inflammatory Bowel Disease [published 2021 Mar]. In: Therapeutic Guidelines [digital]. Melbourne: Therapeutic Guidelines Limited. https://www.tg.org.au

Woo, SD, Luu, QQ, Park, HS. (2020). NSAID-exacerbated respiratory disease (NERD): from pathogenesis to improved care. Frontiers in Pharmacology, 11, 1147. https://doi.org/10.3389/fphar.2020.01147

Wu J, Carter A: Magnesium: the forgotten electrolyte. Australian Prescriber 30:102–105, 2007.

ONLINE RESOURCES

Australian Gastroenterology Institute: http://www.nevdgp.org.au/info/gastro/Helicobacterpylori.htm/ (accessed 22 January 2022)

Crohn's and Colitis Association: http://www.crohnsandcolitis.com.au/ (accessed 22 January 2022)

Crohn's and Colitis New Zealand: http://crohnsandcolitis.org.nz/ (accessed 22 January 2022)

Gastroenterological Society of Australia – Australian guidelines for general practitioners and physicians: inflammatory bowel disease, 4th ed: https://www.gesa.org.au/education/clinical-information/ (accessed 22 January 2022)

International Longevity Centre–UK and Norgine – The burden of constipation in our ageing population: working towards better solutions: http://www.burdenofconstipation.com/wp-content/uploads/2013/09/Constipation-Report.pdf/ (accessed 22 January 2022)

Ministry of Health (New Zealand) – Guidelines for the use of fluorides: http://www.health.govt.nz/publication/guidelines-use-fluorides/ (accessed 17 October 2017)

Ministry of Health (New Zealand) – Water fluoridation: https://www.health.govt.nz/our-work/preventative-health-wellness/fluoride-and-oral-health/water-fluoridation/ (accessed 22 January 2022)

More weblinks at: http://evolve.elsevier.com/AU/Knights/pharmacology/.

CHAPTER 17

DRUGS AFFECTING THE KIDNEY AND BLADDER

Kathleen Knights

KEY ABBREVIATIONS

ADH	antidiuretic hormone
BPH	benign prostatic hyperplasia
CKD	chronic kidney disease
CrCl	creatinine clearance
eGFR	estimated glomerular filtration rate
GFR	glomerular filtration rate
NKCC	Na^+–K^+–2 Cl^- co-transporter
OAB	overactive bladder
SCr	serum creatinine
TALH	thick ascending limb of the loop of Henle

KEY TERMS

Chapter Focus

The kidneys maintain homeostasis, eliminate metabolic byproducts and regulate acid–base balance. Diuretics, widely prescribed for heart failure and hypertension, alter renal function, increasing urine volume and enhancing the excretion of sodium and chloride. Electrolyte imbalance and volume depletion are common and can be minimised by using a low dose and monitoring both clinical response and plasma electrolytes.

Urinary dysfunction (e.g. incontinence) is common, and it is essential to eliminate possible contributing factors such as urinary tract infection, metabolic disorders or drugs with anticholinergic effects prior to drug therapy. In elderly males, benign prostatic hyperplasia causes bladder dysfunction by increasing bladder outlet resistance. Elimination of aggravating factors (e.g. drugs with anticholinergic effects), modification of lifestyle factors (e.g. reducing fluid intake prior to bed) and education (e.g. bladder training) are factors for consideration, in addition to drug therapy.

KEY DRUG GROUPS

Diuretics:

- Loop diuretics: bumetanide, **furosemide** (Drug Monograph 17.1)
- Potassium-sparing diuretics: **amiloride**, amiloride with hydrochlorothiazide
- Thiazide and thiazide-like diuretics: Chlortalidone, **hydrochlorothiazide**, indapamide

Drugs for bladder dysfunction:

- **alfuzosin**, silodosin, tamsulosin, darifenacin, mirabegron, **oxybutynin** (Drug Monograph 17.2), solifenacin

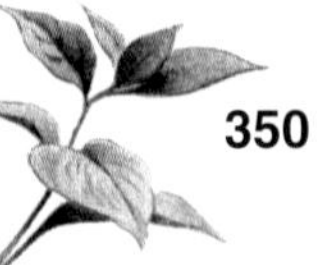

CRITICAL THINKING SCENARIO

Marilyn, a 74-year-old woman with a history of persistent oedema associated with heart failure, presents to hospital with dehydration, dizziness and postural hypotension. On questioning, Marilyn indicates that she feels confused, that she hasn't been drinking very many fluids and that she may have taken too many 'fluid tablets'. You ascertain that she has been prescribed furosemide (frusemide) and her usual daily dose is 400 mg. Discuss the pharmacological/physiological relationship between her current symptoms and the likelihood they are due to an increased dose of frusemide.

Introduction: The kidneys

The kidneys maintain homeostasis by processing salts and water and balancing excretion, hence controlling the volume and ionic composition of the extracellular fluid; regulating blood pH by excreting hydrogen ions (H^+); excreting waste products such as urea, uric acid and creatinine; and modulating blood pressure via the release of renin and activation of the renin–angiotensin–aldosterone system. In addition to these roles, the kidneys synthesise calcitriol (1,25-dihydroxycholecalciferol), an active vitamin D metabolite (Ch 27), and the growth factor erythropoietin, which stimulates red blood cell production (Ch 14).

The functional units of the kidney are the nephrons, the number of which (about 1 million) is determined at birth. Each nephron consists of a glomerulus (the glomerular capillaries and Bowman's capsule) and the renal tubule comprising, in order of the flow through them, the proximal convoluted tubule, the loop of Henle, the distal convoluted tubule and, finally, the collecting duct. Most nephrons (around 80%) have short loops of Henle that penetrate superficially into the medulla and are termed cortical nephrons. The remaining nephrons – with long loops of Henle that almost traverse the medullary region – are called juxtamedullary nephrons and provide the kidney with the ability to concentrate the urine.

The kidneys are highly vascularised, and the complex network of arterioles, capillaries and venules gives rise to the glomerular capillaries, the peritubular capillaries that form a dense plexus surrounding the cortical aspects of the renal tubule, and the vasa recta, the long hairpin loop-shaped capillaries that supply the renal medulla. The peri-tubular capillaries reunite to form the peritubular venules, and blood finally leaves the kidney through a single renal vein. Control of renal blood flow is a complex process involving myogenic (intrinsic) responses, tubuloglomerular feedback via the juxtaglomerular apparatus, the renin–angiotensin–aldosterone system (Ch 11), the sympathetic nervous system and vasoactive agents including renal prostaglandins that play a role in vasodilation in compromised kidneys, leukotrienes and nitric oxide. The interface between the vascular network and the renal tubule provides the basis for the three main renal processes: glomerular filtration, tubular secretion and tubular reabsorption.

Glomerular filtration

Glomerular filtration occurs as a result of ultrafiltration of water and solutes through pores of the glomerular capillaries into the capsular space of the Bowman's capsule. In the absence of disease, the glomerular membrane does not allow molecules larger than 6–7 nanometres in diameter, which includes plasma proteins such as haemoglobin and albumin, to pass through. Cardiac output creates pressure in the blood vessels, which in turn provides the force necessary to accomplish glomerular filtration. Blood flow to the kidney is normally around 1200 mL/min, which is 20–25% of cardiac output, and the glomerular filtration rate (GFR) is about 125 mL/min. This amounts to approximately 180 L of filtrate formed per day in a healthy person, of which 99% (~178 L) is ultimately reabsorbed throughout the length of the nephron.

Maintenance of glomerular hydrostatic pressure depends on systemic blood pressure and is aided by the ability of the afferent and efferent arterioles to constrict and dilate (Fig 17.1). In the walls of the afferent arteriole are juxtaglomerular cells, which are the primary site of renin storage and release in the body. A reduction in afferent arteriole pressure causes the release of renin from the juxtaglomerular cells into the systemic circulation. The renin released causes increased production of angiotensin II, a powerful vasoconstrictor that increases

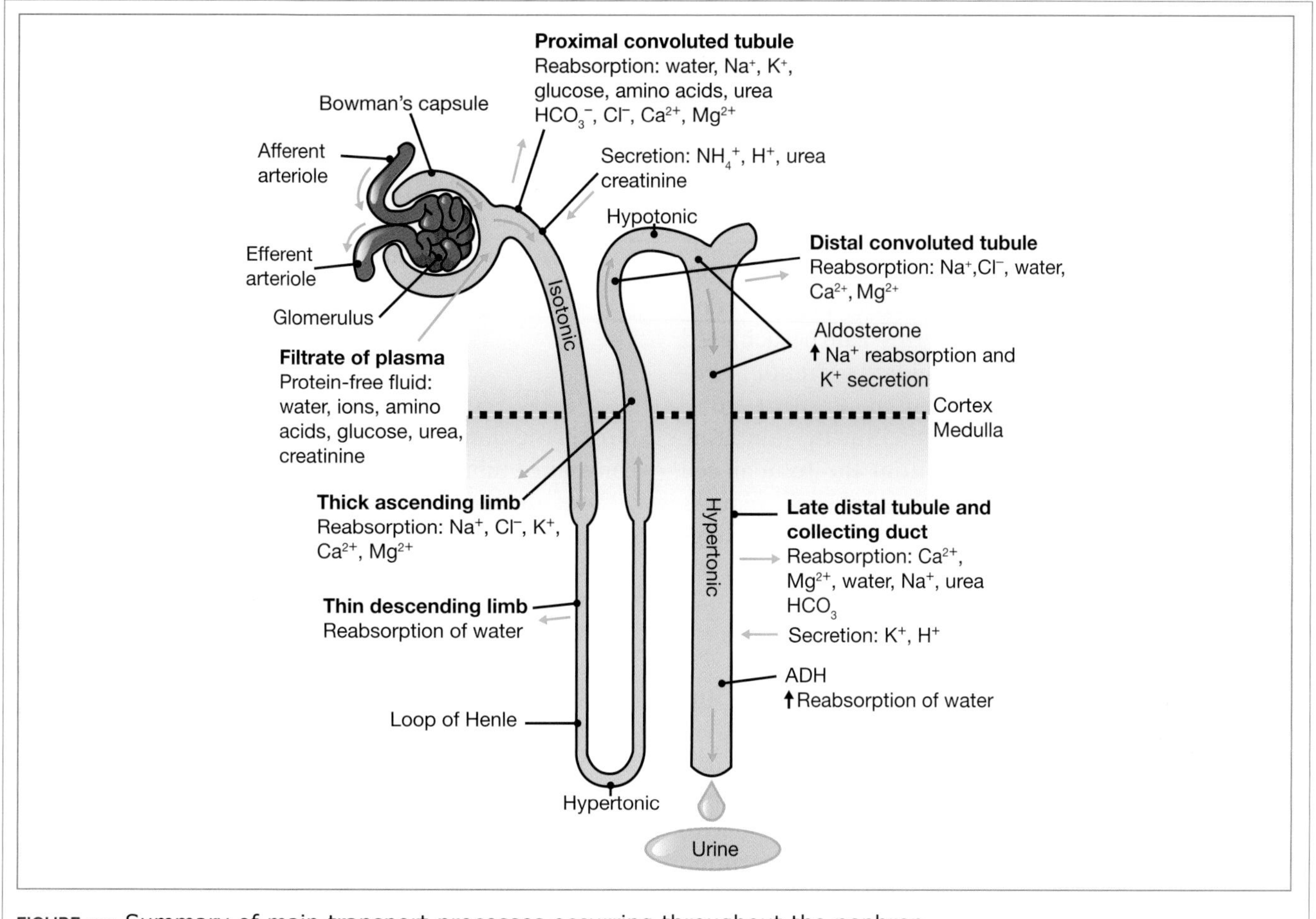

FIGURE 17.1 Summary of main transport processes occurring throughout the nephron

systemic blood pressure. Systemic blood pressure has to be significantly reduced before glomerular filtration is greatly altered. Usually, some degree of filtration will exist if the pressure in the glomerular capillaries remains above 50 mmHg. Renin release is also controlled by specialised tubular cells located in the cortical thick ascending limb of the loop of Henle, where it makes contact with the afferent arteriole. These cells, known as the macula densa, along with the juxtaglomerular cells, form the juxtaglomerular apparatus. The macula densa cells respond to changes in the flow of tubular fluid and sodium chloride concentration. Increases in the luminal concentration of sodium chloride inhibit renin release, whereas a decrease in the luminal concentration stimulates the release of renin from JG cells, which leads to the synthesis of angiotensin II and the release of aldosterone from the adrenal cortex. Aldosterone then promotes sodium reabsorption in the distal tubule and collecting ducts, thus increasing extracellular volume through the retention of water (Fig 11.4).

Tubular secretion

The second main renal process is **tubular secretion**, which is the movement of substances (e.g. endogenous molecules, drugs and/or their metabolites) from peritubular or interstitial capillaries into the renal tubular cells and then into the tubular lumen. The proximal convoluted tubule plays an important role in the secretion of hydrogen ions (H^+) which, coupled with preferential absorption of bicarbonate (HCO_3^-), regulates acid–base balance, and in the secretion of metabolic byproducts (e.g. ammonium ions, creatinine) and certain drugs (e.g. penicillin). Both acidic and basic drugs are taken up from the interstitial fluid into tubular cells via the basolateral uptake 'acid' and 'base' transporters (Ch 4). These include OAT1, 2 and 3 and the organic cation transporters OCT2 and 3. Examples of drugs secreted (effluxed) via the apical (luminal) membrane 'acid' (OAT) transporters include aciclovir, frusemide, penicillins and cefalosporins and methotrexate; those secreted via the 'base' (OCT)

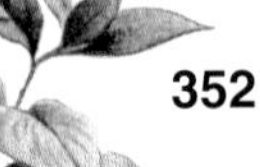

transporters include metformin and ranitidine. The apical membrane of proximal tubular cells additionally expresses efflux transporters, including P-gp, OAT4, MATE1 and 2 and MRP2 and 4, which serve to export compounds from the tubular cell into urine. Another family of transporters found in the kidney, the novel organic cation transporters that are localised on the apical membrane, also appear to contribute to the transfer of organic cations into the tubular lumen. From a clinical perspective, at times reducing the excretion of a drug may be beneficial and this can be achieved by competitively inhibiting tubular secretion. For example, probenecid, which is used to treat gout, reduces the renal excretion of penicillin by inhibiting the efflux of penicillin via OATs from the tubular cell into the lumen of the nephron and hence reduces excretion of penicillin in urine. Clinically, this prolongs the effect of the antibiotic by maintaining a therapeutic plasma concentration for longer.

Tubular reabsorption

Reabsorption of sodium and nutrients leads to the reabsorption of water by osmosis. Of the 180 L of glomerular filtrate delivered to the nephrons per day, most is reabsorbed from the lumen of the proximal convoluted tubule into the peritubular capillaries, with the remainder excreted as urine. This **tubular reabsorption** is a selective process, and the main transport mechanisms that prevail throughout the nephron are:

- simple diffusion and facilitated diffusion; the latter involves carrier-mediated passive transport from a region of high concentration to a region of lower concentration
- primary active transport, principally by the Na^+–K^+-ATPase pump in the basolateral membrane, which transports sodium against an electrochemical gradient
- carrier-mediated (secondary active) transport, in which the transport of sodium down its concentration gradient provides the energy for the active transport of solutes such as glucose against their concentration gradient. Secondary active-transport membrane proteins that move two substrates in the same direction are called symporters, whereas those that transport two substances in opposite directions are called antiporters. The tubular Na^+/H^+ and Na^+/K^+ exchanges are examples of antiport systems.

Within the nephron, competition for transport by a single transporter between ions and drugs often manifests as an adverse effect – for example, hyperuricaemia with some diuretics. As ion transport within the nephron is complex, specific mechanisms will be discussed in those sections detailing the mechanism of action of the various classes of diuretics.

The roles of various segments of the renal tubule in the movement of water and solutes are summarised in the following sections and in Figure 17.1. The final urinary excretion of a substance that is influenced by glomerular filtration, tubular secretion and tubular reabsorption can be summarised as:

$$\begin{aligned}&\text{Amount of substance excreted in urine}\\&= \text{amount of substance filtered}\\&\quad + \text{amount of substance secreted}\\&\quad - \text{amount of substance reabsorbed}\end{aligned}$$

Proximal convoluted tubule

Most of the glomerular filtrate is reabsorbed in the proximal convoluted tubule and returned to the bloodstream. About 70% of the salt and water in the filtrate is reabsorbed, maintaining nearly the same osmolality between the tubular fluid and the interstitial fluid at the end of the proximal convoluted tubule (i.e. the solutions are isotonic). The secretion of H^+ that occurs in the proximal convoluted tubule is linked to the reabsorption of HCO_3^- in the tubular filtrate. This process involves intracellular formation of carbonic acid (H_2CO_3) from carbon dioxide and water. The carbonic acid formed dissociates to give HCO_3^- and H^+. This reversible reaction is catalysed by carbonic anhydrase. The hydrogen ions formed are secreted into the lumen and combine with bicarbonate in the glomerular filtrate to form carbonic acid in the lumen. This, in turn, dissociates into water and carbon dioxide, which diffuses into tubule cells and re-forms H_2CO_3. Dissociation releases bicarbonate, which is then reabsorbed into the blood.

Acid–base balance is maintained in healthy humans by the action of the body's buffer systems, changes in the rate and depth of breathing and excretion of hydrogen ions by the kidneys. As the blood becomes more acidic (decreasing pH), the kidneys will respond by increasing the renal tubule excretion of hydrogen and ammonia, which results in an increase in blood bicarbonate and in pH (towards normal).

Loop of Henle

The loop of Henle is important in regulating urine osmolarity[1] and osmolality[2] of body fluids. The descending limb is highly permeable to water, and movement of water out of the tubule produces a hypertonic (more concentrated) filtrate at the tip of the loop of Henle (the papilla). Permeability to urea and sodium is low in this segment of the loop. In contrast, in the ascending limb of the loop of Henle water permeability is almost nil, whereas

1 Osmolarity is defined as the total number of dissolved particles per litre of solution. Unit = milliosmoles/L (mOsm/L).

2 Plasma osmolality is determined by the total solute content in plasma and the total plasma water mass. Unit = mOsmol/kg H_2O.

sodium and chloride permeability is high. About 20–25% of the sodium chloride in the filtrate is reabsorbed and this is not accompanied by water. Consequently, the tubular filtrate becomes very dilute, or hypotonic (this is often termed 'free water production'), and the medullary interstitium becomes hypertonic, which is necessary for the concentrating capacity of the countercurrent between the renal tubules and the vasa recta. The concentration gradient established across the tubular epithelium becomes multiplied in a longitudinal direction, resulting in a large osmotic gradient between the isosmotic renal cortex and the hyperosmotic medulla and papilla. Potassium is also reabsorbed from the proximal tubules and loop of Henle in percentages equivalent to those for sodium; around 8% of the filtered potassium reaches the distal tubules.

Distal convoluted tubule

Between 5% and 10% of sodium reabsorption takes place actively in the distal convoluted tubule. The net loss of sodium from the filtrate is greater than the reabsorption of water; coupled with reabsorption of chloride, this makes the urine progressively more dilute. Uptake of sodium is largely determined by the presence of the mineralocorticoid aldosterone, produced by the adrenal cortex. When the extracellular fluid volume is decreased, the renin–angiotensin–aldosterone system is activated, stimulating the release of aldosterone, which acts to promote secretion of potassium and also the active reabsorption of sodium. The latter occurs by stimulating both Na^+/H^+ exchange via an action on aldosterone receptors and the insertion of more sodium pumps in the basolateral membrane. Parathyroid hormone and calcitriol also act on this segment of the nephron to increase reabsorption of calcium (Ch 27).

Collecting duct

Composition of the hypotonic fluid entering the collecting duct may be altered in the medullary portion by the action of antidiuretic hormone (ADH, also called vasopressin). ADH is a water-conserving hormone synthesised in the hypothalamus and stored in the posterior pituitary gland. When plasma osmolality increases as a result of dehydration or water deprivation, osmoreceptors in the supraoptic area of the hypothalamus stimulate the release of ADH.

The released ADH increases the expression of aquaporin (water channels) in the apical membrane, thereby increasing permeability of the distal tubule and collecting duct to water, which is passively reabsorbed, increasing plasma volume and thus lowering plasma osmolality. When the ADH concentration is low, a large volume of hypotonic fluid passes from the distal tubule into the collecting ducts, leading to the excretion of dilute urine. In the complete absence of ADH, a condition known as diabetes insipidus occurs and the affected person can excrete as much as 20 L of dilute urine daily.

CLINICAL FOCUS BOX 17.1
Drug-mediated acute kidney injury

A common problem faced in clinical practice is the risk–benefit relationship between use of drugs in seriously ill patients and the potential for nephrotoxicity, particularly acute kidney injury (AKI). It is estimated that as many as two-thirds of patients in an intensive care unit develop AKI, which results not only from drug use but from multiple exacerbating factors, including sepsis, septic shock and multi-organ dysfunction or failure, as well as volume depletion and patient comorbidities (Perazella 2012).

In terms of drug-induced nephrotoxicity, the contributing factors include the innate nephrotoxicity of the drug, altered pharmacokinetics of the drug, changes in renal haemodynamics and the presence of underlying renal disease. Drugs implicated in causing AKI in intensive care include non-steroidal anti-inflammatory drugs (NSAIDs), aminoglycoside antibiotics, antimicrobials (e.g. ciprofloxacin), antifungal drugs, antiretroviral therapy, anti-ulcer drugs, anticonvulsants, diuretics and radiocontrast agents.

Assessment of renal function

Renal function changes with age and in various disease states (Clinical Focus Box 17.1), and often an accurate estimation of renal function or GFR is used clinically to guide management or adjustment of drug dosage (Ch 5). Common measures of renal function include the use of serum creatinine (SCr) and creatinine clearance (CrCl). Serum creatinine concentration represents the balance between production by muscle and excretion or clearance by the kidney. Creatinine clearance by the kidneys is a measure of the 'volume' of serum cleared of creatinine per unit time and has the units of mL/min or mL/second.

Direct determination of CrCl requires simultaneous measurements of both SCr and a timed urine creatinine, usually a 24-hour timed collection. The latter is often not convenient for patients, and an exact 24-hour collection is more frequently unreliable than reliable. The most widely recognised measure of calculating CrCl is the Cockcroft–Gault formula, which relies on knowledge of the person's SCr, age, gender and weight. This formula, in spite of some limitations, is used for estimating renal function when there is a need for adjustment of drug dosage in people with renal impairment.

The Cockcroft–Gault formula is:

$$\text{Creatinine clearance (CrCl) (mL/min)} = (140 - \text{age}) \times (\text{lean body weight in kg}) \times (0.85 \text{ for females}) \div \text{SCr (micromol/L)} \times 0.815$$

An alternative to CrCl is the estimate of glomerular filtration rate (eGFR), which has the units of mL/min/1.73 m^2. The formula used to calculate eGFR was derived during a large clinical study called the Modification of Diet in Renal Disease (MDRD) Study. The MDRD formula is based on the SCr concentration, age, gender and race (if African–American) and is adjusted to an 'average' body surface area. It is important to understand that eGFR is not equivalent to CrCl, because eGFR is not an estimate of a person's actual GFR but instead is an estimate of their GFR adjusted to an 'average' body size. The body surface area of an 'average' person is 1.73 m^2 – hence the use of the number 1.73 m^2 in the units reported.

One problem in clinical practice may be illustrated by considering one person, let's call him David, who weighs 120 kg, which is twice the size of Matthew, who weighs 60 kg. They are both the same gender (male) and age (55 years), and both of them have the same SCr 70 micromol/L. If you do the calculations, Matthew's actual GFR determined by CrCl will be half that of David's but they will both have the same eGFR. If you then calculate the drug dosage based on eGFR, it is likely you will overdose Matthew and underdose David. To further improve the estimation of GFR, the original MDRD formula was modified to the MDRD '175' formula; however, it still underestimates GFR at values greater than 60 mL/min/1.73 m^2.

The Australasian Creatinine Consensus Working Group position statement (Johnson et al. 2012) recommended that the method of calculating eGFR should be changed from the MDRD formula to the Chronic Kidney Disease Epidemiology Collaboration (CKD-EPI) formulae (Clinical Focus Box 17.2). Data from multiple studies have demonstrated that the CKD-EPI formulae are as accurate as the MDRD formula when GFR is less than 60 mL/min/1.73 m^2 and that there is improved precision when GFR is greater than 60 mL/min/1.73 m^2 (Johnson et al. 2012). The Consensus Working Group recommended the following:

- All laboratories should report precise values for eGFR up to at least 90 mL/min/1.73 m^2.
- There should not be any age-related intervals for eGFR in adults, because an eGFR under 60 mL/min/1.73 m^2 was found to be associated with an increased risk of death (all causes), end-stage renal disease, acute kidney injury and progression of chronic kidney disease, irrespective of age.
- If using eGFR to guide drug dosing in the presence of reduced renal function, body size should be considered and reference also made to the approved product information for guidance.
- For drugs with a narrow therapeutic index, drug effect should be monitored using therapeutic drug monitoring or a valid biological marker of drug effect.
- Serum creatinine should continue to be used to determine renal function in pregnant women, as the validity of using eGFR in pregnancy has not been validated.
- Routine calculation of eGFR should not be undertaken in children and people under 18 years of age because of limited and conflicting data on its value in detecting renal disorders.
- Evaluation of both eGFR and urinary albumin should be used for optimal risk stratification of people with chronic kidney disease.

Chronic kidney disease

Chronic kidney disease (CKD) is a major health issue with tens of millions of sufferers worldwide. The major underlying contributing factors include diabetes and diabetic nephropathy, hypertension and glomerulonephritis. The general consensus is that CKD is defined by an eGFR

CLINICAL FOCUS BOX 17.2
CKD-EPI formulae used for calculating eGFR[a]

For females with SCr ≤ 62 micromol/L:

eGFR (mL/min/1.73 m^2)
$= 144 \times (\text{SCr in micromol/L} \times 0.0113/0.7)^{-0.329} \times (0.993)^{\text{age in years}}$

For females with SCr > 62 micromol/L:

eGFR (mL/min/1.73 m^2)
$= 144 \times (\text{SCr in micromol/L} \times 0.0113/0.7)^{-1.209} \times (0.993)^{\text{age in years}}$

For males with SCr ≤ 80 micromol/L:

eGFR (mL/min/1.73 m^2)
$= 141 \times (\text{SCr in micromol/L} \times 0.0113/0.9)^{-0.411} \times (0.993)^{\text{age in years}}$

For males with SCr > 80 micromol/L:

eGFR (mL/min/1.73 m^2)
$= 141 \times (\text{SCr in micromol/L} \times 0.0113/0.9)^{-1.209} \times (0.993)^{\text{age in years}}$

CKD-EPI = Chronic Kidney Disease Epidemiology Collaboration; eGFR = estimated glomerular filtration rate (mL/min/1.73 m^2); SCr = concentration of creatinine in serum.
[a] Coefficients for race are not included in these formulae.
Source: Johnson et al. 2012

less than 60 mL/min/1.73 m^2 or evidence of renal dysfunction (e.g. proteinuria) for more than 3 months (Kidney Health Australia – see 'Online resources'). Many people with CKD will die of cardiovascular disease, often before end-stage renal disease develops. Hence, one aspect of care involves managing cardiovascular risk factors that may include the use of antihypertensive drugs (e.g. ACE inhibitors, angiotensin-receptor blockers), diuretics (loop and thiazide), low-dose aspirin and the statin lipid-lowering drugs. Glycaemic control is achieved by the use of drugs such as metformin (dependent on GFR), oral hypoglycaemic drugs and insulin (Ch 28). Other complications of CKD include anaemia, which may be treated with iron supplements (e.g. oral ferrous fumarate with folic acid, iron polymaltose or iron sucrose IV) and erythropoiesis-stimulating drugs such as epoetin alpha and beta and darbepoetin (Ch 14).

Changes in bone metabolism are a common feature of CKD and include an increase in bone fragility and diminished bone mineralisation (renal osteodystrophy). Hyperphosphataemia and hyperparathyroidism are also contributing factors to adverse vascular changes (e.g. calcification), and current clinical practice guidelines recommend treatment. This includes restricting dietary phosphate intake, administration of a phosphate binder at meal times (e.g. calcium carbonate, lanthanum carbonate, sevelamer), vitamin D supplementation or administration of a calcimimetic (e.g. cinacalcet, see Ch 27). The routine use of bisphosphonates (Ch 27) is not recommended because of limited efficacy and safety data.

Haemodialysis and peritoneal dialysis add further management complexities involving the use of drugs such as the anticoagulant enoxaparin (Ch 13), while following transplantation the most commonly used drugs are the immunosuppressants (e.g. prednisolone [Ch 29] and mycophenolate mofetil, tacrolimus and ciclosporin [Ch 34]).

KEY POINTS

The kidneys

- The kidneys regulate electrolytes, water, the pH of blood via excretion of hydrogen ions, excrete metabolic waste products such as urea and creatinine, modulate blood pressure via release of renin and synthesise calcitriol and the growth factor erythropoietin.
- The functional unit of the kidney is the nephron, which comprises the glomerulus, the renal tubule and the collecting duct.
- The three main renal processes are glomerular filtration and tubular secretion and reabsorption.
- The glomerular membrane filters water, ions, glucose, amino acids and urea, but not plasma proteins.
- GFR is 125 mL/min. About 180 L of filtrate is formed per day in healthy people.
- Tubular secretion involves movement of substances such as ammonium ions, creatinine and certain drugs from the blood into the lumen of the nephron.
- About 99% of the filtrate is reabsorbed, and differential reabsorption of water and ions occurs along the length of the renal tubule.
- Reabsorbed substances include glucose, amino acids, water, bicarbonate, sodium, potassium and chloride ions.
- ADH and aldosterone regulate salt and water reabsorption in the distal convoluted tubule and collecting duct.
- Renal function changes with age and in various disease states.
- Estimation of renal function, or GFR, is used clinically to guide management or adjustment of drug dosage.
- An alternative to measurement of creatinine clearance is the estimate of GFR, or eGFR.
- eGFR has the units mL/min/1.73 m^2.
- CKD is defined by an eGFR under 60 mL/min/1.73 m^2, or by evidence of renal dysfunction for more than 3 months.
- Management of CKD is complex, involving the use of antihypertensive drugs, lipid-lowering drugs, drugs for diabetes, diuretics, erythropoiesis-stimulating drugs, iron supplements, anticoagulants and drugs for managing renal bone disease. After transplantation, the most commonly used drugs are the immunosuppressants.

Diuretics

Diuretics modify renal function and induce diuresis (increased formation and excretion of urine) and **natriuresis** (enhanced excretion of sodium chloride). The increase in urine volume is achieved primarily by inhibiting reabsorption of sodium and chloride in the nephron. The increased excretion of salt leads to an increase in the excretion of water. The three main classes of diuretics are:

- loop diuretics (e.g. frusemide)
- thiazide diuretics (e.g. hydrochlorothiazide)
- potassium-sparing diuretics (e.g. amiloride).

Carbonic anhydrase inhibitors were introduced as diuretics during the 1940s–1950s, but their diuretic action was weak and they were ineffective over the long term. Acetazolamide is now reserved for treating open-angle glaucoma and for menstrual-related epilepsy.

Figure 17.2 shows the various sites of action of diuretic drugs on the nephron, the main mechanisms of ion absorption and the percentages of ions filtered.

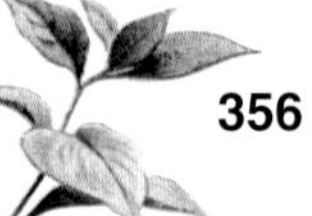

Loop diuretics

The drugs commonly referred to as loop diuretics are bumetanide and frusemide (Drug Monograph 17.1). The pharmacological effects of all the loop diuretics are similar – all produce a rapid and intense diuresis and in general have a short duration of action (4–6 hours).

Mechanism of action

These powerful diuretics are actively secreted into the lumen of the nephron via the organic anion transporters OAT1 and OAT3, located in the basolateral membrane of the proximal tubule cells. On reaching the thick ascending limb of the loop of Henle, they inhibit the Na^+–K^+–2 Cl^- co-transporter (NKCC), thus preventing reabsorption of sodium and chloride from the lumen into the epithelial cells. As this site accounts for 15–25% of the reabsorption of sodium and chloride, their diuretic effect is greater than that reported with the other diuretics. The mechanism by which they inhibit the co-transporter is not known, but evidence suggests that they bind to the chloride-binding site of NKCC. Blockade of NKCC diminishes potassium secretion through the luminal membrane, reabsorption of chloride through the basolateral membrane and paracellular reabsorption of calcium and magnesium. This explains why loop diuretics increase the excretion of all of these ions.

In addition to diuresis, loop diuretics exert direct vascular effects. In particular, frusemide acutely causes venodilation, but the duration of this effect is short, occurring before the onset of diuresis. The mechanisms of the vascular actions are not fully understood but include reduced responsiveness to angiotensin II and noradrenaline, both vasoconstrictors.

Drug Monograph 17.1
Furosemide

Furosemide, a sulfamoylbenzoic acid, is a commonly prescribed loop diuretic. The degree of diuresis depends on the amount of drug reaching the tubular lumen, not the plasma concentration, as furosemide is active from inside the lumen of the thick ascending limb of the loop of Henle (TALH). Hence, adequate urine concentration of furosemide via glomerular filtration and active secretion is essential for maximal diuresis. Furosemide is actively secreted by the renal organic anion transporter OAT3 and, to a lesser extent, by OAT1.

Mechanism of action

There are two isoforms of NKCC in mammalian kidney. NKCC1 is predominantly a 'secretory' transporter, while NKCC2 is an 'absorptive' transporter specific to the luminal membrane of the TALH. The affinity of loop diuretics is greater for NKCC2 than for NKCC1. In the TALH the movement of sodium, potassium and chloride from the lumen into the epithelial cells of the TALH is driven by NKCC2. Translocation of these ions depends on their simultaneous binding to all three ion-binding sites on the luminal side of the membrane. Furosemide inhibits NKCC2, blocking its function and virtually halting transport of sodium, potassium and chloride in the TALH. The mechanism of inhibition has not been fully elucidated but it is thought that furosemide binds to the chloride binding site of NKCC2. Inhibition of NKCC2 also alters the transepithelial electrochemical gradient between the luminal and the basolateral membranes of the epithelial cells. This change in potential difference reduces the driving force for the reabsorption of calcium and magnesium. Hence, furosemide increases the urinary excretion of sodium, chloride, potassium, calcium and magnesium. Acutely it enhances excretion of uric acid, but chronic administration reduces uric acid excretion. This may be explained by increased uric acid reabsorption due to volume depletion or competition between uric acid and furosemide for active secretion in the proximal convoluted tubule.

Prolonged use of furosemide can lead to 'loop diuretic resistance'. The underlying mechanism has not been fully established but may involve rebound sodium retention resulting from significant reabsorption of sodium in the distal nephron. Strategies to deal with this problem include fluid and salt restriction, use of intravenous furosemide, increasing the dose, and use in combination with a thiazide diuretic that blocks sodium reabsorption in the distal tubule.

Pharmacokinetics

Furosemide is highly protein-bound (> 95%). Renal excretion of unchanged drug is the predominant clearance mechanism for furosemide in humans, accounting for about 65% of the dose. The remaining 35% is metabolised predominantly by human kidney UGT1A9 (with a minor contribution from hepatic UGT1A1) to furosemide 1-*O*-acyl glucuronide. The oral bioavailability ranges from 43% to 73% (average about 50%) and the elimination half-life in normal subjects is 1.5–2 hours. The peak effect occurs within 30 minutes when given intravenously and in approximately an hour following oral administration.

Drug interactions

See listing in Drug Interactions 17.1, which is relevant to all loop diuretics.

Adverse reactions

Common adverse reactions are:

- electrolyte disturbances, including hyponatraemia, hypokalaemia, hypomagnesaemia, hyperuricaemia
- dizziness and postural hypotension

- increases in low-density lipoprotein (LDL) cholesterol and triglycerides with a fall in high-density lipoprotein (HDL) cholesterol plasma levels
- ototoxicity (e.g. tinnitus, vertigo and deafness increased with high IV doses). This risk is further increased if furosemide in used in combination with other drugs that also cause ototoxicity (e.g. aminoglycosides).

Warnings and contraindications

Furosemide is contraindicated:

- in states of severe sodium and fluid depletion
- where there is an existing history of allergy to furosemide and sulfonamides.

Dosage and administration

Because the oral bioavailability of furosemide is about 50% in general, 20 mg IV is equivalent to 40 mg oral. However, oral bioavailability can be lower in severe heart failure and renal disease; hence, the dose varies according to the condition being treated and current drug information sources should be consulted.

Clinical Uses of Loop Diuretics

- Treatment of oedema associated with:
  - heart failure
  - hepatic cirrhosis
  - renal impairment and nephrotic syndrome.
- As adjunct therapy:
  - in people with acute pulmonary oedema
  - in conditions refractory to the other diuretics.
- In severe hypercalcaemia to promote calcium excretion.

Loop diuretics should be used with caution in people with diabetes mellitus, gout, hearing impairment, hepatic and renal impairment, and in those in whom hypokalaemia might precipitate dysrhythmias, such as people taking digoxin. These drugs should be avoided in people with known hypersensitivity to loop diuretics, anuria or severe kidney disease or significant renal impairment. As they may cause electrolyte disturbances in the fetus their use in pregnancy should be avoided. These drugs are often included in multiple drug regimens and are subject to numerous drug interactions (Drug Interactions 17.1).

DRUG INTERACTIONS 17.1
Loop diuretics

DRUG	POSSIBLE EFFECTS AND MANAGEMENT
Angiotensin-converting enzyme (ACE) inhibitors	In people on high-dose loop diuretics, increased risk of severe first-dose hypotension. Begin with a low dose of ACE inhibitor and withhold (or reduce dose of) loop diuretic for at least 1 day if possible before commencing ACE inhibitor. Monitor blood pressure.
Aminoglycosides	Increased risk of ototoxicity and nephrotoxicity. Care required in dosing people with renal impairment. Combination with frusemide is not recommended.
Digoxin	Increased risk of digoxin-induced dysrhythmia in people with diuretic-induced hypokalaemia and hypomagnesaemia. Monitor serum potassium concentration and use a supplement if indicated.
Lithium	Increased risk of lithium toxicity because of reduced renal clearance. Monitor closely and adjust lithium dose if necessary.
NSAIDs	Reduce the effect of loop diuretics; predispose to renal failure in the presence of pre-existing hypovolaemia. Monitor blood pressure and renal function.
Sartans	Treatment with loop diuretics increases the risk of severe first-dose hypotension. Begin with a low dose of sartan and withhold (or reduce dose of) loop diuretic for at least 1 day if possible before commencing sartan.
Sevelamer	May reduce the absorption of frusemide; administer 1 hour before or 3 hours after sevelamer.
SGLT2 inhibitors	May increase diuretic effects, increasing the risk of electrolyte disturbances. Assess volume status and correct prior to administration of SGLT2 inhibitor. Concomitant administration of loop diuretic with dapagliflozin is discouraged by the manufacturer.
Thiazide diuretics	Combination with loop diuretics may cause profound diuresis and electrolyte disturbances. Monitor blood pressure, renal function and electrolytes.

Thiazide diuretics

The thiazide diuretics were synthesised during the 1950s and the current drugs include chlortalidone, hydrochlorothiazide and the thiazide-like drug indapamide.

Mechanism of action

These drugs are actively secreted into the lumen of the nephron via OAT1 and OAT3 in the basolateral membrane of the proximal tubule cells. They are then transported to the distal convoluted tubule where they inhibit reabsorption of sodium and chloride by binding to the chloride-binding site of the Na^+–Cl^- symporter (Fig 17.2). This symporter is in the luminal membrane and, using the free energy in the electrochemical gradient of sodium, the Na^+–Cl^- symporter moves chloride into the epithelial cell against its electrochemical gradient. Inhibition of the Na^+–Cl^- symporter increases the excretion of sodium and chloride. However, because the maximum portion of the sodium load they can affect at the distal tubule is about 5%, thiazides are considered only moderately potent diuretics in comparison with the loop diuretics. Like the loop diuretics, inhibitors of the Na^+–Cl^- symporter also increase potassium excretion by the same mechanism discussed for frusemide.

The thiazide diuretics promote the renal excretion of water, sodium, chloride, potassium and magnesium, whereas excretion of uric acid and calcium is decreased with chronic administration. When an increased sodium load is presented to the distal tubule, there is a corresponding increase in potassium secretion. In addition, as the extracellular fluid volume decreases, plasma renin activity and aldosterone concentration increase, with resulting potassium loss (Fig 17.3), which occurs in 14–60% of ambulatory-hypertensive people. This loss is dose-related, occurring early in treatment (first month) and more frequently with larger diuretic doses or with the long-acting type of diuretics (e.g. chlortalidone).

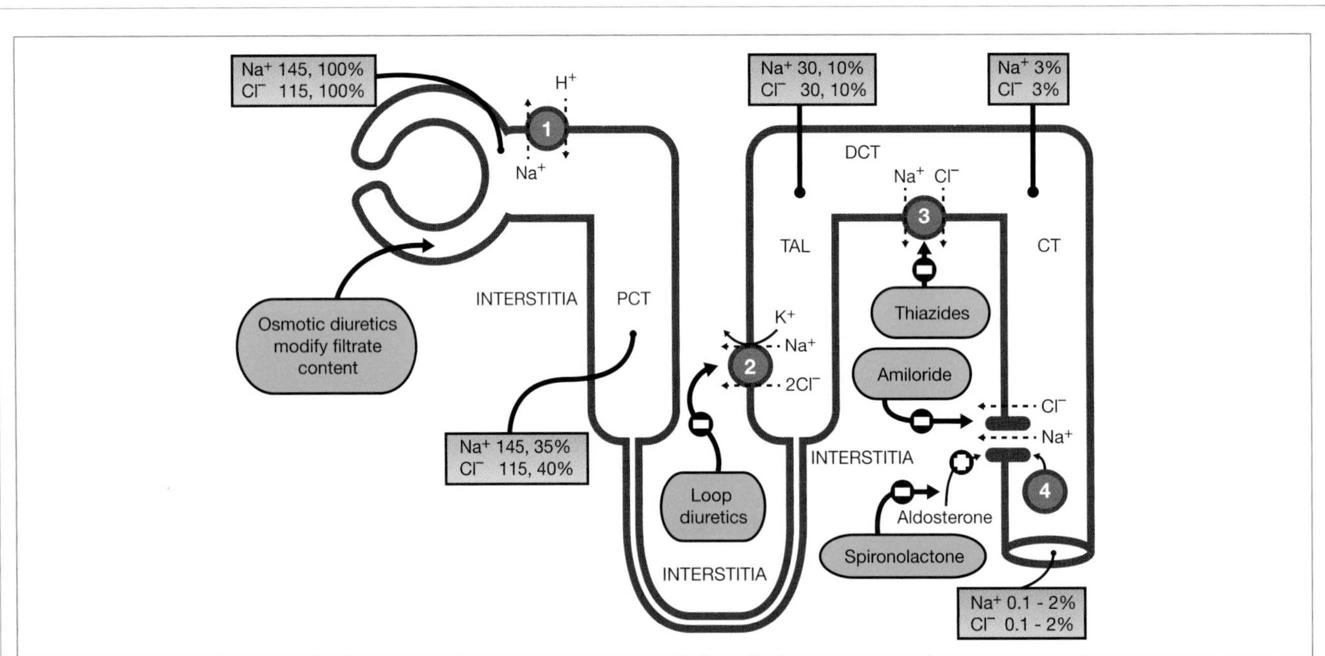

FIGURE 17.2 Schematic showing the absorption of sodium and chloride in the nephron and the main sites of action of drugs

Mechanisms of ion absorption at the apical margin of the tubule cell (not, of course, shown to scale): **1** Na^+/H^+ exchange; **2** $Na^+/K^+/2\ Cl^-$ co-transport; **3** Na^+/Cl^- co-transport; **4** Na^+ entry through sodium channels. Sodium is pumped out of the cells into the interstitium by the Na^+–K^+-ATPase in the basolateral margin of the tubular cells (not shown). Chloride ions may pass out of the tubule through the paracellular pathway. The numbers in the boxes give the concentrations of ions as millimoles per litre of filtrate and the percentages of filtered ions remaining in the tubular fluid at the sites specified. CT = collecting tubule; DT = distal tubule; PCT = proximal convoluted tubule; TAL = thick ascending loop.

Source: Data from Greger 2000, reproduced from Rang et al. 2012, Figure 29.4.

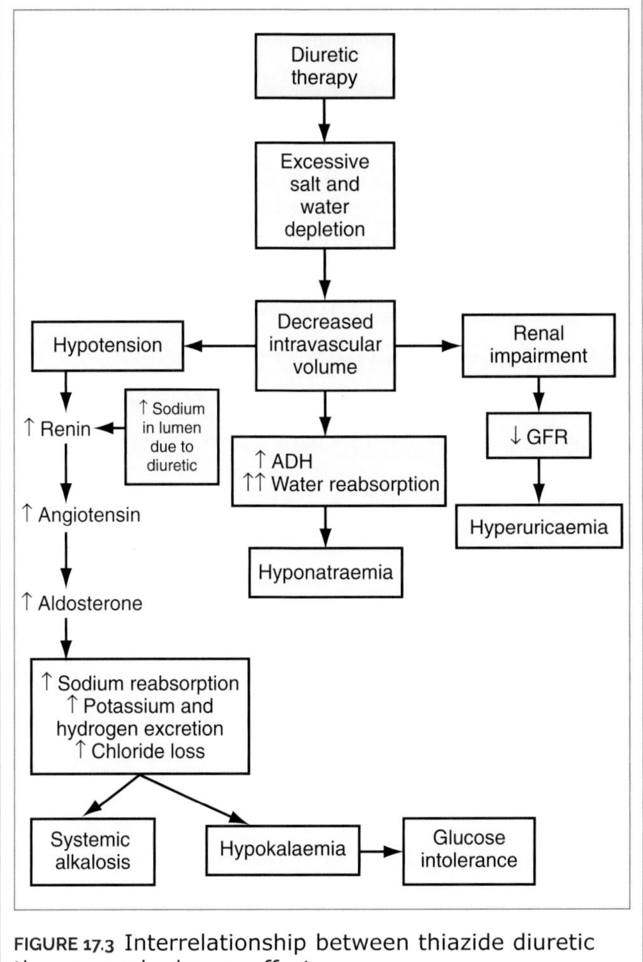

FIGURE 17.3 Interrelationship between thiazide diuretic therapy and adverse effects

Clinical Uses of Thiazide Diuretics

- Treatment of mild-to-moderate hypertension.
- Oedema associated with hepatic cirrhosis or heart failure.
- Treatment of nephrogenic diabetes insipidus (reducing urine volume by as much as 40–50%).

Thiazide diuretics do not lower blood pressure in normotensive people, but in hypertensive people the initial diuresis produces a fall in blood pressure because of decreased blood volume, reduction in venous return and a decrease in cardiac output. During chronic therapy a reduction in total peripheral resistance occurs that may explain the continued antihypertensive effect.

Pharmacokinetics

Hydrochlorothiazide is administered orally and bioavailability is approximately 70%. The maximum plasma concentration occurs 2–2.5 hours after dosing and the plasma half-life is in the order of 2.5 hours but increases in people with renal disease or heart failure. Hydrochlorothiazide is not hepatically metabolised and is excreted almost entirely (> 95%) as unchanged drug in urine. The onset of action is usually within 12 hours, but the duration of action differs between the drugs. For pharmacokinetics and dosages, see Table 17.1.

TABLE 17.1 Selected diuretic pharmacokinetics and dosages[a]

CLASS	ONSET OF ACTION (h)	TIME TO PEAK EFFECT (h)	HALF-LIFE (h)	DOSE RANGE (ADULTS)
Loop diuretics				
Chlortalidone	PO 2–3	8–20	25–69	12.5–25 mg/day (hypertension) 12.5–50 mg/day (oedema, diabetes insipidus)
Hydrochlorothiazide	PO 2	2	2.5	12.5–50 mg/day (hypertension) 25–100 mg/day (oedema)
Indapamide	PO 0.5–2	1–3	15–25	1.25–2.5 mg/day (conventional tablet)
Loop diuretics				
Bumetanide	PO 0.5–1	1–2	1.2–1.5	0.5–8 mg/day; maximum 10 mg/day
Furosemide	PO 0.5–1	0.6–2	0.5–2	20–400 mg/day (oedema)
Potassium-sparing diuretic				
Amiloride	PO 1–2	6–10	17–26	2.5–5 mg/day (prevention of diuretic-induced hypokalaemia) 5–20 mg/day (primary hyperaldosteronism)

[a] Use minimum effective dose and monitor clinical response and plasma electrolytes. Consult current drug information sources to confirm dose ranges.

Sources: Australian Medicines Handbook 2021; Brunton et al. 2018.

Adverse reactions

In addition to electrolyte imbalances, common adverse reactions include dizziness, weakness, muscle cramps and hypotension (Fig 17.3). Infrequently, rash, blurred vision and male impotence have been reported and, rarely, diarrhoea, photosensitivity, agranulocytosis, cholecystitis, jaundice and haemolytic anaemia and thrombocytopenia. In higher doses the thiazide diuretics have been reported to increase plasma levels of LDL cholesterol, total cholesterol and triglycerides, and to reduce HDL cholesterol. The clinical relevance of changes in a person's lipid profile would need to be considered in the context of the overall health status of the person concerned.

Similar to loop diuretics, thiazides are also subject to a number of drug interactions (Drug Interactions 17.2).

Warnings and contraindications

Thiazide diuretics should be used with caution in people with type 1 diabetes, gout, renal or hepatic impairment or dyslipidaemias, and in the elderly. These drugs are contraindicated in severe renal impairment, anuria and Addison's disease, and in people with known thiazide or sulfonamide hypersensitivity.

Diuretic combinations

A number of diuretic combination products are available, which are generally used in people whose hypertension is

DRUG INTERACTIONS 17.2
Thiazide diuretics

DRUG	POSSIBLE EFFECTS AND MANAGEMENT
ACE inhibitors	Increased risk of severe first-dose hypotension. Commence therapy with a low dose of ACE inhibitor. Increased risk of ACE inhibitor-induced renal impairment with combination. Monitor renal function.
Colestyramine	Concurrent administration can decrease gastrointestinal absorption of thiazide diuretics. Schedule administration of diuretics at least 1 hour before or 4–6 hours after administration of colestyramine.
Digoxin	Increased risk of digoxin toxicity in presence of hypokalaemia. Monitor serum potassium concentration and ECG changes.
Lithium	Increased risk of lithium toxicity because of decreased lithium excretion. Monitor plasma lithium concentration and adjust lithium dose if necessary.
Loop diuretics	Combination with thiazide diuretics may cause profound diuresis and electrolyte disturbances. Monitor blood pressure, renal function and electrolytes.
NSAIDs	Decreased natriuresis and reduced antihypertensive effect. In view of increased potential for nephrotoxicity, avoid concurrent use or adjust dose of diuretic.
Sartans	Treatment with thiazide diuretics increases risk of severe first-dose hypotension. Begin with a low dose of sartan and withhold (or reduce dose of) thiazide diuretic for at least 1 day if possible before commencing sartan.

CLINICAL FOCUS BOX 17.3
Adverse effects of thiazide diuretics

Hypokalaemia may precipitate serious dysrhythmias as a result of digitalis toxicity in people who are taking digitalis preparations, and it may predispose people with cirrhosis to hepatic encephalopathy or coma. Potassium loss can be minimised by using the lowest possible dose of thiazide, or by use of a potassium-sparing diuretic or potassium supplements. Potassium replacement can be problematic in the elderly, in those with renal dysfunction, or when used in combination with potassium-sparing diuretics because high plasma potassium concentrations may occur.

Hyperuricaemia may result from either inhibition of tubular secretion of uric acid resulting from competition for the organic acid secretory pump in the proximal tubule or increased uric acid reabsorption. This effect is reversible when thiazides are discontinued. In the absence of gout, hyperuricaemia is usually asymptomatic and requires no treatment; however, in a person with a history of gout, higher doses of thiazides can precipitate an attack that requires treatment (Ch 34).

Hyperglycaemia, or impaired glucose tolerance, has been reported with the thiazides and, rarely, with loop diuretics. This effect is reported most often in the elderly, and thiazides can unmask latent diabetes. The mechanism is not known but may involve a reduction in insulin secretion and alterations in glucose metabolism. With use of low dose thiazides, effects on glucose tolerance are less.

not controlled adequately by a single drug. Fixed-dose combinations can provide additional diuretic activity and decrease potassium depletion, a characteristic of the thiazide diuretics (e.g. amiloride 5 mg plus hydrochlorothiazide 50 mg). Combinations of hydrochlorothiazide with either an ACE inhibitor or an angiotensin-receptor antagonist are also available.

Potassium-sparing diuretics

The potassium-sparing diuretics are amiloride and the aldosterone antagonist spironolactone. Amiloride is only available in combination with hydrochlorothiazide. Both are considered to have limited diuretic efficacy. In addition, spironolactone, a synthetic steroidal compound, is a specific antagonist for the mineralocorticoid receptor. There is clinical evidence that low-dose spironolactone prolongs survival in some patients with severe heart failure by blocking the actions of aldosterone.

Mechanism of action

Amiloride is transported via the organic cation transporter OCT2 into the lumen of the proximal tubule where it flows through to the sites of action in the late distal tubules and collecting ducts (Fig 17.2). This drug inhibits the reabsorption of sodium by blocking epithelial sodium channels in the luminal membrane. The amiloride-sensitive sodium channel is called ENaC, and studies have indicated that amiloride binds to a critical domain in ENaC that then alters activity of the channel. Blockade of sodium channels hyperpolarises the luminal membrane and the consequential reduction in the lumen-negative potential leads to a decrease in the excretion of potassium.

Spironolactone blocks the action of aldosterone, which results in inhibition of the sodium-retaining property of aldosterone and a concomitant reduction in its potassium-secreting property. The effectiveness of spironolactone is directly related to the circulating plasma concentration of aldosterone: if the concentration is high, the effect of spironolactone is greater. It does not interfere with renal tubule transport of sodium and chloride and does not inhibit carbonic anhydrase. When used alone all of these drugs have the potential to cause life-threatening hyperkalaemia.

Pharmacokinetics

Amiloride has poor oral absorption (15–25%), whereas spironolactone is moderately well absorbed from the gastrointestinal tract (30–70%). Amiloride is principally excreted as unchanged drug in urine. Spironolactone is extensively metabolised to the active metabolite canrenone, which has a plasma half-life of 18–20 hours. The actions of spironolactone are largely attributable to canrenone. For pharmacokinetic and dosage information, see Table 17.1.

The potassium-sparing diuretics are indicated for the prevention and treatment of diuretic-induced hypokalaemia. They are also used as adjunct therapy in the treatment of oedema due to heart failure and hepatic cirrhosis. Spironolactone is used to treat primary hyperaldosteronism, hirsutism in females, refractory oedema associated with secondary hyperaldosteronism and severe heart failure.

Adverse reactions

Refer to Drug Interactions 17.3 for interactions with potassium-sparing diuretics. Common adverse reactions include electrolyte disturbances, particularly hyperkalaemia, hyponatraemia and hypochloraemia (worsened by the combination with hydrochlorothiazide), nausea, vomiting, dizziness, constipation, impotence and headache. As spironolactone is structurally similar to progesterone, it binds to progesterone and androgen receptors, and hence its use for prolonged periods or at high dose is associated with endocrine adverse effects. These endocrine adverse effects, which include gynaecomastia, decreased libido, impotence and menstrual irregularities, tend to limit the usefulness of spironolactone.

Potassium-sparing diuretics are contraindicated in situations of pre-existing hyperkalaemia (potassium > 5 mmol/L) and renal failure. Caution should also be exercised in people with type 1 diabetes, renal or hepatic impairment and debilitating cardiopulmonary disease, and in the elderly, who are prone to hyperkalaemia and hypotension. Both amiloride and spironolactone should be avoided in pregnant women; amiloride can cause electrolyte disturbances in the fetus and spironolactone can cause feminisation of the male fetus.

Osmotic diuretics

Osmotic diuretics such as mannitol reach the tubular lumen via glomerular filtration. They are pharmacologically

DRUG INTERACTIONS 17.3
Potassium-sparing diuretics

DRUG	POSSIBLE EFFECTS AND MANAGEMENT
ACE inhibitors, sartans, potassium supplements	Increased risk of hyperkalaemia. Avoid combined use.
NSAIDs	Increased risk of hyperkalaemia and increased risk of renal failure with NSAIDs. Use with caution and monitor serum potassium concentration.
Digoxin	Spironolactone increases risk of digoxin toxicity. Monitor digoxin concentration and reduce dose if necessary

inactive but cause diuresis by adding to the solutes already present in the tubular fluid; they are particularly effective in increasing osmolality of the tubular fluid because they are not reabsorbed by the tubules. Passive water reabsorption is reduced in their presence; as more fluid remains in the lumen, this alters electrochemical gradients so less sodium and chloride are reabsorbed in the proximal tubule. Urine volume increases, but there is only a small increase in sodium excretion. The availability of other highly effective diuretics has resulted in relegation of these agents for use in non-diuretic indications such as cerebral oedema, reducing intraocular pressure before and after intraocular surgery and for acute closed-angle glaucoma.

KEY POINTS

Diuretics

- Diuretics modify renal function and induce diuresis (increased rate of urine flow) and natriuresis (enhanced excretion of sodium chloride).
- The three main classes of diuretics are: the loop diuretics (e.g. frusemide), the thiazide diuretics (e.g. hydrochlorothiazide) and the potassium-sparing diuretics (e.g. amiloride).
- Loop diuretics are potent inhibitors of the reabsorption of sodium and chloride in the thick ascending limb of the loop of Henle.
- Drug interactions with the loop diuretics include ACE inhibitors, angiotensin-receptor antagonists, aminoglycosides, NSAIDs and thiazide diuretics.
- Thiazide diuretics inhibit absorption of sodium and chloride in the proximal (diluting) segment of the distal convoluted tubule and are considered less potent than the loop diuretics.
- Thiazide diuretics primarily promote the renal excretion of water, sodium, chloride, potassium and magnesium, whereas excretion of uric acid and calcium is decreased.
- Hyperglycaemia, or impaired glucose tolerance, has been reported with high-dose thiazide diuretics but rarely with loop diuretics.
- The potassium-sparing diuretics are amiloride and the aldosterone antagonist spironolactone. Both are considered to have limited diuretic efficacy.
- Common adverse reactions associated with loop and thiazide diuretics include electrolyte disturbances (e.g. hyponatraemia, hypokalaemia, hypomagnesaemia).

Drugs for bladder dysfunction

Once formed, urine flows via the ureters to the urinary bladder. The ureters enter the bladder through the detrusor muscle in the floor of the bladder (the trigone area). The normal tone of the detrusor muscle prevents backflow of urine from the bladder to the ureters. The urethra exits from the bladder at the tip of the trigone, with the detrusor muscle forming the internal sphincter, and passes through the floor of the pelvis. In this region, the outer wall of the urethra contains a circular muscle band that forms the external urethral sphincter, which is under voluntary control and normally prevents urination until socially acceptable circumstances are achieved.

The micturition reflex

The storage of urine and emptying of the bladder involve complex neural integration between the central nervous system, the spinal cord and peripheral nerves. The bladder has somatic, parasympathetic and sympathetic innervation. Sympathetic innervation via the release of noradrenaline acts on β_3 receptors on the detrusor muscle, mediating smooth muscle relaxation and increasing bladder compliance. Stimulation of α_{1A}-adrenoceptors in the bladder neck and proximal urethra mediates smooth muscle contraction and increases bladder outlet resistance. The average capacity of the bladder is about 500 mL in an adult. Volume expansion increases tension in the wall of the bladder, triggering stretch receptors in the detrusor muscle and the transmission of sensory impulses by parasympathetic afferent fibres. Reflex parasympathetic discharge via motor efferent fibres releases acetylcholine that acts on M_3 muscarinic receptors causing contraction of the detrusor muscle and relaxation (opening) of the internal urethral sphincter. This reflex arc initiates a conscious desire to urinate and, when impulses from the cerebral cortex of the brain inhibit activity in motor neurons to the external sphincter, voluntary relaxation occurs and the bladder contents are expelled. When the bladder is empty the nerve signals reverse and the bladder is able to fill with urine again.

Micturition may be initiated and stopped voluntarily because of control exerted at the level of the cerebral cortex. The specific mechanisms within the central nervous system are not fully understood but may include neurotransmitters such as dopamine, serotonin and endorphins. A lack of voluntary control is referred to as incontinence, while failure to either completely or normally urinate may lead to urine retention.

Nocturnal enuresis

Persistent bed wetting in children (involuntary voiding of urine) or nocturnal enuresis in the absence of other urinary symptoms or disease is concerning if it persists beyond the age when control of micturition is normally achieved. Factors contributing to the development of nocturnal enuresis include physiological factors (e.g. nocturnal polyuria, reduced functional bladder capacity and failure to arouse in response to full bladder signals), genetic factors and stressful early life events. Following exclusion of structural or organic causes, desmopressin (Ch 28) may be used to treat children with nocturnal enuresis. The condition is much rarer in adults (1–3%) and may be the first indication of some significant underlying pathology. It can be divided into three main categories: persistent primary, recurrent and recent onset nocturnal enuresis. Persistent primary is often a continuation of an earlier childhood problem, as is recurrent nocturnal enuresis, and both are commonly due to nocturnal polyuria and overactivity of the detrusor muscle. As in children, the treatment is desmopressin with or without anticholinergic drugs.

Urinary Incontinence

Urinary incontinence is a common and embarrassing problem that afflicts a significant proportion of the general population – in particular, the elderly. Before instituting drug treatment, potential contributing factors should be eliminated. These include the possibility of a urinary tract infection, excessive fluid intake, metabolic disorders (e.g. hyperglycaemia) and the administration of certain drugs (Table 17.2). Incontinence can be categorised into a number of types including:

- *Overactive bladder (detrusor overactivity):* characterised by urgency to void that is difficult to ignore, increased frequency (> 8 voids per day) and nocturia, which is present in about 50% of both men and women reporting overactive bladder (OAB) symptoms occurring with or without **urge incontinence**, the involuntary leakage of urine with the feeling of urgency to urinate. The severity of OAB increases with ageing, progresses more rapidly after age 60 years and has a negative impact on the quality of life.
- *Stress incontinence:* failure to prevent urine loss due to an increase in intraabdominal pressure (e.g. during coughing).
- *Overflow incontinence:* due to emptying failure resulting in urine retention and bladder distension. This condition may arise from obstruction of the outlet (e.g. prostatic hyperplasia) or as a result of neurogenic bladder (the inability to contract the detrusor muscle).

In addition to the above descriptions of incontinence the International Continence Society has subdivided lower urinary tract symptoms into three groups:

- storage symptoms that include increased daytime frequency, nocturia, urgency and urinary incontinence
- voiding symptoms that include splitting or spraying, slow or intermittent stream, hesitancy, straining and terminal dribble
- post-micturition symptoms that include a sense of incomplete emptying, and post-micturition dribble.

In clinical practice the complex of lower urinary tract symptoms is most commonly described as overactive bladder, and guidelines from the American Urological Association and the Society of Urodynamics, Female Pelvic Medicine and Urogenital Reconstruction. Gormley and colleagues (2015) recommend that the first-line treatment for overactive (non-neurogenic) bladder in adults is bladder training, bladder control strategies, pelvic floor muscle training and fluid management. For patients whose symptoms are not improved by either behavioural therapies or drug treatment alone, a combination of the two has proven beneficial. In terms of drug therapy, the first-line drugs are muscarinic receptor antagonists; however, as they are associated with the typical anticholinergic adverse effects of, in particular, dry mouth, blurred vision and constipation, adherence to therapy is often poor.

TABLE 17.2 Drug therapy that may contribute to urinary incontinence

DRUG CLASS	MECHANISM	CONSEQUENCE
α-Adrenoceptor antagonists	Decreased urethral pressure	Stress incontinence
Anticholinergics	Incomplete bladder emptying	Overflow incontinence
Antidepressants	Detrusor overactivity	Urge incontinence
Antiparkinsonism agents	Incomplete bladder emptying	Overflow incontinence
Antipsychotics	Decreased urethral pressure	Stress incontinence
β-Adrenoceptor antagonists	Incomplete bladder emptying	Overflow incontinence
Benzodiazepines	Decreased urethral pressure	Stress incontinence
Diuretics	Excessive urine production	Urge incontinence
Hormone replacement	Detrusor overactivity	Urge incontinence

Source: Adapted from Tsakiris et al. 2008.

Muscarinic receptor antagonists (anticholinergics)

Acetylcholine is the neurotransmitter that controls the detrusor muscle. Overactivity or spontaneous involuntary contraction of the detrusor muscle that leads to urge incontinence can be controlled by drugs that block the action of acetylcholine (muscarinic receptor antagonists; Fig 17.4) on the detrusor M_3 receptor. This reduces contractility of the bladder muscle, which leads to an increase in bladder capacity. In some people, these drugs may cause voiding difficulties including hesitancy and

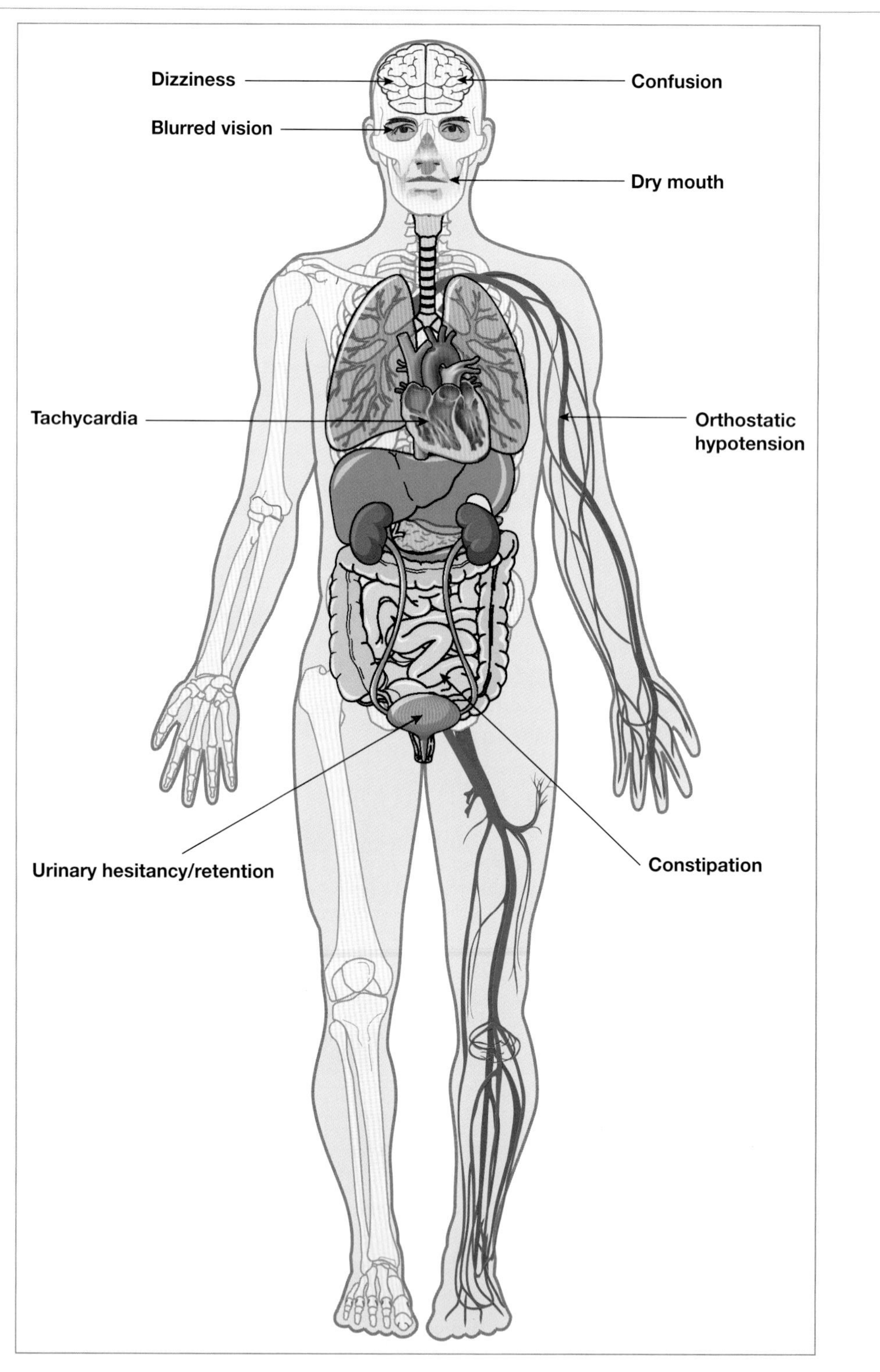

FIGURE 17.4 Adverse effects of muscarinic receptor antagonists

retention. Drugs in this class include darifenacin, oxybutynin (Drug Monograph 17.2), solifenacin and tolterodine. Oxybutynin is generally considered a first-line drug because of its safety, efficacy and tolerability. Imipramine, a tricyclic antidepressant (Ch 22), has significant anticholinergic effects, but it also stimulates β_3 receptors on the detrusor causing relaxation. As imipramine also causes drowsiness, it tends to be used to treat nocturia or nocturnal enuresis.

Darifenacin and solifenacin are drugs with high affinity for the M_3 receptor. This greater receptor selectivity tends to lessen impairment of cognitive and cardiac function. Although superior to placebo, these drugs have adverse effects due to muscarinic receptor blockade and in several studies have been shown to be less well tolerated than tolterodine.

Pharmacokinetics

Both drugs are well absorbed (90–98%) and extensively metabolised in the liver by CYP3A4 (solifenacin) and CYP2D6/CYP3A4 (darifenacin) and excreted in urine (60–70%) and faeces (20–40%). Unchanged drug in urine accounts for only 3–10% of the dose. Due to the involvement of CYP3A4, darifenacin and solifenacin are subject to a significant number of drug interactions involving inhibitors of CYP3A4 (e.g. itraconazole), which may inhibit the metabolism of both drugs. The dose of either darifenacin or solifenacin is reduced when

Drug Monograph 17.2
Oxybutynin

Oxybutynin is a competitive antagonist at muscarinic M_1 and M_3 receptors and has been used for more than 30 years to treat OAB. In addition, oxybutynin has a direct antispasmodic effect on the detrusor muscle as well as local anaesthetic actions. However, both of these effects are around 500 times weaker than the antimuscarinic actions of oxybutynin.

Pharmacokinetics

Oxybutynin is a racemic drug comprising equal proportions (50:50) of *R*-oxybutynin and *S*-oxybutynin. Pharmacological activity resides with the *R*-isomer. It is metabolised in both the intestinal wall and the liver by CYP3A4 and the primary metabolite is *N*-desethyloxybutynin (DEO). The absolute bioavailability is about 60% and the plasma concentration of DEO tends to be 5–12 times greater than that of the parent drug. It has been proposed that many of the anticholinergic adverse effects of oxybutynin may be attributable to DEO. Less than 1% is excreted as unchanged drug. Time to maximal drug concentration varies with the formulation – for example, about an hour with the tablet and 24–48 hours with the transdermal patch. Again, half-life varies – 2–3 hours for the tablet and patch, and 12–13 hours with an extended-release formulation.

Drug interactions

Similar to solifenacin, oxybutynin is subject to drug interactions involving inhibitors of CYP3A4 – for example, itraconazole.

Adverse reactions

Current data suggest that many of the antimuscarinic effects are less frequent with the transdermal patch than the oral formulations. These include:

- dry mouth, constipation
- somnolence, dizziness, agitation, hallucinations, memory impairment.

However, rash, itch and erythema are commonly reported with the patch.

Warnings and contraindications

Oxybutynin is best avoided in:

- combination with other anticholinergic drugs (additive effects)
- people with dementia (it may worsen symptoms)
- situations of pre-existing urinary retention or significant bladder outlet obstruction (it may worsen).

Dosage and administration

The usual adult oral dosage is 2.5–5 mg 2–3 times daily to a maximum daily dose of 20 mg. In the elderly, commence with 2.5 mg at night and, if required, increase the dose slowly. A patch is applied every 3–4 days and in a different area to lessen patch site reactions.

Sources: Australian Medicines Handbook 2021, Kennelly 2010.

administered with potent inhibitors of CYP3A4. The combination of darifenacin and imipramine (a CYP3A4 substrate) should be avoided, as darifenacin may increase the concentration of imipramine and the active metabolite, desipramine, leading to the increased risk of adverse effects. Similarly, tolterodine is metabolised by CYP3A4 and CYP2D6 and the same precautions regarding dose reduction apply when administered concomitantly with inhibitors of CYP3A4 (e.g. itraconazole).

Adverse reactions

In addition to metabolic drug interactions, the main synergistic interactions are with other drugs that have anticholinergic properties. These include tricyclic antidepressants (e.g. amitriptyline), antihistamines (e.g. promethazine) and butyrophenones (e.g. haloperidol). For common adverse reactions related to muscarinic receptor blockade see Figure 17.4. These drugs should not be used in people with narrow-angle glaucoma, partial or complete gastrointestinal tract obstruction, severe colitis, urinary obstruction, myasthenia gravis or unstable cardiac rhythms. Caution should be exercised in patients with hepatic impairment if considering use of either darifenacin or solifenacin.

β_3-Adrenoceptor agonist

Mirabegron is the first β_3-adrenoceptor agonist to be introduced into clinical practice to treat OAB. Stimulation of β_3 receptors located in the detrusor muscle results in relaxation of the detrusor muscle and an increase in bladder compliance thus improving bladder storage capacity. Its pharmacological efficacy is similar to the anticholinergics and it is a viable alternative if the anticholinergics are not well tolerated, ineffective or contraindicated.

Mirabegron is administered orally and about 10% is metabolised by CYP3A4 and CYP2D6 to inactive metabolites. The remainder of the drug is excreted unchanged in urine (55%) and faeces (34%). The drug is well tolerated and adverse effects include hypertension, nasopharyngitis and urinary tract infection.

α_1-Adrenoceptor antagonists (α-blockers)

α-adrenoceptors are present in the bladder neck. The two subtypes of most importance appear to be the α_{1A} and α_{1D}-adrenoceptors. It has yet to be fully established what the individual roles of the two subtypes of α_1-adrenoceptors are, but it has been suggested that the α_{1A}-adrenoceptors may be associated more with obstructive symptoms while the α_{1D}-adrenoceptors may play a role in OAB. Stimulation of the α_{1A}-adrenoceptors in the bladder neck promotes an increase in smooth muscle tone of the bladder neck, which increases bladder outlet resistance. Conversely, the use of α_1-adrenoceptor antagonists results in relaxation of the smooth muscle of the bladder neck, thus decreasing muscle tone. As a consequence, urethral pressure decreases, bladder outlet resistance is reduced and the obstruction to urine outflow is lessened.

Benign prostatic hyperplasia (BPH), a condition occurring frequently in elderly males, can cause bladder dysfunction by increasing bladder outlet resistance. Symptoms include voiding difficulties (e.g. intermittent stream, hesitancy, straining) and bladder storage symptoms (e.g. nocturia, urgency). Selective α_1-adrenoceptor antagonists include alfuzosin, prazosin, silodosin and tamsulosin. Alfuzosin, silodosin and tamsulosin are only indicated for BPH, while prazosin is used to treat hypertension.

Alfuzosin is relatively selective for α_1-adrenoceptors in the genitourinary tract compared with α-adrenoceptors of the vasculature, while tamsulosin and silodosin have a degree of selectivity for α_{1A} receptors favouring an effect on prostatic, bladder neck and urethra α_{1A} receptors. All three drugs are used only to treat benign prostatic hyperplasia.

Pharmacokinetics

Administered orally, the bioavailability of alfuzosin is 49–64% and, as absorption is increased by food, it is recommended to take the drug immediately after a meal. Alfuzosin is metabolised predominantly by hepatic CYP3A4, with a minor contribution from CYP1A2, to inactive metabolites that are excreted via the biliary route into the faeces (~75–91%), with the remaining 11% excreted as unchanged drug in urine. Tamsulosin is extensively metabolised by CYP3A4 and CYP2D6 and less than 10% is excreted in urine as unchanged drug. Silodosin is metabolised by alcohol and aldehyde dehydrogenase, by glucuronidation and oxidative metabolism (CYP3A4). The major metabolite silodosin glucuronide is excreted in urine and the remainder in faeces (54.9%). The half-life of alfuzosin is about 9 hours, silodosin about 13 hours and tamsulosin about 7 hours, and all are administered once daily as a controlled release tablet. As alfuzosin and silodosin are metabolised by CYP3A4, if drugs such as the CYP3A4 inhibitors atazanavir, darunavir and ritonavir are given concomitantly the plasma concentration of alfuzosin and silodosin may increase, predisposing to adverse cardiovascular effects such as hypotension and dizziness, which are major issues in elderly males. As the dose of alfuzosin cannot be reduced, either alfuzosin or the interacting drug should be stopped. Similarly for tamsulosin, inhibitors of CYP3A4 and CYP2D6 may decrease the metabolism and clearance of tamsulosin, predisposing to the adverse effects of α-receptor blockade.

Adverse effects

Penetration of alfuzosin into the brain is poor, which may explain the lower incidence of central nervous system–related adverse effects (e.g. dizziness and somnolence). The safety profile of alfuzosin is similar to silodosin and tamsulosin. All have similar incidences of dizziness (~7%), whereas the incidence of postural hypotension is slightly less common with alfuzosin (~1%) than tamsulosin (~3%). Other adverse effects include headache and tachycardia, which tend to occur within the first 4 weeks. Ejaculatory dysfunction has been reported in about 22% of men prescribed with silodosin and it is sufficiently troublesome to lead to discontinuation of therapy.

α_1-Adrenoceptor antagonists have been trialled in women with OAB. Current evidence indicates that women using α-blockers are five times more likely than non-users to experience urinary dysfunction, including stress incontinence, and women with symptoms of OAB may develop urge incontinence.

KEY POINTS

Drugs for bladder dysfunction

- Micturition (voiding of urine) can be initiated and stopped voluntarily through conscious control at the level of the cerebral cortex. A lack of voluntary control over micturition is referred to as incontinence.
- Urinary incontinence is common and embarrassing and afflicts a significant proportion of the general population – in particular, the elderly.
- Incontinence is categorised into three main types: urge incontinence, stress incontinence and overflow incontinence.
- Muscarinic receptor antagonists (anticholinergic drugs) are the main group of drugs used to treat urinary urge incontinence.
- β_3-adrenoceptors are located in the detrusor muscle and mediate detrusor relaxation and thus increased bladder capacity. Mirabegron is the first clinically available β_3-adrenoceptor agonist.
- α-adrenoceptors are present in the bladder neck, and the two subtypes of most importance appear to be the α_{1A} and α_{1D}-adrenoceptors.
- α_1-adrenoceptor antagonists relax the smooth muscle of the bladder neck, thus decreasing muscle tone. As a consequence, urethral pressure decreases, bladder outlet resistance is reduced and the obstruction to urine outflow is lessened.
- Benign prostatic hyperplasia occurs in elderly males, causing bladder dysfunction by increasing bladder outlet resistance. Symptoms include voiding difficulties (e.g. intermittent stream, hesitancy, straining) and bladder storage symptoms (e.g. nocturia, urgency).
- Selective α_1-adrenoceptor antagonists include alfuzosin, prazosin, silodosin and tamsulosin. Alfuzosin, silodosin and tamsulosin are only indicated for benign prostatic hyperplasia, while prazosin is used to treat hypertension.

DRUGS AT A GLANCE

Drugs affecting the kidney and bladder

PHARMACOLOGICAL GROUP AND EFFECT	KEY EXAMPLES	CLINICAL USE

Loop diuretics
• Inhibit NKCC1 co-transporter
• ↓ reabsorption of sodium and chloride in TALH
• ↑ excretion of water, sodium, chloride, potassium, calcium, magnesium
	Furosemide
	Bumetanide
		• Oedema associated with:
		  • heart failure
		  • hepatic cirrhosis
		  • nephrotic syndrome
		  • renal impairment

Thiazide/thiazide-like diuretics • Inhibit Na^+–Cl^- symporter • ↓ reabsorption of sodium and chloride in proximal segment of the distal convoluted tubule • ↑ excretion of water, sodium, chloride, potassium, calcium, magnesium • ↓ excretion of uric acid and calcium	Chlortalidone (thiazide-like)	• Hypertension • Oedema (due to heart failure or hepatic cirrhosis)
	Hydrochlorothiazide Bendroflumethiazide[NZ]	• Hypertension • Oedema (due to heart failure, hepatic cirrhosis, nephrotic syndrome) • Hypercalcuria (prevention of renal calculi)
	Indapamide (thiazide-like)	• Hypertension
Potassium-sparing diuretic • Block sodium channels • ↓ reabsorption of sodium in distal tubule • ↓ potassium excretion	Amiloride	• Hypertension • Oedema (due to heart failure, hepatic cirrhosis, nephrotic syndrome) • Prevention of diuretic-induced hypokalaemia

Aldosterone antagonist • Antagonises action of aldosterone in distal tubule • ↓ sodium reabsorption • ↓ potassium excretion • ↑ sodium and water excretion	Spironolactone (potassium sparing)	• Primary hyperaldosteronism • Hypertension (resistant) • Refractory oedema associated with secondary hyperaldosteronism
Muscarinic receptor antagonists (Anticholinergics, genitourinary) • Antagonise action of acetylcholine on detrusor M_3 receptors • ↓ bladder contractility • ↑ bladder capacity	Darifenacin[AUS] Oxybutynin Solifenacin Tolterodine	• Treatment of urinary urge incontinence
β_3-Adrenoceptor agonist • Stimulates β_3 receptors on detrusor smooth muscle • Relaxation of detrusor muscle • ↑ bladder capacity	Mirabegron[AUS]	• Treatment of urinary urge incontinence
α_1-Adrenoceptor antagonists • Antagonise the action of NA on α_1-adrenoceptors • Relaxation of bladder neck smooth muscle • ↓ urethral pressure and bladder outlet resistance • ↑ urine outflow	Alfuzosin[AUS] Tamsulosin	• Symptomatic relief of benign prostatic hyperplasia

[AUS] Australia only
[NZ] New Zealand only
TALH = thick ascending limb of the loop of Henle

REVIEW EXERCISES

1. Mrs MB, a 76-year-old female with a long history of heart failure, has been prescribed frusemide by her GP. She asks you as her healthcare nurse to explain how the drug will affect her kidneys and whether she should expect any adverse effects. Prepare a drug information sheet for Mrs MB that will answer her questions.
2. Mr GE, a 69-year-old male, has recently been diagnosed with hypertension. He has been commenced on hydrochlorothiazide 12.5 mg daily. At his next visit the GP informs Mr GE that his blood glucose level is elevated and that he will be changing his medication to a different antihypertensive. Explain how a thiazide diuretic may cause hyperglycaemia.
3. Alfuzosin was prescribed for Mr DL's benign prostatic hyperplasia but when prescribed for Mrs AT's overactive bladder symptoms it was found to worsen her condition. Explain why the drug is effective for treating Mr DL but worsens Mrs AT's symptoms.

REFERENCES

Australian Medicines Handbook. Adelaide: Australian Medicines Handbook Pty Ltd. 2021.

Brunton LL, Hilal-Dandan R, Knollmann BC. Goodman & Gilman's The pharmacological basis of therapeutics. 13th ed. New York: McGraw-Hill Education; 2018.

Gormley EA, Lightner DJ, Faraday M, et al. Diagnosis and treatment of overactive bladder (non-neurogenic) in adults: AUA/SUFU Guideline amendment. Journal of Urology 2015;193:1572–80.

Greger R Physiology of sodium transport. The American Journal of the Medical Sciences 2000;319:51–62.

Johnson DW, Jones GRD, Mathew TH, et al. Chronic kidney disease and automatic reporting of estimated glomerular filtration rate: new developments and revised recommendations. A position statement from the Australasian Creatinine Consensus Working Group. Medical Journal of Australia 2012;197:1–5.

Kennelly MJ. A comparative review of oxybutynin chloride formulations: pharmacokinetics and therapeutic efficacy in overactive bladder, Nature Reviews Urology 2010;12:12–19.

Perazella MA. Drug use and nephrotoxicity in the intensive care unit. Kidney International 2012;81:1172–78.

Rang HP, Dale MM, Ritter JM, et al. Rang and Dale's pharmacology. 7ed. Edinburgh: Elsevier Churchill Livingstone; 2012.

Tsakiris P, Oelke M, Michael MC. Drug-induced urinary incontinence. Drugs Aging 2008;25:541–49.

ONLINE RESOURCES

Kidney Health Australia – CARI Guidelines: diagnosis, classification and staging of chronic kidney disease: https://www.cariguidelines.org/guidelines/chronic-kidney-disease/early-chronic-kidney-disease/diagnosis-classification-and-staging-of-chronic-kidney-disease/ (accessed 11 January 2022)

More weblinks at: http://evolve.elsevier.com/AU/Knights/pharmacology/.

CHAPTER 18

CENTRAL NERVOUS SYSTEM OVERVIEW AND ANAESTHETICS

Shaunagh Darroch

KEY ABBREVIATIONS

ACh	acetylcholine
CNS	central nervous system
CSF	cerebrospinal fluid
EAA	excitatory amino acids
EMLA	eutectic mixture for local anaesthesia
GA	general anaesthesia
5-HT	5-hydroxytryptamine (serotonin)
IV	intravenous
LA	local anaesthetic
MAC	minimum alveolar concentration (for anaesthesia)
NMJ	neuromuscular junction
NMDA	*N*-methyl-D-aspartate
PABA	*p*-aminobenzoic acid
PNS	peripheral nervous system
RAS	reticular activating system
TIVA	total intravenous anaesthesia

Chapter Focus

The central nervous system, comprising the brain and spinal cord, regulates all body functions, allowing the person to adapt, consciously and subconsciously, to the internal and external environments and to carry out complex functions such as integration, reasoning, memory, behaviour and expression of mood and personality. A broad knowledge of the physiology and neurochemistry of the central nervous system is necessary for understanding the many groups of drugs used to treat diseases affecting this system.

Anaesthesia is the loss of sensations of pain, pressure, temperature or touch, in a part or the whole of the body. Anaesthetic drugs cause unconsciousness or insensitivity to pain by a reversible action; that is, cells return to normal when the drug is eliminated from the cells. The two major categories of anaesthetic agents are the general anaesthetics, which depress consciousness and cause generalised loss of sensation, and the local anaesthetics, which block nerve conduction and pain in a limited area when applied locally or to nerve pathways. Many adjuncts to anaesthesia are also used during surgery to maintain the patient in a stable physiological state and to relieve or prevent pain, anxiety and postoperative nausea, and will also be referred to in the following chapters.

KEY TERMS

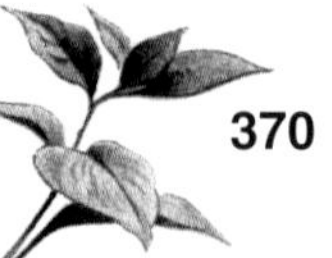

KEY DRUG GROUPS

Adjuncts to anaesthesia:

- Analgesics: **fentanyl**
- Neuromuscular blockers:
  - depolarising: **suxamethonium**
  - non-depolarising: atracurium, **rocuronium**

General anaesthetics:

- Inhaled:
  - gases: **nitrous oxide** (Drug Monograph 18.1)
  - volatile liquids: **methoxyflurane**, **sevoflurane** (Drug Monograph 18.2)
- Intravenous:
  - **ketamine**, **midazolam**, **propofol** (Drug Monograph 18.3), thiopental

Local anaesthetics:

- **cocaine**, **lidocaine (lignocaine)** (Drug Monograph 18.4), **prilocaine**
- Long-acting: **bupivacaine**

CRITICAL THINKING SCENARIO

A 4-year-old boy is brought to the emergency department with a swollen, painful and deformed left forearm after falling off a trampoline. He is otherwise in good health with no known allergies. He has a past medical history of infrequent episodic asthma. His weight is 19 kg. Plain film x-rays reveal displaced mid-shaft fractures of his left radius and ulna, with a moderate degree of angulation. He is administered pain relief. After fasting for 2 hours since his last snack of food or liquid, he has procedural sedation in the emergency department using a mix of 60% inhaled oxygen and 40% inhaled nitrous oxide for approximately 20 minutes, while the fractured bones are set in plaster. He is monitored closely throughout the procedure for asthma symptoms, with suction equipment and medications close by in case of nausea/vomiting. He makes a good recovery with rapid return to his normal conscious state; the attending doctor confirms good neurovascular supply to his hand as the plaster is setting and cooling, and the boy is discharged home.

A review appointment is made with the fracture outpatients' clinic for the following week.

1. What is procedural sedation?
2. Why was nitrous oxide with oxygen used?
3. What is the mechanism of action of this drug?
4. What possible medications are available for nausea and vomiting and how do they work?

Source: Acknowledgments to Dr Philippa Shilson, paediatrician.

Introduction: The central nervous system

The nervous system consists of the **central nervous system** (CNS) and the peripheral nervous system (PNS; Fig 18.1). Drugs with central actions are of particular importance in pharmacology; the main drug groups affecting the CNS are summarised in Clinical Focus Box 18.1. Not only are they frequently prescribed for treatment of common clinical conditions (pain, headache, anxiety, epilepsy, sleeplessness, depression, psychoses), but they are also the most common self-administered

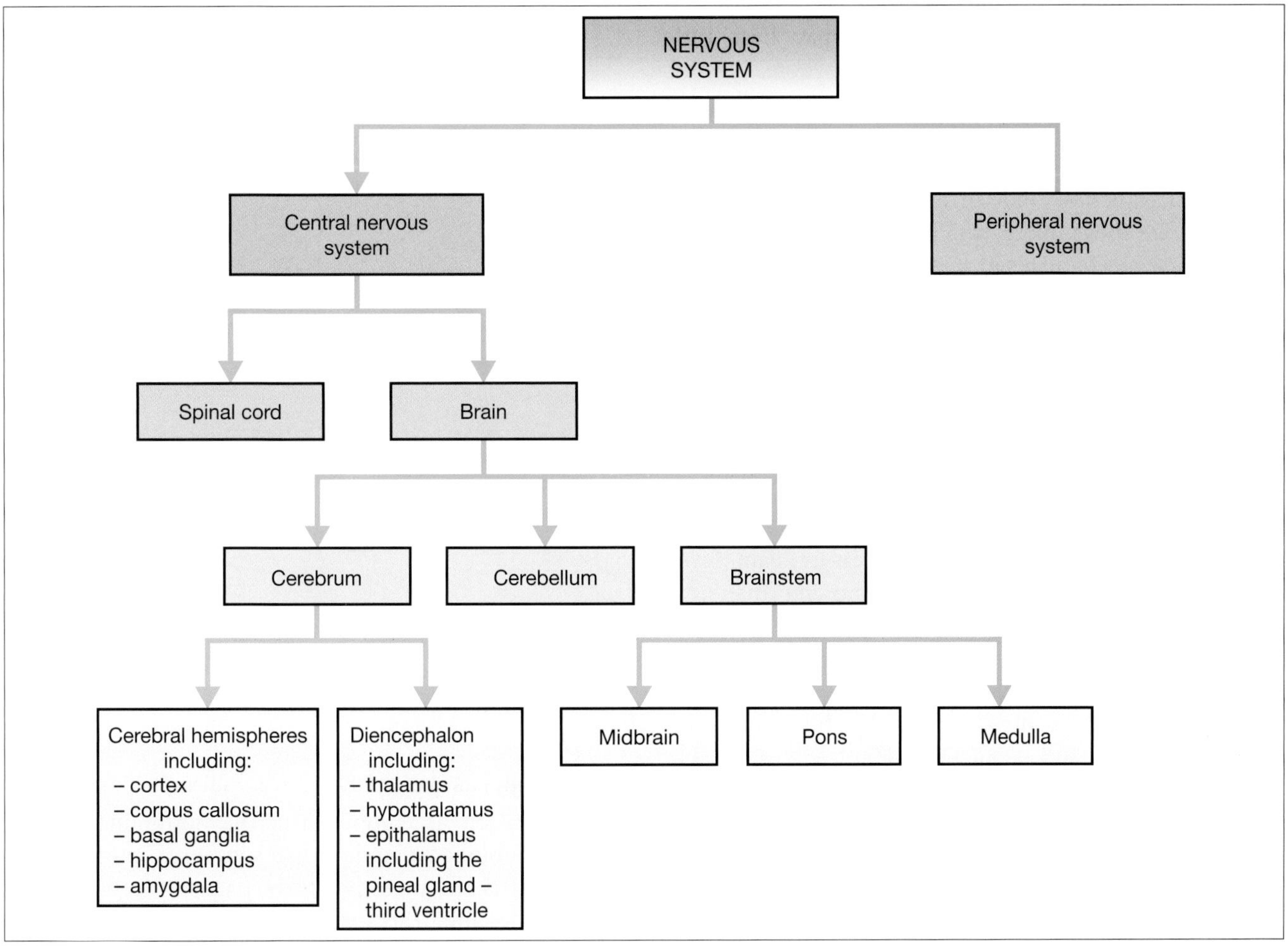

NERVOUS SYSTEM

- Central nervous system
  - Spinal cord
  - Brain
    - Cerebrum
      - Cerebral hemispheres including: – cortex – corpus callosum – basal ganglia – hippocampus – amygdala
      - Diencephalon including: – thalamus – hypothalamus – epithalamus including the pineal gland – third ventricle
    - Cerebellum
    - Brainstem
      - Midbrain
      - Pons
      - Medulla
- Peripheral nervous system

FIGURE 18.1 Organisation of the nervous system, showing the major anatomical subdivisions of the central nervous system

(Details of the peripheral nervous system subdivisions are shown in Ch 9, Fig 9.1.)

Source: Salerno 1999, Figure 11.1; used with permission.

CLINICAL FOCUS BOX 18.1
Drugs affecting the CNS

The major drug groups with actions on the CNS include:

- anxiolytics, especially the benzodiazepines, such as diazepam and midazolam
- sedatives/hypnotics, also used as anticonvulsant and antiepileptic agents
- antipsychotics (tranquillisers, antischizophrenic agents)
- antidepressant and antimanic drugs (e.g. tricyclics, lithium)
- antiparkinson drugs (e.g. levodopa, anticholinergics)
- CNS stimulants (e.g. amphetamines, caffeine)
- general anaesthetics (e.g. ketamine, propofol, sevoflurane)
- opioid analgesics (e.g. morphine)
- drugs for preventing or treating headaches and migraine (e.g. sumatriptan)
- miscellaneous drugs, including anticholinesterases, appetite suppressants and centrally acting muscle relaxants.

Other drugs may be administered to prevent or treat general pathologies to brain tissue – for example, cytotoxic agents for tumours, antibiotics for infections or anti-inflammatory agents in cerebral oedema. Many drugs given for peripheral effects may cross the blood–brain barrier and have side effects on the CNS – for example, autonomic drugs, antihistamines and local anaesthetics (LAs). Drugs are also taken for social, rather than medical, reasons (e.g. tobacco, alcohol, marijuana, stimulants, psychedelics and cocaine).

drugs – for example, analgesics, tobacco, alcohol and caffeine. Actions at the cellular level may bear little obvious relationship to effects on the whole person's complex functions such as emotions, memory, thought processes, personality and behaviour. Consequently, some of the most commonly used CNS-active drugs, such as general anaesthetics and drugs affecting mood and behaviour, are those about which we understand little in terms of their mechanisms of action. For this reason, there is much ongoing research into the mechanism of action and clinical use of these drugs.

CNS structure and function

Composed of the brain and spinal cord, the CNS essentially controls all functions in the body. Sensory information from the periphery is transmitted via PNS afferent pathways,[1] alerting the CNS to internal and external changes such as muscle tension, joint position, blood pressure, pain, fever, sound, smell, taste, touch and sight. This information is integrated in the CNS, and messages are then relayed via peripheral efferent pathways to appropriate cells or tissues to produce the necessary actions and adjustments to ensure effective balanced control of body functions (i.e. homeostasis). Refer to Chapters 8 and 9.

Brain

The human brain weighs about 1400 g and is estimated to contain around 100 billion neurons, each of which connects with around 10,000 others in branching networks. The brain is suspended in cerebrospinal fluid (CSF) and surrounded and protected by membranes called the meninges. CSF helps keep the brain in a very stable environment, acts as a fluid shock-absorber and circulates chemical messengers such as neurotransmitters and other modulators or mediators. The parts of the brain can be described in various ways; a simplified approach is to consider the major component areas (Fig 18.2):

- the brainstem (continuous above the spinal cord), consisting of medulla oblongata, pons and midbrain, and including the reticular formation
- the cerebellum
- the diencephalon, comprising the thalamus, hypothalamus and pineal gland
- the two cerebral hemispheres, each subdivided by fissures into parietal lobe, frontal lobe, occipital lobe and temporal lobe.

In the following sections, the major areas of the brain are described briefly, especially those areas affected by drug therapies. The 'special senses' (sight, hearing, smell) and drugs affecting the eye or the ear are discussed in Chapter 40.

1 A little Latin (or Italian) knowledge is helpful here: 'afferent' comes from the Latin *ad ferens*, carrying towards; and 'efferent' from *ex ferens*, carrying away from.

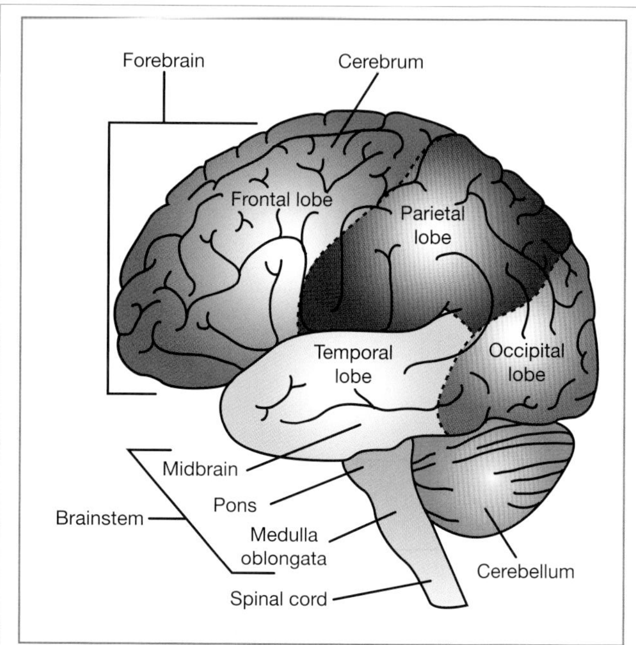

FIGURE 18.2 The human brain, left lateral view
Source: Salerno 1999, Figure 11.2; used with permission.

Brainstem

The brainstem is composed of the midbrain, pons and medulla oblongata and is the source of cranial nerves III–XII. It is the most primitive part of the brain and is essential for life; tests for brain death – for example, after severe CNS trauma or anoxia – all involve testing of brainstem functions such as the gag and cough reflexes, ocular and vestibular reflexes and spontaneous breathing.

The midbrain serves as a relay station between higher areas of the brain and the spinal cord; centres for visual and auditory reflexes are located here. The pons helps bridge the left and right sides of the cerebellum, and contains ascending sensory and descending motor tracts. The upper pons and medulla contain the reticular activating system (RAS).

The medulla oblongata contains several vital centres necessary for survival: the respiratory, vasomotor, cardiac and vomiting centres. Other essential functions also originate here, such as the sneezing, coughing and swallowing reflexes.

Cerebellum

Located in the posterior cranial fossa behind the brainstem, the cerebellum contains more neurons than all the rest of the brain, with centres for muscle coordination, maintenance of posture and muscle tone. It may also have a role in cognitive functions. A lesion or damage to it leads to ataxia (postural instability). Drugs that disturb the cerebellum or vestibular branch of the eighth cranial nerve – such as alcohol and some drugs used in mental disorders – cause dizziness and loss of equilibrium.

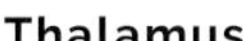

Thalamus

The thalamus is composed of sensory nuclei and serves as the major centre for relaying sensations such as pain, temperature, pleasure and touch to the cerebral cortex. The thalamus plays a role in the acquisition of knowledge and (with the RAS) in arousal or alerting signals. Drugs that depress neurotransmission in the thalamus may relieve pain.

Hypothalamus

The hypothalamus is a major controller of homeostasis of many body functions. It is a link between higher centres in the brain and both the autonomic nervous system and the endocrine system. Functions of the hypothalamus can be summarised as:

- control of the autonomic nervous system, including regulation of smooth muscle tone, body temperature, cardiovascular and gut functions
- control of the pituitary gland, thereby controlling most endocrine functions, including growth, reproductive and sexual functions, and thyroid and adrenal cortex hormones
- regulation of emotional and behavioural patterns, partly through the appetite centre and pleasure or reward centres
- regulation of hunger and thirst, carbohydrate and fat metabolism, and water balance
- regulation of circadian rhythms and sleep.[2]

Drugs affecting the hypothalamus, such as tricyclic antidepressants and other psychotherapeutic agents, induce autonomic symptoms such as weight loss, anorexia, decreased libido and insomnia, and may cause hypothalamic side effects including breast engorgement, lactation, amenorrhoea, appetite stimulation and alterations in temperature regulation.

Cerebrum

The cerebrum, the largest and uppermost section of the brain, is the highest functional area, where sensory, integrative, emotional, language, memory and motor functions are controlled. The cerebrum consists mainly of right and left hemispheres connected by thick fibrous tracts; each hemisphere is involved in functions and sensations of the opposite side of the body – that is, contralateral control. The superficial, massively folded layer of the cerebrum is called the cerebral cortex (Latin: bark, rind) or grey matter of the brain, and covers the four lobes into which each hemisphere is divided. (These lobes are named for the bones of the skull under which they lie: frontal, parietal, occipital and temporal; see Fig 18.2, above.) The white matter is so-called as it is largely made up of myelinated axons, whereas the grey matter comprises dendrites, cell bodies and supportive tissues.

The cortex can be broadly classified into motor areas and sensory areas. The frontal lobe contains the motor and speech areas and areas for intellectual functions, affective behaviour (mood) and abstract thinking. The sensory areas are located in the parietal lobe, the auditory cortex and memory areas in the temporal lobe and the visual cortex in the occipital lobe. Large parts of the cortex are concerned with higher mental activity – reasoning, creative thought, judgement and memory.[3] The limbic lobe is the most primitive component of the cerebral cortex (see 'Limbic system', below) and is responsible for emotions, activities and drives required for the survival of the individual and the species.

Even simple tasks require simultaneous interactions among many parts of the brain, plus general functions of consciousness, attention and decision making. Drugs that depress cerebral cortical activity (CNS depressants such as general anaesthetics and alcohol) may decrease acuity of sensation and perception, inhibit motor activity, decrease alertness and concentration, depress both higher mental functions such as cognition and memory and autonomic functions such as cardiovascular control and respiration and promote drowsiness and sleep. Drugs that stimulate the cortical areas (e.g. caffeine or amphetamines) may induce more vivid impulses to be received, autonomic stimulation, greater awareness of the surrounding environment, increased muscle activity and restlessness.

Spinal cord

The spinal cord is a thick band of nerve fibres surrounded by the three meningeal membranes (dura mater, arachnoid mater, pia mater) that surround the entire CNS; it lies within the spinal canal formed by the protective vertebrae. It functions in the transmission of impulses to and from all parts of the brain and is also a centre for reflex activity. Ascending tracts of afferent nerves in the dorsal (posterior) horns of the grey matter conduct impulses up from peripheral receptors and nerves to the brain, and descending tracts (motor and autonomic) conduct efferent impulses down from the brain to synapse with peripheral motor and autonomic nerves. (See the transverse section of the spinal cord in Fig 18.3.) (Refer to Ch 19 for a discussion of the gate theory of pain and see Fig 19.4.) Through this pathway, the perception of pain can be blunted by stress, stoic determination, the 'heat of battle' (fight-or-flight response) or analgesic drugs. Small doses of spinal stimulants may increase reflex excitability; larger doses may cause convulsions.

2 Circadian rhythms and sleep patterns are determined by complex interactions among the hypothalamus, pineal gland (which secretes melatonin) and tracts linked to the retina that sense light. This system becomes disturbed by long-distance air travel, Arctic/Antarctic extremes of day/night cycles and total blindness.

3 Some of the greatest mysteries of medicine relate to the higher functions of the cerebrum – for example, how memory works, and how personality is formed and controlled. It has been suggested that the human brain is the most complex object in the known universe, so we are unlikely ever to understand how it functions.

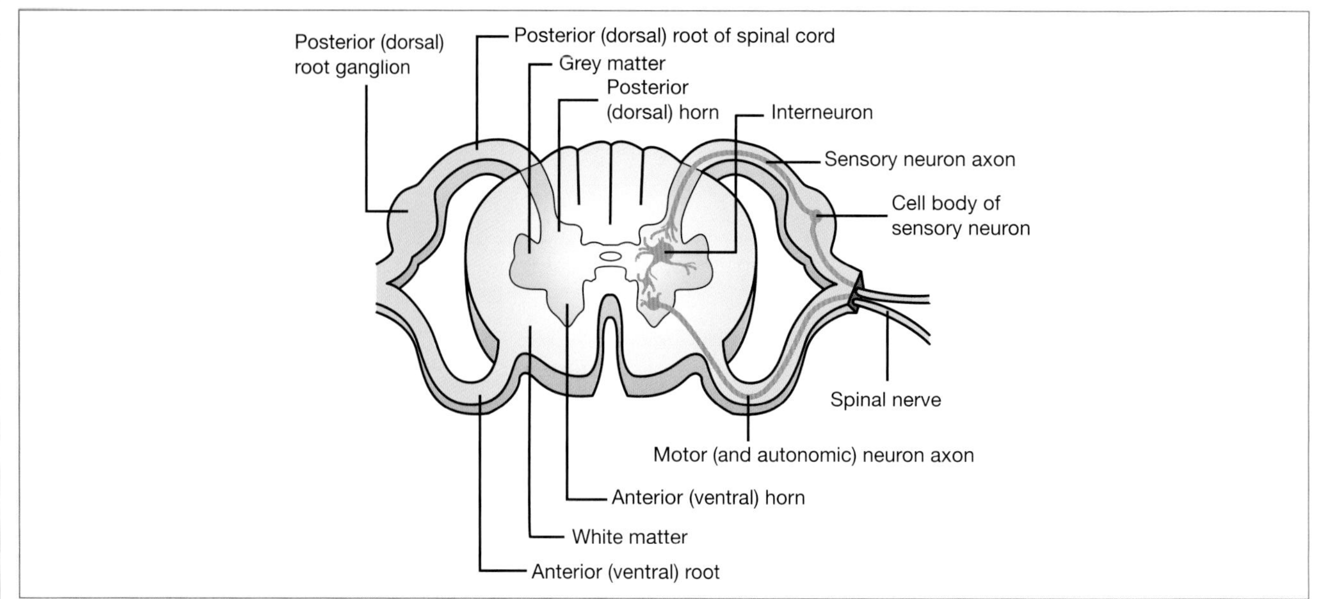

FIGURE 18.3 Transverse section of the spinal cord; neural components of a spinal reflex are shown in darker blue on the right-hand side.
Source: Salerno 1999, Figure 11.3; used with permission.

CNS functional systems

Specific types of signals are processed in particular brain regions, described not so much by anatomical boundaries as by overall functional aspects. Generally, sensory areas receive and interpret information from receptors for touch, temperature, pain and proprioception; motor areas integrate all voluntary movements, including speech; and association areas have complex integrative functions in memory, emotions, willpower, intelligence and personality. Four major CNS functional systems affected by CNS-active drugs include the RAS, the limbic system, the extrapyramidal system and the basal ganglia.

Reticular activating system

The RAS is a diffuse system of nuclei in the reticular formation of the brainstem that permits communication between the spinal cord, thalamus and cerebral cortex. The primary functions of the RAS are:

- consciousness and arousal from sleep, requiring an external signal such as a pain stimulus, an alarm clock or bright light[4]
- a filtering process that allows for concentration on a specific stimulus at a given time
- involvement in regulation of muscle tone and spinal reflexes
- a centre for pain perception
- centres for cardiovascular regulation via descending sympathetic pathways.

Inactivation of the RAS results in sleep, and injury to the RAS or disease may produce a lack of consciousness or a comatose state. 5-hydroxytryptamine (5-HT; serotonin) is a neurotransmitter in many pathways in the RAS.

Many drugs act on the RAS: anaesthetics dampen its activity and induce sleep, whereas amphetamines stimulate or activate the system. Lysergic acid diethylamide (LSD; Ch 25) and other hallucinogenic agents may act on the RAS by interacting with serotonergic pathways, thus interfering with its ability to filter out stimuli; hence a person taking this substance is bombarded by stimuli. In contrast, the phenothiazine tranquillisers such as chlorpromazine (Ch 22) have a depressant activity on the RAS, thus reducing hallucinations in psychotic patients or people taking LSD.

Limbic system

The limbic system is a border of subcortical structures that surround the corpus callosum around the top of the brainstem (Fig 20.2, in Ch 20); components are the olfactory bulbs, hippocampus, cingulate gyrus, hypothalamic nuclei and amygdala. Its functioning is extremely complex, interacting with other parts of the brain to influence or normalise expressions of emotions, such as anger, fear, anxiety, pleasure and sorrow, to affect the biological rhythms, sexual behaviour and motivation of a person, and to assist in learning and memory.

Drugs that affect the limbic system include the benzodiazepines and opioids. The benzodiazepines act at various subtypes in the CNS, affecting the limbic system,

4 The alerting reaction is not, however, stimulated by smell in humans; hence the need for electronic smoke alarms in buildings to detect smoke and change the chemical stimulus to one to which the human RAS responds – for example, sound or light.

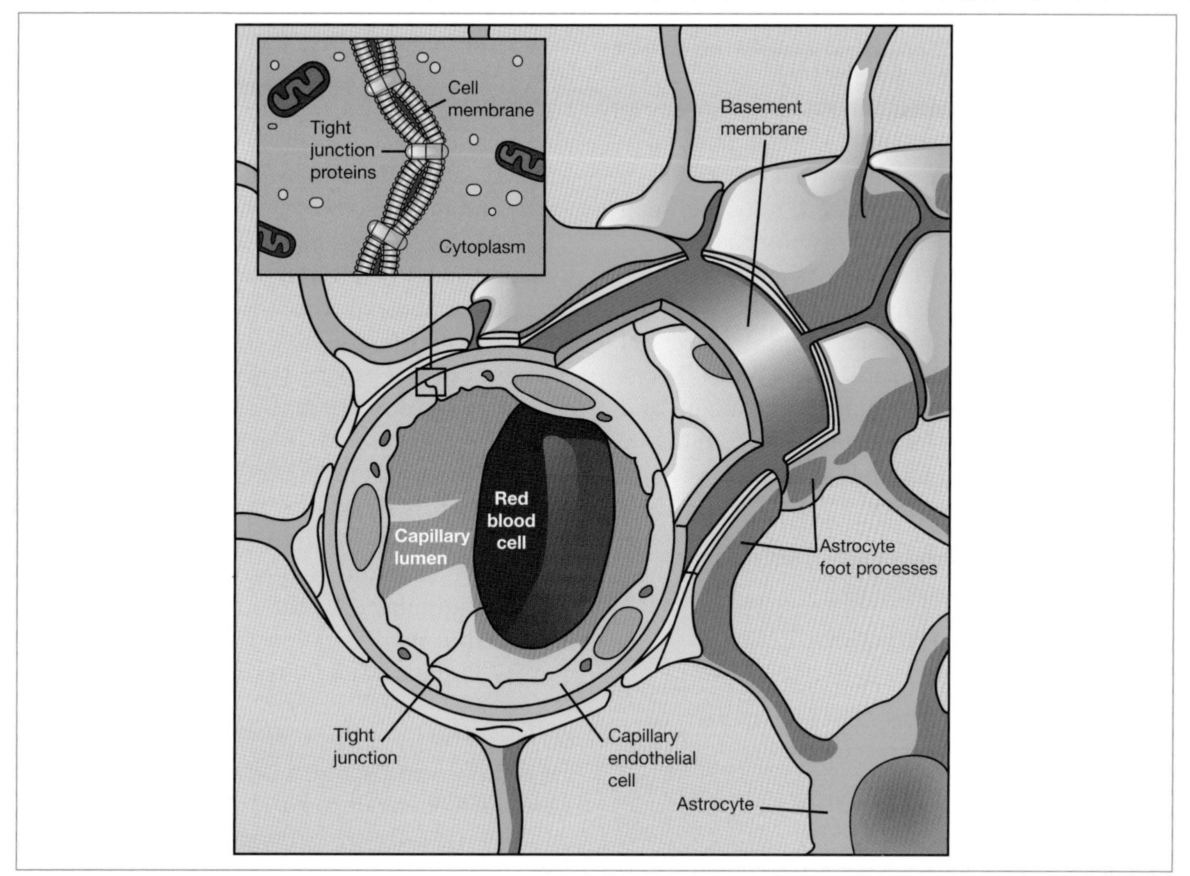

FIGURE 18.4 The blood–brain barrier, showing tight junctions between capillary endothelial cells and astrocyte foot processes

Source: netterimages.com; used with permission.

preventing it from activating the reticular formation, causing drowsiness and sleep and having anxiolytic actions. Morphine is thought to alter subjective reactions to pain as well as abolishing pain stimuli received by special areas within the limbic system.

Extrapyramidal system

The extrapyramidal system is a series of indirect CNS motor pathways that are outside the main motor pathways that traverse the pyramids in the thalamus (hence the term 'extrapyramidal'). The pathways or tracts coordinate posture and movements of muscles in the limbs, head and eyes. Antipsychotic agents that block dopamine receptors may produce adverse effects related to this system; these are referred to as extrapyramidal side effects and may mimic the signs of Parkinsonism (Ch 22, Fig 22.1 and Ch 24).

Basal ganglia

The **basal ganglia** are a series of paired nuclei in each cerebral hemisphere that coordinate gross automatic muscle movements and regulate muscle tone; the main components are the corpus striatum, the globus pallidus and the substantia nigra. They are connected with the cerebral cortex, thalamus and hypothalamus, and regulate the tone and characteristics of all voluntary movements; thus, damage to the basal ganglia, such as occurs commonly in Parkinson's disease, can lead to increased muscle tone, rigidity and tremors (Ch 22, Fig 22.1 and Ch 24).

The blood–brain barrier

The **blood–brain barrier** is a selectively permeable filter between the blood circulation and the cells of the brain and spinal cord, maintaining a highly stable chemical environment and protecting against neurotoxins and pathogens in the CNS. The existence of a barrier between the blood and the brain, preventing easy passage of molecules from the systemic circulation into the CNS, was postulated to account for the fact that acidic dyes (after being injected intravenously into animals to stain tissues for histological studies) did not stain the brain cells.

The blood–brain barrier is now attributed to tight junctions between endothelial cells in the cerebral capillaries, a covering formed from the foot-like processes of the glial cells (astrocytes) that encircle the brain's capillary walls, and the almost complete absence of fenestrations and pinocytotic vesicles in the capillary endothelial cells (Fig 18.4).

The barrier is not absolute but is selectively permeable because it will allow small molecules (e.g. water, alcohol, oxygen and carbon dioxide), lipid-soluble substances, gases and substances essential to energy supply to penetrate but excludes most water-soluble and large molecules. There is also active transport and secretion of compounds between the brain and blood: nutrients such as d-glucose and precursors to neurotransmitter substances (e.g. choline and the amino acids phenylalanine, tyrosine and dopa [dihydroxyphenylalanine]) pass across or are actively transported. Some important clinical aspects of the blood–brain barrier are summarised in Clinical Focus Box 18.2. The barrier is less efficient in young infants and in conditions where there is focal damage to CNS tissue such as ischaemic stroke and multiple sclerosis.

KEY POINTS

Central nervous system function

- The CNS is a complex system that monitors and regulates all body functions, allowing adaptation to changes in both the internal and the external environments.
- The CNS integrates information received from the PNS and then transmits messages via the PNS to body organs to maintain homeostasis and control higher functions.
- The CNS is composed of the brain (cerebrum, cerebellum and brainstem) and the spinal cord; component anatomical areas and functional systems have specific and interrelated neurophysiological effects.
- Major CNS functional systems are the reticular formation, limbic system, extrapyramidal system and basal ganglia. These are responsible for many functions: consciousness and attention; personality, emotions and behaviour; learning, memory and decision making; sensory perception; and motor control, muscle tone and coordination. All of these systems may be affected by drugs.
- The blood–brain barrier maintains the CNS in a highly stable chemical environment, allowing passage of required nutrients, transmitters and lipid-soluble substances while excluding large water-soluble and potentially toxic compounds. The barrier is less efficient in young infants and in conditions of focal damage to CNS tissue.

Nerve cells and synaptic transmission in the CNS

The two major cell types in the CNS are neurons, or nerve cells, and glial cells (neuroglia). The functions of the glial cells are not fully understood: they do not conduct action potentials but may express a range of receptors and transporters, serve to nurture, support and assist neurons in the transfer and integration of information in the CNS, and assist in forming myelin, protecting against disease and helping to form the blood–brain barrier. Glial cells play a role in neural plasticity, in protection from or recovery after injury (by taking up excitatory amino acids) and may also be crucial to memory formation.

There are an estimated 100 billion neurons in the human brain. Neurons in the CNS have the same basic structure as those in the PNS: dendrites, cell body, axon and nerve terminals. Between each nerve terminal and the next cell is a gap, or synapse, and electrical impulses cannot jump directly across. In the process known as synaptic transmission, **neurotransmitters** are released from the terminal end of the first neuron (the presynaptic side) and cross the gap to receptors in the membrane of the cell on the postsynaptic side, which may be a neuron or (in the PNS) another effector cell that carries out some function stimulated by the nerve. (Neurotransmission is described in more detail in Ch 8, and shown in Figs 8.3 and 8.7 in the context of transmission in the PNS.)

Action potentials and ion channels

Most information transmitted in the CNS is due to alterations in electrical currents. The electrical properties of all nerve cells are generated by various ions, pumps and ion channels located in the cell membrane. Channels are described as *voltage-gated* if they open in response to changes in membrane potential (voltage) – for example, during the generation and conductance of action potentials. By comparison, a *ligand-gated channel* opens and closes in response to a specific chemical stimulus. (A ligand is something that binds – for example, a neurotransmitter, hormone or drug that binds to a specific receptor or channel.) Refer to Chapter 8 for examples of ion channels associated with receptor activity.

Many drugs act either directly on the ion channels or via receptors that affect ion channels; for example, LAs enter nerve cells and physically block sodium channels, reducing sodium influx and preventing generation of the action potentials and conduction of nerve impulses, especially in neurons that carry messages from pain receptors. Sedative drugs such as benzodiazepines and barbiturates modulate the binding of the inhibitory transmitter GABA to the $GABA_A$ receptor and thus enhance opening of the chloride channel, producing inhibitory postsynaptic potentials and synaptic inhibition.

CNS neurotransmission

In the CNS there are widely divergent networks of interconnecting neurons, with hundreds or thousands of presynaptic terminals impinging on a postsynaptic cell; thus, each CNS neuron may synapse directly or indirectly with around 10,000 others, allowing integration of complex functions.

CLINICAL FOCUS BOX 18.2
Clinical aspects of the blood–brain barrier

The blood–brain barrier protects the brain from toxic substances within the peripheral circulation, maintaining homeostasis and preventing drug delivery to the CNS to treat neurodegenerative diseases (see below). Its structure involves vascular endothelial cells with tight junctions and pericytes surrounding the endothelial cells, astrocytic end feet and basement membrane. The barrier is 'broken down' in most focal injuries to the brain – for example, inflammation, convulsions, trauma, tumours or infection; this allows useful drugs such as antibiotics to penetrate infected or inflamed tissue. The blood–brain barrier becomes damaged in acute neurological disorders and in neurodegeneration (e.g. multiple sclerosis, ischaemic stroke, Alzheimer's disease). Therapies to alleviate blood–brain barrier damage include stem cell therapy for repair, sealing the barrier, eliminating the consequences of its breakdown (e.g. toxin accumulation) and enhancing its clearance function.

The barrier is underdeveloped at birth; hence, infants are at risk of CNS side effects from any drugs administered, or indeed from drugs taken by the mother during pregnancy or while breastfeeding. Infants are also at risk of accumulating bilirubin, a breakdown product of cell metabolism, in the brain; the neonate's liver is too immature to deal with large amounts of bilirubin, which can pass across into the brain and cause kernicterus and permanent brain damage. (Jaundiced infants are often placed under a UV lamp, which helps to break down bilirubin and prevent its accumulation.)

As a general summary rule, the drugs that do pass the blood–brain barrier are uncharged compounds (not ionised) that have high lipid solubility and are not highly protein-bound; an exception is alcohol (ethanol), which is a very water-soluble molecule, but so small that it crosses membranes as readily as does water.

A focus of current research is on methods to increase the permeability of the blood–brain barrier to specific therapeutic agents, such as antibiotics to treat localised brain infections, antineoplastic agents needed for brain tumours and drugs for neurodegenerative disorders such as Parkinson's disease.

Traversing the blood–brain barrier is a challenge for CNS drug delivery. Several strategies allow drugs to traverse the barrier and include nanomaterial formulations and novel administration routes for nano-sized particles:

- colloidal carrier-based drug delivery systems involving nanoparticles
- use of carrier mediated transport systems (see the use of L-DOPA [levodopa] in Parkinson's disease in Ch 24)
- molecular trojan horses are peptides fused to antibodies to receptor-mediated transport systems, allowing delivery of drugs across the blood–brain barrier
- viral vector-mediated gene delivery to CNS involves viral capsid proteins with novel variants that can deliver genes to the CNS for treatment of neurodegenerative diseases.

Virtually all central neurons have numerous excitatory and inhibitory synapses, which facilitates the balancing of cell excitability between too much (possibly leading to seizures) and too little (reduced consciousness or coma). The monoamines noradrenaline (NA), dopamine (DA) and 5-HT, and acetylcholine (ACh), may all have either excitatory or inhibitory effects (see below).

In the CNS there are many inhibitory synapses, where binding of an **inhibitory transmitter** (gamma-aminobutyric acid [GABA] or glycine) causes hyperpolarisation of the cell membrane (the cell interior becomes more negative) and generates an inhibitory postsynaptic potential; this reduces the likelihood of generation of an action potential and reduces the responsiveness of the cell.

Criteria for central neurotransmitter status

The criteria for a chemical to be classed as a CNS neurotransmitter are as follows:

- The chemical precursor(s) to the transmitter molecule must be present in the neuron or capable of being transported across the blood–brain barrier and neuronal membrane into the neuron.
- The transmitter must be synthesised (if not already present) in the presynaptic (first) neuron; this process requires that the precursor chemicals and enzymes for synthesising the transmitter also be present.
- The transmitter is taken up into and stored in packages (vesicles) in an inactive form in the nerve terminal.
- Electrical stimulation of the neuron releases quanta (bursts) of active transmitter into the synapse in a calcium-dependent manner.
- There are appropriate receptors on the postsynaptic (second) neuron, specific for the transmitter.
- Interaction of the substance with its receptor induces changes in the membrane potential of the postsynaptic neurons and thereby a physiological response (e.g. propagation of an action potential).
- There is a system for removal of the transmitter from the synapse (e.g. a reuptake process, an enzyme to degrade the transmitter or rapid diffusion away from the receptors).
- Experimental application of the substance at the synapse produces an identical response to that of stimulating the neuron.

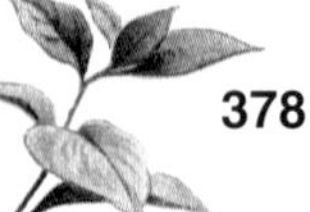

CNS neurotransmitters

There are more than 40 types of CNS neurons (classified by neurotransmitter) that use chemical transmitters for rapid communication across synapses. Some of the chemicals that have been identified as CNS neurotransmitters are:

- monoamines – NA, adrenaline, DA, 5-HT and histamine
- ACh
- amino acids – excitatory: glutamate, aspartate; inhibitory: glycine, GABA; also possibly alanine, taurine, serine
- neuroactive peptides – opioids such as enkephalins and endorphins; gastrointestinal peptides such as cholecystokinin (CCK); substance P; hypothalamic-releasing factors, including somatostatin and thyrotropin-releasing hormone; and other hormones and peptides including oxytocin,[5] calcitonin, bradykinin, galanin, neuropeptide Y, Orexin-A, gastric inhibitory polypeptide, gastrin-releasing peptide and relaxin
- fatty acid neurotransmitters, including anandamide
- gas neurotransmitters such as nitrous oxide.

Pathways (tracts) of neurons containing a particular transmitter have been identified in brain areas (Fig 18.5). For example, there are dopaminergic pathways (neurons that use DA as a transmitter) from the substantia nigra to the striatum, involved in motor control; from the ventral tegmental area to the limbic system and the frontal cortex, involved in cognition and emotion; and from the hypothalamus to the pituitary, controlling release of pituitary hormones.

Monoamines

As noted earlier, the **monoamine** transmitters are NA, adrenaline,[6] 5-HT, DA and histamine. In the CNS, NA is mainly inhibitory; cell bodies for noradrenergic neurons are found in the pons and medulla. NA present in central autonomic pathways, particularly in the hypothalamus and medullary centres, is involved in autonomic control, arousal, mood and reward systems (Fig 18.5A).

Important **5-HT** pathways run between the midbrain and cortex, with extensive innervation of virtually all parts of the CNS; cell bodies are especially prevalent in the raphe nuclei of the brainstem (Fig 18.5B).

5-HT appears to coordinate complex cognitive, sensory, behaviour, mood and motor patterns; 5-HT is involved in sleep–wake cycles; activity levels are highest during waking arousal and lowest during REM (rapid eye movement) sleep. Clinical conditions influenced by 5-HT levels include affective disorders, ageing and neurodegenerative disorders, anxiety, developmental disorders, eating disorders, vomiting, migraine, obsessive–compulsive disorder, pain sensitivity, sexual disorders, sleep disorders and substance abuse. 5-HT is also involved in many interactions with dopaminergic and glutamatergic pathways, to modulate states of consciousness and contribute to psychotic disorders.

Dopamine is particularly involved in motor control, behaviour, reward systems and endocrine control and is present in high concentrations in the ventral tegmental area, the substantia nigra and the caudate nucleus (Fig 18.5C).

Although the effects of **catecholamines** (NA, DA and adrenaline) injected into the CNS are slight in comparison with their effects due to autonomic nervous system activity, rises in levels of catecholamines and 5-HT do cause cerebral stimulation. Drugs such as reserpine (previously used as an antihypertensive agent) and methyldopa, which deplete the 5-HT and NA levels in the brain, have a cerebral depressing effect. Centrally acting α_2-adrenoceptor stimulants such as clonidine paradoxically reduce blood pressure by inhibiting peripheral sympathetic stimulation. The roles of monoamine transmitters in psychiatric disorders (schizophrenia and depression) and the effects of psychotropic drugs on monoaminergic transmission are discussed in greater detail in Chapter 22, and the role of DA in Parkinson's disease in Chapter 24.

Acetylcholine

Acetylcholine (ACh) was the first identified and is the best-known chemical transmitter of nerve impulses. As noted in Chapter 8, in the PNS, ACh is the neurotransmitter at all autonomic ganglia, at parasympathetic (and sympathetic cholinergic) neuro-effector junctions and at the neuromuscular junction. The CNS areas with high concentrations of cholinergic neurons are the reticular formation, the basal forebrain, basal ganglia and anterior spinal roots (Fig 18.5D). In the CNS, ACh is mainly excitatory and is involved in cognition, memory, consciousness and motor control. Muscarinic M_1 receptors appear to be involved in memory functions in the hippocampus; ACh levels are low in Huntington's disease and in dementias such as Alzheimer's disease. There is extensive overlap between the organisation and functions of the nicotinic cholinergic and dopaminergic systems, especially in the basal ganglia, which has implications for treatment of Parkinson's disease (Ch 24).

Amino acid transmitters

Amino acids are probably the most ancient (from an evolutionary viewpoint) type of neurotransmitter, being particularly prevalent in the spinal cord. For example, GABA is an important inhibitory transmitter in many interneurons in the spinal cord and in the cerebellum and hippocampus. GABA is involved particularly in motor

5 Researchers have identified three brain neurotransmitters involved in human love: dopamine, phenylethylamine (similar to noradrenaline) and oxytocin. These transmitters are apparently released in the early stages of courtship and for about 18 months – long enough for a couple to meet, fall in love, mate and produce a child (Young & Alexander 2012).

6 Reminder: in the American literature, noradrenaline and adrenaline are known as norepinephrine and epinephrine, respectively, from an old name for the adrenal gland, the epinephric gland. From April 2016, medicines containing adrenaline and noradrenaline include the international names 'epinephrine' and 'norepinephrine' on labels and information leaflets (Therapeutic Goods Administration 2021).

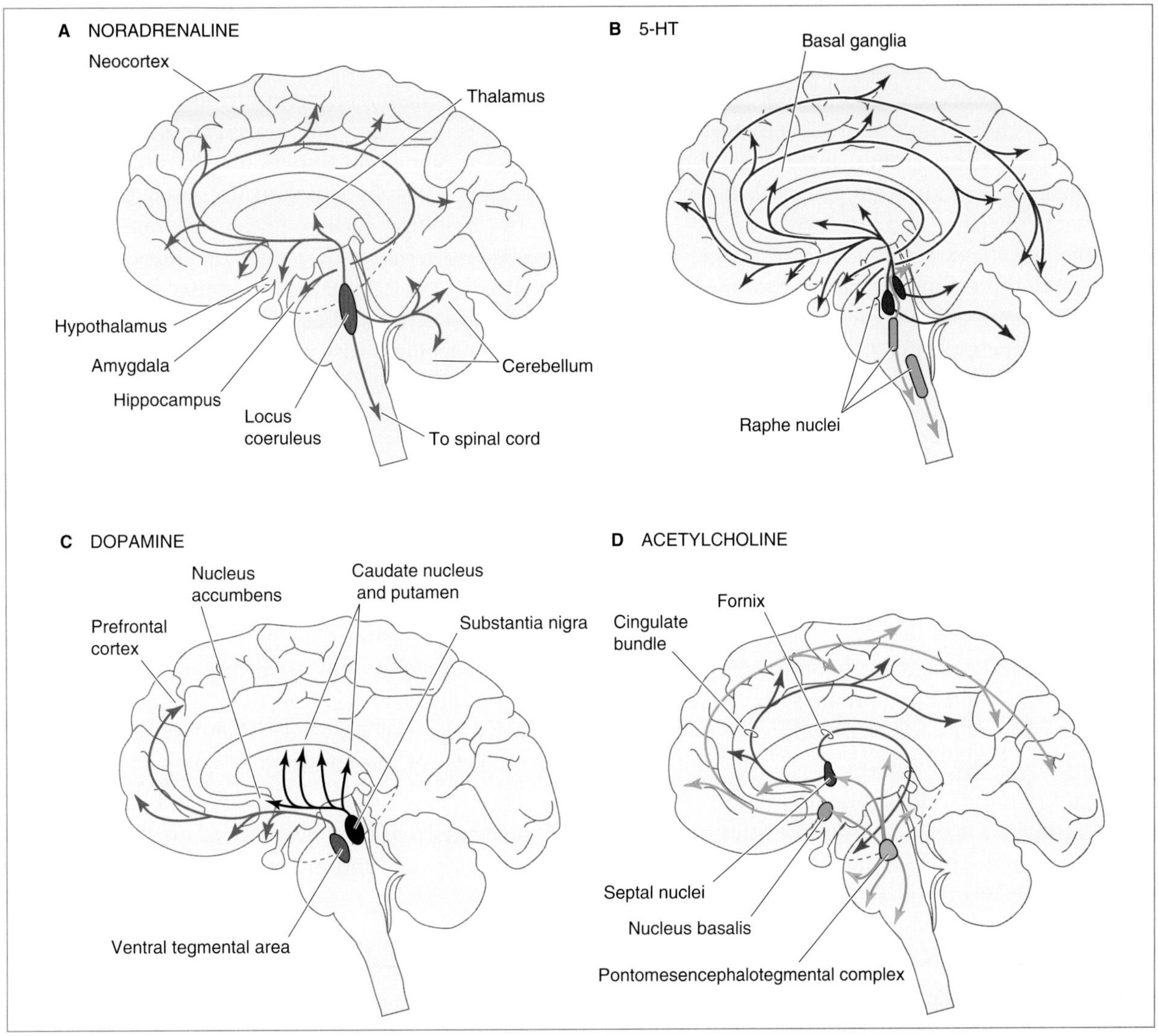

FIGURE 18.5 Sagittal sections of the brain, indicating simplified versions of major pathways of central neurons utilising important neurotransmitters

A Noradrenaline; **B** 5-HT (serotonin); **C** dopamine; **D** acetylcholine

Source: Boron & Boulpaep 2005; used with permission.

control, in spasticity and in sleep/wakefulness. Inhibitory control is necessary to avoid such excessive excitation as occurs during seizures and epilepsy.

The excitatory amino acids (EAAs) glutamate and aspartate are present in virtually all regions and are implicated in the neuronal injury involved in many neurological disorders. Overactivation of receptors for L-glutamate, the major excitatory transmitter, mediates excitotoxicity leading to neuronal death in both acute brain injury such as stroke and chronic disorders such as motor neurone disease. Monosodium glutamate (MSG), a flavour enhancer present in many Asian foods and meals, causes in susceptible people the 'Chinese restaurant syndrome', with CNS stimulation, flushing and nausea. Other excitotoxins may be involved in chronic degenerative diseases such as Huntington's chorea, in dysfunction after CNS viral infections and in neurological syndromes linked to plant neurotoxins.

Neuropeptides

Neuroactive peptides are derived from secretory proteins formed in the cell body; more than 100 have been discovered. Neuropeptides may be considered as neuromodulators, neurohormones or neurotransmitters; they may cause excitation or inhibition of target neurons. Neuropeptide receptors are almost all of the G-protein-coupled receptor (GPCR) type.

The parenteral or intracerebral injection of these chemicals causes potent behavioural effects. Some of these peptides also exist in tissues other than the CNS, primarily in the gastrointestinal tract cells.

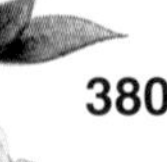

There are several families of neuropeptides: peptides in the same family contain long stretches of identical amino acid chains. Examples are vasopressin and oxytocin, the secretins, the tachykinins (e.g. substance P, neurokinin A, neuropeptide K), cholecystokinin, the somatostatins and the opioid peptides. (The opioids, including enkephalins and endorphins, are considered in greater detail in Ch 19, in the context of pain and analgesic drugs.) Other neuropeptides are neuropeptide Y, cortistatin, orexin, neurotensin and thyrotropin-releasing hormone. In the process of co-transmission, classic neurotransmitters and several neuroactive peptides may be released simultaneously from the same neuron – for example, ACh and adenosine triphosphate and vasoactive intestinal polypeptide (VIP), enkephalin, substance P and galanin. They appear to become 'active' when the nervous system is challenged – for example, in disease states or by stress, injury or drug abuse.

Many CNS neuropeptides currently have no specific pharmacological antagonists, so it is difficult to identify their functions.

- Some neuropeptides mediate communication between the CNS and the immune system, such as corticotrophin-releasing factor and adrenocorticotrophic hormone.
- Cholecystokinin (as well as its action in the gastrointestinal tract) is a neurotransmitter in brain regions associated with fear and panic, and interacts with other transmitters involved with anxiety including 5-HT, GABA and noradrenaline.
- Relaxin-3 (existing in a two-chain structure designated the A-chain and B-chain) is a neuropeptide highly conserved across mammalian species and is a member of the relaxin peptide family, an offshoot of the insulin family. It acts at the Relaxin-3/RXFP3 receptor, a GPCR. Neural networks of Relaxin-3/RXFP3 receptors may represent an ascending arousal system, modulating responses to stress, memory, feeding, motivation and reward and sleep–wake rhythms. Neuropeptides such as relaxin-3 may also be involved in neuropsychiatric conditions including migraine, chronic and neuropathic pain, anxiety, sleep disorders, depression and schizophrenia (Ma et al. 2017).

Other CNS neurotransmitters

Other chemicals that may act as neurotransmitters or neuromodulators include endocannabinoids (marijuana-like compounds), eicosanoids such as prostaglandins and purine nucleotides such as adenosine triphosphate and adenosine. Nitric oxide undoubtedly has neurotransmitter-like functions in the CNS but does not fit the 'classical' criteria listed above. There may indeed be many other chemicals with neurotransmitter functions in the CNS, as yet unidentified.

Receptors for neurotransmitters

The effect of a transmitter at any synapse is determined by the nature of the receptor to which it binds; thus, ACh may have fast excitatory effects at nicotinic receptors and slower effects via G-proteins and second messengers at muscarinic receptors. Some transmitters may have inhibitory effects – for example, by hyperpolarising postsynaptic membranes or by inhibiting further release of transmitter from the presynaptic terminal by actions on autoreceptors.

The field of CNS neurotransmitter receptor types is one of the most active and rapidly developing in all of the fields of pharmacology: vast numbers of types and subtypes of receptors for many CNS transmitters have been discovered, cloned and, for many, the amino acid sequence identified, and chemicals acting as specific agonists or antagonists synthesised. The pharmacological significance and clinical importance of these discoveries are still being elucidated. Table 18.1 summarises some of the better-known receptors and pharmacologically relevant data in this field.

- Several types of receptors for EAAs such as glutamate have been identified, including the *N*-methyl-D-aspartate (NMDA), α-amino-3-hydroxy-5-methyl-4-isoxazolepropionic acid (AMPA) and kainate (a constituent of seaweed) receptors; these may be involved in the aetiology of epilepsy (Ch 21).
- The $GABA_A$ receptor has sites for binding GABA and also sites that bind benzodiazepines, barbiturates, neurosteroids and picrotoxin, a GABA antagonist.
- DA receptors have been classified into several subtypes (D_{1-5}); development of agonists or antagonists specific for the different receptor types will be beneficial clinically and assists research into dopaminergic mechanisms.
- There are at least seven main types of 5-HT receptors, including 13 G-protein-coupled receptors and one family of ligand-gated ion channels their actions may be excitatory or inhibitory (Andrade et al. 2019).

Autoreceptors and heteroceptors

Release of some transmitters can be modulated by the transmitter acting on presynaptic autoreceptors (on nerve endings, dendrites and axons [analogous to α_2-adrenoreceptors in the sympathetic nervous system]; see Fig 9.4, in Ch 9). The mechanisms by which a transmitter inhibits its own release have not been fully elucidated. Presynaptic receptors may also be involved in modulating the release of other transmitters, and these are known as heteroreceptors; for example, NA release can be inhibited by agonists acting on muscarinic, opioid and DA presynaptic heteroreceptors and can be facilitated by agonists on ACh-nicotinic acetylcholine and angiotensin (AT_1) heteroreceptors. There are also presynaptic DA autoreceptors that inhibit DA synthesis and release, and thus slow the firing of dopaminergic neurons; these may be involved in the on–off effects in levodopa therapy for Parkinson's disease. The presynaptic inhibitory and

TABLE 18.1 Summary of types of receptors for CNS neurotransmitters, emphasising those involved in pharmacological activity of clinically important CNS-active drugs[a]

TRANSMITTER	RECEPTOR TYPE	OTHER[a] AGONISTS AND MODULATORS	ANTAGONISTS AND CHANNEL BLOCKERS
ACh (cholinergic)	Muscarinic M_1 (some auto-inhibitory)	Anticholinesterases	Anticholinergic (atropinic) agents
ACh (cholinergic)	Nicotinic Nn (neuronal) (ionotropic) Ca^{2+} channel	Nicotine	Mecamylamine (not registered in Australia), Mg^{2+}, many general anaesthetics
Noradrenaline (CA)	α, β-receptors (mainly inhibitory; increases cAMP levels)	Noradrenaline (norepinephrine), adrenaline (epinephrine) (TCAs block reuptake), amphetamines	Propranolol (β) Prazosin (α_1)
Noradrenaline (CA)	α_2-receptors (auto-inhibitory)	Clonidine	Yohimbine
Dopamine (CA)	D_1, D_5 (increases cAMP)	Dopamine	Haloperidol
Dopamine (CA)	D_2, D_3, D_4 (decreases cAMP)	Dopamine, apomorphine, bromocriptine (D_2, D_3)	Phenothiazines (chlorpromazine), haloperidol
5-HT (indoleamine)	$5\text{-HT}_{1A,B,D,E,F}$ (decreases cAMP)	5-HT_{1A} only: buspirone, partial agonist (not registered for use in Australia – see special access scheme) 5-HT_{1D}: triptans (SSRIs block reuptake)	Ergotamine (partial agonist) HT_{1A} antagonists – pizotifen, sertindole, risperidone
5-HT (indoleamine)	$5\text{-HT}_{2A,C}$ (increases IP_3, DAG)	LSD (SSRIs block reuptake)	Pizotifen, risperidone
5-HT (indoleamine)	5-HT_3 (ligand-gated cation channel)	(SSRIs block reuptake)	Ondansetron
5-HT (indoleamine)	5-HT_4 (increases cAMP)	Metoclopramide (SSRIs block reuptake)	Tropisetron
Histamine (a monoamine)	H_1, H_3 (GPCR) autoreceptors		H_1-antihistamines
L-glutamate (EAA)	AMPA, ionotropic glutamate receptor	AMPA, glutamate	Polyamine ions, some general anaesthetics
L-glutamate (EAA)	Kainate, metabotropic, ionotropic glutamate receptor	Kainate, glutamate	Polyamine ions
L-glutamate (EAA)	NMDA, ionotropic glutamate receptor	Glutamate, glycine, aspartate, NMDA general anaesthetics	Ketamine, memantine
GABA (IAA)	$GABA_A$ ligand-gated Cl^- channel	Benzodiazepines, muscimol, many general anaesthetics	Flumazenil, picrotoxin
GABA (IAA)	$GABA_B$ GPCR (decreases cAMP levels)	Baclofen	
Glycine (IAA)	Ligand-gated Cl^- channel, co-agonist at NMDA receptors	Glycine, some general anaesthetics	Strychnine (tetrodotoxin prevents glycine release)
Adenosine (purine)	A_1, A_2 (GPCR), heteroreceptors		(Methyl)xanthines- theophylline
Cannabinoids	Cannabinoid CB_1	Anandamide, cannabinoids (Δ^9-THC, nabilone)	
Enkephalins, endorphins	μ-opioid	Opioids (e.g. morphine, fentanyl, codeine)	Naloxone, naltrexone

[a] Note that the neurotransmitter itself is the main endogenous agonist at each receptor.
5-HT = 5-hydroxytryptamine (= serotonin); A = adenosine; ACh = acetylcholine; AMPA = α-amino-3-hydroxy-5-methyl-4-isoxazolepropionic acid; CA = catecholamine; cAMP = cyclic adenosine monophosphate; D = dopamine; DAG = diacylglycerol; EAA = excitatory amino acid transmitters; GABA = gamma-aminobutyric acid; GPCR = G-protein-coupled receptor; H = histamine; IAA = inhibitory amino acid transmitters; IP_3 = inositol triphosphate; LSD = lysergic acid diethylamide; NMDA = N-methyl-D-aspartate; SSRI = selective serotonin reuptake inhibitors; TCA = tricyclic antidepressants; THC = tetrahydrocannabinol.

facilitatory receptors on the same nerve terminals are thought to allow for fine-tuning of transmitter release in various physiological (and pharmacological) situations.

Neurotransmitter imbalances in disease states

In many disorders of the CNS, it appears there are imbalances between levels of different neurotransmitters in particular parts of the brain. In some conditions, chemical analysis of the brains of patients who have died from a disease has shown that tracts or neurons had degenerated in particular areas. To describe an overview of these conditions, the following simplistic scheme can be proposed (Fig 18.6):

- The effects of monoamines (NA, DA, adrenaline, 5-HT) are envisaged to 'balance' (as on a see-saw; not in strict molecular equivalents) the effects of ACh, particularly on motor control, mood and thought processes. Thus, in depression there is a relative deficiency of NA and 5-HT in areas of the brain related to mood (affect) and an excess of ACh. The depressed mood can be improved by antidepressant drugs such as the selective serotonin reuptake

inhibitors (SSRIs), tricyclic antidepressants (TCAs) and monoamine oxidase inhibitors (MAOIs), all of which, by differing mechanisms, increase the levels of monoamines at synapses in the CNS.
- In Parkinson's disease there appears to be damage to DA-containing neurons and a relative deficiency of DA and excess of ACh. The main drugs used in treatment of Parkinson's disease either increase the levels of DA or block the actions of ACh (atropinic drugs).

These concepts (Fig 18.6) will be referred to again in later chapters on the clinical use of drugs in neurological and psychiatric disorders.

How drugs modify neurotransmission

After neurochemical transmission, binding of the transmitter to specific receptors elicits a chain of events in the postsynaptic cell. These transduction mechanisms include second messenger systems, G-proteins, ion channels, intracellular enzymes, transport systems (carriers and pumps), transcription factors that activate genes, the genes that code for synthesis of all the proteins involved, the enzymes involved in the biosynthetic pathways and the receptors themselves (Ch 3). Virtually every step above can be affected by other chemicals – that is, by drug actions. There are many drugs that have actions (therapeutic and/or adverse effects) on neurotransmission. Wherever possible in the following chapters, the actions of drugs will be related back to the level of the synapse and to the effects of the drugs on neurochemical transmission and transmitter receptors. Refer to Clinical Focus Box 18.1 for an overview of drugs affecting the CNS.

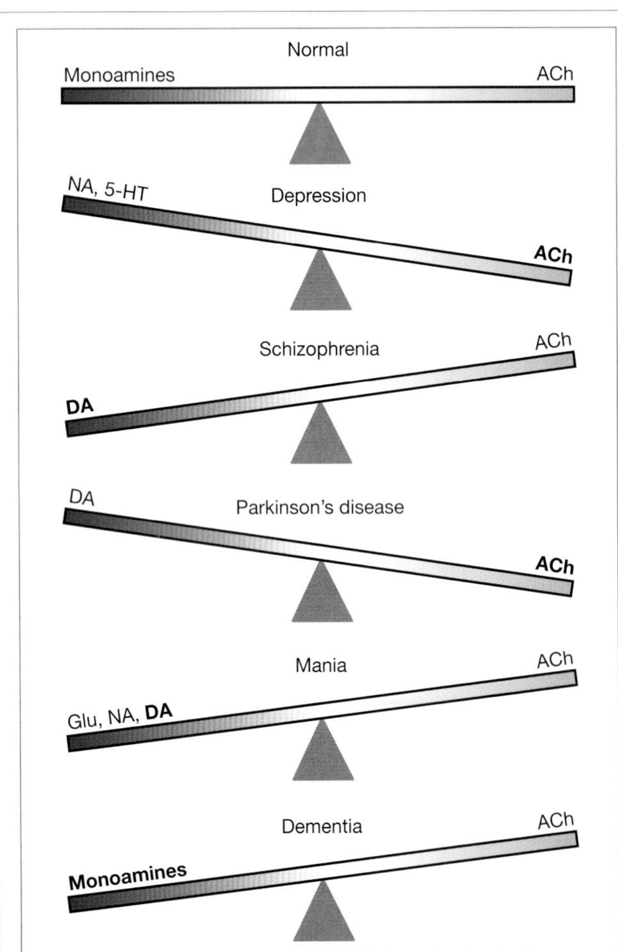

FIGURE 18.6 Neurotransmitter balances in central nervous system disorders

In the normal state, the effects of monoamine transmitters are 'balanced' by those of acetylcholine. In various CNS disorders, imbalances occur and drugs are used in attempts to bring the levels back into balance.

5-HT = 5-hydroxytryptamine (serotonin); ACh = acetylcholine; DA = dopamine; Glu = glutamate; NA = noradrenaline

KEY POINTS

Neurotransmission, and neurotransmitters and receptors

- Action potentials generated in nerve cells are propagated along the axon to nerve terminals, where a synapse intervenes between adjacent neurons.
- Messages are transmitted across synapses by neurotransmitters that are synthesised, stored, then released at nerve terminals to cross the synapse and initiate an action at receptors in the postsynaptic neurons to increase or decrease their activity.
- Neurochemical transmission leads to stimulation of specific receptors and initiates a chain of events in the postsynaptic cell.
- Of the many chemicals proposed as neurotransmitters in the CNS, the most important in the context of drug actions are ACh and the five monoamines, which include 5-HT, histamine and the three catecholamines – DA, NA and adrenaline. Also included are some amino acids and neuroactive peptides. Other neurotransmitters include endocannabinoids and eicosanoids such as prostaglandins.
- There are vast numbers of types and subtypes of receptors for many CNS transmitters.
- In many disorders of the CNS, it appears there are imbalances between levels of different neurotransmitters in particular parts of the brain. There are many drugs that have actions (therapeutic and/or adverse effects) on neurotransmission and specific receptors.

General anaesthesia

A **general anaesthetic** is a drug that produces a reversible state of unconsciousness, with absence of pain sensation over the entire body and immobility; such agents have been described as the drugs that remove the most precious of human attributes – consciousness. Before the development of effective anaesthetics and analgesics, as well as blood transfusions and antibiotics, successful major surgery was virtually impossible owing to the devastating effects of pain, blood loss and infection; the patient was usually tied or held down, or rendered unconscious by hypoxia, concussion or high doses of natural CNS depressants such as alcohol or opium. The discovery of anaesthesia and the development of anaesthetic drugs proved invaluable in limiting pain and suffering during surgical procedures and have resulted in many advances in modern surgical techniques.

Nowadays, anaesthetists are said to be the medical profession's best clinical pharmacologists because they administer a wide range of potent and specific drugs, often in emergency or intensive care situations, continually monitoring the patient for pharmacological effects and adverse reactions, and anticipating potential drug interactions.

For a drug to be useful as a general anaesthetic, its actions must be of rapid onset, extendable for the duration of the surgical procedure, then rapidly reversible; only CNS depressants that have short half-lives and can be continually administered are useful as general anaesthetics. (Hence, depressants such as alcohol and most barbiturates and benzodiazepines are not useful.) General anaesthesia (GA) is usually induced by IV injection of anaesthetic agent such as thiopental or propofol, and then maintained by inhalation of a gas (nitrous oxide) mixed with the vapour of a volatile liquid (desflurane or sevoflurane).

Depressant effects of general anaesthetics

General anaesthetics depress all excitable tissues of the body at concentrations that produce **anaesthesia**. The pattern of depression is irregular and descending and reversible, with higher cortical functions (conscious thought, memory, motor control, perception of sensations) depressed first and medullary centres depressed last, which is fortunate as the medulla contains vital centres maintaining cardiovascular and respiratory control. It should be noted that a drug may have useful anaesthetic actions without being a good analgesic (pain reliever), and vice versa.

Stages of general anaesthesia

The four stages of CNS depression during GA were first described in detail by American anaesthetist Dr Arthur Guedel,[7] who observed the effects on the eyes of slowly deepening unconsciousness induced with early anaesthetics such as ether and chloroform. However, the stages of anaesthesia vary with the choice of anaesthetic, speed of induction and skill of the anaesthetist. Stages 1 and 2 constitute induction of anaesthesia. It is now recognised that stage 2 (excitation) can be dangerous, so current practice is to induce GA rapidly with an intravenously administered anaesthetic, then maintain the stage of surgical anaesthesia (stage 3) by inhaling an anaesthetic gas.

Stage 1: analgesia

- Begins with the onset of anaesthetic administration and lasts until loss of consciousness.
- Senses of smell and pain are reduced first; vivid dreams and auditory or visual hallucinations may be experienced; speech becomes difficult and indistinct; numbness spreads gradually, hearing is the last sense lost. (Hence, a quiet environment should be maintained.)
- There is adequate analgesia for venepuncture and minor dental or obstetric procedures.

Stage 2: excitement

- Stage 2 varies greatly with individuals and depends on the amount and type of premedication, anaesthetic agent used and level of external sensory stimuli.
- Most reflexes are still present and may be exaggerated, particularly with sensory stimulation such as noise; swallowing reflex is abolished and there is risk of aspiration.
- The patient may struggle, talk or laugh; autonomic activity, muscle tone, eye movement, dilation of pupils and rapid irregular breathing increase (causing uneven inhalation of anaesthetic); vomiting and incontinence sometimes occur.

Stage 3: surgical anaesthesia

This stage is divided into four planes of increasing depth: most operations are done with the patient in plane 2 or in the upper part of plane 3; by plane 4 the blood pressure drops and the pulse weakens. The anaesthetist continually monitors the patient's respirations, eye movements, pupil size and degree to which reflexes (e.g. responses to painful stimuli) are present.

Stage 4: medullary paralysis (toxic stage)

This is the stage of impending overdose, respiratory arrest and vasomotor collapse. Respiration ceases before the heart action does, so artificial respiration is required in the reversal of this stage.

These stages may appear complicated, so the scheme has been simplified to the following three levels: anaesthesia is inadequate, surgical or deep. More simply still, 'the patient is awake, asleep or at risk'.

7 Dr Arthur Guedel (1883–1956) became known as 'the motorcycle anaesthetist of World War I', as he roared on his motorcycle through the mud of battlefields in France visiting field hospitals. His painstaking observations of changes in pupil dilation and eyeball oscillation in response to general anaesthetics, in the days before electronic monitoring equipment, allowed surgeons to operate safely while the patient was anaesthetised with open-drop ether, administered by nurses and orderlies trained by Guedel (Calmes & Guedel 2002).

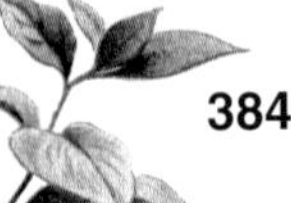

Mechanisms of action of general anaesthetics

No general anaesthetic receptor

General anaesthetics have been studied and used for more than 150 years and many theories of anaesthesia have been proposed. General anaesthetics vary widely in their chemical structures and in the concentration necessary to produce anaesthesia and in mechanism of action; there is no simple chemical structure–activity relationship among general anaesthetics, and so no one 'anaesthetic receptor' or no antagonist to general anaesthetics. The potency of anaesthetic effect is strongly correlated with the lipid solubility of the compound, with very lipid-soluble compounds being very potent. Indeed, the inverse correlation between lipid solubility and dose (expressed as minimal alveolar concentration [MAC] to achieve anaesthesia) is one of the most powerful correlations in biology, extending over a 100,000-fold dose range, across species ranging from goldfish to humans. For any given general anaesthetic, there is a narrow band of concentrations at which consciousness is lost. (Early theories of general anaesthetic mechanisms of action vaguely suggested that general anaesthetics either increase the 'fluidity of lipid membranes' or stabilise membranes by forming 'water crystals' in them.)

Targets for general anaesthetic actions

There is still much ongoing research into the mechanisms of action of general anaesthetics. These drugs act at a number of modulatory sites to produce the various components of anaesthesia. Research using 'knock-out' mice with mutations in particular genes has indicated that transmitter-gated ion channels are important in general anaesthetic actions. At the molecular and receptor level, there appear to be three main targets to which general anaesthetics bind (Table 18.1, earlier) (Hao et al. 2020; Hemmings et al. 2019).

- $GABA_A$ receptors, both those at synapses and those at extrasynaptic receptors – anaesthetic binding at sites other than the GABAs binding site potentiates the depressant actions of GABA via opening of chloride channels; anaesthetics interact with the same site as propofol, the barbiturates and neuroactive steroids (Table 18.1)
- two-pore-domain potassium channels – opening of potassium channels mediates the effects of some volatile general anaesthetics
- NMDA receptors that mediate slow components of synaptic transmission and are inhibited by most inhalational general anaesthetics.

Other potential molecular targets for general anaesthetics include glycine receptors (inhibitory in the lower brainstem and spinal cord), cyclic nucleotide-gated cation channels, presynaptic inhibition of some sodium channels and neuronal nicotinic receptors. Different general anaesthetics appear to have varying selectivities for the above molecular targets.

Transmitter receptors and pathways

Overall, general anaesthetics cause loss of consciousness by decreasing the functions of excitatory neurotransmitters, including ACh (at nicotinic receptors), 5-HT, glutamate and NMDA; by increasing the functions of inhibitory transmitters, including GABA and glycine; and also possibly by interacting with peptidergic transmission, opioid receptors and the nitric oxide–cyclic guanosine monophosphate signal transduction pathway. The most sensitive targets are sensory pathways from the thalamus to the cortex, leading to inhibition of arousal pathways and potentiation of sleep pathways (hence, loss of consciousness); and the hippocampus (causing amnesia). Immobility is mediated primarily via multiple molecular targets in the spinal cord.

Rapidly controllable actions

The concentration of anaesthetic in the CNS tissues should equilibrate rapidly with the concentration in lungs or blood. This increases the speeds of both induction and recovery of anaesthesia, and allows the anaesthetist to control quickly the depth of anaesthesia, which depends on the partial pressure of the anaesthetic gas, or the concentration of an injected drug, in the brain. Study of the ideal pharmacokinetics of anaesthetic gases is complicated, involving consideration of the solubility of the agent both in blood and tissues (the blood–gas partition coefficient) and in lipids (the oil–gas partition coefficient), as well as physiological factors that determine the efficiency of respiration and circulation.

In summary:

- High lipid solubility enhances anaesthetic potency.
- High lipid solubility delays recovery, as the agent forms a depot in fat tissues in the body (following a two-compartment pharmacokinetic model) and may take hours to be cleared from the body, leading to a 'hangover' effect.
- High blood–gas partition coefficient (solubility of agent in blood) implies a longer time for equilibration of gas to tissues, as higher levels have to be reached.
- Low blood and tissue solubility speeds equilibration of the agent from the lungs to the blood and tissues and hence shortens onset time, recovery time and time to resumption of normal activities.
- Alveolar ventilation is the most important factor in equilibration of a gaseous agent into the blood, especially for agents having high blood solubility.
- Low blood flow to fatty tissues slows equilibration of drugs into them.
- Overall, the optimal anaesthetic agent has low blood and tissue solubility, with high potency; sevoflurane and desflurane are good examples (Fig 18.7), whereas nitrous oxide is weak but rapid and ether is potent but slow.

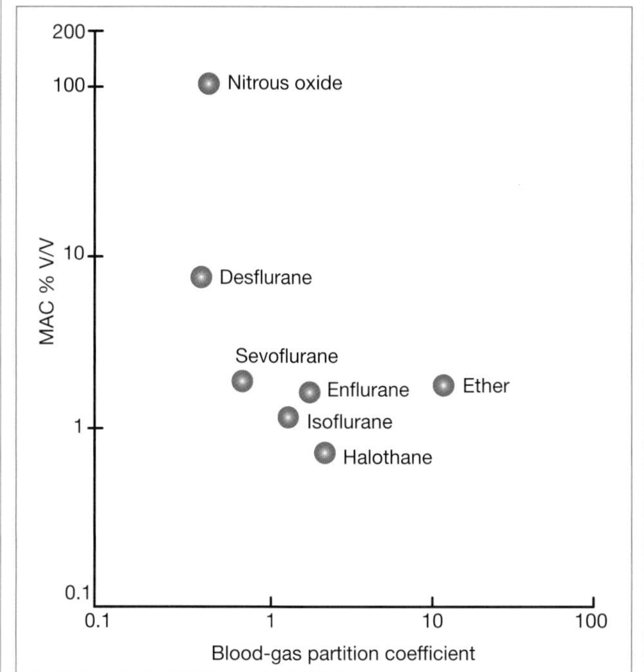

FIGURE 18.7 Potency and solubility of inhaled general anaesthetics

The minimal alveolar concentration (% v/v) required to produce anaesthesia in 50% of patients (MAC) is plotted against the solubility of the anaesthetic drug in blood (expressed as the blood–gas partition coefficient). Drugs with high blood solubility (e.g. ether) are relatively slow in onset and recovery, whereas drugs that have lower blood solubility (desflurane, nitrous oxide) are rapid in onset and recovery. The most potent anaesthetics (halothane, isoflurane) are those with low MAC values, whereas nitrous oxide requires more than 100% concentration for anaesthesia so is usually used at 50% concentration as an analgesic and carrier gas. Note: Data are plotted with logarithmic scale on each axis.

Sources: Data from Speight & Holford 1997; Oberoi & Phillips 2000.

Types of general anaesthetics

General anaesthetics are divided into two groups: (1) inhalation anaesthetics, which include gases and volatile liquids; and (2) intravenous (IV) general anaesthetics, such as thiopental and propofol.

Inhalation anaesthetics

Inhalation anaesthetics are gases or volatile liquids that can be administered by inhalation when mixed with oxygen. These rapidly reach a concentration in the blood and brain sufficient to depress the CNS and cause anaesthesia, expressed as the **minimum alveolar concentration** (MAC) for anaesthesia, which is inversely related to potency and also lipid solubility. MAC provides a correlation between anaesthetic dose and immobility. It is the MAC of inhaled anaesthetic at sea level required to suppress movement to a surgical incision in 50% of the patients. Inhalation anaesthetics have the following characteristics:

- They provide controllable anaesthesia, as depth of anaesthesia is readily varied by changing the inhaled concentration.
- As the route of administration (and most excretion) is via the airways, lung function is critical to effective use of inhaled agents.
- The agents are good anaesthetics and thus can abolish superficial and deep reflexes. However, they may not have useful analgesic actions, so they are used in combination with an adjunct analgesic such as an opioid.
- Rapid recovery can occur as soon as administration ceases because the anaesthetic is excreted in expired air.
- Allergic reactions to these agents are uncommon.

Early inhaled anaesthetics included ether and chloroform as volatile liquids, and cyclopropane and nitrous oxide as gases.

Nitrous oxide

Of the early anaesthetics, only nitrous oxide is still in clinical use today in developed countries with advanced facilities (Drug Monograph 18.1). It is commonly used for analgesia during childbirth, referred to simply as 'gas', and is simply and safely administered (50% in oxygen) by the mother and/or midwife.

Volatile liquid anaesthetics

Volatile liquid anaesthetics now in use include safer analogues of the halogenated hydrocarbon series: desflurane, isoflurane and sevoflurane (Table 18.2). Sevoflurane has become the drug of choice for most procedures owing to its fast action and low toxicity (Drug Monograph 18.2). Historically drugs such as ether or chloroform were originally administered by placing a pad soaked in the liquid over the patient's mouth and nose, so that the fumes were inhaled. This unpleasant procedure caused struggling, skin reactions, uncertain levels of dosage and absorption and a slow progression through the stages of anaesthesia. The more civilised technique used now involves controlled vaporisation of the volatile liquid into a flow of gas (oxygen with or without nitrous oxide), so a known concentration of volatile agent in oxygen is administered via a mask or endotracheal tube. All volatile agents require the use of a vaporiser. Desflurane has a boiling point close to room temperature. This may result in a large variation in concentrations. A heated, temperature-controlled vaporiser is therefore required.

Chloroform is hepatotoxic, and ether and cyclopropane are highly flammable; they were replaced after 1956 by halothane. However, halothane was associated with hepatic dysfunction and failure, so the safer desflurane, isoflurane and sevoflurane are used.

Methoxyflurane as an analgesic

Methoxyflurane is a halogenated ether. Renal toxicity limits its regular use as an anaesthetic; however, it is a

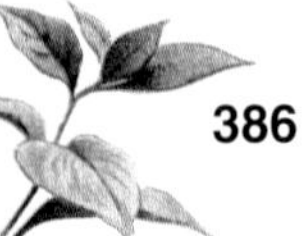

Drug Monograph 18.1
Nitrous oxide

Nitrous oxide is a simple inorganic molecule with the chemical formula N_2O. It should not be confused with nitric oxide, now recognised as a gas generated in many body cells involved in vasodilation and immune responses, and as a chemical mediator in the CNS in neurotransmission and neurodegeneration.

Mechanism of action

Its analgesic action may be mediated via opioid receptors, while the hypnotic/anxiolytic action is mainly due to enhancement of GABA-mediated CNS depression and the anaesthetic action due to NMDA receptor inhibition

Indications

Nitrous oxide is commonly used for dental surgery, minor surgery and obstetric analgesia. It is indicated for induction and maintenance of GA. It is a powerful analgesic, useful anxiolytic but a weak anaesthetic, so is often combined with other (volatile) anaesthetics to enhance its effects. It is presented as a compressed gas – for example, in a 50:50 mixture with oxygen (Entonox), in blue (ultramarine) and white cylinders (Table 22.1, in Ch 22).

Pharmacokinetics

Nitrous oxide is inhaled and absorbed via the lungs; it has low solubility in blood and tissues, so has a rapid onset of action and recovery time. It is excreted 100% unchanged through the lungs.

Adverse effects and drug interactions

It is non-irritant and virtually without odour. Its few adverse effects are hypoxia, mild cardiac depression and postoperative nausea, vomiting or delirium; it has no known significant drug interactions. Prolonged inhalation (> 6 hours) can cause adverse haematological and neurological effects. It may be abused; escaped gas should be scavenged to avoid occupational exposure and contribution to the greenhouse effect. It is considered safe in pregnancy and is widely used as an inhaled analgesic in childbirth, as it can be administered by the mother (and/or midwife) during painful contractions, and does not accumulate or cause respiratory depression in the neonate.

Warnings and contraindications

There is risk of hypoxia if inadequate oxygen is provided. Precaution advised in instances of heart failure and there is a risk of increased volume in air-containing cavities in conditions such as abdominal distension and pneumothorax, At the termination of nitrous oxide anaesthesia, the rapid movement of large amounts of nitrous oxide from the circulation into the lungs may dilute the oxygen in the lungs (diffusion hypoxia). To prevent this, the anaesthetist usually administers supplementary oxygen for 3–5 minutes to clear the nitrous oxide from the lungs.

Dosage and administration

For GA (with another anaesthetic agent), the recommended dosage is 70% nitrous oxide with 30% oxygen for induction and 30–70% for maintenance. In obstetrics, women self-administer a 50:50 mixture of $N_2O:O_2$, and in dental procedures a 25% concentration may be used.

TABLE 18.2 Volatile liquid anaesthetic agents

AGENT	MAC[a] (%)	INDUCTION/ RECOVERY	METABOLISM	EXCRETION	ADVERSE REACTIONS AND NOTES
Desflurane	6.7	Fast	Minimal	Primarily via lungs	Airway irritation: low boiling point, requires vaporiser. Dose-dependent hypotension and respiratory depression
Isoflurane	1.2	Medium	Less than 1% by liver	Via lungs	Marked respiratory depression; pungent odour leading to irritation of mucous membrane
Sevoflurane	2.1 Titrated according to age; MAC decreased with increasing age and dependent on clinical status	Fast	5% by liver	Primarily via lungs	Well tolerated, drug of choice, possible risk of fluoride toxicity. Dose-dependent cardiorespiratory depression. Most adverse effects mild to moderate in severity and are transient

[a] MAC = minimum alveolar concentration (% in oxygen) for anaesthesia; inversely proportional to potency. Higher concentrations may be needed in some patients: generally highest in very young children, lower with increasing age, pregnancy, hypotension or concurrent use of CNS depressants. Note that all these volatile agents are non-flammable liquids, are absorbed through the lungs, may cause some cardio-vascular depression and are potential triggers for **malignant hyperthermia**. Methoxyflurane is not included here as it is usually self-administered by inhalation as an emergency analgesic, at sub-anaesthetic concentrations.

Drug Monograph 18.2
Sevoflurane

Indications
Sevoflurane is an inhaled general anaesthetic non-irritant volatile liquid with a pleasant smell and rapid onset of action and recovery, so it is indicated for induction and maintenance of GA, particularly in children and in day surgery.

Pharmacokinetics
Sevoflurane has a faster uptake, distribution and rate of elimination than isoflurane (but slightly slower than desflurane). About 5% is metabolised in the liver to an inactive derivative that is rapidly eliminated. Inorganic fluoride released during metabolism has an elimination half-life of 15–23 hours.

Adverse effects
Cardiac and respiratory depression, shivering and salivation can occur, as well as agitation during recovery and postoperative nausea and vomiting. Post operative cognitive dysfunction may occur with use.

Drug interactions
Few significant interactions have been reported; concurrent administration of other CNS depressants (opioid analgesics, benzodiazepines) allows reduction in sevoflurane dosage.

Warnings and contraindications
Sevoflurane is contraindicated in patients with susceptibility to malignant hyperthermia (Clinical Focus Box 18.3) and used with caution in those with renal failure. A fluoro-ether derivative of sevoflurane (compound A), formed after passage of the exhaust gas over lime absorbers for carbon dioxide, is potentially toxic; levels can be minimised by using high gas flow rates. In the maintenance phase an increase in concentration leads to a dose dependent decrease in blood pressure and a cardiac depressant effect.

Dosage and administration
Sevoflurane is administered from a vaporiser in a stream of oxygen, with or without nitrous oxide. The induction dose is individualised (e.g. according to age and clinical status, ≤ 5% with or without nitrous oxide; the usual dose for maintenance is 0.5–3% in adults and ≤ 7% for children; surgical anaesthesia is achieved in less than 2 minutes).

powerful analgesic administered to stable, conscious patients by paramedics in pre-hospital settings, such as during acute trauma and patient transport, and by nurses during wound dressing. It is administered via a hand-held 'puffer' in which 3 mL of the solution is vaporised and then inhaled; onset of analgesia occurs after a few breaths, and intermittent use provides effective pain relief for 20–30 minutes. Drowsiness and amnesia may occur, but there are few cardiovascular adverse effects. Due to renal toxicity, it should not be used on consecutive days or in renal impairment.

Intravenous anaesthetics
IV anaesthetic agents are used for induction or maintenance of GA, for conscious sedation, to induce amnesia and as adjuncts to inhalation-type anaesthetics. The major groups are ultrashort-acting barbiturates (thiopental) and non-barbiturates (propofol; (Drug Monograph 18.3). and ketamine (Drug Monograph 18.4). The benzodiazepine midazolam is mainly a sedative–antianxiety agent, and is frequently used as an adjunct to IV anaesthesia. IV anaesthetics are valuable in allaying emotional distress (many patients fear having a tight mask placed over the face while they are conscious) and in reducing the amount of inhalation anaesthetic required.

Advantages and disadvantages
Advantages of IV anaesthetics are that they:

- rapidly induce unconsciousness and suppress reflexes, allowing external control of airways
- are readily controllable
- have amnesic effects (especially midazolam)
- reduce the amount of inhalational agent required
- allow prompt recovery with minimal doses
- are simple to administer and provide pleasant induction (most patients prefer an IV line to a mask)
- do not pose hazard of fire or explosion.

Disadvantages of IV anaesthetics are that they:

- have minimal muscle relaxation and analgesic effects (except ketamine, a good analgesic)
- are subject to elimination by hepatic metabolism and renal excretion
- commonly cause hypersensitivity reactions (to drug or vehicle)
- cause tissue irritation if drug or vehicle infiltrates tissue or if arterial injection occurs
- cause hypotension, laryngospasm and respiratory failure after overdosage or prolonged administration.

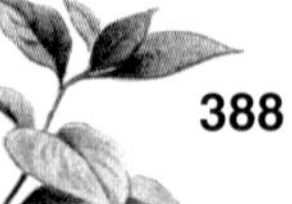

Drug Monograph 18.3
Propofol

Propofol is a rapidly acting, non-barbiturate hypnotic with no analgesic effects. It is formulated in an emulsion[1] for IV injection or infusion and can be used for TIVA.

Mechanism of action

Its CNS depression is probably mediated through GABA receptors. It may also shorten channel opening times at nicotinic receptors and sodium channels in the CNS.

Indications

Propofol is used for the induction and maintenance of GA and for conscious sedation, especially in day-surgery procedures.

Pharmacokinetics

Propofol has a rapid onset of action within 30 seconds and duration of effect of only 3–5 minutes, owing to rapid redistribution from the brain to other tissues; hence, there is a short recovery period and few hangover effects. It is almost completely metabolised to the glucuronide, with a long terminal elimination half-life of 3–8 hours.

Adverse effects

Propofol is a respiratory and cardiac depressant and can produce apnoea, bradycardia and hypotension, depending on dose, rate of administration and drugs concurrently administered. Pain on injection, nausea, vomiting and involuntary muscle movement are commonly reported.

Drug interactions

Sedative and bradycardic effects of other drugs are increased. Bradycardia and cardiac arrest may occur after treatment with suxamethonium and neostigmine; the emulsion is physically incompatible with atracurium or mivacurium.

Warnings and contraindications

Raised intracranial pressure can occur; there is potential for abuse. Respiratory depression is prolonged in those with muscular disorders, and may affect the fetus or neonate if used on pregnant women (Category C).

Propofol infusion syndrome is a rare syndrome affecting patients receiving high doses over a long period. One or more of rhabdomyolysis, metabolic acidosis and cardiac and kidney failure may occur.

IV induction dose for propofol in adults under 55 years by slow bolus injection or infusion is usually 2–2.5 mg/kg. Dosage regimen for TIVA in adults is 4–12 mg/kg/hour as required.

[1] This white emulsion is fondly referred to as 'milk of amnesia' by anaesthetists.

Drug Monograph 18.4
Ketamine

Ketamine is a non-barbiturate, rapidly acting sedative and general anaesthetic agent, producing profound analgesia, usually with normal muscle tone, cardiovascular stimulation with raised blood pressure but little respiratory depression. It causes 'dissociative anaesthesia', with amnesia and dissociation from surroundings, before producing sensory blockade.

Indications

It is frequently used (including by paramedics) as a procedural sedative during short painful diagnostic and operative procedures, especially useful in children, as an induction agent and in chronic and postoperative pain and for pre-hospital pain management, intubation and sedation in the case of aggressive and agitated patients. It allows use of lower doses of opioids, and minimises hyperalgesia and some other opioid adverse effects. It has antidepressant actions and may cause hallucinations, hence its abuse potential (as 'Special K', 'Vitamin K'; Ch 25). It has also been used in epilepsy, asthma and migraine.

Mechanism of action

Ketamine is a non-competitive antagonist and allosteric modulator at NMDA receptors, leading to increased extracellular glutamate in the prefrontal cortex. It has been referred to as the 'pharmacologist's nightmare' due to its complex interactions with many CNS receptors including opioid, 5-HT, NA, DA and muscarinic.

Pharmacokinetics

Ketamine is rapidly and extensively distributed, 20–50% bound to plasma proteins. It is metabolised in the liver to many metabolites, one active. The initial anaesthetic phase of elimination lasts 10–15 minutes; the second phase has a half-life of about 2.5 hours. About 90% of a dose is excreted in the urine as metabolites. Elimination is delayed by hepatic impairment.

Drug interactions

Co-administration of ketamine with other CNS depressants, hypertensive agents or drugs causing neuromuscular blockade (e.g. atracurium) causes synergistic effects.

Adverse reactions

Common adverse reactions include unpleasant emergent reactions postoperatively. Ketamine has abuse and dependence potential. Cardiovascular and respiratory system functions may be either increased or decreased; raised intracranial and intraocular pressures are possible; urinary tract symptoms may be severe following chronic misuse.

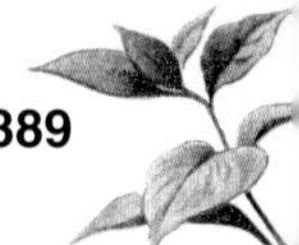

Precautions and contraindications

Ketamine is contraindicated in patients in whom raised blood pressure would be dangerous, and in those hypersensitive to it. Current drug information sources should be consulted regarding many other precautions and contraindications. Ketamine is classified in the Pregnancy Safety Category B3; ketamine crosses the placenta and is not recommended in pregnancy or in breastfeeding mothers. It is a Controlled Drug, Schedule 8.

Dosage and administration

Ketamine is formulated in acidic solution for slow IV infusion, in strength 100 mg/mL, to be diluted before injection; it can also be administered intramuscularly and intranasally. Dosage (same for children and adults) is determined by individual responses; average amount for 5–10 minutes of surgical anaesthesia has been 2 mg/kg administered over 60 seconds. Doses may be repeated as needed for maintenance of anaesthesia.

Pharmacokinetics

IV anaesthetics are rapidly taken up by brain tissue because of their high lipid solubility. Equilibrium between brain and blood levels occurs within one arm–brain circulation time (patients asked to count backwards from 10 as the agent is injected rarely reach 4 or 3). Short action results from the drug being quickly redistributed into the fat depots of the body; due to two-compartment distribution of the drug, the greater the amount of body fat, the briefer the effect of a single IV dose. With prolonged administration or large doses, however, saturation of fat depots leads to prolonged drug action and delayed recovery as drug is slowly released back into the circulation to be eliminated (10–15% per hour). Consequently, patients administered IV anaesthetic agents for short-stay procedures must be advised that they cannot drive or take public transport home, and need a responsible person to care for them for 24 hours.

Pharmaceutics

IV anaesthetic agents present an interesting pharmaceutical formulation problem: an IV anaesthetic agent must be highly lipid-soluble (to cross the blood–brain barrier and act) yet sufficiently water-soluble to be formulated as a solution that can be safely injected IV. This problem has been solved for some drugs with very low water solubilities by formulating them as oil-in-water emulsions (similar to milk) – for example, diazepam or propofol in a soya oil/egg lecithin/glycerol emulsion.

Total intravenous anaesthesia

Surgical procedures can be carried out under **total intravenous anaesthesia** (TIVA), using thiopental or propofol throughout with no inhaled agent. A constant plasma drug level is achieved with a bolus initial dose, then an infusion that can be altered depending on the patient's responses. Computer-controlled infusion pumps can be programmed to take into account mathematically modelled pharmacokinetic parameters of the drug, patient parameters such as weight, age, liver and renal functions, desired blood concentrations of drug, adjunct analgesics and type of surgical operation.

Ultrashort-acting barbiturates

The prototype ultrashort-acting barbiturate-type agent is thiopental (also known as thiopentone), a CNS depressant that potentiates the inhibitory transmitter GABA and thus produces hypnosis and anaesthesia without analgesia. GA with ultrashort-acting barbiturates is believed to result from suppression of the RAS, with respiratory and cardiovascular depression.

Thiopental is often combined with a muscle relaxant and analgesic in balanced anaesthesia. Being very lipid-soluble, it has a rapid action, then short duration due to redistribution mainly to muscle tissues. Thiopental also has anticonvulsant effects and reduces intracranial pressure; it is particularly useful in emergency anaesthesia.

The most common adverse effects during recovery are shivering and trembling and additive effects with other CNS depressants; also nausea, vomiting, prolonged somnolence and headache. Serious adverse reactions include emergence delirium (increased excitability, confusion and hallucinations), cardiac dysrhythmias or depression, allergic responses, bronchospasm and respiratory depression.

Non-barbiturates

Non-barbiturate IV anaesthetic agents include the short-acting hypnotics propofol (the prototype drug of this group; Drug Monograph 18.3) and ketamine (Drug Monograph 18.4), and the benzodiazepines midazolam and diazepam. The opioid analgesics fentanyl, and alfentanil (Ch 19) are sometimes included as IV anaesthetics as they can be used in high doses to induce anaesthesia.

Ketamine (Drug Monograph 18.4) is an effective analgesic and anaesthetic, causing amnesia without loss of respiratory function or reflexes; it can be administered IV or intramuscularly and is useful for brief procedures such as changing burns dressings. It has been called a dissociative anaesthetic as it produces a cataleptic state in which the patient appears to be awake but is detached from the environment and unresponsive to pain; it can cause cardiovascular and respiratory stimulation. Because dreams and hallucinations can occur (e.g. during emergence reactions), it is sometimes subject to abuse (Ch 19).

Benzodiazepines (midazolam, diazepam, lorazepam)
Benzodiazepines are given intravenously for induction of anaesthesia, for their amnesic actions and for seizure control. These drugs enhance the inhibitory actions of GABA (the group is considered in detail in Ch 19; see Table 19.1) and as premedication (antianxiety and sedative effects). Diazepam is not readily water-soluble, so the solution for injection can cause local irritation and thrombosis; it must only be injected very slowly into large veins. Diazepam has a very long elimination half-life; hence, it is long-acting, with prolonged recovery time.

IV midazolam is commonly used in conjunction with propofol and fentanyl in day-surgery procedures where only minimal or moderate sedation is required, and in induction of GA. Midazolam is carried by ambulances and frequently administered by paramedics to treat seizures, agitation and overdose with stimulants, and for sedation for procedures such as intubation and cardioversion.

Concurrent use of benzodiazepines with alcohol or CNS-depressant drugs may result in hypotension and enhanced respiratory depression; a reduction in drug dosage and close monitoring are indicated.

KEY POINTS

General anaesthetics

- GA is the loss of all sensations and consciousness; it can be achieved by inhalation or injection of rapidly acting, reversible CNS depressants.
- General anaesthetics are lipid-soluble agents that act by modulation of transmitter-gated ion channels; the main mechanisms are enhancement of GABA-mediated CNS inhibition and inhibition of NMDA-mediated excitation.
- Speed of onset of and recovery from anaesthetic action depends on the solubility of the agent in lipids and in blood, and on the person's alveolar ventilation.
- There are four stages of induction with a general anaesthetic: analgesia, excitement, surgical anaesthesia and medullary paralysis.
- Inhalation agents include the gas nitrous oxide, methoxyflurane and volatile agents such as desflurane and sevoflurane.
- IV anaesthetics include propofol, thiopental, ketamine and the benzodiazepines midazolam and diazepam.
- Benzodiazepines are given intravenously for induction of anaesthesia and for their amnesic actions and as premedication for their antianxiety and sedative effects.

Clinical aspects of general anaesthetic use

Thanks to recent advances in drugs, monitoring devices and delivery systems, GA is now well tolerated in virtually all patients, allowing new surgical techniques to be made available. As most drugs used are both potent and potentially toxic, drugs and administration techniques must be chosen carefully; patients must be monitored and managed well before, during and after the operation; and concurrent diseases and drug regimens must be considered.

Administration

Most patients will be administered a maintenance anaesthetic by inhalation, so the first rule of anaesthesiology is to keep a clear airway. Airway obstruction leads to anoxia and impaired gas intake, hence to decreased absorption of anaesthetic drugs and risk of the patient regaining consciousness too early.

A typical setup of equipment for administration of gas and volatile liquid anaesthetics via the mouth and larynx is shown diagrammatically in Figure 18.8. In an emergency situation the analgesic methoxyflurane is administered via a hand-held inhaler.

Endotracheal intubation
Airways obstruction can be caused by the tongue falling back, laryngeal spasm, airways disease or mechanical faults. To maintain a reliable airway, most patients will be intubated; that is, have an endotracheal tube passed via the larynx into the upper part of the trachea. The tube is usually cuffed to help prevent inhalation of secretions or vomit. A dose of a skeletal muscle relaxant (see below, 'Adjuncts to Anaesthesia' – 'Muscle Relaxants') is normally administered to facilitate intubation. Supraglottic airway devices are used to keep the upper airway open to provide unobstructed ventilation. First-generation supraglottic airway devices rapidly replaced endotracheal intubation and face masks. A newer, second-generation, supraglottic airway device known as the iGEL is employed in some ambulance services.

Laryngeal mask airway
A laryngeal mask airway can be used as an alternative to either an endotracheal tube or a face mask; it incorporates a curved steel tube sheathed in silicone accommodating a tracheal tube, plus a laryngeal mask and a guiding handle. It can be used with spontaneous or positive pressure ventilation, and is relatively easy to insert even in patients with difficult airways.

Balanced anaesthesia

No single anaesthetic drug can produce rapid, maintained, reversible anaesthesia as well as analgesia, relief of anxiety, muscle relaxation, amnesia and suppression of reflexes,

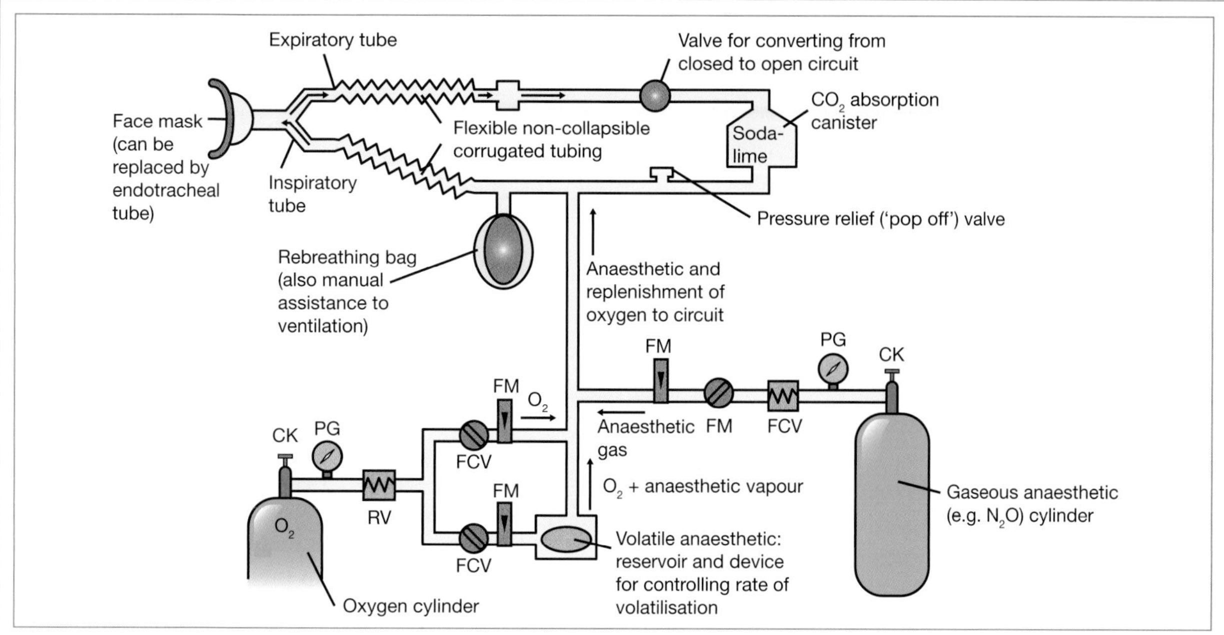

FIGURE 18.8 Diagrammatic representation of the typical equipment for general anaesthesia
Gases from the cylinders are admitted by opening the cylinder keys (CK); pressures are measured with gauges (PG) and lowered by reduction valves (RV). Flows of gases are controlled by flow control valves (FCV) and monitored by flow meters (FM). Gases other than those shown may be available (e.g. 5% CO_2 in O_2); there may be additional volatilisers for generating anaesthetic vapour in the replenishment line or in the circuit; an endotracheal tube or a laryngeal mask may replace a face mask.
Source: Bowman & Rand 1980; used with permission.

while maintaining fluid, electrolyte and metabolic homeostasis. Anaesthesia with a combination of drugs each used for its specific effect, rather than potentially toxic doses of a single CNS depressant, is termed **balanced anaesthesia** or multimodal anaesthesia. The specific drugs and dosages used depend on the procedure to be carried out, the physical condition of the patient and the patient's responses. The advantages of balanced anaesthesia include a safer induction, quicker recovery and lower reported incidence of postoperative nausea, vomiting and pain.

Day-surgery procedures

A typical IV sedative/analgesic regimen for minor day procedures such as colonoscopy, and those in which the patient needs to remain conscious, is propofol and midazolam (for induction/sedation) and fentanyl (for analgesia). There is potential for synergistic respiratory depressant effects, and patients must be warned not to drive, sign important documents or operate machinery for at least 24 hours.

Procedural sedation in children

Procedural sedation and analgesia is particularly important for children requiring relief of pain and anxiety during diagnostic or therapeutic procedures, especially in an emergency department. Typical situations include fracture reduction, laceration repair, lumbar puncture, incision and drainage. Drug combinations most commonly used are midazolam plus fentanyl, ketamine or morphine; these can be administered by non-anaesthetists (e.g. in a pre-hospital setting) and adverse effects are rare and include hypoxia and vomiting (see relevant guidelines for exclusion criteria). The area of paediatric sedation continues to evolve (Mason & Seth 2019).

Adverse effects and toxicity of general anaesthetics

Adverse effects common to all general anaesthetics are depression of the cardiovascular and respiratory systems and reflexes; general anaesthetics may also cause postoperative convulsions, headache, nausea and vomiting, kidney or liver toxicity (hepatotoxicity especially with the superseded general anaesthetics chloroform and halothane), malignant hyperthermia (Clinical Focus Box 18.3). They may have long lasting effects in the young and elderly (Wu et al. 2019). They are relatively contraindicated during pregnancy; however, they may be carefully administered when required, as maintenance of the mother's health is important to the wellbeing of the fetus. Each individual drug also has its particular adverse effects.

Studies on chemical series of halogenated hydrocarbon compounds have shown that, overall, fluorinated compounds are more potent and less toxic than others. Two drugs, sevoflurane and desflurane, appear to have optimal properties as anaesthetics, compared with earlier agents such as ether, chloroform and halothane.

CLINICAL FOCUS BOX 18.3
Malignant hyperthermia

Malignant hyperthermia, or hyperpyrexia, is a rare but potentially fatal condition occurring in susceptible patients with an inherited abnormality of calcium regulation in muscle sarcoplasmic reticulum, due to mutations in the ryanodine receptor gene (which codes for the muscle cell Ca^{2+}-release channel). It appears to be precipitated by the combination of a depolarising neuromuscular blocking agent (suxamethonium [or succinylcholine]) with a halogenated general anaesthetic agent (e.g. sevoflurane, desflurane), leading to acutely accelerated metabolism in skeletal muscle, with rapid fever, hyperthermia, acidosis, hyperkalaemia, tachycardia, muscle rigidity and rhabdomyolysis and dysfunction of many organ systems. It can occur during anaesthesia or in the early postoperative period. Trigger drugs include all volatile general anaesthetics, xanthines (including caffeine), phenothiazines and possibly sympathomimetics; safe drugs include nitrous oxide, benzodiazepines, barbiturates and non-depolarising neuromuscular blockers.

The predisposition to the condition can be diagnosed by muscle biopsy, genetic testing for susceptibility and in-vitro testing by challenge with caffeine and halothane (the CHCT test). While it occurs in only one in 6000 to 200,000 people, mortality is 70% if specific treatment is not given. Emergency treatment consists of stopping the inhalational agent, substituting the volatile GA agent with propofol infusion, actively cooling the patient with normal saline at 4°C and administering dantrolene (a direct inhibitor of muscle contractions), bicarbonate, an antidysrhythmic agent (amiodarone, lignocaine) and appropriate electrolyte and fluid replacements. The patient needs to be cared for and monitored in an intensive care unit for at least 24 hours.

Significant drug interactions
Anaesthetists need to be familiar with the significant interactions between anaesthetics and the maintenance drug therapies used in a wide range of illnesses; interactions are also possible with other drugs used during GA – in particular, between anticholinesterases or aminoglycoside antibiotics and neuromuscular blocking agents.

As a general guideline, if a drug is needed for treatment preoperatively, it should be continued through surgery; other drugs are discontinued for a wash-out period before surgery at least five times the half-life of the drug. Drugs having significant interactions with anaesthetic agents are replaced, where possible, with an alternative medication. An overview of potentially significant drug interactions is given in Drug Interactions 18.1; reference texts (e.g. the *Australian Medicines Handbook*) should be consulted for specific combinations. Not all drug interactions are adverse: the additive CNS-depressant effects of opioid analgesics and general anaesthetics can be useful in allowing lower doses of the general anaesthetic, provided the interaction is anticipated and monitored.

Other surgery-related problems
Many problems related to the anaesthetics used can occur during surgical procedures, such as:

- oxygen toxicity, if the oxygen concentration is too high (Ch 15)
- awareness (patient becoming conscious) can occur despite apparently adequate anaesthesia, leading to pain and enduring memories of the procedure, with adverse psychological sequelae
- occupational hazards – the patient may suffer injury or burns from equipment-related problems, and fire was a potential problem because of the use of electrocautery in the presence of flammable gases and volatile liquids. In addition, the staff in the operating theatre are subject to potentially harmful levels of waste gases, even though exhaust gases are extracted from anaesthetic circuits (see Clinical Focus Box 18.5, later).

Special anaesthesia considerations
Many disease states and risk factors can alter a person's response to anaesthesia, so preoperative assessment of the patient's health status should consider acute and chronic medical conditions.

Predisposition to allergies
Taking a clear history on allergic reactions is necessary to prevent anaphylactic reaction to drugs used during operations: anaesthetists ask the patient prior to surgery about allergies and previous reactions to drugs, but it is not unknown for patients to have first reactions to drugs while on the operating table! The most likely causes of anaphylaxis are penicillin and cephalosporin antibiotics used in trauma or as prophylactic cover against infection, muscle relaxants such as rocuronium or non-steroidal anti-inflammatory drugs (NSAIDs) used as analgesics. Other (non-drug) causes could include latex in materials used, and antiseptics such as chlorhexidine used to clean the area of surgery (Dr Alan Ch'ng, personal communication, 2017; Crilly & Rose 2014).

Young age
The physical characteristics of a neonate predispose to upper airway obstruction or laryngospasm during anaesthesia or resuscitation. A (relatively) large body water compartment, immature liver and kidneys, rapid metabolic rate and undeveloped blood–brain barrier all contribute to the susceptibility to adverse reactions to CNS-active drugs and indicate the need for careful monitoring of the infant or paediatric patient. Drug dosages and administered fluids must be carefully calculated, using recommended paediatric dose regimens. Infants and neonates usually require relatively higher concentrations of inhaled anaesthetic

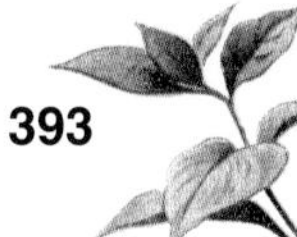

DRUG INTERACTIONS 18.1
General anaesthetics

DRUG OR DRUG GROUP	LIKELY EFFECTS AND MANAGEMENT
Anticoagulants such as heparin and warfarin	Usually discontinued 6 and 48 hours (respectively) before surgery to reduce the risk of haemorrhage.
CNS depressants such as alcohol, antihistamines, antianxiety agents, opioids and sedatives/hypnotics	Intensify the cardiovascular-, respiratory- and CNS-depressant effects of general anaesthetics; monitor carefully and reduce general anaesthetic dose if necessary. Chronic use may increase anaesthetic requirements.
Antidysrhythmic agents	May exacerbate cardiovascular system depression and hypotension caused by general anaesthetics.
Calcium channel blockers, β-blockers, angiotensin-converting enzyme inhibitors (commonly known as ACE inhibitors) (Ch 10) and sartans	Enhance cardiovascular suppression; monitor blood pressure and reduce general anaesthetic dose if necessary. ACE inhibitors and sartans withheld on day of surgery.
Corticosteroids taken chronically	Produce adrenal gland suppression, may result in hypotension during surgery and lack of ability to respond to stress; corticosteroids are usually resumed in patients who have recently stopped exogenous corticosteroid therapy. If chronic steroid use, give steroid replacement and IV hydrocortisone intraoperatively and a day or two postoperatively.
Drugs that inhibit CYP3A4 enzymes – for example, azole antifungals, protease inhibitors, macrolide antibiotics	May inhibit metabolism of midazolam and enhance its CNS-depressant actions; dose of midazolam reduced. Give 1–2 mg at a time and titrate for effect.
Drugs that affect blood pressure or heart rate	Interact with ketamine, which increases blood pressure and heart rate; monitor carefully.
Non-depolarising neuromuscular blockers	Neuromuscular blockade is enhanced by desflurane, isoflurane, sevoflurane or suxamethonium; dose of neuromuscular blocker may need to be reduced.

agents. Neonates are usually more sensitive to the non-depolarising muscle-relaxing agents.

Advanced age

Ageing results in a generalised decline in organ function, decreased organ reserve capacities and often the existence of chronic disease processes and polypharmacy, with many drugs taken to treat concurrent diseases; there is greater potential for drug interactions and adverse effects, and higher mortality rates after major surgery. Generally, increased and prolonged drug effects are seen in the elderly; postoperative drug-induced confusion is more likely (especially after midazolam).

Pregnancy and childbirth

Because CNS-active drugs are lipid-soluble, they are likely to cross the placenta and reach significant levels in the fetal bloodstream, or be secreted in the milk of lactating mothers; expected drug benefits should be considered against the possible risk to the fetus. General anaesthetics, LAs, analgesics and sedatives must be dosed and monitored carefully if used during pregnancy.

For analgesia during childbirth, nitrous oxide ('gas') is commonly safely self-administered by the mother, with assistance from the midwife and/or doctor. Opioid analgesics used during childbirth can cause respiratory depression in the neonate, so doses are kept to a minimum and adverse effects reversed by administration of naloxone to the infant. Caesarean section may require GA, but can be carried out under **epidural anaesthesia** with lidocaine (lignocaine) (Drug Monograph 18.5) and fentanyl, allowing the mother to remain conscious throughout the birth.

Concurrent disease conditions

Whenever possible, concurrent diseases should be treated and pathologies corrected before surgery. Implications of common diseases for drug use in anaesthesia are summarised below.

- *Cardiovascular diseases:* heart failure, recent heart attack, major vascular surgery, dysrhythmias, valve disease and hypertension predispose patients to stress-induced tachycardia, hypoxia and ischaemia, myocardial infarction and stroke, and cardiac complications after surgery; epidural analgesia is protective in the postoperative period.
- *Respiratory diseases:* asthma and chronic obstructive airways diseases impair inhalation of anaesthetics and exacerbate hypoxia and respiratory depression from CNS depressants and opioids; pre- and postoperative physiotherapy, bronchodilators and epidural analgesia assist postoperative care and coughing.
- *Renal disease:* may cause anaemia, and impaired blood pressure control, fluid and electrolyte balance and drug clearance; severe kidney dysfunction prolongs some drug half-lives; active opioid metabolites are retained, and non-narcotic analgesics (NSAIDs) can further damage kidneys.
- *Liver disease:* in mild cirrhosis there is CNS tolerance to depressant drugs, but in severe alcoholic cirrhosis, hepatic metabolic pathways may be impaired, the blood–brain barrier may be more permeable and encephalopathy present, so CNS depressants should be avoided; blood clotting and drug protein binding may also be impaired.

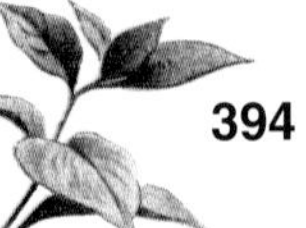

Drug Monograph 18.5
Lidocaine (lignocaine)

Mechanism of action
Lidocaine (lignocaine) is an amide-type LA that prevents the initiation and propagation of nerve impulses. It also has antidysrhythmic properties because it stabilises all potentially excitable membranes, including the conduction system of the heart.

Indications
Lidocaine (lignocaine) is used commonly for production of local anaesthesia by topical, infiltration, nerve block, epidural and intrathecal, spinal, ophthalmic, dermal (patches, cream, ointment) and IV regional anaesthesia routes. It is also used to treat or prevent ventricular dysrhythmias.

Pharmacokinetics
Onset of action is rapid (5–10 minutes) and duration of nerve blockade is 1–1.5 hours. After absorption into the general circulation or after IV injection, the drug is redistributed rapidly to tissues, especially the heart. Metabolism occurs in the liver and excretion via the kidneys; less than 10% is excreted unchanged. The elimination half-life is 90–120 minutes.

Adverse effects
Excessive dosage, rapid absorption or delayed elimination can lead to toxic depressant effects in the central, autonomic and peripheral nervous systems and the cardiovascular and respiratory systems. Allergic reactions are rare.

Drug interactions
Other antidysrhythmics, phenytoin and alcohol may potentiate the cardiovascular effects of lidocaine (lignocaine). The clearance of lidocaine (lignocaine) may be reduced by drugs including β-blockers, cimetidine, erythromycin and itraconazole.

Warnings and contraindications
Reduced doses should be given to children, elderly patients and those with cardiac, neurological, liver or kidney disease; cardiovascular function should be monitored during IV administration. Lidocaine (lignocaine) is contraindicated in patients with hypersensitivity to amide LAs, inflammation or sepsis at the site of injection, severe shock or hypotension, diseases of the CNS or supraventricular dysrhythmias.

Dosage and administration
Lidocaine (lignocaine) is formulated as an oral liquid (2%), oral paint (2.5%), topical liquid (4%), injection (0.5–2%), gel (2%), ointment (5%), cream (4%), spray (5%) and in various combination products. For local anaesthesia, the lowest effective dosage should be used, depending on the area to be anaesthetised, technique to be used, vascularity of the tissues and patient factors. The typical maximum safe dose is 3 mg/kg (solution without adrenaline) or 7 mg/kg with adrenaline; the specific dose depends on the route and usage.

Lifestyle factors
Obesity
Overweight and obese patients may have cardiac insufficiency, respiratory problems, atherosclerosis, hypertension or an increased predisposition to diabetes, liver disease or thrombo-phlebitis. Obtaining the desired depth of anaesthesia and muscle relaxation may be a problem. Generally, highly fat-soluble anaesthetics, especially those such as methoxyflurane with toxic metabolites, should be avoided.

Smoking
People who smoke have increased risks of coronary heart disease, peripheral vascular disease and compromised respiratory functions (e.g. bronchitis, emphysema or carcinoma) and increased sensitivity to muscle relaxants. Postoperative complications are six times more common in smokers than in non-smokers.

Alcohol intake
Heavy or regular drinkers of alcohol may have associated disease states including liver dysfunction, pancreatitis, gastritis and oesophageal varices. Anaesthetic requirements may be increased because of the increase in liver drug-metabolising enzymes and the development of cross-tolerance. Alcoholic patients need to be monitored closely during the post-anaesthetic period for alcohol withdrawal syndrome, as its onset may be delayed by the administration of analgesics. Diazepam or other sedatives may be required to prevent withdrawal symptoms.

Preoperative management
The preoperative visit to the patient by the anaesthetist and care of the patient by other health professionals should include taking a thorough medical history and ascertaining any relevant information such as drug allergies and concurrent disease. Questions (in words the patient can understand) are asked about:

- respiratory and circulatory systems, kidney and liver functions, general medical history
- diabetes, seizures and faints, bleeding problems
- previous drug reactions and drug use (including alcohol, tobacco and anaesthetics)
- fasting period (solids and fluids)
- current conditions and medications (most can and should be continued)
- possibility of pregnancy and/or infectious disease.

Preoperative management also includes general aspects such as correct identification of the patient and obtaining written consent; providing information on the proposed procedures, risks and equipment; allaying of anxieties; and teaching of exercises for breathing, coughing and movement postoperatively.

Premedication

Premedication (i.e. preoperative medication) was introduced in the early days of anaesthetic practice to prevent or treat some of the problems associated with ether and chloroform; it is no longer considered essential. Rationales for 'premed' include to: allay anxiety (allows lower doses of anaesthetics); decrease secretions (salivary, gastric and bronchial); reduce postoperative vomiting; overcome CNS depression; and provide prophylactic analgesia and sedation. Table 18.3 gives an overview of the common agents used.

Adjuncts to anaesthesia

Anaesthetic adjuncts are used to augment specific components of anaesthesia, permitting lower doses of general anaesthetics with fewer side effects. Opioid analgesics are used including morphine and fentanyl. Adjuncts also include neuromuscular blockers (muscle relaxants – see below).

Procedural sedation

Dexmedetomidine is a sedative and analgesic drug, related to the α_2-adrenoceptor agonists such as clonidine, and with similar pharmacological properties. It acts on α_2-adrenoreceptors in the CNS to reduce noradrenergic activity. It is used for procedural sedation and postsurgical and intensive care sedation of intubated patients and is administered intravenously. Refer to Chapter 20 for more information (see also procedural sedation in children earlier).

Muscle relaxants

Many surgical procedures, especially those on the abdomen, require inhibition of voluntary muscle tone and reflexes to stop muscles contracting when stimulated, to provide surgeons with easier access or to aid intubation. This can be achieved with deep GA or with nerve block regional anaesthesia, but both these techniques carry risks. Alternatively, neuromuscular blocking agents (see also Ch 8) can be administered once the patient is lightly anaesthetised and adequate analgesia provided. Artificial mechanical ventilation must be administered, as the respiratory muscles are paralysed by skeletal muscle relaxants.

These drugs are commonly carried in ambulances and administered by paramedics: suxamethonium to aid endotracheal intubation, and rocuronium to maintain skeletal muscle paralysis and allow mechanical ventilation in intubated patients. Continuous monitoring of vital signs, including blood gases, is essential.

The pharmacology of these drugs is considered in detail in Chapter 8; the two main groups of drugs used are summarised below.

Non-depolarising neuromuscular blockers

Non-depolarising neuromuscular blockers:

- are competitive antagonists of ACh nicotinic receptors at the neuromuscular junction
- do not directly depolarise the end-plate
- cause a flaccid paralysis, lasting 20–30 minutes
- are reversible with anticholinesterase drugs such as neostigmine
- are based on the natural arrow-poison curare.

Examples include rocuronium (Ch 8), cis- and atracurium, vecuronium and mivacurium.

Depolarising neuromuscular blockers

Depolarising neuromuscular blockers:

- activate the nicotinic ACh receptor at the NMJ, depolarising the end-plate
- cause initial muscle twitching, then paralysis, lasting 3–5 minutes
- are useful for short procedures (e.g. intubation and electroconvulsive therapy)
- are enhanced, rather than reversed, by anticholinesterase drugs.

The only example is suxamethonium (succinylcholine); suxamethonium is a powerful trigger for malignant hyperpyrexia/hyperthermia (Ch 8, Drug Monograph 8.5 and Clinical Focus Box 18.3) and also hyperkalemia in children and adolescents.

TABLE 18.3 Premedication agents

DRUG CLASSIFICATION	AGENTS USED	DESIRED EFFECT
Opioid analgesics	Morphine, fentanyl, oxycodone	Sedation to decrease anxiety; provide analgesia (if required) and decrease amount of anaesthetic used
Benzodiazepines	Midazolam, diazepam, lorazepam, oxazepam	Anxiolytic, sedative, rapid induction, amnesia
Anticholinergics	Glycopyrronium bromide (glycopyrrolate)	Inhibition of secretions (antisialogogue); reduced vomiting and laryngospasms; modify parasympathetic response to induction
Dissociative anaesthetic	Ketamine	Anxiolysis, sedation
H_2-receptor antagonists	Cimetidine, ranitidine	Reduce acidity of stomach contents
Antacids	Sodium citrate	Reduce acidity; for procedures such as emergency C-section

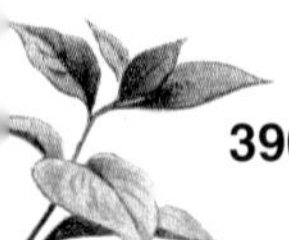

Postoperative aspects

Recovery

As soon as administration of the anaesthetic ceases, recovery begins and consciousness starts to return, following the stages of anaesthesia in reverse; however, it may be some hours before the patient is fully conscious with stable cardiovascular and respiratory functions. There are many potential complications following surgical operations:

- Nausea and vomiting can be induced by pain, drugs (especially opioids), ketosis or dehydration. If nausea and vomiting are severe, antiemetics (metoclopramide, ondansetron) can be given.
- Postoperative pain is common, particularly after procedures involving the thorax or abdomen, episiotomy and after childbirth. Adequate pain relief must be maintained to facilitate recovery and ease of coughing and defecation; remifentanil (an opioid analgesic) and NSAIDs (e.g. parecoxib) are useful.
- Respiratory depression often follows the use of narcotic analgesics (opioids); treatment may be with the opioid antagonist naloxone. Chest complications are exacerbated in smokers and patients with chronic obstructive pulmonary disease and by sputum retention, dehydration, ongoing use of opioids and pain that inhibits coughing. Physiotherapy and rehydration are helpful.
- The inactivity caused by long surgical procedures and prolonged bed rest predisposes the patient to thrombosis; early ambulation and antithrombotic drugs (aspirin) or anticoagulants help prevent thrombosis and embolism.

More general aspects of postoperative care include monitoring of cardiovascular and respiratory functions and fluid balance, supportive nursing and provision of adequate information. Doses of concurrent drugs may need to be lower than usual in the postoperative period.

Reversal of non-depolarising neuromuscular blockade

Neuromuscular blockade by suxamethonium is usually so short lasting as to need no reversal. However, non-depolarising neuromuscular blockade needs to be reversed to hasten spontaneous breathing, usually with an anticholinesterase such as neostigmine.

A new drug used postoperatively is sugammadex, which reverses the neuromuscular blockade caused by the non-depolarising neuromuscular blockers rocuronium and vecuronium. It is a modified cyclodextrin that forms a complex with these drugs (but not with other neuromuscular blockers) and thus reduces their binding to nicotinic receptors and speeds recovery from muscle relaxation. It is injected IV and has a rapid effect; recovery of muscle function occurs within 5 minutes, compared to 50 minutes after reversal with neostigmine. Adverse effects include disturbances in taste and allergic reactions; interactions are likely to occur with flucloxacillin and sodium fusidate (antibacterials), toremifene (an estrogen blocker) and progestogens; and women using hormonal contraception should be warned to take extra contraceptive precautions for 7 days after sugammadex administration.

Refer to Clinical Focus Box 18.4 for an overview of drugs typically found in the anaesthetist's trolley or paramedic's bag.

KEY POINTS

Clinical aspects of general anaesthetic use

- Most patients will be administered a maintenance anaesthetic by inhalation, so the first rule of anaesthesiology is to keep a clear airway.
- To maintain a reliable airway, most patients will be intubated. A dose of a skeletal muscle relaxant is normally administered to facilitate intubation.
- Supraglottic airway devices, including the laryngeal mask airway, are used to keep the upper airway open to provide unobstructed ventilation.
- Balanced anaesthesia is the use of a combination of agents to achieve unconsciousness, analgesia, muscle relaxation and amnesia.
- Common adverse effects and drug interactions are the potentiation of CNS depression and the risk of malignant hyperthermia from suxamethonium plus a general anaesthetic.
- As many disease states and risk factors can alter a person's response to anaesthesia, preoperative assessment of the patient's health status should be undertaken. Factors such as age, concurrent disease states, medications, lifestyle factors and possibility of pregnancy should be taken into consideration.
- Premedication may include an antianxiety agent (e.g. midazolam) and atropine to suppress secretions. Adjuncts to anaesthesia include depolarising and non-depolarising neuromuscular blockers. Antiemetics and opioids are used for postoperative nausea and pain.
- Postoperative care includes the administration of antiemetics for nausea and vomiting, opioid analgesics and NSAIDs for pain and aspirin to prevent postoperative thrombosis.

Local anaesthesia

Local anaesthesia refers to the direct administration of a drug to tissues to induce the absence of pain sensation in a part of the body. Unlike GA, local anaesthesia does not

CLINICAL FOCUS BOX 18.4
In the anaesthetist's drug trolley or paramedic's bag

A typical anaesthetic drug trolley (and nearby refrigerator and drug safe) may contain supplies of the following drugs, for use by the anaesthetist or, depending on the clinical practice guidelines of the particular ambulance service, selected drugs used by the paramedic. Drugs shown in **bold type** are also among those listed as commonly carried in ambulances and administered by paramedics in pre-hospital settings.

- induction agents (propofol)
- analgesics (**morphine, fentanyl**, alfentanil or remifentanil, all kept in a drug safe; **methoxyflurane**, parecoxib)
- local anaesthetics (**lidocaine [lignocaine]**, **bupivacaine**)
- muscle relaxants (**suxamethonium**, **rocuronium**; most kept refrigerated)
- sedatives (**midazolam**; usually kept in a drug safe; propofol, dexmedetomidine, ketamine, clonidine)
- reversal drugs (neostigmine, flumazenil, **naloxone**, **glucagon**)
- resuscitation agents (**adrenaline [epinephrine]**, **atropine**)
- cardiovascular drugs (antihypertensives (metoprolol), **antidysrhythmics**, sympathomimetics, **inotropic agents**, **antianginal drugs**)
- coagulants (tranexamic acid)
- anticoagulants (heparin) and antiplatelet agents (**aspirin**)
- vasoconstrictors (ephedrine, phenylephrine, metaraminol)
- renal drugs (vasodilators, **diuretics**)
- **electrolyte replacements** (calcium, bicarbonate; potassium no longer kept on trolleys due to accidental therapeutic mishaps)
- antiasthma drugs (**salbutamol**, dexamethasone, hydrocortisone, **ipratropium bromide**)
- antiemetics (metoclopramide, **ondansetron**, **prochlorperazine**)
- IV fluids (normal saline, Hartmann's solution, **glucose [dextrose]** 5%, 10%)
- stabilising/analgesic agents (clonidine, dexmedetomidine)
- antibiotics (gentamicin, metronidazole, cefalexin, **ceftriaxone**)
- miscellaneous (eyedrops, nasal drops, non-opioid analgesics).

Note that most anaesthetic drugs and adjuncts are given intravenously. It would be a useful pre-examination exercise for the student to 'play anaesthetist or paramedic' and consider the actions, indications for use and common adverse effects of all these drugs, and attempt to predict any potentially major drug interactions and problems in elderly or renal-impaired patients.

Source: Acknowledgment to Dr Alan Ch'ng and Dr Melanie Van Twest; Dr Sally Tsang

CLINICAL FOCUS BOX 18.5
Waste anaesthetic gases as a workplace health hazard

Chronic exposure of staff in hospital operating rooms, ambulances, dental surgeries and veterinary clinics to waste anaesthetic gases (nitrous oxide and vapours from volatile halogenated agents) presents a workplace health hazard. Potential adverse effects include nausea, dizziness, headaches, cancers, liver and kidney disease, impaired mental performance, fatigue and irritability. Studies have demonstrated an increased incidence of miscarriages among women exposed to nitrous oxide in the workplace, as well as among women whose male partners are exposed, and liver disease in children There is a risk of mutagenicity and genotoxicity.

Operating theatre staff and paramedics should be aware of the potential risks and protect themselves by avoiding the area within about 20 cm of the patient's mouth and nose when the breath contains exhaled anaesthetic agents. Institutions need to ensure that all exhaust gases are scavenged and vented to the outside air, and establish exposure monitoring programs to detect unsafe levels caused by faulty equipment or unsafe practices. Internationally there is a push to reduce the use of desflurane due to its significant contribution to greenhouse gas emissions. Some departments within Australian hospitals have already removed this general anaesthetic from operating theatres.

Source: Safety and health topics: waste anesthetic gases (see 'Online resources').

depress consciousness. As most sensations are not lost, the term 'anaesthesia' (total lack of sensation) is strictly speaking inappropriate, and some pharmacologists prefer the term 'local analgesia'. However, 150 years of usage sanction the terms 'local anaesthesia' and 'local anaesthetic'. LA drugs reversibly prevent both the generation and the conduction of impulses in excitable membranes, particularly in sensory nerves, and hence decrease the sensitivity to pain. They are used in many surgical procedures and for pain relief.

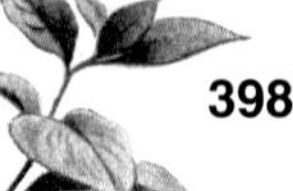

Local anaesthetic drugs

LA drugs were developed following the introduction of the natural compound cocaine into medicine and ophthalmic surgery in the 1870s and 1880s. The main problems with cocaine were its CNS actions, acute toxicity and addictive properties, so other benzoic acid esters were studied for LA activity (Clinical Focus Box 18.6). The amide compound lidocaine (lignocaine), developed in 1943, rapidly became widely used and is still considered the prototype LA. A long-acting drug from the bupivacaine-type group is used when longer duration of activity is required, and more recently a combination of lidocaine (lignocaine) and prilocaine (EMLA: eutectic mixture for local anaesthesia) has been formulated as a cream and a patch for topical application (see under 'Formulations of Local Anaesthetics and Topical Anaesthesia' later).

An ideal LA would produce nerve blockade only in sensory nerves when administered topically or parenterally (by injection) and would be rapidly reversible, non-toxic to both local tissue and major organs, with rapid, painless onset of action for a reasonable operating time. While no LA is perfect, two that are commonly used are lidocaine (lignocaine; Drug Monograph 18.4) and the longer acting bupivacaine.

Chemistry and dissociation of local anaesthetic drugs

Chemically, LA drugs have similar structures: they generally have at one end an aromatic (phenyl) group, joined through an intermediate chain of carbons to an amine (nitrogen-containing) group. The aromatic group helps make that end of the molecule lipid-soluble (lipophilic) and the amine group makes the other end water-soluble (hydrophilic). This allows the LA molecules to align and act within nerve cell membranes, which can be considered as phospholipid bilayers.

Esters and amides

The intermediate carbon chains contain either an ester link (O=C–O-) or an amide link (O=C–N-). The ester-type LAs (cocaine, procaine, tetracaine [amethocaine] and benzocaine) are metabolised rapidly by plasma esterase enzymes to p-aminobenzoic acid (PABA) metabolites, which can cause allergic reactions in some patients; ester LAs are not often used now. Amide anaesthetics (e.g. lidocaine [lignocaine], prilocaine, bupivacaine and ropivacaine) are not metabolised to PABA derivatives, and rarely induce allergic reactions.

Amines can be charged or uncharged

Because the LAs are all amines (except benzocaine), they can exist in solution as the uncharged tertiary amine form (NR_3, analogous to ammonia, NH_3) or as the charged quaternary amine form (N^+R_3H like the ammonium ion, N^+H_4). The forms are in equilibrium, as shown in the dissociation reaction at the top of Figure 18.9. The proportion of each form depends on the chemistry of the individual LA molecule and the pH of the solution or tissue it is in.

Clinically, this is important for the following reasons:

- The basic form (NR_3, where R stands for any substituent radical bonded to nitrogen) is non-ionised, non-polar and lipid-soluble; this form can diffuse across membranes and enter cells. At physiological pH (around 7.4), sufficient basic form is present to enter cells, where it can then pick up a hydrogen ion (H^+) to become charged and active.
- The cation form (N^+R_3H) is ionised, polar and water-soluble; this active form of the LA blocks sodium ion channels from inside the neuron.
- At highly acidic pH (in inflamed tissue), the equilibrium shifts towards the charged form and virtually all LA molecules exist as the cation form,

---

CLINICAL FOCUS BOX 18.6

Cocaine: the original local anaesthetic

Cocaine comes from the leaves of the plant *Erythroxylon coca*; it has been used for more than 2000 years in Central America, where the leaves are chewed or sucked to relieve pain, cause central stimulation and facilitate heavy work at high altitudes.

The dried leaves contain about 1% pure cocaine alkaloid, extractable as flaky crystals – hence the street name 'snow'.

- The famous Austrian physician and psychotherapist Sigmund Freud described how 50–100 mg cocaine injected subcutaneously decreased fatigue, sleep and appetite, increased power and caused euphoria; Freud's friend Köller introduced cocaine as an LA (in the eye); however, this led to corneal damage, as protective reflexes were suppressed.
- The peripheral actions of cocaine are as an LA. It also inhibits reuptake of NA into nerve terminals; hence, it has indirect sympathomimetic effects, including vasoconstriction.
- Unlike other LAs, cocaine has marked central actions: initially it acts as a stimulant, causing excitement, talkativeness, tremors and vomiting, and increases respiration; it induces powerful psychological dependence, with 'reward' feelings and exhilaration.
- The toxic effects are psychosis, hallucinations and paranoia, then CNS depression, with cardiotoxicity and respiratory depression.
- Cocaine is still occasionally used medically in nasal and ophthalmic surgery, and to aid intubation; it may be formulated extemporaneously by hospital pharmacists.

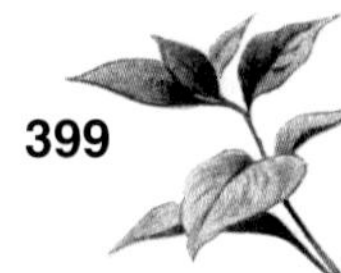

CLINICAL FOCUS BOX 18.7

Calculating the safe dose of a local anaesthetic

The strength of a solution of an LA formulated for injection is usually expressed in percentage terms or in mg/mL – for example, lidocaine (lignocaine) 2% weight in volume (w/v) means there are 2 g solid drug dissolved in 100 mL solution. It follows that each 1 mL contains 20 mg of drug. Adrenaline (epinephrine) concentration is usually expressed differently – for example, as 1 in 200,000, meaning that 1 g is present in 200,000 mL solution, or 1 mg in 200 mL.

Doses of LAs depend on many factors, including the drug, type of regional anaesthesia intended, weight, age and state of the patient, and whether a vasoconstrictor is present, degree of muscle relaxation or duration of anaesthesia; doses quoted are guidelines.

The minimum dose that results in effective anaesthesia should be used. The average dose of an LA is usually quoted in mL solution, rather than mg/kg body weight; thus the typical dose recommended for epidural block in an average 70 kg adult is 10–20 mL of a 1% lidocaine (lignocaine) solution (up to 200 mg).

As a vasoconstrictor localises the LA in tissues and prevents a rapid bolus of drug being absorbed into the bloodstream, larger doses can be used than are safe in the absence of the vasoconstrictor. Thus the maximum dose of lidocaine (lignocaine) in the presence of adrenaline (epinephrine) is 7 mg/kg.

Source: Dosages quoted from Australian Medicines Handbook 2021.

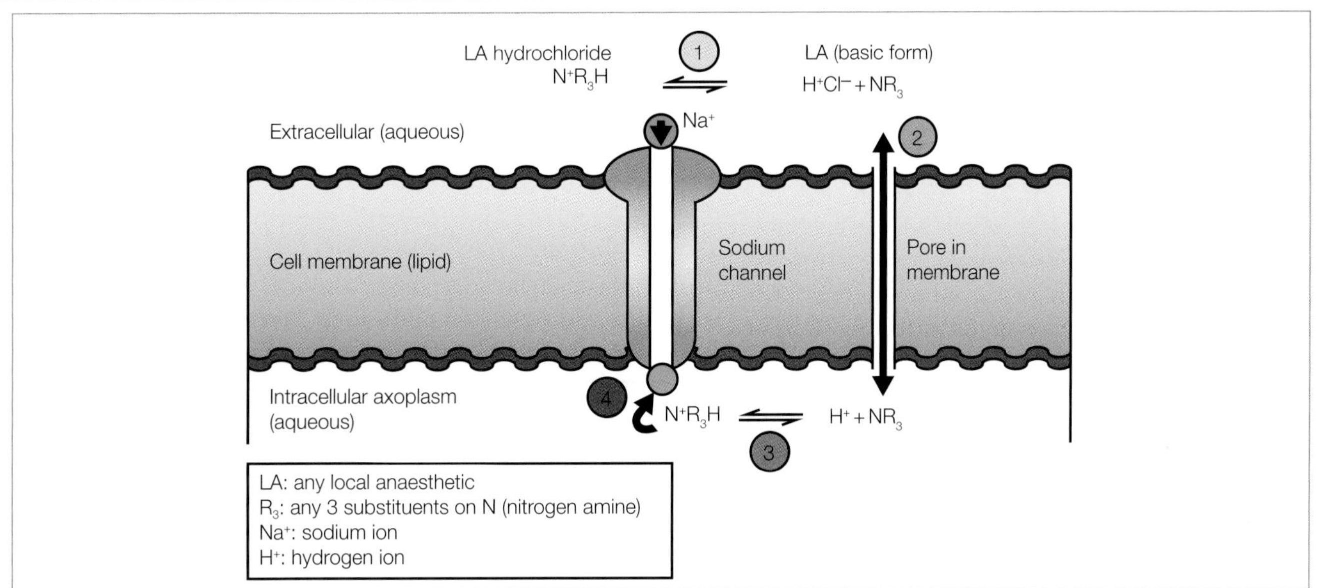

FIGURE 18.9 Mechanism of action of local anaesthetics

(1) The local anaesthetic (LA) is injected into tissues as a solution of the salt form, usually the hydrochloride; this positively charged quaternary amine form (N^+R_3H) is in equilibrium with the basic uncharged tertiary amine form (NR_3). (2) The non-polar uncharged form can diffuse readily through cell membranes. (3) Inside the neuronal cell, LA picks up hydrogen ions from intracellular fluid and is in equilibrium again with the ionised cation form. (4) The cation is the active LA form, which blocks sodium (Na^+) channels from the inside and prevents development of the action potential, thus reducing electrical activity in excitable cells (nerve and muscle) and blocking nerves.

unable to enter cells to act; this explains why LAs are less effective in inflamed tissues.

Mechanism of action

LAs reversibly prevent the generation and conduction of impulses in excitable membranes and thus decrease sensitivity to pain. The basic mechanism of action of these drugs has been studied in detail: as above, the non-ionised form enters the cell by diffusion through membranes, where it readily becomes ionised and binds to a modulatory site in the voltage-dependent sodium channel (Fig 18.9), blocking the channel and interfering with their transient opening, thus preventing the transient inrush of sodium. Hence, threshold potential is not reached, the cell membrane is not depolarised, the development of the action potential and its propagation are prevented and the nerve is blocked.

The LA drugs are said to be ion channel modulators or membrane stabilisers. Other drug groups with similar actions are the antidysrhythmic agents and anticonvulsants.

(Lidocaine [lignocaine] is in fact used for these effects.) Natural toxins, such as those of the puffer fish (tetrodotoxin), blue-ringed octopus (maculotoxin) and marine organisms (saxitoxin), also block nerve transmission, particularly in skeletal muscle, often causing fatal paralysis.

Autonomic and sensory nerves are blocked preferentially

All potentially excitable membranes are affected, so LAs have actions not only on sensory nerve cells but also on autonomic and motor nerves, muscle cells (cardiac, smooth, skeletal), secretory cells and neurons in the CNS.

The susceptibility of a nerve to LA action depends on the fibre diameter, myelination, tissue pH and length of nerve fibre exposed to LA solution. Autonomic and sensory fibres are blocked preferentially because they are thinner, unmyelinated and more easily penetrated by drugs. Loss of pain is followed in sequence by loss of responses to temperature, proprioception (position of body parts), touch and pressure. Motor fibres may also be anaesthetised if adequate concentration of the drug is present over sufficient time.[8]

Pharmacokinetics

An LA is administered for local analgesic action in the tissue or nerve pathway into which it is injected. It is only later that the drug is absorbed from the tissues into the bloodstream and distributed around the body, where it affects other systems and is metabolised and excreted.

Local disposition and action

An injected LA will first undergo local disposition (i.e. moving around) in the tissue. Onset of action is determined by the speed with which it diffuses into nerve cells, depending on its lipid solubility, which, as noted above depends in turn on the pH of the tissue and the degree of ionisation of the LA molecules (a function of the pK_a [negative logarithm of the ionisation constant] of the drug). Binding of the LA to tissue proteins and the presence of a vasoconstrictor in the solution help retain the drug in the tissues for longer action. Other potential factors include the volume and concentration of solution injected, speed of injection and local blood flow.

Diffusion, distribution and metabolism

Local action is terminated by diffusion away, dilution and uptake into the vasculature (i.e. systemic absorption from the tissue) and distribution around the body. Lipid solubility is again the major determining factor, and a vasoconstrictor will decrease the rate of absorption into the general circulation.

Metabolism of amide LAs occurs on first pass through the liver; this explains why LAs are inactive if taken orally. (Oral administration would not allow for localised actions except in the upper gastrointestinal tract.) Inactive metabolites are excreted via the kidneys.

Duration of action

Overall, the onset and duration of action of an injected LA depend on pharmacokinetic factors. The half-lives of LAs are generally short (1–2 hours); however, the bupivacaine-type LAs have longer durations of action. The choice of LA for a particular procedure depends largely on the duration of drug action desired; Table 18.4 summarises the properties of several commonly used short-, intermediate- and long-acting LAs. Some others are available in eyedrop formulations for use as ocular LAs.

Long-acting local anaesthetics

Bupivacaine was the first long-acting LA developed, soon followed by others with high lipid solubility and high protein-binding, giving them longer durations of action – up to 14 hours for major nerve blocks. Bupivacaine and ropivacaine differentiate well between sensory and motor blockade; however, bupivacaine is more cardiotoxic. Most are indicated for infiltration, nerve block, epidural and intrathecal anaesthesia; bupivacaine and ropivacaine are each also formulated combined with fentanyl for epidural anaesthesia/analgesia, and bupivacaine with adrenaline (epinephrine) for more prolonged action.

Clinical aspects of local anaesthetic use

Indications and contraindications

LAs are indicated for surgical procedures when the patient's cooperation and consciousness are required or desired, for minor superficial and body surface procedures when GA would be unnecessary or hazardous, and for sympathetic blockade or postoperative analgesia.

Contraindications to the use of local anaesthesia include extensive surgery that would require potentially toxic doses, known allergy or hypersensitivity to the LA agent, lack of cooperation from the patient and local inflammation, infection or ischaemia at the injection site. As usual, precautions may be required in paediatric, elderly or pregnant patients and in patients with liver disease.

Dosage

The lowest effective dose should be used, noting that maximum safe doses are only guides (Clinical Focus Box 18.7). Because

8 This sequence can be remembered by recalling the experience of having 'an injection' (i.e. of LA) at the dentist's surgery. Loss of pain occurs very rapidly, allowing dental procedures within about 5 minutes. Some time afterwards there may still be lingering loss of sensations of pressure, heat and pain, so it can be dangerous to attempt to drink a hot drink or chew food; chewing is possible since motor function has not been lost. Loss of sense of proprioception accounts for the phenomenon of feeling as if the face is grossly swollen when in fact it looks surprisingly normal.

TABLE 18.4 Properties of commonly used local anaesthetics

NAME (MAXIMUM DOSE[a])	TYPE/METABOLISM; HALF-LIFE	USES	TOXICITY/NOTES
Short-acting (30–60 min)			
Benzocaine	Ester/plasma; short (minimal systemic absorption)	Topical: drops, gel, lozenges, paint, suppositories	Relatively non-toxic; very low potency; only active topically (not an amine)
Cocaine (1.5 mg/kg)	Ester/plasma; approx. 1 h (acute)	Topical (ENT surgery)	Rapid onset, rapidly absorbed; cardiotoxic; sympathomimetic, CNS stimulant
Intermediate duration (0.5–4 h)			
Lidocaine (lignocaine) (3 mg/kg; with adrenaline/ epinephrine 7 mg/kg	Amide/liver; 2 h	Infiltration, nerve block, spinal epidural, IV, topical	Prototype LA, potency = 1; more cardiotoxic than prilocaine; rapid onset
Prilocaine (6 mg/kg; with adrenaline/ epinephrine 8 mg/kg)	Amide/liver; 2 h	Infiltration, nerve blocks, caudal, epidural, IV	Rapid onset; lower systemic toxicity than and equipotent with lidocaine (lignocaine); products of liver metabolism may cause methaemoglobinaemia; little vasodilator activity
Lidocaine (lignocaine)/prilocaine cream or patch (EMLA)	Amides/liver	Topical (venepuncture, cannulation, minor skin surgery)	Local irritation; risk in infants < 6 months (methaemoglobinaemia); toxic if swallowed by small children
Mepivacaine (Adults 66 mg cartridges, maximum 3 cartridges)	Amide/liver; 3 h	Dental anaesthesia	Less toxic than and equipotent with lidocaine (lignocaine); avoid use in pregnancy; decrease dose according to age and physical condition
Long duration (3–10 h)			
Bupivacaine (2 mg/kg); levobupivacaine (2 mg/kg); ropivacaine (3 mg/kg)	Amides/liver; 2–3 h	Infiltration, caudal, epidural, nerve blocks	Bupivacaine: More cardiotoxic than lidocaine (lignocaine); potency 4 × lidocaine (lignocaine); slow onset; less motor blockade
Tetracaine (amethocaine) (1 mg/kg)	Ester/plasma; 1 h	Topical anaesthesia; venous cannulation; eyedrops	Potency 5 × lidocaine (lignocaine); slow onset, very long acting; high systemic toxicity

[a] Guideline maximum adult doses quoted are for plain solution, as single dose for infiltration, nerve block or topical route.

Source: Australian Medicines Handbook 2021.

a dose that is safe when injected subcutaneously may be toxic if injected intravenously, the dose should be injected slowly, with frequent aspirations (applying suction to syringe) to avoid intravascular injection. Doses for epidural, spinal or ophthalmic blocks are determined by specialist anaesthetists.

Use of a vasoconstrictor

Most LAs produce vasodilation by direct action on blood vessels and by anaesthetising sympathetic fibres to vasculature. This can cause rapid absorption of the drug into the systemic circulation; when the rate of absorption exceeds the rate of elimination, toxic effects can occur. Vasoconstrictors such as adrenaline (epinephrine) or felypressin may be formulated in the LA solution to decrease systemic absorption and detain the drug in local tissue, prolonging the duration of action of the anaesthetic and reducing the risk of systemic toxicity.

Vasoconstrictors are not used for penile blocks, and only with caution in other areas where there are end-arteries (fingers, toes, ears, nose) because ischaemia may develop, resulting in gangrene. Other potential risks include cardiovascular stimulation (from stimulation of cardiac β_1-adrenoceptors by adrenaline [epinephrine]), so caution is required in patients with cardiovascular or thyroid disease or those taking antidepressants.

Some LAs do not require the use of a vasoconstrictor: cocaine itself has vasoconstrictor actions (due to its sympathomimetic effects).

Formulations of local anaesthetics

Interestingly, there are no formulations for oral administration and systemic absorption (although there are topical formulations for mouth and gastric ulcers). This is because LAs are rapidly metabolised in the circulation or liver (first-pass effect) and because it would be impossible to localise their effects once absorbed into the systemic circulation.

Parenterals

For injection by infiltration and nerve block techniques, the LA must be formulated as a parenteral solution that is sterile, particle-free, stable and preferably isotonic and buffered to the pH of body solutions. Particular cases are those of LA solutions with added vasoconstrictor (e.g. adrenaline [epinephrine], 1 in 200,000); and heavy solutions (for spinal anaesthesia) such as Marcain Spinal 0.5% Heavy Injection, a hyperbaric bupivacaine solution containing glucose at 80 mg/mL. Parenteral solutions of LA may also be formulated with an opioid analgesic such as fentanyl or pethidine.

Topicals

For topical administration, almost every dose form known to pharmaceutical science has been used, including creams, jellies, paints, lotions, ointments, adhesive ointments, sprays, dressings, lozenges, eye/eardrops, viscous solutions, emulsions and suppositories. Some interesting topical combination formulations are lidocaine (lignocaine) with chlorhexidine in a gel, for use as a lubricant in urological procedures, lidocaine (lignocaine) with benzalkonium chloride in a skin spray for sunburn relief, and benzocaine and clove oil for application to a tooth cavity to relieve throbbing persistent toothache (Oral-Eze). LAs formulated for use as eyedrops are tetracaine (amethocaine), oxybuprocaine (also known as benoxinate) and proxymetacaine (Ch 40).

Techniques for local anaesthesia

There are several techniques by which LAs are administered (Fig 18.10 and Table 18.5). Applied to an area (topical) or injected into tissues (infiltration), they produce their effect in the immediate area only; hence the term 'local anaesthesia'. Injected around a nerve or nerve trunk (e.g. nerve block, spinal or epidural techniques), they anaesthetise a large region of the body (**regional anaesthesia**). The LA should be injected slowly, with frequent aspirations (gentle 'sucking back' on the syringe) to ensure the needle tip is not in a blood vessel; pauses between bolus injections allow monitoring for systemic effects.

Topical or surface anaesthesia

Topical local anaesthesia is used to relieve pain and itching; for damaged skin surfaces, wounds and burns; to anaesthetise mucous membranes of the eye, nose, gums, throat or urethra for minor surgical procedures; to facilitate instrumentation; and before venepuncture or split skin grafting. As noted above, many dose forms are available, including eyedrops, eardrops, solutions, ointments, gels, creams, sprays and impregnated dressings.

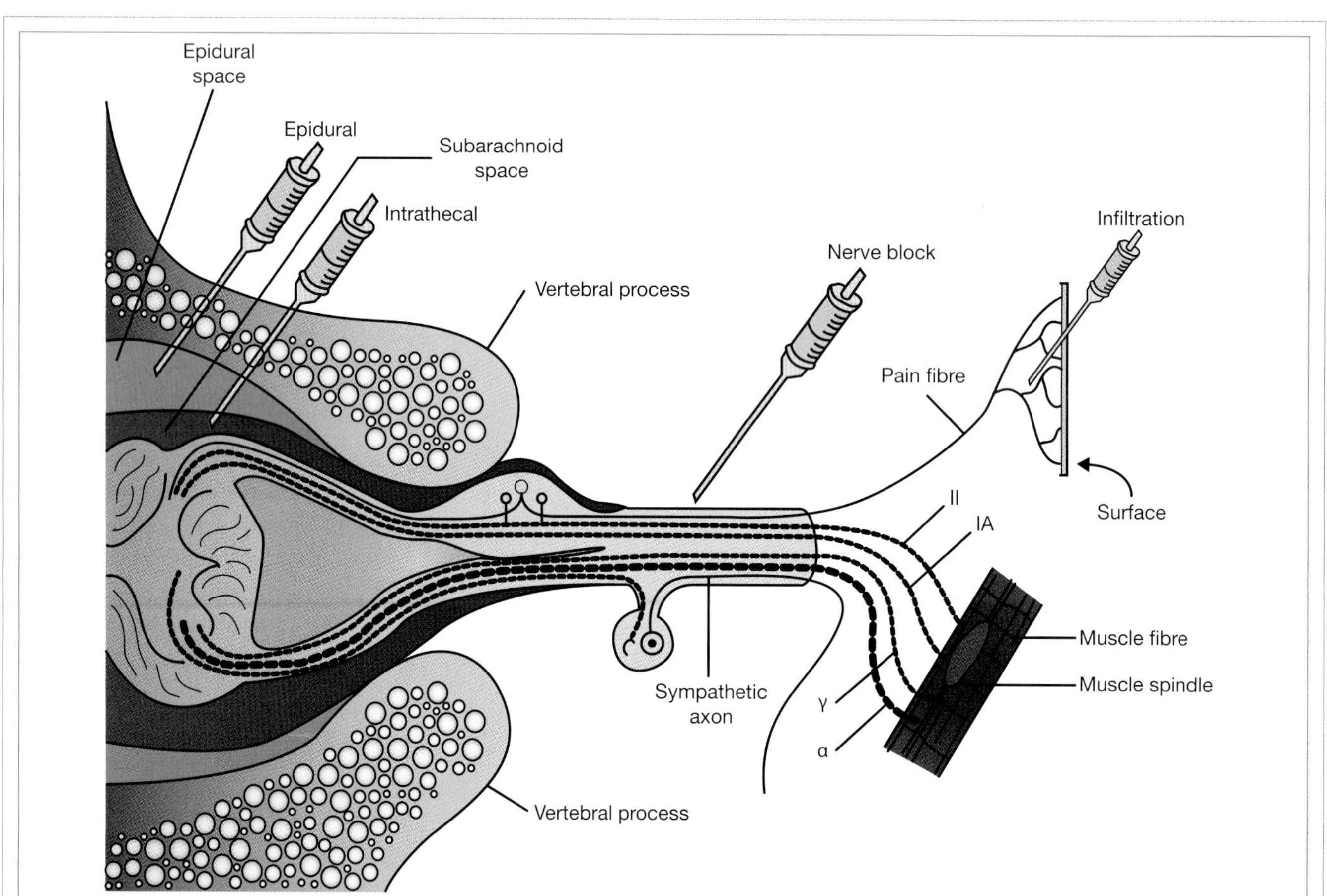

FIGURE 18.10 The routes of administration of local anaesthetic drugs

Half of a cross-section of the spinal column is shown with a mixed spinal nerve composed of examples of the main types of efferent and afferent fibres. IA, II = afferent axons from ending of muscle spindle; α = α axon (lower motor neuron) to extrafusal muscle fibres; γ = γ-efferent axon to intrafusal fibres of muscle spindle. Note that intrathecal injection into the subarachnoid space (spinal anaesthesia) is made in the lumbar region *below the termination of the spinal cord* (not as is shown here for convenience).

Source: Bowman & Rand 1980; used with permission.

TABLE 18.5 Local anaesthetic techniques

METHOD	TISSUE AFFECTED	DOSE FORM USED	EXAMPLES OF DRUGS USED	THERAPEUTIC INDICATIONS
Topical	Sensory nerve endings in mucous membranes and dermis	Solution, ointment, cream, eyedrops, spray, etc.	Cocaine, benzocaine, lidocaine (lignocaine), tetracaine (amethocaine), prilocaine	Relief of pain or itching; examination of conjunctiva; minor surgery; instrumentation
Infiltration	Sensory nerve endings in subcutaneous tissues or dermis	Injection	Prilocaine, lidocaine (lignocaine)	Minor surgery; skin lesions
Nerve block	Nerve trunk	Injection	Articaine, prilocaine, lidocaine (lignocaine), bupivacaine	Dental, eye and limb surgery; sympathetic block; obstetrics; postoperative pain relief
Epidural block	Spinal roots	Injection	Lidocaine (lignocaine), bupivacaine, levobupivacaine, ropivacaine	Thoracic and abdominal surgery; labour pain; caesarean section; postoperative pain relief
Spinal (subarachnoid) block	Spinal roots	Injection	Bupivacaine, levobupivacaine, ropivacaine	Abdominal surgery; surgery of the lower extremities; muscle relaxation
Intravenous regional anaesthesia	Upper limb	Injection	Prilocaine	Surgery on upper limb

Topical anaesthetics do not effectively penetrate unbroken skin, except for tetracaine (amethocaine) 4% gel or the combination cream EMLA (see above), which contains 25 mg/g each of lidocaine (lignocaine) and prilocaine. Cocaine in a 4–10% solution is still used topically for nasal anaesthesia.

Topical LAs occasionally cause dermatitis and allergic sensitisation, which necessitates their discontinuance. Absorption is increased from mucous membranes and broken skin (e.g. abrasions, trauma and ulcers), possibly causing systemic effects; deaths have occurred from absorption via the urethra. When they are used in the oral cavity (mouth and pharynx), aspiration or interference with swallowing may occur; a returning gag reflex is assessed by gentle touching of the back of the pharynx with a tongue blade. All food and fluids are withheld until the reflex returns.

Topical local anaesthesia may also be achieved by cooling because low temperatures in living tissues produce diminished sensation; hence the use of ice-packs to relieve pain, as in the first-aid acronym RICE: Rest, Ice, Compression, Elevation. This form of anaesthesia is sometimes used for minor operative procedures. However, tissues that are cooled too intensely for too long can be destroyed.

Infiltration anaesthesia

Infiltration anaesthesia is the use of LAs in a small area that circles the operative field; it is produced by injecting dilute solutions of the agent, usually with adrenaline, into the skin and then subcutaneously into the region to be anaesthetised. Repeated injection extends the anaesthesia as long as needed. Sensory nerve endings are anaesthetised, but not motor nerves. This method is used for minor surgery such as for skin lesions, skin incision and drainage, or excision of a cyst, and sometimes for more major procedures including dental extractions.

Intravenous regional anaesthesia

Intravenous regional anaesthesia (Bier's block) is a specialised technique for anaesthesia of the upper limb; the technique is as follows (Fig 18.11):

1 A tourniquet is placed on the upper part of the arm to be anaesthetised.

2 A vein distal to the tourniquet is cannulated – for example, a vein in the dorsum of the hand.

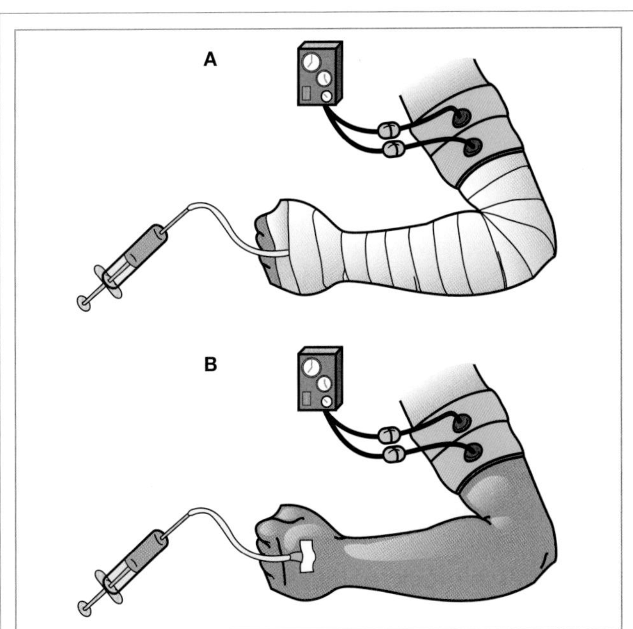

FIGURE 18.11 Technique for Bier's block: IV regional anaesthesia of the upper limb
A Cuff has been positioned, IV cannula inserted, and limb exsanguinated by winding an Esmarch bandage proximally up the arm. **B** Cuff has been inflated and the bandage removed, allowing injection of local anaesthetic.

3 The field of operation is exsanguinated by wrapping an Esmarch bandage up the arm or by elevation for 4–5 minutes.
4 The tourniquet is inflated to a pressure greater than the patient's pulse pressure to occlude arterial flow and kept inflated; the Esmarch bandage is then removed.
5 The LA solution (prilocaine or lidocaine [lignocaine], without adrenaline [epinephrine] or preservative) is injected slowly IV distal to the cuff.
6 The procedure is then carried out.
7 After the procedure the tourniquet must be released only gradually to avoid a bolus of LA rapidly entering the systemic circulation; during this time the patient's pulse, blood pressure and electrocardiogram (ECG) are monitored.

Keeping the tourniquet tight during the operation localises the LA and facilitates tissue binding. The injected LA diffuses from the vein into adjacent arteries and tissues, causing analgesia and muscle relaxation within 10–15 minutes; the whole limb distal to the cuff is thus anaesthetised, allowing major surgery. This technique is considered safer than a major nerve block of the upper limb. It is not used in children, who do not tolerate well the discomfort of the tourniquet, but is very useful in emergency situations – for example, treatment of Colles' fracture – and in developing countries.

In theory, Bier's block can also be used for the lower limb, but the large muscle masses in the leg make the method unsatisfactory in practice.

Nerve (conduction) block anaesthesia

In a **nerve block**, LA injected in the vicinity of a nerve trunk inhibits conduction of impulses to and from the area supplied by that nerve, the region of the operative site. A single nerve may be blocked, or LA may be injected where several nerve trunks emerge from the spinal cord (paravertebral block). During peripheral nerve block, motor nerves are usually blocked as well as sensory pathways. A concentrated solution is required because of the thickness of nerve trunk fibres; overall, less LA is needed than for the infiltration technique. This method of anaesthesia is often used for foot and hand surgery, eye surgery, obstetric procedures (pudendal block) and for postoperative pain relief.

Central nerve block: epidural and spinal anaesthesia

Epidural and spinal blocks are specialised central nerve blocks in which spinal roots are blocked where they emerge from the spinal canal. These techniques are used for abdominal, pelvic and lower limb surgery. Autonomic nerves may also be blocked, so there is a risk of autonomic adverse effects. To enhance analgesia, an opioid such as morphine, pethidine or fentanyl is often co-administered by these techniques. Central nerve block is contraindicated if there is systemic anticoagulation, coagulation abnormality or raised intracranial pressure.

Dermatome assessment

Dermatome assessment is used to monitor the level and extent of analgesia, using a standard dermatome chart (showing the areas of skin supplied with afferent nerve fibres by a single posterior root). Sensory block is assessed to ensure that the spinal/epidural/caudal LA is covering the patient's pain, and that the block is not so extensive as to cause complications. Since pain and temperature nerves are blocked similarly, reaction to temperature stimulation indicates that pain is still felt. Cold stimulation can be done with an ice-block on the skin, starting with an area away from the area likely to be affected (e.g. face or forearm), then testing areas likely to be blocked, plus areas above and below, to establish the level of block on both sides of the body. Anaesthetised areas are indicated on a dermatome chart – for example, R: T8–L1; L: T10–L2.

Epidural (extradural) anaesthesia

An epidural is an injection of LA into the space between the dura mater and the ligamentum flavum, at spinal cord levels C7–T10. The 'space' is actually filled with loose adipose tissue, lymphatics and blood vessels; LA solution tends to remain localised at the level where it is injected. Epidural anaesthesia is commonly used for obstetrics, urology and thoracic, abdominal and perineal surgery. The solution does not contact the spinal cord or CSF, so there is less risk of CNS infection than with spinal injection. The dose is determined by the number of spinal segments to be blocked. Postoperative urinary retention is common, due to blockade of parasympathetic nerves. To provide additional analgesia with epidural anaesthesia, ropivacaine 2 mg/mL is formulated with the opioid analgesic fentanyl (2 or 4 micrograms/mL).

Caudal anaesthesia is an epidural procedure in which the anaesthetic solution is injected into the caudal canal, the sacral part of the vertebral canal containing the cauda equina or the bundle of spinal nerves that innervate the pelvic viscera. It is used in obstetrics and for pelvic or genital surgery.

Spinal (subarachnoid) anaesthesia

In **spinal anaesthesia** (also called **subarachnoid**, intradural or intrathecal block), the LA is injected into the CSF in the subarachnoid space, below the level of termination of the spinal cord (i.e. at L3–4 or L4–5) and affects the lower part of the spinal cord and nerve roots. As the needle and solution come into contact with the CSF, sterility and aseptic procedures are essential to prevent infections such as meningitis. The onset of anaesthesia usually occurs within 1–2 minutes of injection; duration is 1–3 hours, depending on the anaesthetic used. Spinal anaesthesia is used for surgical procedures on the lower abdomen, inguinal area or lower extremities and is often the method of choice for elderly patients or those with severe respiratory problems or liver, kidney or metabolic disease, in whom GA is contraindicated. The specific gravity of the LA solution and the patient's position determine the level of anaesthesia: a solution with a specific gravity greater than that of CSF will tend to diffuse downward. The success and safety of spinal anaesthesia depend primarily on the anaesthetist's skill and knowledge.

Disadvantages of this method include marked hypotension, decreased cardiac output and respiratory depression due to depression of medullary centres and sympathetic pathways. Hypotension may be treated with sympathomimetic agents such as ephedrine or metaraminol. Postoperatively, headache is the most common complaint; it may be accompanied by difficulty in hearing or seeing, or may be postural and occur only in certain positions. Headache may be due to the opening in the dura made by the large spinal needle; the opening may persist for days or weeks, permitting loss of CSF and risk of infection (meningitis). Paraesthesias such as numbness and tingling may occur, usually limited to the lumbar or sacral areas and disappearing within a relatively short time.

Adverse drug reactions and drug interactions

Adverse drug reactions

Because LAs are potentially toxic drugs, dosage must be determined carefully. Adverse reactions can occur very quickly, so patients must never be left alone; equipment for resuscitation and airways management should be available. Most reactions to LAs result from overdosage, inadvertent IV administration and rapid absorption into systemic circulation or individual hypersensitivity or allergic response. Procaine is the least toxic LA and cocaine the most toxic.

Adverse reactions can be classified as:

- local complications at the site of injection – for example, inflammation, haematoma, nerve injury, abscess formation, necrosis
- psychogenic reactions – hyperventilation or vasovagal syncope (fainting) secondary to the injection stress (these may occur even before injection)
- adverse drug reactions specific to the individual LA – for example, prilocaine causing methaemoglobinaemia and cyanosis
- systemic effects of the vasoconstrictor – for example, sympathetic or central stimulation
- local effects of the vasoconstrictor, such as ischaemia, necrosis, gangrene
- reactions specific to epidural and spinal LAs – headache, hypotension, infections, neuropathies, paraesthesias and autonomic dysfunction
- allergies and hypersensitivity reactions such as rash, bronchospasm, anaphylaxis (more common with esters than amides; can also occur in response to preservatives in the solution)
- systemic effects of the LA after absorption – numbness of tongue, CNS stimulation (tremor, visual disturbances, irritability, convulsions, due to blockade of inhibitory pathways) then CNS depression, relaxation of smooth and skeletal muscle, cardiovascular and respiratory depression; hypotension and inhibition of sympathetic pathways contribute to the risk of fainting.

Adverse reactions may require treatment. For minor reactions, conservative resuscitation and first-aid efforts are effective. For major reactions, oxygen, assisted ventilation and IV infusion of fluids and drugs to counteract convulsions, cardiovascular and respiratory depression may be necessary.

Accidental overdose with an LA may prove fatal due to cardiotoxicity leading to cardiac arrest resistant to the usual resuscitation measures. IV administration of a lipid emulsion (e.g. Intralipid, normally used to provide parenteral nutrition) is an effective antidote, acting as a 'lipid sink' absorbing excess LA and counteracting toxic effects on the myocardium.

Significant drug interactions

Significant drug interactions and unexpected responses can occur (Drug Interactions 18.2), so close observation is needed.

Anaesthetics containing a vasoconstrictor are used with caution in patients receiving antihypertensives, monoamine oxidase inhibitors and tricyclic antidepressants, as the combination may produce hypertension.

Reversal of local anaesthesia

Recovery of sensation after local anaesthesia (administered plus a vasoconstrictor) can be accelerated by administration of phentolamine, an α-adrenoceptor antagonist (α-blocker). This is particularly important in dental practice, to reduce the number of soft tissue injuries in children from biting their lips or tongue, and to reduce difficulties eating, drinking and speaking. Phentolamine injected by infiltration into the same site as the LA overcomes the vasoconstriction, enhances the clearance of lidocaine (lignocaine) from oral tissues and markedly reduces the time to recovery of full lip sensation (not currently available in Australia or New Zealand) (Moore et al. 2008).

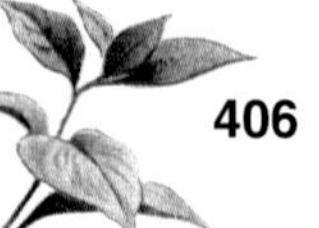

DRUG INTERACTIONS 18.2
Local anaesthetics

DRUG OR DRUG GROUP	LIKELY EFFECTS AND MANAGEMENT
Drugs that depress the cardiovascular system, including phenytoin	Additive cardiovascular depressant effects if LA is significantly absorbed; use LA cautiously and monitor effects
Antihypertensive agents	Enhanced hypotension with epidural or spinal LA
Drugs that predispose to methaemoglobinaemia (sulfonamides, primaquine, sodium nitroprusside)	Exacerbate methaemoglobinaemia from prilocaine; use cautiously
Drugs that cause dysrhythmias or prolong QT interval	Effects exacerbated by LA; avoid combination
Ciprofloxacin, fluvoxamine	Increase concentration, duration of action and toxicity of ropivacaine; avoid prolonged administration of the LA
Cimetidine, erythromycin, fluvoxamine, itraconazole, metoprolol, propranolol	May inhibit metabolism of lidocaine (lignocaine) and/or increase its concentration (depends on route of LA administration); monitor for effects and toxicity and decrease LA dose if necessary
Suxamethonium	Lidocaine (lignocaine) IV may decrease plasma cholinesterase activity and prolong muscle relaxation; monitor respiratory function
Anticholinesterase drugs	May inhibit the metabolism of ester-type LAs (procaine, cocaine)

KEY POINTS

Local anaesthesia

- Local anaesthesia is used to render a specific region of the body insensitive to pain.
- LAs such as lidocaine (lignocaine) inhibit action potential transmission in all excitable tissues, especially in sensory nerves, by blocking voltage-dependent sodium channels and interfering with the transient opening of these channels.
- The non-ionised form enters the cell by diffusion through membranes, where it readily becomes ionised and binds to a modulatory site in the voltage-dependent sodium channel.
- The drugs are said to be ion channel modulators or membrane stabilisers.
- The susceptibility of a nerve to LA action depends on the fibre diameter, myelination, tissue pH and length of nerve fibre exposed to LA solution. Autonomic and sensory fibres are blocked preferentially because they are thinner, unmyelinated and more easily penetrated by drugs.
- The LA drug acts locally in the tissue to which it is administered before being absorbed into the general circulation; ester-type agents are metabolised in the bloodstream and amides in the liver.
- A vasoconstrictor agent may be added to the solution to localise and prolong the action of the drug and minimise systemic adverse effects; adrenaline (epinephrine) is commonly used in the proportion of 1:200,000.
- Local anaesthesia is achieved by various techniques, including topical application or by subcutaneous infiltration of the selected operative area. Regional anaesthesia is the injecting of an LA drug near a peripheral nerve trunk (nerve block) or around the spinal column to anaesthetise spinal nerve roots (epidural or subarachnoid techniques).
- Adverse drug reactions to LAs include allergies (especially to ester-type drugs) and systemic depressant effects on the heart, CNS and respiratory system if large amounts of the drug are absorbed.
- Drug interactions occur particularly with other drugs that depress cardiovascular functions and with drugs that inhibit metabolism of LA agents.

DRUGS AT A GLANCE
Anaesthetics

PHARMACOLOGICAL GROUP AND EFFECT	KEY EXAMPLES	CLINICAL USE
Induction and maintenance agents (IV) Gases	Nitrous oxide (induction; inhaled)	• Adjuncts to inhaled anaesthetics • Induction and maintenance of anaesthesia • Conscious sedation • Day surgery procedures
Barbiturates • Modulate the binding of the inhibitory transmitter GABA to the $GABA_A$ receptor and increase duration of opening of Cl^- channels, producing inhibitory postsynaptic potentials and synaptic inhibition	Thiopental (IV)	
Non-barbiturates	Propofol (IV; induction and maintenance)	
Benzodiazepines • As above except increases frequency of opening of Cl^- channel, producing inhibitory postsynaptic potentials and synaptic inhibition	Midazolam, diazepam	Analgesia

Propofol • GABA receptors activation. It may also shorten channel opening times at nicotinic receptors and sodium channels in the CNS Dissociative anaesthetic • Non-competitive antagonist and allosteric modulator at NMDA receptors General anaesthetic	Ketamine (see also premedication)	Anxiety, induction of anaesthesia, premedication
Maintenance agents (inhaled general anaesthetics) Gases • General anaesthetic action may be mediated via opioid receptors • Hypnotic/anxiolytic action is mainly due to enhancement of GABA-mediated CNS depression • Anaesthetic action due to NMDA receptor inhibition	Nitrous oxide	Dental surgery, minor surgery, obstetric analgesia
Volatile liquid anaesthetics Proposed action at: • GABAA receptors • two-pore-domain potassium channels – opening of potassium channels • NMDA receptors that mediate slow components of synaptic transmission	Sevoflurane, desflurane, isoflurane, methoxyflurane	General anaesthesia for medical procedures
Adjuncts to anaesthesia Dexmedetomidine Acts on a_2- adrenoreceptors in the CNS to decrease noradrenergic activity		Procedural sedation and postsurgical and intensive care sedation of intubated patients
Premedications		Premedications allay anxiety (allows lower doses of anaesthetics); decrease secretions (salivary, gastric and bronchial); reduce postoperative vomiting; overcome CNS depression; and provide prophylactic analgesia and sedation.
Sedative–antianxiety agents Benzodiazepines • Modulate the binding of the inhibitory transmitter GABA to the $GABA_A$ receptor and increase frequency of opening of Cl^- channel, producing inhibitory postsynaptic potentials and synaptic inhibition Barbiturates • As above except increase duration of opening of Cl^- channel Ketamine (see under induction and maintenance agents)	Midazolam Thiopental	
Antisecretory agents Anticholinergics • Block muscarinic receptors on glandular tissues and decrease secretions H_2 receptor antagonists Block histamine receptors in GIT and decrease acid secretion	Atropine, hyoscine Cimetidine	
Analgesics Opioid analgesics • Act at μ-opioid receptors in descending pain pathways	Morphine, fentanyl, oxycodone	Sedation to decrease anxiety; provide analgesia (if required) and decrease amount of anaesthetic used
Skeletal muscle relaxants Competitive, non-depolarising relaxants • Blockade of nicotinic receptors at the NMJ preventing contraction of skeletal muscle Depolarising relaxants • Stimulation of nicotinic receptors at the NMJ and subsequent relaxation of skeletal muscles	Rocuronium Suxamethonium	• Inhibition of voluntary muscle tone and reflexes • Maintenance of skeletal muscle relaxation • Facilitation of intubation, mechanical ventilation

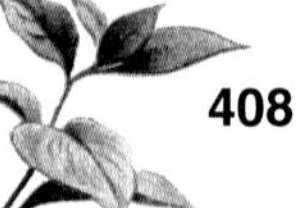

Antiemetics Dopamine antagonists Blockade of D_2 receptors in vomiting centre in CNS 5-HT antagonists • Specific and selective serotonin $5\text{-}HT_3$ receptor antagonist acts at vagus nerve and vomiting centre	 Metoclopramide Ondansetron	Postoperative nausea and vomiting
LOCAL ANAESTHETICS		Act particularly in sensory nerves to decrease the sensitivity to pain in surgical procedures and for pain relief
Esters • Prevent the generation and conduction of impulses in excitable membranes via blockade of sodium ion channels in the nerve	Procaine, tetracaine (amethocaine) Cocaine	
Amides As above	Lidocaine (lignocaine) Prilocaine	

REVIEW EXERCISES

1. Ms JC, a 40 year old, is undergoing a laparoscopic cholecystectomy. Her premedication includes fentanyl and glycopyrrolate and her induction agent includes rocuronium. Discuss the actions, mechanism of action and clinical uses of her:
   - premedication agents
   - neuromuscular-blocking drugs.
2. Ms PQ, a 10 year old, is undergoing a dental procedure at the local children's hospital. She is quite anxious about the procedure and her mother agrees to the use of nitrous oxide. Prior to the procedure the local anaesthetic, 5% lignocaine ointment is applied to the gum area surrounding the tooth and lidocaine (lignocaine) 2% is administered as an injection. Describe the properties of lidocaine (lignocaine) that lead to its being so commonly used. Why is it first administered topically? What are the mechanisms of action and durations of action of nitrous oxide and lidocaine (lignocaine)?

REFERENCES

Andrade R, Barnes NM, Baxter G, et al. 5-Hydroxytryptamine receptors (version 2019.4) in the IUPHAR/BPS Guide to Pharmacology Database. IUPHAR/BPS Guide to Pharmacology CITE. 2019; 2019(4). Available from: https://doi.org/10.2218/gtopdb/F1/2019.4.

Australian Medicines Handbook 2021, ***Australian medicines handbook 2021***, Adelaide, AMH.

Boron WF, Boulpaep EL: Medical physiology: a cellular and molecular approach, Updated edn, Philadephia, PA, 2005, Elsevier Saunders.

Bowman WC, Rand MJ: Chapters 7, 16. Textbook of pharmacology, ed 2, Oxford, 1980, Blackwell.

Calmes SH, Guedel A. MD and the eyes signs of anaesthesia. American Society of Anaesthesiologists Newsletter. 2002; 66(9):17–19.

Crilly H, Rose M: Anaphylaxis and anaesthesia: Can treating a cough kill? Australian Prescriber. 2014;37(3):74–76.

Hao X, Ou M, Zhang D, et al. The Effects of General Anesthetics on Synaptic Transmission. Current Neuropharmacology. 2020;18(10):936–965. doi: 10.2174/1570159X18666200227125854. PMID: 32106800; PMCID: PMC7709148.

Hemmings HC Jr, Riegelhaupt PM, Kelz MB, et al. Towards a Comprehensive Understanding of Anesthetic Mechanisms of Action: A Decade of Discovery. Trends in Pharmacological Science. 2019;40(7):464–481. doi: 10.1016/j.tips.2019.05.001

Ma S, Smith CM, Blasiak A, et al. Distribution, physiology and pharmacology of relaxin-3/RXFP3 systems in brain. British Journal of Pharmacology. 2017 May;174(10):1034–1048. doi: 10.1111/bph.13659. Epub 2016 Dec 4. PMID: 27774604; PMCID: PMC5406293.

Mason KP, Seth N. Future of paediatric sedation: towards a unified goal of improving practice. British Journal of Anaesthesia. 2019 May;122(5):652–661. doi: 10.1016/j.bja.2019.01.025. Epub 2019 Mar 2. PMID: 30916013.

Moore PA, Hersh EV, Papas AS, et al: Pharmacokinetics of lidocaine with epinephrine following local anesthesia reversal with phentolamine mesylate, Anesthesia Progress. 2008; 55:40–48.

Oberoi G, Phillips G: Anaesthesia and emergency situations: a management guide, Sydney, 2000, McGraw-Hill.

Salerno E: Pharmacology for health professionals, St Louis, 1999, Mosby.

Speight TM, Holford NHG, editors: Avery's drug treatment, ed 4, Auckland, 1997, Adis.

Therapeutic Goods Administration 2021. Changes to adrenaline and noradrenaline labels [online] Available at: https://www.tga.gov.au/changes-adrenaline-and-noradrenaline-labels [Accessed 9 Oct 2021].

Wu L, Zhao H, Weng H, et al. Lasting effects of general anesthetics on the brain in the young and elderly: 'mixed picture' of neurotoxicity, neuroprotection and cognitive impairment. Journal of Anesthesia. 2019 Apr;33(2):321–335. doi: 10.1007/s00540-019-02623-7. Epub 2019 Mar 11. PMID: 30859366; PMCID: PMC6443620.

Young L, Alexander B: The chemistry between us: love, sex and the science of attraction, New York, 2012, Current, Penguin.

ONLINE RESOURCES

New Zealand Medicines and Medical Devices Safety Authority: https://www.medsafe.govt.nz/ (medicine data sheets) (accessed 22 October 2020)

Waste anaesthetic gases: https://www.osha.gov/waste-anesthetic-gases (accessed 11 January 2022)

More weblinks at: http://evolve.elsevier.com/AU/Knights/pharmacology/.

CHAPTER 19

ANALGESICS

Shaunagh Darroch

KEY ABBREVIATIONS

5-HT	5-hydroxytryptamine (serotonin)
CNS	central nervous system
COX	cyclooxygenase
DOR	δ-opioid receptor
EO	endogenous opioids
GABA	gamma-aminobutyric acid
KOR	κ-opioid receptor
M6G	morphine-6-glucuronide
MOR	μ-opioid receptor
NMDA	*N*-methyl-D-aspartate
NSAID	non-steroidal anti-inflammatory drug
OR	opioid receptor
PG	prostaglandin

KEY TERMS

acute pain 412
adjuvant analgesic 435
analgesic 411
chronic pain 412
cyclooxygenase 430
endogenous opioids 418
endorphin 418
enkephalins 418
equianalgesic dose 423
gate control theory 418
neuropathic pain 412
nociceptive pain 413
non-steroidal anti-inflammatory drugs 430
opioid 421
opioid analgesic 420
opioid receptor 419
opium 421
pain 411
patient-controlled analgesia 437
prostaglandin 413
salicylate 430
stepwise management of pain 416
substance P 418
tolerance 423

Chapter Focus

Pain is a distressing and incapacitating symptom experienced by most people at some stage. Many chemical mediators are potentially involved. Pain can be classified depending on its aetiology and duration. Fortunately, the main analgesics currently available – opioids such as morphine and non-steroidal anti-inflammatory drugs including aspirin and paracetamol – are safe and effective when properly selected and administered, based on individual patient needs and responses and on individual drug's actions and pharmacokinetics.

KEY DRUG GROUPS

Adjuvant/adjunct analgesic medications:

- gabapentinoids (e.g. gabapentin, pregabalin)
- antiepileptic drugs
- psychotropics; tricyclic antidepressants (amitriptyline) and serotonin-noradrenaline reuptake inhibitors (duloxetine, venlafaxine)
- topical local anaesthetics (lidocaine [lignocaine])
- general anaesthetics (ketamine)

Non-steroidal anti-inflammatory drugs:

- **Aspirin**, ibuprofen, **paracetamol** (Drug Monograph 19.3)

Opioid analgesics:

- **Codeine**, **morphine** (Drug Monograph 19.1), **fentanyl** (Drug Monograph 19.2)

Partial agonists:

- **buprenorphine**

Opioid/SSRI activity:

- Tramadol

Opioid antagonists:

- **Naloxone**, **naltrexone**

Other analgesic drugs:

- **Capsaicin**, **clonidine**, **cannabinoids, methoxyflurane**

CRITICAL THINKING SCENARIO

A 4-year-old boy is brought to the emergency department with a swollen, painful and deformed left forearm after falling off a trampoline. He is otherwise in good health with no known allergies. He has a past medical history of infrequent episodic asthma. His weight is 19 kg. While in the waiting room, he is given a single oral dose of the hospital's combined paracetamol–codeine liquid preparation PainStop for Children, containing 120 mg of paracetamol and 5 mg of codeine phosphate per 5 mL. Clinical examination finds no additional injuries. Plain film x-rays reveal displaced mid-shaft fractures of his left radius and ulna, with a moderate degree of angulation. After fasting for 2 hours since his last snack of food or liquid, he has procedural sedation in the emergency department while the fractured bones are set in plaster. He makes a good recovery with rapid return to his normal conscious state; the attending doctor confirms good neurovascular supply to his hand as the plaster is setting and cooling, and the boy is discharged home.

His parents ask about pain relief for him for the next few days. They are reminded that immobilising and elevating the injured limb will provide initial analgesia (including overnight) and are given prescriptions for paracetamol 15 mg/kg qid and ibuprofen 10 mg/kg tds, regularly for 48 hours, then on a 'prn' basis. A review appointment is made with the fracture outpatients clinic for the following week.

Discuss the choice of medications for his pain.

Source: Acknowledgments to Dr Philippa Shilson, paediatrician.

Introduction

Pain is defined by the International Association for the Study of Pain as 'an unpleasant sensory and emotional experience associated with actual or potential tissue damage, or described in terms of such damage'. This definition emphasises the dual aspects of pain (sensory and emotional); only the person suffering can tell how much pain is being experienced. Pain is an important protective mechanism, warning of potential injury from the environment or from inside the body. Because of the differences in an individual's response to pain and the difficulties in measuring and describing pain, it is important that treatment focuses on the individual. There is increased recognition that sociopsychobiomedical (biopsychosocial) factors can worsen or prolong the pain experience, and pain can have an impact on these factors.

This chapter describes the classification of pain, its assessment, associated physiology, the main groups of analgesic drugs, non-pharmacological management and some general principles related to the treatment of pain. Pain management is a highly specialised and continually evolving area of medicine. The latest Australian *Therapeutic Guidelines: Analgesic* (2021) includes specific recommendations for first-choice drugs and dosing regimens in specific conditions: examples include acute pain (mild, moderate and severe), acute neuropathic pain, postsurgical pain, chronic pain (nociceptive with or without neuropathic pain), acute pain in opioid-tolerant people and procedure-related pain in adults. Indicated drugs and dosages suggested in this chapter are guidelines only; specialist advice or local protocols should be consulted and followed.

Pain and suffering

Understanding the actions of **analgesics** (pain-relieving drugs) requires first an understanding of how pain is generated. The physical component, the sensation of pain (nociception), involves peripheral and central nerve pathways; and the psychological component, the emotional response to pain, involves factors such as a person's anxiety level, previous pain experiences, age, sex and culture. Pain and suffering (a broader term referring to physical, emotional and spiritual aspects) may be addressed by interdisciplinary teams in pain management programs, hospices and palliative care centres.

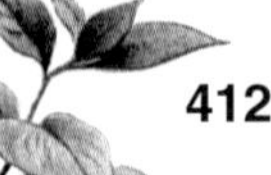

People have a relatively constant pain threshold; for example, heat applied to the skin at an intensity of 45–48°C will initiate the sensation of pain in most people. By contrast, pain tolerance – the point beyond which pain becomes unbearable – varies widely among individuals and in a single person under different circumstances. Pain tolerance is lowered (pain is made worse) by anxiety, anger, depression, isolation, fatigue, communication difficulties, previous pain experiences and adverse reactions to analgesic drugs. Tolerance to pain is increased by many medications (analgesics, anaesthetics, adjuncts; e.g. antianxiety agents, antidepressants) as well as by coping strategies such as distraction, sleep, rest and empathy from carers.

Pain classification

Pain can be classified in various ways: on the basis of its time course as acute or chronic (Table 19.1); or on the basis of its origin – that is, as nociceptive, neurogenic, psychogenic or nociplastic.

Acute pain

Acute pain, the sensation of severe discomfort, has a sudden onset usually with an obvious cause related to an injury, surgery or disease, and often has a protective function; it usually lasts only a short time and subsides with treatment. Examples include burn, acute myocardial infarction, or gall bladder or kidney stones. Treatment of acute pain is warranted to reduce the risk of chronic pain.

Progression to chronic pain is facilitated by neuronal plasticity, upregulation of *N*-methyl-D-aspartate (NMDA) receptors, hyperalgesic priming by inflammatory mediators or opioids, or nerve damage leading to **neuropathic pain**. Treatment of acute pain aims to prevent this and relieve suffering.

Chronic pain

Chronic pain, such as that accompanying cancer, osteo- or rheumatoid arthritis, is a persistent or recurring pain that continues for more than 3 months or after completion of healing, and may be difficult to relieve with simple pain treatments. Chronic pain has a significant impact on function and quality of life.

It is very common. A major health survey in New Zealand found that 19.6% of the population (one in five adults) experiences chronic pain; it was more prevalent in adults 55–64 years (one in five), in men than in women, in Māori than other Pacific/Asian people and in those from deprived areas (Ministry of Health 2020). Similar statistics are found in Australia, with approximately one in five Australian children and adults experiencing chronic pain, and this increases to one in three adults over 65 years of age.

People with chronic severe pain experience an adaptation process; they may become trapped within a chronic pain disability cycle in which ineffective treatments increase anxiety and contribute to pain persisting. The primary goal of treatment then becomes not total relief from pain, but minimisation of pain-related disabilities, improving coping skills and quality of life, and avoidance of unnecessary investigations and ineffective therapies. The principles of the 'analgesic ladder' (Fig 19.3, later) should be followed, with a multidisciplinary approach and regular reviews. The biopsychosocial aspects of pain should be taken into consideration and a multidimensionary approach should be undertaken.

TABLE 19.1 Comparisons between acute and chronic pain

	ACUTE PAIN	CHRONIC PAIN
Onset	Usually sudden	Long duration (> 3 months)
Characteristics	Generally sharp, localised, may radiate	Dull, aching, persistent, diffuse
Physiological responses	Autonomic responses: raised blood pressure, respiratory and heart rate; sweating, pallor, dilated pupils; increased muscle tension, tremor Long-term physical changes if no relief (e.g. changes in muscle mass, fatigue)	Often absent: normal blood pressure, respiratory and heart rates, and pupil size
Emotional/ behavioural responses	Increased anxiety and restlessness; focuses on pain, rubs affected part; cries, grimaces, protects part	Person may be angry, depressed, withdrawn, expressionless and exhausted; physical inactivity or sleep; no report of pain unless questioned Long-term without relief psychological changes (e.g. hyperalgesia) and social changes (adoption of a 'sick role', isolation, loss of employment)
Therapeutic goals	Cure of cause; relief of pain; prevent transition to chronic pain; sedation often desirable	Restore functions; tolerance of some pain; improve quality of life; sedation not usually wanted
Drug administration	NSAIDs and/or opioids: dependent on severity (mild, moderate, severe) and type (neuropathic or nociceptive)	Paracetamol, NSAIDs, opioids and/or adjuvants
Timing	Start as soon as possible; assess regularly; patient-controlled analgesia is useful	Regular preventive schedule
Dose	Standard dosages are often adequate; dose reviewed frequently	Individualise according to response
Route	Parenteral (IV or SC) or oral	Oral or transdermal

Chronic non-cancer pain

First-line therapy for pain encompasses social, psychological and physical activity with attention to sleep and nutrition.

As second-line therapy paracetamol, antidepressants and anticonvulsants are used; non-steroidal anti-inflammatory drugs (NSAIDs) should be avoided in older people, and opioids are reserved for pain unresponsive to other treatments. Parenteral and short-acting oral opioids should be avoided (Analgesic, Pain and Analgesia Expert Group 2020; Mills et al. 2019). (Treatment of cancer pain and palliative care are discussed in Ch 33.)

Indicators of effective analgesia include:

- improved analgesia
- increased activity
- improved affect
- limited or tolerable adverse effects of drugs
- no aberrant behaviours.

Nociceptive pain

Nociceptive pain is 'physiological' pain, arising from stimulation of superficial or visceral (deep) nociceptors by noxious stimuli such as tissue injury or inflammation.

- Somatic nociceptive pain originates especially in the skin, mucosal surfaces, bones and joints, pleura and peritoneum; it is usually well localised. It is described as being sharp, shooting, throbbing, burning, stinging or cutting. Examples are the pain from burns, wounds, arthritis, bony metastases of cancer or minor surgery. Somatic pain responds best to treatment with paracetamol and NSAIDs.
- Visceral nociceptive pain originates in the walls of visceral organs such as the liver and pancreas. It is described as being deep, aching, diffuse, cramping and nagging, and may be associated with nausea, vomiting or sweating. Examples include pain from bowel obstruction, ischaemic muscle or major surgery. The pain may be referred such as the pain of an acute myocardial infarction felt initially in the left arm or shoulder. Visceral pain usually responds well to opioid analgesics.
- Muscle spasm nociceptive pain originates in skeletal or smooth muscle, is mediated by **prostaglandins** (PGs) and is worse on movement or when smooth muscle is stretched (colic). It usually responds to muscle relaxants and NSAIDs.

Neuropathic pain

Neuropathic pain arises from a primary lesion or dysfunction in the somatosensory nervous system pathways, such as inflammation, trauma or degeneration, and occurs in post-herpetic neuralgia, trigeminal neuralgia and diabetic neuropathy. This pain is described as burning, shooting and/or tingling, is often associated with paraesthesia ('pins and needles'), hyperalgesia and allodynia (pain due to a stimulus that does not usually cause pain, such as pressure from clothing), and may be accompanied by sympathetic nervous system dysfunction.

Neuropathic pain responds less well to opioid analgesics or NSAIDs, and often requires the addition of adjuncts/adjuvants and other analgesics such as:

- a tricyclic antidepressant or a serotonin–noradrenaline (norepinephrine) reuptake inhibitor (Ch 22) to enhance noradrenaline- and 5-hydroxytryptamine (5-HT)-mediated descending inhibition of pain stimuli
- an anticonvulsant such as pregabalin or gabapentin to enhance gamma-aminobutyric acid (GABA)-mediated inhibition (Ch 21)
- a local anaesthetic such as lidocaine (lignocaine) to reduce sodium-channel-mediated transmission of nociception (Ch 18)
- tramadol, which has both opioid and selective serotonin reuptake inhibitor activities
- topical capsaicin, which gradually depletes substance P levels
- ketamine, a general anaesthetic and NMDA antagonist implicated in the afferent pathways (Ch 18).

Refer to adjuvant analgesics later in this chapter.

Specific pain syndromes

More specific types of pain are treated whenever possible with specific therapies (directed analgesia). Tension headaches, for example, usually respond to over-the-counter analgesics such as aspirin and paracetamol, while migraine headaches require specific vasoactive drugs such as sumatriptan (Ch 24). Dental pain and toothache usually require treatment of the underlying dental or oral disease; since most dental pain is caused by inflammation, NSAIDs are the preferred analgesics. Cancer pain relief requires a multimodal approach of palliative care (Ch 33), possibly involving analgesics and anaesthetics, other cancer therapies (radiotherapy, hormones, surgery, chemotherapy) and physical therapies.

Psychogenic pain has psychological, psychiatric or psychosocial causes as its primary aetiology: anxiety, depression and fear of dying have been known to cause severe pain. Drug therapy alone does not usually bring relief; a multimodal approach with psychotherapy is indicated.

Acute postoperative pain

Approximately 75% of patients who undergo surgery experience acute postoperative pain, which is often medium–high in severity. Severe pain is likely after joint replacement surgery, moderate pain after operations on the thorax or abdomen, and less severe pain after operations on limbs. Multimodal analgesic methods are recommended, appropriate for the person's level and type of pain, including opioids delivered by patient-controlled analgesia, local anaesthetic infusions, peripheral nerve blocks, and oral analgesics from different pharmacological groups – low dose clonidine and ketamine and lidocaine (lignocaine), paracetamol, NSAIDs, alpha-2 agonists and gabapentin/pregabalin (Horn & Kramer 2021; Yang et al. 2019). Treatment of acute pain is warranted to reduce the risk of chronic pain.

Breakthrough pain

Pain occurring between doses of regular analgesics in people with severe chronic pain is referred to as breakthrough pain or incident pain. It is usually managed with extra doses of short-acting oral (morphine liquid) or transmucosal (fentanyl lozenge) opioids. See the relevant expert texts.

Pain management

Assessment of pain

Measurement of clinical pain

As 'pain is what the patient says hurts', it is important to take a careful history and examination to assess the time course, type, site and extent of pain and its associations and effects. Pain assessment charts and scales are useful for monitoring pain intensity during treatment and to assess the need for ongoing analgesia. Doses are titrated depending on clinical responses and adverse effects; after opioid doses, depth of sedation indicates likely depth of respiratory depression. A Pain Assessment Chart or the 'PQRST' approach helps the patient describe the pain:

P: Palliative or provocative factors – What makes the pain better or worse?
Q: Quality – What is the pain like? Burning, nagging, shooting?
R: Radiation – Where does it hurt? Does the pain go anywhere else?
S: Severity – How severe is it? How much does it hurt?
T: Timing – Does the pain come and go? What brings it on? How long has it hurt?

With respect to locating the pain, a body chart such as that shown in Figure 19.1 (see 'I. Location: client or nurse mark drawing') can be helpful. For an estimate of the severity of the pain, scales such as those in Figure 19.2 help clients indicate the intensity and distress levels of the pain. Physical examination, with attention to tender spots, patient's responses to movement and stretch and non-verbal behaviours, helps accurate diagnosis. Regular reassessment of pain is essential, to monitor both the disease process and analgesic therapy, and to assess whether other therapy is required.

Pain assessment in children

Children are often inadequately treated for pain, resulting in needless suffering, due to an incorrect belief that children do not 'feel pain' in the same way that adults do. Assessing pain in young children is more difficult than in an older child or adult. Assessment should be based on the procedure or event that caused the pain and the child's non-verbal behaviour.

Pain in a child needs to be assessed in the context of the child's age, developmental stage, family and cultural situation and previous pain experiences. In infants and toddlers, observers can estimate pain by various scales taking into account behaviours, vital signs, sleep patterns and consolability. In older children, a pictorial scale can be used, with faces to 'show how much it hurts' (Fig 19.2, 'III. Faces Pain Scale').

General principles of pain management

Some important principles in pain management, based on the World Health Organization Guidelines on Analgesic Use and still current, are summarised below: Treat the cause of pain where possible, not just the symptom.

1 Make accurate assessment of pain extent and type to ensure appropriate analgesic prescription.
2 Keep the patient pain-free: patients recover faster if pain is anticipated and relieved, and they should not have to suffer pain before being allowed the next dose of analgesic. Analgesic effect should be optimised, starting with a low oral dose and titrating upwards depending on the patient's response and adverse effects. In prescription notation, the dose should be 'qs' (sufficient quantity) to prevent pain, not 'prn' (only when necessary).
3 Dose at regular specified intervals: particularly for chronic pain, analgesics should be given prophylactically on a regular basis to prevent pain, to optimise drug blood levels and analgesia and to reduce the conditioning reaction in which pain leads to drug-seeking behaviours (e.g. dose every 6 hours, not prn).
4 Avoid the chronic pain cycle, disability and 'sick role' by integrating analgesia into a comprehensive patient management plan with a multidisciplinary approach and involvement of a pain-control team if appropriate. An antidepressant may help stabilise sleep patterns and enhance analgesia, whereas sedatives may impair participation in pain management programs.

Access to opioid medications for pain control is an enormous problem worldwide. More than 80% (84.25%) of the world's population lacks adequate access to opioid medications for pain control. Australia, Canada,

Date: __________

Client's Name: __________ Age: _____ Room: _____

Diagnosis: __________ Physician: __________

Nurse: __________

I. Location: Client or nurse mark drawing

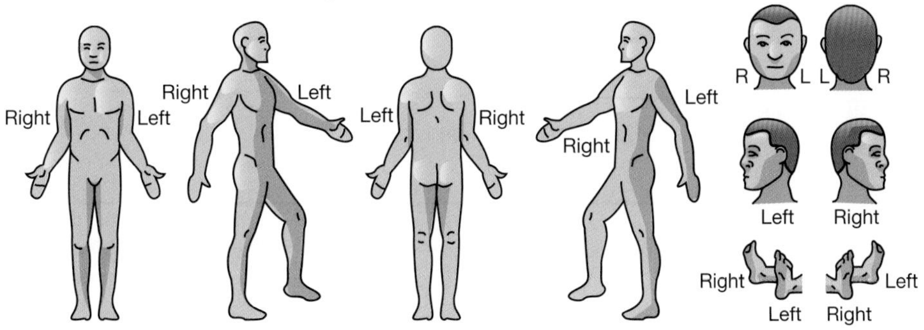

II. Intensity: Client rates the pain. Scale used: __________
- Present: __________
- Worst pain gets: __________
- Best pain gets: __________
- Acceptable level of pain: __________

III. Quality: (Use client's own words, e.g. prick, ache, burn, throb, pull, sharp): __________

IV. Onset: duration variations, rhythms: __________

V. Manner of expressing pain: __________

VI. What relieves the pain?: __________

VII. What causes or increases the pain?: __________

VIII. Effects of pain (note decreased function, decreased quality of life)
- Accompanying symptons (e.g. nausea) __________
- Sleep __________
- Appetite __________
- Physical activity __________
- Relationship with others (e.g. irritability) __________
- Emotions (e.g. anger, suicidal, crying) __________
- Concentration __________
- Other __________

IX. Other comments: __________

X. Plan: __________

FIGURE 19.1 Pain assessment chart

Source: Developed by McCaffery & Pasero 1999; from Salerno 1999.

New Zealand, the United States and several European countries accounted for more than 90% of the global consumption of opioid analgesics, while Low-and-Middle-Income Countries (LMICs) consumed only 10% of global opioids (Bhadelia et al. 2019).

Stepwise management

The analgesic ladder was first proposed by the World Health Organization in 1986 to provide adequate pain relief for those living with cancer. It is useful as a foundational model and as a simple guideline to pain management even

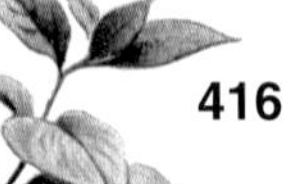

I. Pain Intensity Scale
0–10 Numerical Pain Intensity Scale*
0 No pain
1
2 Mild pain
3
4
5 Moderate pain
6
7
8 Severe pain
9
10 Worst possible pain
II. Pain Distress Scale
Simple Descriptive Pain Distress Scale*
None
Annoying
Uncomfortable
Bad
Dreadful
Agonising, unbearable
III. Faces Pain Scale
0 NO HURT
1 HURTS LITTLE BIT
2 HURTS LITTLE MORE
3 HURTS EVEN MORE
4 HURTS WHOLE LOT
5 HURTS WORST

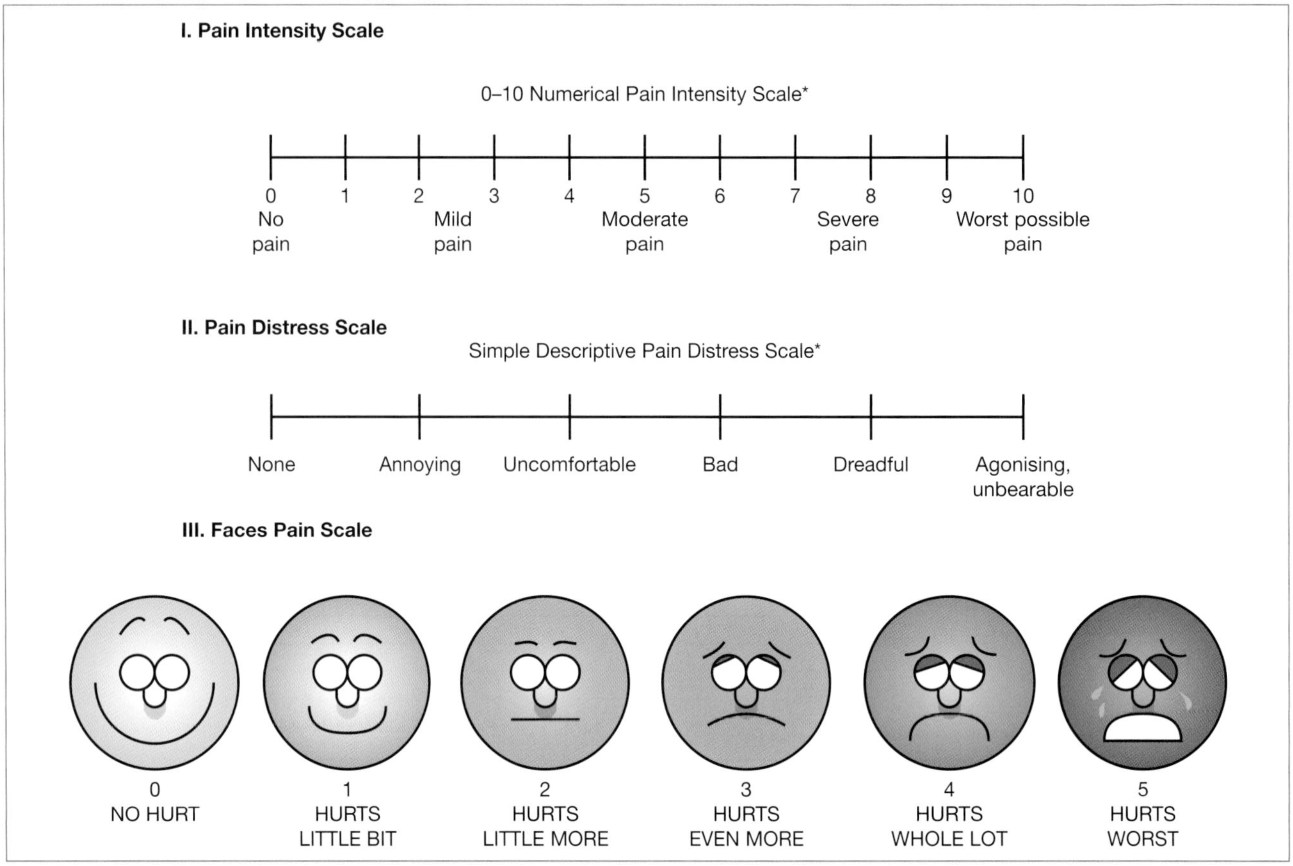

FIGURE 19.2 Scales for rating the intensity and distress of pain
In the Faces Pain Scale used for paediatric patients, the gradation in 'hurt' or 'pain' is explained to the child, with increasing pain shown from left to right; the child is asked to point to the face that shows how much she/he hurts now.
Sources: ***I:*** *Adapted from Salerno 1999;* ***II:*** *Adapted from Carr et al. 1992;* ***III.*** *Adapted from Wong et al. 2001; reproduced with permission.*

today. The original suggestion was that doses and types of opioid analgesics, for example, should be stepped up the 'analgesic ladder' (Fig 19.3) as required for increasing pain or development of tolerance. However, it is important to note that for the treatment of some types of pain (e.g. neuropathic), the ladder may not be entirely suitable. It may be important to adopt a therapeutic approach focused on the mechanisms of pain and the mechanisms of the drug and to adopt the biopsychosocial model of pain treatment. As examples, the tricyclic antidepressant amitriptyline may be used for migraine and small fibre pain and the antiepileptic topiramate used for chronic migraine. Also, it is important to note that the ladder should be bidirectional. See later Refer to expert texts (Anekar & Cascella 2021).

The stepwise management of pain is as follows:

- Step 1 – for mild pain, start with non-opioids (soluble aspirin [NSAID], paracetamol) with or without adjuvant drugs (dependent on specific circumstances; antidepressants, anticonvulsants, antipsychotics, antispasmodics).
- Step 2 – for mild to moderate pain, substitute or add an oral low dose opioid (codeine, tramadol).
- Step 3 – for moderate to severe pain use a strong opioid (morphine as slow-release tablets/capsules or IV or SC, fentanyl SC or patch, oxycodone; increase the dose of opioid, plus adjuvant drugs.
- Step 4 – adjuvants: invasive and minimally invasive treatment.

For opioids, prevent adverse effects of opioids rather than allowing them to occur and then treating them. Constipation commonly requires a bowel management program with attention to high-fibre diet, high fluid intake and laxatives. An antiemetic and analgesic may prevent the postoperative patient from vomiting and opening up a wound. Respiratory depression may be problematic in patients with asthma or chronic obstructive airways disease. Tolerance and dependence can occur even after 1 week on continuous opioid therapy, and higher doses may be needed. Addiction is not an issue in terminal care.

The original World Health Organization ladder was unidirectional, starting from the lowest step of NSAIDs, including COX-inhibitors and paracetamol and heading up towards the strong opioids and adjuvants, depending on the

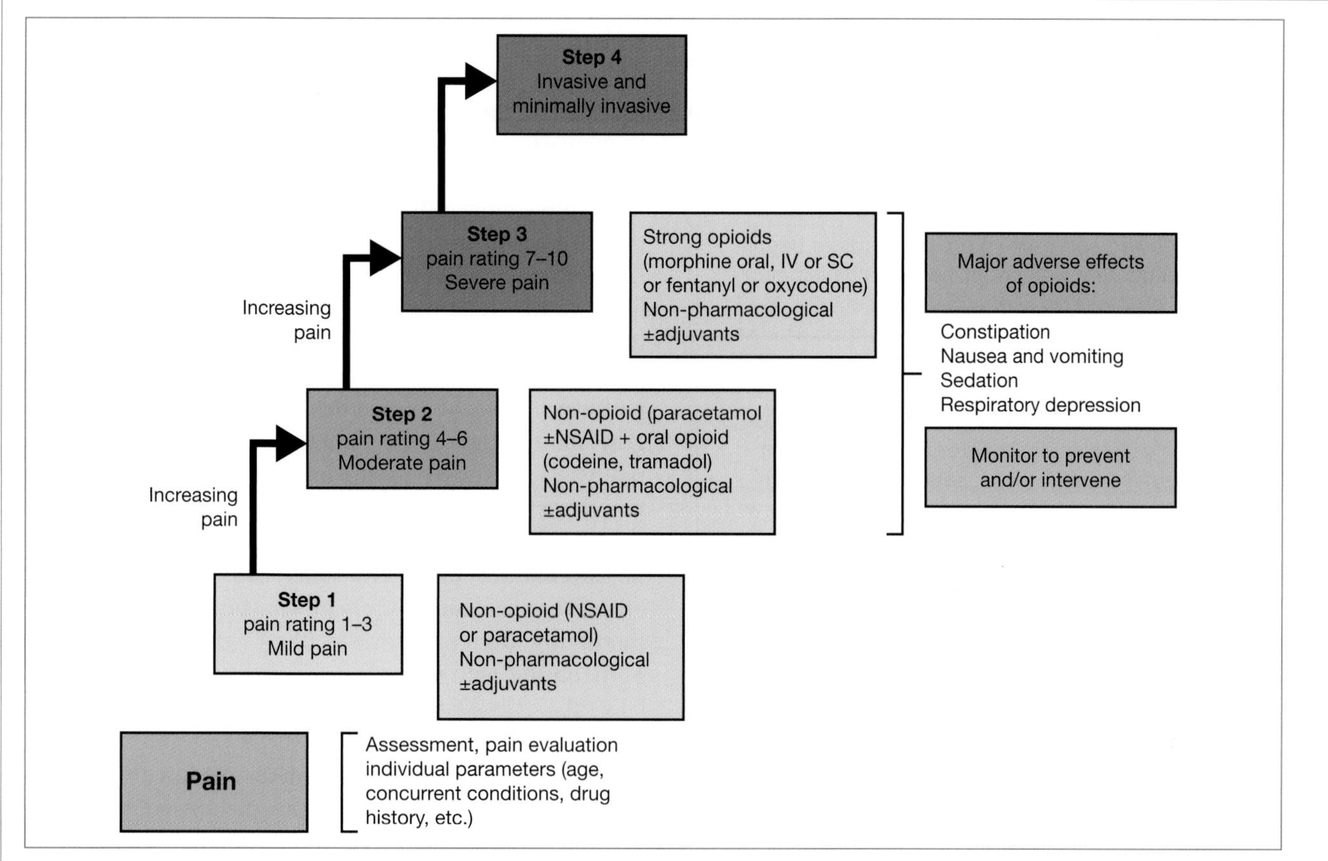

FIGURE 19.3 Flowchart for the 'stepwise' pharmacological management of pain

Analgesic dosage is commenced at the lower end of the range and is increased depending on the patient's responses. Adjuvants may include antidepressants, anti-inflammatories, antianxiety agents and local anaesthetics; non-pharmacological techniques include physiotherapy, acupuncture, psychotherapeutic methods and complementary and alternative therapies. IV = intravenous; NSAID = non-steroidal anti-inflammatory drugs; SC = subcutaneous

Sources: Adapted from Anekar et al. 2021; Salerno & Willens 1996; Therapeutic Guidelines Limited 2021.

patient's pain. The revised model (Fig 19.3) integrates a fourth step with interventional treatment involving invasive and minimally invasive treatment as above. It is also bidirectional, allowing for deprescribing. Neuropathic pain may require antidepressants or anticonvulsants, and specific drugs such as immune modulators are required in certain rheumatological clinical conditions.

Avoid under-treatment of pain

Despite healthcare providers being legally as well as morally responsible for pain relief, and although effective pain management techniques are available, many people still suffer pain. Some reasons for under-treatment of pain are summarised in Clinical Focus Box 19.1.

Endpoints of treatment

The aim of treatment is to maintain comfort for the patient, avoiding peaks and troughs of pain relief and relapses. When administration is initiated in hospital, the cessation date and/or date for review should be specified and a letter sent to the patient's general practitioner outlining a discharge and weaning plan. If adequate pain relief cannot be achieved, the patient should be referred to a multidisciplinary pain or palliative care clinic.

Physiology of pain

Neural mechanisms and the generation and transmission of pain (nociception)

As described above, pain is a subjective experience involving both physiological and emotional responses. Nociception, or the perception of noxious stimuli, is only one component of pain. There is much ongoing research into the physiological mechanisms of pain. Pain is detected by nociceptors (pain receptors). Tissue injury in the periphery releases many mediators, such as bradykinin, PGs, adenosine triphosphate and histamine, which can enhance or initiate firing of the nociceptive fibres (Fig 19.4). These nociceptive fibres are A-delta (δ) fibres (mediating sharp, transient, fast pain) or C-fibres (mediating burning, aching, slow, visceral pain). Signals are transmitted to the spinal cord via these primary (first-order) afferent fibres terminating in the dorsal horn of the spinal cord (substantia gelatinosa). Several neuropeptides

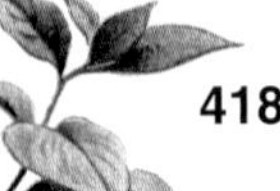

CLINICAL FOCUS BOX 19.1

Misconceptions about pain and pain management

Many mistaken ideas contribute to the mismanagement of pain:

- *Fear of inducing addiction to opioids* leads to people being inadequately treated for pain and developing a pattern of drug-seeking behaviours ('pseudo-addiction') to achieve adequate pain control. The risk of addiction in hospitalised patients with severe pain receiving opioids at regular intervals is minimal.
- *Tolerance to opioids* (the need to increase the dose of an analgesic to maintain the desired effect) is not usually seen in 'opioid-naive' patients with severe acute or chronic pain from a physical cause such as trauma, tumour growth or surgery; increase in pain is usually due to disease progression or complications.
- *Respiratory depression:* rarely develops if opioids are carefully prescribed and monitored; in patients with severe pain requiring very large doses of opioids, tolerance develops to respiratory depressant effects.
- *Under-assessment of pain severity* may lead to under-treatment, especially in children, women, elderly people and minority groups.
- *Inadequate reporting of pain* due to stoicism, dementia or other cognitive impairment leads to inadequate treatment.
- *Legal regulation of opioids* due to their potential for abuse and illegal diversion may limit prescribing, leading to under-treatment of pain even in patients with severe pain.
- *The wish to reserve strong analgesics for later use:* patients need to be reassured that it will be possible to treat more severe pain with higher doses and/or combinations of analgesic methods.

are released from neurons; **substance P** (a neurokinin) and calcitonin gene-related peptide are present, especially in nociceptive primary afferent neurons (Fig 19.4).

Voltage-gated calcium channels are opened, and the transmitter glutamate is released and crosses the synaptic gap, activating AMPA (at the first synapse). Activation of NMDA receptors is a slower response and associated with activity-dependent plasticity, a progressive increase in the response of dorsal horn nociceptive neurons to repeated stimuli. (Known as 'windup', this greatly increased sensitivity is associated with hyperalgesia.) The ascending nerve axons (second-order neurons) continue upwards in the anterolateral spinothalamic tracts (see the left-hand side of Fig 19.4) to the ventral and medial parts of the thalamus where they synapse with third-order neurons connecting to specific areas of the limbic system and somatosensory cortex, where the messages are perceived as pain.

Descending inhibitory controls: the gate control theory

Although there are further developments in the understanding of pain, the **gate control theory** of pain transmission put forward by Melzack and Wall in 1965 greatly enhanced the understanding of pain. It proposes that a physiologically analgesic spinal 'gate' mechanism in the dorsal horn of the spinal cord can modify the transmission of painful sensations from peripheral nerve fibres to the thalamus and cortex of the brain. The gate is influenced by descending inhibition from the higher centres of the brain: efferent anti-nociceptive (analgesic) pathways from the cortex descend via the periaqueductal grey matter down the spinal cord. (These descending pathways are shown on the left-hand side of Fig 19.4, and the descending pain control system in Fig 19.5.) The important transmitters in this pathway are 5-HT, noradrenaline, enkephalins and GABA. In the dorsal horn areas, they act directly on or via the short interneurons modifying afferent impulses, thus reducing transmission of incoming pain sensation.

Modulation of pain

Modulation of the chemical mediators involved in pain and the use of opioids are the mechanisms for many methods of pain relief. NSAIDs, local anaesthetics, GABA agonists, NMDA antagonists (cannabinoids, calcium-channel blockers [Kreutzwiser & Tawfic 2019]), α_2-adrenergic agonists and antidepressants are some of the drugs used. The individual drug classes will be discussed throughout this chapter.

Endogenous opioids

The **enkephalins** (pentapeptides), **endorphins** (larger polypeptides: the name implies '**end**ogenous m**orphin**es'), and dynorphins are all known as **endogenous opioids** (EOs). For example, the dynorphins ('powerful endorphins'), dynorphin A and dynorphin B, are stored in large vesicles in parts of the central nervous system (CNS) (hypothalamus, medulla, pons, midbrain and spinal cord) and have varying functions involved in analgesia, hypothermia, endocrine and reproductive functions, mood, learning and memory, control of appetite and other physiological functions. They are important natural analgesics, acting via κ-opioid receptors (KORs) and mediating analgesia, addiction, tolerance to opioids, drug-seeking behaviours and stress (Bodnar 2016) See Table 19.2, later.

There are precursors for EOs and other peptides. Pro-opiomelanocortin, a 241-amino-acid polypeptide, is a precursor in the body to a wide range of peptides: various cleavage stages produce melanocortins, lipotropins, corticotropin, endorphins and met-enkephalin. Other precursor polypeptides are proenkephalin, cleaved to met- and leu-enkephalin, adrenorphin and amidorphin; and

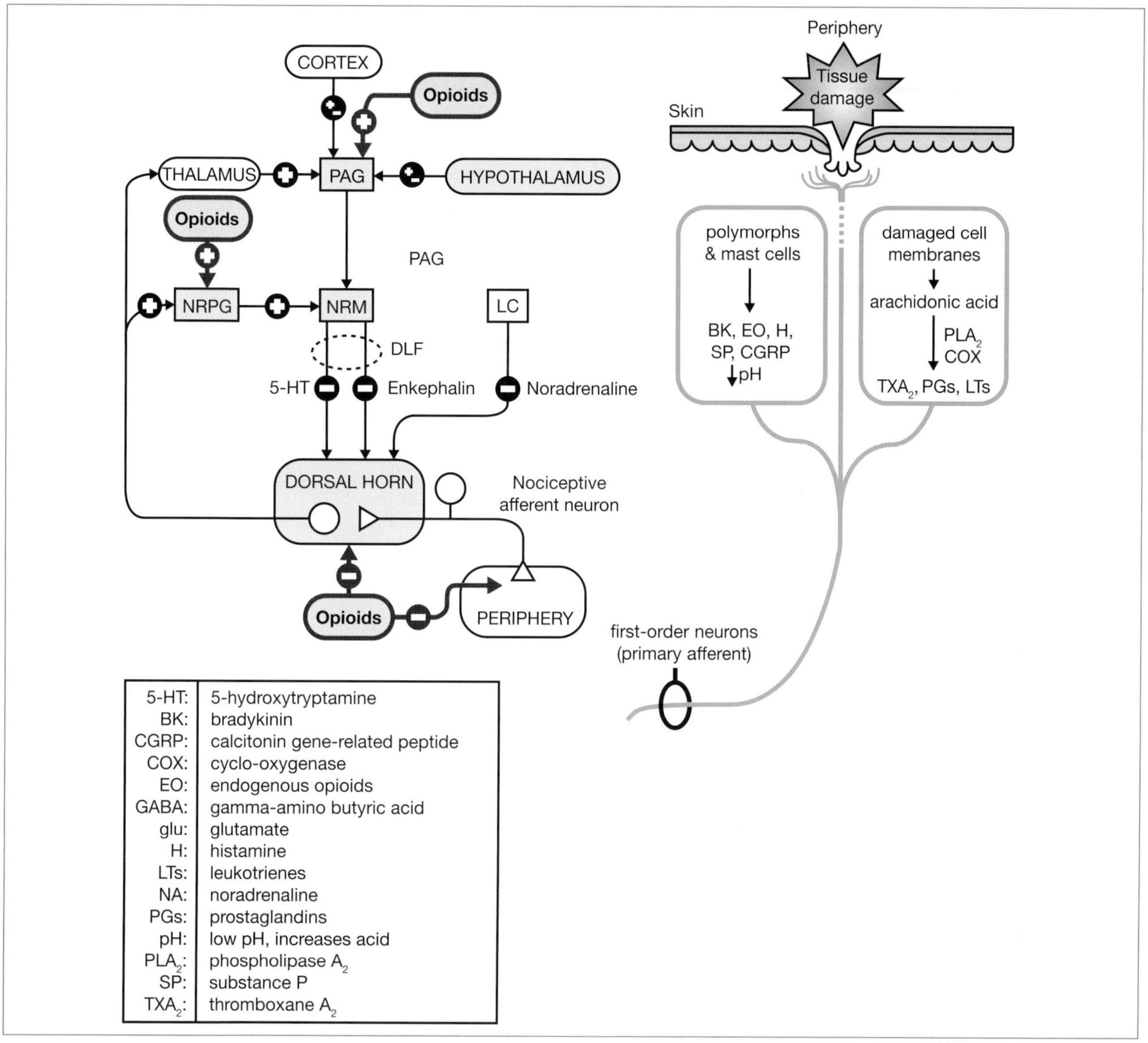

Periphery
Tissue damage
Skin
polymorphs & mast cells
BK, EO, H, SP, CGRP ↓pH
damaged cell membranes
arachidonic acid
PLA_2 COX
TXA_2, PGs, LTs
first-order neurons (primary afferent)
CORTEX
Opioids
THALAMUS
PAG
HYPOTHALAMUS
Opioids
PAG
NRPG
NRM
LC
DLF
5-HT
Enkephalin
Noradrenaline
DORSAL HORN
Nociceptive afferent neuron
Opioids
PERIPHERY

5-HT:	5-hydroxytryptamine
BK:	bradykinin
CGRP:	calcitonin gene-related peptide
COX:	cyclo-oxygenase
EO:	endogenous opioids
GABA:	gamma-amino butyric acid
glu:	glutamate
H:	histamine
LTs:	leukotrienes
NA:	noradrenaline
PGs:	prostaglandins
pH:	low pH, increases acid
PLA_2:	phospholipase A_2
SP:	substance P
TXA_2:	thromboxane A_2

FIGURE 19.4 Right-hand side: periphery – some mediators, neurotransmitters and nerve pathways involved in pain sensation Left-hand side: the descending control system, showing the main sites of action of opioids. 5-HT = 5-hydroxytryptamine; BK = bradykinin; COX = cyclooxygenase; DLF = dorsolateral funiculus of spinal cord; EO = endogenous opioids; H = histamine; LC = locus coeruleus; LTs = leukotrienes; NRM = nucleus raphe magnus; NRPG = nucleus reticularis paragigantocellularis; PAG = periaqueductal grey matter; PGs = prostaglandins; low pH = increasing acidity; PLA_2 = phospholipase A_2; SP = substance P; TXA_2 = thromboxane A_2

Sources: Adapted from Argoff 2011; Rang et al. 2007; used with permission.

prodynorphin (aka proenkephalin B), cleaved to dynorphins A and B, leu-enkephalin, nociceptin and neoendorphin.

There are high concentrations of **opioid receptors** (ORs) in many areas of the CNS involved in pain transmission or perception, at interneurons in the dorsal horn areas, particularly in the periaqueductal grey matter of the midbrain and in the limbic system. The substantia gelatinosa, for example, is rich in ORs and EOs. These areas are important sites of action for morphine-like drugs; the EOs act at the receptors to produce analgesia and other effects.

In early research on the actions of opiate drugs, pharmacologists spoke of actions at 'morphine receptors'; however, it is now recognised that morphine and other similar analgesics act at receptors for the body's EOs – that is, ORs – where they enhance inhibitory effects and thus mediate analgesia. Endorphin release in the body is stimulated by acupuncture and transcutaneous electrical nerve stimulation (and possibly by placebos), and effects of both may be reversed by the use of naloxone, an opioid antagonist.

Pain measurement in the laboratory

To test analgesic activity, there must be some standard (mild) pain stimulus. The traditional laboratory method was to place white mice gently onto a heated metal surface

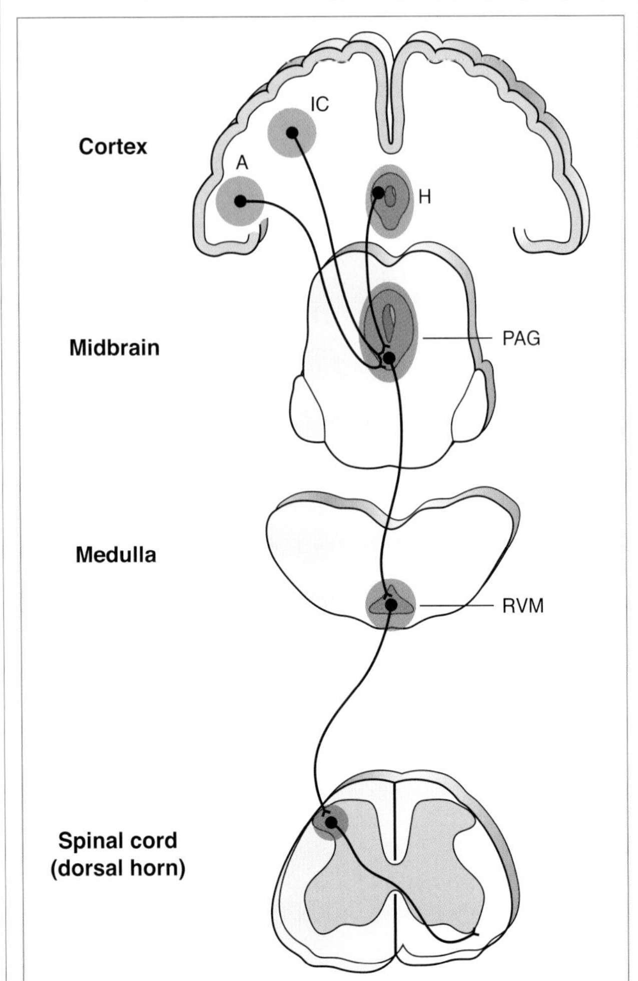

FIGURE 19.5 The descending pain control system and sites of action of opioids to relieve pain
A- = anterior cingulate cortex; IC = insular cortex; H = hypothalamus; PAG = periaqueductal gray; RVM = rostral ventromedial medulla

(a 'hot plate' at 55°C) and measure the time taken for the mouse to show some evidence of discomfort such as lifting or licking its paws or trying to hop off the plate. Groups of mice previously administered analgesics might show longer times before heat elicited a response. This method obviously raises ethical issues – should animals have to suffer pain for us (and them) to have access to better analgesic drugs?

A newer method with fewer ethical problems is that of the 'third molar model', in which (human) patients undergoing a standard dental procedure, extraction of third molars (wisdom teeth), are recruited into trials comparing new analgesics or new routes of administration without causing extra pain. This situation allows prospective clinical trials to investigate the onset, depth and duration of analgesic activity of drugs such as local anaesthetics and analgesics. Since patients may return subsequently for extraction of other wisdom teeth, cross-over studies may be possible, in which the patient acts as his/her own control (Christensen et al. 2008).

Prostaglandins and non-steroidal anti-inflammatories

Damage to tissue may directly activate sensory nerves and also sets in train the process of inflammation (Fig 19.4), in which inflammatory mediators are released – so many that this has been referred to as the 'inflammatory soup'. Of particular importance in pain mechanisms is arachidonic acid, produced from damaged cell membranes and metabolised by the cyclooxygenase (COX) enzyme system to the tissue hormones; example PGs, which lower the threshold of nociceptors to other mediators (discussed in greater detail in Ch 34). The second main group of analgesic agents, the NSAIDs, inhibit production of PGs (see later).

KEY POINTS

Pain

- Pain is a common health problem, with sensory and emotional components contributing to suffering that disables and distresses people.
- Pain may be classified by its time course and origin, and assessed by its severity.
- Clinical principles of pain management emphasise the importance of adequate, regular doses of appropriate analgesics, stepping up the analgesic ladder as necessary with adjunctive care.
- Assessment tools, pain scales and clinical guidelines are the basis for an effective pain management program.
- Pain is often inadequately or inappropriately treated because of attitudes, fears and biases of health professionals, patients and family.
- Physiological theories of pain involve mediators of pain, including PGs, nociceptors, ascending afferent pathways of sensory nerves and substance P, spinothalamic tracts, and descending efferent pathways from the cortex which modulate dorsal-horn 'gating' mechanisms.

Analgesic drugs

Opioid analgesics

Opioids are the first main group of pain-relieving drugs discussed in this chapter. Morphine, a natural alkaloid present in opium, is still the 'gold standard' **opioid analgesic** most commonly used clinically. The actions and clinical uses of morphine are described as the prototype opioid analgesic (Drug Monograph 19.1, later); other opioids will be mentioned briefly, highlighting the main aspects in which they differ from morphine.

History and background

Opium is the dried extract of seed capsules of the opium poppy *Papaver somniferum* (meaning 'the poppy bringing sleep'). Opium contains many pharmacologically active alkaloids (nitrogenous compounds), including morphine, codeine and papaverine. The term 'opiate' strictly refers only to opium derivatives, whereas '**opioid**' means any opium-like compound and includes endogenous pain-relieving substances as well as synthetic drugs mimicking opiates.

The medicinal effects of opium have been known in many cultures for over 6000 years. Opium (which contains 8–14% morphine) was almost literally 'the panacea for all ills', as it is effective against pain, diarrhoea, cough and sleeplessness. A Latin synonym for opium preparations was 'laudanum', meaning 'praiseworthy'. Opium was widely advertised and available well into the 20th century for even mild conditions such as coughs and infants' teething pains.

Opium preparations were standardised in terms of their morphine content (see 'Standardisation of drugs' in Ch 1). It is now considered preferable to administer pure forms of single drugs (e.g. morphine) rather than crude extracts (opium) that contain varying amounts of several active ingredients plus unknown amounts of contaminants.

Narcotic analgesics

The term 'narcotic' has also suffered misuse and confusion: literally, it means a compound causing numbness or stupor; hence, 'narcotic analgesics' was the group name for the morphine-like drugs, which cause pain relief with sedation, to distinguish them from the non-narcotic (aspirin group) analgesics. (Morphine was named after Morpheus, the Greek god of sleep and dreams.) The term 'narcotic' was later extended to refer to all drugs causing addiction and likely to be abused, so it now includes stimulants such as cocaine as well as sedatives such as morphine. The term is probably best avoided in the medical context. Because of their addictive potential, opium and opioids are tightly controlled worldwide. Most opioids (except low-dose codeine, pholcodine, diphenoxylate and tramadol preparations) are 'Controlled Drugs' (Schedule 8) in Australia and New Zealand, requiring strict controls on storage and supply.

Mechanism of action of opioids

The mechanism of the analgesic action of opioids is still not totally clear despite decades of intensive study. The gate control theory of pain goes some way to describing the mechanism of action of the opioids. At the spinal cord level, stimulation of ORs inhibits release of substance P from dorsal horn neurons, and opioids act to 'close the gate' in the dorsal horn, thus inhibiting afferent transmission (see Fig 19.4 earlier).

At supraspinal levels, opioids activate ORs widely distributed in the CNS, especially in the limbic system, thalamus, hypothalamus and midbrain. Pain perception and emotional responses are altered; thus, people have reported they could still feel the pain, but it no longer worried them (Bannister & Dickenson 2020).

Opioid receptors

Endogenous opioid peptides involved in nociception and sensory pathways have been described earlier. High-affinity binding sites for the enkephalins, endorphins and dynorphins are widely located in the CNS (also in peripheral tissue, especially in the gut) and respond to various opioid agonists. On the basis of their actions at ORs, drugs may be classed as opioid agonists (natural or synthetic agents that have a full morphine-like effect), antagonists or partial agonists such as buprenorphine, having a less than maximal effect at μ (mu) receptors.

ORs are G-protein-coupled trans-membrane receptors, activation of which inhibits adenylate cyclase and reduces cyclic adenosine monophosphate (cAMP) levels. G-protein coupling also promotes opening of potassium channels and inhibits opening of calcium channels, which reduces neuronal excitability and inhibits release of excitatory (pain) transmitters, leading to inhibitory effects at the cellular level. Effects that appear to be excitatory are probably actually due to suppression of firing of inhibitory neurons. Tolerance to opioid effects may be due to both a gradual loss of inhibitory functions and an increase in excitatory signalling. Withdrawal effects may be due to a rebound increase in cAMP formation activated via delta ORs by chronic administration of opioid.

Opioid receptor subtypes

Subtypes of ORs are classified by responses to different agonists and antagonists (just as there are several subtypes of noradrenaline receptors). The main CNS ORs are named by the Greek letters μ (m; mu), κ (k; kappa) and δ (d; delta): MOR, KOR and DOR, respectively (Borsodi et al. 2019). Analgesia and constipation have been associated with all three receptors, while euphoria (feeling good) is associated mainly with actions at MOR, and dysphoria (feeling bad) with actions at KOR. What were formerly thought to be specific sigma (σ) OR are now considered general 'psychotomimetic receptors', associated with unwanted effects such as dysphoria, hallucinations and confusion.

Agonists and antagonists

The agonist analgesics (e.g. morphine, pethidine) activate both the μ and the κ receptors, while partial agonist agents such as buprenorphine activate one type of OR (μ receptors; agonist effect) and have minimal effects on other

TABLE 19.2 Opioid receptor responses

RECEPTOR	DRUG EXAMPLES	RESPONSE
mu (μ) MOR	*Strong agonists:* morphine, hydromorphone, fentanyl, methadone, β-endorphin *Partial agonist:* buprenorphine *Weak agonist:* pethidine	Supraspinal analgesia, euphoria, respiratory depression, sedation, constipation, miosis, drug dependence
	Antagonists: naloxone, nalorphine, naltrexone	Reverses opioid effects, induces acute withdrawal in opioid dependency
kappa (κ) KOR	*Agonists:* morphine, β-endorphin, dynorphins *Little or no activity:* methadone (partial agonist), pethidine	Spinal and peripheral analgesia, sedation, miosis, dysphoria, respiratory depression
	Antagonists: naloxone, naltrexone, buprenorphine	Reverses opioid effects, induces acute withdrawal in opioid dependency
delta (δ) DOR	*Agonists:* enkephalins, β-endorphin, tramadol	Spinal analgesia, respiratory depression, constipation; neuroprotection, cardioprotection
	Antagonist: naltrexone, naloxone, buprenorphine	Reverses opioid effects, induces acute withdrawal in opioid dependency

receptors. They may induce undesirable effects. Pure antagonists (naloxone, naltrexone) antagonise all ORs. A summary of OR responses is shown in Table 19.2; the situation is complicated by the fact that some drugs show varying effects in different tissues or species.

Pharmacological effects of opioids

Considering the widespread distribution of ORs in peripheral and central tissues, it is not surprising that opioids have a broad spectrum of actions. (Aspects of opioid actions relevant to drug dependence and social pharmacology are discussed in Ch 25.)

Central effects

Effects of opioids in the CNS include:

- analgesia – the main clinical use
- suppression of the cough reflex – another useful effect (e.g. codeine or pholcodine cough linctuses)
- suppression of the respiratory centre in the medulla – a major adverse effect leading to toxicity; the commonest cause of death from overdose
- sedation and sleep, hence the term 'narcotic analgesics'; a useful clinical effect if pain is keeping the patient awake, but not helpful with daytime activities
- euphoria, the feeling of contentedness and wellbeing, which contributes to the analgesic actions and dependence
- dysphoria (unpleasant feelings, hallucinations, nightmares)
- miosis (pupillary constriction); 'pinpoint pupils' are a diagnostic sign of an opioid-dependent person
- nausea and vomiting – mediated through the chemoreceptor trigger zone; tolerance develops to these effects
- prolongation of labour – not usually a problem clinically
- hypotension and bradycardia occurring after large doses, mediated via the medulla
- tolerance and dependence or addiction, mediated by μ receptors; tolerance develops after a few doses of morphine; physical dependence is shown by a marked withdrawal syndrome after doses are missed for 1–2 days.

Peripheral effects

Effects of opioids in the peripheral nervous system include:

- significant analgesic and anti-inflammatory effects in peripheral inflamed tissues
- actions via ORs in the gut, leading to decreased motility and increased tone in smooth muscle; severe constipation is a common adverse effect; these effects may be useful in treating diarrhoea – the antidiarrhoeal agent loperamide is a mild opioid (Ch 16)
- spasms of sphincter muscles, which can lead to delayed gastric emptying, biliary colic or urinary retention
- suppression of some spinal reflexes
- release of histamine, causing bronchoconstriction and severe itching.[1] (This effect of morphine is not mediated by ORs; it is via a direct action on mast cells.)

Adverse drug reactions and drug interactions

The most serious adverse effects of opioids are respiratory depression, excessive sedation, dysphoria, constipation, nausea and vomiting, tolerance and dependence. The cause of death from acute toxicity after an overdose of an opioid such as heroin is usually respiratory failure.

1 The sensation of having ants crawling over the body, known as formication – a word that has to be pronounced and spelt carefully!

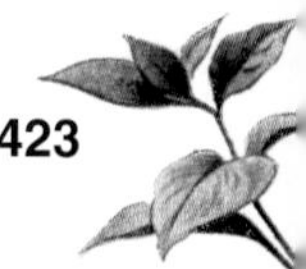

Tolerance to opioid analgesics

Drug **tolerance** is defined as the gradual decrease in the effectiveness of a drug given repeatedly over a period of time.

If tolerance develops, higher doses are required to achieve the same effect. Morphine and other opioids are classic examples of drugs to whose effects tolerance develops: prolonged administration causes cellular adaptations leading to tolerance and dependence, and also opioid-induced hyperalgesia, the mechanisms of which are still not well understood (Srivastava et al. 2020).

If tolerance is not recognised and higher doses are not given, tolerant patients may be under-treated. The dose of an opioid may therefore be gradually increased to large amounts (doses potentially fatal in 'opioid-naive' people) to control increasing pain in those living with cancer without producing severe respiratory depression or excessive sedation.

Tolerance usually develops to the analgesic effects and to sedation, nausea and vomiting. Unfortunately, tolerance does not develop to the accompanying constipation, confusion, nightmares and hallucinations, so these adverse reactions may become more of a problem as doses are increased; laxatives should be taken prophylactically from the start of treatment.

A change to another opioid (e.g. fentanyl or methadone) sometimes minimises the adverse CNS effects. (Treatment of chronic pain is a specialised aspect of pain management: see Pain and analgesia Expert Group 2020 for protocols.)

Pharmacokinetic aspects

Opioids generally are not well absorbed after oral administration and have a low and variable bioavailability due to extensive first-pass metabolism in the liver.[2] Even after parenteral administration, there is variability in plasma concentrations, metabolism and rates of elimination, so doses need to be individualised.

People with liver damage may accumulate the active drug and are very sensitive to the depressant effects of opioids. Renal disease can extend the half-lives of opioids that are excreted in an active form and cause respiratory depression, especially from methadone, morphine-6-glucuronide (M6G – an active metabolite of morphine) and norpethidine. Codeine is not recommended as a first-choice analgesic as it is a prodrug (Ch 5) subject to variable metabolism.

Morphine is not highly protein-bound (35%) and is relatively hydrophilic, so it crosses only slowly into the CNS. By comparison, fentanyl and its analogues are highly lipophilic and so have rapid onset and short duration of action and can be administered transdermally.

In the elderly and in infants under 1 year, doses need to be reduced because of increased CNS sensitivity and decreased clearance. In patients with hypovolaemia (e.g. from burns or trauma), intramuscular medications are poorly absorbed.

Equianalgesic dosing

Some patients experience intolerable adverse effects from a particular opioid agent and need to be switched to a different analgesic. Doses of other opioids are compared with standard morphine 10 mg IM/IV/SC or 30 mg orally, and quoted in terms of **equianalgesic doses** – see Table 19.3. Switching requires careful assessment of pain levels, adverse effects and tolerance that has developed. It is recommended that the initial dose of the new agent should be only half of that indicated by comparing doses, as tolerance developed to the previous agent may not fully extend to the new agent. (Note that switching from morphine to methadone is complicated and expert advice should be sought; see Australian Medicines Handbook 2021.)

Drug interactions with opioids

Some clinically important drug interactions occurring when morphine or other opioids are given with concomitant drugs are listed in Drug Interactions 19.1.

Opioid receptor agonists

Morphine

Morphine is the prototype opioid analgesic; all new analgesics are compared with morphine for potency and for therapeutic effects or adverse reactions, particularly in the palliative care situation. Morphine is available in many dosage forms, including injection, oral mixture, modified-release capsules and tablets (Drug Monograph 19.1); and slow-release epidural injection.

Other opioids

Codeine

Codeine (see Ch 15 in the context of use for cough) is absorbed well after either oral or parenteral administration. Codeine, the 3-methyl ether of morphine, is actually a prodrug, being rapidly metabolised in most people to morphine (by CYP2D6). Inter-individual variation in pharmacokinetics leads to variable effectiveness, so codeine is not generally recommended. Constipation is a frequent adverse effect and may limit clinical usefulness.

Codeine is often combined with a non-opioid analgesic such as aspirin, paracetamol or ibuprofen in compound analgesic tablets to provide stronger relief than the NSAID alone can achieve; however, misuse of combination products can lead to toxicity. Since 1st February 2018, medicines that contain low-dose codeine are no longer available without prescription.

Fentanyl

Fentanyl, a very potent opioid with a good adverse-effect profile, has become popular for use as a component of

2 Hence, opium was traditionally smoked; while on the street scene, morphine and heroin are usually injected ('shot up') – an interesting example of pharmacokinetic principles being applied in everyday practice.

TABLE 19.3 Selected opioid dosage forms

DRUG/DOSE FORM	USUAL DOSE	FREQUENCY OF ADMINISTRATION (HOURLY OR PER DAY)	NOTES
Morphine			The 'gold standard'; analgesic for severe pain, acute and chronic pain; has an active metabolite M6G
Oral solution	5–20 mg	4-hourly	30 mg oral morphine is considered equivalent to 10 mg parenteral morphine
Tablets	15–30 mg	4–6-hourly	
CR tablets	5–30 mg	12-hourly	
IM/SC/IV	0.5–10 mg 5–20 mg (MIMS)	4–6-hourly	
Epidural, IT	100–200 micrograms intrathecal 2–3 mg epidural	12–24-hourly	Slow-release form for anaesthetist-only use in hospital; patient requires close monitoring for 48 hours
Buprenorphine			For chronic pain or opioid dependence; slow onset; partial agonist, low dependence liability
IM, IV	0.3–0.6 mg	6–8-hourly	Also 8 mg and 16 mg oral fast-dissolving tablets
Sublingual film	0.4, 2 and 8 mg	6–8-hourly	
Transdermal patch	5, 10, 15, 20, 25, 30 and 40 micrograms/h	Every 7 days	For moderate-to-severe pain
Codeine			Weak opioid, metabolised to morphine; for mild-to-moderate pain; cough suppression; diarrhoea
Oral Linctus	30–100 mg 5 mg/mL	4–6 hourly maximum 240 mg in 24 hours	Combination formulations contain sub-therapeutic doses
Fentanyl			Highly potent (dosed in micrograms); for moderate-to-severe pain, during anaesthesia, chronic pain, breakthrough pain. Note: various preparations are not equivalent.
Orally disintegrating	100, 200, 300, 400, 600 and 800 micrograms		
Sublingual tablets	100, 200, 300, 400, 600 and 800 micrograms		Sublingual tablets: Initial dose may be repeated after 30 minutes if necessary (but 2 hours should elapse before retreatment of breakthrough pain)
SC/IV, epidural (obstetric analgesic slow IV), IT	50–100 micrograms	1–2 hourly	
Transdermal patch	12–100 micrograms/h	Every 3 days	Patches release 12–100 micrograms/h; not for opioid-naive
Lozenge ('lollipop')	200–1600 micrograms	6–8 hourly. Max. 4 doses per day	Absorbed via buccal mucosa; for breakthrough pain and children
Intranasal	Child 1.5 microgram/kg to max. 100 micrograms		If needed second dose of 0.75–1.5 microgram/kg to max. of 100 micrograms may be given after 5–10 minutes
Hydromorphone			Less sedative
Oral:			Morphine 30 mg oral is equivalent to 6 mg hydromorphone
Solution	1 mg/mL dose 2–4 mg	4-hourly	
Tablets	2, 4 and 8 mg	4-hourly	
CR tablets	4, 8, 16, 32 and 64 mg	Every 24 hours	
IM/SC/IV	1–2 mg	4–6-hourly	Morphine 10 mg IM/SC is equivalent to hydromorphone 1.5–2 mg IM/SC
Methadone			Severe postoperative or chronic pain; maintenance of dependence; long half-life, so risk of accumulation
Oral:			
Tablets	5–10 mg	6–8 hourly, short term Chronic: max. 12 hourly	
Syrup	5 mg/mL dose 10–20 mg (max. 80 mg) per day	6–8 hourly, short term Chronic: max. 12 hourly	
IM/IV/SC	5–10 mg	6–8-hourly	
Oxycodone			Oral bioavailability variable, 50–90%
Oral:			
Tablets	5 mg only	6-hourly	
CR tablets	10, 20, 30, 40 and 80 mg	12-hourly	CR formulations have longer duration of action (12–24 h)

TABLE 19.3 Selected opioid dosage forms—cont'd

DRUG/DOSE FORM	USUAL DOSE	FREQUENCY OF ADMINISTRATION (HOURLY OR PER DAY)	NOTES
Capsules	5, 10 and 20 mg	4–6-hourly	
Liquid	5 mg/5 mL Dose 5 mg	4–6-hourly	
SC	2.5–10 mg	4–6-hourly	1 mg parenteral = 2 mg oral
Slow IV	Dose 1–5 mg (max. 10 mg)	4-hourly	
Rectal	30 mg	6–8-hourly	Rectal bioavailability also variable
Pethidine			Risk of excitement, poor oral efficacy; useful in labour, renal and biliary colic pain; interactions with drugs affecting 5-HT levels
IM/SC	25–100 mg	3–4-hourly	
Slow IV	25–50 mg	3–4-hourly	
Epidural	25–50 mg	Single dose duration of action 2–5 hours	Obstetric analgesia
Tramadol			Weak opioid; moderate-to-severe pain; monoamine uptake inhibitor, useful for neuropathic pain; low misuse potential
Oral:			
Capsules	50–100 mg	4–6-hourly	
CR formulation	100, 150 and 200 mg	12–24 hours	
IM, IV	50–100 mg	Every 12 hours hourly	

CR = controlled-release; IM = intramuscular; IT = intrathecal; IV = intravenous; SC = subcutaneous
Note: Doses need to be titrated depending on age, level of pain, tolerance and renal or hepatic impairment; doses for high-potency opioids buprenorphine and fentanyl are in micrograms or fractions of a mg.
Source: Adapted from information in MIMS Online and Australian Medicines Handbook 2021.

DRUG INTERACTIONS 19.1
Opioids

DRUG	POSSIBLE EFFECTS AND MANAGEMENT
Alcohol or other CNS depressants (other opioids, anaesthetics, sedatives, psychotropics)	May result in enhanced CNS depression, respiratory depression and hypotension. Reduce dosage and monitor closely.
Buprenorphine (partial agonist)	May result in additive effect of respiratory depression if given concurrently with low doses of μ- or κ-receptor agonists; avoid concurrent usage. Partial agonists given with an opioid agonist may reduce the analgesic effects of the full agonist or precipitate withdrawal symptoms.
Monoamine oxidase inhibitors (MAOIs) (phenelzine, tranylcypromine; moclobemide and selegiline)	Intensify the effects of opioids (especially pethidine, tramadol and fentanyl) and may cause serotonin syndrome.[3] Caution should be exercised and dosages of opioids reduced.
Opioid antagonists (naltrexone, naloxone)	Will produce withdrawal symptoms in those dependent on opioid medications. Avoid concurrent administration.
Diltiazem, erythromycin and fluconazole	May inhibit metabolism and increase concentration of alfentanil, thus exacerbating respiratory depression. Dose may need to be decreased.
Rifampicin	May enhance metabolism and decrease concentration of morphine, codeine and alfentanil, thus reducing their effects. Effects should be monitored, and dose may need to be increased or another analgesic substituted.
Many drugs (including anticonvulsants, antivirals, antifungals, rifampicin and St John's wort)	May enhance metabolism and decrease concentration of methadone, thus reducing its effects. Effects should be monitored, and dose may need to be increased.

3 Serotonin syndrome is an adverse effect due to excessive stimulation of 5-HT_{2A} receptors caused by drugs such as antidepressants; it is characterised by mental state changes (confusion, delirium and hypomania), gastrointestinal tract effects (diarrhoea), neuromuscular hyperactivity (hyperreflexia, incoordination and tremor), autonomic instability, sweating, fever and shivering (see Ch 22 for more detail).

Drug Monograph 19.1
Morphine

Morphine is a strong analgesic with central actions on pain perception; it mimics the actions of enkephalins and endorphins at ORs.

Mechanism of action of opioids

See text for specific mechanisms of action.

Indications

Morphine is indicated for treating opioid-responsive moderate-to-severe acute and chronic pain, such as after trauma or surgery or for cancer pain. It may be given to suppress an unproductive nagging cough and to those living with lung cancer to treat pain aggravated by coughing, when the sedative and euphoriant actions are also useful. Morphine increases gastrointestinal tract (GIT) tone, and decreases peristalsis and glandular secretions so is useful in treating diarrhoea. In the prehospital and emergency situation, morphine is commonly carried in ambulances and administered by paramedics IV, IM or by IV infusion, for acute pain relief, sedation to enable and maintain intubation.

Pharmacokinetics

Morphine may be administered by many routes – PO (i.e. by mouth), IM, IV, SC, epidural, intrathecal and rectal. It is rapidly absorbed and is subject to extensive first-pass metabolism in the liver, leading to poor bioavailability (about 40% when taken orally), so the oral dose may need to be 2–6 times the parenteral dose (Table 19.3). The main metabolites are active M6G and morphine-3-glucuronide.

Morphine is distributed widely in most body tissues, but only a small fraction crosses the blood–brain barrier. Metabolites are excreted primarily via the kidneys, with 7–10% undergoing enterohepatic circulation, which extends the half-life. The mean elimination half-life is 2–3 hours, but this is increased with slow-release preparations (tablets, capsules, oral suspension), such that the peak morphine concentrations during chronic use occur 4–8 hours after dosing and therapeutic effects may extend for 16–24 hours.

Drug interactions

See Drug Interactions 19.1.

Adverse reactions

The most common adverse reactions reported are constipation, nausea and vomiting, itch, urinary retention, sedation, circulatory and respiratory depression and miosis (pin-point pupils); overdose with opioids can cause cessation of respiration. Tolerance occurs to analgesia as well as to depressant effects (but not to constipation), requiring higher dosages. Constipation should be pre-empted with prophylactic laxative or a diet high in fibre. Respiratory depression, dependence and withdrawal reactions are not usually problems when opioids are used clinically for relief of severe pain.

Warnings and contraindications

- Avoid the use of opioids in people with known opioid drug hypersensitivity, or a history of drug abuse, acute alcoholism or head injury.
- Use opioids with caution in patients with acute respiratory depression, acute asthma, chronic obstructive pulmonary disease or other respiratory impairment, and in patients with elevated intracranial pressure (may be exacerbated).
- Use with caution in biliary colic or pancreatitis (may cause spasm of biliary tract muscle and sphincter), acute abdominal conditions or severe inflammatory bowel disease (risk of obscuring the diagnosis, or risk of toxic megacolon).
- Doses need to be reduced in patients with renal or liver impairment and in the elderly and children.
- Administration during pregnancy may result in dependence in the infant; use during labour may cause respiratory depression in the infant, treated with naloxone.

Dosage and administration

Standard morphine doses are 10 mg IV/IM/SC or 30 mg orally; higher doses are required for tolerant patients.

anaesthesia in day-surgery procedures, for prehospital use and in breakthrough pain in cancer therapy. Fentanyl is formulated for IM or slow IV injection, intranasal use, as a topical patch or lozenge ('lollipop') for absorption via the oral mucosa and, in combination with bupivacaine or ropivacaine, for epidural administration for postoperative or obstetric analgesia (Drug Monograph 19.2). Analogues of fentanyl include alfentanil and remifentanil and are indicated for intravenous use by specialist anaesthetists and their trainees as an analgesic supplement and an anaesthetic induction agent (Ch 18).

Hydromorphone

Hydromorphone is a semisynthetic opioid with a faster onset and shorter duration of action than morphine. It is prescribed for its analgesic and antitussive effects, and is administered as tablets, oral liquid or injection.

Methadone

Methadone is an orally effective analgesic with properties similar to those of morphine. To control pain, methadone is administered once or twice daily, based on the

Drug Monograph 19.2
Fentanyl

Fentanyl is a strong opioid analgesic with a mechanism and actions similar to morphine. Its clinical potency ranges from 50 to 100 times that of morphine, and it mimics the actions of endogenous enkephalins and endorphins at ORs.

Indications

Fentanyl is indicated for the treatment of opioid-responsive acute and chronic pain, as an adjunctive analgesic during general anaesthesia, for breakthrough pain in those living with cancer (lozenge formulation) and in epidural anaesthesia in combination with bupivacaine or ropivacaine. In the prehospital and emergency situation, fentanyl is administered by paramedics by IV injection or intranasal inhalation for analgesia and sedation to facilitate intubation.

Pharmacokinetics

The plasma-protein binding of fentanyl is about 84%. Fentanyl is rapidly and extensively metabolised primarily by CYP3A4 in the liver to a number of pharmacologically inactive metabolites. The minimum effective analgesic serum concentration of fentanyl ranges from 0.3 to 1.2 ng/mL, while surgical anaesthesia and profound respiratory depression occur at serum levels of 10–20 ng/mL. Elderly or debilitated patients may have a reduced clearance of fentanyl and so its terminal half-life may be prolonged in this patient group. Within 72 hours of IV fentanyl administration, approximately 75% of fentanyl is excreted in the urine, and about 9% in the faeces, mostly as inactive metabolites.

Drug interactions

See Drug Interactions 19.1. In addition, as fentanyl can contribute to serotonin toxicity, it is contraindicated with MAOIs or other drugs implicated in serotonin syndrome (see under 'Pethidine', and Ch 22). Azole antifungals can impair the metabolism of fentanyl, leading to prolonged half-lives and risk of adverse effects.

Severe and unpredictable potentiation by MAOIs has been reported with opioid analgesics, and the use of fentanyl in patients who have received MAOIs within 14 days is not recommended. Due to additive pharmacological effect, the concomitant use of benzodiazepines or other CNS depressants increases the risk of respiratory depression, profound sedation, coma and death.

Adverse reactions

The most common adverse reactions are bradycardia and rash and itch at the site of administration, constipation, nausea, somnolescence and headache. The most serious potential adverse reactions associated with opioid use are respiratory depression, hypotension and shock.

Warnings and contraindications

- Fentanyl should only be used by experienced doctors and in patients who are under constant supervision.
- Respiratory depression is the most marked and dangerous side effect, and fentanyl should be used with caution in patients with severe impairment of pulmonary function. The respiratory depressant effect of fentanyl persists longer than the measured analgesic effect. Respiratory depression can be reversed by opioid antagonists; however, appropriate surveillance should be maintained. Safe conditions for use in children 2 years of age or younger have not been established.
- Fentanyl should be used with caution in impaired hepatic or renal function or in patients susceptible to respiratory depression.
- Fentanyl may induce hypotension, particularly in hypovolaemic patients, and may produce bradycardia and possibly asystole.
- Contraindications include known hypersensitivity or intolerance to fentanyl, other opioid analgesics or to any of the excipients, bronchial asthma, head injuries and increased intracranial pressure.
- Fentanyl may cause muscle rigidity, particularly involving the muscles of respiration. This effect is related to the dose and speed of injection and may be reduced by slow intravenous injection.
- Profound sedation, respiratory depression, coma and death may result from the concomitant use of fentanyl with benzodiazepines or other CNS depressants.
- Fentanyl can produce drug dependence and therefore has the potential for being abused. Patients on chronic opioid therapy or with a history of opioid abuse may require higher doses to achieve an adequate therapeutic effect.
- Elderly patients may be more susceptible to adverse effects, such as respiratory depression and cardiovascular effects. They may also have age-related kidney function impairment, resulting in lower clearance rates of fentanyl.

Dosage and administration

Doses may vary widely depending on the indication for which it is given, the route of administration, tolerance developed, level of pain, age and opioid familiarity/naivety of the patient.

Sources: Based on information from Australian Medicines Handbook 2021; Medsafe NZ database – see 'Online resources'.

individual's response. Accumulation can occur, and steady-state concentrations may not be reached for several days. Cardiac dysrhythmias may occur with high doses.

Because of its oral bioavailability and extended half-life, methadone is approved for use in opioid detoxification and maintenance programs in people who are physiologically dependent on heroin or other opioids and in intractable cancer pain. Oral administration in liquid form is preferred, as this removes the need for injections (Ch 25).

Oxycodone

Oxycodone is a potent synthetic opioid about 10 times more potent than codeine; it is available in many different strength tablets, as capsules and oral liquid. It is well absorbed through the rectal mucosa, making the suppository dosage form (30 mg) useful for night-time analgesia and in people who cannot swallow. Doses may need to be reduced in renal impairment.

Controlled-release combinations with naloxone (an opioid antagonist) are indicated for moderate-to-severe chronic pain when constipation is refractory to treatment with regular laxatives.

Pethidine

Pethidine (known as meperidine in the United States) is an effective analgesic for short-term use but is unsuitable for oral administration because of low bioavailability. It is less likely than morphine to release histamine or raise biliary tract pressure so is useful for patients with acute asthma, biliary colic or pancreatitis. A metabolite (norpethidine) is neurotoxic and can accumulate, so pethidine is used only in acute pain such as for obstetric analgesia. Pethidine has serotonergic actions, and concurrent use of MAOIs may result in unpredictable life-threatening reactions, including serotonin syndrome. Pethidine is often requested by illicit drug users (who may very effectively mimic the signs and symptoms of severe pain), and prescribers are warned of this drug-seeking behaviour.

Tramadol

Tramadol is a relatively new centrally acting synthetic analgesic that is not chemically related to the opioids but binds to MORs; it also inhibits reuptake of noradrenaline and 5-HT so is referred to as an opioid–SNRI (serotonin noradrenaline reuptake inhibitor) analgesic. It is indicated in treatment of moderate-to-severe chronic pain and neuropathic pain, but is less effective and more expensive than morphine; it may have less potential for respiratory depression and drug dependency. Common adverse reactions include nausea, dizziness, hypertension and seizures; precautions are needed in elderly patients as hallucinations are possible. Tramadol is a prodrug, activated by CYP2D6; there are many interactions with other drugs inducing or inhibiting CYP2D6, and with other drugs affecting 5-HT levels, contributing to serotonin syndrome.

A chemically related drug is tapentadol; it appears to have similar mechanisms of action, indications, adverse effects and contraindications. Modified release tablets are available. Tapentadol is recommended for severe pain.

Pholcodine

Pholcodine (see Ch 15, for use as a cough suppressant), an opioid chemically similar to the opium alkaloid papaverine, has virtually no analgesic effects but retains other morphine-like effects, including suppressing cough and respiration and causing mild sedation, nausea and vomiting, dependence and constipation. It is used mainly as a cough suppressant, as are dextromethorphan and dihydrocodeine.

Dextropropoxyphene

Dextropropoxyphene is a synthetic analgesic structurally related to methadone, previously indicated for treatment of mild-to-moderate pain. It has significant dysphoric effects, accumulation and cardiotoxicity can occur and it has no marked advantages over safer analgesics such as codeine, aspirin or paracetamol, so is not recommended. It has been removed from the market in many countries (UK in 2004, EU in 2009, US and NZ in 2010).

Heroin

Pharmacologically, heroin is a prodrug: when administered it is rapidly converted in the liver to morphine and morphine metabolites, which provide its analgesic effects. Due to its greater lipid solubility, heroin crosses the blood–brain barrier faster than morphine, inducing a greater 'rush'; hence, it is preferred by opioid-dependent people. It has a shorter duration of action than morphine.

The case is often put for legalisation of heroin for treating intractable pain because of its analgesic and euphoric effects. Some advocates believe it is more potent, faster acting and produces more prolonged euphoric effects than other opioids (Ch 25).

Partial agonists

Partial agonists produce less than maximal effects at a receptor; for example, buprenorphine is a partial agonist at MORs and antagonist at KORs (Table 19.2, earlier). Generally, these drugs are less effective analgesics with lower dependency potential and less severe withdrawal symptoms than full opioid agonists. However, their use as analgesics is not recommended, as they may precipitate pain or withdrawal reactions in those taking other opioids, their actions may not be reversible with an antagonist (naloxone), and people taking a partial agonist may not respond adequately if a full agonist needs to be given.

Buprenorphine

Buprenorphine is a partial agonist at MORs, a full agonist at nociceptin opioid receptors (NOPs) and an antagonist at KORs and DORs. It is available as sublingual film, injection or patches, and is indicated for relief of moderate-to-severe pain and for treatment of opioid dependence. As it has a prolonged onset of action, it is not suitable for acute pain; and as a partial agonist, it may precipitate withdrawal in people who depend on other opioids, and its effects are not readily reversed by naloxone (Hale et al. 2021).

Opioid antagonists

The search for pure morphine antagonists produced naloxone and naltrexone, opioid antagonists that competitively displace opioid analgesics from their receptor sites, thus reversing their effects. The drugs are believed to bind to all three receptor types, but their greatest affinity is for μ receptors.

Antagonism of EOs (enkephalins and endorphins) released during inflammatory reactions and acupuncture can lead to a state of hyperalgesia (exacerbated pain).

Naloxone and naltrexone

Antagonists block subjective and objective opioid effects and can precipitate withdrawal symptoms in people physically dependent on opioids. Naloxone and naltrexone are used to reverse the adverse or toxic effects of opioid agonists such as morphine and heroin. Respiratory difficulties in newborn babies, caused by opioids given to the mother for pain relief during childbirth, can also be treated. Respiratory depression induced by non-opioids (e.g. barbiturates), CNS depression or respiratory disease is unlikely to respond.

Naloxone, a short-acting antagonist administered parenterally, is used mainly for treating an overdose or for reversing opioid depressant effects. (The serum half-life of naloxone is approximately 0.5–1 hour, whereas that of morphine is 1.5–2 hours; hence, frequent doses of naloxone may be necessary to prevent the person slipping back into the overdose state.) Naltrexone, a long-acting antagonist given orally, is used mainly for treating alcohol or opioid dependence and for rapid opioid detoxification (Ch 25). Adverse reactions include nausea, dizziness, nervousness, headache and fatigue.

Antagonists for reversal of opioid-induced constipation

Methylnaltrexone is useful in treating opioid-induced constipation as it is a relatively selective antagonist for peripheral ORs. Injected SC, it causes a bowel motion within 4 hours in most patients, with little change in pain scores. At present, its use is reserved for palliative care patients for whom laxatives have been ineffective.

Alvimopan and naloxegol (not available in Australia) were designed as a peripherally acting MOR antagonist to accelerate GIT recovery following bowel surgery (e.g. for postoperative ileus).

KEY POINTS

Analgesia and the opioids

- The enkephalins (pentapeptides), endorphins, dynorphins and nociceptin are all known as endogenous opioids (EOs).
- High-affinity binding sites (ORs) for the EOs are widely located in the CNS (also in peripheral tissue, especially in the gut) and are responsive to various opioid agonists.
- Opioid agonists (natural or synthetic agents) are strong analgesic drugs, acting centrally on ORs. Morphine is the prototype opioid analgesic.
- In pain pathways, stimulation of ORs at the spinal cord level inhibits release of substance P from dorsal-horn neurons, 'closing the gate' in the dorsal horn, thus inhibiting afferent transmission.
- At supraspinal levels, opioids activate ORs widely distributed in the CNS, especially in the limbic system, thalamus, hypothalamus and midbrain.
- Opioid receptors are G-protein-coupled trans-membrane receptors. The main CNS ORs are named by the Greek letters μ (m; mu), κ (k; kappa) and δ (d; delta): MOR, KOR and DOR, respectively.
- Subtypes of ORs are classified by responses to different agonists and antagonists.
- Agonist analgesics (e.g. morphine) activate both the μ and κ receptors.
- Non-selective antagonists (naloxone, naltrexone) antagonise all ORs.
- Due to the widespread distribution of ORs in peripheral and central tissues, opioids have a broad spectrum of actions. In the CNS, these include analgesia, suppression of the cough reflex and of the respiratory centre function, and sedation. Peripheral effects include severe constipation.
- Serious adverse drug reactions include respiratory depression, excessive sedation, dysphoria, tolerance and dependence.
- If tolerance develops to the analgesic effects, higher doses are required to achieve the same effect.

- Other opioid analgesics include fentanyl (with a clinical potency ranging from 50 to 100 times that of morphine), oxycodone, pethidine (an effective analgesic for short-term use) and codeine (a mild opioid). Partial agonists include buprenorphine.
- Opioid antagonists are used to treat adverse effects, overdoses or dependence, and include naloxone.

Non-opioid analgesics: the NSAIDs

Pharmacological actions and clinical uses

Non-opioid (non-narcotic) analgesics constitute the second main group of pain-relieving drugs. These drugs have significant anti-inflammatory actions and thus reduction of inflammation leads to analgesia. These and antipyretic (anti-fever) actions are typified by aspirin. As these drugs do not possess the steroidal chemical structure of anti-inflammatories such as cortisone, they are also known as **non-steroidal anti-inflammatory drugs** and antipyretic analgesics.[4] The drugs also inhibit platelet aggregation and thus decrease the risk of thrombosis (e.g. low-dose aspirin) (Chs 13 and 34). These drugs block the enzyme COX pathway thereby preventing the formation of inflammatory mediators such as PGs and thromboxanes. Only paracetamol will be considered in this chapter; other NSAIDs, including indometacin and ibuprofen, and the newer specific cyclooxygenase-2 (COX-2) inhibitors, such as celecoxib, are covered in Chapter 34.

NSAIDs are effective for mild-to-moderate pain (Step 1 in the stepwise management of pain, Fig 19.3 earlier). They have useful opioid-sparing effects, allowing reduction of opioid dosage when combined with opioid analgesics in people with moderate pain (Step 2). These agents are some of the most commonly used of all drugs for treatment of mild-to-moderate pain, fever and inflammation caused by rheumatoid arthritis, osteoarthritis and other acute and chronic musculoskeletal and soft tissue inflammations (Ch 34). No particular NSAID has been shown to be generally more effective as an analgesic than others.

Mechanism of action: inhibition of prostaglandin formation

Salicylates are extracts from the bark of the willow tree *Salix alba* and from the herb meadowsweet (*Filipendula ulmaria*).

4 There is considerable confusion in terminology in this area, especially as to whether paracetamol (known as acetaminophen in North America) should be included among the NSAIDs. Admittedly, paracetamol has very little anti-inflammatory effect in many tissues, but aspirin, paracetamol and other NSAIDs all act by the same mechanism (inhibition of PG synthesis) and show varying levels of analgesic, anti-inflammatory, antipyretic and antiplatelet actions. Hence, we are using the term 'NSAID' in the broad sense and including aspirin (as the prototype NSAID) and paracetamol.

History

In the 18th century in England, the Reverend Edward Stone searched for a remedy for 'the ague' (fevers, shivering, rigor and rheumatism), and tested extracts of willow bark with great success. Salicin, the bitter glycoside of the *Salix* species, was extracted in 1827 and found to contain saligenin, an active ingredient from which salicylic acid was prepared. Sodium salicylate was first used in 1875, and acetylsalicylic acid was introduced into medicine in 1899 as aspirin. The trade name Aspro was popularised by the Nicholas drug company in Australia. Many other derivatives of salicylic acid have been synthesised and trialled; still in use are methyl salicylate (present in oil of wintergreen), salicylamide and choline salicylate.

Despite **salicylates** from willow trees having been used for thousands of years for the relief of pain, fever and inflammation, their mechanism of action was discovered only relatively recently (Vane 1971; 2000). NSAIDs inhibit arachidonic acid breakdown via **cyclooxygenase** isoenzymes (Ch 34), and thus reduce production at the site of injury of PGs that sensitise nociceptors to the algesic actions of bradykinin and other pain mediators. As shown in Ch 34, Fig 34.2, metabolic products of arachidonic acid such as PGs and leukotrienes play important roles in both pain and inflammation, so NSAIDs are particularly useful in pain of inflammatory origin. COX inhibition accounts for most of the analgesic effects – and also adverse effects – of the non-opioid analgesics. (Selective COX-2 inhibitors are preferred for anti-inflammatory effects and for reduced GIT adverse effects.)

The analgesic action is peripheral, and non-opioids do not cause tolerance or dependence, or modify psychological reactions to pain. They may, however, also have a central analgesic action in the spinal cord. The antipyretic action is due to inhibition of PG synthesis in the hypothalamus, the temperature-regulating centre of the body.

Adverse drug reactions and drug interactions

Common adverse drug reactions to non-opioid analgesics include GIT disorders (dyspepsia, nausea and vomiting, diarrhoea/constipation and gastritis) due to reduced synthesis of mucoprotective PGs by systemically absorbed NSAIDs; hence, NSAIDs are contraindicated in peptic ulcer disease. Other adverse effects include renal damage (due to inhibition of renal vasodilating PGs – particularly a problem in elderly people on long-acting NSAIDs), allergic reactions such as asthma rashes and urticaria, and sodium retention and consequent heart failure and hypertension in predisposed clients.

Individual NSAIDs may cause specific adverse effects; for example, salicylates generally can cause tinnitus and impaired acid–base imbalances, whereas a large overdose of paracetamol can cause acute liver damage if not promptly treated. General drug interactions are shown in Drug Interactions 34.1.

Paracetamol

Paracetamol (known as acetaminophen in the US) inhibits PG synthesis in the CNS and hence is an effective antipyretic analgesic. Although its anti-inflammatory effects are minimal, paracetamol does appear to inhibit COX in some tissues in some species, so its exact mechanisms of action are not clear. There is recent evidence that paracetamol also acts as a prodrug, with one of its metabolites, AM404, being active at cannabinoid receptors in the CNS, thus mimicking the analgesic actions of marijuana (Drug Monograph 19.3).

Drug Monograph 19.3
Paracetamol

Paracetamol, having little anti-inflammatory action, is rather different from the other NSAIDs, but is safer than aspirin as an analgesic.

Mechanism of action

Paracetamol's analgesic and antipyretic (anti-fever) actions are thought to be due to inhibition of PG synthesis in CNS tissues via cyclo-oxygenase inhibition; it may also modulate inhibitory descending serotonin (5-HT) pathways, and a metabolite may activate cannabinoid receptors.

Indications

Paracetamol is indicated for relief of fever and mild to moderate pain associated with headaches, muscular aches, period pain, acute sinusitis, otitis media, arthritis, migraine and postoperative pain. It is the recommended first-line treatment for osteoarthritis.

Pharmacokinetics

After oral administration, paracetamol is rapidly and completely absorbed from the GIT; peak plasma concentration is reached in 10–60 minutes, and pain relief begins after 30 minutes. Absorption is delayed by food in the GIT. Distribution via the bloodstream is uniform, with an apparent volume of distribution of 1–1.2 L/kg, implying some sequestration (binding) of paracetamol in tissues. There is negligible plasma protein binding. Paracetamol does cross the placenta in small amounts and so can affect the fetus. It is excreted in only small amounts in the milk of lactating women; hence it is the analgesic of choice in breastfeeding mothers.

The metabolism of paracetamol occurs in the liver by hepatic microsomal enzymes. In adults the main metabolites (65–85%) are the glucuronide and sulfate conjugates, whereas in children it is the sulfate derivative. Excretion is via the urine as metabolites (95%) within 24 hours. The elimination half-life is 1–3 hours; hence, doses must be given regularly every 3–4 hours to maintain therapeutic blood levels.

Adverse drug reactions

In normal doses, paracetamol rarely causes adverse effects except in at-risk patients; dyspepsia (stomach upsets), allergy, raised aminotransferase levels and blood disorders may occur. Because of the high therapeutic index (safety margin), accidental overdose is rare. If taken in acute overdose, it is potentially fatal, with acute liver failure occurring 2–3 days later. As there may be few symptoms in the early stages (vomiting, abdominal pain, hypotension, sweating and CNS effects), treatment is instituted as soon as overdose is suspected, with attempts to remove the drug by gastric lavage or activated charcoal and administration of the specific antidote acetylcysteine.

Drug interactions

There are few clinically significant drug interactions. Paracetamol is a substrate for CYP1A2, so may interact with inducers of this enzyme (e.g. phenytoin, tobacco) or inhibitors (amitriptyline, warfarin). Thus paracetamol may prolong bleeding times in people previously stabilised on warfarin.

Precautions and contraindications

Caution should be used before administering paracetamol to people with renal or hepatic dysfunction, as the drug or its metabolites may accumulate. Paracetamol is considered safe in pregnancy (Category A) and in breastfeeding. Products may contain appreciable amounts of sodium or aspartame.

Dosage and administration

Paracetamol is available in a multitude of formulations (oral and IV infusion), and mixed with other active ingredients, so it is important to check the total paracetamol dose in people taking more than one formulation. The standard adult dose is 1–2 tablets, capsules or suppositories, each containing 500 mg paracetamol, administered every 3–4 hours, not exceeding a maximum of 4 g per day (8 standard tablets). Formulations suitable for children include infant drops, elixirs, suspensions and suppositories; dose recommendations on the basis of the child's age and weight should not be exceeded (children 1 month to 12 years, medically unsupervised: maximum 60 mg/kg daily for up to 48 hours, not to exceed 4 g daily). Small elderly people should have doses lower than 1 g four times daily.

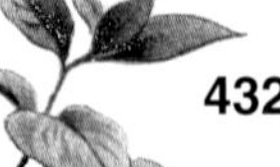

In normal dose, paracetamol is a safer over-the-counter analgesic than aspirin:

- Adverse effects and allergic reactions are rare with therapeutic doses.
- There is very low risk of gastric upset, peptic ulceration or bleeding, tinnitus or renal impairment compared with aspirin and other NSAIDs; hence it can be used when other NSAIDs are contraindicated.
- Plasma protein binding is negligible; hence there is no risk of displacement causing drug interactions.
- There are few serious adverse drug interactions; low doses may be used by people taking anticoagulant medications.
- It may be used by children with mild fevers, colds and flu symptoms because it is not associated with Reye's syndrome, as is aspirin.
- It is safe to use during pregnancy and lactation.

Paracetamol is an effective analgesic provided that adequate regular doses are maintained.

Paracetamol is recommended particularly for treatment of mild pain and fevers in children, and in adults in a wide range of conditions causing mild-to-moderate pain (especially of non-inflammatory origin), fever, migraine and tension headache and some forms of arthritis (osteoarthritis).

Pharmacokinetics of paracetamol

Paracetamol taken orally is rapidly absorbed, with bioavailability approximately 90%, reaching peak serum levels in 15–60 minutes; its elimination half-life is 1–3 hours. It is metabolised in the liver, and glucuronide and sulfate metabolites are excreted by the kidneys.

Dosage and formulation

Paracetamol is available in infant, paediatric and adult strengths, as tablets, capsules, chewable tablets, elixirs, suppositories (not recommended due to erratic absorption) and as an injection. Modified-release tablets are available, containing 655 mg paracetamol in a formulation that maintains therapeutically active levels of drug for up to 8 hours after oral administration. The tablets must not be crushed.

Adverse drug reactions

As noted in Drug Monograph 19.3, adverse effects are rare with paracetamol in normal therapeutic doses, although in some instances nausea and rash have occurred. Ingestion of 20 or more tablets (10 g) can cause potentially fatal damage to the liver and kidneys and hypoglycaemia, due to buildup of a toxic metabolite (Fig 19.6). Even normal doses (4 g/day) can cause hepatotoxicity, especially in people who are fasting, have regular excessive alcohol use or are taking drugs that induce CYP2E1. Inadvertent overdose can also occur by exceeding the recommended daily dose in attempts to manage increasing pain or by additive effects of paracetamol present in more than one over-the-counter preparation. (See Clinical Focus Box 19.2 for management of deliberate paracetamol overdose; and Ch 15, under 'Other mucolytics', for a discussion of the use of acetylcysteine as a mucolytic agent in respiratory disorders.)

Compound analgesics

Simple analgesics (500 mg paracetamol or 300–500 mg aspirin) are sometimes formulated with other drugs (e.g. mild opioids, other NSAIDs, antihistamines, caffeine, decongestants, antiemetics, muscle relaxants or antacids) to combine the pharmacological actions of two or more drugs. An example is Panadeine Forte (500 mg paracetamol and 30 mg codeine).

Such combinations suffer the disadvantages of all fixed-dose combinations: it is impossible to titrate the dose of either individual drug; effects of the drug with the shorter half-life may wear off first or the drug with the longer half-life may accumulate; the drug with more severe adverse effects may become toxic; and combinations may be more expensive and no more effective than taking the individual drugs at the appropriate intervals and dosages (Murnion 2010). There are some situations in which NSAID–other drug combinations are clinically useful:

- Paracetamol with another NSAID: adequate analgesic doses of paracetamol may allow decreased dosing of the other (anti-inflammatory) NSAID, with a decrease in incidence of adverse effects.
- A simple analgesic (aspirin or paracetamol) with a mild opioid (codeine, at 8 or 30 mg) provides an intermediate step in the 'analgesic ladder'.

A 'classic' Australian compound analgesic formulation in the early–mid 20th century, APC powders or tablets contained standard doses of aspirin, phenacetin and caffeine. Many people suffering repetitive strain injuries, headache or muscular tissue pain followed the common advice, 'Have a cup of tea, an APC and a good lie-down', and took the compound analgesics regularly in high doses for relief of pain and inflammation (aspirin and phenacetin) and for mild CNS stimulation (caffeine). Unfortunately, the aspirin and phenacetin components caused gastric upsets and pain, leading to more doses of APC being taken; caffeine withdrawal as drug levels decreased caused a rebound headache; and regular use of NSAID analgesics, especially phenacetin, caused chronic nephritis, renal tubular necrosis and eventually renal

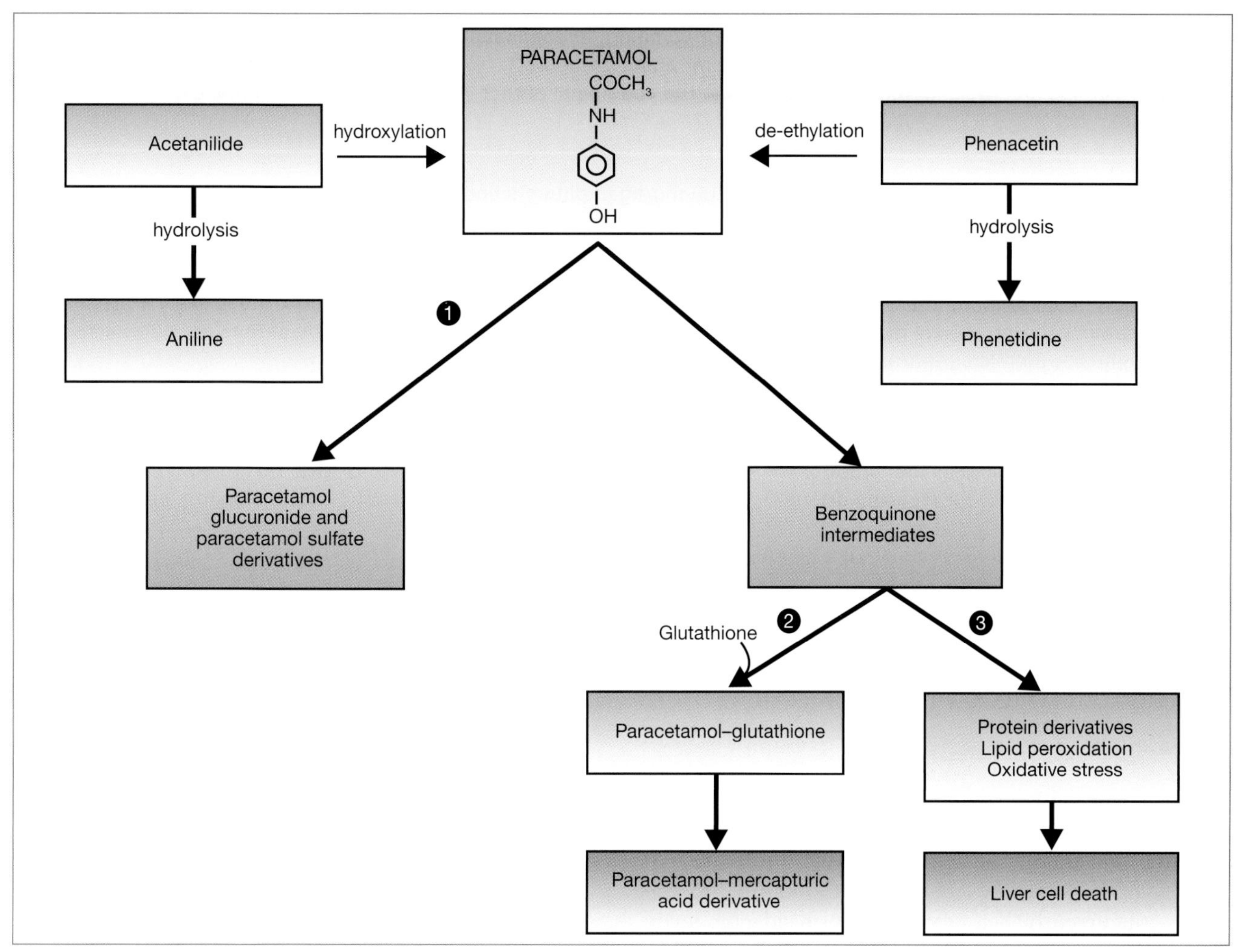

FIGURE 19.6 Metabolic pathways involving paracetamol

In normal doses, paracetamol is conjugated (pathway 1) to non-toxic glucuronide and sulfate derivatives. In higher doses, pathway 1 becomes saturated and a benzoquinone intermediate (BQI) is produced. Combination of the BQI with glutathione (GSH, a gamma-glutamyl-cysteinyl-glycine tripeptide involved in amino acid transport in cells) via pathway 2 produces mercapturic acid metabolites. In large overdoses, GSH reserves are used up and BQIs are diverted via pathway 3, in which toxic derivatives cause potentially lethal reactions in liver cells. Paracetamol overdose is treated with acetylcysteine, a precursor of the natural compound GSH; this replenishes GSH supplies and avoids formation of toxic BQI metabolites.

CLINICAL FOCUS BOX 19.2
Managing deliberate paracetamol overdose

Paracetamol is widely available and responsible for a large proportion of accidental and deliberate cases of poisoning. Paracetamol poisoning is common, but rarely causes severe liver injury or death. Patients suspected of taking an overdose of paracetamol are notoriously unreliable as to the amount taken and the time of ingestion, and may appear well for 1–2 days after an eventually fatal overdose. It is important that any patient with possible paracetamol overdose be tested for plasma paracetamol levels. Measure liver biochemistry and serum paracetamol concentration urgently. There is a specific antidote (acetylcysteine, which replaces depleted glutathione, see Fig 19.6). Activated charcoal is also given. Acetylcysteine given within 8 hours of paracetamol ingestion prevents hepatotoxicity in most cases. Indications for acetylcysteine therapy depends on the time since ingestion, the serum paracetamol concentration and the serum ALT concentration (in some situations).

More than 200 mg paracetamol per kg body weight (about 20 standard 500 mg paracetamol tablets for an average adult) or 10 g total paracetamol is potentially a toxic dose. People with previously impaired liver function (e.g. by alcohol abuse) are more susceptible to liver damage and have a lowered threshold for toxicity.

Symptoms

- Early symptoms are sweating, anorexia, nausea or vomiting, abdominal pain or cramping and/or diarrhoea; these usually occur 6–14 hours after ingestion and last for about 24 hours.
- Late symptoms are swelling, tenderness or pain in the abdominal area 2–4 days after ingestion (indicates hepatic damage).

Treatment

- For immediate release preparations: if 10 g (or 200 mg/kg in patients under 50 kg) give activated charcoal and lavage within 2 hours. If more than 30 g (or 500 mg/kg in patients under 60 kg) of a solid preparation give gastric lavage or activated charcoal within 4 hours.
- A plasma sample should be obtained for liver function tests and coagulation studies. Determine paracetamol serum levels at 4 hours or more after ingestion, then start acetylcysteine administration. Hepatotoxicity is likely if plasma paracetamol concentration is more than 200 microgram/mL at 4 hours, 150 microgram/mL at 6 hours, 100 microgram/mL at 8 hours, 50 microgram/mL at 12 hours or 5 microgram/mL at 24 hours.
- Administer acetylcysteine IV in 5% glucose from 4 hours after overdose, with a loading dose, then maintenance dose continuing for 21 hours. (See current *Australian Medicines Handbook* or other reference for the nomogram to determine likelihood of paracetamol toxicity from plasma levels, and dosage instructions.)
- Perform liver function tests and prothrombin time determinations to monitor hepatotoxicity. Institute supportive measures as indicated for bleeding disorders, renal failure, cardiac toxicity and hepatic encephalopathy and hepatic encephalopathy.
- Children younger than 6 years are less susceptible to paracetamol toxicity

failure requiring regular dialysis or kidney transplantation. (Phenacetin has long been withdrawn from use.)

NSAIDs and polypharmacy

NSAIDs are often included in commercial products such as pain relievers, cough and cold remedies, sedatives and medicines for allergy or (pre)menstrual problems, so clients may be unaware that they are taking several NSAIDs concurrently[5] – for example, for headache, fever, arthritis and prophylaxis of acute myocardial infarction or stroke. Taking more than one of these products at the same time, or with a prescribed NSAID, can lead to toxicity. Elderly people with impaired renal function are particularly at risk of adverse drug reactions and interactions, especially from NSAIDs with long half-lives.

5 A tactful review of the family's drug cabinet or questioning about all the medicines currently being taken, including those bought in pharmacies or supermarkets, often reveals a potentially toxic cocktail of many NSAID preparations.

KEY POINTS

Non-opioid (non-narcotic) analgesics – the NSAIDs

- Non-opioid (non-narcotic) analgesics constitute the second main group of pain-relieving drugs. They are typified by NSAIDs such as aspirin.
- NSAIDs have significant anti-inflammatory actions and these actions are combined with antipyretic (anti-fever) actions in the hypothalamus.
- NSAIDS inhibit arachidonic acid breakdown and PG release by blocking COX isoenzymes. Prostaglandins sensitise nociceptors to the algesic actions of bradykinin and other pain mediators.
- Non-opioid analgesics do not cause tolerance or dependence, or modify psychological reactions to pain. Common adverse drug reactions include GIT disorders (e.g. dyspepsia and gastritis) and renal damage.
- Individual NSAIDs may cause specific adverse effects. For example, a large overdose of paracetamol can cause acute liver damage if not promptly treated.
- Compound analgesics include simple analgesics such as NSAIDs together with drugs such as decongestants to combine their pharmacological actions.
- NSAIDs are often included in commercial products such as pain relievers, and cough and cold remedies. Clients may therefore be unaware that they are taking several NSAIDs concurrently, and toxicity can ensue.

Other analgesic drugs

Pregabalin and gabapentin

Newer analgesics unrelated to opioids or NSAIDs are pregabalin and gabapentin. Pregabalin (an analogue of the neurotransmitter GABA) reduces the release of various transmitters via interference with the calcium channels in nerve terminals. Pregabalin is indicated in neuropathic pain in diabetic neuropathy and post-herpetic neuralgia, but a person's response is variable. It is also useful as adjunctive therapy in partial seizures. The related gabapentin, an anticonvulsant drug (Ch 21), is also effective in the relief of neuropathic pain and blocks Ca^{2+} channels. Adverse reactions include dizziness, sedation and incoordination, ocular dysfunctions and weight gain. Doses need to be reduced in renal impairment, and prescribers are warned against stopping the drugs abruptly.

Other drugs useful for their analgesic effects

The following drugs are also useful:

- Local anaesthetics – for example, lidocaine (lignocaine), EMLA cream (Ch 18).
- General anaesthetics – for example, sevoflurane, nitrous oxide, ketamine and methoxyflurane (Ch 18).
- Cannabinoids – that is, derivatives of the marijuana plant *Cannabis sativa*, main active ingredient Δ^9-tetrahydrocannabinol (THC; see Ch 25): its psychopharmacological actions include analgesia mediated via the inhibition of neurotransmitter release, via cannabinoid receptors in areas involved in pain transmission and modulation (e.g. periaqueductal grey, rostral ventromedial medulla and spinal cord dorsal horn). THC enhances the analgesic potency of morphine, and allows lower doses of opioids to be used in pain syndromes resistant to opioids alone. An oromucosal spray formulation is being trialled in cancer pain.
- Specific antimigraine drugs, including 5-hydroxytryptamine (5-HT, serotonin) agonists (sumatriptan) and vasoconstrictors (ergot alkaloids) (Ch 24).
- Natural remedies in addition to opium and willow bark (which provide morphine and aspirin, respectively) include clove oil, feverfew and kava and sugar solutions for infants (described later).

Capsaicin

Capsaicin, an alkaloid found in chilli peppers, is formulated into topical creams for treating neuralgias, arthritic pain, and pain associated with cystitis and HIV infection. It is known as a counterirritant. It is said to activate capsaicin receptors (transient receptor potential vanilloid 1 (TRPV1) ion channel); on application, it causes an initial release and then a depletion of substance P from nerve fibres, which eventually results in a decrease in pain transmission.

Adjuvant analgesics

Adjuvant medications are used in combination with opioid or NSAID analgesics to enhance pain relief or to treat symptoms that exacerbate pain (Fig 19.3, earlier). Commonly used **adjuvant analgesic** medications include anticonvulsants (topiramate), tricyclic (and SNRI) antidepressants (amitryptiline; duloxetine and venlafaxine respectively) and the gabapentinoids (gabapentin, pregabalin), corticosteroids, local anaesthetics (lidocaine [lignocaine]), psychostimulants and clonidine may be used. Some important points to note:

- Tricyclic and SNRIs antidepressants and membrane-stabilising agents (e.g. some anticonvulsants and antidysrhythmic agents) may be useful in neuropathic pain and are often used in combination with opioids for cancer-associated nerve pain; the mechanism is via inhibition of 5-HT reuptake and blockade of sodium channels, respectively. The analgesic effects of the antidepressants (in neuropathic pain) are independent of their mood-altering effects.
- The analgesic actions of gabapentin may be due to blockade of calcium channels.
- Corticosteroids such as dexamethasone help relieve pain associated with inflammation and swelling and space-occupying lesions – for example, for cancer pain that originates in a restricted area such as intracranially, alongside a nerve root or in pelvic, neck or hepatic areas.
- Psychoactive drugs, including phenothiazines and benzodiazepines, may be useful for their sedating, antianxiety and muscle-relaxing properties.
- Clonidine, a centrally acting α_2-adrenergic agonist and antihypertensive agent, has been tried for the treatment of pain associated with reflex sympathetic dystrophy, diabetic neuropathy, post-herpetic neuralgia, spinal cord injury, phantom pain and pain in those living with cancer who are opioid-tolerant. Clonidine is effective in treating opioid withdrawal reactions by reducing autonomic hyperactivity.
- Ketamine, a general anaesthetic (Ch 18), is an antagonist at NMDA receptors and, in sub-anaesthetic doses, helps relieve chronic neuropathic pain; other NMDA receptor antagonists are being developed.

Recent approaches

New pharmacological approaches to pain management include:

- conopeptides (cone snail venom peptides)
- orexin-A, orexin-B (excitatory neuropeptides) (Roohbakhsh et al. 2018) and drugs that:
  - enhance the inhibitory effects of adenosine on nociceptors
  - mimic the actions of analgesic neuropeptides – for example, nociceptin/orphanin FQ, the natural ligand of the OR-like 1 (nociceptin) receptor, avoiding adverse effects of the opioids
  - inhibit the enzymes inactivating enkephalins or endorphins (opiorphin)
  - inhibit fatty acid amide hydrolase, and thus prolong the actions of endogenous cannabinoids.

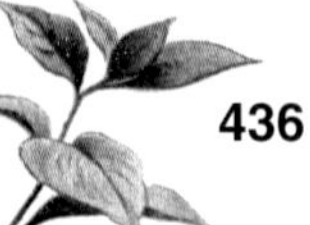

Non-pharmacological analgesic techniques

Non-pharmacological analgesic methods include:

- first-aid techniques: RICE (rest, ice, compression, elevation); heat packs and cold packs
- physiotherapy: exercise techniques that improve strength and flexibility, muscle relaxation techniques, massage, trigger-point therapy and hydrotherapy
- counterirritants: scratching, liniments, rubefacients (substances that redden the skin by causing vasodilation)
- transcutaneous electrical nerve stimulation: passing small electrical currents into the spinal cord or sensory nerves via electrodes applied to the skin
- acupuncture: a technique from traditional Chinese medicine in which needles are inserted into the skin at specific points; acupuncture releases endorphins and enkephalins and may also block gates in the dorsal horn regions (possibly via inhibitory 5-HT pathways); excitatory amino acid and autonomic neurotransmitters and inflammatory mediators are also affected, and there is a major placebo effect
- psychotherapeutic methods: hypnosis, behaviour modification, biofeedback techniques, assertiveness training, art and music therapy, meditation and the placebo effects induced by various methods
- surgery: neurosurgical techniques in chronic pain resistant to other management procedures; neurectomy (removal of part of a nerve), leucotomy (removal of part of the white matter of the CNS), sympathetic chain ablation, cortical ablation (removal of part of the cerebral cortex) and neurotomy by radiofrequency
- community support groups, family therapy and support, occupational therapy to assist with activities of daily living, and use of orthoses
- complementary and alternative medicine (CAM; see Clinical Focus Box 19.3) in acute and chronic pain and cognitive behaviour therapy.

KEY POINTS

Other pharmacological analgesics and non-pharmacological analgesic techniques

- Newer analgesics, unrelated to opioids or NSAIDs, are pregabalin and gabapentin. They are useful in treating neuropathic pain and reduce the release of various transmitters via interference with the calcium channels.
- Capsaicin, an alkaloid found in chilli peppers, activates capsaicin receptors and is useful in post-hepatic neuralgia.
- Other drugs useful for their analgesic effects include local and general anaesthetics, cannabinoids, specific antimigraine drugs and sugar solutions for infants and natural remedies including clove oil, feverfew and kava.

CLINICAL FOCUS BOX 19.3
Herbal remedies for pain

The most important herbal remedies for pain are, of course, morphine and codeine in opium extracts from the poppy (*Papaver somniferum*) and salicylates from the bark of the willow tree *Salix alba* and from the herb meadowsweet (*Filipendula ulmaria*).

Many other plants also have analgesic properties, including the following, which have been clinically tested and proven:

- cloves, the dried flower buds of *Eugenia* species, containing the oil eugenol, which has analgesic, anti-inflammatory, antimicrobial and antiplatelet activities; clove oil has traditional use in dentistry as an analgesic and antiseptic; it depresses nociceptors and inhibits PG synthesis
- feverfew, the leaves and flowering tops of the plant *Tanacetum parthenium*, containing many active ingredients including the terpene parthenolide; feverfew has long been used to treat headaches, arthritis and fever, and is effective prophylactically against migraine headache
- kava kava, a beverage prepared by Pacific Islands people from the root of *Piper methysticum*; the lipid-soluble lactones and flavonoids have mainly CNS effects (sedative and anxiolytic, via various transmitter receptors) as well as analgesic actions (via inhibition of COX enzymes) and local anaesthetic effects
- St John's wort, used since ancient times to rid the body of evil spirits and treat neuralgia, neuroses and depression; the herb is mainly used for its antidepressant actions, which mimic those of the serotonin selective reuptake inhibitors such as fluoxetine; analgesic actions are due to modulation of both ORs and COX enzyme expression
- other natural extracts and supplements with analgesic properties, such as devil's claw, ginger, ginseng, lemon balm, stinging nettle and shark cartilage
- in Australian Indigenous bush medicine, several traditional remedies are available to relieve the symptoms of headaches: the leaves of small-leaf clematis (*Clematis microphylla*), stinkwood (*Ziera* spp.) or *Melaleuca* species are crushed and the vapour inhaled, or leaves bound around the head to relieve pain.

Source: Adapted from Braun & Cohen 2010, inter alia.

- Adjuvants are combined with opioid or NSAID analgesics to enhance pain relief and include anticonvulsants, antidepressants, corticosteroids and NMDA receptor antagonists such as ketamine.
- Non-pharmacological analgesic methods include first-aid techniques, physiotherapy, counterirritants, acupuncture and psychotherapy.

Routes of administration of analgesics

If it is possible to deliver an analgesic drug directly to the site of pain or to the sensory nerve pathway, this will localise the effects, minimise the dose required and reduce the time to onset of action. Examples are epidural administration of local anaesthetics and opioids, intraarticular administration of corticosteroids and topical administration of local anaesthetics and NSAIDs. Generally, analgesics must be administered systemically to be circulated to the required site of action, whether in the painful tissues or in the CNS.

Oral route

The oral route is preferred as being the most acceptable and has the advantage of minimising IV drug-related problems. Opioid drugs may undergo significant hepatic metabolism after oral administration (first-pass effect), so higher doses are required than for parenteral administration; however, if the metabolites are pharmacologically active, they contribute to the analgesic effects. Modified-release preparations (e.g. morphine sulfate controlled-release tablets) help prolong the half-life of morphine from 3–4 hours to 12–24 hours, and are useful for stable, chronic pain.

Parenteral routes

IV injection is obviously the fastest route for rapid pain control and dosage titration, as it avoids the absorption phase. IM and SC injection routes are common for opioid analgesics, the latter having a slower onset of action. Relatively poor lipid solubility delays the onset of analgesia when morphine is administered by epidural or intrathecal injection. The risk of inducing respiratory depression is greater by the intrathecal route than by epidural administration, so patients must be monitored for at least 24 hours after intrathecal administration.

Continuous infusion of opioids

Continuous opioid infusions by SC or IV routes may be used when there is intractable vomiting; for severe pain not relieved by oral, rectal or intermittent parenteral dosing; or for pain management in the postoperative period.

Opioids may be infused by a microdrip infusion set and pump or by a **patient-controlled analgesia** unit. Patient-controlled analgesia is commonly ordered in a hospital or hospice setting, usually after surgery or for chronic cancer pain. It is a microprocessor-controlled injector programmed to deliver a predetermined IV opioid dose when the patient triggers the pump mechanism. The dose is based on the prescriber's order and a lock-out interval (5–20 minutes), which protects the patient from overdosing. The unit may record all patient dosing attempts so the prescriber can evaluate the need for analgesia. For children or other patients unable to control their own dose regimen, nurse-controlled analgesia setups can be used.

Other routes for systemic absorption

The rectal route is useful in patients who cannot swallow or who are vomiting, and for slower absorption; absorption from the rectal route is variable, so oral administration is the preferred route. Transdermal administration is effective for lipid-soluble drugs: fentanyl patches are available for patients with stable chronic pain who cannot tolerate oral morphine. Additional analgesics may be prescribed to cover rising levels of pain (breakthrough pain). Nitrous oxide and other gaseous and volatile general anaesthetics are administered by inhalation.

KEY POINTS

Routes of administration of analgesics

- Both oral and parenteral administration of analgesics is available. Generally, analgesics must be administered systemically to be circulated to the required site of action.
- The oral route is preferred, and has the advantage of minimising IV drug-related problems. Modified-release preparations extend the half-life of analgesics.
- Parenteral routes include intravenous, epidural or intrathecal injection.
- The rectal route is useful in patients who cannot swallow or who are vomiting, and for slower absorption. Transdermal administration is effective for lipid-soluble drugs (e.g. fentanyl patches).

Analgesic use in special groups

Pregnancy, labour and delivery

During pregnancy, the analgesic of choice for mild to moderate pain is paracetamol or codeine. In late pregnancy, NSAIDs should be avoided because of increased risk of bleeding (especially after aspirin); adverse effects on the fetal cardiovascular, respiratory and renal systems; and prolongation of gestation and labour.

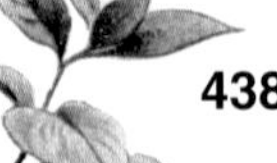

Labour and lactation

Most women experience pain during childbirth; ideally, the analgesic used provides pain relief without interference with labour and without increasing risk to mother or baby. Inhaled nitrous oxide is commonly used (Ch 18, under 'Inhalation anaesthetics'), or injected pethidine. For more severe pain, epidural administration of combined local anaesthetic and opioid is effective and allows the mother to remain conscious even through caesarean section. Morphine is a potent analgesic when used during labour but is associated with greater neonatal respiratory depression than pethidine and has a slower onset of action. Both drugs cross the placenta to enter fetal circulation. Naloxone, an opioid antagonist, should be available to treat the mother or neonate if excessive CNS or respiratory depression occurs.

If an opioid analgesic or methadone is administered to a woman who is breastfeeding a baby, the dose should be given immediately after a feed to minimise the quantity of drug passed on to the infant in breast milk.

Opioid dependence

A concern with the use of opioids during pregnancy (particularly in an addicted woman) is that these agents may lead to physical drug dependence in the fetus, causing severe withdrawal reactions in the baby after birth. Pregnant women dependent on an opioid and/or enrolled in methadone maintenance programs may present with fetal distress syndrome in utero and often deliver an underweight baby. Such infants are usually lethargic, with difficulty breathing, high-pitched cry and poor feeding and sleeping patterns; the infant will require small doses of morphine postnatally to prevent potentially fatal opiate withdrawal effects and may require special-care nursing for weeks while being weaned off the opioids.

Children

Doses of analgesics for children must be calculated carefully, especially in those who are malnourished, dehydrated or with serious illness. Paracetamol is the most commonly used analgesic, orally or IV in hospital where parenteral formulations can be prepared. Local protocols or *Therapeutic Guidelines: Analgesic* should be consulted for specific dosage regimens.

Guidelines for analgesic use in children

- As with adults, it is best to medicate a child early for pain rather than waiting until pain is severe.
- Young infants are especially sensitive to CNS-adverse drug effects, including respiratory depression.
- In some situations, the pain of a local anaesthetic injection may be more severe than that of a quick procedure (e.g. venepuncture or bladder aspiration); a local anaesthetic cream (EMLA, see Ch 18) is useful in such cases.
- Children may deny pain to avoid being given an injection; alternative analgesic dose forms, such as suppositories and liquid oral preparations, can be considered.
- Aspirin should not be used in children because of its association with Reye's syndrome.
- Paracetamol is the analgesic of choice, but children are often underdosed; ibuprofen is equally effective.
- Codeine has variable metabolism and efficacy in young children, and is not recommended.
- Preterm neonates are often given parenteral opiate analgesia to minimise fluctuations in heart rate and blood pressure after frequent invasive procedures such as heel pricks for blood sampling.
- Non-organic (psychogenic) pain in children usually resolves spontaneously but may mask more serious problems such as child abuse or depression.

Infants and neonates

Painful procedures often need to be carried out on neonates: injections, heel pricks or venepuncture for blood sampling or placement of a peripheral venous or arterial line, dressings and suture or adhesive tape removal. Medicating a child under 2 years who cannot verbally report pain is justified if the child displays increased irritability, restlessness, crying, anorexia and decreased activity. The approach should be individualised based on the child's age and stage of development and the various assessment tools available. Reassurance, establishing rapport and non-pharmacological means of analgesia such as (breast)feeding, swaddling, calming and warming are important; during painful procedures a young child can be distracted with toys, bubble-blowing, games, singing, stories, clowns and breathing-blowing exercises (see Beggs 2008; Murtagh 2006).

Sweet solutions

A simple pharmacological technique for infants that can be easily implemented by nurses is oral administration of a sweet solution, such as more than 24% sucrose or more than 30% glucose. Of a total dose of 1–2 mL of solution, one-quarter is given a couple of minutes before the procedure, then the rest incrementally as needed, dropped onto the front of the tongue from a syringe (with no needle). This reduces stress from painful procedures, as evidenced by reduced crying time and grimacing behaviours, but is not sufficient analgesia for lengthy or significantly painful procedures (see HANDI 2013; Royal Children's Hospital Melbourne, under 'Online resources'). The mechanism of action is thought to be an increase in EOs (Beggs 2008).

Elderly people

Analgesic use in elderly people usually requires careful adjustment of dosage and dosing interval according to the person's liver and kidney functions, therapeutic responses and development of undesirable adverse effects (increased pain, confusion or respiratory depression). The elderly often show enhanced drug responses and may not tolerate adverse effects well. Elderly people may have comorbidities (multiple medical problems) and several medications prescribed for them (polypharmacy).

Elderly people often report pain differently from younger people because of the belief that pain is a part of old age, because they do not want to cause difficulties to their carer or because they deny their discomfort as a cultural and ethnic issue. In such instances, non-verbal communication and behaviours should be carefully assessed, such as increased irritability, loss of appetite, decreased activity, crying easily or tightly gripping an object. Confusion or dementia may make pain assessment difficult; methods are available for assessing pain in people with dementia.

It is common practice to start the opioid dosage at 25–50% of the usual adult dose, and titrate upwards carefully, with frequent monitoring. The elderly may have impaired circulatory function, resulting in slower absorption of drugs administered IM or SC; administering additional doses may result in unpredictable or increased drug absorption, increasing adverse reactions.

Analgesics inappropriate for use in the elderly because of toxicity include pethidine; safer analgesics are available. All NSAIDs are relatively dangerous in the elderly because of gastrointestinal, renal and cardiovascular adverse effects; those with long half-lives, such as naproxen and piroxicam, must be avoided.

Opioid-tolerant people

Managing acute pain in people taking long-term opioids for chronic pain or with an opioid-dependence disorder is difficult, due to tolerance and/or blockade of ORs by antagonists or partial agonists used in treatment. Pain and the addictive disorder must be carefully assessed, and prescribers need to be alert to drug-seeking behaviours. The usual opioid drug (same dose and formulation) is continued to avoid withdrawal symptoms, and extra analgesics added as required. Other techniques of pain management (other analgesics, adjuvants, non-pharmacological methods) are used whenever possible.

KEY POINTS

Analgesic use in special groups

Pregnancy, labour and delivery

- During pregnancy, the analgesic of choice for mild to moderate pain is paracetamol or codeine. In late pregnancy, NSAIDs should be avoided because of increased risk of bleeding (especially after aspirin).
- During labour, ideally the analgesic used will provide pain relief without interference with labour and without increasing risk to the mother or baby. Inhaled nitrous oxide is commonly used, or injected pethidine.

Analgesic use in children

- Specific guidelines exist for analgesic use in children. Doses of analgesics for children must be calculated carefully, especially in those who are malnourished, dehydrated or with serious illness. Paracetamol is the most commonly used analgesic.
- Oral administration of a sweet solution reduces stress from painful procedures but is not sufficient analgesia for lengthy or significantly painful procedures.

Analgesic use in elderly people

- Careful adjustment of dosage and dosing interval is required in the elderly according to the person's liver and kidney functions, therapeutic responses, comorbidities and polypharmacy.
- Analgesics inappropriate for use in the elderly include pethidine and NSAIDs.

Analgesic use in opioid-tolerant people

- Acute pain treatment in opioid-tolerant people is difficult due to tolerance and/or blockade of ORs. Pain and the addictive disorder must be carefully assessed, and prescribers need to be alert to drug-seeking behaviours. Other techniques of pain management are used whenever possible.

DRUGS AT A GLANCE
Analgesics

PHARMACOLOGICAL GROUP AND EFFECT	KEY EXAMPLES	CLINICAL USE
Opioid analgesics		
• Act as agonists at μ (m; mu), G-protein-coupled trans-membrane receptors • Activation inhibits adenylate cyclase and reduces cyclic adenosine monophosphate (cAMP) levels • Also opens potassium channels and inhibits opening of calcium channels, reducing neuronal excitability and inhibiting release of excitatory (pain) transmitters	Morphine, fentanyl, codeine	Analgesia Suppression of cough reflex

Opioid antagonists		
Opioid receptor antagonists • Competitively block μ (m; mu) receptors to reverse action of opioids	Naloxone	Reversal of opioid overdose, constipation refractory to treatment with regular laxatives
Non-opioid analgesics		
Antipyretic analgesics • Inhibit PG synthesis in the hypothalamus, the temperature-regulating centre of the body	Paracetamol	Pain, fever and mild anti-inflammatory effect
NSAIDs • Block the enzyme COX pathway thereby preventing the formation of inflammatory mediators such as PGs and thromboxanes	Aspirin, ibuprofen	Treatment of mild to moderate pain due to inflammation
Counterirritants • Capsaicin activates capsaicin receptors (transient receptor potential vanilloid 1 (TRPV1) ion channel), causing an initial release and then a depletion of substance P from nerve fibres	Capsaicin	Shingles; neuropathic pain
Adjuvant drugs		
Tricyclic antidepressants • Inhibit 5-HT reuptake at nerve terminals Serotonin–norepinephrine (noradrenaline) reuptake inhibitors • Inhibit 5-HT and noradrenaline reuptake at nerve terminals	Amitriptyline Duloxetine, venlafaxine	Neuropathic pain
Membrane stabilising agents Antiepileptics/anticonvulsants • Increase activity of GABA, blocking sodium channels to reduce the frequency of action potentials, and inhibit a subtype of glutamate receptors Local anaesthetics • Block neuronal sodium channels to reduce sodium-channel-mediated transmission of nociception	Topiramate Lidocaine (lignocaine)	Neuropathic pain
GABA analogues (gabapentinoids) • Enhance gamma-aminobutyric acid (GABA)-mediated inhibition	Gabapentin, pregabalin	Neuropathic pain
NMDA receptor antagonists • Block NMDA receptors implicated in the afferent pathways	Ketamine	Acute postoperative pain Analgesia Adjunct/adjuvant

REVIEW EXERCISES

1. Mr JP, a 25 year old, was found lying on the ground in a local park. An ambulance was called, and it was noted that he was he was drowsy but arousable, appeared cyanotic, with a respiratory rate of 10 breaths per minute, and oxygen saturation of 80%. He had pinpoint pupils and shallow breathing. The person who found him stated that he was known to use heroin and had recently returned from rehabilitation and was now on a methadone program. Paramedics administered intranasal naloxone and he became alert and oriented although agitated. Describe the mechanisms of action of heroin and methadone. Why did the paramedics administer naloxone? What is its mechanism of action? What dosage considerations should the paramedics make when administering naloxone?
2. Mr BR is a 59-year-old man with metastatic disease of unknown origin. He reports his pain as 9 on a scale of 1 (least pain) to 10 (most severe pain). His prescriber ordered Panadeine Forte (paracetamol 500 mg with codeine phosphate 30 mg) 1–2 tablets every 6 hours as required for pain. Two hours after receiving two tablets of this medication, Mr BR is still in very severe pain. Was this order appropriate for the reported pain level? How might the prescription be improved? What adjuvant medications and non-pharmacological interventions would you suggest, and why?
3. Further questions related to the Critical Thinking Scenario at the beginning of the chapter.
   a. Would you need to change your plans for procedural sedation and post-injury analgesia if the child had experienced more severe and unpredictable asthma attacks recently?
   b. What are the advantages and disadvantages of combined oral liquid preparations for children, such as PainStop for Children?
   c. After the setting of his broken arm what signs will you be observing closely? How will you assess any breakthrough pain?

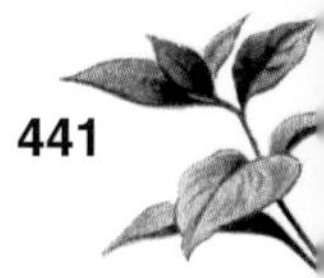

REFERENCES

Anekar AA, Cascella M, 2021. WHO Analgesic Ladder. [Updated 2021 May 18]. In: StatPearls [Internet]. Treasure Island (FL): StatPearls Publishing. Available from: https://www.ncbi.nlm.nih.gov/books/NBK554435/

Argoff C, 2011: Mechanisms of pain transmission and pharmacologic management. Current Medical Research and Opinion 27(10):2019–2031.

Australian Medicines Handbook, 2021. Australian medicines handbook 2021, Adelaide, AMH.

Bannister K, Dickenson AH, 2020. Central Nervous System Targets: Supraspinal Mechanisms of Analgesia. Neurotherapeutics. 17(3):839–845. doi:10.1007/s13311-020-00887-6

Beggs S, 2008: Paediatric analgesia. Australian Prescriber. 31(3):63–65.

Bhadelia A, De Lima L, Arreola-Ornelas H, et al., 2019. Solving the global crisis in access to pain relief: lessons from country actions. American Journal of Public Health. 109(1), 58–60. https://doi.org/10.2105/AJPH.2018.304769

Bodnar RJ, 2016: Endogenous opiates and behavior: Peptides. 75:18–70.

Borsodi A, Bruchas M, Caló G, et al., 2019. Opioid receptors (version 2019.4) in the IUPHAR/BPS Guide to Pharmacology Database. IUPHAR/BPS Guide to Pharmacology CITE. 2019(4). Available from: https://doi.org/10.2218/gtopdb/F50/2019.4.

Braun L, Cohen M, 2010: Herbs and natural supplements: an evidence-based guide, ed 3, Sydney, Elsevier Churchill Livingstone.

Carr DB, Jacox AK, Chapman CR, et al., 1992: Acute pain management: operative or medical procedures and trauma. Clinical practice guideline. AHCPR Pub. No. 92-0032. Rockville, MD: Agency for Health Care Policy and Research, Public Health Service, US Department of Health and Human Services.

Christensen KS, Cohen AE, Mermelstein FH, et al., 2008: The analgesic efficacy and safety of a novel intranasal morphine formulation (morphine plus chitosan), immediate release oral morphine, intravenous morphine, and placebo in a postsurgical dental pain model. Anesthesia & Analgesia; 107(6): 2018–24. doi: 10.1213/ane.0b013e318187b952.

Hale M, Garofoli M, Raffa RB, 2021. Benefit-risk analysis of buprenorphine for pain management. Journal of Pain Research. 14:1359–1369. doi:10.2147/JPR.S305146

HANDI (Handbook of Non Drug Intervention) Project Team: Sweet solutions for procedural pain in infants. Australian Family Physician. 2013;42(8):572.

Horn R, Kramer J, 2021. Postoperative pain control. [Updated 2020 Jun 28]. In: StatPearls [Internet]. Treasure Island (FL): StatPearls Publishing. Available from: https://www.ncbi.nlm.nih.gov/books/NBK544298/

Kreutzwiser D, Tawfic QA, 2019. Expanding Role of NMDA Receptor Antagonists in the Management of Pain. CNS Drugs. 33(4): 347–374. doi: 10.1007/s40263-019-00618-2. PMID: 30826987

Melzack R, Wall PD, 1965: Pain mechanisms: a new theory. Science 150:971–979.

Mills SEE, Nicolson KP, Smith BH, 2019. Chronic pain: a review of its epidemiology and associated factors in population-based studies. British Journal of Anaesthesia. 123(2): e273–e283. doi: 10.1016/j.bja.2019.03.023. Epub 2019 May 10. PMID: 31079836; PMCID: PMC6676152.

Ministry of Health, 2020. Annual Data Explorer 2019/20: New Zealand Health Survey [Data File]. URL: https://minhealthnz.shinyapps.io/nz-health-survey-2019-20-annual-data-explorer/

Murnion BP, 2010: Combination analgesics in adults, Aust Prescr. 33(4):113–115.

Murtagh JE, 2006: Managing painful paediatric procedures. Australian Prescriber. 29:94–96.

Pain and Analgesia, [published 2021 Mar]. In: Therapeutic Guidelines [digital]. Melbourne: Therapeutic Guidelines Limited; 2021 Mar. https://www.tg.org.au

Rang HP, Dale MM, Ritter JM, et al., 2007: Pharmacology, ed 6, Edinburgh, Churchill Livingstone.

Roohbakhsh A, Alavi MS, Azhdari-Zarmehri H, 2018. The Orexinergic (Hypocretin) System and Nociception: an update to supraspinal mechanisms. Current Medicinal Chemistry. 25(32):3917–3929. doi: 10.2174/0929867324666170529072554. PMID: 28552056.

Salerno E, Willens JS, 1996: Pain management handbook, St Louis, MO, Mosby.

Salerno E, 1999: Pharmacology for health professionals, St Louis, MO, Mosby.

Srivastava AB, Mariani JJ, Levin FR, 2020. New directions in the treatment of opioid withdrawal. Lancet. 395(10241): 1938–1948. doi: 10.1016/S0140-6736(20)30852-7. PMID: 32563380; PMCID: PMC7385662.

Therapeutic Guidelines Limited, 2021. Pain and Analgesia [published 2021 Mar]. In: Therapeutic Guidelines [digital]. Melbourne: Therapeutic Guidelines Limited https://www.tg.org.au

Vane JR, 1971: Inhibition of prostaglandin synthesis as a mechanism of action for aspirin-like drugs. Nature New Biology. 231:232–239.

Vane JR, 2000: The fight against rheumatism: from willow-bark to COX-1 sparing drugs. Journal of Physiology and Pharmacology. 51(4 Pt 1):573–586.

Wang C, Meng Q, 2021. Global research trends of herbal medicine for pain in three decades (1990–2019): a bibliometric analysis. Journal of Pain Research. 14:1611–1626. Published, 2021 Jun 4. doi:10.2147/JPR.S311311bhade

Wong D, Hockenberry-Eaton M, Wilson D, et al., 2001: Wong's essentials of pediatric nursing, ed 6, St Louis, MO, Mosby.

Yang MMH, Hartley RL, Leung AA, et al., 2019. Preoperative predictors of poor acute postoperative pain control: a systematic review and meta-analysis. BMJ Open. 9(4): e025091. doi: 10.1136/bmjopen-2018-025091. PMID: 30940757; PMCID: PMC6500309.

ONLINE RESOURCES

MIMS Online: https://www.mimsonline.com.au/Login/Login.aspx?ReturnUrl=%2fdefault.aspx (accessed 20 January 2022)

NPS MedicineWise – Pain management in patients with a history of opioid dependence. Information for health professionals: https://www2.health.vic.gov.au/Api/downloadmedia/%7BA97F0E38-B1E3-4293-A061-7D0362BB8CC6%7D (accessed 20 January 2022)

Royal Children's Hospital Melbourne – information on reducing pain and distress in children: https://www.rch.org.au/comfortkids (accessed 20 January 2022)

More weblinks at: http://evolve.elsevier.com/AU/Knights/pharmacology/.

— CHAPTER 20 —

ANTIANXIETY, SEDATIVE AND HYPNOTIC DRUGS

Shaunagh Darroch

KEY ABBREVIATIONS

CAM complementary and alternative medicine
CNS central nervous system
EEG electroencephalograph
GABA gamma-aminobutyric acid
REM rapid eye movement
SNRIs serotonin noradrenaline reuptake inhibitors
SSRIs selective serotonin reuptake inhibitors
TCA tricyclic antidepressant

KEY TERMS

anterograde amnesic effect 452
antianxiety (anxiolytic) agents 445
anxiety 444
benzodiazepines 448
gamma-aminobutyric acid 444
hypnotics 446
insomnia 444
melatonin 457
non–rapid eye movement (non-REM) sleep 443
orexin 458
psycholeptics 448
rapid eye movement (REM) sleep 443
sedatives 446
sleep hygiene 446
Z-drugs 456

Chapter Focus

Anxiety and insomnia are common health problems that occur across the life span. When anxiety or fear is in response to a threat or danger, this is a normal physiological response to a threatening situation. However, excessive anxiety or panic that interferes with daily functioning and sleep is counterproductive and usually requires medical intervention and treatment. Insomnia is a common sleep disorder and is often a concern in the elderly. This chapter reviews the antianxiety, sedative and hypnotic drugs available to treat these disorders. Barbiturates were previously used extensively as sedative–hypnotic agents, but because of their low therapeutic index and relative non-selectivity they have largely been replaced by the safer benzodiazepines and newer related agents that have specific anxiolytic (antianxiety) actions. Antidepressants (Ch 22) are now recommended as first-line treatment for anxiety disorders.

KEY DRUG GROUPS

Barbiturates:

- Phenobarbital (phenobarbitone)

Benzodiazepines:

- **Diazepam** (Drug Monograph 20.1), **lorazepam**, **midazolam** (Drug Monograph 20.2)

Benzodiazepine antagonists:

- **Flumazenil**

Other sedatives/hypnotics:

- Buspirone, **chloral hydrate**, **melatonin**, **promethazine**, suvorexant

Z-drugs:

- **Zolpidem**, **zopiclone**

CRITICAL THINKING SCENARIO

Millie, aged 3 years, is attending a remote health service clinic with her two parents in preparation for upcoming cleft palate surgery. A specialist clinic appointment and CT scan has been scheduled at the nearest regional hospital. This appointment will require a 4-hour road trip and an overnight stay for the family.

Her parents are reminded that, to facilitate the scan, Millie may need to be still for 20–30 minutes, and short-term sedation using a drug named chloral hydrate may be required. The parents mention that their daughter becomes distressed during her frequent medical procedures and that the long road trips are also a cause of agitation. They have heard that a drug named Phenergan™ could be used to calm their daughter during the road trip.

1. What is the mechanism of action of chloral hydrate?
2. What is the recommended clinical use for chloral hydrate? Note potential adverse reactions, contraindications and special precautions.
3. What advice would you give about using Phenergan™ for the road trip?
4. What is Phenergan's generic name and mechanism of action?
5. What are potential adverse reactions, contraindications and special precautions for use as a sedative in paediatrics?
6. What are other clinical uses for this drug?

Introduction: Sleep and anxiety

Sleep: Physiology and purposes

Sleep is a recurrent, natural, reversible condition of inertia, reduced consciousness and reduced metabolism, during which a person is no longer in sensory contact with the immediate environment, and stimuli no longer attract attention or exert a controlling influence over voluntary and involuntary movements or functions. Some of the proposed purposes of sleep are to regulate glucose homeostasis and appetite, consolidate synaptic circuits to maintain memory and regulate hormone levels and circadian rhythms. A person's normal sleep pattern can vary from night to night and is influenced by their emotional and physical state. The sleep pattern is controlled from the ascending reticular activating system in the brainstem, as noted in Chapter 18. The main neurotransmitters involved in sleep are histamine, noradrenaline (norepinephrine), serotonin and the orexins.

Stages of sleep

The stages of sleep are based on electrical activity that can be observed in the brain by means of an electroencephalograph (EEG). The EEG is also used to detect abnormal brainwaves in epilepsy, for example (Fig 21.1, in Ch 21). Sleep consists of two fundamental states that occur cyclically: non–rapid eye movement (non-REM) sleep and rapid eye movement (REM) sleep. Periods of REM and non-REM sleep alternate throughout the night. The individual moves through three stages of **non-REM sleep** (stage 1, stage 2 and combined stages 3 and 4) into progressively deeper stages of sleep during which brainwaves are seen to be of high amplitude and low frequency (Fig 20.1). The individual then passes into **REM sleep**, which is characterised by rapid eye movements, dreaming and low-amplitude, high-frequency waves on an EEG (similar to the awake state).

REM sleep is not synonymous with light sleep: it takes a more powerful stimulus to arouse a person from REM sleep than from synchronous slow-wave sleep.

The sleep–wake cycle varies with age: infants spend more time asleep, and a much greater proportion of sleep time in REM sleep, than do adults. Adolescents usually prefer to go to sleep later, whereas elderly people tend to go to sleep earlier, and spend more time

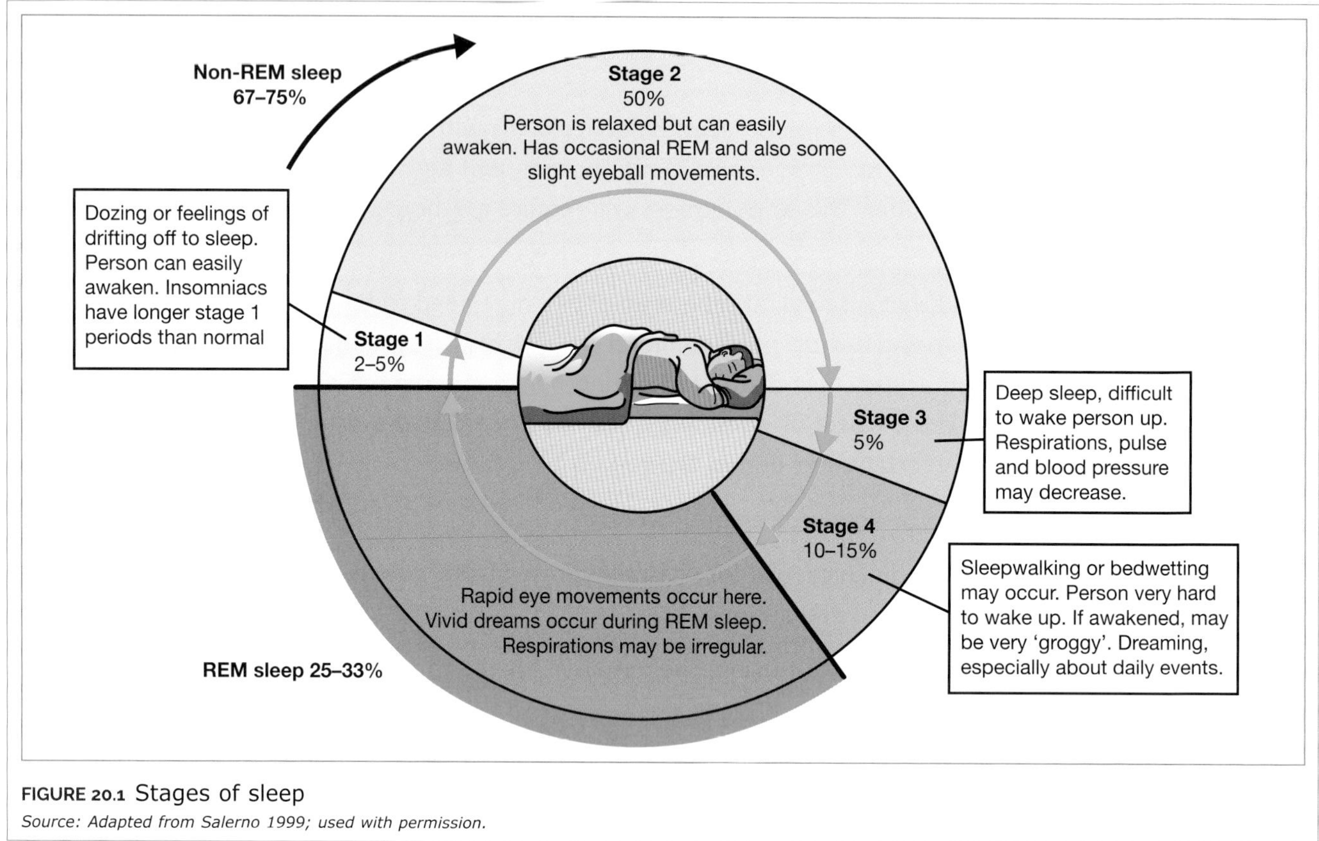

FIGURE 20.1 Stages of sleep
Source: Adapted from Salerno 1999; used with permission.

in stages 1 and 2 of non-REM sleep with frequent arousals.

Sleep disorders

A person's sleep patterns can be affected by their emotional and physical states and can vary from night to night. There are various sleep disorders caused by neurological disorders or lifestyle factors. Sleep-related respiratory disorders include obstructive sleep apnoea and Cheyne-Stokes respiration associated with congestive cardiac failure. Shift workers whose regular circadian rhythms are often disrupted may suffer from adverse effects on hormonal and metabolic patterns. Narcolepsy is an uncommon neurological disorder that affects sleep–wake cycles and causes episodes of unpreventable sleep throughout the day.

Insomnia

Insomnia is the inability to obtain adequate sleep, whether from difficulty in falling asleep, frequent nocturnal waking or early awakening. It can be classified as a standalone disorder or associated with other disorders (e.g. depression). Excessive intake of central nervous system (CNS) stimulants such as caffeine-containing drinks can cause insomnia, as can anxiety disorders, depression, alcohol abuse, environmental factors (heat, cold and noise), pain, cardiac or respiratory disorders and jet lag. Furthermore, shift workers often suffer adverse effects on hormonal and metabolic patterns. It is important to treat the causes of insomnia individually.

Disorders of excessive daytime sleepiness may be due to inadequate sleep at night, excessive use of CNS depressants (including antidepressants, antihistamines and alcohol), and narcolepsy (sudden sleep attacks) or sleep apnoea causing disturbed sleep at night. Clinical Focus Box 20.1 lists some drugs that can cause insomnia or sedation.

Anxiety

Anxiety is a state of apprehension, agitation, uncertainty and fear resulting from the experience or anticipation of some stress or danger. It may impact on sleep cycles and may interfere with day-to-day activities. Anxiety is thought to be mediated in the limbic system (Fig 20.2); neurotransmitters particularly involved are noradrenaline, 5-hydroxytryptamine (5-HT [serotonin]) and **gamma-aminobutyric acid** (GABA), while the neuropeptide cholecystokinin appears to be a modulator in panic disorder. The orexin neuropeptides are

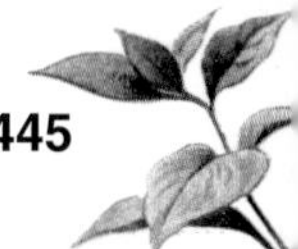

CLINICAL FOCUS BOX 20.1

Drugs associated with inducing insomnia or causing sedation

Drugs liable to induce insomnia or sleep disturbances

- ACE inhibitors (e.g. perindopril)
- Alcohol
- β-adrenoceptor antagonists (e.g. propranolol)
- CNS stimulants (amphetamines, caffeine)
- Corticosteroids
- Levodopa
- Methyldopa
- Metoclopramide
- Monoamine oxidase inhibitors
- Nicotine (cigarettes, gum, patches)
- Phenytoin
- Thyroid hormones
- Xanthines (caffeine, theophylline)

Withdrawal from CNS depressants can induce insomnia; these depressants include alcohol, barbiturates, benzodiazepines, tricyclic antidepressants, hypnotics and opioids.

Drugs liable to induce sedation or CNS depression

- Alcohol
- All CNS depressants (e.g. benzodiazepines, barbiturates, antiepileptics, general anaesthetics)
- Antihistamines
- Antipsychotics (phenothiazines)
- Cannabis (marijuana)
- Clonidine
- Melatonin
- Methyldopa
- Opioids
- Tricyclic antidepressants (high doses)

Effects of alcohol

It is notable that alcohol can induce insomnia or sleep disturbances and sedation. Alcohol is a CNS depressant; hence, it acts as a hypnotic, and is taken by many people as a 'nightcap'. However, it also disrupts sleep, delaying and reducing time spent in REM sleep, suppressing breathing and increasing snoring due to its muscle relaxant and nasal congestant effects (from additives in red wines, especially). It is recommended that alcohol not be drunk within about 2 hours of bedtime.

produced in discrete groups of neurons in the hypothalamus and are involved in regulation of the sleep–wake and activity cycles, feeding and reward-seeking, as well as anxiety and depressive behaviours. Orexin receptor antagonists are being investigated for their role in reducing panic/anxiety and promoting sleep (see under 'Miscellaneous Anxiolytics, Sedatives and Hypnotics' later).

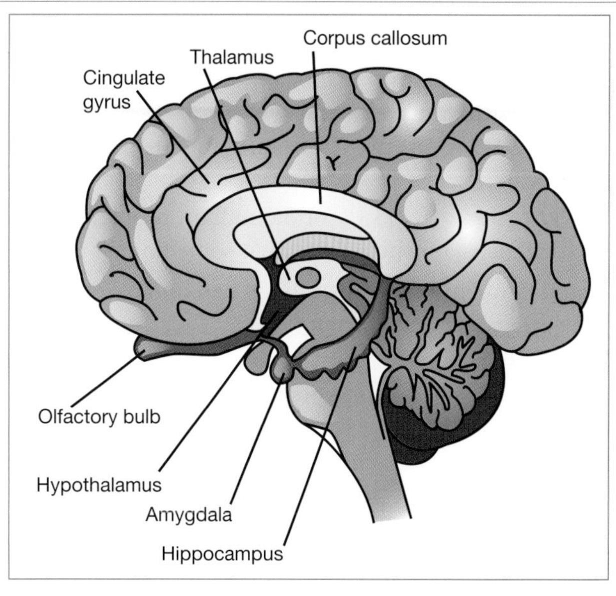

FIGURE 20.2 Sagittal section of the human brain, showing components of the limbic system

Anxiety is usually a natural psychological and physiological response to a personally threatening situation such as a threat to one's health, loved ones, job or lifestyle. Generally, this anxiety effectively stimulates the person to take constructive actions to counteract the perceived threats. In its extreme form, anxiety can be characterised by autonomic nervous system responses including rapid heart rate, dry mouth, sweaty palms, insomnia, loss of appetite, muscle tremor, diarrhoea and dyspnoea.

When excessive anxiety interferes with daily functioning, it may be necessary to seek help. Many non-pharmacological treatments such as counselling and behaviour modification therapies are available, while **anxiolytic** drugs (**antianxiety agents**) are commonly prescribed for the short-term treatment of anxiety. These drugs reduce feelings of excessive anxiety, such as apprehension, fear and panic, and reduce the physiological responses, such as dyspnoea and insomnia, thus improving sleep patterns. Hence, both directly and indirectly, anxiolytic drugs are also sedatives/hypnotics. The drug classes to be discussed in this context include benzodiazepines as well as antidepressants and atypical antipsychotics.

Generalised anxiety disorder

Generalised anxiety disorder exists when a person has symptoms of excessive anxiety, uncontrollable worry, irritability, muscle tension and sleep disturbances for a period of 6 months or longer. It is common, affecting up to 5% of the population. In 2022 the Australian Bureau of Statistics released the results of the National Study of Mental Health and Wellbeing.

In 2020–21, of the 19.6 million Australians aged 16–85 years:

- Over two in five (43.7% or 8.6 million people) had experienced a mental disorder at some time in their life.
- 16.8 per cent of all Australians had an anxiety Disorder (see also Chapter 22)

Anxiety particularly affects young to middle-aged adults, those separated/divorced/widowed, people living in rural areas and those with no tertiary qualifications or who are unemployed; concurrent other affective, anxiety, substance abuse or personality disorders are frequent (Australian Bureau of Statistics 2018).

The most effective drugs used for treatment are the selective serotonin reuptake inhibitor antidepressants (SSRIs) and selective noradrenaline reuptake inhibitors, described fully in Chapter 22 (see review by Lampe 2013; Bandelow et al. 2017).

Related disorders

Panic is an acute condition characterised by intense fears, with palpitations, sweating and chest pain, sensations of choking or smothering, and feelings of unreality or dizziness. It is often associated with anxiety about being in particular situations (alone, or in an enclosed space such as in a lift, in a crowd, on a bridge, in a vehicle). Panic disorder involves recurrent and unexpected disabling panic attacks not associated with a situational trigger, with persistent concerns and behaviour changes.

Other associated disorders include adjustment disorder with anxious mood, obsessive–compulsive disorder, phobic disorders and post-traumatic stress disorder. For most of these conditions, drug therapy is not the preferred option. Recommended primary therapies include counselling, relaxation techniques and cognitive behaviour therapy. Short-term use of anxiolytic or antidepressant drugs is sometimes required.

Treatment of sleep disorders

Cognitive behaviour therapy is initially recommended followed by treatment of comorbidities and short-term use of drugs that promote sleep such as the sedatives and hypnotics. All are CNS depressants. **Sedatives**, including the benzodiazepines and Z-drugs, reduce alertness, consciousness, nervousness or excitability by producing a calming or soothing effect. **Hypnotics** induce sleep. The main difference between a sedative and a hypnotic is the degree of CNS depression induced: the same drug might be used in small doses for a sedative effect and in larger doses for hypnotic effects. Sedatives were previously called the minor tranquillisers to distinguish them from the antipsychotic drugs (major tranquillisers) used in treating schizophrenia and include the benzodiazepines and barbiturates. Antipsychotics and tricyclic antidepressants (TCAs) are not recommended for treating insomnia; however, the SSRIs, such as escitalopram, are indicated if the causative factor is a severe anxiety disorder (e.g. panic disorder, obsessive–compulsive disorder) (Ch 22). Orexin antagonists such as suvorexant may be used to manage insomnia by acting as antagonists in the arousal centre (see later: 'Miscellaneous Anxiolytics, Sedatives and Hypnotics').

Management of sleep disorders requires careful attention to specific sleep history and patterns, drug history (including use of 'social' drugs such as caffeine and alcohol) and discussion of lifestyle and psychological factors that might impair good sleep cycles. As above, any physical or depressive or anxiety disorders that might disturb sleep need treating.

The aim of any treatment of sleep disorders is to restore normal sleep architecture. Owing to the risk of dependence, sedative/hypnotic drugs should be used only for limited periods – for example, 2–4 weeks – to assist with anxiety, or impaired sleep cycles following jet lag or shift-work changes, or in one-off doses as preoperative medication. They are not recommended for people aged over 60 years, those who need to drive or make important decisions the next day or those who live alone.

Sleep hygiene

Non-pharmacological treatments include promotion of good sleep patterns (**sleep hygiene**). For example:

- Avoid evening activities that stimulate the CNS or impair sleep, including consuming caffeinated drinks, smoking cigarettes or taking strenuous exercise; taking diuretic drugs (including excessive alcohol); and having computers, TV or pets in the bedroom.
- Encourage regular sleep–wake patterns, exercise during the day, relax before retiring, have a snack or warm non-caffeinated drink before bed, use behavioural therapy to reduce anxiety, and ensure a quiet and dark bedroom (Psychotropic Expert Group 2021).

Paediatric and geriatric use of sedatives and hypnotics

Paediatric sedative use

Because young children are more sensitive than adults to the CNS-depressant effects of antianxiety, sedative or hypnotic drugs (Clinical Focus Box 20.2), use of these agents is not recommended, and counselling and psychotherapy are usually tried first. However, sedation may be indicated for particular situations and the drug

> **CLINICAL FOCUS BOX 20.2**
> **Paediatric implications**
>
> Antianxiety agents and sedatives
>
> - To minimise excessive CNS-depressant effects, the manufacturer's dosage instructions should be followed carefully, and concurrent administration of other CNS-depressants avoided, including those in over-the-counter medications.
> - Benzodiazepines should be avoided except to treat convulsive disorders (Ch 21), and for short-term use in specific conditions such as night terrors or sleepwalking; close monitoring and assessment are required.
> - Children should be monitored for excessive sedation, lethargy and lack of coordination, and doses adjusted accordingly.
> - In neonates and infants, profound CNS depression can result because of the lower rate of drug metabolism by the immature liver.
> - Paradoxical reactions (reactions contrary to the expected reaction) such as excitability, hostility, confusion and hallucinations have been reported in children with the use of antihistamines and barbiturates.
> - Benzodiazepines should not be used to treat a hyperactive or psychotic child.
> - Chronic use of clonazepam (an antiepileptic) can result in impaired physical, endocrine or mental functions in the developing child, which may not become apparent until years later.
> - Newer sedative drugs such as buspirone (under the Special Access Scheme in Australia) and the Z-drugs have not been widely studied in children, so they are not recommended.

and dosage are carefully selected for the individual child. Antihistamines are generally safe for mild sedation.

Young children may need sedation for medical indications, including before medical, surgical, dental or diagnostic procedures, or when they are in intensive care to minimise the risk of removal of catheters. Clinical and risk assessments must be undertaken prior to sedation. Drugs used in these situations include propofol, intravenous (IV) induction anaesthetic agents, oral midazolam and inhaled nitrous oxide.

Geriatric sedative use

Sleep disturbance is one of the most frequent concerns of elderly people, who have more fragmented sleeping patterns than do younger adults; they may have reduced daytime activity, may take multiple daytime naps, tend to go to bed earlier and may have difficulty in falling asleep. Anxiety may interrupt their sleep, and they tend to wake earlier. There is some evidence that, in elderly people, the circadian sleep–wake pattern is advanced to earlier hours by earlier secretion of melatonin. Primary sleep disorders, including sleep apnoea and restless legs syndrome, and other factors such as retirement, death of a close friend or spouse, social isolation and polypharmacy, also contribute to disturbed sleep.

Hypnotic/sedative drugs are used about three times more pro rata by elderly people than by younger adults. Before these drugs are prescribed, elderly people should be evaluated for pre-existing health conditions that can alter sleep patterns, such as arthritic pain, cardiac dysrhythmia, paroxysmal nocturnal dyspnoea and the need to urinate.

Drug interactions and increased sensitivity to CNS effects of drugs combine to cause frequent problems. The use of TCAs, sedating antihistamines, chloral hydrate or antipsychotics is not recommended for insomnia in the elderly due to limited evidence for effectiveness and the risk of adverse reactions and toxicity (Ch 41).

Paradoxical reactions (i.e. increased excitability, rage, hostility, confusion and hallucinations) have been reported in elderly people taking barbiturates and, in rare instances, the benzodiazepines; these agents should be monitored.

Altered pharmacokinetics in geriatrics

As described in Chapter 6, pharmacokinetic characteristics of drugs are frequently different in older adults, leading to delayed elimination and hence increased accumulation, with risk of toxicity. For example, the half-life of diazepam is about 20 hours in 20-year-old adults but 90 hours in people in their eighties. With sedative/hypnotics, careful drug selection and dosage is necessary to avoid producing excessive CNS depression in the elderly. Some factors to consider are:

- Because elimination half-lives may be extended, drugs with shorter half-lives and no active metabolites (which might accumulate and cause toxicity) are safer for elderly people.
- Barbiturates commonly cause confusion and ataxia in elderly people, so short-acting benzodiazepines such as oxazepam, temazepam and alprazolam are safer for those who require a sedative (Table 20.1).
- Intake of hypnotic drugs should be limited to three or four times a week, allowing people to select the nights on which they most need to take their medication. This schedule usually results in enhanced effectiveness, less daytime drowsiness or sedation and a decreased potential for inducing tolerance to the medication.
- Regular and careful monitoring and re-evaluation of the need for hypnotics are recommended.

KEY POINTS

Sleep and anxiety

- Sleep is a recurrent, natural, reversible condition of inertia, reduced consciousness and reduced metabolism.
- A person's sleep pattern is influenced by their emotional and physical state and is controlled from the ascending reticular activating system in the brainstem. The main neurotransmitters involved are histamine, noradrenaline (norepinephrine), serotonin and the orexins.
- The stages of sleep are monitored via an EEG and consist of two fundamental states that occur cyclically: non-REM and REM sleep.
- Sleep disorders, including insomnia, disorders of excessive daytime sleepiness, narcolepsy and sleep apnoea, cause many physiological dysfunctions. They are common, particularly in elderly people.
- Anxiety is a state of apprehension, agitation, uncertainty and fear resulting from the experience or anticipation of some stress or danger. It can impact on sleep cycles and may interfere with day-to-day activities.
- Anxiety is thought to be mediated in the limbic system. The neurotransmitters particularly involved are noradrenaline, 5-HT and GABA.
- Anxiety disorders include generalised anxiety, panic, obsessive–compulsive, phobic and post-traumatic stress disorders.
- Anxiolytic drugs (antianxiety agents) are commonly prescribed for the short-term treatment of anxiety. Drugs used for anxiety include benzodiazepines (sedatives and hypnotics), antidepressants and antipsychotics.
- Treatment of sleep disorders includes the sedatives and hypnotics; all are CNS depressants.
- Sedatives, including the benzodiazepines, reduce alertness, consciousness, nervousness or excitability. Hypnotics induce sleep.
- Non-pharmacological treatments for sleep disorders include promotion of good sleep patterns (sleep hygiene).
- Owing to the risk of dependence, sedative/hypnotic drugs should be used only for limited periods.
- In paediatric clients, caution is advised in using anxiolytics, sedatives or hypnotics, due to their CNS-depressant effects.
- In geriatric clients, sleep disturbance is one of the most frequent concerns. Hypnotic/sedative drugs are used, although drug interactions, altered pharmacokinetics and increased sensitivity to CNS effects combine to cause frequent problems.

Sedatives, hypnotics and anxiolytics

A psychoactive drug that acts on the central nervous system and has a sedating effect is named **psycholeptic**. Psycholeptics include benzodiazepines, barbiturates, phenothiazines and opioids.

Benzodiazepines

The **benzodiazepines** are among the most widely prescribed drugs in clinical medicine, primarily because of their advantages over older sedative/hypnotic agents such as barbiturates, chloral hydrate and alcohol, and their action as anxiolytics. These advantages include:

- specific dose-related anxiolytic action
- lower fatality rates following acute toxicity and overdose
- lower potential for abuse
- more favourable adverse effect profiles
- fewer potentially serious drug interactions when administered with other medications
- the availability of a specific antidote (flumazenil).

Diazepam (well known as Valium; see Drug Monograph 20.1) is the prototype benzodiazepine. It was the most prescribed for many years until newer and safer (shorter acting) benzodiazepines such as temazepam and alprazolam were released. As the various benzodiazepines have similar pharmacodynamic effects, they will be discussed as a group; pharmacokinetic differences are summarised in Table 20.1.

Pharmacological effects

Benzodiazepines are not general CNS-depressants: specific actions include sedative, hypnotic, antianxiety, muscle-relaxant, antiepileptic and memory-impairing effects.

Mechanism of action

Benzodiazepines act via effects on receptors for the inhibitory CNS neurotransmitter GABA. This is the main inhibitory transmitter in the brain, at about 30% of all CNS synapses, in many pathways and brain areas (Table 18.1, in Ch 18). There are 11 different confirmed subtypes of $GABA_A$ receptors; all are ligand-gated chloride channels, composed of five sub-units, in the membranes of postsynaptic cells, and they mediate fast inhibition: when activated by GABA, there is an increase in chloride permeability and influx of chloride into the cell causing hyperpolarisation and decreased excitability of the neuron.

$GABA_A$ receptors have several modulatory sites at which drugs can act; particular sites have been identified as involved with different actions – for example, sedative, anxiolytic, muscle relaxant or affecting cognition. The natural endogenous ligand is (obviously) GABA, but other

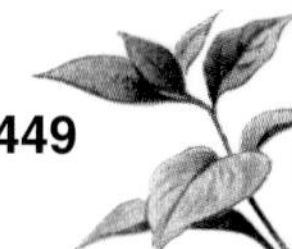

Drug Monograph 20.1
Diazepam

Diazepam is the prototype benzodiazepine and, as such, has anxiolytic, sedative–hypnotic, muscle relaxant and antiepileptic actions.

Mechanism of action

Diazepam acts as an agonist at an allosteric modulatory site (sometimes confusingly referred to as the benzodiazepine receptor) to facilitate GABA binding to the $GABA_A$ receptors, changing conformation of the active site and thus enhancing the frequency of chloride channel opening, leading to more neuronal inhibition. This results in anxiolytic, sedative, hypnotic, muscle relaxant as well as antiepileptic effects.

Indications

Diazepam is indicated for short-term (a few days) management of anxiety, acute withdrawal from alcohol or benzodiazepines, acute behavioural disturbance, muscle spasm and spasticity, premedication and conscious sedation, and febrile seizures and epilepsy (as adjunctive treatment or for acute treatment of seizures such as in status epilepticus).

Pharmacokinetics

Diazepam is one of the longest-acting benzodiazepines because it is very lipid-soluble and has active metabolites, some of which themselves are administered as benzodiazepines (Table 20.1). However, owing to its metabolism to active derivatives and hence very long duration of action, other benzodiazepines may be indicated when short-acting sedatives are required or for the elderly.

Adverse reactions

All benzodiazepines can cause excessive CNS depression, dependence and neurological dysfunction.

Diazepam is likely to cause fatigue, drowsiness and muscle weakness. Less common adverse effects include disturbances of memory, gastrointestinal tract function, genitourinary functions and vision and skin reactions.

Paradoxical CNS stimulation can occur. Tolerance and dependence develop readily.

Drug interactions

Diazepam has additive CNS-depressant effects with all other CNS depressants, including alcohol, other sedative–hypnotics, antihistamines, anaesthetics, antidepressants and antiepileptic agents.

Many drugs can inhibit the metabolism of diazepam and hence prolong its effects; examples are cimetidine and fluconazole (see also Drug Interactions 20.1).

Warnings and contraindications

Diazepam is contraindicated in people with chronic obstructive airways disease, severe respiratory or liver disease, sleep apnoea, myasthenia gravis and dependence on other substances or hypersensitivity to benzodiazepines.

It should be prescribed only for short periods. Dependence develops readily and a long withdrawal period may be necessary to avoid withdrawal seizures.

Diazepam should be used only with caution in people with glaucoma, impaired kidney or liver function, depression or other psychosis, elderly or very young people, or during pregnancy or lactation. In pregnancy consider the use of shorter acting benzodiazepines.

Dosage and administration

Dosage should be individualised depending on the person's liver and kidney functions, age and the indication for which the drug is prescribed

- agitation and anxiety: diazepam is normally given orally, the adult dose being 2–5 mg up to a maximum of 10 mg daily; it can also be administered IV or by rectal solution
- premedication: IV, 0.1–0.2 mg/kg
- acute severe anxiety, agitation, behaviour disturbance: IV, 5–10 mg, repeated if necessary every 5–10 minutes to a maximum of 30 mg.

endogenous ligands have been identified, including some neuropeptides and steroid metabolites. These could be considered the body's 'natural diazepam', by analogy with endorphins being named as the body's endogenous morphine.

Benzodiazepines do not act as agonists by occupying the entire $GABA_A$ receptor or at the active site but act at an allosteric modulatory site (sometimes confusingly referred to as the benzodiazepine receptor) to facilitate GABA binding to the $GABA_A$ receptors, changing conformation of the active site and thus enhancing the frequency of chloride channel opening, leading to more neuronal inhibition. The limbic system (Fig 20.2),

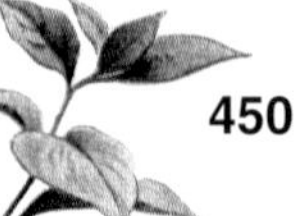

TABLE 20.1 Pharmacokinetic overview: benzodiazepines

NAME	DURATION OF ACTION	HALF-LIFE (h)	ACTIVE METABOLITES (HALF-LIFE [h])	MAIN INDICATIONS
Midazolam	VS	1–3	1-hydroxymidazolam (1–3)	Sedation, premedication, induction anaesthetic, status epilepticus
Alprazolam	S	11–16	4-hydroxyalprazolam and α-hydroxyalprazolam (10–15)	Anxiety, panic
Oxazepam	S	5–15	None	Anxiety, alcohol withdrawal
Temazepam	S	5–15	None	Insomnia
Bromazepam	M	12–24	3-hydroxybromazepam (20)	Anxiety
Lorazepam	M	10–20	None	Anxiety, insomnia, premedication
Clobazam	L	18–48	N-desmethyl-clobazam (2–5 days)	Anxiety, insomnia, epilepsy
Clonazepam	L	18–50	None	Epilepsy
Diazepam	L	20–70	Desmethyldiazepam (30–100) Temazepam (8–15) Oxazepam (5–15)	Anxiety, alcohol withdrawal, agitation, muscle spasm, premedication, sedation, status epilepticus
Flunitrazepam	L	20–30	7-amino-flunitrazepam and *N*-desmethyl-flunitrazepam (10–16, 23–33)	Insomnia
Nitrazepam	L	25	None	Insomnia, infantile spasms, myoclonic epilepsy

L = long-acting; M = medium-acting; S = short-acting; VS = very short-acting

associated with the regulation of emotional behaviour, contains a highly dense area of GABA binding sites in the amygdala, suggesting that the antianxiety effects occur there. People with pathological anxiety have reduced numbers of GABA–benzodiazepine receptor complexes.

Other drugs also can bind to $GABA_A$ receptors; these include the Z-drugs (more selective at the alpha sub-unit) and the barbiturates, which have hypnotic/antiepileptic actions by acting as channel modulators. Barbiturates increase the duration of channel opening. Flumazenil (see later discussion) is an antagonist at the benzodiazepine binding site on the $GABA_A$ receptor, where it decreases the binding of GABA so the chloride channels remain closed. Flumazenil is anxiogenic and is used to treat benzodiazepine overdoses.

Indications for clinical use

The most common indications for benzodiazepines include anxiety disorders, panic disorders, insomnia and sleep disturbances, seizure disorders, alcohol withdrawal, muscle spasm, preoperative medication and to calm aggressive patients (see Fig 20.3, later). They are also used to induce amnesia during cardioversion and endoscopic procedures. The choice of benzodiazepine depends on pharmacokinetic characteristics (Table 20.1), with longer-acting (long half-life) agents such as diazepam preferred for treating anxiety and epilepsy and short-acting agents such as temazepam and midazolam (Drug Monograph 20.2) preferred for induction of anaesthesia or sleep and for treating insomnia. Medium-acting sedative drugs are useful for ensuring early-morning wakefulness.

Anxiety disorders

Diazepam or medium-acting (lorazepam) or long-acting benzodiazepines (clonazepam and flunitrazepam) are commonly used as antianxiety agents. There is overuse and abuse of these drugs (known previously as 'mother's little helpers') when preferably the causes of anxiety should be addressed, and long-term coping methods encouraged. Antidepressants are also effective in generalised anxiety disorders but have significant unwanted adverse effects.

Panic disorders

First-line treatment for panic attacks and panic disorder is non-pharmacological: many people respond to cognitive behaviour therapy and lifestyle changes, particularly control of caffeine and alcohol use. Benzodiazepines are effective, but the requirement for chronic administration (6–12 months) and the likelihood of dependence and sedation limit their usefulness. Various types of antidepressant drugs are also effective.

Sleep disorders

Generally, sedative drugs are indicated only for short-term treatment of insomnia (2–4 weeks), after sleep hygiene is addressed, owing to the risk of dependence developing and broken sleep after withdrawal. The preferred hypnotics

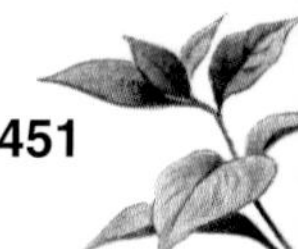

Drug Monograph 20.2
Midazolam

Midazolam is a very short-acting benzodiazepine, with powerful anxiolytic, sedative–hypnotic and muscle-relaxant effects.

Mechanism of action

As for all benzodiazepines, it acts as an agonist at an allosteric modulatory site to facilitate GABA binding to the $GABA_A$ receptors, changing conformation of the active site and thus enhancing the frequency of chloride channel opening, leading to more neuronal inhibition.

Indications

Midazolam is indicated for premedication and conscious sedation, and for induction of general anaesthesia. It has rapid onset of action and, because of rapid metabolic transformation, short duration.

The anterograde amnesic effect may last longer than sedation, so patients may not remember advice given soon after recovery from anaesthetic.

It is commonly carried in ambulances and administered by paramedics to treat seizures and agitation, and for sedation for intubation and cardioversion procedures.

Pharmacokinetics

Midazolam is one of the shortest-acting benzodiazepines (Table 20.1). After intramuscular (IM) injection, absorption from the muscle tissue is rapid and complete. Maximum plasma concentrations are reached within 30 minutes. The absolute bioavailability after IM injection is over 90%. Midazolam has been shown to cross the placenta slowly and to enter fetal circulation. Small quantities of midazolam are found in human milk.

Midazolam is almost entirely eliminated by biotransformation; 60–80% of the dose is excreted in urine as conjugates. In healthy volunteers, the elimination half-life is between 1 and 3 hours. In adults over 60 years of age, the elimination half-life may be prolonged up to four times.

Adverse reactions

Because of its low toxicity, midazolam has a wide therapeutic range. All benzodiazepines can cause excessive CNS depression, dependence and neurological dysfunction. Midazolam is likely to cause hypotension, hiccup and cough. Less common adverse effects include pain on injection, rash, bronchospasm, nausea and vomiting, confusion and respiratory and cardiovascular dysfunctions. Paradoxical CNS stimulation can occur in children.

Drug interactions

See Drug Interactions 20.1. Midazolam has additive CNS-depressant effects with all other CNS depressants.

Drugs that inhibit CYP3A4 can inhibit the metabolism of midazolam and hence prolong its therapeutic and adverse effects for several hours. (Individual combinations should be checked for safety in reference books or databases.)

Warnings and contraindications

Midazolam is contraindicated in people with severe liver disease and before and during childbirth (Category C); precautions should be taken in people with respiratory or musculoskeletal disease, renal impairment, debilitated or chronically ill people, the elderly and children.

Dosage and administration

Dosage should be individualised depending on the client's characteristics, route of administration and the indication for which the drug is prescribed; it should be administered slowly while monitoring effects closely. It can also be administered IM or by rectal or intranasal solution, or via the buccal mucosa in seizures.

for sleep disorders such as insomnia are the short-acting agents such as temazepam, alprazolam, oxazepam and the Z-drugs zolpidem or zopiclone.

Seizure disorders

Clonazepam, midazolam and clobazam are used as anticonvulsants (Ch 21). Parenteral diazepam is indicated for intractable, repetitive seizures, such as in status epilepticus, when its rapid onset of action is useful. Oral diazepam may be used for short-term adjunctive therapy (1–2 weeks) with other antiepileptics for treating convulsions.

Preoperative medication and procedural sedation

Diazepam, lorazepam and parenteral midazolam are used preoperatively, particularly in day surgery and endoscopic procedures, to reduce anxiety and help induce general anaesthesia and to reduce the dose of anaesthetic needed

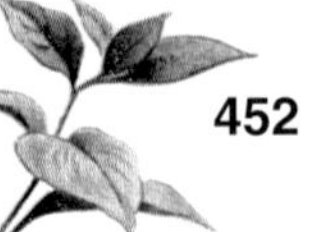

DRUG INTERACTIONS 20.1
Benzodiazepines

DRUG OR DRUG GROUP	LIKELY EFFECTS AND MANAGEMENT
CNS depressants such as alcohol, antihistamines, antianxiety agents, opioids, other sedatives/hypnotics, psychotropic agents (especially clozapine) and antidepressants	Enhanced CNS-depressant effects, sedation and respiratory depression; monitoring is necessary because the dosage of one or both drugs may need adjustment
Many drugs can inhibit the metabolism of benzodiazepines (especially drugs that inhibit CYP3A4); examples are azole antifungals (itraconazole), cimetidine, verapamil, omeprazole, macrolide antibiotics (erythromycin, clarithromycin), fluoxetine and some antivirals used against HIV infection	CNS depression and respiratory depression effects of benzodiazepines are prolonged; reduce dose or substitute a non-interacting drug
Drugs can increase benzodiazepine metabolism (carbamazepine, phenytoin, rifampicin, St John's wort)	Higher dose of benzodiazepine may be required
Stimulant drugs such as theophylline may reduce the sedative effects of benzodiazepines	Increase benzodiazepine dose if necessary
Drugs that lower the seizure threshold, including many antipsychotics, antivirals and antimicrobials	Benzodiazepines used cautiously, if at all

(Ch 18). They can also produce a useful **anterograde amnesic effect**; that is, they minimise the person's memory of the procedure.

Muscular spasms

Benzodiazepines, especially diazepam, are useful as adjunct medications for treating skeletal muscle spasms, caused by muscle or joint inflammation, or spasticity resulting from upper motor neuron dysfunction, such as cerebral palsy and paraplegia.

Withdrawal from CNS depressants

Acute withdrawal from regular use of CNS depressants such as alcohol, barbiturates or benzodiazepines can lead to acute agitation, anxiety, tremors and headache, and may require treatment with more CNS depressants. The withdrawal should be gradual. Withdrawal symptoms can include anxiety, dysphoria, irritability, insomnia, nightmares, sweating, memory impairment, hallucinations, tachycardia, psychosis, tremors and seizures. The benzodiazepines most often used to treat alcohol withdrawal syndromes are diazepam and oxazepam.

Pharmacokinetics

The pharmacokinetic properties of the benzodiazepines vary widely and determine the choice between the drugs in this group. For example, half-lives range from about 2 to 70 hours, and there are many metabolic interconversions to active metabolites with long half-lives (Table 20.1). The injectable benzodiazepines include diazepam and midazolam. The onset of sedative, anticonvulsant, antianxiety and muscle-relaxant effects of these agents after intravenous administration occurs at 1–5 minutes.

Absorption and distribution

Most benzodiazepines are lipid-soluble and readily absorbed from the gastrointestinal tract; diazepam and flunitrazepam are the most rapidly absorbed and produce a prompt and intense onset of action. The benzodiazepines become widely distributed in the body and brain. Redistribution from the CNS to peripheral tissues can reduce the duration of action; for example, although diazepam has a long half-life, it has only a short duration of antiepileptic action after IV administration. Midazolam is water-soluble, so is readily formulated for injection. It has a short action because its (active) metabolite has a shorter half-life than the parent drug.

After multiple doses, benzodiazepines accumulate in the body's fluids and tissues, which act as storage depots and account for the prolonged sedative actions even after the drugs have been discontinued. These drugs are mostly highly protein-bound ($>85\%$); protein binding is reduced in newborns, in those with alcoholism and in those with cirrhosis or impaired liver function.

Elimination

The gastrointestinal tract and the liver are the sites of metabolism. Benzodiazepines are often hydroxylated or demethylated to active derivatives, including desmethyldiazepam, a long-acting metabolite (30–100 hours). The long-acting benzodiazepines such as diazepam with active metabolites oxazepam and temazepam are more apt to accumulate, especially in the elderly, resulting in higher risk of falls and hip fractures (Clinical Focus Box 20.3). Oxazepam and lorazepam are metabolised to inactive metabolites and are preferred agents in elderly people and people with liver disease. Metabolites are generally excreted by the kidneys.

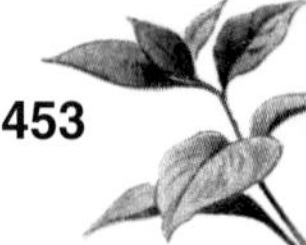

CLINICAL FOCUS BOX 20.3
Falls and fractures in the elderly

Studies have shown that each year about 30% of people aged over 65 have a major fall, with the rate even higher in nursing homes; many falls lead to fractures, particularly hip fractures with severe associated morbidity and mortality (Westaway et al. 2019). Tracing links between medications and falls reveals:

- a twofold increased risk of falls and fractures in elderly people taking psychotropic drugs, especially antidepressants and benzodiazepines
- other drugs commonly taken by elderly people that increase risk of falls include cardiovascular drugs, non-steroidal anti-inflammatory drugs, antiepileptics, antiparkinson drugs, opioids and diuretics
- antipsychotic drugs are more commonly prescribed in nursing homes than for elderly people in other locations
- the greater the use of CNS depressants such as benzodiazepines, antidepressants, antipsychotics and opioids, the worse is the decline in cognitive function over 5 years
- higher doses and increased number of CNS medications increase the risk of falls, with an extra two falls per year likely
- in middle-aged and older adults, polypharmacy, including antidepressant or benzodiazepine use, is associated with injurious falls and a greater number of falls.

It is recommended that hypnotics should be reserved to treat acute insomnia and, when prescribed, limited to short-term or intermittent use to avoid the development of tolerance and dependence. Further, psychotropic drug use in the elderly should be minimised and monitored, especially in nursing home residents. Refer to Chapter 41 for drugs in aged care.

Drug interactions

Significant drug interactions can occur when benzodiazepines are used in combination with other CNS depressants or with drugs that affect their metabolism (Drug Interactions 20.1, earlier). Effects are often unpredictable, so patients should be monitored closely. Drug metabolism interactions occur particularly with alprazolam, diazepam and midazolam; there are relatively fewer metabolic interactions with lorazepam, oxazepam and temazepam. (Reference sources such as *Australian Medicines Handbook* should be consulted for interactions with specific benzodiazepines.)

Adverse drug reactions

Excessive CNS depression

As a group, the benzodiazepines commonly cause excess CNS depression: drowsiness, ataxia, diplopia, vertigo, lassitude, memory loss, slurred speech and loss of dexterity. Less frequently, headaches, decreased libido, anterograde amnesia, muscle weakness and hypotension can occur, as well as increased behavioural problems (anger and impaired ability to concentrate), seen mostly with children. Neurological reactions include paradoxical insomnia, increased excitability, hallucinations and apprehension (Fig 20.3). There is a greater risk of falls and motor vehicle crashes, particularly in the elderly.

General points

Because elderly people are more sensitive to these agents than younger adults and are at risk of accumulating active drugs and of falls, non-pharmacological approaches are recommended to treat their sleep disturbances. Both paediatric and geriatric patients are at risk of paradoxical-type reactions (CNS stimulation, rather than depression) from sedative drugs. It is recommended that prescriptions for these agents be limited in these groups, with close monitoring.

Many other drugs can cause sedation and CNS depression, including anaesthetics, alcohol, antipsychotics and antidepressants, opioid analgesics, melatonin and antihistamines. Insomnia can also be an adverse effect of drugs, especially CNS stimulants such as the amphetamines and caffeine-containing drinks.

Management of benzodiazepine overdose

Benzodiazepine overdose is manifest as CNS depression, ranging from confusion and drowsiness through to coma, hypotonia, hypotension and respiratory depression.

Overdose is not usually life-threatening unless multiple other CNS depressant drugs have been taken. Supportive treatment is necessary, and may include maintaining an adequate airway with oxygen for depressed respiration, monitoring vital signs and promoting diuresis by administering IV fluids. Hypotension must be monitored and might require vasopressors such as noradrenaline (norepinephrine) or dopamine. Dialysis is of limited value in treating a benzodiazepine overdose.

Flumazenil

Intravenous administration of flumazenil, a specific benzodiazepine antagonist, is sometimes required to treat a benzodiazepine overdose or reverse the sedative effects of benzodiazepines after surgical or diagnostic procedures to avoid intubation and intensive care admission. It may precipitate withdrawal symptoms and seizures in people taking benzodiazepines to control epilepsy, or in mixed overdoses with benzodiazepines and proconvulsant drugs such as antidepressants or CNS stimulants.

Flumazenil is administered IV, with antagonistic effects (reversal of sedation) occurring within 2 minutes and duration of action of 1–3 hours. Because most

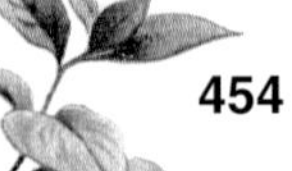

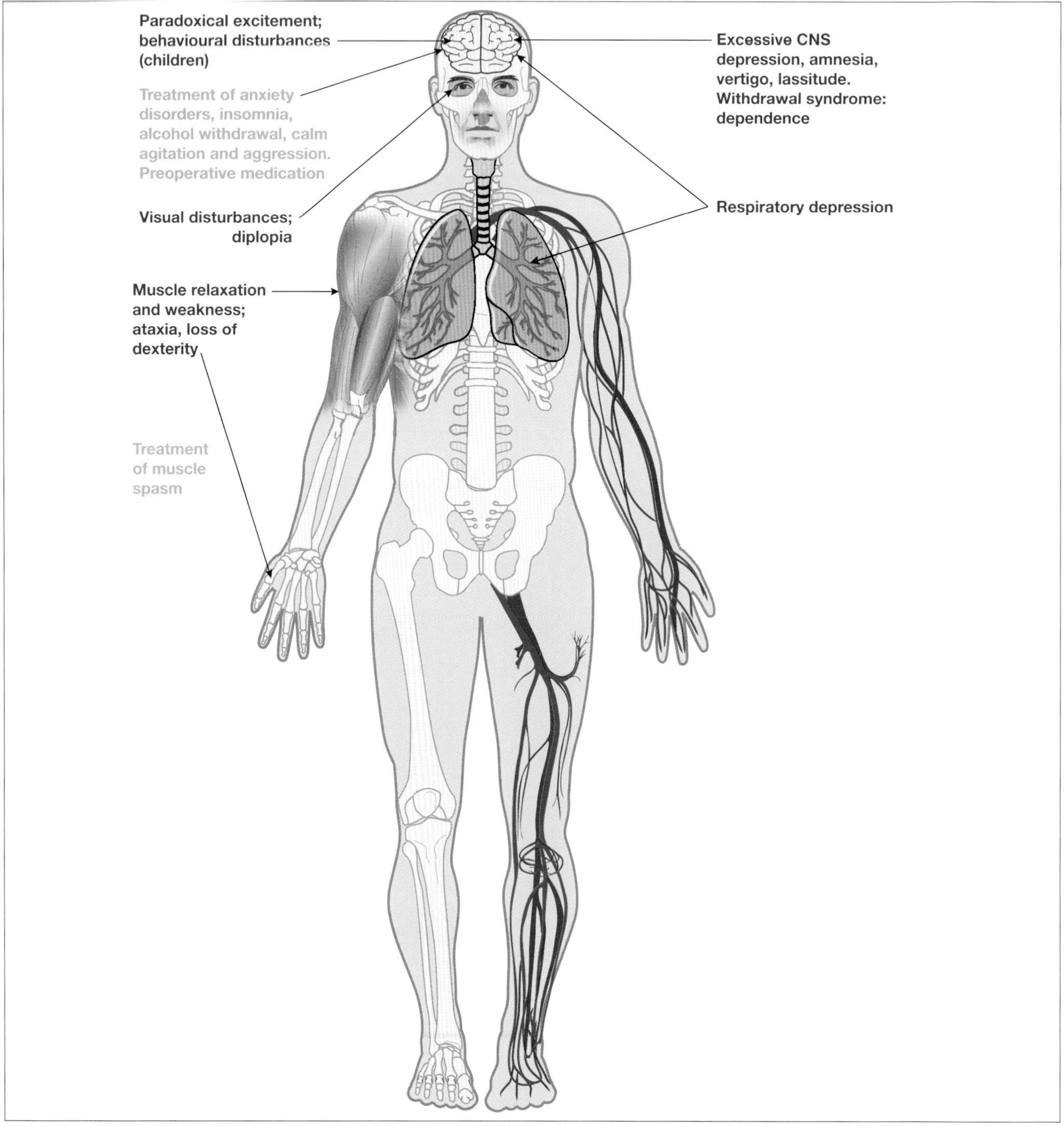

Paradoxical excitement; behavioural disturbances (children)

Treatment of anxiety disorders, insomnia, alcohol withdrawal, calm agitation and aggression. Preoperative medication

Visual disturbances; diplopia

Muscle relaxation and weakness; ataxia, loss of dexterity

Treatment of muscle spasm

Excessive CNS depression, amnesia, vertigo, lassitude. Withdrawal syndrome: dependence

Respiratory depression

FIGURE 20.3 Pharmacological effects of benzodiazepines

benzodiazepines have a half-life longer than an hour, repeated injections of flumazenil are necessary. The drug is metabolised in the liver and excreted by the kidneys. Adverse reactions reported with this drug include headache, visual disturbance, increased anxiety, nausea and light-headedness.

Tolerance and dependence associated with benzodiazepine use

With chronic administration, tolerance develops to the sedative effects but less often to the anxiolytic effects. Dependence is common and leads to craving, overuse and abuse of these drugs, and drug-seeking behaviours.

Dependence can develop after only a few days' use of benzodiazepines, and withdrawal from chronic use of the drugs can be difficult. Addiction (compulsive use despite adverse effects) is induced via activation of dopaminergic neurons in the mesocortical limbic reward system.[1] Withdrawal is characterised by CNS stimulation: anxiety, sleep disorders, aching limbs, palpitations and nervousness; seizures can occur in people who previously were taking high doses.

Withdrawal from hypnotic drugs is recommended for chronic users, especially for older people who are at greater risk of harm. Withdrawal should be gradual – for example, dose reduced by 10–20% per week, with a few days to stabilise at each dose level. Rebound insomnia is likely, but usually lasts only 2–3 days (National Prescribing Service 2010; Royal Australian College of General Practitioners 2022).

Warnings and contraindications

Benzodiazepines are contraindicated in people with respiratory depression or sleep apnoea, severe hepatic impairment or myasthenia gravis. They should be used with caution in children and in the elderly, in women during pregnancy or lactation, in debilitated people and in those with renal impairment.

KEY POINTS

Benzodiazepines

- Benzodiazepines, such as diazepam, are the most common drugs used to treat anxiety and insomnia. They are also used as preoperative medication, for seizure disorders and to calm aggressive people and also for muscle relaxation.
- The mechanism of action of the benzodiazepines is binding at an allosteric site on the $GABA_A$ receptor complex to facilitate GABA binding to its active site, thus changing its conformation, enhancing the frequency of chloride channel opening, leading to more neuronal inhibition. Their action is due to facilitation of GABA-mediated CNS inhibitory pathways.
- The limbic system, associated with the regulation of emotional behaviour, contains a highly dense area of GABA binding sites in the amygdala, suggesting that the antianxiety effects occur there.
- Because of their safety and effectiveness and the variety of conditions in which benzodiazepines are effective, they have largely replaced the barbiturates, chloral hydrate and other earlier sedatives.
- Pharmacokinetic properties of benzodiazepines vary widely; half-lives range from 2 to 60 hours; and many benzodiazepines are converted to pharmacologically active metabolites that prolong the sedative effects. Short-acting agents are used to induce anaesthesia or sleep, and longer acting agents to treat anxiety or epilepsy.
- Drug interactions frequently occur with other CNS depressants and with drugs that affect the metabolism of benzodiazepines.
- Common adverse reactions include excessive CNS depression, tolerance and dependence.
- Benzodiazepine overdose is manifest as CNS depression, ranging from confusion and drowsiness through to coma, hypotonia, hypotension and respiratory depression.
- Overdose is not usually life-threatening unless multiple other CNS-depressant drugs have been taken. Supportive treatment is necessary.
- Intravenous administration of flumazenil, a specific benzodiazepine antagonist, is sometimes required to treat a benzodiazepine overdose or reverse the sedative effects of benzodiazepines.
- With chronic administration, tolerance develops to the sedative effects of the benzodiazepines but less often to the anxiolytic effects. Dependence is common and leads to craving, overuse and abuse of these drugs and to drug-seeking behaviours. Withdrawal from chronic use of the drugs can be difficult.

Other anxiolytic and sedative/hypnotic agents

As shown earlier in Clinical Focus Box 20.1, many drugs from diverse pharmacological groups can depress the CNS and hence cause sedation. However, for most of them, CNS depressant actions are too general to be clinically useful. In specific conditions, the sedative side effects may be therapeutic; for example, the serotonin noradrenaline reuptake inhibitors (SNRIs), TCAs and SSRIs such as escitalopram, and SNRIs are indicated for treatment of generalised anxiety disorder. (The antidepressant effects also help to reduce anxiety.) Generalised anxiety in elderly

1 Alprazolam, commonly known as Xanax, has been referred to as the 21st century's equivalent of Valium in terms of popularity as a 'downer', usually in combination with methadone or cocaine. It is implicated in the deaths of celebrities Heath Ledger and Michael Jackson. Its short onset time brings the quick 'fix' sought by drug abusers (Ch 25).

people is often associated with depression. In this situation, antidepressant medication is more effective and safer than use of benzodiazepines, which carry an increased risk of oversedation, confusion, respiratory depression, short-term memory impairment and falls (Clinical Focus Box 20.3, earlier).

Other sedative/hypnotics related to benzodiazepines are described below.

Drugs related to benzodiazepines

Barbiturates

The barbiturates were once the most commonly prescribed class of medications for hypnotic and sedative effects; they are derivatives of barbituric acid, so named because it was discovered in 1863 on St Barbara's Day. The first active drug in this group, barbitone, was used medically in 1903 and hundreds of 'me-too' barbiturates soon followed. With few exceptions, barbiturates have been replaced by the safer benzodiazepines and more specific antiepileptic agents. Phenobarbital (phenobarbitone), the prototype drug for this classification, is now used mainly as an antiepileptic (Ch 21), and thiopental to induce general anaesthesia (Ch 18).

The Z-drugs

The '**Z-drugs**' are agonists at the $GABA_A$ receptors and are more selective at the alpha sub-unit than the benzodiazepines. Most of their generic names begin with the letter 'Z' – for example, zolpidem and zopiclone.

Zopiclone

Although chemically unlike the benzodiazepines, zopiclone also potentiates inhibitory effects of GABA, so it has very similar pharmacological properties. It is a hypnotic indicated for short-term treatment of insomnia. It is rapidly absorbed, distributed and metabolised, with only one metabolite having weak CNS-depressant activity. The half-life is short (5–7 hours) but may be extended in the elderly and in people with impaired liver function.

The adverse reactions profile is similar to that of the benzodiazepines: CNS depression, possibility of dependence and withdrawal reactions, and increased risk of sleepwalking and related risky behaviours. In addition, zopiclone can interfere with thyroid hormone balance. It alters taste sensation, causing bitter taste. Use during pregnancy or lactation and in children is not recommended.

Zolpidem

Zolpidem tartrate is another non-benzodiazepine that is more selective in its binding to a sub-unit of the $GABA_A$ receptor than the benzodiazepines; thus, it has some sedative properties similar to those of benzodiazepines but lacks the anticonvulsant, muscle-relaxant and antianxiety properties associated with the benzodiazepines. It is approved for short-term treatment of insomnia and is available as tablets. It has a rapid onset of action, short half-life and no active metabolites so should be taken immediately before going to sleep. Adverse effects, drug interactions and precautions are similar to those of the benzodiazepines. In addition, zolpidem is likely to cause diarrhoea and myalgia, and has been reported to cause bizarre CNS effects such as hallucinations, amnesia, sleepwalking and related inappropriate behaviours, particularly when taken with other psychoactive drugs including alcohol, and increased risk of suicide.

KEY POINTS

Other anxiolytic and sedative/hypnotic agents

- Many drugs from diverse pharmacological groups can depress the CNS and hence cause sedation. In specific conditions, the sedative side effects may be therapeutic.
- Drugs other than the benzodiazepines can bind to $GABA_A$ receptors and potentiate the inhibitory effects of GABA; these include the barbiturates and the Z-drugs.
- The barbiturates have hypnotic/antiepileptic actions and increase the duration of chloride channel opening. They were once the most commonly prescribed class of medications for hypnotic and sedative effects. They are also used to treat epilepsy. With a few exceptions barbiturates have been replaced by the safer benzodiazepines. Phenobarbital (phenobarbitone), the prototype drug for this classification, is now used mainly as an antiepileptic (Ch 21), and thiopental is used to induce general anaesthesia.
- The Z-drugs are agonists at the $GABA_A$ receptors and are more selective at the alpha sub-unit than the benzodiazepines. They potentiate the inhibitory effects of GABA, similar to the pharmacological actions of benzodiazepines. Most of their generic names begin with the letter 'Z' – for example, zolpidem and zopiclone.

Miscellaneous anxiolytics, sedatives and hypnotics

Buspirone

Buspirone is not closely related pharmacologically to the other drugs discussed in this chapter. It is an anxiolytic with less sedative effect than the benzodiazepines and little anticonvulsant or muscle-relaxant activity. The exact mechanism of action is unknown, but the drug has a high affinity for and partial agonist activity at 5-HT_{1A} receptors and a moderate affinity for and agonist activity at dopamine D_2 receptors in the CNS. It does not affect GABA, nor does it have any significant affinity for the benzodiazepine site on GABA receptors.

Buspirone is indicated for treating anxiety disorders and is considered equivalent in efficacy to the benzodiazepines but usually with less sedation. It appears to have little risk of causing dependence and withdrawal reactions. Common adverse effects are CNS and gastrointestinal tract disturbances. Due to its affinity for brain dopamine receptors, it can cause dystonias, akathisia, tardive dyskinesia, parkinsonian symptoms and endocrine disturbances; serotonin toxicity can be increased with other serotonergic agents and with grapefruit juice. Buspirone is indicated for generalised anxiety disorders (only available in Australia under the special access scheme).

Dexmedetomidine

Dexmedetomidine is a sedative and analgesic drug, related to the α_2-adrenoceptor agonists such as clonidine and with similar pharmacological properties. It acts on α_2-adrenoceptors in the CNS to reduce noradrenergic activity; hence, it is likely to cause bradycardia and hypotension. Stimulation of imidazoline-1 receptors (I_1) results in a central hypotensive and antiarrhythmic action. It does not affect GABA receptors or have anticholinergic or respiratory depressant effects. It is used specifically by IV infusion for procedural sedation and postsurgical and intensive care sedation of intubated people. Refer also to Chapter 18. There are many precautions to its use, particularly in people with autonomic or behavioural disturbances; continuous infusion duration should not exceed 24 hours. It has cardiovascular and CNS adverse effects that should be monitored closely.

Melatonin

Melatonin, *N*-acetyl-5-methoxytryptamine, is a natural body hormone, chemically related to 5-HT. It is secreted in darkness hours by the pineal gland, acts on melatonin receptors, MT_1 and MT_2 receptors, in the anterior hypothalamus and promotes sleepiness; it may help reset the body's circadian rhythm 'clocks'. It is a Schedule 3 drug for short-term use as monotherapy in primary insomnia in people aged over 55 years. Its use has recently included treatment of insomnia in children and adolescents aged 2–18 years with autism spectrum disorder or Smith-Magenis syndrome, where sleep hygiene measures have been insufficient. Adverse effects include nausea, arthralgia, headaches, hypothermia and hangover. It is available as modified-release tablets up to 2 mg strength and 1 mg and 5 mg prolonged release tablets for children and adolescents.

Dozens of medical uses for melatonin have been proposed – and many people take melatonin (readily available over the counter in some countries) to regularise sleep patterns after long-distance flights or shiftwork. It is also included in many 'relaxation drinks' (along with other natural compounds such as kava kava, valerian and tryptophan), with marketing designed to appeal to young people to mimic the effects of alcohol and other less safe drugs (Stacy 2011).

Antihistamines

The older antihistamines (histamine H_1-antagonists) have significant sedative effects via blockade of histamine (as well as muscarinic and other receptors) in the CNS, producing sedation. As well they are useful in suppressing allergic reactions (Ch 34) and as antiemetics. Examples of antihistamines effective as sedatives are promethazine, doxylamine and diphenhydramine.

They are non-prescription medications and antihistamine mixtures are sometimes used as mild sedatives for children. When used as antiemetics to protect children against travel sickness, their sedative effects are appropriate only to reduce the child's distress, not for the convenience of the parents or other passengers; the primary focus must be the safety and wellbeing of the child (see the Clinical Thinking Scenario at the beginning of the chapter). There are significant hangover effects after antihistamine-induced sedation.

Chloral hydrate

Chloral hydrate (trichloroethanediol) is a simple chemical substance related structurally to both chloroform and ethanol (Fig 20.4). It is essentially a 'prodrug' that is converted in the body to active trichloroethanol, which has a rapid, powerful hypnotic action. Its exact mechanism of action is unknown. It has a general CNS-depressant effect similar to that of alcohol.

Chloral hydrate was formerly frequently used as a sedative and hypnotic and as premedication, particularly in children and the elderly, as both oral and rectal forms are rapidly absorbed. It is now mainly used as a mild hypnotic or preoperative sedative, particularly in children's hospitals to sedate children for diagnostic procedures and in intensive care units so that catheters are not pulled out; continuous monitoring is required. Its use as a sedative may be superseded by less toxic agents. A mixture form is available, containing 1 g/10 mL sweetened with sucrose and saccharin (see Clinical Thinking Scenario at the beginning of the chapter).

Chloral hydrate is considered relatively safe but can be toxic in overdose, especially in combination with alcohol, causing cardiac and respiratory failure; deaths have occurred. This mixture, used historically with criminal intent and known as a 'Mickey Finn' or knock-out drops, is particularly dangerous because not only are the

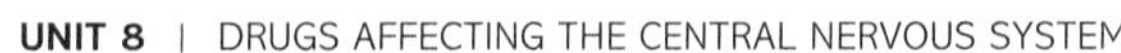

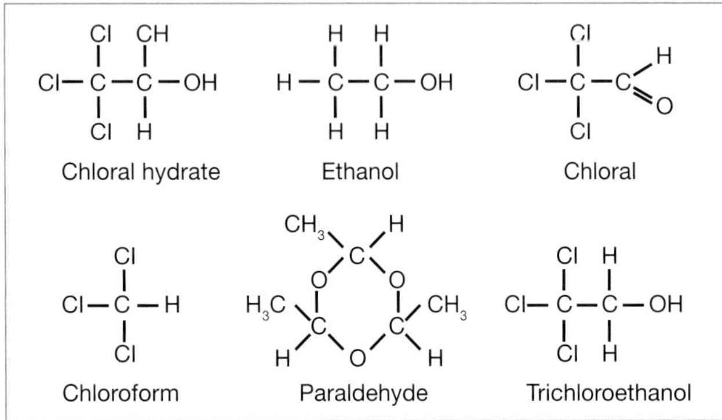

Chloral hydrate Ethanol Chloral

Chloroform Paraldehyde Trichloroethanol

FIGURE 20.4 Chemical structures of some simple sedative drugs showing close structural relationships between the sedative chloral hydrate, anaesthetic chloroform, depressant ethanol (alcohol) and sedative paraldehyde, which can be visualised as three molecules of ethanol joined in a cyclical ether formation.

CNS-depressant effects additive but trichloroethanol also inhibits the metabolism of alcohol and prolongs its actions.

Orexin antagonists

Orexin neuropeptides are produced in discrete groups of neurons in the hypothalamus; they are involved in regulation of the sleep–wake and activity cycles, feeding and reward-seeking. They activate two G-protein-coupled receptors (OX_1R and OX_2R), the relative roles of which are still being established. Orexin receptor antagonists are being investigated for their role in reducing panic/anxiety and promoting sleep (Han et al. 2019).

These antagonists inhibit the action of the wakefulness-promoting orexin neurons of the arousal system reducing activity and promoting sleep; OX_2R antagonists mainly increase non-REM sleep and may be useful in treating insomnia, while dual antagonists such as suvorexant increase REM sleep.

Older drugs

Bromides

Bromide salts such as potassium bromide were used in medicine as antiepileptic agents and as sedative–hypnotics from the mid-1850s to the mid-20th century (Lampe 2013). Bromide ion is absorbed in the body and replaces chloride (biologically the more common halide ion) in extracellular fluids. Bromide acts in the CNS as a depressant and sedative, and in (not much) larger doses it depresses motor activity and reflexes. At toxic levels it causes ataxia, delirium, coma and death and is particularly toxic as a cumulative poison, so it has been replaced by safer drugs.

Paraldehyde

Paraldehyde is a polymer of acetaldehyde (Fig 20.4); it is a colourless liquid with a strong odour and taste. The CNS-depressant effects of paraldehyde are similar to those of alcohol, barbiturates and chloral hydrate; it depresses various levels of the CNS, including the ascending reticular activating system. It is used when other agents are inappropriate or ineffective. It may also be used to treat convulsive episodes arising from tetanus, status epilepticus and poisoning by convulsive drugs, and in reducing the anxiety associated with withdrawal from drugs such as narcotics or barbiturates, or delirium tremens due to alcohol withdrawal. Paraldehyde was used in the past as a sedative–hypnotic agent but has been superseded by safer and more effective drugs.

Complementary and alternative sedatives and anxiolytics

Many natural products and techniques from complementary and alternative medicine (CAM) have been used to attain sleep or relieve stress and anxiety. For treating insomnia, the natural products melatonin, valerian, kava kava, lavender, lemon balm, passionflower, hops, withania and L-tryptophan have been shown to be clinically effective.

In the treatment of anxiety, music therapy, massage, acupuncture, selenium and many herbs (Baical skullcap, ginger, *Ginkgo biloba*, ginseng, licorice and St John's wort) as well as the Chinese herb *Suan Zao Ren Tang* have been shown to be effective.

KEY POINTS

Miscellaneous anxiolytics, sedatives and hypnotics

- Miscellaneous anxiolytics, sedatives and hypnotics include the following:
  - Buspirone is indicated for treating generalised anxiety disorders (only available in Australia under the special access scheme). Its exact mechanism of action is unknown.
  - Dexmedetomidine is used for procedural sedation. It is related to the α_2-adrenoceptor agonists such as clonidine, and exhibits similar pharmacological profiles.
  - Melatonin (*N*-acetyl-5-methoxytryptamine) is chemically related to 5-HT and is a hormone secreted by the pineal gland in darkness hours. It acts on melatonin receptors in the hypothalamus and may help reset the body's circadian rhythm 'clocks'.
  - The older antihistamines (histamine H_1-antagonists, e.g. promethazine) have significant sedative effects, as well as being useful in suppressing allergic reactions (and as antiemetics). These are non-prescription medications, and antihistamine mixtures are sometimes used as mild sedatives for children.

- Chloral hydrate is related structurally to both chloroform and ethanol and is now used mainly as a mild hypnotic or preoperative sedative. Its use as a sedative has been superseded by less toxic agents.
- Orexin receptor antagonists promote sleep; mainly increasing non-REM sleep. Suvorexant is an example of a dual antagonist.
- Older drugs include the bromides and paraldehyde. Although bromides are no longer used, paraldehyde is used when other agents are inappropriate or ineffective.
- Many natural products and techniques from CAM have been used to attain sleep or relieve stress and anxiety.

DRUGS AT A GLANCE
Antianxiety, sedative and hypnotic drugs

PHARMACOLOGICAL GROUP AND EFFECT	KEY EXAMPLES	CLINICAL USE
Antianxiety/sedative agents		
Benzodiazepines • Act at an allosteric modulatory site to facilitate GABA binding to the $GABA_A$ receptors, changing conformation of the active site and enhancing the frequency of chloride channel opening, leading to more neuronal inhibition		
• Long acting	Diazepam	Sedation, anxiety
• Short acting	Alprazolam	Insomnia, anxiety
• Very short acting	Midazolam	Insomnia
Other sedative/hypnotics		
Barbiturates • Act at an allosteric modulatory site (distinct from benzodiazepine site) to facilitate GABA binding to the $GABA_A$ receptors, changing conformation of the active site and increasing the duration of chloride channel opening, leading to more neuronal inhibition	Phenobarbital (phenobarbitone)	Sedation
Z drugs • Agonists at the $GABA_A$ receptors and more selective at the alpha sub-unit than the benzodiazepines (see benzodiazepine actions above)	Zopiclone[NZ, AUS]	Insomnia
Miscellaneous sedatives, anxiolytics, hypnotics		
• High affinity for and partial agonist activity at $5\text{-}HT_{1A}$ (serotonin) receptors and a moderate affinity for agonist activity at dopamine D_2 receptors in the CNS	Buspirone	Generalised anxiety disorders
• Related to α_2-adrenoceptor agonists; acts in CNS to stimulate imidazoline –1 receptors (I_1) resulting in a central hypotensive and antiarrhythmic	Dexmedetomidine	Procedural sedation
Acts on melatonin MT_1 and MT_2 receptors, in the anterior hypothalamus and promotes sleepiness; it may help re-set the body's circadian rhythm	Melatonin	Jet lag, insomnia
• Histamine 1 receptor antagonists; significant sedative effects by blocking histamine (as well as muscarinic and other receptors) in the CNS	Diphenhydramine, doxylamine, promethazine	Sedation
• Exact mechanism of action is unknown. It has a general CNS-depressant effect similar to that of alcohol.	Chloral hydrate	Mild hypnotic or preoperative sedative (paediatric)
Orexin antagonists • OX_1R and OX_2R antagonists inhibit wakefulness, promoting orexin neurons of the arousal system	Suvorexant[AUS]	Insomnia
Benzodiazepine antagonists		
• Antagonism of action of GABA and benzodiazepines at the GABA receptor complex	Flumazenil	Benzodiazepine overdose

[AUS] = Australia only
[NZ] = New Zealand only

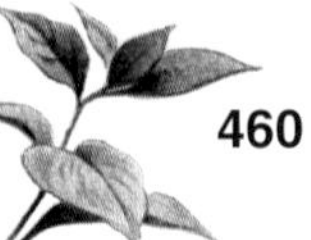

REVIEW EXERCISES

1. Mrs BD, a 75-year-old, attends her GP clinic where she discussed her issues with insomnia. She states that she has had trouble sleeping since her husband passed away 6 months ago. She was prescribed 10 mg of temazepam nightly and advised to return for a follow-up visit in a month's time. Discuss the class of drug, mechanism of action and pharmacokinetic aspects of this medication. What are the adverse reactions she should be aware of?
2. Mr JP, a 30-year-old, is brought to the emergency department by ambulance. He has overdosed on flunitrazepam, which he has been prescribed for anxiety-related insomnia. What are the adverse reactions associated with overdose? What is the antidote for this overdose? Explain how this drug works and the precautions associated with its use.
3. Mr XY is a 35-year-old professional athlete. He has been prescribed 10 mg of zolpidem to address jet lag–induced insomnia; his attendance at international competitions several times a year has potentiated this insomnia. He was found wandering confused around his neighbourhood at night. Explain the mechanism of action and known adverse reactions of a 'Z-drug' such as zolpidem. His doctor prescribed melatonin 2 mg and asks him to return to the clinic in 3 months. What is the mechanism of action of melatonin and how will it relieve his insomnia?

REFERENCES

Australian Bureau of Statistics (2022) National Study of Mental Health and Wellbeing. https://www.abs.gov.au/statistics/health/mental-health/national-study-mental-health-andwellbeing/ 2020-21 (accessed 2022)

Australian Bureau of Statistics (2018). First insights from the National Study of Mental Health and Wellbeing: 2017–18 financial year. Accessed 3 March 2022. https://www.abs.gov.au/statistics/health/mental-health/mental-health/latest-release#articles

Bandelow B, Michaelis S, Wedekind D. Treatment of anxiety disorders. Dialogues in Clinical Neuroscience. 2017; Jun;19(2):93–107. doi: 10.31887/DCNS.2017.19.2/bbandelow. PMID: 28867934; PMCID: PMC5573566.

Han Y, Yuan K, Zheng Y, et al. Orexin receptor antagonists as emerging treatments for psychiatric disorders. Neuroscience Bulletin. 2020 Apr;36(4):432–448. doi: 10.1007/s12264-019-00447-9.

Lampe L 2013: Drug treatment for anxiety, Australian Prescriber 36(6):186–189.

National Prescribing Service: Addressing hypnotic medicines use in primary care, Medicinewise New 67:2010.

Psychotropic Expert Group: Therapeutic guidelines: Neurology, version 8, Melbourne, 2021 Therapeutic Guidelines Limited. eTG complete [digital]. <https://www.tg.org.au

Royal Australian College of General Practitioners 2022. Prescribing drugs of dependence in general practice Part B: Benzodiazepines – Chapter 5 Discontinuing benzodiazepines: https://www.racgp.org.au/clinical-resources/clinical-guidelines/key-racgp-guidelines/view-all-racgp-guidelines/drugs-of-dependence/part-b/discontinuing-benzodiazepines. Accessed 24 February 2022.

Salerno E 1999: Pharmacology for health professionals, St Louis, Mosby.

Stacy S 2011: Relaxation drinks and their use in adolescents, Journal of Child and Adolescent Psychopharmacology. 21(6):605–610.

Westaway K, Blacker N, Shute R, et al. 2019. Combination psychotropic medicine use in older adults and risk of hip fracture. Australian Prescriber; 42:93–6. https://doi.org/10.18773/austprescr.2019.01

ONLINE RESOURCES

New Zealand Medicines and Medical Devices Safety Authority: https://www.medsafe.govt.nz/ (accessed January 2022)

More weblinks at: http://evolve.elsevier.com/AU/Knights/pharmacology/.

CHAPTER 21

ANTIEPILEPTIC DRUGS

Shaunagh Darroch

KEY ABBREVIATIONS

AED antiepileptic drug
CA carbonic anhydrase
GABA gamma-aminobutyric acid

KEY TERMS

Chapter Focus

Epilepsy is one of the most common chronic neurological illnesses, involving recurrent epileptic seizures that may affect parts or the whole of the cerebral hemispheres and that cause muscle twitching and impaired consciousness. Approximately 50 million people worldwide have epilepsy, affecting one in every 200 adults in Western societies, although mild seizures in children are much more common. This chapter discusses classifications of the types of epilepsy and the various antiepileptic drugs available to treat this disorder. Clinical aspects of therapy of epilepsies, including choice of drug, compliance, therapeutic drug monitoring, lifestyle aspects and drug use in particular patient groups, are considered.

KEY DRUG GROUPS

Antiepileptic drugs:

- Acting by blockade of sodium channels: **phenytoin** (Drug Monograph 21.2), **carbamazepine**, **lacosamide**, **lamotrigine**, **oxcarbazepine**, **sodium valproate**
- Acting by enhancement of GABA inhibition
  - barbiturates: **phenobarbital (phenobarbitone)**
  - benzodiazepines: **clonazepam**, **diazepam**, **midazolam**
  - other drugs: **primidone**, **tiagabine**, **topiramate** (Drug Monograph 21.1), **vigabatrin**
- Acting by other mechanisms:
  - inhibition of calcium channel function
  - inhibiting glutamate release
  - antagonism of AMPA-induced neuronal excitability; **ethosuximide**, **gabapentin**, **pregabalin**, **levetiracetam**
  - carbonic anhydrase inhibitors; **zonisamide**

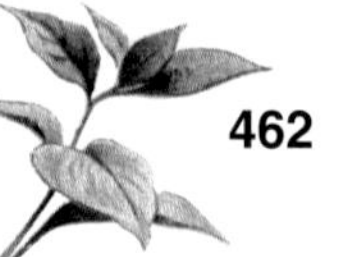

CRITICAL THINKING SCENARIO

Julia is a 23-year-old primiparous woman with a history of generalised (tonic–clonic) epilepsy. Her seizures are well controlled on carbamazepine. She is on the combined oral contraceptive pill (levonorgestrel 150 microgram, ethinylestradiol 30 microgram) and is not planning to become pregnant again. However, she misses her next two periods and is found to be 7 weeks' pregnant. After discussion with her supportive partner, she decides to continue the pregnancy. The antiepileptic drug dose is continued in order to minimise the dangers from uncontrolled epilepsy and because the risk to the baby does not necessarily reduce if the mother's antiepileptic drug is stopped at this stage.

Her GP starts her on high-dose folic acid (5 mg daily). At her routine 20-week morphology ultrasound, however, a mild spina bifida is noted. She delivers vaginally 1 week after her due date, and the healthy baby is given 1 mg vitamin D intramuscularly because enzyme inducers during pregnancy can cause vitamin D deficiency in the fetus leading to increased risk of bleeding in the neonate. The baby undergoes corrective spinal surgery at 1 month of age, with no long-lasting neurological deficits.

1. Why are the contraindications in pregnancy with the use of antiepileptics in general? Is this contraceptive pill appropriate for someone also taking carbamazepine? If not, what are the recommended contraceptive methods?
2. Why did the patient's doctor suggest that she take high-dose folic acid?
3. In order to benefit most from taking the high-dose folic acid, when should Julia have started taking it?
4. How do practitioners of your profession respond to a person with status epilepticus?

Source: Acknowledgments to Dr Alison Bryant-Smith, Consultant Obstetrician and Gynaecologist.

Introduction: Epilepsy

Epilepsy is a group of chronic neurological disorders consisting of many syndromes or diseases. It is characterised by sporadic, recurrent episodes of convulsive seizures resulting from occasional excessive disorderly discharges in neuronal pathways across the cerebral cortex. It has been known for more than 3000 years, in ancient Babylonian and Chinese civilisations, and described as 'the falling sickness'.[1]

About 5% of people will suffer seizures at some stage in their lives, while about 1% of people are diagnosed with recurrent epilepsy. Around 50 million people worldwide have epilepsy. Between 4 and 10 per 1000 people in the general population are estimated to have active epilepsy (i.e. continuing seizures or with the need for treatment), and rates are even higher (between 7 and 14 per 1000 people) in low- and middle-income countries. According to the International League Against Epilepsy (ILAE; see 'Online resources'), epilepsy is a disease of the brain defined by any of the following conditions:

- at least two unprovoked (or reflex) seizures occurring more than 24 hours apart
- one unprovoked (or reflex) seizure and a probability of further seizures similar to the general recurrence risk (at least 60%) after two unprovoked seizures, occurring over the next 10 years
- diagnosis of an epilepsy syndrome (Fisher et al. 2017b).

The seizures can lead to loss of consciousness, muscle jerking, sensory disturbances and abnormal behaviour. Although nearly 70% of seizures do not have an identifiable cause (**primary, or idiopathic, epilepsy**), around 30% have an underlying cause (**secondary epilepsy**) that may be treatable – for example, traumatic head injury, cerebrovascular infarct or haemorrhage, infection, brain

1 The Roman general and emperor Julius Caesar apparently suffered; as Shakespeare dramatised it: '*Casca*: He fell down in the market-place, and foam'd at mouth, and was speechless. *Brutus*: 'Tis very like. He hath the falling sickness.' (*Julius Caesar*, 1.ii.)

tumour, drug toxicity or a metabolic imbalance. There is evidence of genetic links, particularly in familial focal epilepsy (Fisher et al. 2017a).

The aim of therapy is to avoid factors that tend to trigger attacks and to find the drug or drugs that will effectively control the seizures and restore physiological homeostasis with a minimum of undesirable side effects or drug interactions.

Triggers to seizures

Idiopathic epilepsy has no known organic cause, but many factors are likely to act as triggers to an attack: hyperventilation, trauma, lack of sleep, poor nutrition, excess alcohol, fever, stress, bright lights – especially flashing lights of a TV set or strobe lights such as in a nightclub – or changes in blood levels of hormones, fluids or electrolytes. A wide variety of drugs have been implicated as potentially able to trigger convulsions or to lower the seizure threshold.

Drugs that may cause seizures

Drugs that reduce the seizure threshold via their action in the central nervous system (CNS) are potentially dangerous in people predisposed to or who have epilepsy. Groups of drugs known to have this effect include some anticholinesterases, antipsychotics, antihistamines, interferons, monoamine oxidase inhibitors, quinolone antibiotics and some other antimicrobials, selective serotonin reuptake inhibitors and other serotonergic drugs, tricyclic antidepressants, general anaesthetics, vaccines, narcotic analgesics, bronchodilators, social drugs (alcohol, caffeine, cocaine, cannabis) and even some **antiepileptic (anticonvulsant) drugs** (AEDs) themselves (clonazepam, sodium valproate) plus many individual drugs. Metabolites of drugs can also cause seizures – for example, norpethidine. Such drugs should be used cautiously, if at all, in conjunction with AEDs.

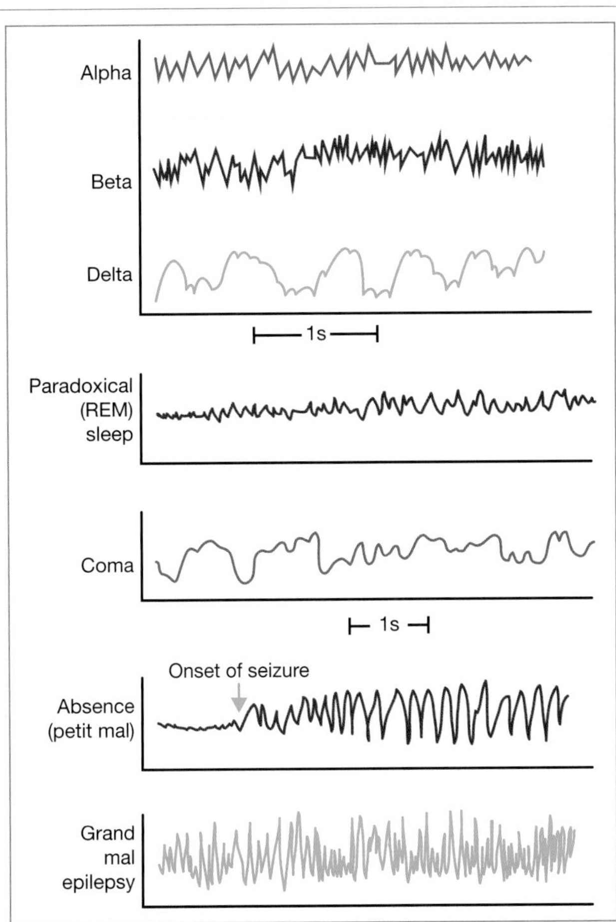

FIGURE 21.1 Electroencephalograms during sleep and in epilepsy

Alpha waves: awake, eyes closed (8–13 cycles/second). Beta waves: mental activity (14–30 cycles/second). Delta waves: deep sleep (1–5 cycles/second). REM sleep: EEG pattern similar to that for alpha waves when awake. Coma: similar to delta waves. Epilepsy – generalised absence (petit mal) seizure: EEG tracing shows spikes and waves (3 cycles/second). Epilepsy – generalised tonic–clonic seizure (grand mal): tracing shows spikes of clonic phase.

Sources: Adapted from Rang et al. 2016; Dale & Rang 2007, inter alia.

Classification of seizures

The choice of appropriate AEDs for treating individuals has depended on accurate diagnosis and classification of the seizure type, although there has been a recent shift to treatment with first-line agents and then classification. The types of seizures are outlined below. A full medical history, laboratory tests, a neurological examination and electroencephalogram (EEG; Fig 21.1) are necessary for classification. Computed tomography (CT) scans and magnetic resonance imaging (MRI) may also be used to detect anatomical defects or to locate small focal brain lesions. Identifying specific seizure types is critical in developing a treatment plan.

The classification of epileptic seizures is complex and still evolving. The ILAE provides definitions for key concepts and classification schemes. Figure 22.2 shows earlier terminologies, as well as a revised operational (practical) classification recently introduced by the ILAE (Fig 22.3 and Scheffer & Mullen 2013). The purpose of the update is to enable transparency and clarification of nomenclature, classification of some seizure types as either focal or generalised and indication when onset is unknown.

It may take some time for these classifications to be adopted by the clinical community. In practice, many health professionals still use the former common terms: grand mal, Jacksonian, psychomotor partial and petit mal epilepsy.

Focal onset seizures

Focal onset seizures (formerly known as partial) originate within CNS networks limited to one hemisphere and are

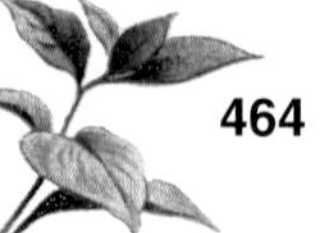

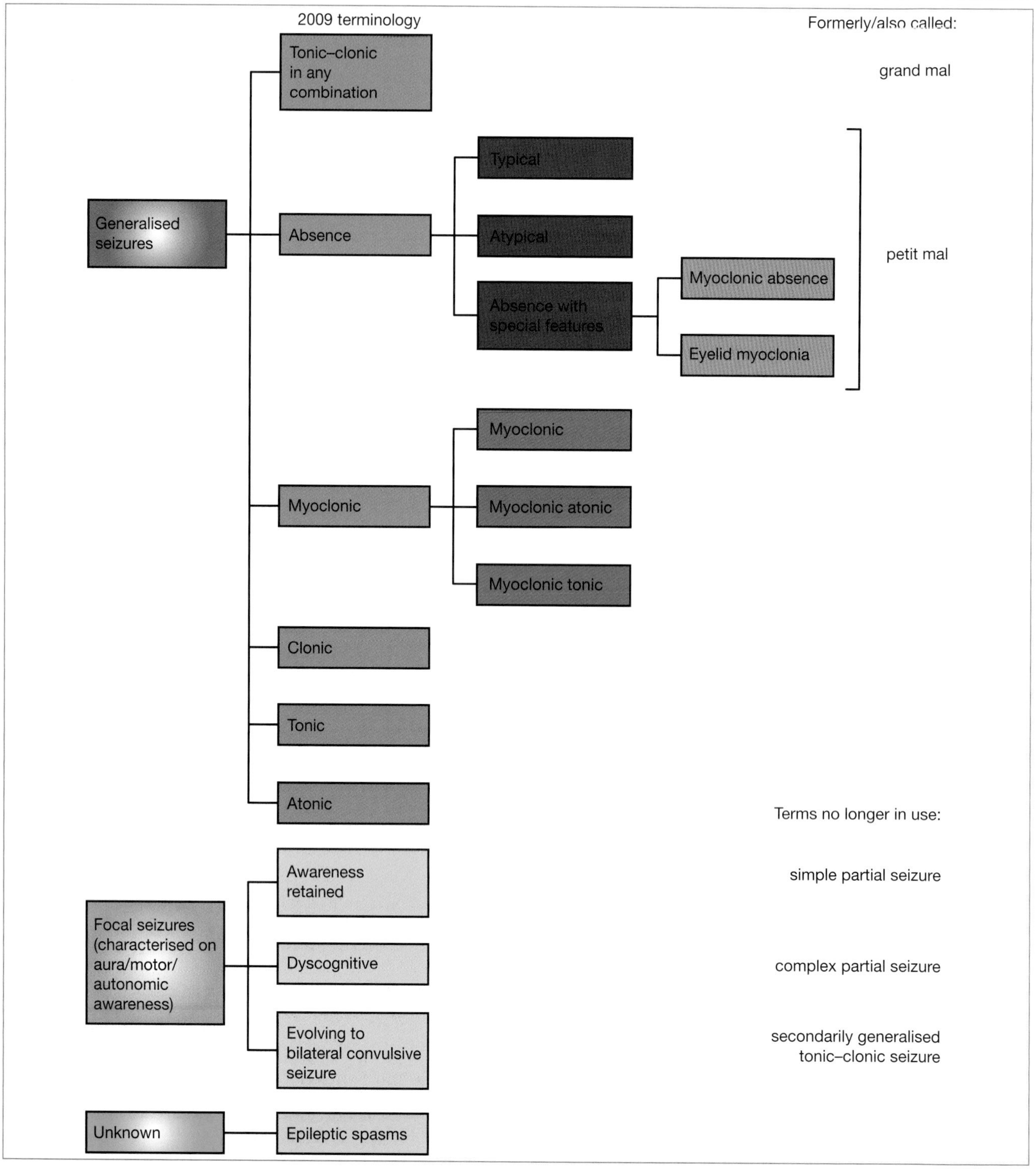

2009 terminology

Formerly/also called:

Generalised seizures
- Tonic–clonic in any combination — grand mal
- Absence — petit mal
  - Typical
  - Atypical
  - Absence with special features
    - Myoclonic absence
    - Eyelid myoclonia
- Myoclonic
  - Myoclonic
  - Myoclonic atonic
  - Myoclonic tonic
- Clonic
- Tonic
- Atonic

Terms no longer in use:

Focal seizures (characterised on aura/motor/autonomic awareness)
- Awareness retained — simple partial seizure
- Dyscognitive — complex partial seizure
- Evolving to bilateral convulsive seizure — secondarily generalised tonic–clonic seizure

Unknown
- Epileptic spasms

FIGURE 21.2 Classification of seizures, based on the system proposed by the International League Against Epilepsy (ILAE) and showing some earlier terminology. See also the classification diagram at www.epilepsy.org.au/about-epilepsy/.
Source: Fisher et al. 2017a; with permission of John Wiley & Sons.

associated with irritation of a specific part of the brain. A single body part such as a finger or an extremity may jerk, and such movements may end spontaneously or spread over the whole musculature. Consciousness may not be lost unless the seizure develops into a generalised convulsion.

Dyscognitive seizures are characterised by brief alterations in consciousness and may include unusual, stereotyped movements (e.g. chewing or swallowing movements) repeated over and over, changes in temperament, confusion and feelings of unreality. These

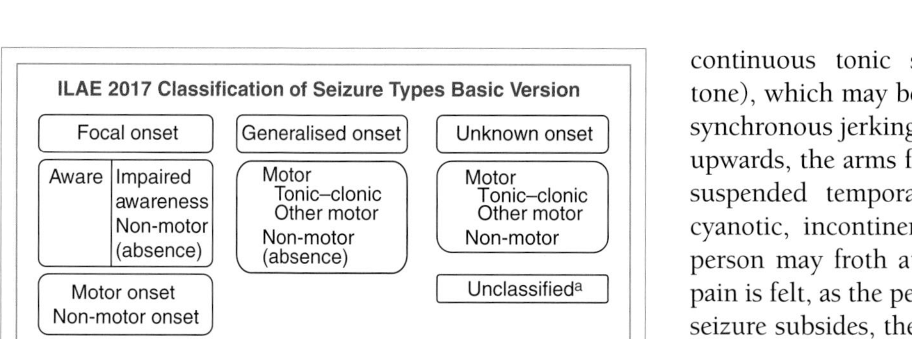

FIGURE 21.3 Basic International League Against Epilepsy 2017 operational classification of seizure types

[a] Due to inadequate information or inability to place in other categories.

Source: Adapted from Fisher et al. 2017a.

seizures may spread and evolve to generalised tonic–clonic seizures, and are likely to be resistant to therapy with drugs.

Generalised onset seizures

Generalised onset seizures arise within the CNS and rapidly involve bilaterally distributed networks in the brain. They start in both hemispheres simultaneously. Generalised non-motor or '**absence**[2] **seizures**', simple or complex (formerly known as petit mal), are most often seen in childhood and consist of temporary lapses in consciousness that last a few seconds. Children may appear to stare into space or daydream, are inattentive and may exhibit a few rhythmic movements of the eyes (slight blinking), head or hands, but they do not convulse. They may have many attacks in a single day. The EEG records a 3/second spike-wave pattern (Fig 21.1). Sometimes an attack of generalised absence seizures is followed by a generalised **tonic–clonic seizure**. When the child reaches adulthood, other types of seizures may occur.

Myoclonic seizures, a type of generalised onset motor seizure, are characterised by sudden shock-like muscle jerks, often with loss of consciousness. They may be atonic (with loss of muscle tone), tonic (with sudden muscle stiffening) or tonic–clonic (alternating muscle stiffening and jerking).

Tonic–clonic generalised epilepsy (formerly known as grand mal) is the type most commonly seen and may constitute a medical emergency. Such attacks may be characterised by a warning aura (numbness, visual disturbance or dizziness) and a sudden loss of consciousness and motor control. The person falls forcefully due to continuous tonic spasm (stiffening, increased muscle tone), which may be followed by a series of clonic (rapid, synchronous jerking) muscular contractions. The eyes roll upwards, the arms flex and the legs extend. Respiration is suspended temporarily, the skin becomes sweaty and cyanotic, incontinence may occur, saliva flows and the person may froth at the mouth and bite the tongue. No pain is felt, as the person is deeply unconscious. When the seizure subsides, the person regains partial consciousness, may complain of aching and then tends to fall into a deep sleep. High frequency of tonic–clonic seizures is associated with a high risk of sudden unexplained death in epilepsy due to seizure-induced respiratory or cerebral depression, cardiac dysrhythmias and autonomic dysfunction; a warning should be given against risky behaviours such as swimming or driving alone.

Status epilepticus is a clinical emergency. It is the state of continuous seizure activity or repeated seizures without an intervening period of consciousness. A 10–20% mortality rate results from anoxia in this state. The major cause of status epilepticus is noncompliance with an AED regimen; other causes include cerebral infarction, CNS tumour or infection, trauma or low blood concentration of calcium or glucose (Trinka et al. 2015).

Relation of age to seizures

A relationship exists between age and onset of an epileptic seizure state. Most people with epilepsy have their initial seizure before the age of 20; however, seizures may have an onset at any age in life. Idiopathic (of no defined aetiology, or genetic in origin or cause) seizures are often diagnosed between the ages of 5 and 20. Onset before or after this age period is often from identifiable causes and is termed 'symptomatic' (acquired, organic) epilepsy.

Neonates

Neonatal seizures occur in children younger than 1 month. Among the more common causes of neonatal seizures are congenital defects or malformation of the brain, infections (meningitis, encephalitis and abscess) within the CNS, hypoxia (in utero or during delivery), premature birth, defects in metabolism, hypoglycaemia, hypocalcaemia and pyridoxine deficiency and electrolyte disturbances. Differential diagnosis is difficult, but emphasis is on stopping seizures quickly.

Infants

In infants younger than 2 years, the seizure types most frequently described are sudden, brief contractions of the head, neck and trunk in runs lasting several minutes. The more common causes of infant seizures are as for neonatal seizures, plus infection, exposure to toxins (in utero, caused by maternal exposure to or use, misuse or abuse of drugs), maternal exposure to X-rays and postnatal

2 To be pronounced with a French accent! There are many French terms in neurology (e.g. grand mal, petit mal, migraine, Guillain-Barré syndrome, contrecoup, tic douloureux, Duchenne's muscular dystrophy, Gilles de la Tourette syndrome and Charcot joint) due to the important early work in this area by French neuroscientists. Even nicotine is named after Jean Nicot, who popularised tobacco smoking in France in the 16th century as a treatment for headache.

trauma. Infantile spasms may lead to atonic epileptic seizures seen in later development (ages 2–5 years).

Children

In children 2–5 years of age, the seizure types often diagnosed include generalised tonic–clonic seizures and atonic seizures. The causes are similar to those mentioned above for newborns and infants, with the addition of chronic diseases involving the CNS. Febrile convulsions are frequently associated with a fever from a source outside the CNS.

In children 6 years or older, the most common seizure types are absence seizures and generalised tonic–clonic seizures, which may be idiopathic in origin. Sometimes the convulsive seizure is associated with a brain tumour or infection, vascular disease, head trauma (accident or sport), fever, presence of a toxin or drug withdrawal. (See Clinical Focus Box 21.1 for more information on paediatric implications.)

Young adults

Within the 16–25-year age group, **generalised seizures** may be idiopathic in origin. The **focal seizure** and generalised seizures may result from the use of alcohol; social or recreational drug use, misuse or withdrawal; or head injury. Young adults who had been previously stabilised on antiepileptic therapies may require monitoring and review of treatment as pharmacokinetic parameters change. Teenagers often become embarrassed about taking medications for chronic conditions and compliance with drug therapy may drop.

Elderly

People over 60 years of age are at greater risk of seizure episodes. Common causes of seizures in the elderly include trauma, brain tumours, vascular disease, embolic stroke and Alzheimer's disease. In this population, osteoporosis and cerebrovascular disease are common and therefore seizures may lead to fractures, intracranial bleeding, neurological deficit, cognitive impairment and severe limitation in daily functioning. (See Clinical Focus Box 22.2 for more information on the geriatric implications of AED therapy.)

Clinical trials and treatment of children or elderly patients

Clinical trials of drugs do not usually include children or elderly patients as subjects, so these groups often do not benefit from the advantages of new drugs until some years after their general acceptance as drugs of choice. However, systematic reviews of clinical trials and published results show that efficacy results in adults can usually be extrapolated to other groups. (See Clinical Focus Boxes 21.1 and 21.2, respectively, for paediatric and geriatric aspects of AED therapy.)

CLINICAL FOCUS BOX 21.1
Paediatric implications of antiepileptic drug therapy

The following are important paediatric implications for antiepileptic drug therapy:

- Febrile seizures occur commonly with mild infections and fevers. While distressing to parents, these do not indicate that the child will develop epilepsy. They are not prevented by use of cooling. Although paracetamol reduces fever symptoms in children, it does not prevent febrile convulsions. Febrile convulsions generally do not require AED treatment.
- Treatment of seizures in neonates depends on aetiology and may include pyridoxine, phenobarbital (phenobarbitone), phenytoin or clonazepam (midazolam or diazepam in seizures lasting more than 5 minutes).
- Young children receiving sodium valproate, especially those up to 2 years of age or those receiving multiple AEDs, are at a greater risk of developing serious hepatotoxicity; this risk decreases with advancing age.
- Neonates whose mothers received phenytoin during pregnancy (not recommended) may require vitamin K to treat hypoprothrombinaemia.

Problems related to phenytoin use in children include:

- Whenever possible, antiepileptics other than phenytoin should be considered first: sodium valproate, lamotrigine, clonazepam and phenobarbital are less likely to cause the adverse effects induced by the hydantoins.
- Chewable phenytoin tablets are not indicated for once-daily administration.
- If skin rash develops with use of phenytoin, discontinue drug immediately and notify prescriber.
- Coarse facial features and excessive body hair growth occur more frequently as adverse drug reactions in young people.
- Avoid intramuscular phenytoin injections.
- Young people are more susceptible to gingival hyperplasia (gum overgrowth), which usually starts during the first 6 months of drug therapy, although severe hyperplasia is unlikely at dosages under 500 mg/day. A dental program of teeth cleaning and plaque control started within 7–10 days of initiating drug therapy helps to reduce the rate and severity of this condition.
- Impaired school performance is associated with long-term high-dose phenytoin therapy.

CLINICAL FOCUS BOX 21.2

Geriatric implications of antiepileptic drug therapy

- The prevalence of epilepsy is as high as 1% in the elderly, often precipitated by stroke, systemic diseases or chronic neurological conditions; focal impaired awareness seizures are common.
- The prognosis for complete seizure control is good. Drug therapy should be initiated cautiously, with low doses.
- Therapeutic drug monitoring is important in the elderly to ensure drug accumulation and ensuing toxicity do not occur. The elderly tend to metabolise and excrete AEDs more slowly.
- Serum albumin levels may also be lower in geriatric clients, resulting in decreased protein binding of highly bound drugs such as phenytoin and sodium valproate.
- Administer intravenous doses at a rate slower than the rate recommended for a younger adult.
- If skin rash develops with the use of phenytoin, discontinue drug immediately and notify the prescriber.
- Drug interactions are common because of the likelihood of multiple pathologies and polypharmacy.

KEY POINTS

Epilepsy

- Epilepsy is characterised by sporadic recurrent episodes of convulsive seizures and is classified by extent (generalised/focal) and signs exhibited (loss of consciousness; muscle tone and twitching).
- The seizures may be idiopathic, triggered by external events or internal changes, or secondary to head injury or focal brain damage.
- Different types of seizure are more likely at particular life stages.

Antiepileptic drug therapy

Clinical aspects

The main goal of antiepileptic drugs is to control or prevent the recurrence of the seizure disorder while ensuring the unwanted effects of the treatment do not handicap the person more than further seizures would. When deciding whether to treat epilepsy with drugs the severity of the seizures and the person's circumstances are taken into consideration. Factors to consider when choosing an antiepileptic drug include:

- efficacy in treating the syndrome
- certainty of syndrome diagnosis
- pregnancy
- adverse effects including body weight changes, impaired cognition and sedation, cosmetic changes such as hirsutism, gingival hyperplasia
- age
- cost
- ease of use
- need for measuring serum drug concentration
- pharmacokinetics
- drug interactions
- preparations available.

Lifestyle aspects, including issues related to emergency management of seizures, sleep patterns, employment, driving and other hazardous activities, use of social drugs, sport, relationships and pregnancy, also need to be discussed with clients. While secondary epilepsy usually responds to correction of the underlying condition and perhaps short-term use of drugs, primary generalised epilepsy requires long-term AED therapy (*Therapeutic Guidelines: Neurology*, 2021).

Monotherapy and subsequent therapy

If possible, epilepsy is controlled with one AED (monotherapy) introduced slowly; approximately 70% of patients become seizure-free with the first AED tried. In Australia, the drugs of first choice are levetiracetam and sodium valproate for all seizures. If maximum tolerated doses of one drug are not effective, another drug is added and the first drug is gradually withdrawn. If seizure control cannot be achieved with the two drugs, a different drug may be tried. Up to 70% of children and adults with epilepsy can be successfully treated (i.e. their seizures completely controlled) with AEDs. About 14% become seizure-free with the second or third drug. Furthermore, after 2–5 years of successful treatment and being seizure-free, drugs can be withdrawn in about 70% of children and 60% of adults without subsequent relapse.

Choice of antiepileptic drug

As stated earlier, different types of seizure may respond to particular antiepileptic agents, although levetiracetam and sodium valproate are first-line treatment. Specific subsets of epilepsy require individualised treatment (e.g. in absence seizures in childhood ethosuximide is better tolerated and therefore is the drug of first choice). Drug treatment should be individualised according to the seizure type, comorbidities, current drug treatment and the preferences of the individual. The currently

TABLE 21.1 First and second-line antiepileptic agents for seizure disorders in adults[a]

	GENERALISED TONIC–CLONIC (GRAND MAL)*	ABSENCE SEIZURES (PETIT MAL)*	FOCAL SEIZURES (SIMPLE OR COMPLEX PARTIAL)*	MYOCLONIC
1st line	Sodium valproate Levetiracetam	Sodium valproate Levetiracetam	Sodium valproate Levetiracetam	Sodium valproate Levetiracetam
2nd line	Carbamazepine	Ethosuximide	Phenytoin	Lamotrigine, levetiracetam
	Gabapentin	Clonazepam Clobazam	Carbamazepine	Clonazepam Clobazam
	Lamotrigine, phenytoin	Lamotrigine	Gabapentin, lamotrigine	Phenobarbital (phenobarbitone)

[a] For children, barbiturates, lacosamide, lamotrigine, pregabalin, vigabatrin and zonisamide are not recommended. For prolonged febrile seizures in children, diazepam or midazolam are administered. For infantile spasms, tetracosactrin (ACTH) and prednisolone are the first-line drugs, then sodium valproate or a benzodiazepine.

* Older naming conventions. If the possibility of pregnancy, avoid sodium valproate; see specialist texts for use.

Sources: Adapted from Australian Medicines Handbook 2021; Therapeutic Guidelines Limited 2021.

recommended drugs are listed in Table 21.1; other second-line agents may be tried if the first-line drugs are not successful in controlling seizures. (See tables in *Therapeutic Guidelines: Neurology* 2021 for details and dose regimens.)

Drug-resistant epilepsy

Drug-resistant (refractory or uncontrolled or pharmacoresistant) epilepsy is defined as a failure of adequate trials of two (or more) tolerated, appropriately chosen and used AED regimens (whether administered as monotherapy or in combination) to achieve freedom from seizures. About 75% of patients can be well controlled with drugs; the other 25%, especially those who had many seizures before treatment, had inadequate response to the first drug tried or in whom there was a known cause of epilepsy, may remain refractory to treatment for a period and should be referred to a specialist epilepsy centre for careful re-examination and treatment. Reasons for the failure of first AED treatment are commonly lack of efficacy or intolerable side effects, particularly severe skin reactions. The most extensively studied mechanisms are transporter proteins. There are reported associations between drug-resistant epilepsy and increased expression of the gene for the drug-efflux transporter P-glycoprotein 170, a protein involved in transporting a wide range of compounds across cell membranes, including across the blood–brain barrier (Brodie et al. 2012; Kwan et al. 2011; Leandro et al. 2019) (see also Ch 18). The over-expression ion of the transporters may be due to, for example, oxidative stress and genetic polymorphisms. Thus, personalisation of treatment for refractory epilepsy remains important. Treatment may include resective surgery, immunotherapy (there is a purported role of inflammation in epilepsy), metabolic therapy (as metabolic conditions may play a small role) and identification of specific genetic causes.

Compliance

Good compliance with chronic, life-long therapy is often difficult. Lack of compliance can lead to drug withdrawal symptoms, including lack of seizure control and onset of convulsions. Therapeutic monitoring is usually carried out regularly (see below), partly to facilitate adjustment of doses and also to check compliance and toxicity. Compliance is improved if the client, family, teachers and carers understand the condition and the importance of regular therapy. (See epilepsy support groups' websites under 'Online resources'.)

Special situations

Epilepsy in women

In some women, seizure frequency increases during menstruation. AEDs may reduce the effectiveness of the oral contraceptive pill due to enzyme-inducing capabilities of these drugs, leading to breakthrough bleeding, pill failure and pregnancy. (See Drug Interactions 21.1 later and Critical Thinking Scenario at the beginning of this chapter.). The risks of antiepileptic drug therapy to the fetus, and the risks of suboptimally treated epilepsy to the mother and fetus, should be considered and discussed with the patient (Stephen et al. 2019).

- Many AEDs are potentially teratogenic or can affect cognitive development of the child; fetal abnormalities are two to three times more likely in babies whose mothers took AEDs during pregnancy. Treatment of epileptic women of childbearing age must include consideration of these risks. In women planning a pregnancy only continue treatment if needed to prevent seizures (Veroniki et al. 2017; Weston et al. 2016).
- Use monotherapy if possible.
- Minimise the dose of antiepileptic drug. All of the 'old' AEDs are implicated, especially high-dose sodium valproate, which has negative effects on cognitive performance of children exposed to sodium valproate in utero. Recommendations for sodium valproate now include a lower maximum daily dose of 600 mg for females of childbearing potential. At this dose the teratogenic risk is similar to that of other antiepileptic drugs.

Some of the second-generation AEDs, such as tiagabine, gabapentin, pregabalin and levetiracetam, appear to be safer. Increasing the intake of folic acid (5 mg/day) in women

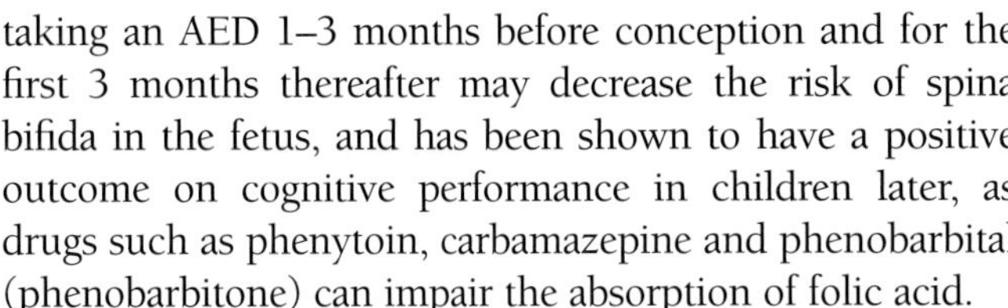

taking an AED 1–3 months before conception and for the first 3 months thereafter may decrease the risk of spina bifida in the fetus, and has been shown to have a positive outcome on cognitive performance in children later, as drugs such as phenytoin, carbamazepine and phenobarbital (phenobarbitone) can impair the absorption of folic acid.

Overall, seizure control is of the highest priority because seizures during pregnancy pose a greater risk to mother and fetus than do AED adverse effects (Vajda et al. 2020).

Although breastfeeding is not usually contraindicated in mothers taking AEDs, CNS-depressant drugs may pass into breast milk, so the infant should be monitored for drowsiness or feeding difficulties.

Eclampsia – toxaemia of pregnancy

Eclampsia is a serious complication of pregnancy and is estimated to complicate 2–8% of pregnancies. Dangerous seizures occur with a high maternal and fetal mortality. It is always preceded by pre-eclampsia, a condition characterised by elevated blood pressure, oedema of the extremities (hands, feet and ankles) and proteinuria (see discussion in Ch 30). The treatment plan for pre-eclampsia is to control the elevated blood pressure (antihypertensives), prevent seizures (AEDs), maintain renal function and generally provide optimal conditions for the fetus.

In eclampsia the seizures are usually self-limiting. If the seizure is prolonged intravenous diazepam (2 mg/minute to maximum of 10 mg) or clonazepam (1–2 mg over 2–5 minutes) may be given while the magnesium sulphate is being prepared if the seizure is prolonged. To prevent further seizures, treatment should begin with magnesium sulphate given as a 4 g loading dose (diluted in normal saline over 15–20 minutes) followed by an infusion (1–2 g/hour, diluted in normal saline). Magnesium sulfate has useful CNS-depressant effects and reduces the incidence of initial and recurrent seizures in women compared with use of anticonvulsants, such as phenytoin and diazepam, by reducing neuromuscular transmission and, hence, muscular contractions. Decreased muscle tone and respiratory depression may, however, be seen in neonates. This approach is primarily symptomatic because the only real cure for the syndrome is delivering the baby. The mother should be monitored for up to 2 days after delivery, as seizures may still occur in the immediate postpartum period.

Status epilepticus

Generalised convulsive status epilepticus results from failure of normal mechanisms that terminate an isolated seizure. First-line drugs are fast-acting benzodiazepines, such as diazepam given IV or rectally, clonazepam (IV), midazolam (IV, IM, intranasal, buccal), then a long-acting AED such as IV phenytoin, sodium valproate, phenobarbital or levetiracetam. If these are ineffective, general anaesthetics are required (thiopental, midazolam or propofol), with assisted ventilation.

If status epilepticus persists, give thiopental, midazolam or propofol; assisted ventilation is usually required because of the risk of severe respiratory depression (Australian Medicines Handbook 2021).

Maintenance therapy

After a drug regimen is found that successfully controls seizures without significant adverse effects, it is continued until the person has been seizure-free for 2–5 years. Plasma drug levels are occasionally monitored to check compliance (noncompliance being the commonest cause of failure of seizure control). Carers should watch for signs of delayed adverse effects such as gum hypertrophy, poor school performance or liver failure.

Therapeutic drug monitoring

Epilepsy is not a stable condition and seizures may occur at irregular intervals; hence, it is difficult to control clinically. Clinical response to treatment is the mainstay of monitoring, in line with ILAE guidelines. Clients should be encouraged to keep a simple diary, recording all drugs taken and seizures experienced. As with other conditions in which relapses and remissions occur, therapeutic monitoring can be useful in optimising drug therapy while minimising adverse drug reactions.

It is important to individualise epilepsy treatment to achieve seizure control with the least adverse effects (optimal therapy regimen). Therapeutic drug monitoring involves measuring serum concentrations of drugs to determine the relationship between dosage/concentration in body fluids and pharmacological effect. Measurement of plasma antiepileptic drug concentrations is only recommended in a few specific cases, especially for carbamazepine, phenobarbital and phenytoin. It is a valuable tool for assessing individual variability in responses to doses and noncompliance, and for studying variations in pharmacokinetics.

Routine haematological and biochemical monitoring is discouraged because there is no clear evidence of value in predicting adverse reactions in asymptomatic people. In the emergency setting they may be used to check concordance with therapy. Plasma concentrations of some AEDs, especially carbamazepine, lamotrigine and phenytoin, may fall during pregnancy, putting the mother and fetus at risk. Baseline measurements should be taken before or early in pregnancy and then regularly to maintain drug level close to optimum (Jacob & Nair 2016). Published therapeutic plasma 'reference ranges' of various AEDs are used as a guide to therapy.

Parenteral use of antiepileptics

Antiepileptic drugs are administered parenterally (usually IV or IM) in acute conditions involving seizures, such as eclampsia, status epilepticus, severe recurrent seizures, tetanus, seizure during neurosurgery, and in toxicity due to convulsant drugs. Phenobarbital, phenytoin and the

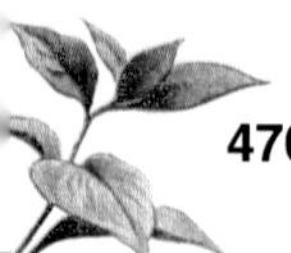

benzodiazepine diazepam are given by injection; there is variable absorption of diazepam after IM injection, depending on the muscle mass injected. If it is impossible to administer the drugs by injection because of severe convulsions, the rectal route may be used.

Discontinuing antiepileptic therapy

A diagnosis of epilepsy no longer implies a lifetime of drug therapy: as noted before, AEDs may be safely withdrawn from up to 70% of people who are seizure-free for at least 2 years. In long-term studies, seizures recurred in about 50% of people, particularly in those who had:

- an onset of seizures after 12 years of age
- a family history of seizure activity
- previous 2–6-year period before seizure control was achieved
- a large total number of seizures
- an abnormal EEG even with therapy
- the presence of an organic neurological disorder or mental retardation.

Withdrawal from phenytoin or sodium valproate is associated with a higher rate of recurrence than for other drugs.

Abrupt discontinuation of an AED may provoke seizures or status epilepticus, so medications should be tapered down slowly (in a non-emergency situation) to avoid risks. If the person is taking more than one AED, each drug is withdrawn separately and slowly over several months.

Use of antiepileptics in neuropathic pain

Antiepileptic agents are sometimes used in conditions other than epilepsy, notably in pain syndromes such as neuropathic pain and fibromyalgia that do not respond to the usual analgesic drugs (Ch 19). In particular, carbamazepine, lamotrigine and phenytoin are used in trigeminal neuralgia, sodium valproate in migraine headache (Ch 24), antiepileptics such as gabapentin and pregabalin in neuropathic pain (Dosenovic et al. 2017) and lamotrigine in spinal cord injury pain.

KEY POINTS

Antiepileptic drug therapy

- Antiepileptic drug therapy to control seizures may be lifelong; the choice of drug is determined by the type of seizure, likely adverse drug reactions, other drugs that may interact and individual aspects such as pregnancy and compliance.
- Therapeutic monitoring is regularly carried out for some AEDs by measuring drug concentration in plasma samples. This helps in checking whether levels are in the therapeutic range, and in monitoring adverse drug reactions and compliance. It is important to individualise epilepsy treatment to achieve seizure control with the least adverse effects (optimal therapy regimen).

Antiepileptic drugs

The ideal antiepileptic drug

Although there is no ideal antiepileptic drug, the following characteristics would be desirable:

- highly effective, but with a low incidence of toxicity
- effective against more than one type of seizure and for mixed seizures
- long-acting and non-sedating so the person is not inconvenienced by the need for multiple daily drug dosing or by excessive drowsiness
- not highly protein-bound and not involved in significant drug interactions
- inexpensive, as clients may have to take it for years or for the rest of their lives
- not resulting in the development of tolerance to the therapeutic effects.

The major drugs used in the treatment of focal seizures and generalised tonic–clonic seizures are sodium valproate and levetiracetam as first-line treatment.

Refer to Table 21.1 earlier for first- and second-line antiepileptic agents for seizure disorders in adults.

AEDs include gabapentin, lamotrigine, vigabatrin, tiagabine, topiramate and levetiracetam. Typical AEDs will be discussed briefly, with more detailed drug monographs on topiramate (Drug Monograph 21.1) and phenytoin (Drug Monograph 21.2) as examples from different groups.

As no one antiepileptic agent is ideal, there is considerable current research into new mechanisms of action of AEDs. It is very expensive to carry out large-scale, high-powered clinical trials, particularly in a chronic condition such as epilepsy in which the manifestations (seizures) occur occasionally and randomly, so there is little level-one evidence on the comparative efficacy and safety of the newer AEDs from randomised controlled clinical trials.

Mechanisms of action of currently used antiepileptics

The aim of using a drug to prevent seizures is to decrease the likelihood of excessive neuronal transmission in CNS pathways; however, most CNS depressants are too sedating to be clinically useful in epilepsy. For those that are effective AEDs, the exact modes and sites of action are complex and incompletely understood. A common mechanism of action relates to stabilisation of the nerve cell membrane by altering cation transport, especially that of sodium, potassium or calcium (e.g. sodium valproate, phenytoin or carbamazepine) and enhancement of the effect of **gamma-aminobutyric acid** (GABA) (e.g. benzodiazepines).

The main mechanisms of action of currently used antiepileptics are:

- enhancement of GABA inhibition
- inhibition of sodium channel function
- other mechanisms, including inhibition of calcium channel function, inhibiting glutamate release, antagonism of AMPA-induced neuronal excitability and inhibition of carbonic anhydrase in the CNS causing intracellular acidification.

Note that some drugs may have more than one proposed mechanism of action. Refer to Tables 21.2 and 21.3 for the properties of long-established and newer antiepileptic drugs.

Antiepileptics that enhance GABA inhibition

Neuronal activity is reduced by drugs that enhance GABA-mediated inhibition – for example, by facilitating GABA-mediated opening of chloride channels; by inhibiting GABA-transaminase, the enzyme that inactivates GABA; or by inhibiting the GABA reuptake processes. The benzodiazepines such as midazolam, clobazam and clonazepam, and barbiturates (phenobarbital) act by, for example, facilitating GABA-mediated opening of chloride channels (Ch 20). Vigabatrin, tiagabine and topiramate act by mechanisms highlighted below. Drugs such as the gabapentinoids pregabalin and gabapentin are also being used in conditions of acute, neuropathic and chronic pain (with a neurological component; Ch 19).

Benzodiazepines

The benzodiazepines used as AEDs are those with long half-lives, such as clonazepam, diazepam and midazolam. These drugs are the standard sedative–hypnotic and antianxiety agents (see Drug Monograph 20.1, in Ch 20, for details on diazepam). Their mechanism of action is to occupy specific allosteric or benzodiazepine-binding sites in the GABA receptor and hence facilitate GABA-mediated inhibition of neural activity via activation of chloride ion channels (Ch 20). This suppresses the propagation of seizure activity produced by foci in the cortex, thalamus and limbic areas. Long-term use is not recommended due to sedative effects, dependence, tolerance and withdrawal reactions after cessation.

Clonazepam is a long-acting benzodiazepine used when epilepsy is refractory to other antiepileptic drugs to treat absence seizures, myoclonic seizure disorders and status epilepticus. It has been used alone but more often it is prescribed as an adjunct to other AEDs to establish seizure control. Clonazepam is given orally or by slow IV injection (for status epilepticus).

Diazepam can be given orally or IV, or rectally when IV injection is not possible – for example, in prolonged convulsions in children. It has rapid onset but short duration of antiepileptic action because it redistributes rapidly out of the CNS, then has a long elimination half-life.

Midazolam has the advantage that it can be administered by IM, buccal or intranasal routes when IV access is difficult due to convulsions. For buccal or intranasal administration, a 5 mg/mL plastic ampoule can be opened, and the solution dripped into the mouth or nostrils; each drop contains about 0.3 mg midazolam.

Drug interactions with other CNS depressants (including alcohol, which is contraindicated) are common. Severe withdrawal reactions and an increase in seizures may follow abrupt withdrawal of benzodiazepines. Dosage is usually individualised and titrated for each patient and increased as necessary.

Barbiturates

The mechanism of action for barbiturates is non-selective depression of the CNS due to facilitation of chloride entry into cells via $GABA_A$ receptors (acting at a different site from those where GABA or benzodiazepines bind), hence enhancement of inhibitory systems that use GABA as a neurotransmitter (Ch 20). There is a selective depressant action on the motor cortex even in small doses, which explains their use as AEDs.

Barbiturates, especially phenobarbital (phenobarbitone), have been used for many decades to treat generalised tonic–clonic and focal seizures and for neonatal febrile convulsions and status epilepticus. It is considered as effective in monotherapy as phenytoin or carbamazepine; however, its use is limited by initial sedative effects and tolerance to anticonvulsant activity. It has the most relatively low cost and favourable cost–efficacy ratio of drug treatments for epilepsy in low- and middle-income countries.

Primidone, while strictly speaking not a barbiturate, has two active metabolites, phenobarbital (phenobarbitone) and phenyl-ethylmalonamide, which contribute to antiepileptic activity. Primidone has been used for control of generalised tonic–clonic and complex seizures but is less well tolerated than phenobarbital (phenobarbitone) alone and so is dropping out of use.

Adverse drug reactions and interactions

Barbiturates have a much lower therapeutic index (safety margin) than do the benzodiazepines. Large doses, especially when administered intravenously, depress the respiratory and vasomotor centres. Elderly or debilitated patients are especially sensitive and can exhibit confusion and disorientation. Physical dependence on the drugs is common. Phenobarbital (phenobarbitone) parenteral solutions are highly alkaline and can cause local tissue necrosis. (See Ch 20 for use as a sedative.)

Drug interactions are frequent, especially with other CNS depressants, including alcohol. The barbiturates induce hepatic drug-metabolising enzymes (Drug Interactions 21.1, later).

Vigabatrin (a fatty acid derivative)

Vigabatrin also enhances GABA-mediated inhibition but by a very different mechanism: it is an irreversible inhibitor of GABA transaminase, the enzyme that inactivates GABA, and thereby allows a buildup of the neurotransmitter in synapses. It is indicated for adjunctive (add-on) treatment, especially of focal seizures. It has a specific adverse effect on vision: it can cause an irreversible visual field constriction in 20–40% of patients taking the drug, so visual fields should be tested before starting therapy, then every 3–6 months. Vigabatrin should be prescribed for adults only when other treatments have proved unsuccessful. Use in young children is limited because performing adequate visual field tests is difficult.

Topiramate and tiagabine

These AEDs are indicated as adjunctive therapy in seizures not well controlled by other drugs. Topiramate has four useful mechanisms of action (Drug Monograph 21.1) and is used for focal and generalised seizures in adults (monotherapy). The main adverse reactions are CNS-depressant effects.

Drug Monograph 21.1
Topiramate

Mechanism of action

Topiramate stabilises neuronal membranes by blocking sodium channels, thus reducing the frequency of action potentials. It enhances GABA inhibition, and therefore enhances inhibitory neuronal activity. Topiramate antagonises the action of kainate at excitatory glutamate receptors. It is a weak carbonic anhydrase inhibitor. (See 'Carbonic anhydrase inhibitors' for a description of the mechanism of action.) Topiramate is considered safer than some of the older AEDs; however, the newer drugs are currently considerably more expensive.

Indications

Used for monotherapy and as add-on therapy in the treatment of focal (partial) onset seizures, and as monotherapy or as adjunctive treatment of primary generalised tonic–clonic seizures, and in Lennox-Gastaut syndrome. It is also used for prophylaxis of migraine headaches in adults, although its mechanism of action in migraine is unknown.

Pharmacokinetics

Topiramate is administered orally, and is well and rapidly absorbed. It is distributed to the total body water, with low protein binding, reaching peak plasma concentration by 2–3 hours. It is not extensively metabolised unless metabolism has been enhanced by enzyme-inducers and metabolites are inactive. Topiramate is not a potent inducer of drug-metabolising enzymes. It is mainly cleared by the kidneys, with a long half-life of approximately 21 hours; steady state is not reached for several days.

Drug interactions

As with all AEDs, there are potential additive effects with other CNS depressants. Metabolism may be increased by drugs that induce drug-metabolising enzymes, including other AEDs such as carbamazepine and phenytoin, necessitating dose increase. It may increase the concentration of phenytoin in plasma.

Adverse reactions

The most common adverse effects are due to CNS depression and include cognitive impairment, ataxia and speech disorders; clients need to be warned against driving or operating machinery.

Psychiatric disorders also occur, including confusion, mood disturbances and depression, and amnesia. As for any AED, clients should be monitored for any emergence or worsening of depression, suicidal thoughts or behaviour or any unusual changes in mood or behaviour.

Other possible adverse effects include fatigue, diarrhoea, weight loss, reduced sweating and hyperthermia, nephrolithiasis, myopia and secondary angle-closure glaucoma, and metabolic acidosis. Serious skin reactions (Stevens-Johnson syndrome and toxic epidermal necrolysis) have been reported in people receiving topiramate, usually when concurrently taking AEDs associated with these disorders.

Warnings and contraindications

Precautions are required before prescribing to people predisposed to the adverse effects, especially renal stone formation, psychiatric disturbances, metabolic acidosis or glaucoma and serious skin reactions. In those with reduced renal function, the half-life of topiramate may be even longer.

The drug is classified D with respect to pregnancy safety, due to increased risk of cleft lip/palate.

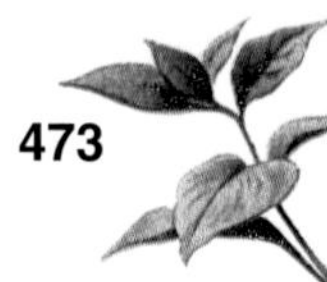

Dosage and administration

Topiramate is available as tablets and as 'sprinkle capsules', which may be opened and the contents sprinkled on soft food before swallowing without chewing. The usual starting monotherapy dose in adults is 25 mg/day, taken at night, gradually increasing to a maximum of 500 mg. Some people with refractory forms of epilepsy may tolerate 1000 mg/day daily; dosage in children aged over 2 years is 0.5–1 mg/kg once daily at bedtime, increasing to 3–6 mg/kg/day in two divided doses, to maximum 500 mg daily.

Tiagabine is a potent and selective inhibitor of both neuronal and glial GABA uptake, resulting in an increase in GABA-ergic mediated inhibition in the brain and is indicated as adjunctive therapy in those with focal seizures. Adverse reactions occur most commonly in the CNS and gastrointestinal tract (GIT).

KEY POINTS

Antiepileptics that enhance GABA inhibition

Drugs that act by enhancement of GABA inhibition include:

- barbiturates (phenobarbital [phenobarbitone]) and benzodiazepines (clonazepam, midazolam) that act to facilitate the action of GABA at the GABA receptor complex
- vigabatrin, which inhibits the enzyme that breaks down GABA transaminase
- topiramate, which has four mechanisms of action and tiagabine, which inhibits the reuptake of GABA.

Antiepileptics that inhibit sodium channel function

Drugs that inhibit sodium channel function appear to block preferentially the excitation of cells that are firing repetitively. Refer to Tables 21.2 and 21.3 for the properties of long-established and newer antiepileptic drugs.

- Phenytoin blocks sodium channels and possibly also calcium influx, thus stabilising cell membrane excitability and reducing the spread of seizure discharge.
- Carbamazepine also inactivates sodium channels, which alters neuronal excitability and decreases synaptic transmission.
- Other examples of drugs acting by this mechanism are oxcarbazepine, sodium valproate and lamotrigine* and lacosamide,* oxcarbazepine, rufinamide and zonisamide (* = other mechanisms also).

Phenytoin

The prototype hydantoin drug is phenytoin (diphenylhydantoin; Drug Monograph 21.2), which was developed from a search for an AED that would cause less sedation than the barbiturates. Phenytoin is recommended for treating all types of epilepsy except absence seizures. It blocks voltage-dependent sodium channels, decreasing the propagation of seizures. It is particularly interesting from the pharmacokinetic point of view, as it has **non-linear pharmacokinetic** parameters, which often make clinical use of phenytoin difficult. There is a genetic variability in metabolism.

Phenytoin and enteral feeds

People with chronic neurological conditions who require phenytoin often also need to be given nutrition via enteral feeds – that is, a nutritionally complete feed directly into the stomach, duodenum or jejunum, via a nasogastric, nasojejunal or percutaneous endoscopic gastrostomy (PEG) tube. There are numerous reports of drug–nutrient interactions in these individuals, showing dramatic decreases in phenytoin absorption, bioavailability and serum concentrations, potentially leading to increased risk of seizures. The mechanism of the interaction is not well understood; it may relate to altered GIT transit time, the nitrogen source, calcium content or pH of the feed, or the dosage form or dilution of the phenytoin formulation. Current recommendations are that the enteral feed be stopped for 2 hours before and 2 hours after phenytoin administration, the phenytoin oral liquid be diluted with water, and the feeding tube be well flushed through with water before and after phenytoin. IV phenytoin may be preferred if enteral feeding cannot be interrupted (Australian Medicines Handbook 2021; Phelps 2012).

Carbamazepine (a carboxamide derivative)

Carbamazepine also blocks sodium channels, thus preventing repetitive neuronal discharges and decreasing the propagation of seizures. The effects of the drug are somewhat similar to those of phenytoin. Carbamazepine is indicated in the treatment of generalised tonic–clonic seizures, focal impaired awareness seizures and psychomotor seizures and for mixed seizure patterns. It is also indicated for treating neuropathic pain such as that associated with trigeminal neuralgia, and for bipolar disorder and mania.

Pharmacokinetics

Oral absorption is slow, and onset of action may range from hours to days, depending on the individual. Due to

TABLE 21.2 Properties of long-established antiepileptic drugs

DRUG	SITE OF ACTION: SODIUM CHANNEL	SITE OF ACTION: GABA$_A$ RECEPTOR	SITE OF ACTION: CALCIUM CHANNEL	SITE OF ACTION: OTHER	MAIN USES	MAIN UNWANTED EFFECT(S)	PHARMACOKINETICS
Carbamazepine[a]	+				All types (except absence seizures) Especially temporal lobe epilepsy Also trigeminal neuralgia Most widely used antiepileptic drug	Sedation, ataxia, blurred vision, water retention, hypersensitivity reactions, leukopenia, liver failure (rare) (Table 21.4)	Half-life 12–18 h (longer initially) Strong induction of liver enzymes, so risk of drug interactions
Phenytoin	+				All types except absence seizures	Ataxia, vertigo, gum hypertrophy, hirsutism, megaloblastic anaemia, fetal malformation, hypersensitivity reactions (Table 21.4)	Half-life ~24 h Saturation kinetics therefore unpredictable plasma levels Plasma monitoring often required
Sodium valproate[b]	+	?+	+	GABA transaminase inhibition	Most types, including absence seizures	Generally less than with other drugs Nausea, hair loss, weight gain, fetal malformations (Table 21.4)	Half-life 12–15 h
Ethosuximide			+		Absence seizures May exacerbate tonic–clonic seizures	Nausea, anorexia, mood changes, headache	Long plasma half-life (~60 h)
Phenobarbital (phenobarbitone)	?+	+			All types except absence seizures	Sedation, depression (Table 21.4)	Long plasma half-life (> 60 h) Strong induction of liver enzymes, so risk of drug interactions (e.g. with phenytoin)
Benzodiazepines (e.g. clonazepam, clobazam,[c] lorazepam, diazepam)		+			Lorazepam used intravenously to control status epilepticus	Sedation Withdrawal syndrome (Table 21.4)	See Chapter 20

[a] Oxcarbazepine, recently introduced, is similar; claimed to have fewer adverse effects.
[b] Sodium valproate is effective against both focal and generalised seizures, including absence seizures.
[c] In children clobazam is used as an adjunctive therapy in those with partial refractory and Lennox-Gastaut epilepsy types who are not adequately stabilised with their current anticonvulsant therapy.
Source: Adapted from Dale & Rang 2007.

auto-induction of metabolism (i.e. it induces higher levels of the enzymes that metabolise it) it may take a month to reach a stable therapeutic serum level. Carbamazepine is metabolised in the liver (it has one active metabolite) and excreted primarily by the kidneys.

Adverse reactions and drug interactions

These include CNS depression, possible severe hypersensitivity reactions including skin reactions (particularly in people of Asian ancestry) and depressed white cell counts, GIT disorders and antidiuretic hormone-like effects.

Again, there are many clinically significant drug interactions with carbamazepine. Its half-life is prolonged by drugs that inhibit CYP3A4 enzymes and by grapefruit juice. It enhances the metabolism and thus decreases the effectiveness of many drugs, including anticoagulants (warfarin), other AEDs and carbamazepine itself, corticosteroids and oral contraceptives (see a typical example in the Critical Thinking Scenario at the beginning of the chapter). Plasma concentration should be monitored whenever any of these medications is added or discontinued in people receiving carbamazepine, as dosage adjustment may be necessary.

Oxcarbazepine

Oxcarbazepine, an analogue of carbamazepine, has been developed to overcome some of the problems of the latter. Oxcarbazepine is less toxic and has fewer drug interactions; it is useful in adults and children with focal

TABLE 21.3 Properties of newer antiepileptic drugs

DRUG	SITE OF ACTION: SODIUM CHANNEL	GABA$_A$ RECEPTOR	CALCIUM CHANNEL	OTHER	MAIN USES	MAIN UNWANTED EFFECT(S)	PHARMACOKINETICS
Vigabatrin				GABA transaminase inhibition	All types Appears to be effective in those resistant to other drugs	Sedation, behavioural and mood changes (occasionally psychosis) Visual field defects	Short plasma half-life, but enzyme inhibition is long-lasting
Lamotrigine	+		?+	Inhibits glutamate release	All types	Dizziness, sedation, rashes	Plasma half-life 24–36 h
Gabapentin				Increases GABA levels, inhibits glutamate release	Focal seizures	Few side effects, mainly sedation	Plasma half-life 6–9 h
Pregabalin			+	Inhibits release of some excitatory neurotransmitters			
Tiagabine				Inhibits GABA uptake	Focal seizures	Sedation Dizziness, lightheadedness	Plasma half-life ~7 h Liver metabolism
Topiramate	+	?+	?+	AMPA receptor block. Carbonic anhydrase inhibitor	Focal and generalised tonic–clonic seizures Lennox–Gastaut syndrome	Sedation Fewer pharmacokinetic interactions than phenytoin Fetal malformation	Plasma half-life ~20 h Excreted unchanged
Levetiracetam			+	Binds to SV2A protein. Inhibits presynaptic Ca^{2+} channels	Focal and generalised tonic–clonic seizures	Sedation (slight)	Plasma half-life ~7 h Excreted unchanged
Zonisamide	+	?+	+	Carbonic anhydrase inhibitor	Focal seizures	Sedation (slight) Appetite suppression, weight loss	Plasma half-life ~70 h
Rufinamide	+			?+ Inhibits GABA reuptake	Partial seizures	Headache, dizziness, fatigue	Plasma half-life 6–10 h
Lacosamide	+				Focal seizures	Nausea, vomiting, dizziness, visual disturbances, impaired coordination, mood changes	Plasma half-life ~13 h
Perampanel				Non-competitive AMPA antagonist	Focal seizures	Dizziness, weight gain, sedation, impaired coordination changes in mood and behaviour	Plasma half-life 70–100 h

SV2A = synaptic vesicle protein 2A

Source: Rang et al. 2016, Table 45.2.

and generalised seizures uncontrolled by other drugs and has been used as both adjunctive and monotherapy. Hyponatraemia (low sodium concentrations) can develop, so it is recommended that plasma sodium concentration be monitored. As with carbamazepine, there is a risk of hypersensitivity reactions, severe skin reactions and cross-sensitivity with several other AEDs.

Sodium valproate (a fatty acid derivative)

The mechanism by which sodium valproate exerts its antiepileptic effects has not been fully established. It may enhance brain levels of GABA and also block sodium, potassium and/or calcium channels. By competitive inhibition, it may prevent the reuptake of GABA by glial cells and axonal terminals.

Indications

As can be seen from Table 21.1 (earlier in the chapter), sodium valproate is one of the most generally useful AEDs. It is indicated for use as therapy in treating absence seizures, including generalised absence seizures (although in children ethosuximide is now first-line therapy for childhood and juvenile absence seizures) and in people with multiple seizure types, including partial (simple and complex), generalised, myoclonic or atonic seizures, and also in bipolar disorder and migraine. Adult doses start at

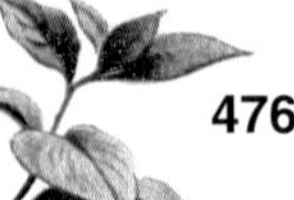

Drug Monograph 21.2
Phenytoin

Mechanism of action and indications

Phenytoin acts by blocking voltage- and use-dependent sodium channels; it is more effective for generalised and focal seizures than for generalised absence seizures. It is also frequently prescribed in combination with phenobarbital (phenobarbitone) and may be prescribed for patients to prevent seizures after surgery on the brain, after head trauma and for status epilepticus.

Pharmacokinetics

Because of saturable metabolism, the non-linear pharmacokinetics of phenytoin means that the dose–plasma concentration relationship is not linear, and a small rise in dose may cause an unexpectedly large rise in plasma drug levels.

Oral absorption of phenytoin is slow and variable (poor in neonates); it is highly bound to plasma albumin.
The time to peak serum level is 1.5–3 hours and the half-life varies with dose and serum level, ranging from 7 to 42 hours, with an average of about 24 hours. Steady-state levels are achieved after 7–10 days. It is inactivated in the liver and metabolites are excreted in the bile and in urine.

Drug interactions

There are many important drug interactions with phenytoin (Drug Interactions 21.1 and Australian Medicines Handbook 2021). In particular, many drugs (including chloramphenicol, cimetidine, disulfiram, isoniazid, oral anticoagulants, allopurinol, omeprazole, imipramine, azole antifungals and sulfonamides) may inhibit the metabolism of phenytoin and hence prolong the half-life, leading to neurotoxic effects. Enteral feeds reduce absorption; see text.

Adverse reactions

There are many dose-related neurotoxic effects (drowsiness, dizziness, confusion) at plasma concentrations higher than 80 micromol/L (20 mg/L), as well as idiosyncratic reactions such as hirsutism, gingival hyperplasia with bleeding, sensitive gum tissue or overgrowth of gum tissue, acne and facial coarsening.

Signs of overdose or toxicity include blurred or double vision, slurred speech, clumsiness, dizziness, confusion and hallucinations.

Other signs of toxicity with intravenous phenytoin include cardiovascular collapse, CNS depression, ischaemia of distal extremities and hypotension. The rate of IV administration (25–50 mg/min in adults) is critical, as severe cardiotoxic reactions and fatal outcomes have been reported with faster infusions.

Warnings and contraindications

- Use with caution in pregnancy (Category D) and in people with drug allergies, diabetes mellitus, cardiac arrhythmias or liver or renal impairment.
- Women relying on estrogen-containing contraceptives may require higher doses or should use non-hormonal contraception.
- Regular dental care is important to detect gum problems.
- Avoid use in people with hydantoin hypersensitivity, and exercise caution when used in combination with similar compounds such as phenobarbital (phenobarbitone) and carbamazepine.
- In long-term use, bone mineral density should be monitored, and vitamin D and calcium supplements may be required.

Dosage and administration

The usual adult dosage is 200–500 mg daily; the target dose can be started, or a loading dose given. However, careful monitoring and titration of dose is required to keep the plasma concentration within the therapeutic range, quoted as 40–80 micromol/L (10–20 mg/L).

Free phenytoin levels may need to be measured at steady state in patients with impaired protein binding (e.g. infants, or renal failure, hypoalbuminaemia, pregnancy).

Dosage adjustment is facilitated by the availability of various formulations of phenytoin. It should be noted for dosage calculations that 100 mg phenytoin sodium contains approximately 92 mg phenytoin. In status epilepticus in adults, phenytoin is given IV 15–20 mg/kg and an additional 5 mg/kg is given after 12 hours if necessary.

Phenytoin has very low water solubility and is provided in specially formulated IV solutions, which should not be administered IM or mixed with other drugs or glucose solutions.

DRUG INTERACTIONS 21.1
Antiepileptics

DRUG	POSSIBLE EFFECTS AND MANAGEMENT
Barbiturates, benzodiazepines, phenytoin	Can cause raised plasma concentrations of other AEDs and of many other drugs, and increase toxicity. Dosages of these drugs may need to be lowered.
Barbiturates, carbamazepine, phenytoin, oxcarbazepine, primidone, topiramate	Can induce drug-metabolising enzymes and cause lowered plasma concentrations of other AEDs and even of themselves (and of other drugs, including hormones, cardiovascular drugs and antimicrobial agents) and reduce seizure control. Drug dosages may need to be raised; increased metabolism of vitamin D increases risk of fractures. Induce hepatic enzymes and increase metabolism of many hormonal contraceptives, excluding the levonorgestrel intrauterine device and medroxyprogesterone depot, which are preferred hormonal contraceptives.
Drugs that lower the convulsive threshold (including antidepressants, antipsychotics and anticholinesterases) – usually contraindicated in epilepsy	Potential danger; AED requirements are altered.
Drugs that inhibit CYP3A4, including cimetidine, conazole antifungals, protease inhibitors, grapefruit juice and fluoroquinolone antibiotics	May inhibit metabolism of some benzodiazepines, carbamazepine and tiagabine, and prolong their effects. Reduce dose of AED.
Drugs that induce CYP3A4, including corticosteroids, rifampicin, some antivirals and St John's wort	May increase metabolism of some benzodiazepines, carbamazepine and tiagabine, and reduce their effects. Increase dose of AED or use another drug.
Sodium valproate	May reduce platelet aggregation and prolong bleeding time. Monitor effects if giving with other drugs that affect bleeding times. Regular use increases concentration and toxicity of lamotrigine, phenobarbital (phenobarbitone), zidovudine and phenytoin.
Phenytoin and enteral feeds	Absorption, bioavailability and serum levels of phenytoin may be markedly reduced, leading to loss of epilepsy control. Stop enteral feed for 2 hours either side of phenytoin administration through tube, or change to IV administration of drug.

300 mg twice daily, and can be increased gradually up to a maximum of 2.5 g/day.

Pharmacokinetics

Sodium valproate is converted in the stomach to valproic acid, which is rapidly absorbed from the GIT; food delays absorption. Sodium valproate has variable onset time and half-life (6–16 hours), depending on the formulation administered.

Adverse effects and drug interactions

These include drowsiness, tremors, mild gastric distress, hair thinning, weight gain, irregular menstruation, skin reactions and hepatotoxicity (especially in infants), or pancreatitis. Drug interactions occur, particularly with CNS depressants (alcohol, general anaesthetics, barbiturates), anticoagulants and aspirin (increased risk of bleeding), carbapenem antibiotics (reduce sodium valproate levels and increase risk of seizures), drugs that lower the seizure threshold and with combinations of AEDs because of drug metabolism interactions. (Levels should be monitored to check toxicity or compliance.) Sodium valproate causes an increased risk of congenital malformations, including spina bifida, and is in Pregnancy Safety Category D.

Lamotrigine

Lamotrigine is believed to stabilise seizures by blocking sodium channels and thus inhibiting the release of excitatory neurotransmitters (glutamate and aspartate). It is indicated as adjunctive therapy for treating focal seizures and generalised epilepsy. It has a long half-life (30 hours) that may be reduced by enzyme-inducing drugs and female sex hormones but increased by sodium valproate. Dosage regimens are complicated, depending on whether or not other drugs affecting the metabolism of lamotrigine are being taken.

Early clinical experience with lamotrigine has shown that there is a high risk of severe, potentially life-threatening skin reactions, including toxic epidermal necrolysis – in particular, with high dosage or when drug interactions prolong the half-life. Administration must be ceased if any rashes or skin reactions occur.

Lacosamide

Lacosamide has been approved in Australia for adjunctive therapy in focal seizures; it enhances slow inactivation of voltage-gated sodium channels and also binds to a protein (CRMP2) involved in neuronal differentiation, outgrowth and epileptogenesis. In clinical trials in patients poorly

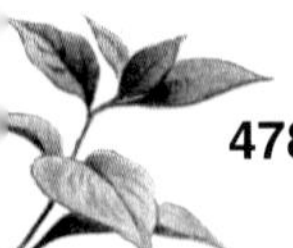

controlled on at least two other anticonvulsants who had added 200 or 400 mg oral doses of lacosamide, seizure frequency decreased by 35–40%. Adverse reactions were dizziness, altered vision, headache and vomiting. As the drug is still relatively new, there is little experience yet with its use in children or pregnant or lactating women (pregnancy safety Category B3). Lacosamide is not indicated for monotherapy in children and is not recommended for use in children below the age of 4 because there is limited data on safety and efficacy in these age groups.

KEY POINTS

Antiepileptics that inhibit sodium channel function

- Drugs that inhibit sodium channel function appear to block preferentially the excitation of cells that are firing repetitively.
- Phenytoin blocks sodium channels and possibly also calcium influx, thus stabilising cell membrane excitability and reducing the spread of seizure discharge.
- Carbamazepine also inactivates sodium channels, which alters neuronal excitability and decreases synaptic transmission.
- Other examples of drugs acting by this mechanism are oxcarbazepine, sodium valproate, lamotrigine and lacosamide.

Antiepileptics that act by other mechanisms

There are other antiepileptics whose mechanisms of action vary. These antiepileptics include zonisamide, ethosuximide, levetiracetam, gabapentin, pregabalin and some drugs that are more commonly used in other clinical conditions but have useful membrane-stabilising actions (the diuretic acetazolamide, magnesium sulfate, sulthiame and adrenocorticotrophic hormone [ACTH]).

Zonisamide

Zonisamide prevents repetitive neuronal discharges by blocking some sodium and calcium channels, and modulating GABA-ergic inhibition. A weak carbonic anhydrase inhibitor, it is indicated as adjunctive therapy in focal seizures. Zonisamide carries risks of AED hypersensitivity syndrome, metabolic acidosis, nephrolithiasis, allergic reactions (cross-reactivity with other sulfonamides) and reduced sweating. The main other adverse effects are CNS depression and GIT disorders. People taking carbamazepine, phenytoin or other CYP3A4 inducers may need higher-than-normal doses.

Ethosuximide

Ethosuximide is the only surviving member of the succinimide group of AEDs; it is indicated in absence seizures. It produces a variety of effects: by decreasing calcium conductance in the motor cortex, it increases the seizure threshold and reduces the EEG spike-and-wave pattern of absence seizures. Ethosuximide has a long half-life, allowing once-daily administration. Common adverse reactions are disturbances in CNS and gastrointestinal functions. Other AEDs may increase the metabolism of ethosuximide, decreasing its effectiveness, or may change the pattern of seizures.

Gabapentin

Gabapentin is an AED that was designed as a GABA analogue but unexpectedly appears not to mimic the actions of GABA. The mechanism for its antiepileptic action is not yet established; however, it raises brain GABA levels and inhibits glutamate synthesis. It is indicated for treating focal seizures with or without secondary generalisation and also for neuropathic pain such as in diabetic neuropathy and post-herpetic neuralgia (Ch 19). Absorption is reduced with high doses and by antacids.

Levetiracetam

Levetiracetam is indicated as monotherapy in seizures, and adjunctive therapy for those whose focal seizures are not well controlled with other drugs. Its mechanism of action is as yet unknown; however, it binds to synaptic vesicle glycoprotein SV2A and inhibits presynaptic calcium channels, thus reducing neurotransmitter release. It is well tolerated. Common adverse effects include somnolence, headache and altered behaviours, but long-term safety has not yet been established. There are few significant drug interactions. In mood disorders such as in severe depression it should not be used as it can enhance symptoms.

Pregabalin

Pregabalin is another GABA analogue that appears not to act via GABA-ergic mechanisms; it binds to calcium channels and also inhibits release of some excitatory transmitters. It has useful anticonvulsant, analgesic and anxiolytic actions, and is indicated for focal seizures and neuropathic pain. It is excreted almost 100% unchanged, so dosage is adjusted depending on renal clearance, and there are few drug interactions. The main adverse effects are CNS depression, weight gain and oedema.

Carbonic anhydrase inhibitors

Acetazolamide is a carbonic anhydrase (CA) inhibitor usually prescribed to treat open-angle glaucoma. Its membrane-stabilising activity may be due to inhibition of carbonic anhydrase in the CNS, resulting in an increase in carbon dioxide that retards neuronal activity. Systemic

metabolic acidosis may also play a part in its action. It is occasionally used in combination with other AEDs.

Sulthiame, another older AED, is a carbonic anhydrase inhibitor and also reduces sodium channel currents. It is indicated mainly for childhood epilepsy and for temporal lobe and myoclonic seizures. Zonisamide and topiramate also have weak CA inhibitory actions. Evidence for clinical efficacy of acetazolamide and sulthiame is limited and they are not in common use in Australia.

Miscellaneous and new drugs

Drugs may reduce CNS neuronal excitation by blocking the excitatory amino acid transmitter glutamate at its ionotropic receptors involving calcium channels.[3] Three types of glutamate receptors are of interest: NMDA (N-methyl-D-aspartate) receptors, kainate receptors and AMPA (alpha-amino-3-hydroxy-5-methyl-4-isoxazole propionic acid) receptors (Ch 18, Table 18.1). Antagonists of these receptors are being assessed for clinical efficacy in neurodegenerative conditions and in epilepsy, anxiety, hyperalgesia and psychosis.

Magnesium sulfate

Magnesium sulfate has a depressant effect on the CNS and reduces striated muscle contractions. It is used to treat toxaemia of pregnancy. (See discussion of use under 'Eclampsia – toxaemia of pregnancy' earlier and in Ch 30.)

New drugs

Since there is no ideal AED, the search is always on for new, safer drugs; more recent discoveries include third-generation drugs eslicarbazepine (a prodrug for an oxcarbazepine metabolite) and perampanel (a selective non-competitive antagonist of AMPA receptors). These drugs have been trialled and approved in various countries. The orphan drugs include stiripentol (a GABA-enhancer used in the treatment of Dravet syndrome) and rufinamide (possibly a sodium-channel blocker), which is an effective, well-tolerated adjunct to treatment of Lennox–Gastaut syndrome, a serious paediatric epilepsy syndrome for which there are few treatment options.

KEY POINTS

Antiepileptics that act by other mechanisms

- Newer drugs act by other mechanisms, including calcium channel blockade. Some of the mechanisms are yet to be elucidated.
- Zonisamide acts by blocking some sodium and calcium channels, and modulating GABA-ergic inhibition.
- Ethosuximide acts by decreasing calcium conductance in the motor cortex.
- Gabapentin's mechanism of action is not yet established; however, it raises brain GABA levels and inhibits glutamate synthesis.
- Levetiracetam's mechanism of action is not yet established; however, it binds to synaptic vesicle glycoprotein SV2A and inhibits presynaptic calcium channels, thus reducing neurotransmitter release.
- Pregabalin binds to calcium channels, and also inhibits release of some excitatory transmitters.
- CA inhibitors are weak diuretics, usually prescribed to treat open-angle glaucoma. Acetazolamide has membrane-stabilising activity, which may be due to inhibition of carbonic anhydrase in the CNS.

3 Glutamate is infamous for its involvement in 'Chinese restaurant syndrome'. Many people are sensitive to the stimulant effects of monosodium glutamate (MSG), added to dishes of Asian food to enhance the flavours. Excessive amounts can cause flushing, nausea and CNS stimulation.

General considerations

Adverse drug reactions are common with AEDs; in particular, CNS depression is likely (Table 21.4) and there are behavioural and cognitive effects. While each drug has its own adverse-effect profile, common reactions include excessive sedation, ataxia and confusion, and depression of the cardiovascular and respiratory centres. Paradoxical reactions (excitation rather than depression) sometimes occur with benzodiazepines and barbiturates, especially in children and the elderly. A possible association between some AEDs and suicidal thoughts or behaviours has been flagged, and should be monitored.

Some AEDs enhance metabolism of vitamin D and reduce bone mineral density. Along with the increased risk of falls with seizures and with the CNS depressant effects of AEDs, this compounds the risk of fractures, so levels of calcium and vitamin D may need monitoring. Adverse effects on the GIT and haematological system are also possible.

Antiepileptic hypersensitivity syndrome

Antiepileptic hypersensitivity syndrome is a rare but potentially serious reaction related to the CYP450 metabolites of barbiturates, carbamazepine and analogues and phenytoin. It can occur after 1–4 weeks' treatment and involves fever, rash that can develop into Stevens-Johnson syndrome, toxic epidermal necrolysis and impairment of systemic organs. Administration of the offending drug must be stopped.

TABLE 21.4 Central nervous system adverse effects of some antiepileptic drugs

DRUG	BEHAVIOURAL ALTERATIONS	COGNITIVE EFFECTS
Phenobarbital (phenobarbitone)	Physical dependence, altered mood; may cause a paradoxical effect, especially in children or the elderly (e.g. increased activity or excitement, irritability, altered sleep patterns, increased tiredness)	Confusion, impaired judgement, short-term memory impairment, decreased attention span
Carbamazepine	Drowsiness, anorexia, increased irritability, insomnia, behavioural changes (especially in children), depression	Less than phenytoin, phenobarbital (phenobarbitone) or primidone
Clonazepam	Drowsiness, dizziness, ataxia, impaired speech and vision, hysteria; tolerance; dependence and withdrawal symptoms after cessation; paradoxical reactions (excitement, insomnia, agitation)	Anterograde amnesia, memory impairment, confusion, impaired concentration
Lamotrigine	Dizziness, ataxia, somnolence, hyperkinesia	
Phenytoin	Insomnia/sedation, fatigue, increased clumsiness, mood alterations, agitation, vertigo	Decreased attention span, decreased ability to solve problems, impaired learning, confusion
Sodium valproate	Sedation, ataxia, depression, increased appetite and weight, tremor; hyperactivity and aggression in children	Stupor (associated with excess dosage or polytherapy)

Drug interactions

Many AEDs are metabolised by CYP450 enzymes, and/or either induce or inhibit these enzymes, so drug interactions with AEDs are common, variable and unpredictable. Interactions need to be anticipated. A good general rule is 'see an antiepileptic, think **drug interactions**'. Regular monitoring is important whenever adding or withdrawing an antiepileptic drug, as drug concentrations and efficacies may be increased or reduced (Johannessen et al. 2020). Typical examples are shown in Drug Interactions 21.1. As an example, drug interactions may occur when tiagabine is given in combination with other AEDs such as carbamazepine, phenytoin, primidone or phenobarbital. It has been reported that tiagabine clearance is increased by nearly 60% when combined with these AEDs; therefore, tiagabine dosage increase may be necessary. As it is difficult to generalise drug interaction effects with AEDs, a reference text should be consulted for details of adverse drug interactions with individual antiepileptic agents; see, especially, *Australian Medicines Handbook 2021* (Fisher et al. 2017b).

KEY POINTS

General considerations for antiepileptic drugs

- While all CNS-depressant drugs may reduce seizure incidence, most are too sedating to be useful. The major drugs used to treat seizures act by enhancing GABA-mediated inhibition of neural transmission or inhibit neurotransmission by blocking sodium channel functions.
- The most common adverse effects are those of CNS depression; antiepileptic hypersensitivity syndrome is a more rare but serious reaction affecting particularly the skin.
- Drug interactions are common because of the effects of antiepileptic agents in increasing or decreasing the metabolism of other drugs. The possibility of drug interactions must always be borne in mind by health professionals providing care for people with epilepsy.

DRUGS AT A GLANCE

Antiepileptic drugs

PHARMACOLOGICAL GROUP AND EFFECT	KEY EXAMPLES	CLINICAL USE
Antiepileptic drugs (= anticonvulsants)		
GABA inhibition enhancers Benzodiazepines	Clobazam, clonazepam, diazepam, midazolam	Treatment of acute seizure activity and status epilepticus
Barbiturates • Occupy specific allosteric binding sites in the GABA receptor complex to facilitate GABA-mediated inhibition of neural activity via activation of chloride ion channels	Phenytoin	

Others		
• Blocks sodium channels • Enhances GABA inhibition • Antagonises the action of kainate at excitatory glutamate receptors • Weak carbonic anhydrase inhibitor	Topiramate	Management of seizure activity (preventative)
• Selective inhibitor of both neuronal and glial GABA (gamma-aminobutyric acid) uptake, resulting in an increase in GABA-ergic mediated inhibition in the brain	Tiagabine[AUS]	
• Irreversible inhibitor of GABA transaminase, thereby allows a buildup of the neurotransmitter in synapses	Vigabatrin	
Sodium channel function inhibitors • Blocks neuronal sodium channels decreasing excitability	Sodium valproate, phenytoin, carbamazepine, lamotrigine	Management of seizure activity (including acute and preventative)
Miscellaneous/others • Prevents repetitive neuronal discharges by blocking some sodium and calcium channels, and modulating GABA-ergic inhibition	Zonisamide	Management of seizure activity (preventative)
• Raises CNS GABA levels and inhibits glutamate synthesis	Gabapentin	Management of seizure activity (preventative), neurogenic pain
• Binds to synaptic vesicle glycoprotein SV2A and inhibits presynaptic calcium channels, thus reducing neurotransmitter release	Levetiracetam	Management of seizure activity (preventative)
• Binds to calcium channels and also inhibits release of some excitatory transmitters	Pregabalin	Management of seizure activity (preventative), neurogenic pain
Inhibition of CNS carbonic anhydrase		
• Carbonic anhydrase (CA) inhibitor has membrane-stabilising activity which may be due to inhibition of carbonic anhydrase in the CNS, resulting in an increase in carbon dioxide that retards neuronal activity.	Zonisamide and topiramate (weak activity)	Management of seizure activity (preventative)

AUS = Australia only

REVIEW EXERCISES

1 Mr SD, aged 40, has developed generalised seizures after acquiring a head injury in a motor vehicle crash 2 years ago. Although previously well controlled on sodium valproate, he currently experiences several seizures per month. It is decided to now include carbamazepine and gabapentin in his regimen. His seizures resolve.
   a. What are the mechanisms of action of his three medications?
   b. What are possible adverse reactions to each of these drugs?
   c. Why does sodium valproate no longer control his seizures?
   d. What are the potential drug interactions between these drugs?

2. Miss PQ, aged 10, and Mr JS, aged 80, both have focal onset (partial) seizures. They have both been prescribed carbamazepine. Explain what is paradoxical in the reaction in children and the elderly. Briefly describe any important pharmacokinetic differences between children and the elderly that may lead to adverse reactions to AEDs.

REFERENCES

Australian Medicines Handbook 2021: Australian medicines handbook. Adelaide: AMH.

Brodie MJ, Barry SJE, Bamagous JD, et al. 2012: Patterns of treatment response in newly diagnosed epilepsy. Neurology 78(2):1548–1554.

Dale MM, Rang HP 2007: Rang & Dale's pharmacology, Edinburgh, Churchill Livingstone.

Dosenovic S, Jelicic Kadic A, Miljanovic M, et al. 2017: Interventions for neuropathic pain: an overview of systematic reviews. Anesthesia and Analgesia 125(2):643–652.

Fisher RS, Cross JH, D'Souza C, et al. 2017a: Instruction manual for the International League Against Epilepsy: operational classification of seizure types, Epilepsia 58:531–542. doi:10.1111/epi.13671.

Fisher RS, Cross JH, French JA, et al. 2017b: Operational classification of seizure types by the International League Against Epilepsy: Position Paper of the ILAE Commission for Classification and Terminology. Epilepsia 58:522–530. doi:10.1111/epi.13670.

Jacob S, Nair AB 2016: An updated overview on therapeutic drug monitoring of recent antiepileptic drugs. Drugs in R&D 16:303.

Johannessen Landmark C, Johannessen SI, et al: 2020. Therapeutic drug monitoring of antiepileptic drugs: current status and future prospects. Expert Opinion on Drug Metabolism & Toxicology. Mar;16(3):227–238. doi: 10.1080/17425255.2020.1724956. Epub 2020 Feb 13. PMID: 32054370.

Kwan P, Schachter SC, Brodie MJ 2020: Drug-resistant epilepsy. New England Journal of Medicine 365(10):919–926.

Leandro K, Bicker J, Alves G, et al. ABC transporters in drug-resistant epilepsy: mechanisms of upregulation and therapeutic approaches. Pharmacological Research [Internet]. 2019 Jun [cited 2021 Oct 5]; 144:357–76. Available from: https://search.ebscohost.com/login.aspx?direct=true&AuthType=shib&db=mnh&AN=31051235&site=ehost-live

Phelps N 2012: Management of phenytoin with enteral tube feeding. Mental Health Clinician 2(5):108–109.

Rang HP, Dale MM, Ritter JM, et al. 2016: Rang & Dale's pharmacology, ed 8, Edinburgh, Churchill Livingstone.

Scheffer IE, Mullen SA 2013: Epilepsy in 2012: advances in epilepsy shed light on key questions. Nature Reviews Neurology 9:66–68.

Stephen LJ, Harden C, Tomson T, et al. 2019. Management of epilepsy in women. Lancet Neurology. 2019 May;18(5): 481–491. doi: 10.1016/S1474-4422(18)30495-2. Epub 2019 Mar 8. PMID: 30857949.

Therapeutic Guidelines Limited 2021. Neurology [published 2021 Mar]. In: Therapeutic Guidelines [digital]. Melbourne: Therapeutic Guidelines Limited https://www.tg.org.au.

Trinka E, Cock H, Hesdorffer D, et al. 2015. A definition and classification of status epilepticus—Report of the ILAE Task Force on Classification of Status Epilepticus. Epilepsia. Oct;56(10):1515–23. doi: 10.1111/epi.13121. Epub 2015 Sep 4. PMID: 26336950.Au

Vajda FJE, O'Brien TJ, Graham JE, Hitchcock AA, Lander CM, Eadie MJ 2020. The outcome of altering antiepileptic drug therapy before pregnancy. Epilepsy Behav. Oct;111:107263. doi: 10.1016/j.yebeh.2020.107263. Epub 2020 Jul 22. PMID: 32759062.

Veroniki AA, Cogo E, Rios P, et al. 2017. Comparative safety of anti-epileptic drugs during pregnancy: a systematic review and network meta-analysis of congenital malformations and prenatal outcomes. BMC Medicine 15(1): 95. 10.1186/s12916-017-0845-1

Weston J, Bromley R, Jackson CF, et al. 2016. Monotherapy treatment of epilepsy in pregnancy: congenital malformation outcomes in the child. Cochrane Database of Systemic Reviews 11(11): CD010224. 10.1002/14651858.CD010224.pub2

ONLINE RESOURCES

Epilepsy Action Australia: https://www.epilepsy.org.au/ (accessed January 2022)

Epilepsy foundation: https://www.epilepsy.org (accessed January 2022)

Epilepsy support groups (Australia): https://www.epilepsy.org.au/how-we-can-help/our-services/ (accessed January 2022)

International League Against Epilepsy – an organisation of more than 100 national chapters: https://www.ilae.org/ (accessed January 2022)

New Zealand Medicines and Medical Devices Safety Authority: https://www.medsafe.govt.nz/ (accessed January 2022)

More weblinks at: http://evolve.elsevier.com/AU/Knights/pharmacology/.

CHAPTER 22
PSYCHOTROPIC AGENTS
Shaunagh Darroch

KEY ABBREVIATIONS

ECT	electroconvulsive therapy
5-HT	5-hydroxytryptamine (serotonin)
MAO	monoamine oxidase
MAOI	monoamine oxidase inhibitor
RIMA	reversible inhibitor of MAO-A
SNRI	serotonin noradrenaline (norepinephrine) reuptake inhibitor
SSRI	selective serotonin reuptake inhibitor
TCA	tricyclic antidepressant

KEY TERMS

affective disorders 500
anticholinergic effects 494
antidepressant 503
antipsychotics 492
atypical antipsychotic 492
bipolar affective disorder 501
depression 501
dopamine 486
electroconvulsive therapy 491
extrapyramidal effects 486
extrapyramidal tracts 486
5-HT (serotonin) 486
mania 510
mental health 484
monoamine oxidase inhibitors 501
neuroleptic 492
neuroses 484
phenothiazines 488
psychoanaleptics 486
psycholeptic 486
psychoses 484
psychotropic 486
reversible inhibitors of MAO-A 501
schizophrenia 492
selective serotonin reuptake inhibitors 501
serotonin noradrenaline (norepinephrine) reuptake inhibitors 501
serotonin syndrome 509
tardive dyskinesia 486
tranquilliser 492
tricyclic antidepressants 501
typical antipsychotics 492
tyramine reaction 508

Chapter Focus

People with a major psychosis such as in schizophrenia, depression or mania are usually prescribed drug therapy. To optimise treatment, health professionals must be familiar with the role of the central nervous system in mood and emotions, the potential pathological changes that occur in psychiatric disorders and the mechanisms of action, main effects and adverse effects of psychotropic drugs. This is one of the more complex and rapidly changing areas of pharmacology.

Relationships between neurotransmitter levels in the brain and mood, emotions and behaviour are described, and the pathogenesis of the major psychoses is discussed. This background assists understanding of the pharmacological properties of psychotropic drugs: antipsychotic agents used in schizophrenia and antidepressants and antimanic drugs used in affective disorders. Actions of these agents on many receptor types can induce some serious adverse reactions and drug interactions.

KEY DRUG GROUPS

Antidepressants:

- Monoamine oxidase inhibitors: non-selective: **phenelzine**, **tranylcypromine;** selective: reversible inhibitors of monoamine oxidase (RIMAs): (MAO A): **moclobemide**
- Selective serotonin reuptake inhibitors: **escitalopram**, **fluoxetine** (Drug Monograph 22.3)
- Serotonin noradrenaline (norepinephrine) reuptake inhibitors: **duloxetine**, **venlafaxine**
- Tricyclics: **imipramine**, **nortriptyline**

Antimania drugs: lithium (Drug Monograph 22.4)

Antipsychotic agents:

- Atypical: **aripiprazole** (Drug Monograph 22.2), **clozapine**, **olanzapine**, **risperidone**
- Conventional:
  - butyrophenones: **droperidol**, **haloperidol**
  - phenothiazines: **chlorpromazine** (Drug Monograph 22.1), periciazine
  - thioxanthines: **flupentixol**

CRITICAL THINKING SCENARIO

Serge and his daughter Anna are attending for a renewal of Serge's prescriptions. Serge is a 78-year-old man who was diagnosed with dementia (probable Alzheimer's disease) 4 years ago and has experienced a rapid decline in cognition. He lives with Anna, who is his primary carer. He is an ex-smoker, BMI 18, BP 140/90, taking perindopril erbumine 4 mg daily for hypertension. His only other diagnosis is prostatic hyperplasia, for which he takes prazosin 2 mg twice daily. Seven months ago, Serge had a violent episode after which he was started on risperidone (current dose 1 mg/day). Anna reports that Serge has had no outbursts of verbal or physical aggression in the last 2 months, but she notes that since starting on risperidone he has difficulty stopping and starting walking, with a tendency to shuffle. As Serge's symptoms have been stable for some time, and in view of the apparent adverse effects, a trial of dose reduction to risperidone 0.5 mg/day, and ultimately withdrawal of risperidone, is instituted.

1. What are the issues in reviewing Serge's medications?
2. What else can be done to assist Anna in Serge's dementia care?
3. If you, as a health professional (nurse, pharmacist, physiotherapist, doctor, podiatrist, optometrist), are looking after Serge, what signs of his condition and effects of his drugs will you monitor? What drug interactions should you be wary of?

Source: Based on Case Review in National Prescribing Service News *2011; see also Rummel-Kluge et al. 2012; Fulde & Preisz 2011.*

Introduction: Psychiatry and central nervous system neurotransmitters

Psychiatry and mental health

Psychoses and neuroses

Psychiatry is the branch of medicine that deals with treating disorders of the mind. Traditionally, such disorders were classified into two main areas:

- **Psychoses** are characterised by hearing voices or seeing visions (auditory or visual hallucinations), having fixed but false beliefs (delusions) or displaying bizarre or unusual behaviours – the main conditions affecting a person's whole mind and mental state. There are several mental illnesses that can include psychosis as a symptom (see below).
- **Neuroses** is where a person's mental state is only partly changed. It is a non-psychotic mental illness that includes anxiety, obsessive–compulsive disorder and phobias; in these disorders, responses to stress are at the extreme of the normal range rather than abnormal. This classification is no longer in use, and the neuroses are identified by individual disorders such as anxiety, dissociative, mood or somatoform disorders.

In the two main types of psychosis – schizophrenia and the affective disorders (depression, depression with psychotic features, mania and bipolar affective disorder) – clinical features are disordered thought, perception, emotion, behaviour, intellect and personality. These conditions are not static but are defined in terms of relationships and the person's responses to the environment, and usually have a remitting/relapsing course. There is often a high risk of suicide, hence the importance of early effective treatment. Most people with a psychosis can live in the community but may require long-term treatment; unfortunately, adverse effects make treatment and compliance difficult.

Psychiatrists may also see clients with organic mental disorders (dementias, delirium and drug-related disorders), developmental disorders (autism spectrum disorders, intellectual disability and specific disorders of speech, attention, etc.) and personality disorders involving maladaptive responses to circumstances and unusual behaviour patterns – some of these are discussed in other chapters.

Mental health

The more general term '**mental health**' is preferred by some health professionals who see 'psychiatry' as having negative connotations. Mental health is defined by the World Health Organization (2018) as 'a state of well-being

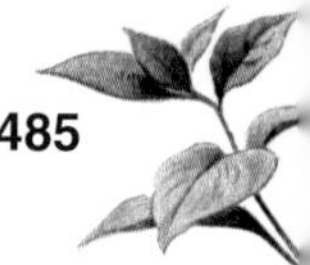

in which the person realises his or her own abilities, can cope with the normal stresses of life, can work productively and fruitfully, and is able to make a contribution to his or her community'; this definition involves subjective, sociological and philosophical aspects. Mental health problems are experienced in the major psychiatric disorders and in such conditions as chronic pain (Ch 19), anxiety and sleep disorders (Ch 20), behavioural disorders (Ch 22), epilepsy (Ch 21), dementia (Ch 24) and drug dependence (Ch 25).

Prevalence of mental illness

Mental illness in Australia

In 2022 the Australian Bureau of Statistics released the results of the National Study of Mental Health and Wellbeing.

In 2020–21, of the 19.6 million Australians aged 16–85 years:

- Over two in five (43.7% or 8.6 million people) had experienced a mental disorder at some time in their life.
- One in five people (21.4% or 4.2 million people) had a 12-month mental disorder (that is, they had experienced a mental disorder at some time in their life and had sufficient symptoms of that disorder in the 12 months prior to the survey).
- 16.8 per cent of all Australians had an anxiety disorder, 7.5 per cent had an affective disorder such as depression, 3.3 per cent had a substance use disorder.
- 15.4% of Australians aged 16–85 years experienced high or very high levels of psychological distress, an increase from 13.0% or 2.4 million in the period 2017–2018.

Previous surveys showed that economically disadvantaged or homeless people, people who had never been married, current smokers and people with a disability restricting their core activities were all more vulnerable to mental disorders. For help with mental disorders, people were most likely to seek the services of a general practitioner, then a psychologist before a psychiatrist. (A GP's referral is required before seeing a psychiatrist, who is a medically trained specialist.)

Mental illness in New Zealand

The New Zealand Health Survey update 2020–21 reported that nearly one in 10 adults (9.6%) had experienced psychological distress in the 4 weeks prior to the 2020–21 survey, an increase from 7.5% in 2019–20. The rate for Māori was 15.9% compared with 9.1% for non-Māori adults. Māori and Pacific adults were 1.6 and 1.4 times as likely to have experienced psychological distress as non-Pacific and non-Māori adults respectively (after adjusting for age and gender differences). Adults living in the most socioeconomically deprived areas were 2.2 times as likely to have experienced psychological distress as those in the least deprived areas, after adjusting for age, gender and ethnicity.

An overview of the history of modern psychiatry

Historically, treatment for people perceived as being 'mad' or insane included being committed to custodial care in jails or so-called 'lunatic' asylums. Physical restraints (stone walls, straitjackets, tranquilliser chairs); shock therapy with water, icepacks, insulin or electricity; or major central nervous system (CNS) surgery such as lobotomy were the only ways to deal with severe mental illness. As sedating medicines became available, sufferers could be given narcotics (opioids) or early hypnotics (bromides, alcohols, paraldehyde, chloral hydrate and the barbiturates).

Psychiatry as a specialist branch of medicine started in the late 19th century, and scientific psychiatry in the 1920s, with studies to define and classify types of mental illness and relate them to inheritance or traumatic events. Electroconvulsive therapy (ECT) was discovered as an effective form of treatment of severe depression in 1938.

The first specific drug treatment was discovered in 1949: lithium was recognised by Dr John Cade, a Melbourne psychiatrist, as being effective in mania (Cade 1979). The first safe 'major tranquilliser', or neuroleptic drug (chlorpromazine), was developed in 1952 and an effective antidepressant drug (imipramine) soon afterwards.

With research into mental illness and its treatment this enabled people to remain in their families, jobs and communities. Safer and more effective, and more specific, drugs are continually being developed and used clinically.

Models used in psychiatry

Various models are used in psychiatry to help describe conditions and rationalise therapy. They include:

- biological model, in which genetic, biochemical and physiological factors are considered
- behavioural model, which emphasises that symptoms are learned habits that can be corrected
- social model, which considers disruptive circumstances, relationships and family situations
- psychoanalytical model (based on Sigmund Freud's work), in which inborn drives are considered to conflict with outside demands.

Overall, an eclectic approach that borrows from all models where relevant is most useful. In the context of pharmacology, the biological model is inevitably emphasised, considering how psychoactive drugs may affect balances in CNS neurotransmitter levels.

Drugs used in psychiatry

'Psychotropic' literally means 'affecting the mind'. 'Psychotropic agents' could therefore include drugs used in major psychiatric disorders, plus all sedatives/hypnotics, antianxiety agents, CNS stimulants, general anaesthetics and social drugs, including alcohol,

marijuana and caffeine. In this text, the term '**psychotropic**' is used in the narrower sense for drugs used to treat the major psychoses. '**Psycholeptic**' refers to a drug that produces a 'calming effect upon a person' and includes antipsychotics and anxiolytics/sedatives/hypnotics. '**Psychoanaleptics**', or analeptics, refer to drugs that have a stimulant effect on the body and comprise antidepressants, psychostimulants (Ch 23), nootropics and antidementia drugs (Ch 24) and also includes combinations with psycholeptics.

The main emphasis in this chapter will be on antipsychotic drugs used to treat schizophrenia and antidepressant and antimanic drugs used in mood disorders.

The central nervous system, the mind and emotions

It is difficult in practice to separate the functions of the mind from those of the body. Anatomical and physiological aspects of the CNS are discussed in Chapter 18. The CNS is responsible for consciousness, behaviour, memory, recognition, learning and the more highly developed integrative and creative processes such as imagination, abstract reasoning and creative thought. It also serves to coordinate regulatory functions such as blood pressure and heart rate. Neuronal networks and functional systems produce patterns of behaviour that can be modified by conscious choice, external situations, internal adjustments or drugs, allowing adaptations to changes in external and internal environments.

Relevant neurotransmitter mechanisms implicated in schizophrenia and affective disorders

It should be noted that the causes and pathophysiology of the various CNS disorders and diseases are still relatively poorly understood, and that research continues. To understand the actions of psycholeptics and psychoanaleptics, it is important to review current knowledge of the anatomy, physiology and functions of the various components of the CNS. (See, for example, in Ch 18; Figs 18.1, 18.2 and 18.5 for brain structures and relevant neurotransmitter pathways, Fig 18.6 for neurotransmitter imbalances [catecholamines, 5-hydroxytryptamine and acetylcholine] in various disorders and Table 18.1 for the various neurotransmitters and neurochemicals. Refer also to Fig 20.2, in Ch 20, for components of the limbic system – important in behaviour and mood.)

Monoamine neurotransmitters

The monoamine neurotransmitters are particularly involved in the aetiology, pathogenesis and pharmacological treatment of schizophrenia and depression. While there may be evidence that a transmitter is depleted in a condition (e.g. 5-HT in depression) or is present in increased levels (e.g. dopamine in schizophrenia) or that enhancement of a transmitter improves the patient (e.g. selective serotonin reuptake inhibitors [SSRIs] in depression), many links in the cause–effect–cure chain remain to be completed. Interactions between transmitter systems are also important – for example, in schizophrenia between glutamate/*N*-methyl-D-aspartate signalling, muscarinic receptors and the glycine transporter.

Dopamine

Dopamine is present in high concentrations in the striatum (due to increased synthesis), ventral tegmental area, caudate nucleus, basal ganglia and **extrapyramidal tracts** (Fig 18.5C), and both a neurotransmitter in its own right and a precursor for noradrenaline. It is particularly important in major psychoses: in schizophrenia, the density of D_2 receptors in the caudate and putamen brain regions is consistently high. D_1 and D_2 receptors are the main types involved with movement disorders in the basal ganglia and are influenced by antipsychotic agents (Table 18.1) with **extrapyramidal effects** due to dopamine receptor antagonism. Similarly, **tardive dyskinesia**, a severe adverse effect of chronic treatment with antipsychotic agents, may be due to supersensitivity of D_2 receptors to dopamine receptor antagonism (see later – adverse effects). Newer antipsychotic agents with low affinity for D_2 receptors but high affinity for D_4 receptors, such as clozapine, are less apt to cause extrapyramidal effects (see later). Further research in this field may produce more specific agents with fewer adverse effects.

Noradrenaline

Noradrenergic pathways are thought to have global activating functions in responses to sensory stimuli. Noradrenaline has important roles in arousal, autonomic control and mood and reward systems. High concentrations of noradrenaline are located in neurons in the hypothalamus, pons (locus coeruleus), medulla and cranial nerve nuclei; noradrenergic neurons innervate virtually the entire CNS from the cerebral cortex to all spinal levels (Fig 18.5A). Many antidepressants enhance noradrenergic transmission by inhibiting reuptake of noradrenaline into nerve terminals.

5-hydroxytryptamine (5-HT; serotonin)

CNS areas rich in **5-HT**-containing neurons include the hypothalamus, pineal gland and midbrain, with pathways projecting to the spinal cord, limbic system and thalamus (Fig 22.5B, later). 5-HT usually decreases the discharge rate and hence is inhibitory. At least 15 distinct types of 5-HT receptors have been cloned, with more than eight

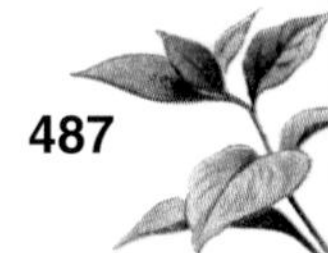

types found in brain regions (Table 18.1). For example, 5-HT_1-type receptors are involved particularly in thermoregulation, regulation of the cardiovascular system and hypotension, sexual behaviour and serotonin syndrome (see later); 5-HT_2 receptors mediate excitation, rather than inhibition.

Many drugs that mimic or block actions of 5-HT produce changes in mood and behaviour: hallucinogenic agents such as lysergic acid diethylamide (LSD) are chemically related to 5-HT, and ecstasy (3,4-methylenedioxy-methamphetamine [MDMA], a neurotoxic 'party drug') decreases 5-HT turnover in the brain and causes a loss of 5-HT-containing axons in animal models. The efficacy of the SSRIs in treating major depression is good evidence that 5-HT function is impaired in depressive illness. Although not directly involved in the pathogenesis of schizophrenia, many antipsychotics have an action at both dopamine and 5-HT receptors.

Histamine

Histamine, although not a catecholamine, is included among the monoamine transmitters. Histamine-containing neurons in the posterior hypothalamus send long projecting fibres to many areas, including the cortex, hippocampus, striatum and thalamus. Histamine may be involved in food and water intake, thermoregulation, autonomic activity and hormone release; its effects are mediated by histamine H_1, H_2 and H_3 receptors. Systemically administered antihistamines cause CNS effects (sedation, hunger), evidence for roles of histamine in the brain. Many antipsychotics and antidepressants have antagonistic activity on histamine receptors; hence, they frequently cause sedation, weight gain and antiemetic effects.

Acetylcholine

Acetylcholine is the neurotransmitter in many short interneurons in the CNS, especially in the spinal cord. There are also two major cholinergic tracts in the brain, starting in the basal forebrain and the pons–tegmental areas (Fig 18.5D). Acetylcholine may participate in pain perception, and cholinergic dysfunction has been implicated in schizophrenia (reduced levels of M_1 and M_4 muscarinic ACh receptors) and some degenerative diseases, including Huntington's chorea and Alzheimer's disease (Ch 24). Treatment of schizophrenia has included modulation of the cholinergic system by use of anticholinergic drugs to treat adverse effects of older antipsychotics. (There is evidence that in some forms of schizophrenia there are deficits in muscarinic receptors and that drugs targeting these, such as positive allosteric modulators, could prove useful.)

KEY POINTS

Psychiatry and CNS neurotransmitters

- There are several individual disorders, such as anxiety, schizophrenia and the affective disorders (e.g. depression, mania and bipolar affective disorder), that require pharmacological intervention.
- Various models are used in psychiatry to help describe conditions and rationalise therapy. They include the biological model, behavioural model, social model and psychoanalytical model. In the context of pharmacology, the biological model is inevitably emphasised.
- Psychoactive drugs may affect balances in CNS neurotransmitter levels, especially the monoamines noradrenaline (norepinephrine), dopamine and 5-HT (serotonin). These neurotransmitters are involved in the pathogenesis and clinical manifestations of the major psychoses, schizophrenia and bipolar affective disorder.
- There may be evidence that a transmitter is depleted in a condition (e.g. 5-HT in depression) or that enhancement of a transmitter improves the condition (e.g. SSRIs in depression). A neurotransmitter may be present in increased levels (e.g. dopamine in schizophrenia), and hence blockade of receptors alleviates symptoms. Adverse effects of dopamine antagonism include tardive dyskinesia and extrapyramidal effects.
- Psychotropic drugs are used to treat the major psychoses. 'Psycholeptic' refers to a drug that produces a 'calming effect upon a person' and includes antipsychotics and anxiolytics/sedatives/hypnotics.
- 'Psychoanaleptic' refers to drugs that have a stimulant effect on the body and includes antidepressants, psychostimulants, nootropics and antidementia drugs, as well as combinations with psycholeptics.
- Although not directly involved in the pathogenesis of schizophrenia, many antipsychotics have an action at both dopamine and 5-HT receptors.
- Many antipsychotics and antidepressants have antagonistic activity on histamine receptors; hence, they frequently cause sedation, weight gain and antiemetic effects.
- Anticholinergic drugs are used to treat adverse effects of older antipsychotics (extrapyramidal effects).

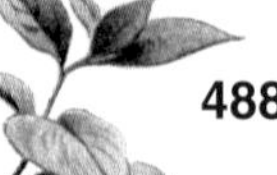

Clinical aspects of drug therapy in psychiatry

Prescribing of drugs

This is a highly specialised and rapidly changing area of pharmacotherapy; general guidelines are described below, and comparative information is given later in the chapter in Tables 22.1 and 22.2. Specialised references such as *Therapeutic Guidelines: Psychotropic* (Psychotropic Expert Group 2021) and the latest *Australian Medicines Handbook* (2021) should be consulted for individual clinical situations and drugs.

Guidelines for drug therapy

People with mild mental disorders may be treated successfully with non-drug psychotherapies; however, those with moderate-to-severe disorders usually require drugs or ECT. Drug therapy reduces mood and behaviour symptoms and allows the patient to participate in other forms of treatment.

The following are general guidelines for prescribing psychotropic drugs:

- Thorough diagnostic assessment is necessary.
- Drugs should be used only if essential, not in place of other therapies.
- Drug therapy needs to be tailored to the specific patient (young/elderly/pregnant/concurrent disease/past responses).
- The patient should be informed of the expected time-course of response and likely adverse effects.
- The simplest and lowest effective dose regimen and regular follow-up enhance compliance.

Current research into genetic bases for varying aetiologies of psychoses and responsiveness to antipsychotic therapies may soon enhance prescribing for individuals; however, at present, pharmacogenetic studies are rarely applied to psychotropic agents in individuals.

Informed consent

Informed consent is usually taken to imply that the patient has agreed to participate in particular treatment after being given adequate information to assist in making the decision. In the context of mental illness, however, the concept of informed consent can be difficult. Patients need to be assisted to make wise and balanced decisions about their treatment; and the patient's involvement in and 'owning' of the treatment plan will improve compliance with it. Negotiations should be documented, which may involve signing of appropriate consent forms.

Improving compliance

Compliance with long-term antipsychotic drug therapy is sometimes an issue due to the wide-ranging side effects of these drugs. Many of these medications have unpleasant and disabling adverse effects, and the treatment might seem to the patient to be worse than the disease. (It is noteworthy in this context that animals in the laboratory situation will self-administer many drugs for reward, including alcohol, cocaine, opioids, nicotine and amphetamines but will not self-administer antipsychotic agents such as **phenothiazines**.) In many countries over the past two decades or more, mental health care has been 'de-institutionalised', with patients moved from custodial or institutional care into the community. While this has improved many aspects of the patients' quality of life, in the clinical context, patients may not have sufficient insight into their own condition to recognise the need for medication. Compliance can be improved by:

- patients and doctors agreeing on management plans
- discussions about the goals, advantages and disadvantages of treatments
- simple once-daily drug regimens
- effective case management and regular visiting by community mental health nurses
- involvement of family and friends in therapy
- clear, concise written information and instructions, and use of reminders
- regular monitoring of compliance by means of tablet counts or assay of drug levels in plasma
- administration of long-acting depot preparations (e.g. intramuscular injections of oily preparations of antipsychotics every 2–4 weeks).

Discontinuation of therapy and rebound effects

After discontinuing therapy, there are often withdrawal effects related more to rebound phenomena[1] than to any dependence on the drug. For example, after discontinuing antipsychotics, there may be nausea, vomiting, restlessness and excessive cholinergic stimulation effects; after cessation of antidepressant therapy, there may be agitation and insomnia; and after abrupt withdrawal of lithium, relapse of mania. These effects may be avoided by slow tapering off of the drug. Many patients eventually relapse and require renewed drug treatment (Henssler et al. 2019).

Psychotropic therapy in special groups

Mental illness in childhood

It is estimated that 15% of children at some stage show symptoms of psychosocial impairment. Common conditions are anxiety, depression, attention deficit hyperactivity (ADHD), autism-spectrum and conduct disorders; girls are

1 A simple way to envisage this is to use the see-saw analogy again (Fig 18.6). If drugs that increase the levels of monoamine transmitters to treat depression are suddenly withdrawn, the balance is tilted to the opposite extreme so that again cholinergic effects outweigh monoaminergic effects.

more likely to have emotion-type problems and boys to have behaviour-type problems. Contributing factors include genetic factors, family history, socioeconomic problems, family disruption, child abuse, poor coping skills and stressful life experiences. The prevalence of some disorders decreases with age (e.g. ADHD), whereas for others it increases with age (e.g. depression, schizophrenia, substance abuse).

The increasing use of psychotropic medications in children and adolescents is of concern (Shafiq & Pringsheim 2018) (see Clinical Focus Box 22.1 and discussion of ADHD in Ch 23).

Mental illness in the elderly

Multiple pathologies can exist in the elderly, and polypharmacy can confound diagnosis of mental illness, as can progressive neurodegenerative or endocrine disorders, anxiety or depression. For example, antipsychotic medications are commonly used to manage the behavioural and psychological symptoms of dementia. Inappropriate prescribing exposes older people to adverse reactions and drug interactions detrimental to cognitive and functional health status. Psychotropic drugs need to be used with caution because of the likelihood of impaired renal function, prolonged half-lives and possible drug toxicity (Clinical Focus Box 22.2).

CLINICAL FOCUS BOX 22.1
Paediatric psychiatric therapy

Children are at a greater risk than adults of developing neuromuscular or extrapyramidal adverse effects from antipsychotic agents, especially dystonias; use should be limited to severely disturbed children and monitored closely. Extrapyramidal effects may be confused with CNS signs of encephalopathy or Reye's syndrome; phenothiazine antiemetic drugs should be avoided.

Children and young adolescents may suffer depression; however, antidepressants are not recommended first-line for children, in whom an acute overdose can be fatal. Adverse effects include changes in electrocardiogram patterns, increased nervousness, sleep disorders, complaints of tiredness, hypertension and gastrointestinal tract (GIT) distress. Adolescents often require a lower dose because of sensitivity to antidepressants. Compliance with long-term medication regimens can be a problem, particularly with teenagers, who may not like feeling different from their peer group. (The side effects of SSRIs in adolescents are discussed later under 'Selective Serotonin Reuptake Inhibitors'.)

Lithium may decrease bone density or bone formation in children. If it must be used, serum levels and signs of toxicity must be closely monitored.

CLINICAL FOCUS BOX 22.2
Geriatric psychiatric therapy

Elderly people prescribed antipsychotic and antidepressant drugs may develop higher plasma drug levels because of decrease in lean body mass, less total body water, less serum albumin for binding, a relative increase in body fat, hyponatraemia and impaired renal and hepatic clearance mechanisms. They often require a lower drug dose and more gradual dose changes than younger patients.

Geriatric patients are more prone to adverse effects such as sedation, orthostatic hypotension and anticholinergic or extrapyramidal effects. They should be assessed before therapy and if an antipsychotic agent is necessary, generally receive only half the recommended adult dose. When clinical improvement is noted, attempts at tapering and discontinuing the drug should be made.

Tricyclic antidepressants may cause increased anxiety in geriatric patients, and increased risk of inducing dysrhythmias, tachycardia, stroke, congestive heart failure, myocardial infarction and falls. Lithium is more toxic, so lower lithium dosages, a lower lithium plasma level and very close monitoring are critical in this age group. Generally, excessive thirst and polyuria may be early adverse effects of lithium toxicity, and CNS toxicity, lithium-induced goitre and clinical hypothyroidism may develop.

Sources: See publications by the Schizophrenia Fellowship of New Zealand (www.sfnat.org.nz/) and the Mental Illness Fellowship of Australia (www.wellways.org.au).

Mental health issues specific to women

Some gender issues in mental health are psychosocial: for example, in certain societies, girls and women may have inferior status and roles, less opportunity for education, paid employment or healthcare, and may be more at risk of violence and abuse. Biological differences in hormones and stresses due to menstruation, pregnancies, breastfeeding, childcare and menopause increase the risk of mental illness.

The following syndromes are specific to women:

- Premenstrual syndrome and premenstrual dysphoric disorder (see Ch 30 under 'Disorders of Menstruation') – anxiety, depression and insomnia may occur, and retained fluid can alter pharmacokinetic parameters of drugs being taken. Non-steroidal anti-inflammatory drugs (NSAIDs) or oral contraceptive formulations are first-line therapy.
- A major postpartum psychosis, a rare disorder, can occur within 1–4 weeks of childbirth with an incidence of 1–2 per 1000 births; mood disorders are more common than schizophrenia.

- Postnatal depression, with persistent severe lowering of mood, has a prevalence of 15–25% in the first postnatal year; milder postpartum blues affecting 60–70% of new mothers may not require treatment.
- Stillbirth, habitual miscarriage or infertility can cause grief and psychological symptoms.
- Menopausal changes, including vasomotor symptoms and insomnia, can trigger perimenopausal depression.

The ageing population and women's longer life span mean that in Western societies about two-thirds of people over 80 years of age are women; depression, anxiety and dementia (usually from Alzheimer's disease) are common diagnoses. Older women with continuing social links, interests and support are least at risk of mental illness.

Pregnancy and breastfeeding

Drugs should be avoided during pregnancy if possible; however, if the mother's psychiatric condition is so serious as to warrant medication during pregnancy or breastfeeding, then the safest drugs should be used at the lowest effective doses. Depression occurs during pregnancy, approximately 10% of pregnant women experience depression, as well as postpartum, and suicide is the leading cause of death in pregnant women (in Australia) and in the 12 months following birth. The health of the mother and baby are paramount; mild-to-moderate depression should be treated with psychological methods, and for more serious depression SSRIs (except paroxetine, which is associated with fetal heart defects) are generally considered safest in pregnancy. Current experience with SSRIs suggests that, after exposure during pregnancy and lactation, cognitive development of the infant is normal, but behavioural problems may be increased albeit transiently (Ornoy & Koren 2019).

There is no clear evidence for safest antipsychotics in pregnancy; most cross the placenta and can cause extrapyramidal signs or withdrawal symptoms in the neonate. They will be secreted in breast milk and are sedating, so the infant should be monitored for lethargy and delayed development. Atypical antipsychotics have been associated with birth defects and close monitoring is advised. Decision making requires balancing the risks and benefits of proposed interventions against those of untreated depression or anxiety (Anderson et al. 2020).

Mental illness in indigenous populations

Indigenous communities worldwide have suffered disruptions after colonisation of their lands, with subsequent discrimination, dispossession, poverty, poor health, suppression of traditional cultures and family supports and lack of educational and employment opportunities. These are all established risk factors for psychological distress and mental illness, particularly for depression, anxiety and substance abuse.

Australia

In Australia, Indigenous Australians are the most disadvantaged group in socioeconomic terms and frequently have unequal access to health services, education and employment. There is different understanding of health and illness: spiritual factors, family groups and relationship with the land are important; hence, Western psychiatric classifications and treatment methods may not be appropriate. Depression, psychological stress, substance abuse, post-traumatic stress disorder and reactions to perceived racism are much more prevalent in Indigenous Australian communities than in the general population, while rates of schizophrenia and bipolar disorder are similar. In remote communities, in young adult Indigenous Australian men, psychotic disorders are common, often along with high rates of diabetes, substance misuse and intellectual impairment (Hunter et al. 2011; Hunter 2014). Mental health services need to be sensitive to cultural differences and provide appropriate training, policies, resources and ongoing programs to 'close the gap' in mental health.

New Zealand

In New Zealand, Māori people place high values on spiritual and family dimensions in life and health; in the traditional community, people with mental illness and epilepsy were not shunned. After dispossession of land and culture, near-extinction, then more supportive public health policies, Māori people still suffer disadvantage. Māori adults were 1.9 times as likely to have experienced psychological distress as non-Māori adults after adjusting for age and gender. Māori men have much higher rates of readmission to psychiatric hospitals than Māori women or non-Māori men, and youth suicide rates are almost double those in the non-Māori community. Drug and alcohol misuse and rates of psychological distress are much higher in Māori and Pacific Islander communities than in other people; the prevalence of diagnosis of common mental disorders (depression, bipolar disorder, anxiety disorder) are higher in Māori versus non-Māori populations. High prevalence of mental illness is closely associated with living in deprived neighbourhoods (refer to the Health of New Zealand Adults 2019–20 Survey – see 'Online resources').

Māori participation in mental health services is being encouraged and increased, with assessments and treatments that acknowledge the importance of traditional culture, spirituality and the extended family.

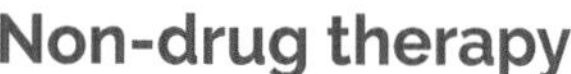

Non-drug therapy

In mild mental disorders, non-drug therapies are used first; indeed, drugs may be no more effective than placebos. Most patients taking psychotropic drugs have already experienced non-drug therapies, so these modalities are described briefly.

Psychotherapies

Psychotherapies include treatments based on a relationship between a person needing help for psychological distress or disturbed behaviour, and a trained health professional (e.g. psychologist, psychiatrist, social worker, occupational therapist) who uses interventions without drugs to deal with a crisis, improve specific symptoms, facilitate self-awareness or provide long-term supportive help.

Types of therapies include psychoanalysis (frequent long, intense sessions over a prolonged period), group psychotherapy, self-help groups, counselling, behaviour modification therapy, cognitive therapy and cognitive behaviour therapy, which challenges patterns of negative thought and behaviour to improve thinking, mood and relationships.

Electroconvulsive therapy

Electroconvulsive therapy is used mainly as a safe, effective treatment for severe depression that is unresponsive to drugs, and also for mania and schizophrenia. It was originally introduced (in the 1930s) for schizophrenia, on the rationale that inducing a series of epileptic-type fits would help the disordered CNS functions. Early techniques were primitive and potentially dangerous; however, in current practice anaesthetics and muscle relaxants are used, dosage of the electrical current is more accurately determined and applied and the electroencephalogram is routinely monitored. The convulsion induced by the current is essential; ECT is thought to act by causing readjustment in monoamine levels in the brain.

There is a higher positive response from ECT (80%) than from antidepressants (60%) in severe depression, especially when associated with psychotic features, suicidal ideas, psychomotor slowing and weight loss. ECT is relatively contraindicated in people with severe cardiovascular and respiratory disorders, or in conditions with raised intracranial pressure. The main adverse effects are memory impairment and confusion, plus muscle pains. Individualising treatments improves outcomes and newer techniques include brief and ultra-brief pulse stimulation leading to fewer adverse cognitive effects. More studies are warranted.

Psychosurgery

In the early 20th century, prefrontal lobotomy was used to treat severe schizophrenia by severing the connections between the frontal lobes and the rest of the brain. Limbic system surgery, sometimes currently used in severe cases of depression and obsessive–compulsive disorder unresponsive to other treatments, targets connections between the frontal lobes and particular components of the limbic system.

KEY POINTS

Clinical aspects of drug therapy in psychiatry

- For the prescribing of drugs, specialised reference texts such as *Therapeutic Guidelines: Psychotropic* (Psychotropic Expert Group 2021) and the latest *Australian Medicines Handbook* should be consulted for individual clinical situations and drugs.
- Drug therapy reduces mood and behaviour symptoms and allows the patient to participate in other forms of treatment.
- General guidelines for prescribing psychotropic drugs include:
  - thorough diagnostic assessment
  - drugs only being used if essential, not in place of other therapies
  - tailoring drug therapy to the specific patient (young/elderly/pregnant/concurrent disease/past responses)
  - informing the patient of the expected time-course of response and likely adverse effects.
- Compliance can be enhanced by using the simplest and lowest effective dose regimen and using regular follow-up. Clinical aspects of psychotropic drug use include informed consent and compliance with therapy; the frequency of serious adverse drug reactions and interactions; concomitant non-drug therapy such as psychotherapy, ECT and psychosurgery.
- Compliance with long-term antipsychotic drug therapy is sometimes an issue due to the wide-ranging side effects of these drugs.
- After discontinuing therapy, there are often withdrawal effects related more to rebound phenomena than to any dependence on the drug. The effects may be avoided by slow tapering off of the drug.
- People with mild mental disorders may be treated successfully with non-drug psychotherapies; however, patients with moderate-to-severe disorders usually require drugs and/or ECT.
- Psychotropic therapy is tailored, especially when working with specific groups.

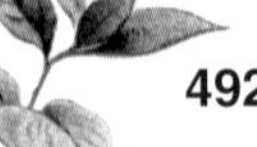

Antipsychotic agents

Schizophrenia

Schizophrenia (sometimes erroneously referred to as split personality) is manifested by disordered emotion, speech, thought, perception and volition, leading to delusions, withdrawal and loss of insight possibly due to abnormalities in brain circuitry or neurotransmission. It has an insidious onset in young adults (aged 15–35 years) and a prevalence of about 1% in virtually all societies. It causes considerable morbidity, lost work time and mortality from suicide.

The following causative factors are proposed:

- Altered neurotransmission: implicated are 5-HT, due to the similarity between psychoses and the hallucinations produced by serotonergic drugs such as LSD (Ch 25), and dopamine in mesolimbic pathways, as many antipsychotic drugs are dopamine antagonists. Also gabaergic, glutaminergic and cholinergic neurotransmission has been implicated.
- Genetic vulnerability and hereditary tendencies: implicated are genes coding for proteins involved in dopamine, glutamate and gamma-aminobutyric acid (GABA) pathways, and also immune and signalling networks.
- Environmental associations with perinatal complications (first few days of the person's life) or other stressful life events or relationships.
- A defect in early brain development.
- Use of cannabis (marijuana) in adolescence increases the risk of developing schizophrenia; the related condition, schizophreniform psychosis, has an acute onset related to drugs or trauma (physical or emotional).
- The main clinical features of schizophrenia include positive and negative symptoms.
- Positive symptoms (excessive, or hyper-behaviours): include hallucinations, delusions (paranoid, bizarre, religious); and disorganised thinking, communication and behaviour (agitation, anxiety, hyperactivity and hostility).
- Negative (reduced, or hypo-behaviour) symptoms: such as flat affect (mood), withdrawal, lack of motivation, poor hygiene and dress, social inadequacy and diminished speech patterns.
- Impaired cognitive powers: poor insight, memory, planning and mental flexibility.

Antipsychotic drug groups

Antipsychotic, or **neuroleptic**, agents, classified under psycholeptics, are the mainstay of treatment of schizophrenia, and in acutely disturbed people in the manic phase of bipolar disorder or in acute agitation or delirium. The first effective **tranquilliser** (to calm an agitated or anxious person) without serious sedating actions was chlorpromazine (Largactil); it revolutionised treatment when released in the early 1950s and is still the prototype antipsychotic. Hundreds of phenothiazines were developed as 'me-too' drugs; a few remain in use (Table 22.1). More recent antipsychotics tend to be grouped as 'second-generation' or 'atypical' agents.

Classification of antipsychotics

Antipsychotics are classified using various criteria, but it is difficult to generalise because there are many differences between agents within a group.

High–low potency

Antipsychotic drugs have been classified (based on average dose required) as low-potency, intermediate-potency and high-potency drugs. For example, 100 mg chlorpromazine (low-potency agent) is considered about equivalent to 5 mg trifluoperazine or 2 mg haloperidol (high-potency agents). Trifluoperazine is not marketed in Australia however, it may be available in the Special Access Scheme. Low-potency agents tend to have predominant sedating, hypotensive and anticholinergic effects with fewer extrapyramidal side effects, whereas high-potency drugs cause more problems with extrapyramidal side effects but are less sedating, hypotensive or anticholinergic (Table 22.1).

Typical–atypical

Based on chronology, antipsychotics are classified as **typical antipsychotics**, classical or conventional first-generation (older) antipsychotics such as the phenothiazines, thioxanthines and haloperidol-type drugs; and the **atypical antipsychotics**, second-generation agents, such as clozapine, olanzapine and risperidone, which appear to have rather different profiles of actions (Table 22.1). These atypical antipsychotics are less likely to induce extrapyramidal side effects but more likely to cause metabolic effects such as weight gain and diabetes.

Most antipsychotic agents produce useful effects on the positive symptoms, but negative symptoms and cognitive impairments are usually less responsive. They decrease hallucinations, delusions, initiative, emotion, aggression, responses to external stimuli and thought disorder, and can prevent relapses. The person may become drowsy, but is readily arousable without confusion. Later atypical antipsychotic drugs such as clozapine and risperidone appear to be more effective than other neuroleptic agents against the negative symptoms.

Chemistry

First-generation antipsychotics such as the phenothiazines are also sometimes classified chemically into subgroups

TABLE 22.1 Properties of some antipsychotic agents: typical maintenance doses (in schizophrenia and psychoses) and major effects

		FREQUENCY OF EFFECTS AND ADVERSE EFFECTS[a]					
CHEMICAL, GENERIC NAME	DAILY DOSE RANGE (mg)	ANTIEMETIC	SEDATION	HYPOTENSION[b]	ANTICHOLINERGIC	EXTRAPYRAMIDAL[c]	WEIGHT GAIN
Phenothiazines							
Chlorpromazine	25 mg 3 times daily increased, if necessary, by 25 mg 2–3 times daily up to 600–800 mg per day	3	3	3	2–3	1 (2 if higher doses)	2
Periciazine	15–75 mg daily in divided doses Elderly 10–30 mg depending on symptoms		3	3	3	1	
Thioxanthines							
Flupentixol	20–40 mg IM every 2–4 weeks (usual max. dosage 100 mg every 2 weeks)	–	1	1	1	3	
Zuclopenthixol	Acute (oral) 10–50 mg/day up to 75 mg (severe): Chronic 20–40 mg/day orally 200–400 mg depot IM every 2–4 weeks	–	3	1	2	2	
Butyrophenones							
Droperidol	IMI repeat every 4–6 hours 5–25 mg single dose Slow IV infusion: 50–125 mg/day in 2 divided 250 mL 20 min infusions	–	1	1	1	3	
Haloperidol (for chronic psychoses)	2–15 mg; max. 30 mg daily; depot dose adults: initially 10–15 times previous daily dose of oral haloperidol, max. 100 mg; adjust dose by 50 mg every 4 weeks as necessary to max. 300 mg	2	1	1	1	3	1
Atypical agents							
Amisulpride	oral 50–300 mg once daily	–	1	1	0–1	1–2	1
Aripiprazole	Oral 10–15 mg once daily IM 400 mg once monthly	–	(possibly insomnia)	1	0–1	1	0–1
Asenapine	Sublingual 5–10 mg twice daily	–	1	1	0–1	1	1
Clozapine	Initial 12.5 mg, increase gradually in divided doses to 200–600 mg (use lowest effective dose)	1	3	3	3	1	1
Olanzapine	5–10 mg/day; may increase to 20 mg once daily; max. 20 mg once daily (wafer 2.5–10 mg)	–	2	1	1–2	1	3
Paliperidone	3–12 mg once daily	–	1–3	2	0–1	1–2	2
Quetiapine	400–800 mg daily	–	1–2	2	1	0–1	2
Risperidone	4–6 mg to a max. of 30 mg	–	1	2	0–1	1	2
Ziprasidone	40–80 mg twice daily	–	1–2	1–2	0–1	1	0–1

[a] Grading: 1 = low; 2 = moderate; 3 = high
[b] Orthostatic hypotension
[c] Extrapyramidal side effects include akathisia, dystonia, parkinsonism and tardive dyskinesia.
Note: Doses are typical total daily oral dose (regular formulation) unless otherwise indicated; higher doses may be needed for acute severe psychoses; drugs with short half-lives require twice-daily dosing (or controlled-release formulations).
Refer to expert texts for further dosages.
Sources: Australian Medicines Handbook 2021; Psychotropic Expert Group 2021.

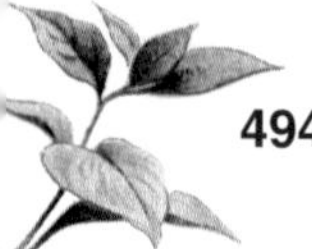

depending on the type of side chain in the molecule; for example, the piperidine compounds (e.g. periciazine) and the piperazine compounds (e.g. prochlorperazine and trifluoperazine) are structurally related to antihistamines such as promethazine. Many second-generation antipsychotics such as dibenzodiazepines (clozapine), thiobenzodiazepines (olanzapine) and dibenzothiazepines (quetiapine) are chemically related to tricyclic antidepressants.

Formulations and routes

Most antipsychotics are administered orally, as regular tablets or capsules, oral liquid or sublingual wafers. Controlled-release tablets are useful for drugs with short half-lives. Some are available only as parenterals; for example, droperidol in a short-acting injection for acute psychosis or as an adjunct to anaesthesia, and flupentixol as a long-acting depot preparation for chronic psychoses, are useful if the person has been stabilised on an oral formulation but has poor compliance due to forgetfulness or impaired insight.

Mechanisms of action and therapeutic actions of antipsychotics

Mechanisms of action

There is good evidence that antipsychotics act by antagonism of dopamine receptors, especially first-generation agents, by acting at the D_2 type. These subtypes mediate the main inhibitory central effects of dopamine in nigrostriatal, mesolimbic and tuberoinfundibular pathways. This antidopaminergic action leads to useful therapeutic effects (slower thinking and movements and antiemetic actions) and also common adverse reactions, including extrapyramidal effects (Fig 22.1, later) and hyperprolactinaemia, which infrequently results in swelling of the breasts and milk secretion. The second-generation agents also act at the D_2 type, and may – combined with antagonism 5-HT_{2A} and partial agonism of 5-HT_{1A} receptors – contribute to the clinical effects seen. Adverse effects are mainly due to antagonism at α-adrenoceptors (hypotension) and muscarinic ACh receptors (**anticholinergic effects**).

Therapeutic actions

In clinical use, antipsychotic drugs may take many weeks before their actions are most effective, even though in-vitro biochemical actions and sedation may be immediate. The in-vivo delay may be due to a transient increase in dopaminergic activity, which changes after about 3 weeks to inhibition, causing antipsychotic effects to 'kick in'.

Other indications for antipsychotic agents

There are several other conditions in which the antipsychotic drugs are indicated: as shown in Table 22.1, conventional antipsychotics have useful antiemetic actions (presumably due to antidopamine actions in the CNS); most commonly prescribed as antiemetics are prochlorperazine (now used only as an antiemetic) and haloperidol. Chlorpromazine and haloperidol are used in the short-term management of severe anxiety and for intractable hiccups. Haloperidol is also indicated for treating choreas (repetitive behaviours) such as tics (facial grimaces and blinking) and Tourette's syndrome, a rare CNS disorder presenting as involuntary, rapid and repetitive motor movements, tics and vocal noises. Drugs such as aripiprazole, olanzapine, risperidone or quetiapine are used to treat bipolar disorder or mania.

Behavioural emergencies and delirium

In behavioural emergencies, when a person is threatening assault or self-harm or is excessively agitated, hostile, aggressive or intimidating, medical intervention may be necessary (as may physical assistance from security staff or police). Pharmacological management includes use of sedatives, such as diazepam or midazolam, or antipsychotics, such as chlorpromazine, haloperidol, trifluoperazine or risperidone. Drugs may have to be administered by IM or IV injection, and close monitoring of the person's vital signs is necessary.

Delirium is a state characterised by impaired cognitive function and ability to maintain attention, often with agitation, delusions and disturbed sleep patterns. Aetiologies include CNS infections, metabolic disturbances and drug toxicity (especially from alcohol, anticholinergic drugs or narcotic analgesics). Haloperidol is indicated, but antipsychotics with major anticholinergic actions should be avoided.

Childhood psychoses

Schizophrenia is rare in children; other disorders that may indicate the need for antipsychotic agents include disruptive behaviours and some developmental disorders. Risperidone is used in severe behavioural disorders associated with autism, intellectual disabilities or Tourette's syndrome.

Conventional (typical) antipsychotics

Phenothiazine derivatives

Chlorpromazine

Chlorpromazine was the first – and is still the prototype – phenothiazine antipsychotic drug; details are shown in Drug Monograph 22.1, and brief comparative information is given on other phenothiazines.

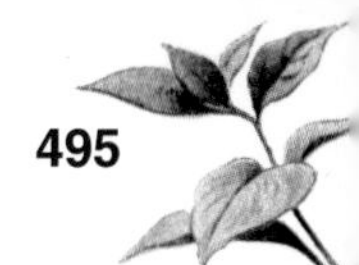

Drug Monograph 22.1
Chlorpromazine

Mechanism of action
Chlorpromazine is a dopamine inhibitor, and the antagonism of central dopaminergic function may be related to the therapeutic effect in psychotic conditions.

Indications
Chlorpromazine is indicated in schizophrenia and other acute and chronic psychoses, intractable hiccups (if non-drug treatment fails), short-term management of anxiety, agitation or disturbed behaviour in non-psychotic disorders and nausea and vomiting in terminal illness.

Pharmacokinetics
Phenothiazines are lipid-soluble so are well absorbed orally and concentrate in the CNS. Chlorpromazine is subject to first-pass metabolism, and oral bioavailability ranges from 10% to 80%. Peak plasma levels are reached 1–4 hours after oral administration. Onset of antipsychotic effect is achieved gradually over several weeks, and peak effects occur between 6 weeks and 6 months. Duration of action varies from 6 to more than 24 hours, depending on dosage and frequency. Chlorpromazine is metabolised in the liver; metabolites are generally inactive and are excreted primarily by the kidneys.

Adverse effects
Common adverse effects include orthostatic hypotension, sedation, anticholinergic and extrapyramidal effects (see general discussion on adverse effects, Table 22.1 and Fig 22.1) and tardive dyskinesia; there is no known effective treatment for tardive dyskinesia, so early assessment and diagnosis are crucial. Chlorpromazine can cause cholestatic jaundice and phototoxic skin reactions. IM and SC injections are not recommended, as they are painful and can cause muscle necrosis. Neuroleptic malignant syndrome incidence is greater in young men and may be seen after months or years of treatment. Metabolic effects include increased blood glucose, weight gain and dyslipidaemia.

Drug interactions
See Drug Interactions 22.1, later in the chapter. Chlorpromazine is a substrate of CYP2D6, so interactions with inducers, inhibitors or other substrates of this enzyme are likely. Lithium can decrease the concentration of chlorpromazine, whereas propranolol and chlorpromazine can increase the concentration of each other.

Warnings and contraindications
Use with caution in clients with breast cancer, cardiovascular disease, moderate-to-severe liver impairment, hyperthyroidism, Parkinson's disease, chronic respiratory disease or epilepsy, in glaucoma and other conditions involving problems of parasympathetic control, in children and the elderly (Clinical Focus Boxes 22.1 and 22.2). Avoid use in clients with phenothiazine hypersensitivity, phaeochromocytoma, profound CNS depression or alcohol abuse, in pregnant women, during lactation and in people often exposed to sunlight.

Dosage and administration
Dosage of antipsychotic agents varies according to the individual, indication for treatment and the person's response to the medication. It is best to titrate from a low dose, increasing when necessary for therapeutic response. When stopping antipsychotic therapy, dosage should be reduced gradually over 2 or 3 weeks; otherwise, rebound nausea, vomiting, dizziness, tremors and dyskinesias may occur. Chlorpromazine is available in tablet, oral liquid and injection (not recommended, as the solution is highly irritant) formulations. For acute and chronic psychoses in adults the oral dose is 25–100 mg three times daily adjusted according to response. The dosing range is not well defined but up to 500–600 mg daily is generally adequate. For chronic use it can be given as a single daily dose. For a child aged over 5 years with a behaviour disorder, one-third to half of the appropriate adult dosage may be given. Syrup is available for clients who refuse tablets or have difficulty in swallowing. Avoid giving IM or SC, as the solution is highly irritant and may cause necrosis.

Other phenothiazines
Table 22.1 summarises the properties of various phenothiazines. Periciazine is a low-potency drug recommended in low doses for behavioural disturbances in children, the elderly and in dementias.

Prochlorperazine, as a first-generation antipsychotic, and is mainly used for its antiemetic actions: it is more effective than antihistamines in severe vomiting, especially in vertigo due to Ménière's syndrome and labyrinthitis and also in migraine, and is available as tablets, injections and suppositories (see Ch 16).

Thioxanthine derivatives: flupentixol and zuclopenthixol
The thioxanthines resemble the piperazine phenothiazines in their antipsychotic effects, with high affinity for D_1 and D_2 receptors, including a high incidence of extrapyramidal effects. Their antipsychotic indications, adverse effects,

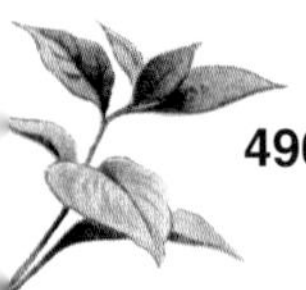

precautions and drug interactions are similar to those for the phenothiazines.

Butyrophenone derivatives: haloperidol and droperidol

Haloperidol and droperidol are highly potent antipsychotic agents. Although structurally different from the other antipsychotic agents, they have similar properties in terms of antipsychotic efficacy, adverse effects and drug interactions. Haloperidol appears to have a selective CNS effect, competitively blocking D_2 receptors in the mesolimbic system and causing increased turnover of brain dopamine. It is useful in chronic psychoses, and in alcoholic hallucinations. It is associated with a significant degree of extrapyramidal effects but has less effect on noradrenergic receptors (e.g. decreased incidence of orthostatic hypertension). Use should be avoided in pregnant and breastfeeding women.

Droperidol is used as an adjunct in anaesthesia, in nausea and vomiting and in short-term management of disturbed behaviour and severe anxiety. It is available only as an injection.

Atypical antipsychotic agents

The atypical antipsychotics, as above, are better at treating the negative symptoms of schizophrenia than earlier neuroleptics. They also have less potential to cause extrapyramidal effects, tardive dyskinesia, neuroleptic malignant syndrome or sedation, so are now more commonly prescribed; however, they are more likely to prolong the cardiac QT interval, cause metabolic adverse effects or weight gain. They are not a homogeneous class, having widely differing adverse effect profiles; clozapine and olanzapine are most likely to cause hyperglycaemia and weight gain (Table 22.1). Efficacy and safety in children, pregnancy or lactation are not well established due to insufficient data. Epidemiological data suggest that antipsychotics are not associated with an increased risk of congenital malformations; however, there are limited data for other outcomes. Gestational diabetes may occur in pregnancy so monitoring for metabolic changes is important (Betcher et al. 2019).

Aripiprazole

Aripiprazole is a partial agonist at D_2 and 5-HT_{1A} receptors, and antagonist at 5-HT_{2A}; it is one of the safest atypical antipsychotics (DM 22.2).

Clozapine

Clozapine differs from other neuroleptics by antagonising D_1, D_2 and D_4 dopamine receptors, with less affinity for D_2 receptors, so is less apt to induce extrapyramidal effects. Clozapine also antagonises 5-HT_{2A}, α_1-adrenoceptors and histamine H_1 receptors. It has been suggested to be more effective than all other antipsychotics, particularly to treat negative symptoms or in treatment-resistant people.

Clozapine is reserved for treatment-resistant schizophrenia or for when adverse effects of other drugs preclude their continued use as it can cause neutropenia, agranulocytosis, seizures, cardiomyopathies and potentially life-threatening constipation. Treatment is closely monitored for 18 weeks when first started.

Common adverse effects include drowsiness and seizures orthostatic hypotension when treatment is started and type 2 diabetes.

In Australia, there is a national distribution system requiring registration of doctors, pharmacists and patients involved with clinical use of clozapine.

Olanzapine and risperidone

Olanzapine and risperidone (see the Critical Thinking Scenario at the beginning of the chapter) also block both 5-HT_{2A} and dopamine D_2 receptors. Compared with clozapine, they are less sedating, cause fewer anticholinergic effects and do not have the same potential to cause agranulocytosis.

There are clinically significant drug interactions with CNS depressants, antihypertensives, dopamine agonists, the new antidepressants and drugs that inhibit or enhance drug-metabolising enzymes.

Olanzapine has also been approved for IM use in acute manic episodes associated with bipolar disorder, maintenance treatment of schizophrenia in adults sufficiently stabilised during acute treatment with oral olanzapine, agitation and behavioural symptoms in dementia and in acute aggressive or violent behaviour.

It is available as tablets (including orally disintegrating) and IM injection, and in wafer form for acutely psychotic people.

Other antipsychotics

Other atypicals include amisulpride (an antagonist at $D_2/D_3/5\text{-HT}_7$ receptors) and paliperidone (an active metabolite of risperidone), asenapine (an antagonist at D_2 and 5-HT_2 receptors; it is approved for treating schizophrenia and bipolar disorder), quetiapine (an antagonist at many CNS neurotransmitter receptors), ziprasidone and lurasidone.

New drugs on the horizon

None of the many drugs developed to treat schizophrenia is ideal: there are still many concerns over safety and efficacy, so new agents and formulations are required. The biological complexity of mental health disorders has limited the research into this area. Apart from dopamine D_2 receptors newer drugs target glutamate receptors,

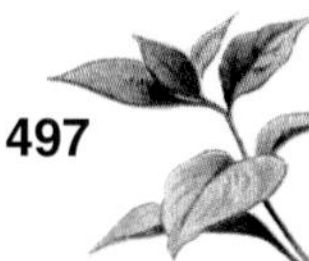

Drug Monograph 22.2
Aripiprazole

Mechanism of action

Aripiprazole is a partial agonist at D_2 and 5-HT_{1A} receptors, and antagonist at 5-HT_{2A} receptors.

Indications

Aripiprazole is indicated to treat schizophrenia; also as monotherapy in bipolar disorder in adults it is a maintenance treatment to prevent the recurrence of manic or mixed episodes of bipolar I disorder.

Pharmacokinetics

Aripiprazole is highly lipid-soluble, so is well absorbed orally (delayed by food) with peak plasma levels reached in 3–5 hours; oral bioavailability is about 87%. It is widely distributed, highly bound to plasma proteins (88–99%) and is extensively metabolised, mainly by CYP3A4 and CYP2D6.

The main metabolite, dehydroaripiprazole, is active with similar affinity for D_2 receptors as the parent drug, thus prolonging action.

Some unchanged drug is excreted via the faeces, and metabolites via urine and faeces. The half-life of the main active metabolite is about 100 hours; steady state is not reached for about 14 days.

No dosage adjustment is required in severe renal or hepatic impairment.

Adverse effects

Common adverse effects include headache and light-headedness, akathisia (motor restlessness) and constipation; less common is orthostatic hypotension (see earlier summary and Table 22.1).

Rare cases of neuroleptic malignant syndrome, seizures or metabolic disturbances have occurred. A small weight gain (1–3 kg) is likely over 52 weeks, especially for people with a low body mass index to start.

Drug interactions

Aripiprazole may interact with inhibitors of enzymes CYP3A4 and CYP2D6 (including fluoxetine and paroxetine), which can decrease its metabolism and increase effects and toxicity, thus requiring reduced dosage.

Inducers of CYP3A4 (notably carbamazepine) can enhance metabolism of aripiprazole and thus require higher doses.

Warnings and contraindications

Elderly clients with dementia-associated psychosis are at increased risk of fatal cardiovascular events from atypical antipsychotics; use with caution in those with recent history of myocardial infarction or with unstable heart disease.

It is contraindicated in those who are hypersensitive to the drug or any tablet ingredients. Use with caution in children (Clinical Focus Box 22.1), in the elderly (Clinical Focus Box 22.2), in pregnant women or during lactation.

Dosage and administration

Modified release

Long-acting modified release IM injections are initially given at 400 mg once a month; reduce dose to 300 mg once a month if this is not tolerated (minimum 26 days between injections).

Oral

In schizophrenia the typical dosage (oral tablets) is 10–15 mg once daily; at least 2 weeks should be allowed for reaching steady state. Tablets are available in strengths of 10, 15, 20 or 30 mg, allowing close titration of dose.

The dose of aripiprazole in bipolar disorder is 15–30 mg once daily.

People can be safely switched from another antipsychotic to aripiprazole without a washout period.

glycine transporters or the α-7-nicotinic acetylcholine receptor (Huhn et al. 2019; Meltzer 2017; Yang & Tsai 2017).

Those in the pre-marketing stage include cariprazine, relatively selective for partial agonism at D_2R and D_3 receptors, which has been through clinical trials and has recently received approval from the Therapeutic Goods Administration in Australia. Other potential drugs include the neurosteroid pregnenolone in anxiety, depression and psychosis-related disorders.

Adverse effects of antipsychotics

The monoamine neurotransmitters and acetylcholine are also neurotransmitters in the peripheral nervous system, particularly in the autonomic and enteric nervous systems, so it is inevitable that drugs given for CNS

disorders will have adverse peripheral effects. This is compounded by the fact that many antipsychotic and antidepressant drugs affect several transmitters and their receptors. Adverse effects on blood pressure (orthostatic hypotension), GIT functions (dry mouth, constipation and weight gain), sexual function (impotence, decreased libido) and eye functions (blurred vision) are common with psychotropic drugs.

Adverse drug reactions to typical antipsychotics

Because typical antipsychotic drugs also block receptors for a wide range of receptors (ACh [muscarinic], noradrenaline [α-], histamine [H_1], 5-HT and dopamine), there are wide-ranging adverse CNS and peripheral effects. For example, the phenothiazines are known as 'dirty drugs', due to their effects at multiple receptors. Adverse effects include movement disorders, dizziness, constipation, dry mouth, confusion and drowsiness. Partly because of their unpleasant adverse effects, there is no abuse potential.

Adverse effect profiles of various antipsychotic agents can be compared to aid in drug selection (Table 22.1). For example, if a drug with a strong sedative property is desired, chlorpromazine might be prescribed, whereas haloperidol is less likely to cause daytime drowsiness. However, sedative effects impair psychomotor performance, driving skills, ability to operate machinery and reaction times to dangerous stimuli.

Extrapyramidal effects

Common adverse effects from antipsychotics are the extrapyramidal effects, due to blockade of D_2 receptors and subsequent overactivity of cholinergic (motor) pathways or extrapyramidal pathways. Motor effects, including dystonias, akathisia, parkinsonism and dyskinesia, are described in Figure 22.1. Akathisia can be associated with typical and atypical antipsychotics, antiemetics and antidepressants. An anticholinergic drug (e.g. benzatropine) is sometimes required to reduce excessive motor stimulation. If extrapyramidal/parkinsonian effects are troublesome, one of the atypical agents might be chosen.

Neuroleptic malignant syndrome

This rare but potentially fatal adverse effect occurs in 0.5–1% of people on typical antipsychotics, with incidence highest in young men. It may occur months or years after starting treatment with the drug, then progress rapidly over 1–3 days. It involves high temperature, muscle rigidity, altered consciousness and impaired autonomic homeostasis. Treatment requires withdrawal of the drug, hydration and sometimes bromocriptine (a dopamine agonist) and dantrolene to control muscle spasms.

Tardive dyskinesia

Dyskinesia refers to involuntary muscle movements that can range from slight tremor to uncontrollable movement of the entire body. The tardive dyskinesia form of dyskinesia gets its name from the slow (or tardive) onset of movements of the tongue, lips, face, trunk and extremities that occur in people treated with long-term dopaminergic antagonist medications (Fig 22.1) (Cornett et al. 2017).

Other adverse effects

All groups of antipsychotics can cause metabolic disturbances such as weight gain, diabetes and dyslipidaemia; clozapine, olanzapine and quetiapine particularly are associated with weight gain and type 2 diabetes, and clozapine with serious constipation. Weight gain and its sequelae (hyperglycaemia, hypertension, hyperlipidaemia and metabolic syndrome) need to be monitored and managed with appropriate education, lifestyle changes and monitoring of blood glucose levels.

Atypical antipsychotics are sometimes prescribed for behavioural disturbances in people with dementia, but this use is associated with increased risk of morbidity and mortality from stroke. Other antipsychotics have individual adverse reactions profiles; for example, chlorpromazine is associated with skin reactions and photosensitivity, and several agents with prolonged cardiac QT interval, sexual problems or prolactin increases.

Drug interactions

With all antipsychotics, there is a multitude of potential drug interactions and long lists of potential interactions with psychiatric drugs. (Common interactions are listed in Drug Interactions 22.1. Consult tables in the *Therapeutic Guidelines: Psychotropics* and *Australian Medicines Handbook* for specific interactions, especially those involving altered metabolism.)

It is impossible for anyone – health professional or student – to learn all these potential drug interactions. It is safer to understand the general principles and to look up databases for specific interactions between drugs prescribed concurrently.

Antipsychotic drugs are likely to interact with all other drugs affecting the central or autonomic nervous systems; for example, those that depress the CNS (opioids, anxiolytics, anaesthetics, sedatives, antiepileptics, antiemetics), alter the cardiac QT interval, cause hypotension, lower the seizure threshold, are dopamine agonists or antagonists, have anticholinergic effects, affect blood glucose concentration or either inhibit or enhance the metabolism of the antipsychotic agent (e.g. social drugs such as alcohol and tobacco).

Elderly clients are particularly at risk, because of polypharmacy to treat multiple pathologies and renal impairment, leading to prolonged half-lives of drugs.

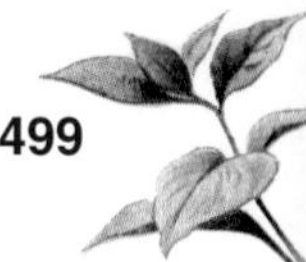

AKATHISIA

Description: Motor restlessness; person unable to sit or stand still, feels urgent need to move, pace, rock or tap foot. Can also present as apprehension, irritability, general uneasiness, insomnia and aggressive behaviour; may be mistaken for worsened agitation. More common in females than males; usually occurs within a few weeks of starting drug therapy, particularly with haloperidol and thioxanthines.

Treatment: Lower dose of neuroleptic agent, switch to an atypical antipsychotic or administer an antiparkinson drug such as benztropine or diazepam.

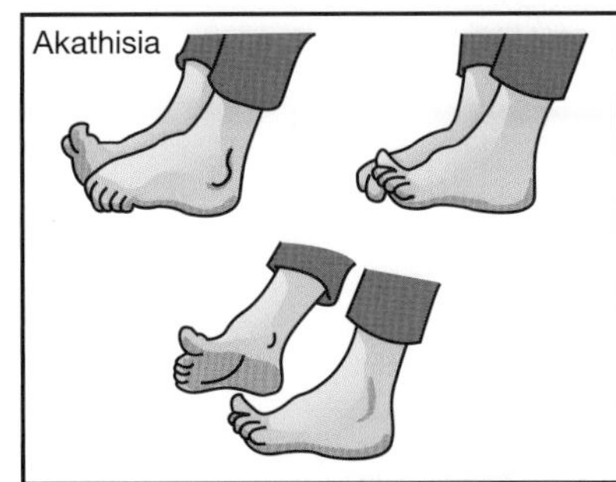

DYSTONIA

Description: Acute reaction requiring immediate intervention. Person exhibits muscle spasms of face, tongue, neck, jaw and/or hands, hyperextension of neck and trunk and arching of back; oculogyric crisis may occur (fixed upward gaze and/or eye muscle spasms); laryngeal spasm is potentially fatal. Occurs more often in males than females; usually after large doses of neuroleptics, within a week of drug therapy especially with phenothiazines, thioxanthines, risperidone and haloperidol.

Treatment: Depending on the severity of reaction, lower neuroleptic dose, administer benztropine IM or IV.

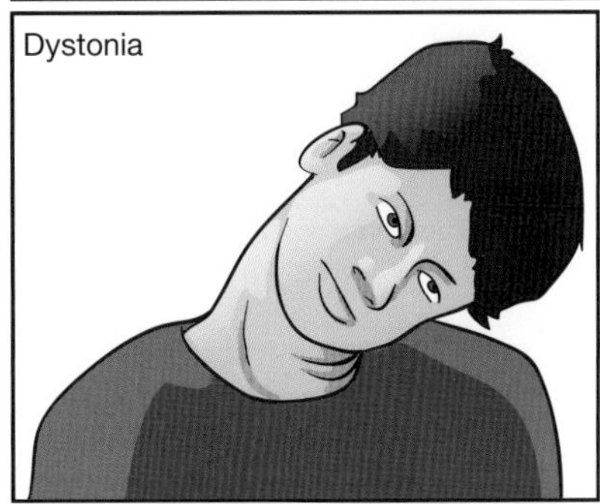

DRUG-INDUCED PARKINSONISM

Description: Symptoms similar to Parkinson's disease: shuffling gait, drooling, tremors, increased rigidity (cogwheel), bradykinesia (slow movements) and akinesia (immobility).

Treatment: Add antiparkinson drug (benztropine or benzhexol); possibly switch to a newer atypical agent.

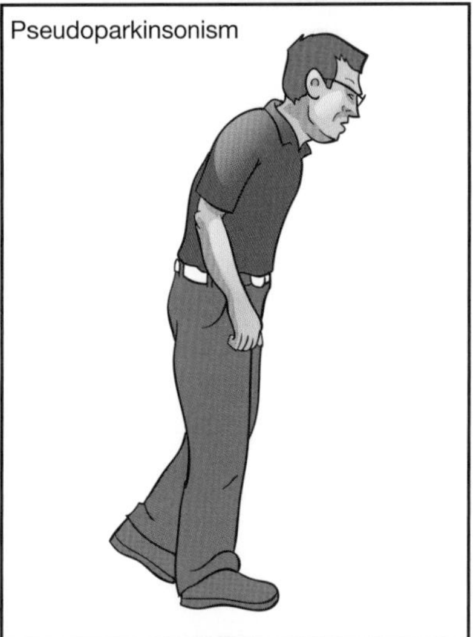

TARDIVE DYSKINESIA

Description: A late-developing serious adverse reaction in about 20% of people, especially older women; involuntary repetitive hyperkinetic movements, usually of mouth and face, possibly also of arms and legs; possibly due to supersensitivity to dopamine following upregulation of receptors.

Treatment: Prevention is vital, as there is no effective treatment and it may be irreversible. Monitor for early signs, and reduce or cease neuroleptic agent as soon as possible.

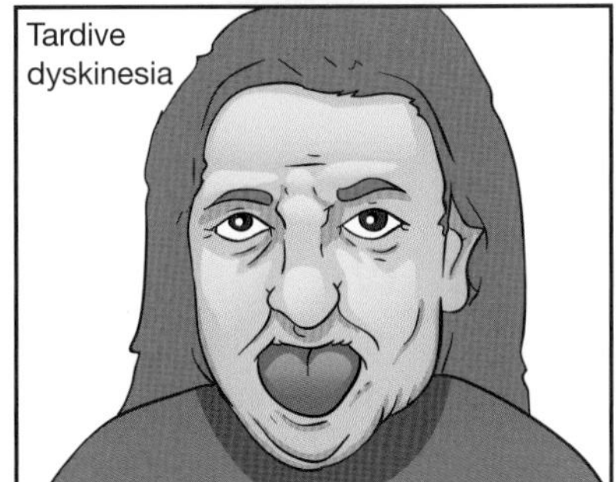

FIGURE 22.1 Antipsychotic extrapyramidal adverse effects

DRUG INTERACTIONS 22.1
Antipsychotic drugs

DRUG	POSSIBLE EFFECTS AND MANAGEMENT
CNS depressants such as benzodiazepines, anaesthetics, lithium, antihistamines, opioids and alcohol	Additive CNS depression (may be useful in acutely disturbed people), respiratory depression and hypotensive effects. The drug dosage should be reduced
Drugs that lower seizure threshold	May cause seizures – avoid combination
Levodopa (L-dopa), other dopamine agonists	Concurrent use with antipsychotic agents can render levodopa ineffective in controlling Parkinson's disease and antipsychotics ineffective in schizophrenia
Antihypertensive agents	Concurrent drug use with the antipsychotics may result in an exacerbation of hypotensive effects
Drugs with anticholinergic effects	Concurrent drug use may result in an increase in anticholinergic adverse effects, including delirium
Drugs that prolong the QT interval, such as antidysrhythmic agents, many antimicrobials (e.g. clarithromycin), tyrosine kinase inhibitors (antineoplastics)	Additive prolongation with antipsychotics droperidol, haloperidol, amisulpride, sertindole, ziprasidone – potentially fatal ventricular dysrhythmia
Drugs affecting blood glucose concentrations	Many antipsychotic drugs cause hyperglycaemia, so alter the actions of other drugs

KEY POINTS

Antipsychotic agents

- The main antipsychotic (antischizophrenic) agents are the phenothiazine derivatives, thioxanthines and atypical antipsychotics, acting mainly by dopamine blockade in specific areas of the CNS. Receptors for many other neurotransmitters are also likely to be blocked.
- Major adverse effects of antipsychotics occur in the central, autonomic and motor nervous systems, including sedation, hypotension, behaviour changes, extrapyramidal effects such as dystonias, parkinsonism and akathisia. Serious adverse effects are tardive dyskinesia and neuroleptic malignant syndrome.
- There are many potential drug interactions with antipsychotics, affecting both the CNS and the peripheral nervous system.

Treating affective disorders

Affective disorders, or mood disturbances, include depression (the most common) and mania; bipolar affective disorder involves mood swings between these conditions.

Epidemiology and pathology

As noted earlier, In 2020–21, of the 19.6 million Australians aged 16–85 years:

- Over two in five (43.7% or 8.6 million people) had experienced a mental disorder at some time in their life. Previous Australian surveys have shown that about 6.2% of people have had an affective disorder with depressive symptoms in the previous 12 months, including about 4% with a depressive disorder and 1.8% with bipolar affective disorder.

The New Zealand Health Survey update 2020–21 reported that nearly one in 10 adults (9.6%) had experienced psychological distress in the 4 weeks prior to the 2020–21 survey. Depression and bipolar affective disorder are recognised as serious public health issues due to considerable morbidity and high risk of suicide (10–19% in people with bipolar affective disorder). Globally, an estimated 264 million people are affected by depression. More women are affected than men.

- In in the period 2020-21, of the 19.6 million Australians aged 16-85 years:
  16.8 per cent of all Australians had an anxiety disorder and 7.5 per cent had an affective disorder such as depression (Australian Bureau of Statistics 2018).

Aetiologies of affective disorders

No single factor has been identified as the cause. Aetiological models include the following:

- *Psychosocial theories:* stressful events or mental conflicts that preceded the onset of depression (divorce, death of a parent or partner, inadequate parenting, physiological stressors, illness, infection, weight gain, immune system impairment or childbirth).
- *Biological theories:* refer to reduced levels of catecholamine (noradrenaline, dopamine, adrenaline) and indoleamine (5-HT) transmitters in the CNS in depression; or changes in hormones or sodium levels, or vitamin D deficiency; an excess of dopamine or noradrenaline is believed to be related to mania.
- *Genetic theories:* functional polymorphisms in the promoter region of the serotonin transporter gene

moderate the influences of stressful life events on a person's liability to suffer depression or tendency to suicide.

A combination of genetic, psychosocial and biological factors probably leads to common pathways that result in an affective disorder.

Many drugs themselves can evoke depression, probably by altering monoamine neurotransmitter levels in the CNS. Drug groups implicated include sedatives (alcohol, benzodiazepines and barbiturates), antipsychotics, antihypertensives (β-blockers), hormones (corticosteroids, oral contraceptives), opioids and hallucinogens.

Depression and bipolar disorder

Depression

Many classifications of **depression** have been used, such as the time during life at which depression occurred (childhood, adolescent, postnatal or senile depression) or the reason for the depression (exogenous [from outside; reactive or secondary] or endogenous [from within] depression). Exogenous depression may be a person's response to a loss, serious illness or disappointment, manifest as lack of pleasure or interest in activities and everyday living; it generally improves within a few weeks or months without the need for antidepressant medications. Mobilisation of support systems and psychotherapy is useful, and benzodiazepines can treat associated anxiety. Endogenous depression has no obvious external causes.

Major affective disorders are now defined as unipolar depressive disorders (single or recurrent major depressive episodes) or bipolar affective disorders (including one or more manic or hypomanic episodes). There are also atypical affective disorders, and depression can occur concurrently with neurotic and personality disorders or schizophrenia.

Criteria for major depressive disorder include the presence of:

- mood changes (sadness, guilt feelings, self-pity, pessimism and loss of interest in life and social activities); often worse in the morning
- psychological symptoms (low self-esteem, poor concentration, hopeless or helpless feelings, indecisiveness and suicidal tendencies or increased focus on death)
- physiological manifestations (sleep disturbances, decreased interest in sex, loss of energy, menstrual dysfunction, headaches, palpitations, constipation, loss of appetite and weight loss or gain)
- thought alterations (a decrease in ability to concentrate, poor memory, confusion; delusions relating to health, persecution or religion).

Bipolar affective disorder

Bipolar (affective) disorder, previously called manic–depressive psychosis, involves wild mood swings between depression and manic episodes. Mania, the opposite pole of depression, is characterised by excessive energy, high pressure of speech, extravagant gestures and gifts and seeming lack of need for sleep. Bipolar disorder is the sixth leading cause of disability worldwide, with a lifetime prevalence of 1–4%, a major burden of illness on people's lives and a high suicide risk (Rowland & Marwaha 2018).

Measures to treat depression include reduction of environmental stressors and treatment with ECT, psychotherapy, drugs and transcranial magnetic stimulation. In some people with treatment-resistant depression adjunct measures include combinations of the antidepressant drugs and the use of non-antidepressants treatment. (A carefully planned course of benzodiazepines or the Z-drugs may help insomnia and/or anxiety in the early phase of antidepressant treatment). Herbal remedies such as St John's wort have become popular. Referral to a specialist psychiatrist is advisable in severe depression when the person has not responded to other measures.

Antidepressant drugs

The first antidepressant drugs were discovered by serendipity (sheer good luck): iproniazide, an antitubercular agent, and imipramine, a drug being tested as an antischizophrenic, were found to elevate the mood. This led to studies of the actions and mechanisms of similar drugs, which came to be called the 'first-generation' antidepressants, such as **monoamine oxidase inhibitors** (MAOIs, iproniazide-like) and the **tricyclic antidepressants** (TCAs, such as imipramine), respectively. Second-generation antidepressants include the SSRIs, **serotonin noradrenaline reuptake inhibitors** (SNRIs) and **reversible inhibitors of MAO-A** (RIMAs). Third-generation antidepressants are considered to be those not confined to serotonin reuptake inhibition. These include venlafaxine, reboxetine and mirtazapine.

Mechanisms of action of antidepressants

The storage, release, action on receptors and inactivation of monoamine neurotransmitters are shown diagrammatically in Chapter 9, Figure 9.4 (in the peripheral nervous system); proposed mechanisms of action of antidepressants are shown in Figure 22.2. Although there are inconsistencies in the monoamine theory of depression (e.g. why is cocaine not an effective antidepressant, and why and how are 5-HT_2 and 5-HT_3 receptor antagonists effective?), the following mechanisms of action are generally accepted:

- Many antidepressants (including the tricyclics) act by inhibiting the reuptake of noradrenaline or 5-HT, which increases the amount of monoamine neurotransmitter available. These drugs have many sympathetic nervous system side effects; they also have significant anticholinergic actions, and can cause sleepiness, weakness and impaired cognition.

A: NA in CNS
B: 5-HT in CNS
synthesis from tyrosine
pre-synaptic terminals
synthesis from tryptophan
DA
MAO
NA
MAO
5-HT
metabolites
5-HT
α_2
NET
T
5-HT
ENT
COMT
NA
circulation
α
β
5-HT
5-HT
1A, 1B, 1D
2, 3
Post-synaptic neurons
COMT: catechol O-methyl transferase
DA: dopamine
α,β: NA receptors
ENT: extraneuronal transporter
NET: NA uptake transporter (formerly called uptake$_1$ process)
NA: noradrenaline
MAO: monoamine oxidase
5-HT: 5-hydroxytryptamine
5-HT$_{1A, 1B, 1D}$, 5-HT$_2$, 5-HT$_3$: 5-HT receptor subtypes
T : 5-HT reuptake transporter (SERT)

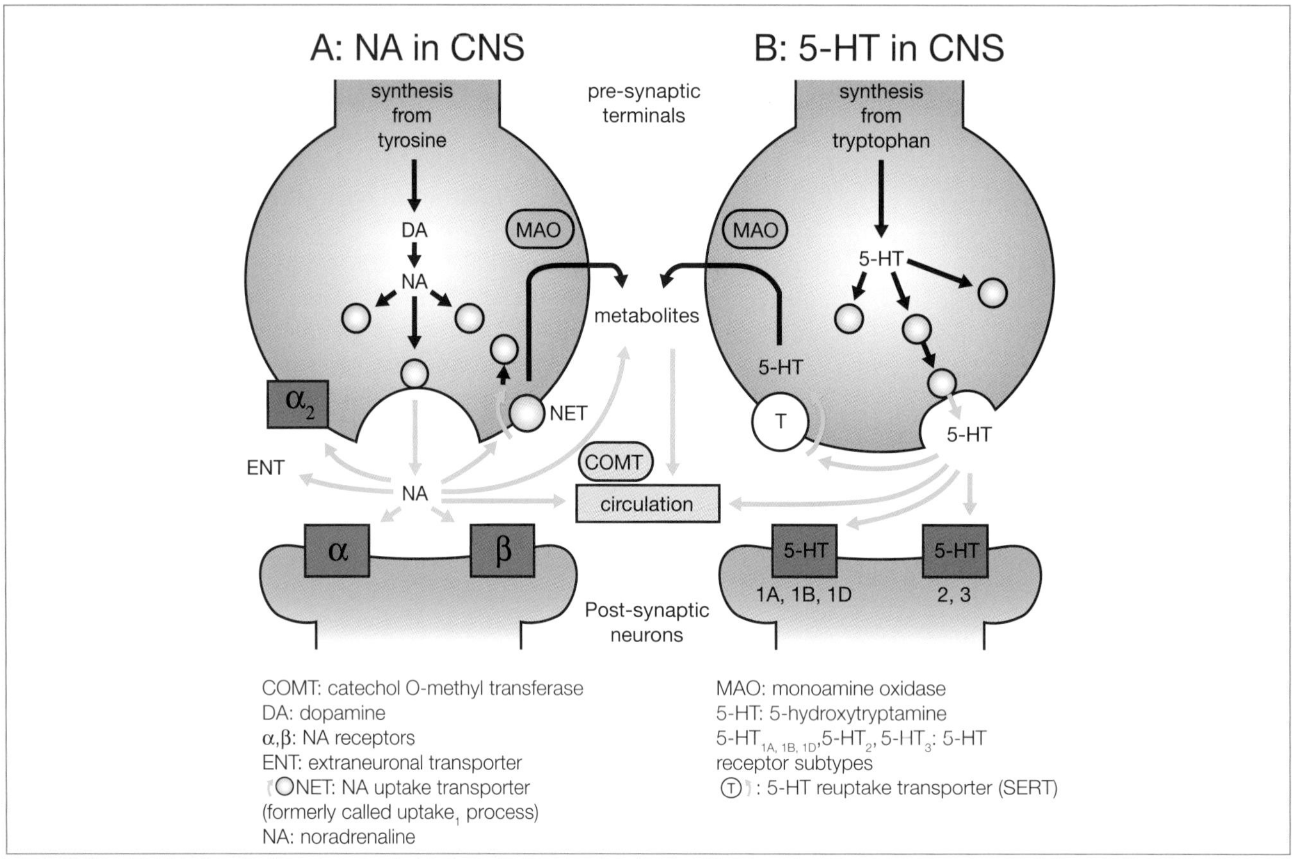

FIGURE 22.2 Proposed mechanisms of action of antidepressant drugs

A Noradrenaline (NA), synthesised from dietary tyrosine, is stored in vesicles at the nerve ending; it is released by the arrival of a nerve impulse, diffuses across the synaptic cleft and acts on α- and β-adrenoceptors on the postsynaptic nerve or other cell; activation leads to wakefulness and is involved in autonomic regulation. Noradrenaline is inactivated mainly by reuptake back into the nerve ending by the noradrenaline transporter (NET, formerly called the uptake 1 process) and stored again in vesicles. Noradrenaline may also be metabolised by enzymes catechol-O-methyltransferase (COMT) in the synaptic cleft or MAO within the nerve terminal. Noradrenaline that diffuses into the circulation is taken up into non-neuronal cells by the extraneuronal transporter (ENT, uptake 2). Activation of α_2-adrenoceptors (autoreceptors) on the presynaptic nerve terminal reduces release of noradrenaline. Dopamine neurotransmission is closely analogous to noradrenaline:dopamine released from dopaminergic neurons acts on dopamine receptors (mainly D_1 and D_2), is involved in motor control and endocrine functions, is taken up back into the presynaptic neuron by a specific dopamine transporter and is metabolised by MAO and COMT. **B** 5-HT, synthesised from tryptophan, is stored and released similarly in serotonergic nerves, and acts on 5-HT receptors, activation of which is involved in mood, sleep and appetite. It is inactivated by reuptake via a specific 5-HT transporter (SERT), and by MAO and other enzymes. Tricyclic antidepressants block the reuptake of released noradrenaline and 5-HT, preventing them from re-entering the nerves; thus, there is more transmitter available to act on receptors. MAO inhibitors block MAO located on the surface of the mitochondria within the cell, leaving more noradrenaline or 5-HT available for release. Selective serotonin reuptake inhibitors selectively block the 5-HT transporter reuptake process, thus allowing more 5-HT to act on postsynaptic 5-HT receptors. Serotonin noradrenaline reuptake inhibitors block both NET and T, thus increasing available noradrenaline and 5-HT for receptor actions. Other drugs acting on monoamine transmission in the CNS include reserpine, which blocks vesicular storage of catecholamines and hence inhibits aminergic transmission; cocaine, which is a powerful inhibitor of NET; amphetamine and tyramine, which are accumulated by NET and stored in vesicles, displacing noradrenaline, which is free to act; and entacapone, a COMT inhibitor used in Parkinson's disease.

- SSRIs (e.g. fluoxetine), a relatively new group of drugs, are more potent inhibitors of 5-HT reuptake than noradrenaline, so they have fewer cardiovascular effects and are less lethal in overdose than the TCAs. These drugs now dominate antidepressant prescribing in Australia and New Zealand.
- SNRIs (e.g. venlafaxine) act by inhibiting reuptake of both 5-HT and noradrenaline (norepinephrine).
- MAOIs (e.g. moclobemide) inhibit MAO enzymes found in the mitochondria of nerve cells that are responsible for metabolising noradrenaline, dopamine and 5-HT, thus allowing a buildup of neurotransmitter available for release.
- Agomelatine – mode of action unclear; it is a melatonin receptor (MT_1 and MT_2) agonist and 5-HT_{2C} receptor antagonist.

Other antidepressants

Mianserin, a tetracyclic antidepressant, increases central noradrenergic neurotransmission by blocking presynaptic α_2-adrenergic receptors. It also antagonises some postsynaptic 5-HT receptors.

Mirtazapine, a tetracyclic related to mianserin, blocks 5-HT_2 and 5-HT_3 receptors, and also presynaptic noradrenaline α_2-autoreceptors.

Reboxetine, a highly selective and potent inhibitor of noradrenaline reuptake, has only a weak effect on the 5-HT reuptake and does not affect the uptake of dopamine.

Vortioxetine inhibits the serotonin transporter, and acts as an antagonist at some 5-HT receptor subtypes and as an agonist at others. It is thought to increase serotonin activity in the CNS.

Antidepressant drug therapy: clinical aspects

Indications for antidepressant drugs

Antidepressants are administered in moderate-to-severe depressive disorder to relieve psychological and physical symptoms, improve general functioning and reduce the likelihood of self-harm or suicide. They are also indicated in post-traumatic stress disorder, neuroses (some anxiety disorders, panic disorder, obsessive–compulsive disorder and eating disorders), premenstrual syndrome, and as adjunctive therapy in neuropathic pain, migraine and ADHD in children (see Chs 23 and 24 respectively). They may also be used in nocturnal enuresis in children (due to their action antagonist at muscarinic receptors). People with mild depressive disorder are unlikely to benefit from antidepressant drugs.

Selecting an antidepressant

Moderate-to-severe depression does benefit from drug therapy. All antidepressants are administered orally.

Antidepressants appear to have similar efficacies, although there is a wide variability in individual patient responses. The *Australian Medicines Handbook* (2021) and *Therapeutic Guidelines: Psychotropic* (2021) recommend as first-line therapy for the treatment of major depression the SSRIs (citalopram, fluoxetine) or the tetracyclic antidepressants (mirtazapine), for second-line therapies the SNRIs (desvenlafaxine and venlafaxine) and others such as agomelatine, and third-line therapies RIMA (moclobemide).

Selecting an antidepressant is empirical, taking into consideration any concurrent conditions and medications of the person, the adverse effect or drug interaction potential of the drug and the person's previous responses. A sedating antidepressant (amitriptyline, doxepin or mianserin) might be selected for an agitated depressed person, whereas a drug less likely to cause sedation or hypotension (nortriptyline, or an SSRI or MAOI) is safer for an elderly person. Potential toxicity in overdose is also important, especially if suicide is a risk – SSRIs are safer than TCAs.

Delayed onset of action

Antidepressants have a long-delayed onset of action. Some improvement in clinical symptoms may be apparent in 2–3 weeks and full effects may not appear for 6–8 weeks; this time corresponds with inhibition rather than facilitation of monoaminergic transmission. The initial drug should be tried with low dose, increasing over 2–4 weeks, then in recommended doses for an adequate period and compliance checked before changing to another class. During this period, clients are at great risk of deepening depression ('nothing is ever going to help me') and increased suicidal thoughts, and might need adjunct treatment with psychotherapy or ECT.

After symptoms improve, therapy for a major depressive episode should be continued for at least 6 months.

Change-over or withdrawal

When changing antidepressants, consider the following factors:

- Gradual withdrawal, then a drug-free interval ranging from 1–2 days up to 2–5 weeks is recommended.
- Therapy should be monitored carefully.
- Drugs with a long half-life (especially fluoxetine) take weeks to clear from the body.
- The actions of irreversible MAOIs continue for 2–3 weeks after cessation.

Rebound effects may occur on withdrawal; thus, withdrawal from TCAs with strong anticholinergic actions leads to typical parasympathetic effects (salivation, urination, diarrhoea), while withdrawal from SSRIs, SNRIs or mirtazapine may lead to anxiety, agitation and confusion. Withdrawal effects may occur after missing just 1 or 2 doses of drugs with a short half-life.

Plasma levels and compliance with TCAs

Plasma levels of TCAs can vary widely between individuals, and, with the possible exceptions of nortriptyline and imipramine, levels often do not correlate with dose or therapeutic response. A lower-than-expected plasma level indicates the need to interview the person to verify compliance with the prescribed schedule. Possible reasons (such as intolerable adverse effects, misunderstanding of directions, potential drug interaction or inadequate finances to purchase prescriptions) can then be identified.

If compliance is verified but plasma concentration remains low, dosage adjustments may be necessary or the prescriber

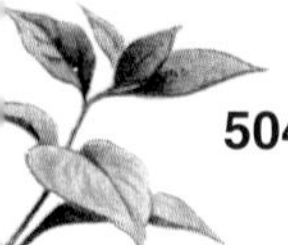

might consider switching drugs – for example, from a noradrenaline-potentiating to a 5-HT-potentiating drug.

Antidepressant therapy in special groups

In children, antidepressants should be reserved for those with severe conditions not manageable with psychotherapy, and supervised by a specialist child psychiatrist – there have been few trials of antidepressants in children; however, SSRIs are considered the first-line drugs (Clinical Focus Box 22.1, earlier).

Elderly people often have reduced levels of liver drug-metabolising enzymes, and so prescribed doses can lead to higher plasma drug concentrations and a greater potential for adverse effects. Many prescribers start geriatric clients at one-third to half the usual adult dosage, adjusting as necessary according to therapeutic response or presence of undesirable effects (Clinical Focus Box 22.2, earlier). Claims that the newer antidepressants are better tolerated in the elderly are not well supported by evidence.

In the context of safety in pregnancy and breastfeeding, the risks of depression to both mother and baby must be considered, as well as the risks from antidepressants. With respect to safety in pregnancy, most antidepressants are classified as C; however, some are considered safer – for example, mianserin and moclobemide. Paroxetine is contraindicated, and the SNRI antidepressants are not recommended due to possible withdrawal effects in the neonate. Postnatal or perinatal depression affects about 10–20% of mothers, who may need drug treatment. The SSRIs (except fluoxetine) appear to be safest with respect to transfer into breast milk.

As antidepressants generally elevate the mood and raise levels of 'stimulating' CNS neurotransmitters, they can cause unwanted effects in people with other conditions. For example, many antidepressants lower the seizure threshold and can precipitate epileptic seizures, provoke manic episodes in people with bipolar disorder and cause dysrhythmias or angina in those with cardiac disease. People with insomnia or anxiety may benefit from adjunct therapy with an antianxiety drug (e.g. a benzodiazepine), while those with psychotic depression may require antipsychotic therapy.

Selective serotonin reuptake inhibitors

SSRIs are as effective as other antidepressants and considerably safer than TCAs because they increase levels of 5-HT with less effect on noradrenaline levels; hence, they have fewer autonomic effects.

Mechanism of action

SSRIs block reuptake of serotonin (5-HT) via the SERT. The first, fluoxetine (Drug Monograph 22.3), was so successful that it rapidly took over the market for antidepressants. Fluoxetine was soon followed by sertraline, fluvoxamine, paroxetine and citalopram, then the active S-isomer of the latter, escitalopram. Sertraline appears to show good balance between benefits, acceptability and cost. Citalopram has been associated with cardiac QT prolongation; recommended doses have been reduced and ECG monitoring advised. Escitalopram is frequently administered for generalised anxiety disorder (Ch 20) as well as mood disorders.

Indications and actions

SSRIs are indicated to treat depression and anxiety disorders such as obsessive–compulsive disorder and panic disorder, eating disorders and premenstrual syndrome, and paroxetine also for post-traumatic stress disorder. They have similar delayed onset of action to the TCAs. Unlike the TCAs, which often cause weight gain, the SSRIs (except paroxetine) can cause anorexia and weight loss. They have little affinity for receptors for dopamine, acetylcholine, histamine or noradrenaline and are the least toxic antidepressants in overdose.

Adverse drug reactions

Adverse effects of SSRIs are summarised in Table 22.2. Early suggestions that the use of fluoxetine is associated with enhanced suicidal behaviour have not been supported by later studies.

Adverse drug reactions in adolescents

Unfortunately, suicide is a real risk in people with depression, including in children and adolescents, so drug therapy is often indicated. TCAs appear not to be effective in adolescents; hence, SSRIs are drugs of first choice in this group, in whom adverse effects may present differently. The most common are physical effects: headache, nausea, vomiting, abdominal pain and insomnia or sedation. Mental health side effects are mania, hypomania and elevated mood or deepening depression, agitation, anxiety and panic. Increased suicidal behaviours do occur and must be monitored; risk is increased by about 60%. Serotonin syndrome can occur with the use of SSRIs, as described below.

Drug interactions

There are potential drug interactions, especially with other antidepressants and with drugs implicated in serotonin syndrome. SSRIs can also inhibit the metabolism of many drugs (Drug Interactions 22.2).

Serotonin noradrenaline reuptake inhibitors

Mechanism of action

The relatively new SNRIs have a mechanism similar to that of the old TCAs, inhibition of reuptake of noradrenaline and 5-HT into nerve terminals via blockade of the SERT and NET, but they are more specific. This

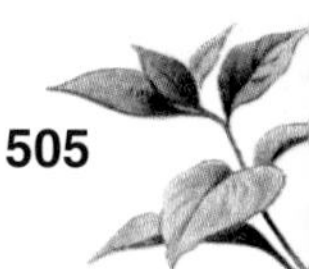

Drug Monograph 22.3
Fluoxetine

Mechanism of action

Fluoxetine (well known by its original trade name, Prozac) is an SSRI antidepressant, inhibiting reuptake of 5-HT (serotonin) more than of noradrenaline. It is less effective at antagonism of acetylcholine, histamine and α-adrenergic receptors than are the tricyclic antidepressants.

Indications

Fluoxetine is indicated in major depression, obsessive–compulsive disorder and premenstrual syndrome. It can also be used for bulimia nervosa, panic disorder and post-traumatic stress disorder. It helps to elevate mood, relieve other symptoms and reduce social impairment.

Pharmacokinetics

Fluoxetine is readily absorbed after oral administration and reaches peak plasma levels after about 6–8 hours. It is highly protein-bound and has a very high volume of distribution. It is extensively metabolised in the liver but has non-linear kinetics as it inhibits its own metabolism. With chronic administration the half-lives of fluoxetine and norfluoxetine are, respectively, 4–6 and 9–16 days; hence, it takes some weeks to achieve steady-state concentration or to eliminate the active metabolite after discontinuation of the drug, and there is an extended period for drug interactions. Metabolites are excreted via the kidneys.

Drug interactions

Fluoxetine inhibits metabolism by the CYP2D6 and CYP3A4 isoenzymes; hence, it raises plasma levels of drugs metabolised by these enzymes, including many antiepileptic drugs, antipsychotics, benzodiazepines, tricyclic antidepressants and St John's wort. There are protein-binding interactions with warfarin and interactions with serotonergic drugs implicated in serotonin syndrome (Drug Interactions 22.2).

Adverse reactions

Common reactions include rashes, anxiety, dizziness, weight loss, nausea and headaches; seizures are rare. There is some debate as to whether antidepressants increase the risk of suicide in depression, or whether this and worsening symptoms occur while waiting for the drug's effects to begin.

Warnings and contraindications

Clients need to be warned of possible adverse effects, of the delay before therapeutic effects and of caution required if driving or operating machinery. The dose needs to be reduced in severe liver disease. Fluoxetine is in pregnancy Category C, as it crosses the placenta and can lead to withdrawal reactions in the neonate. It is not recommended during lactation due to its lipid solubility and long half-life. Antidepressants are not generally indicated for treating childhood depression.

Dosage and administration

The usual starting dose in adults is 20 mg/day taken in the morning, which may be increased after several weeks' trial gradually to a maximum of 80 mg/day in divided doses. It is available in capsule and dispersible tablet formulations.

group includes duloxetine, venlafaxine and its metabolite desvenlafaxine; reboxetine only weakly inhibits 5-HT reuptake and is sometimes classed as a noradrenaline reuptake inhibitor. The precise mechanisms of action of SNRIs differ; they do affect various other neurotransmitters (though less than do the TCAs).

They are indicated in major depression, and some also in generalised anxiety and panic disorder; duloxetine is indicated in diabetic neuropathy (effective first- and second-line therapy for neuropathic pain).

Adverse effects include autonomic, CNS and sexual dysfunctions (Table 22.2); they may provoke manic episodes or seizures, and reduced platelet aggregation can cause GIT bleeding. Venlafaxine has been associated with stress cardiomyopathy as an adverse effect. In theory, there might be fewer drug interactions with desvenlafaxine than with the parent drug; however, the precautions are similar for both drugs. There are now warnings associated with the use of duloxetine.

Tricyclic antidepressants

Tricyclic antidepressants were the first major group of drugs successful in treating depression and tend to have names ending in -mipramine or -tryptyline (e.g. imipramine and amitriptyline, respectively); their chemical structures have three rings, hence their group name.

Mechanism of action

All TCAs act by the same mechanism, inhibition of reuptake of noradrenaline and 5-HT into nerve terminals, and appear to have similar efficacies, leading to improved mood.

TABLE 22.2 Adverse effect profiles of some antidepressant drugs

	ADVERSE EFFECTS					
DRUG	ANTICHOLINERGIC EFFECTS	SEDATION	INSOMNIA OR AGITATION	ORTHOSTATIC HYPOTENSION	GASTROINTESTINAL DISTRESS	WEIGHT GAIN (> 6 kg)
Tricyclic/tetracyclic antidepressants						
Amitriptyline, doxepin, trimipramine	3–4+	3–4+	2–3+	3/4+	0	3+
Nortriptyline	1+	1–2+	0	1+	0	1+
Clomipramine, dosulepin (dothiepin), imipramine	2–3+	2+	2–3+	2+	0	2+
Selective serotonin reuptake inhibitors						
Citalopram	0	0–1+	1+	0	3+	0+
Escitalopram	0	0	2+	0	3+	0
Fluoxetine, paroxetine, sertraline	0	0	0–1+	0	3+	1+
Monoamine oxidase inhibitors						
Phenelzine, tranylcypromine	0–1+	1+	2+	2+	1+	2+
Moclobemide (RIMA)	2+	–	2+	–	2+	0
Serotonin noradrenaline reuptake inhibitors						
Venlafaxine, desvenlafaxine	0–1+	–	2+	(increase blood pressure)	3+	0
Other						
Mirtazapine	0	3+	0 (lowers seizure threshold)	Rare (peripheral oedema)	–	1+

0 = absent or rare; 1+ = least common; 2+ = uncommon; 3+ = relatively common; 4+ = most common; – indicates not relevant or not established

Sources: Adapted from Australian Medicines Handbook 2021; Brunton et al. 2011; Psychotropic Expert Group 2021.

DRUG INTERACTIONS 22.2
Antidepressants

DRUG	POSSIBLE EFFECTS AND MANAGEMENT
Other serotonergic drugs	With TCAs, SSRIs, SNRIs or MAOIs: risk of serotonin syndrome; implicated drugs must be discontinued
Other CNS depressants	Enhanced CNS depression and orthostatic hypotension
Drugs that lower seizure threshold	With TCAs, SNRIs or SSRIs: may cause seizures; avoid combination
Other drugs with sympathomimetic effects	With TCAs or MAOIs: additive effects, including hypertension
Drugs with anticholinergic effects	With TCAs: concurrent drug use may result in an increase in anticholinergic adverse effects, including delirium
Other drugs that prolong the QT interval	With TCAs: increased risk of cardiac dysrhythmias; avoid combination
Other drugs affecting blood glucose	With SSRIs: can increase blood glucose concentration; monitor blood glucose level. MAOIs may decrease blood glucose concentrations affecting control of diabetes
Drugs affecting platelet aggregation	With SSRIs or SNRIs: added risk of bleeding
Other drugs that lower blood pressure	With MAOIs: can cause hypotension; monitor closely when co-administered
Tyramine-containing foods and drinks	Potentially dangerous drug–food interactions with MAOIs; avoid those foods and drinks
Fluoxamine and fluvoxamine	Interact with many drugs at specific liver enzymes, increasing concentration and toxicity; consult reference lists for specific interactions

Other actions include antagonism of receptors for other transmitters, acetylcholine (muscarinic), histamine H_1, noradrenaline α_1 and 5-HT, leading to adverse drug reactions in many body systems, including anticholinergic effects, sexual dysfunction, weight gain and sedation, and are particularly unsafe in overdose (Table 22.2).

TCA toxicity

TCA toxicity manifests as dilated pupils, extrapyramidal signs, CNS excitement or depression, life-threatening dysrhythmias and seizures; the cause of death from overdose is usually cardiac failure secondary to dysrhythmias, hypoxaemia and acidosis. TCAs have been largely overtaken by safer drugs such as the SSRIs; they are currently used as second-line agents.

There are many drug interactions (Drug Interactions 22.2) affecting all the neurotransmitters mentioned above, with other antidepressants and antipsychotics, all CNS depressants, drugs inhibiting or inducing drug metabolism, and other drugs with serotonergic actions (risk of serotonin toxicity).

Indications and precautions

The TCAs are indicated in treatment of major depression and also as adjunct therapy in pain management, in prophylaxis of migraine, for nocturnal enuresis and urge incontinence, and as third-line therapy for ADHD.

Precautions need to be taken in people with other conditions, including other psychoses; seizure disorders; prostatic hypertrophy and urinary retention; cardiac, liver, renal or thyroid disease; glaucoma; in the elderly; and during pregnancy or breastfeeding. Dosage is started low and gradually increased while monitoring therapeutic and adverse effects.

Other tricyclic antidepressants

Nortriptyline is less likely to cause sedation, hypotension or anticholinergic effects, so is safer in the elderly. Dosulepin (dothiepin) is thought to be the most toxic in overdose, and doxepin is the most sedating. Clomipramine, an analogue of imipramine, is a more selective inhibitor of 5-HT reuptake (over noradrenaline) compared to the other TCAs; hence, it may have fewer autonomic effects but is more likely to provoke serotonin syndrome. It is indicated for treating obsessive–compulsive disorders and premenstrual tension.

The herbal remedy St John's wort has been shown to have a similar mechanism of action to the TCAs, acting by inhibition of monoamine reuptake and metabolism;

CLINICAL FOCUS BOX 22.3

St John's wort and other complementary and alternative therapies in mental disorders

Extracts of the plant St John's wort (*Hypericum perforatum*) have been used for more than 2000 years for their medicinal properties ('wort' is an old English word for herb). It is believed to be the most widely prescribed herbal medicine worldwide; about 450 products containing St John's wort are listed in Australia. St John's wort has been shown to block reuptake of monoamine neurotransmitters, bind to GABA receptors, upregulate 5-HT receptors and inhibit MAO and COMT enzymes.

Double-blind, randomised controlled trials subjected to meta-analysis have shown St John's wort to be more effective than placebo in depression but less effective than tricyclic antidepressants. Rates of adverse effects are low, but serotonin syndrome and drug interactions can occur, so it should not be taken with other antidepressants. Hypericum extracts are potent inducers of hepatic drug-metabolising enzymes and can reduce the levels and efficacy of important drugs such as warfarin, digoxin, theophylline, antiretroviral agents, ciclosporin and oral contraceptives.

Frequent problems arising with the use of natural products and complementary therapies in mental disorders are:

- The purity and strength of the active ingredient are often not stated and can vary between preparations.
- Other ingredients or contaminants are seldom listed or identified.
- Diagnostic criteria in clinical trials are often poorly defined.
- It may be impossible to design double-blind trials – for example, of herbal extracts.
- There is a placebo-response rate of about 50% in trials of treatments of depression.

Clients and consumers should be asked about their use of all remedies – prescription, non-prescription and complementary.

Other complementary and alternative therapies used in mental illnesses include folate, tryptophan, tyrosine, 5-adenosylmethionine, phenylalanine N-acetyl cysteine, acupuncture, aromatherapy, prayer, tai chi exercise and homeopathy as adjuncts to antidepressants; *Ginkgo biloba* for dementia; kava for anxiety; valerian for insomnia and stress; and omega-3 polyunsaturated fatty acids as mood stabilisers. In schizophrenia treatment, some trials show clinical benefit from administration of eicosapentaenoic acid (in fish oil), or folate + vitamin B12 + vitamin B6 (pyridoxine); also hypnotherapy, movement therapies, acupuncture and dietary interventions. Cognitive behaviour therapy is significantly effective in depression, insomnia, anxiety and panic disorders.

Sources: Braun & Cohen 2014; Sarris 2014.

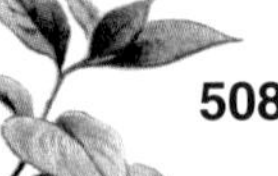

hence, it has some similar actions, adverse reactions and interactions. It has been shown to block reuptake of monoamine neurotransmitters, bind to GABA receptors, upregulate 5-HT receptors and inhibit MAO and COMT enzymes (Clinical Focus Box 22.3).

Monoamine oxidase inhibitor antidepressants

MAO, an enzyme found in mitochondrial membranes in nerve terminals, the liver and the brain, inactivates and degrades various monoamines. Tyramine, catecholamines (noradrenaline, adrenaline and dopamine), 5-HT and several amine drugs are all substrates for the enzyme. MAOIs inhibit the enzyme and thus impair inactivation of amine neurotransmitters and may potentiate their actions, particularly the vasopressor effects, causing high blood pressure.

Two types of MAO enzymes have been identified: MAO-A and MAO-B. MAO-A[2] preferentially metabolises 5-HT, noradrenaline, adrenaline and dopamine and is located throughout the body. MAO-B is contained mainly in human platelets; about equal amounts of both types are found in the liver and brain. Dopamine and tyramine (a sympathomimetic amine found in many foodstuffs) are inactivated by both MAO-A and MAO-B. Hence, an inhibitor that selects for the MAO-A form is likely to be better clinically as an antidepressant, as it will raise the levels of neurotransmitter amines while allowing inactivation of tyramine and other potentially toxic monoamines (Fig 22.2).

MAO inhibitors (irreversible non-selective MAOIs)

The early MAOIs were irreversible and non-selective in their inhibitory effects; that is, they inhibited both MAO-A and MAO-B for 2–3 weeks. They also desensitise the α_2- or β-adrenoceptors and 5-HT receptors (downregulation). Examples are the drugs phenelzine and tranylcypromine. They raise levels of monoamines, but there is a long delay in mood improvement. There are many serious adverse reactions, including autonomic and sexual dysfunction, orthostatic hypotension or severe hypertension, serotonin syndrome and insomnia. Because of serious adverse drug reactions and interactions, the old non-selective MAOIs are now indicated only as second- or third-line antidepressants for depression that does not respond to other, safer drugs. Some people, however, respond only to MAOIs.

Drug–drug and drug–food interactions

MAOIs impair the metabolism of many amines and drugs, including adrenaline and sympathomimetic amines, dopamine (including that formed after administration of levodopa), methyldopa and pethidine, and enhance the activity of drugs that cause release of amine transmitters. Interactions can occur with prescription-only and over-the-counter medications, caffeine and tyramine-containing foods and beverages, causing sudden and possibly severe hypertension that if untreated can progress to vascular collapse and death.

The tyramine, or 'cheese', reaction

People taking non-selective MAOIs are at risk of the **tyramine reaction** if they take tyramine-containing foods or drinks, as tyramine (usually inactivated by MAO-B) levels increase and raise the blood pressure by a sympathomimetic action. Advise to avoid:

- cheeses – especially mature and aged (e.g. blue, Brie, Emmenthaler, Gruyère, Parmesan, Roquefort, Stilton)
- aged, cured and pickled meats and fish – game, caviar, herring, sausages (kabana, pepperoni, salami), bacon, hot dogs
- vegetables – overripe avocado, broad bean pods, pickled vegetables, soy products
- fruit – overripe figs, bananas and raisins
- meat or yeast extracts (Vegemite, Bonox) and stock cubes or packet soups
- alcoholic beverages – red wines, especially Chianti; sherry, beer, liqueurs.

Some foods that contain tyramine or other pressor amines, if eaten in moderation when fresh, are safer, including yoghurt, sour cream, cream cheese, cottage cheese, chocolate and soy sauce.

Reversible inhibitors of MAO-A (RIMAs)

Moclobemide

Moclobemide is an example of a selective inhibitor. It is a **reversible inhibitor of MAO-A** (RIMA), a newer antidepressant drug group. It is relatively selective for MAO-A. It increases synaptic concentrations of serotonin, noradrenaline and dopamine.

Moclobemide is much less likely to cause tyramine reactions, as tyramine and other amines can still be inactivated by MAO-B. MAO activity is restored within 1–2 days of stopping administration of the drug. Nausea, headache and insomnia are adverse effects; there may be adverse interactions with SSRIs, SNRIs, TCAs, sympathomimetic amines and pethidine. A tyramine-free diet is not required, although large quantities of tyramine-rich foods should be avoided. Moclobemide is relatively safe in overdose.

Other miscellaneous antidepressants

Other new antidepressants act by various mechanisms affecting amine neurotransmitter levels. Future treatment

2 The gene encoding MAO-A has been called the 'warrior gene', as an association has been found between males who have variant versions of the gene, leading to low levels of MAO-A, and antisocial behaviour and high levels of violent aggression on provocation.

may involve glutamatergic drugs because glutamate receptors are implicated in the pathophysiology of mood disorders (Henter et al. 2021).

Mianserin and mirtazapine

These have been referred to as NaSSA-type antidepressants: noradrenergic and specific serotonergic antidepressants.

Mianserin has a tetracyclic chemical structure, rather than tricyclic. It does not inhibit the reuptake of monoamine transmitters but enhances postsynaptic 5-HT_{1A} receptor signalling. It shares some of the other properties of the TCAs, as it antagonises α_1-adrenoreceptors and histamine H_1 receptors, but has less anticholinergic action so has fewer cardiovascular adverse effects. A rare adverse effect unrelated to the antidepressant actions is reversible neutropenia, monitored by blood counts before and during therapy.

Mirtazapine, also a tetracylic, was released for general use in mid-2001. It is chemically related to mianserin and has different mechanisms of action from those of the TCAs and MAOIs. Mirtazapine, by selective blockade of histamine H_1 receptors, α_2-adrenoceptors and 5-HT_{2A}, 5-HT_{2C} and 5-HT_3 receptors, enhances noradrenergic activity and 5-HT_{1A} activity, which gives it better antidepressant efficacy and fewer peripheral and central adverse effects. It is safer in overdose, has fewer anticholinergic effects and does not cause nausea or diarrhoea, insomnia or sexual dysfunction. However, markedly increased appetite and carbohydrate cravings can lead to serious weight gain.

Agomelatine

This relatively new antidepressant has a very different mechanism from all the others: it is melatonergic – that is, an agonist at melatonin MT_1 and MT_2 receptors; it also blocks 5-HT_{2c} receptors. It is indicated in major depression in adults including prevention of relapse. It is contraindicated in liver disease, as it can raise aminotransferase levels and interact with drugs that inhibit CYP1A2 enzymes; liver function tests are required. Other main adverse effects are headache, dizziness, GIT dysfunctions and sedation. (See 'Melatonin' under 'Miscellaneous Anxiolytics, Sedatives and Hypnotics', in Ch 20.) There is as yet little data on safety in pregnancy or breastfeeding.

Adverse drug reactions of antidepressants

As noted, antidepressants have many adverse effects, as they enhance monoamine neurotransmission in many areas of the peripheral, enteric and central nervous systems (Table 22.2, earlier). (The relative places of newer drugs in such comparative tables are not yet well established.) Other common adverse effects are gastrointestinal and sexual dysfunctions and precipitation of manic episodes in people with bipolar disorder.

Due to the risk of suicide, adverse effects of antidepressants can be dangerous. Least toxic in overdose are the SSRIs, reboxetine, mirtazapine, mianserin and moclobemide; most toxic, and to be avoided in high-risk people, are the TCAs and MAOIs.

Serotonin syndrome

Excessive stimulation of 5-HT_{2A} receptors by serotonergic drugs can cause **serotonin syndrome**, or serotonin toxicity, characterised by mental state changes (confusion, delirium and hypomania), GIT effects (diarrhoea), neuromuscular hyperactivity (hyperreflexia, incoordination, tremor and ocular clonus), autonomic instability, sweating and fever and shivering. It occurs particularly when MAOIs are combined with SSRIs or SNRIs. Other drugs that enhance 5-HT transmission, including antimigraine drugs, opioid analgesics, CNS stimulants, St John's wort and many illicit drugs, can also cause or exacerbate the syndrome. Implicated drugs must be stopped immediately as the syndrome is serious and deaths have occurred. Moderate-to-severe cases require hospitalisation for CVS and temperature stabilisation, sedation and hydration. 5-HT antagonists such as cyproheptadine or chlorpromazine may be administered.

Treatment of adverse drug reactions

Simple strategies may help manage adverse effects: for example, for dry mouth – adequate fluid intake, lip balm, sugarless gum; for constipation – adequate fluid and fibre intake and physical activity; for orthostatic hypotension – care when standing or sitting up suddenly; for insomnia – taking medication in the morning; for weight gain – taking medications at bedtime, encouraging healthy eating and physical activity.

Overdosage (usually in attempted suicide cases) produces potentially fatal cardiotoxicity. Correction of the accompanying acidosis may be life-saving: paramedics can administer an IV hypertonic solution of sodium bicarbonate 8.4%, which increases pH and reduces metabolic acidosis.

Drug interactions

With antidepressants, there are potentially many drug interactions due to their interactions with multiple neurotransmitter systems (Drug Interactions 22.2, earlier). Reference texts should be consulted for specific interactions, especially for effects on CYP drug-metabolising enzymes.

Treating mania

Bipolar affective disorder involves mood swings between the poles of depression and mania; people with unipolar mania are rare. Bipolar disorders are much less common than unipolar depression. The peak age of onset of bipolar illness is in the late 20s, about 15 years earlier than unipolar depression; however, it may occur in adolescents. In predisposed people, mania can be provoked by many drugs, including the antidepressants, corticosteroids, angiotensin-converting-enzyme (ACE) inhibitors, dopaminergic agents and various illicit and stimulant drugs.

Mania is characterised by speech and motor hyperactivity, reduced sleep requirements, grandiose or paranoid ideas, elated or angry mood, poor judgement, aggressiveness and hostility, overspending and possibly promiscuity. (The milder hypomanic state may cause social problems, with overactivity, uncompleted tasks, irritability, excessively untidy and brightly coloured clothing, poor judgement and increased sexual interest.) People with bipolar disorder may then suffer a mood swing to depression, which can persist for several months.

Treating bipolar disorder

Counselling, psychotherapy and drug therapy are useful for treating bipolar disorders. ECT may be required for severe mood disturbance or for suicidal depression. Antipsychotic drugs, benzodiazepines and some antiepileptic drugs are useful for sedation and control of the mania symptoms, and antidepressants with lithium in the depressive phases for at least 6 months.

Lithium is specific for acute mania and prevention of recurrences of manic episodes (Drug Monograph 22.4). Other mood-stabilising drugs include the antipsychotics for rapid relief from acute symptoms of mania. Other drugs used in conjunction with the antipsychotics and long term are the antiepileptic drugs sodium valproate, carbamazepine (Ch 21), sometimes used in combination with lithium, or as alternatives if lithium is not tolerated. Clients need to be monitored for compliance, suicidal ideas, substance abuse and adverse effects of therapy.

Drug Monograph 22.4
Lithium

Mechanism of action

The mechanism of action of lithium has still not been established. Sodium in cells has been reported to increase by as much as 200% in manic patients. Lithium and sodium are both actively transported across cell membranes, but lithium cannot be pumped out of the cell as effectively as sodium can. Lithium can impair sodium actions in many physiological processes. It inhibits or slows down G-protein coupling with receptors, adenylate cyclase activity, phosphoinositol cycling and various phosphokinase activities and affects neuroprotective proteins. Overall, it inhibits transmitter release (especially dopamine) at synapses, increases the turnover of noradrenaline and 5-HT in the brain and decreases postsynaptic receptor sensitivity, with the result that the presumed overactive catecholamine systems in mania are corrected. It has little effect in people not suffering from mania.

Indications

Lithium is indicated for preventing manic or depressive episodes in bipolar affective disorder and to treat acute mania, and as adjunctive therapy in schizophrenia and treatment-resistant depression. It is a difficult drug clinically due to its low therapeutic index; it must be monitored closely. Lithium has little or no psychotropic effect in people who don't experience such episodes.

Pharmacokinetics

Apart from the slow-release dosage form, lithium is rapidly absorbed and reaches peak plasma concentrations in 1–3 hours. It has a long half-life: in adults, 24 hours; in adolescents, 18 hours; and in geriatric patients, up to 36 hours – hence, steady-state plasma concentrations are not reached for 5–7 days. Lithium is excreted unchanged by the kidneys; it is partly reabsorbed from the proximal tubule along with sodium.

Therapeutic drug monitoring

Lithium has a very narrow therapeutic range: concentrations only 1.5 times therapeutic concentration can cause severe toxicity, so plasma levels must be monitored regularly. Samples are taken 8–12 hours post-dose to measure trough levels. Therapeutic plasma concentrations for treatment of bipolar disorder are: acute, 0.8–1.2 mmol/L; maintenance, 0.6–0.8 mmol/L. A clinical response is usually reported in 1–3 weeks. Levels are monitored weekly during dosage adjustment, then every 3 months once stabilised, more frequently during illnesses or other changes.

Drug interactions

Lithium has specific interactions with other drugs affecting the kidneys, such as diuretics, sodium salts and non-steroidal anti-inflammatory agents (Drug Interactions 22.3). In addition, there can be interactions with drugs affecting thyroid function or 5-HT levels, and pharmacokinetic interactions based on altered metabolism or excretion.

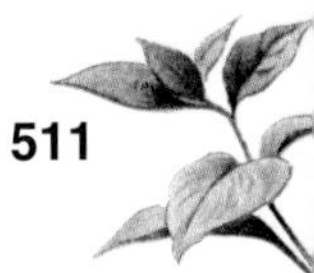

Adverse effects

These include tremors of the hands, thirst, nausea, increased urination, diarrhoea and irregular pulse rate. Long-term effects include acne, psoriasis, hypothyroidism, weight gain, hyperparathyroidism and renal damage. A specific adverse reaction is nephrogenic diabetes insipidus, in which lithium inhibits the actions of antidiuretic hormone on the distal tubule cells, leading to polyuria. Early signs of toxicity include confusion, vomiting, tremors, slurred speech and drowsiness. Later signs are blurred vision, convulsions, severe trembling, ataxia, dysrhythmias and increased production of urine. Prolonged toxic levels can lead to irreversible brain damage, and even relatively low plasma levels can be fatal. Treatment of toxicity is by gastric lavage, forced diuresis and dialysis.

Warnings and contraindications

Lithium should be used with caution in people with diabetes mellitus, hypothyroidism, goitre or psoriasis, and in pregnant or severely debilitated people or those on a sodium-restricted diet. Avoid use in people with a history of lithium hypersensitivity or with severe dehydration or renal impairment, and during lactation. Calcium levels should be monitored for hyperparathyroidism.

Lithium levels are elevated by renal dysfunction, diarrhoea, vomiting, fluid or salt loss, diuretics, dehydration, low-salt diets, excess sweating, high fever or strenuous exercise. Conversely, lithium levels are lowered by high intake of sodium chloride, sodium bicarbonate or potassium citrate, theophylline or during pregnancy.

Dosage and administration

Lithium, as the carbonate salt, is available as tablets and controlled-release tablets.

Acute mania

For Lithicarb the oral dose is initially day 1: 500–1000 mg; day 2: 1250–1750 mg; day 3: 1500–2000 mg. Adjust dosage according to serum concentration. Once remission occurs (7–14 days) gradually decrease to 500–1000 mg/day (taken in 1 or 2 doses) based on serum lithium.

It is most important not to exceed a level of 2 mmol/L. The dose is adjusted according to the person's response. Geriatric patients require a much lower dosage (one-third to half).

DRUG INTERACTIONS 22.3
Lithium

DRUG	POSSIBLE EFFECTS AND MANAGEMENT
Antithyroid drugs or iodides	Can enhance the hypothyroid goitrogenic effects of lithium or these medications; monitor closely for lethargy or intolerance to cold
Non-steroidal anti-inflammatory agents; ACE inhibitors; sartans; topiramate	Can decrease excretion of lithium, leading to raised lithium levels and toxicity; monitor closely for blurred vision, confusion and dizziness
Phenothiazines, fluoxetine, haloperidol	Lithium levels may be altered, with risk of neurotoxicity; monitor physical symptoms and drug serum levels
Diuretics (loop; thiazide)	Decreased lithium excretion results in a raised lithium level and toxicity; a reduction in lithium dosage may be indicated; monitor closely
Drugs increasing 5-HT levels	Enhanced risk of serotonin toxicity
Ziprasidone	Interacts with lithium to augment the prolongation of the cardiac QT interval

Note: See also Tables 22.1 and 22.2; Drug Interactions 22.1 and 22.2.

KEY POINTS

Treatment of affective disorders

- The major affective disorders are depression and bipolar affective disorder. The monoamine theory suggests that during depressive episodes, levels of monoamines – especially noradrenaline and 5-HT – are low in parts of the brain related to mood.
- Antidepressant drug groups include the SSRIs, SNRIs, TCAs and MAOIs. All appear to act by increasing brain levels of 5-HT and noradrenaline, and have multiple adverse effects on transmitter systems.
- Lithium is the drug of choice for prophylaxis and treatment of mania or bipolar affective disorder.
- All psychotherapeutic medications can produce undesirable adverse effects. Patient education and close monitoring are necessary to improve compliance and clinical outcomes, and to avoid or reduce the potential for unwanted and potentially serious adverse effects and drug interactions.

DRUGS AT A GLANCE

PHARMACOLOGICAL GROUP AND EFFECT	KEY EXAMPLES	CLINICAL USE
Antipsychotic agents		
Phenothiazines – conventional (typical) • Antagonism of D_1 and D_2 dopamine receptors	Chlorpromazine	Schizophrenia Behavioural emergencies
Thioxanthine derivatives • Antagonism of D_1 and D_2 dopamine receptors	Flupentixol	Schizophrenia
Butyrophenone derivatives (haloperidol type) • Competitively antagonises D_2 receptors in the mesolimbic system	Haloperidol	Schizophrenia
Atypical antipsychotics		Schizophrenia
• Partial agonist at D_2 and 5-HT_{IA} receptors, and antagonist at 5-HT_{2A} receptors	Aripiprazole	
• Antagonises D_1, D_2 and D_4 dopamine receptors, with less affinity for D_2 receptors, so is less apt to induce extrapyramidal effects • Antagonist at α_1-adrenoceptors and histamine H_1 receptors	Clozapine	
• Antagonists at both 5-HT_{2A} and dopamine D_2 receptors	Olanzapine, risperidone	
Other • Antagonist at D_2/D_3/5-HT_7 receptors • Antagonist at 5-HT_{2A} and dopamine D_2 receptors	Amisulpride Paliperidone	
Antidepressants		
Tricyclic antidepressants (TCAs) • Block reuptake of noradrenaline and 5-HT into nerve terminals	Imipramine Amitriptyline Nortriptyline	Mood disorders: • Depression • Bipolar disorder • Generalised anxiety disorder
Selective serotonin reuptake inhibitors (SSRIs) • Block reuptake of serotonin (5-HT) into nerve terminal via the transporter (SERT)	Fluoxetine (es)citalopram	Mood disorders: • Depression • Bipolar disorder • Generalised anxiety disorder
Serotonin noradrenaline reuptake inhibitors (SNRIs) • Block reuptake of noradrenaline and 5-HT into nerve terminals via blockade of the serotonin transporter (SERT) and NET	Venlafaxine, desvenlafaxine[AUS]	Mood disorders: • Moderate to severe depression • Bipolar disorder • Generalised anxiety disorder
Monoamine oxidase inhibitors (MAOIs); non-selective • Inhibit both MAO-A and MAO-B enzymes for 2–3 weeks • Desensitise the α_2- or β-adrenoceptors and 5-HT receptors (downregulation) • Increase levels of monoamine neurotransmitters	Tranylcypromine	Mood disorders: • Moderate to severe depression • Bipolar disorder
Reversible (selective) inhibitors of MAO-A (RIMAs) • Relatively selective inhibitor (MAO-A). It increases synaptic concentrations of serotonin, noradrenaline (norepinephrine) and dopamine	Moclobemide	Mood disorders: Moderate to severe depression Bipolar disorder
Others • Melatonin receptor agonist and 5-HT_{2C} receptor antagonist • Enhances postsynaptic 5-HT_{1A} receptor signalling	Agomelatine,[AUS] mianserin	Mood disorders: Moderate to severe depression Bipolar disorder
Antimanic agents		
Lithium • Mechanism generally unknown. It inhibits G-protein coupling with receptors, adenylate cyclase activity, phosphoinositol cycling and various phosphokinase activities • Inhibits transmitter release (especially dopamine) at synapses, increases the turnover of noradrenaline and 5-HT in the brain, and decreases postsynaptic receptor sensitivity		Mania
Mood stabilisers • Various mechanisms as per antiepileptics including blockade of sodium channels to reduce neuronal firing	Antiepileptic drugs, sodium valproate	Acute mania

AUS = Australia only

REVIEW EXERCISES

1. Mrs JD is a 45-year-old who has been diagnosed with major depression. She has previously been prescribed an SSRI (fluoxetine) but has experienced agitation and insomnia. Her GP decides she should be prescribed the MAOI tranylcypromine. Describe the mechanism of action of both drugs. What advice should she be given about starting the new medication, adverse reactions and dietary considerations?
2. Mr XY, a 25-year-old, has been transported to the emergency department with an intentional overdose of his antidepressant medication, amitriptyline. An ECG undertaken by the treating paramedics indicates he is suffering from a dangerous arrhythmia. Is this arrhythmia a result of his medication? What is this class of medication, its mechanism of action and what would have been safer antidepressant for Mr XY?

REFERENCES

Anderson KN, Ailes EC, Lind JN, et al. 2020. Atypical antipsychotic use during pregnancy and birth defect risk: National Birth Defects Prevention Study, 1997-2011. Schizophrenia Research. 215:81–88. doi:10.1016/j.schres.2019.11.019

Australian Bureau of Statistics (2022) National Study of Mental Health and Wellbeing. https://www.abs.gov.au/statistics/health/mental-health/national-study-mental-health-and-wellbeing/2020-21 accessed 09/08/2022

Australian Medicines Handbook 2021. Australian Medicines Handbook. Adelaide: AMH.

Betcher HK, Montiel C, Clark CT 2019. Use of antipsychotic drugs during pregnancy. Current Treatment Options in Psychiatry. Mar;6(1):17–31. doi:10.1007/s40501-019-0165-5. Epub 2019 Jan 30. PMID: 32775146; PMCID: PMC7410162

Braun L, Cohen M 2014: Herbs and natural supplements: an evidence-based guide, 4th ed, Sydney, Elsevier Mosby.

Brunton LL, Chabner B, Knollman B, editors 2011: Goodman and Gilman's The pharmacological basis of therapeutics, ed 12, New York, McGraw-Hill.

Cade JF: Mending the mind 1979: a short history of twentieth century psychiatry, Melbourne, Sun Books.

Cornett EM, Novitch M, Kaye AD, et al. 2017. Medication-induced tardive dyskinesia: a review and update. Ochsner Journal. 17(2):162–174.

Fulde G, Preisz P 2011: Managing aggressive and violent patients. Australian Prescriber 34(4):115–118.

Henssler J, Heinz A, Brandt L, et al. Antidepressant withdrawal and rebound phenomena. Deutsches Ärzteblatt International. 2019; May 17;116(20):355–361. doi:10.3238/arztebl.2019.0355. PMID: 31288917; PMCID: PMC6637660.

Henter ID, Park LT, Zarate CA Jr 2021. Novel glutamatergic modulators for the treatment of mood disorders: current status. CNS Drugs. 35(5):527–543. doi:10.1007/s40263-021-00816-x

Huhn M, Nikolakopoulou A, Schneider-Thoma J, et al. 2019. Comparative efficacy and tolerability of 32 oral antipsychotics for the acute treatment of adults with multi-episode schizophrenia: a systematic review and network meta-analysis [published correction appears in Lancet. Sep 14; 394(10202):918]. Lancet. 2019;394(10202):939–951. doi:10.1016/S0140-6736(19)31135-3

Hunter E, Gynther B, Anderson C, et al. 2011: Psychosis and its correlates in a remote indigenous population. Australasian Psychiatry 19(5):434–438.

Hunter E 2014: Mental health in Indigenous settings: challenges for clinicians. Australian Family Physician 43(1–2):26–32.

Meltzer HY. New trends in the treatment of schizophrenia. 2017. CNS & Neurological Disorders – Drug Targets. 16(8):900–906. doi:10.2174/1871527316666170728165355. PMID: 28758583.

National Prescribing Service 2011: Depression: challenges in primary care, NPS News 74:3.

New Zealand Ministry of Health 2021. New Zealand Health Survey. https://www.health.govt.nz/nz-health-statistics/national-collections-and-surveys/surveys/current-recent-surveys/new-zealand-health-survey.

Ornoy A, Koren G 2019. SSRIs and SNRIs (SRI) in Pregnancy: Effects on the course of pregnancy and the offspring: How far are we from having all the answers? International Journal of Molecular Sciences, May 14;20(10):2370. doi:10.3390/ijms20102370. PMID: 31091646; PMCID: PMC6567187.

Psychotropic Expert Group: Therapeutic guidelines: psychotropic, version 7, Melbourne, 2021 Therapeutic Guidelines Limited. *eTG complete* [digital]. Melbourne: Therapeutic Guidelines Limited; 2019 Jun. https://www.tg.org.au

Rowland TA, Marwaha S 2018. Epidemiology and risk factors for bipolar disorder. Ther Adv Psychopharmacol. 8(9):251–269. Published Apr 26. doi:10.1177/2045125318769235

Rummel-Kluge C, Komossa K, Schwarz S, et al 2012: Second-generation antipsychotic drugs and extrapyramidal side effects: a systematic review and meta-analysis of head-to-head comparisons. Schizophrenia Bulletin 38(1):167–177.

Sarris J 2014: Nutrients and herbal supplements for mental health. Australian Prescriber 37(3):90–93.

Shafiq S, Pringsheim T 2018. Using antipsychotics for behavioral problems in children. Expert Opinion on Pharmacotherapy. Sep;19(13):1475–1488. doi:10.1080/14656566.2018.1509069. Epub 2018 Aug 13. PMID: 30102079.

World Health Organization 2018. Mental health: strengthening our response. Online. https://www.who.int/news-room/fact-sheets/detail/mental-health-strengthening-our-response

Yang AC, Tsai SJ 2017. New targets for schizophrenia treatment beyond the dopamine hypothesis. International Journal of Molecular Sciences. Aug 3;18(8):1689. doi:10.3390/ijms18081689. PMID: 28771182; PMCID: PMC5578079.

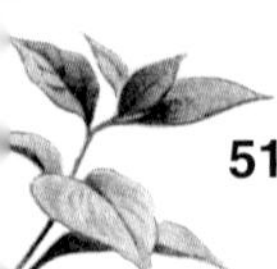

ONLINE RESOURCES

Australian Bureau of Statistics, 2018: https://www.abs.gov.au/statistics/health/mental-health/mental-health/latest-release (accessed January 2022)

Australian Health Survey – first results, 2017–18: https://www.abs.gov.au/ausstats/abs@.nsf/Lookup/4364.0.55.001main+features12011-12

Beyond Blue, the national depression initiative: https://www.beyondblue.org.au/home

Mental Illness Fellowship of Australia: https://www.mifa.org.au/en/ (accessed January 2022)

New Zealand Medicines and Medical Devices Safety Authority: www.medsafe.govt.nz

Schizophrenia Fellowship of New Zealand: http://sfnat.org.nz/ (accessed January 2022)

Wellways Australia Limited: a leading not-for-profit mental health and disability support organisation with services in Queensland, New South Wales, the Australian Capital Territory, Victoria and Tasmania: https://www.wellways.org/ (accessed January 2022)

More weblinks at: http://evolve.elsevier.com/AU/Knights/pharmacology/.

CHAPTER 23

CENTRAL NERVOUS SYSTEM STIMULANTS

Shaunagh Darroch

KEY ABBREVIATIONS

ADHD	attention deficit hyperactivity disorder
cAMP	cyclic adenosine monophosphate
CNS	central nervous system
MAO	monoamine oxidase
TCAs	tricyclic antidepressants

KEY TERMS

Chapter Focus

Central nervous system (CNS) stimulant drugs such as amphetamine and caffeine may produce dramatic effects by increasing the activity of CNS neurons; however, their therapeutic usefulness is limited because of their many general and adverse effects in the body. Chronic use and misuse occur with amphetamines, resulting in drug tolerance, drug dependence and drug abuse problems. This chapter reviews the CNS-stimulant drugs that are available for clinical use. Their approved indications are for treating attention disorders and narcolepsy, and to suppress the appetite. The amphetamines have clinical applications in attention deficit hyperactivity disorder and narcolepsy, and as anorectic agents, but are widely abused for their stimulant effects. The methylxanthines (caffeine, theophylline and theobromine) are mainly taken in beverages (coffee, tea, cocoa and soft drinks) to increase alertness, and are administered in respiratory disorders.

KEY DRUG GROUPS

Amphetamines:

- **Dexamfetamine** (Drug Monograph 23.1), **lisdexamfetamine**

Amphetamine-like drugs:

- **Atomoxetine**, **methylphenidate**, **modafinil**

(Methyl)xanthines:

- **Caffeine** (Drug Monograph 23.2)

CRITICAL THINKING SCENARIO

Isaiah, a 30-year-old marketing executive, presents to his GP complaining of a pounding heart and chest pains. He appears highly agitated with palpitations, sweating and dyspnoea. On examination he is found to have a heart rate of 160 bpm and low blood pressure. An ambulance was called, and paramedics diagnosed, by ECG, supraventricular tachycardia. On questioning, Isaiah stated he had been working long hours and to stay awake and alert had been drinking about five coffees per day. Yesterday a friend had given him a couple of 'energy drinks' to help with his fatigue. He noted that he thought the energy drink had 'kicked off' this current problem.

1. What would be the cause of Isaiah's palpitations and chest pain?
2. What would cause the agitation seen?
3. Discuss the mechanism of action of the causative agent.

Introduction: History and uses of stimulants

The central nervous system (CNS) stimulants (amphetamines and methylxanthines) exert their main effects on the cerebrum, medulla and brainstem, and on the hypothalamic or limbic regions. Amphetamines are mainly stimulants of the cerebral cortex, whereas anorectic (appetite-reducing) agents suppress the appetite, possibly by a direct stimulant effect on the satiety centres in the hypothalamic and limbic regions, and **analeptics** (respiratory stimulants) primarily affect centres in the medulla and the brainstem. CNS stimulants act by increasing the neuronal discharge in excitatory pathways or by blocking inhibitory pathways.

Cerebral stimulants were commonly prescribed in the past for obesity, to counteract CNS-depressant over-dosage and to increase alertness in people trying to stay awake during long shiftwork or boring tasks (today, such use is considered inappropriate). Although CNS stimulants such as phentermine suppress appetite and are used as an adjunct to lifestyle modifications, tolerance develops to the anorectic effect, usually before the weight reduction goal is reached. Treating over-dosage of CNS depressants with stimulants is discouraged because close monitoring and simple supportive measures have been found to be successful, avoiding undesirable adverse reactions to stimulants.

These drugs may also affect other parts of the nervous system, including the autonomic nervous system, so adverse effects are common. With their narrow therapeutic range between effectiveness and toxicity, CNS stimulants may induce cardiac dysrhythmias, hypertension, convulsions and violent behaviour. They therefore have limited use in practice today and are primarily used for the treatment of 'alertness disorders' such as attention deficit hyperactivity disorder (ADHD) and narcolepsy, and as appetite suppressants. They are also being examined for their effectiveness in improving functional recovery after brain injuries such as stroke or traumatic brain injury.

Amphetamines

Pharmacodynamics

Relationships to neurotransmitters

Amphetamine itself (α-methylphenethylamine) is closely related chemically to noradrenaline (norepinephrine), adrenaline (epinephrine) and many other sympathomimetic amines (Ch 9). There are also trace amounts of similar amines in the brain, such as octopamine, tyramine and phenylethylamine, which may act as neuromodulators as well as participating in reactions in the biosynthetic pathways for neurotransmitters. The amphetamine-like analogues have fewer hydroxyl (–OH) groups than do the catecholamines; they therefore have higher lipid solubilities and so cross the blood–brain barrier and have CNS activities. The generic term 'phenylethylamines' is sometimes used to refer to all the drugs in this group, including drugs described in this section: dexamfetamine, lisdexamfetamine, methylphenidate and phentermine (an anorectic); however, as they are all related chemically to the prototype amphetamine, we will refer to the group as the **amphetamines**.

Mechanisms of action

The proposed mechanisms of action for the amphetamines include:

- noradrenaline accumulation due to inhibition of the noradrenaline transporter (NET), and the release of noradrenaline, from storage sites in nerve terminals (hence, an indirect sympathomimetic effect), direct stimulating effects on α- and β-adrenoceptor sites
- inhibition of the dopamine transporter (DAT) enhancing dopaminergic transmission; it facilitates the movement of dopamine out of vesicles and into the cytoplasm; and promotes DAT-mediated reverse-transport of dopamine into the synaptic cleft
- modulation of the 5-HT (serotonin) transporter (SERT) enhancing serotonergic transmission.

  Methylphenidate also stimulates 5-HT_{1A} receptors.

(See also Table 18.1, in Ch 18, and Fig 22.2 in Ch 22, noting that amphetamines are not used for depression).

The primary action centrally appears to be in the cerebral cortex and, possibly, the reticular activating system. Stimulation results in increased mental alertness and motor function, decreased sense of fatigue and, usually, a euphoric effect. These effects are probably mediated through effects on central adrenoceptors. The stereotyped behaviours in animals (compulsive gnawing and sniffing, and circling) and paranoid psychosis in humans, similar to an acute schizophrenic attack, can be reversed by antipsychotic drugs and thus are most likely related to actions on dopaminergic pathways. Amphetamines can also contribute to serotonin toxicity.

Indirect actions at glutamate receptors have also been implicated in the mechanism of action of amphetamines and related CNS stimulants. Agonists at the glutamatergic AMPA receptor, associated with fast and slow ligand-gated cation channels (Table 18.1), termed ampakines, have CNS-stimulant actions and have been reported to enhance attention span and facilitate learning; they are being trialled in many conditions involving mental disturbances, including ADHD, Alzheimer's and Parkinson's diseases, and schizophrenia. Behavioural actions of amphetamines are blocked by antagonists at both types of glutamate receptors, and glutamate-receptor blockers may be useful in treatment of psychostimulant toxicity.

Central actions

Amphetamine-like drugs have four main effects on the CNS:

- euphoria ('feel-good' excitement – people become hyperactive and talkative fatigue is reduced and sex drive is said to be enhanced; however, overconfidence may mask impaired performance[1])
- locomotor stimulation (increased alertness and activity; animals are described as appearing busier, rather than brighter)
- anorexia (appetite suppression)
- stereotyped behaviours (repeated inappropriate actions, such as animals gnawing, sniffing or moving the head; in humans, choreas can develop, with repeated involuntary, purposeless movements).

Tolerance and dependence

Tolerance develops readily to the peripheral and anorectic effects of amphetamines; indeed, the anorectic effects wear off a few days after taking these drugs, which detracts from their clinical usefulness in weight reduction. Addiction to and dependence on amphetamines can develop, possibly due to users taking more of the drugs to overcome the unpleasant mood swing (depression and tiredness) after the effects of a dose wear off, leading to 'binge' drug-taking behaviour. (These aspects of amphetamine abuse are covered in Ch 25.) Because of their potential for abuse, dexamfetamine and methylphenidate fall under the Australian Poisons and Controlled Substances Regulations into the 'Controlled Drug' classification, Schedule 8.

Adverse drug reactions

Signs and symptoms of psychostimulant overdose include tachycardia, dilated pupils, euphoria, insomnia, confusion and tremors, through to delirium, convulsions, psychosis, cerebrovascular accidents and death. Important adverse reactions can be seen in Drug Monograph 23.1 and Fig 23.1. The acute neurotoxicity of amphetamines, which causes potentially irreversible cellular necrosis and loss of CNS neurons, is thought to be due to the formation of active free radicals and hence mitochondrial malfunction. The pregnancy category of methylphenidate has now been updated to Category D in Australia. In chronic abuse of amphetamines, there is a strong association with psychoses and especially schizophrenia; whether this is a causal effect (amphetamines causing psychosis) and/or a 'dual diagnosis' effect (people with schizophrenia being more likely to use or abuse drugs) is at present unclear.

In the peripheral nervous system, amphetamines and related phenylethylamines such as pseudoephedrine have

1 Amphetamines may improve performance in endurance sporting events and may increase alertness and reduce fatigue; hence, they are prohibited by the World Anti-Doping Agency. Pharmacological folklore includes many anecdotes of university students who sat for examinations while 'high' on amphetamines (taken to keep them awake while studying) and spent the entire 3-hour exam time writing out their names!

Drug Monograph 23.1
Dexamfetamine

Dexamfetamine, the (+) or dexamfetamine of amphetamine, is the prototype CNS stimulant. It is indicated for use in ADHD in children, and in narcolepsy.

Mechanism of action

As an amphetamine, dexamfetamine causes noradrenaline accumulation due to inhibition of the noradrenaline transporter (NET) and the release of noradrenaline from storage sites in nerve terminals (hence, an indirect sympathomimetic effect). It has direct stimulating effects on α- and β-adrenoceptor sites. As noted, it also inhibits the DAT, enhancing dopaminergic transmission; it facilitates the movement of dopamine out of vesicles and into the cytoplasm. It also modulates the SERT, enhancing serotonergic transmission.

Pharmacokinetics

Amphetamines are well absorbed from the gut, with peak plasma concentrations reached 2 hours after oral administration. They are widely distributed to body tissues with a V_d of 2–3 L/kg body weight, with especially high concentrations in the brain and cerebrospinal fluid, lungs and kidneys. Thirty to 40% of dexamfetamine is metabolised in the liver, and the remainder is excreted unchanged by the kidneys.

Excretion (and, therefore, half-life) is pH-dependent; excretion is increased in acidic urine and decreased in more alkaline urine. Approximate half-lives are 6–8 hours in acidic urine with pH under 5 (e.g. after taking ammonium chloride); or 16–31 hours in alkaline urine of pH over 7.5 (e.g. after taking sodium or potassium citrate).

Drug interactions

See Drug Interactions 23.1.

Adverse reactions

Important adverse reactions include:

- CNS – euphoria, increased irritability, insomnia, headache, nausea, visual disturbance, dizziness, anorexia, dyskinesia and Tourette's syndrome
- cardiovascular system – tachycardia, angina
- autonomic nervous system – excessive sweating, dry mouth
- gastrointestinal system – nausea or vomiting
- endocrine system – impotence, alterations in libido.

With high dosage or prolonged consumption, mood changes, including depression, increased agitation, choreas and psychosis, may occur. Drug dependence and tolerance may also develop.

Treating amphetamine overdose consists of symptomatic and supportive care, as described in the text.

Warnings and contraindications

Amphetamines have a high liability for abuse. The CNS stimulation and the rebound depression after withdrawal both impair abilities to drive or operate machinery.

Avoid use in people with amphetamine hypersensitivity, hyperthyroidism, hypertension, glaucoma, history of drug abuse, cardiovascular disease, severe agitation, severe arteriosclerosis and Tourette's syndrome. Amphetamines are contraindicated during pregnancy because they cause increased risk of malformations, premature delivery and withdrawal symptoms in the infant (Category B3).

Dosage and administration

Dosage depends on the indications for which the drug is prescribed and is adjusted individually to the lowest effective dose. It is not taken in the evenings because of the CNS excitation effects. Typical doses for school-age children are initially 2.5–10 mg daily, increasing at weekly intervals to a maximum of 40 mg/day in ADHD, taken in divided doses in the morning and early afternoon. For narcolepsy in adults, dosage starts at 5 mg in the morning, increasing to a maximum of 60 mg/day in divided doses.

indirect sympathomimetic actions by causing the release of noradrenaline; hence, they have vasoconstrictor and hypertensive effects.

Managing psychostimulant poisoning

Drugs from both the legal psychostimulant group (dexamfetamine, methylphenidate, caffeine and some decongestant and weight loss drugs) and the illicit stimulants (other amphetamines, designer drugs including 'ecstasy' and cocaine) can cause acute toxicity as well as drug abuse problems. There is no specific antidote for an overdose of amphetamines, so symptomatic relief and supportive measures should be instituted. De-escalation (calming and support) is helpful, with physical restraint if

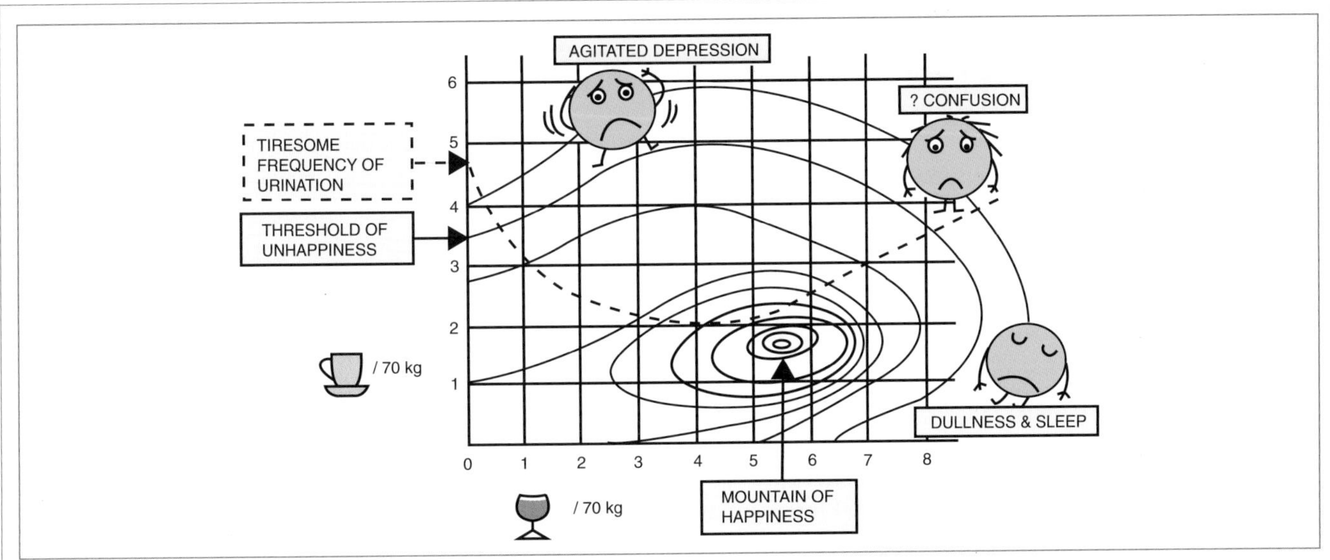

FIGURE 23.1 Drug interactions between caffeine and alcohol

The scenario is a dinner party, restaurant or nightclub: alcohol is consumed during the evening, and coffee before leaving. Doses of alcohol (measured in glasses of wine per 70 kg adult) are plotted along the *x*-axis, and doses of caffeine (measured in cups of coffee per 70 kg adult) up the *y*-axis. The CNS-depressant effect of alcohol taken alone leads to dullness and sleep, whereas the CNS-stimulant effect of caffeine alone causes agitation and depression. These effects are antagonistic, causing CNS confusion at high doses of both taken together. Unfortunately, the diuretic effects of the two drugs are additive, leading to a tiresome frequency of urination.

Source: Figure adapted from Andrew Herxheimer, in Laurence 1973.

necessary. Vital signs, cardiac and respiratory functions, hydration and nutrition should be monitored frequently.

Medications usually used for hypertension are nitrites; for dysrhythmias: lidocaine (lignocaine) IV; to decrease dopaminergic effects, seizures and hyperthermia: diazepam, the antipsychotics haloperidol or droperidol; and for serotonin toxicity: IV hydration, active cooling and assisted ventilation.

Drug interactions with amphetamines

Adverse drug interactions are common: typical interactions and possible outcomes are shown in Drug Interactions 23.1.

Clinical uses

Attention deficit hyperactivity disorder

The syndrome of **attention deficit hyperactivity disorder** (ADHD) is considered a psychiatric disorder of childhood and occurs in 5–7% of school-aged children. (Previously, these children were probably just considered naughty or unmanageable.) It is characterised by persistently short attention span, impulsive behaviour and hyperactivity; the child may be moody and irritable and have low self-esteem and learning disabilities. Most children with ADHD also have other concurrent disorders, such as

DRUG INTERACTIONS 23.1
Amphetamines

DRUG OR DRUG GROUP	LIKELY EFFECTS AND MANAGEMENT
Tricyclic antidepressants; other CNS stimulants; sympathomimetics including inotropes	Effects of these drugs are enhanced, which may result in adverse cardiovascular and CNS effects, such as dysrhythmias, tachycardia or severe hypertension; avoid, or a potentially serious drug interaction may occur. Chronic users of amphetamines may require higher doses of sympathomimetic inotropes in an emergency, due to tolerance.
Non-selective monoamine oxidase (MAO) inhibitors, and reversible inhibitors of MAO-A (RIMAs)	Avoid concurrent usage because effects of catecholamines are increased; headaches, dysrhythmias, vomiting, sudden severe hypertension or hyperpyrexia may result. Avoid, or a potentially serious adrenergic crisis may occur.
α-adrenergic blocking drugs (systemic and ophthalmic) and other autonomic antihypertensive agents	Amphetamines may overcome adrenoceptor antagonism by α- or β-blockers, causing sympathomimetic effects resulting in loss of blood pressure control and hypertension.
Digoxin	May result in an increase in cardiac dysrhythmias.
Thyroid hormones	Concomitant administration may result in enhanced effects of thyroid hormones or amphetamines.

conduct, anxiety, learning or depressive disorders. Improper functioning of the monoamine neurotransmitter systems (noradrenergic, dopaminergic and serotonergic) has been implicated in ADHD. Other risk/predisposing factors suggested include:

- genetic mechanisms (especially monoamine oxidase [MAO] deficiencies)
- high sugar intake, food additives and preservatives
- extreme low birth weight or prematurity
- maternal alcohol or tobacco use during pregnancy
- early exposure to chemicals and toxins.

Symptoms of ADHD may present from infancy, and ADHD usually becomes apparent between the ages of 3 and 7 years, with boys affected more often than girls by a ratio ranging from 4:1 to 10:1. Usually, professional intervention is unnecessary until the child enters the school setting, when symptoms may start to cause functional impairment. Paradoxically, CNS-stimulant medications tend to decrease the distractibility and hyperactivity, resulting in a lengthened attention span and improved cognitive performance and social behaviour. ADHD may persist into adulthood, with higher incidences of substance abuse, antisocial personality disorders, anxiety and depression, lower education and unemployment being observed in comparisons with control groups (Kooij et al. 2019; Psychotropic Expert Group 2021).

Behavioural management

Managing this disorder requires a behavioural modification program (family support, directed activities, special educational programs, speech and/or occupational therapy and psychotherapy) with use of pharmacological therapy as an adjunct if necessary. Around 15–20% of children do not respond, or their symptoms increase with the stimulant drugs; in these cases, therapy with tricyclic antidepressants (TCAs) or with clonidine may be tried.

Use of amphetamine-related drugs

Psychostimulants

The amphetamine-related drugs approved for treatment of ADHD in Australia are dexamfetamine (Drug Monograph 23.1), lisdexamfetamine and methylphenidate, which is more selective at blocking dopamine transporters. Use of these psychostimulants helps improve academic performance, vocational success and social and emotional development, and has been shown to be cost-effective compared to no treatment, placebo or behavioural therapy; however, there is no strong evidence for long-term improvement in life outcomes. Response is usually rapid and obvious. Dexamfetamine doses are started low and gradually increased to a maximum of 40 mg per day (in up to three divided doses), provided effective responses are obtained. Lisdexamfetamine is a prodrug of dexamfetamine, with a longer half-life; it is approved for use in children and adults with ADHD. It is given 30 mg orally, in the morning, increasing the dose according to response and tolerability in increments of 20 mg at weekly intervals until optimal response is obtained or a daily dose of 70 mg is reached.

Methylphenidate is also available in modified-release formulations, providing both immediate-release and delayed-release drug, for up to 8–12 hours. These formulations have the advantage of once-daily dosing, which improves the privacy of people taking them and minimises the likelihood of the drugs being diverted or abused.

If one of the drugs is not effective or tolerated, another drug should be tried. The prescriber needs to work closely with the child, the parents, carers and school staff in evaluating results and planning dosages. There are as yet no clear guidelines as to how long therapy should be continued; drug-free trials are recommended at yearly intervals, at periods of low stress.

Non-stimulant drugs

Atomoxetine

A non-stimulant drug now recommended as second-line treatment for ADHD in children is atomoxetine. It is used when treatment with stimulants is not suitable or not tolerated or there is a risk of misuse of stimulants or tics or severe anxiety. This compound inhibits the reuptake of noradrenaline (as do cocaine, amphetamines, TCAs, serotonin noradrenaline reuptake inhibitors [SNRIs] and selective serotonin reuptake inhibitors [SSRIs]). However, it appears not to cause CNS stimulation and does not cause dependence; hence, it is not a controlled (S8) drug. It is well absorbed but has variable bioavailability; the half-life varies from 5 to 22 hours. Clinical placebo-controlled trials in children showed its efficacy in reducing ADHD symptoms; it was approximately equiactive with (but not better than) methylphenidate. As expected, autonomic adverse effects are common.

Clinical experience has shown that, in children and adolescents taking atomoxetine regularly, there may be increased risk of suicidal ideation. They should be closely monitored for clinical worsening or changes in behaviour such as agitation, panic attacks, irritability, insomnia or (hypo)mania. Precautions also need to be taken in those with cardiovascular diseases, hepatic impairment, glaucoma and history of seizures. There are potential drug interactions with other drugs that raise monoamine levels, including MAOI, SNRI and SSRI antidepressants. It is metabolised by CYP2D6 enzyme, so interactions with drugs that inhibit or induce this enzyme are common.

Narcolepsy and idiopathic hypersomnolence

Narcolepsy is a condition characterised by excessive drowsiness and uncontrollable sleep attacks during the daytime, even while eating, driving or talking.[2] In addition, the person may exhibit a sleep paralysis (inability to move that occurs immediately on falling asleep or on awakening), cataplexy (stress-induced generalised muscle weakness) and hypnagogic illusions or hallucinations (vivid auditory or visual dreams occurring at onset of sleep). It is a specific, permanent neurological disorder, coming on in early adulthood and causing great distress to the sufferers. The aetiology is unclear; loss of neurons producing orexin-type neuropeptides (which regulate activity and sleep/wake cycles) has been proposed.

Although narcolepsy is essentially incurable, education about the condition assists the person to recognise the symptoms and adapt their daily schedule.

CNS stimulants such as modafinil, dexamfetamine and methylphenidate are useful in controlling the daytime drowsiness and excessive sleep patterns, TCAs and SSRIs are used in conjunction with the stimulants for cataplexy and sleep paralysis. Other drugs that have been approved outside Australia and New Zealand are sodium oxybate and gamma-hydroxybutyrate (GHB), a GABA receptor agonist.

Modafinil

A non-amphetamine drug, modafinil, has been shown to be clinically effective in treating excessive sleepiness associated with narcolepsy and idiopathic hypersomnolence, with significantly increased scores on tests for maintenance of wakefulness and sleep latency. It may also be used for obstructive sleep apnoea, and in disturbed sleep patterns due to shiftwork changes when non-pharmacological methods have been unsuccessful. The r-isomer of modafinil, armodafinil, is also used.

Mechanism of action

Modafanil's mechanism of action is unclear: it does not appear to bind with receptors for the usual monoamine transmitters, but may be involved with histaminergic and orexinergic systems. It improves alertness and opposes the impaired cognitive functioning caused by lack of sleep, while not affecting appetite, behaviour, nocturnal sleep or the autonomic nervous system.

Dosage

An oral single dose of 200 mg is taken in the morning or modafinil 100 mg orally, twice daily, in the morning and at midday (maximum daily dose 400 mg).

2 A colleague explained the condition to his students thus: 'If you fall asleep during my lectures, that's normal. If I do, that's narcolepsy.'

Pharmacokinetics

Modafinil is slowly absorbed and eliminated mainly by metabolism in the liver to inactive metabolites which are excreted via the kidneys. The elimination half-life is approximately 10–12 hours.

The main adverse effects are central: headache, nausea, nervousness, exacerbation of psychiatric disorders and possibly euphoria; hence, the drug might be abused. Potentially life-threatening multi-organ hypersensitivity reactions have occurred with high doses. There are potential drug interactions with other drugs metabolised by CYP3A4; in women, combined oral contraceptives may be inactivated faster, so other contraception should be used. Precautions are advised in those with psychiatric or substance abuse disorders, and cardiovascular or hepatic disease.

Amphetamines as anorectic agents

Anorectic drugs (also called appetite suppressants or anorexiants) include some indirectly acting sympathomimetics and phenylethylamine-like or amphetamine-like drugs used for the short-term treatment of obesity (Ch 42). Their exact mechanism of action is unknown, but they appear to reduce hunger by effects in the hypothalamus and limbic areas of the brain. In the past, many such drugs were readily available to treat obesity by decreasing appetite; however, the amphetamines are liable to be abused because of their dependence potential, and tolerance develops rapidly. Analogues fenfluramine and dexfenfluramine were withdrawn in Australia because of adverse cardiovascular effects (particularly pulmonary hypertension). Also withdrawn was sibutramine, a serotonin and SNRI that induces the sensation of satiety (fullness). Some other SSRIs (e.g. fluoxetine) used as antidepressants have also been shown to reduce appetite. Significant weight loss and anorexia, especially in underweight depressed people, may be an undesirable result of treatment with fluoxetine hydrochloride.

Phentermine

The only remaining amphetamine-related compound indicated as an anorectic is phentermine. It acts mainly on adrenergic pathways and, while causing some CNS stimulation and mild euphoria, is less liable to lead to dependence than other amphetamines. It is an anorectic agent indicated in the management of obesity as a short-term adjunct in a medically monitored comprehensive regimen of weight in obese people with a body mass index of 30 kg/m^2 or greater. Actions, adverse effects and drug interactions are generally similar to those of dexamfetamine. See Chapter 42 for a discussion of its role in obesity.

KEY POINTS

Amphetamines

- The CNS-stimulant drugs have a limited use in clinical practice today as mild stimulants, appetite suppressants and in treating 'alertness disorders'.
- The amphetamines and related drugs have sympathomimetic actions (indirect and direct), and may also act through effects on dopamine and glutamate receptors.
- The main actions of the amphetamines are to cause euphoria, locomotor stimulation, anorexia and stereotyped movements. In overdose or chronic use, they may lead to developing tolerance, dependence and psychoses, as well as acute cardiovascular and neurological toxicity.
- The amphetamine-related stimulants dexamfetamine and methylphenidate are approved for use in the treatment of ADHD and narcolepsy.
- When used as an appetite suppressant, phentermine is usually recommended as an adjunct to other regimens that include physical exercise, behaviour modification, diet and exercise.

Methylxanthines

The **methylxanthines** – such as caffeine (Drug Monograph 23.2), theophylline, theobromine and the herbal medicine *Paullinia cupana* (commonly known as guarana) – are naturally occurring chemicals found in beverages such as coffee, tea, cocoa and cola drinks. Xanthine itself occurs naturally in our bodies, as a metabolite of the purine base adenine (a constituent of DNA and RNA); excessive breakdown of cells or impaired excretory pathways produces excess uric acid (hyperuricaemia) which deposits in joints in gout.

Caffeine

Caffeine is also present in many foods, over-the-counter drugs, prescription drugs and 'energy drinks'; it is probably the most commonly used stimulant worldwide. A large daily intake of caffeine-containing products may increase alertness but may also induce insomnia and heart dysrhythmias in some people, especially the elderly. Aspects of caffeine related to the social use of, and dependence on, caffeine-containing products are discussed in Chapter 25. The clinical use of methylxanthines as bronchodilators is considered in Chapter 15 (Drug Monograph 15.3).

Mechanism of action

The mechanism of action of caffeine was initially postulated to involve raising of cyclic adenosine monophosphate (cAMP) levels through blocking of the enzyme phosphodiesterase leading to smooth muscle relaxation and other effects. However, it is now recognised that the concentrations required for this action are probably not reached in clinical (or social) doses (Drug Monograph 23.2).

The effects of caffeine are primarily due to non-selective antagonism of adenosine receptors. Adenosine is an endogenous nucleoside and a neuromodulator that is structurally similar to caffeine. Adenosine mediates CNS depression, has cardiac depressant and bronchoconstrictor effects, inhibits platelet aggregation and is an important regulator of blood flow (vasodilator in most regions, including the coronary circulation, but vasoconstrictor in the renal and cerebral circulations). Adenosine is used clinically in supraventricular tachycardias: rapid IV injection decreases atrioventricular conduction and effectively converts the dysrhythmia to sinus rhythm.

By antagonising adenosine A_1 and A_{2A} receptors, methylxanthines oppose these effects and indirectly lead to cardiac stimulatory effects, increased cAMP levels and contraction of the smooth muscle of coronary vessels and relaxation of smooth muscle in the airways – hence the pharmacological effects described.

Some of the behavioural effects of caffeine may be mediated by dopamine. By antagonising inhibitory effects of adenosine on dopamine receptors, caffeine may indirectly stimulate dopamine activity. This mechanism could explain the similarities between the behavioural effects of caffeine, amphetamines and cocaine; the interplay between adenosine and dopamine receptors in reward and addiction is being investigated.

Pharmacological effects of caffeine

Because caffeine has effects on many body functions and is so widely used, both its short-term and possible long-term effects are important. Overall, moderate habitual coffee intake is not a health hazard; consumption of up to 400 mg caffeine/day in healthy adults is not associated with adverse effects (Reyes & Cornelis 2018).

Central nervous system stimulation

Although all levels of the CNS may be affected, regular doses of caffeine (100–150 mg) will stimulate the cortex and produce increased alertness but decreased motor reaction time to both visual and auditory events. The mechanism is thought to be via antagonism of adenosine receptors and consequent enhancement of dopamine activity. Drowsiness and fatigue generally disappear. Larger doses may affect the medullary, vagus, vasomotor and respiratory centres, and the effects are dose-dependent (Temple et al. 2017).

Caffeine is thus useful for counteracting fatigue in shiftworkers and as a cognitive enhancer (but can cause anxiety). Caffeine also lifts the mood and may enhance

Drug Monograph 23.2
Caffeine

Indications

Caffeine is used to treat fatigue or drowsiness and as an adjunct to analgesics to enhance relief of pain; it is indicated as a respiratory stimulant in premature infants with respiratory difficulties and to aid in extubation.

Pharmacokinetics

Caffeine is rapidly and totally absorbed after oral administration. It is only 35–40% protein-bound and is distributed to all body compartments. It crosses the blood–brain barrier and enters the CNS, and passes readily through the placenta. The peak plasma level is achieved within 50–75 minutes, with therapeutic plasma levels in apnoea of prematurity of 8–20 mg/L.

Caffeine is metabolised in the liver. In adults, it is metabolised to paraxanthine, theophylline and theobromine, and thence via xanthine derivatives to uric acid; in the neonate, only a small portion is metabolised to theophylline. The half-life of caffeine is 3–10 hours (average 5 hours) in adults and 65–130 hours in neonates. In adults, caffeine metabolites are excreted by the kidneys, with only 1–2% excreted unchanged; in neonates, it is excreted by the kidneys, with about 85% excreted unchanged.

Drug interactions

The following effects may occur when caffeine is taken with other drugs: caffeine antagonises the antidysrhythmic actions of adenosine, so larger doses of adenosine may be needed, and the actions of dipyridamole (a phosphodiesterase inhibitor) when used in cardiac stress testing. Caffeine increases blood pressure and heart rate, so potentiates these effects of other drugs. When caffeine is taken along with other CNS-stimulating drugs, or other caffeine-containing medications or drinks, increased CNS stimulation, nervousness and dysrhythmias can occur.

Adverse reactions

Common adverse reactions include increased nervousness or anxiety and irritation of the gastrointestinal tract, resulting in dyspepsia and nausea. Adverse reactions in neonates include abdominal swelling or distension, vomiting, body tremors, tachycardia or nervousness, feed intolerance, irritability and reduced weight gain.

The toxic dose also depends on the development of tolerance with regular use of caffeine.

Significant effects in poisoning are rare, except after massive ingestions and the toxic dose is unclear. Ingestions of more than 15–30 mg/kg can cause mild to moderate toxicity; more than 100 mg/kg can cause severe and life-threatening toxicity.

Signs of overdose include raised temperature, headache, confusion, increased irritability and sensitivity to pain or touch, tinnitus, insomnia, palpitations, fine tremor, increased urination, dehydration, nausea and vomiting, abdominal pain and convulsions. A withdrawal syndrome of irritability, headache and increased weakness has been reported when users of more than 600 mg/day (about six cups of coffee) decrease or eliminate their intake.

Warnings and contraindications

Use with caution in people with insomnia, nervousness and tachycardia. Avoid use in people with caffeine or xanthine hypersensitivity; severe anxiety, including agoraphobia or panic attacks; severe cardiac disease; liver function impairment; or hypertension.

Dosage and administration

The maintenance dose in apnoea of prematurity is 5 mg/kg PO or IV, once daily after a loading dose. Caffeine is not recommended for use in children up to 12 years of age (except in neonatal respiratory distress). The adult dose is 100 mg orally, repeated in 3–4 hours if necessary to a maximum of 500 mg daily. (A standard cup of coffee contains 50–150 mg caffeine; espresso up to 600 mg.) Caffeine is present in some 'tonic' preparations in combination with vitamins and glucose; the usual dose of caffeine in these formulations is 100 mg.

the effects of antidepressants in major depression and has antidepressant effects; it has been shown to reduce the risk of suicide. Caffeine withdrawal leads to headaches, fatigue, decreased alertness and irritability;[3] it has therefore been used clinically to relieve postoperative caffeine withdrawal symptoms and for post-dural-puncture headaches. A study in Australian long-distance commercial vehicle drivers showed that those who consumed caffeinated products for the express purpose of staying awake had a 63% reduced likelihood of crashing compared with other drivers. However, commentators noted that 'coffee is no substitute for sleep' (Sharwood et al. 2013).

Caffeine is used in analgesic products, in combination with paracetamol or aspirin, in

3 This contributes to the morning 'hangover' in people who insist that they are not fit to be spoken to until they have had their morning 'hit' of coffee.

combination with paracetamol and phenylephrine in cold and flu preparations and in combination with ergotamine for treating migraine and other headaches, to enhance pain relief in these conditions (Ch 24). The enhanced effect of ergotamine may be a result of better absorption of the ergotamine in the presence of caffeine; caffeine itself may also have some direct antimigraine action.

Respiratory effects

Although the mechanism of action is not clearly defined, caffeine appears to stimulate the medullary respiratory centre and normalise autonomic function. Thus, it may be useful for treating apnoea in preterm infants and Cheyne-Stokes respiration in adults, as an adjunct to non-drug measures and as an alternative to theophylline. The methylxanthines are an important group of bronchodilator agents; in particular, aminophylline, a derivative of theophylline (Drug Monograph 15.3, in Ch 15), is used in Australia as an IV preparation for life-threatening asthma where the person is not responding to other therapy and in New Zealand is given via IV infusion or slow IV injection for chronic obstructive pulmonary disease and for paroxysmal dyspnoea associated with left heart failure.

Cardiovascular system

In low doses, caffeine is thought to enhance vagal stimulation and thus slow the heart. In higher doses, caffeine stimulates the myocardium, increasing both heart rate and cardiac output. Overstimulation may cause tachycardia and cardiac irregularities.

Depending on the dose, caffeine may cause either vasodilation or a reflex increase in systemic vascular resistance and vasoconstriction, which can cause a rise in blood pressure. This latter effect may be secondary to stimulation of the sympathetic nervous system and blockade of adenosine-induced vasodilation. Overall, caffeine has a weak vasodilator action, with little effect on blood pressure.

Musculoskeletal system

Caffeine affects voluntary skeletal muscles to increase the force of contraction and decrease muscle fatigue. These effects are via activation of the 'ryanodine receptor' family, activation of which opens calcium channels in the sarcoplasmic reticulum of skeletal muscle cells, causing calcium release and contraction of the muscle. The inherited predisposition for malignant hyperthermia, after being administered general anaesthetics combined with skeletal muscle relaxants, can be diagnosed by testing the effectiveness of caffeine in causing calcium release in a small sample of skeletal muscle removed at biopsy. Caffeine also has a general thermogenic action, increasing heat production, possibly via the hypothalamus or by enhancing catecholamine effects.

In animals, abnormalities of fetal bone and joint development have been shown in relation to high doses of caffeine. In humans, there is some evidence that high caffeine intake may increase urinary excretion of calcium, decreasing bone mineral density. This could have important implications for the development of osteoporosis, especially in postmenopausal women.

Other actions

In the gastrointestinal tract, caffeine increases secretion of pepsin and hydrochloric acid from the parietal cells; hence, coffee may cause dyspepsia, and intake is contraindicated in those who have a gastric or duodenal ulcer.

The methylxanthines produce a mild diuretic effect by increasing renal blood flow and glomerular filtration rate and by decreasing the tubular reabsorption of sodium and water. Theophylline is the only xanthine still used for this diuretic effect; however, the effect is well known to coffee drinkers and is additive with the diuretic effects of alcohol (Fig 23.2).

Caffeine also increases metabolic activity and may reduce the risk of metabolic syndrome, inhibits uterine contractions, transiently raises glucose levels by stimulating glycolysis, and raises catecholamine levels in plasma and urine. It is a marker drug for activities of various enzymes, including CYP1A2, *N*-acetyltransferase and xanthine.

KEY POINTS

Caffeine and methylxanthines

- Caffeine and other methylxanthine alkaloids are CNS stimulants that are present in many beverages and medications. They have diverse pharmacological effects and are used as mild CNS stimulants, bronchodilators and social drugs.
- The mechanism of action of caffeine may involve raising of cAMP levels through blocking of the enzyme phosphodiesterase, leading to smooth muscle relaxation and other effects. Studies indicate that the effects of caffeine are primarily due to antagonism of adenosine receptors.

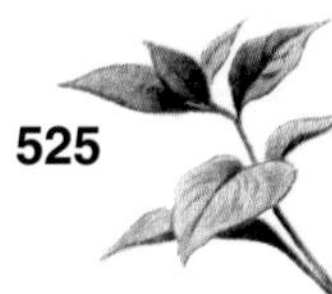

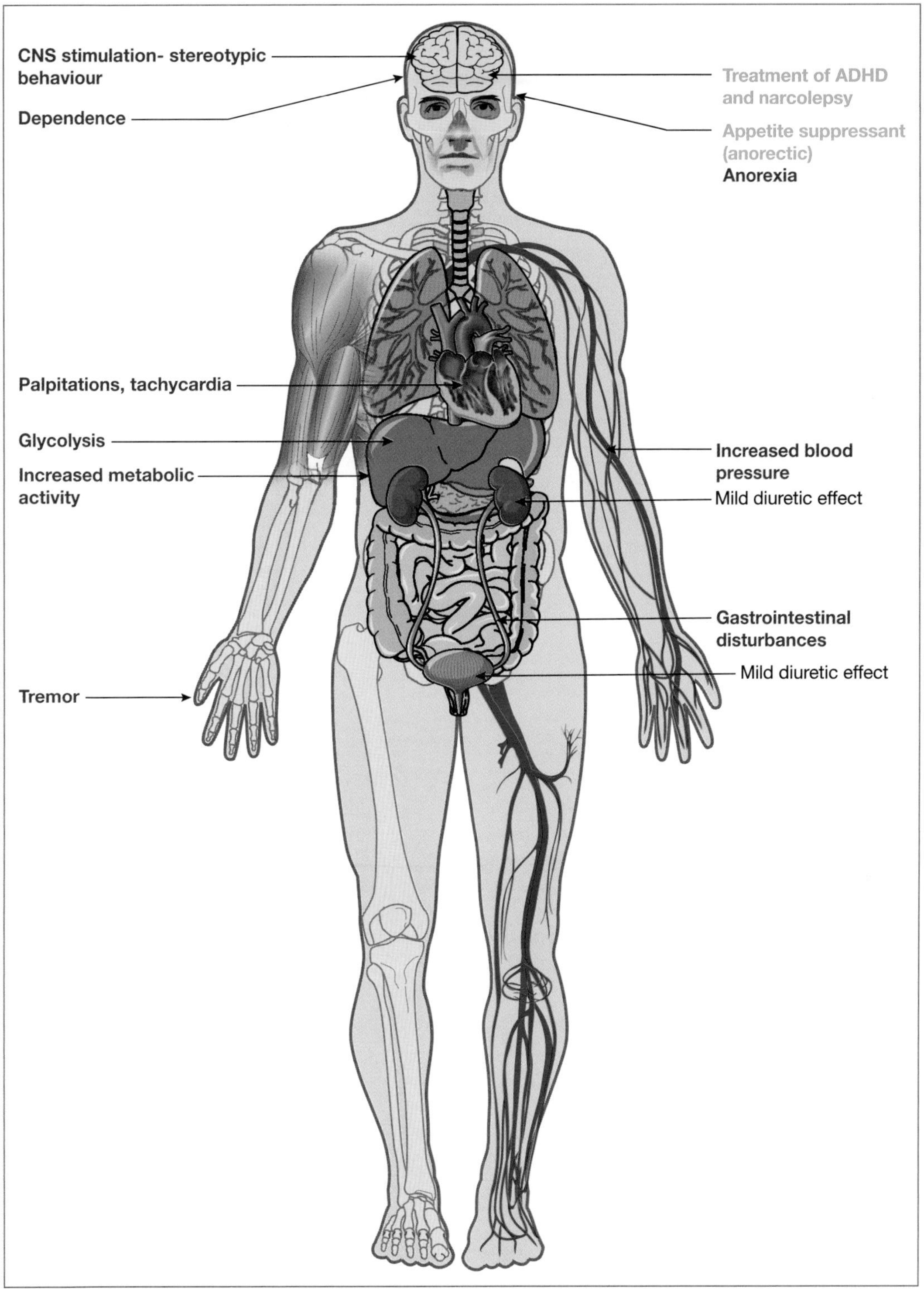

CNS stimulation- stereotypic behaviour
Dependence
Treatment of ADHD and narcolepsy
Appetite suppressant (anorectic)
Anorexia
Palpitations, tachycardia
Glycolysis
Increased metabolic activity
Increased blood pressure
Mild diuretic effect
Gastrointestinal disturbances
Mild diuretic effect
Tremor

FIGURE 23.2 Clinical uses and adverse effects of stimulants

DRUGS AT A GLANCE
Central nervous system stimulants

THERAPEUTIC GROUP AND EFFECT	KEY EXAMPLES	CLINICAL USE
CNS stimulants Amphetamines: • Inhibit the noradrenaline transporter (NET) and the release of noradrenaline from storage sites in nerve terminals (hence, an indirect sympathomimetic effect) • Directly stimulate α- and β-adrenoceptor sites • Inhibit the dopamine transporter (DAT) enhancing dopaminergic transmission • Facilitate the movement of DA out of vesicles and into the cytoplasm • Modulate the 5-HT (serotonin) transporter (SERT), enhancing serotonergic transmission	Dexamfetamine Lisdexamfetamine Methylphenidate	ADHD Narcolepsy
Non-amphetamine like drugs • May be involved with histaminergic and orexinergic systems. It improves alertness	Modafinil	Excessive sleepiness associated with narcolepsy and idiopathic hypersomnolence
Anorectics	Phentermine	Weight loss
Methylxanthines • Antagonise adenosine A_1 and A_{2A} receptors, and resultant cardiac stimulatory effects, increased cyclic adenosine monophosphate (cAMP) levels	Caffeine	Combined with aspirin/paracetamol preparations for migraine Social drug, cognition enhancer
	Theophylline	Bronchodilator

REVIEW EXERCISES

1 JB, a 7-year-old boy, has been having difficulty at school. His teacher has reported learning difficulties compounded by behaviour issues; he is easily distracted in the classroom. JB is diagnosed with ADHD. As well as seeing a psychologist for behavioural issues he is prescribed dexamfetamine at a starting dose of 0.5 mg in the morning for 1 week. What is the pharmacological class and mechanism of action of this drug? How is it useful in the treatment of ADHD?

2 Ms PQ is a 30-year-old shop assistant who seeks advice from her GP regarding her inability to lose weight despite trying to reduce her food intake. She has a knee injury and is currently unable to exercise. She currently weighs 100 kg and has a body mass index of 30 kg/m². She wishes to try pharmacological management. Her GP prescribes phentermine 15 mg at breakfast. Why has phentermine been promoted as being advantageous over previous anorectic drugs that were removed from the market, such as fenfluramine?

REFERENCES

Kooij JJS, Bijlenga D, Salerno L, et al. Updated European Consensus Statement on diagnosis and treatment of adult ADHD. European Psychiatry. 2019; Feb; 56:14–34. doi: 10.1016/j.eurpsy.2018.11.001. Epub 2018 Nov 16. PMID: 30453134.https://doi.org/10.1016/j.eurpsy.2018.11.001.

Laurence DR: Clinical pharmacology, ed 4, Edinburgh, 1973, Churchill Livingstone

Psychotropic Expert Group: Therapeutic guidelines: psychotropics. Melbourne: Therapeutic Guidelines Limited, 2021. Etg complete

Reyes CM, Cornelis MC. Caffeine in the diet: country-level consumption and guidelines. nutrients. 2018; Nov 15; 10(11):1772. doi:10.3390/nu10111772. PMID: 30445721; PMCID: PMC6266969.

Sharwood LN, Elkington J, Meuleners L, et al: Use of caffeinated substances and risk of crashes in long distance drivers of commercial vehicles: case-control study. BMJ; 2013; 346: f1140 (published online)

Temple JL, Bernard C, Lipshultz SE, et al. The safety of ingested caffeine: a comprehensive review. Frontiers in Psychiatry. 2017. 8. 80. https://www.frontiersin.org/article/10.3389/fpsyt.2017.00080

ONLINE RESOURCES

New Zealand Medicines and Medical Devices Safety Authority: https://www.medsafe.govt.nz/ (accessed January 2022)

Pharmaceutical Benefits Scheme – to review the use of PBS-listed medicines used in the management of ADHD: https://www.pbs.gov.au/info/industry/listing/participants/public-release-docs/2015-06/attention-deficit-hyperactivity-disorder-2015-06-prd

Food Standards Australia & New Zealand – Caffeine report 2019: https://www.foodstandards.gov.au/Documents/CaffeineReport2019.pdf (accessed January 2022)

More weblinks at: http://evolve.elsevier.com/AU/Knights/pharmacology/.

CHAPTER 24

DRUGS FOR NEURODEGENERATIVE DISORDERS AND HEADACHE

Shaunagh Darroch

KEY ABBREVIATIONS

ACh	acetylcholine
COMT	catechol-O-methyltransferase
DA	dopamine
DDC	dopa decarboxylase
DDCI	dopa decarboxylase inhibitor
GABA	gamma-aminobutyric acid

KEY TERMS

akinesia 533
Alzheimer's disease 542
amyloid 543
anticholinergics 537
anticholinesterase agents 529
bradykinesia 531
delirium 544
dementia 541
dopa decarboxylase 532
dystonia 531
dyskinesia 533
headache 548
migraine 545
motor neurone disease 540
multiple sclerosis 538
myasthenia gravis 539
on–off syndrome 535
Parkinson's disease 531
restless legs syndrome 539
skeletal muscle relaxant 529
spasms 528
spasticity 529
stroke 545

Chapter Focus

This chapter covers drugs used in treating neurodegenerative disorders such as Parkinson's disease, myasthenia gravis, multiple sclerosis and dementias, including Alzheimer's disease. Drugs with centrally mediated actions on skeletal muscle are also discussed; these medications are used to treat muscle spasm and spasticity. The actions of the drugs are related to neurotransmitter imbalances, especially of dopamine and acetylcholine in motor function. Also discussed are drugs used to treat headache, along with the role of 5-hydroxytryptamine in the pathogenesis of migraine and the use of 5-HT agonists and antagonists in treatment and prophylaxis.

KEY DRUG GROUPS

Anticholinesterase:

- **Pyridostigmine**

Antimigraine agents:

- 5-HT agonists triptans: **sumatriptan** (Drug Monograph 24.4)
- 5-HT antagonists: **methysergide**
- CGRP receptor antagonists: erenumab
- Monoclonal antibodies: fremanezumab and galcanezumab

Antiparkinson agents:

- Anticholinergics: **benzatropine, trihexyphenidyl (benzhexol)**
- Dopamine agonists: **apomorphine**, pramipexole, **rotigotine**, cabergoline, bromocriptine
- Drugs raising dopamine levels: **amantadine**, **entacapone**, MAO-B inhibitors: **selegiline** (Drug Monograph 24.3)
- **Levodopa** with dopa decarboxylase inhibitor
- **Carbidopa** (Drug Monograph 24.2) or benserazide

Drugs for dementias:

- Centrally acting anticholinesterases: **donepezil**, **galantamine**, **rivastigmine**
- NMDA antagonist: **memantine**

Drugs for movement disorders:

- Amyotrophic lateral sclerosis: **riluzole**
- Multiple sclerosis: **glatiramer**, **natalizumab**
- Huntington's chorea, senile chorea and tardive dyskinesia: tetrabenazine
- Restless legs syndrome: ropinirole

Skeletal muscle relaxants:

- Centrally-acting: **baclofen** (Drug Monograph 24.1), peripherally-acting: **botulinum toxin**, **dantrolene**

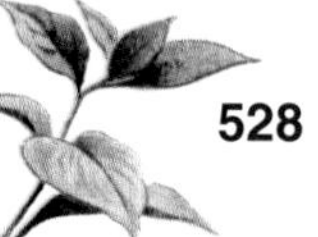

CRITICAL THINKING SCENARIO

Johan is a 70-year-old retired accountant who complains that over the past year he has had occasional falls, a shuffling gait and a trembling hand. Parkinson's disease is diagnosed, and his doctor discusses the option of taking a levodopa-benserazide combination. He says he would prefer to take a medication that he only needs to take once daily as he is already taking tranylcypromine for his bipolar disorder and propranolol for his hypertension. He is prescribed pramipexole controlled release tablets to a final dose of 1.5 mg.

One month later, he returns for follow-up. On discussion it becomes apparent that he is quite anxious about his increasingly obsessive behaviours; he spends much of the time in gaming venues, describing his compulsion to spend on the poker machines. He also notes that he sometimes has trouble staying awake when performing his daily duties.

1. What is the mechanism of action of pramipexole?
2. Discuss the possibility of drug interactions as a cause of his behaviours.
3. What other drugs could he be prescribed to treat his Parkinson's disease?

Introduction

Neurodegenerative pathologies

The neurodegenerative disorders include conditions such as Parkinson's disease, myasthenia gravis, multiple sclerosis, other movement and neuromuscular disorders, such as motor neurone disease and the dementias, including Alzheimer's disease and stroke-related cognitive impairments. Pathological processes occurring in these dysfunctions are not completely understood, and good animal models of the diseases and specific drug therapies are not always available.

Currently, there are no cures for these conditions, so drug therapies are used to minimise the symptoms. In some conditions, novel techniques involving transplantation of neurons, stem cell therapy and gene therapy are being trialled.

The motor nervous system

Central and peripheral control of motor function and skeletal muscles are discussed in Chapters 8 and 18 (in sections on central nervous system [CNS] functional systems and neurotransmitters); these areas are background to drugs used in neurodegenerative conditions and movement disorders. Drugs may affect central control of motor activity via actions on gamma-aminobutyric acid (GABA) or dopamine (DA) receptors. (Psychotropic agents are also considered in Ch 22.) In the periphery, drugs affecting transmission at the neuromuscular junction via acetylcholine (ACh) receptors are used in many clinical contexts – for example, as skeletal muscle relaxants during surgical operations, to stimulate ACh receptors in muscle weakness and to relieve spasticity and spasms in skeletal muscle.

Movement and neuromuscular disorders

Movement disorders may be classified as hyperkinetic, with excessive movement – for example, tremor or tics; or hypokinetic, with inadequate movement, such as in bradykinesia. Movement is also impaired in neuromuscular disorders, muscle cramps, muscular dystrophies, various types of myositis, myasthenia gravis, palsies and motor neurone disease. The most common movement disorders are restless legs syndrome, essential tremor and Parkinson's disease.

Skeletal muscle spasm and spasticity

Skeletal muscle **spasms**, or cramps, result when there is an involuntary contraction of muscles accompanied by pain or limited function. Most are caused by local injuries, but some result from low calcium or sodium levels, epileptic myoclonic seizures or disease of the spinal nerves and their roots as a result of degenerative osteoarthritis, herniated discs or spondylosis. Skeletal muscle injuries and strains are usually self-limiting and can be treated with rest, physiotherapy or immobilisation by use of casts, neck collars, crutches or arm slings. When tissue damage and oedema and pain are present, anti-inflammatory drugs and weak opioid analgesics such as codeine can be used.

Spasticity (a form of muscular hypertonicity with increased resistance to stretch) occurs when gamma motor neurons, which tonically control muscle spindle contractile activity, become hyperactive as the result of stroke, closed head injuries, cerebral palsy, multiple sclerosis, spinal cord trauma and other neurological disorders. Spinal spasticity can be identified by a marked loss of inhibitory influences with hyperactive tendon stretch reflexes, clonus (alternating contraction and relaxation of muscles), primitive flexion withdrawal reflexes and a flexed posture. Varying degrees of spasm of the smooth muscle of the bladder and bowel can also occur. Cerebral spasticity is associated with less reflex excitability, increased or impaired muscle tone and no primitive flexion withdrawal reflexes or flexed posture. Spasticity may require long-term use of muscle-relaxing agents.

Drug treatment of movement disorders

Drugs affecting skeletal muscles

Anticholinesterases

The **anticholinesterase agents** enhance cholinergic actions by inhibiting cholinesterase enzymes that inactivate ACh at cholinergic nerve terminals (Ch 8: Figs 8.5 and 8.6; Drug Monograph 8.3 neostigmine). This permits the accumulation of ACh and enhanced effects at autonomic ganglia, parasympathetic neuroeffector junctions and neuromuscular junctions. In degenerative neuromuscular conditions such as myasthenia gravis they may improve muscle weakness. They are also used for reversal of neuromuscular blockade agents. Anticholinesterases that are lipid-soluble and cross the blood–brain barrier are used for central effects on cholinergic transmission, especially in dementias (see later section). In conditions such as myasthenia gravis drugs used do not cross into the CNS.

Anticholinesterases are divided into three groups based on their duration of action, determined by the type of binding to the enzyme (Ch 8). Of the medium-acting agents, pyridostigmine has better oral bioavailability than neostigmine, a longer half-life and fewer gastrointestinal tract (GIT) adverse reactions, so it is the first-line drug for myasthenia gravis (antimyasthenic; discussed later, see Fig 24.3).

Overdose or poisoning with an anticholinesterase causes toxic effects in the peripheral nervous system ('SLUD syndrome') and CNS (Ch 8; Table 8.4 and Clinical Focus Box 8.2). These agents are rapidly absorbed through the skin, so they have been used as chemical warfare agents and insecticides. The antidote is atropine, a drug commonly carried in ambulances and administered by paramedics; after intravenous (IV) administration, effects peak within 5 minutes.

Skeletal muscle relaxants

Centrally and direct- (peripherally) acting skeletal muscle relaxants

Centrally and directly- acting **skeletal muscle relaxants** are used in muscle spasticity and spasms that do not respond to other therapy. These drugs include the centrally acting baclofen (Drug Monograph 24.1) and diazepam (Drug Monograph 20.1, see Ch 20) and the direct-acting dantrolene (they are more effective in the treatment of spinal spasticity than cerebral spasticity; concurrent physiotherapy is always required for optimal treatment).

Centrally-acting skeletal muscle relaxants

Baclofen and benzodiazepines

The main centrally acting antispastic agents are baclofen and diazepam, both of which act via enhancing GABA inhibitory transmission, inhibiting motor neurons mainly in the spinal cord. (A related compound, gamma-hydroxybutyric acid, previously used as an anaesthetic agent, is subject to abuse as a street drug – see under 'Hallucinogens' in Ch 25.)

Tetrabenazine

Tetrabenazine is a centrally acting skeletal muscle relaxant that acts via DA pathways. It releases monoamine neurotransmitters and depletes brain DA levels, and thus causes sedation and muscle relaxation. It was formerly used as a neuroleptic agent, but causes parkinsonism, extrapyramidal effects and depression, so is now used only occasionally in the treatment of movement disorders such as Huntington's chorea and tardive dyskinesia.

Adverse reactions

Tetrabenazine causes CNS depression in the brainstem, thalamus, basal ganglia and spinal cord, resulting in relaxation of striated muscle; CNS depression accompanies the muscle relaxation. Adverse reactions of drowsiness, blurred vision, light-headedness, headache and feelings of weakness, lassitude and lethargy make their long-term use undesirable. Excessive muscle relaxation can cause serious adverse reactions of dysphagia (difficulty in swallowing) and choking.

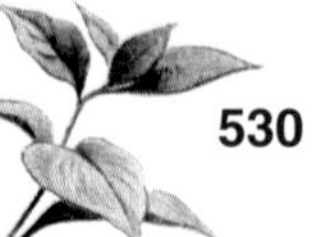

Drug Monograph 24.1
Baclofen

Effects of baclofen are mediated via GABA receptors. Baclofen is a selective agonist at presynaptic $GABA_B$ receptors; by inhibition of adenylyl cyclase it blocks calcium channels and thus inhibits the release of transmitters from many types of nerve terminals; it has an antispastic action via the spinal cord, inhibiting activation of motor neurons.

Indications

Baclofen is used orally in the treatment of spasticity resulting from multiple sclerosis and spinal cord lesions or from injuries to the spinal cord or head injury; it may be effective in spasticity associated with cerebral palsy, but not in epilepsy. It may also reduce pain in people with spasticity by inhibiting substance P release in the spinal cord.

Pharmacokinetics

Absorption after oral administration (with meals) is generally good (bioavailability 70–80%) but can vary among individuals.

Baclofen crosses the blood–brain barrier and acts centrally. The time to peak plasma concentration is 2–3 hours. The onset of action is variable and can occur in hours or may take weeks. Baclofen has a half-life of 2.5–6 hours and is partly metabolised in the liver. It is excreted in the kidneys 70% unchanged.

Drug interactions

Enhanced CNS-depressant and hypotensive effects can occur when baclofen is given with other CNS-depressant medications (including alcohol), antihypertensive agents or monoamine oxidase inhibitors (MAOIs) or tricyclic antidepressants (TCAs). With levodopa, there is increased risk of psychotic reactions.

Adverse reactions

Common adverse effects include: transient drowsiness, headache, vertigo, confusion, muscle weakness, nausea, hallucinations, respiratory and cardiovascular depression, urinary disorders, tinnitus and GIT upset.

Warnings and contraindications

- Severe withdrawal syndrome may occur if baclofen is withdrawn suddenly.
- Use with caution in people with cerebral lesions, cerebrovascular accident, diabetes mellitus, seizure disorders, kidney impairment, hepatic impairment, respiratory disease or a history of psychiatric problems, and in the elderly. Not recommended for cerebral palsy.
- In cases of renal impairment, the dose is initially 5 mg once daily; titrate dose cautiously according to response and give after dialysis. Toxicity (e.g. encephalopathy) has occurred after low doses in people with renal impairment.
- Use with extreme caution in children under 16 years.
- There is limited data available for use in pregnancy. An increased risk of congenital malformations has been associated with baclofen, and neonatal seizures (due to baclofen withdrawal) have been reported following in utero exposure
- Avoid use in people with peptic ulcer or known baclofen hypersensitivity.
- Drug withdrawal must be slow and gradual over 1–2 weeks to avoid rebound spasticity and CNS disturbances.

Dosage and administration

Baclofen is given orally, initially 5 mg three times daily; increasing gradually by 15 mg daily every fourth day until therapeutic effect is obtained. The usual range is 10–25 mg three times daily. Doses up to 100 mg daily may be given in hospitalised people.

In the elderly baclofen is given initially 5–10 mg daily in divided doses; increase by smaller increments and at longer intervals.

Peripherally acting skeletal muscle relaxants

Neuromuscular blocking agents

Neuromuscular blocking agents are clinically the most important skeletal muscle relaxants; they are discussed in detail in Chapter 8 and Chapter 18, under 'Adjuncts to Anaesthesia' – 'Muscle Relaxants'. The two groups are:

- non-depolarising drugs, which compete with ACh at the neuromuscular junction end-plate and antagonise nicotinic receptors and thus cause flaccid paralysis as exemplified by curare and rocuronium (Drug Monograph 8.5).
- depolarising blockers (suxamethonium, Drug Monograph 8.5), which activate the nicotinic receptors, leading to loss of excitability, and cause muscle twitching followed by short-duration paralysis.

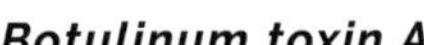

Botulinum toxin A

The type A toxin from the bacterium *Clostridium botulinum* has long been known to be poisonous, causing botulism from food poisoning when the anaerobic organisms multiply in poorly preserved or refrigerated food. The toxin blocks release of ACh from cholinergic nerves and thus causes a chemical denervation (Ch 8). It has a permanent toxic effect, decreasing muscle tone and contractility, leading to flaccid paralysis and atrophy of the affected muscles. It is a protein toxin and extraordinarily potent: it is estimated that less than 10–12 g (1 picogram) will kill a mouse.

These effects are used clinically in parenteral administration of the toxin to specific muscle groups undergoing involuntary spasm – for example, in blepharospasm (uncontrollable winking or sustained tight closure of the eyes due to spasm of the eyelid muscles; see Drug Monograph 40.3), equinus foot deformity or other focal muscle **dystonias**. Botulinum toxin is also used to paralyse superficial facial muscles to (apparently) reduce wrinkles: the toxin is injected subcutaneously (SC) to the muscle and relieves muscle spasm for several months until new motor end-plates sprout and re-innervation occurs.

Botulinum toxin A is contraindicated in myasthenia gravis, which it exacerbates, and has adverse interactions with aminoglycoside antibiotics and other drugs that impair ACh release and cause neuromuscular blockade. Adverse reactions include muscle weakness in muscle groups adjacent to the site of injection.

Dantrolene

Dantrolene, a direct-acting relaxant, is used in the treatment of spasticity, especially upper motor neuron disorders such as multiple sclerosis, cerebral palsy, spinal cord injury and cerebrovascular accident, and in prophylaxis and treatment of malignant hyperthermia that may occur during surgery.

It directly relaxes skeletal muscle by inhibiting release of calcium from the sarcoplasmic reticulum to the myoplasm, dissociating excitation–contraction coupling and decreasing muscle contraction in response to the action potential. It acts by antagonising ryanodine receptors. Dantrolene reduces both monosynaptic- and polysynaptic-induced muscle contractions.

Available orally (for chronic spasticity) and parenterally (for malignant hypothermia), oral absorption is incomplete and slow; the onset of action when dantrolene is used to treat the spasticity of upper motor neurons can take 1 week or more. When given concurrently with other CNS depressants, an increase in CNS-depressant effects can result.

Adverse effects include diarrhoea, dizziness, sleepiness, unusual fatigue, muscle weakness, bladder dysfunction, hepatotoxicity, respiratory and cardiovascular effects and, haematological and CNS changes. Potentially fatal hepatitis can occur, so liver function should be monitored. Use with caution in people with myopathy, pulmonary function impairment and neuromuscular diseases and in people over 35 years of age (especially women) as they have increased potential for hepatotoxicity. Caution against driving or other hazardous occupations.

Parkinson's disease

Parkinson's disease is a progressively debilitating movement disorder particularly affecting the basal ganglia, a series of paired nuclei in the cerebral hemispheres including the corpus striatum (caudate nucleus and putamen; see Ch 18, Fig 18.5C) and globus pallidus, which regulate the tone and characteristics of all voluntary movements. There is loss of dopaminergic neurons in the basal ganglia and degeneration in the substantia nigra. It is characterised by tremors at rest, **bradykinesia** (abnormal slowing of all voluntary movements and speech), forward flexion of the trunk, muscle rigidity, loss of postural reflexes and muscle weakness. Other associated disabling symptoms include depression, anxiety, autonomic dysfunctions (GIT and bladder) and sleep disturbances. Specialist neurologists are usually involved in long-term management of people.

It is estimated that 1–2 per 1000 people in Australia have Parkinson's disease, with the incidence increasing to 1 per 100 over the age of 60 (Parkinson's Western Australia 2022). The number of people with Parkinson's in New Zealand has increased by 60 per cent over the past 14 years, from an estimated 7,000 in 2006 to 11,000 in 2020 (New Zealand Brain Research Institute 2022). It occurs usually between the ages of 50 and 80 years, affecting both sexes equally.

Aetiologies

The cause of DA deficiency in motor-associated areas is unknown, with head injury, genetic factors, viral influences, oxidative damage and environmental contaminants having been suspected. Parkinsonism is classified as idiopathic (no known cause), postencephalitic (particularly after viral encephalitis), degenerative (e.g. due to arteriosclerosis) or drug-induced (Pajares et al. 2020).

Drug-induced parkinsonism

Movement disorders, extrapyramidal effects, including parkinsonian symptoms, are induced by chronic administration of DA receptor antagonists such as the antipsychotic agents phenothiazines (chlorpromazine) and haloperidol (for drug-induced parkinsonism, see Ch 22, Fig 22.1 and Table 22.1); the atypical antipsychotics are less likely to produce extrapyramidal adverse effects. Other drugs causing parkinsonism include antidepressants, calcium channel blockers, antihistamines and some antiepileptics) (Bondon-Guitton et al. 2011) and 'designer drugs' (i.e. chemical variations of illegal or controlled substances), which are usually not yet illegal but are produced to mimic the psychoactive effects of various illegal products (see example below).

Effect of MPTP on DA pathways

The designer drug 1-methyl-4-phenyl-1, 2, 3, 6-tetrahydropyridine (MPTP), initially a contaminant of a pethidine analogue from clandestine laboratories, has been sold as synthetic heroin, cocaine or other 'street drugs'. MPTP may induce a severe degenerative CNS disorder characterised by tremors and muscle paralysis similar to the symptoms of Parkinson's disease; the paralysis may become permanent. MPTP causes irreversible destruction selectively of the nigrostriatal dopaminergic pathways in animal species, and is used as a model of parkinsonism in which to study the actions of drugs and other potentially useful treatments (Langston 2017).

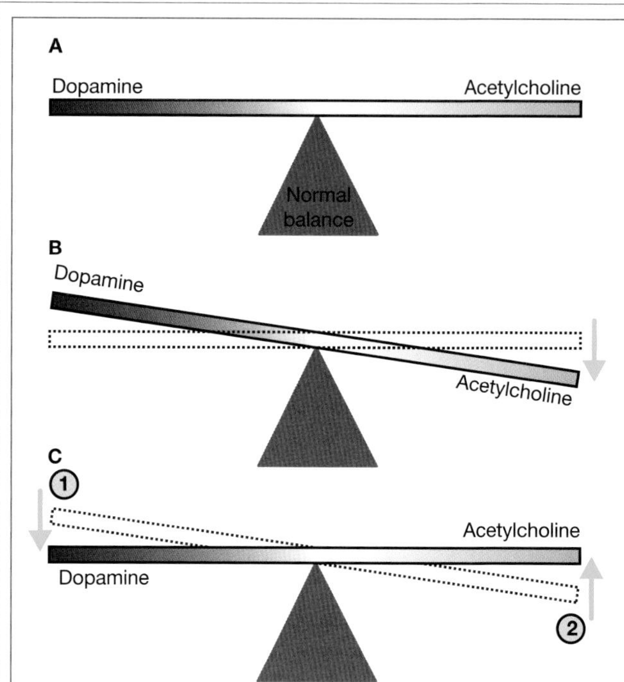

FIGURE 24.1 Central acetylcholine/dopamine balance
A Normal 'balance' of ACh and DA. **B** In Parkinson's disease, a decrease in dopamine results in an ACh–DA imbalance: cholinergic effects outweigh dopaminergic. **C** Drug therapy for Parkinson's disease focuses on (1) increasing the availability of DA or stimulating DA receptors, which restores the ACh–DA balance towards normal, and/or (2) blocking ACh receptors with anticholinergic agents.

Pathology: dopamine deficiency

The CNS has five main types of DA receptors (Ch 18, Table 18.1). The exact roles of some are not currently known (although D_1 receptor activation is necessary for maximal expression of D_2 receptor activity), but D_2 – and especially D_{2A}–receptors are particularly involved with motor effects.

The biosynthetic pathways for catecholamine neurotransmitters are shown in Chapter 9. The essential amino acids phenylalanine and tyrosine are converted in adrenergic nerves to dopa (dihydroxyphenylalanine), which is rapidly metabolised to DA by the enzyme **dopa decarboxylase** (DDC), a general aromatic amino acid decarboxylase and then to noradrenaline (norepinephrine) in specific neurons.

Most of the signs and symptoms of Parkinson's disease are caused by a DA-deficiency state in the extrapyramidal motor system (Ch 18, Fig 18.5C), particularly in the nigrostriatal tracts; levels of DA, an inhibitory transmitter, in the basal ganglia fall to as low as 20% of normal levels. This produces a DA/ACh imbalance, with a relative increase in ACh (an excitatory neurotransmitter) and thus impaired regulation of posture, muscle tone and voluntary movement (Figs 18.6 and 24.1). Ongoing inflammation contributes to progression of the condition. The anatomical and physiological pathways are considerably more complex and there is much research into the aetiology and treatment of Parkinson's disease (Pajares et al. 2020).

Amounts of other neurotransmitters (noradrenaline, 5-HT, somatostatin, substance P and enkephalins) are also decreased in Parkinson's disease. Altered 5-HT transmission plays an important role in many of the non-motor features and treatment-related complications (Qamhawi et al. 2015). Nicotinic cholinergic receptors interact with DA in the basal ganglia, and there is some evidence that nicotine protects against neurotoxin-induced nigrostriatal damage. Selective estrogen receptor modulators may also be neuroprotective. Increased glutamate levels have been detected in people with Parkinson's disease and hence a role for glutamate in the pathological processes is proposed (Zhang et al. 2019). There may be a role for NMDA receptor antagonists. Parkinsonian symptoms are present in other disorders, including dementia with Lewy bodies (see later section).

Gene therapy and cell transplantation techniques

The goals of gene and transplantation therapy in Parkinson's disease have been pursued since the 1970s. In animal models, DA-producing cells can be grown from stem cells and transplanted into brains of mature animals, where they appear to function as normal nigrostriatal-type cells. Similar work in humans has produced functioning dopaminergic neurons from cell culture of human embryonic or postnatal fibroblast cells or stem cells, by providing in cell cultures the requisite transcriptional factors and directing expression of the two genes involved in DA neuron generation (Maiti et al. 2017).

Transplantation into human adult brains of human fetal mesencephalic DA-rich tissue can generate fully functioning and safe midbrain DA neurons; however, there are few long-term results and demonstrated lack of efficacy in treating the disease. There has been subsequent occurrence of **dyskinesias** in operated patients, grafted neurons showing disease-related pathologies or being destroyed by the disease and non-motor symptoms. Technologies are improving, and some people with grafts that are functioning well have exhibited long-term recovery of motor control (Kordower & Olanov 2016; Parmar et al. 2020). Newer therapies undergoing clinical trials include electrical stimulation, grafts and growth factor administration (Troncoso-Escudero et al. 2020).

Pharmacotherapy

No agents have yet been found that cure the condition or slow its progression. Non-drug therapies that have been tried include physiotherapy, deep brain stimulation, surgery to specific tracts in the CNS and transplantation of dopaminergic neuronal tissue from fetal CNS.

Drug treatment is usually not started until symptoms become disturbing to the person. It focuses on symptomatic relief by correcting the DA–ACh imbalance via raising DA levels or blocking ACh effects. The classes of drugs used in treatment include: (1) drugs that raise brain DA levels or stimulate DA receptors to enhance dopaminergic mechanisms; (2) drugs with central anticholinergic activity (anticholinergics and antihistamines); and (3) other drugs as adjuncts and for symptomatic relief, such as anti-inflammatory agents, decongestants, laxatives and antipsychotics. Choice of drugs depends on which symptoms are most troublesome; severe tremor requires use of anticholinergic agents. Initial treatment is usually with levodopa plus a dopa decarboxylase inhibitor (DDCI), or a DA agonist (rotigotine).

This is an exciting area of pharmacological research, with many new molecules undergoing development and clinical trials: esterified forms of levodopa, DA reuptake inhibitors and new formulations of older drugs (Müller 2021). In addition, efforts are being made to treat dyskinesias and to halt or reverse disease progression with neuroprotective agents (Parkinson's Foundation – see 'Online resources').

Drugs enhancing brain dopamine activity

Three classes of drugs enhance the action of brain DA: (1) those that raise brain levels of DA, (2) those that release DA and (3) directly acting dopaminergic agonists. Drugs enhancing brain DA mainly improve bradykinesia (slowed movements), **akinesia** (difficulty in initiating muscle movement, manifesting as mask-like facial expression, impairment of postural reflexes and, eventually, inability for self-care) and rigidity; but are less effective in relieving tremor.

Drugs that raise brain levels of dopamine

Levodopa: a prodrug

Levodopa is the first-line treatment for most people with Parkinson's disease; it is a precursor to DA that is not active if given systemically to 'top up' stores in the CNS (Fig 24.2). For this reason, large doses of levodopa used to be given, leading to major peripheral adverse reactions, including constipation, difficult urination, orthostatic hypotension, irregular heart rate and severe nausea or vomiting.

Drugs that inhibit breakdown of dopamine

Dopa decarboxylase inhibitors

Compounds have been developed that inhibit the DDC enzyme in the peripheral nervous system, allowing a greater proportion of the levodopa dose to enter the CNS. The DDCIs themselves do not pass the blood–brain barrier, so the enzyme is not inhibited in the CNS and DA is synthesised there. CNS dopaminergic pathways are replenished, DA release is facilitated and functional receptors are 'flooded' with DA. The dose of levodopa required when administered together with a DDCI is only 20% to 25% of that previously needed.

Carbidopa (Drug Monograph 24.2) or benserazide is administered orally in combination with levodopa; both are structural analogues of DA and competitive inhibitors of the decarboxylase enzyme. This strategy has been so successful in reducing the dose of levodopa required and the peripheral adverse reactions that levodopa is no longer available in Australia and New Zealand without a DDCI. CNS adverse effects are a greater risk with the combination because more levodopa reaches the brain to be converted to DA. Some tolerance develops to the adverse effects in the GIT.

Entacapone, a catechol-O-methyltransferase (COMT) inhibitor

The other main enzyme involved in metabolism of the catecholamines is COMT (see Fig 9.2, in Ch 9). Thus, a COMT inhibitor, analogous to an MAOI, will also inhibit inactivation of DA and levodopa and prolong clinical response to levodopa, increasing the 'on' time for motor response. Entacapone, a peripherally acting reversible and specific COMT inhibitor, is used as an adjunct to a

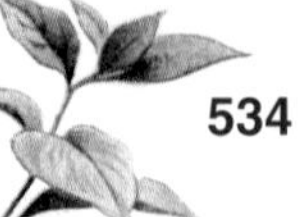

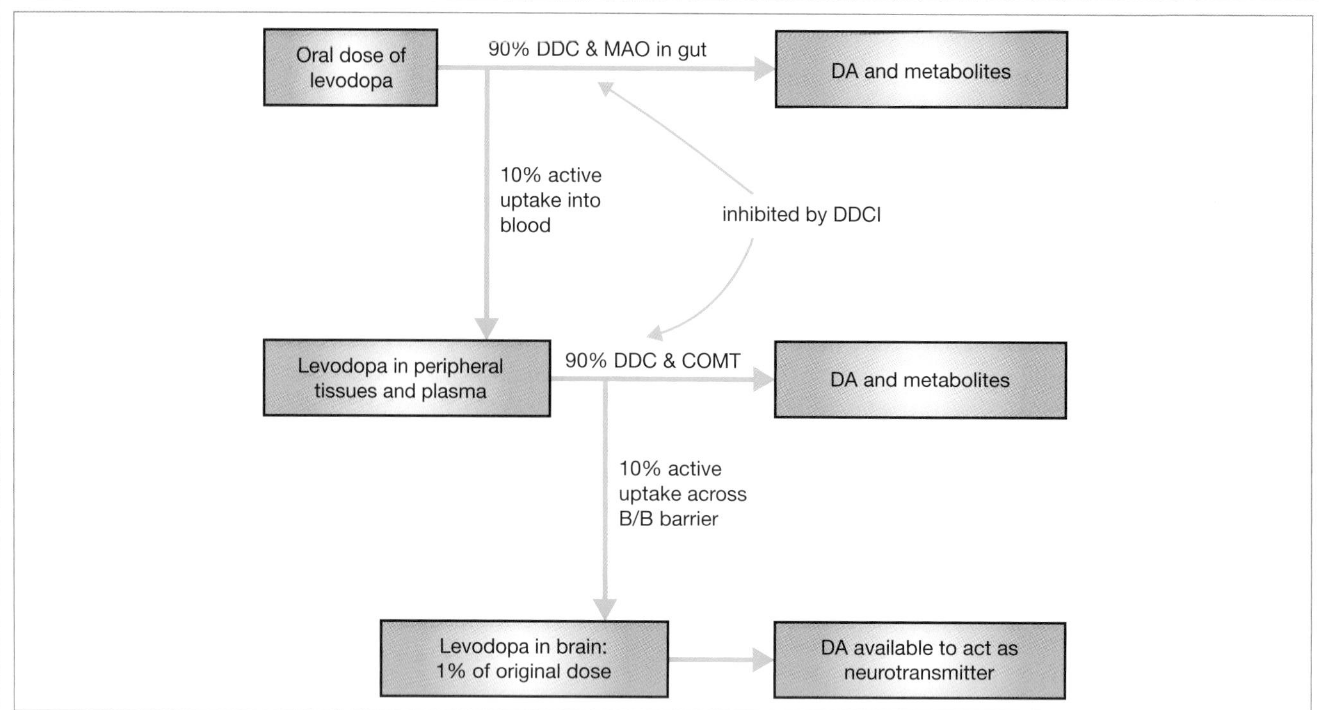

FIGURE 24.2 Levodopa in Parkinson's disease

Of the orally administered dose, about 99% is metabolised in the periphery by the enzymes DDC, MAO and catechol-O-methyltransferase (COMT), allowing only 1% to cross the blood–brain barrier and be converted to DA. In the presence of a DDCI that does not pass the blood–brain barrier, the enzyme in the periphery is inhibited, thus allowing a much greater proportion of administered dose to reach the CNS and be converted to active DA.

Drug Monograph 24.2
Levodopa-carbidopa

This combination formulation consists of **levodopa plus carbidopa** in a 4:1 or 10:1 ratio.

Indications

Levodopa-carbidopa is indicated in idiopathic, postencephalitic and symptomatic Parkinson's disease. It is particularly effective against rigidity and bradykinesia; tremor is less well treated.

Pharmacokinetics

Levodopa is absorbed by active transport; much is metabolised in the gut by MAO and DDC; 99% is metabolised. The drug is distributed to most body tissues; in the absence of a DDCI, the CNS receives less than 1% of the dose and it is metabolised in the brain to DA. Levodopa has a half-life of 1–3 hours. Duration of action is up to 5 hours. Metabolites, principally homovanillic acid, are excreted by the kidneys.

Usually, improvement is seen within 2–3 weeks, although some people require levodopa for up to 6 months to obtain maximal therapeutic effect.

Drug interactions

See Drug Interactions 24.1.

Adverse reactions

Large doses must be given (as it is extensively metabolised; see above). Adverse reactions include peripheral dopaminergic effects (nausea and vomiting, postural hypotension, irregular heart rate, difficult urination, dark discolouration of urine and sweat) and CNS effects (confusion [especially in the elderly], anxiety, nightmares, and mood changes, involuntary movements of the body and sudden loss of mobility [the 'off' stage – see 'On–off syndrome', later]). A withdrawal syndrome can occur, resembling the 'neuroleptic malignant syndrome' related to decreased dopaminergic transmission. Eyelid spasms or closing (blepharospasm) may be an early sign of drug overdose.

Adverse reactions due to levodopa–carbidopa are similar to those for levodopa.

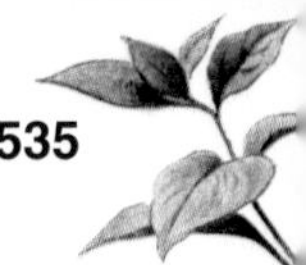

Warnings and contraindications

- Caution is required in severe cardiovascular, pulmonary, renal, hepatic, psychiatric and endocrine diseases, in peptic ulcer and during pregnancy (Category B3). Monitoring should be carried out for mental and behavioural changes, and for arrhythmias.
- The combination is contraindicated in closed-angle glaucoma; monitor for intraocular pressure changes.
- Levodopa should not be stopped abruptly, due to risk of sudden drop in DA levels and a withdrawal syndrome resembling neuroleptic malignant syndrome. DA agonists are contraindicated during lactation, as DA inhibits secretion of prolactin, and during treatment with typical antipsychotic agents.

Dosage and administration

- Levodopa dosage for adults is initiated with 50–100 mg two-three times a day, increasing gradually until a therapeutic response is achieved, to a maximum of 2 g/day in divided doses.
- Food reduces absorption of levodopa; it is recommended that the drug be given with food initially to minimise GIT discomfort, but later doses be given on an empty stomach to minimise fluctuations in plasma level and effects.
- Varying dosage forms permit greater flexibility in titrating the dose–response of both levodopa and carbidopa. Controlled-release formulations can minimise the on–off swings, but have lower oral bioavailability, so higher levodopa doses may be required. There are also formulations containing three drugs: levodopa, carbidopa and entacapone (a COMT inhibitor) for Parkinson's disease with motor fluctuations. Conversions between different formulations must be initiated cautiously.

DRUG INTERACTIONS 24.1
Levodopa plus a dopa decarboxylase inhibitor

OTHER DRUG OR DRUG GROUP	LIKELY EFFECTS AND MANAGEMENT
DA antagonists including antipsychotics and metoclopramide	Can result in decreased levodopa effects, due to blockade of DA receptors in the brain; if possible, avoid the combination with levodopa
Antihypertensives	Increased risk of postural hypotension; decrease dose.
MAOIs (type A)	This combination can result in a hypertensive crisis. MAOIs should be discontinued 2–4 weeks before starting levodopa therapy
MAOIs (type B) (selegiline)	This combination may be used (see later), but can result in increased levodopa-induced nausea and CNS effects; levodopa dose should be reduced
Iron (ferrous sulfate or ferrous gluconate) may decrease absorption of levodopa and carbidopa	Control of Parkinson's disease may be impaired; administration times should be separated by as long an interval as possible.
Other drugs with dopaminergic activity, including methyldopa	Increased adverse effects; monitor and reduce levodopa dose if necessary
Phenytoin, tetrabenazine	May reduce action of levodopa and worsen symptoms; reduce dose or avoid

levodopa-DDCI combination in Parkinson's disease with motor fluctuations. The dose of levodopa needs to be decreased by 10–30%.

Drug interactions are similar to those for other drugs that increase dopaminergic activity – that is, with MAOIs, catecholamines and TCAs. Adverse effects include GIT, CNS and skin disorders. Entacapone is contraindicated in hepatic impairment, and liver functions are monitored as a similar drug was withdrawn from use due to severe hepatic reactions.

Monoamine oxidase B inhibitors

Drugs such as selegiline irreversibly inhibits MAO-B (which metabolises mainly DA), thus preventing breakdown of DA, and blocks DA reuptake (Drug Monograph 24.3 for selegiline). Selegiline enhances antiparkinson effects of levodopa, allowing lowering of the daily dose. Another MAO-B inhibitor, rasagiline, is prescribed with special authority; its role in the management of Parkinson's disease is indicated for the symptomatic treatment of idiopathic Parkinson's disease, as monotherapy (without concomitant levodopa/decarboxylase inhibitor therapy) or as adjunct therapy (with concomitant levodopa/decarboxylase inhibitor therapy).

On–off syndrome

The effectiveness of the combination of levodopa plus DDCI often declines with chronic administration, resulting in the '**on–off syndrome**' of fluctuations in motor control, from being symptom-free ('on') to

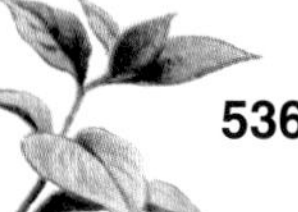

Drug Monograph 24.3
Selegiline

Mechanism of action
Selegiline is an irreversible MAO-B inhibitor used as adjunctive therapy in Parkinson's disease, in combination with levodopa or levodopa-carbidopa.

Pharmacokinetics
Selegiline is well absorbed orally, reaching peak plasma level in 30 minutes to 2 hours. It is rapidly metabolised and has three active metabolites, including L-amphetamine and methamphetamine (with half-lives of 2–20 hours), so has low bioavailability. It readily crosses the blood–brain barrier; metabolites are excreted slowly via the kidneys.

Drug interactions
- In usual doses (< 10 mg/day), selegiline can be given with levodopa, and without dietary tyramine restrictions.
- Adverse effects are enhanced by other DA agonists or oral contraceptives.
- When used with serotonergic drugs, including other MAOIs, serotonin selective reuptake inhibitors including fluoxetine and sertraline, sumatriptan or pethidine, a reaction similar to the serotonin syndrome (confusion, restlessness, hyperreflexia, sweating, shivering, tremors, diarrhoea, ataxia and fever) can occur; these combinations should be avoided.

Adverse reactions
These are typical dopaminergic effects, including nausea, vomiting, insomnia, dizziness, GIT distress, dyskinesias and mood alterations.

Warnings
Use with caution in people with movement or cardiovascular disorders, psychoses, history of peptic ulcer disease or selegiline hypersensitivity.

Dosage and administration
The usual adult dose of selegiline is 2.5 mg once daily increasing gradually to a dose of 5 mg twice daily. If after 2–3 days of treatment with selegiline levodopa related adverse effects occur, consider reducing dose of levodopa by about 10–30%.

demonstrating full-blown Parkinson's symptoms ('off'). These effects can last from minutes to hours, and may be due to decreased delivery of DA centrally, alteration in sensitivity of DA receptors, variation in the amount and rate of drug absorption and/or interference from a DA metabolite. Levodopa plus DDCI may have only a few years of usefulness.

Doses of levodopa and the frequency of administration eventually need to be increased to maintain therapeutic effect. Addition of a direct-acting DA agonist or a COMT inhibitor (entacapone) may help reduce 'off' times. After a drug holiday of several days, some people demonstrate an improved response to therapy, possibly because of the re-establishment of DA receptor sensitivity. Symptoms can worsen during the drug-free period, so this should be instituted in a hospital setting.

Dopamine-releasing drugs
Amantadine
Amantadine is a synthetic antiviral compound used occasionally to treat influenza. Other actions include releasing DA and other catecholamines from neuronal storage sites, blocking uptake of DA into presynaptic neurons, accumulating peripheral and central DA and inducing elevation of mood, plus useful antimuscarinic and anti-NMDA receptor activities in the glutamatergic pathway from subthalamic nucleus to globus pallidus. It is less effective than levodopa in Parkinson's disease but produces more rapid clinical improvement and causes fewer adverse reactions.

Amantadine is indicated for use as an antidyskinetic agent in treatment of mild Parkinson's disease It is well absorbed orally and is excreted by the kidneys unchanged, so doses need to be reduced in people with kidney impairment. Precautions are required in many concurrent conditions, including epilepsy, glaucoma, heart failure, hypotension and psychiatric disorders.

Adverse reactions are typical anticholinergic (atropinic) effects and effects of DA agonists (GIT, mood and cardiovascular changes). With chronic therapy, amantadine can cause unusual purple-red skin spots (livedo reticularis). There are clinically significant drug interactions with DA antagonists (which oppose its effects) and other drugs with anticholinergic actions (additive).

Dopaminergic adverse effects
Drugs that mimic brain DA may cause confusion and hallucinations in the elderly. Tachyphylaxis (gradual reduction in efficacy) develops for all the DA-enhancing

agents, making long-term treatment difficult. If withdrawn rapidly, neuroleptic malignant syndrome may be induced.

DA antagonists used in schizophrenia can cause parkinson-like (extrapyramidal) symptoms as adverse effects, drugs increasing DA levels used to treat Parkinson's disease can tilt the DA–ACh 'see-saw' in the opposite direction and cause drug-induced psychosis with GIT disorders, hallucinations and impulse control disorders such as pathological gambling, overspending and hypersexuality; patients and their carers need to be warned of these possibilities.

Directly acting dopaminergic agonists

Non-ergot-derived dopaminergic agonists

Pramipexole, an orally administered non-ergot DA agonist indicated in Parkinson's disease and restless legs syndrome, acts at D_2 and D_3 receptors. When added to levodopa therapy, it improves motor functions and reduces 'off' time. Adverse dopaminergic effects include hallucinations, nausea, insomnia and/or somnolence and dyskinesia. A similar drug, **rotigotine**, is formulated as a skin patch; it improves motor functions and activities of daily living, with similar adverse effects. Both drugs can cause sudden sleepiness and compulsive behaviours.

Apomorphine is a morphine derivative with very little analgesic activity; its four-ring structure contains the DA backbone, and it acts as a DA agonist, stimulating central DA receptors. By stimulating the medullary chemoreceptor trigger zone, it acts as a powerful emetic in animals that can vomit (including dogs and humans). In the past it was used as an emetic to treat poisoning by orally ingested (non-corrosive) substances.

Apomorphine injected SC is used in people severely disabled by fluctuations in levodopa response that are non-responsive to other treatment (see On-off syndrome) Adverse reactions are similar to dopaminergic effects of levodopa or the ergot alkaloids, especially vomiting, hypotension and mental disturbances. Apomorphine is contraindicated in cardiovascular diseases, respiratory or CNS depression, dyskinesias and psychiatric disorders. Because of its low therapeutic index and the need to determine an effective dose range during an 'off' motor period, the drug is best administered in a hospital setting under specialist supervision. An antiemetic such as domperidone (which acts on the chemoreceptor trigger zone that is peripheral to the blood–brain barrier) must be given prophylactically 48–72 hours before apomorphine; use of a centrally acting DA antagonist antiemetic such as prochlorperazine or metoclopramide would be counterproductive as it would block the dopaminergic effects of levodopa. The 'cocktail' of domperidone (peripheral DA antagonist), apomorphine (central DA agonist), carbidopa (peripheral dopa-decarboxylase inhibitor) plus levodopa (central DA precursor) is a powerful one. It is administered parenterally (SC) or sublingually, as it has little effect if taken orally.

Ergot derivatives

The ergot alkaloids come from a fungus, *Claviceps purpurea*, which grows on damp rye grains and can cause outbreaks of poisoning (ergotism). Ergot alkaloids are renowned for affecting a variety of receptors. Ergot derivatives for uses other than Parkinson's disease include ergometrine (used as an oxytocic agent, Drug Monograph 30.6), methysergide (5-HT receptor antagonist not a first-line treatment in migraine) and lysergic acid diethylamide (LSD, the classic hallucinogenic agent; see Ch 25).

Ergot derivatives used in Parkinson's disease are bromocriptine (a central DA agonist, also used in hyperprolactinaemia) and cabergoline. They stimulate central DA receptors and thus improve bradykinesia and rigidity, but are less effective than levodopa so are no longer first-line drugs. Adverse reactions are similar to those for levodopa, including effects in the CNS, GIT, cardiovascular and central nervous systems. The peripheral DA antagonist domperidone is usually given 30–60 minutes before, to minimise nausea and hypotension. The drugs should be used with caution in people with arrhythmias and psychosis. Their DA-agonist actions inhibit lactation, so they are contraindicated in breastfeeding women. Cabergoline is also used as a lactation inhibitor and to treat hyperprolactinaemia (Ch 30).

Drug interactions can be expected with DA antagonists such as phenothiazines, thioxanthines, haloperidol and metoclopramide. Drugs that produce hypotension can have an additive hypotensive effect when administered concurrently with ergot alkaloids.

Drugs with central anticholinergic activity

Symptoms of Parkinson's disease caused by an excess of cholinergic activity include muscle rigidity and muscle tremor. Increased muscle tone appears as 'ratchet resistance' or 'cogwheel rigidity': the affected muscle initially moves easily, then meets resistance or remains fixed in the new position. Muscle tremors have a to-and-fro movement caused by the sequence of contractions of agonistic and antagonistic muscles involved. The tremors are usually worse at rest and are commonly manifested as a pill-rolling motion of the hands and bobbing of the head. **Anticholinergics** are more useful early in the course of the disease because the adverse reactions to DA depletion are not prominent at this stage. (See Clinical Focus Box 24.1 for a discussion on the implications of anticholinergic drugs in the elderly.)

Anticholinergics that readily cross the blood–brain barrier can block central cholinergic excitatory pathways, returning the DA–ACh balance especially in the basal ganglia to normal (Fig 24.1, earlier) and producing some

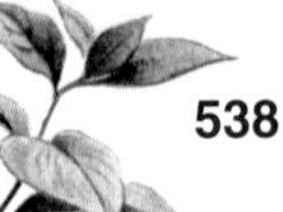

CLINICAL FOCUS BOX 24.1
Geriatric implications of anticholinergic drugs

Elderly people are highly susceptible to the adverse effects of anticholinergic drugs, especially constipation, dry mouth and urinary retention (usually in men). These drugs should be avoided in people with narrow-angle glaucoma or a history of urinary retention.

Other adverse effects more common in the elderly are memory impairment, paradoxical excitation (hyperexcitability, agitation, confusion and sedation), reduced flow of saliva (leading to oral discomfort, periodontal disease and candidiasis), overheating resulting in heat stroke during vigorous exercise or periods of hot weather, and blurred vision and/or increased sensitivity to light.

Anticholinergic dosing in the elderly should begin with a low dose, with gradual increases until maximum improvement is noted, or intolerable adverse effects occur.

improvement in functional capacity and relief of tremor. There is less effect on the rigidity and akinesia.

The belladonna alkaloids atropine (Drug Monograph 8.2, in Ch 8) and hyoscine were early agents to treat parkinsonism; they have been superseded by synthetic anticholinergics with fewer adverse effects, such as benzatropine and trihexyphenidyl (benzhexol). Their usefulness is limited by peripheral anticholinergic (atropinic) adverse reactions and by their tendency to be less effective with continued use. They are also used to control extrapyramidal reactions, such as rigidity, akinesia (difficulty in or lack of ability to initiate muscle movement), tremor and akathisia, induced by antipsychotic drugs.

CLINICAL FOCUS BOX 24.2
Bulgarian snowdrops for Alzheimer's disease

Galantamine is one of the cholinesterase inhibitors approved by the Therapeutic Goods Administration in Australia for dementias. It has been used for hundreds of years in a traditional European herbal remedy from snowdrops (*Galanthus nivalis*, *Galanthus woronowii*). There are reports that in the 1950s a Bulgarian pharmacologist noticed people rubbing the common snowdrop on their foreheads to ease nerve pain, and giving an infusion of the bulbs to relieve poliomyelitis-associated paralysis. Russian pharmacologists identified anticholinesterase activity in extracts and determined the chemical structure of the active ingredient galantamine in 1952; it is a complex polycyclic alkaloid. It was soon introduced into Russian medicine as an antidote to neuromuscular blockade and for many neurological conditions including myasthenia gravis.

Perhaps because its pharmacology was originally studied in Russia during the Cold War period, it was some decades before galantamine made its appearance in the West. In Australia, it is now marketed in capsules (8, 16 or 24 mg), and subsidised for use in mild-to-moderate Alzheimer's disease. Galantamine has dual mechanisms of action: inhibiting acetylcholinesterase and enhancing binding of ACh to nicotinic receptors. Clinically, galantamine improves cognitive performance (memory, attention, reasoning and language) and performance in activities of daily living. Its adverse reactions, as with other cholinomimetic agents, include gastrointestinal stimulation, depression and weakness.

Drug treatment of other movement disorders

Multiple sclerosis

Multiple sclerosis is the most common cause of progressive neurological disability in the 20–50 years age group. Its incidence varies with latitude, being higher further from the equator; in Australia, the incidence in Tasmania is seven times that in north Queensland. This may be due to seasonal changes in sunlight exposure influencing vitamin D levels or pathogens prevalent in these regions. There is widespread demyelination of neurons in the brain (white matter) and spinal cord, and inflammation and glial activation. This leads to muscle weakness, sensory and visual disturbances, urinary and GIT dysfunctions, anxiety and depression. Environmental and genetic factors have been implicated in triggering the autoimmune reaction against CNS myelin. There is usually a relapsing–remitting course of progressive disability over a period of about 40 years.

There are three main treatments for the disease:

- relapse treatment
- disease-modifying treatment
- symptom treatment (no treatment fully reverses the progressive neurological deterioration). The choice of drug depends on the individual person, their history and severity of multiple sclerosis and the route of administration and adverse effects of the drug. The aim is to start treatment early to slow the progression of the disease.

Preventative immunomodulators are used long term for relapsing forms of multiple sclerosis to reduce the frequency of relapses and slow progressive deterioration. These include the parenteral therapies interferons β-1a, β-1b and glatiramer, monoclonal antibodies (the newer natalizumab, alemtuzumab and ocrelizumab [a B-cell targeted therapy]). The oral therapies include the new drugs ozanimod, siponimod and cladribine and the older drugs fingolimod, teriflunomide and dimethyl fumarate. Also, immunosuppressants (e.g. corticosteroids) are used for acute relapses. Centrally acting antispasticity drugs such as baclofen (Drug Monograph 24.1, earlier), diazepam and dantrolene are used, as well as anticonvulsants, antidepressants (for sensory disturbances, pain and depression) and autonomic drugs (to relieve urinary problems).

Immunomodulators

First-line therapy of multiple sclerosis is directed at damping-down excessive immune response in the CNS, reducing the frequency and severity of attacks and the number and size of lesions. Symptoms are not reversed and the disease is not cured.

Relapses are commonly treated with intravenous methylprednisolone at a dose of 1 g/day or 500 mg/day for 3–5 days with or without oral tapering. In case of persistent severe relapse symptoms, a second cycle can be applied with dosages up to 2 g/day for 5 days. Other immunomodulators used include β-interferons (Ch 34) and the cytotoxic immunosuppressants methotrexate, azathioprine and mitozantrone (Ch 33).

Newer immunomodulators more specific to use in multiple sclerosis may selectively modify cytokine actions during relapses. These include:

- glatiramer, an unusual synthetic polypeptide that blocks T-lymphocyte actions against myelin antigens and reduces relapses in multiple sclerosis
- natalizumab, a monoclonal antibody that binds to integrins on the surface of leucocytes and slows entry of T-cells through cerebral capillaries into the CNS, reducing inflammation and demyelination; administered IV every 4 weeks (see above).

Restless legs syndrome

Restless legs syndrome affects from 5% to 15% of the population; it can begin at any age, and may have a hereditary aetiology or be secondary to various metabolic, neurological or drug-induced conditions. People complain of limb discomfort (usually leg, possibly also arm) after lying quietly, with an urge to move the affected part (which temporarily relieves the discomfort) and unpleasant sensory sensations deep in muscle or bone. The condition is usually chronic and progressive.

Some people do not require treatment, and good 'sleep hygiene' (referred to in Ch 20) may relieve mild symptoms. For more severe symptoms, dopaminergic drugs are first-line therapy, and initially 90% of people obtain relief from levodopa or DA agonists such as ropinirole, pramipexole or rotigotine. Adverse reactions are typical of dopaminergic agonists, plus there is a risk of augmentation of symptoms, impulse control disorders and rebound after the drug effects have worn off. Other drugs tried include benzodiazepines (clonazepam), opioid analgesics and neuropathic pain relievers (gabapentin); drugs with anticholinergic actions may worsen the condition by enhancing restlessness and agitation.

Myasthenia gravis

Although this condition is uncommon – occurring with a worldwide prevalence of about 200–400 cases per million population – it has long been of interest to pharmacologists because of the interesting pharmacological concepts exemplified.

Pathology

Myasthenia gravis is a progressive, incurable disease characterised by the loss of or decrease in ACh nicotinic motor end-plate receptors by antibodies specific to the receptor (AChR-Ab MG) (or, more rarely, for muscle-specific tyrosine kinase (MuSK-Ab MG). The autoimmune process results in skeletal muscle weakness. The thymus gland is believed to be involved in causation, through production of antibodies directed against ACh receptor proteins; nearly 15% of people with myasthenia gravis have a tumour of the thymus gland. It is a fluctuating but treatable condition, until the number of functioning ACh receptors drops too low; treatment may include thymectomy, plasmapheresis to remove antibodies and drug therapy.

Clinical signs, symptoms and implications are shown in Figure 24.3. Common early reported symptoms are ptosis and diplopia, shoulder fatigue after lifting the arm, hand weakness and finding it difficult to perform repetitive tasks such as playing the piano. The most serious consequences of myasthenia gravis are dysphagia and respiratory muscle weakness, since these can result in aspiration pneumonia or respiratory failure.

The condition is exacerbated by many drugs that impair neuromuscular transmission or unmask autoimmune disorders, including neuromuscular blockers; botulinum toxin; aminoglycosides, fluoroquinolone and macrolide antibiotics; quinine, interferons; magnesium and lithium; calcium channel blockers and β-blockers; statins; iodinated contrast agents and D-penicillamine.

Pharmacotherapy

Drug therapy includes anticholinesterases (edrophonium for diagnosis and neostigmine and pyridostigmine for treatment). Immunosuppressants are also used (Narayanaswami et al. 2021). Anticholinesterases reduce the breakdown of ACh by cholinesterases, ACh binds to the remaining functional nicotinic receptors and competes with autoantibodies for binding sites (Ch 8). The drug of choice is pyridostigmine, a reversible inhibitor of

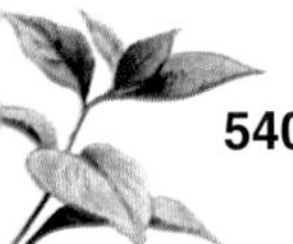

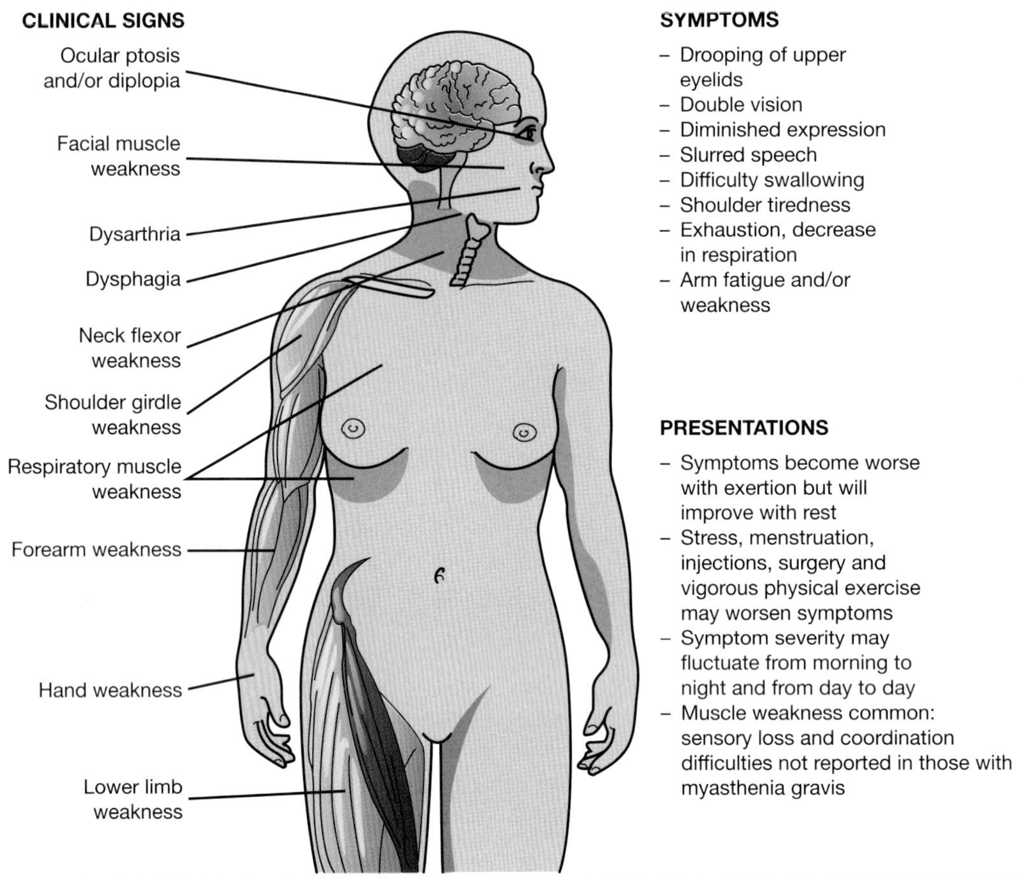

CLINICAL SIGNS

Ocular ptosis and/or diplopia
Facial muscle weakness
Dysarthria
Dysphagia
Neck flexor weakness
Shoulder girdle weakness
Respiratory muscle weakness
Forearm weakness
Hand weakness
Lower limb weakness

SYMPTOMS

- Drooping of upper eyelids
- Double vision
- Diminished expression
- Slurred speech
- Difficulty swallowing
- Shoulder tiredness
- Exhaustion, decrease in respiration
- Arm fatigue and/or weakness

PRESENTATIONS

- Symptoms become worse with exertion but will improve with rest
- Stress, menstruation, injections, surgery and vigorous physical exercise may worsen symptoms
- Symptom severity may fluctuate from morning to night and from day to day
- Muscle weakness common: sensory loss and coordination difficulties not reported in those with myasthenia gravis

FIGURE 24.3 Signs, symptoms and presentations of myasthenia gravis

acetylcholinesterase, as described earlier. It is given orally, and is slower in onset but longer acting than neostigmine. It has fewer cholinergic adverse effects and is the first-line drug treatment for myasthenia gravis. An old drug is edrophonium, used for diagnosis and monitoring of myasthenia gravis or to differentiate between under- and over-treatment. It is available in Australia through the Special Access Scheme and in New Zealand.

Immunosuppressants such as corticosteroids (prednisolone) and azathioprine, ciclosporin, methotrexate (although studies are limited), mycophenolate; or tacrolimus are used (Ch 34). The monoclonal antibody eculizumab may be used for severe refractory myasthenia gravis. Rituximab is an early therapeutic option in muscle-specific tyrosine kinase type who have an unsatisfactory response to initial immunotherapy and in refractory ACHR antibody if other agents are not tolerated.

Motor neurone disease (amyotrophic lateral sclerosis)

Motor neurone disease is a progressive neuromuscular disorder, leading to bulbar palsy and atrophy of skeletal muscles. It is eventually fatal, due to respiratory failure and/or choking. The disease is possibly due to accumulation of glutamate in affected neurons. Muscle cramps may respond to baclofen, and muscle pain to non-steroidal anti-inflammatory drugs (NSAIDs); physiotherapy and speech therapy are helpful.

Riluzole, a neuroprotective agent that specifically inhibits the release of glutamate and blocks NMDA receptors and is thought to inactivate voltage dependent sodium channels, significantly slows deterioration in muscle strength and prolongs life by a few months. High-fat meals reduce absorption, so it is taken on an empty stomach. Common adverse effects are weakness, nausea and decreased lung function; liver function and white cell counts require monitoring.

Other movement disorders

Hyperkinetic movement disorders include tremor, chorea, tics and myoclonus. The term ‘Parkinson-plus disorders’ or atypical parkinsonian variants has been coined to refer to conditions including multiple system atrophy, supranuclear palsy and corticobasilar ganglionic degeneration; some people with these

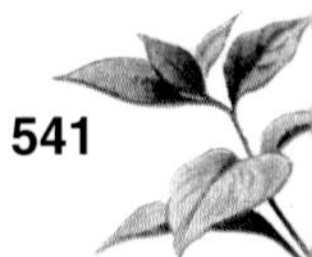

diseases respond to antiparkinson therapies plus symptomatic treatment of autonomic dysfunctions. Tetrabenazine, a DA-depletor describer earlier, is indicated for treatment of many movement disorders, dystonias and dyskinesias.

Tremor (muscle contractions in the frequency range 4–12 Hz) may be reduced after drinking alcohol; other drugs tried include β-blockers, benzodiazepines, primidone and gabapentin. Choreas (abnormal involuntary movement disorders characterised by brief, irregular muscle contractions) may resolve spontaneously; drugs used include DA antagonists (neuroleptics) and anticonvulsants. Dystonias (movement disorders in which involuntary sustained muscle contractions cause twisting and repetitive movements or abnormal postures) may respond to botulinum toxin or anticholinergics, GABA agonists and DA agonists or antagonists.

Drug-induced movement disorders

As discussed in Chapter 22, antipsychotic drugs commonly cause movement disorders (dystonias, akathisia, tardive dyskinesia) due to their DA-blocking actions. Anticholinergics are the first-line drugs for treating acute syndromes, whereas for tardive dyskinesia, withdrawal of the offending drug is important, and tetrabenazine is used.

KEY POINTS

Drug treatment of Parkinson's disease and other movement disorders

- Skeletal muscle relaxants are drugs of choice in the treatment of muscle spasticity and have central actions (e.g. baclofen, diazepam) or peripheral actions (botulinum toxin A, dantrolene).
- The neuromuscular blocking agents used in surgery (e.g. curare and suxamethonium) act at the neuromuscular junction.
- People with Parkinson's disease are treated with dopaminergic agents (to raise brain levels of DA) and/or with drugs that have central anticholinergic effects.
- The main dopaminergic agents are levodopa with a decarboxylase inhibitor, the ergot derivatives, and apomorphine, amantadine and selegiline; all tend to have adverse reactions on DA receptors in the CNS and GIT.
- Centrally acting anticholinergic drugs (e.g. benzatropine) inhibit ACh-mediated motor activity but have adverse reactions in the autonomic nervous system.
- Multiple sclerosis is characterised by widespread demyelination of neurons in the brain (white matter) and spinal cord. There are three main treatments for the disease: relapse treatment; disease-modifying treatment; and symptom treatment.
- Immunomodulators are the first-line therapy of multiple sclerosis and include the interferons β-1a and β-1b. Cytotoxic immunosuppressants such as methotrexate and azathioprine, and also corticosteroids, are used. Other drugs include centrally acting antispasticity drugs, as well as symptomatic treatment.
- Restless legs syndrome with more severe symptoms is treated with dopaminergic drugs, benzodiazepines, opioid analgesics and neuropathic pain relievers.
- Myasthenia gravis is a progressive, incurable autoimmune disease characterised by the loss of or decrease in ACh nicotinic motor end-plate receptors and resulting in skeletal muscle weakness. Drug therapy includes anticholinesterases and immunosuppressants.
- Motor neurone disease is a progressive neuromuscular disorder possibly due to accumulation of glutamate in affected neurons, and may be treated with the neuroprotective agent riluzole.
- Hyperkinetic movement disorders include tremor, chorea, tics and myoclonus.
- Tremor may be treated with β-blockers, benzodiazepines, primidone and gabapentin. Choreas may be treated with DA antagonists and anticonvulsants, and dystonias may respond to botulinum toxin or anticholinergics, GABA agonists and DA agonists or antagonists.
- Drug-induced movement disorders may occur due to antipsychotic drug use (due to their DA-blocking actions). Anticholinergics are the first-line drugs for treatment of acute syndromes, whereas for tardive dyskinesia, withdrawal of the offending drug is important.

Dementias, delirium and stroke

Dementia

Prevalence

Dementia is a syndrome associated with more than 100 diseases; it is a progressive mental disorder characterised

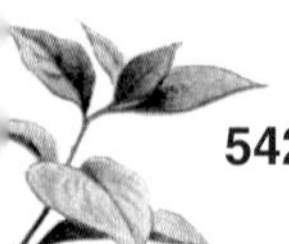

by chronic personality disintegration, confusion and deterioration of intellectual capacity and impulse control. In Australia, dementia is in the top 10 leading causes of disease burden in the community, accounting for 3.8% of total disability-adjusted life years, ranking ahead of diabetes and asthma (Australian Institute of Health and Welfare 2021).

In 2021, there were an estimated 472,000 Australians living with dementia. The number of people with dementia is expected to increase to almost 1.1 million by 2058 with Alzheimer's disease accounting for up to 70% of diagnosed cases (Australian Institute of Health and Welfare 2021). The prevalence in remote-living Indigenous Australians is among the highest in the world and prevalence in Aboriginal and Torres Strait Islander populations three to four times higher than the general population; it is associated with older age, male gender, no formal education, current smoking, previous stroke, epilepsy, head injury, poor mobility, incontinence and falls. Interventions aimed at managing modifiable factors could reduce dementia risk (Australian Institute of Health and Welfare 2021; Radford et al. 2019).

In New Zealand the most common form of dementia is Alzheimer's disease, accounting for 60–80% of cases of dementia in that country. The second most common cause is vascular dementia. More than 170,000 New Zealanders will be living with dementia by 2050 (Neurological Foundation 2019).

Aetiologies and pathogenesis

Many degenerative conditions are common causes of dementia including Alzheimer's disease (50–70%); frontotemporal dementias, dementia with Lewy bodies and Parkinson's disease (all around 10%). Other types are vascular dementia, including multi-infarct dementia (formerly known as cerebrovascular arteriosclerosis), which accounts for 10–20%; and alcohol- or AIDS-related dementia (5%). Cognitive impairment can also occur in hypothyroidism, deficiencies of vitamin B, in various CNS disorders, and as an adverse reaction to many CNS depressants and anticholinergic drugs (Psychotropic Expert Group 2021).

Dementia develops over a period of months or years. Intellectual (cognitive) ability is usually the first to decline, especially affecting short-term memory, language and decision-making ability, with loss of orientation to time, place and person, and of ability to concentrate or perform complex tasks. Other early signs include depression, anxiety, irritability and agitation. Personal habits and personality change; the person may become loud, obscene or violent, or quieter and withdrawn. Helplessness, total dependency and loss of manual skills occur, with loss of speech and mobility; the person may be bedridden, with loss of bladder and sphincter control.

Management

Possible reversible causes of dementia should be considered and managed first, and other conditions treated. Management of cognitive symptoms includes anticholinesterases and the NMDA antagonist memantine. Pharmacological treatment of other symptoms, after non-pharmacological management has been used, includes low-dose antipsychotic agents for severe agitation, delusions and hallucinations, or antidepressants for severe depression. Supportive care should include occupational therapy and assistance with activities of daily living, proper nutrition, moderate exercise if permitted, vitamins if indicated, plus support for the person's carers.

Alzheimer's disease

Alzheimer's disease (described in 1906 by the German neuropathologist Alois Alzheimer) is a dementia of insidious onset and gradually progressive course, characterised by confusion, memory failure, disorientation, restlessness, speech disturbances and impaired cognitive abilities. It is currently incurable, and accounts for more than half of people with dementia and more than half of all nursing home admissions. Although not an inevitable consequence of biological ageing, there is a linear incidence with age, so that about 50% of the population over 85 years shows some evidence of Alzheimer's disease.

Aetiological factors

Researchers are still searching for the cause of Alzheimer's disease. Many aetiologies are proposed, and the latest studies investigate:

- the integrated stress response and aberrant phosphorylation of eukaryotic initiation factor-2α (eIF2α), important factors in neuronal death and memory loss (Khoury et al. 2018)
- the role of the gene TREM2 in microglial function and microgliosis and inflammation in neurodegeneration (Gratuze et al. 2018).

Other research has focused on:

- accumulation of β-amyloid protein[1] in the CNS, especially the Aβ56 protein, and its aggregation into fibrils

1 A technique for blood tests to quantify biological markers associated with amyloid-beta, showing that they reach abnormal levels at least 17 years before the onset of dementia symptoms, was announced by Australian scientists early in 2013; it is hoped that identifying people at risk of developing Alzheimer's disease will allow early interventions before irreversible damage occurs. A recent study has indicated that those with elevated glial fibrillary acidic protein (GFAP) in the blood also have increased amyloid beta in the brain and the role of TREM 2 (Chatterjee et al. 2021).

- hyper-phosphorylation of tau protein, contributing to neurofibrillary tangles
- deficiency in the neurotransmitter ACh, and perhaps other neurotransmitters in the brain
- slow viral or other infection that attacks selected brain cells
- defective gene producing apolipoprotein E, a cholesterol carrier
- genetic predisposition (estimated variously from 10% to 70% of risk), especially mutations related to Aβ, tau, apolipoprotein E and presenilin proteins
- failure of the metal transport functions of **amyloid** and tau proteins (iron) and presenilins (copper, zinc), leading to accumulation of the metals within protein aggregates
- an autoimmune theory (that the body fails to recognise host tissue and attacks itself)
- the role of glutamate from astrocytes activating extrasynaptic NMDA receptors and triggering apoptosis (Wang & Reddy 2017)
- the link between type 2 diabetes and Alzheimer's disease.

Postulated pathogenesis

Accumulation of amyloid plaques is, in part, due to inappropriate activity of some metalloproteinase enzymes in the CNS and dysfunctions in clearance. Amyloid precursor protein, a transmembrane cell-surface protein formed in central neurons with unknown function, is cleaved by secretase enzymes to small proteins including a 42-amino-acid residue called amyloid-beta 42 (Aβ42). This peptide is the most amyloidogenic form of the peptides and spontaneously forms oligomers and then larger amyloid plaques, which accumulate and cause death of neurons. Abnormal Aβ accumulation in the brain causes neurodegeneration, neuroinflammation, impaired neuronal function and ultimately cognitive decline. Loss of cholinergic neurons particularly from the basal forebrain to the hippocampus and cerebral cortex causes impairments in memory and learning. There is also reactive gliosis (glial scarring), and formation of dendritic plaques and tangles, especially in the grey matter.

Life expectancy

Knowing likely life expectancy after diagnosis is of great interest to patients and carers, and is important to health planners and caregivers. As with other dementias, Alzheimer's is associated with shortened but variable life expectancy of between 3 and 10 years after diagnosis; some, however, will live beyond 20 years. A median expectancy is 7–10 years for people diagnosed in their 60s and early 70s, compared with 2–3 years or less for those diagnosed in their 90s (Liang et al. 2021).

Pharmacotherapy

Current pharmacotherapy focuses on improving cognitive functioning or limiting disease progression and symptom control, as no medication cures or prevents Alzheimer's disease. Centrally acting reversible anticholinesterases, which raise and prolong ACh levels in cholinergic pathways, in some people enhance cognitive functioning and slow decline. Other drugs may relieve behavioural disturbances and mood changes, especially antipsychotics.

New therapies currently under trial include newer anticholinesterases. Further therapies include immunotherapy such as monoclonal antibodies aducanumab, donanemab and lecanemab removing amyloid plaques and therapies that target tau phosphorylation or aggregation. With an increasing understanding of the role of immune/inflammatory pathways in AD the roles of anti-inflammatory drugs in Alzheimer's disease are being elucidated. Antioxidants such as vitamin E, and also the spice curcumin, are also under trial.

Centrally acting anticholinesterases

As noted, earlier, anticholinesterases are known as antidotes to neuromuscular blockade and for many neurological conditions including myasthenia gravis (Ch 8). Donepezil, galantamine (available as a prolonged-release formulation; and rivastigmine available as a capsule and a patch for daily transcutaneous administration, which improves compliance) enhance neurotransmitter actions of ACh in CNS pathways. Galantamine is a polycyclic alkaloid extracted from the flowering bulb 'snowdrops' (*Galanthus nivalis*, *Galanthus woronowii*). It has dual mechanisms of action: inhibiting acetylcholinesterase and enhancing binding of ACh to nicotinic receptors. Clinically, galantamine improves cognitive performance (memory, attention, reasoning and language) and performance in activities of daily living (Clinical Focus Box 24.2)

The pharmacokinetic properties of the three anticholinesterases approved for use in Alzheimer's disease are compared in Table 8.5 (Ch 8). Clinical benefits are small; however, the drugs may delay deterioration in cognition by 6–18 months and hence may delay movement of the person into nursing care. Currently, in Australia, there are strict guidelines for subsidised prescribing of the drugs.

As ACh is also the neurotransmitter at neuroeffector junctions in the parasympathetic and motor nervous systems, these drugs have many adverse reactions, especially in the GIT and heart. (The mechanism is discussed earlier and in Ch 8.) They should be used only cautiously in people with asthma, chronic obstructive pulmonary disease, peptic ulcers, cardiac conduction disorders and cardiac arrhythmias. The enhanced vagal effect on the heart (bradycardia) can lead to arrhythmias and syncope, especially in older people; rates of hip fractures are increased, and some people have required hospitalisation and insertion of a pacemaker.

Memantine, an NMDA antagonist

Memantine, a non-competitive antagonist at glutamate NMDA-type receptors, may reduce neuronal degradation due to excess glutamate. (Glutamate is an excitatory amino acid that can cause excitotoxicity and neuronal degradation – see Table 18.1 in Ch 18.) Memantine is approved for use in moderate-to-severe dementia and can be used in combination with an anticholinesterase; adverse CNS effects are common. Functional status should be monitored and the drug discontinued if ineffective.

Symptom management

Due to the widespread prevalence of dementias, and the limited benefits from anticholinesterase agents, the search is on for better drugs. Other drugs under clinical investigation include biologics, disease modifying small molecules and symptomatic agents:

- donepezil once-weekly transdermal patch in people with Alzheimer's disease
- rivastigmine intranasal spray
- 5-HT_6 receptor antagonists for cognitive and behavioural effects and angiotensin receptor blockers.

Drugs for managing psychological and behavioural symptoms in Alzheimer's disease

Drugs may be required if the person with dementia exhibits symptoms such as aggression, agitation or psychosis:

- Antipsychotic agents, such as risperidone or olanzapine, for management of behavioural disturbances, including delusions and hallucinations; adverse reactions should be monitored, as antipsychotic agents or medications with anticholinergic effects could worsen cognitive functioning.
- Low doses of antidepressants with a low anticholinergic profile, such as desipramine or nortriptyline, may be required.
- Antianxiety agents, especially those with short-to-intermediate half-lives such as lorazepam, oxazepam or alprazolam, help people with severe anxiety or agitation; a paradoxical reaction (increase in activity, restlessness and agitation) that might be confused with increasing dementia may occur. Use with caution.

Non-pharmacological methods of improving cognitive reserve are mental activities, physical activity and exercise and good social networks; there are negative associations with alcohol intake, smoking and obesity. Most studies show no benefit from vitamin supplements, antioxidants, statins or most antihypertensive drugs (except in the treatment of relevant diagnosed disorders).

Other dementias

Dementia with Lewy bodies is another common dementia, often difficult to distinguish from Alzheimer's; post-mortem autopsy shows the presence of Lewy bodies (accumulated deposits of alpha-synuclein protein) in nuclei of neurons from brain areas associated with memory and motor control. Two of the following symptoms must be present: visual hallucinations, parkinsonian tremors and stiffness, and fluctuation in mental state; other symptoms may include impaired concentration, extreme confusion and difficulty judging distances. Progression is usually fairly rapid, leading to death within about 7 years. Anticholinesterases may be helpful; antipsychotics can help reduce hallucinations, but worsen parkinsonian symptoms.

Delirium

Delirium is defined as an acute, transient disturbance of attention and consciousness accompanied by a change in cognition and having a fluctuating course; the pathophysiology is not well understood, and delirium is seriously underdiagnosed. Delirium is common in hospitals, especially in critically ill, older and postoperative people. It can be induced by drugs or by withdrawal of drugs. Reversible impairment of cognition can be caused by many factors, including:

- drugs (anticholinergics; amphetamines and other CNS stimulants; CNS-depressant drugs such as butyrophenones, phenothiazines, benzodiazepines, anticonvulsants, alcohol; high-dose corticosteroids; opioid analgesics; diuretics and other antihypertensives; hallucinogens; NSAIDs; dopaminergic agents; sotalol and propranolol)
- withdrawal from drugs (alcohol, other CNS depressants)
- metabolic or endocrine disorders (hyperglycaemia, hypothyroidism, hypopituitarism)
- poor nutrition (deficiency of vitamin B12, folic acid, niacin)
- release of inflammatory mediators such as interleukins
- other causes – emotional problems, trauma, infections and fever, brain tumours or metastases, and cerebrovascular disorders.

Prevention and management

Good nursing care, monitoring vital signs and attending to hydration, nutrition, pain relief and environment (noise, light and visitors) help minimise episodes. Risk factors should be identified, especially any drugs likely to exacerbate the condition. Most people with delirium do not need pharmacological management; however, if the

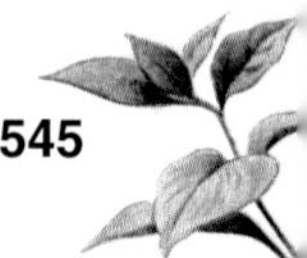

condition is causing distress, threatens treatment or others, then an antipsychotic drug such as haloperidol, olanzapine or risperidone is used; a single dose is often adequate, and the person's vital signs should be monitored (Psychotropic Expert Group 2021).

Stroke

Treatment

Stroke (cerebrovascular accident) may lead to progressive mental dysfunction resembling dementia. A stroke is characterised by sudden onset of neurological dysfunction due to insufficient blood supply to the brain; the major types are ischaemic (85%), due to embolism or infarction, and haemorrhagic (15%), due to intracerebral or subarachnoid haemorrhage. Stroke is the third most common cause of death in Western countries; there are about 40,000 strokes per year in Australia, leading to long-term neurological disability. In 2018, an estimated 387,000 people had had a stroke at some time in their lives, based on self-reported data from the Australian Bureau of Statistics (2019) 2018 Survey of Disability, Ageing and Carers. The estimated prevalence of stroke has declined slightly between 2003 and 2018 (1.7% and 1.3% respectively).

Transient ischaemic attacks are transient episodes of neurological dysfunction caused by focal ischaemia without infarction; they are associated with a 10% risk of stroke within the next 2 weeks unless treatment ensues.

Prevention

The main risk factors for stroke are atrial fibrillation, hypertension, smoking, diabetes, cardiovascular disease and hypercholesterolaemia; the drugs used to reduce these risk factors are warfarin, low-dose aspirin and other antiplatelet agents; antihypertensive agents, antidiabetes drugs and statins (all covered in other chapters). Cessation of smoking is the most important modifiable risk factor, and surgery for carotid artery stenosis reduces the risk of stroke in suitable patients.

Treatment of acute stroke

Development of acute stroke is a medical emergency. Aspirin administered within 48 hours of onset of stroke (100–300 mg orally daily, except in people with haemorrhagic stroke) has been shown to have moderate benefit. Thrombolytic therapy with the recombinant tissue plasminogen factor (tPA) alteplase is indicated in specific people (dependent on whether it is an ischaemic or haemorrhagic stroke) and is effective when given within 4.5 hours of onset of acute stroke. Secondary prevention of ischaemic stroke and transient ischaemic attack includes the anticoagulant (warfarin). Other drugs include antiplatelet agents such as aspirin, dipyridamole or clopidogrel; statins; reperfusion therapies; neuroprotective agents. After haemorrhagic stroke, urgent neurosurgery may be required to drain blood and evacuate haematomas and treatment for the underlying predisposing condition; in hypertensive people, aggressive lowering of blood pressure with an angiotensin-converting enzyme inhibitor and a diuretic or β-blocker or, for example, a β-blocker with a calcium channel blocker significantly reduces further risk. Nimodipine is the recommended antihypertensive agent for complications of subarachnoid haemorrhage.

KEY POINTS

Drug treatments of Alzheimer's disease, dementia, delirium and stroke

- There is no current medication to cure or prevent Alzheimer's disease or other dementias. Centrally acting anticholinesterases (e.g. donepezil) slow cognitive decline by enhancing ACh functions. Other pharmacotherapy is used for symptom control and to manage agitation, delusions and hallucinations.
- Delirium, a transient disturbance of attention and consciousness, is common in critically ill, older and postoperative hospital patients; it is also frequently induced by psychotropic and anticholinergic drugs.
- Stroke may lead to progressive mental dysfunction resembling dementia. It is characterised by sudden onset of neurological dysfunction due to insufficient blood supply to the brain. The main types of stroke are ischaemic and haemorrhagic.
- Treating risk factors is important in acute stroke (a medical emergency). An anticoagulant (warfarin) or thrombolytic therapy with tPA is indicated in specific people (depending on whether it is an ischaemic or haemorrhagic stroke).

Drug treatment in migraine and other headaches

Migraine

Pathology and prevalence

Migraine is a severe intermittent headache with at least two of the following features: pain affecting one side of the head only, pulsating in quality, moderate or severe in intensity, aggravated by exertion; plus nausea with or without vomiting and sensitivity to light and sound.

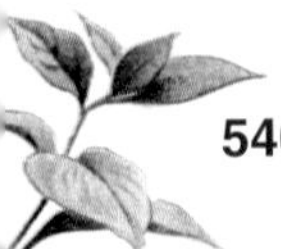

The nature of the attacks varies between people, and within an individual at different times.

The prevalence of migraine in the community is about 7% in males and 16% in females (during reproductive non-pregnant years). Migraine often first appears in young children, adolescence or early adulthood; prevalence rises from about 3% in 7-year-olds to 9% in 15-year-olds. In Australia, it is estimated that a quarter of people suffering migraines require medical attention, and about 70% have some positive family history of migraines. It affects the greatest number of people between 35 and 45 years of age. In adolescents and adults, the disease disproportionately affects women (22% vs 10% lifetime prevalence).

Migraine has been described for thousands of years; it has been considered a bad headache, a spontaneous 'concussion', an inflammatory disorder, a vascular disorder, a form of epilepsy or a platelet disorder. The fact that dilation of cerebral blood vessels is involved was proved by showing that if people are (gently) centrifuged feet-outwards, the head pain is relieved, by taking the blood to the periphery.

A typical migraine attack begins with the prodrome or aura phase, during which there is vasoconstriction of the intracranial vessels. This impairs blood flow to the brain, starting in the visual cortex and causing the sensation of flashing lights, pin-pricking, impaired speech and weakness. The second phase is headache, thought to be due to protective reflex vasodilation, with severe unilateral pulsating pain, during which blood flow to the brain and head is increased by about 20%. The nervous system is over-reactive, with sensations of flashing lights, spectra, double vision and increased sensitivity to light (photophobia), smells and noise. Autonomic effects include nausea and vomiting, diarrhoea, fluid retention and, afterwards, diuresis, along with CNS effects of vertigo, ataxia, incoordination and impaired consciousness.

Aetiology and trigger factors

While the exact aetiology is unknown, many people realise that particular factors trigger an attack. Some common 'triggers' are:

- mechanical – a blow to the head or pressure on the head
- environmental changes – hot winds (the sirocco of the Mediterranean, the sharav in Israel and hot north winds in Melbourne), changes in barometric pressure or the weather
- stress (emotions, glare, loud noise, flashing lights) or relaxation after stress
- hormone-level changes, such as at puberty, pre- and during menstruation (the declining estrogen phase)
- drugs – estrogens, vasodilators including nitrates, caffeine
- foods (chocolate, cheese, oranges, preservatives) and alcohol, especially red wines; however, placebos (inactive substances) have also triggered attacks
- dehydration; sunstroke
- changes in sleep patterns, especially in REM sleep.

Neurotransmitters involved

It is now generally considered that migraine is a syndrome of unstable cerebral blood vessels, probably mediated by 5-HT. During the early phase there is release of 5-HT, which causes the vasoconstriction, aura and pain. Later, 5-HT levels are low, allowing vasodilation. GIT symptoms are due to the effects of 5-HT on receptors in the gut. The headache is due to both arterial dilation and sensitisation to pain by released 5-HT and bradykinin. Spontaneous discharge along trigeminal nerve pathways releases other neurotransmitters (substance P, calcitonin, gene-related peptide), which contribute to pain, vasodilation and visual and GIT disturbances. Another theory is that about half of migraine sufferers are deficient in magnesium, and may benefit from magnesium supplements.

As the main neurotransmitter involved in migraine is 5-HT, specific drugs involved in treatment are 5-HT agonists (triptans) in the acute attack and, apparently paradoxically, 5-HT antagonists in prophylaxis.

Non-pharmacological treatment

Before pharmacological treatment of migraine is commenced, it is important that the diagnosis be confirmed and other causes of severe headache excluded. Trigger factors need to be avoided; severe attacks may be pre-empted if the person can remove to a quiet dark room, avoid movement, take mild analgesics (aspirin or paracetamol) and sleep off the attack. Behavioural therapies are useful.

Treatment of the acute attack

Analgesics and antiemetics

Mild analgesics should be tried early in the attack and in sufficient doses, with stronger drugs tried as necessary, moving up the analgesic ladder (Fig 19.3, in Ch 19). Suitable analgesics are paracetamol in children and, in adults, aspirin (600–900 mg, repeated in 4 hours if necessary) or paracetamol (1–1.5 g every 4 hours, to a maximum of 4 g/day). An NSAID (naproxen or ibuprofen, or rectal ketoprofen) can be added. Opioids including codeine combinations and pethidine should be avoided as they exacerbate the GIT symptoms and cause potential problems with dependence.

To enhance absorption of the antimigraine drug, and reduce vomiting if nausea is severe, an antiemetic such as ondansetron, metoclopramide, domperidone or prochlorperazine may be given (Ch 16); parenteral administration may be necessary. Non-oral drugs can be given; prochlorperazine is carried in ambulances and is administered IV or IM by paramedics to treat severe nausea and vomiting, including in people previously diagnosed with migraine.

Triptans

If the above therapies have been ineffective in relieving previous attacks, one of the 'triptan' drugs may be prescribed: sumatriptan (Drug Monograph 24.4), eletriptan, naratriptan, rizatriptan or zolmitriptan. They came into use in the 1990s and revolutionised treatment of migraine, relieving headache in 50–75% of cases within 2–4 hours of oral administration. Triptans are structural analogues of 5-HT, selective agonists at 5-$HT_{1B/1D}$ receptors and effective vasoconstrictors, especially on cerebral arteries.

They should be given when the headache is beginning to develop and can be administered orally (but have low bioavailability), parenterally, as a wafer for buccal absorption or as a nasal spray. Individuals may respond differently to different triptans. Serotonin syndrome is a risk as an adverse reaction; triptans should be used only cautiously in people concurrently taking lithium, MAOIs or serotonin noradrenaline/selective reuptake inhibitors.

Ergot alkaloids

A drug previously used to treat migraine was ergotamine, a powerful vasoconstrictor and partial agonist at both

Drug Monograph 24.4
Sumatriptan

Mechanism of action

Sumatriptan selectively constricts cranial vessels by agonist actions at 5-$HT_{1B/1D}$ receptors. It is also thought to inhibit the abnormal activation of trigeminal nociceptors.

Indications

It is indicated for treatment of an acute migraine attack in those unresponsive to or intolerant of other therapies, and also by injection for acute relief of cluster headache pain. This medication is most effective if taken when the headache is beginning to develop, and not earlier (e.g. during aura) or later (when headache more severe).

Pharmacokinetics

After oral administration, absorption of sumatriptan is rapid but high first-pass metabolism leads to low bioavailability. After SC administration, the peak plasma concentration is reached in about 30 minutes, and doses are considerably lower (6 mg compared with 50–100 mg orally).

Intranasal administration as a spray has a quicker onset of action than if given orally, and hence is useful to relieve pain and slow development of the attack, especially in people with severe nausea and vomiting, but has a shorter duration of action.

Drug interactions

The triptan drugs interact significantly with other drugs that raise serotonin levels, especially MAOIs including moclobemide and SSRIs.

There is increased risk of adverse drug reactions including serotonin syndrome and ischaemia, so effects should be monitored. They are contraindicated with ergot alkaloids.

Adverse reactions

Minor reactions include dizziness, fatigue, drowsiness, chest pain, nausea and vomiting, feelings of heaviness and rash.

Rarely, there have been reports of arrhythmias, stroke, anaphylactic reactions, seizures, and even acute myocardial infarction and death.

Warnings and contraindications

- Sumatriptan should be taken as monotherapy; that is, other antimigraine preparations should be avoided.
- Caution is advised in the elderly and during pregnancy.
- The drug is contraindicated in ischaemic diseases (ischaemic heart disease, myocardial infarction, coronary vasospasm, peripheral vascular disease) and hypertension. It should not be used during lactation or in severe liver disease, and is not licensed for use in children.
- Overuse can lead to recurrent or rebound headaches and withdrawal syndrome.

Dosage and administration

Sumatriptan is available as a tablet, nasal spray or injection. The oral dose is 50–100 mg as soon as possible in the attack, repeating after at least 1 hour if necessary to a maximum of 300 mg/day. The SC dose regimen is 6 mg, repeating after 1 hour to a maximum of 12 mg/day. For intranasal administration the dose is 10–20 mg into one nostril, repeating after 2 hours to a maximum of 40 mg/day.

α-adrenoceptors and 5-HT_1 receptors. Caffeine or diphenhydramine were sometimes given concurrently with ergotamine (with doubtful pharmacological rationale). However, ergot alkaloids have many adverse reactions and rebound headaches occur after cessation of administration, so this drug and the dihydro-derivative have been withdrawn from use in Australia.

Methysergide

Methysergide is an ergot derivative that is a potent 5-HT_2 antagonist. It suppresses migraine headache in about 25% of people, but is ineffective in treatment of acute attacks.

There is a high incidence of adverse reactions, especially in the CNS, GIT and cardiovascular systems, with behavioural changes and peripheral vascular disease. Methysergide is contraindicated in many conditions: CVS disease, hyperthyroidism, collagen disease, urinary tract disorders, renal or liver disease, in children, and during pregnancy or lactation. It can be used episodic and chronic migraine and for episodic and chronic cluster headaches however it is currently not registered for use in Australia, New Zealand, the USA or Canada.

Prevention of migraine attacks

If triggering factors are avoided and non-pharmacological treatments applied, but the person still suffers more than one severe attack per month, the following prophylactic agents are some of the drugs tried:

- Newer drugs include erenumab, fremanezumab and galcanezumab. They inhibit calcitonin gene-related peptide (CGRP) induced vasodilation. CGRP is a highly potent vasodilator associated with sensory nerve endings (in pain pathways). It acts at the calcitonin-like receptor (CLR) and a single transmembrane protein, RAMP1. Fremanezumab and galcanezumab, monoclonal antibodies, bind to CGRP and erenumab blocks the CGRP receptors.
- Amitriptyline has been shown to be effective in preventing migraine, especially when associated with tension headache; it should be started with a low dose at bedtime and gradually increased. Nortryptiline is another TCA that is also used (Ch 22). Candesartan, an ACE inhibitor, may be used (with no effect on blood pressure in normotensive people).
- β-blockers with no intrinsic sympathomimetic actions (propranolol, metoprolol, atenolol) reduce frequency of attacks; their clinical efficacy may be due to effects at 5-HT receptors rather than β-blocking actions; they are contraindicated in asthma.
- Pizotifen, an anti-serotonin/antihistamine/antimuscarinic agent, is poorly tolerated, due to adverse effects of drowsiness and weight gain.
- Anticonvulsants (topiramate, sodium valproate, gabapentin); caution is required in women due to potential teratogenic effects.
- Methysergide, a potent 5-HT antagonist (see above).
- Botulinum toxin for prophylaxis of chronic migraine.

Only one preventive drug should be used at a time. It may take 1–3 months for a prophylactic effect to be evident; during this time, treatment of acute attacks is still required. Note that the possibility of adverse effects and comorbidities influence the use of this and other drugs.

Drugs used in other headaches

Normal headaches

Headaches can be triggered in a wide variety of conditions:

- excess stimulation of the nerves of the scalp (wearing a tight hat or goggles)
- 'ice-cream headache', from eating very cold food or drinks
- 'Chinese restaurant syndrome', from monosodium glutamate (MSG)
- hangover headache, from dehydration, aldehydes and acetate after excessive alcohol consumption
- fasting, from low blood glucose levels
- drug-induced headache, from vasodilators, oral contraceptives or hormone replacement therapy, tetracyclines, indometacin, amphetamines, pethidine, histamine H_2-antagonists or epidural anaesthesia
- rebound or medication overuse headache, after withdrawal from drugs such as analgesics, caffeine, nicotine and β-blockers
- mountain sickness, from changes in fluid balance and low oxygen levels at high altitudes
- exertional vascular headaches, from strenuous exercise, coughing, straining or sexual intercourse (due to increased blood pressure, vasodilation, muscle contractions)
- low-pressure headache (from cerebrospinal fluid leak after lumbar puncture)
- other pain conditions, including neuralgias, sinusitis, neck pain, neuropathic pain and toothache.

In most of these types of headache simple analgesics provide adequate pain relief. Appropriate doses are aspirin 600 mg orally every 4 hours to a maximum of 4 doses in 24 hours, or paracetamol 0.5–1 g orally every 3–6 hours, with a maximum of 4 g/day. In medication overuse headache, the causative drug must be withdrawn.

Although most headaches are mild and self-limiting, there are potentially serious causes of headaches that need to be checked: a space-occupying lesion (e.g. intracranial haemorrhage, inflammation due to meningitis or encephalitis, cerebral oedema or tumour), vascular insufficiency, temporal arteritis, severe hypertension or headache after head injury.

Tension headache

Tension headache is the commonest form of headache, without aura or vomiting, affecting both sides of the head, with a feeling of heaviness or tightness, often with depression or anxiety. It affects women more frequently than men. It has been suggested that it is a syndrome of low 5-HT levels; lack of sleep is a common trigger. Physical management includes relaxation, exercises and massage, and avoidance or reduction of caffeine intake. Drug treatments tried are simple analgesics/NSAIDs (ibuprofen, diclofenac or naproxen), then amitriptyline (an antidepressant) and diazepam (an antianxiety agent).

Cluster headache

Cluster headache is a severe one-sided pain, centred on one eye with tearing and redness of the eye, often with one blocked or runny nostril and decreased sympathetic function on the affected side, recurring within 24 hours. Multiple attacks may occur each day; it has been called 'migrainous neuralgia'. Men are affected more frequently than women; it is triggered particularly by vasodilators, including alcohol.

Treatment is with inhaled oxygen (100% for up to 15 minutes) and SC sumatriptan. Prevention is with prophylactic use of corticosteroids and lithium or calcium channel blockers.

KEY POINTS

Drug treatment in migraine and other headaches

- Migraine is a severe unilateral headache involving fluctuating levels of 5-HT causing vasoconstriction, then vasodilation, of cerebral blood vessels. For treatment of acute attacks, analgesics and 5-HT agonists (triptans) are used.
- To prevent attacks, 5-HT antagonists, antidepressants (amitryptiline), β-blockers and various other drugs are used prophylactically. Individuals need to identify and avoid triggering factors.
- Other headaches ('normal', tension and cluster headaches) are treated with simple analgesics, plus antidepressants, antianxiety agents or antimigraine drugs as required.

DRUGS AT A GLANCE

Drugs for neurodegenerative conditions and headaches

THERAPEUTIC GROUP AND EFFECT	KEY EXAMPLES	CLINICAL USE
Drugs affecting skeletal muscle		
Skeletal muscle stimulants Anticholinesterases • Block the enzyme that breaks down ACh leading to increased levels of neurotransmitter	Pyridostigmine	Myasthenia gravis Reversal of neuromuscular blockade
Centrally acting skeletal muscle relaxants GABA agonists		
• Enhance GABA inhibitory transmission, inhibiting motor neurons mainly in the spinal cord	Baclofen	Spasticity
• Benzodiazepines act at GABA^A receptors to facilitate GABA binding and open calcium channels decreasing excitability	Diazepam	Seizures
Dopamine agonists • Direct action at DA D_2, D_3 and D_4 receptors in motor pathways	Ropinirole	Restless legs syndrome
Direct (peripherally) acting skeletal muscle relaxants: Inhibitors of ACh release • Block release of ACh from cholinergic nerve terminals	Botulinum toxin	Dystonias, blepharospasm, migraine, cosmetic procedures
Inhibitors of calcium release • Block release of calcium in skeletal muscles promoting relaxation	Dantrolene	Spasticity, multiple sclerosis, cerebral palsy, spinal cord injury, stroke and malignant hypothermia

Antiparkinson agents		
Drugs enhancing brain dopamine Drugs that raise brain DA levels: Dopa-decarboxylase (DDC) inhibitor • Block the peripheral breakdown of L-dopa allowing it to enter the CNS before conversion to DA MAO-B inhibitors: • Block the breakdown of monoamines by MAO-B thereby raising levels in CNS COMT inhibitors: • Block the breakdown of monoamines by COMT inhibitors thereby raising levels in CNS	Levodopa plus carbidopa or benserazide Selegiline Entacapone	Parkinson's disease Parkinson's disease and depression
Direct-acting dopamine agonists Non-ergot derivatives: • Direct action at DA D_2, D_3 and D_4 receptors in motor pathways Ergot derivatives: • Direct action at DA D_2, D_3 and D_4 receptors in motor pathways	Pramipexole, rotigotine, apomorphine Cabergoline, bromocriptine	Parkinson's disease
Drugs that release dopamine • Release of DA from nerve terminals	Amantadine	Parkinson's disease
Drugs that block cholinergic receptors • Block central cholinergic excitatory pathways, returning the DA–ACh balance, especially in the basal ganglia to normal	Benzatropine	Parkinson's disease
Drugs for multiple sclerosis		
Immunomodulators • Preventative immunomodulators are used long term for relapsing forms of multiple sclerosis	Natalizumab, Fingolimod, Interferon beta Glatiramer	
Drugs used in dementias		
Centrally acting anticholinesterases • Block the enzyme that breaks down ACh leading to increased levels of neurotransmitter and activation of central cholinergic receptors	Donepezil Galantamine Rivastigmine	Alzheimer's disease, dementias
N-methyl-D-aspartate (NMDA) antagonists	Memantine	
Antimigraine drugs		
Drugs for acute treatment Analgesics/NSAIDs • Block COX enzymes and prevent formation of inflammatory mediators 5-HT agonists Triptans • Stimulate 5-$HT_{1B/1D}$ receptors on vasculature-effective vasoconstrictors, especially on cerebral arteries	Aspirin Paracetamol Naproxen Sumatriptan	Migraine (aura phase) Prophylaxis and treatment of migraine
Drugs for prophylaxis 5-HT antagonists Block 5-HT_2 receptors and cause vasodilation	Methysergide	Methysergide

REVIEW EXERCISES

1 Mr PQ, aged 45, visited his GP complaining of intermittent muscle weakness in his shoulder and hands, spasms and sometimes blurred vision. He was sent to a neurologist and was diagnosed with myasthenia gravis, using the drug edrophonium and muscle biopsy. He was prescribed a one 'timespan' tablet (180 mg) once daily of pyridostigmine. What class of drugs are edrophonium and pyridostigmine? In relation to the pathogenesis of myasthenia gravis how are these drugs useful? Describe the duration of action of each of these drugs and its relevance in treatment.

2 Mrs MK is a 75-year-old who was diagnosed with Alzheimer's disease two years ago. She was prescribed donepezil 5 mg daily however her symptoms seem to be worsening. Her doctor wishes to increase her dose to 10 mg. What is the rationale for anticholinesterase treatment in Alzheimer's disease? What are the adverse reactions Mrs MK should be aware of, especially if her dose is being increased?

3 Ms JC, a 24-year-old student, suffers from migraine, especially when she is anxious about her examinations. Recently, she has been experiencing 2 or more severe attacks per month. What drug could she be prescribed as prophylaxis for recurrent attacks? What is the mechanism of action of this drug? Her doctor has prescribed her sumatriptan in case of acute attack. When should she take this drug? Describe the involvement of 5-HT in the pathogenesis of migraine and define the mechanism of action of the triptans.

REFERENCES

Australian Bureau of Statistics 2019. Disability, Ageing and Carers, Australia: Summary of Findings [https://www.abs.gov.au/ausstats/abs@.nsf/mf/4430.0], accessed 7 October 2021

Australian Institute of Health and Welfare 2021. Dementia in Australia [Internet]. Canberra: Australian Institute of Health and Welfare, [cited 2021 Oct. 27]. Available from: https://www.aihw.gov.au/reports/dementia/dementia-in-aus

Bondon-Guitton E, Perez-Lloret S, Bagheri H, et al. 2011: Drug-induced parkinsonism: a review of 17 years' experience in a regional pharmacovigilance center in France. Movement Disorders. 26(12):2226–2231

Chatterjee, P, Pedrini, S, Stoops, E et al. 2021. Plasma glial fibrillary acidic protein is elevated in cognitively normal older adults at risk of Alzheimer's disease. Translational Psychiatry. 11, 27. https://doi.org/10.1038/s41398-020-01137-1

Gratuze, M, Leyns, CE, Holtzman, DM 2018. New insights into the role of TREM2 in Alzheimer's disease. Molecular Neurodegeneration. 13, 66.

Khoury R, Grysman N, Gold J, et al. The role of 5 HT6-receptor antagonists in Alzheimer's disease: an update. Expert Opinion on Investigational Drugs. Jun;27(6):523–533. doi: 10.1080/13543784.2018.1483334. Epub 2018 Jun 18. PMID: 29848076.

Kordower JH, Olanov CW 2016: Fetal grafts for Parkinson's disease: decades in the making. Proceedings of the National Academy of Sciences of the United States of America. 113(23):6332–6334.

Langston JW 2017. The MPTP Story. Journal of Parkinson's Disease. 7(s1): S11–S19. doi: 10.3233/JPD-179006. PMID: 28282815; PMCID: PMC5345642.

Liang, C-S, Li, D-J, Yang, F-C, et al. 2021. Mortality rates in Alzheimer's disease and non-Alzheimer's dementias: a systematic review and meta-analysis. Lancet Healthy Longev, 2 (8) e479–e488. ISSN 2666-7568, https://doi.org/10.1016/S2666-7568(21)00140-9.

Maiti P, Manna J, Dunbar GL 2017: Current understanding of the molecular mechanisms in Parkinson's disease: Targets for potential treatments. Translational Neurodegeneration. 6:28

Müller T 2021. Experimental dopamine reuptake inhibitors in Parkinson's disease: a review of the evidence. Journal of Pharmacology and Experimental Therapeutics. Mar 29; 13:397–408. doi: 10.2147/JEP.S267032. PMID: 33824605; PMCID: PMC8018398.

Narayanaswami P, Sanders DB, Wolfe G, et al. 2021. International Consensus Guidance for Management of Myasthenia Gravis: 2020 Update. Neurology. Jan 19;96(3):114–122. doi: 10.1212/WNL.0000000000011124. Epub 2020 Nov 3. PMID: 33144515; PMCID: PMC7884987.

Neurological Foundation 2019. Alzheimer's disease and dementia. Available from: https://neurological.org.nz/what-we-do/awareness-and-education/brain-disorders-and-support/alzheimers-disease-and-dementia/?

New Zealand Brain Research Institute 2022; Prevalence and Incidence of Parkinson's in New Zealand: https://www.nzbri.org/Labs/parkinsons/Epidemiology/

Pajares MI, Rojo A, Manda G, et al. 2020. Inflammation in Parkinson's disease: mechanisms and therapeutic implications. Cells. Jul 14;9(7):1687. doi: 10.3390/cells9071687. PMID: 32674367; PMCID: PMC7408280.

Parkinson's Western Australia 2022: What Is Parkinson's & What Does It Do. Online. https://www.parkinsonswa.org.au/

Parmar M, Grealish S, Henchcliffe C 2020. The future of stem cell therapies for Parkinson disease. Nature Reviews Neuroscience. Feb;21(2):103–115. doi: 10.1038/s41583-019-0257-7. Epub 2020 Jan 6. PMID: 31907406.

Psychotropic Expert Group 2021: Therapeutic guidelines: psychotropic, version 7, Melbourne, Therapeutic Guidelines Limited. eTG complete [digital]. Melbourne: Therapeutic Guidelines Limited; 2021 Jun. https://www.tg.org.au

Qamhawi Z, Towey D, Shah B, et al. 2015: Clinical correlates of raphe serotonergic dysfunction in early Parkinson's disease. Brain. 138(10):2964–2973.

Radford K, Lavrencic LM, Delbaere K, et al. 2019. Factors associated with the high prevalence of dementia in older Aboriginal Australians. Journal of Alzheimer's Disease. 70(s1): S75–S85. doi:10.3233/JAD-180573

Troncoso-Escudero P, Sepulveda D, Pérez-Arancibia R, et al. 2020. On the right track to treat movement disorders: promising therapeutic approaches for Parkinson's and Huntington's disease. Frontiers in Aging Neuroscience. 12:571185. Published 2020 Sep 3. doi:10.3389/fnagi.2020.571185

Wang R, Reddy PH 2017. Role of glutamate and NMDA receptors in Alzheimer's disease. Journal of Alzheimer's Disease. 57(4):1041–1048. doi:10.3233/JAD-160763

Zhang Z, Zhang S, Fu P, et al. 2019. Roles of glutamate receptors in Parkinson's disease. International Journal of Molecular Sciences. 20(18):4391. Published 2019 Sep 6. doi:10.3390/ijms20184391

ONLINE RESOURCES

Australian Myasthenic Association in NSW: https://www.myasthenia.org.au/ (accessed January 2022)

Dementia Australia: https://www.dementia.org.au/ (accessed January 2022)

Migraine and Headache Australia: https://www.headacheaustralia.org.au/ (accessed January 2022)

Motor Neurone Disease (MND) Australia: https://www.mndaust.asn.au/ (accessed January 2022)

Multiple Sclerosis Australia: https://www.msaustralia.org.au/ (accessed January 2022)

New Zealand Medicines and Medical Devices Safety Authority: https://www.medsafe.govt.nz/ (accessed January 2022)

NPS MedicineWise – Managing migraine: https://www.nps.org.au/australian-prescriber/articles/migraine-management/ (accessed January 2022)

Parkinson's Foundation: https://www.parkinson.org/ (accessed January 2022)

Parkinson's Australia: https://www.parkinsons.org.au/ (accessed January 2022)

Parkinson's Western Australia: https://www.parkinsonswa.org.au/ (accessed January 2022)

More weblinks at: http://evolve.elsevier.com/AU/Knights/pharmacology/.

CHAPTER 25

DRUG DEPENDENCE AND SOCIAL PHARMACOLOGY

Mary Bushell

KEY ABBREVIATIONS

DA	dopamine
GHB	gamma-hydroxybutyrate
5-HT	5-hydroxytryptamine (serotonin)
LSD	lysergic acid diethylamide
MDMA	3,4-methylenedioxy-methamphetamine
THC	tetrahydrocannabinol
UNODC	United Nations Office on Drugs and Crime

KEY TERMS

addiction 555
alcohol 552
alcoholism 570
dependence 554
designer drugs 574
drug abuse/misuse 553
drug-seeking behaviour 564
ethanol 568
hallucinogen 580
harm minimisation 563
illicit drugs 555
'legal highs' 574
methadone 552
reinforcement 557
tolerance 555
withdrawal syndrome 555

Chapter Focus

Drugs likely to produce dependence have three characteristics: they act fast, make you feel good or stop you feeling bad. Substance and drug abuse is widespread in societies despite legislation, enforcement, medical treatments and educational efforts to curb abuse. Patterns of drug abuse and policies related to abuse in Australia and New Zealand are described in this chapter. Drugs most commonly abused are opioids (e.g. heroin, morphine, codeine), central nervous system depressants (e.g. alcohol, benzodiazepines), central nervous system stimulants (e.g. cocaine, amphetamines, ecstasy, nicotine, caffeine) and psychotomimetics (cannabis and hallucinogens). This chapter describes misuse and abuse of these drugs, the pharmacological basis of dependence and tolerance, effects of drug abuse on individuals and society and issues that affect health professionals. Treatment of acute overdose, detoxification, substitution, withdrawal and maintenance programs are discussed.

KEY DRUG GROUPS

Central nervous system depressants:

- **alcohol** (Drug Monograph 25.1)
- drugs for alcohol abuse: **acamprosate**, **thiamine** (Drug Monograph 25.3)
- **benzodiazepines**, **gamma-hydroxybutyrate**, **inhalants**, **kava**

Central nervous system stimulants:

- amphetamines, **caffeine**, **cocaine**
- designer drugs, **ecstasy**, 'legal highs'
- **nicotine** and smoking
- drugs for nicotine dependence: **nicotine** (Drug Monograph 25.4), **varenicline**, **bupropion**

Opioids:

- morphine, codeine, **heroin**
- drugs for opioid dependence: buprenorphine, **methadone** (Drug Monograph 25.1), naltrexone

Psychotomimetics:

- cannabinoids: **cannabis**, **marijuana**, Δ^9-tetrahydrocannabinol (Drug Monograph 25.5)
- hallucinogens: ketamine, lysergide, **mescaline**

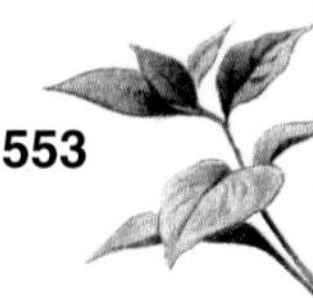

CRITICAL THINKING SCENARIO

Greg, a 45-year-old male, was recently diagnosed with alcohol use disorder. Each day Greg starts the day with a drink and a smoke and consumes at least another eight standards drinks, and 15 cigarettes. Greg has tried several times in the past to cut back or reduce his drinking and smoking. Greg's GP has encouraged him to enter a psychosocial treatment program and has prescribed disulfiram 100 mg orally daily for 1–2 weeks and then 200 mg daily ongoing and bupropion initially 150 mg once daily in the morning for 3 days, then 150 mg twice daily for 7 weeks.

1. Describe the hazards of use and toxic effects of smoking and excessive alcohol intake.
2. Explain why the GP has commenced Greg on disulfiram and bupropion. Describe the pharmacological action of both medicines.
3. If Greg continues to drink alcohol while taking disulfiram, what are some of the expected side effects and why?

Three months later, while travelling the Northern Territory of Australia, Greg is diagnosed with giardiasis, an infection mainly of the small intestine caused by a parasite. Greg visits a local GP, where he is prescribed the antibiotic metronidazole 2 g orally once daily for 3 days. Greg presents to the emergency department with confusion and psychotic reactions.

4. Explain the relationship between Greg's medicines and his signs and symptoms.

Introduction

The harms associated with the misuse and abuse of drugs are widespread and include health impacts to the person (e.g. tolerance, adverse effects, overdose, hospitalisation, death), society (e.g. violence, crime to support drug habits, trauma) and the economy (e.g. cost of health care, social welfare and law enforcement).

Many of the drugs likely to be abused – such as opioid analgesics, benzodiazepine antianxiety agents, amphetamine-type stimulants and the local anaesthetic cocaine – have been discussed in other chapters for their detailed pharmacology and medical uses. Other drug groups – alcohol, tobacco, caffeine, cannabis – are primarily known as 'social drugs'.

In this chapter, we consider factors leading to drug abuse and dependence, policies for minimising problems and the fascinating pharmacology of the drugs themselves.

Drug abuse and dependence

Drug abuse

Drug abuse refers to self-administration of a drug in chronically excessive quantities, in a manner that deviates from approved medical or social patterns in a given culture, resulting in physical or psychological harm. Abuse is therefore defined by what is accepted in a society based on its laws, history, religion and ethos. It depends on accepted medical practice: opiates are approved on medical prescription for pain but not for relief of anxiety; β-blockers are approved in cardiovascular disease but banned in some sporting events. (The term **drug misuse** simply refers to inappropriate or indiscriminate use of drugs.)

Drug abuse may take a variety of forms:

- experimental – using drugs in an exploratory way, then continuing or abandoning use
- social or recreational – for example, with alcohol, nicotine, caffeine, marijuana and 3,4-methylenedioxymethamphetamine (MDMA)
- compulsive – irrational, irresistible dependence on a drug
- self-medication – a person's search for relief of physical, psychological, social or financial problems
- ritualistic – related to religious practices such as with psychotomimetic or hallucinogenic drugs
- polydrug or multiple drugs – marijuana, alcohol and other depressants are often used together or alternately with central nervous system (CNS)

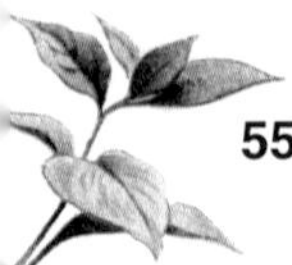

stimulants; many people in Western societies have coffee in the morning (caffeine) and alcohol in the evening

- abuse in sport – anabolic steroids, stimulants, narcotic analgesics and diuretics are banned or restricted in sporting competitions.

Drugs commonly abused

The drugs most abused in Western societies are legal drugs: nicotine and ethanol (alcohol). Others may be prescription medicines (opioid analgesics, benzodiazepines, ketamine, amphetamines) or illicit drugs (ecstasy, heroin, cocaine, 'ice', cannabis [legal in some situations for medical use], LSD [lysergic acid diethylamide]) or household chemicals. Table 25.1 summarises several aspects of the main drugs of abuse. (Therapeutic uses are discussed in other chapters.)

Drug dependence

In drug **dependence**, administration of a drug is compulsively sought in the absence of a therapeutic indication and despite adverse psychological, social or physical effects; dependence may lead to disturbed behaviour to ensure further supplies. Drug abuse does not always entail dependence on the drug: people may abuse simple analgesics or megadoses of vitamins. Dependence does not always cause problems; a person may be dependent on caffeine, which is safe and cheap, without breaking laws or suffering serious adverse or withdrawal reactions.

There are two main types of dependence:

- *psychological dependence*, characterised by out-of-control craving for the pleasurable effects of the drug, plus denial of excessive drug use and continuing abuse of the drug despite personal, social or legal difficulties

TABLE 25.1 Drugs commonly abused, symptoms and hazards

DRUG CATEGORY	SOME STREET NAMES	METHODS OF USE	SIGNS AND SYMPTOMS OF USE	HAZARDS OF USE AND TOXIC EFFECTS
Marijuana/hashish and 'synthetic cannabis'	Bhang, charas, chronic, Columbian, cone, dagga, dope, ganja, grass, green, gunga, hemp, hooch, joint, K2 kiff, Mary Jane, mull, pot, reefer, sinsemilla, skunk, weed	Most often smoked; can also be swallowed in solid form, baked in cookies etc.	Sweet, burnt odour; neglect of appearance; loss of interest and motivation; possible weight loss; red eyes	Impaired memory, perception and psychological maturation; psychological dependence; increased risk of schizophrenia Toxicity: tachycardia and postural hypotension, possible panic, disorientation, hyperemesis
Alcohol	Amber fluid, booze, grog, hooch, juice, piss, plonk, turps	Swallowed in liquid form	Impaired muscle coordination, slurred speech and impaired judgement	Heart and liver damage, injury or death from accidents; addiction, unsafe sex
Stimulants				
Amphetamines[a] Dexamfetamine Methamphetamine	Bennies, black beauties, crystal, dexies, ice, meth, pep pills, purple hearts, speed, uppers, vitamin A	Swallowed in pill or capsule form, injected into veins, dissolved in drinks, administered rectally, inhaled or snorted	Excess activity, irritability; nervousness, mood swings, needle marks, violence	Dysrhythmias, loss of appetite, hallucinations, paranoia, euphoria, convulsions Toxicity: circulatory collapse, hyperactive reflexes, pupils dilated, fever, sweating, shallow respirations, delirium
Designer drugs: ecstasy, 'legal highs', 'new psychoactive substances'	Adam, E, eccies, love drug, XTC	Taken as tablets	Increased confidence, paranoia, dry mouth, hangover, 'burnout'	High blood pressure, heart rate and temperature; thirst and over-hydration
Cocaine	Blow, Charlie, coke, crack, line, rock, snow, toot, vitamin C	Most often inhaled (snorted); also injected or swallowed in powder form, smoked	Restlessness, anxiety, intense short-term high followed by dysphoria	Intense dependence, euphoria, anxiety, nasal passage and lung damage Toxicity: insomnia, agitation; raised blood pressure, heart rate and temperature; anorexia; hallucinations, seizures, death
Nicotine/tobacco	Butt, cancer stick, ciggie, coffin nail, death stick, durry, fag, gasper, smokes, tar	Smoked in cigarettes, cigars and pipes; snuff; chewing tobacco	Smell of tobacco, high carbon monoxide blood levels, stained fingers and teeth	Cancers of the lung, throat, mouth and oesophagus; cardiovascular disease; emphysema
Depressants				
Barbiturates Benzodiazepines	Barbs, blues, downers, yellow jackets benzos, downers, moggies, tranx	Swallowed in pill form or injected into veins	Drowsiness, confusion, impaired judgement, slurred speech, needle marks, constricted pupils	Infection after parenteral use, addiction with severe withdrawal symptoms, loss of appetite, nausea

TABLE 25.1 Drugs commonly abused, symptoms and hazards—cont'd

DRUG CATEGORY	SOME STREET NAMES	METHODS OF USE	SIGNS AND SYMPTOMS OF USE	HAZARDS OF USE AND TOXIC EFFECTS
				Toxicity: depressed blood pressure and respiration; ataxia, slurred speech, confusion, depressed reflexes, coma
Gamma-hydroxybutyrate	Date rape drug, fantasy, Georgia Home Boy, GHB, grievous bodily harm, liquid X/E/G	Orally, mixed with alcohol; injected IV	Sedation, sleep, loss of memory	Neurotoxicity, coma, convulsions, respiratory depression; delayed onset, so risk of overdosing; risk of drug-assisted sexual assaults
Ketamine	K, special K, vitamin K	Injected	Analgesia with dissociation from surroundings; increased blood pressure, heart rate and muscle tone	Hallucinations, irrational behaviour; excess secretions
Opioids				
Methadone, morphine, pethidine Heroin Codeine	Big O, dreamer, junk, metho, monkey Brown, H, hammer, Harry, horse, junk, skag, smack Cody, loads, school boy	Swallowed in pill or liquid form, injected, smoked	Drowsiness, lethargy; miosis, needle marks, intense high	Addiction with severe withdrawal symptoms, loss of appetite, constipation, tolerance Toxicity: depressed blood pressure and respiration, hypercapnia, fixed pinpoint pupils, pulmonary oedema, hypothermia, rhabdomyolysis, coma
Hallucinogens				
PCP (phencyclidine)	Angel dust, killer weed, peace pill, supergrass	Most often smoked; can also be inhaled (snorted); injected or swallowed in tablets	Distorted sensations, slurred speech; blurred vision, incoordination, confusion, agitation, aggression	Anxiety, depression, impaired memory and perception, psychological dependence
LSD (Lysergide) Mescaline Psilocybin	Acid, trip, cubes, purple haze, purple pyramids, smiley buttons, cactus Mesc Magic mushrooms	Injected or swallowed in tablets Usually ingested in their natural form	Dilated pupils, delusions; hallucinations, mood swings	Breaks from reality, emotional breakdown, flashbacks Toxicity: elevated blood pressure, hyperactive reflexes, piloerection, sweating, dilated pupils, anxiety, hallucinations, death from accidents or overdose
Inhalants				
Solvents: gasoline, glue, paint thinner, lighter fluid, nail polish remover Nitrites: amyl, butyl	Chroming, gas, glue sniffing, poppers, quicksilver, rush Poppers, locker room, rush, snappers	Inhaled or sniffed, often with use of paper or plastic bag or rag Inhaled or sniffed from gauze or ampoules	Initial high, then CNS depression; poor motor coordination; impaired vision and thought processes; abusive, violent behaviour; slowed thought; headache	Severe weight loss; brain, liver and bone marrow damage; anaemia Toxicity: high risk of sudden death by anoxia

[a] Includes lookalike drugs resembling amphetamines that may contain caffeine, phenylpropanolamine and ephedrine.

- *physical dependence*, causing physiological disturbances when administration of the drug ceases (the **withdrawal syndrome**).

People with chronic conditions may be in a state of medical dependence on a drug required for effective therapy; for example, people with type 1 diabetes are said to be 'insulin-dependent'.

Governments regulate most drugs of dependence (Ch 2); however, some drugs (alcohol, nicotine, caffeine) are considered differently and are readily available in most countries. In Australia, drugs of dependence are generally listed in Schedule 8: Controlled Drugs of The Poisons Standard (SUSMP), subject to the strictest controls of availability, storage, labelling and prescribing. (An exception is codeine, available on prescription in compound analgesics.) Thus, most drugs of dependence are **illicit** (illegal) outside of approved medical use on prescription.

Addiction (a term sometimes used synonymously with 'dependence') is a behavioural pattern of drug use with overwhelming involvement in procurement and use of the drug and a high tendency to relapse back into dependence.[1] Addiction involves impairment in three functional systems: motivation–reward, affect (mood) and behavioural inhibition.

Tolerance is a physical state in which repeated doses of the drug cause decreasing effects, or doses must be

1 The class of addictive disorders includes addiction to psychoactive drugs; bulimia nervosa (binge eating with excessive exercise and/or dieting or self-induced vomiting); pathological gambling or shopping; addiction to the internet; and sexual addictions–all characterised by recurrent failure to control the behaviour and continuation despite harmful consequences.

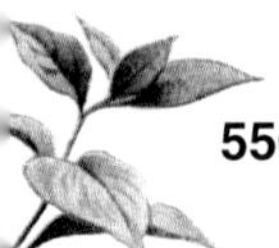

increased to maintain the same effects. Not all drugs of dependence induce tolerance; tolerance develops rapidly to most effects of morphine (but not to constipation or miosis), whereas there is little tolerance to marijuana.

Mechanisms of dependence and tolerance

Dependence and addiction

Addiction begins with recreational or therapeutic use that may progress through excessive consumption to compulsive drug seeking, with a shift from positive reinforcement (rewards) to negative reinforcement (abstinence and withdrawal syndromes) driving behaviours (drug craving and compulsive seeking).

Currently, the theory explaining dependence involves the mesolimbic dopaminergic pathway from the substantia nigra through the nucleus accumbens to the frontal cortex; activation of this pathway is critical for rewarding and reinforcing properties. Dopamine (DA) has a pivotal role in signalling incentives (reward, novel stimuli), driving motivated behaviour and consolidating memory. Drug seeking and relapse appear to be mediated by a more complex network of circuits including the prefrontal cortex (involved in motivation, response to drug, behavioural inhibition); the locus coeruleus (withdrawal); ventral tegmental area (reward); nucleus accumbens (reward, dysphoria); and striae terminalis (negative reinforcement, relapse).

Drug-induced effects lead to regulatory changes at the mRNA or protein level, causing neuroadaptations and altered behaviours.[2] Interactions between many molecular pathways, mediators and transmitters may be involved, including 5-hydroxytryptamine (serotonin) (5-HT), noradrenaline (norepinephrine), gamma-aminobutyric acid (GABA), glutamate, endocannabinoids, corticosteroids, phosphodiesterases 4, 7 and 10A, peroxisome proliferating activator receptors, the Toll-like receptor 4, and various neuropeptides including endorphins, melanocortins, galanin, orexin, hypocretin, leptin, nociception and neurokinin. Pharmacological studies on these targets may lead to new drugs to treat addictive behaviours (Ubaldi et al. 2016).

Tolerance

Tolerance, the tendency for successive doses to have lesser effects, may exist with either psychological or physical dependence. In receptor-site (pharmacodynamic) tolerance, receptor synthesis may be downregulated, receptors may be lost or desensitised, or there may be exhaustion of chemical mediators or transmitters. Neuroadaptations contributing to tolerance may exist also at the cellular, nerve network and body systems levels.

In metabolic (pharmacokinetic) tolerance, prolonged exposure increases drug clearance. With repeated ingestion of barbiturates (CNS depressants), steady-state blood concentrations fall progressively because of increased hepatic microsomal enzymes, which increase the metabolism and inactivation of many other drugs administered concurrently (see 'Pharmacokinetic Drug Interactions', Ch 7).

Factors leading to drug abuse and dependence

Sociocultural factors

Societies allow, restrict or ban drugs depending on the particular society's religious rules, typical ethos (aggressive/meditative), history and traditional medicine practices; drug taking is clearly seen as very different from other forms of self-gratification. There are double standards here: most governments condemn abuse of alcohol and tobacco products but do not ban them, for civil liberty reasons and because enormous revenue is received from taxes. (In 2021 the Australian Government collected more than $13.8 billion in revenue from tobacco products.)

The popularity of a drug may depend on its availability, ease of sharing, peer-group pressures and wide publicity of drug abuse in the mass media. There are differing patterns of drug abuse in various sections of society – for example, between men and women, Indigenous and non-Indigenous people, adolescents and adults, and different religious or ethnic groups. Where particular drugs are illegal and in short supply, criminals are motivated to obtain and sell the substances.

Personality factors

Models proposed as to why some people abuse drugs include the:

- moralistic model – the person lacks moral willpower to 'just say no'
- disease model – the person suffers a psychopathology or is genetically predisposed
- poor environment model – the social victim suffers from disadvantage.

Psychological theories to explain drug abuse include:

- cognitive behaviour theory – dependence is due to a learned (reinforced) set of dysfunctional behaviours
- psychoanalytical theory – behaviours are determined by unconscious forces; drugs are used in self-medication
- poor self-care theory – people struggling to cope tend to abuse drugs
- dual-diagnosis theory – the person concurrently suffers both psychiatric difficulties and substance dependence.

The three most important predictors of a person becoming dependent on drugs are rebelliousness,

2 Dopaminergic CNS-active drugs affect behaviour in many ways, notably inducing circling in test animals due to asymmetry in dopaminergic activity between the left and right sides of the brain. It can be induced by opiates and amphetamines. Farmers in northern Tasmania had occasionally noticed unusual circles in their fields of (legally grown) opium poppies; the mystery was solved when a farmer noticed wallabies acting strangely in his fields: eating some poppies, hopping off, returning for more and circling in the paddocks.

tolerance of deviance and low school performance. The 'alcoholic personality' has a higher-than-average incidence of depression and antisocial tendencies plus a genetic predisposition to dependence.

Many drug-dependent people are in denial, believing myths such as:

- 'Recreational use of drugs isn't harmful.'
- 'Only weak people become addicts.'
- 'If you drink milk (or eat yoghurt) before drinking alcohol, you won't get drunk.'
- 'Marijuana isn't dangerous.'
- 'Taking "speed" pills or drinking strong coffee will metabolise the alcohol at a faster rate.'
- 'Growing and pushing drugs is okay because it's one way poor people can make money.'

Pharmacological factors: CNS effects

Drugs that activate the mechanisms leading to dependence and addiction have desirable effects in the CNS: providing relief from problems or the achievement of pleasure. All drugs likely to be abused have three characteristics: they act fast, make you feel good or stop you feeling bad.[3] (Obviously there is little temptation to abuse a drug that takes hours to act.) The pharmacological effects of some mind-altering drugs (on spiders) are graphically illustrated in Fig 25.1 (Noever et al. 1995).

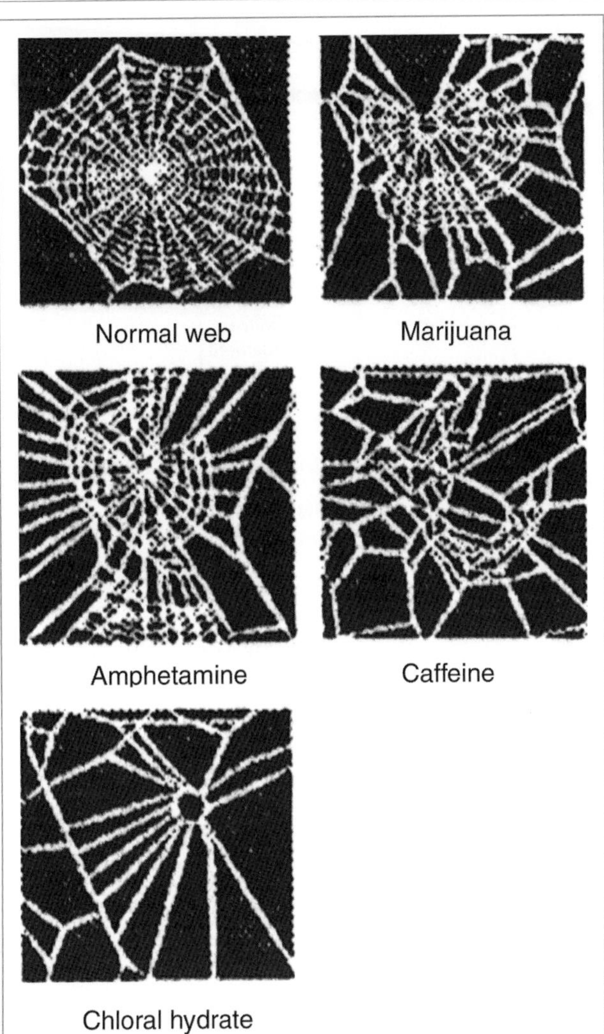

FIGURE 25.1 Effects of mind-altering drugs on spiders
In a technique developed to test toxicity of chemicals, household spiders were sprayed with solutions and the shapes of webs subsequently spun were analysed. The figure shows the effects of marijuana (a drug causing relaxation and impairment of motor coordination and memory), amphetamine and caffeine (CNS stimulants) and chloral hydrate (a sedative drug). The technique was developed as an alternative to toxicity testing in higher animals, which is subject to ethical concerns, expensive and time-consuming. The head of the research team, Dr David Noever, was quoted as saying that he did not expect complaints from animal rights groups: 'We're all concerned about tests on warm and fuzzy creatures, but in this case, they are only fuzzy.'
Source: Noever et al. 1995; used with permission.

Euphoria

Euphoria includes 'feel-good' effects, enhanced alertness, and relief from anxiety or pain. Legal drugs that may induce euphoria and alter states of perception include opioids, stimulants, anticholinergics, corticosteroids, psychotropic agents, pregabalin, quetiapine and levodopa.

Reinforcement and reward

Drugs of dependence produce **reinforcement** (conditioning) or reward in animals or humans: subjects will carry out work to obtain further doses. Strong reinforcers include opioids, barbiturates, alcohol and cocaine. Weak reinforcers in animals include caffeine and nicotine. (However, some human drug addicts have found it easier to give up heroin than to quit smoking.) Non-reinforcers include cannabis: animals (non-human) will not bother to self-administer marijuana.

An unpleasant withdrawal syndrome after stopping drugs that cause physical dependence can encourage addicts to seek another dose (Fig 25.2, later). Craving may also be stimulated by stress, or by the people and situations in which the person has previously taken the drug.

Problems associated with drug abuse

The scale of trafficking and abuse of drugs

Illicit drugs comprise 10% of all international trade: the big four groups (opioids, cocaine, cannabis and amphetamines) comprise an industry worth more than US$350 billion a year, making drugs one of the most 'valuable' commodities.

3 Edgar Allan Poe, the American writer (1809–49), famously wrote: 'I have absolutely no pleasure in the stimulants in which I sometimes so madly indulge. It has not been in the pursuit of pleasure that I have periled life and reputation and reason. It has been the desperate attempt to escape from torturing memories, from a sense of insupportable loneliness and a dread of some strange impending doom.' (Many writers, musicians and artists of the day took cocaine and opioids regularly.)

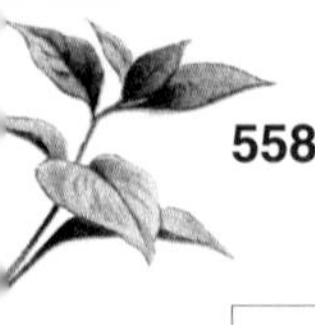

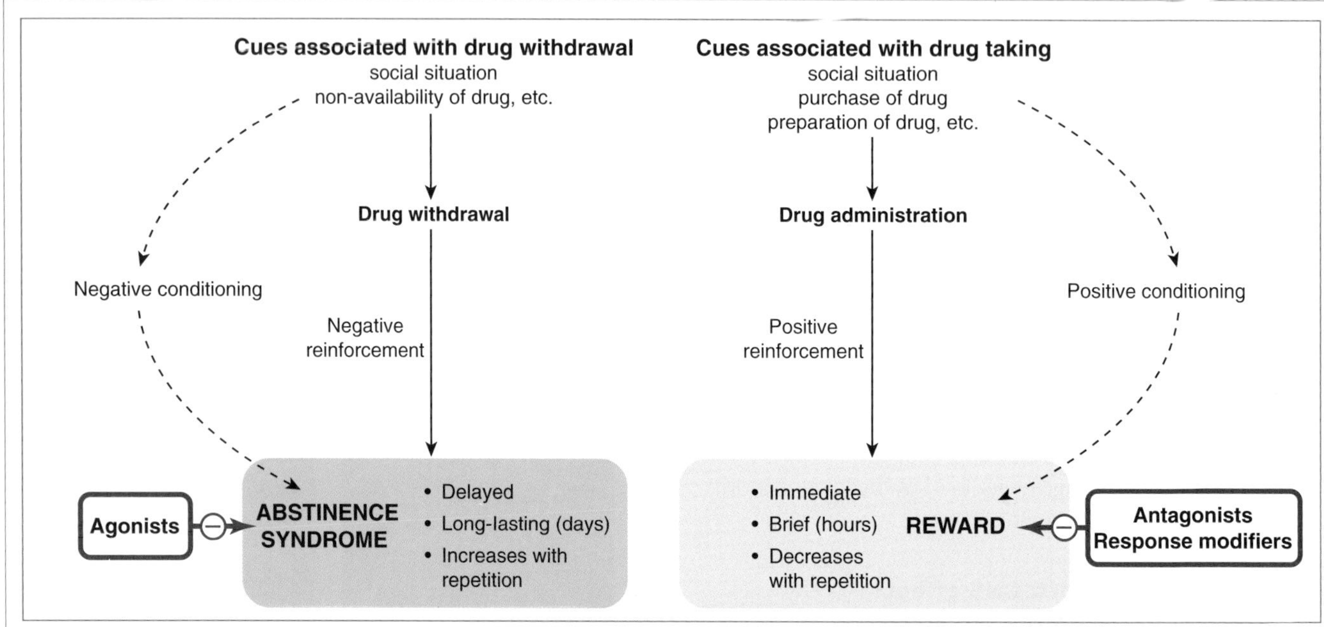

FIGURE 25.2 A simplified scheme of some of the psychological factors involved in drug dependence
Source: Rang et al. 2016, Figure 49-2.

The economic cost of drug abuse in Australia, including tangible and intangible costs (drains on legal, health and policing systems; lost productivity and income; and indirect costs to families), was estimated at more than A$228.96 billion in 2015–16. About 56% was due to tobacco, 27% to alcohol and only 15% to illicit drugs. Legal drugs (alcohol and tobacco) therefore cause the most medical and economic harm in our community.

Patterns of drug abuse worldwide

The United Nations Office on Drugs and Crime (UNODC) produces regular reports; quoting from its recent summary: 'The *2020 World Drug Report* provides a global overview of the supply and demand of opiates, cocaine, cannabis, amphetamine-type stimulants and new psychoactive substances, as well as their impact on health. It also reviews the scientific evidence on polydrug use, treatment demand for cannabis and developments since the legalization of cannabis for recreational use in some parts of the world.' Some of the report's findings are:

- Around 5% of the adult population, or nearly 269 million people between the ages of 15 and 64, used at least one (illicit) drug in 2018.
- The number of people suffering from drug use disorders has increased from 29 million to approximately 35.6 million.
- Around 15.3 million people inject drugs. Sharing of needles is a contributor to blood-borne virus transmission, including HIV and hepatitis B and C. Globally, 50%, 8.3% and 10% of people who inject drugs is living with hepatitis C, hepatitis B and HIV respectively.
- Overall, opioids continue to pose the highest potential harm among major drug groups: heroin use, and related overdose deaths, has increased sharply over recent years; heroin continues to be the drug that kills the most people.
- Cannabis remains the most commonly used drug at the global level, with an estimated 192 million people having used it in 2019.
- There are links between the use of stimulants (including new psychoactive substances not under international control) and engaging in risky injecting and sexual behaviours that can result in higher risk of HIV infection.
- There are high levels of drug use, including opiates and injected drugs, in prisons, which remain a high-risk environment for infectious diseases such as HIV, hepatitis and tuberculosis. Among convicted prisoners, 18% are in prison for drug-related offences.
- Men are three times more likely than women to use cannabis, cocaine or amphetamines, whereas women are more likely than men to use opioids and tranquillisers non-medically; women are more likely to be the victims of drug-related violence.
- There is a strong link between poverty and aspects of the drug problem such as social and economic disadvantage, marginalisation and social exclusion, unemployment and low levels of education.
- The drug trade is generally seen to flourish where state presence is weak, where the rule of law is unevenly applied and where opportunities for corruption exist.[4]

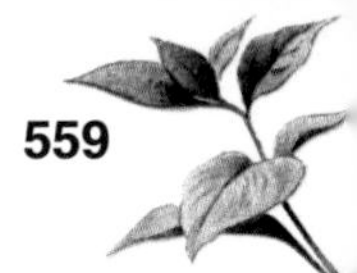

Patterns of drug abuse in Australia

To estimate the extent of drug abuse, attitudes and behaviours in Australia, large-scale population surveys have been carried out every 3–4 years since 1985. Data collected underpin policies for Australia's response to drug-related issues.[5]

Some emerging facts and trends are:

- Australians are reducing their alcohol intake, with 5.4% of the population drinking daily (down from 6.2% in 2016).
- Fewer Australians are smoking tobacco daily (down from 24% in 1991, to 12.2% to 2016 to 11% in 2019). However, more Australians are using e-cigarettes, with 11.3% of the population having ever used an e-cigarette in 2019 (up from 8.3% in 2016).
- 17.4% of Australians had used an illicit drug at some time in 2019, with marijuana the most common, then ecstasy, meth/amphetamines and cocaine (up from 15.6 in 2016).
- Non-medical pharmaceutical use is down (from 4.8% in 2016 to 4.2% in 2019).
- Public support remains high for reduction of alcohol use (to reduce drink-driving) and tobacco use.
- The people most likely to experience drug-related risks are residents of remote and very remote areas, Aboriginal and Torres Strait Islander people and people who are unemployed, homosexual or bisexual.
- Other studies[6] show that approximately 75% of people in Australian custodial institutions have used illicit substances before imprisonment. Drugs most likely to be misused or diverted to unintended uses or users in prisons are benzodiazepines, opioids, GABA analogues, anticholinergics, nicotine patches and sedatives.

Tobacco and alcohol

The most commonly abused drugs are in fact legal (licit): alcohol and tobacco. Daily smoking among the general population has more than halved since 1991 (down from 24.3% to 11% in 2019). This is mainly the result of younger people not taking up smoking. Many smokers are reducing their daily cigarette consumption. In 2019 the average number of cigarettes smoked a day was 13, compared with 16 in 2010. The ever-increasing cost of cigarettes is associated as a motivational reason to quit. Over a decade ago, in 2011, Australia became the first country in the world to introduce and legislate plain packaging of cigarettes. The intervention, aimed to reduce the attractiveness of smoking, saw all tobacco products packaged in a certain colour (drab green) and free from branding logos and text, has worked at reducing smoking rates (White et al. 2019). Interestingly, the use of e-cigarettes is increasing. In large part, they are perceived to have less harmful health impacts.

While more Australians are abstaining or reducing alcohol intake, 25% still drink to risky levels on a single occasion at least monthly. The most recent Alcohol Harm Snapshot Survey, conducted in 2019, showed that 13% of emergency department presentations in Australia were alcohol-related; this has remained constant since 2016. In contrast, 16% of emergency department presentations in New Zealand were alcohol-related. This has decreased from 23% in 2016 (Australasian College for Emergency Medicine 2020).

Illicit drugs

Cannabis is the most widely used illicit drug, with about 11.6% of Australians admitting to having used it in the previous 12 months. In some states, laws against cannabis have been relaxed, and medical marijuana may now be prescribed. New 'legal high' drugs are flooding the markets; law enforcement agencies cannot keep up with this new wave of drugs.

With respect to 'recent use' of other illicit drugs in Australia: about 3% of the population admit to having recently used ecstasy, 1.3% amphetamines, 4.2% cocaine. Illicit drugs were most commonly obtained from friends or acquaintances (70%), heroin from dealers (64%), steroids from gyms and sports clubs (65%) and 'legal highs' from tobacconists and 'adult shops' (Australian Institute of Health and Welfare 2022).

Therapeutic drugs

The extent of non-medical use of therapeutic drugs (prescribed and over-the-counter, or OTC) is difficult to determine; sudden deaths of famous entertainers attributed to overdoses of prescription drugs have raised the level of awareness. Surveys suggest that 4.8% of Australians have misused prescription drugs. Opioid analgesics are most frequently abused (3.3%), then benzodiazepines (1.6%) – these are renowned for causing dependence.

Prescribers and pharmacists need to be aware that people can become very persuasive in faking symptoms to get certain drugs prescribed, and often 'shop around' to augment their supply (Dobbin & Liew 2020). Prescription drugs are also frequently 'diverted' from their intended uses or users, and also may be sourced from family members, friends, overseas pharmacies, the internet or dealers.

There have been several recent strategies implemented by the Australian Government to reduce the misuse of prescription medications. One strategy was the up-scheduling of analgesics containing codeine from Pharmacist-Only to Prescription-Only medicines. This strategy, introduced in 2018, is associated with a reduction in codeine-related

---

4 For the full report and media content, see: wdr.unodc.org/wdr2020

5 Results from the 2019 survey are available from the Australian Institute of Health and Welfare: www.aihw.gov.au/reports/australias-health/illicit-drug-use.

6 Analysis of samples from sewage systems can give estimates of drug usage: cocaine, alcohol, tobacco, ecstasy and methamphetamine can all be measured; demographic trends discovered are that regional Victorians use more 'ice', alcohol and nicotine, while Melburnians use more cocaine.

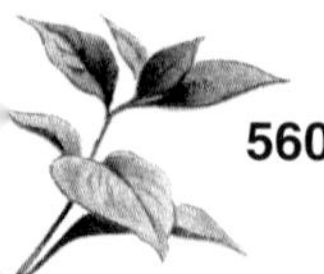

hospitalisation and misuse in Australia (Cairns et al. 2020). Another strategy is the Real Time Prescription Monitoring computer system, which monitors the prescribing and dispensing of controlled medicines in Australia.[7]

Patterns of drug abuse in New Zealand

The 2019–20 New Zealand Health Survey reported that most New Zealanders report being in good health; however, Māori, Pacific Islander peoples and those living in the most deprived areas generally report poorer health. Results relating to use of specific drugs are summarised below.

- Alcohol is the most commonly consumed drug in New Zealand: 81.5% of adults consumed alcohol in the past year. One in five adults drank alcohol in a way that could harm themselves or others.
- Smoking: The 2019–20 Health Survey showed that 13.4% of adults were current smokers; approximately 31.4% of Māori adults, 22.4% of Pacific Islanders.
- Marijuana is the most popular illegal drug in New Zealand, with 14.9% of people having used cannabis in the past year.
- Amphetamines: In 2019–20, 1.1% of adults self-reported using amphetamines in the preceding year. Pseudoephedrine is used as a precursor substance in the manufacture in clandestine home laboratories of methamphetamine or 'P' (known also as 'speed', 'pure', 'burn' and 'ice'; the name 'P' is used only in New Zealand).

Individual, family and society problems

While deaths from overdose of illicit drugs such as heroin are tragic and newsworthy, the vast majority of drug-related deaths in Australia are due to tobacco or alcohol. In 2018–19, of clients attending specialist drug treatment services, about 34% of problems are related to alcohol, 28% amphetamines, 20% cannabis and 5% heroin (Australian Institute of Health and Welfare 2021). The signs and symptoms of acute drug intoxication are summarised in Table 25.1.

The harm done may be directly to the individual from adverse drug reactions such as alcoholic liver cirrhosis, psychosis from amphetamines or cannabis, or cancers and cardiovascular disease from smoking. There are also indirect effects: IV drug abuse (opioids, amphetamines and cocaine) may lead into the subculture of 'shooting up', with the risk of blood-borne infections (including HIV, hepatitis B and C). Families of drug-dependent people may have to cope with aggressive behaviour, destructive relationships, reduced earnings and resources, increased medical expenses and increased dependence on state welfare for support.

Withdrawal syndromes

The withdrawal syndrome after drug cessation is due to uncompensated adaptive changes induced by chronic drug administration; it frequently manifests as a rebound in the systems affected. Thus, withdrawal from benzodiazepines (CNS depressants) may lead to anxiety and agitation, whereas withdrawal from amphetamines (CNS stimulants) leads to depressed mood and drowsiness.

Crime and drink-driving

Craving for further doses may dominate a person's life, leading to an unacceptable lifestyle or a life of crime to support dependence. Escalating crime in the community necessitates increased policing, court procedures and prisons to deal with offences related to production, supply and possession of illicit drugs. Alcohol-related intoxication increases violence, drink-driving, risk taking, injuries and deaths.

Appendix K of the Poisons Standard outlines all drugs that are required to be labelled with a sedation warning. Medicines in this list can reduce alertness and cause driving impairment. It is important for health professionals to counsel people not to drink alcohol while taking medications from the list, as impairment can be further enhanced (Drug Interactions 25.1).

Drug abuse during pregnancy and breastfeeding

Most drugs of dependence, being lipid-soluble, can cross the placental barrier and adversely affect the fetus, potentially causing altered gene expression, birth of drug-dependent infants or long-term behavioural and psychiatric disorders. Illicit drugs such as heroin, cannabis and ecstasy do not have pregnancy safety classifications, nor do non-scheduled substances such as caffeine, alcohol and tobacco. Drug abusers often use many different drugs, and lifestyle factors may contribute to poor antenatal care.

With respect to use of social drugs during pregnancy, the following should be noted:

- Alcohol intake (moderate to high) leads to risk of fetal alcohol syndrome.
- Tobacco use leads to poor pregnancy outcomes (increased risk of spontaneous abortion, preterm delivery, low birthweight). Nicotine is in Pregnancy Safety Category D; however, nicotine substitution is considered safer than smoking.
- Cocaine use leads to poor outcomes and is teratogenic (genitourinary tract malformations).
- Opioids use can cause opioid withdrawal in the neonate, with CNS excitability (Clinical Focus Box 25.1, later); for heroin-dependent women, methadone maintenance is the preferred treatment.

---

7 For more information, see: www.health.gov.au/initiatives-and-programs/national-real-time-prescription-monitoring-rtpm

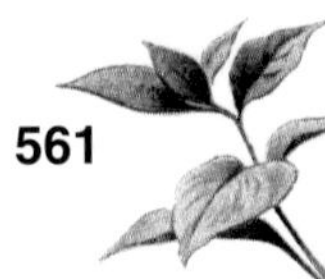

DRUG INTERACTIONS 25.1
Alcohol

SUBSTANCES INTERACTING WITH ALCOHOL	MECHANISM	POSSIBLE EFFECTS
All CNS depressants, including antihistamines, antidepressants, opioid analgesics, hypnotics, antianxiety agents, antipsychotics, chloral hydrate	Additive	Enhanced CNS-depressant effects
Disulfiram, some cefalosporins, oral antidiabetic agents, griseofulvin, metronidazole, procarbazine, tinidazole, chloral hydrate	Inhibition of alcohol metabolism by aldehyde dehydrogenase, leading to acetaldehyde accumulation (a 'disulfiram-type reaction')	Most severe effects seen with disulfiram and alcohol: flushing, stomach pain, head throbbing, raised heart rate, hypotension, sweating, nausea and vomiting; with antidiabetic agents, mild-to-severe hypoglycaemia
Phenytoin, warfarin	Increase or decrease in liver metabolism	Chronically: possible decrease in effect due to enzyme induction; acutely: possible decrease in metabolism, causing raised serum level and toxicity
Salicylates	Additive	Increased gastrointestinal irritability and bleeding
Nitrates, glyceryl trinitrate	Additive	Vasodilation leading to hypotension, syncope
Anticholinergics, antispasmodics	Slowed gastrointestinal functions	Slowed absorption of alcohol
Paracetamol	Additive	Enhanced hepatic toxicity of paracetamol
Acitretin (an oral retinoid)	Alcohol may increase metabolism of acitretin to etretinate, which is teratogenic	Women of child-bearing age should avoid alcohol while taking acitretin and for 2 months afterwards

Source: Adapted from Australian Medicines Handbook 2021; inter alia.

- Cannabis and the hallucinogens have not been shown to be teratogenic.
- Caffeine appears safe in moderate amounts, but caffeine clearance decreases during pregnancy.

Benefits of breastfeeding generally outweigh any potential risks to the baby from drugs a mother takes, so moderate amounts of caffeine, alcohol and tobacco may be preferable to withdrawal syndromes or to weaning the infant (Ch 30). 'Hard' illicit drugs are of such risk to the infant that breastfeeding is not advised.

Problems among health professionals

Career pressures, long working hours and easy accessibility to drugs place health professionals, particularly anaesthetists and other doctors, pharmacists, nurses and dentists, at risk of drug abuse. Studies among health professionals in the United States have shown that health professionals who abused medications generally used more than four substances, including prescription drugs (opioid analgesics and benzodiazepines), alcohol, tobacco and nitrous oxide.

Policies related to drug abuse and its management

History of legislation

Opium, the source of alkaloids with analgesic, sedative (narcotic) and antidiarrhoeal activities, has been used medically for thousands of years, and has been the cause of crime and wars. An international Opium Convention was set up in 1912 to curb opium trade, and was ratified after World War I. Other drugs of addiction were added to the charter, including cannabis in 1925. The responsibility for worldwide control of 'narcotics' (by then defined to include cocaine and cannabis) was handed over to the United Nations after World War II (1946). The main international treaties are the:

- 1961 Single Convention on Narcotic Drugs
- 1971 Convention on Psychotropic Substances
- 1988 Convention against the Illicit Traffic in Narcotic Drugs and Psychotropic Substances.

  (See Ch 2, under 'International Drug Controls'.)

Policy approaches

A former head of UNODC noted: 'Each country gets the drug problem that it deserves.' Thus, a country that wages 'war on drugs', focusing on prohibition, spends most of its illicit drugs' budget on law enforcement, with little left for treatment and harm reduction.

Worldwide

The UNODC has promulgated International Standards on Drug Use Prevention. Most countries attempt to keep their official drug legislation in line with that of the UN, but this can be problematic if a country wishes to trial an alternative policy, such as supervised injecting facilities or decriminalisation of marijuana.

The UN Commission on Narcotic Drugs, composed of 53 elected member states, is the central policymaking body for drug-related matters, including the monitoring of global trends of illicit drug trafficking and abuse, resolutions on agreed policies to address drug issues and scheduling of substances. The International Narcotics Control Board is a permanent and independent body that monitors implementation of the conventions, administers statistical control of drugs data, assesses world requirements of licit drugs, gathers information on illicit trafficking and reports annually on developments in the world situation.

UNODC Reports (2009, 2013) recommend:

- policies to improve access to treatment for drug addicts, to reduce demand
- shifting the focus of law enforcement from drug users to drug traffickers
- addressing the problems of slums and dereliction in 'cities out of control', especially by assisting youth with jobs, education and sport
- ratifying UN Conventions against organised crime and against trafficking of people and arms, especially targeting money-laundering and cyber-crime.

Prevention policies ('prohibition') have proved to be enormously expensive, but the extent of drug trafficking and abuse has changed little over several decades. Most studies show that relaxing drug laws does not markedly increase abuse or deaths from drugs but allows governments to implement harm reduction policies and reduces profits for criminals.

New Zealand drug policies

Some aspects of New Zealand policies related to drug abuse are as follows:

- There is a wide range of controlled and illegal drugs, which the *Misuse of Drugs Act 1975* classifies according to the level of risk of harm they pose:
    - Class A (very high risk): methamphetamine, magic mushrooms, cocaine, heroin, LSD ('acid')
    - Class B (high risk): cannabis oil, hashish, morphine, opium, ecstasy and many amphetamine-type substances
    - Class C (moderate risk): cannabis seed, cannabis plant, codeine.
- Maximum penalties for possession (having control or custody of a drug) are: Class A: 6 months' imprisonment and/or NZ$1000 fine; Classes B&C: 3 months' imprisonment and/or NZ$500 fine.
- There are also severe penalties for supply or manufacture, possession of instruments for drug taking and cultivation or possession of prohibited plants.[8]
- Temporary Class Drug Notices: Many stimulant or mood-altering 'legal highs' were not banned by old laws covering the misuse of drugs; more than 50 synthetic cannabis and amphetamine products are now illegal, as the Ministry of Health has issued numerous Temporary Class Drug Notices that make it illegal to import, export, manufacture, sell or supply any product containing substances under notice.
- The upper legal limit of alcohol for licensed drivers aged over 20 years is 80 mg of alcohol per 100 mL of blood (0.08%) or 400 micrograms/L of breath on a breathalyser; limits for drivers under 20 are lower.
- In 2013 New Zealand became the second country in the world to introduce laws enforcing plain-packaging of cigarettes.
- Pseudoephedrine and pseudoephedrine-containing products became controlled drugs from 2004 to minimise risk of pseudoephedrine being diverted to manufacture amphetamines; parcels containing 2000–20,000 pseudoephedrine tablets have been seized by customs officers.
- Information on alcohol and illicit drugs can be found on the NZ Police website (see 'Online resources').

Australian drug policies

Australia has been a signatory to three international drug treaties (1961, 1971, 1988), requiring it to impose criminal sanctions on people convicted of trafficking any of now 250 listed drugs – that is, the 'prohibition model' of 'zero tolerance' for illicit drug abuse. The fundamentals are reduction of demand, supply and harm by national, state and territory ministers for health, law enforcement and education (see Australian National Drug Strategy in 'Online resources').

Currently, Australia spends much more on policing drug policies than on treatment services. The huge rewards for manufacturers and dealers mean that forces driving drug consumption are likely always to outstrip law enforcement.

Drug law reformers recommend that health and social interventions gradually replace criminal justice measures, and that emphasis moves to improving treatment systems and life opportunities for disadvantaged communities. Medically supervised safe injecting centres operate in Sydney and Melbourne. Currently, legal requirements for prescriptions for Controlled (Schedule 8) Drugs vary between states and territories, causing confusion for prescribers, pharmacists and patients, especially when moving between states. Standardising legal S8 requirements would minimise ambiguity and simplify practice.

8 See: www.police.govt.nz/advice/drugs-and-alcohol

In recognition that some people will continue to abuse drugs and need protection, the following practical advice for **harm minimisation** has been promulgated:

- Use only one drug at a time.
- Inhaling is safer than injecting.
- If using ecstasy, take frequent rest and water breaks.
- Don't use drugs when alone.
- Practise safe sex.
- If injecting, use clean syringes, needles and water; dispose of used equipment safely.
- If someone collapses, put them in the recovery position, call an ambulance immediately and stay with the person.

Other possible drug policies

In the Netherlands and some other European countries, policies are based on normalisation and destigmatisation, whereby less harmful 'soft drugs' may be ignored by police; for example, cannabis can be ordered in a coffee shop. Portugal has decriminalised many previously illicit drugs and switched efforts to treatment, harm reduction and counselling. In Switzerland, it has been found cheaper to prescribe heroin than to prosecute users of it. Supervised injecting facilities have been demonstrated to operate well in some German cities, leading to decreased public nuisance, fewer heroin overdose deaths and decreased frequency of drug-related infections. In 2021, in the United States, 17 states had fully legalised marijuana for adult use. Thirty-seven states had legalised medical marijuana. Since June 2018 the adult use of marijuana has been legal in Canada.

Treating drug dependence: general aspects

Methods for treating drug abuse are determined by whether it is a case of acute toxicity, chronic abuse or long-term management. The primary goal should be to reduce harm, rather than reduce supply or punish offenders. A combination of therapeutic approaches is useful, including antagonists and other drugs to block the reward and modify responses, agonists to substitute for the drug and overcome the withdrawal syndrome, as well as aversive therapies to block cravings, behavioural modifications, and drugs to treat adverse effects of the drug of dependence (Fig 25.2).

Some general points relevant to treatment are:

- For any treatment to work, the person must first acknowledge that drug abuse has become a problem.
- Pharmacological approaches to treatment of addictive disorders focus on substitution-based methods, use of antagonist drugs or targeting endogenous neurotransmitters.
- Other treatment modalities include education and information, self-help strategies, psychological therapies including counselling and complementary and alternative medicine methods.
- Multiple drug abuse is common, so a full drug screen should be carried out.
- 'Dual diagnosis' means psychiatric problems such as depression, psychoses, anxiety disorders and personality disorders often occur along with drug abuse; all problems need to be addressed.
- Intravenous drug users run extra risks of contracting blood-borne viral diseases such as hepatitis B or C or HIV infection through sharing of equipment; needle exchange programs and supervised injecting rooms reduce these risks.
- Drug abusers become very skilled at 'conning' doctors into prescribing more of the drugs they crave; pethidine is particularly in demand (see 'Drug-Seeking Behaviours', below).

Treating acute overdose

Despite the low prevalence of their abuse, the highest mortality rate from illicit drug overdose in Australia is from opioids, the second highest from amphetamines. A high rate of hospitalisation for illicit drug overdose is from cannabis substances but they appear not to have caused a fatality. Three common 'toxidromes' (toxicity syndromes) are recognised, caused by sympathomimetic-type compounds (amphetamines, cocaine, MDMA), opioids and cannabis (Table 25.1).

The primary aim of treatment is first aid and resuscitation of the person, then establishing what drugs have been taken, elimination of the drug if possible and treatment of toxic effects. A full history should be taken when possible, including comorbidities and previous psychiatric disturbances and drug taking.

Treatment is specific for drugs taken: sedatives/antipsychotics for overdose with stimulants or cannabis, oxygen plus opioid antagonist for opioid overdose and flumazenil for benzodiazepine overdose. Antidepressants, sedatives, α_2-agonists or β-blockers may be useful for withdrawal syndromes. Symptomatic treatment of cardiovascular adverse effects, seizures, hypo-/hyperthermia, hypo-/hyperglycaemia, agitation and nausea/vomiting is administered.

Treating chronic abuse

Initially, a comprehensive assessment of the person is required, with a full history and drug screening. Goals of treatment are to achieve total withdrawal from the drug, detoxification and treatment of any withdrawal reactions, possibly best carried out in a hospital or 'detox' facility. Antagonists (e.g. naltrexone at opioid receptors) will suppress the harmful effects of agonist drugs but also suppress the euphoriant effects and provide no reinforcement, so compliance with them is

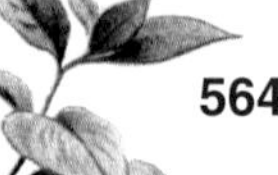

poor. Naltrexone is also prescribed to treat alcohol use disorder.

Long-term maintenance

The preferred scenario is to achieve abstinence from any drug abuse; however, this is difficult because withdrawal causes distress and resumption of drug-taking behaviours. A more realistic goal is harm minimisation. A milder substitute drug may help maintain effects while reducing harms – for example, methadone substituted for morphine or heroin, and nicotine patches for cigarettes.

A novel approach still undergoing research and trials is developing vaccines to stimulate the immune system to produce antibodies to block the pharmacological effects of a drug of dependence. To date, vaccines have been developed against nicotine and cocaine, with some limited success (John et al. 2020).

Drug-seeking behaviours

Health professionals have to remain alert for **drug-seeking behaviours**. Many dependent people 'shop around' among prescribers to obtain prescriptions, particularly seeking pethidine, codeine, oxycodone, amphetamines, benzodiazepines, pregabalin and newer antipsychotics (quetiapine and olanzapine). A study in Australia revealed that over 850 people had each seen more than 50 different doctors in one year, and more than 20,000 people had seen 15 or more doctors.

While it is important that people with genuine need for a drug are not denied it, drug-seekers need to be referred for treatment. Signs of drug-seeking behaviours include:

- requesting a specific drug (of dependence) and refusing other suggestions
- reporting inconsistent symptoms
- reporting a recent move into the area, with a (forged?) letter of support
- manifesting signs of drug intoxication or withdrawal, especially impaired cognitive functions, injection-site marks and constricted or dilated pupils.

Prescribers are encouraged to register with the Prescription Shopping Information Service. This service enables the prescriber to check a person's prescribing history before making a decision about how to treat a person.

KEY POINTS

Drug abuse and dependence

- Drug dependence may be psychological and/or physical; related problems are addiction, tolerance and withdrawal syndromes. Trafficking in illicit drugs leads to problems in individuals, families and societies; government policies attempt to reduce supply and demand and minimise harm arising from drug dependence.
- Drug abuse may be influenced by sociocultural aspects that dictate which drugs are prohibited or allowed, personality factors that predispose to drug dependence and pharmacological factors that cause some drugs to be reinforcing or rewarding. Most drugs of abuse affect central dopaminergic pathways.
- Drugs of dependence may be legal (alcohol, caffeine, nicotine) and prescribed (opioids, benzodiazepines, amphetamines), or illicit (heroin, cocaine).
- Drug groups commonly abused are opioids, including heroin; CNS depressants, including alcohol, the benzodiazepines and inhalants; CNS stimulants (cocaine, amphetamines, caffeine and nicotine); and psychotomimetics (cannabis and hallucinogens).
- Treating drug dependence involves managing the acute overdose situation or withdrawal reaction, attempts to detoxify, reduce dependence and maintain abstinence, or maintenance of dependence with a less harmful substitute drug.

Dependence on opioids

Opioid abuse and dependence

Morphine and codeine are opium alkaloids from natural sources (Fig 1.3A); related are many semi/synthetic drugs including heroin and oxycodone. The term 'opioid' refers to products with morphine-like agonist effects on enkephalin (opioid) receptors. (For mechanisms and clinical uses, see Ch 19.)

Tolerance develops to analgesia, euphoria, sedation and respiratory depression but not to constipation or miosis (constricted pupils). Tolerance may involve μ-opioid receptor-mediated alterations in regulatory events, and recycling of μ-opioid receptors.

Opioids rapidly relieve pain and anxiety, change or elevate mood, and produce feelings of peace and euphoria, so they are particularly likely to lead to dependence, abuse and chronic adverse effects, potentially criminal behaviour to support the habit, uncertainty about strength and purity of procured drugs, issues related to IV injecting and withdrawal reactions. Prior to 2018, codeine was available without prescription and was often taken with other opioids and CNS depressants, leading to many deaths from codeine overdose in Australia.

Opioids generally have low oral bioavailability and so are abused by sniffing (snorting), subcutaneous injection

Lethargy, unresponsiveness or loss of consciousness
Vomiting making choking sounds
Bluish purple skin (in people with light-coloured skin)
Greyish or ashen skin (in people with dark-coloured skin)
Small pupils
Respiratory failure, slow or shallow breathing
Hypotension
Slow, erratic pulse
Poor circulation

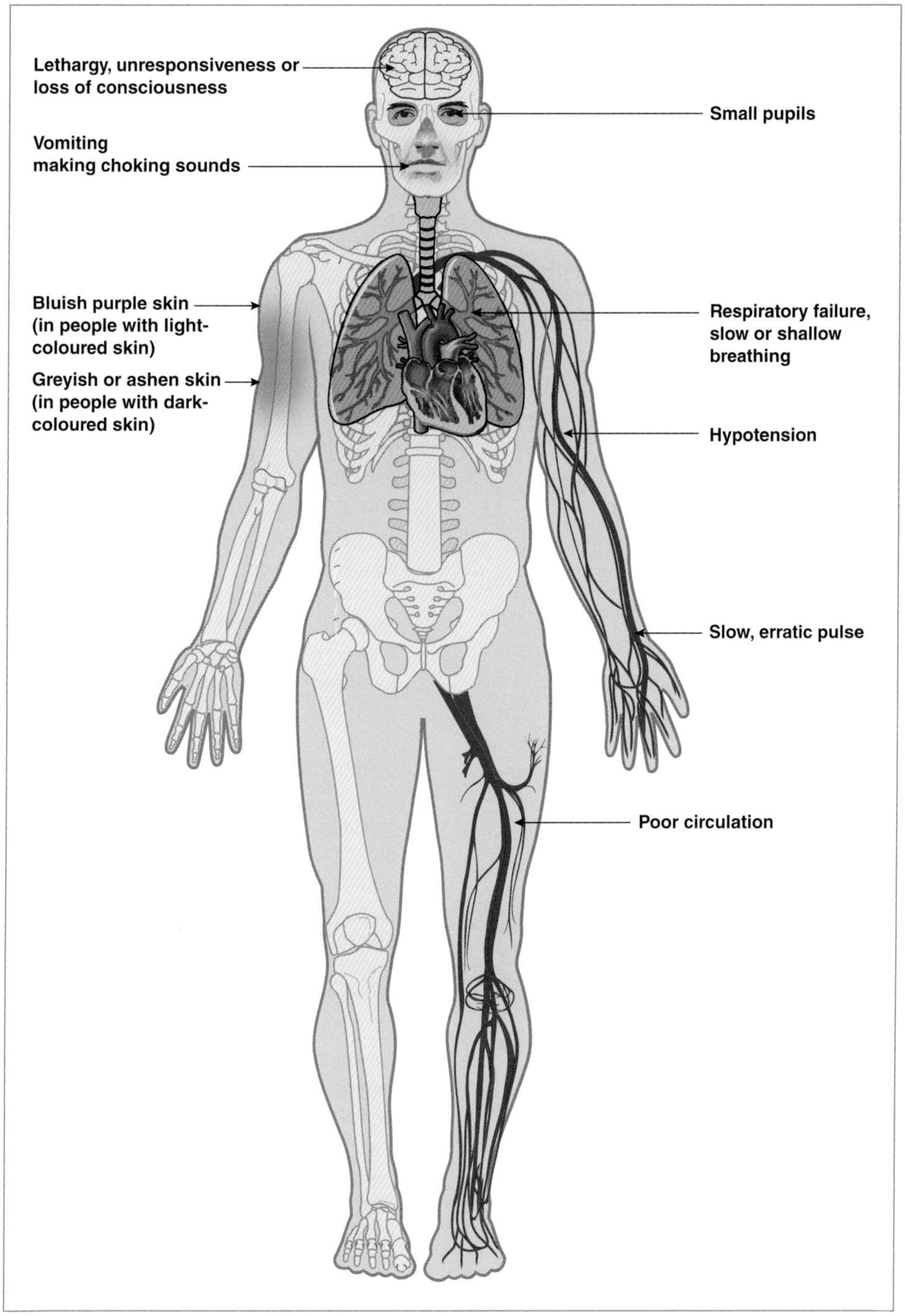

FIGURE 25.3 Signs and symptoms of opioid overdose

(skin popping) or direct IV injection (mainlining, 'shooting up'), which produces almost immediate effects.

Heroin abuse

Diacetylmorphine (heroin, diamorphine) was initially introduced into medicine as a cough suppressant and to treat morphine addiction but is banned in most countries. Heroin is highly lipid-soluble, so it quickly passes the blood–brain barrier producing a rapid, intense 'rush'. It is highly addictive, and tolerance develops rapidly. Controlled studies comparing heroin and morphine do not support the belief that heroin is 'better'.

Heroin is a prodrug, rapidly converted in the liver to morphine, with a short half-life requiring frequent doses. The purity of heroin supplies varies widely – from 25% to 90% pure – so it is easy for addicts to overdose fatally. The mortality rate is 1–2% of users per annum. Impurities injected along with the opioid can cause collapsed veins, infections and organ damage.

Acute over-dosage

The signs and symptoms of acute opioid overdose are shown in Fig 25.3. The lethal dose depends on the tolerance.

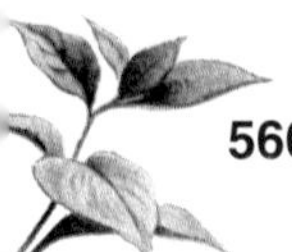

Thrombophlebitis, scarred veins and puckered scars from injections help identify a person with opioid dependence.

The treatment of choice for acute over-dosage is administration of an antagonist (e.g. naloxone), respiratory and cardiovascular support and rehydration. Naloxone is commonly administered by paramedics to treat opioid overdose; it is now available OTC as a Pharmacist-Only drug, and can safely be administered IM by laypeople in emergencies (Jauncey & Nielsen 2017). Onset of effect after IM or IV injection is 1–3 minutes. As naloxone duration of action (30–45 minutes) may be shorter than that of the opioid, multiple doses of naloxone may be required; adverse effects are those of acute opioid withdrawal.

Withdrawal syndrome

In a person who is physically dependent on opioids, sudden withdrawal or abrupt reversal with an opioid antagonist may precipitate acute withdrawal, with excitation and diarrhoea, 'cold turkey' skin and pupil dilation. While unpleasant, the withdrawal symptoms are not usually dangerous. Milder symptoms (craving and sleep disturbances) may continue for many months, and psychological dependence for much longer.

Babies born to women who are dependent on an opioid may suffer an immediate withdrawal reaction (Clinical Focus Box 25.1).

Treating opioid dependence

The main aim is to keep users alive; withdrawal is difficult and stressful, and repeated relapses occur. Abrupt complete withdrawal (known as 'going cold turkey', due to the 'goose-bumps' induced) is dangerous, especially in people with a co-existing illness. Therapeutic community programs (e.g. Odyssey House – see 'Online resources') have been established offering group psychotherapy and self-help approaches. Chilling statistics report that, on average after 10 years, 30–40% of former users remain abstinent, 40–50% are active users or imprisoned and 10–20% have died.

There are various regimens for treatment:

- Rapid detox programs: an opioid antagonist (e.g. naltrexone) is administered under close medical supervision while the opioid-dependent person is under anaesthesia or sedation; naltrexone precipitates an acute withdrawal syndrome within a few minutes. Counselling and support are usually necessary to help the person remain committed to opioid abstinence and ongoing naltrexone treatment; serious adverse effects are uncommon as naltrexone has no intrinsic agonist activity.
- Gradual reduction, then continuing total abstinence: successively tapering the dosage over several days may be accomplished with close medical supervision and treatment of withdrawal symptoms.
- Substitution, then gradual withdrawal: methadone is substituted for the opioid (e.g. heroine), then withdrawn over a 3-week period. Methadone is a synthetic agonist opioid, effective orally (Drug Monograph 25.1); it has a slower onset of action than heroin and a longer half-life. Methadone dependence is safer than heroin; it can replace euphoriant effects and craving without injections and risk of infection. Relapse from methadone withdrawal programs is common.

CLINICAL FOCUS BOX 25.1

An overdose in an opioid-dependent newborn baby

Opioid pharmacology in pregnant women and newborn babies is complex. A dependent woman often requires increasing doses of methadone as the pregnancy progresses due to placental metabolism (e.g. requiring up to 120 mg/day); sudden withdrawal must be avoided to prevent miscarriage or fetal stress. After birth, opioid withdrawal symptoms will develop in the newborn at variable times depending on the opioid used during pregnancy. Clinical features of neonatal narcotic abstinence syndrome include high-pitched crying, irritability, tremors, poor feeding, vomiting and diarrhoea, increased sweating, exaggerated reflexes and unstable temperature.

An infant was born at a large regional hospital at 34 weeks' gestation to a mother who was taking prescribed methadone and illicit heroin. Routine medical and nursing care of the infant included supportive treatment of anticipated opioid withdrawal: swaddling, frequent small feeds and 4-hourly narcotic abstinence syndrome scoring to monitor withdrawal symptoms. Scores increased rapidly over the first 48 hours, indicating seizures could be imminent. The baby was started on 4-hourly doses of oral morphine (0.5 mg/kg/day in six divided doses) to manage the withdrawal syndrome. Unfortunately, the baby received two 6-fold overdoses of morphine, due to administration errors: the morphine dose was documented as 0.5 mg/kg *per dose* rather than *per day*. The infant's withdrawal symptoms stopped immediately, but the baby developed sedation and respiratory depression and overdose was diagnosed. Oxygen was administered and the senior paediatrician was called in.

Normally, an opioid antagonist such as naloxone would be contraindicated in this situation, but the baby needed an antagonist to overcome adverse effects of the morphine overdose. Naloxone was administered IV and IM, carefully titrating effects on opioid receptors of the antagonist (naloxone) against the agonists (morphine, plus any methadone or heroin in the baby's system). The baby survived the iatrogenic morphine overdose, the abstinence syndrome was controlled over the coming days using oral morphine, and then the slow process of weaning the baby off oral morphine began, determined by the baby's abstinence scores.

Source: Acknowledgments to Dr Philippa Shilson, Paediatrician.

Drug Monograph 25.1
Methadone oral syrup

Indications

Methadone is a synthetic orally active opioid agonist formulated as a syrup for short-term management of withdrawal symptoms during opioid detoxification programs or long-term use in methadone maintenance programs. (It is also used as tablets or parenteral solution for pain relief; for mechanism of action, see Ch 19.) Oral administration reduces IV drug habits, removes the opioid taker from the 'street drug' scene and can be readily supervised.

Pharmacokinetics

Methadone is well absorbed orally and has good bioavailability but variable pharmacokinetics. Peak plasma levels are reached in 1–5 hours; it is widely distributed via the bloodstream, with protein binding in the range 60–90%. Metabolism occurs in the liver to at least two inactive metabolites; auto-induction of metabolising enzymes leads to a shorter half-life and tolerance. Methadone and metabolites are excreted in urine and faeces. The half-life is long (15–60 hours), so steady-state levels take several days.

Adverse drug reactions

The adverse-reaction profile of methadone is typical of opioids: euphoria, CNS and respiratory depression, gastrointestinal tract (GIT) and cardiovascular disturbances and spasm of biliary and renal tract smooth muscle. Tolerance develops in a few weeks to most adverse effects, so people on methadone maintenance can usually resume a normal lifestyle.

Drug interactions

Persons on a methadone (or buprenorphine) maintenance program should alert health professionals so that other drugs can be prescribed appropriately. Other CNS depressants have additive effects. Enzyme inducers, including many antiepileptic drugs and antivirals, can precipitate a withdrawal syndrome, requiring higher methadone doses. There is increased risk of dysrhythmias with other drugs that prolong the cardiac QT interval (i.e. the time between the start of the Q wave and the end of the T wave in the heart's electrical cycle). (For general drug interactions with opioids, see Ch 19.)

Warnings and contraindications

Methadone is contraindicated in respiratory depression, acute alcoholism, head injury and severe hepatic or gastrointestinal diseases. Prolonged use leads to dependence, but it is usually easier to wean off methadone than off heroin or morphine. There are cautions against driving or operating machinery. Methadone is in Category C with respect to pregnancy safety classification; higher doses may be required in pregnancy because of faster metabolism.

Dosage and administration

Methadone syrup is classified as Schedule 8 and there are strict regulations as to prescribing, dispensing and administration. The strength of the formulation is 5 mg/mL. Initial oral dose is 10–20 mg/day, with dosage increased gradually to the minimum required maintenance dose, usually 30–50 mg/day to a maximum 80 mg/day. Some people can eventually come off methadone by gradually reducing their daily dosage, but many remain on methadone programs indefinitely.

- Substitution and ongoing maintenance with another less dangerous opioid such as methadone or buprenorphine.

During the withdrawal phases, drugs may be required to treat symptoms: antidiarrhoeal agents, antispasmodics, non-steroidal anti-inflammatories and antianxiety sedatives such as diazepam.

Methadone or buprenorphine maintenance

Methadone or buprenorphine maintenance programs are cost-effective harm-minimisation options. In Australia, programs must comply with requirements of the state health department. The person attends the pharmacy for supervised oral dosing of methadone (daily) or buprenorphine (daily or alternate days). Maintenance doses that avoid withdrawal syndrome and deter cravings are in the order of 30–50 mg/day oral methadone or 12–24 mg/day sublingual buprenorphine. The dose of methadone is gradually decreased until total withdrawal is achieved.

Buprenorphine is a partial agonist at μ- and antagonist at κ-opioid receptors so is safer in overdose and can block effects of any heroin taken simultaneously; it also helps suppress craving and withdrawal symptoms. Due to its longer half-life it is a useful alternative to methadone. Sublingual 'film' formulations also contain a low dose of naloxone to deter IV usage: if injected, naloxone can precipitate an unpleasant withdrawal reaction.

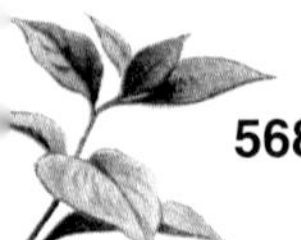

Similar programs operate in New Zealand to minimise harms associated with misuse of opioid drugs. The *New Zealand Practice Guidelines for Opioid Substitution Treatment 2014* emphasise moving from maintenance treatment to recovery while deterring substance misuse and diversion (see 'Online resources').

Analgesia for people with opioid abuse disorders

Providing adequate analgesics to manage acute pain in people with an opioid dependence disorder is difficult: they may be tolerant to opioids, in remission or withdrawal or showing drug-seeking behaviours to obtain doses. Aims are to provide effective relief of acute pain, prevent opioid withdrawal and assist with discharge planning and long-term care. Continuation of usual medications is required, with short-term use of additional opioid if indicated, plus maximisation of non-opioid analgesics and adjuvant therapies. Opioids cannot be readily used for those on naltrexone programs.

KEY POINTS

Opioid dependence and its treatment

- Most opioids are subject to abuse and dependence, particularly heroin, codeine and pethidine.
- In the treatment of opioid dependence, naloxone is used as an opioid antagonist to treat acute toxicity, naltrexone for detoxification and methadone or buprenorphine as an opioid substitute or for long-term maintenance.

Central nervous system depressants

Alcohols

The term 'alcohol' simply refers to a hydrocarbon derivative in which one or more of the hydrogen atoms (–H) has been replaced by a hydroxyl group (–OH; see Fig 1.3E). In a medical or social context, the term usually refers to ethanol (ethyl alcohol). Methyl, propyl, butyl and amyl alcohols are related alcohols, toxic when taken orally. Alcohols are naturally produced by the fermentation of cereals and fruits: wine from grapes, beer from grains, and spirits distilled after fermentation of sugar cane, grains, fruits or vegetables.

Strength of solutions

The strengths of alcoholic solutions could scientifically be expressed in SI units – for example, in g/L, mg/mL or even molar terms; however, the unit % v/v is most commonly used – that is, the number of mL of pure ethanol per 100 mL solution. 'Proof spirit' is an old term originally defined as 'a solution of alcohol of such strength that it will ignite when mixed with gunpowder' (an important concept in naval warfare); and more recently as 'the alcoholic solution that weighs 12/13 of an equal measure of distilled water'. Proof spirit contains about 57% v/v ethanol.

Alcoholic beverages contain varying amounts of ethanol, ranging from about 1–5% v/v for beers, 9–15% for wines, 16–23% for fortified wines (sherry and port) to 40–55% for spirits. The standard measures of alcoholic drinks take these varying strengths into account; hence the large beer glass, medium-sized wine glass and small 'shot glass' for spirits contain roughly the same 'dose' of pure alcohol, 10–20 g.

Ethanol (ethyl alcohol, 'alcohol')

Uses

Ethanol (**alcohol**) is the only alcohol used extensively in medicine and in alcoholic beverages. Therapeutically, ethanol has been used as an appetite stimulant, a mild hypnotic, an antidote for acute methanol or ethylene glycol poisoning and in many oral pharmaceuticals as a solvent, preservative or component of flavoured vehicles. Ethanol denatures proteins by precipitation and dehydration, hence its effects as a skin antiseptic and disinfectant. It is used in sclerotherapy (to cause hardening and closure of varicose veins) and to cause lesions to sensory nerves in neuralgias.

Ethanol is taken in alcoholic drinks, and a low level of alcohol intake has been shown (in some studies, but not all) to be protective against some cardiac conditions.[9] However, the Australian Heart Foundation does not recommend alcoholic drinks, as harms outweigh any potential benefits. As ethanol is a very commonly taken drug, it is here discussed in the usual format (Drug Monograph 25.2).

Pharmacological mechanisms and actions of ethanol

Mechanisms of action

Alcohol impairs transmission of nerve impulses at synaptic connections; a proposed mechanism for the euphoria, feelings of reward, relief of stress and pain, is release of endorphins in the nucleus accumbens and activation of mesolimbic dopaminergic pathways. Alcohol also inhibits calcium entry into nerve cells, possibly by enhancing GABA- and glycine-mediated inhibition and/or antagonising excitatory amino acid transmitters (e.g.

9 This protective effect is known as the 'French paradox', as the mortality from cardiovascular disease is lower than expected in France and other Mediterranean countries, where drinking red wine with meals is common. The flavonoids (polyphenolic compounds) present in red wines are thought to have antioxidant, anti-inflammatory, antithrombotic, vasodilator and possibly antitumour effects.

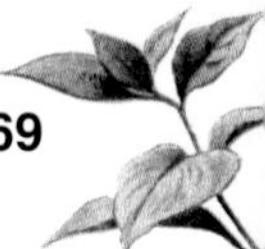

Drug Monograph 25.2
Alcohol (ethanol)

Taken orally, alcohol is a sedative and euphoriant. Alcohol is the most commonly used and abused drug in Australia, usually taken in the form of alcoholic drinks. (For actions and mechanisms, see text.)

Pharmacokinetics

Being a very small molecule (molecular weight 46), ethanol does not require digestion before absorption; despite being very water-soluble, it diffuses as readily as water through lipid membranes and into cells. Most is absorbed from the small intestine; peak blood alcohol levels are reached after 30–60 minutes. Alcohol is distributed into every tissue; the volume of distribution is about 35 L for a 70 kg adult. Analysis of the blood alcohol level gives a rough indication of the quantity consumed and of alcohol levels in the brain.

About 90% of alcohol absorbed is metabolised in the liver by alcohol dehydrogenase to acetaldehyde, which is oxidised to acetic acid, and thence to carbon dioxide and water. Remaining alcohol is excreted via lungs, sweat and kidneys. The amount excreted in 2 L of expired air – as measured by 'breathalysers' – is about equivalent to that in 1 mL blood.

As plasma ethanol levels rise, the hepatic alcohol dehydrogenase pathway becomes saturated; the maximum rate of metabolism is about 120 mg/kg/h, and clearance and half-life are dose-dependent. Hence, blood alcohol levels remain high if the person keeps drinking steadily. Plasma levels tend to be higher in women than in men after equivalent doses because women have lower levels of dehydrogenase enzymes and a relatively smaller volume of distribution for water-soluble drugs. Chronic administration (i.e. in people who have a dependence on alcohol) initially increases the rate of metabolism, but as liver damage and cirrhosis develop, metabolism becomes impaired.

Adverse drug reactions

See text for pharmacological effects.

Drug interactions

Ethanol interacts with many prescription and OTC drugs – in particular, with other CNS depressants; hence, there are frequent adverse drug interactions (DI 25.1).

Warnings and contraindications

Women are advised to avoid alcohol throughout pregnancy due to a 10% risk of fetal alcohol syndrome (mental retardation, craniofacial dysgenesis and growth retardation) if consumption exceeds 2 g ethanol/kg/day during the first trimester. In breastfeeding women, ethanol partitions into milk and causes CNS depression in the infant. Alcohol is not recommended for people with liver disease or psychiatric problems, or people taking any of the many drugs with which it interacts.

Dosage and administration

The standard 'measures' of alcoholic drinks are such that an average drink contains in the range 5–20 grams of ethanol: the stronger the drink, the smaller is the typical glass. It is generally recommended that men drink no more than four standard drinks per day on a maximum of 3–4 days per week, and women no more than two standard drinks.

glutamate). Other proposed targets are receptors for N-methyl-D-aspartate (NMDA), 5-HT_3, acetylcholine (nicotinic), adenosine A_1 and A_{2A}, several neuropeptides and some potassium channels.

Signalling pathways mediating the effects of alcohol include several receptor and intracellular kinases. Ethanol also regulates the functions of scaffolding proteins, gene expression and addictive behaviours via modulation of DNA and expression of microRNAs (small, non-coding RNA molecules involved in gene expression).

CNS depression

Alcohol causes progressive depression of the cerebrum, cerebellum, medulla and spinal cord. What may appear as behavioural stimulation results from depression of higher faculties and loss of inhibitions. Pharmacological effects vary with the blood alcohol level, the person's tolerance, the presence or absence of extraneous stimuli, the rate of ingestion and gastric contents, as described below.

- Small or moderate quantities (blood alcohol 30–50 mg/100 mL) produce a feeling of wellbeing (euphoria) and increased confidence, with slight deterioration in motor function, coordination and mental acuity.
- At blood alcohol 100–200 mg/100 mL, there is emotional instability, decreased inhibitions, muscular incoordination, slowing of responses, signs of intoxication; finer powers of concentration, judgement, memory and visual acuity are lost.
- At blood alcohol 200–300 mg/100 mL, there is confusion, disturbance of sensation, decreased pain sense, staggering gait, slurred speech.

- At 300–400 mg/100 mL: stupor, marked decrease in response to stimuli, muscular incoordination approaching paralysis, impaired intelligence.
- Above 400 mg/100 mL: complete unconsciousness, depressed reflexes and respiration, subnormal temperature, anaesthesia, impairment of circulation, coma, possible death.

(Note: A blood alcohol level of 0.05%, the legally safe driving limit in most states of Australia – that is, 0.05 g/100 mL – equates to 50 mg/100 mL; in New Zealand blood alcohol level of 0.08%, the legally safe driving limit – that is, 0.08 g/100 mL – equates to 80 mg/100 mL.)

Effects on other systems

Some effects of alcohol on other body systems are:

- *Cardiovascular system – depression:* vasodilation; chronically: hypertension, dysrhythmias and cardiomyopathy; possible protective effect against ischaemic heart disease.
- *Gastrointestinal system:* secretion of saliva and gastric juice rich in acid; nutritional deficiencies, gastritis, thiamine deficiency, pancreatitis; fatty liver, hepatitis, irreversible fibrosis and cirrhosis.
- *Endocrine system:* raised levels of adrenocorticotrophic hormone; lowered levels of antidiuretic hormone (ADH; hence diuresis and dehydration), oxytocin (delayed labour during childbirth) and testosterone (feminisation and impotence).
- *The fetus:* risk of fetal alcohol syndrome via acetaldehyde.

Methanol (methyl alcohol, wood alcohol)

Methanol is a CNS toxin: the fatal dose is 100–200 mL and as little as 10 mL can cause permanent blindness. The reason for severe toxicity is that, whereas ethanol is metabolised to acetaldehyde and then acetate, methanol is metabolised to formaldehyde (formalin) and formate, which are more toxic, causing metabolic acidosis, ocular toxicity, abdominal pain, coma and respiratory failure.

There are several forms of 'methylated spirits', all consisting largely of ethyl alcohol that has been purposely contaminated with other solvents (methanol, acetone or pyridine) to render it unfit for human consumption. It is used clinically for skin disinfection. Sadly, some 'skid-row alcoholics' in desperation resort to drinking 'metho' and suffer severe toxicity.

Poisoning by methanol or ethylene glycol (antifreeze) is treated with ethanol, which competitively inhibits the dehydrogenase enzyme, preventing formation of toxic metabolites. Fomepizole (an alcohol dehydrogenase inhibitor) is used for the same mechanism and effects.

Alcohol abuse

Alcohol is the most widely used recreational drug in Australia: see earlier section, 'Patterns of drug abuse in Australia' – 'Tobacco and alcohol'.

Problems from alcohol abuse

Levels of alcohol use and misuse have been classified as:

- social drinking – no regular excessive drinking, problems or symptoms
- heavy drinking – habitual excessive drinking, no problems or symptoms
- problem drinking – problems for self, family or work; intoxication but no symptoms of addiction
- alcoholic addiction – strokes, blackouts, loss of control, impairment to health and intellect.

Problem drinking and addiction lead to social isolation, increase in self-destructive behaviours, suicide and motor vehicle crashes (the risk increasing rapidly above 100 mg ethanol/dL blood); neuropathies and myopathies; chronic hepatotoxicity and cirrhosis; gastrointestinal or haematological toxicity; Korsakoff's psychosis, alcohol dementia and cerebellar degeneration; and fetal abnormalities. It is estimated that one in seven of all presentations to Australasian hospital emergency departments involve alcohol use, that 15–25% of all male hospital admissions are due to alcohol-related causes and that 5% of all cancers are due to chronic long-term drinking (due to DNA damage to stem cells) (Egerton-Warburton et al. 2014).

Tolerance and dependence

Tolerance develops to most effects of chronic low doses of ethanol: pharmacokinetic tolerance, due to induction of drug-metabolising enzymes, and pharmacodynamic tolerance due to adaptation to depressant effects and increased endogenous opioid neurotransmission.

Alcoholism is physical or psychological dependence on alcohol, with a compulsion to consume despite adverse effects. Genetic factors contribute to more than 50% of the risk for alcoholism, along with environmental factors and dysfunctional behavioural choices. Genes implicated include those coding for receptors for $GABA_A$, mu-opioids, DA and 5-HT transporter.

Hangover and alcohol withdrawal syndrome

A 'hangover' is a mild withdrawal syndrome after acute intoxication. The symptoms are craving for alcohol, headache, nausea, tremor, anxiety, vertigo, pallor, tachycardia and nystagmus (rapid jerky eye movements). A more severe withdrawal reaction includes hallucinations, flushes, GIT disturbances and in severe cases delirium tremens ('DTs') requiring hospitalisation. Symptoms are caused by hypoglycaemia, dehydration, electrolyte imbalances and persistence of lactic acid and acetaldehyde in the bloodstream. The withdrawal reaction can be 'cured' by another dose of the drug of dependence – that is, alcohol – known colloquially as taking 'the hair of the dog that bit you'.

Treating alcohol abuse

Acute withdrawal

Acute alcohol withdrawal syndrome is treated with a benzodiazepine sedative: diazepam or oxazepam (Ch 20). The α_2-adrenergic agonists clonidine and dexmedetomidine reduce sympathomimetic over-activity. Supportive care for the acute phase includes fluid, electrolyte and glucose replacement, adequate nutrition, thiamine to prevent development of Wernicke's encephalopathy (Drug Monograph 25.3) and antiemetics; hospitalisation may be necessary.

Long-term treatment

Long-term treatment of ethanol withdrawal and abuse must be continued for many months or years; it includes the person admitting that they need help, motivation to stop drinking, plus symptom relief, treating complications, psychotherapy to prevent relapses, developing long-term rehabilitation plans and drug treatment (Crowley 2015). There are currently three drugs that work by different modes of action that are used to treat ethanol withdrawal: naltrexone, acamprosate and disulfiram. Duration of treatment should be 6 months or more.

- Naltrexone is an opioid antagonist that blocks the effect of endogenous opioids released following alcohol intake. Drinking alcohol then becomes less pleasurable. Naltrexone may reduce craving and assist abstinence.
- Acamprosate is chemically related to the neurotransmitters GABA, glutamate and taurine, and may restore inhibitory neurotransmission in these pathways. Acamprosate reduces symptoms (craving, anxiety, irritability and insomnia) but does not cause unpleasant effects if alcohol is consumed. It is dosed at 4–6 × 333 mg tablets daily.

Drug Monograph 25.3
Thiamine

Thiamine is the water-soluble vitamin B1, commonly administered to people with alcohol abuse, which causes malabsorption of the vitamin and general malnutrition.

Indications

Thiamine is indicated for prophylaxis and treatment of all thiamine deficiencies: in chronic alcohol misuse, prolonged fasting, total parenteral nutrition, faddist diets, haemo- and peritoneal dialysis and the deficiency state beri-beri. Deficiency leads to peripheral neuritis, paraesthesias, sensory loss, Wernicke's encephalopathy, cardiovascular impairments, oedema and eventually irreversible neurological damage and Korsakoff's psychosis.

Mechanism of action

Thiamine (in the diphosphate form) is an essential coenzyme in carbohydrate metabolism, in the decarboxylation of some organic acids to acetaldehyde and carbon dioxide. It is also involved in conduction of action potentials in peripheral nerves and in neuromuscular transmission.

Pharmacokinetics

Orally administered thiamine is partly absorbed in the small intestine by active and passive transfer; absorption is impaired in alcoholism. It is widely distributed in tissues, with some storage in skeletal muscles, heart, liver, kidneys and brain. It is metabolised in the liver to the active pyrophosphate form; excess amounts of thiamine and its metabolites are excreted in the urine.

Drug interactions

There are no significant drug interactions.

Adverse reactions

Adverse reactions are rare, but may include warmth, pruritis, sweating and nausea.

Precautions and contraindications

Hypersensitivity reactions occur rarely, mainly after IV administration. Multiple vitamin deficiency states are common in chronic alcoholics, and should be checked. Thiamine is safe in pregnancy and breastfeeding.

Dosage and administration

Most varied diets provide adequate thiamine (0.8–1.5 mg/day); this is the preferred source. Adult doses to treat deficiency are 50–300 mg/day in divided doses; in severe deficiency, thiamine can be administered IV. Requirements may be increased in burns, chronic fever, hyperthyroidism and various gastrointestinal disorders. Available formulations include 100 mg tablets and 100 mg/mL injections.

- Disulfiram[10] is an alcohol-sensitising drug that, co-administered with alcohol, produces such a severe drug interaction the person is deterred from drinking. Disulfiram inhibits aldehyde dehydrogenase, permitting acetaldehyde to accumulate and cause vasodilation, hyperventilation, raised pulse rate, pounding headache and copious vomiting.
- Other methods being trialled include baclofen (Drug Monograph 24.1) and topiramate (Drug Monograph 21.1; both enhancers of GABA activity), drugs desensitising nicotinic receptors, antagonising histamine H_3 receptors, targeting glutaminergic transmission, inhibiting aldehyde dehydrogenase and novel antiepileptic and anxiolytic agents.

Other central nervous system depressants

Benzodiazepines, barbiturates and Z-drugs

Benzodiazepines are commonly prescribed for anxiety, insomnia, convulsive disorders and musculoskeletal problems, but it can take as little as 2 weeks of regular use to become dependent. It is estimated that there are four times more Australians dependent on 'benzos' than on heroin; benzodiazepines are the prescription drugs causing most overdose deaths. Men tend more to abuse alcohol, while women are more likely to abuse benzodiazepines ('mother's little helpers'). Tolerance develops to the sedating effects but not to respiratory depression. Patients may 'shop around' to obtain supplies. Alprazolam is a particular problem, being highly addictive and potentially lethal when combined with opioids; it is a Schedule 8 Controlled Drug. Use and abuse of older CNS depressants – barbiturates and chloral hydrate-type – has declined in recent years (for general information, see Table 25.1, Chs 21 and 22, Drug Monograph 21.1 and 22.2). Z-drugs (zolpidem, zopiclone) can also induce dependence, managed as for benzodiazepines.

Treating dependence

Managing benzodiazepine dependence should include gradual drug withdrawal. Flumazenil is a specific benzodiazepine-receptor antagonist that is administered intravenously to reverse sedation from benzodiazepines used during anaesthesia, and (rarely) for benzodiazepine toxicity; it may precipitate withdrawal seizures. As flumazenil has a short half-life (50 minutes), several doses may be required to overcome a benzodiazepine. Withdrawal is difficult; maintenance therapy with a long-acting benzodiazepine may be the alternative.

Ketamine

Ketamine ('K', 'special K') is a non-barbiturate, rapidly acting general anaesthetic agent, producing 'dissociative anaesthesia', with amnesia and detachment from surroundings (Table 25.1). It is an NMDA receptor antagonist, and an effective analgesic, especially in the prehospital setting and in day procedures, reducing the doses of opioids required. Overdose can cause CNS stimulation and delirium. Long-term use is limited by adverse effects: dependence, flashbacks and hepatic and renal disorders. Due to its hallucinogenic and antidepressant actions, it has become a drug of abuse and is now a Schedule 8 Controlled Drug.

Kava

Kava (*yaqona*, 'grog') is an intoxicating drink made by fermenting the roots of *Piper methysticum*, a plant native to the South Pacific region. Traditional uses include at religious and welcoming ceremonies, to calm tensions and to improve socialising, as a panacea for various complaints, a contraceptive, a poultice for wounds and to improve male sex drive. Many active constituents have been identified – in particular, the kava lactone kawain and various dihydro-derivatives. Kava has serotonergic activity, modulates GABA activity, inhibits monoamine oxidase-B (MAO-B) and inhibits uptake of noradrenaline (NA) and DA. CNS effects are similar to benzodiazepines or alcohol.

Adverse effects

Chronic use causes scaly skin rash, nausea, reduced appetite and weight loss, raised levels of some liver enzymes, and associations with gastritis, hepatitis, red eyes, impotence and general poor health. Kava has fewer detrimental effects than alcohol on cognitive functions but can cause dependence. In many Pacific countries, the main problems caused by kava are social ones: heavy consumers (usually men) tend to suffer sedative and de-motivating effects that harm families and communities.

Gamma-hydroxybutyrate

Gamma-hydroxybutyrate (GHB), originally used as a general anaesthetic and to treat insomnia, depression, narcolepsy, alcohol withdrawal and fibromyalgia, has become a drug of abuse, especially among bodybuilders and athletes, because it stimulates release of growth hormone. GHB (GBH, 'grievous bodily harm'; sodium oxybate) is a naturally occurring metabolite of the inhibitory neurotransmitter GABA; their structures are very similar:

- GHB: $CH_2OH–(CH_2)_2–COOH$
- GABA: $CH_2NH_2–(CH_2)_2–COOH$.

GHB is a weak agonist at $GABA_B$ receptors (inhibitory) and stimulates 5-HT systems and DA release; higher concentrations inhibit DA release. GHB increases levels of

10 Disulfiram is finding a new use in treatment of HIV/AIDS: it 'wakes up' dormant viral cells, making them more susceptible to antiretroviral treatments.

glutamate (excitatory) in the brain, so GHB can have both CNS-depressant and stimulatory effects. Injected IV, GHB causes a long-lasting unconsciousness (1.5–3 hours), longer if taken orally mixed with alcohol. It has weak analgesic actions but enhances the actions of narcotic analgesics and neuromuscular blocking agents.

Abuse of GHB

GHB comes in a clear liquid form and is used in the rave dance scene as an alternative or additive to alcohol, to 'spike' drinks and as a 'date-rape' drug (see Table 25.1 for effects). Risks with GHB are the fine line between the dose required to give the desired effect and that causing an overdose; the delayed onset of effect; unpredictability of effects and interactions; risk of dependence; risks associated with driving or of drug-assisted sexual assaults; and fatal overdoses.

Inhalants

Other CNS-depressant substances abused are volatile solvents, aerosols, anaesthetics and nitrates. Chemically, they are hydrocarbons (halogenated, aliphatic or aromatic), ketones, esters or ethers. They are general CNS depressants with pharmacological properties similar to alcohol and general anaesthetics such as chloroform and sevoflurane (Ch 18; Drug Monograph 18.2). When abused, they are inhaled, known as 'chroming' or 'glue sniffing' (Table 25.1). This type of substance abuse is most common among children and teenagers (6–15 years of age), and in economically depressed populations.[11]

Adverse effects and toxicity

Inhaled agents produce a rapid general CNS depression; at high doses, confusion and coma occur. Generally, treatment is with removal of the inhaled agent and bed rest. Chronic inhalant abuse will lead to dependence and tolerance, neuro-, hepatic and renal toxicity and blood dyscrasias; deaths from cardiac dysrhythmia, vagal inhibition, anoxia and respiratory failure (inhaling from a plastic bag and suffocating) have occurred.

KEY POINTS

Dependence on CNS depressants

- Alcohol abuse is very common in Australian society and ranges from occasional problem drinking through to chronic alcoholism; treatment is with thiamine, acamprosate, disulfiram or naltrexone.
- Other CNS depressants abused are prescription sedatives such as benzodiazepines, ketamine, kava and inhaled solvents.

11 As depicted graphically in the 2009 Australian movie *Samson and Delilah*.

Central nervous system stimulants

CNS stimulants commonly abused are amphetamines (and related 'designer drugs' such as ecstasy), nicotine, cocaine, caffeine and (more rarely) methylphenidate and modafinil. Mechanisms of actions of stimulants involve the DA transporter (reuptake process), especially in reinforcer and behavioural stimulant effects, and also transmitters NA, 5-HT, GABA and glutamate. (See Ch 23 for mechanisms and clinical aspects.) Stimulants are banned in sports in-competition (Drug Monograph 23.1).

Amphetamines

Amphetamines exemplify well the rule that 'drugs likely to be abused ... act fast, make you feel good, or stop you feeling bad'. Amphetamines have rapid euphoriant effects and are strongly addictive. Natural amphetamine-type compounds include ephedrine from *Ephedra sinica* and cathinone (khat) from *Catha edulis*.

Actions and pharmacokinetics

Chemically, amphetamines are similar to the natural catecholamines adrenaline, NA (Fig 1.4A) and DA but have fewer hydroxyl groups so are more lipid-soluble and CNS-active. They cause release of catecholamines from nerve terminals and inhibit their reuptake. Central effects include increases in alertness and mental and physical capacities, and decreased appetite and sleep, euphoria and stereotyped behaviours also occur. There is a rapid fall-off in drug effects, followed by periods of sleep; on waking the person feels hungry, lethargic and profoundly depressed (anhedonia, 'crashing'), which enhances intense craving and rapidly leads to addiction and risk of suicide.

Amphetamines are generally taken orally but can also be inhaled after vaporisation, inhaled as fine powders ('snorted') or injected; they cause rapid marked euphoria – a 'rush'.

Dexamfetamine is a basic drug with a pK_a of 9.9; therefore, alkaline urine with a pH more than 7 reduces excretion of dexamfetamine and extends its half-life. People who abuse amphetamines can enhance effects by taking oral sodium or potassium citrate, whereas doctors treating dexamfetamine overdose know that giving oral ammonium chloride will acidify the person's urine to a pH of 4.5–5.5 and hasten dexamfetamine excretion.

Abuse of amphetamines

Amphetamines were widely used during World War II by servicemen to enhance alertness and reduce battle fatigue, quickly becoming popular drugs of abuse – amphetamine as 'benzedrine', and methamphetamine or methedrine as 'speed' or 'ice' (Table 19.1). They were readily available in

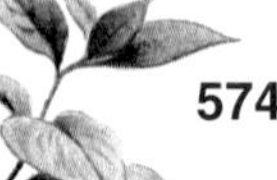

the 1950s and 1960s but are now indicated only for narcolepsy and attention deficit hyperactivity disorder (ADHD) (Ch 23). They are frequently abused by people wanting the CNS-stimulant effects (e.g. long-distance drivers and sportspeople), and children prescribed stimulants for ADHD have been known to sell them on. Pseudoephedrine, another amphetamine-type stimulant, is available in cough and cold medicines; however, real time online monitoring of sales through Project Stop helps to ensure that the product sold is for legitimate use. As pseudoephedrine can be used to synthesise the more dangerous amphetamines, each time a product containing pseudoephedrine is sold the pharmacist will record the sale in the Real Time Prescription Monitoring system. This alerts both the pharmacist and the police if someone is purchasing multiple products from multiple pharmacies (known as pseudo running).

Users often take depressants or 'downers', such as alcohol, marijuana, benzodiazepines, barbiturates or heroin, to offset overstimulation. Treatment of acute toxicity requires detoxification plus anticonvulsants and antihypertensive agents.

Abuse in Australia

Amphetamine use more than doubled over the period from 2002 to 2014, now causing major problems with violent behaviours, especially in many regional towns where young people are targeted by dealers. Most amphetamines are produced in illegal backyard laboratories, with no controls over the manufacturing practices or the purity or strength of the product, and sold illegally. Due to the unknown strength of street products, overdose is common and potentially fatal.

Designer drugs, new psychoactive substances and 'legal highs'

'**Legal highs**' refers to hundreds of new psychoactive substances, semi/synthetic drugs designed to mimic the actions of cannabis or amphetamines; people designing the drugs aim to keep a step ahead of drug policymakers and law-enforcement officers. New psychoactive substances are based on the phenylethylamine molecule (as are catecholamines and amphetamines) or on cocaine, tryptamine, phencyclidine or cannabinoids; their number more than doubled between approximately 2005 and 2015 (Milano et al. 2016). They all increase DA signalling in the nucleus accumbens, causing reward and dependence. They are available readily from 'head shops', the internet, the 'dark net', on the street or at festivals; toxicologists cannot keep up with overseas products flooding markets.

The classic **designer drug** is MDMA (better known as 'ecstasy'), originally synthesised in 1914 as an appetite suppressant. Related compounds have varying chemical substituents (methoxy-, methyl-, halogen or sulfur) on the phenyl ring of the amphetamine. Examples are methylenedioxypyrovalerone (MDPV), methadrone (MPDT, 'miaow miaow') and mephedrone (4-MMC, MCAT), all cathinone derivatives and primary ingredients in 'bath salts'. Their cute street names aim to mislead young people into thinking they are harmless.

Abuse of designer drugs

The typical scenario for abuse of designer drugs is at nightclubs and music festivals, to produce euphoria, feelings of closeness and confidence (Table 25.1). Unwanted effects include jaw clenching and teeth grinding, paranoia, confusion, mild hallucinations, impaired cognition, bizarre behaviour and possibly psychosis. Complex mixtures of synthetic drugs with unknown additives and side effects pose new threats: they are highly addictive, causing long-lasting severe toxicities. Overdoses can result in hypertension, tachycardia and hyperthermia; many deaths have occurred from excess CNS and autonomic stimulation.

Nicotine and tobacco smoking

Acetylcholine is the neurotransmitter at all autonomic ganglia, where its effects were originally described as nicotinic because they most closely mimicked those of nicotine. (See Ch 8 for the mechanism of action.)

Nicotine is the chief alkaloid in the tobacco plant *Nicotiana tabacum*; it is an oily liquid that turns brown on exposure to air and is freely soluble in both organic solvents and water. Nicotine has no therapeutic use (other than in nicotine replacement therapy for smokers trying to quit) but is of great pharmacological and public health importance. Nicotine is most commonly self-administered by smoking cigarettes (which contain about 1 g of nicotine each), cigars or pipes and liquid nicotine vaping (electronic cigarettes). Tobacco smoking was introduced into European societies from Central America in the 16th century; smoking has major toxic effects, while the absorbed nicotine causes addiction to the products.

Pharmacological effects of nicotine

Peripheral effects

Autonomic

- Low doses stimulate all sympathetic and parasympathetic ganglia, while higher doses depress responses at all autonomic pathways.
- Effects on the cardiovascular system are complex: heart rate may be slowed then accelerated; small blood vessels constrict but later dilate; the blood pressure rises then falls.
- Nicotine has an antidiuretic action and decreases gastrointestinal motility.

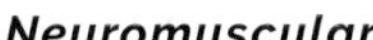

Neuromuscular

- At neuromuscular junctions, nicotine exerts a curare-like action (flaccidity) on skeletal muscle.
- Large doses may cause tremor; death may result from respiratory failure due to paralysis of the diaphragm.

CNS effects

- Nicotine stimulates acetylcholine receptors in medullary centres (respiratory, emetic and vasomotor); convulsions may occur.
- Stimulation is followed by depression; first-time smokers become anxious and nauseated.[12]
- Repeated administration of nicotine causes dependence; tolerance develops to some effects, particularly to nausea, sweating and antidiuretic effects, so habitual smokers find smoking pleasurable.
- Central effects commonly reported are euphoria and antidepressant effects; increased alertness and concentration, and reduced boredom and anxiety; learning and performance may improve.
  (See also Table 25.1.)

Potential beneficial effects

- Chronic smokers have a lower-than-average prevalence of Alzheimer's disease and Parkinson's disease; nicotine may enhance cholinergic and dopaminergic activity in central pathways.
- Nicotine acts as an appetite suppressant by activating receptors in the pro-opiomelanocortin cells in the hypothalamus, causing sensation of satiety and reduced eating; antidepressant effects may also help reduce food intake.

Overall, however, stopping smoking has major health benefits for all smokers.

Toxic effects

- Nicotine has both short- and long-term toxic effects in public health terms.
- Small children have died from nicotine toxicity after ingesting tobacco products, as have farm workers after percutaneous absorption of insecticides containing nicotine.

Tobacco smoking

Tobacco smoke is an aerosol containing about 4×10^9 particles per mL, about 10–80 mg per cigarette; nicotine accounts for about 0.14–1.21 mg. Burning tobacco generates around 4000 chemicals, including 60 known carcinogens such as tars, formaldehyde, hydrogen cyanide, benzene and nitrosamines, implicated in causing cancers of the lung, bladder, buccal cavity, oesophagus and pancreas. Other smoking-related problems include the following:

- Smoking causes illnesses such as pulmonary emphysema, chronic bronchitis, coronary heart disease, strokes, myocardial infarction, chronic dyspepsia, peripheral vascular disease such as thromboangiitis obliterans (Buerger's disease) and vasospasm in retinal blood vessels.
- Male smokers have about one-third the sperm count of non-smokers, and increased impotence, due to microvascular damage.
- Mothers who smoke usually deliver infants with lower birthweights and a higher incidence of congenital abnormalities; prematurity and stillbirth are more common.
- Smoking is responsible for more than 50% of all domestic fires.
- Smoking is a considerable financial outlay.

Passive smoking

Passive smoking refers to the inhalation of environmental tobacco smoke by non-smokers. Reports from studies in Australia, the United States and the United Kingdom all indicate that:

- Environmental tobacco smoke can cause cancers and cardiac diseases in non-smokers.
- Children of parents who smoke have a greater incidence of asthma, respiratory tract symptoms, infections and middle ear disease than children from a non-smoking family, and a greatly increased likelihood of becoming smokers.
- Environmental tobacco smoke exposure is causally linked to sudden infant death syndrome.

Dependence on nicotine

Tobacco is Australia's worst 'killer' drug, said to kill more people than alcohol, drugs, murder, suicide, road, rail and air crashes, poisoning, HIV, drowning, fires, falls, lightning, electrocution, snakes, spiders and sharks put together. A 2019 national survey of drug use found that about 11.6% of Australians aged 15 years and over smoked daily. Rates are much higher (37%) among Aboriginal and Torres Strait Islander Australians, in whom smoking accounts for 20% of all mortality.

The addictive component of tobacco is nicotine. Monkeys trained to press a bar to receive an IV injection of nicotine will self-administer until adverse effects outweigh rewards. The powerful addiction is mediated via dopaminergic systems in the mesolimbic pathway and

12 It is an indication of the strong 'rewarding' effect and addictive potential of nicotine – and of the aggressive advertising practices and peer pressures encouraging smoking – that anyone goes on to smoke a second cigarette.

amygdala. Nicotine also has an antidepressant action, and ex-smokers who successfully quit often suffer clinical depression.

The dose of nicotine absorbed from one cigarette is about 10–40 micrograms/kg body weight, and smokers tend to maintain their plasma nicotine concentration at about 10–50 ng/mL.

Drug interactions

Pharmacodynamic interactions can occur between nicotine and any drug affecting acetylcholine functions in the autonomic, motor or central nervous systems (DI 25.2). Tobacco smoking induces the drug-metabolising enzymes CYP1A2 and CYP2B6, causing numerous pharmacokinetic drug interactions with other inducers, inhibitors or substrates of the enzymes. Heavy smokers have greater rates of clearance of many drugs, and those who have to stop smoking abruptly may have altered metabolism of other drugs (see databases for individual potential interactions) (Australian Medicines Handbook 2021; Lucas & Martin 2013).

Treating nicotine dependence

Treatment of nicotine dependence aims to relieve symptoms of nicotine withdrawal, help smokers to 'quit' smoking and reduce morbidity and mortality. Drug therapy is recommended for those who smoke more than 10 cigarettes daily. Treatment may be by replacement with a less harmful related drug (varenicline), another stimulant/antidepressant (bupropion) or with nicotine delivered in a less harmful formulation such as a gum (Drug Monograph 25.4), lozenge or patch; nicotinic antagonists are not effective. Smoking cessation programs need to be flexible and tailored to specific communities (e.g. for Indigenous populations).

Cessation of smoking, 'quitting'

Smoking is notoriously hard to quit; the withdrawal syndrome, consisting of craving, irritability, hunger, anxiety and headaches, continues for several days; the craving can persist for years. Medical advice, behavioural therapy, combination pharmacotherapy with follow-up by QuitLine (see 'Online resources') can significantly enhance quit rates. Anti-smoking campaigns effectively reduce the prevalence of smoking, and by preventing thousands of cases of cancers, cardiovascular and pulmonary diseases can bring significant healthcare savings.

Nicotine by other routes

Nicotine replacement therapy doubles the cessation rate of advice or behavioural therapy alone. Nicotine patches, gum, lozenges, sublingual tablets, oral spray or inhaler are formulated in a range of doses; the dose is tapered off over several weeks. Many are available in supermarkets (unscheduled) and some are subsidised on the Pharmaceutical Benefits Scheme.

Electronic (e-) cigarettes are designed to mimic the act of smoking while delivering a small dose of nicotine but not burning tobacco and may help with quitting. E-cigarettes are Schedule 4 prescription only in Australia. That is, they can only be legally supplied by a pharmacist on presentation of a prescription and evidence of Therapeutic Goods Administration approval (under the

DRUG INTERACTIONS 25.2
Nicotine (or tobacco)

DRUG	POSSIBLE EFFECTS AND MANAGEMENT
CYP substrates: paracetamol, duloxetine, fluvoxamine, imipramine, caffeine, oxazepam, melatonin, propranolol, clozapine, mirtazapine, zolmitriptan, olanzapine, methadone and theophylline (and others)	Cigarette smoking induces the activity CYP 1A2, and increases the metabolism of substrates, lowering substrate blood concentrations and efficacy. Higher or more frequent drug dosing of CYP1A2 substrates may be required.
Adrenergic agonists or blocking agents, catecholamines, corticosteroids	Smoking and nicotine raise catecholamine and cortisone levels; therapy with adrenoceptor agonists or antagonists or corticosteroids may require dosage adjustment.
Insulin	Smoking cessation may result in an increased insulin effect; dosage reduction may be necessary; monitor closely for symptoms of hypoglycaemia.
Autonomic drugs, including antihypertensives, bronchodilators and vasodilators	Effects of nicotine on autonomic ganglia are complicated and dose-dependent; doses of other autonomic drugs may need adjusting.
Vasoconstrictors	Nicotine decreases myocardial oxygen supply and increases demand, effects compounded by other vasoconstrictors.
Acidic beverages (coffee, soft drinks)	May decrease buccal absorption of nicotine.
Nicotine (in other forms, e.g. cigarettes, patches)	Additive effects, leading to chest pains and palpitations.

Sources: Australian Medicines Handbook 2021; Lucas & Martin 2013.

Drug Monograph 25.4
Nicotine gum

When used medically in nicotine replacement therapy by smokers trying to quit, nicotine facilitates smoking cessation and decreases severity of the withdrawal syndrome. An effective treatment for heavy smokers is a combination of patch (providing steady nicotine replacement) with gum or inhaler to provide a euphoriant boost. Dependence on nicotine replacement therapy is considered easier to break than the smoking habit.

Actions and mechanism of action

Nicotine released from the gum mimics the actions of nicotine absorbed from smoking. (For the mechanism of action and effects, see text.)

Indications

Nicotine is used in various regimens: in a 'cold turkey' Quit Now program; while gradually reducing the number of cigarettes smoked over several weeks; or as combination therapy with patches, gradually withdrawing patches then gum use. When the person has a strong craving to smoke, a stick of gum is chewed instead, which relieves withdrawal. Usage is reduced over a 2- to 6-month period.

Pharmacokinetics

Nicotine is very lipid-soluble so is rapidly absorbed across lipid membranes of the mouth, airways and GIT. When chewed as a gum, it is steadily released and absorbed through buccal mucosa more slowly than if inhaled while smoking. When saliva containing nicotine is swallowed, the drug is absorbed from the GIT. Peak plasma concentration is reached at 45–60 minutes.

Nicotine is metabolised primarily in the liver. Most metabolites are inactive, but cotinine, the main oxidation product, may have antidepressant and psychomotor stimulant properties. The half-life is 1–3 hours. Elimination is primarily renal with 10% excreted unchanged; the drug is excreted in breast milk.

Drug interactions

Cimetidine slows the elimination of nicotine. Nicotine potentiates the effect of adenosine.

While cigarette smoke induces hepatic enzymes CYP1A1, CYP1A2 and 2E1, nicotine has no effect on the enzymes. Simply put, tobacco (smoking) has many more drug interactions than nicotine alone.

Adverse reactions

Adverse effects of nicotine have been described in the text; reactions to nicotine gum include local injury to mouth, teeth or dental work, and jaw muscle ache. Some signs and symptoms may be due to stopping smoking, rather than to nicotine gum. Early signs of overdose are nausea and vomiting, increased salivation and abdominal pain, diarrhoea, cold sweat, severe headache and dizziness, disturbed hearing and vision, confusion and severe weakness; signs of toxicity include circulatory collapse, difficulty breathing and convulsions.

Warnings and contraindications

Use with caution in people with cardiovascular disease, insulin-dependent diabetes mellitus, hyperthyroidism, peptic ulcer disease or phaeochromocytoma. Avoid use in people with nicotine hypersensitivity, and moderate hepatic or renal impairment. Use is not recommended in pregnancy or breastfeeding; however, nicotine replacement therapy is less dangerous than smoking. Nicotine is not used in children under 12 (very toxic), or in non-smokers; in children 12–17 years, it is used only under professional health care. The gum contains significant amounts of sodium.

Dosage and administration

Nicotine gum comes in two strengths, 2 mg or 4 mg nicotine per piece, and various flavours. The person should be instructed to stop smoking before using nicotine replacements. The gum is chewed intermittently when the person has the craving to smoke, controlling the dose by biting the gum to release nicotine. Dosage is 2 or 4 mg as chewing gum, repeated as needed to a maximum of 40 mg/day, tapering off over several weeks.

Special Access Scheme B or authorised prescriber scheme). This is controversial, due to evidence that 'vaping' is safer than legal tobacco smoking. E-cigarettes containing nicotine, or nicotine liquid, are being accessed illegally via the internet from overseas.

Varenicline or bupropion

Varenicline is a partial agonist at neuronal nicotinic receptors; hence, it substitutes for nicotine and helps reduce withdrawal symptoms, with fewer adverse effects (analogous to buprenorphine, a partial opioid agonist, in heroin addiction). Patients start taking varenicline 1–2 weeks before stopping smoking; other nicotine products should be avoided. A typical course is 0.5 mg once daily, increasing dose gradually to 1 mg twice a day for 3–6 months as required, then gradual reduction. Adverse effects (nausea, dizziness, GIT disturbances, insomnia) may also be related to nicotine withdrawal.

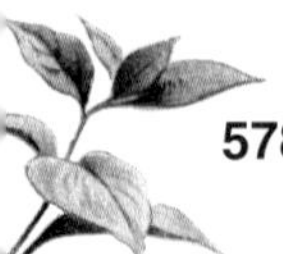

Bupropion, which inhibits neuronal reuptake of DA and NA by the NA transporter, was previously used as an antidepressant. Used along with counselling and nicotine replacement therapy, it improves quit rates; antidepressant effects contribute. Adverse effects (sleep disturbance, dizziness, headache, anxiety, suicidal ideation) may be related to withdrawal from nicotine. Initial dose is 150 mg daily, increasing to 150 mg twice daily maximum; it is contraindicated in people with psychiatric or seizure disorders, and can cause severe cardiovascular adverse events.

Cocaine

Pharmacological properties and mechanisms

Cocaine is an alkaloid related to the belladonna alkaloids atropine and hyoscine; it is an ester-type local anaesthetic with vasoconstrictor effects. Its sympathomimetic effects are due to inhibited reuptake of catecholamines NA, adrenaline and DA into nerve terminals. Cocaine has central stimulant properties, causing excitement, talkativeness, tremors, vomiting and increased respiration and blood pressure (Table 25.1).

Use and abuse of cocaine

Topically and parenterally, cocaine now has limited local anaesthetic use in a few nasal and ophthalmic surgical procedures. Orally administered cocaine is readily absorbed but subject to extensive first-pass inactivation and short half-life (about 1 hour). When abused, cocaine is taken as a snuff ('snorted') or by injection; when coca leaves are chewed, cocaine is absorbed via the buccal mucosa. The free-base form ('rock' or 'crack') is smoked for a rapid, intense effect.

Cocaine is a powerful reinforcer, rapidly producing sensations of reward and exhilaration, and hence dependence; it is a Controlled Substance Schedule 8. While abuse of cocaine in Australia is nowhere near the problem it is in the United States, availability and abuse are increasing: use in males aged 14 and older increased from 1.1% of the population in 1995 to 4.2% in 2019. There is no typical withdrawal syndrome, but rebound effects are fatigue and depression, with anxiety disorders, suicidal thinking and self-harm.

Caffeine

Xanthine alkaloids

The xanthine alkaloids caffeine, theophylline and theobromine are found naturally in plants used for making the stimulating beverages coffee, tea and cocoa. Xanthines have medical uses as CNS stimulants and bronchodilators, with mild diuretic and cardiac-stimulant effects, used to treat respiratory failure in premature infants. Caffeine, the most powerful CNS stimulant of the xanthine alkaloids, is present in many OTC medications, in some prescribed medicines and in coffee, tea, cocoa, cola and 'energy drinks'. Theophylline and aminophylline are used in asthma.

Pharmacological mechanisms and effects

Chemically, xanthines are closely related to the purine bases adenine and guanine (building blocks for DNA and RNA), and are thought to act through antagonist effects on adenosine receptors, thus disinhibiting effects of endogenous adenosine on ascending DA and arousal systems. At higher concentrations, xanthines also inhibit phosphodiesterase, raising intracellular levels of cyclic adenosine monophosphate (cAMP).

Caffeine is a mild stimulant, reducing fatigue and improving concentration, intellectual and motor tasks. Large doses (300–600 mg) can cause insomnia, anxiety, palpitations, tremor, headache, increased gastric secretion and seizures.

Social use of caffeine

Caffeine is the most widely used psychoactive substance worldwide; about 20% of the world's population drink a caffeinated beverage every day. Typical daily caffeine intake of adults is 180–250 mg. Tea accounts for about 43% of caffeine consumption worldwide. Caffeine is metabolised by CYP1A2, with a half-life of 4–5 hours; habitual consumers and smokers are faster metabolisers. Two to three cups of strong coffee are sufficient to raise caffeine levels in the plasma or brain to approximately 100 microM, a concentration at which adenosine-receptor blockade and some phosphodiesterase inhibition occurs. Caffeine is also present in many foodstuffs, which may not be noted on the labelling if it is 'natural' as in cocoa or coffee/tea/chocolate/guarana products. The maximum recommended daily intake for caffeine is 300–400 mg.

Dependence on caffeine?

Habitual moderate coffee intake does not represent a health hazard; caffeine does not activate dopaminergic structures related to reward and addiction, or cause euphoria, stereotyped behaviours or psychoses. Animals cannot be trained to self-administer caffeine, implying that it does not produce reward (or they do not like the bitter taste). Some tolerance and dependence may develop and an acute withdrawal syndrome (possibly a mild irritability and headache). Caffeine use does not warrant legislation or treatment and is usually self-limiting because of the negative adverse effects (diuresis, insomnia and dyspepsia) and lack of positive reward.

High regular intakes of caffeine have been associated with increased incidence of cancers (breast, pancreatic, urogenital), possibly due to carcinogens from roasted coffee beans, which contain more than 1000 chemicals. Caffeine has also been implicated in female infertility and in low-birthweight infants, but moderate caffeine intake appears safe in pregnant women.

Diterpenes (present in unfiltered coffee brews, as in Turkish or Greek coffees) have been shown to raise cholesterol levels in the blood. Moderate caffeine-drinking may be protective against liver disease, neurodegenerative diseases and non-melanocytic skin cancers.

Tea may be protective, as the tannins and flavonoids are antiatherosclerotic, and polyphenols delay cancer onset in humans and have antioxidant properties. Studies of chocolate consumption have shown reduced risk of cardiovascular disease and stroke; 'chocoholics' are more likely 'addicted' to the sugar and flavours than to caffeine or theobromine.

Caffeinated energy drinks

Gaining prominence in the soft-drink market are pre-mixed 'formulated caffeinated beverages', marketed to 'sustain energy levels' and 'improve mental acuity'. These drinks may also contain guarana, another natural source of caffeine, and can cause agitation, palpitations, tremor and GIT upset, also serious effects of hallucinations, dysrhythmias and seizures.

KEY POINTS

Dependence on CNS stimulants

- CNS stimulants including amphetamines, ecstasy and similar designer drugs, 'legal highs' and cathinone derivatives, cocaine and caffeine are commonly abused for their euphoriant effects.
- The most problematic drug of dependence is nicotine, taken by smoking; smoking-related cardiovascular disease and cancers are a major public health problem.
- Nicotine dependence is treated by substituting nicotine by less dangerous routes, such as gum, patches or inhalers; or with bupropion or varenicline, a partial agonist at nicotinic receptors.
- Caffeine is very commonly consumed in beverages such as coffee, tea and sports/energy drinks; if use becomes excessive, it can lead to adverse effects.

Psychotomimetics

Psychotomimetics are drugs that produce or mimic psychotic reactions, and could include cocaine, amphetamines, centrally acting anticholinergics, corticosteroids and even some antimicrobial agents. They are drugs with a history of religious and social use to alter perception or cause hallucinations. The main groups are cannabinoids and hallucinogens.

Cannabis drugs (marijuana, hashish)

The cannabis drugs are derived from hemp plants (*Cannabis sativa*), probably originally native to Central Asia. The plants have historically been grown for their strong fibres and fast growth (up to 5 m in length), and for weaving into fabric ('canvas'), for twisting into ropes (hemp) and for making paper. Hempseed is used as birdseed and a source of oil. There are also dermatological preparations (oils, soaps, lotions) and foods and fabrics based on cannabis. The active drugs used for mental relaxation and euphoria are from the resin of the plant, exuded from the leaves and flowering tops.

Preparations and active constituents

Marijuana (cannabis prepared for smoking) and hashish (the compressed form of the plant resin) are the most common forms. Cannabis plants contain chemicals termed phytocannabinoids, with complex three-ring structures. The main psychoactive ingredient is Δ^9-tetrahydrocannabinol (THC); typical leaves contain 3–10% THC, hashish 7–12% and marijuana cigarettes about 0.5–2 g. Others are cannabidiol and cannabinol. Cannabis smoked for recreational use is high in Δ^9-THC.

Administration and pharmacokinetics

Cannabinoids are highly lipid-soluble so are readily absorbed; they are most potent when inhaled. Cannabis may be smoked in pipes or cigarettes, with smoke retained in the lungs for maximal absorption; about 15–50% of THC is absorbed, with peak plasma level occurring within minutes. THC is highly protein-bound, so only a small proportion enters the CNS; it persists in adipose tissue (for over 4 weeks) and in lungs and liver, with a long half-life. It is metabolised in the liver by CYP 2C9 and 3A4 enzymes to hydroxylation products, some pharmacologically active. Metabolites are excreted in urine, bile and faeces. The long half-lives of cannabinoids make it difficult to correlate blood cannabinoid concentration with impaired driving performance.

Mechanism and pharmacological effects

Cannabinoid receptors

Cannabinoid (CB) receptors have been isolated, and the search for a 'natural' endogenous cannabinoid (endocannabinoid) produced anandamide and 2-arachidonoyl glycerol, arachidonic acid derivatives related to the eicosanoids and prostaglandins. Endocannabinoids are agonists at G-protein-coupled

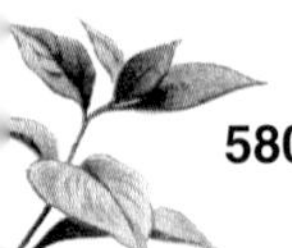

receptors, inhibiting adenylyl cyclase to regulate transcription factors, CB1 mainly in presynaptic membranes of neurons regulating transmitter release including glutamate and GABA, and CB2 in immune and haemopoietic cells.

The actions of cannabinoids have been extensively studied: Δ^9-THC is a partial agonist at CB1 and CB2 receptors, mainly causing euphoria and distorted perceptions. Cannabidiol is an agonist at CB2R and antagonist at CB1R, causing relaxation and is used for pain management; it does not impair cognition and may have antipsychotic effects. Cannabinol is an agonist preferentially at CB2R with no psychoactive effects. Synthetic cannabinoids including dexanabinol, dronabinol, nabilone and nabiximols.

Effects

Cannabinoids act as CNS depressants similar to ethanol and as mild hallucinogens; responses are subjective, with a high placebo reaction. THC has effects on lipid membranes similar to general anaesthetics: at low doses, relief of anxiety, disinhibition and excitement, then anaesthesia; at high doses, respiratory and vasomotor depression occur.

Cannabinoids can affect most systems of the body:

- CNS – euphoria, reduced anxiety, distorted perceptions, loss of concentration, impaired decision making, increased risk of fatal road crashes, tremors, incoordination, sedation; antiemetic, anticonvulsant and analgesic effects; hypothermia; with high doses hallucinations, anxiety, acute psychoses, increased risk of schizophrenia
- cardiovascular system – palpitations, tachycardia then bradycardia, postural hypotension, atherosclerosis
- GI tract – dry mouth and throat, decreased gastrointestinal motility, enhanced appetite and flavour appreciation, gum overgrowth
- respiratory tract – bronchodilation, sore throat, bronchitis, emphysema and increased risk of lung cancer from heavy long-term smoking
- ocular effects – reddening of eyes, ptosis (drooping of eyelids), decreased intraocular pressure (useful antiglaucoma effect)
- endocrine system – diuretic effect, estrogenic effects (reduced fertility and libido in male chronic users)
- other actions – reported antibacterial, immunosuppressant and antineoplastic effects
- toxic effects – low acute toxicity, with few if any human deaths ever attributed solely to its use; for adverse effects see Drug Monograph 25.5 and 'Marijuana abuse' (below).

Medical uses of cannabinoids

Synthetic cannabinoids have been tested in treatment of nausea and vomiting induced by cancer, symptomatic relief in neuropathic and cancer pain, as an adjunct in treating people with wasting conditions, and in chronic pain syndromes, migraine, insomnia, anorexia, epilepsy, opioid withdrawal, glaucoma, asthma and neurological diseases with spasticity such as stroke and multiple sclerosis (Drug Monograph 25.5).

All Australian states have legalised the use of medical marijuana for defined groups of people, including those with a terminal illness and children with intractable epilepsy. The use of social marijuana remains illegal in all Australian jurisdictions, with the exception of the ACT.

Problems with chronic use

With regular low doses no tolerance develops to cannabis. Approximately 9% of users develop dependence; withdrawal causes mild rebound anxiety, sleep disturbances, muscle weakness and tremor. Craving can recur intermittently for months.

Overall health risks from regular use of cannabinoids are less than from some legal drugs of dependence, notably alcohol and tobacco. Heavy daily use over many years may cause cannabis dependence, cognitive and occupational impairment (secondary school teachers say they can readily identify regular users), diseases associated with smoking including cancers, higher risk of birth defects and leukaemia in offspring exposed in utero, two to three times increased risk of moving on to other drugs (tobacco, amphetamines, ecstasy, cocaine) and increased risk of developing schizophrenia (see below).

High-risk groups for adverse effects are adolescents, pregnant women and their offspring; people with pre-existing diseases, especially cardiovascular, respiratory or psychotic conditions; and drug-dependent people.

Cannabis and psychosis

There is strong evidence associating cannabis use with psychosis, as CB1 agonists increase activity of dopaminergic neurons. Acute cannabis intoxication can cause brief psychotic symptoms, and in people with established psychosis use of cannabis causes more frequent relapses. Endocannabinoids function as crucial molecular signallers in the development of the fetal nervous system; heavy smoking by pregnant women causes cognitive impairments in children.

Hallucinogens

A **hallucinogen** is a drug that produces auditory or visual hallucinations. Hallucinogens are lysergic acid diethylamide (LSD) and its variants, mescaline, psilocybin and PCP (phencyclidine); drugs such as ecstasy based on amphetamine; cathinone and ketamine (Clinical Focus Box 19.9, Fig 19.5).

Drug Monograph 25.5
Cannabis extract for oromucosal spray

Cannabis extract is from the leaves and flowers of *Cannabis sativa*; it is legally prescribed for medicinal purposes in Australia and New Zealand as the S8 Controlled Drug nabiximols. It consists of a mixture of phytocannabinoids Δ^9-THC and cannabidiol (CBD). It is supplied in a metered spray nebuliser; each 100 microlitre spray delivers 2.7 mg THC and 2.5 mg CBD.

Indications

Cannabis extract is indicated as adjunct therapy for symptoms of moderate–severe spasticity in multiple sclerosis in people who respond in an initial trial but who are unresponsive to other medicines. In clinical trials, cannabis extract reduced spasticity and showed no abuse potential.

Mechanism of action and effects

See text.

Pharmacokinetics

See text. Pharmacokinetic parameters are highly variable both within and between people using cannabis extract. After spray onto oral mucosa, cannabis extract is rapidly absorbed, reaching maximum concentration in plasma within 1–2 hours.

Drug interactions

Interactions are possible with other antispasticity agents and muscle relaxants (e.g. baclofen and benzodiazepines), and with other drugs inhibiting or enhancing CYP 2C9 and 3A4 enzymes; also with sedatives/hypnotics, including alcohol.

Adverse reactions

The most commonly reported adverse reactions in clinical trials of cannabis extract spray were: dizziness and risk of falls; appetite increased or decreased; and impaired GIT and CNS functions. Higher than recommended usage of extract (18 sprays over 20 minutes twice daily) caused significant psychoactive effects and cognitive impairments (see text for other pharmacological effects).

Precautions and contraindications

Treatment with cannabis extract requires regular reviews by a clinician familiar with its use. It is not recommended for children; elderly people may be hypersensitive to its effects. It should be used only with caution in people hypersensitive to cannabinoids, and in those with a history of psychiatric illness, epilepsy, seizures or substance abuse. People using this spray should not drive or operate machinery. Both men and women (of child-producing potential) should use effective contraception during therapy and for 3 months after cessation.

Dosage and administration

The extract is sprayed onto the oral mucosa, starting with one spray per day and gradually titrating the dose upwards (according to manufacturer's dose regimen) over 2 weeks to a maximum of 12 sprays per day, with at least 15 minutes between sprays. It may take some days for optimum dose to be determined.

Source: Based on information in NPS and Medsafe (NZ) on nabiximols product; see 'Online resources'.

Various psychoactive hallucinogens have been used in religious ceremonies, in the hippie scene in the 1960s and are again popular for the vivid dreams produced. There is an illicit market for capsules purportedly containing such drugs but no guarantee as to what they actually contain.

Possible mechanisms and effects

Many hallucinogenic agents have chemical structures related to central neurotransmitters or are methylated derivatives of the transmitters so may act by altering transmitter actions. This has led to the 'methylated amine hypothesis' of schizophrenia, as it raises the fascinating possibility that some psychiatric disturbances may be due to altered metabolic pathways producing endogenous methylated transmitters in the CNS, or to high levels of transmitters being shunted down unusual metabolic paths. Unwanted effects include agitation and paranoia, possibly leading to self-harm, and 'bad trips', flashbacks and psychosis.

LSD

Lysergide is a potent hallucinogenic drug usually available illicitly in doses of around 200 micrograms. LSD is related to the ergot alkaloids (Ch 30) and can affect many neurotransmitters and body systems. After oral administration it causes a central sympathomimetic effect within 20 minutes: hypertension, dilated pupils, hyperthermia, tachycardia and enhanced alertness. Psychoactive effects are heightened perceptions, distortions of body image and visual hallucinations; mood changes range from euphoria to severe depression, panic, paranoia

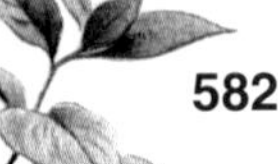

and 'bad trips' resulting in homicidal or suicidal thoughts. Long-term effects include psychosis and flashback phenomena, in which unfavourable reactions induced by LSD recur weeks, or even years, after using the drug.

Other hallucinogens

Mescaline is the chief alkaloid extracted from mescal buttons (flowering heads) of the peyote cactus. It produces hallucinogenic effects but has only about 0.02% of the potency of LSD. The trimethoxy- and dimethoxy-derivatives of mescaline are also hallucinogenic. It is usually ingested as crystalline powder that is dissolved into teas or encapsulated. The usual dose is 300–500 mg, which produces gastrointestinal disturbances and sympathomimetic effects, then vivid visual hallucinations. The half-life of mescaline is about 6 hours, and it is excreted in the urine.

Psilocybin and psilocyn are derived from Mexican mushrooms; they produce subjective hallucinogenic effects within 30–60 minutes after ingestion, similar to mescaline but of shorter duration. A dose of 20–60 mg may produce apprehension, poor critical judgement and impaired performance ability, also hyperkinetic compulsive movements, laughter, mydriasis, vertigo, muscle weakness and drowsiness.

PCP (also known as 'angel dust') was originally used as an anaesthetic similar to ketamine but was discontinued because of its hallucinogenic effects and many suicides and violent crimes. Common effects include flushing, profuse sweating, eye disorders, analgesia, sedation, perceptual distortions and symptoms that mimic schizophrenia. Toxic pressor effects may cause hypertensive crisis, intracerebral haemorrhage, convulsions, coma and death.

Other drugs of abuse

Over-the-counter and prescription drugs

Abuse of prescription drugs for non-medical purposes (i.e. non-therapeutic, or other than as directed by a registered health professional) is on the rise in Australia: pharmaceuticals most often abused are analgesics, including opioids and ketamine, sedatives and stimulants. In 2019, drug-induced deaths were more likely to be due to non-medical use of prescription drugs than illicit drugs (see Australian Institute of Health and Welfare in 'Online resources'). There is diversion and abuse of opioids (especially oxycodone, morphine and fentanyl) prescribed for pain relief or in methadone/buprenorphine substitution programs. There is also diversion and subsequent sale of benzodiazepines and amphetamines (especially dexamphetamine and methylphenidate) prescribed for ADHD treatment. Antipsychotics quetiapine and olanzapine are also subject to trafficking. People abusing prescription drugs tend to be older than those using illicit drugs; cannabis is often used concurrently.

KEY POINTS

Abuse of psychotomimetics, hallucinogens and prescription drugs

- The illicit drug most frequently abused is cannabis/marijuana and its synthetic derivatives. It is used to produce euphoria, distorted perceptions and freedom from anxiety. Chronic use can precipitate psychotic episodes.
- Medical marijuana/cannabis is used to treat spasticity related to movement disorders, and has been used to treat severe vomiting, pain, glaucoma and epilepsy.
- Hallucinogens include lysergide (LSD), mescaline and various designer drugs, amphetamines and natural products; these can produce 'bad trips', flashback phenomena and psychoses.
- Prescription drugs most likely to be abused are amphetamines, opioids, benzodiazepines and some antipsychotics.

DRUGS AT A GLANCE

Drug dependence and social pharmacology

PHARMACOLOGICAL GROUP AND EFFECT	KEY EXAMPLES	CLINICAL USE
Opioids • ↓ pain • Euphoria	Heroin	• Drug of abuse
	Morphine	• Acute or chronic severe pain
	Codeine	• Acute or chronic pain
	Methadone, buprenorphine	• Severe chronic pain • Management of opioid dependence
Opioid antagonists	Naltrexone	• Treatment of alcohol dependence • Maintenance of opioid abstinence
	Naloxone	• Opioid overdose antidote

Alcohols • CNS depressant • Sedative • Euphoria	Ethanol (= 'alcohol')	• Legal recreational drug • Antidote for methanol and antifreeze poisoning
Drugs for alcohol use disorder	Acamprosate	• Maintenance of abstinence in alcohol use disorder
	Disulfiram	• Deters alcohol use
	Thiamine	• Vitamin B1 • Coenzyme in carbohydrate metabolism. Prevents Wernicke's encephalopathy
Benzodiazepines • CNS depressant, ↑ inhibitory effects of GABA = anxiolytic, sedative, hypnotic, muscle relaxant, antiepileptic	Alprazolam, diazepam, oxazepam	• Acute alcohol withdrawal • Anxiety • Panic disorder
	Temazepam	• Insomnia
Benzodiazepine antagonists	Flumazenil	• Benzodiazepine antidote, used in benzodiazepine overdose and to reverse sedation/anaesthesia brought on by benzodiazepines
Amphetamines • Potent CNS stimulant	Methamphetamine, amphetamine	• Drug of abuse
	Dexamfetamine	• ADHD • Narcolepsy
Stimulant • Elevate mood, ↑ alertness, energy	Cocaine	• Drug of abuse
Tobacco • Nicotinic agonists • CNS stimulant	Smoking	• Legal recreational drug
Drugs for nicotine dependance	Nicotine replacement therapy, bupropion, varenicline	• Aid to stopping smoking (with counselling)
(Methyl)xanthines • CNS stimulant	Caffeine	• ↑ mental alertness, reduce fatigue
Cannabinoids • Psychotomimetic • Euphoria, distorted perceptions	Marijuana, Δ^9-THC	• Recreational drug, mild hallucinogen
	Nabiximols	• To ↓ spasticity in multiple sclerosis
Hallucinogens • Euphoria, distorted perceptions	Lysergide (= lysergic acid diethylamide, LSD)	• Drug of abuse
	Ketamine	• Induction and maintenance of anaesthesia

REVIEW EXERCISES

1 Ms PE experiences an accidental overdose of heroin. Describe the signs and symptoms Ms SB is likely to have. What antidote should be administered? How is this antidote administered and who can administer it?

2 Mr TO has recently purchased some e-cigarettes from an online store and is vaping regularly to reduce stress. Is vaping legal in the jurisdiction you live in? Are there any harms associated with smoking e-cigarettes? Compare these harms with tobacco smoking. List five drug interactions between the nicotine in e-cigarettes and commonly prescribed medicines. Explain why these interactions occur.

3 Mr EL has alcohol use disorder. Review the pharmacological effects of ethanol on the central nervous, cardiovascular and gastrointestinal systems, both in short-term use and in chronic alcohol consumption. Name at least three major drug interactions between alcohol and other drugs.

REFERENCES

Australasian College for Emergency Medicine, Alcohol and Methamphetamine Harm in Emergency Departments: Findings from the 2019 Snapshot Survey. 2020, ACEM: Melbourne

Australian Institute of Health and Welfare 2021. Alcohol & other drug treatment services. Online. www.aihw.gov.au/reports-data/health-welfare-services/alcohol-other-drug-treatment-services/reports.

Australian Institute of Health and Welfare 2022. Illicit drug use. Online. https://www.aihw.gov.au/reports/australias-health/illicit-drug-use.

Australian Medicines Handbook 2021. Australian Medicines Handbook. Adelaide: AMH

Cairns R, Schaffer AL, Brown JA, et al., Codeine use and harms in Australia: evaluating the effects of re-scheduling. Addiction, 2020. 115(3): 451–459.

Crowley, P., Long-term drug treatment of patients with alcohol dependence. Australian Prescriber, 2015. 38(2): 41–43.

Dobbin, M. and D.F. Liew, Real-time prescription monitoring: helping people at risk of harm. Australian Prescriber, 2020. 43(5): 164.

Egerton-Warburton D, Gosbell A, Wadsworth A, et al., Survey of alcohol-related presentations to Australasian emergency departments. Medical Journal of Australia, 2014. 201(10): 584–587.

Jauncey, M.E. and S. Nielsen, Community use of naloxone for opioid overdose. Australian prescriber, 2017. 40(4): 137.

John ALS, Choi HW, Walker QD, et al., Novel mucosal adjuvant, mastoparan-7, improves cocaine vaccine efficacy. NPJ Vaccines, 2020. 5(1): 1–9.

Lucas, C. and J. Martin, Smoking and drug interactions. Australian Prescriber, 2013. 36(3): 102–4.

Miliano C, Serpelloni G, Rimondo C, et al., Neuropharmacology of new psychoactive substances (NPS): focus on the rewarding and reinforcing properties of cannabimimetics and amphetamine-like stimulants. Frontiers in Neuroscience, 2016. 10: 153.

Noever, D.A., R.J. Cronise, and R.A. Relwani, Using spider-web patterns to determine toxicity. 1995. NASA Tech Briefs, 19, 4.

Rang, H., Dale MM, Ritter JM, et al., Rang and Dale's Pharmacology.[Edinburgh etc.]. 2016, Elsevier, Churchill Livingstone.

Ubaldi, M., N. Cannella, and R. Ciccocioppo, Emerging targets for addiction neuropharmacology: from mechanisms to therapeutics. Progress in Brain Research, 2016. 224: 251–284.

White VM, Guerin N, Williams T, et al., Long-term impact of plain packaging of cigarettes with larger graphic health warnings: findings from cross-sectional surveys of Australian adolescents between 2011 and 2017. Tobacco Control, 2019. 28(e1): e77.

ONLINE RESOURCES

- Alcohol and Drug Foundation: https://www.adf.org.au/ (accessed 10 August 2021)
- Australian Government National Drugs Campaign: https://campaigns.health.gov.au/drughelp/about-this-campaign/ (accessed 10 August 2021)
- Australian Institute of Health and Welfare (AIHW): National Drug Strategy Household Survey Detailed Report: 2013. Drug statistics series no. 28. Cat. no. PHE 183. Canberra: AIHW: https://www.aihw.gov.au/reports/australias-health/illicit-drug-use/ (accessed 10 August 2021)
- Australian Institute of Health and Welfare (AIHW): https://www.aihw.gov.au/publications/ (accessed 10 August 2021) [For many relevant reports and publications, follow links to Drugs and substance abuse, then to Program/Initiatives, Publications, Tobacco control, National Drug Strategy, etc.]
- Commonwealth of Australia Department of Health Drugs: https://www.health.gov.au/health- topics/drugs?utm_source=health.gov.au&utm_medium=redirect&utm_campaign=digital_transformation&utm_content=drugs (accessed 10 August 2021)
- Family drug support Australia: https://www.fds.org.au/ (accessed 10 August 2021)
- New Zealand Police: https://www.police.govt.nz/advice/drugs-and-alcohol/ (accessed 10 August 2021)
- Odyssey House Australia: https://www.odyssey.org.au/ (accessed 10 August 2021)
- Prescription Shopping Programme: https://www.humanservices.gov.au/organisations/health-professionals/services/medicare/prescription-shopping-programme (accessed 10 August 2021)
- Quit organisation: https://www.quit.org.au/ (accessed 10 August 2021)
- Turning Point Alcohol and Drug Centre: https://www.turningpoint.org.au/ (accessed 10 August 2021)
- United Nations Office on Drugs and Crime (UNODC): World Drug Report 2020: https://www.unodc.org/unodc/en/data-and-analysis/wdr2021.html (accessed 10 August 2021)

More weblinks at: http://evolve.elsevier.com/AU/Knights/pharmacology/.

CHAPTER 26
THE NEUROENDOCRINE SYSTEM AND PITUITARY GLAND

Mary Bushell

KEY ABBREVIATIONS

ADH	antidiuretic hormone (argipressin)
GH	growth hormone (somatropin)
GHRIF	growth hormone release-inhibiting factor
IGF-1	insulin-like growth factor 1
IU	International Units
PRIF	prolactin release-inhibiting factor

KEY TERMS

adenohypophysis 589
argipressin (antidiuretic hormone) 597
endocrine gland 586
growth hormone (and somatropin) 594
hormone 586
hypothalamic factor 589
negative feedback 588
neurohypophysis 589
oxytocin 597
pituitary gland 591
prolactin 594
releasing factor/hormone 590
replacement therapy 587

Chapter Focus

The endocrine system comprises glands that produce hormones necessary for a variety of vital functions in the body. Neuroendocrine interactions between the brain (hypothalamus) and the endocrine system (at the pituitary gland), via secretion of hypothalamic releasing factors and release-inhibiting factors (anterior pituitary) or by neural stimuli from the hypothalamus (posterior pituitary), help control the functions of the pituitary gland and hence of many other endocrine glands. Negative feedback control of anterior pituitary functions via raised levels of target gland hormones also maintains homeostasis.

Disorders of the pituitary gland commonly manifest as hyper- or hyposecretion of target gland hormones. Hypothalamic factors may be used in treatment, along with surgery and irradiation of tumours.

Although the pituitary gland secretes many hormones, detailed discussion in this chapter is limited to two anterior pituitary hormones – growth hormone (and its release-inhibiting factor, somatostatin) and prolactin – and the posterior pituitary hormones antidiuretic hormone and oxytocin. Other hormones will be discussed in the appropriate chapters more directly involved with target endocrine glands.

KEY DRUG GROUPS

Anterior pituitary hormones and analogues:
- Growth hormone, somatropin (Drug Monograph 26.2), prolactin

Hypothalamic release-inhibiting factors and analogues:
- Somatostatin, octreotide (Drug Monograph 26.1)

Posterior pituitary hormones and analogues:
- Argipressin, desmopressin (Drug Monograph 26.3), oxytocin, carbetocin

Prolactin release-inhibiting factor analogues:
- Bromocriptine, quinagolide

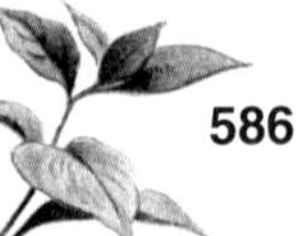

CRITICAL THINKING SCENARIO

Harry, a 33-year-old man, has recently been diagnosed with acromegaly due to an adenoma in his pituitary gland leading to excessive growth hormone (GH) secretion. Diagnosis was confirmed by both a random GH test and measurement of insulin-like growth factor-1 (IGF-1). Harry has been prescribed a long-acting injectable somatostatin analogue.

1. Why was a random GH test alone insufficient for the diagnosis of acromegaly?
2. List the somatostatin analogues that are available. Why are they all injectable preparations?
3. Explain the mode of action, expected effects and adverse effects of Harry's medication.

Introduction

Hormones

Hormones are natural chemicals secreted into the bloodstream from **endocrine glands** (Fig 26.1) that initiate or regulate the activity of an organ or group of cells in another part of the body. They have specific physiological effects on metabolism, growth, homeostasis and integration of bodily functions.

FIGURE 26.1 Locations of the major endocrine glands

Source: Salerno 1999; used with permission.

The list of major hormones includes the hypothalamic factors, which stimulate or inhibit release of anterior pituitary hormones, the hormones from the anterior and posterior pituitary glands, the thyroid hormones, parathyroid hormone, pancreatic insulin and glucagon, several potent steroids from the adrenal cortex and the gonadal hormones of both sexes. The hormones and their functions are summarised in Table 26.1 and in Table 26.3 (later in the chapter). Each hormone will be discussed in greater detail, and its uses in endocrine medicine described in this and the following five chapters 27–31.

Chemical classes of hormones

The main types of hormones are the steroid hormones, amino-acid-derived hormones and polypeptides and simple proteins. The chemical class of a hormone affects

TABLE 26.1 The major endocrine glands (excluding the pituitary), their hormones and main functions

GLAND	HORMONES	FUNCTIONS
Adrenal cortex	Glucocorticoids, mineralocorticoids and some sex hormones	Regulates carbohydrate and protein metabolism and fluid balance; also involved in inflammatory and immune responses
Corpus luteum, placenta	Progesterone	Menstrual cycle, pregnancy
Ovary, placenta	Estradiol	Female sex organs and characteristics; menstrual cycle, pregnancy
Pancreas	Insulin; glucagon	Glucose uptake, fat synthesis; gluconeogenesis
Parathyroid	Parathyroid hormone	Calcium balance
Testes	Testosterone	Male sex organs, characteristics and behaviour
Thyroid	Thyroxine, tri-iodothyronine; calcitonin	Metabolism, growth, protein synthesis; calcium balance and bone resorption

CLINICAL FOCUS BOX 26.1
Melatonin, hormonal messenger of darkness?

Many organs not usually considered as endocrine glands do secrete into the bloodstream 'hormones' that act on distant tissues. For example, the pineal gland, in the centre of the brain but on the vascular side of the blood–brain barrier, secretes melatonin, a chemical isolated in 1958 and so named because it lightens tadpoles' skin by contracting their melanocytes. Chemically, it is closely related to the neurotransmitter 5-HT. It acts via stimulation of two G-protein-coupled receptors, MT_1 and MT_2 (Hardeland & Poeggeler 2012).

The metabolic activity of the pineal gland is sensitive to light and darkness, melatonin being secreted during periods of darkness and serotonin during exposure to light. Melatonin has been called 'the endocrine messenger of darkness' and 'the darkness hormone'. Secretion is reduced by daylight, blue light, alcohol, caffeine and some other common drugs.

Because it entrains the body's circadian rhythms, melatonin has been trialled in sleep management – for example, for treating jet lag, insomnia, narcolepsy and sleep disorders in blind people and neurologically impaired children. It is available in Australia as a Pharmacist-Only medicine (Schedule 3) as melatonin 2 mg controlled-release tablets, indicated for short-term (up to 13 weeks) treatment of primary insomnia in people over 55 years. It has a short half-life ($<$ 1 hour), being 90% cleared on first pass through the liver.

Reductions in melatonin secretion occur in ageing and in disorders including cardiovascular diseases, Alzheimer's disease, diabetes and migraine, but the role of melatonin in their pathophysiology has not been established.

Melatonin is not without adverse effects, causing tolerance, somnolence, increased dreaming and fatigue, so it is recommended that only the lowest effective hypnotic dose should be taken, and use on consecutive nights should be avoided (Australian Medicines Handbook 2021; Hardeland & Poeggeler 2012).

how it is administered: peptide and protein hormones would be digested in the gastrointestinal tract, so they are administered by injection (parenterally) or sometimes as nasal sprays or sublingual tablets or wafers.

Steroid hormones are secreted by the adrenal cortex and the sex glands (testes and ovaries). They are lipid-soluble cholesterol derivatives whose physiological effects generally begin when the steroid enters the cell nucleus and binds to its specific receptor. Steroid hormones are usually secreted as they are synthesised.

Amino acid derivatives include the thyroid hormones, which are iodinated tyrosine derivatives (Ch 27).

Polypeptide hormones ($<$ 20 amino acid residues) include the posterior pituitary hormones, oxytocin and antidiuretic hormone and some of the hypothalamic releasing factors. Protein hormones ($>$ 20 amino acids) include insulin, growth hormone (GH) and parathyroid hormone, and other releasing factors. Peptide and protein hormones are generally stored in cells' membrane-bound vesicles and released by exocytosis.

Many other active chemicals released into the bloodstream could be classified as hormones, ranging from ions such as sodium and calcium, through the neurotransmitters noradrenaline (norepinephrine), 5-hydroxytryptamine (5-HT) and related melatonin (Clinical Focus Box 26.1), to steroids such as vitamin D, as well as local hormones (autacoids) such as prostaglandins, histamine and nitric oxide.

General functions of hormones

Hormones from the various endocrine glands function together to regulate vital processes, including:

- secretory and motor activities of the digestive tract
- energy production and storage
- composition and volume of extracellular fluid
- adaptation, such as acclimatisation and immunity
- growth and development
- reproduction and lactation.

Interactions among hormones provide homeostasis of growth and development, blood pressure, glucose levels, responses to stress, bone strength and conception, development and breastfeeding of a baby.

Hormones as drugs

Pharmacological use of hormones

In medicine, hormones are generally used in three ways:

- for **replacement therapy**, in hyposecretory states when the gland is not producing adequate amounts of the hormone, exemplified by dosing physiological amounts of insulin in diabetes or adrenal steroids in Addison's disease
- for pharmacological effects beyond replacement, as in higher doses of glucocorticosteroids for anti-inflammatory or immunosuppressant effects

- for endocrine diagnostic testing – for example, in the 'dexamethasone suppression test' of the functionality of the hypothalamic–pituitary–adrenal axis.

The endogenous hormones themselves may be used as drugs; or, if they have very short half-lives, are expensive or are difficult to extract, then synthetic analogues with similar activities but better pharmacokinetic properties may be administered. Drugs may act as 'antihormones' to antagonise the actions of excess hormones in hypersecretory states.

Receptor mechanisms of action

Receptors specific for particular hormones are situated in target organs in the cell membranes or inside nuclei. Most steroid hormones act intracellularly by binding to specific steroid receptors in the cytoplasm, then translocating into the nucleus and binding to response elements in target genes, leading to altered transcription of DNA and thence synthesis of proteins that cause the actions of the hormone.

Water-soluble hormones, such as the amino acids and proteins, act through receptors located in the cell membranes, activating second messenger systems such as adenylate cyclase or inositol triphosphate, which activate protein kinases and phosphorylate other enzymes, leading to physiological responses.

Transport of hormones

A hormone transported in blood is usually bound to a specific binding protein, such as thyroxine-binding globulin. The process is analogous to protein binding of drugs: binding increases transportability of the hormone in blood, decreases its movement across membranes and acts as a reserve depot in the blood.

Onset and duration of actions

Some hormones exert their physiological effects immediately, while others require minutes or hours before taking effect. Some effects end immediately the hormone disappears from the circulation, while other responses persist for days or weeks. Steroid hormones typically have prolonged actions because they induce synthesis of new proteins, and have long half-lives, being retained in the enterohepatic circulation.

Hormones are not 'used up' in exerting their physiological effects but must be inactivated or excreted. Most hormones are metabolised rapidly, having a half-life in blood of 10–30 minutes; metabolites are excreted primarily via the urine and, for steroids, the bile. However, thyroid hormones have half-lives measured in days.

Negative feedback effects

The anterior pituitary and some of the target glands have a **negative feedback** relationship, as shown in Figure 26.2. As the level of the target-gland hormone builds up in the bloodstream, it inhibits further secretion of both the specific hypothalamic releasing factor and the trophic hormone by the pituitary (the long negative feedback loops), thereby preventing excessive hormone effects. Exogenous hormones given as drugs can also activate this negative feedback effect; for example, chronic administration of corticosteroids 'switches off' the hypothalamic–pituitary–adrenal axis, leading to immune suppression and risk of infections. Secretion of the specific hypothalamic factor may also be inhibited by high levels of the anterior pituitary hormone whose release it stimulates (the short negative feedback loop).

Dosing: international units or milligrams?

In the past, hormones produced for therapeutic use were extracted from animal (or human) cadaver tissues, then purified and tested biologically for pharmacological activity. Activity of the extract was compared in biological assays with international standard preparations, and the strength of the new preparation was quoted in terms of 'International Units' (IU) of activity. Thus, most insulin preparations are still standardised to contain 100 IU hypoglycaemic activity per millilitre of solution (see 'Bioassays' in Ch 1).

Although hormone preparations are now prepared purely synthetically or by recombinant DNA technology, and are therefore 100% pure, such preparations may still have doses quoted in IU rather than in absolute amounts (mg or microgram).

KEY POINTS

Hormones as drugs

- The endocrine system is composed of specialised glands that secrete into the bloodstream hormones that act on specific target cells to integrate and regulate body functions.
- Hormones may be steroids, amino acids, peptides or proteins; they act via receptors in cell membranes or inside nuclei.
- Pathological endocrine conditions usually involve the overproduction or underproduction of hormones, and are treated by surgery, antihormones, replacement hormone therapy or hypothalamic factors.

Neuroendocrine controls: hypothalamic factors and related drugs

Control by the neuroendocrine system

To maintain balance in the internal environment (homeostasis), physiological functions must be regulated;

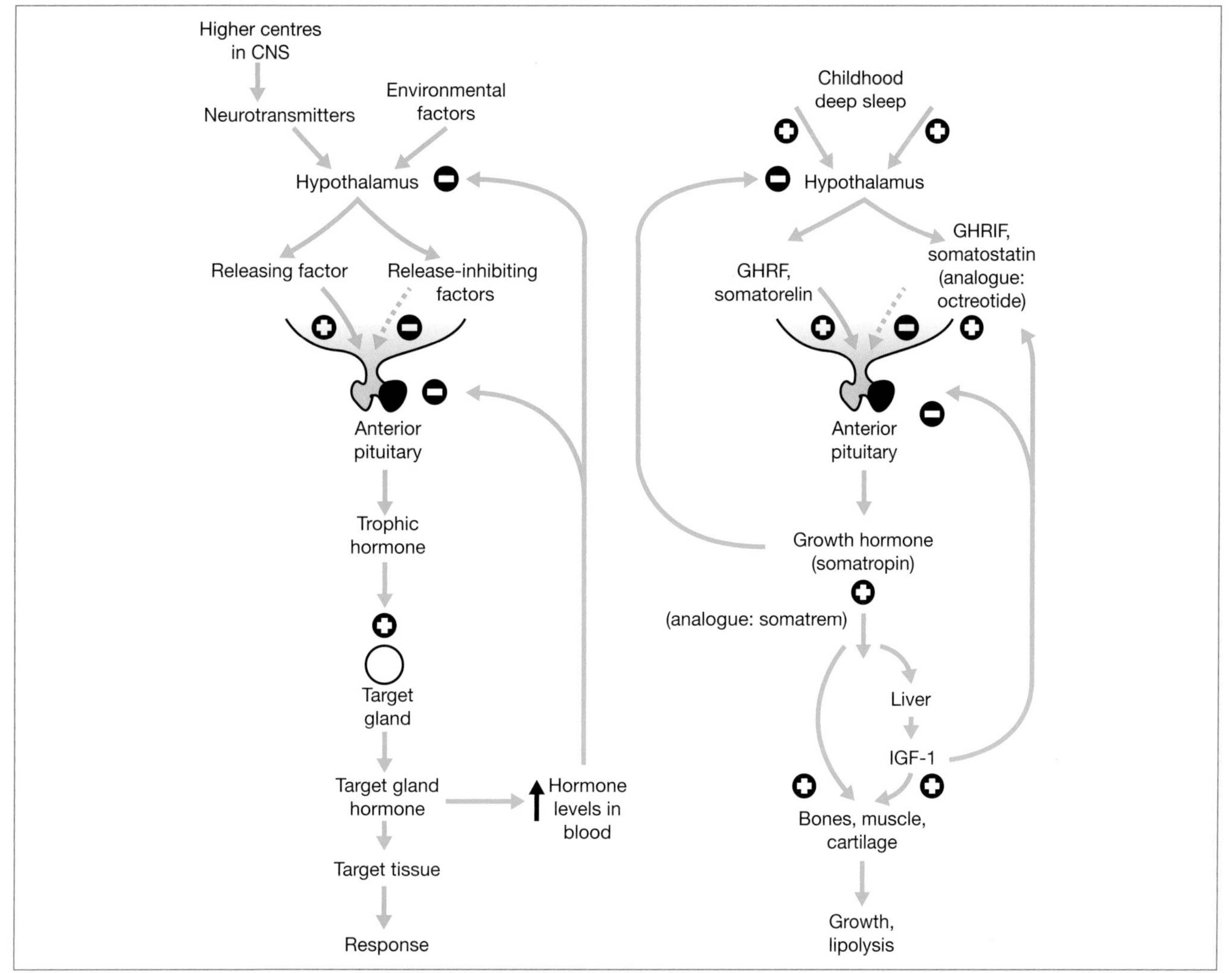

FIGURE 26.2 Levels of control of growth hormone secretion
A General negative feedback control systems. **B** Growth hormone controls
(+) indicates stimulation or increase, and (−) inhibition or decrease
GHRF = growth hormone-releasing factor; GHRIF = growth hormone release-inhibiting factor; IGF-1 = insulin-like growth factor 1

in the endocrine system there are multiple levels of control (Fig 26.2). At the highest level, environmental, cognitive, emotional, chemical and neuronal factors may influence hormone concentrations; this interaction between the brain and endocrine glands is known as the neuroendocrine system. The hypothalamus secretes into the hypothalamic–hypophyseal portal system active peptides known as **hypothalamic factors** (or hormones) that either stimulate or inhibit release of hormones from the *anterior* pituitary gland, also known as the **adenohypophysis**. (The hypothalamic control of the *posterior* pituitary gland, **neurohypophysis**, is neuronal; its hormones are released from nerve endings in response to neural stimuli.)

The neuroendocrine control process can be summarised as follows:

- Central monoamine-containing neurons secrete neurotransmitters.
- The neurotransmitters stimulate hypothalamic neuroendocrine transducer cells.
- These cells secrete releasing factors (or release-inhibiting factors) into the portal system.
- These factors stimulate (or inhibit) anterior pituitary secretion of trophic hormones.
- Pituitary hormones circulate to target glands.
- Target glands are stimulated to respond and/or produce further hormones.

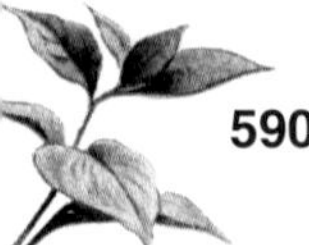

This is a 'cascading amplifier' process: minute amounts of monoamine neurotransmitter may eventually lead to dramatic changes in behaviour or growth.

Hypothalamic factors

Several hypothalamic factors have been identified and synthesised, as have analogues with better pharmacokinetic properties:

- growth hormone-releasing factor (GHRF, somatorelin) and analogue sermorelin
- growth hormone release-inhibiting factor (GHRIF, somatostatin) and analogues octreotide (Drug Monograph 26.1) and lanreotide
- thyrotrophin-releasing hormone (TRH) and analogue protirelin
- corticotrophin-releasing factor (CRF)
- gonadotrophin-releasing hormone (GnRH, gonadorelin) and analogues goserelin, leuprorelin, nafarelin and triptorelin (these are also luteinising hormone-releasing hormone [LHRH] agonists)
- prolactin release-inhibiting factor (PRIF = dopamine)
- melanocyte-stimulating hormone (MSH)-releasing factor and release-inhibiting factor.

The hypothalamic **releasing factors** are peptides, ranging in size from a tripeptide to large proteins. Their specificity of action is not absolute: TRH causes release of prolactin as well as thyrotrophin, while GHRIF inhibits the release of GH, thyroid-stimulating hormone (TSH), insulin, glucagon, gastrointestinal tract hormones and various autacoids.

Medical uses of hypothalamic factors and antagonists

The medical uses of some hypothalamic factors are summarised in Table 26.2; the use of dopamine agonists (as PRIF analogues) is discussed later under 'Prolactin'. Other releasing factors are sometimes used by specialist

Drug Monograph 26.1
Octreotide

Mechanism of action

Octreotide is a synthetic octapeptide analogue of GHRIF (somatostatin), inhibiting secretion of GH and many gastrointestinal hormones.

Indications

Octreotide is indicated for lowering blood levels of GH and IGF-1 to normal in people with acromegaly who are unable to have or have not responded to surgery or radiotherapy. It is also used to treat bleeding oesophageal varices, hypoglycaemia and symptoms associated with carcinoid tumours, and to prevent complications following pancreatic surgery.

Pharmacokinetics

It is rapidly absorbed after subcutaneous (SC) injection, with peak levels reached after 0.4 hour, duration of action up to 12 hours and an elimination half-life of about 1.5 hours; about 32% is excreted in the urine unchanged. A long-acting form is available for monthly intramuscular (IM) injections.

Drug interactions

Due to its effects on fluid, electrolyte and glucose balance, octreotide can interact with many drugs; glucose, fluid and electrolyte levels should be monitored, especially if other drugs increasing blood glucose concentrations are being taken (Table 30.2). Absorption of ciclosporin or cimetidine may be reduced or delayed, and clearance of CYP3A4 substrates (e.g. diazepam, oxycodone) may be reduced.

Adverse reactions

Adverse effects include local injection-site reactions and gastrointestinal disorders including nausea and vomiting, abdominal pain, steatorrhoea and hypoglycaemia. Blood glucose levels may be increased or decreased. Severe gallstone formation may necessitate cholecystectomy.

Warnings and contraindications

Use with caution in people with diabetes mellitus, gastrointestinal tract tumours or severe kidney impairment, and in pregnancy; contraindicated in gall bladder disease and during breastfeeding. Thyroid and gall bladder functions require monitoring during long-term treatment.

Dosage and administration

Octreotide and lanreotide, a similar GHRIF analogue, are available formulated in both medium- and long-acting forms, for SC or IM injection. Dosage depends on clinical use and on formulation administered; for example, in acromegaly the maintenance dose of octreotide is 0.2–0.3 mg daily.

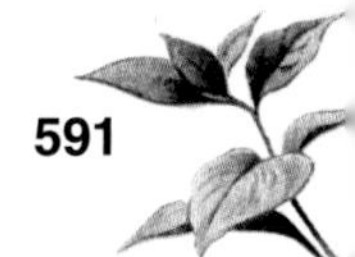

TABLE 26.2 Hypothalamic factors and antagonists in medical use

HYPOTHALAMIC FACTOR	CHARACTERISTICS	CLINICAL USES
GHRIF (somatostatin); also octreotide, pasireotide and lanreotide, analogues with longer half-lives	14-amino-acid peptide, inhibits release of GH; also inhibits release of TSH, insulin, glucagon and gastrointestinal hormones	Used in acromegaly and in therapy of various endocrine tumours (Drug Monograph 26.1: Octreotide)
PRIF	Dopamine	Dopamine agonists used in prolactin-secreting tumours and galactorrhoea (Clinical Focus Box 26.2, later)
GnRH analogues (also known as LHRH analogues): goserelin, leuprorelin, nafarelin, triptorelin	Synthetic analogues of GnRH, cause release of FSH and LH	Used in diagnosis, and in infertility, uterine disorders, pituitary downregulation, prostate and breast cancers
GnRH antagonists: cetrorelix, degarelix, ganirelix	Reduce release of FSH and LH	Cetrorelix and ganirelix prevent premature ovulation, before controlled ovarian stimulation; degarelix reduces androgen synthesis in treatment of prostate cancer

FSH = follicle-stimulating hormone; GH = growth hormone; GHRIF = growth hormone release-inhibiting factor; GnRH = gonadotrophin-releasing hormone; LH = luteinising hormone; LHRH = luteinising hormone-releasing hormone; PRIF = prolactin release-inhibiting factor; TSH = thyroid-stimulating hormone

endocrinologists in diagnostic tests of pituitary or target gland functions. Antagonists to some releasing factors have been developed – for example, cetrorelix (an LHRH antagonist) and ganirelix (a GnRH antagonist); these are discussed in Unit 10, 'Drugs affecting the reproductive system'.

KEY POINTS

Hypothalamic factors and related drugs

- The neuroendocrine system (interactions between the hypothalamus in the brain and the pituitary gland) helps coordinate central nervous system and endocrine functions via hypothalamic factors (to the anterior pituitary) and neuronal signals (to the posterior pituitary).
- Hypothalamic factors may stimulate or inhibit release of anterior pituitary hormones.
- Some hypothalamic factors, and their agonists and antagonists, are used in medicine to diagnose endocrine disorders or to treat dysfunction of the target glands.
- Octreotide is similar to somatostatin, the GH-inhibiting agent; it is used in acromegaly and in gastrointestinal tract tumours.
- Prolactin is hypersecreted in pituitary adenomas and as an adverse effect of antidopamine drugs. It can be suppressed by dopamine agonist drugs that mimic the prolactin release-inhibiting factor.

Anterior pituitary gland hormones and related drugs

The **pituitary gland** exerts important effects in regulating the function of other endocrine glands and hormones. In an adult human it is about the size of a pea, occupying a niche in the sphenoid bone at the base of the skull, and attached to the hypothalamus. The pituitary gland consists of two main lobes: anterior (adenohypophysis) and posterior (neurohypophysis), which are histologically and functionally distinct.

Anterior pituitary hormones

The hormones of the anterior part of the pituitary gland regulate secretion of many other hormones (Fig 26.3). Note that four of the hormones – adrenocorticotrophic hormone (ACTH; corticotrophin), TSH (thyrotrophin) and the gonadotrophins, FSH and LH – regulate the functions of other target endocrine glands.[1] The other three (GH, MSH and prolactin) act directly on target organs.

Pharmacological uses

The main functions of the hormones are listed in Table 26.3; common pathological conditions related to gland or hormone dysfunction are also indicated. The hormones, and drugs that mimic them, are generally used as replacement therapy for deficiencies or to diagnose gland disorders. Analogues of the natural hormones can be synthesised, often now by recombinant technologies, to improve pharmacokinetic properties or to make antagonists.

The pharmacology of GH and prolactin will be discussed in detail in this section; TSH, ACTH and the gonadotrophins are considered in subsequent chapters.

1 There is some confusion as to whether the suffix 'tropic' or 'trophic' is correct. Trophic comes from the Greek root meaning 'nutrition' or 'feeding', whereas tropic comes from the root meaning 'to turn' or 'to change'. In the context of endocrinology, the terms are sometimes used interchangeably. We have standardised on 'trophic' except where the approved name of the hormone used as a drug is definitely otherwise, as in somatropin (recombinant or biosynthetic growth hormone) and follitropin (recombinant human follicle-stimulating hormone). The natural hormones are somatotrophin, urofollitrophin, gonadotrophins, etc.

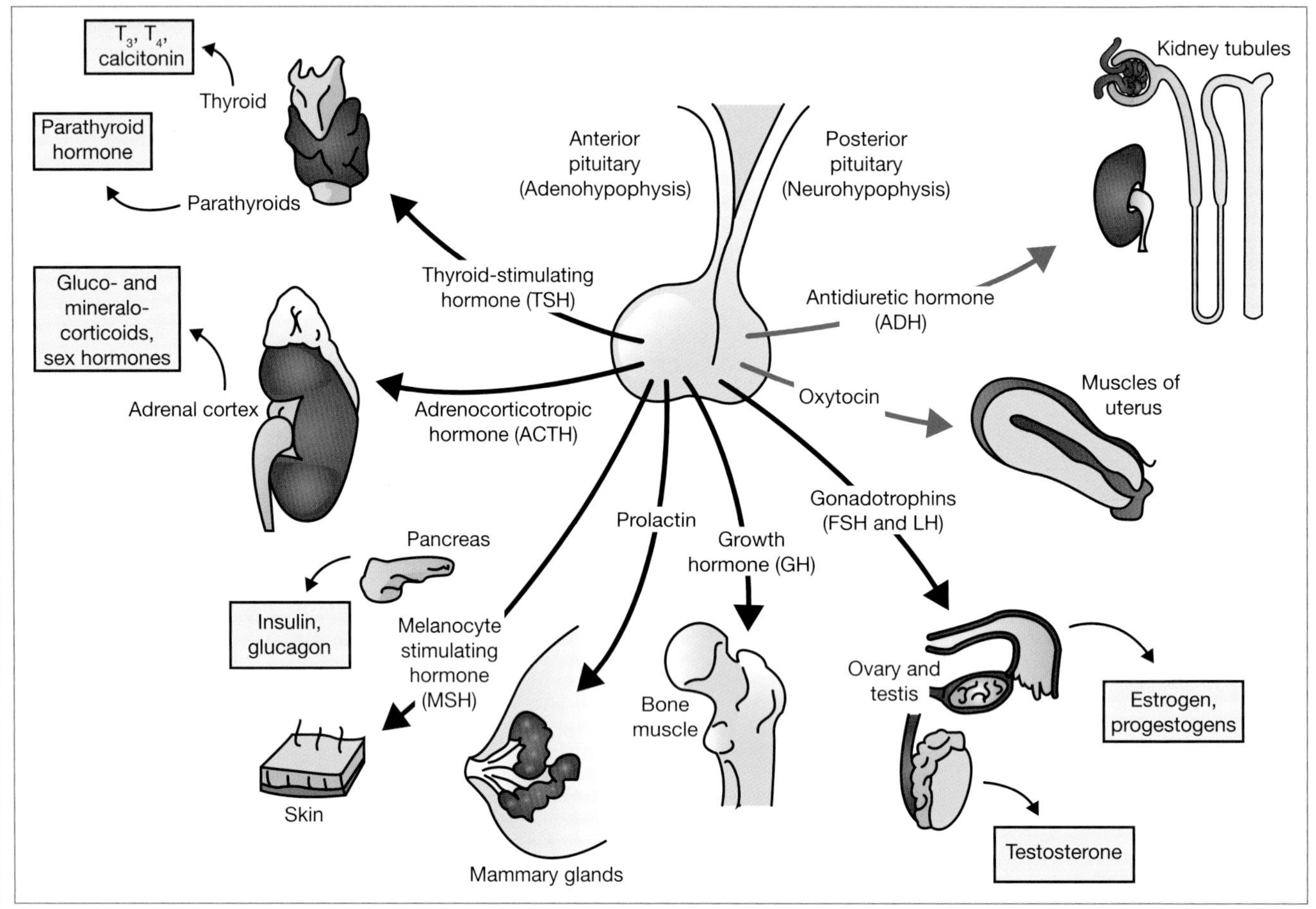

FIGURE 26.3 Pituitary hormones

Major hormones of the adenohypophysis and neurohypophysis and their principal target organs; hormones produced by target glands are shown in boxes. Note that there are no pituitary trophic hormones for the pancreas or parathyroid glands, and that some target glands do not produce further hormones.

FSH = follicle-stimulating hormone; LH = luteinising hormone; T_3 = tri-iodothyronine; T_4 = tetra-iodothyronine

Source: Salerno 1999; used with permission.

TABLE 26.3 The hormones secreted by the anterior pituitary gland, their functions and related pathological conditions

ANTERIOR PITUITARY HORMONE	FUNCTIONS	RELATED PATHOLOGIES
Thyroid-stimulating hormone (thyrotrophic hormone, thyrotrophin)	Stimulates the thyroid gland to produce thyroid hormones, hence regulates metabolic rate, growth and maturation; also affects central nervous system and cardiovascular functions; and calcium metabolism	Graves' disease, hyperthyroidism
Adrenocorticotrophic hormone (corticotrophin)	Stimulates the cortex of the adrenal gland to produce glucocorticoids, mineralocorticoids and precursors to sex hormones; hence, regulates metabolism and fluid balance	Cushing's disease, Addison's disease
Growth hormone (somatotrophin)	Promotes growth in most tissues; regulates metabolism	Pituitary adenomas, acromegaly and gigantism, dwarfism
Follicle-stimulating hormone	Stimulates the growth and maturation of the ovarian follicle, regulates menstruation or spermatogenesis	Dysmenorrhoea, infertility
Luteinising hormone, also known (in the male) as interstitial cell-stimulating hormone	Regulates reproduction (ovulation, formation of the corpus luteum, or spermatogenesis; secretion of sex hormones)	Dysmenorrhoea, infertility
Prolactin	Proliferation and secretion of the mammary glands	Pituitary adenomas, galactorrhoea, gynaecomastia
Melanocyte-stimulating hormone	Functions in humans are not defined; does darken skin	

Hyperpituitarism

Hypersecretion of anterior pituitary hormones is most commonly due to a pituitary adenoma (a hormone-secreting tumour). The clinical manifestations are both those of the 'space-occupying lesion' effects (raised intracranial pressure, compression of the brainstem and optic nerves) and those of excess hormone levels (pituitary and/or target-gland hormones). Thus, prolactin-secreting adenomas manifest as gynaecomastia, galactorrhoea and infertility (Clinical Focus Box 26.2), and GH-secreting adenomas as gigantism or acromegaly.

First-line treatment is usually surgical removal of the tumour. Then pharmacological treatment may involve administering the relevant hypothalamic release-inhibiting factor, or of a target gland hormone antagonist. Thus, acromegaly (Fig 26.4) is treated with surgery, somatostatin

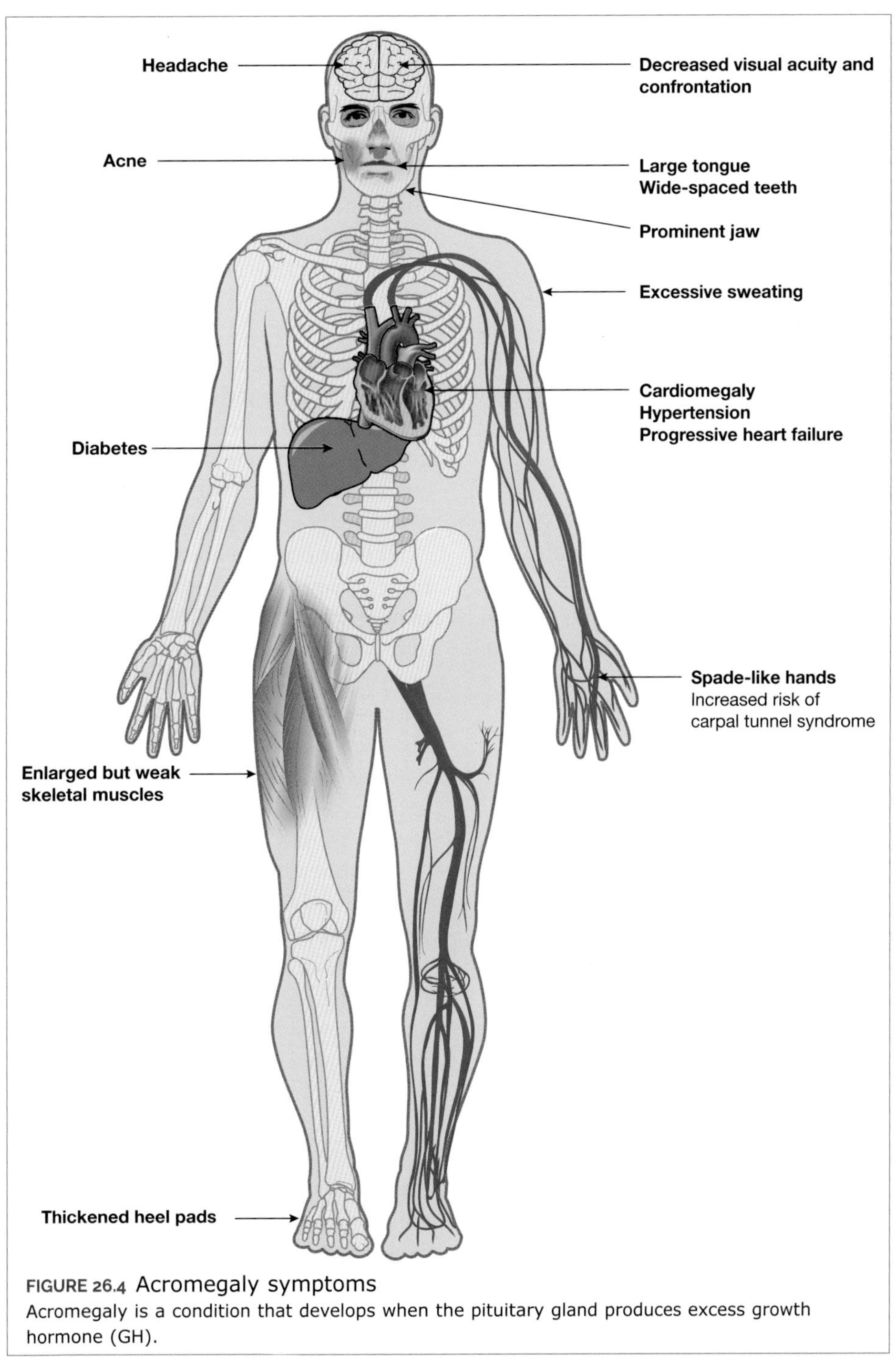

FIGURE 26.4 Acromegaly symptoms
Acromegaly is a condition that develops when the pituitary gland produces excess growth hormone (GH).

analogues such as octreotide (Drug Monograph 26.1) or pegvisomant, a GH antagonist.

Hypopituitarism

Deficiencies of pituitary hormones are most commonly due to tumours impairing hormone production; combination deficiencies are common. For diagnosis, levels of both pituitary hormones and target-gland hormones are measured to distinguish between primary pituitary hyposecretion and target-gland hypofunction or negative feedback effects. Treatment is usually lifelong and requires replacing all target-gland hormones; imbalance in adrenal cortex hormones is corrected first with IV hydrocortisone, as this deficiency can be life-threatening.

Growth hormone

Growth hormone (GH) is the main growth factor influencing the development of the body. A 191-amino-acid protein, it promotes skeletal, visceral and general growth. The anterior lobe of the pituitary gland in the average adult usually contains about 5–10 mg GH, the greatest amount of all pituitary hormones. Formerly produced for medical use from cadaver material, it is now synthesised by recombinant techniques.

Mechanism and pharmacological actions

The anabolic (growth-increasing) effects of GH are indirect, via the mediator (somatomedin) insulin-like growth factor 1 (IGF-1). This is produced in the liver and is directly responsible for skeletal and soft tissue growth, increased protein synthesis in cartilage and bone, tissue hypertrophy and wound healing.

GH has many metabolic effects including:

- decreases insulin sensitivity and may also affect glucose transport
- increases lipolysis
- promotes cellular growth through retention of phosphorus, sodium and potassium
- enhances protein synthesis through increased nitrogen retention.

Secretory system

The amount of GH secreted is very high in the newborn and decreases progressively throughout childhood, puberty and adulthood. The levels of control of GH secretion are shown in Fig 26.3B, and the sites of action of hormones and analogues used in pharmacological treatment of disorders of GH secretion are indicated. Normally, release of GH is pulsatile during the 24-hour cycle, high at night: levels can vary by factors of 10–100-fold. Secretion is increased by GHRF and during deep sleep in children and decreased by GHRIF (somatostatin). Reduced levels of signalling by GH and IGF-1 in ageing may contribute to cognitive decline. GH expression occurs in non-pituitary tissues and may have autocrine roles in disease states, including cancers.

Hyposecretion of GH

Congenital GH deficiency leads to hypopituitary dwarfism, with early-onset growth failure and delayed onset of puberty. Treatment is with GH and appropriate gonadotrophins; dosage is individualised (Drug Monograph 26.2). Treated children grow at a normal or faster-than-normal rate, and 'catch-up' growth brings them up to natural stature. There are questions related to the best age of starting treatment and duration of treatment, and ethical issues related to patient selection, risk of off-label use and diversion to illicit use such as in athletes. (GH is banned in sport; see Ch 42.)

The use of GH to increase height in short children is controversial (unless there are medical reasons for the short stature). The short height usually concerns the parents more than the child.

(In Australia, somatropin as a subsidised drug can be prescribed only on written authority.)

Hypersecretion of GH

Chronic GH hypersecretion causes excessive production of IGF-1, with over-growth of bone and soft tissues and generalised systemic disorders. GH-secreting pituitary adenomas cause the classical clinical syndromes of acromegaly and gigantism.

If this occurs in adults (in whom the epiphyses of long bones have already fused), acromegaly results, with manifestations including enlargement of the hands, feet and organs, and coarsening of facial features, with arthritis, hypertension and diabetes (Fig 26.4). GH hypersecretion in childhood and adolescence leads to gigantism, with striking acceleration of linear growth and features of acromegaly. Despite being very tall, pituitary giants are not abnormally strong because of thyroid, cardiovascular, joint and vision problems.

Treatment is with trans-sphenoidal surgery, radiation therapy and a somatostatin (GHRIF) analogue: octreotide (Drug Monograph 26.1), lanreotide or pasireotide. If there is insufficient shrinkage of the tumour and reduction in GH secretion, other drugs can be added. Pegvisomant, an antagonist at the GH receptor, is a protein administered SC daily; it effectively normalises IGF-1 levels in about 70% of patients (Freda et al. 2015).

Prolactin

Prolactin is the lactogenic hormone involved in proliferation and secretion of the mammary glands of mammals. Human prolactin is a protein hormone (198 amino acids in a single peptide chain), closely related chemically to GH and the placental hormone human chorionic gonadotrophin (human placental lactogen). Females have about 1.5 times the male concentration of prolactin; in males, lower than

Drug Monograph 26.2
Somatropin, recombinant hGH

Somatropin is used to stimulate linear growth in people who lack sufficient endogenous GH. Somatropin products are all synthesised by recombinant DNA technology and are identical to human GH; however, products are not interchangeable between brands.

Mechanism of action
Somatropin mimics hGH mechanism and actions (see text).

Indications
Somatropin is indicated for the treatment of growth failure in children caused by a pituitary GH deficiency, or in Turner's syndrome, Prader-Willi syndrome or chronic renal insufficiency; also in severe GH deficiency in adults. It is sometimes abused by people seeking increased size and strength.

Pharmacokinetics
Being a protein, GH can only be administered parenterally. Maximum serum level occurs at about 5 hours and the elimination half-life of parenteral (SC) somatropin is about 4 hours.

Drug interactions
When somatropin is given concurrently with glucocorticoids or ACTH, the growth-promoting effects of GH may be impaired. Doses of other replacement hormones require careful adjustment and monitoring. There may be interactions with other substrates of CYP3A4, including anticonvulsants and ciclosporin; reference texts should be consulted for individual combinations.

Adverse reactions
Antibodies to GH have been reported, but it is rare for a person not to respond to therapy. An allergic-type reaction (rash and itching) and lipodystrophy have been reported at the site of injection. Hypothyroidism, arthralgia, 'growing pains', fluid retention, diabetogenic effects and intracranial hypertension can occur. Excessive doses may produce gigantism and acromegaly.

Warnings and contraindications
Use with caution in patients with acute critical illness, hypothyroidism, diabetes or cancer. Avoid use in patients with GH hypersensitivity, intracranial tumour or closed epiphyses, and during pregnancy or lactation.

Dosage and administration
The dosage of somatropin for children is individualised, 0.7–1 mg/m^2/day SC for 6–7 days per week (usually in the evening). The growth rate response is monitored after 3–6 months to determine whether dosage adjustment is necessary. Therapy is usually continued until epiphyseal closure occurs or there is no further response. Available products range from 0.4 mg/0.25 mL to 24 mg/3.15 mL. (1 mg somatropin is equivalent to 3 IU.)

normal prolactin levels are associated with erectile dysfunction and premature ejaculation. Peptide fragments of prolactin hormone, known as vasoinhibins, inhibit blood vessel growth, vasodilation and vascular permeability.

Physiological actions (in females)
Prolactin causes an increase in the amount of breast tissue during pregnancy (via actions of estrogens) and in milk production, and possibly 'nest-building behaviour'. Gonadotrophin release and ovulation are suppressed, which tends to have natural contraceptive effects in breastfeeding women.[2] Prolactin is also secreted and has autocrine roles in other tissues, and signalling may be involved in reproductive cancers (breast and prostate).

2 While this is effective on a mass scale, such that the birth rate is generally low in countries in which women customarily breastfeed for extended periods, it is not sufficiently reliable as a contraceptive in individual women, as a woman can ovulate and become pregnant despite breastfeeding.

Secretory system
The main hypothalamic control over prolactin release is inhibitory, via PRIF, which appears to be the central nervous system neurotransmitter dopamine. Stimuli for release of prolactin include estrogens, suckling by a baby, dopamine antagonists (notably the neuroleptic agents used in schizophrenia) and TRH. Prolactin inhibits its own secretion by stimulating dopamine production in the brain, a short-feedback loop (Grattan 2015).

Dopamine agonists as PRIF agents
Secretion is decreased by dopamine agonists acting as PRIF analogues; thus, prolactin-secreting tumours are treated with bromocriptine, cabergoline or quinagolide (Clinical Focus Box 26.2) (Chen & Burt 2017). The main adverse effects are nausea, vomiting, hypotension and headache; impulse control disorders (including pathological gambling) may occur at higher

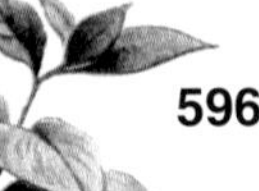

CLINICAL FOCUS BOX 26.2
Dopamine and lactation

Galactorrhoea (excessive production of milk other than after pregnancy) can occur in both men and women, and is due to hyperprolactinaemia, usually caused by low levels of the hypothalamic inhibitory factor PRIF (dopamine). This can occur in hypothalamic lesions and tumours, and also after use of dopamine-blocking agents such as antipsychotic drugs.

Treatment is with dopamine agonists, to mimic PRIF and hence decrease synthesis and release of prolactin. Dopamine agonists used include apomorphine, levodopa and bromocriptine, cabergoline or quinagolide. They are useful in pituitary adenomas (e.g. those causing male infertility) and in preventing lactation; also in Parkinson's disease (Ch 24).

Conversely, when stimulation of lactation is required in a breastfeeding mother, a dopamine antagonist (e.g. domperidone) can be administered to inhibit PRIF, an example of two negatives making a positive. However, natural methods facilitating breastfeeding are preferred.

Because dopamine is a neurotransmitter in many pathways in both the central and the peripheral nervous systems, there are many adverse reactions and adverse drug interactions whenever dopamine agonists or antagonists are used. Adverse effects occur particularly in the central nervous system, motor nervous system, cardiovascular system, endocrine glands and gastrointestinal tract.

doses due to dopaminergic actions in the central nervous system. Quinagolide is a non-ergot-derived selective dopamine D_2-receptor agonist, used in hyperprolactinaemia for its specific effects; doses are given once daily at bedtime with food, starting at 25 micrograms/day, increasing gradually to the usual maintenance dose of 75–150 micrograms/day.

KEY POINTS

Anterior pituitary hormones and related drugs

- The functions of the anterior pituitary gland are controlled by hypothalamic factors and by negative feedback loops from target-gland hormones; seven main hormones are secreted.
- Somatropin (growth hormone) is used to treat pituitary dwarfism and short stature.
- Prolactin enhances functions of the mammary glands; its release is inhibited by dopamine.

Posterior pituitary gland hormones and related drugs

Posterior pituitary hormones

The posterior lobe of the pituitary gland, the neurohypophysis, consists almost entirely of glial cells and neurons, with their cell bodies in the paraventricular and supraoptic nuclei of the hypothalamus. The hormones oxytocin and antidiuretic hormone (ADH) are synthesised there and stored in secretory granules that are transported down the axons to the nerve endings in the neurohypophysis, from where they are released in response to neural stimuli.

Oxytocin and antidiuretic hormone are both nonapeptides (9-amino-acids), with very similar chemical structures: pure oxytocin has some ADH activity, and vice versa. The hormones are released together[3] into the circulation but in varying proportions depending on the stimulus: during uterine contractions in childbirth, and in response to suckling by the infant, mainly oxytocin is released, whereas in response to fluid loss mainly ADH is released.

Antidiuretic hormone

Antidiuretic hormone, also known as vasopressin or arginine vasopressin, is released in response to raised plasma osmotic pressure. This may occur after haemorrhage, water deprivation, excessive diuresis or decrease in the circulating blood volume. Originally named because of its pressor effects (raising blood pressure), its antidiuretic effect is much more potent. ADH levels and effects are greater in males than females.

ADH is not often used in medicine now that potent, specific analogues have been synthesised: felypressin predominantly a vasoconstrictor) and desmopressin (1-desamino-8-D-arg-vasopressin, DDAVP, a specific V_2-receptor agonist with potent ADH activity; Drug Monograph 26.3) have very little oxytocic activity.

Pharmacological aspects

Mechanisms and actions

Antidiuretic hormone activates vasopressin V_1 receptors (via inositol phosphate production) and V_2 receptors (via adenylate cyclase). Via V_2 receptors it increases the

3 It is interesting to note that ethanol (alcohol) inhibits release of both ADH and oxytocin; hence, its diuretic effect and effects in slowing uterine contractions and milk letdown. Nicotine, on the other hand, increases secretion of ADH, thus decreasing urine production - formerly a useful drug interaction for drinkers who smoked, especially while listening to long after-dinner speeches (before smoking indoors at public functions was banned).

Drug Monograph 26.3
Desmopressin nasal spray

Desmopressin has a longer duration of activity than argipressin or felypressin. The nasal spray comes in a solution 0.1 mg/mL desmopressin acetate; each spray delivers 0.1 mL, 10 microgram dose.

Indications

Desmopressin spray is used to treat pituitary diabetes insipidus and primary nocturnal enuresis.

Pharmacokinetics

About 3–5% of an intranasal dose becomes bioavailable; it is distributed in two-compartment mode. The terminal half-life is about 2.8 hours. The drug is excreted by the kidneys, about 50% unchanged. Metabolism does not involve CYP450 enzymes.

Adverse reactions and interactions

The most serious adverse effect is hyponatraemia, which can cause headache, nausea, mild stomach cramps, dizziness and convulsions. (For drug interactions, see text.)

Warnings and contraindications

Desmopressin is contraindicated in other causes of polyuria, and in cardiac or renal insufficiency, in fluid or electrolyte imbalances and in raised intracranial pressure. Fluid intake must be restricted for 1 hour before administration and 8 hours afterwards in nocturnal enuresis. Precautions are needed in concurrent illnesses such as fever. Desmopressin appears safe in pregnancy and breastfeeding.

Dosage and administration

The intranasal adult dose to treat central diabetes insipidus is 10–20 micrograms 1–2 times daily. The dose for children with nocturnal enuresis (child > 6 years) is initially 10 micrograms at bedtime. This dose may be gradually increased if needed up to a maximum of 40 micrograms.

permeability of renal distal tubule walls to water, causing reabsorption and decreased urine volume with a higher osmolarity. The mechanism is via an aquaporin (water channel) in the epithelial cells: antidiuretic hormone binding to its cell-surface receptor activates a signalling pathway causing vesicles to fuse with the plasma membrane, increasing reabsorption of water. Mutations in the VP gene or the aquaporin 2 gene lead to diabetes insipidus, with large volumes of dilute urine excreted.

In 100-fold higher doses, vasoconstrictor effects occur via V_1 receptors, useful in treating haemorrhage but causing raised blood pressure. Antidiuretic hormone has many other non-renal actions, including platelet aggregation, raised factor VIII levels (hence its use in haemorrhage and haemophilia), increased release of ACTH and hydrocortisone and neuromodulator actions.

Clinical uses and drug interactions

Argipressin and its analogues are used as replacement therapy in pituitary diabetes insipidus, in bleeding conditions, for antidiuretic effects in nocturnal enuresis (bedwetting) and as vasoconstrictors in formulations of local anaesthetics. Being peptides, they are rapidly metabolised by peptidases, so are administered intranasally, sublingually or by injection.

There are interactions with any drugs that raise blood pressure, impair renal functions or affect bleeding – for example, with non-steroidal anti-inflammatory drugs. Additive antidiuretic effects occur with drugs that may cause the syndrome of inappropriate secretion of ADH (SIADH), such as some antidepressants (tricyclics, selective serotonin reuptake inhibitors), sulfonylurea antidiabetic agents, chlorpromazine and carbamazepine.

Antidiuretic hormone antagonists

A new class of drugs, the 'vaptans', are vasopressin receptor antagonists, targeting VP-mediated impairment of water excretion; they may become useful in treating hyponatraemia (Palmer 2015). Tolvaptan was approved in Australia in 2017 to treat some types of chronic kidney disease.

Oxytocin

Oxytocin means 'rapid birth', reflecting its ability to contract the pregnant uterus. The non-pregnant uterus is relatively insensitive to oxytocin; however, during pregnancy, uterine sensitivity gradually increases until

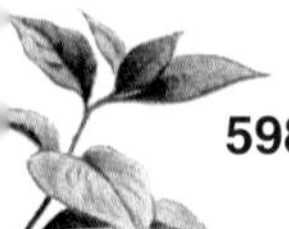

term. When released (or administered) during childbirth it causes regular coordinated contractions towards the cervix, with relaxation in between. A positive feedback mechanism may be operating: more forceful contractions of uterine muscle and greater stretching of the cervix and vagina result in more oxytocin release; the cycle is ended by the birth of the baby. Oxytocin also transiently impedes uterine blood flow and stimulates the mammary glands to increase milk excretion; release during suckling by the infant helps reduce the uterus to pre-pregnancy size. Oxytocin also has weak ADH-like actions but may have transient vasodilator (not vasoconstrictor) action. There is no distinct clinical syndrome related to oxytocin deficiency.

Oxytocin has been called the 'love hormone' and the 'moral molecule', as it appears to be involved in personal relationships, trust, altruism and generosity, parenting, postnatal depression, autism and the immune system (Zik & Roberts 2015). Mammals deprived of social contact when young have reduced levels of oxytocin and get less pleasure from rewarding stimuli; oxytocin has been suggested as a possible treatment for addictive behaviours.

Pharmacological aspects

Oxytocin is used clinically to induce or enhance labour when uterine muscle function is inadequate, and to prevent and treat postpartum haemorrhage (Clinical Focus Box 26.3). Uterine motility and fetal heart rate must be monitored. It is contraindicated if there is fetal distress or if vaginal delivery is contraindicated. It is usually given by IV infusion, when its onset of action is immediate; being a peptide, it is inactivated rapidly. An inhalable form is being developed.

Adverse reactions include nausea, vomiting, hypotension, tachycardia and irregular heart rate; prolonged therapy may cause water intoxication. Careful monitored use of oxytocin has contributed significantly to the safety of childbirth; it has an Australian pregnancy safety classification of A. (See also Ch 30 for drugs used in childbirth.)

Carbetocin, a new synthetic analogue of oxytocin, is an octapeptide with similar therapeutic actions but prolonged duration. It is given by single slow IV injection after caesarean section to prevent excessive postpartum haemorrhage. Carbetocin has a Pregnancy Safety Category C, as it is only indicated for use post-delivery.

CLINICAL FOCUS BOX 26.3
Oxytocin in childbirth

Mrs SS is a 36-year-old pregnant woman who has previously had four normal vaginal deliveries at term; she is not on any regular medications. She is currently 3 days overdue with her fifth baby, and has described decreased fetal movements over the past day. Given that this is concerning for impending fetal death, her obstetric team decides that she requires induction of labour (artificially stimulating the uterus to commence labour).

Upon admission to the labour ward, her cervix is found to be 2 cm dilated. Her waters are broken, and oxytocin infusion commenced at 0.12 U/hour. A cardiotocograph (to monitor uterine contractions and fetal heart rate) is commenced and continued throughout her labour.

Her midwife up-titrates the oxytocin infusion every half-hour, increasing the hourly dose until Mrs SS is having four strong contractions in 10 minutes. After 3.5 hours, Mrs SS is feeling the 'urge to push': vaginal examination reveals the cervix to be fully dilated, so she starts pushing. A baby boy is born 25 minutes later, with a further 10 U oxytocin administered when the baby's shoulders have been delivered. A perineal tear is repaired in theatre, and 40 U oxytocin given by infusion over 4 hours, to reduce the risk of postpartum haemorrhage.

Source: Acknowledgment to Dr Alison Bryant-Smith, MRCOG (personal communication).

KEY POINTS

Posterior pituitary hormones and related drugs

- The posterior lobe (neurohypophysis) secretes two hormones synthesised in the hypothalamus, under neural control.
- Antidiuretic hormone analogues such as desmopressin are used for central diabetes insipidus and to treat primary nocturnal enuresis or haemorrhage; felypressin is used as a vasoconstrictor.
- Oxytocin is administered to induce or manage uterine contractions during childbirth, and to prevent or treat postpartum haemorrhage.

DRUGS AT A GLANCE

PHARMACOLOGICAL GROUP AND EFFECT	KEY EXAMPLES	CLINICAL USE
Hypothalamic factors		
Somatostatin/growth hormone release-inhibiting factor analogues • Inhibits release of GH/somatostatin	Octreotide Lanreotide	• Acromegaly • Reduce symptoms of gastroenteropancreatic neuroendocrine tumours
Prolactin release-inhibiting factor mimetics (dopamine agonists) • Stimulate centrally located dopaminergic receptors • Inhibit prolactin secretion • Suppress GH	Bromocriptine cabergoline	• Treatment of galactorrhoea due to hyperprolactinaemia • Prevention of onset of lactation • Parkinson's disease • Acromegaly
Gonadotrophin-releasing hormone agonists • Initially increase FSH and LH synthesis • Repeated administration inhibits gonadotrophin production and decreases estrogen and testosterone levels	Goserelin	• Pituitary down regulation, for controlled ovarian stimulation • Prostate cancer • Advanced breast cancer
Gonadotrophin-releasing hormone antagonists • Block GnRH at the receptor • Inhibit the release of LH, inhibit gonadotrophin production	Cetrorelix, ganirelix	• Prevents premature ovulation during IVF • Prostate cancer • Reduce pain related to endometriosis
Anterior pituitary hormones and analogues		
Growth hormone • Induces growth in human body tissues and organs • Stimulates lipolysis	Somatropin	• Paediatric growth failure • GH deficiency
Posterior pituitary hormones and analogues		
Oxytocics • Stimulate uterine muscle contraction	Oxytocin	• Stimulates uterine muscle contraction
	Carbetocin	• Prevents postpartum haemorrhage
Antidiuretic hormone agonists • Increases tubular reabsorption of water • Vasoconstrictor	Argipressin	• Diabetes insipidus

FSH = follicle-stimulating hormone; LH = luteinising hormone

REVIEW QUESTIONS

1. Mr BI, hoping to improve his athletic capability, has been abusing the synthetic growth hormone somatropin. How does somatropin work? Why is it only available in injectable formulations (IM, SC)? What adverse effects might Mr BI experience? What are the legal indications for synthetic somatropin?
2. Ms SJ presents to her GP with extreme thirst and a history of passing large amounts of odour and colourless urine. She is later diagnosed with central (cranial) diabetes insipidus and prescribed desmopressin 100 micrograms orally, three times daily. What is desmopressin an analogue for? How will it work to reduce Ms SJ's urine output? What are some of the more serious adverse effects of desmopressin? What other formulations of desmopressin are available?
3. Mr HA has recently been diagnosed with hyperprolactinaemia secondary to a protein-secreting tumour. Mr HA is prescribed the dopamine agonist bromocriptine 2.5 mg three times a day. Describe how the drug bromocriptine reduces prolactin levels. Discuss some of the adverse effects of bromocriptine. Name another drug that works by the same mode of action that could be used in place of bromocriptine.

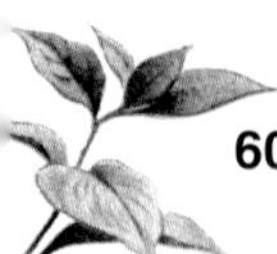

REFERENCES

Australian Medicines Handbook 2021. Australian medicines handbook. Adelaide: AMH.

Chen, A.X. and M.G. Burt, Hyperprolactinaemia. Australian Prescriber, 2017; 40(6): 220.

Freda, P.U., Gordon, M.B., Kelepouris, N., et al., Long-term treatment with pegvisomant as monotherapy in patients with acromegaly: experience from ACROSTUDY. Endocrine Practice, 2015. 21(3): 264–74.

Grattan, D.R., 60 years of neuroendocrinology: the hypothalamo-prolactin axis. Journal of Endocrinology, 2015. 226(2): T101–T122.

Hardeland, R. and B. Poeggeler, Melatonin and synthetic melatonergic agonists: actions and metabolism in the central nervous system. Central Nervous System Agents in Medicinal Chemistry, 2012. 12(3): 189–216.

Palmer, B.F., Vasopressin receptor antagonists. Current Hypertension Reports, 2015. 17(1): 1.

Salerno E, Pharmacology for health professionals. 1999, St Louis, Mosby.

Zik, J.B. and D.L. Roberts, The many faces of oxytocin: implications for psychiatry. Psychiatry Research, 2015. 226(1): 31–37.

ONLINE RESOURCES

Growth hormone program: https://www.humanservices.gov.au/organisations/health-professionals/enablers/growth-hormone-program (accessed 29 August 2021)

New Zealand Medicines and Medical Devices Safety Authority: https://www.medsafe.govt.nz/ (accessed 29 August 2021)

More weblinks at: http://evolve.elsevier.com/AU/Knights/pharmacology/.

CHAPTER 27

THE THYROID GLAND, THE PARATHYROID GLANDS AND BONE DISORDERS

Kathleen Knights

KEY ABBREVIATIONS

PTH parathyroid hormone
RANKL receptor activator of nuclear factor-kappa B ligand
T_3 tri-iodothyronine (liothyronine)
T_4 tetra-iodothyronine (thyroxine)
TRH thyrotrophin-releasing hormone
TSH thyroid-stimulating hormone (thyrotrophin)

KEY TERMS

Chapter Focus

This chapter is divided into two sections because of the differing metabolic roles of the thyroid and parathyroid glands and the pharmacological management of their respective disease pathologies.

The thyroid hormones thyroxine and tri-iodothyronine increase oxygen consumption and basal metabolic rate; accelerate carbohydrate, lipid and protein metabolism; increase sensitivity to sympathetic stimulation and promote growth, and are required for normal development of the central nervous system. Replacement thyroid hormones are useful in treating hypothyroidism, and iodine (iodide ion), radioactive iodine and antithyroid thioureylene drugs in treating hyperthyroidism.

The parathyroid glands have an important role in controlling the body's calcium and bone mineral concentrations via actions of parathyroid hormone and interactions with calcitonin and vitamin D. Various hormones and analogues (parathyroid hormone, calcitonin), vitamin D, bisphosphonates and other drugs are used to treat disorders of parathyroid function and bone pathologies.

KEY DRUG GROUPS

Thyroid gland:

- Antithyroid drugs: thioureylenes: **carbimazole** (Drug Monograph 27.2), **propylthiouracil**
- Iodine: **radioactive iodine** (Drug Monograph 27.3)
- Thyroid hormones: **thyroxine** (Drug Monograph 27.1), **liothyronine**

Parathyroid glands and bone disorders:

- Bisphosphonates: **alendronate, risedronate, zoledronic acid**
- Calcimimetics: **cinacalcet** (Drug Monograph 27.6)
- Calcitonin preparation: **calcitonin salmon** (salcatonin) (Drug Monograph 27.5)
- Calcium supplements
- Monoclonal antibodies: **Denosumab, romosozumab**
- Selective estrogen receptor modulator: **raloxifene**
- Parathyroid hormone and analogues: **teriparatide**
- Vitamin D analogues: **calcitriol** (Drug Monograph 27.4), **colecalciferol** (vitamin D3)

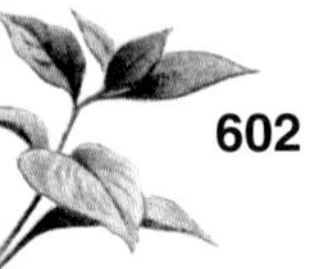

CRITICAL THINKING SCENARIO

Edith, a 58-year-old woman, has presented to the local hospital after a fall, which has resulted in a fractured wrist. Previously diagnosed with osteoporosis (T score $\leq$ 2.5 at the spine and hip) she indicated that she had stopped taking that 'horrible' weekly tablet about 3 months ago. After discussion regarding the need for her to be treated for osteoporosis she was administered denosumab 60 mg subcutaneously and advised that she would require a further dose in 6 months. On her next visit to her local clinic the GP expressed concern of the timing of denosumab in relation to when she stopped taking alendronate. Discuss the pharmacological/biochemical basis for the GP's concerns.

Introduction

The thyroid gland, one of the most richly vascularised tissues of the body, is located in the throat region, in front of the trachea. It has right and left lateral lobes, linked by a narrow central section, the isthmus (Fig 27.1). The thyroid lobules contain follicles filled with a thick colloid containing thyroglobulin and lined with follicular cells, which produce the thyroid hormones **thyroxine** (tetra-iodothyronine [T_4]) and **tri-iodothyronine** (T_3). The thyroid also contains parafollicular (C) cells, which produce the hormone calcitonin, which is discussed in the following section on the parathyroid glands. In 1914, the main thyroid hormone, T_4, was purified and crystallised, allowing detailed studies of its physiological actions. It was not until 1952, however, that T_3 was discovered, and not until 1961 that the actions of calcitonin were demonstrated.

T_4 and T_3 are essential for normal growth and development and functioning of the CNS. The growth-promoting actions of thyroid hormones are said to be 'permissive' – that is, a normal T_4 level permits the cells of the body to function properly. Children who develop hypothyroidism after birth have increasingly slow bodily growth and delayed maturity. Additionally, thyroid hormone secretion determines basal metabolic rate by altering carbohydrate, lipid and protein metabolism; promotes normal gastrointestinal tract (GIT), cardiovascular, reproductive and temperature regulation functions; and increases sensitivity to sympathetic stimulation through increased expression of β-adrenoceptors.

Thyroid hormones

Synthesis, storage and secretion

T_4 and T_3 are amino acid hormones, being iodinated derivatives of tyrosine. The synthesis, storage, secretion and circulation of the hormones are complicated. During the process, the scene of action moves from the bloodstream into the follicle cell, thence into the follicle lumen, back into the cell and finally into the blood again. A summary of the processes involved is given below and in Figure 27.2.

1 *Iodide trapping:* Iodide is extracted from the blood by the sodium–iodide symporter into the thyroid follicular cells and concentrates to many times the level found in plasma. Thus the thyroid gland normally contains virtually all of the iodide in the body. Around 1 mg of iodine is required by an adult each week; most of this is ingested in food, water and iodised table salt. The ratio of iodide in the thyroid gland to that in the plasma is expressed as the T/S ratio; normally, this ratio ranges from 20:1 to 39:1. In hypoactivity of the gland, the ratio may be 10:1; in hyperactivity, it may be as great as 250:1.
2 *Synthesis of thyroglobulin in follicle cells:* Thyroglobulin is a large glycoprotein with about 115 tyrosine residues per molecule of thyroglobulin, which is released into the lumen of the follicle as the main component of the thick colloid gel.
3 *Oxidation of iodide (I^-) to iodine (I_2):* Oxidation occurs in the follicle cells and is catalysed by the enzyme thyroperoxidase, followed by transfer of iodine into the lumen.
4 *Iodination of tyrosine residues in thyroglobulin:* Initially, one or two iodine atoms bind to tyrosine residues (yielding mono- or di-iodinated tyrosine, MIT or DIT).
5 *Coupling of MIT and DIT:* These occur as pairs: MIT + DIT gives T_3; and MIT + MIT gives T_4. The thyroid hormones are thus incorporated into thyroglobulin molecules, about 90% as T_4.
6 *Storage of T_3 and T_4:* T_3 and T_4 are stored in thyroglobulin in the lumen of the follicle. About 30% of the thyroid mass is thyroglobulin, which contains enough thyroid hormone to meet normal requirements for 2–3 months without any further synthesis.

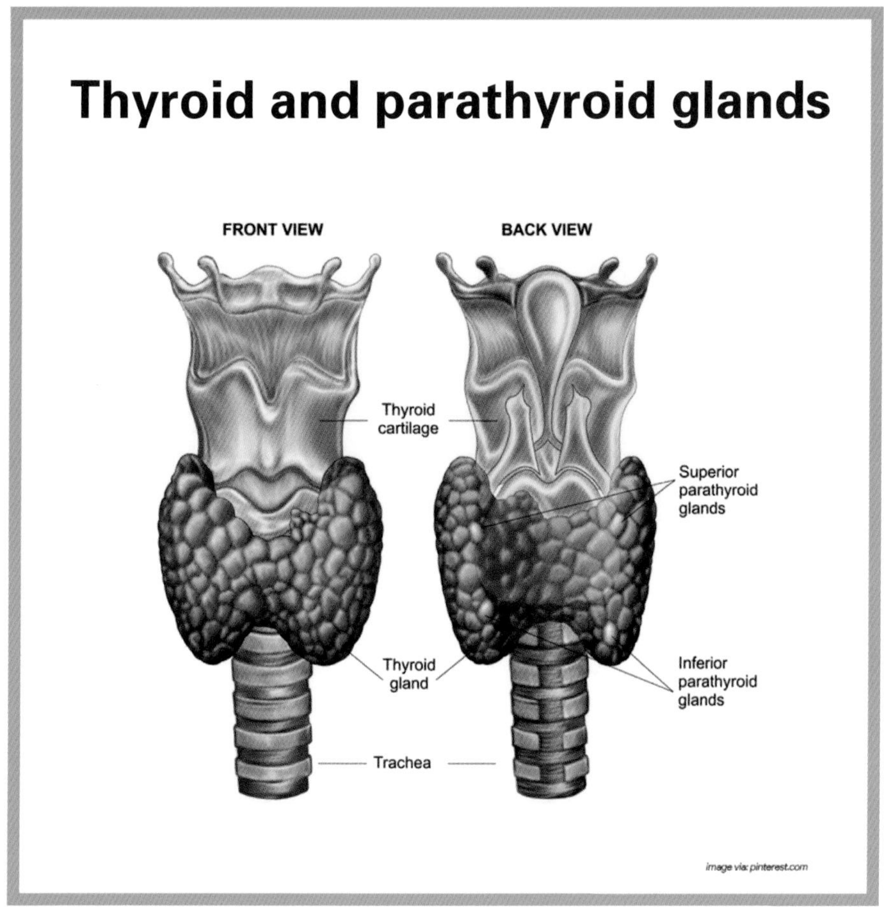

FIGURE 27.1 Thyroid gland
The thyroid gland is located in the throat region in front of the trachea, with the right and left lateral lobes linked by the isthmus. The small parathyroid glands are located on the posterior surface of each lobe of the thyroid gland.
Source: Getty Images/Stocktrek Images.

7 *Release of active T_3 and T_4*: This is accomplished by proteolytic digestion of colloid in the follicle cells; iodine, MIT, DIT and peptide residues are reused.

8 *Secretion of T_3 and T_4*: As lipid-soluble amino acids, they can diffuse from thyroid cells into the bloodstream.

9 *Circulation:* T_4 is present as a large pool in the circulation, 99.95% protein-bound to thyroxine-binding globulin and other proteins. T_4 has a low turnover rate, with a half-life of about 6–7 days; as it circulates and enters cells, most T_4 is converted to T_3. T_3 is present as a small pool, mainly stored intracellularly; it is more potent than T_4, less strongly protein-bound and has a faster turnover rate, with a half-life of about 2 days.

Regulation

Control of thyroid hormone concentrations is complex. High concentrations of circulating thyroid hormones activate typical negative-feedback loops, by inhibiting the synthesis of genes for both hypothalamic **thyrotrophin-releasing hormone** (TRH) and anterior pituitary **thyroid-stimulating hormone** (TSH, thyrotrophin) at the transcriptional level (Fig 27.3). This inhibits synthesis and release of TSH, thus overall reducing production of thyroid hormones. In contrast, low concentrations of circulating thyroid hormones increase the release of TSH from the pituitary gland and appear to influence the secretion of TRH from the hypothalamus.

TSH binds to TSH receptors, which are G-protein-coupled receptors, on thyroid cells (and cells of thyroid tumours) and, via activation of adenylyl cyclase and phosphorylation of enzymes, then stimulates many aspects of thyroid gland function, including increasing:

- thyroid cell utilisation of glucose and oxygen
- blood flow to the thyroid gland
- iodide trapping by the gland
- iodination of thyroglobulin, thus increasing synthesis of hormones
- proteolysis of thyroglobulin and, hence, release of hormones.

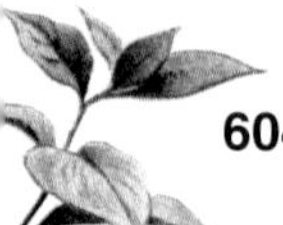

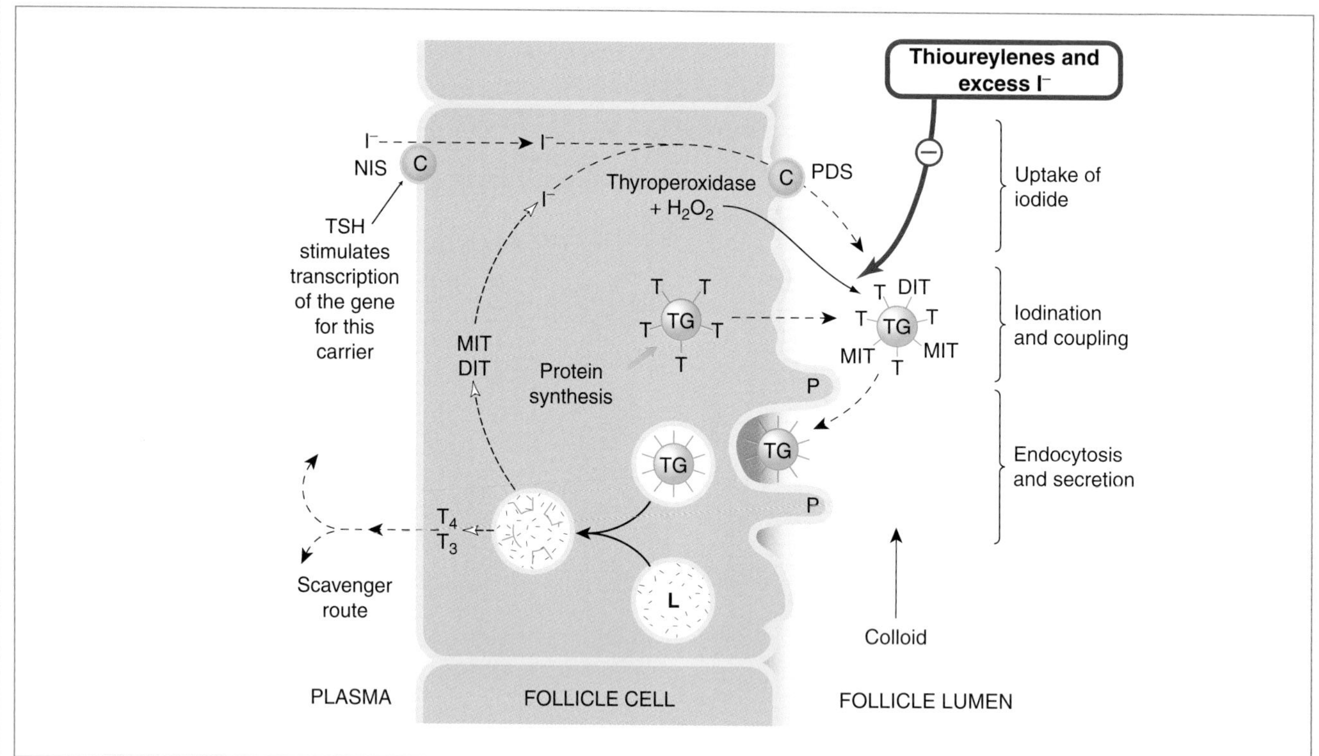

FIGURE 27.2 Diagram of thyroid hormone synthesis and secretion, with the sites of action of drugs used in the treatment of thyroid disorders Iodide in the blood is transported by the carriers NIS and pendrin (PDS) through the follicular cell and into the colloid-rich lumen, where it is incorporated into thyroglobulin under the influence of the thyroperoxidase enzyme. The hormones are produced by processing of the endocytosed thyroglobulin and exported into blood.
DIT = di-iodotyrosine; L = lysosome; MIT = monoiodotyrosine; P = pseudopod; T = tyrosine; T_3 = tri-iodothyronine; T_4 = thyroxine; TG = thyroglobulin; TSH = thyroid-stimulating hormone
Source: Adapted from Rang et al. 2012, Figure 33-1; reproduced with permission from Elsevier Churchill Livingstone.

In the long term, an increase in TSH leads to both thyroid hypertrophy (greater size of cells) and hyperplasia (greater number of cells). Thyrotropin alfa, a recombinant form of human TSH, is used in testing for remnants of thyroid cancers after thyroidectomy surgery. TSH is commonly measured in thyroid function tests, to diagnose and monitor dysfunction (Clinical Focus Box 27.1).

Another factor regulating thyroid function is changes in iodide concentration: reduced plasma iodide concentration reduces thyroid hormone synthesis and increases TSH secretion, while excessively high concentrations switch off production via negative feedback and possibly by inhibiting the iodination of **thyroglobulin**.

Mechanism of thyroid hormone actions

T_4 (which is converted to T_3 on entering the cell) and T_3 enter the nucleus of target cells, where they bind to specific nuclear receptors. These then bind to thyroid response elements on genes. Transcription is then altered as a result of activation or repression of various genes. Hence, synthesis of specific proteins – for example, Na^+–K^+-ATPase – is altered. T_3 is more potent than T_4 and has a greater affinity for thyroid receptors.

CLINICAL FOCUS BOX 27.1
Thyroid function tests

Thyroid function tests are commonly carried out to determine the exact site of thyroid dysfunction - and, hence, to optimise therapy by monitoring treatment and adjusting dosage (Mortimer 2011). Note that many drugs can alter thyroid state and function test results and affect thyroxine absorption and metabolism.

The hormone that is usually measured is TSH, a sensitive marker of thyroid function because it is influenced (inversely) by small changes in free T_4 concentration. A low TSH usually indicates hyperthyroidism. A raised TSH usually means primary hypothyroidism due to thyroid dysfunction: TSH basal concentrations are raised, and the pituitary is hyper-reactive to TRH stimulation, but T_3 and T_4 concentrations remain low.

There are several other thyroid function tests, including the free T_4 index (FTI), free T_3 and T_3 resin uptake (T_3RU) test, thyroglobulin concentration and concentrations of thyroid-related autoantibodies (to thyroperoxidase, thyroglobulin or TSH receptor).

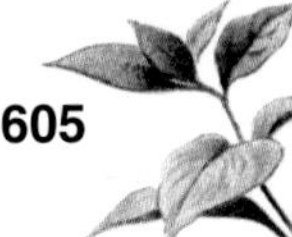

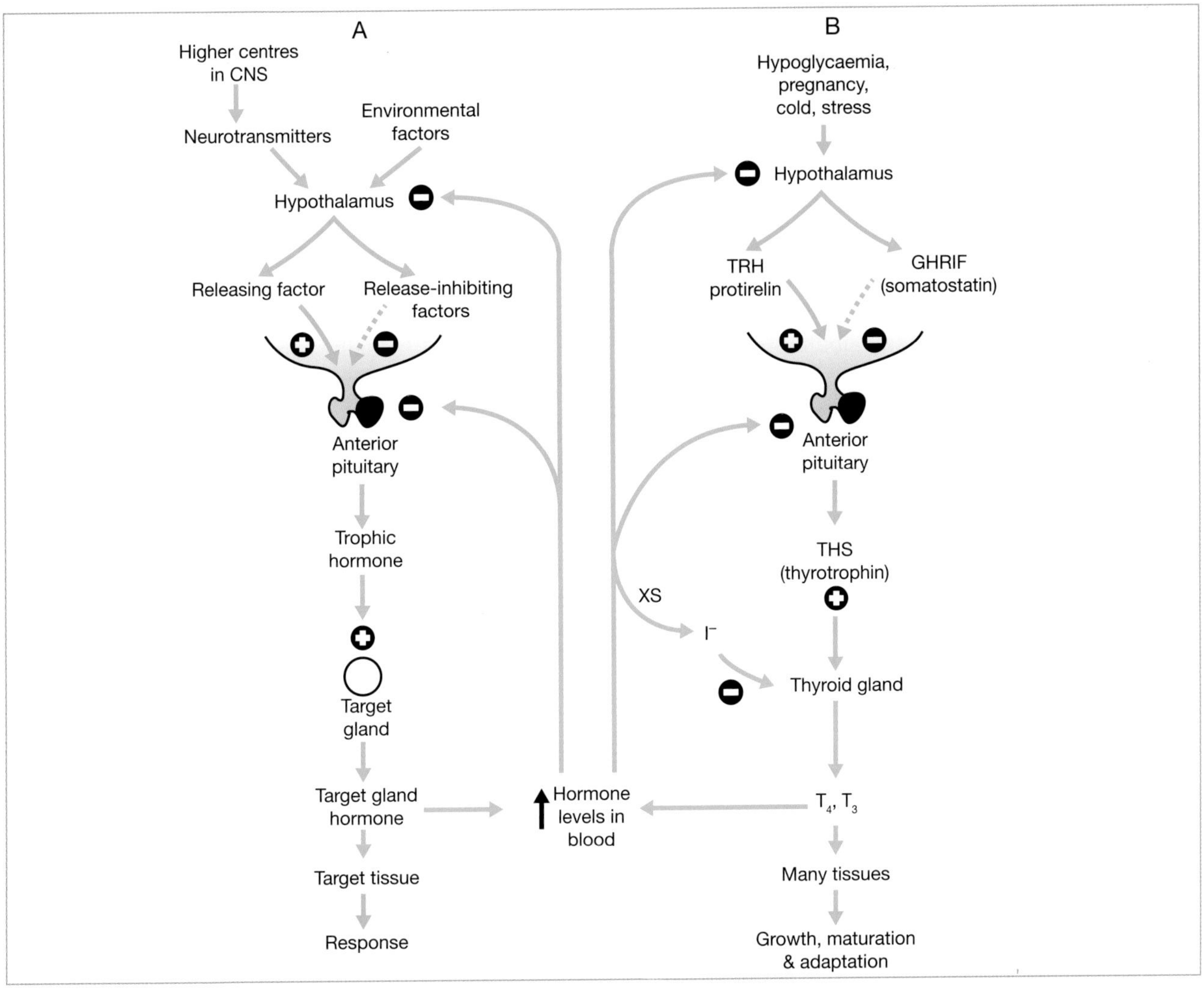

A

Higher centres in CNS

Neurotransmitters

Environmental factors

Hypothalamus

Releasing factor

Release-inhibiting factors

Anterior pituitary

Trophic hormone

Target gland

Target gland hormone

Target tissue

Response

Hormone levels in blood

B

Hypoglycaemia, pregnancy, cold, stress

Hypothalamus

TRH protirelin

GHRIF (somatostatin)

Anterior pituitary

THS (thyrotrophin)

XS

I⁻

Thyroid gland

T_4, T_3

Many tissues

Growth, maturation & adaptation

FIGURE 27.3 Secretion and control of thyroid hormones

A General control mechanisms for hormone secretion. **B** Control mechanisms for thyroid hormone secretion. Environmental factors influence secretion of the hypothalamic factors thyrotrophin-releasing hormone (TRH) and growth hormone release-inhibiting factor (GHRIF, somatostatin) to increase or decrease release from the anterior pituitary of thyrotrophin (TSH), which stimulates production in the thyroid glands of thyroxine (T_4) and T_3.

KEY POINTS

The thyroid gland

- The thyroid gland has an important homeostatic role in growth and development, metabolism and energy balance and cardiovascular and nervous system functions.
- The hormones produced by the thyroid gland include T_4 and T_3 and calcitonin.
- Iodine is actively taken up from the circulation by the thyroid gland and incorporated in T_3 and T_4, which are stored in the thyroid follicles, bound in thyroglobulin.
- The synthesis, storage and secretion of thyroid hormones is a multi-step process.
- High concentrations of circulating thyroid hormones activate negative-feedback loops by inhibiting the synthesis of genes for both hypothalamic TRH and anterior pituitary TSH at the transcriptional level, thus overall reducing production of thyroid hormones.
- Low concentrations of circulating thyroid hormones increase the release of TSH from the pituitary gland and appear to influence the secretion of TRH from the hypothalamus.
- T_4 and T_3 bind to nuclear receptors, altering transcription – and hence protein synthesis – by activation or repression of various genes.

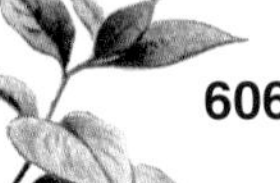

Pharmacotherapy of thyroid disorders

Iodine deficiency and simple or non-toxic goitre

Iodine deficiency is inevitably a result of decreased dietary iodine intake, leading to insufficient synthesis of thyroid hormones and impairment of thyroid functions. During the first two trimesters of pregnancy, the fetus is dependent on placental transfer of maternal T_4 for normal brain development (Haugen 2009). If iodine deficiency is untreated during pregnancy and in the first few months of life, congenital hypothyroidism leads to severe brain damage, neurological disorders and 'cretinism', which have been described since the Middle Ages. It is recognised by the World Health Organization as the most common preventable cause of brain damage. In iodine-deficient areas and where access to iodised salt is low, extra iodine supplementation in pregnancy and infancy is recommended.

Since 2009, there has been mandatory fortification of bread with iodised salt and the expectation of consumption of three slices of bread/day. Despite the requirement for commercial bread to contain iodised salt, pregnant and breastfeeding women are advised to take supplements containing 150 micrograms/day, as well as adequate intake from dietary sources. However, the margin between too much iodine and too little is narrow, so excessive iodine-rich foods should not be eaten. Iodine is not abundant in most foods, with the exception of fish and seafood. The World Health Organization and UNESCO have therefore committed to a public health program of mandatory fortification of iodine in the food supply via staple dietary components. The recommendation is for the regular use of iodised salt (25–40 mg iodine per kilo salt), to provide about 200 micrograms of iodine daily.

Endemic goitre is usually due to low soil iodine concentrations, especially common in inland hilly areas, leading to prolonged low concentrations of iodine in the food chain and decreased synthesis of thyroid hormones. Compensatory increased hypothalamic TRH and pituitary TSH results in enlargement of the thyroid gland, known as a simple **goitre**. The enlarged thyroid scavenges residual traces of iodine from the blood. This type of goitre can be prevented by providing an adequate supply of iodine (described earlier). Note that the presence of goitre is not necessarily diagnostic of simple goitre, as an enlarged thyroid gland may also be due to excessive stimulation of the gland in thyrotoxicosis.

Hypothyroidism

Pathology

Hypothyroidism is estimated to be present in up to 2% of the population, especially in middle-aged and elderly women; it is associated with autoimmune disorders, previous Graves' disease (and antithyroid therapy) and Down syndrome. Aetiological factors include post-thyroidectomy or radiation therapy, iodine deficiencies (simple non-toxic goitre), Hashimoto's thyroiditis (development of autoantibodies to thyroglobulin and some components of thyroid tissue), use of antithyroid drugs or lithium or amiodarone. Patients with primary hypothyroidism have low T_3 and T_4 concentrations despite an elevated TSH level. The condition can easily be missed, as it has very variable and non-specific presentations and development is usually insidious. The TSH stimulation test is diagnostic (Clinical Focus Box 27.1, earlier).

Clinical manifestations

Clinical manifestations are illustrated in Figure 27.4. Severe hypothyroidism in the adult is called myxoedema, referring to the thickened skin caused by acid mucopolysaccharide accumulation. In the last stage of longstanding, inadequately treated or untreated hypothyroidism, coma sets in accompanied by hypotension, hypoventilation, hypothermia, hyponatraemia and hypoglycaemia.

In children

Hypothyroidism in a young child (formerly known as cretinism) is characterised by slowed physical and mental development, which leads to dwarfism and mental retardation. The condition may result from faulty development or atrophy of the thyroid gland during fetal life and may be caused by lack of iodine in the mother. In congenital hypothyroidism, thyroid hormone concentrations equal to or above those required for the adult must be established immediately after birth to prevent permanent mental and physical retardation (Fig 27.5).

In elderly people

In the elderly, hypothyroidism is the second most common endocrine disease; it is often overlooked or misdiagnosed. Only one-third of geriatric people exhibit the typical signs and symptoms of cold intolerance and weight gain; more often, the symptoms are non-specific, such as failing to thrive, stumbling and falling episodes and incontinence. If neurological involvement has occurred, a misdiagnosis of dementia, depression or a psychotic episode may be made. Laboratory tests for plasma T_4 and TSH are used to confirm hypothyroidism.

Treatment

The goal of treating people with hypothyroidism or myxoedema is to eliminate their symptoms and restore them to a normal physical and emotional state (i.e. render them euthyroid). Therapy is simple: for lifelong thyroid replacement the thyroid hormones are safe, stable, cheap and available orally; dosage regimens can

Confusion,
forgetfulness
Hair loss
Slow speech
Generalised
cold intolerance
Non-toxic goitre
Husky voice
Thickened skin
Bradycardia
Low metabolic rate
Infertility
Muscle pain
Generalised fatigue
and lethagy

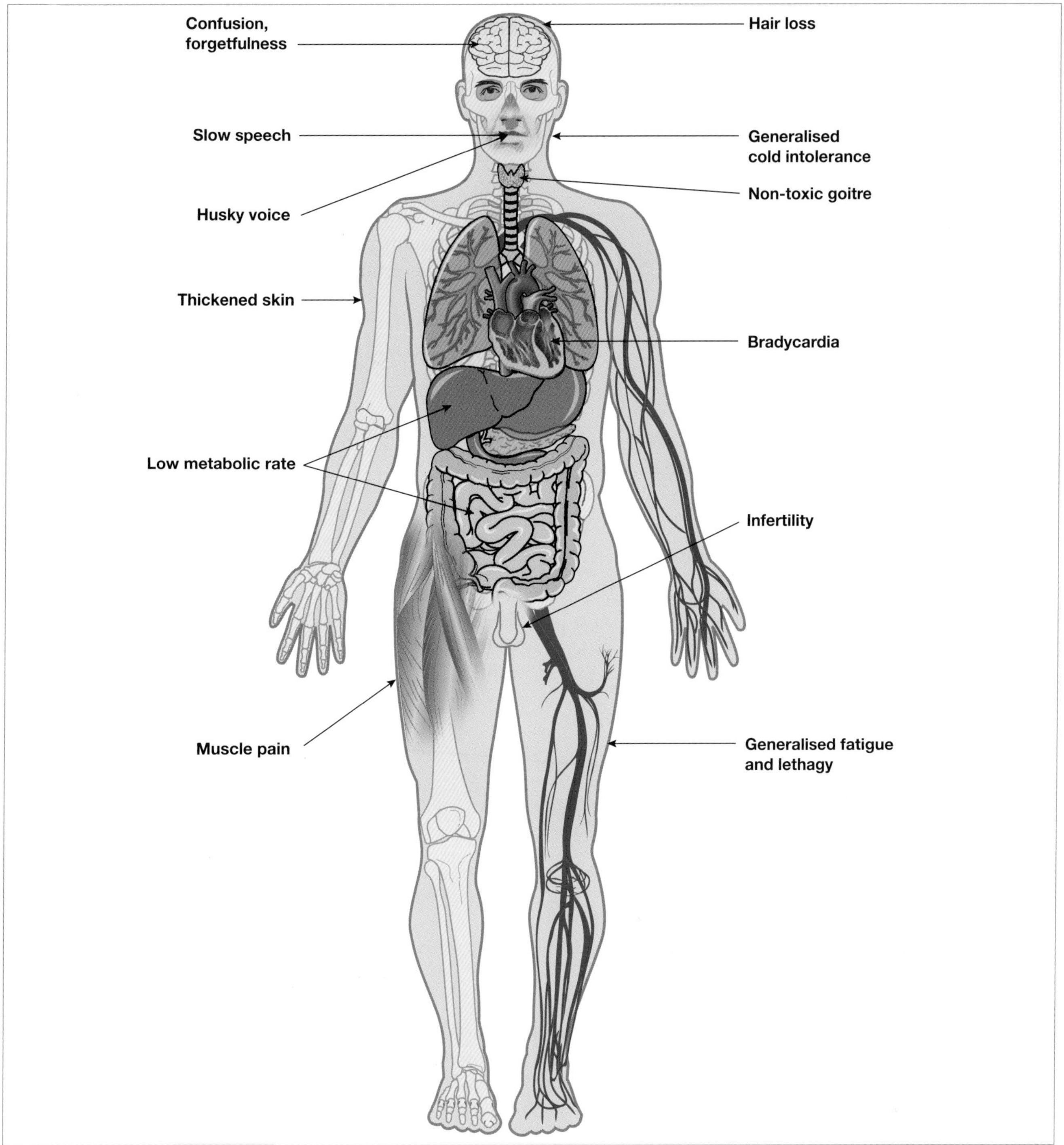

FIGURE 27.4 Clinical manifestations of hypothyroidism

be adjusted in response to thyroid function test results. For many years, natural extract or desiccated thyroid tissue was used for replacement therapy, but the pure synthetic thyroid hormones available today are better standardised and are more stable formulations. The preparations available in Australasia are: thyroxine (levothyroxine, T_4; Drug Monograph 27.1), which is the drug of choice for replacement therapy, and liothyronine (T_3); the latter hormone is more potent and has a shorter half-life so is preferred for emergency use. Liothyronine is not recommended in pregnant women because of the requirement of the fetal brain for T_4. Table 27.1 illustrates the usual adult dosing schedules for thyroid products.

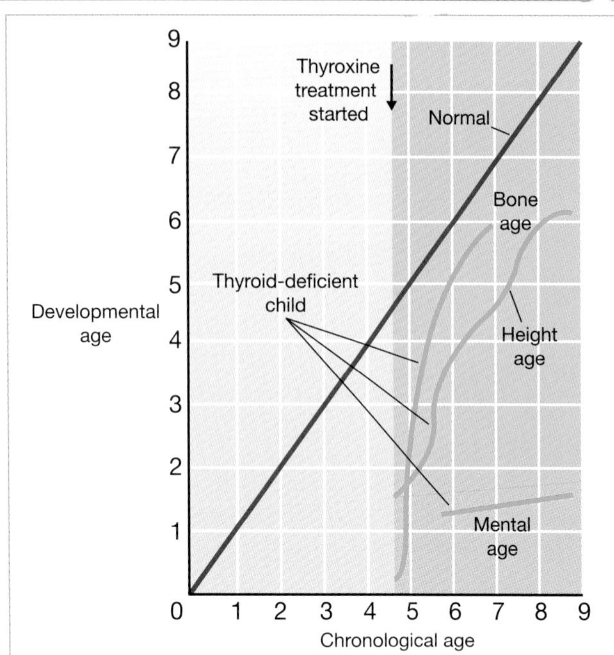

FIGURE 27.5 Effect of thyroid hormone treatment on development of a thyroid-deficient child

Apparent developmental age is shown (dark green) compared with that of normal child (red line). Thyroxine therapy initiated at 4.5 years caused catch-up growth in height and bone age but little improvement in mental age.

Source: Boron & Boulpaep 2012, Figure 49-7; reproduced with permission from Elsevier Saunders.

Clinical response is more important than blood hormone concentrations; determination of TSH is used to assess adequacy of therapy and compliance, to maintain TSH concentration at about 0.4–5 mIU/L. Because of the long half-life and long duration of effect of T_4, plasma TSH concentrations are measured 2, 4 and 10 months after initiation of therapy, and annually thereafter for adults. In children who develop hypothyroidism, the delay in growth and maturity can be reversed by administration of T_4. There is a rapid catch-up growth spurt, and eventually the expected adult height is attained (Fig 27.5).

Hyperthyroidism (thyrotoxicosis)

Pathology

Excessive formation of the thyroid hormones and their release into the circulation result in thyrotoxicosis, which occurs in conditions such as multinodular goitre, toxic hot nodule (adenoma), Graves' disease and subacute thyroiditis, and as an adverse reaction to some drugs (iatrogenic causes), including thyroid hormones, excess iodine and amiodarone. (Amiodarone [see Drug Monograph 10.3] is an antidysrhythmic agent with two atoms of iodine per drug molecule; the high iodine content inhibits the enzyme 5′-deiodinase. It can cause either hypothyroidism, by blocking release of T_3 and T_4; or

Drug Monograph 27.1
Levothyroxine sodium

Synthetic levothyroxine (thyroxine) given exogenously as a drug has all the chemical and pharmacological properties of natural thyroxine.

Indications

Thyroid supplements are indicated for the treatment of hypothyroidism, treatment and prevention of goitre, replacement therapy after thyroid block in hyperthyroidism and treatment of thyroiditis and thyroid carcinoma (high doses for suppressive effects). Thyroid hormones are also used as replacement therapy after thyroidectomy (near-total or total) as treatment for thyroid cancers: T_4 not only replaces missing hormone but also activates the negative-feedback loop and thus suppresses pituitary release of TSH, which would stimulate any remaining thyroid cancer cells.

Pharmacokinetics

Levothyroxine is adequately absorbed from the GIT (48–80%) and is more than 99.9% bound in the circulation to thyroxine-binding globulin, thyroxine-binding prealbumin and albumin. The plasma half-life of T_4 is 6–7 days and T_3 1–2 days in euthyroid people. The duration of biological effect is much longer, so steady state may not be reached for 3–4 weeks; response to altered dosage is slow. It is converted in the liver and kidney to T_3, and conjugated and de-iodinated metabolites are excreted in bile and urine. There is some enterohepatic recycling. Levothyroxine can be dosed once daily and is given on an empty stomach, usually before breakfast.

Drug interactions

See Drug Interactions 27.1. The clearance of many drugs is reduced in hypothyroidism but not of anticoagulants, which may require higher doses. Current drug information sources should be consulted.

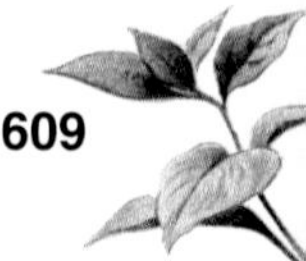

Adverse reactions

- Adverse effects associated with excessive dosages generally correspond to symptoms of hyperthyroidism: tachycardia, elevated temperature, diarrhoea, hand tremors, increased irritability, weight loss and insomnia.
- A rare adverse reaction is an allergic skin rash.
- Suppression of TSH by exogenous levothyroxine may reduce bone density and cause osteoporosis; excessive doses may cause osteoporotic fractures, especially in the elderly.
- Elderly people are usually more sensitive to, and experience more adverse reactions (particularly cardiovascular effects) to, thyroid hormones than other age groups, so it is recommended that thyroid replacement doses be individualised, with lower doses than usual and slower dosage adjustments.
- Adverse effects are dose-related and may occur more rapidly with T_3 than with T_4, mainly because the former has a faster onset of action.
- The general signs of under-dosage are those of hypothyroidism: coldness, dry skin, constipation, lethargy, headaches, drowsiness, tiredness, weight gain and muscle aching. During the early period of treatment, hair loss may occur in children.

Warnings and contraindications

Use with caution in people with diabetes mellitus, adrenocortical or pituitary insufficiency, cardiac disease and malabsorption problems. Avoid use in people with hyperthyroidism, thyrotoxicosis or thyroid hypersensitivity. Requirements increase during pregnancy, and dosage should be adjusted depending on TSH concentration.

Dosage and administration

See Table 27.1. Levothyroxine tablets are available in a range of doses (25, 50, 75, 100, 125 and 200 micrograms), which allows easy adjustment of doses. The stability of levothyroxine tablets is limited, and 'use-by' dates should be heeded. With the exception of Eltroxin, storage at 2–8°C is generally recommended. Not all brands are bioequivalent, so care should be exercised if changing brands.

TABLE 27.1 Thyroid preparations: adult dosage schedules

DRUG	ADULT DOSAGE SCHEDULES
Levothyroxine (thyroxine)	Orally: initially 50–200 micrograms once daily on an empty stomach. Dose changes should be considered only every 6–8 weeks, based on TSH results. Initial dose is lower in elderly people or those with ischaemic heart disease (25–50 micrograms once daily). Fine dosage adjustments can be achieved with alternating doses of 50-, 75-, 100-, 125- or 200-microgram tablets. Dose for children (1–12 years) is 2–6 micrograms/kg once daily, adjusted every 2–4 weeks.
Liothyronine	Orally: 20–60 micrograms daily, in 2–3 divided doses. For myxoedema coma, treatment may be initiated (under specialist supervision) using IV liothyronine (available through the Special Access Scheme). For maintenance therapy of myxoedema, thyroxine is preferred.

DRUG INTERACTIONS 27.1
Thyroid hormone preparations

DRUG	POSSIBLE EFFECTS AND MANAGEMENT
Colestyramine, ciprofloxacin, calcium carbonate, ferrous sulfate, orlistat, proton pump inhibitors, raloxifene, sevelamer, simethicone and sucralfate	These drugs reduce the absorption of levothyroxine from the GIT. A 4-hour interval is recommended between administration of these drugs and levothyroxine.
Imatinib, phenobarbital (phenobarbitone), phenytoin, rifampin (rifampicin), ritonavir and sunitinib	May increase metabolism of levothyroxine; dose may need to be increased.
Warfarin	Thyroid hormones affect metabolism of clotting factors, thereby enhancing the therapeutic effects of warfarin: a decrease in anticoagulant oral dosage may be required. Monitor international normalised ratio.

hyperthyroidism, by causing focal thyroiditis or excess thyroid hormone synthesis. Amiodarone is used by paramedics as an emergency antidysrhythmic agent; however, such use in the acute situation is unlikely to cause adverse thyroid effects.)

Graves' disease, or autoimmune hyperthyroidism, is the most common type of hyperthyroidism in patients under age 40, affecting about 0.4% of the population, women more often than men, and causing 'exophthalmic goitre'. Smoking exacerbates Graves' disease. There are two main types of autoantibodies against thyroid antigens: thyroid-stimulating antibodies, which lead to the signs of hyperthyroidism; and thyroid-growth antibodies, which stimulate growth and hence lead to goitre. The first symptoms noticed may be fullness in the neck, difficulty in doing up the collar button and grittiness in the eyes; other signs and symptoms are as described for hyperthyroidism. The classic sign, exophthalmos (i.e. protruding eyes), is due to fat deposition behind the eyeballs and oedema of the muscles controlling eye movements, leading to excessive fibrosis and eyelid retraction; corneal ulceration can occur. As well as therapy of the thyroid dysfunction to render the person euthyroid, immunosuppressants are required to minimise the autoimmune processes.

Clinical manifestations

Primary hyperthyroidism is characterised by elevated concentrations of T_3 and T_4 despite a decreased level of TSH. In pituitary (secondary) hyperthyroidism, concentrations of TSH, T_3 and T_4 all rise. Hyperthyroidism leads to symptoms the opposite of those seen in myxoedema. The metabolic rate is increased, sometimes as much as 60% or more. Body temperature is frequently above normal, appetite increases and body weight decreases. Other symptoms include restlessness, anxiety, emotional instability, insomnia, muscle tremor and weakness, sweating and exophthalmos. The raised T_4 concentrations can cause cardiomegaly, dysrhythmias, congestive heart failure and hepatic damage. Drug clearance may be increased, so doses of other drugs might need to be increased. In thyroid storm, a sudden onset of exaggerated hyperthyroid symptoms occurs, especially those affecting the nervous and cardiovascular systems, because of elevated T_4 concentrations. Thyroid storm is a life-threatening condition, potentially leading to heart failure and coma.

Beta-adrenoceptor antagonists (e.g. propranolol) are frequently used as adjunctive therapy to provide relief of hyperthyroid symptoms due to the peripheral effects of excess T_4, including tachycardia, tremor and sweating. Both cardioselective and non-selective β-blockers are effective; they should be used with caution in cardiovascular disease and are contraindicated in asthma. (These drugs are covered in more detail in Ch 9.)

Treatment

The aims of treatment are to decrease thyroid hormone overproduction and block peripheral effects of excess T_4. Before the advent of antithyroid drugs, treatment was surgical, by subtotal resection of the hyperactive gland. Antithyroid drugs lower the basal metabolic rate by interfering with the formation, release or action of thyroid hormones; some occur naturally and are known as goitrogens – for example, chemicals found in cabbages, turnips and celery seeds. Those used clinically are the thioureylene derivatives, iodine (iodide ion) and radioactive iodine. Corticosteroids and lithium also impair thyroid hormone release, and may be used in severe uncontrolled cases of hyperthyroidism, including that induced by amiodarone.

Thioureylenes

The oral thioureylene drugs carbimazole (Drug Monograph 27.2) and propylthiouracil inhibit thyroid hormone synthesis by competitively inhibiting the iodination of tyrosine residues in thyroglobulin. Propylthiouracil (but not carbimazole) also inhibits the conversion of T_4 to T_3 in peripheral tissues, which may make it more effective for treatment of thyroid crisis or storm. These drugs all contain a sulfur–carbon–nitrogen linkage; they are closely related chemically to the sulfonamide antibacterials and the sulfonylurea hypoglycaemic agents. (Both of these drug groups may also interfere with thyroid function.)

High doses of thioureylenes are given initially to control severe hyperthyroidism, reducing the dose gradually after 3–4 weeks. A course of 12–18 months may be necessary for sustained remission of Graves' disease.

Iodine/iodide

Iodine

Iodine, which is converted in the body to iodide (I^-), is the oldest antithyroid drug available. Although a small amount of iodine is necessary for normal thyroid function and synthesis of thyroid hormones, large amounts of iodine depress TRH and TSH release (Fig 27.3), thus causing inhibition of thyroid hormone synthesis and release. High doses of iodides such as in Lugol's solution are generally used for 7–10 days before thyroid surgery to decrease the gland's size and vascularity, resulting in diminished blood loss and a less complicated surgical procedure (Clinical Focus Box 27.2).

Radioactive Iodine

Radioactive iodine (radioiodine, ^{131}I) is the preferred antithyroid drug for people who are poor surgical risks, such as debilitated or elderly people and those with advanced cardiac disease. It is also used for people who have not responded adequately to drug therapy or who have had recurrent hyperthyroidism after surgery. The ^{131}I radioactive isotope of iodine is chemically identical to iodine, so it has the same pharmacokinetic parameters. After oral administration, it is taken up actively by thyroid cells and accumulates in thyroid tissue, where the ionising beta-radiation emitted selectively damages thyroid cells (Drug Monograph 27.3). It is an interesting example of radiopharmaceuticals, where dosage is in units of radioactivity rather than milligrams of active drug.

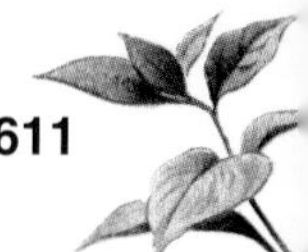

Drug Monograph 27.2
Carbimazole

Actions
Carbimazole acts as an antithyroid drug by inhibiting synthesis of the thyroid hormones (see text).

Indications
The thioureylenes are indicated for the treatment of hyperthyroidism, either as a short course in thyroid storm or before surgery or radiotherapy, or as a long course as adjunct therapy for the treatment of thyrotoxicosis.

Pharmacokinetics
Thioureylenes are readily absorbed from the GIT. Carbimazole is a prodrug; it is rapidly converted in the body to the active metabolite methimazole. The half-life of each drug is relatively short (2–6 hours); however, maximal effects may take some weeks to occur, as the body may already have large stores of preformed thyroid hormones. Thus, the peak effect occurs in about 7 weeks with carbimazole and 17 weeks with propylthiouracil. Metabolised in the liver and excreted by the kidneys, thioureylenes cross the placenta and can cause fetal hypothyroidism and goitre. As they are excreted in breast milk, the lowest effective doses with monitoring should be used during breastfeeding.

Drug interactions
See Drug Interactions 27.2. Current drug information sources should be consulted.

Adverse reactions
These include rash, pruritus, dizziness, loss of taste, nausea, vomiting, leucopenia, paraesthesias and stomach pain. Fever, mouth ulcers and sore throat may be early indications of serious agranulocytosis, which necessitates cessation of the drug and appropriate antibiotic treatment. Overall, signs of thyrotoxicosis indicate inadequate dosing, and signs of hypothyroidism indicate possible over-dosage.

Warnings and contraindications
Use with caution in individuals with a low leucocyte count. The lowest effective dose should be used during pregnancy, with regular monitoring. Avoid use in people with a history of carbimazole or propylthiouracil hypersensitivity or liver impairment. Regular blood tests and liver and thyroid function tests are recommended.

Dosage and administration
Dosage depends on usage: after an initial 3–4 weeks of high-dose antithyroid therapy, the dosage is either regularly adjusted to maintain euthyroid status, or high dosage is maintained and thyroxine added to restore thyroid function to normal ('block-and-replace' regimen).

The carbimazole oral adult dosage is initially 10–45 mg daily (in severe cases, up to 60 mg daily) in divided doses, reducing to a usual maintenance dose of 5–15 mg daily (though this can vary from 2.5 to 40 mg daily). In the 'block-and-replace' regimen, the initial dose is continued with the addition of levothyroxine 100–150 micrograms if T_4 is in the normal range. Treatment is continued with monitoring for about 2 years, as remissions may occur. Relapse, however, is frequent.

DRUG INTERACTIONS 27.2
Thioureylene antithyroid drugs

DRUG	POSSIBLE EFFECTS AND MANAGEMENT
Anticoagulants (warfarin)	Treatment with carbimazole or propylthiouracil may alter metabolism of clotting factors and decrease the anticoagulant effect of warfarin. Monitor closely and adjust warfarin dose based on international normalised ratio results.
Sodium iodide ^{131}I	Thyroid uptake of ^{131}I may be decreased by antithyroid agents. Antithyroid drug should be stopped at least 4 days before and for 3 days after ^{131}I therapy.
Theophylline	May be metabolised faster by hyperthyroid people; theophylline concentration and effects should be monitored when either carbimazole or propylthiouracil are commenced, and the dose of theophylline adjusted if necessary.

CLINICAL FOCUS BOX 27.2
Lugol's solution

Lugol's solution, or Iodine Solution Aqueous BP, was first documented in 1829. It is a mixture of 5% iodine and 10% potassium iodide in water; the total iodine content is 130 mg/mL. After oral administration, the iodine is converted to iodide in the GIT before systemic absorption. Iodine solution is indicated to protect the thyroid gland from radiation before and after the administration of radioactive isotopes of iodine or in radiation emergencies, and in people with hyperthyroidism, to suppress thyroid function and vascularity prior to thyroidectomy. The adult dose of Lugol's solution is 0.3–0.9 mL/day (in divided doses, administered in a full glass of water, fruit juice or milk) for 7 days immediately prior to thyroid surgery.

It is used with caution in patients with tuberculosis, iodine or potassium iodide hypersensitivity, bronchitis, hyperkalaemia or kidney impairment, and in pregnancy. Adverse reactions include diarrhoea, nausea, vomiting, stomach pain, rash, swelling of the salivary gland and a metallic taste in the mouth.

The primary disadvantage of using surgery or radioiodine therapy, in addition to the risks involved with surgery and radiation, is the induction of hypothyroidism. However, it is now recognised that, in the long term, definitive therapy that produces hypothyroidism, followed by replacement with adequate thyroxine ('block–replace'), is an easier regimen for maintaining a euthyroid state than frequent changes of antithyroid drug doses.

Other drugs causing thyroid dysfunction

The following drugs have been implicated in causing thyroid dysfunction (whether hypothyroidism or hyperthyroidism):

- Amiodarone contains two iodine atoms that are released during metabolism of amiodarone. Approximately 3 mg of inorganic iodine is released per 100 mg of amiodarone ingested. Amiodarone impairs de-iodination of T_4 and, hence, conversion of T_4 to T_3.
- Glucocorticoids suppress TSH secretion at the level of the hypothalamus.

Drug Monograph 27.3
Radioactive iodine

Indications
^{131}I is indicated for treating hyperthyroidism and thyroid carcinoma, and is also used in diagnostic thyroid function tests.

Pharmacokinetics
Administered orally (usually as sodium iodide in a capsule), it has an onset of effect within 2–4 weeks; the peak therapeutic effect occurs between 2 and 4 months. It is mainly excreted by the kidneys, 50% within 24 hours. It has a radionuclide half-life of about 8 days; principal types of radiation are beta and gamma rays.

Adverse reactions
These include sore throat, neck swelling or pain, temporary loss of taste, nausea, vomiting, gastritis and painful salivary glands. After treatment for hyperthyroidism, the person may experience increased or unusual irritability or tiredness. After treatment for thyroid carcinoma, the person may experience fever, sore throat, chills (due to leucopenia) and increased bleeding episodes (thrombocytopenia). There is a small suspected increased risk of subsequent thyroid cancer. If hypothyroidism occurs after treatment, symptoms should be monitored, and thyroid function tests carried out for replacement therapy.

Warnings and contraindications
Use with caution in individuals with diarrhoea, vomiting, kidney function impairment or severe thyrotoxic cardiac disease, especially the elderly. Avoid use in people with hypersensitivity to radiopharmaceutical preparations, and in pregnancy and breastfeeding. Precautions for radioactivity safety must be observed; after high doses all excretions (e.g. faeces, urine) are collected for safe disposal.

Dosage
Dosage depends on the indications for which it is being administered, and the size and activity of the gland; dosage is in millicuries (mCi) or in the SI units megabecquerels (MBq, where 1 Bq = 2.7×10^{-11} Ci). For example, 5–15 mCi may be prescribed for hyperthyroidism, whereas 50–100 mCi is required for thyroid carcinoma.

- Other drugs that suppress TSH include dopamine and the dopamine agonist bromocriptine and the antiepileptic drug carbamazepine (Chung & Van Hul 2012).

KEY POINTS

Pharmacotherapy of thyroid disorders

- Simple or non-toxic goitre is due to iodine deficiency, which leads to decreased synthesis of thyroid hormones. Compensatory increased hypothalamic TRH and pituitary TSH, and enlargement of the thyroid gland, is treated by increasing iodine intake - for example, iodised salt.
- Hypothyroidism characterised by decreased basal metabolic rate is treated by administration of oral levothyroxine, which mimics the actions of T_4, and in emergency situations by IV liothyronine, which has the same actions as endogenous T_3.
- Hyperthyroidism (thyrotoxicosis) leads to increased basal metabolic rate.
- Pharmacotherapy of hyperthyroidism involves use of oral drugs, including:
  - carbimazole and propylthiouracil, which reduce thyroid hormone synthesis by inhibiting iodination of thyroglobulin
  - ^{131}I, which is sequestered by thyroid cells that are selectively damaged by the ionising beta-radiation emitted.
- Regular testing of thyroid function is required to monitor disease progression and therapy, and to optimise dosage regimens.

Pharmacotherapy of parathyroid disorders

The small parathyroid glands are located on the posterior surface of each lobe of the thyroid gland (Fig 27.1). There are usually two pairs, but the number can range from two to six, and ectopic parathyroid tissue can occur elsewhere in the body. The primary function of the parathyroid glands, which are composed largely of chief cells, is to secrete parathyroid hormone (PTH), which maintains adequate concentration of calcium in the blood and extracellular fluid. The parathyroid glands are not subject to higher control from the pituitary gland or hypothalamus (Fig 26.4) but respond directly to, and help control, blood calcium concentration (analogous to the pancreas responding to and controlling blood glucose). Removal of the parathyroid glands during thyroid surgery, before the significance of the parathyroid glands was recognised, resulted in severe hypocalcaemia, leading to tetany and death.

Parathyroid hormone

PTH is a polypeptide of 84 amino acids. Active PTH has a half-life of 2–4 minutes; smaller peptide fragments produced in the liver and kidneys have longer half-lives. PTH has multiple effects, culminating in raised plasma calcium concentration (Fig 27.6). It also reduces phosphate concentration, permitting more calcium mobilisation. The main effects are as follows:

- In the kidneys, PTH increases reabsorption of calcium in distal convoluted tubules; reabsorption of phosphate and bicarbonate is inhibited.
- In the GIT, calcium absorption is increased – an indirect effect via increased renal activation of vitamin D.
- In bone, PTH stimulates bone resorption by osteoclasts, thus mobilising calcium from bone.

Mechanism of action

The mechanism of PTH action in bone or kidney is incompletely understood; in osteoblasts, PTH activates Wnt signalling (Wnt proteins are signalling molecules that regulate cell-to-cell interactions) and increases osteoblast differentiation, numbers and survival. By integrated effects in various tissues, PTH increases inflow of calcium into extracellular fluid and protects against hypocalcaemia. The 'bottom line' in calcium balance is the concentration of calcium in blood, as this provides the source for all calcium functions; in this context, bone acts as a depot of calcium to be mobilised.

Calcium-sensing receptors

Parathyroid cells have in their membranes specialised calcium sensors (G-protein-coupled receptors) that are master regulators of PTH secretion and calcium concentrations. When calcium concentrations in extracellular fluid are low, the parathyroids are stimulated to synthesise and secrete PTH, which acts to conserve calcium. When plasma calcium concentrations are high, binding of calcium to the receptors activates G-proteins, leading to activation of phospholipase C enzymes and inhibition of further PTH secretion. Mutations in the calcium-sensing receptor gene lead to familial disorders of calcium balance: inactivating mutations cause hypercalcaemia, while activating mutations cause hypocalcaemia.

Calcium-sensing receptors are present in other tissues, where their functions are less clear; other cations can also bind. Complex feedback loops involving calcium,

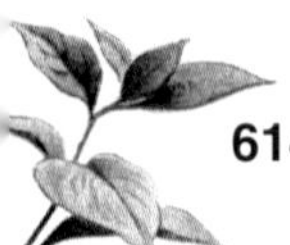

↓Plasma Ca
Parathyroids
Kidneys
Thyroid
↑PTH release
↑Vitamin D activation
↓Calcitonin release
Intestine
Kidney
Bone
Remodelling
Bone
↑Ca absorption
↑Ca reabsorption
↓Ca excretion
↑Bone resorption
↑Bone deposition
Ca mobilisation
↓PTH
Activation Ca-sensing receptors on parathyroid cells
↑Plasma Ca
↑Calcitonin

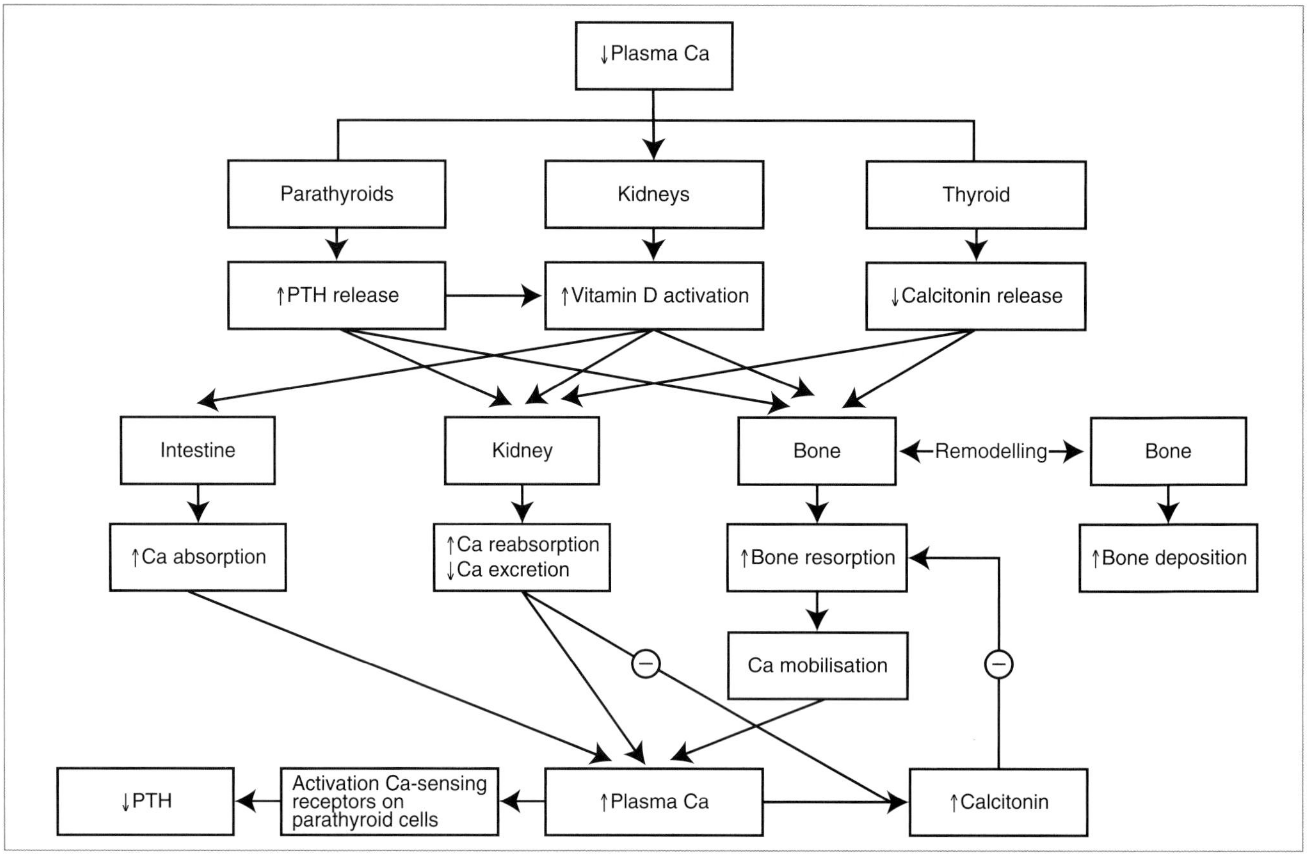

FIGURE 27.6 The main factors regulating plasma calcium concentration

Low plasma calcium concentration triggers release of PTH and vitamin D and inhibits release of calcitonin, leading to conservation of calcium from the intestine, kidneys and bone, hence raising plasma calcium. Increased plasma calcium concentration leads to activation of calcium-sensing receptors and decreased PTH secretion, and increased secretion of calcitonin from the thyroid gland, which decreases bone resorption and inhibits calcium reabsorption by the kidney.

Ca = calcium; PTH = parathyroid hormone; ⊖ = inhibition

phosphorus, PTH and vitamin D all participate in controlling calcium concentrations.

Calcitonin

Calcitonin, the third main hormone product of the thyroid gland, was discovered in 1961. It is a polypeptide secreted by thyroid C cells when there is a high blood calcium concentration, especially when this is due to conditions of increased bone resorption. Calcitonin has several actions including:

- inhibiting osteoclastic bone resorption, decreasing rate of bone turnover
- inhibiting calcium reabsorption in the kidney
- promoting bone and collagen formation
- not affecting GIT absorption of calcium (but has other GIT effects, including inhibiting secretion of gastric acid and pancreatic enzymes)
- having analgesic activity and relieves bone pain, possibly mediated by endorphins
- leading to rapid lowering of plasma calcium concentrations; long-term effects may decrease bone formation.

Calcitonin can thus be considered as a natural antagonist of the actions of PTH and vitamin D (Fig 27.6).

Mechanism of action

Calcitonin (like other peptide hormones of the calcitonin family) acts via specific G-protein-coupled receptors on cell membranes of target tissues; it forms dimers with receptor activity modifying proteins, thus mediating many effects that reduce plasma calcium concentration.

Hypoparathyroidism/hypocalcaemia

Pathology and clinical manifestations

Hypoparathyroidism may be surgical (after surgery on the throat), autoimmune, familial or idiopathic. Manifestations of **hypocalcaemia** (decreased serum calcium concentration) include hyperexcitability of nerves, which manifest as paraesthesias ('pins and needles'), muscle spasms (including dysrhythmias, dysphonia and dysphagia) and tetany. Serum phosphate concentration is raised due to loss of the phosphaturic effect of PTH.

Treatment

In acute severe hypocalcaemia, symptoms of tetany are relieved by administration of IV calcium gluconate. The individual is initially hospitalised because frequent assessment of blood calcium and phosphate concentrations are essential. PTH itself has too short a half-life to be useful clinically. Moderate hypocalcaemia can be controlled with the vitamin D analogue calcitriol (Drug Monograph 27.4) plus a calcium supplement.

Hyperparathyroidism/hypercalcaemia

Pathology and clinical manifestations

Primary **hyperparathyroidism** is the third most common endocrine disorder, with highest incidence in postmenopausal women; hyperactivity of parathyroid glands causes excessive PTH secretion. It is generally caused by a parathyroid adenoma or spontaneous hyperplasia. PTH elevations produce increased resorption of calcium from the skeletal system and increased absorption of calcium by the kidneys and the gastrointestinal system. Elevated plasma concentration of calcium with high urine phosphate concentration can lead to renal stones, bone pain with skeletal lesions and pathological fractures. Secondary hyperparathyroidism occurs commonly in renal osteodystrophy associated with chronic renal insufficiency, and often requires parathyroidectomy. Other causes of **hypercalcaemia** include Paget's disease of bone (see later section); excess vitamin D, causing excess calcium to be retained; and occurrence in various malignancies of osteolytic bone metastases, with increased bone turnover. Excess calcium may be consumed in other medications, including antacids.

Clinical manifestations are weakness, dysrhythmias, nausea, vomiting, constipation and ectopic calcification – for example, as kidney stones.

Drug Monograph 27.4
Calcitriol

There are several forms of vitamin D available. Vitamins D2 and D3 require activation in the liver and kidney, and have a slow onset (4–8 weeks) and long duration of action (8–16 weeks). They are useful for preventing vitamin D deficiencies in people with adequate kidney function. Calcitriol (1,25-dihydroxycolecalciferol) is the active metabolite of calcifediol.

Indications

Calcitriol is indicated for treatment of hypocalcaemia in hypoparathyroidism, hypophosphataemic rickets, vitamin D deficiencies associated with renal osteodystrophy, chronic renal dialysis (which may remove calcium or vitamin D) and post-menopausal and corticosteroid-induced osteoporosis.

Pharmacokinetics

Calcitriol is well absorbed from the intestine, requiring bile salts for absorption. It enters the enterohepatic circulation and metabolites (some active) are excreted in faeces and urine; some are stored in fat. It has a rapid onset of action (1–3 days) and short duration (< 1 week). Elimination half-life is about 3–6 hours, but effects of a single dose last for several days. It is transported across the placenta and into breast milk; hence, high doses are contraindicated during pregnancy and lactation. Seek advice from one of the pregnancy drug information centres.

Adverse drug reactions and interactions

The main adverse effects are as follows:

- Hypercalcaemia (see above) – that is, gastrointestinal disturbances, polyuria and ectopic calcification.
- In the presence of hypercalcaemia, significant interactions occur with digoxin (dysrhythmias).
- Colestyramine impairs absorption, and phenytoin and phenobarbital (phenobarbitone) increase metabolism of vitamin D; hence, the dose may need to be increased.
- Calcium supplements or thiazide diuretics increase plasma calcium concentration, increasing the risk of hypercalcaemia.

Dosage and administration

Calcitriol is usually administered orally (an injectable formulation is available through the Special Access Scheme). It is highly potent, average dosage being 0.25 micrograms daily. Concurrent multivitamin preparations and calcium supplements should be avoided due to the risk of hypercalcaemia.

People with renal osteodystrophy, hypoparathyroidism or hypophosphataemia may require higher doses due to inadequate renal activation of vitamin D: for adults, initially 0.25 micrograms once daily, increasing every 2–4 weeks by 0.25 micrograms per day as needed up to 0.5–1 micrograms daily. For people with hypocalcaemia due to renal dialysis, an IV bolus dose of 0.5 micrograms is given three times each week at the end of dialysis, increased as needed by 0.25–0.5 micrograms every 2–4 weeks.

Treatment

Surgery is usually the first-line treatment to remove tumours. High serum concentration of calcium may require immediate treatment with initial rehydration. Other drugs used to treat hypercalcaemia include IV bisphosphonates (pamidronate or zoledronic acid) and, in life-threatening situations, parenteral calcitonin salmon (salcatonin, Drug Monograph 27.5). In situations of primary hyperparathyroidism and parathyroid cancer where surgical intervention is not possible or is unsuccessful, the calcimimetic drug cinacalcet (Drug Monograph 27.6) is used under specialist supervision.

KEY POINTS

Pharmacotherapy of parathyroid disorders

- The parathyroid glands synthesise and secrete PTH, a peptide hormone that maintains the calcium concentration in extracellular fluid.
- Calcium-sensing receptors on parathyroid cells respond to the extracellular calcium concentration to increase or decrease secretion of PTH.
- In hypoparathyroidism, severe hypocalcaemia and tetany can occur; moderate hypocalcaemia is treated with the vitamin D analogue calcitriol and a calcium supplement.
- In hyperparathyroidism, the primary approach is usually surgery; hypercalcaemia also responds to rehydration, calcitonin and bisphosphonate drugs.
- The calcimimetic drug cinacalcet is used for primary hyperparathyroidism and parathyroid cancer when surgery either is not possible or is unsuccessful.

Pharmacotherapy of bone disorders

Bone mineral homeostasis

Bone remodelling

Bone has three main functions:

- It provides rigid support for the body and cavities.
- It acts as levers and sites of attachment for muscles in locomotion.

Drug Monograph 27.5

Calcitonin salmon (salcatonin)

Synthetic calcitonin salmon has the same physiological actions as human calcitonin. Synthetic human calcitonin has now also been produced.

Indications

Calcitonin salmon is indicated for the treatment of hypercalcaemia (and rarely now for Paget's disease of bone).

Pharmacokinetics

Calcitonin salmon (a peptide) cannot be administered orally; it is usually given SC, but also IM and IV. Elimination half-life is 60–90 minutes, but the biological half-life is considerably longer. Peak effect in clinical hypercalcaemia occurs in 2 hours, and duration of action is 6–8 hours. Tachyphylaxis develops over several days. Excretion of metabolites is via the kidneys.

Onset of the therapeutic effect in Paget's disease may take from 6 to 24 months of regular treatment, although some improvement (measured by a decrease in serum alkaline phosphatase concentration) may occur within the first few months.

Adverse reactions and drug interactions

No significant drug interactions have been reported. Adverse effects may include:

- flushing or a tingling sensation of the face and hands
- increased urinary frequency
- nausea, vomiting and pain or swelling at the injection site
- allergic reactions, antibody development and visual disturbances.

Contraindications

Avoid use in people with a history of protein allergy or calcitonin hypersensitivity. Few data are available on use in children, pregnancy or lactation.

Dosage and administration

The usual calcitonin salmon adult dosage for Paget's disease is SC/IM 50–100 units daily for 3–6 months; for hypercalcaemia 5–10 units/kg daily by slow IV infusion or injection (2–4 doses). To reduce occurrence of nausea or flushing, administer after meals or at bedtime; if necessary, an antiemetic may be administered.

Drug Monograph 27.6
Cinacalcet

Calcimimetics are a newer class of drugs that increase affinity of calcium-sensing receptors for calcium, hence inhibiting parathyroid cell proliferation, PTH synthesis and secretion. Calcimimetics reduce calcium, PTH and phosphate concentrations, and are useful in treating primary and secondary hyperparathyroidism. Cinacalcet is the first such agent in clinical use; it can be considered an anti-PTH agent.

Indications

Cinacalcet is indicated in some cases of primary hyperparathyroidism in patients not amenable to or refractory after surgery, of parathyroid carcinoma, and in patients with chronic kidney disease on dialysis with secondary hyperparathyroidism.

Pharmacokinetics

There is low bioavailability (25%) from tablets; this is increased by taking with or after food. Maximum plasma concentrations are reached after 2–6 hours, and steady state after about 7 days. Cinacalcet is 97% plasma-protein bound and has extensive distribution in tissues, with a volume of distribution (> 1000 L). The terminal elimination half-life is 30–40 hours; once-daily dosing is effective. The drug is oxidatively metabolised by CYP1A2, CYP2D6 and CYP3A4, and the metabolites eliminated via conjugation and excretion by the kidneys.

Adverse drug reactions

Common adverse effects include:

- hypocalcaemia, weakness and paraesthesias
- nausea, vomiting, anorexia, dizziness
- reduced testosterone concentrations
- hypersensitivity and rash.

Drug interactions

There are potential interactions with CYP2D6 substrates (e.g. metoprolol, flecainide and most tricyclic antidepressants) and strong CYP3A4 inhibitors (e.g. erythromycin, -conazole antifungals) or inducers of CYP enzymes (phenytoin, rifampin (rifampicin), St John's wort).

Warnings and contraindications

Precautions are advised in:

- hypocalcaemia (contraindicated)
- cardiac and hepatic impairment
- pregnancy, lactation and children.

Calcium and PTH concentrations should be monitored.

Dosage and administration

Dosage needs to be titrated according to response; typical starting doses are 30 mg twice daily in primary hyperparathyroidism or parathyroid carcinoma, and 30 mg once daily in dialysis patients with secondary hyperparathyroidism. Doses can be increased gradually to maximum 180 mg daily for renal disease and 90 mg three–four times daily for parathyroid cancer.

- It provides a reservoir of ions, especially calcium, phosphate, magnesium and sodium.

Bone is constantly renewing itself by remodelling, where old bone is resorbed by osteoclast cells and new bone is deposited by osteoblasts (Fig 27.7). Until the age of about 20–25, bone mass increases and stabilises; thereafter, during adulthood, bone is lost slowly until after menopause in women, when the rate of bone loss due to osteoclast activity increases. Elderly people are likely to suffer from osteoporosis, leaving them at higher risk of fractures.

Calcium balance

Bone remodelling is integrated by many endocrine and other factors, including vitamin D, PTH, calcitonin and plasma calcium concentration (Fig 27.6). Ninety-nine per cent of body calcium is in bone and the daily turnover of calcium in and out of adult bone is estimated to be at least 500 mg – that is, about half the average daily dietary requirements for calcium. Increased bone resorption (stimulated by PTH and vitamin D) leads to mobilisation of calcium from bone into extracellular fluid where it plays important roles in cellular physiology and metabolic regulation including:

- stabilising excitable cell membranes
- release of neurotransmitters and formation of secretions
- second-messenger functions inside cells
- muscle contractility
- exocytosis of hormones and other regulators
- blood coagulation and platelet aggregation.

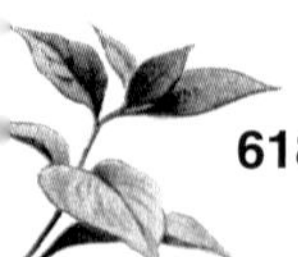

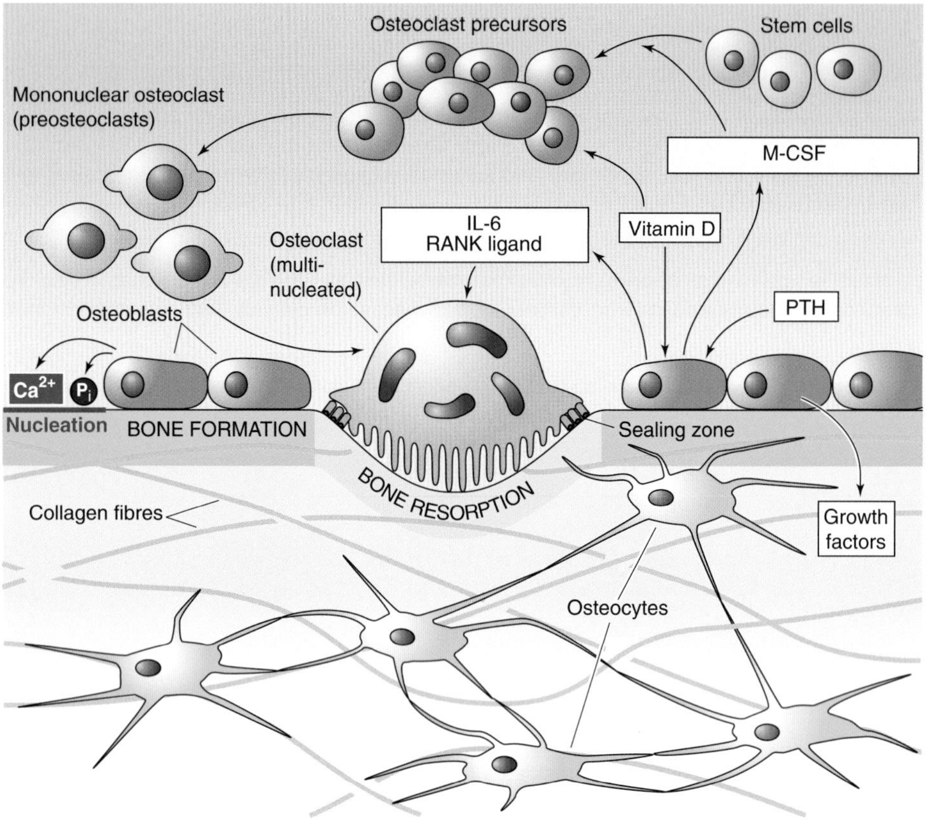

FIGURE 27.7 Bone formation and resorption

PTH and vitamin D stimulate osteoblastic cells to secrete factors such as macrophage colony-stimulating factor (M-CSF). This and other agents induce stem cells to differentiate into osteoclast precursors, mononuclear osteoclasts and, finally, mature multinucleated osteoclasts. Osteoblasts also secrete Ca^{2+} and P_i, which nucleate on the surface of bone. PTH indirectly stimulates bone resorption by osteoclasts. Osteoclasts do not have PTH receptors. Instead, PTH binds to receptors on osteoblasts and stimulates the release of factors, such as IL-6 and RANK ligand, and the expression of membrane-bound RANK ligand. These factors promote bone resorption by osteoclasts.

Source: Boron & Boulpaep 2012, Figure 52-4; reproduced with permission from Elsevier Saunders.

Concentrations of extracellular and intracellular calcium are tightly controlled (the concentration of calcium inside cells is only 1/10,000 of that outside) despite varying amounts absorbed from the diet and excretion via kidneys and faeces.

Clinical Use of Calcium

- Physiological supplementation in acute hypocalcaemia and hypocalcaemic tetany
- Treatment of osteoporosis, osteomalacia and rickets
- Hyperphosphataemia in situations of renal failure (calcium carbonate)
- Severe hyperkalaemia unrelated to digoxin toxicity (calcium gluconate)
- Toxicity due to magnesium (calcium gluconate)
- Symptomatic relief of dyspepsia and oesophageal or peptic ulcer disease (as antacids).

The recommended daily dietary intake of calcium for adults (including pregnant and breastfeeding women) is 1000 mg/day; for postmenopausal women and men over 70 years old, requirements are higher, at 1200 mg/day. The available calcium in a product depends on total calcium ion (elemental) present; as some calcium salts contain only a small proportion of calcium (e.g. calcium gluconate: 9% calcium), it is important to check the dose on product labels as *mg calcium* rather than mg calcium salt (Table 27.2). There is some evidence that rates of cardiovascular disease are higher in women receiving calcium supplementation, so cardiovascular health should be considered before recommending supplements.

Phosphate balance

Bone resorption also mobilises phosphate from calcium phosphate present in bone hydroxyapatite. Phosphate is involved in many biochemical pathways: energy balance and phosphorylation of enzymes; component of nucleic acids, phospholipids and proteins; buffering systems in body fluids; and in many cell-signalling reactions. Specific

TABLE 27.2 Calcium supplements

CALCIUM SALT IN TABLET	CALCIUM (mg/g SALT)	CALCIUM (meq/g SALT)	% CALCIUM	CALCIUM (OR SALT) IN TABLET (mg)	APPROXIMATE NO. TABLETS NEEDED TO PROVIDE 1200 mg CALCIUM
Calcium carbonate	400	20	40	80 (200)	15
				40 (100)	30
				500 (1250)	2
				600 (1500)	2
Calcium citrate	211	10.5	21.1	164 (780)	7
				250 (1190)	5
Calcium gluconate	90	4.5	9	45 (500)	26
				1.8 (20)	666
Calcium lactate	130	6.5	13	42 (325)	29
Calcium phosphate				115 (500)	10
– dibasic ($CaHPO_4$)	230	11.5	23	140 (600)	9
– tribasic ($Ca_3(PO_4)_2$)	380	19	38	16 (40)	> 75
				220 (570)	6
				1000 (2580)	1.2

The approximate calcium (Ca) contents of typical Ca supplements are listed as milligrams Ca per gram of the Ca salt, milliequivalents Ca per gram salt or percentage of Ca in the salt. The average number of tablets providing 1.3 g calcium (RDI for postmenopausal women) is also shown.

mechanisms regulating phosphate concentrations are not well identified: vitamin D and PTH tend to increase calcium reabsorption from kidney tubules while increasing phosphate excretion, thus conserving calcium but removing phosphate. Fibroblast growth factor 23 (FGF23), a protein hormone involved in maintenance of the skeleton, also has phosphaturic activity. Mutations in the FGF23 gene are responsible for disorders of phosphate metabolism such as hypophosphataemic rickets and tumour-associated osteomalacia.

Phosphate is present in many foods, milk and dairy products, so phosphate supplements are rarely needed. Hypophosphataemia can occur in severe kidney disorders, fluid and electrolyte abnormalities, after excess use of antacids or phosphate-binding resins, in re-feeding syndrome, alcohol withdrawal, trauma, major sepsis and X-linked hypophosphataemic rickets.

Bone morphogenetic proteins

Bone morphogenetic proteins are cytokines that induce formation of bone and cartilage and are important during embryonic skeletal development and bone repair after fracture. It has long been known that bone has great capacity for regeneration and repair; at least 20 bone morphogenetic proteins have been discovered, several belonging to the transforming growth factor beta superfamily of proteins. They are present in bone matrix and act via specific cell surface receptors in several types of tissue, with signal transduction via serine/threonine kinase receptors and subsequent actions in the cell nucleus involving gene transcription and protein synthesis.

Bone morphogenetic proteins are used clinically in spinal fusion and fracture fixation operations, in cases of delayed healing and non-union, in craniofacial and periodontal applications and in chronic kidney disease.

Other bone-regulating factors

Receptor activator of nuclear factor-kappa B (RANK), its ligand (RANKL) and osteoprotegerin are all members of the tumour necrosis factor receptor superfamily, with roles in bone remodelling and mineral balance. Their role in conditions such as osteoporosis, bone loss and rheumatoid arthritis are still being elucidated. RANKL is considered the principal mediator of osteoclastic bone resorption.

Many other bone-regulating growth factors and peptides are still being identified and studied, including Wnt proteins (which play important roles in osteoclastogenesis), PTH-related protein (a paracrine regulator of bone formation), leptin (secreted by adipocytes, with negative effects on osteoblasts), osteocalcin (a bone-derived hormone with positive effects on bone mineral density that also regulates energy metabolism via effects on insulin and adiponectin), cathepsin K (a lysosomal protease expressed by osteoclasts) and vitamin K (via carboxylation of osteocalcin). Drugs affecting these mediators will no doubt in the future prove interesting and useful in various bone diseases.

Bone pathologies

Paget's disease of bone (osteitis deformans)

Pathology and clinical manifestations

Paget's disease is more common in those aged over 40 years, and clusters occur in some families. It is a disorder of bone remodelling, with focal areas of greatly increased bone turnover and disorganised remodelling, leading to

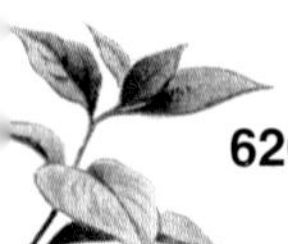

soft, poorly mineralised bone, hypercalcaemia, bone pain, limb deformities, fractures, deafness, osteoarthritis and nerve compression problems. The aetiology is unknown; however, mutations in four genes involved have been identified, and possible triggers include a viral infection and deficiency of dietary calcium (Willems et al. 2017). It is estimated to affect 3–4% of middle-aged to elderly Australians, but only a small proportion of those affected may require treatment.

Treatment

Treatment is with bisphosphonates (see later section); calcitonin is rarely used. Analgesics and non-steroidal anti-inflammatory drugs (Ch 34) may be used to control pain due to secondary arthritis. Serum and urine markers of bone turnover are monitored; surgery may be necessary to free entrapped nerves or in cases of spinal cord compression.

Rickets and osteomalacia

Pathology and clinical manifestations

In various pathological conditions (e.g. obesity, malabsorption, liver disease, kidney failure) and in countries where people are not exposed to sufficient sunlight (due to long winters, high latitudes or use of highly protective clothing or sunscreens), sufficient active vitamin D cannot be produced, and hypocalcaemia can result. This leads to the conditions **rickets** (in children) and osteomalacia (in adults), marked by defects in bone mineralisation, with bone weakness, bending and distortion (Clinical Focus Box 27.3).

Vitamin D is involved in calcium, phosphate and magnesium metabolism in bone and the GIT. The mechanism of action of vitamin D is generally similar to that of steroid hormones: it enters the nucleus, activates vitamin D receptors (present in more than 36 cell types) and sets in train a series of reactions leading to gene transcription and synthesis of calcium-binding proteins and bone matrix proteins. It raises plasma calcium concentration by increasing calcium absorption (in the GIT), by re-absorption (in kidney distal tubules) and mobilisation (from bone) – actions similar to those of PTH. Vitamin D also has a permissive role in PTH actions.

Many sterol sources and tissues are involved in the production of vitamin D:

- In skin, 7-dehydrocholesterol is converted to vitamin D_3 (colecalciferol) by the action of UV rays in sunlight.
- In the diet, a plant ergosterol derivative is present in some foods and added to fortified dairy products such as some milk varieties (0.5–2 microgram vitamin D/100 mL).
- Ergocalciferol (vitamin D_2) is absorbed from the GIT into the bloodstream.

> **CLINICAL FOCUS BOX 27.3**
> **Rickets and vitamin D**
>
> Nutritional rickets, thought to have been cured in the early part of the 20th century when vitamin D and its role in bone strength were discovered, has made an unexpected return throughout the world, even in sunny countries. The risk of nutritional rickets in Australia is thought to be due to low dietary intake of vitamin D and decreased sunshine exposure (including regular use of high-SPF sunscreens), particularly in children and women who wear protective hats/clothing, in children of recent immigrant families from Africa or the Middle East, in elderly people house-bound or in residential care and in people with dark skin pigmentation.
>
> A large-scale study of Australian children under age 15 showed an incidence of 4.9/100,000/year; 98% of the children identified as vitamin D deficient had dark or intermediate skin pigmentation, and most were refugees from African countries.
>
> A report from the New Zealand Ministry of Health in 2020 stated that the incidence of vitamin D-deficient rickets from 2010 to 2013 in children under 15 years old was 2.2/100,000 and 10.5/100,000 in children under 3 years old (New Zealand Ministry of Health – see 'Online resources'). Adequate intake for people with no/minimal sun exposure aged older than 70 years is 20 micrograms (800 IU)/day.

- In the liver, vitamin D is hydroxylated to 25-hydroxyvitamin D (25[OH]D, calcifidiol).
- In body fat, 25-hydroxyvitamin D is stored as the depot form.
- In kidneys, vitamin D is converted to its most active form, calcitriol (1,25-dihydroxycolecalciferol; see Drug Monograph 27.4).

Treatment

Rickets and osteomalacia are prevented or treated with vitamin D, which is effective in relieving hypocalcaemia but cannot correct already deformed bones. The treatment regimen for moderate–severe vitamin D deficiency involves administration of colecalciferol 75–125 micrograms (3000–5000 IU) daily for 6–12 weeks, thereafter reducing to a daily oral dose of 25–50 micrograms (1000–2000 IU).

Osteoporosis

Osteoporosis refers to increased bone fragility due to distortion of bone microarchitecture, and consequent risk of fracture due to reduced bone density – the lower the bone density, the greater the risk of low-trauma bone fracture, especially of vertebrae, hip or forearm.

CLINICAL FOCUS BOX 27.4

Prevalence of osteoporosis in Australia and New Zealand

It is estimated that of the population over 50 years old, 1.04 million Australians have osteoporosis and 3.69 million have osteopenia. This is expected to increase to 6.2 million by 2022, a 31% increase since 2012. In 2013, one fracture occurred every 3.6 minutes, equating to 2765 fractures/week. By 2020 a fracture is expected to occur every 2.9 minutes – that is, 3521 fractures/week. By 2022 the cost to the healthcare system was estimated to reach $3.84 billion (Osteoporosis Australia Medical and Scientific Advisory Committee – see 'Online resources').

In New Zealand ~3700 people sustain a hip fracture annually and a further 13,800 are hospitalised with other fragility fractures. In 2014 the estimated cost of hip fractures to the New Zealand health system was $171 million and the total cost for all fractures was over $300 million per year (Osteoporosis New Zealand – see 'Online resources').

Osteoporosis is an important health problem, and adequate dietary intake through the life span of calcium, vitamin D and vitamin K enhances bone density and reduces risk of osteoporosis later in life. Unfortunately, bone strength is lost progressively during the adult years, so osteoporosis has an increasing prevalence as the proportion of the population aged 65 years and over increases. Not unexpectedly, fractures contribute significantly to morbidity, mortality and growing healthcare costs (Clinical Focus Box 27.4).

Risk and other contributing factors

There are many risk factors for osteoporosis in women: late menarche (first menstrual period), episodic amenorrhoea and early menopause, all indicating the protective effect that estrogens normally have on bones. Men also experience bone loss with ageing and declining sex steroid concentrations, so osteoporosis and hip fractures also occur in older men. Malabsorption syndromes, hyperparathyroidism and other endocrine disorders can impair calcium balance. Low calcium intake and excessive phosphate are contributing factors.

Several drug groups and lifestyle factors are also detrimental to strong bones. High-fat diets lead to obesity, which impairs response of the growing skeleton to mechanical loading and reduces trabecular bone mass. The mechanism is thought to be via inhibition of Wnt signalling and activation of the PPAR-gamma pathway (see under 'Thiazolidinediones' in Ch 28). Chronic alcohol consumption has similar effects, with oxidative stress leading to reduced bone formation. Conversely, dietary components such as fluoride, vitamin K, vitamin D and (phyto)estrogens have the potential to beneficially improve bone health (Willems et al. 2017).

Glucocorticoids are well known to increase the risk of osteoporosis. Osteoporosis-related fractures occur in 30–50% of people receiving long-term glucocorticoids in daily doses equivalent to 2.5 mg prednisolone. Several mechanisms have been proposed: glucocorticoids chronically impair transcription of the collagenase gene and block induction of the osteocalcin (calcium-binding) gene by vitamin D, alter the ratio between osteoprotegerin and RANKL, reduce intestinal calcium absorption, increase urinary excretion of calcium and inhibit functions and replenishment of osteoblasts, overall leading to increased bone resorption.

Other drug groups (Pitt & Kearns 2011; Watts 2017) with potentially adverse effects on bone include:

- antiepileptic drugs (phenytoin, carbamazepine)
- aromatase inhibitors (anastrozole, letrozole, exemestane) used as adjunct therapy in breast cancer, which reduce estrogen production and hence predispose to osteoporosis
- gonadotrophin-releasing hormone agonists (used in the treatment of endometriosis)
- medroxyprogesterone acetate (a depot contraceptive agent)
- proton-pump inhibitors (omeprazole)
- selective serotonin reuptake inhibitors (antidepressants)
- SGLT2 inhibitors (dapagliflozin)
- thiazolidinediones (oral hypoglycaemic agents, agonists at PPAR-gamma receptors).

Treatment

Management involves assessing risk factors and contributing conditions, reducing the risk of falls, monitoring bone mineral density by densitometry techniques, regular exercise and attention to diet, especially intake of vitamin D, to maintain a serum 25[OH]D concentration of 75 nmol/L or greater. Calcium and vitamin D supplementation is not recommended in active community living individuals as the benefit in terms of reducing fracture risk is low. However, in institutionalised patients, supplementation with calcium and vitamin D may be beneficial in those receiving drug treatment for osteoporosis. Current recommendations (The Royal Australian College of General Practitioners and Osteoporosis Australia 2017) for treating osteoporosis include:

- bisphosphonates (alendronate, risedronate and zoledronic acid)
- denosumab
- raloxifene.

Initiation of estrogen therapy in post-menopausal women should be carefully considered: balancing benefit versus risk, long-term use is not recommended.

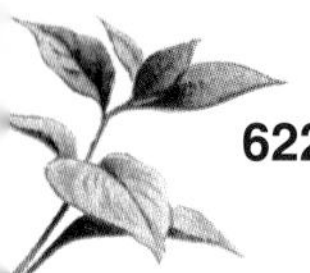

Bisphosphonates

Bisphosphonates are drugs specifically designed to decrease bone turnover, hence increasing bone mass and reducing the incidence of fractures. They are analogues of pyrophosphate (basic structure P–O–P), which plays a role in regulating bone resorption. The bisphosphonates have the general structure P–C–P, with two phosphonate groups linked by carbon rather than oxygen, making them more resistant to enzymatic inactivation.

Mechanism of action

Bisphosphonates are incorporated into bone where they form a depot for months to years. They inhibit normal and abnormal resorption, primarily by decreasing activity of osteoclasts at the site of bone resorption, and inhibit pathological calcification. Nitrogen-containing analogues (alendronate, ibandronic acid, pamidronate, risedronate and zoledronic acid) inhibit bone resorption without also inhibiting bone formation. There are many proposed sites of action, including inhibition of a key enzyme (farnesyl pyrophosphate synthase) in the mevalonate pathway, which leads to an inhibition of the synthesis of many GTP-binding proteins important in the regulation of osteoclast functions.

Clinical Uses of Bisphosphonates

- Treatment of osteoporosis – alendronate, risedronate and zoledronic acid
- Paget's disease of bone – alendronate, pamidronate, risedronate and zoledronic acid
- Bone metastases and hypercalcaemia of malignancy – ibandronic acid, pamidronate, zoledronic acid

Many cancers, especially metastases from breast, prostate, lung and other solid tumours, cause hypercalcaemia and osteolytic bone disease, due to secretion of PTH-like protein from tumour cells.

Formulations and administration

All bisphosphonates have extremely low oral bioavailability (< 1%). For those taken orally (e.g. alendronate), the tablet or capsule must be taken with a full glass of plain water at least 30 minutes before eating, and the person should remain upright until after eating. (This is because bisphosphonates, including alendronate, tended to cause acid regurgitation, oesophageal ulceration and oesophagitis.) Pamidronate and zoledronic acid are only formulated for administration by IV infusion.

Due to the unusual pharmacokinetic properties of bisphosphonates, various formulations are available – for example, risedronate once-daily (5 mg), once-a-week (35 mg) and once-a-month (150 mg) tablets and as combination products with other drugs affecting bone, so it is important that patients understand their dosage regimen.

Adverse drug reactions and interactions

There are many adverse effects, especially in the GIT, including gas production, acid regurgitation, oesophageal ulceration, gastritis, dysphagia, constipation and diarrhoea. Hypocalcaemia, muscle pain and headaches are common, as are flu-like symptoms after IV injection. Intravenous administration of zoledronic acid and pamidronate has led to cases of nephrotoxicity, characterised by tubular necrosis and glomerulosclerosis; ibandronic acid appears to be safer. Bisphosphonates may increase risk of renal impairment, atrial fibrillation and heart failure.

Antacids, minerals and food reduce the oral absorption of bisphosphonates and these drugs should not be taken within 2 hours of a bisphosphonate. The risk of gastric ulceration is increased with concomitant administration of non-steroidal anti-inflammatory drugs.

A rare (0.1–0.3% risk) but potentially severe adverse effect is osteonecrosis of the jaw. This is apparently triggered in susceptible people by dental extractions, periodontal disease or oral trauma, especially after IV administration of pamidronate or zoledronic acid. People especially at risk are those with cancer (particularly multiple myeloma or bony metastases), poor oral hygiene, anaemia or periodontal disease or receiving chemotherapy, radiotherapy or corticosteroid treatment. Individuals should have a dental assessment and any required treatment before starting bisphosphonate therapy, and regular dental checks thereafter.

Denosumab

The antiresorptive agent denosumab is a fully human monoclonal antibody that binds to RANKL (a cytokine involved in activation of osteoclasts). It decreases the formation and activation of osteoclasts, and thus reduces bone resorption and risk of fractures. Administered SC, bioavailability is approximately 60%, and a reduction in bone turnover markers occurs within 1 day.

It is indicated in postmenopausal osteoporosis and osteopenia in men to increase bone mass following androgen deprivation therapy for prostate cancer; the recommended dosage is 60 mg SC every 6 months. A much higher dose (120 mg SC every 4 weeks) is indicated for preventing skeleton-related events in adults with bony metastases. It is contraindicated in hypocalcaemia, renal impairment and pregnancy, due to evidence of teratogenicity in animal studies.

Common adverse effects include back pain, pain in extremities, eczema, hypercholesterolaemia and skin infections. There are concerns with respect to osteonecrosis of the jaw, pancreatitis and immune suppression causing increased infections. Hypocalcaemia is a known risk and can be fatal; serum calcium concentration should be monitored. Calcium and vitamin D supplementation may be required in some individuals (e.g. people with bone metastases in the absence of hypercalcaemia).

Romosozumab

Recently approved in Australia, romosozumab is a new monoclonal antibody that inhibits the action of sclerostin. Sclerostin is produced by osteocytes and is involved in increasing bone resorption while decreasing bone formation. Inhibition of sclerostin by romosozumab has been shown to increase bone density in the lumbar spine and hip in both males and females.

Disadvantages of the drug include the need for twice-monthly SC injections, the 3-month delay before reaching a steady-state concentration and the decline in effectiveness over a 12-month period.

Common adverse effects reported in clinical trials included injection site reactions, headache, arthralgia and muscle spasms and hypocalcaemia. Of a more serious issue were reports of osteonecrosis of the jaw and serious cardiovascular adverse effects including death. Romosozumab is contraindicated in people with a history of stroke or myocardial infarction in the previous year.

Raloxifene

The selective second-generation estrogen receptor modulator (SERM) raloxifene has partial agonist and partial antagonist estrogenic properties. It has positive effects on bone (stimulating osteoblast and inhibiting osteoclast activity) and lipid metabolism and antagonist effects on the uterus and breast, minimising the risk of estrogen-dependent cancers. Current clinical evidence indicates efficacy in reducing vertebral fractures only. Use for the treatment of osteoporosis is further complicated by evidence of venous thromboembolism and the risk–benefit relationship should be considered.

Administered orally, it is well absorbed but undergoes extensive first-pass metabolism resulting in a bioavailability in the region of 2%. It is metabolised by UGT1A1 and UGT1A9, forming a number of glucuronide metabolites. The average half-life for raloxifene is 32 hours but ranges from 16 to 87 hours.

The main adverse effects are typical estrogenic actions: hot flushes, leg cramps, peripheral oedema and increased risk of venous thromboembolism.

Lasofoxifene, a third-generation SERM, is currently in clinical trials in postmenopausal osteoporosis (https://lasofoxifene.com/). It appears to be as effective as raloxifene at increasing total hip bone mineral density, with greater effect on lumbar spine bone mineral density.

Teriparatide

Teriparatide, a recombinant PTH analogue, is an anabolic agent stimulating bone formation. It is used in severe osteoporosis only when the risk of fracture is extremely high, or if other effective therapies are unsuitable. Treatment duration is limited to a lifetime maximum of 18 months because of the potential risk of osteosarcoma, which has been observed in animal studies.

KEY POINTS

Pharmacotherapy of bone disorders

- Bone undergoes continual remodelling. Bone resorption leads to mobilisation of both calcium and phosphate from bone components.
- Impaired bone formation and remodelling leads to the pathological states of Paget's disease, osteoporosis, rickets and osteomalacia. Dietary deficiencies and administered drugs (e.g. glucocorticoids) can also lead to bone disorders.
- Calcium is important for physiological processes and in bone structure. Calcium balance is tightly controlled by PTH, calcitonin and vitamin D.
- Drugs for the treatment of bone disorders include calcium, colecalciferol, vitamin D, the bisphosphonate group of drugs (antiresorptive drugs), denosumab (a fully human monoclonal antibody that binds to RANKL), raloxifene (a SERM) and teriparitide (a PTH analogue).
- Raloxifene and teriparatide are reserved for situations where the risk of fracture is extremely high, or if other effective therapies are unsuitable.

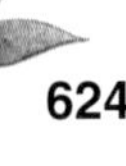

DRUGS AT A GLANCE
Drugs affecting the thyroid and parathyroid glands and bone

PHARMACOLOGICAL GROUP AND EFFECT	KEY EXAMPLES	CLINICAL USE
Thyroid hormones • Control growth and development • Regulate metabolism and energy balance • Promote normal cardiovascular and nervous system functions	Levothyroxine (T_4)	• Hypothyroidism • Thyroid cancer • Euthyroid goitre
	Liothyronine (T_3)	• Severe hypothyroidism (e.g. myxoedema coma)
Iodine therapy • Inhibition of thyroid hormone release	Iodine; iodine solution aqueous	• Before surgery for Graves' disease
	^{131}I (radioiodine)	• Hyperthyroidism • Thyroid carcinoma • Diagnostic thyroid function tests
Antithyroid agents • Inhibits thyroid hormone synthesis • Inhibits peripheral conversion of T_4 to T_3 (propylthiouracil)	Carbimazole Propylthiouracil	• Graves' disease • Before thyroid surgery • Before/after radioiodine • Thyroid storm
Calcium salts • Important role in cellular physiology and metabolic regulation • Important in bone homeostasis	Calcium	• Supplementation in osteoporosis, osteomalacia, rickets • Acute hypocalcaemia • Hypocalcaemic tetany
Vitamin D analogues	Calcitriol	• Hypocalcaemia in hypoparathyroidism • Hypophosphataemic rickets • Osteoporosis • Chronic renal dialysis • Renal osteodystrophy
	Colecalciferol	• Prevention/treatment of vitamin D deficiency • Osteoporosis (fixed-dose combination with either alendronate or calcium)
Calcitonin analogue • Inhibits osteoclatic bone resorption • Inhibits calcium reabsorption in kidney • Lowers plasma calcium concentration	Calcitonin salmon	• Hypercalcaemia • Paget's disease of bone (rarely used)
Calcimimetic agent • Increase affinity of calcium-sensing receptors for calcium • Consequential reduction in parathyroid hormone (PTH) synthesis and secretion and serum calcium concentration	Cinacalcet	• Primary hyperparathyroidism (when surgery is not an option) • Hypercalcaemia associated with parathyroid carcinoma • Hyperparathyroidism in end-stage renal disease in individuals on dialysis
Drugs treating osteoporosis Bisphosphonates • Inhibit osteoclast activity reducing bone resorption	Alendronate Risedronate Zoledronic acid	• Osteoporosis • Hypercalcaemia of malignancy • Paget's disease of bone
PTH analogue • Recombinant PTH analogue that stimulates bone formation	Teriparatide	• Osteoporosis (postmenopausal females and males with high fracture risk) • Corticosteroid-induced osteoporosis with high fracture risk
RANKL antibody • Inhibits activation of RANK receptor decreasing formation and activity of osteoclasts • Reduces bone resorption	Denosumab	• Postmenopausal osteoporosis • Corticosteroid-induced osteoporosis with high fracture risk • In males with osteopenia from androgen deprivation therapy • Giant cell tumour of bone
Sclerostin antibody • Inhibits sclerostin reducing bone resorption	Romosozumab[AUS]	• Osteoporosis in both males and females
SERM • Partial agonist/antagonist at estrogen receptors • Inhibits osteoclast activity • Stimulates osteoblast activity	Raloxifene	• Postmenopausal osteoporosis

Note: Drugs are not exclusive to each therapeutic group; for example, colecalciferol is used in a fixed dose combination with alendronate for the treatment of osteoporosis; and the bisphosphonates, being strongly alkaline, are usually present as their sodium or disodium salts. For simplicity, the drugs are referred to by just the basic form, '-dronate'.
[AUS] Australia only

REVIEW EXERCISES

1 Mrs FG is 62 years old. Her routine annual blood test revealed low free T_3 and T_4 and elevated TSH consistent with hypothyroidism. Discuss the advantages of levothyroxine and her dosage regimen in light of her history of cardiovascular disease.

2 Mr MN has been diagnosed with hyperthyroidism (Graves' disease) and is treated with oral carbimazole. When collecting his prescription, he asks you (the pharmacist) to explain to him how the drug works and what he may expect in the way of adverse effects. What explanation will you provide?

3 Mrs TB, a 61-year-old, had undergone a number of tests to determine if she has osteoporosis. At her most recent visit to her GP she was advised that her bone mineral density was indicative of osteoporosis and her bone markers indicated significant bone resorption. She was commenced on alendronate 70 mg once a week. Discuss why alendronate is effective for treating osteoporosis and why the drug has a long half-life in bone.

REFERENCES

Boron WF, Boulpaep EL, editors: Medical physiology, ed 2, Philadelphia, 2012, Elsevier Saunders.

Chung PY, Van Hul W. Paget's disease of bone: evidence for complex pathogenetic interactions. Seminars in Arthritis and Rheumatism 2012; 41(5):619–41.

Haugen BR. Drugs that suppress TSH or cause central hypothyroidism. Best Practice & Research Clinical Endocrinology & Metabolism 2009;23:793–800.

Hynes KL, Seal JA, Otahal P, et al. Women remain at risk of iodine deficiency during pregnancy: The importance of iodine supplementation before conception and throughout gestation. Nutrients 2019;11:172. Online. Available: http://dx.doi.org/10.3390/nu11010172.

Mortimer RH. Thyroid function tests, Australian Prescriber 34(1):12–15, 2011.

Pitt CJ, Kearns AE. Update on medications with adverse skeletal effects. Mayo Clinic Proceedings 2011;86(4):338–43.

Rang HP, Dale MM, Ritter JM, et al: Pharmacology, Edinburgh, 2012, Elsevier.

The Royal Australian College of General Practitioners and Osteoporosis Australia. Osteoporosis prevention, diagnosis and management in postmenopausal women and men over 50 years of age. 2nd edn. East Melbourne, Vic: RACGP, 2017. Online. Available

Watts NB. Adverse bone effects of medications used to treat non-skeletal disorders. Osteoporosis International 2017;28:2741–76.

Willems HME, van den Heuvel EGHM, Schoemaker RJW, et al. Diet and exercise: A match made in bone. Current Osteoporosis Reports 2017;15:555–63.

ONLINE RESOURCES

American Association of Clinical Endocrinologists/American College of Endocrinology – Clinical practice guidelines for the diagnosis and treatment of postmenopausal osteoporosis (2020): https://pro.aace.com/sites/default/files/2020-05/Vol%2026%20Supplement%201%20(May%202020)%20GL-2019-0524_0.pdf (accessed 13 April 2020)

Guidance on the diagnosis and management of osteoporosis in New Zealand. Online. Available https://osteoporosis.org.nz/clinical-guidance/ (accessed 13 April 2021)

New Zealand Ministry of Health – Companion statement on vitamin D and sun exposure in pregnancy and infancy in New Zealand: https://www.health.govt.nz/publication/companion-statement-vitamin-d-and-sun-exposure-pregnancy-and-infancy-new-zealand (accessed 13 April 2021)

Osteoporosis Australia Medical and Scientific Advisory Committee: https://www.osteoporosis.org.au/ (accessed 13 April 2021)

Osteoporosis New Zealand – Annual report 2017: https://osteoporosis.org.nz/wp-content/uploads/ONZ-2017-Annual-Report-WEB.pdf (accessed 13 April 2021)

CHAPTER 28

THE ENDOCRINE PANCREAS AND DIABETES MELLITUS

Mary Bushell

KEY ABBREVIATIONS

BGL blood glucose level
DPP4 dipeptidyl peptidase-4
GLP glucagon-like peptide
NPH neutral protamine Hagedorn
OHA oral hypoglycaemic agent
SGLT2 sodium-glucose co-transporter 2

KEY TERMS

antihyperglycaemic drugs 633
basal release 627
blood glucose level 630
diabetes mellitus 631
glucagon 630
hyperglycaemia 631
incretins 631
insulin 627
ketoacidosis 632
macro/microvascular disease 633
type 1/type 2 diabetes 631

Chapter Focus

Insulin and glucagon, hormones secreted by the pancreas, have major roles in regulation of blood glucose levels and nutrient storage. Inadequate production of insulin and/or resistance to insulin causes diabetes mellitus, a disorder of carbohydrate metabolism affecting approximately 8.5% of the adult population. Serious long-term complications include cardiovascular disease, stroke, kidney failure (diabetic kidney disease), blindness (diabetic retinopathy) and nerve damage (diabetic neuropathy) that may lead to lower limb amputation.

People with type 1 diabetes are dependent on parenteral insulin (injections, pumps); many formulations of human and bovine insulin are available. People with type 2 diabetes may be managed with lifestyle modifications, such as diet and exercise, and/or treated with antihyperglycaemic drugs. Many people with type 2 diabetes will eventually require insulin. Hypoglycaemia is a potential adverse effect of insulin and most antihyperglycaemic drugs. Hypoglycaemia can be treated with hyperglycaemic medications such as glucose or glucagon.

KEY DRUG GROUPS

- **Glucagon** (Drug Monograph 28.1)

Insulins:

- **Human insulin** (Drug Monograph 28.2)
- **Insulin lispro**, insulin isophane, **insulin glargine**

Oral hypoglycaemic agents:

- **Metformin** (Drug Monograph 28.3)
- Sulfonylureas: **glibenclamide**, **glipizide**
- Thiazolidinediones: **pioglitazone**, **rosiglitazone**
- Incretin-based drugs: exenatide, sitagliptin
- Sodium-glucose co-transporter 2 inhibitors: dapagliflozin
- **Acarbose**

CRITICAL THINKING SCENARIO

Annie (aged 67 years) was diagnosed with type 2 diabetes 15 years ago. When first diagnosed, Annie was prescribed lifestyle modification and metformin. When glycaemic control was not achieved after 3 months, a sulfonylurea (gliclazide) was added. About 2 years ago, the dipeptidyl peptidase-4 (DPP-4) inhibitor sitagliptin was also added. To overcome therapy inertia with the three existing oral hypoglycaemic agents, last month Annie's prescriber ceased the sulfonylurea and added insulin (insulin glargine 100 units/mL). The insulin is injected subcutaneously once daily in the evening. Annie continues to take metformin plus the (DPP-4) inhibitor orally. Her last HbA_{1C}, recorded 2 weeks ago, was 7.8%.

Over the past week, Annie has been trying to lose weight for her daughter's wedding and has been increasing the intensity and frequency of her gym workouts. Today she skipped her breakfast and lunch. She is now dizzy, sweating, hungry, and has headaches and had a sudden change in mood.

1. Explain the normal changes that occur to blood glucose levels when a person eats a carbohydrate-rich meal. In your answer, include the normal range of blood glucose levels for both before (i.e.'fasting') and after (i.e. post-prandial) meals.
2. Explain the rationale for adding oral hypoglycaemic agents (metformin, sulfonylureas and dipeptidyl peptidase-4 (DPP-4) inhibitor). Explain the rationale for adding insulin.
3. Explain what was happening physiologically for Annie when she became dizzy, was sweating, hungry, and had headaches and a sudden change in mood. What treatment should she take to reduce her symptoms?
4. Annie becomes unconscious. What treatments should now be administered to treat her? Ensure you cover what routes of administration the treatments can be given.

Introduction

The pancreas is a mixed gland, with both endocrine and exocrine functions (Fig 16.1). Exocrine secretions (i.e. pancreatic juice) contain digestive enzymes, enzyme precursors and electrolytes, and are discharged into the pancreatic ducts and subsequently into the gastrointestinal tract (GIT) (Ch 16).

The endocrine tissue of the pancreas, the islets of Langerhans, consists of clumps of cells scattered throughout the organ. They make up about 2% of the weight of the pancreas and produce hormones (insulin, glucagon and somatostatin) that control blood glucose levels (BGLs) and some gastrointestinal functions. Insulin is produced by beta (or B) cells, glucagon by alpha (or A) cells, and somatostatin by delta (or D) cells. (Somatostatin inhibits release not only of growth hormone but also of insulin and glucagon.) Pathologies of pancreatic endocrine functions cause widespread and serious disorders including diabetes mellitus and metabolic syndrome.

Pancreatic hormones and diabetes

Insulin from the pancreas

Insulin is a protein hormone consisting of two polypeptide chains joined by disulfide bridges (Fig 28.1). Insulin was the first protein for which the amino acid sequence was determined, and the first synthesised by genetic engineering technologies, showing its importance in medicine (Clinical Focus Box 28.1).

Insulin release and circulation

Insulin is synthesised from a larger protein, proinsulin, which acts as the storage form. There is a low basal release in pulses every 15–30 minutes into the portal

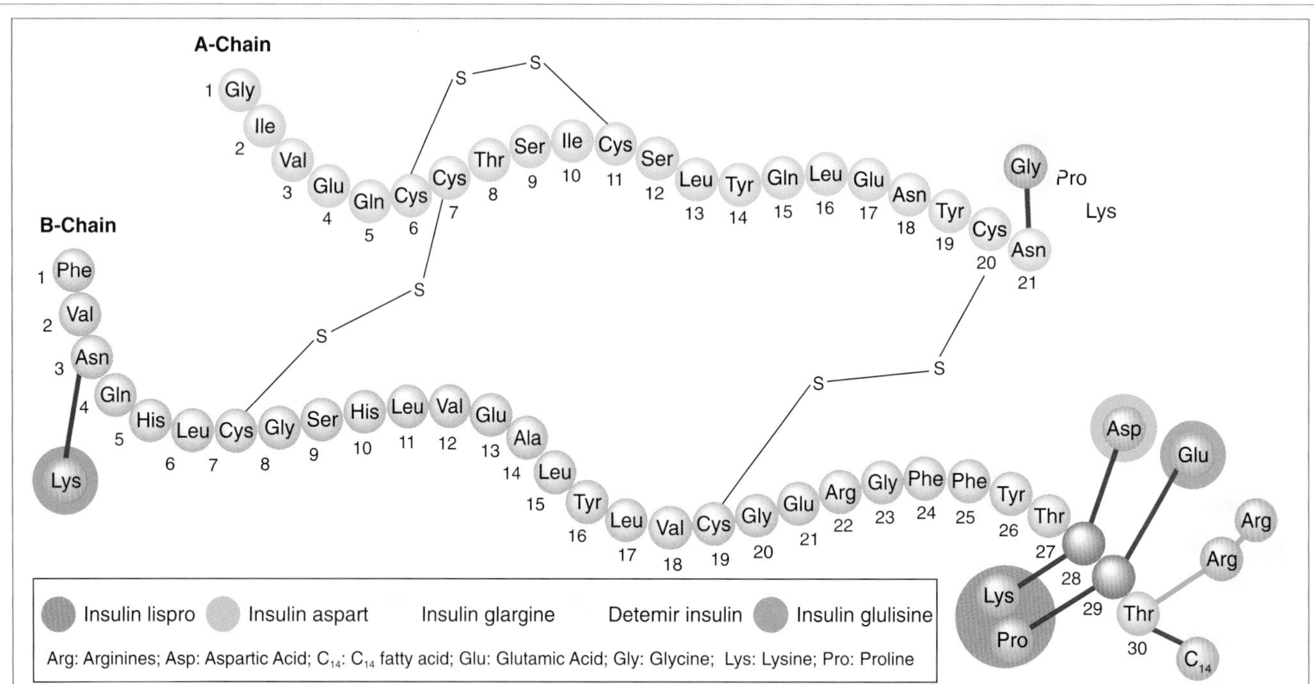

FIGURE 28.1 Structure of human insulin, and modifications to make insulin analogues

Purple line denotes substitution of an amino acid; green line denotes addition.

Source: Adapted from Heile & Schneider 2012.

CLINICAL FOCUS BOX 28.1

History of diabetes and insulin

The condition has been known for thousands of years; early Egyptian references describe flesh melting into urine, unquenchable thirst and inevitable early death.

1788

Involvement of the pancreas described.

1889

Minkowski and von Mering demonstrated that a pancreatectomised dog produced large volumes of sugary urine.

1900

People with diabetes were shown to have pancreatic lesions in the islets of Langerhans.

1904

The concept of hormones secreted from a gland into the bloodstream developed.

1921

Toronto scientist Banting and medical student Best extracted from islet tissue an active hypoglycaemic fraction (later called insulin), successfully treating pancreatectomised dogs and then people with diabetes.

1923

Insulin purified from cattle pancreas was available clinically. Banting and McLeod, a professor of physiology, received the 1923 Nobel Prize for Medicine.

1936 onwards

Intermediate-acting and long-acting insulin formulations were developed; long-term renal, vascular and retinal complications of diabetes were noted.

1945–55

The amino acid sequence and structure of insulin were determined by English biochemist Frederick Sanger, who was awarded the 1958 Nobel Prize (and another in 1980 for determining the base sequences in nucleic acids).

1954

The first oral hypoglycaemic agent, a sulfonylurea, became available.

1982

Recombinant human insulin was produced by genetic engineering techniques.

1990s onwards

Rapid-acting and long-acting analogues of human insulin produced; computer-controlled insulin pumps developed. Thiazolidinediones (glitazones) available to treat type 2 diabetes.

2005

Incretin-based therapies introduced.

2013

3D pictures of the binding of insulin to its receptors were published by 17 scientists, including some from Melbourne, utilising the cyclotron in Clayton, Victoria.

SGLT2 inhibitors (-agliflozins) introduced for type 2 diabetes.

2022

The primary cause of type 1 diabetes is still not known.

circulation to the liver. Release is increased within 30–60 seconds after absorption of glucose from a meal, a rapid initial rise due to release of stored insulin, then a slower delayed phase over 60–90 minutes when newly synthesised insulin is also released.

Other factors that stimulate insulin secretion include:

- raised blood amino acid levels
- glucagon
- incretins (glucose-dependent insulinotropic peptides, glucagon-like peptides) released from the digestive tract in response to food
- vagal stimulation, due to increased parasympathetic activity in response to a meal
- β-adrenoceptor stimulation
- some antihyperglycaemic drugs (e.g. sulphonylureas).

Insulin release is inhibited by falling blood glucose levels, fasting, somatostatin, adrenaline (epinephrine; via α_2-receptors) and drugs such as the thiazide diuretics. Deficiencies of release occur in pancreatic disorders: diabetes mellitus, pancreatitis and tumours.

Insulin circulates bound to a β-globulin. As a protein, it is rapidly digested in the gut if given orally, with a half-life of only a few minutes, so it must be administered parenterally to treat diabetes. Its biological duration of action is longer, 2–4 hours, as it is bound to receptors in tissues where it acts.

Insulin actions and mechanism

Insulin is the body's primary fuel storage hormone: it facilitates removal of glucose from the blood into muscle and fat cells via biochemical reactions affecting uptake, utilisation and storage of carbohydrates, fats and amino acids in liver, adipose and muscle cells. Nutrients are stored as glycogen, triglycerides, fatty acids and proteins. Insulin therefore controls intermediary metabolism, promotes the anabolic state (building up) and has long-term effects on cell proliferation and growth regulation. Glycogenolysis, lipolysis and proteolysis are inhibited.

The actions of insulin are physiologically antagonised by the catabolic hormones – that is, adrenocorticotrophic hormone (ACTH), glucocorticoids, adrenaline, growth hormone and thyroxine. Hence, low insulin levels (and diabetes) can occur secondary to other endocrine disorders, including acromegaly and Cushing's disease.

Mechanism of action

The mechanism of action of insulin is via binding to specific membrane receptors on target cells and activation of a tyrosine kinase enzyme. This initiates a cascade of phosphorylation reactions leading to many kinase and phosphatase activities, as well as DNA transcription and cell replication. Intracellular vesicles containing a glucose transporter (GLUT-4) fuse with the plasma membrane and the transporter is inserted, leading to a rapid 10- to

30-fold increase in glucose uptake into the cell, where it is 'trapped' as glucose-6-phosphate. Cells in the brain, exercising muscle and liver are not dependent on insulin-mediated glucose uptake.

Control of blood glucose levels

Insulin and glucagon

Carbohydrate metabolism and **blood glucose levels** are controlled by finely balanced interactions between the anterior pituitary, pancreas, adrenal and thyroid glands, maintaining the plasma glucose level around the optimum. These processes are summarised in Figure 28.2 and its legend.

Glucagon is a 29-amino-acid polypeptide hormone secreted by alpha cells of islets of Langerhans in response to hypoglycaemia and high-protein meals, and stimulated by exercise, stress and infections. It is a fuel-mobilising hormone and has been called an 'anti-insulin'. Its actions include:

- stimulating hepatic glycogenolysis gluconeogenesis (the conversion of glycerol and amino acids to glucose), lipolysis and ketogenesis

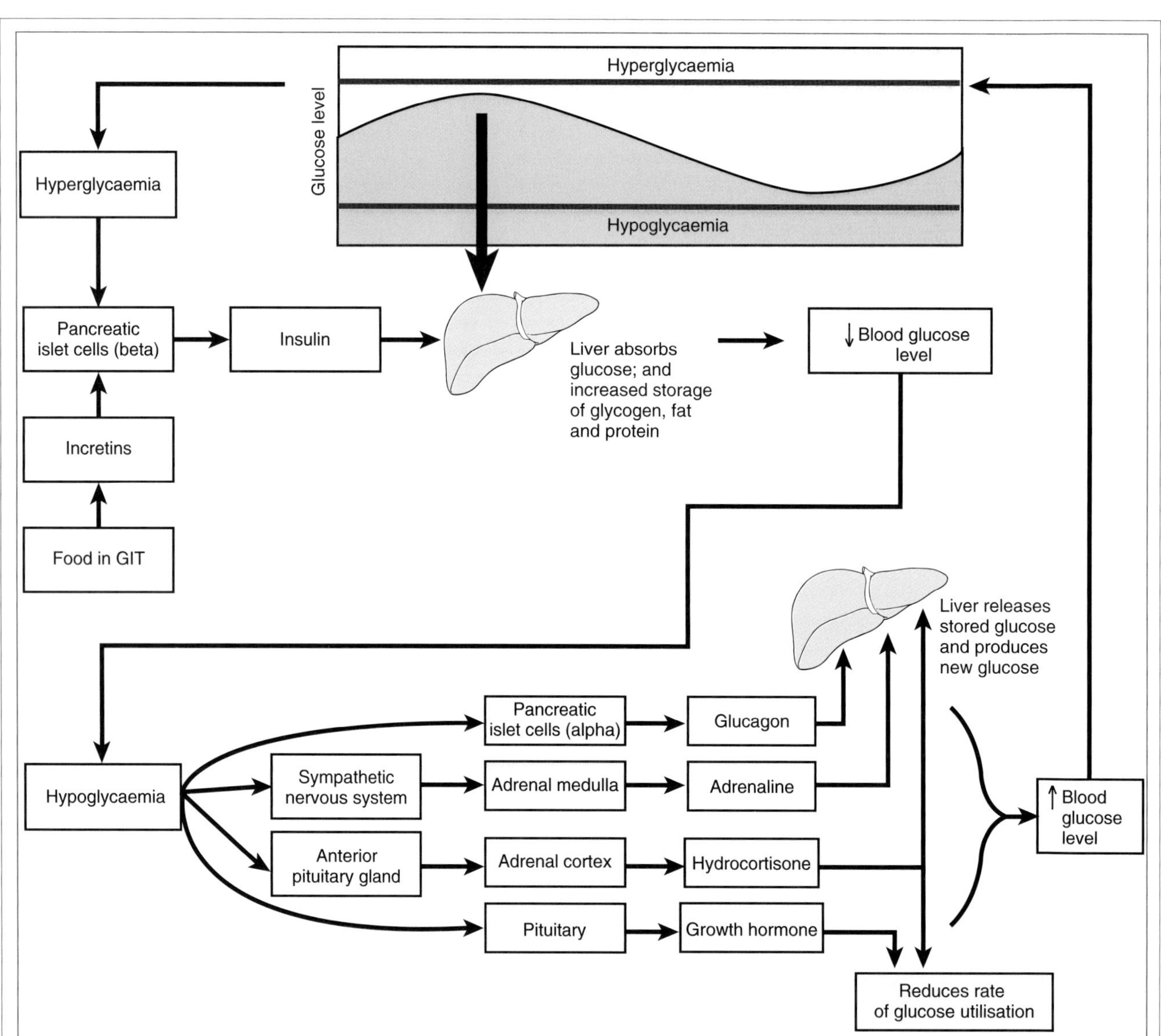

FIGURE 28.2 Control of blood glucose levels

Raised blood glucose levels and the presence of food in the GIT (via incretins) cause the pancreas to release insulin, which causes the liver to absorb excess blood glucose and leads to storage of glycogen, fat and protein. When blood glucose levels are low, the A cells in the islets of Langerhans secrete glucagon, which stimulates liver glycogenolysis and gluconeogenesis. The sympathetic nervous system signals the adrenal medulla to secrete adrenaline (epinephrine), while the anterior pituitary gland signals the adrenal cortex to release hydrocortisone. Both substances enhance gluconeogenesis, while adrenaline also increases glycogenolysis, and hydrocortisone slows down the rate of glucose utilisation and raises the plasma level of amino acids available for glucose production. The pituitary secretes growth hormone, which decreases cellular glucose utilisation and promotes glycogenolysis.

TABLE 28.1 Features of type 1 and type 2 diabetes

FEATURE	TYPE 1	TYPE 2
Synonyms (former)	Insulin-dependent diabetes, juvenile-onset	Non-insulin-dependent diabetes, maturity-onset
Age of onset	Usually < 20 years	Usually > 35 years
Onset of symptoms	Sudden (symptomatic)	Gradual
Body weight	Usually non-obese	Obese (80%)
Aetiology	Predisposition inherited; viral infection may cause auto-immune onset	Family history often positive; risk factors: advancing age, obesity, cardiovascular disease, metabolic syndrome, tobacco use
Incidence (% all diabetes)	5%	90–95%
Insulin levels	Low, then absent	May be low, normal or high (insulin resistance)
Insulin-dependent	Yes	Usually not (may progress to be)
Insulin resistance	No	Yes
Insulin receptors	Normal	Usually low or defective
Complications	Frequent	Frequent
Ketoacidosis	Prone to	Rare
Dietary modifications	Mandatory	Mandatory
Treatment	Insulin essential	Diet, exercise, antihyperglycaemic drugs, possibly insulin

- inhibiting glycogen synthesis
- stimulating release of catecholamines, hence inhibiting tone and motility in GIT smooth muscle, plus other sympathomimetic effects
- increasing release of growth hormone and ACTH, and (paradoxically) of insulin.

Secretion is inhibited by insulin, hyperglycaemia and incretins. (In diabetes, the lack of insulin leads to increased release of glucagon, which contributes to raised blood glucose levels and eventually to the state of ketosis.) Glucagon is used clinically to treat insulin-induced hypoglycaemia (Drug Monograph 28.1, later).

Incretins

Incretins are peptide hormones secreted from the intestinal mucosa into the circulation in the presence of food. The incretins currently known are glucagon-like peptide-1 (GLP-1) and glucose-dependent insulinotropic polypeptide (GIP). They increase insulin secretion via G-protein-coupled receptor activation, raised cyclic adenosine monophosphate (cAMP) levels and calcium-induced exocytosis, mediating much of the B-cell response to an ingested meal. Incretins regulate islet hormone secretion, glucose concentrations, lipid metabolism, gut motility, appetite and body weight, plus non-glycaemic effects in many tissues. Response to incretins is reduced in people with type 2 diabetes; drugs enhancing incretin actions are used in this condition.

Central nervous system influences

Availability of nutrients is sensed in the arcuate nucleus of the hypothalamus, which contains high densities of insulin receptors; neural signals are relayed via efferent vagal fibres to the liver where glucose production is inhibited. The antiobesity hormone leptin improves insulin sensitivity in the arcuate nucleus, partly by activating neurons producing melanocortins with anorectic (appetite suppressant) actions. In type 2 diabetes and obesity, the brain incorrectly perceives and responds to peripheral signals of nutrient availability.

Diabetes mellitus

Diabetes mellitus[1] is characterised by polyuria associated with a chronic disorder of carbohydrate and lipid metabolism and an inappropriate rise in glucose level in the blood, due to defects in insulin secretion, insulin action, or both. Other pathological conditions in the pancreas, such as pancreatitis and pancreatic cancer, also impair its endocrine functions, causing impaired glucose tolerance, **hyperglycaemia** and a wide range of metabolic and cardiovascular problems.

The two main types of diabetes are **type 1** (formerly known as insulin-dependent diabetes mellitus, IDDM, or juvenile-onset), in which there is complete lack of insulin, and **type 2** (non-insulin-dependent diabetes mellitus, NIDDM, maturity-onset), where there is a relative lack of insulin or defects of the insulin receptors. Features of the two types are summarised in Table 28.1, and epidemiological data are summarised in Clinical Interest Box 28.2.

Pathologies

Lack of insulin produces a complex disorder of carbohydrate, fat and protein metabolism, leading to cardiovascular diseases (increasing risk of stroke and myocardial infarction), blindness, end-stage renal disease, neuropathies, accelerated atherosclerosis and lower limb amputations.

General aspects of the pathology of diabetes include:

- *Hyperglycaemia:* Lack of insulin means glucose cannot be taken up into cells. Without treatment the

1 The term 'diabetes mellitus' refers to the 'copious urine, sweet or honey-tasting', distinguishing it in earlier times (when doctors diagnosed by tasting a person's urine) from diabetes insipidus, in which the copious urine was dilute and tasteless.

CLINICAL FOCUS BOX 28.2

Diabetes prevalence

Globally:

- The World Health Organization estimates that 422 million adults are living with diabetes, a global prevalence of 8.5% (2016).
- In 2016, diabetes was the seventh-leading cause of death.
- Prevalence is increasing rapidly, especially in low- and middle-income countries, and projected to double by 2030.
- Risk factors include disadvantaged socioeconomic status, overweight and obesity, energy-dense but low-nutrient foods, increasing age, tobacco use, hypertension and sedentary lifestyles.
- In developing countries, the mortality rate is unacceptably high, often due to inadequate access to medical care and expensive and irregular supplies of insulin.

Australia:

- Approximately 1.2 million (4.9%) Australians have diabetes.
- One million hospitalisations were associated with diabetes – 10% of all hospitalisations.
- Diabetes is a contributing factor in almost 10% of all deaths.
- Prevalence is twice as high in the lowest socioeconomic group compared with the highest.
- Prevalence of type 2 diabetes is four times higher in the Indigenous Australian and Torres Strait Islander population compared with non-Indigenous Australians.
- Prevalence is twice as high in remote and very remote areas than in major cities.

New Zealand:

- Diabetes is a major and increasing health problem; prevalence is highest (15%) in adults 65 years and older.
- According to the New Zealand Health Survey 2014–15, 6.1% of adults (6.8% men, 5.4% women) have doctor-diagnosed diabetes (excluding pregnancy-associated diabetes).
- Prevalence is highest in Pacific Islander people (13%), then Māori (7.2%), Asian (6.4%) and European/others (5.1%).
- Adults in the most deprived areas were three times more likely to be diagnosed with diabetes than others.

Sources: World Health Organization; Diabetes Australian Institute of Health and Welfare; New Zealand Health Survey 2014–15 – see 'Online resources'.

blood glucose level rises rapidly (hyperglycaemia) and excess glucose is secreted by the kidneys (glycosuria).

- *Signs and symptoms of diabetes:* These include increased appetite (polyphagia) and thirst (polydipsia), increased urine output (polyuria), fruity breath odour (ketosis), anorexia and weight loss, abdominal pain, nausea and vomiting, dry mouth, rapid deep breathing, weakness (fatigue) and recurrent infections.
- *Diagnosis of diabetes:* Diagnosis is by signs and symptoms, by measurement of high BGL (random > 11.1 mmol/L, fasting > 7.0 mmol/L), by glucose tolerance testing, 75 gram of glucose administered orally, after overnight fasting (fasting glucose ≥ 7.0 mmol/L or 2 hr glucose ≥ 11.1 mmol/L) and/or by glycated haemoglobin levels (HbA_{1C} ≥ 6.5%; 48 mmol/mol).
- *Prediabetes state:* The prediabetes state is indicated by impaired fasting plasma glucose or glucose tolerance, and commonly associated with metabolic syndrome (see later) and obesity.
- *Type 1 diabetes:* Type 1 usually occurs before the age of 20. High breakdown of proteins and fats causes ketone bodies (acetoacetic acid, acetone and β-hydroxybutyric acid) to accumulate, resulting in ketosis and acidosis. Diabetic **ketoacidosis** with associated cerebral oedema is a medical emergency. Regular two to three times daily injections of exogenous insulin are required lifelong for survival.
- *Type 2 diabetes:* Patients generally have some functioning islet cells. There is impaired insulin secretion (especially the early phase after glucose load) and/or insulin resistance because of receptor and post-receptor defects.
- *Gestational diabetes:* This category includes women in whom diabetes or impaired glucose tolerance is first detected during pregnancy. Insulin resistance develops during the second and third trimesters in approximately 5% of pregnancies, notably in older women. High BGLs in mother can lead to fetal hyperinsulinism; this may cause increased fetal growth, organomegaly and neonatal hypoglycaemia. If BGL cannot be controlled with diet and exercise, mild diabetes may be treated first with metformin, then insulin added or substituted as required. Moderate–severe gestational diabetes requires immediate insulin therapy. Following childbirth, maternal impaired glucose tolerance or diabetes may resolve; breastfeeding the baby is advantageous (Clinical Focus Box 28.3, later).

- *Diabetes in childhood:* Incidence of diabetes in children under age 15 is steadily rising; a specialist paediatrician should be involved in medical management. Hypoglycaemic episodes must be avoided due to risk of injury to the developing brain. Intensive insulin therapy, dietetic advice, frequent monitoring of BGL, specialist clinics, family support and regular screening for diabetic complications are recommended.

Course and complications

The course of untreated diabetes is progressive, and without treatment will result in dehydration, ketosis, acidosis and diabetic coma.

Long-term complications lead to increased morbidity and mortality, despite treatment with insulin (type 1) or diet modification and oral hypoglycaemic agents (OHAs) (type 2). **Microvascular disease** leads to ischaemia, neuropathies, nephropathy and diabetic retinopathy, with possible retinal detachment and blindness. **Macrovascular disease** (atherosclerosis and thrombosis of larger vessels) may result in coronary artery disease, strokes, peripheral vascular disease, cardiomyopathy and heart failure. Other complications include polycystic ovary syndrome, non-alcoholic fatty liver disease, some cancers and eating disorders. There is increased risk of infections and impaired wound healing; even minor foot infections may lead to osteomyelitis and gangrene requiring amputation. There is a high likelihood of polypharmacy with escalating adverse reactions and drug interactions.

General management plans

The general aims of treatment are to replace insulin to physiological levels; to obtain metabolic control with insulin, **antihyperglycaemic drugs** or exercise and dietary regimens; and to avoid or delay acute symptoms and long-term complications. Type 2 diabetes often occurs in association with hypertension and hyperlipidaemia, so absolute cardiovascular risk factors need to be assessed, lifestyle factors improved (especially diet, exercise and smoking) and treatment with antihypertensives and lipid-lowering drugs optimised. Diabetes Australia has specified maximum levels for fasting blood glucose (6–8 mmol/L), glycated haemoglobin (6.5–7.5%), cholesterol and lipoproteins, blood pressure, body mass index, albumin excretion and alcohol intake.

Standard pharmacological treatment plans are for type 1: daily insulin, with regimen and doses determined by monitored BGLs; and for type 2: dietary and weight control and/or an antihyperglycaemic drug with insulin as necessary. People need to be taught to self-monitor BGL and self-administer insulin and/or antihyperglycaemic drug(s).

The treatment plan for diabetes preferably involves a multidisciplinary team, including an endocrinologist, specialist nurse, pharmacist, podiatrist, optometrist, diabetes educator and dietitian. Regular monitoring is recommended of eyes, blood pressure, feet, blood lipids and kidney functions, and specialised care is required during concurrent illness, surgery, pregnancy, travel and other stressful times.

Adherence with therapy

In diabetes, adherence to strict injection/administration regimens and dietary restrictions is essential to maintain blood glucose control and avoid long-term complications; however, overall adherence rates with antidiabetic and cardiovascular medications is only about 70%.

Adherence of young people with type 1 diabetes is particularly important but often worsens in adolescents. Factors reducing adherence are large numbers of injections, tablets or other treatments per day; adverse drug reactions (especially weight gain from some OHAs); barriers such as embarrassment at injecting in public; and depression, denial or behaviour problems.

Blood glucose monitoring

Large-scale trials have shown that tight control of BGLs reduces microvascular risks of retinopathy, nephropathy and neuropathy and other cardiovascular complications. To maintain euglycaemia (normal BGL: 3.5–8 mmol/L), BGLs are regularly determined by blood glucose monitoring (self-monitored blood glucose), test strips and blood glucose meters. Continuous glucose monitoring is a novel way of recording BGLs without constant finger pricks. Patients have a disposable sensor inserted under their skin, which measures the BGLs in the interstitial fluid. Patients then make necessary adjustments with medication, diet and exercise. Urine tests are used mainly for detecting ketone bodies in the urine.

A better indicator of long-term management of diabetes is glycosylated (glycated) haemoglobin (HbA_{1C}), which reflects average BGL over the preceding 3 months; normal value is less than 6%. Levels of HbA_{1C} above 6.5% (48 mmol/mol) are correlated with diabetes complications.

Prescribed, over-the-counter and social drugs can all affect BGL and alter diabetic control (Table 28.2), leading to many potential drug interactions with insulin and antihyperglycaemic agent(s).

Hyperglycaemia and sugar intake

Chronic hyperglycaemia can lead to diabetic ketoacidosis and hyperosmolar coma; treatment is with rehydration and insulin. Carers of children with diabetes need to be aware of the sugar content of medicines[2] as well as that of

---

2 Many medicines formulated for children have a high sugar content to encourage adherence. As Mary Poppins sang so engagingly, 'A spoonful of sugar helps the medicine go down'.

TABLE 28.2 Some drugs reported to cause hyperglycaemia or hypoglycaemia

HYPERGLYCAEMIA	HYPOGLYCAEMIA
(Hence, insulin requirements may need to be increased)	(Hence, insulin requirements may need to be reduced)
Antipsychotics (some)	Angiotensin-converting enzyme inhibitors
Calcineurin inhibitors	α-blockers
Glucagon	Anabolic steroids (some)
Glucocorticosteroids	Aspirin (analgesic doses)
Growth hormones	β-blockers (non-selective)
Loop diuretics	Disopyramide
Phenytoin	Growth hormones
Progestogens (oral contraceptives)	Insulins
Protease inhibitors	Monoamine oxidase inhibitors
Sympathomimetics (adrenaline [epinephrine], high-dose salbutamol)	Oral hypoglycaemics
Thiazide diuretics	Quinine
Thyroid hormones	Sulfonamides
Tricyclic antidepressants	
Social drugs: amphetamines, cocaine, psychedelics, caffeine drinks (large amounts), marijuana, tobacco/nicotine	Social drugs: ethanol (alcohol)

Note: Growth hormone and its analogues can either increase or decrease blood glucose concentrations. β-blockers may mask the symptoms of hypoglycaemia.
Sources: Australian Medicines Handbook 2021; MIMS Annual Online (see 'Online resources').

foods and drinks; syrup and elixir formulations frequently have 50–70% weight per volume sucrose plus other calorigenic sweetening agents. 'Sugar-free' formulations are available for some antibiotic mixtures and lozenges, analgesics, antiepileptic agents, antihistamines and antiasthma drugs.

Hypoglycaemia

Hypoglycaemia (BGL $<$ 3.5 mmol/L) can occur rapidly from excess insulin and is also a common adverse effect of treatment with a sulfonylurea or dipeptidyl peptidase-4 inhibitor (DPP4) inhibitor (Amiel et al. 2019). Hypoglycaemia can also occur from unexpectedly high levels of exercise, inadequate food intake or as an adverse effect of various drugs (Table 28.2). People (and their carers) need to detect early symptoms of a 'hypo': faintness, anxiety, blurred vision, cold sweating, pallor, confusion, difficulty in concentrating, drowsiness, headache, nausea, increased pulse rate, shakiness, weakness and increased appetite (Fig 28.3). Unless treated with an oral rapidly absorbed glucose source, this can lead to coma and death. Chronic hypoglycaemia is particularly dangerous for young people with diabetes, as the developing brain is dependent on glucose as an energy source; management of children with diabetes thus errs on the side of hyperglycaemia.

Treatment is with hyperglycaemic agents:

- In mild-to-moderate hypoglycaemia, a readily available sugar source such as jellybeans, honey or a sweet drink can be administered, followed by slowly absorbed complex carbohydrates such as bread or dried fruit.
- Glucose can be administered orally, in adults 10–20 g, repeated in 10 minutes if necessary.
- In severe hypoglycaemia, if the person is unconscious or cannot take oral glucose, glucagon is administered SC or IM (Drug Monograph 28.1).
- People at risk of developing hypoglycaemia may carry a glucagon injection kit, and their families or carers should know how to administer it. Glucagon is commonly carried in ambulances and administered by paramedics.

Insulin replacement

By the time type 1 diabetes is diagnosed, those affected usually have no functioning pancreatic islet tissue remaining, so are dependent on an exogenous source of insulin as lifesaving, lifelong therapy (hence the term 'insulin-dependent diabetes mellitus'). Other antihyperglycaemic drugs cannot be used in these people because their actions depend on there being some remaining normally functioning islet tissue and/or insulin receptors.

Insulin formulations

Sources

Early sources of insulin were beef (bovine) or pig (porcine) pancreas. Preparations available in Australia

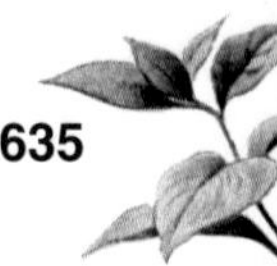

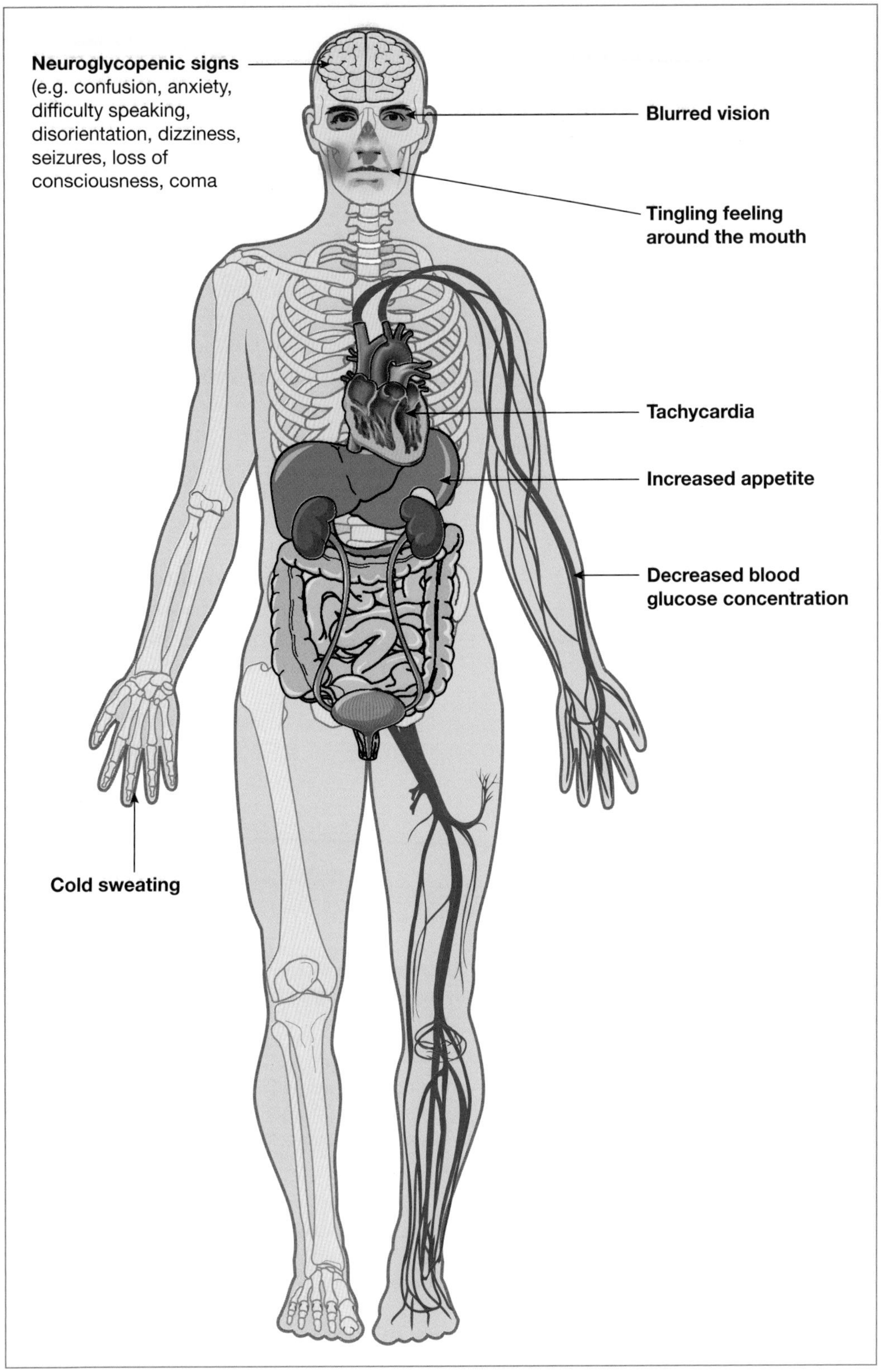

Neuroglycopenic signs (e.g. confusion, anxiety, difficulty speaking, disorientation, dizziness, seizures, loss of consciousness, coma

Blurred vision

Tingling feeling around the mouth

Tachycardia

Increased appetite

Decreased blood glucose concentration

Cold sweating

FIGURE 28.3 Signs of hypoglycaemia

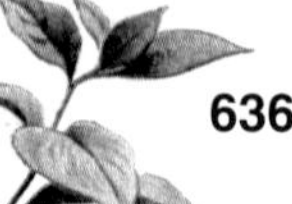

KEY POINTS

Insulin, glucagon and diabetes mellitus

- The primary hormones of the pancreas, insulin and glucagon, are involved in the regulation of blood glucose levels and storage of nutrients as fuels.
- Glucagon release is increased when blood glucose levels fall, which facilitates the breakdown of liver glycogen to raise and restore blood glucose levels. Glucagon also stimulates insulin secretion, inhibits further release of glucagon and maintains carbohydrate homeostasis.
- Glucagon and glucose are hyperglycaemic agents for treating hypoglycaemia.
- Insulin facilitates the uptake of glucose into cells and promotes storage of glycogen, lipids and protein.
- Incretins increase insulin secretion and regulate many gastrointestinal metabolic functions.
- Diabetes mellitus is a disorder of carbohydrate metabolism resulting from insulin deficiency or resistance. Diabetes mellitus is classified as type 1 (insulin-dependent diabetes or juvenile-onset diabetes) or type 2 (non-insulin-dependent diabetes or maturity-onset diabetes).
- Prevalence of diabetes is increasing worldwide. Long-term complications can be severe and the risk minimised by tight control of blood glucose levels.

now are either human insulin (synthesised by chemical alteration of porcine insulin or by recombinant DNA technology) or bovine insulin (rarely used now), which differs from human insulin by three amino acids. Insulins produced by recombinant DNA technology are identified by the suffixes *rys*, recombinant yeast *Saccharomyces cerevisiae*, or *rbe*, recombinant bacteria *Escherichia coli*; they are identical to insulin produced by the human pancreas; see Drug Monograph 28.2.

Time-course of formulations

Insulins have been formulated in different ways to alter their pharmacokinetic properties. In the very-short- and new long-acting analogues, minor changes are

Drug Monograph 28.1
Glucagon

Indication
Treatment of severe hypoglycaemia.

Mechanism
Glucagon is a 29-amino-acids protein (peptide hormone), released from pancreatic A cells. It increases plasma levels of glucose by decreasing glycogen synthesis and promoting glycogenolysis, gluconeogenesis, fat breakdown and degradation of protein.

Indications
Glucagon is indicated in severe hypoglycaemia in people with diabetes, and to terminate insulin coma. It is ineffective for chronic hypoglycaemia, starvation and adrenal insufficiency, when liver glycogen is unavailable. It is also used as an adjunct for gastrointestinal radiography as it produces relaxation and decreases peristalsis; and in acute overdose of β-blockers or calcium channel blockers.

Pharmacokinetics
Glucagon must be parenterally administered (IM, IV or SC). It has a half-life of 5–10 minutes; onset of hyperglycaemic action depends on route of administration: IV, 5–20 minutes; IM, 15 minutes; and SC, 30–45 minutes. Its duration of action is 1.5 hours. It is bound in the liver, kidneys and other organs, and is metabolised in the blood and organs.

Adverse reactions
No significant drug interactions are reported. Adverse effects are mild and may include nausea or vomiting and an allergic reaction. It is safe in pregnancy and lactation, but is contraindicated in people with glucagon hypersensitivity, phaeochromocytoma or a history of insulinoma. The adolescent and adult dose for hypoglycaemia is 1 mg IM, IV or SC, and for a child under 25 kg: 0.5 mg. If there is no response within 10 minutes, IV glucose is required. When a person regains consciousness, complex carbohydrates are administered orally.

Dosage and administration
Glucagon is presented as an emergency kit with syringe, 1 mg glucagon plus sterile water for injections.

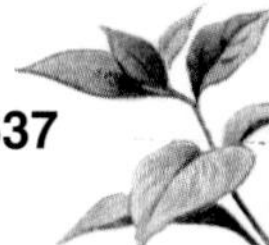

Drug Monograph 28.2
Human insulin

Indications

Insulin is indicated in type 1 diabetes, and in type 2 diabetes during emergencies, in stress situations, during pregnancy or as an adjunct to treatment with OHAs. The wide variety of insulins available (including combination mixtures) allows titration of dose to achieve tight blood glucose control depending on the person's needs and lifestyle.

Pharmacokinetics

The onset, time to peak and duration of action depend on types and proportions of insulin used. Insulin injected SC is gradually leached from the injection site into the bloodstream and will circulate to tissues where it acts, especially in liver, muscles and fat. Insulin is metabolised and inactivated rapidly in most tissues of the body; the disulfide bonds are cleaved, then the peptide chains are broken down into amino acids. However, biological activity continues much longer.

Drug interactions

Many drugs (prescribed, OTC and social) can affect BGL and thus interact with insulin and impair diabetes control – in particular, corticosteroids, β-blockers, thiazide diuretics and ACE inhibitors (Table 28.2); dosage adjustments of insulin may be necessary. β-blockers can mask the symptoms of hypoglycaemia and prolong it by blocking gluconeogenesis.

Adverse reactions

Rare with human insulin; allergic reactions and lipodystrophy (breakdown of subcutaneous fat) can occur. Overdose is indicated by symptoms of hypoglycaemia: faintness, sweating and tremor (see earlier description).

Warnings and contraindications

Insulin requirements may increase in acute trauma or illness, and during prolonged surgery. Insulin is contraindicated in those with hypoglycaemia or hypersensitivity to human insulin solutions. Changes in type, brand or species of insulin should be made cautiously. Insulin is safe in pregnancy and breastfeeding.

Dosage and administration

Dosage depends on the person's weight, diet and lifestyle and on the type of insulin and regimen used; dosage is individualised by monitoring blood glucose levels. Typical dose is 0.5–0.8 IU/kg body weight/day (see later under 'Dosage Regimens').

made in the amino acid sequences of the protein (Fig 28.1); pharmacodynamic actions and mechanisms are unaltered. Most contain 100 IU/mL. The range of formulations available allows titration of dosage to optimise BGL control and minimise fluctuations (Table 28.3 and Fig 28.4). (Note that the time-course of action may vary among individuals, or at different times in the same person, and is dependent on site of injection, blood supply, body temperature, physical activity, etc.)

Formulations are described as very- or ultra-short-acting (or rapid), short-acting, intermediate-acting or long-acting.

- *Ultra-short-acting synthetic analogues:* Insulin lispro, insulin aspart and insulin glulisine; also called 'post-prandial', very-short or rapid. Two or three amino acids in human insulin have been changed. Rapid onset of action, so administered as a 'bolus' immediately before or after a meal. Short duration of action (3–5 hours). People with type 1 diabetes usually require concurrent use of an intermediate- or long-acting product to provide basal insulin activity.
- *Short- and intermediate-acting (the early insulins):* Neutral insulin, isophane insulin (also known as neutral protamine Hagedorn, NPH).
- *'Basal'/long-acting insulins:* Their long, flat absorption profiles give them a more reproducible effect than older formulations. *Insulin glargine* has a slightly different amino acid sequence; after injection, microcrystals form in the tissues and insulin is slowly released. It may cause pain on injection and must not be mixed with other insulins. *Insulin detemir* has a fatty acid compound attached to the insulin molecule, providing slow release. Detemir formulations may cause local reactions but are less likely than other insulins to cause weight gain.
- *Premixed commercial combination formulations:* These are 30/70 or 50/50 mixtures of short-acting plus intermediate-acting insulins, or ultra-short plus long-acting insulins, providing varying pharmacokinetic characteristics dependent on proportions in the mixture. They suffer the disadvantage of all fixed-dose combinations: the dose of an individual component cannot be varied when needed.

TABLE 28.3 Characteristics of insulin preparations after subcutaneous administration

INSULINS	ONSET (h)	PEAK EFFECT (h)	DURATION OF ACTION (h)
Ultra-short-acting (rapid)[a]			
Insulin lispro and insulin aspart	0.25	1–3	3–5
Insulin glulisine	0.25	1	3–5
Short-acting[a]			
Neutral insulin	0.5	2–3	6–8
Intermediate-acting			
Isophane insulin (NPH insulin)	1–2.5	4–12	16–24
Long-acting			
Insulin glargine (basal insulin analogue) (100 IU/mL)	1–2	(no peak)	24
Insulin glargine (basal insulin analogue) (300 IU/mL)	1–6	(no peak)	24–36
Insulin detemir	1–2	3–14	12–24
Typical combination#			
Neutral human insulin (30%) and isophane insulin (70%) (Humulin 30/70)	0.5–1	2–12	16–24

[a] These soluble insulins may be administered IV under medical supervision. Intravenously, the onset of action is within 10–30 minutes, peak effect is within 15–30 minutes, and duration of action is 30–60 minutes. # Other combinations have properties combining those of the constituents.

Sources: Australian Medicines Handbook 2021; MIMS Annual Online (see 'Online resources'); product information from Novo Nordisk.

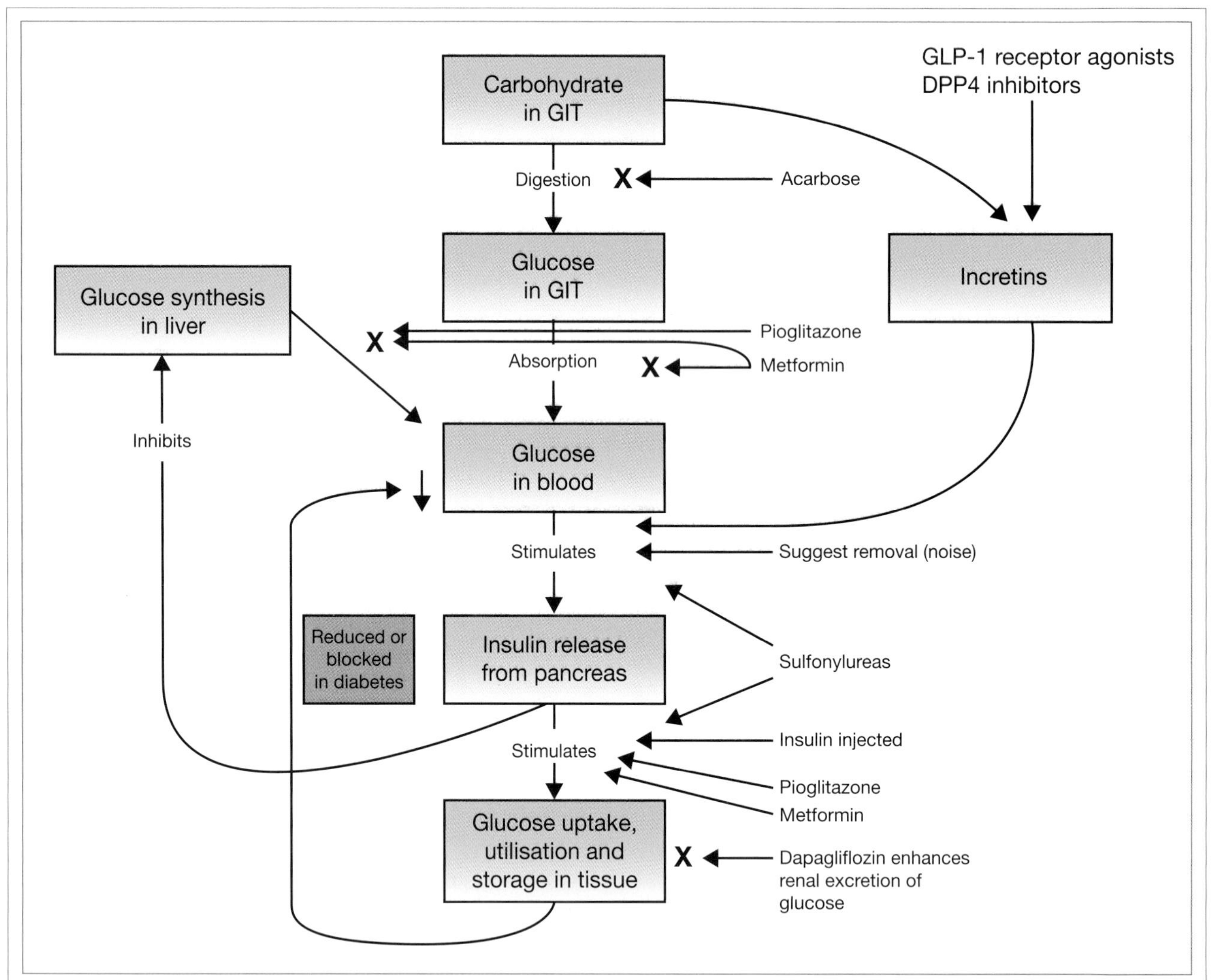

FIGURE 28.4 Mechanisms of action of oral antihyperglycaemic drugs (and injected insulin and GLP-1 receptor agonists)

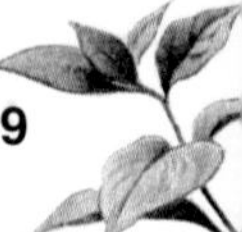

Insulin administration

Routes of administration

Insulins are supplied in vials, usual strength 100 IU/mL, for use with a syringe, or prepacked in cartridge 'pens', facilitating injection and improving convenience and adherence. Vials or cartridges of insoluble preparations should be rotated and inverted gently before a dose is withdrawn, to resuspend the protein; vigorous shaking or freezing could denature the protein. Insulin stocks not in use should be refrigerated (2–8°C), but the vial or cartridge currently in use is stable at room temperature (Khurana & Gupta 2019). The older-type insulin formulations were all chemically compatible and could be mixed, but some newer forms cannot, especially insulins detemir and glargine.

Insulin (short-acting) is usually administered 'ac, SC' – that is, before meals (15–30 minutes before), subcutaneously. Injection sites are alternated, rotating around the abdomen and thighs, to minimise adverse local effects from injections. In an emergency (diabetic ketoacidosis), short-acting insulins can be administered IV by infusion or IM.

Portable battery-operated, computer-programmed pumps delivering insulin via an implanted SC catheter may improve diabetic control. The insulin pump does not monitor the BGL but is programmed based on the person's estimated daily insulin needs, diet and physical exercise. Pumps are expensive, subject to mechanical failure and require careful maintenance.

Insulin dosage and regimens

There is no standard dose of insulin in diabetes; requirements depend on lifestyle, weight, diet, exercise levels, stress, illness and pregnancy. People are taught to carry out self-monitoring of blood glucose, and to adjust their insulin doses to avoid hypoglycaemia or hyperglycaemia and prevent long-term complications. A typical daily dose might be in the order of 0.7 IU/kg (reflecting the average pancreatic production of about 50 IU per day) split into two to four injections and, possibly, two or three different types of insulin. Treatment programs need to be reviewed and adjusted regularly, depending on physical growth, illness, surgery, development of anti-insulin antibodies, concomitant administration of drugs, changes in lifestyle, missing a meal or doing unexpected exercise.

'Basal–bolus' regimen

A bolus dose of short-acting insulin is given before each meal, plus some intermediate- or long-acting insulin at bedtime. This regimen is preferred; it is demanding, requiring multiple daily injections, but mimics well the body's natural rhythms of insulin release.

'Split–mixed' regimen

The total daily dose in units is estimated, and this is split between 1/3 short-acting and 2/3 intermediate- or long-acting insulins, with 2/3 of the total mixture given before breakfast and the other 1/3 before the evening meal.

Dosage in altered circumstances

As well as regular self-monitoring of BGL and subsequent adjustment of insulin dosage, there are many clinical situations in which dosage is altered:

- pregnancy – insulin is usually the drug of choice to control diabetes; insulin requirements may drop for 24–72 hours after delivery and slowly return to pre-pregnancy levels in about 6 weeks (Clinical Focus Box 28.3)
- exercising – requires increased caloric intake and/or reduced insulin dose

---

CLINICAL FOCUS BOX 28.3

Insulin in gestational diabetes

Mrs MG is a 32-year-old woman having her third child. She has no background risk factors for diabetes. She has a routine oral glucose tolerance test at 28 weeks' gestation, which diagnoses gestational diabetes mellitus. She is referred to a dietitian at the hospital and attends hospital-run diabetes education classes about changes she can make to her diet and exercise routines. She meets with a diabetes educator, who teaches her how to measure her blood glucose levels via a finger-prick test four times a day. Every time she returns to antenatal clinic, her blood glucose readings are reviewed. Up until 32 weeks' gestation, they remain within the desired range (< 5.5 mmol/L fasting sugar first thing in the morning, and < 6.7 mmol/L 2 hours after each meal). At her 32-week visit, however, several results are above these limits, so she is commenced on metformin (oral 1 g twice daily). By 34 weeks' gestation, her blood glucose levels are again above the recommended ranges, so low-dose insulin is commenced: 4 units of NovoRapid (insulin aspart) with each meal. Her blood glucose readings are reviewed at each weekly antenatal visit and insulin requirements adjusted as needed. By the time she delivers, at 39 weeks' gestation, she is on 12 units of NovoRapid with each meal and 20 units of Protophane (isophane) at night. She eventually has a forceps delivery of a healthy 3.8 kg baby boy. She is discharged into the care of her GP; repeating the glucose tolerance test at 6 weeks postpartum is normal.

Source: Acknowledgments to Dr Alison Bryant-Smith, MRCOG (personal communication). See also Endocrinology Expert Group; National Institute for Health and Care Excellence (UK) and Australasian Diabetes in Pregnancy Society – see 'Online resources'.

- other illnesses – metabolic instability can lead to hyperglycaemia and diabetic ketoacidosis; insulin requirements usually increase by 15–20%
- vomiting – sugary drinks should replace solid food; if vomiting lasts more than 6 hours, the person should be admitted to hospital care
- fasting – some basal insulin is still required, plus some IV glucose
- surgical procedures – may be covered with IV glucose and IV or SC insulin
- international travel – people on insulin are advised to take copies of prescriptions and medical records, plus double their anticipated insulin needs and carbohydrate snacks.

KEY POINTS

Insulin

- People with type 1 diabetes require lifelong insulin replacement; BGL, diet and lifestyle factors must be controlled, and a multidisciplinary clinical team is usually involved.
- Various formulations of human or bovine insulins are available, with differing pharmacokinetic characteristics; dosage regimen is determined by results of self-monitored blood glucose estimations.
- Dosing may need to be altered in times of stress and pregnancy.

Management of type 2 diabetes

Type 2 diabetes

Type 2 diabetes was previously known as maturity-onset diabetes, as patients were typically middle-aged to elderly; however, with increasing obesity and physical inactivity in populations, young people – and even children – are developing it. Males and females are affected equally. About 85% of people with diabetes have type 2; they generally have some functioning pancreatic islet cells, so are not fully dependent on insulin for survival. There is reduced insulin production and secretion (especially the early phase after glucose load) and/or insulin resistance (the body does not respond to insulin effectively) because of receptor and post-receptor defects.

Risk factors include advancing age, obesity, positive family history, cardiovascular disease, hypokalaemia following the use of thiazide diuretics and polycystic ovary syndrome in women. The condition comes on gradually, with glucose intolerance often associated with hypertension and hyperlipidaemia. Although usually older at the time of diagnosis, people with type 2 diabetes are still at risk of long-term complications and of hyperosmolar coma, but diabetic ketoacidosis is rare.

Lifestyle factors in type 2 diabetes

Weight reduction with diet control and increased exercise are of primary importance and may be all that is required to prevent progression from impaired glucose tolerance to overt type 2 diabetes. If symptoms persist after weight reduction, people may also need antihyperglycaemic drugs; the target BGL is 4 to 8 mmol/L (fasting and pre-prandial) and below 10 mmol/L (postprandial). People with type 2 diabetes benefit from tight control of blood glucose, blood pressure and hyperlipidaemia. Lifestyle changes suitable for preventing type 2 diabetes (healthy eating, regular exercise, healthy body weight, limited alcohol intake and ceasing cigarette smoking) will bring about major improvements in control of most cardiovascular diseases – a 'type 2 lifestyle plan'. Recommended exercise levels are: 210 minutes (3.5 hours) moderate-intensity or 125 minutes (about 2 hours) vigorous-intensity exercise per week.

Metabolic syndrome

The 'metabolic syndrome' was first defined by the World Health Organization in 1998; the definition now specifies five risk factors: high serum triglycerides, low high-density lipoprotein cholesterol level, hypertension, elevated fasting blood glucose and abdominal obesity (increased waist circumference) – a combination of any three of these is diagnostic. Metabolic syndrome is an insidious inflammatory state, with impaired inflammation, endothelial function and coagulation, predisposing people to cardiovascular disease. Obesity, inactivity, ageing, foodstuffs including *trans* fats, branched-chain amino acids, alcohol and fructose promote insulin resistance and excessive insulin secretion, leading eventually to insulin deficiency, type 2 diabetes and increased morbidity and mortality from chronic cardiovascular and kidney disease.

Prevalence has been estimated to be as high as one-third of the adult Australian population. In adolescents, high consumption of fast foods and sugar-sweetened drinks and low levels of physical activity are particularly linked with obesity, insulin resistance and metabolic syndrome.

Treatment

It is recommended that large-scale community intervention programs focus on increasing physical activity and healthier food options (fruit, vegetables, whole grains, dairy products and unsaturated fats), especially for children. Weight-reduction surgery is very effective in treatment, emphasising the central role of obesity. Concomitant drugs that exacerbate central obesity should be reviewed, including certain antipsychotics, antidepressants, anticonvulsants and β-blockers.

Drugs trialled include orlistat (for obesity), OHAs (for insulin resistance and hyperglycaemia), statins and fibrates (for dyslipidaemia) and antihypertensive drugs. Dietary supplements and alternative therapies that have some benefit include eicosapentaenoic acid and docosahexaenoic acid (in fish oils), soy proteins, dietary fibre, polyphenolic compounds, modest wine intake and green tea.

Drugs for type 2 diabetes

Oral antihyperglycaemic drugs for type 2 diabetes were first used in diabetes therapy in the 1950s; they are not useful in type 1 diabetes, as they depend for their action on some residual insulin secretion or functioning insulin receptors. Adjunctive drugs used may alter the absorption of carbohydrates, help reduce obesity or treat cardiovascular risk factors.

Metformin is recommended as first-line therapy unless contraindicated (as in renal, hepatic or cardiac impairment, and in the very elderly). If glycaemic management is not achieved a second antihyperglycaemic treatment should be introduced. Antiglycaemic treatments for type 2 diabetes include sulfonylureas, DPP4 inhibitor, GLP-1 analogues, SGLT2 inhibitors, acarbose and pioglitazone. Combination products with two antihyperglycaemic drugs are available.

Antihyperglycaemic drugs act by various mechanisms, summarised in Figure 28.4; they may stimulate further insulin release, lower insulin resistance, sensitise cells to the actions of insulin, reduce glucose load, enhance functions of incretins or alter absorption of carbohydrates. They are classified as insulin sensitisers (metformin, thiazolidinediones), insulin secretagogues (sulfonylureas), incretin-mimetics (GLP-1 analogues), incretin enhancers (DPP4 inhibitor) or may reduce carbohydrate absorption or enhance renal excretion of glucose. (See Table 28.4 for a summary of antihyperglycaemic drugs, their pharmacokinetic parameters and usual adult doses.)

The choice of drug depends on several factors, including the person's weight, pancreatic, renal and liver functions and response to trialled drugs. Any antihyperglycaemic drug's effectiveness may decrease over time (secondary failure), due to increased severity of disease or decreased responsiveness to the drug; dosage may need adjustment. It is estimated that 50% of type 2 diabetics will require insulin within 10 years of diagnosis; typically, the person is stabilised on an antihyperglycaemic drug, and an intermediate- or long-acting insulin is administered at night.

Metformin, the last biguanide standing

Metformin, a biguanide, is the first-line treatment of type 2 diabetes (Drug Monograph 28.3). The first drug in this drug class, phenformin, was withdrawn due to its association with potentially life-threatening lactic acidosis. Metformin subsequently fell from favour, but it has been associated only rarely with this complication and is the drug of first choice for all those with type 2 diabetes in many countries. Metformin is usually continued lifelong in people with type 2 diabetes unless contraindicated.

Actions, mechanisms and indications

Its mechanism of action is not completely understood; however, it is known to:

- increase glucose uptake and utilisation in skeletal muscle (thus reducing insulin resistance)
- reduce glucose production in the liver (gluconeogenesis)
- reduce low- and very-low-density lipoproteins
- increase insulin sensitivity, via increased number of receptors and affinity for receptors.

It does not affect the pancreatic B cells, so it does not increase insulin release and is unlikely to cause hypoglycaemia. Metformin is available in combination formulations with other antihypertensives (DPP4 inhibitors, SGLT2 inhibitors, sulfonylureas) emphasising the pivotal role of metformin as first-line therapy.

Currently, metformin is contraindicated in those at risk of lactic acidosis – that is, those with liver disease, acidosis, the elderly and those taking alcohol or drugs that raise metformin levels. It can be administered cautiously in low doses to those with mild renal disease provided treatment is closely monitored.

Sulfonylureas

Mechanisms and actions

The sulfonylureas were developed from sulfonamide antibacterial agents, when it was noticed that some people taking sulfonamides had lowered BGL. Their mechanism of action is to bind to receptors and block ATP-sensitive potassium channels (K-ATP), thus blocking potassium efflux and causing cell depolarisation, calcium entry and insulin secretion from pancreatic B cells. Sulfonylureas also increase the number of insulin receptors, decrease insulin uptake by peripheral tissues and reduce hepatic glycogenolysis. Hence, they reduce BGL in people with a functioning pancreas and, over the long term, diabetic complications.

Second-generation sulfonylureas include glibenclamide, glipizide, gliclazide and glimepiride. All are taken just before or with meals to minimise hypoglycaemia. Choice is made on pharmacokinetic parameters, as those with long half-lives (e.g. glimeperide) are riskier in elderly people. Those excreted as active drug or metabolites are riskier in those with renal disease, and those eliminated mainly by hepatic inactivation are riskier in people with liver disease.

Adverse reactions and interactions

Common adverse effects include hypoglycaemia, weight gain, GIT and taste disturbances and rashes. Serious blood disorders and allergic reactions occur rarely. Interactions are common with drugs involved with

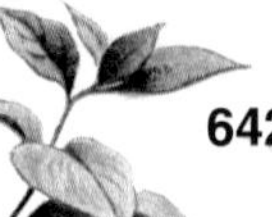

Drug Monograph 28.3
Metformin

Metformin is a biguanide, an oral antihyperglycaemic agent. (For actions and mechanisms, see text.) It rarely causes hypoglycaemia or weight gain.

Indications
Metformin is indicated for treating uncomplicated type 2 diabetes in adults and children aged over 10 years, when diabetes is not controlled by diet and exercise; it may be given as adjunct therapy with insulin or another OHA. It reduces the risk of diabetes-associated complications or mortality. It is being used to treat anovulatory infertility due to polycystic ovary syndrome, and is being trialled in some cancers.

Pharmacokinetics
Metformin is absorbed after an oral dose along the length of the GIT. It has a short half-life (5–10 hours) and is excreted unchanged in the urine (Table 28.4).

Drug interactions
Drug interactions occur with alcohol (increased risk of lactic acidosis) and any drugs that impair glucose tolerance, cause hyper- or hypoglycaemia or reduce clearance of metformin (including cimetidine, dolutegravir, topiramate, trimethoprim and warfarin). Blood glucose levels should be monitored whenever another drug is introduced, as dosage adjustment may be necessary (see also Table 28.2).

Adverse reactions
Adverse reactions include gastrointestinal upsets such as nausea, vomiting, anorexia and diarrhoea (common) and, rarely, lactic acidosis, acute hepatitis or vitamin B12-deficiency anaemia.

Warnings and contraindications
Use with caution in people with renal or GIT problems and conditions affecting blood glucose levels. Use is avoided in people with metformin hypersensitivity, severe liver or kidney disease, lactic acidosis, cardiac disorders, severe burns, dehydration or severe infections, in people in diabetic coma or with ketoacidosis and in those who have recently had major surgery or trauma. The Australian Pregnancy Safety classification is C; it is recommended that pregnant and lactating women requiring hypoglycaemic therapy use insulin.

Dosage and administration
Doses are taken orally with meals; dosage is individualised and based on BGL. Initial dosage is low to minimise GIT adverse effects: 500 mg once or twice daily, gradually increasing to 1 g three times daily if necessary, then reducing; or extended-release form once daily, increasing to maximum of 2 g/day.

CYP2C9 metabolic pathways (see Australian Medicines Handbook 2021, Table D1 – 4 Drugs and CYP enzymes), alcohol, drugs that compete for protein-binding sites, and drugs affecting BGL (Table 28.2).

Incretin-based antihyperglycaemic agents
Incretins are peptide hormones that are released from the GIT in response to food; those currently known are GIP and GLP-1 (see earlier under 'Control of Blood Glucose Levels' and Fig 28.2). People with type 2 diabetes have a markedly lowered response to incretins, so drugs that enhance incretin actions provide a different mode of action. In Australia, they are currently only approved as add-on therapy, usually with metformin. Due to limited data, they are not recommended for use in pregnancy or lactation.

Incretin-enhancers (DPP-4 inhibitors or 'gliptins')
Sitagliptin, linagliptin, saxagliptin, vildagliptin and alogliptin inhibit DPP4, the enzyme that inactivates GLP-1 and GIP; they have long half-lives and can be administered orally once daily. DPP4 inhibitors increase incretin levels and B-cell glucose sensitivity in those with type 2 diabetes to normal levels, and reduce glucagon secretion and preserve B-cell mass. They are usually used in combination with another oral antihyperglycaemic drugs (e.g. metformin). They appear to have few adverse effects (mainly gastrointestinal and musculoskeletal complaints) and the risk of hypoglycaemia with DPP4 inhibitors is low (Deacon 2020).

Incretin-mimetics (GLP-1 analogues)
Dulaglutide, liraglutide, exenatide and semaglutide are all GLP-1 analogues. GLP-1 analogues are small peptides that bind to and activate the GLP-1 receptor but are resistant to inactivation by the DPP4 enzyme so have long-lasting activity. As peptides, they must be given by injection. All GLP-1 analogues are given by subcutaneous injection. Exenatide was the first incretin-mimetic; liraglutide has a longer half-life and is also indicated as adjunct therapy in obesity (Ch 42). They are proving safe

and effective in those unable to maintain glycaemic control with diet, exercise and standard OHAs. They are used as adjunct therapy with basal insulin and/or metformin or another OHA. The GLP-1 agonists delay gastric emptying, and so slow glucose absorption and reduce appetite; they induce weight loss but frequently cause transient nausea, dyspepsia and diarrhoea; hypoglycaemia can occur, and immune reactions against the peptides. Pancreatitis is a serious potential adverse event that is being monitored (Nauck et al. 2021).

Thiazolidinediones ('glitazones')

Mechanisms and actions

Pioglitazone is a thiazolidinedione. Its mechanism of action is via activation of the peroxisome proliferator-activated (PPAR)-gamma receptor, a nuclear receptor that regulates gene transcription, especially in adipocytes, via proteins including GLUT-4 (the principal glucose transporter protein), lipoprotein lipase and transporter and binding proteins for fatty acids. They enhance the sensitivity of peripheral tissues and the liver to insulin and thus reduce insulin resistance. Circulating free fatty acid levels and hepatic glucose output are reduced.

Reductions in BGLs occur soon after starting treatment, but the full effect on insulin sensitivity is not seen for several weeks. Pioglitazone can be used in combination with metformin and/or sulfonylureas or insulin.

Adverse effects include anaemia, peripheral oedema, weight gain and increased risk of heart failure and peripheral limb fractures; liver enzymes should be monitored. Pioglitazone appears to be safer with respect to cardiovascular risk factors, but prolonged use may be associated with increased risk of bladder cancer.

Alpha-glucosidase inhibitor: acarbose

Acarbose is an oligosaccharide that inhibits α-glucosidase and thus delays digestion and absorption of carbohydrates in the small intestine, reducing glucose load. It is indicated as an adjunct to diet for the treatment of type 2 diabetes; it may be given alone or in combination with a sulfonylurea. It does not increase insulin secretion or cause lactic acidosis or weight gain.

It is taken orally (initial dose 50 mg) before or at the beginning of a meal; absorption of acarbose is intentionally minimal (around 2%) as its actions are confined in the gut. Later, metabolites (35%) may be absorbed from the GIT (for pharmacokinetics, see Table 28.4). Drug interactions occur particularly with drugs that affect absorption in the intestine, such as digestive enzymes and cholestyramine. The most frequent adverse reactions are disturbed gut functions. If hypoglycaemia occurs, it should be treated with glucose rather than sucrose, as the absorption of sucrose will be impaired by the drug. As the drug is relatively new, use in pregnancy and renal impairment is not advised.

SGLT2 inhibitors: ('-flozin')

Dapagliflozin, empagliflozin and ertugliflozin are selective, reversible inhibitors of the sodium-glucose co-transporter 2 (SGLT2). SGLT2 causes reabsorption of glucose in the renal tubules. Inhibiting SGLT2 produces glycosuria (excess sugar in the urine) and osmotic diuresis, reduces hyperglycaemia and reduces weight and fluid load. SGLT2 inhibitor actions affect renal function and do not depend on insulin secretion or sensitivity. Potential risks include urinary and genital tract infections, thirst, hypovolaemia, increased haematocrit and bone

TABLE 28.4 Antihyperglycaemic drugs: pharmacokinetics and usual adult doses

DRUG	ROUTE	PEAK IN PLASMA (h)	HALF-LIFE (h)	PROTEIN BINDING	USUAL ADULT MAINTENANCE DOSE[a]	COMMENTS
Biguanide						
Metformin	Oral	2–3	3	Not bound	500–1000 mg bd or tid	Risk of lactic acidosis. Take with food to reduce nausea and vomiting. (R) Not metabolised
Sulfonylureas						
Glibenclamide	Oral	2–6	2–10	99%	2.5–20 mg/day	(H) (R) (A)
Gliclazide	Oral	4–6	12	94%	30–320 mg/day (max single dose 160 mg)	(H) (R)
Glimepiride	Oral	2.5	5–8	> 99%	1–4 mg once/day	(R) (A)
Glipizide	Oral	2	2–4	98%	5–40 mg before meals in divided doses	(H) (R)
Dipeptidylpeptidase-4 (DPP-4) inhibitors (gliptins)						
Alogliptin	Oral	1–2	21	20%	25 mg/day	Used in combination with other antihyperglycaemic agents or as monotherapy; lower dose in moderate-to-severe renal failure (D: saxagliptin)
Linagliptin	Oral	1.5	3-phase	90%	5 mg/day	
Saxagliptin	Oral	2	2.5	Not bound	5 mg/day	
Sitagliptin	Oral	1–4	12.4	Low (38%)	100 mg/day	
Vildagliptin	Oral	1.75	2–3	9%	50–100 mg/day	

Continued

TABLE 28.4 Antihyperglycaemic drugs: pharmacokinetics and usual adult doses—cont'd

DRUG	ROUTE	PEAK IN PLASMA (h)	HALF-LIFE (h)	PROTEIN BINDING	USUAL ADULT MAINTENANCE DOSE[a]	COMMENTS
Glucagon-like peptide-1 (GLP-1) receptor agonists						
Dulaglutide	Subcutaneous	48 h	120	N/A	1.5 mg once weekly	Used in combination with other antihyperglycaemic agents; avoid in severe kidney impairment.
Exenatide	Subcutaneous	2.1	2.4	N/A	5–10 microgram bd	
Liraglutide	Subcutaneous	8–12	13	98%	0.6–1.8 mg/day SC	
Thiazolidinediones (TZD)						
Pioglitazone	Oral	2–4	5–23	> 99%	15–45 mg/day	
Sodium-glucose co-transporter 2 (SGLT2) inhibitors						
Dapagliflozin	Oral	2	13	91%	10 mg once daily with or without meals	Efficacy is reduced in renal impairment
Empagliflozin	Oral	1.3–3	21	20%	10–25 mg/day	
Ertugliflozin	Oral	0.5–1.5	11–17	94–96%	5–15 mg daily	
Alpha 1 glucosidase inhibitor						
Acarbose	Oral	1	2	< 2% absorbed	50–200 mg tid with meals	Most effective if given with high-fibre diet

A = active metabolites; bd = twice daily; H = hepatic impairment leads to increased risk of hypoglycaemia; N/A = not available or not applicable; R = renal impairment leads to increased risk of hypoglycaemia; tid = three times daily.
D = May be given as divided doses.
Source: Adapted from data in Medsafe website and Australian Medicines Handbook 2021. Product information sheets should be consulted for detailed dosing advice.

fractures risks. Monitoring of renal function is recommended. SGLT2 inhibitors are contraindicated in moderate–severe renal impairment, severe hepatic impairment, pregnancy and lactation.

KEY POINTS

Pharmacological management of type 2 diabetes

- Type 2 diabetes is managed by lifestyle modification (diet and weight reduction) and, if necessary, antihyperglycaemic drugs.
- Antihyperglycaemic drugs acting by different mechanisms are available: metformin, sulfonylureas, incretin mimetics and enhancers and SGLT2 inhibitors; thiazolidinediones ('glitazones') and acarbose.
- Choice of treatment is made depending on the person's weight, response and liver and kidney functions.
- Many people with type 2 diabetes will be taking two or more antihyperglycaemic drugs to achieve glycaemic targets.
- People with type 2 diabetes may require insulin at some stage.

DRUGS AT A GLANCE
Antihyperglycaemic drugs

PHARMACOLOGICAL GROUP AND EFFECT	KEY EXAMPLES	CLINICAL USE
Insulins • Increase the uptake of glucose into cells = increased glucose metabolism • Decrease the body's production of glucose • Decrease lipolysis	Ultra-short-acting -aspart, -lispro	Treat type 1, type 2 and gestational diabetes mellitus Control blood glucose concentration
	Short-acting -neutral	
	Intermediate-acting -isophane	
	Long-acting (basal) - detemir, -glargine,	
	Biphasic insulins (mixed) combinations with various ratios of ultra-short/neutral/isophane insulins	

Biguanide • Decreases glucose production in the liver • Increases peripheral utilisation of glucose	Metformin	Treat type 2 diabetes mellitus Treat diabetes in children aged over 10 years
Sulfonylureas • Increase secretion of insulin from the pancreas • Decrease insulin resistance	Glibenclamide, gliclazide, glimepiride, glipizide	Treat type 2 diabetes mellitus
DPP4 inhibitors (gliptins) • Increase incretins • Increase glucose dependent insulin secretion • Decrease glucagon production	Alo-, lina-, saxa-, sita-, vildagliptin	
Sodium-glucose co-transporter 2 (SGLT2) inhibitors (gliflozins) Decrease glucose reabsorption in the kidney = increase excretion in urine	Dapa-, empa-, ertugliflozin	
GLP-1 receptor agonists Incretin mimetic Increase glucose dependent insulin secretion • Decrease glucagon production • Slow gastric emptying = slows glucose absorption from the GIT	Dulaglutide, exenatide, liraglutide	
Thiazolidinedione • Increases peripheral tissues sensitivity to insulin • Increases peripheral utilisation of glucose • Decreases glucose production in the liver	Pioglitazone	
• Delays carbohydrate digestion and glucose absorption • Decreases spikes in BGLs after eating	Acarbose	

[a] See also Figure 28.1 and summaries in Table 28.3 (insulins) and Table 28.4 (Antihyperglycaemic Drugs).

REVIEW EXERCISES

1 Mr MS, aged 61 years, has been diagnosed with type 2 diabetes. Mr MS would like you, the health professional, to describe how his diabetes developed (i.e. pathogenesis) and what health complication could occur if he did not control his diabetes mellitus. He would also like to know about the different medications he can take, and how they work, to reduce his risk of getting such complications.

2 HB, a 4-year-old, is diagnosed with type 1 diabetes and started on insulin. What is the action of insulin in treating type 1 diabetes? What are the primary drug interactions and adverse reactions a health professional should be aware of when counselling this drug?

3 HB is also prescribed a glucagon hydrochloride 1 mg injection. What is the mechanism of action of glucagon? How long does it take to have an effect? What is the rationale for prescribing the glucogon for HB?

REFERENCES

Amiel SA, Frier BM, Heller SR, et al. (2019). Hypoglycaemia, cardiovascular disease, and mortality in diabetes: epidemiology, pathogenesis, and management. The Lancet Diabetes & Endocrinology 7(5): 385–396.

Australian Medicines Handbook 2021. Australian Medicines Handbook, Adelaide: AMH.

Deacon, C.F., Dipeptidyl peptidase 4 inhibitors in the treatment of type 2 diabetes mellitus. Nature Reviews Endocrinology, 2020. 16(11): 642–653.

Heile M, Schneider D 2012: The evolution of insulin therapy in diabetes mellitus, Journal of Family Practice 61(Suppl 5): S6–S12.

Khurana, G. and V 2019. Gupta, Effect on insulin upon storage in extreme climatic conditions (temperature and pressure) and their preventive measures. Journal of Social Health and Diabetes, 7(01): 006–010.

Nauck, M.A., Nauck MA, Quast DR, Wefers J., et al. 2021: GLP-1 receptor agonists in the treatment of type 2 diabetes–state-of-the-art. Molecular Metabolism, 46: 101–102.

ONLINE RESOURCES

Australasian Diabetes in Pregnancy Society: http://adips.org (accessed 14 May 2021)

Australian Institute of Health and Welfare: https://www.aihw.gov.au/reports-statistics/health-conditions-disability-deaths/diabetes/overview (accessed 14 May 2021)

Australian type 2 diabetes management algorithm: https://diabetessociety.com.au/20200908%20T2D%20Management%20Algorithm%2003092020.pdf (accessed 14 May 2021)

Diabetes Australia: https://www.diabetesaustralia.com.au/ (accessed 14 May 2021)

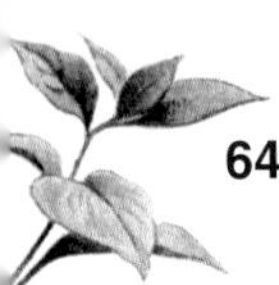

Diabetes Australia – best practice guidelines: www.diabetesaustralia.com.au/for-health-professionals/best-practice-guidelines/ (accessed 14 May 2021)

MIMS Annual Online: https://www.mims.com.au/index.php/products/mims-annual (accessed 14 May 2021)

New Zealand Health Survey 2016–17: https://www.health.govt.nz/publication/annual-update-key-results-2016-17-new-zealand-health-survey (accessed 14 May 2021)

New Zealand Medicines and Medical Devices Safety Authority: https://www.medsafe.govt.nz/ (accessed 14 May 2021)

World Health Organization: https://www.who.int/news-room/fact-sheets/detail/diabetes (accessed 14 May 2021)

More weblinks at: http://evolve.elsevier.com/AU/Knights/pharmacology/.

CHAPTER 29

THE ADRENAL CORTEX AND CORTICOSTEROIDS

Kathleen Knights

KEY ABBREVIATIONS

ACTH	adrenocorticotrophic hormone (corticotrophin)
CRF	corticotrophin-releasing factor
GR	glucocorticoid receptor
GRE	glucocorticoid response elements
HPA	hypothalamic–pituitary–adrenal (axis)
RAAS	renin–angiotensin–aldosterone system

KEY TERMS

Addison's disease 650
adrenocorticotrophic hormone 650
aldosterone 650
Conn's syndrome 650
corticosteroids 651
Cushing's syndrome 650
glucocorticoid 650
hypothalamic–pituitary–adrenal axis 651
mineralocorticoids 650

Chapter Focus

This chapter describes the endocrine functions of the adrenal glands, including the synthesis and secretion of glucocorticoids and mineralocorticoids. The glucocorticoids affect numerous normal and pathological processes in the body and are often used for their replacement, anti-inflammatory and immunosuppressant effects. The routes of administration, clinical use, major adverse effects and potentially serious drug interactions with glucocorticoids are discussed along with the clinical use of synthetic analogues of the mineralocorticoids.

KEY DRUG GROUPS

Corticotrophins:

- **Tetracosactride**

Glucocorticoids:

- **Dexamethasone**, **hydrocortisone**, **prednisolone/prednisone** (Drug Monograph 29.1)

Mineralocorticoids:

- **Fludrocortisone** (Drug Monograph 29.2)

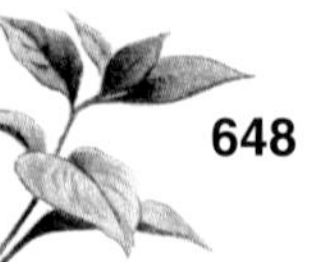

CRITICAL THINKING SCENARIO

Bernie, a 65-year-old with a long history of severe asthma, had presented at the local emergency department with an acute exacerbation of his asthma. In addition to his usual drug therapy he was prescribed prednisolone 40 mg daily for 10 days. When he was reviewed by his GP after 7 days, he complained of feeling anxious, depressed and having difficulty sleeping. As his lung function had improved considerably the GP ceased the prednisolone. Explain why prednisolone is beneficial for treating an acute exacerbation of asthma but causes adverse central nervous system effects.

Introduction

The adrenal glands[1] are located just above the kidneys in the retroperitoneal space, in capsules of connective tissue. Each adrenal gland consists of two regions: the outer cortex, which secretes the adrenal steroids; and the inner medulla. The adrenal cortex is further divided into three layers:

- The outermost layer, the *zona glomerulosa*, is under the control of both the pituitary **adrenocorticotrophic hormone** (ACTH, corticotrophin) and the renin–angiotensin–aldosterone system (RAAS) and secretes the **mineralocorticoids** (primarily **aldosterone**), which help to maintain blood volume, promote retention of sodium and water and increase urinary excretion of potassium and hydrogen ions.
- The *zona fasiculata* is under the control of ACTH and secretes the **glucocorticoids** (e.g. hydrocortisone, also called cortisol), which have important metabolic, anti-inflammatory and immunosuppressant effects.
- The innermost layer, the *zona reticularis*, secretes androgens (primarily dehydroepiandrosterone) that are metabolic precursors to the sex hormones.

The adrenal medulla is innervated by preganglionic sympathetic fibres and secretes the catecholamine hormones/neurotransmitters adrenaline and noradrenaline.

In a situation of stress, the adrenal glands help the body to respond and adapt by increasing the release of adrenaline, noradrenaline, hydrocortisone and aldosterone, which operate together to maintain homeostasis and survival. In adrenal insufficiency there is a deficit of both gluco- and mineralo-corticoids. Sodium reabsorption is inhibited and potassium excretion decreases; hyperkalaemia and mild acidosis occur, and a powerful and uncontrolled loss of extracellular fluid can lead to a state of hypovolaemic shock. The corticosteroids have many physiological actions and pathological conditions affecting the adrenal cortex that lead to glucocorticoid deficiencies (**Addison's disease**) or excesses (**Cushing's syndrome**) or mineralocorticoid excess (**Conn's syndrome**) that have widespread and potentially severe clinical manifestations (Clinical Focus Box 29.1). This chapter discusses the corticosteroids with either predominantly glucocorticoid or mineralocorticoid activity; androgens are discussed in Chapter 31.

1 The adrenal glands have also been called the perinephric (meaning 'round about the kidneys') and the epinephric or suprarenal ('over, above or beside the kidneys') glands; hence the American terms 'epinephrine' and 'norepinephrine' for the English terms 'adrenaline' and 'noradrenaline', the hormones from the adrenal medulla.

CLINICAL FOCUS BOX 29.1
Addison's, Cushing's and Conn's

Addison's disease: deficiency of corticosteroids

- *Aetiologies:* autoimmune; tuberculosis (less common now); breast cancer; bilateral adrenalectomy; iatrogenic (resulting from hypothalamic–pituitary–adrenal suppression).
- *Detection:* secretion of hydrocortisone does not increase in response to an injection of ACTH.
- *Manifestations:* muscle weakness, depression, anorexia, weight loss, hypoglycaemia, excessive skin pigmentation, hyperkalaemia, hyponatraemia with or without aldosterone deficiency (hypotension, dehydration). Potentially a life-threatening crisis if there is trauma or severe infection.
- *Treatment:* a glucocorticoid (life-saving). A mineralocorticoid (e.g. fludrocortisone, see Drug Monograph 29.2, later) may be required. Other drugs are used with caution.

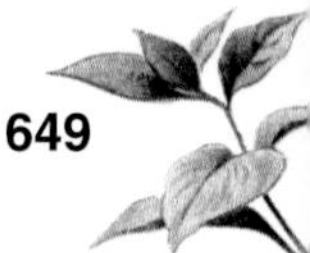

Cushing's syndrome: excess of glucocorticosteroids

- *Aetiologies:* adrenal hypersecretion (e.g. pituitary or adrenal ACTH-secreting tumour); prolonged glucocorticoid administration.
- *Detection:* increased secretion of hydrocortisone is not reduced during the dexamethasone suppression test.
- *Manifestations:* increased fat mass, 'moon face', trunk obesity, 'buffalo hump', thin extremities, skin striae, hirsutism (due to excessive androgenic steroid production), decreased bone mass and osteoporosis, amenorrhoea, impotence, diabetes mellitus, reduced lean mass and stunted growth.
- *Treatment:* depends on aetiology – for example, surgery, radiation therapy or adrenalectomy for tumour, plus replacement corticosteroids afterwards. Steroid biosynthesis inhibitors, somatostatin analogues (pasireotide) and dopamine agonists may be used when surgery has not controlled the disease.

Conn's syndrome: excess of mineralocorticosteroids

- *Aetiologies:* an aldosterone-secreting adenoma.
- *Detection:* a high ratio of aldosterone to plasma renin activity.
- *Manifestations of hyperaldosteronism:* increased potassium excretion and hypokalaemia; acidification of the urine and metabolic alkalosis; hypertension; suppressed plasma renin activity.
- *Treatment:* surgery, such as unilateral adrenalectomy; drug therapy with the competitive aldosterone antagonist spironolactone (also known as a potassium-sparing diuretic).

Corticosteroids

Synthesis and inhibition

Cholesterol is the precursor for the biosynthesis of **corticosteroids**. Conversion to pregnenolone, the rate-limiting step, is under the control of ACTH. Corticosteroids are not stored in the adrenal glands, so the rate of synthesis from plasma cholesterol determines the rate of release. The general pathways for synthesis of the adrenal cortex hormones are shown in Figure 29.1 (and the chemical structures of typical steroids in Fig 26.2).

The synthetic pathways can be blocked if there are deficiencies of the enzymes required, and by enzyme inhibitors such as the drug metyrapone (mainly of research and diagnostic interest), which inhibits the formation of hydrocortisone and, to some extent, aldosterone. Aminoglutethimide inhibits the rate-limiting step for conversion of cholesterol to pregnenolone, thereby blocking the synthesis of all adrenal steroids. It was previously indicated for the treatment of Cushing's syndrome associated with adrenal carcinoma, ectopic ACTH-dependent tumours and adrenal gland hyperplasia; however, there were many adverse effects, and it was frequently abused by athletes. It has been withdrawn in Australasia.

Control of synthesis

Hypothalamic and pituitary control

Corticosteroid synthesis depends on stimulation of the adrenal cortex by ACTH, which is governed by corticotrophin-releasing factor (CRF) from the hypothalamus (Fig 29.2). Corticotrophin secretion fluctuates with a circadian rhythm (see below), with high concentrations in the early morning and trough concentrations in the evening. This rhythm, in turn, determines the circadian rhythm in secretion of corticosteroids. The rhythms are disrupted by long transmeridian airline flights and take several days to be restored.

Corticotrophin is a 39-amino-acid polypeptide. When administered clinically, it tends to be antigenic; hence, a synthetic analogue tetracosactride (24 amino acids) has been developed. It has similar actions to the natural hormone – that is, trophic actions on adrenal cortex cells, increasing the synthesis and release of corticosteroids (mainly glucocorticoids) and regulating enzymes for steroidogenesis. It is administered parenterally in diagnostic tests of adrenal cortex function: administration should result in a rapid rise in cholesterol synthesis and release of hydrocortisone into the bloodstream. A sustained-release depot preparation for intramuscular injection is also available, for treatment of hypsarrhythmia and/or infantile spasms.

ACTH secretion is suppressed by somatostatin (growth hormone release-inhibiting hormone – see Drug Monograph 26.1, 'Octreotide'). The analogue pasireotide, which is more selective for suppression of ACTH secretion, is approved in the treatment of Cushing's disease.

Negative feedback control

Increased concentrations of corticosteroids, in the typical negative feedback fashion, inhibit the release of CRF from the hypothalamus and also inhibit the release of ACTH from the anterior pituitary (Fig 29.2). This is referred to as the **hypothalamic–pituitary–adrenal (HPA) axis**.

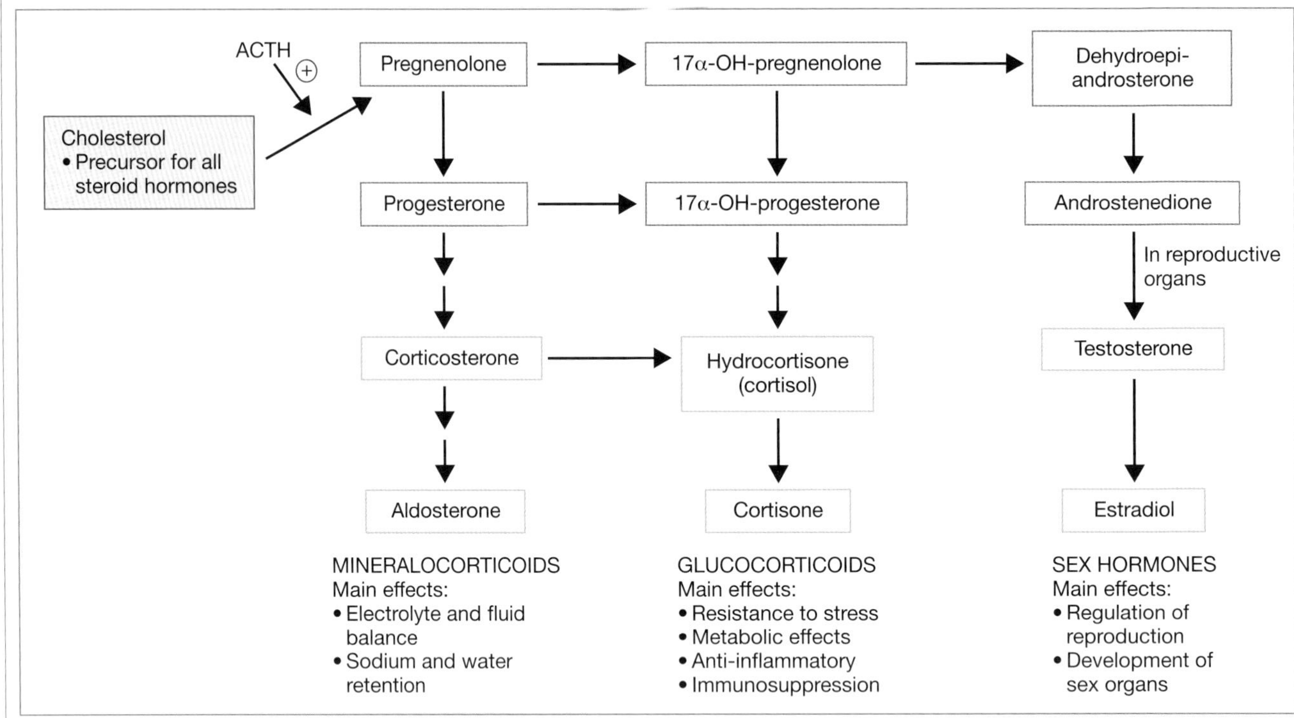

FIGURE 29.1 Biosynthesis of corticosteroids and sex hormones
Metabolic intermediates are shown in blue boxes. The glucocorticoids are produced by cells of the zona fasciculata, while aldosterone is produced in the zona glomerulosa. Physiologically active hormones are shown in gold boxes.

Secretion

Two rhythms appear to influence glucocorticoid release: circadian (diurnal, daily) and ultradian (less than daily) rhythm. A circadian rhythm, a pattern based on a 24-hour cycle with the repetition of certain physiological processes, is controlled by the dark–light and sleep–wakefulness cycles via the limbic system. People living a normal awake-during-the-day–asleep-at-night cycle will have higher plasma hydrocortisone concentrations in the early morning hours that reach a peak after they are awake and very low concentrations in the evening and during the early phase of sleep. The importance of this rhythm is emphasised by the finding that corticosteroid therapy is more potent when given at midnight than when given at noon. To simulate the natural diurnal rhythm when corticosteroids are administered as drugs, daily doses are usually divided, with two-thirds given in the morning and one-third early or late afternoon.

In humans, there are also 4–8 bursts of adrenal glucocorticoid release that occur over each 24 hours, which may follow peaks in the release of CRF and ACTH, and more frequent hourly bursts. Although the basal production rate averages 30 mg every 24 hours, under stressful conditions such as trauma, major surgery or infection, there is a reserve capacity production of up to 300 mg daily. Increases in glucocorticoid production may be proportional to increases in the release of ACTH by the anterior pituitary gland.

KEY POINTS

Corticosteroids

- The adrenal cortex is divided into three layers: the outer *zona glomerulosa*, which is under the control of both pituitary ACTH and the RAAS and secretes the mineralocorticoid aldosterone; the *zona fasiculata*, which is under the control of ACTH and secretes the glucocorticoids; and the innermost layer, the *zona reticularis*, which secretes androgens.
- The adrenal medulla secretes the catecholamine hormones/neurotransmitters adrenaline and noradrenaline.
- Cholesterol is the precursor for the biosynthesis of corticosteroids. Conversion to pregnenolone, the rate-limiting step, is under the control of ACTH.
- Corticosteroids are not stored in the adrenal glands, so the rate of synthesis from plasma cholesterol determines the rate of release.
- Increased concentrations of corticosteroids, in the typical negative feedback fashion, inhibit the release of CRF from the hypothalamus and the release of ACTH from the anterior pituitary. This is referred to as the HPA axis.
- Release of glucocorticosteroids is controlled by CRH and ACTH, and is subject to circadian rhythms.

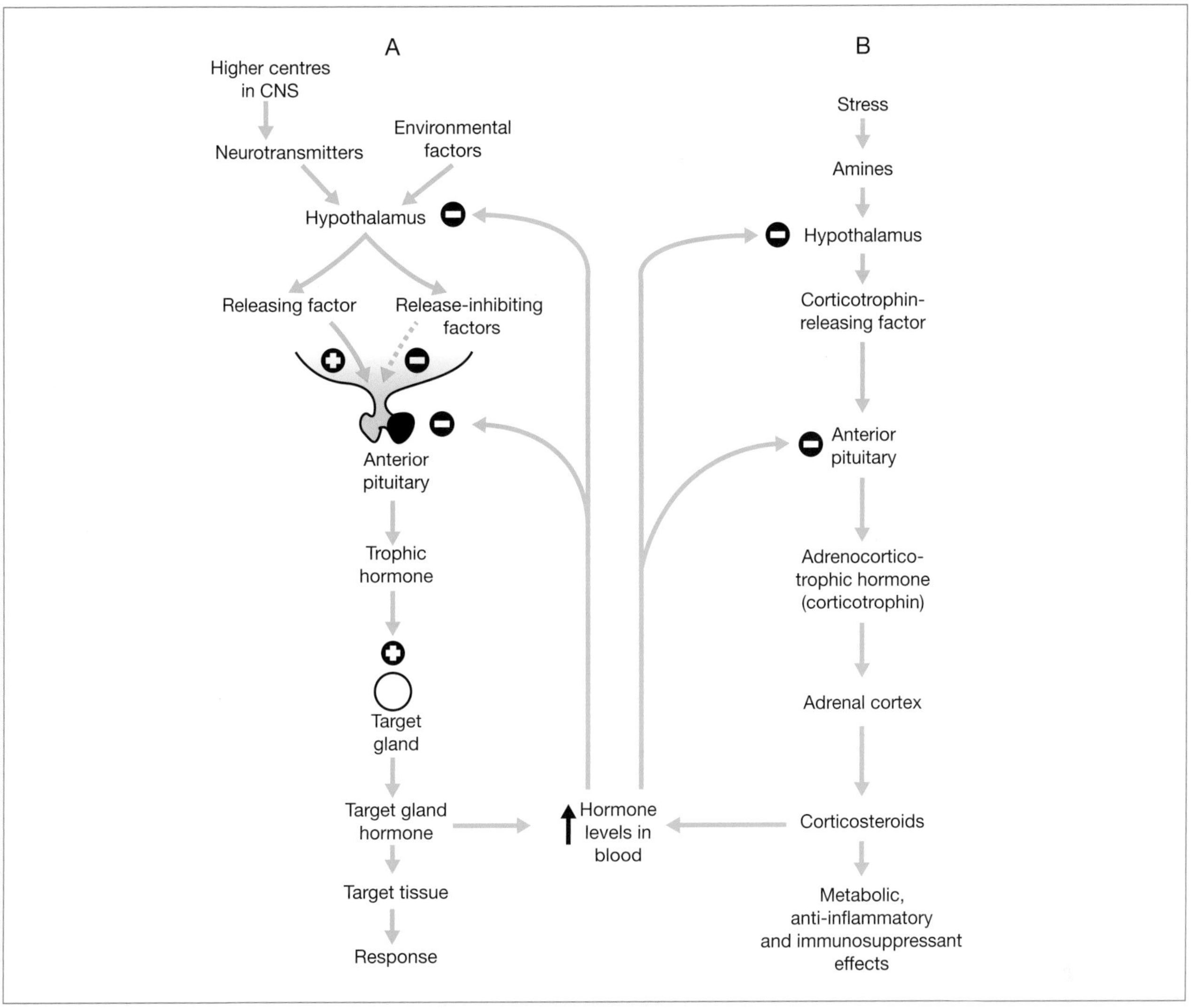

A

Higher centres in CNS

Neurotransmitters

Environmental factors

Hypothalamus

Releasing factor

Release-inhibiting factors

Anterior pituitary

Trophic hormone

Target gland

Target gland hormone

Target tissue

Response

Hormone levels in blood

B

Stress

Amines

Hypothalamus

Corticotrophin-releasing factor

Anterior pituitary

Adrenocortico-trophic hormone (corticotrophin)

Adrenal cortex

Corticosteroids

Metabolic, anti-inflammatory and immunosuppressant effects

FIGURE 29.2 Levels of endocrine control

Various internal and external factors may inhibit or stimulate the hypothalamus to secrete inhibitory or releasing factors, which increase (+) or decrease (−) output of hormones from the anterior pituitary gland and, ultimately, hormone release from target glands. Short and long negative feedback loops 'damp down' further release. **A** Typical pattern of levels of controls. **B** Example in the adrenal cortex, showing negative feedback control of release of hypothalamic corticotrophin-releasing factor (CRF) and of pituitary adrenocorticotrophic hormone (ACTH) by high levels of adrenocorticosteroids.

Glucocorticoids

Mechanism of action

The general mechanism of action of the glucocorticoids is as for most steroids, and is described below:

1 Glucocorticoids enter the target cell and bind to specific receptors in the cytoplasm, mainly glucocorticoid receptor alpha (GRα).

2 The steroid–glucocorticoid receptor (GR) complex undergoes a conformational change that exposes a DNA-binding domain.

3 Dimers of the complex translocate into the nucleus, where they bind with glucocorticoid response elements (GREs) present in the promoters of target genes (Fig 29.3).

4 This binding brings about induction or repression of transcription of specific mRNAs, via interaction with various transcription factors.

5 Hence, the synthesis of specific proteins is increased or decreased.

6 Mediators are generated or suppressed.

In the case of the glucocorticoids, there are many molecular forms of the GR expressed in tissues, both inside the nucleus and extranuclear on cell membranes. Many genes are targeted, and there is increased synthesis of various kinase enzymes and anti-inflammatory

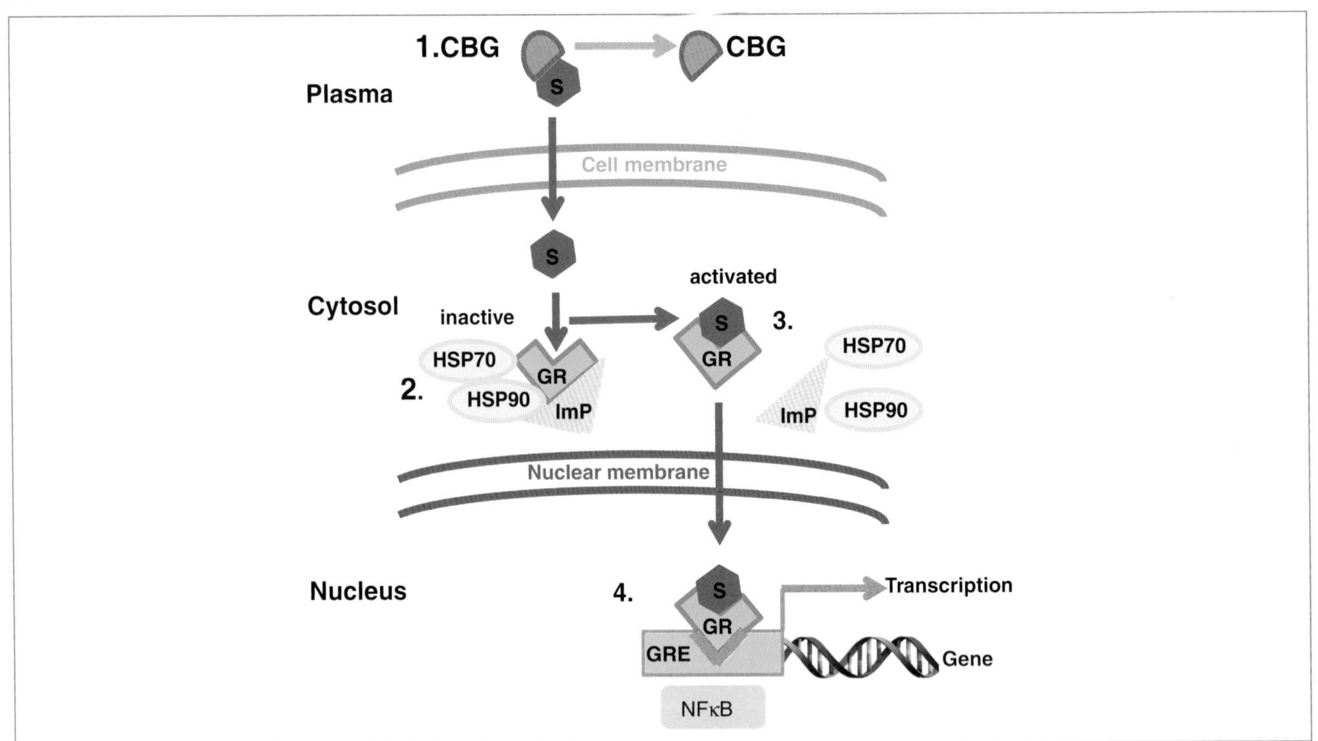

FIGURE 29.3 Mechanism of action of glucocorticoids
1 Steroid (S) bound to corticosteroid-binding globulin (CBG; also called transcortin) in plasma. **2** GR resides in cytoplasm in an inactive form in a complex with heat shock proteins (stress-induced proteins) HSP90 and HSP70 and immunophilin (ImP) (intracellular protein involved in T cell activation). **3** Steroid binding results in dissociation of the complex, receptor activation and translocation to the nucleus. **4** In the nucleus, S+GR interacts with specific glucocorticoid response elements (GRE) that provide for gene transcription and protein–protein interactions. For example, interaction between the GR and the transcription factor NFκB regulates expression of a number of components of the immune system.

mediators, including lipocortin (annexin-1). At the same time, there is decreased synthesis of other enzymes, including cyclo-oxygenase-2 and collagenase, and hence suppression of pro-inflammatory mediators, including histamine, some cytokines, prostaglandins and leukotrienes (Kumar & McEwan 2012). Thus, steroid effects can be mediated both via genes and transcription and via signalling pathways and mediators.

GR antagonists are currently being investigated; such drugs could potentially be useful in therapy of Cushing's disease, diabetes, obesity, neuropathic pain and glaucoma. Early research led to the non-selective GR antagonist RU-486 (mifepristone), used in medical termination of pregnancy.

Steroid resistance

In circumstances in which steroids may be used chronically (e.g. chronic obstructive pulmonary disease, inflammatory bowel disease), some people develop reduced responsiveness to the drugs. This is known as 'steroid resistance', and as a consequence conditions become more difficult to treat. Some proposed mechanisms of development of steroid resistance include:

- mutations in the gene coding for the GR
- altered numbers of GRs
- abnormalities in absorption or metabolism (considered unlikely)
- altered affinity of the steroid for the GR
- reduced affinity of the GR to bind GREs on DNA
- altered expression of transcription factors and/or cytokines
- genetic variations in the disease phenotypes.

Strategies for dealing with steroid resistance include administration of other types of immunosuppressants and/or of drugs targeting other processes in the disease.

Physiological actions of glucocorticoids

Hydrocortisone (cortisol) is considered the prototype glucocorticoid hormone; synthetic analogues have similar effects in the body. These include general metabolic

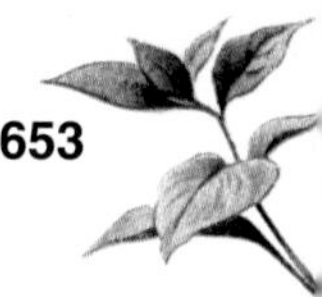

effects, anti-inflammatory and immunosuppressant actions and negative feedback effects on the HPA axis. Some mineralocorticoid effects may also occur from the natural hormones, as the specificity between the two types of corticosteroids is not absolute.

Metabolic effects

Carbohydrate, protein and fat metabolism

Glucocorticoids decrease glucose uptake into cells and glucose utilisation while increasing gluconeogenesis; thus, they help to maintain the blood glucose level and liver and muscle glycogen content. This can produce hyperglycaemia and glycosuria; that is, glucocorticoids are diabetogenic: they can aggravate diabetes, unmask latent diabetes and cause insulin resistance.

Glucocorticoids facilitate the breakdown of protein in muscle and extrahepatic tissues, which leads to increased plasma amino acid levels. Glucocorticoids increase the trapping of amino acids by the liver and stimulate their deamination. Subsequent inhibition of protein synthesis can delay wound healing and cause muscle wasting and osteoporosis. In young people, these effects can inhibit growth.

Glucocorticoids promote mobilisation of fatty acids from adipose tissue, increasing their concentration in the plasma and their use for energy. Despite this effect, people taking glucocorticoids for long periods may accumulate fat stores ('moon face', 'buffalo hump') because of redistribution of fat. The effects of glucocorticoids on fat metabolism are complex and are thought to occur through 'permissive' actions of catecholamines.

Calcium balance

Glucocorticoids tend to decrease calcium absorption from the gut and increase its excretion via the kidneys, causing an overall negative calcium balance. In response, bone is resorbed by osteoclastic activity, raising blood calcium levels. Chronically, this can lead to osteoporosis.

Blood pressure and stress responses

Glucocorticoids potentiate the vasoconstrictor action of noradrenaline, partly by inhibiting extraneuronal uptake of catecholamines. When glucocorticoids are absent, the vasoconstricting action of the catecholamines is diminished and blood pressure falls.

Both CRF and arginine vasopressin are released in response to acute and chronic stress and, via activation of pro-opiomelanocortin in anterior pituitary cells, cause release of ACTH and hence of glucocorticoids, which help maintain homeostasis. This sudden release is believed to be a protective mechanism: without steroid release (or administration), hypotension and shock may occur. Simultaneous release of adrenaline and noradrenaline from the adrenal medulla has a synergistic action with the corticosteroids.

Central nervous system effects

Corticosteroids affect mood and behaviour, and possibly cause neuronal or brain excitability. GR function is impaired in major depression, resulting in reduced negative feedback on the HPA axis and increased secretion of CRF; it is thought that hyperactivity of the HPA is involved in causing depression. Some people on exogenous corticosteroids report mood swings (euphoria and/or depression), insomnia, anxiety and increased motor activity; chronic high doses can lead to psychoses. Prolonged stress during childhood and adolescence may lead to depression and psychotic disorders in adulthood, via increased activity of the HPA, leading to impaired N-methyl-D-aspartate (NMDA) and glutamate functioning in cortical neural networks.

Suppression of the hypothalamic–pituitary–adrenal axis

High levels of circulating corticosteroids have negative feedback effects on secretion of CRF and ACTH, thus suppressing the HPA axis, leading to decreased secretion of glucocorticoids and, in the long term, atrophy of the adrenal cortex. This leaves the body unable to cope rapidly with stress, infection, surgery or challenges to the immune system.

Anti-inflammatory actions

Glucocorticoids, especially hydrocortisone, stabilise lysosomal membranes and prevent movement of neutrophils and release of proteolytic enzymes during inflammation. They can also suppress virtually all vascular and cellular events in the inflammatory response, both immediate events and late processes, including wound healing and repair. By stimulating the production of the mediator protein lipocortin (also called annexin-1), they inhibit phospholipase-A_2 (Fig 34.2), inhibiting the production from damaged cell membranes of many mediators, including prostaglandins, prostacyclin and leukotrienes. Because phospholipase-A_2 is involved much earlier in the pathways for synthesis of inflammatory mediators than are cyclo-oxygenases, the corticosteroids inhibit production of many more mediators than do non-steroidal anti-inflammatory drugs (NSAIDs) (Ch 34).

Immunosuppressant actions

Glucocorticoids can cause atrophy of the thymus and decrease the number of lymphocytes, plasma cells and eosinophils in the blood. By blocking the production and release of cytokines and other mediators, corticosteroids interfere with the integrated roles of T and B lymphocytes, macrophages and monocytes in immune and allergic responses.

KEY POINTS

Glucocorticoids

- On entry to a target cell, steroids bind to specific receptors in the cytoplasm, mainly GRα. The complex undergoes a conformational change that exposes a DNA-binding domain. It then translocates to the nucleus, where it binds to GRE present in the promoters of target genes. This may result in induction or repression of transcription of specific mRNAs, or interaction with various transcription factors that increase or decrease synthesis of specific proteins and either generation or suppression of mediators.
- Steroid resistance can arise from changes within this binding pathway.
- The glucocorticoids have many important effects, including metabolic, anti-inflammatory, immunosuppressant and central nervous system effects.
- The actions of these hormones are vitally important in helping the body to maintain homeostasis, particularly in times of stress.

Glucocorticoids used clinically

When corticosteroids are administered in doses that lead to higher than normal (physiological) concentrations in the body, the doses are said to be 'pharmacological'. Many thousands of steroid compounds have been synthesised and their pharmacological actions assessed in an attempt to enhance particular actions or improve pharmacokinetic properties. The synthesis of steroids with little or no mineralocorticoid activity was an advance, as the most useful clinical effects are those of the glucocorticoids – that is, anti-inflammatory and immunosuppressant actions.

Hydrocortisone (cortisol) is taken as the 'gold standard' glucocorticoid, so relative affinities of other steroids at glucocorticoid receptors can be compared and relative potencies calculated. Many synthetic glucocorticoids have been designed to maximise anti-inflammatory and immunosuppressant activities and minimise mineralocorticoid effects such as hypokalaemia, hypertension and oedema. Three drugs of choice for glucocorticoid (anti-inflammatory) activity are prednisolone (four times the potency of hydrocortisone, Drug Monograph 29.1), dexamethasone (27 times) and betamethasone (27 times) – the latter two drugs with minimal sodium-retaining activity.

For mineralocorticoid activity, the drug of choice is fludrocortisone (150 times the potency of hydrocortisone, Drug Monograph 29.2). Commonly used corticosteroids are compared in Table 29.1, showing typical dosage, relative glucocorticoid and mineralocorticoid potencies, plasma half-life and duration of action.

Topical glucocorticoids

Dozens of topical steroid preparations are available, in many dosage forms (creams, gels, ointments, eyedrops, eardrops, eye ointments, lotions, shampoos, suppositories) and in many combinations (e.g. with antibacterials or keratolytics). For skin disorders, topical glucocorticosteroids are used for inflammatory and pruritic eruptions, hyperplastic conditions, infiltrative disorders such as eczema, and psoriasis. There are many advantages of topical preparations, including broad applicability, rapid action, stable formulations, compatibility and ease of use, with no pain or odour and few systemic adverse effects. Typical drugs include betamethasone, desonide, triamcinolone and methylprednisolone; these are discussed in greater detail in Chapter 39.

Ocular (eye) and otic (ear) formulations of corticosteroids commonly include dexamethasone, fluorometholone, prednisolone, triamcinolone or hydrocortisone, in drops or ointments. An antibiotic is sometimes included in the formulation to treat or prevent infections (see discussion in Table 40.5 and Drug Monograph 40.1).

Inhaled glucocorticoids

The glucocorticoids are extremely useful as preventers in asthma. The available inhaled corticosteroids are: beclometasone (Drug Monograph 26.4), budesonide, ciclesonide and fluticasone. For further information, see Chapter 15 and Table 15.3.

Pharmacokinetics

Absorption and distribution

Glucocorticoids are well absorbed after oral, topical or local administration. Parenterally (IM) and topically, the soluble esters (phosphate and succinate) are rapidly absorbed, while the poorly soluble forms (acetate, acetonide, diacetate, hexacetonide and valerate) are slowly but completely absorbed and act as depots in the tissues for slow release of hormone. If administered rectally, about 20% of the drug is absorbed unless the rectum is inflamed, when absorption may increase by up to 50%. Steroids are transported in the bloodstream reversibly bound to albumin and to corticosteroid-binding globulin. Only unbound corticosteroids diffuse freely into cells.

Metabolism and excretion

The natural hormone cortisone is enzymatically hydroxylated to hydrocortisone before it is active; the same is true for the synthetic analogue prednisone, which is activated to prednisolone. (Thus, cortisone and prednisone are prodrugs.) Steroids are conjugated by sulfation and

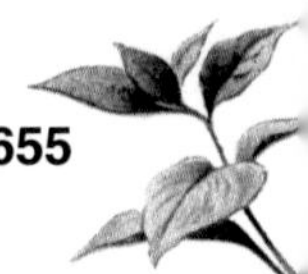

Drug Monograph 29.1
Prednisolone and prednisone

Prednisone is a synthetic prodrug that is inactive until converted to prednisolone. A synthetic glucocorticoid, it is used primarily for anti-inflammatory conditions and as an immunosuppressant. It has reduced sodium-retaining properties. Prednisolone and prednisone are used clinically for inflammatory and immune disorders, acute asthma, croup, chronic obstructive pulmonary disease exacerbation and in treatment protocols for malignancies – for example, multiple myeloma, some leukaemias and lymphoma.

Pharmacokinetics

Prednisone is metabolised by CYP3A4 in the liver to the active metabolite prednisolone within about 60 minutes. Both drugs are well absorbed, and peak plasma concentration occurs in 1.3 hours. The half-life of prednisone is 3.4–3.8 hours, while that of prednisolone is 2.1–3.5 hours. The duration of biological action is in the order of 12–36 hours. Prednisolone is excreted in urine as unchanged drug and as inactive glucuronide metabolites.

Adverse reactions

Adverse effects are widespread (see text), including:

- musculoskeletal, cardiovascular, gastrointestinal, dermatological, neurological, endocrine, immunological, haematological, ophthalmic and metabolic effects
- chronic administration leads to suppression of the HPA and hypokalaemia, and excessive doses to cushingoid effects.

Warnings and contraindications

Use with caution in people with:

- hypertension, heart failure, hyperlipidaemia, liver or kidney disease
- colitis, diverticulitis, open-angle glaucoma, oral herpes lesions
- hypothyroidism, hypoalbuminaemia, psychotic tendencies, osteoporosis, systemic lupus erythematosus
- uncontrolled infections (and many other conditions).

Avoid use in people with corticosteroid hypersensitivity, HIV infection (or AIDS), heart disease, heart failure, severe kidney disease, chickenpox, measles, peptic ulcer, oesophagitis, systemic fungal infection, diabetes mellitus, herpes simplex infection (eye), myasthenia gravis or tuberculosis. Prednisolone and prednisone are preferred for treating maternal disorders because both drugs have limited placental transfer.

Drug interactions

(See also DI 29.1.) Important interactions occur with phenobarbital (phenobarbitone) and ritonavir, both of which increase the metabolism of prednisone.

Dosage and administration

Prednisolone is available as an oral formulation (tablet and liquid) and is also formulated for rectal administration (as suppositories or a retention enema) for use in inflammatory bowel disease (ulcerative colitis, Crohn's disease) and other painful inflammatory conditions of the rectum and anus. Prednisone is available as a tablet. The dosage range for both drugs is 5–60 mg daily (short duration), depending on the disease and the severity of the clinical symptoms.

DRUG INTERACTIONS 29.1
Glucocorticoids

The following drug interactions may potentially occur when a corticosteroid is given with the drugs listed below. Current drug information sources should be consulted for interactions with specific corticosteroids.

DRUG	POSSIBLE EFFECTS AND MANAGEMENT
Amphotericin B (parenteral)	May result in severe hypokalaemia. If given concurrently, monitor serum potassium concentration closely.
Antacids (e.g. magnesium trisilicate); bile-acid-binding resins	When given concurrently, a decrease in steroid absorption may result. Doses should be separated by at least 2 hours, and steroid dosage increase may be necessary.
Antidiabetic drugs (oral) or insulin; other drugs affecting blood glucose concentration (Table 30.2)	Glucocorticoids may elevate serum glucose concentration; hence, dosage adjustment of one or both drugs may be necessary.
Azole antifungal agents (e.g. itraconazole)	Reduce the metabolism and enhance the clinical effects of some glucocorticoids; chronic administration should be monitored, and dosage of glucocorticoid may need to be reduced.

Digoxin	May result in increased potential for toxicity (dysrhythmias) associated with hypokalaemia.
Diuretics	The sodium- and fluid-retaining effects of the corticosteroids may reduce the effectiveness of diuretic agents. Monitor closely for oedema and fluid retention. Potassium-depleting diuretics given with corticosteroids may result in severe hypokalaemia, whereas the effects of potassium-sparing diuretics may be decreased. Monitor serum potassium concentration and clinical response closely.
Hepatic enzyme (CYP3A4)-inducing agents	Carbamazepine, phenytoin and others may decrease the corticosteroid effect because of increased metabolism. Monitor clinical effect and increase corticosteroid dose if necessary.
Non-steroidal anti-inflammatory drugs	Can cause gastrointestinal bleeding, which may be exacerbated by corticosteroids; if necessary, use lowest effective dose of NSAID for shortest possible time.

Drug Monograph 29.2
Fludrocortisone

Fludrocortisone, a synthetic drug, has potent mineralocorticoid activity, for which it is mainly used, with strong glucocorticoid effects as well. Its physiological actions are similar to hydrocortisone but with augmented effects on electrolyte balance. It binds to mineralocorticoid receptors, causing reabsorption of sodium in the renal distal convoluted tubule, enhanced excretion of potassium and hydrogen ions and an increase in blood pressure. It is indicated for treating Addison's disease (adrenocortical insufficiency), renal insufficiency with hyperkalaemia and salt-losing adrenogenital syndrome, and is also used in orthostatic hypotension.

Pharmacokinetics

Fludrocortisone has good oral absorption and peak serum concentration occurs in about 1.7 hours. The half-life of the drug is about 3.5 hours in the plasma, with a biological duration of action of 12–36 hours. It is highly protein-bound, and inactive metabolites produced in the liver and kidneys are excreted by the kidneys.

Drug interactions

The main interactions with fludrocortisone are due to potassium loss and hence hypokalaemia; interactions with amphotericin B, digitalis glycosides, diuretics and potassium supplements are as for glucocorticoids (Drug Interactions 29.1). Potassium levels should be monitored and supplements given as necessary.

Adverse reactions

These include:

- salt and water retention, hypokalaemia, oedema of the lower extremities
- severe or persistent headaches, hypertension, dizziness
- joint pain and increased weakness.

Such adverse reactions should be reported immediately to the prescriber. Heart failure may be exacerbated by fluid and electrolyte disturbances. At the low doses of mineralocorticoids usually used, serious glucocorticoid adverse effects are unlikely.

Warnings and contraindications

Use with caution in people with peripheral oedema, acute glomerulonephritis, liver impairment, hypothyroidism, hyperthyroidism, chronic nephritis, infections or osteoporosis.

Avoid use in those with fludrocortisone hypersensitivity, heart disease, hypertension or kidney function impairment.

During chronic administration, periodic monitoring of serum electrolytes, and dietary sodium restriction and potassium supplementation, are advisable.

Dosage and administration

The adolescent and adult oral dosage is 50–100 micrograms once daily, in the morning. Dosage is adjusted within the range of 50–200 micrograms daily.

glucuronidation to inactive metabolites, which are excreted in urine. The fluorinated corticosteroids are metabolised more slowly than non-fluorinated steroids.

Although the elimination half-lives of the drugs may be short (e.g. the half-life of hydrocortisone is about 90 minutes), the biological half-life and duration of action may be several hours or days. This is because once the steroid binds to the GRE, the actions initiated (e.g. gene expression, protein synthesis) continue in tissues long after the drug has diffused away from the receptor and been eliminated (Table 29.1).

TABLE 29.1 Relative potencies and pharmacokinetic properties of major corticosteroids

CORTICOSTEROID	EQUIVALENT GLUCOCORTICOID DOSE (mg)[a]	RELATIVE GLUCOCORTICOID (ANTI-INFLAMMATORY) POTENCY[b]	RELATIVE MINERALOCORTICOID (NA^+-RETAINING) POTENCY[c]	PLASMA DRUG HALF-LIFE (h)	DURATION OF BIOLOGICAL ACTION (h)
Short-acting – natural steroids					
Cortisone (prodrug)	25	0.8	0.8	0.5	8–12
Hydrocortisone	20	1	1	1.5–2	8–12
Intermediate-acting – synthetic steroids					
Fludrocortisone	–	10	150	0.5–3	12–36
Methylprednisolone	4	5	0[d]	3–4	12–36
Prednisolone	5	4	0.8	2.1–3.5	12–36
Prednisone (prodrug)	5	4	0.8	3.4–3.8	12–36
Triamcinolone	4	5	0[d]	2–5	12–36
Long-acting – synthetic steroids					
Betamethasone	0.75	27	0[d]	3–6.5	36–72
Dexamethasone	0.75	25	0[d]	3–4	36–72

[a] Approximate dosages, applies to PO ('by mouth') only; see also Table 40.5 for ocular corticosteroids.
[b] Refers to anti-inflammatory, immunosuppressant and metabolic effects.
[c] Potassium excretion, and sodium and water retention.
[d] Some hypokalaemia and/or sodium and water retention may occur, depending on dose and individual response.
Sources: Rang et al. 2015, Table 33.2; Brunton et al. 2018, Table 46-3.

Clinical Uses of Glucocorticoids

Glucocorticoids have multiple uses including:

- prevention of organ/tissue transplant rejection
- haematological malignancies such as lymphomas and leukaemia (to suppress white cells, induce lymphopenia and reduce the size of enlarged lymph nodes)
- severe allergic reactions, including asthma, urticaria, anaphylactic shock, and reactions to drugs and venoms
- autoimmune disorders (systemic lupus erythematosus, rheumatoid arthritis)
- chronic inflammatory conditions in the skin, gut, joints, liver, eye, etc.
- neoplastic diseases, to decrease cerebral oedema, and for the euphoric effects
- prevention of postoperative/chemotherapy-induced nausea and vomiting
- replacement therapy in patients with adrenal insufficiency (e.g. Addison's disease, hypopituitarism).

Adverse reactions

There are many adverse reactions from the use of glucocorticoids, especially after prolonged administration (Fig 29.4). Chronic use may result in abdominal pain, gastrointestinal bleeding and peptic ulcers.

Drug interactions

Potentially, adverse interactions can occur between corticosteroids and many drugs; examples are summarised in Drug Interactions 29.1.

Dosage and administration

These drugs have been administered by every imaginable route and formulation, including PO, IM, IV, by inhalation, topically (cutaneous creams and ointments) and locally (by intra-articular, ocular, otic, nasal, intralesional and per rectum routes). Local administration to the site of action is preferred if possible, as this allows lower doses to be used, fewer systemic adverse effects are likely, and a more rapid and direct action occurs.

A typical daily adult dose of hydrocortisone as replacement therapy is 12–25 mg, with two-thirds in the morning and one-third in the early or mid-afternoon. In acute adrenal insufficiency in adults, higher doses (100 mg immediately, followed by 200 mg over 24 hours) may be required IV or IM. Higher doses such as 100–500 mg hydrocortisone three to four times daily are also used for the anti-inflammatory and immunosuppressant effects.

Doses are increased in times of stress (e.g. during inter-current illness, before surgery and after trauma). People already taking corticosteroids prior to surgery – for example, for adrenal insufficiency, immunosuppression or a chronic inflammatory condition such as asthma – will have some level of HPA suppression. To cover against adrenal crisis during the stress of surgery and for

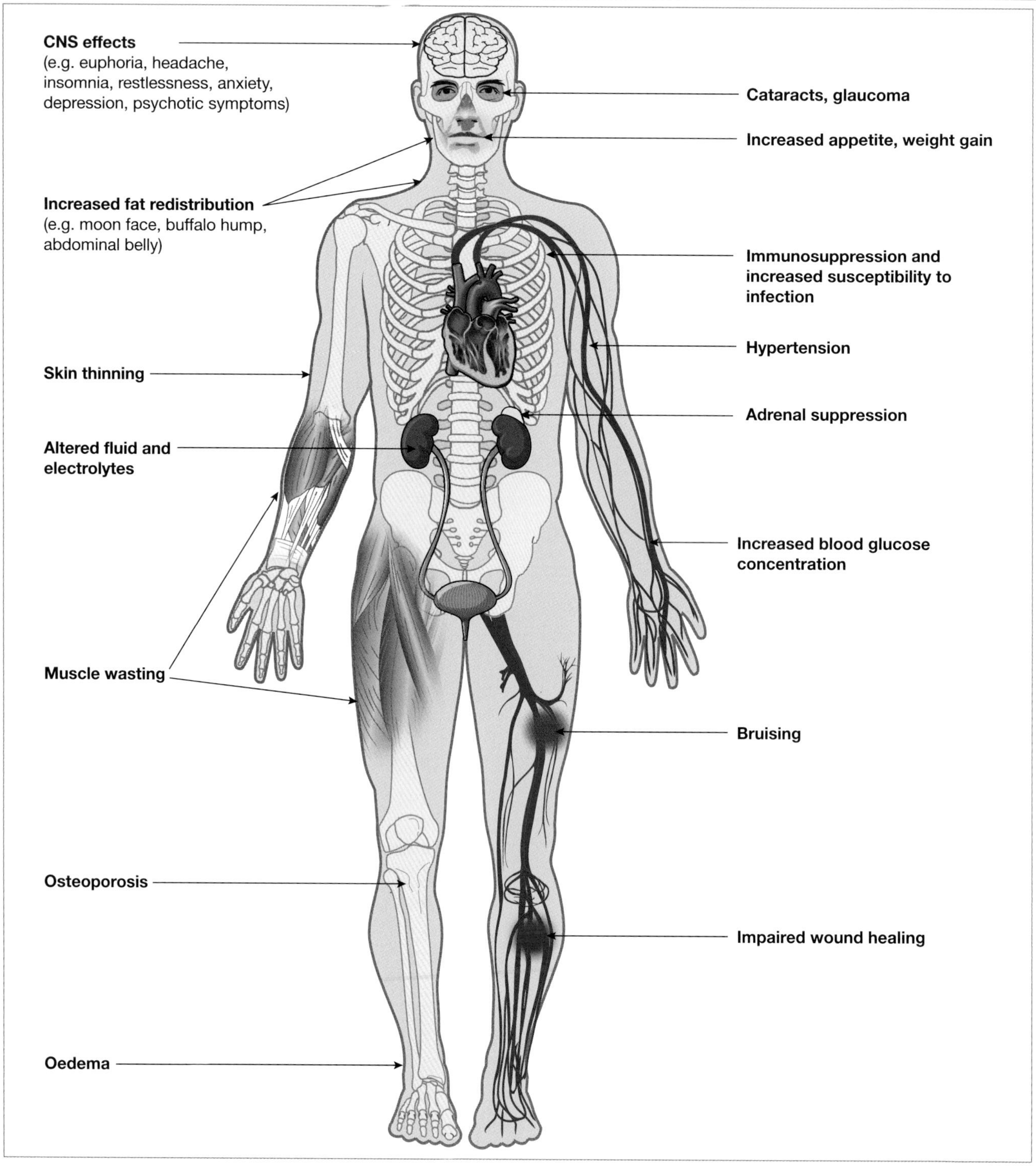

CNS effects
(e.g. euphoria, headache, insomnia, restlessness, anxiety, depression, psychotic symptoms)

Cataracts, glaucoma

Increased appetite, weight gain

Increased fat redistribution
(e.g. moon face, buffalo hump, abdominal belly)

Immunosuppression and increased susceptibility to infection

Hypertension

Skin thinning

Adrenal suppression

Altered fluid and electrolytes

Increased blood glucose concentration

Muscle wasting

Bruising

Osteoporosis

Impaired wound healing

Oedema

FIGURE 29.4 Adverse effects of administered glucocorticoids

1–2 days afterwards the dose may need to be increased depending on the individual and severity of the condition; doses are frequently doubled or trebled, and given more frequently. Critically ill people (e.g. those in intensive care units and with respiratory distress syndrome) may require high-dose corticosteroids due to HPA suppression and to tissue resistance to glucocorticoids. It is recommended that people wear a bracelet and carry a card with details of their corticosteroid dose regimen and emergency procedures.

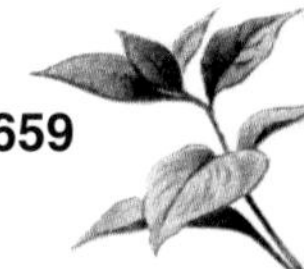

KEY POINTS

Glucocorticoids used clinically

- Common glucocorticoids used systemically include dexamethasone, hydrocortisone and prednisolone.
- Indications for glucocorticoids include replacement therapy (Addison's disease) and as anti-inflammatory/immunosuppressive agents for asthma, allergic reactions, autoimmune diseases, prevention of organ transplant rejection, haematological malignancies, neoplasia, etc.
- Glucocorticoids are available, for example, as oral IM, IV, cream, ointment, eyedrops, nosedrops and eardrops, and as inhaled formulations.
- Glucocorticoids are well absorbed and metabolised predominantly by glucuronidation and sulfation, with the inactive metabolites excreted in urine.
- The elimination half-life of the drugs is short, but the biological effects mediated via altered gene transcription may persist for days.
- Adverse drug reactions include metabolic effects, suppression of HPA, and central nervous system, GIT and mineralocorticoid effects.
- Withdrawal of corticosteroids is undertaken by gradual dose reduction over days/weeks, due to the unpredictability of HPA suppression.
- Current drug information resources should be consulted for details of drug dosages and drug interactions with glucocorticoids.

Mineralocorticoids

Aldosterone is synthesised in the *zona glomerulosa* and is regulated primarily by the RAAS and the concentration of circulating serum potassium (Fig 11.5), rather than by stimulation of the adrenal cortex by ACTH. A rise in plasma potassium concentration directly stimulates the adrenal cortex output of aldosterone, whereas aldosterone secretion is suppressed by an elevation of sodium levels in the blood – for example, by excessive dietary salt intake.

CLINICAL FOCUS BOX 29.2
Withdrawal from corticosteroids

Suppression of the HPA axis is unpredictable. It is less likely in the following cases:

- with doses under 7.5 mg/day of prednisolone or equivalent
- during treatment periods shorter than 3 weeks
- with alternate-day glucocorticoid therapy, if the dose is given in the morning rather than the evening
- with topical or inhaled doses, compared with oral or systemic doses.

After cessation of therapy (sudden withdrawal should be avoided), it can take many months - even up to a year - for HPA functions to recover. During that time the body is at risk because the adrenal gland cannot rapidly respond to the demand for synthesis of steroids. Local protocols should be consulted for phased withdrawal of corticosteroids.

The primary function of aldosterone is to stimulate potassium secretion by the renal tubular cells in the distal and collecting tubules while simultaneously enhancing the cells' reabsorption of sodium and its accompanying anions, chloride and bicarbonate, and thereby maintaining extracellular fluid volume and blood pressure. (See Ch 11 for a discussion of drugs that target the RAAS.)

Clinical uses

Aldosterone is several thousand times more potent as a mineralocorticoid than is hydrocortisone. In adrenal cortex insufficiency, replacement of a glucocorticoid, and sometimes also a mineralocorticoid, is necessary. Aldosterone is not used clinically because of its cost, short half-life and relative unavailability. Instead synthetic analogues such as fludrocortisone are administered (Drug Monograph 29.2) in Addison's disease and orthostatic hypotension. In high doses, aldosterone analogues have a negative-feedback effect on the pituitary secretion of ACTH and on adrenal cortex secretion of endogenous steroids (Fig 29.2).

DRUGS AT A GLANCE
Drugs acting on the adrenal cortex

PHARMACOLOGICAL GROUP AND EFFECT	KEY EXAMPLES	CLINICAL USE
Corticotrophin analogue • Increases synthesis and release of corticosteroids	Tetracosactride[AUS]	• Diagnosis of adrenal insufficiency • Hypsarrhythmia and/or infantile spasms
Corticosteroids (glucocorticoids) • Regulate gene expression • Increase or decrease synthesis of specific proteins	Betamethasone Cortisone[AUS] Dexamethasone Hydrocortisone[a] Methylprednisolone Prednisolone Prednisone Triamcinolone	• Wide range of conditions requiring immunosuppressive and anti-inflammatory effects • Adrenal insufficiency
Corticosteroid (mineralocorticoid)	Fludrocortisone	• Replacement therapy in primary adrenal insufficiency

[a] Hydrocortisone has both gluco- and mineralocorticoid activity.
[AUS] = Australia only

REVIEW EXERCISES

1 Mrs DT advises you that her daughter has been diagnosed with Addison's disease. She asks you to explain why her daughter requires lifelong replacement therapy and what would happen if she ceased taking the steroids. Make a list of the key points you would discuss with Mrs DT.

2 The trainee nurse asks you to explain why Mr GE, who has been prescribed fludrocortisone, has to have his serum sodium and potassium concentration measured and his blood pressure monitored regularly. What explanation will you provide to the trainee?

3 Mr TN, who has come for an appointment with you, casually mentions that he is using a steroid eyedrop. What information should you provide that would allow him to appreciate the benefits and the problems associated with long-term use of steroid eyedrops?

REFERENCES

Brunton LL, Hilal-Dandan R, Knollman BC. Goodman and Gilman's The pharmacological basis of therapeutics, 13th ed, New York, McGraw-Hill; 2018.

Kumar R, McEwan IJ. Allosteric modulators of steroid hormone receptors: structural dynamics and gene regulation. Endocrine Reviews 2012;33:271–99.

Rang HP, Ritter JM, Flower RJ, et al. Rang and Dale's Pharmacology, 8 ed, Edinburgh: Elsevier Churchill Livingstone; 2015.

ONLINE RESOURCES

Endocrine Nurses' Society of Australasia: https://www.ensa.org.au/ (accessed 14 March 2022)

The Endocrine Society of Australia: https://www.endocrinesociety.org.au (accessed 14 March 2022)

More weblinks at: http://evolve.elsevier.com/AU/Knights/pharmacology/.

UNIT 10 Drugs Affecting the Reproductive System

CHAPTER 30

DRUGS AFFECTING THE FEMALE REPRODUCTIVE SYSTEM

Mary Bushell

KEY ABBREVIATIONS

COC	combined oral contraceptive
EE	ethinylestradiol
ER	estrogen receptor
FSH	follicle-stimulating hormone
GnRH	gonadotrophin-releasing hormone
hCG	human chorionic gonadotrophin
HRT	hormone replacement therapy
IUD	intrauterine device
LARC	long-acting reversible contraceptives
LH	luteinising hormone
OC	oral contraceptive
SERM	selective estrogen receptor modulator
SPRM	selective progesterone receptor modulator

Chapter Focus

Many drugs used clinically to affect the female reproductive system are analogues or antagonists of pituitary gonadotrophins (follicle-stimulating hormone and luteinising hormone) or oxytocin, or of the ovarian hormones estrogen and progesterone. They are administered to mimic or suppress the biological effects of endogenous hormones, to supplement inadequate production (e.g. in menopause), to correct hormonal imbalance (e.g. in menstrual disorders), to reverse abnormal processes (endometriosis, anovulation and infertility) and for contraception.

For many people, an important issue in sexual functioning is contraception. The various methods of contraception for women – including drugs, devices and 'natural' methods – are described, and their relative advantages and disadvantages, and rates of use and of failure, are compared.

The physiological changes affecting usage of drugs in pregnancy are discussed briefly, including risks affecting the fetus. Drugs affecting uterine smooth muscle activity include those that induce labour (oxytocics) or inhibit premature labour (tocolytics). Lactation can be affected by drug therapy, as can the infant if drugs pass across into breast milk; guidelines for use of drugs by lactating mothers are described.

KEY TERMS

Australian categorisation system for prescribing medicines in pregnancy 687
combined oral contraceptive 678
contraception 676
dysmenorrhoea 672
emergency contraception 681
endometriosis 673
estrogen receptor 667
estrogens 667
gonadotrophin-releasing hormone 663
hormone replacement therapy 692
infertility 674
intrauterine device 681
lactation 690
menarche 663
menopause 692
menstrual cycle 664
minipill 680
oral contraceptive 667
oxytocics 688
perinatal period 687
phytoestrogens 696
pregnancy 684
progestogen 671
teratogen 685
tocolytic 690

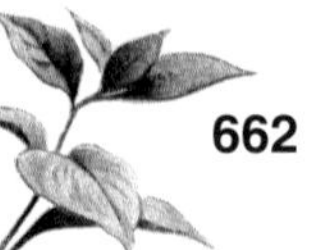

KEY DRUG GROUPS

Antiestrogens:

- **Clomifene** (Drug Monograph 30.3)
- **Tamoxifen**

Antiprogestogens:

- **Mifepristone**

Drugs used in pre-eclampsia:

- **Magnesium sulfate**

Gonadotrophin-releasing hormone analogues:

- **Nafarelin**

Gonadotrophins:

- **Human chorionic gonadotrophin**

Hormone replacement therapy:

- **Estrogens**
- **Progestogens**
- **Tibolone**

Long-acting reversible contraceptives:

- **Depot injections**, **IUD with copper**
- **Vaginal ring**

Estrogens:

- **Estradiol valerate** (Drug Monograph 30.1)
- Ethinylestradiol

Oral contraceptives:

- see estrogens, progestogens

Oxytocics:

- **Ergometrine** (Drug Monograph 30.4)
- **Oxytocin**

Progestogens:

- **Levonorgestrel** (Drug Monograph 30.2)
- **Medroxyprogesterone acetate**
- **Norethisterone**

Prostaglandins:

- **Dinoprostone**
- **Gemeprost**
- **Misoprostol**

Selective estrogen receptor modulators:

- **Raloxifene**

Selective progesterone receptor modulators:

- **Ulipristal**

Tocolytics:

- **Nifedipine**
- **Salbutamol**

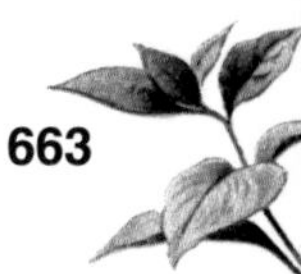

CRITICAL THINKING SCENARIO

Sophie, a 25-year-old early-career lawyer, presents to her local sexual health and family planning centre to speak with a health professional. Sophie is wanting to prevent unwanted pregnancy. Sophie states that she continues to suffer from acne, something she thought she would 'grow out of' and that she suffers from heavy menstrual bleeding, which in the past has led to anaemia. She also describes having breast tenderness, mood swings, headache and oedema 2–3 days before menstruation.

1. Discuss and compare the current contraceptive methods available. Make sure you cover their mode of action and the advantages and disadvantages of each method.

Five years later, Sophie returns to the sexual health and family planning centre. She says she ceased her contraceptive 2 years ago and has been trying to conceive since. Sophie describes that she has gone through a period of great stress and that she is having very irregular cycles. She is diagnosed with anovulatory infertility and subsequently prescribed clomifene, 50 mg once daily for 5 days starting on day 5 of her menstrual cycle.

2. How does this medicine work to induce ovulation?
3. What is the success rate of this medicine?
4. What other drugs are used to assist female infertility and what are their mode of actions?

Introduction: Female reproductive system controls and hormones

There are several levels of control of the female reproductive system (Fig 30.1), involving factors and hormones that can be used to treat gynaecological disorders and affect reproductive functions.

- The hypothalamus secretes a releasing factor (**gonadotrophin-releasing hormone** [GnRH, gonadorelin]), which stimulates the anterior pituitary gland. It helps initiate puberty.
- The anterior pituitary gland releases trophic hormones gonadotrophins (follicle-stimulating hormone [FSH] and luteinising hormone [LH]), which control ovarian function in the menstrual cycle.
- The target gland (gonadal) hormones are estrogens and progesterone, which control female secondary sex characteristics, the reproductive cycle and growth and development of accessory reproductive organs. Periodic cycling of hormone levels results in the menstrual cycle, which normally continues throughout reproductive life from menarche until menopause, except during pregnancy.
- Inhibins, glycoproteins produced in the gonads, decrease secretion of FSH and LH.
- Human chorionic gonadotrophin (hCG) and placental lactogen are secreted by the placenta during pregnancy.
- Prolactin and oxytocin, released from the anterior and posterior pituitary gland respectively (Ch 26), are involved in breast tissue proliferation, breastfeeding and childbirth.

The 'puberty clock'

The prolonged period of childhood in humans allows a long period of learning before onset of reproductive life. After about the age of 10 years, hormonal changes start to occur in both sexes: increased pulsatile output of GnRH from the hypothalamus in girls stimulates the pituitary gland to increase production of FSH and LH, stimulating the ovaries to produce estrogen and progesterone, and causing ovulation, maturation of female reproductive organs, development of secondary sexual characteristics and accelerated growth, followed by closure of the epiphyses of the long bones. The first menstrual period (**menarche**) is closely correlated with a skeletal age of 13 years but may occur some years earlier or later (range 8–15 years).

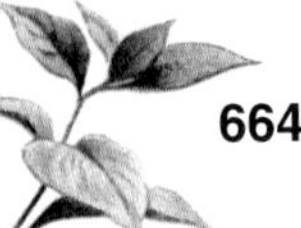

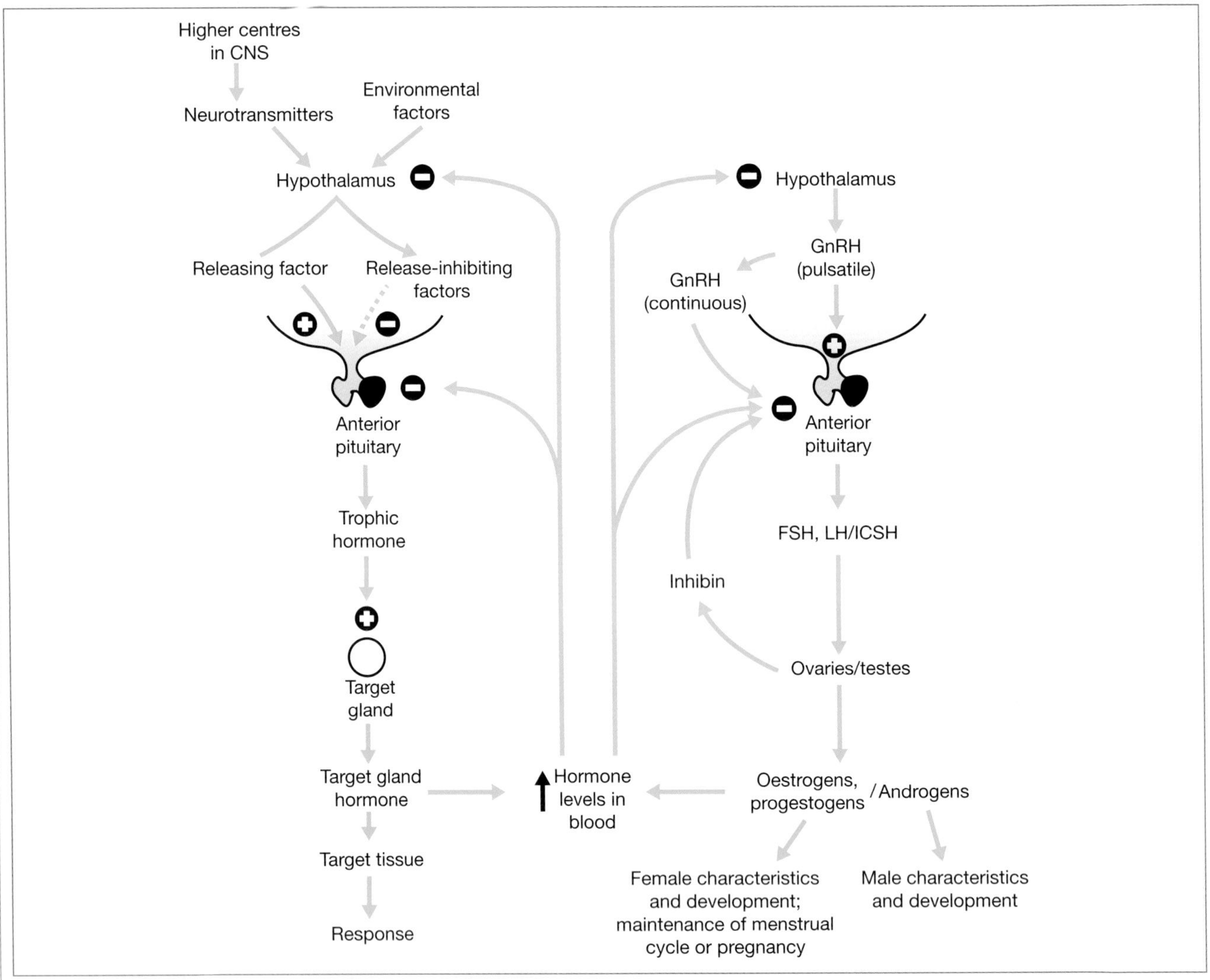

FIGURE 30.1 Sex hormone secretion and control: the hypothalamic–pituitary–gonadal axis

The actual 'clock' that switches on reproductive development and function is unknown; the timing depends mainly (50–80%) on multiple genetic factors, as well as stimuli from the nervous system, metabolic hormones leptin and ghrelin, neurokinin B and kisspeptin peptides, now considered the master regulators of reproductive functions in mammals (Abreu & Kaiser 2016). Puberty is occurring earlier worldwide, possibly associated with increased dietary intake of animal protein and the increasing prevalence of obesity and height gain in childhood.

Delayed puberty (no pubertal changes in girls older than 13 years or boys older than 14) may be due to familial late development, gonadal dysfunction, hypopituitarism or chronic severe illness. Treatment with the appropriate sex hormone(s) accelerates growth rate, development and closure of the epiphyses of long bones, potentially leading to short stature.

The menstrual cycle

The changes occurring during the **menstrual cycle**, and the actions of pituitary gonadotrophins and ovarian hormones, are illustrated in Fig 30.2. The physiological processes of a typical 28-day cycle are summarised below:

- *Days 1–5, menstruation:* Uterine lining is being shed, and FSH is stimulating follicle growth and production of estrogen in the ovary.
- *Days 4–14 (roughly), proliferative stage:* Rising estrogen levels prepare the uterus for a fertilised ovum, and stimulate the pre-ovulatory surge in pituitary LH production (by positive feedback) and, later, the mid-cycle FSH surge.
- *About day 14, ovulation:* Occurs when the mature follicle ruptures and releases its ovum.

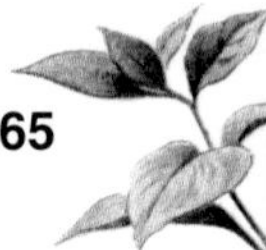

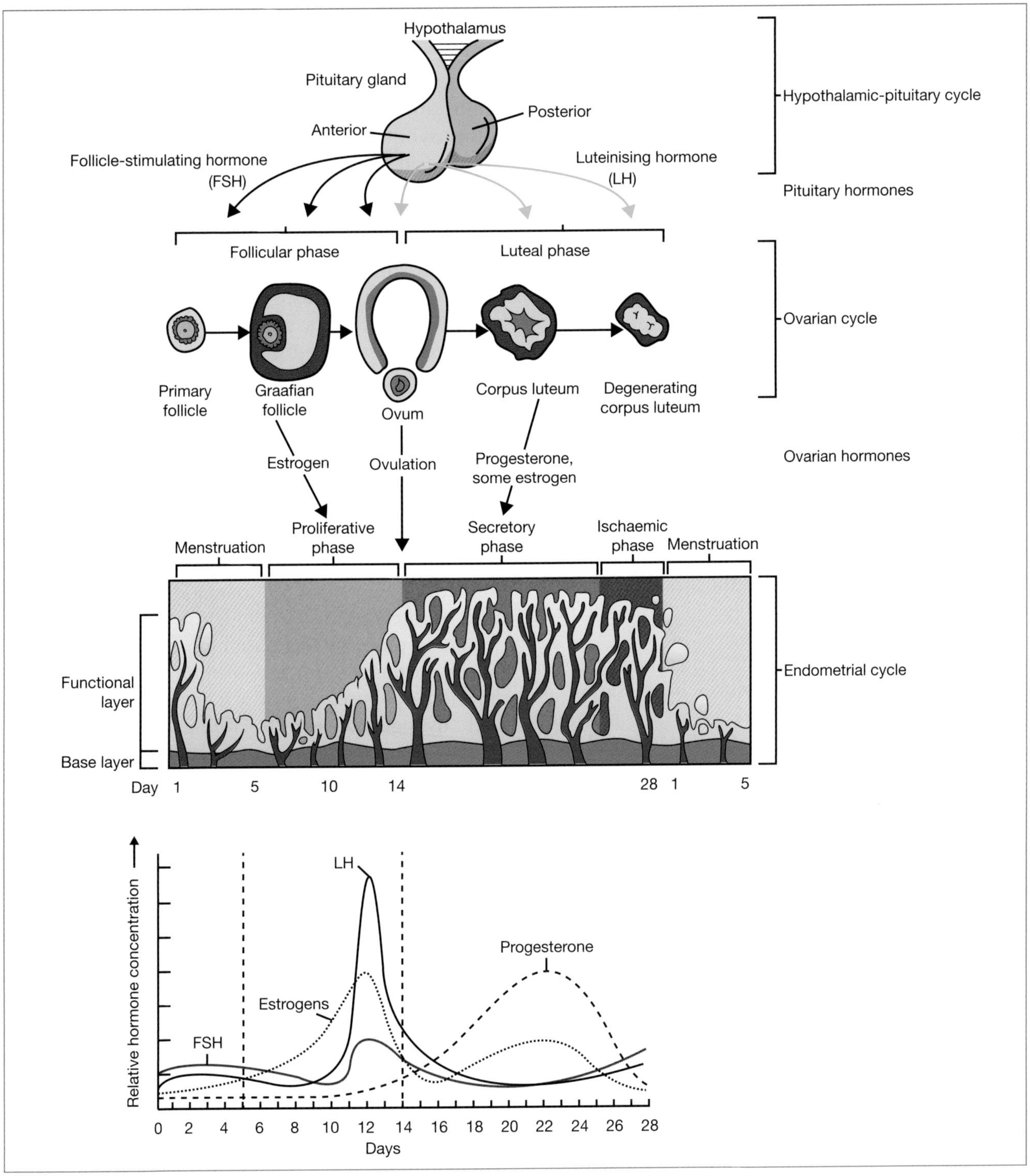

FIGURE 30.2 The menstrual cycle (in the absence of fertilisation and pregnancy)
Source: Adapted from Salerno 1999; used with permission.

- *Days 13–16, fertile period:* The ovum travels through the oviduct to the uterus; if fertilised, it implants in the uterine wall and continues to divide and grow (pregnancy).
- *Days 15–25, secretory phase:* LH causes luteinisation – the ruptured follicle capsule changes into the corpus luteum, which releases estrogen and progesterone. Progesterone maintains the endometrium to facilitate implantation and suppresses further ovulation to prevent subsequent pregnancy. Inhibin from follicle and corpus luteum inhibits secretion of FSH and LH.

- *Days 25–28:* If fertilisation (pregnancy) occurs, the corpus luteum continues to produce progesterone and maintains endometrium and pregnancy, and secretion of hCG begins. Levels of estrogens and progestogens continue to rise, and all changes of pregnancy begin to occur.
  or
- *Days 25–28:* If fertilisation does not occur, then, in the absence of hCG to 'rescue' the corpus luteum, luteal cells become less responsive to LH, levels of estrogen and progesterone fall, the endometrium degenerates and is sloughed off, resulting in menstruation.
- *Day 28 / day 1:* Next menstrual period starts.

Timing of ovulation and length of cycles vary (25–31 days); therefore, ovulation is not always predictable. The cyclical nature of the menstrual periods is regulated by the ovaries, and by the time required for developing the follicle and the functional life span of the corpus luteum, rather than by any cyclical release of hypothalamic or pituitary hormones. Urine test kits used by women to predict time of ovulation detect the LH surge, which indicates that ovulation is likely to occur within the next 24–36 hours.

Later in life, gonadal (ovarian) function decreases, and women experience menopause, or cessation of menses. (Men also have a decrease in sex hormone production, which may lead to physiological and psychological changes – sometimes called the male climacteric.[1])

Drugs used in gynaecological disorders

Gonadotrophins: release and clinical use

Gonadotrophin-releasing hormone

GnRH is a 10-amino-acid peptide; its actions depend on how it is administered. At low (physiological) doses, and given in a *pulsatile* dose schedule, it stimulates pituitary synthesis and release of the pituitary gonadotrophins FSH and LH, and thus overall regulates the female reproductive system.

Continuous administration in higher doses results in desensitisation and *decreased* pituitary production of LH and FSH. This is used to inhibit growth of steroid-dependent tumours. Gonadorelin, a synthetic form of GnRH identical to the natural hormone, has been used to induce ovulation and as an adjunct to diagnose hypogonadism in males and females.

GnRH analogues and inhibitors

Other synthetic GnRH analogues with slightly different amino acid sequences, such as nafarelin, are more potent as LHRH agonists and have longer durations of action (Table 30.1, later). At higher continuous doses, they are used to down-regulate pituitary functions. They can cause an initial 'flare' of symptoms, due to release of stored gonadotrophins.

GnRH inhibitors are used to treat endometriosis and in assisted reproduction programs (described later).

Gonadotrophic hormones

Pituitary gonadotrophins

FSH and LH are glycoprotein hormones responsible for development and maintenance of sexual gland functions. FSH stimulates development of the Graafian ovarian follicles up to the point of ovulation. LH (known in the male as interstitial-cell-stimulating hormone) acts in the female to promote maturation of the follicle, formation of the corpus luteum and secretion of estrogen. These hormones are used clinically in male or female infertility and hypogonadism. Prescribing such hormones is usually restricted to specialists, such as endocrinologists and doctors involved in assisted reproduction clinics, as close monitoring of hormone levels and responses is essential.

Other gonadotrophins

Other gonadotrophins include:

- human chorionic gonadotrophin (hCG), secreted by the chorion (the outer membrane enveloping the fetus): hCG is measurable in urine of pregnant women within a few days of fertilisation and is the antigen detected in pregnancy tests; it has mainly LH-type actions and is used to induce ovulation and treat hypogonadism
- menotropins (human menopausal gonadotrophins, a mixture of FSH and LH extracted from the urine of menopausal women): used to stimulate the ovaries in assisted reproduction procedures
- choriogonadotropin alfa and lutropin alfa: recombinant forms of hCG used for their LH activities
- follitropin-α and follitropin-β: recombinant forms used for their FSH-type actions.

1 The term 'male menopause' is inappropriate because 'menopause' literally means cessation of menstruation.

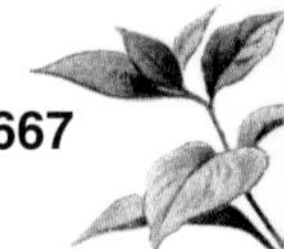

Gonadal hormones and antagonists

Estrogenic, or follicular, hormones (estradiol, estrone, estriol)[2] are produced mainly by cells of the developing Graafian follicle. Progestational, or luteal, hormones (progesterone, hydroxyprogesterone) are produced by the corpus luteum. The main functions of the female sex hormones are to:

- regulate development of accessory sex organs (including breasts, uterus and vagina)
- regulate secondary sexual characteristics (differences in skeletal and muscle size, body fat deposition, distribution of hair, pitch of voice, development of breasts)
- control ovulation and the menstrual cycle or maintain pregnancy.

They are used clinically as drugs in replacement therapies, in contraception and in some cancers. Cyclical secretion of estrogens and progesterone, as occurs during the menstrual cycle, needs to be mimicked when hormones are given exogenously in the **oral contraceptive** (OC) pill or postmenopausal hormone replacement therapy (HRT) formulations.

Estrogens

Sources

Estrogens are secreted by ovarian follicles, synthesised from cholesterol via androgens, and by the corpus luteum, placenta (up to 100 times the pre-pregnancy levels), liver and testes. The 'A' ring of estrogens is aromatic (like benzene), unlike that of most other steroid hormones. Estrogens used as drugs are purified from natural sources – for example, the urine of pregnant mares – in conjugated dosage forms known as conjugated equine estrogens (INN name).

The three natural estrogens (estradiol, estrone and estriol) are rapidly metabolised in the liver, so esterified or semisynthetic orally active derivatives (e.g. **estradiol valerate**, ethinylestradiol [EE], mestranol) are used. The natural estrogens tend to be used in HRT formulations, which require only low doses; whereas synthetic hormones, especially EE, are used in OC preparations (Table 30.2, later).

Actions

The main physiological actions of estrogens are (Fig 30.3):

- assisting in follicle development
- stimulating the mid-cycle LH surge
- stimulating growth of myometrium and endometrium and mucus production
- metabolic actions – retention of salt and fluid, mild anabolic actions, decreased risk of atheroma, increased coagulability of blood and decreased rate of bone resorption
- inhibiting secretion of FSH and LH from the pituitary gland, resulting in inhibition of ovulation and lactation and development of proliferative endometrium.

Estrogens appear to be protective against Parkinson's disease, which is less prevalent in women than men. Estrogens enhance cell proliferation and the humoral immune response; women have a higher prevalence of autoimmune disorders such as rheumatoid arthritis and systemic lupus erythematosus.

Mechanisms: estrogen receptors

Estrogens activate **estrogen receptors** (ERs) in estrogen-responsive target tissues, especially in the uterus, vagina and breast. They diffuse through cell membranes, bind to membrane-associated ERs and induce a conformational change; ligand-receptor dimers then translocate to the nucleus, recruit co-activators of the receptor, and there is interaction with DNA and activation of gene transcription, leading to altered synthesis of proteins. There are also GPCR-type ERs in cell membranes and non-genomic signal-transduction pathways, leading to more rapid responses and roles in cognition, depression and pain processing (Lu & Herndon 2017).

ERs have been classified into ERα and Erβ subtypes, with many different isoform variants; they are members of the nuclear receptor superfamily Class I, which includes receptors for progesterone and adrenocorticosteroids. 17β-estradiol is the main endogenous ligand bonding to ERα/β; estrone and estriol bind with lower affinity. Both types have roles in cardiovascular protection, prevention of atherosclerosis, neuroprotection and central nervous system (CNS) functions. ERα are particularly involved in development of breast and uterus tissue, bone protection, metabolic control and protection against multiple sclerosis, whereas ERβ are more involved in follicle development and ovulation, controlling breast-development actions of ERα and protection against depression. Overall, agonists at ERβ are therefore preferred for their bone protection and lipid-lowering actions, and for being less likely to stimulate breast and uterine tissue.

Clinical uses

A large number of the world's female population take estrogens regularly for many years, either in contraceptive

2 The term 'estrus' is derived from the Greek word meaning the sexual heat period of female mammals.

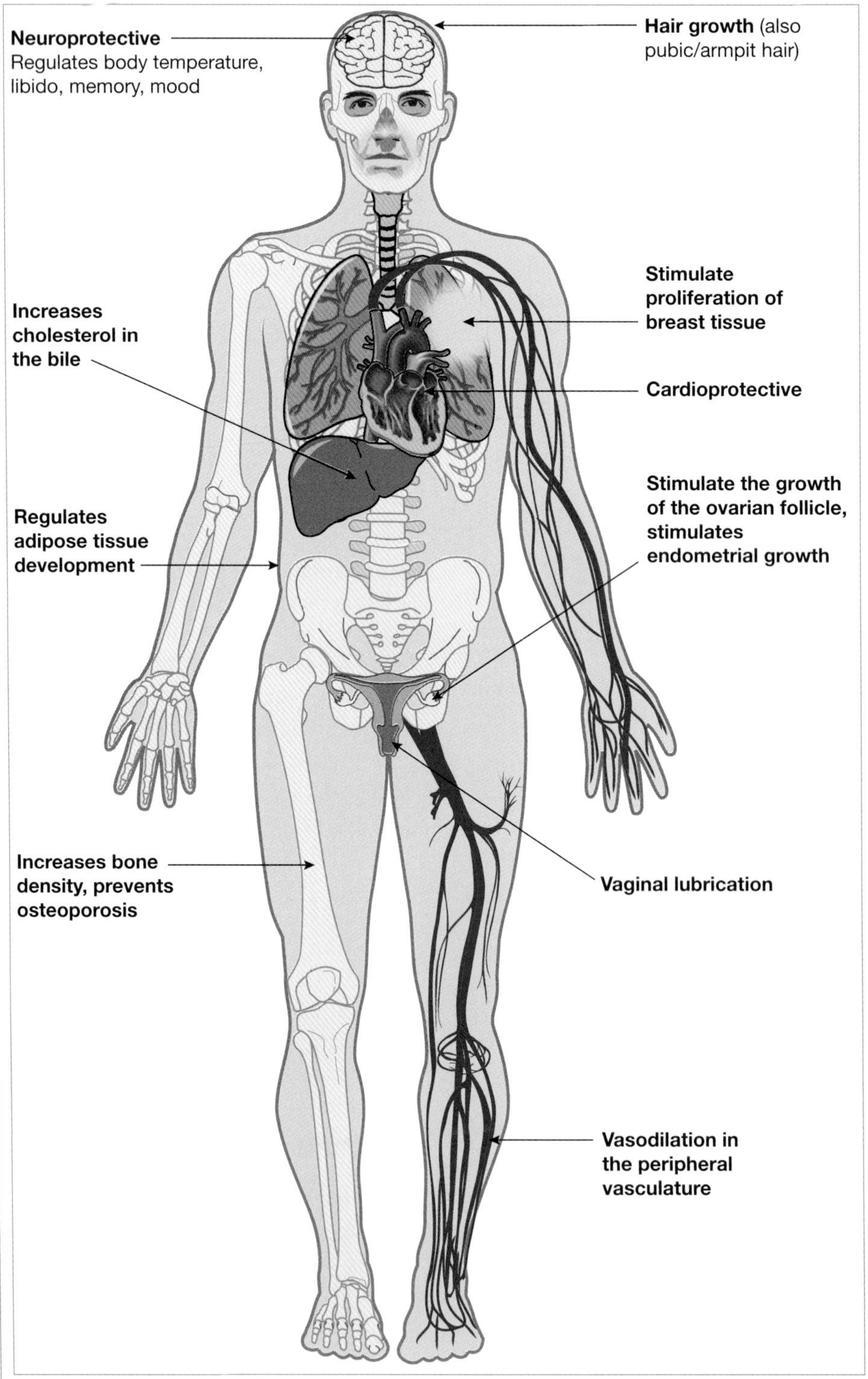

Neuroprotective Regulates body temperature, libido, memory, mood

Hair growth (also pubic/armpit hair)

Stimulate proliferation of breast tissue

Increases cholesterol in the bile

Cardioprotective

Stimulate the growth of the ovarian follicle, stimulates endometrial growth

Regulates adipose tissue development

Vaginal lubrication

Increases bone density, prevents osteoporosis

Vasodilation in the peripheral vasculature

FIGURE 30.3 The effects of estrogen

preparations or as HRT during menopause. Other indications include:

- disorders of menstruation – for example, endometrial hyperplasia, dysfunctional uterine bleeding, amenorrhoea
- replacement therapy (cyclical administration) in estrogen deficiency, atrophic vaginitis or female hypogonadism
- some breast cancers (metastatic breast carcinomas in postmenopausal women with tumour estrogen-negative receptors)

- hirsutism (excessive androgen-dependent hair growth).

Dosages of estrogens must be individualised according to diagnosis, clinical use, route of administration and therapeutic response – for example, for contraception, treatment of breast cancer or vasomotor symptoms associated with menopause (Drug Monograph 30.1 for typical routes, pharmacokinetics, adverse drug reactions and precautions; and Drug Interactions 30.1). In high doses (e.g. as were present in early formulations of the OC pill), there was increased incidence of thromboembolic disorders such as deep vein thrombosis and stroke. Because of this risk, the OC pill is not recommended for women over 35 years who smoke.

SERMs, anti-estrogens and endocrine-disrupting chemicals

Selective estrogen receptor modulators

Selective estrogen receptor modulators (SERMs) are tissue-specific, non-steroidal ER modulators that have Erβ-agonist actions at some ERs, particularly in bone, cardiovascular system, liver and CNS function, but antagonistic actions on other ERs (in breast and uterus). Hence, SERMs are useful in infertility and to protect against menopausal osteoporosis and cardiovascular disease while not increasing (possibly even reducing) the risk of estrogen-dependent breast or uterine cancers. SERMs have potential uses in many estrogen-dependent conditions and are being tested

Drug Monograph 30.1
Estradiol valerate

Indications
Estradiol valerate is used for its estrogenic actions on ovary and uterus in HRT to prevent and treat estrogen-deficiency symptoms after ovariectomy or menopause, and in the COC 'pill' for contraception.

Actions and mechanisms
Estradiol valerate is an ester derivative of the natural hormone. See text.

Pharmacokinetics
Estradiol valerate is a prodrug of estradiol-17β. It is rapidly and completely absorbed (peak plasma concentration within 6 hours), and quickly metabolised in the liver to estradiol, then to various metabolites, of which estriol and estrone have estrogenic activity. Estradiol is highly protein-bound and has a half-life of 18–24 hours. Metabolites are excreted in bile, and undergo enterohepatic recycling.

Drug interactions
See Drug Interactions 30.1.

Side effects and adverse reactions
Typical estrogenic effects are breast pain and enlargement, changes in menstrual bleeding, headaches, nausea, vomiting, a change in libido, oedema of lower extremities, chloasma (darkened patches of skin on the face) and increased risk of thromboembolism. Administration by skin patch can cause irritation and dermatitis.

Warnings and contraindications
Estrogens should be used with caution in smokers and in women with endometriosis, diabetes, migraine or epilepsy. Avoid use in pregnancy and in women with estrogen hypersensitivity, thromboembolic disorders or severe cardiovascular or liver disease, breast cancer and other estrogen-dependent tumours, or hypercalcaemia (see also later discussion of risks with COC or HRT). Estrogens reduce lactation and are excreted in breast milk, so administration to breastfeeding mothers is not recommended.

Dosage and administration
In HRT: a cyclical dosing schedule of 3 weeks estradiol administration (1–2 mg daily by mouth) and 1 week off, possibly with addition of a progestogen for the last 10–14 days of the cycle, most closely approximates the natural menstrual cycle. The progestogen must be added to HRT in postmenopausal women with an intact uterus to avoid endometrial hyperplasia or carcinoma. The prescriber should re-evaluate the person at least annually.

Transdermal estradiol is also used for women with estrogen deficiency, particularly as HRT in menopause (used with a progestogen in women with an intact uterus). Applied topically to intact skin, the patch releases 25–100 micrograms (0.025–0.1 mg) daily. It is usually worn continuously and should be replaced twice weekly. Sensitivity reactions at the application site often occur. Estradiol is also formulated in many COC tablet types (Table 30.2, later) and as a vaginal pessary and transdermal gel.

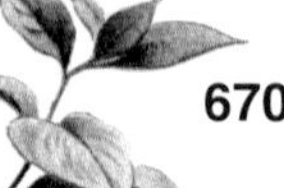

DRUG INTERACTIONS 30.1

Some potentially significant interactions with estrogens

DRUG	POSSIBLE EFFECTS AND MANAGEMENT
Enzyme inducers (barbiturates, some antiepileptics, aprepitant, bosentan, modafinil, some antivirals, rifamycins, St John's wort)	May accelerate metabolism of estrogens and reduce their activity; additional contraception such as condoms should be used if required; effects in HRT may be reduced
Atazanavir, etoricoxib	Increase concentrations of EE and risk of adverse effects; low-dose EE (30 micrograms) OC formulations should be used or a different interacting drug selected
Antibiotics (e.g. ampicillin)	May reduce potency of estradiol because of metabolism by altered gut flora
Tobacco (smoking)	Tobacco smoking increases risk of serious cardiovascular adverse reactions and venous thromboembolism; risk is higher in women over 35 who smoke; OCs not recommended
Orlistat	Orlistat-induced diarrhoea may reduce estrogen levels; additional contraception may be necessary
Selegiline	COCs may increase selegiline concentration, enhancing its effects and adverse effects; reduce selegiline dose or avoid combination
Drugs affecting blood glucose	Estrogens can increase blood glucose levels, thus affecting diabetes control
Thyroid hormones	Estrogens may alter concentrations of thyroid hormones, requiring increased thyroxine dose; thyroid function should be monitored

Notes: (1) See Australian Medicines Handbook 2021, Drug interactions, under 'Combined Oral Contraceptives' and 'Hormone Replacement Therapy'. (2) Doses of estrogens in HRT formulations are considerably lower than in COC, so fewer drug interactions are expected.

against some prostate cancers; each SERM appears to have a unique array of activities and potential uses (Ellis et al. 2015).

Raloxifene was the first clinically used SERM. It increases bone mineral density, improves the blood lipid profile and reduces bone resorption and vertebral fractures, with no stimulation of endometrium or breast tissue; however, hot flushes associated with menopause may be exacerbated. There is a potential increased risk of venous thromboembolism (VTE) and stroke. It is contraindicated in pregnancy (Category X). Related '-ifene' drugs such as toremifene have improved effects in enhancing bone mineral density and reducing cholesterol levels. Tamoxifen, long used as an anti-estrogen in breast cancer (see below), is now recognised as a SERM.

Anti-estrogens

Tamoxifen binds to most ERs but does not stimulate transcription and so has few estrogenic actions. It is mainly used as an estrogen antagonist in postmenopausal estrogen-dependent breast cancers. (In premenopausal women, it would be swamped by the large amounts of circulating estrogens.) However, it has pro-estrogenic effects so can cause endometrial cancer and thromboembolic events.

Fulvestrant, a pure estrogen antagonist, competes for binding with the ER and prevents its dimerisation and nuclear localisation; it therefore abolishes all estrogenic actions, including protective effects. It inhibits growth of ER-positive tumours and is used to treat locally advanced or metastatic breast cancer in postmenopausal women.

Clomifene (Drug Monograph 30.3, later) acts by rather different mechanisms: it inhibits estrogen binding in the hypothalamus and pituitary gland, reducing negative feedback effects of circulating estrogens so that more GnRH is produced, which increases release of gonadotrophins, especially LH (Fig 30.1). The *raised* estrogen levels from the stimulated ovaries induce ovulation. The drug is used to treat female infertility and polycystic ovary syndrome. Major risks are multiple pregnancies, ovarian enlargement and estrogenic adverse effects.

Endocrine-disrupting chemicals

Endocrine-disrupting chemicals present in the environment may have stimulating or antagonistic effects on estrogen or androgen receptors or on GnRH. They include about 800 chemicals found in air, soil, water and food, coming from household and personal products, plastic products and flame-retardants, as well as natural phytoestrogens in plants such as soy, carrots, garlic, coffee and legumes. Chemical types include bisphenols, phthalates, parabens and heavy metals. While a causal relationship is yet to be determined, possible adverse effects include changes in hormone levels, impaired sperm and egg quality, precocious puberty, delayed puberty or sexual differentiation disorders, longer menstrual cycles, endometriosis, increased risk of infertility or miscarriage, earlier menopause and increased risk of some endocrine-dependent cancers.

Progesterone and progestogens

Sources

LH secreted from the anterior pituitary stimulates synthesis and secretion of progesterone from the corpus luteum during the latter half of the menstrual cycle; this is the main naturally occurring **progestogen** (also known as progestin) along with hydroxyprogesterone. Progesterone is also formed during pregnancy (in the placenta, from steroid precursors); it promotes breast development, maintains pregnancy and prevents further ovulation.

Actions and mechanisms

Physiological actions of progesterone are to:

- stimulate the secretory phase of the menstrual cycle
- maintain the endometrium to prepare for implantation and nourishment of the embryo (i.e. 'pro-gestational' effects that sustain pregnancy)
- cause relaxation of uterine smooth muscles at all gestational stages
- decrease levels of LH and ERs
- raise core body temperature[3] (thermogenic).

Progesterone receptors are also members of the nuclear receptor superfamily Class I; the physiological ligand is (obviously) progesterone. The main signalling pathway for cellular genomic response is as described above for estrogens on ERs. Interestingly, progesterone and receptors are synthesised in some CNS neurons when stimulated by circulating estrogens, which partially accounts for the mid-cycle LH surge.

Clinical uses

Progestogens are commonly used clinically in hormonal contraception (both combined with an estrogen and in progestogen-only formulations), in endometriosis (to suppress ovarian functions), in HRT (in women with an intact uterus, to oppose the actions of estrogen) and in assisted reproduction technologies.

Progesterone itself is virtually inactive orally, due to rapid metabolism; it can be administered as a pessary (100 or 200 mg) or vaginal gel (90 mg) to avoid first-pass effects. When used as 'luteal support' in assisted reproductive technologies to treat infertility, the dosage is one or two intravaginal applications daily for up to 12 weeks.

Synthetic derivatives, collectively called progestogens or progestins, provide effective oral or sublingual forms and longer durations of action. Progestogens commonly used include:

- medroxyprogesterone acetate (MPA) – active orally and intramuscularly
- testosterone derivatives – for example, norethisterone, active orally; these have some androgenic and estrogenic actions and may cause androgenic adverse effects (e.g. acne, hirsutism)
- cyproterone, another testosterone derivative, has significant anti-androgenic actions, used mainly as an OC and in HRT in women suffering masculinisation effects
- megestrol, used for its antitumour activity in breast cancer and endometrial cancer.

Others commonly used in combined OC formulations are levonorgestrel (Drug Monograph 30.2), desogestrel, dienogest, gestodene and drospirenone (Table 32.2, latter); the last-named has mild anti-mineralocorticoid effects and hence may cause diuresis and potassium retention.

Antiprogestogens and selective progesterone receptor modulators

Antiprogestogens all appear to be partial agonists/antagonists, and may also be referred to as selective progesterone receptor modulators SPRMs. They are used to treat endometriosis (Clinical Focus Box 30.1), heavy menstrual bleeding due to leiomyomas (fibroids), in emergency contraception and medical termination of pregnancy and for antiproliferative effects in breast cancer (Wagenfeld et al. 2016).

Mifepristone (RU486) blocks LH surge and prevents implantation; it also has antiglucocorticoid activity and sensitises the uterus to prostaglandins (PGs). It is used in combination with a PG agonist (gemeprost or misoprostol) for early termination of pregnancy. It has been trialled for third trimester induction of labour, for ripening of the cervix and to reduce the need for caesarean section (see later discussion of oxytocic agents).

Drug treatment of gynaecological disorders

Many drugs used to treat women's conditions have already been described in this chapter, and in other chapters (on the neuroendocrine system and pituitary gland, analgesics, anti-inflammatory drugs, etc.), so only a brief overview of drug treatments will be given.

3 The basis for attempting to time ovulation in the 'rhythm' method of contraception, by monitoring body temperature: a rise of about 0.5°C occurs after ovulation, due to rising levels of progesterone.

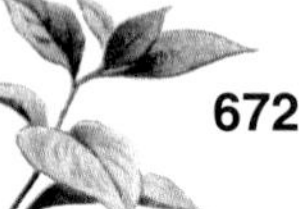

Drug Monograph 30.2
Levonorgestrel

Levonorgestrel is a prototype synthetic progestogen. Levonorgestrel's contraceptive effects are by preventing ovulation and fertilisation if intercourse has taken place in the pre-ovulatory phase, when the likelihood of fertilisation is the highest. (For actions and mechanisms, see text.)

Indications

Levonorgestrel is indicated for oral contraception (alone or combined with an estrogen), emergency contraception, in long-term contraception (as an IUD), in postmenopausal HRT, in treatment of hormonal imbalances in dysmenorrhoea and in specific carcinomas (breast, endometrial, renal cell – specialist oncologist use only).

Pharmacokinetics

Levonorgestrel is rapidly absorbed after oral administration, reaching maximum plasma concentration after 2 hours, with a mean elimination half-life of about 26 hours. It is highly protein-bound to sex-hormone-binding globulin. It is metabolised in the liver, with inactive metabolites excreted in urine and faeces.

Drug interactions

Effectiveness of oral progestogens, and possibly of the IUD, may be reduced by CYP3A4 enzyme-inducing drugs, particularly rifamycins, many anticonvulsants and some antivirals; contraceptive failure may result, so alternative contraception is necessary. (For details, see reference texts such as the *Australian Medicines Handbook*, Appendix B, under 'Combined Oral Contraceptives' and 'Progestogens'.)

Adverse reactions

High doses for emergency contraception may cause breast pain, nausea and vomiting, vaginal bleeding and headache; lower long-term doses may cause reversible ovarian cysts. IUD insertion may cause pain or cramps and irregular bleeding.

Warnings and contraindications

Should be used with caution in women with uterine, genital or urinary tract bleeding (undiagnosed) or malabsorption syndromes. Avoid use in women with progestogen hypersensitivity, breast or genital tract cancer (contraceptive use), severe liver or thromboembolic disease and in pregnancy.

Dosage and administration

Low physiological dosages are used for progestational effects in replacement therapy, and higher doses to suppress ovulation, menstruation and gonadotrophin production. Examples of dosing regimens are:

- in IUD, for contraception or HRT: 52 mg (replaced every 5 years)
- as component of COC: 50–150 micrograms
- as emergency contraceptive: 1.5 mg single dose, taken within 72 hours of unprotected intercourse.

Disorders of menstruation

Uterine smooth muscle undergoes physiological rhythmical contractions, with myometrial cells in the fundus (inner surface of the dome) acting as pacemakers. During the menstrual cycle contractions are weak on days 6–14, become gradually stronger and more prolonged, until during menstruation (days 1–5) coordinated contractions can lead to cramping pain.

Dysmenorrhoea

Painful menstruation (**dysmenorrhoea**) occurs in about 40% of young women and is incapacitating in about 3%. Pain and spasms of uterine muscles are likely due to PGs (e.g. $PGF_{2}\alpha$) released from degenerating endometrium. The most effective treatments for excessive uterine bleeding are:

- the levonorgestrel intrauterine contraceptive system
- OC progestogen formulations used in extended-cycle manner
- COC preparations containing at least 35 micrograms EE.

Also used are tranexamic acid, an antifibrinolytic drug, and non-steroidal anti-inflammatory agents (NSAIDs), especially naproxen, which also has analgesic actions and decreases the contractions, symptoms and blood loss (Bryant-Smith et al. 2018).

Heavy menstrual bleeding

Heavy menstrual bleeding (formerly called menorrhagia) may be ovulatory (earlier in life) or anovulatory (leading up to menopause). Ovulatory bleeding is due to structural cause such as uterine fibroids; treatment may include antianaemic drugs (iron, folic acid), NSAIDs (naproxen) to relieve symptoms, tranexamic acid, the OC pill or depot progestogen; less frequently, GnRH agonists are

CLINICAL FOCUS BOX 30.1
Management of endometriosis

Ms CY is a 23-year-old woman whose GP has made the clinical diagnosis of endometriosis, based on a longstanding history of severe dysmenorrhoea, deep dyspareunia and painful defecation when she has her period. Ms CY initially tries taking regular non-steroidal antiinflammatories during her periods, without much relief. Her GP suggests that she go on the oral contraceptive pill, which somewhat alleviates her symptoms for the next 3 years.

By the time she is 27, her symptoms have worsened again, such that she is very reluctant to have intercourse (due to pain), and has to take several days off work every month due to crippling dysmenorrhoea. She is referred to a gynaecology clinic at her local hospital; the treating specialist prescribes 'Synarel' nasal spray (nafarelin acetate, a GnRH agonist; 200 microgram/dose, twice daily for 6 months). One year later, she is keen to conceive, but her symptoms have returned. Her gynaecologist performs a laparoscopy to excise all visible endometriosis tissue. Her condition markedly improves postoperatively, and she is able to manage symptoms with NSAIDs alone. She successfully conceives 6 months after her operation.

Over the next 10 years, Ms CY uses NSAIDs and the OC pill to control her symptoms between pregnancies. During this time, she requires two additional laparoscopies to remove all visible endometriosis, including an endometriotic ovarian cyst.

Source: Acknowledgment to Dr Alison Bryant-Smith, MRCOG (personal communication).

used. Anovulatory bleeding is when intervals between periods lengthen and uterine lining builds up, leading to heavier periods (formerly called dysfunctional uterine bleeding); treatment usually involves balancing progestogen and estrogen levels with COC or HRT preparations, or progestogen-only IUD.

Heavy menstrual bleeding occurs in about 5% of menstruating women. It is relatively common around puberty and menopause, and in association with platelet dysfunction, cervical cancer, endocrine disorders, or in women with low body-fat mass or who do excessive exercise. Primary causes should be sought and anaemia monitored. Surgical treatments include dilation and curettage of the uterus, laser endometrial ablation and, as a last resort, hysterectomy.

Premenstrual syndrome

Premenstrual syndrome refers to the breast tenderness, backache, depression or anxiety, mood swings, headache, bloating, nausea and oedema suffered by up to 12% of women during the luteal phase, 2–3 days before onset of menstruation, and impairing daily activities. Symptoms may be due to increased sensitivity to cycling estrogen and progesterone, increased aldosterone and plasma renin activity and abnormalities of neurotransmitters, especially serotonin (5-HT) and gamma aminobutyric acid. Symptoms resolve shortly after menstruation. Premenstrual dysphoric disorder is a more severe form, suffered by 2–4% of women.

Low-dose selective serotonin reuptake inhibitor antidepressants (sertraline, escitalopram), a COC preparation, diuretics, dietary modifications, exercise, calcium, vitamin B6 (50–100 mg pyridoxine daily), and cognitive behaviour therapy are useful treatments. Second-line therapies are GnRH analogues with combination patches, and/or HRT preparations and surgery (see RCOG guidelines in 'Online resources'; and review by Hofmeister & Bodden 2016).

Other disorders of menstruation

Other menstrual disorders are listed below. (The debate about whether menstruation should be optional is summarised in Clinical Focus Box 30.2.)

- *Amenorrhoea:* absence of menstruation, which is physiological before menarche, during pregnancy and lactation and after menopause; pathological causes include stress and endocrine tumours.
- *Irregular bleeding* (formerly called metrorrhagia): bleeding from the uterus other than during a normal menstrual period; although strictly speaking not a disorder of menstruation, it is a significant warning sign for cancer of the uterine cervix or endometrium.

Endometriosis

Endometriosis is a chronic condition of endometrial tissue at unusual (ectopic) locations – for example, within oviducts (fallopian tubes), ovaries, myometrium or pelvis; aetiology may involve altered ERs or metabolism, leading to hormone imbalances. It occurs in about 10% of women of reproductive age. Ectopic tissue undergoes cyclical changes and produces menstrual fluid that cannot escape the abdominal cavity or other location. This can lead to ovarian cysts, pain, chronic inflammation, scar formation, infertility, dysmenorrhoea and dyspareunia (painful intercourse). First-line treatment is surgical, to remove ectopic endometrial tissue. Hormonal treatments trialled include levonorgestrel IUD, progestogens such as dienogest, COC preparations, androgens (to inhibit GnRH release and block LH surge) or GnRH analogues (e.g. nafarelin, continuous dose for gonadal suppression). NSAIDs are

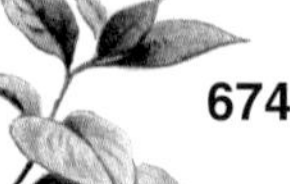

CLINICAL FOCUS BOX 30.2
A short history of the oral contraceptive pill

The rationale for thinking that estrogens and progestogens might act as reversible contraceptive agents was the fact that ovulation does not occur during pregnancy, when levels of estrogens and progestogens are high. Important stages in the development of OCs are as follows:

- In the 1930s, advances in steroid chemistry facilitated chemical synthesis of steroid hormones; research into methods of chemically modifying plant hormones to mass-produce steroids led to the development of some inexpensive orally active preparations.
- In the 1950s, combinations of mestranol (metabolised to EE) and norethynodrel as OCs were tested in large-scale clinical trials in Puerto Rico and Haiti, and provided successful reversible contraception with acceptable levels of adverse reactions.
- In 1960, the first OC preparation was marketed in the United States; it was a combination containing mestranol 150 micrograms and ethynodiol diacetate 10 mg. In 1961, OC were available in Australia.
- Early OC formulations were indeed pills (small spherical masses containing active drugs, prepared by rolling techniques), but now the hormones are formulated into small tablets; the term 'pill' has remained in the OC context.
- Typical early preparations contained EE 100–150 micrograms per tablet plus 1–4 mg norethisterone, now recognised as unnecessarily large amounts of estrogen. Current formulations include only 20–50 micrograms EE plus 0.5–1 mg norethisterone or equivalent.
- The importance of taking a 'pill' every day was recognised, so tablets were soon packaged in 'calendar packs' (Fig 30.3A) with the days marked, and seven placebo (sugar) tablets included in most packs to avoid a break in tablet-taking.

Today there are many formulations of the pill. Monophasic and multiphasic options are available. All COCs contain an estrogen and a progestogen.

Availability of an OC pill heralded not only a pharmacological revolution but also sexual and social revolutions: for the first time, women had a reliable, safe and reversible method of controlling their fertility, which allowed them to be sexually active without fear of pregnancy, to separate career choices from family planning and to compete more equally with men in the workforce.

used to reduce inflammation and pain (Clinical Focus Box 30.2; Brown & Farquhar 2015).

Polycystic ovary syndrome

Polycystic ovary syndrome is present in approximately 5–10% of women of childbearing age; it commonly causes infertility, menstrual irregularities, hirsutism, acne and male pattern alopecia in women. It may be associated with obesity, metabolic syndrome, diabetes mellitus, ovarian dysfunction and hyperandrogenic anovulation. Adipocytes (increased in obesity) synthesise and release mediators (adipokines), including leptin and tumour necrosis factor α, involved in cardiovascular risk and insulin resistance.

The most common therapies are COC tablets, anti-androgens, weight reduction and exercise, and hypoglycaemic agents, especially insulin sensitisers such as metformin and thiazolidinediones. Metformin reduces hyperinsulinaemia, improves cardiovascular risk factors such as high blood pressure and dyslipidaemia, reduces free fatty acids, reduces high androgen levels, promotes weight loss and overall improves the chance of ovulation and outcome of pregnancy.

In women hoping to conceive, ovulation inducers such as clomifene citrate (Drug Monograph 30.3) and aromatase inhibitors are used (see later under 'Treatment of female infertility').

Hirsutism

Hirsutism – excessive growth of coarse pigmented hair in women – can be distressing and require treatment. It may be an inherited trait or a response to drugs, including phenytoin, minoxidil or testosterone-derived progestogens. Androgens from hyperactive ovaries (e.g. polycystic ovaries), from the adrenal cortex or from other virilising endocrine disorders cause relative androgen excess at hair follicles, especially on the lower face and midline of the trunk.

Possible treatments include suppression of ovarian functions with COC preparations, suppression of the adrenal cortex – for example, with dexamethasone – or administration of anti-androgens such as cyproterone or spironolactone (Ch 31).

Female infertility

Fertility in humans requires effective, coordinated and appropriately timed functioning of several reproductive processes and many hormones: production of viable gametes in both woman and man, deposition and motility of sufficient spermatozoa in the female reproductive tract, fertilisation of a mature oocyte, then its implantation and development in the primed uterine mucosa and maintenance of pregnancy. Defects in any step can lead to **infertility**, defined as the absence of conception by a couple after more than 1 year of regular sexual intercourse without contraception. It affects 10–15% of all cohabiting couples wishing to conceive, and can cause great emotional distress.

Effective treatment requires careful assessment of possible causes in both partners. Infertility is attributed to male factors in about 40% of cases, female factors in about 40% of cases and couple factors in 20% of cases. In women, cycles may be anovulatory due to hyperprolactinaemia, hypothalamic or pituitary dysfunction or ovarian

Drug Monograph 30.3
Clomifene citrate

Actions and mechanism
Competitively antagonises ERs in the hypothalamus. By blocking negative feedback effects, it causes ovarian stimulation, maturation of the ovarian follicle, ovulation and development of the corpus luteum.

Indications
Clomifene is indicated to treat anovulatory infertility; it is usually prescribed only by specialist gynaecologists. A course of therapy (5 days) usually results in a single ovulation. If unsuccessful – that is, sexual intercourse or intrauterine insemination does not result in conception – further courses are tried, or the dose is doubled. Assuming there is no other reason for infertility in the couple, about 80% of women will ovulate and 35–40% will conceive after clomifene therapy.

Pharmacokinetics
Clomifene is well absorbed orally, with peak plasma concentrations reached 6–7 hours after oral administration. It is recirculated in the enterohepatic system, hence its long plasma half-life of 5–7 days. Ovulation usually occurs 6–12 days after a course of treatment. Clomifene is metabolised in the liver and metabolites are excreted in the faeces and bile.

Drug interactions
There are no known significant drug interactions.

Adverse reactions
These include hot flushes, abdominal pain or gas, visual disturbances, ovarian enlargement or cyst formation, nausea and vomiting, abnormal uterine bleeding and ovarian hyperstimulation syndrome. There is an increased incidence of multiple pregnancies (8–10%).

Contraindications
Avoid use in women with clomifene hypersensitivity, severe liver function impairment, endometrial carcinoma, ovarian cyst or enlargement that is not associated with polycystic ovary syndrome, abnormal vaginal bleeding (undiagnosed) or fibroid tumours in the uterus; not indicated for use during pregnancy.

Dosage and administration
The dose for female infertility is 50–100 mg orally daily for 5 days, starting on the fifth day of the menstrual period if bleeding occurs, or at any time in women who have no recent uterine bleeding. This cycle is repeated until conception occurs, for a maximum of three to six cycles.

dysfunction; or, if ovulation is normal, conception may be impossible due to tubal damage, endometriosis or uterine or vaginal abnormalities. Weight reduction (in overweight women) and avoidance of smoking or excessive alcohol intake may be helpful.

Drugs for female infertilty
Management of infertility is a highly specialised area of medicine, usually provided in clinics attached to teaching hospitals. Assisted reproduction technologies (e.g. in-vitro fertilisation [IVF], intrauterine insemination, gamete intrafollicular transfer or intracytoplasmic sperm injection) are highly complex, possibly requiring prior pituitary down-regulation, then controlled ovarian hyperstimulation to stimulate development of a single or multiple follicles. Summaries of possible treatments are given below:

- to regularise cycles: OCs or progesterone (supplementation or replacement therapy)
- anovulatory infertility: clomifene citrate, an ER antagonist (Drug Monograph 30.3); gonadotrophins (FSH agonists: hCG)
- treatments for endometriosis or polycystic ovary syndrome
- women with hypopituitarism: FSH and LH
- women with hyperprolactinaemia: dopamine agonists (bromocriptine or cabergoline)
- assisted reproduction technologies: GnRH antagonist to prevent premature ovulation (cetrorelix, ganirelix); GnRH agonist for pituitary down-regulation (Table 30.1); gonadotrophins for controlled ovarian stimulation, to induce ovulation, stimulate follicular development or support luteal phase (hCG, FSH, LH or hMG) (see Australian Medicines Handbook 2021 – Drugs for infertility)
- drugs affecting female sexual functioning.

Female sexual response: hormones and neurotransmitters
In most mammalian animals, sexual behaviour and the sexual response (mating) are more likely during estrus, which coincides with peak levels of LH and ovulation,

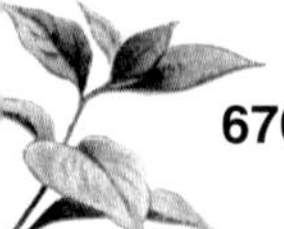

TABLE 30.1 Characteristics of GnRH analogues

Examples	Goserelin, leuprorelin, nafarelin, triptorelin
Administration	Continuous – e.g. SC or IM depot – or nasal spray
Rationale	To suppress pituitary gonadotrophin release
Indications	Treatment of prostate or breast cancers, endometriosis, uterine fibroids and before controlled ovarian stimulation
Half-life (approximate)	3–4 hours
Adverse reactions	Impaired fertility, decreased bone density; males: impotence, gynaecomastia; females: hot flushes, headache, pain, menstrual problems, hypercalcaemia
Precautions	Pregnancy, lactation

implying maximal likelihood of conception. Sexual behaviours in animals may be inhibited by a rise in brain 5-HT levels, whereas dopamine is involved in pleasure and reward pathways. In women, increasing levels of estrogen secretion, especially during the pre-ovulatory period of the menstrual cycle, enhance sexual functioning. Autonomic nervous system influences include parasympathetic (cholinergic) impulses causing arterial dilation, venoconstriction and exudation of lubricating secretions; sympathetic responses include skeletal muscle contractions and increases in heart rate and blood pressure. Catecholamine neurotransmitters are involved in neuroendocrine integration (dopamine acting as the prolactin release-inhibiting factor), in vascular control and pleasurable sensations. Release of oxytocin from the posterior pituitary gland causes rhythmic contractions of vagina, uterus and perineal muscles, which promote passage of sperm and seminal fluid and fertilisation of the ovum. Estrogens and progestogens are involved in sexual behaviour and responsiveness, and androgens in enhancing libido in women as well as in men.

In humans, basic endocrine and neurochemical effects involved in sexual functions are usually overridden by psychological, social, cognitive and emotional influences.

Drugs that may affect sexual functioning

Since so many neurotransmitters and hormones are involved in sexual responses and reproductive behaviours, it is inevitable that many drugs can affect these functions: drugs affecting autonomic, central and somatic nervous systems, catecholaminergic, cholinergic and serotonergic pathways, neuroendocrine and pituitary control systems and all hormones involved in female and male reproduction. Many of these can affect both males and females (e.g. sex hormones, social drugs, antihypertensives and sedatives); others are specific to male issues (e.g. erectile dysfunction). These will all be considered briefly in the next chapter.

KEY POINTS

Drugs used in gynaecological disorders

- Production of female sex hormones (estrogens and progesterone) is under control of gonadotrophins released from the anterior pituitary gland when stimulated by GnRH from the hypothalamus.
- GnRH is used clinically to stimulate or suppress release of pituitary gonadotrophins, depending on whether it is given in low pulsatile doses or high continuous doses.
- The pituitary gonadotrophic hormones FSH and LH regulate development and maintenance of sex gland functions; they are administered clinically to treat hypogonadism and infertility.
- Estrogens stimulate and maintain the regular menstrual cycle, have metabolic actions and inhibit release of pituitary gonadotrophins.
- Estrogens are used in OC preparations; in HRT after menopause; for disorders of menstruation, polycystic ovary syndrome and hirsutism; and for preventing osteoporosis in postmenopausal women.
- Anti-estrogens and SERMs are used in breast cancers, infertility and menopausal problems.
- Progesterone stimulates the secretory phase of the menstrual cycle and facilitates and maintains pregnancy.
- Synthetic progestogens are orally active and are indicated for HRT, treating endometriosis and specific carcinomas, and for preventing pregnancy.
- Antiprogestogens (SPRMs) are used to treat endometriosis, heavy menstrual bleeding, in emergency contraception and medical termination of pregnancy and for antiproliferative effects in breast cancer.
- Anovulatory infertility in women may be treated with ovulatory stimulants, such as clomifene, or with gonadotrophins.

Contraception

For many sexually active men and women, an ongoing problem is not inability to conceive, but the desire to prevent conception and pregnancy after sexual intercourse – that is, **contraception**. The average sexually active woman who wants two children spends about three decades trying to avoid pregnancy and only a few years trying to become or being pregnant (Frost et al.

2008). The average rate of pregnancy following a year in which a couple engages in regular unprotected intercourse is about 85%. About 50% of couples worldwide use some contraceptive technique, yet the rates of abortion and unplanned pregnancies remain high.

An ideal contraceptive technique should be safe, 100% effective, immediately functional, easy to use, rapidly reversible after discontinuation and should not interfere with sex life. Although no technique totally fulfils these criteria, many methods have remarkably low failure rates when used correctly by a highly motivated couple (Table 30.3, later). Most contraceptive techniques, while protecting against pregnancy, do not protect against transmission of sexually transmitted infections (STIs; only condoms do the latter).

Readiness of availability, requirement for prescription or fitting by a doctor, and cost may be significant factors in choice of method; in Australia, preparations subsidised on the Pharmaceutical Benefits Scheme (PBS) are usually significantly cheaper than others.

Contraception in females

The availability of effective and acceptable contraception is critical to women's sexual health. Contraceptive methods in women include oral tablets (usually provided in monthly calendar packs), IUDs, intravaginal rings and diaphragms, intramuscular implants and female condoms. Some typical products are shown in Fig 30.4. Estimates for 'who uses what' in Australian couples suggest that about 30% use the COC, 23% a barrier method, 16% sterilisation (male or female), 5% a long-acting method, and the rest another or no method.

Many factors determine what form of contraception suits a particular woman: age; postpartum, breastfeeding or perimenopause status; whether family is complete; concurrent medical conditions (cancer, cardiovascular disease, liver function, diabetes, pre- or postsurgery, epilepsy); predisposition to thromboembolism, acne or hirsutism; concurrent drugs; adverse reactions to previous

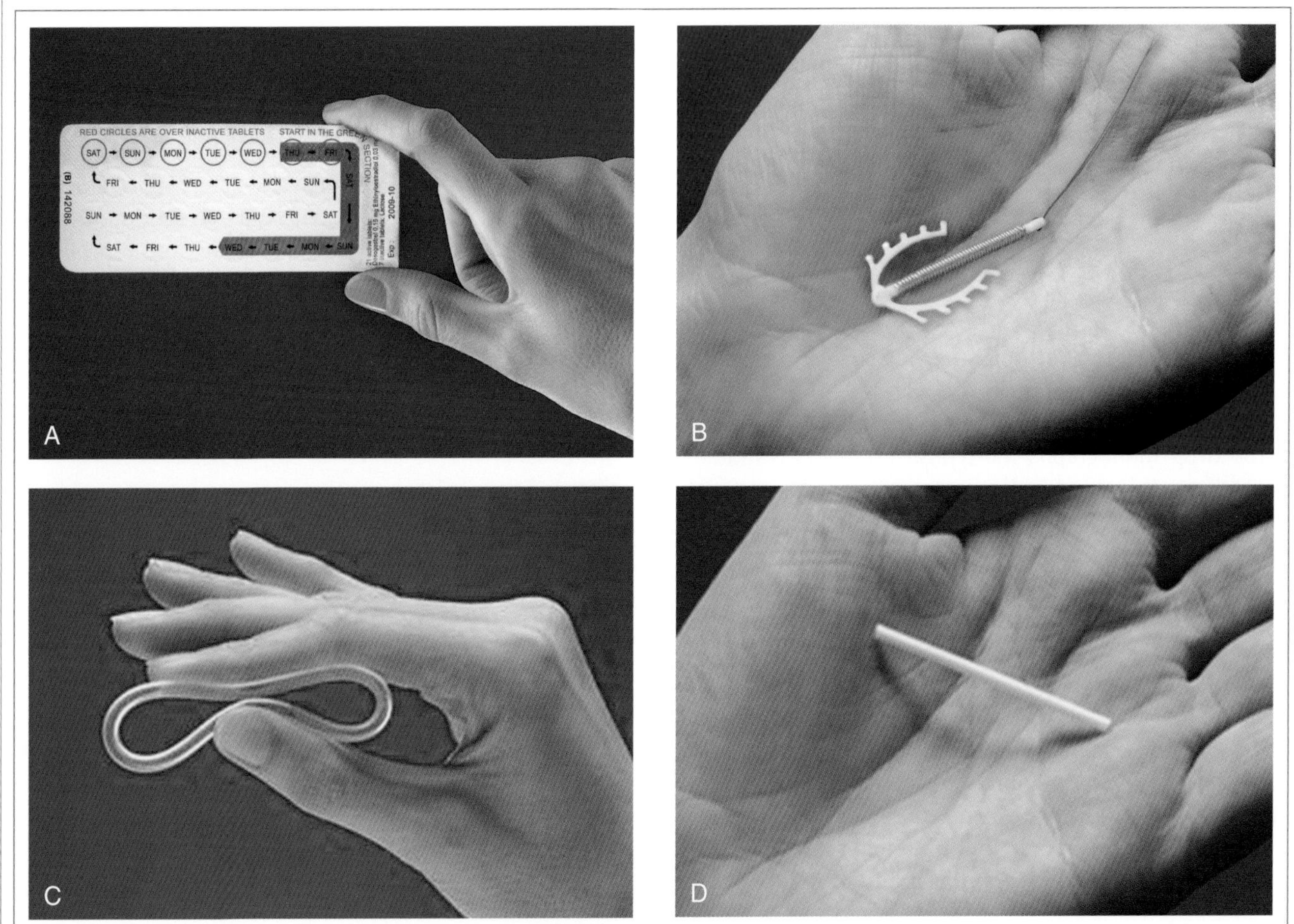

FIGURE 30.4 Different types of female contraceptive products **A** 28-day pack of COC; **B** copper IUD; **C** intravaginal ring; **D** intramuscular implant.
Source: Merck Sharp & Dohme (Australia) Pty Ltd; reproduced with permission.

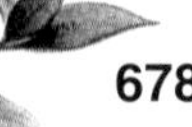

pharmacological contraceptives; smoking status; and individual preferences.

Oral contraceptives

Since the 1960s, millions of women have used **combined oral contraceptives** (COCs; an estrogen–progestogen combination in various doses in a 28-day cyclical regimen), or an oral progestogen-only formulation, for decades during their reproductive lives (Clinical Focus Box 30.2).

Hormone components

The aim of most COC formulations is to mimic closely the sequence and levels of hormones in the menstrual cycle, in which estrogen levels are low early in the cycle, high in mid-cycle and medium late in the cycle; progestogen levels are very low or absent until the mid-cycle surge of gonadotrophins, then rise late in the cycle (Fig 30.2, earlier). The typical 21/7 COC regimen for 1 month contains 21 days of active hormone tablets, then 7 days with placebo or no tablets, which precipitates the withdrawal bleed – that is, the next menstrual cycle.

Note that menstruation can be effectively suppressed by 'tricycling' – that is, taking only the active tablets from 3-monthly packs of COCs for 9 weeks in a row, then placebo (or no) tablets for 7 days. This decreases the frequency of withdrawal bleeds and heavy or painful periods, which is useful when menstruation would be inconvenient. A commercially available 3-month pack (84 tablets with 150 micrograms levonorgestrel plus 30 micrograms EE, followed by seven tablets with 10 micrograms EE) achieves the same results.

Actions and mechanisms

For detailed information on the physiological actions, mechanisms, pharmacokinetics, adverse effects, drug interactions and contraindications of the component drugs, see the drug monographs for typical estrogens (estradiol, Drug Monograph 30.1) and progestogens (levonorgestrel, Drug Monograph 30.2). Relevant to contraceptive effects is that the estrogen component decreases FSH release and thus impairs selection and development of a follicle; this decreases the likelihood of ovulation and implantation. The progestogen component thickens uterine mucus, decreases LH release and impairs ovulation and tubal motility, decreasing the likelihood of fertilisation. Over a few cycles, estrogen–progestogen combinations inhibit secretion of hypothalamic GnRH, pituitary gonadotrophins FSH and LH and endogenous ovarian steroids. Overall, pregnancy does not occur.

The mechanisms of action of female contraceptive methods are compared diagrammatically in Figure 30.5.

Clinical use of oral contraceptives

OCs are indicated in regular and emergency contraception, menstrual disorders and to treat endometriosis and acne. Precautions are needed in women with migraine, unexplained vaginal bleeding, obesity or malabsorption syndromes, early postpartum mothers, women over 40, those on drugs that induce CYP3A4 enzymes and smokers. COCs are contraindicated in women with a history of hypertension, breast cancer, cardiovascular disease or liver disease, at risk of VTE or having major surgery.

Beneficial effects

More than 50 years of worldwide clinical experience have shown the OC pill to be safe and effective. Beneficial effects include: avoidance of unwanted pregnancy and pregnancy-related morbidity and mortality; lower rates of ectopic pregnancies, atheroma, thyroid disease, menstrual problems, anaemia, premenstrual dysphoric disorder, benign cysts, pelvic inflammatory disease, ovarian cancer and endometrial cancer, STIs, acne and hirsutism; and protection against endometriosis and fibroids.

Provided that risk factors are minimised, COCs are safe for most women for most of their reproductive lives. On balance, the life-threatening risks associated with using modern low-dose OC formulations are statistically lower than those in having a baby or driving a car.

Possible disadvantages

Possible adverse effects or disadvantages include: weight gain and fluid retention (anabolic effects); breast tenderness, impaired glucose tolerance and skin changes (estrogenic effects); general symptoms (nausea, depression, chloasma, acne); short-term amenorrhoea after cessation; increased risk of thrombosis and myocardial infarction, especially in smokers, obese women and those aged over 35; breakthrough bleeding; and possible association with breast cancer, cervical cancer, liver cancer, gall bladder disease, inflammatory bowel disease and rheumatoid arthritis.

Adverse effects usually diminish over time, with continued use of the same method.

Counselling points

All women prescribed the contraceptive pill should be appropriately counselled by a health professional. In particular, a woman needs to know:

- when to start taking a pack of tablets (most should be taken within the first 5 days of the cycle – that is, days of menstrual bleeding)
- what to do if one or more active tablets are missed or if she suffers from vomiting or diarrhoea (generally, if more than 24 hours late or a tablet may not have been absorbed, or if pack was started on other than days 1–5 of the cycle, additional contraception methods should be used for 7 days)
- what adverse effects to watch out for and report (severe chest pain or headache, vision changes, leg pain or swelling, acne, weight gain)

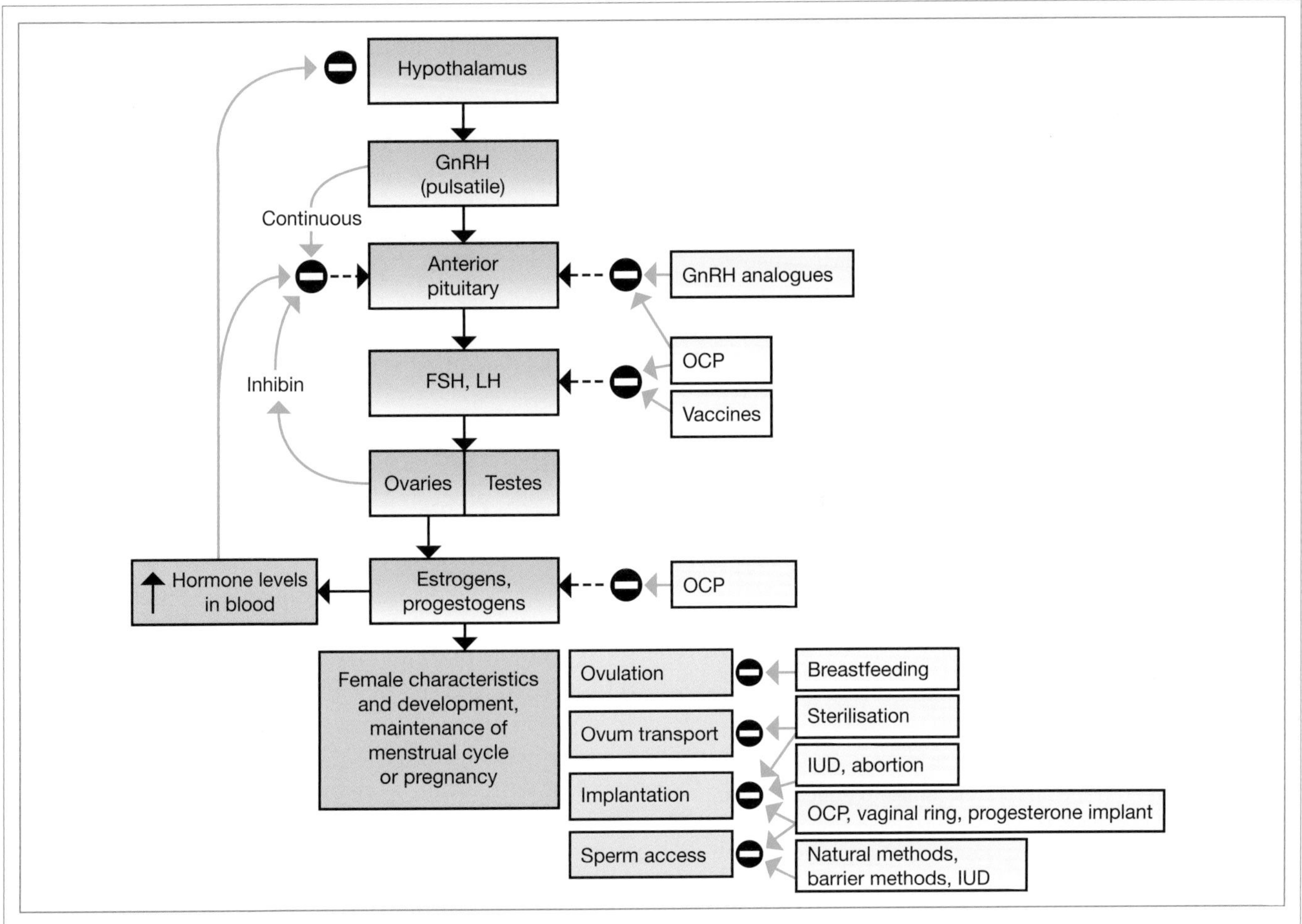

FIGURE 30.5 Sites of action of various contraceptive methods in the female reproductive tract (compare Fig 30.1)
[-] = effect decreased or inhibited; GnRH = gonadotrophin-releasing hormone; IUD = intrauterine device; OCP = oral contraceptive pill

- the greater risks of adverse effects if she is a smoker
- that there are many effective methods of contraception, and many formulations of COCs
- how to change formulations if prescribed (skip the inert tablets for the first cycle and keep taking the active tablets; another contraceptive method may be needed)
- that the pill does not protect against STIs
- if taking the progestogen-only pill (POP or minipill), it needs to be taken at the same time each day
- that many antiepileptic medicines and rifamycin antibiotics may reduce the effectiveness of some COCs due to increased metabolism of EE; a COC with higher EE doses and/or other contraceptive method may be necessary
- that it is possible to delay menstruation temporarily by tricycling.

Combined oral contraceptive formulations

Many different types of COC formulations are available, with different combinations and sequences of semisynthetic hormones selected to optimise activity and minimise adverse effects.

Most formulations in Australia and New Zealand contain an estrogen (EE); other estrogens used are mestranol or estradiol (Drug Monograph 30.1). Several synthetic progestogens are used in COCs: norethisterone, levonorgestrel (Drug Monograph 30.2), desogestrel, gestodene or drospirenone (the latter three are less likely to have androgenic effects), or cyproterone, dienogest or nomegestrol (with anti-androgen activity). Drospirenone also has useful anti-mineralocorticoid actions, and may help reduce blood pressure and body weight; however, it carries increased risk of VTE (Clinical Focus Box 30.3). Formulations containing EE 35 micrograms or less plus norethisterone or levonorgestrel are considered first-line (Stewart & Black 2015).

Monophasic OCs containing a fixed ratio of estrogen and progestogen are taken for 21 (or 24) days of the normal menstrual cycle, then inactive tablets may be taken for the next 7 (or 4) days. Tri- or multi-phasic COCs most closely mimic the normal estrogen and progesterone levels during the menstrual cycle. The dose of estrogen is kept at a low level during the 21-day dosing

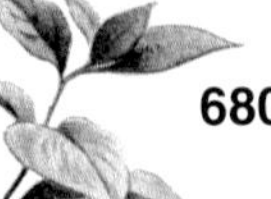

CLINICAL FOCUS BOX 30.3

Combined oral contraceptives and venous thromboembolism risk

VTE is a rare but serious side effect of COCs. That is, blockage of leg and pulmonary vessels by a venous thrombosis (blood clot). A thrombosis in the lower leg, thigh or pelvis vessels is known as a deep vein thrombosis, while a blockage in the pulmonary vasculature is known as pulmonary embolism. A pulmonary embolism can be life-threatening and can cause sudden death.

Different COCs have different thromboembolism risk. Higher estrogen doses are correlated with higher VTE risk, as increased levels of plasma estrogen increase the hepatic synthesis of procoagulant proteins and decrease the synthesis of fibrinolytic and anticoagulant factors, leading to hypercoagulability.

COCs that contain third- and fourth-generation progestogens (desogestrel, dienogest, gestodene or drospirenone) have a higher relative risk of VTE when compared with second-generation progestogens (norethisterone, levonorgestrel). For every 10,000 women taking third- or fourth-generation progestogens, nine to 12 women will develop a VTE in a year. This is reduced to five to seven women taking second-generation progestogens.

It is important for health professionals to educate those who are prescribed the COC to recognise the signs and symptoms of VTE. The most common signs and symptoms of deep vein thrombosis include pain, swelling, heaviness, redness and cramping in the legs. The most common clinical symptoms of pulmonary embolism include shortness of breath, rapid breathing, cough, sharp chest pain that worsens during breathing (pleuritic chest pain) and syncope (fainting).

Other factors that increase VTE risk include cigarette smoking, obesity, increasing age, migraines and a family history of VTE.

period, or may increase ('mid-cycle surge') in the middle of the cycle, while the progestogen is progressively phased up (increased twice) to mimic the natural release of hormones; inactive tablets are taken for the last 7 days. Because of the lower doses, adverse reactions reported are lower than with the monophasic formulations; however, controlled trials show little difference in cycle control.

Table 30.2 lists the compositions, doses and brand names of some typical OCs used in these methods; a typical calendar pack is shown in Fig 30.4A. (However, formulations change frequently, so current references should be consulted.)

Progestogen-only oral contraception

'Minipill'

Low-dosage progestogen-only OCs (the **minipill**) were developed for women unable to take estrogens – for example, during lactation – or with a history of thromboembolic disorders or those who smoke. They are less effective than COCs and have a higher incidence of breakthrough bleeding and menstrual irregularity. They do not cause adverse reactions associated with estrogen therapy or inhibit lactation so can be taken by women who are breastfeeding.

Most postpartum women will not ovulate for at least 6 weeks; however, in approximately one-third of women, the first cycle is *preceded* by ovulation and so they are potentially fertile. In some maternity hospitals, on discharge, all women with a newborn are offered a prescription for the POP (minipill). Midwives in some Australian states are authorised to prescribe OCs for postnatal contraception.

Because the dose is low, the timing of taking the tablet each day is critical; it is recommended that, if administration is delayed by more than 3 hours, an additional method of contraception be used for 48 hours. The minipill may be unreliable in overweight and obese women.

TABLE 30.2 Examples of hormonal contraceptives

BRAND NAME	ESTROGEN (micrograms)	PROGESTOGEN (mg)
Monophasic COC		
Femme-tab ED, Lenest 20 ED, Loette, Microgynon 20 ED, Microlevlen ED, Micronelle 20 ED	EE 20	Levonorgestrel 0.1
Petibelle, Yasmin, Yaz, Yaz Flex	EE 20 or 30	Drospirenone 3.0
Madeline, Marvelon 28	EE 30	Desogestrel 0.15
Valette	EE 30	Dienogest 2.0
Eleanor 150/30 ED, Evelyn 150/30 ED, Femme-Tab 30/150 ED, Lenest 30 ED, Levlen ED, Microgynon 30 ED, Micronelle 30 ED, Monofeme, Nordette	EE 30	Levonorgestrel 0.15
Minulet	EE 30	Gestodene 0.075
Brenda-35 ED, Diane-35 ED, Estelle-35 ED, Jene-35 ED, Juliet-35 ED	EE 35	Cyproterone acetate 2.0
Brevinor, Brevinor-1; Norimin, Norimin-1	EE 35	Norethisterone 0.5 or 1.0
Norinyl-1	Mestranol 50	Norethisterone 1.0
Microgynon 50 ED	EE 50	Levonorgestrel 0.125
Zoely	Estradiol 1.5 mg	Nomegestrol 2.5

TABLE 30.2 Examples of hormonal contraceptives—cont'd

BRAND NAME	ESTROGEN (micrograms)	PROGESTOGEN (mg)
Multiphasic COC		
Triphasil, Logynon ED, Trifeme, Triquilar ED (6/5/10/7 tabs)	EE 30/40/30/0	Levonorgestrel 0.05/0.075/0.125/0
Qlaira (2/5/17/2/2 tabs)	Estradiol 3/2/2/1/0	Dienogest 0/2/3/0/0
Combined, depot		
NuvaRing (vaginal ring, for 3 weeks)	EE 2.7 mg	Etonogestrel 11.7 mg
Progestogen-only (oral)		
Noriday 28	None	Norethisterone 0.35
Microlut	None	Levonorgestrel 0.03
Levonelle-1, NorLevo-1, Postella-1, Postinor-1	None	Levonorgestrel 1.5 (for emergency contraception)
Progestogen-only (depot/IUD)		
Depo-Provera, Depo-Ralovera	None	Medroxyprogesterone acetate 150 mg IM every 3 months
Implanon NXT	None	Etonogestrel 68 mg subdermal every 3 years
Mirena IUD	None	Levonorgestrel 52 mg; replaced every 5 years

Note: Those with EE dose under 30 micrograms or estradiol dose under 1.5 mg are considered low-dose; an EE dose of 30–35 micrograms is standard, and EE 50 micrograms is high-dose.
ED = extended dose
Source: Australian Medicines Handbook 2021

Emergency contraception

The emergency contraceptive pill, sometimes misnamed the 'morning-after pill', is indicated for use within 72 hours of unprotected sexual intercourse or in possible failure of contraceptive method in women not wanting to conceive. The available methods are:

- ulipristal acetate, 30 mg, an SPRM; most effective oral emergency contraceptive pill, effective in 99% of cases up to 5 days after unprotected intercourse
- levonorgestrel, 1.5 mg, within 72 hours of unprotected intercourse; 85% effective; less effective in obese women.

Ulipristal and levonorgestrel as an emergency contraceptive pill are Pharmacist-Only Medicines (Schedule 3) in Australia. **Emergency contraception** has been shown in societies in which it is readily available to reduce the rate of abortion. The main contraindication to these regimens is known pregnancy (see RANZCOG statement in 'Online resources').

(The use of antiprogestogens such as mifepristone, RU486, at a single dose of 200 mg, followed by a PG analogue, to terminate pregnancy is usually classified as medical termination rather than as emergency contraception; mifepristone is not available in Australia or New Zealand for emergency contraception.)

An alternative, non-oral, non-hormonal method of emergency contraception is insertion of a copper-impregnated **intrauterine device** (IUD), which is 99% effective if inserted for up to 5 days after unprotected intercourse. It provides ongoing contraception, and is preferred in women taking liver enzyme-inducing drugs that might reduce effectiveness of hormonal treatments.

Contraindications and interactions

Because OC preparations are taken by millions of women for most of their reproductive lives, it is crucial that long-term safety, risks and benefits be identified and compared with risks associated with pregnancy and childbirth, particularly in countries where obstetric care is inadequate, and with the risks of abortion in the case of unwanted pregnancy. Major long-term studies have demonstrated that the low-dose OCs incur fewer risks than does pregnancy.

Absolute contraindications for OCs are: thromboembolic disease, coronary artery disease, stroke, active liver disease, estrogen-dependent cancers, focal migraine, porphyrias and pregnancy. OC use is relatively contraindicated in hypertension, diabetes, previous cholestasis, undiagnosed vaginal bleeding, elective surgery within 4 weeks, sickle cell disease and severe depression, and in women aged over 35 years with risks for coronary artery disease (see earlier under 'Estrogens' and 'Progestogens').

There are many potential drug interactions with COCs, especially with drugs that induce CYP3A4 enzymes, enhancing clearance of sex hormones (estrogen and progesterone) and leading to contraception failure; barbiturates, many anticonvulsants, some antivirals and rifamycin antibiotics are particularly implicated (see earlier drug monographs, Drug Interactions 30.1 and Australian Medicines Handbook 2021: 'Drug Interactions').

Women taking these drugs are recommended to use IUDs with levonorgestrel or copper, or medroxyprogesterone depot for contraception.

Long-acting reversible contraceptives

The non-oral hormonal methods of contraception (depot injection, vaginal ring, depot IM rod and hormonal IUD) have many advantages over oral formulations, including:

- they avoid problems with impaired gastrointestinal tract (GIT) absorption (e.g. from vomiting or diarrhoea)
- they avoid hepatic first-pass metabolism, so lower estrogen doses are effective
- controlled-release formulations readily achieve steady plasma concentrations
- long durations of action (3–10 years)
- improved compliance and effectiveness, as no daily action (or memory) or regular maintenance is required
- scant or no menstrual bleeding or pain (excluding copper IUD)
- more effective than OCs at preventing unintended pregnancies (in the first year of use, the failure rates of long-acting reversible contraceptives [LARCs] are 0.05–0.8%, compared with 9% with the OC)
- good safety profile with few contraindications.

The main reasons given by women for discontinuing these methods are the irregularity of bleeding and unpredictable return of ovulation.

Combined vaginal ring

The vaginal ring provides controlled release of a progestogen/estrogen combination (Fig 30.4C). It is a flexible polymer ring that slowly releases EE (15 micrograms/24 hours) and etonogestrel (120 micrograms/24 hours). It is inserted by the woman into her vagina and left for 3 weeks, then removed; her next menstrual period usually starts within 2–3 days. Absorption of the steroid hormones through vaginal epithelium is rapid, and first-pass metabolism is avoided. The ring has similar contraceptive efficacy, possible adverse effects, precautions and contraindications as combined estrogen–progestogen products taken orally in the COC pill.

Progestogen-only depot preparations

Injections

Depot injections of progestogen (e.g. medroxyprogesterone acetate [MPA] 150 mg given IM every 3 months) have the lowest failure rate of all reversible contraceptive methods. This method is suitable for women who do not want to take a daily tablet or who cannot take estrogens. There may be a period of infertility for some months after completing the course.

Implant or IUD

A subdermal depot implant containing a progestogen is also available, consisting of a polymer rod (4 cm long, 2 mm diameter) impregnated with 68 mg etonogestrel (Fig 30.4D). It is implanted using aseptic procedures under the skin of the inner aspect of the upper arm, and is left in place for 3 years, during which there is a gradually reducing rate of release of active drug (from 60–70 to 25–30 micrograms/day). Fertility will return after removal of the implant, with rapid return to normal menstrual periods.

A plastic IUD impregnated with 52 mg levonorgestrel, a slow-release progestogen, is also available. It is useful for long-term contraception (5 years), to treat heavy menstrual bleeding and to provide the progestogen content of continuous combined HRT.

Other pharmacological contraceptive methods

Intrauterine devices

IUDs impregnated with copper (Fig 30.4B) or levonorgestrel are used for long-term (5–8 years) reversible contraception. IUDs alter the intrauterine environment to decrease sperm motility and viability, inhibit or decrease ovulation and follicular development and inhibit nidation (attachment of the fertilised ovum in the endometrium). They can cause dysmenorrhoea, pelvic inflammatory disease or uterine perforation, and the IUD can be expelled from the uterus.

In Australia, LARC use is increasing. Approximately, 11% of women use a LARC (6.1% for IUDs and 4.9% for implants).

Non-drug contraceptive methods

Non-drug methods (except for condoms) generally have much lower success rates in preventing pregnancies – see Table 30.3, later, for failure rates for various contraceptive methods.

Barrier methods

Barrier methods of contraception impose a physical barrier between sperm ejaculated during sexual intercourse and an oocyte in the woman's uterine tube. Some offer protection against STIs and cervical cancer; male condoms are especially effective. The female condom, a thin rubber pouch inserted in the vaginal canal, also protects against STIs.

'Diaphragms' or 'caps' inserted in the vagina prevent access of sperm to the cervical canal. They are inserted before intercourse and left in place for at least 6 hours afterwards. Complications include irritation or pain and allergic reactions. They do not prevent STIs.

'Natural' methods

The 'natural' methods of family planning or contraception include total abstinence from sexual activity, periodic abstinence planned to avoid the most fertile days of a woman's cycle ('rhythm methods'), withdrawal of the penis before ejaculation ('coitus interruptus') and reliance on the anti-ovulation effects of prolactin during breastfeeding.

Rhythm method

Natural family planning methods are commonly used by people who prefer not to use devices or drugs to prevent conception. They rely on attempts to predict the day of ovulation and avoidance of intercourse for several days before and after ovulation (as the ovum is viable for about 2 days and sperm for up to 7 days after intercourse). The method works only if the woman has regular periods and can predict the time of ovulation (usually 14 days *before* her next period). The methods require abstinence from sexual intercourse for at least half the cycle (days 8–20 in a 28-day cycle).

Accuracy in predicting the day of ovulation can be improved by measuring the small rise in basal body temperature occurring in response to the mid-cycle rise in progesterone, or by identifying changes in mucus secretions, abdominal pain, breast tenderness or cervix or mood changes before, during and after ovulation.

The unreliability of such methods contributes to the high birth rates and/or high abortion rates in societies or couples relying on these methods.

Sterilisation

Sterilisation is virtually 100% effective as a contraceptive method and is the most widely used form of contraception worldwide. The techniques in women involve ligation or clipping of the fallopian tubes ('tubal ligation') and in men, vasectomy – that is, surgical interruption of the vas deferens to prevent transport of sperm. New Zealand has the highest rate of male vasectomy globally, followed by Australia, with approximately one in four men over the age of 40 having had a vasectomy. Although considered a permanent form of sterilisation, vasectomy can be reversed (vasovasostomy) in most men. Severe complications are rare.

Failure of contraception

Unintended pregnancy despite contraception can be considered an adverse event of failed therapy. More than 50% of women with an unplanned pregnancy report that they had been using some contraceptive method, obviously unsuccessfully. Of women in many countries using the COC pill, 50% admit to having missed at least one pill in the previous 3 months. Common reasons for stopping contraception, leading to 'accidental' pregnancies, include concerns about long-term effects and adverse media stories.

A common way of expressing the ineffectiveness (likely failure rate) of a contraceptive method is the Pearl Index, which gives a statistical estimate of the number of unintended pregnancies in 100 women over 1 year of use. It is calculated as follows:

$$\frac{\text{number of pregnancies} \times 12}{\text{total number of women-months of usage}} \times 100$$

Reported failure rates of methods are shown in Table 30.3.

TABLE 30.3 Failure rates for contraceptive methods

CONTRACEPTIVE METHOD	CONTRACEPTIVE FAILURE RATE (%)
No method	85
Periodic abstinence ('rhythm method')	1–25
Withdrawal ('coitus interruptus')	4–22
Female condom	5–21
Male condom	2–18
Diaphragm	6–12
OC pill: combination	0.3–9
OC pill: progestogen-only	0.3–9
Combined hormone vaginal ring	0.3–9
Depot MPA	0.2–6
IUD + copper	0.6–0.8
Sterilisation (female)	0.2–0.5
IUD + levonorgestrel	0.2
Vasectomy (male)	0.1–0.15
Implant etonogestrel	0.05

Failure rates are expressed as % women with pregnancy during 1 year of use. Ranges are lowest expected rate (perfect use) to typical rate in use.
IUD = intrauterine device; MPA = medroxyprogesterone acetate; OC = oral contraceptive
Sources: Australian Medicines Handbook 2021; Endocrinology Expert Group 2014.

KEY POINTS

Contraception in women

- Contraception is practised by about 50% of couples to limit their fertility or plan their family. Drug and non-drug methods are available for the female or male partner, with varying usage rates, failure rates and degrees of reversibility. 'Barrier' methods are most effective at preventing STIs.
- Oral contraception with combinations of an estrogen and a progestogen is the most widely and frequently used method of female contraception.
- Types of contraceptive formulations include combined continuous and phased preparations, progestogen-only tablets and implants and emergency contraception regimens.
- Risk–benefit analysis shows that, for most women, use of oral contraception is safe, effective, reversible

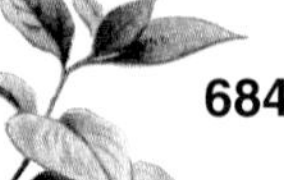

and inexpensive, and protects against many gynaecological problems. Adverse reactions are mild with low- or no-estrogen formulations.

- Because OCs are primarily for self-administration, education is important for accurate and safe administration and for early recognition of adverse reactions, particularly thromboembolism.

Drugs during pregnancy, the perinatal period and lactation

Drug therapy in the pregnant or breastfeeding woman may differ from that in the rest of the adult population. Drugs taken by a pregnant woman or during labour may reach the fetus via the maternal circulation and cause birth defects or adverse reactions. Drugs consumed by a breastfeeding woman may be excreted in breast milk; if the drug concentrations are high, this can cause adverse effects in the breastfed infant.

Drugs during pregnancy

Maternal adaptations

Maternal adaptations to **pregnancy** include anatomical changes due to the expanding fetus and weight gain due to fetus, placenta, amniotic fluid and enlarged uterus. Endogenous hormone levels change markedly from the non-pregnant cycling state, with high levels of chorionic gonadotrophin, placental hormones (progesterone, estrogens, chorionic somatomammotrophin, growth hormone, adrenocorticotrophic hormone and thyroid-stimulating hormone), prolactin and relaxin (a peptide hormone produced by corpus luteum and placenta).

Physiological adaptations may affect pharmacokinetic factors (Ch 5) or how the mother responds to drugs. Cardiac output, stroke volume, heart rate and blood volume all increase by 15–30%, while blood pressure usually falls. Pulmonary function increases to meet oxygen demands of the fetus. Decreased GIT motility and increased nausea and vomiting may reduce absorption of nutrients and drugs. Chronic conditions that the mother suffered before pregnancy, such as diabetes, epilepsy, asthma, hypertension, arthritis, peptic ulcer, migraine, depression, thyroid disorder or urinary tract infection need careful monitoring and treatment to optimise the mother's (and fetus's) health.

Common conditions in pregnancy

Morning sickness

Nausea, heartburn and 'morning sickness' are common and can threaten the health of mother and fetus; treatment in early stages may prevent more serious complications. Dietary measures are tried first (small amounts of cold foods, dry crackers, vitamin B6, herbal teas). If antiemetic drugs are required, those known to be safe include:

- for mild symptoms: ginger (up to 1 g daily), pyridoxine (vitamin B6, 25–50 mg up to three times a day)
- in more severe cases: doxylamine, corticosteroids, metoclopramide, prochlorperazine, promethazine.

Severe vomiting (hyperemesis gravidarum) may require hospitalisation, IV rehydration and antiemetics including ondansetron (Australian Medicines Handbook 2021).

Miscarriage and stillbirth

Miscarriage, or spontaneous abortion, before 20 weeks may be natural rejection of an abnormal embryo or fetus. Threatened abortion (miscarriage) later in pregnancy may be successfully delayed by tocolytic drugs (e.g. salbutamol, nifedipine). Therapeutic termination, sometimes carried out if there is a threat to the life or health of the mother, is facilitated by oxytocic drugs (see later sections). Treatable conditions that contribute to stillbirth are preexisting diabetes and hypertension.

Gestational diabetes mellitus

Gestational diabetes mellitus (glucose intolerance first detected in pregnancy) affects 5–10% of pregnant women, especially older women and those with obesity or family history of diabetes. Blood glucose levels should be monitored frequently. Gestational diabetes may be controlled simply with diet and exercise, but about half of women with gestational diabetes require metformin or insulin therapy (see a typical case in Clinical Focus Box 28.3).

Preeclampsia

Preeclampsia (toxaemia of pregnancy) is a potentially dangerous combination of hypertension, proteinuria and oedema, thought to be due to renal ischaemia. It complicates the second half of 2–8% of pregnancies; control of blood pressure with antihypertensives is essential. (See a typical case in Clinical Focus Box 30.5, later.) Treatment to control convulsions is with magnesium sulfate by IV infusion or slow IM injection. Large doses (several grams over a period of hours) are given and can lead to magnesium toxicity, manifest by loss of reflexes and respiratory and cardiovascular collapse. (Magnesium is also used in migraine, cerebral palsy, dysrhythmias, severe asthma, dysmenorrhoea, leg cramps, metabolic syndrome, dyspepsia and constipation.)

Preeclampsia is a warning sign for the dangerous complication eclampsia, a condition carrying a high maternal and fetal mortality risk. The only safe treatment of eclampsia is delivery of the baby.

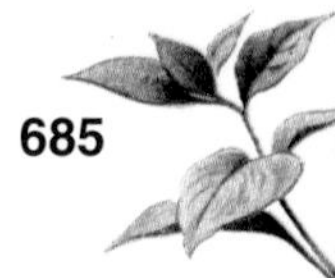

Drug use in pregnancy

During pregnancy, any substance consumed and absorbed may reach the fetus by way of the maternal circulation. Drug use during pregnancy should be avoided or limited to essential treatment and where the benefit to the mother is considered greater than the risk to the fetus. All pregnant women, and women of childbearing age who are not using contraceptives and who are sexually active, should be counselled to avoid exposure to unnecessary drugs (including complementary and alternative medicines) and chemicals, and drugs prescribed carefully, as effects on the embryo may occur before a woman is aware she is pregnant.

With the recent trend towards higher birth rates in the older age group of 35–44 years, it is likely that many women will be on medications for chronic medical conditions (e.g. allergies, hypertension, diabetes, depression) when they become pregnant, increasing the risk of exposure of the fetus to maternal drugs. 'Social drugs' can also affect the infant: alcohol consumption during pregnancy can cause CNS depression and abnormalities, and babies born to smokers are smaller and have increased incidence of jaundice. Babies born to women dependent on narcotic analgesics such as heroin, or on methadone maintenance programs, suffer a withdrawal syndrome after birth, which can be alleviated by administration of an opioid (Clinical Focus Box 25.1).

If it is necessary to administer drug therapy, the most important factors to be considered include:

- the potential for the drug to produce harmful effects in the fetus
- fetal gestational age at the time of drug exposure
- any other drugs or complementary medicines administered concurrently
- the drug dose, dosing intervals and duration of treatment
- risks to the mother and fetus if the mother is *not* treated with necessary drugs.

Vitamins in pregnancy

Anaemias are common due to increased demand for iron and blood cell functions, so iron and folic acid are frequently prescribed. Folic acid protects against many congenital abnormalities (e.g. neural tube defects) and some paediatric cancers. Women planning to conceive, and all pregnant women, should eat a varied nutritional diet and take folic acid supplements (500 micrograms per day) up to 12 weeks' gestation. Women at risk of vitamin D deficiency should take 10 micrograms vitamin D daily.

'Pregnancy multivitamin' formulations may contain 20 or more vitamins and minerals, most of which are only needed by women in low-income and developing countries. There is no evidence of a general need to take supplements of vitamins A, B, C, E or K.

Midwives prescribing

Suitably qualified and authorised Australian midwives are licensed to prescribe a number of Prescription-Only drugs during antenatal, perinatal and postnatal care; the list may vary between states. The PBS list for midwives includes several anti-infective agents (e.g. amoxicillin, cefalexin and nitrofurantoin), pain relievers/anti-inflammatories (diclofenac, ibuprofen, morphine), GIT drugs (metoclopramide, ranitidine) and progestogens for postnatal contraception during breastfeeding (etonogestrel, levonorgestrel); also vitamin K for neonates.

Teratogenesis: causing abnormal fetal development

The first trimester is when the developing embryo is most vulnerable to **teratogenic** effects of any chemicals that the mother is exposed to during this time (Fig 30.6), including prescription and over-the-counter drugs, complementary medicines (which include vitamin, mineral, herbal, aromatherapy and homoeopathic products), social drugs (alcohol and nicotine) and drugs of abuse. Some examples are described below and in Table 30.4.

Diethylstilboestrol

The use of the estrogen diethylstilboestrol during pregnancy initially was not found to cause any problems; however, during the 1970s it was linked to a delayed increased risk of vaginal and cervical cancer in female offspring and to genital abnormalities in both male and female offspring. Diethylstilboestrol taken by the mother during the first trimester of pregnancy presumably accumulated in the fetus, which was unable to metabolise it. The recognition that a drug taken during developmental stages in pregnancy can cause problems in the next generation is still a concern.

Thalidomide

Thalidomide is a well-known example of a drug with teratogenic effects during organogenesis. It was used in Australia and New Zealand as a sedative–hypnotic drug and to treat morning sickness from the 1950s to the early 1960s (Clinical Focus Box 2.1). Every precaution must be taken if it or an analogue is prescribed (to treat multiple myeloma) for a woman of childbearing age.

Alcohol

Alcohol easily crosses the placenta, entering the fetal bloodstream; consumption during pregnancy therefore substantially increases the risk of fetal abnormalities. One drink a week is associated with the possibility of mental health problems, and at the severe end of the spectrum is fetal alcohol syndrome, congenital abnormalities including

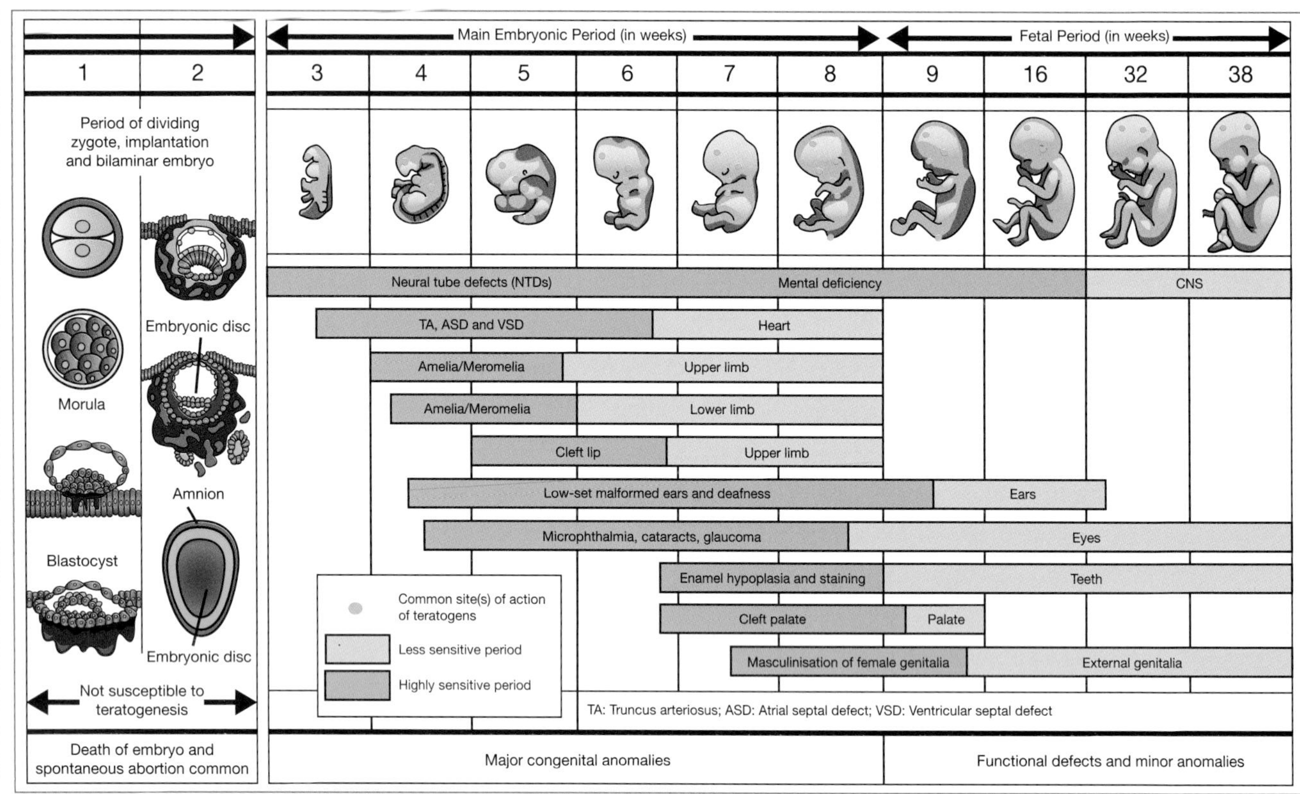

FIGURE 30.6 Schematic illustration of critical periods in human prenatal development
Source: Moore et al. 2016, Figure 20-15; reproduced with permission from Elsevier.

TABLE 30.4 Examples of drugs and teratogenic effects in the human fetus

DRUG	CRITICAL TIME PERIOD	POTENTIAL DEFECT
Alcohol (chronic use)	< 12 weeks > 24 weeks	Fetal alcohol syndrome: heart defects, CNS abnormalities Low birthweight, delay in development
Androgens	> 10 weeks	External female genitalia masculinisation
Angiotensin-converting enzyme (ACE) inhibitors and angiotensin receptor antagonists	1st–3rd trimester	Renal dysgenesis, defects in skull ossification, prolonged renal failure and hypotension in neonates
Carbamazepine	< 30 days after conception	Neural tube defects, craniofacial defects
Clomipramine	3rd trimester	Neonatal lethargy, hypotonia, cyanosis
Cocaine	2nd–3rd trimester 3rd trimester	Abruptio placentae Premature labour and delivery, intracranial bleeding
Cyclophosphamide	1st trimester	CNS malformations, secondary cancer
Isotretinoin	> 15 days after conception	Hydrocephalus, CNS abnormalities, fetal death
Lithium	< 2 months	Ebstein's anomaly and other heart defects
Methotrexate	6–9 weeks after conception	Skull ossification defect, limb and craniofacial defects
Phenytoin	1st trimester	Craniofacial defects, underdevelopment of phalanges or nails, impaired neurological development
Tetracycline antibiotics	> 20 weeks	Stained teeth, bone growth defect
Thalidomide	1st trimester	Phocomelia, internal malformations
Valproic acid	< 1 month after conception 1st trimester	Neural tube defects Craniofacial defects
Vitamin A (high doses and parenteral)	1st trimester	Fetal abnormalities including urinary tract malformations, growth retardation
Warfarin	1st–3rd trimester	CNS and skeletal defects, low birthweight (< 10th percentile), hearing loss

Source: Adapted from Katzung 2012; inter alia.

small head (microcephaly), low birthweight, mental and growth retardation, impaired coordination, irritability in infancy, hyperactivity in childhood, cardiac murmurs, cleft lip or palate, and hernias. Current guidelines recommend that, for women who are pregnant or planning a pregnancy or for women who are breastfeeding, not drinking alcohol is the safest option.

Antiepileptic drugs

Antiepileptic drugs are infamous for potentially causing birth defects or developmental problems in infants of mothers taking antiepileptics during pregnancy; see Table 30.4 (carbamazepine, phenytoin and valproic acid) and discussion in Chapter 14.

Retinoids

These vitamin A derivatives are used to treat severe acne. They are potentially teratogenic (Ch 41 and Drug Monograph 41.2).

Cocaine

The abuse of cocaine during pregnancy can result in spontaneous abortions, fetal hypoxia, premature delivery, congenital abnormalities (skull defects, cardiac abnormality) and cerebral infarction or stroke. At birth, the newborn may exhibit symptoms of cocaine drug withdrawal (irritability, increased respiratory and heart rates, diarrhoea, irregular sleeping patterns and poor appetite). Long-term behavioural patterns, such as poor attention span and a decrease in organisational skills, may also occur in offspring of cocaine-abusing women.

Database for prescribing medicines in pregnancy

The Australian Advisory Committee on Prescription Medicines categorises drugs into Pregnancy Categories A–D and X, on the basis of their potential for harmful effects (Clinical Focus Box 30.4), so that the safest effective drug can be prescribed.

Drugs in the perinatal period

Drugs given to a mother in the **perinatal period** (i.e. around childbirth, defined as from week 28 of pregnancy to the end of the first week of the infant's life) may affect the fetus or infant following drug passage across the placenta or into breast milk. For example, β-blockers depress the infant's cardiovascular system, insulin causes hypoglycaemia and antithyroid drugs can cause goitre. Infants are born with immature hepatic and renal functions, so drugs are cleared more slowly and may reach toxic concentrations, and with an immature blood–brain barrier, allowing passage into the CNS of drugs (and normal metabolites, including bilirubin), which may have adverse effects. (Detailed pharmacokinetic aspects are discussed in Ch 7.)

CLINICAL FOCUS BOX 30.4
Australian categorisation system for prescribing medicines in pregnancy

The **Australian categorisation system for prescribing medicines in pregnancy** has seven categories (A, B1, B2, B3, C, D and X) to indicate the level of risk to the fetus of drugs used at recommended therapeutic doses. Category A drugs are considered the least problematic, whereas drugs in Category X are considered the most dangerous and should not be used in pregnancy or if there is a possibility of pregnancy. The categorisation of B drugs (B1–B3) is based on animal data or contains drugs which have been taken by only a limited number of pregnant women; Category B drugs should not be considered 'safer' than drugs with a Category C designation. Category D drugs have caused, or are suspected to have caused, human fetal malformations.

The categorisation of a particular drug assumes it will be used at normal therapeutic doses in women; if the therapeutic dose is exceeded, the category assigned is no longer valid. A drug may have two categories; for example, isotretinoin is in Category D when used topically, in which case both the dose of the drug and the likely exposure of the fetus are low; however, it is in Category X when used systemically, when the dose and fetal exposure are greater. The categories do not differentiate between different stages of pregnancy (see Kennedy 2014).

Extensive information on this categorisation system and access to the database is available at the Therapeutic Goods Administration website, which is updated regularly and allows searching by either generic name/active ingredient or pharmacological classification/action. Note that accessing the website requires the reader to acknowledge a disclaimer that the material is general information and not specific advice.

The database does not contain all medicines approved for use in Australia because certain classes of medicines are generally exempted from categorisation. Few complementary medicines are included; these have little safety data. A full list of exempt medicines can be found at <www.tga.gov.au/hp/medicines-pregnancy-exempt.htm>.

As of 2015, the US Food and Drug Administration (FDA) discontinued its pregnancy risk categories system (which had been substantially similar to Australia's), and replaced it with the FDA Pregnancy and Lactation Labeling Rule, requiring narrative text describing risk and other data for each drug.

Source: Therapeutic Goods Administration – see 'Online resources'.

Hormones during parturition (labour)

During pregnancy the uterus increases in weight by about 20-fold (50 g to 1000 g), and by 10-fold in length. Control of uterine activity is via sympathetic fibres: noradrenaline (acting at α_2-adrenoceptors) causes excitation and muscle contraction; adrenaline (β_2) causes inhibition (relaxation of uterine muscle).

During the last few weeks of pregnancy, painless uterine contractions become increasingly frequent, and the lower uterine segment and cervix become softer and thinner, preparing the uterus for parturition. The key event stimulating labour is still not determined; it involves complex interactions of several placental, fetal and maternal hormones, including a rise in the estrogen:progesterone ratio (which increases the number of oxytocin receptors), increased sensitivity of the uterus to oxytocin released from the posterior pituitary gland, and PGs produced from amnion and chorion (two membranes surrounding the embryo/fetus).

After labour has been initiated, regular uterine contractions moving downwards from the fundus help expel the fetus. The process of birth usually takes several hours, with the first stage (dilation of the cervix, 6–12 hours) and second (expulsion of the baby, 10 minutes to several hours) taking much longer than the third stage, delivery of the placenta (10–30 minutes). The birth process is stressful on both mother and baby. The fetal adrenal medulla responds by secreting high amounts of catecholamines, and adrenal cortex secretes corticosteroids, which clear the infant's lungs, provide surfactant for breathing, mobilise nutrients and promote increased blood flow to brain and heart, all preparing the infant for independent existence.

Drugs during labour

The pharmacokinetics of drugs may be altered during labour and delivery. During labour, gastric emptying is delayed and vomiting may result, which would alter drug absorption, so parenteral routes are used. Drug metabolism and excretion may be prolonged (Ch 7).

Drugs commonly used during childbirth include:

- oxytocics (see below), which increase uterine contractility and assist in induction of labour and reduction of postpartum haemorrhage (tocolytics decrease contractility – from the Greek stem *tokos*: 'birth')
- analgesics for pain relief: opioids such as morphine and pethidine (IM, IV) are strong analgesics, but can depress respiration in the infant (treated with the narcotic antagonist naloxone) and cause constipation in the mother (Ch 12)
- anaesthetics for pain relief: most common is nitrous oxide ('gas') 50% in oxygen, self-administered by the mother; this has little depressant effect on the infant (Ch 11)
- epidural local anaesthetics such as lidocaine (lignocaine) and bupivacaine: often administered via epidural injection; an opioid and local anaesthetic can be co-administered for effective obstetric analgesia, for caesarean section or vaginal delivery (Ch 11)
- a benzodiazepine such as temazepam, for antianxiety or sedative effects during early labour.

Oxytocics

Agents that stimulate contraction of the smooth muscle of the uterus, resulting in contractions and labour, are **oxytocics**. Those most commonly used are synthetic oxytocin, alkaloids of the plant fungus ergot, and PGs of the E and F series. Oxytocics are used to induce labour, reduce postpartum haemorrhage (PPH) or terminate pregnancy. PPH is a common cause of maternal death in childbirth in both developing and developed countries. Drugs that are nitric oxide donors (isosorbide nitrates, nitroglycerin, sodium nitroprusside) usefully cause cervical ripening, and are being assessed in labour induction.

Oxytocin

Oxytocin is one of two hormones secreted by the posterior pituitary; the other is vasopressin (Ch 28). It is indicated to induce, augment and manage labour, and to treat PPH; it is administered IM or by IV infusion. Carbetocin, an analogue, has longer duration of action and is administered as a single slow IV injection, 100 microgram dose. A case study exemplifying the use of oxytocin in childbirth is described in Clinical Focus Box 28.4.

Ergot alkaloids

Ergot alkaloids are naturally occurring fungal compounds with varied actions on several types of receptors. Ergometrine produces prolonged, strong contractions of the uterus, especially postpartum, and has vasoconstrictor actions, so is useful in the treatment of PPH (Drug Monograph 30.4).

Prostaglandins

PGs are produced in the endometrium and myometrium; $PGF_2\alpha$ is a vasoconstrictor, while PGE_2 and prostacyclin are vasodilators. PGEs and PGFs contract uterine smooth muscle and are implicated in disorders of menstruation. The uterus becomes increasingly sensitive to PGs during pregnancy, so they can be used to produce medical termination.

In obstetrics, PGs are used to soften and dilate the cervix ('uterine priming') and to stimulate uterine contractions, as follows:

- dinoprostone, a PGE_2 analogue, for induction or augmentation of labour at term, given by vaginal gel or pessary (Clinical Focus Box 30.5)
- gemeprost, a PGE_1 analogue, to facilitate first or second trimester termination of pregnancy, given by pessary

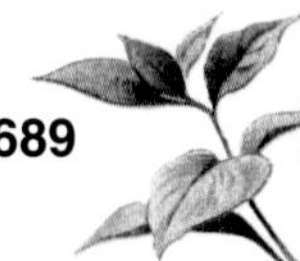

Drug Monograph 30.4
Ergometrine

Actions and mechanism

Ergometrine increases the force and frequency of uterine contractions by direct stimulation of the smooth muscle of the uterine wall. Increased contractions and muscle tone, and vasoconstriction of bleeding vessels at the placental site, arrest PPH.

Indications and contraindications

Ergometrine is administered after delivery of the placenta to contract the uterus and uterine blood vessels, and promote involution of the uterus, to prevent PPH.

Ergometrine is contraindicated to induce labour or during the first two stages because contraction of the cervix would cause fetal distress and compression, and delay birth.

Pharmacokinetics

Ergometrine has unpredictable bioavailability, so is given parenterally. It is formulated for IM administration (or, in emergency, IV) and has rapid onset of action within 1–3 minutes. The duration of uterine contractions after IM injection is about 3 hours. The drug is metabolised in the liver and excreted mainly in faeces.

Drug interactions

Ergometrine has significant interactions with many drugs that also affect receptors for noradrenaline or 5-HT. Effects of other vasoconstrictors are enhanced, whereas those of antianginal vasodilators are antagonised. Drugs that reduce metabolism of ergometrine (e.g. erythromycin, clarithromycin and some antivirals) may cause ergotism and ischaemia if given concurrently.

Adverse reactions

These include nausea, vomiting, hypertension, headache, allergic reactions and, rarely, infarction, pulmonary oedema and gangrene. A dose-related effect is abdominal cramping.

Warnings and contraindications

Use with caution in people with hypocalcaemia. Avoid use in women with ergot alkaloid hypersensitivity, cardiac or vascular disease, eclampsia or preeclampsia, sepsis, or liver or kidney impairment. It is contraindicated in pregnancy (Category C), during the first two stages of labour or to induce labour, or in multiple pregnancies.

Dosage and administration

To prevent PPH, a dose of 200 micrograms is administered IM; in emergencies or in those with excessive uterine bleeding 25–50 micrograms repeated up to total 250 micrograms by slow IV route is recommended. Ergometrine 0.5 mg/mL is also formulated in combination with oxytocin 5 IU/mL (Syntometrine) for active management of the third stage of labour and prevention of PPH.

CLINICAL FOCUS BOX 30.5
Dinoprostone gel for induction of labour

Ms AC is a 39-year-old primiparous woman whose pregnancy has been uneventful. At 38 weeks' gestation her blood pressure in the antenatal clinic is noted to be 140/95. Blood pressure is monitored over 4 hours and is consistently elevated. A spot urine test reveals a slightly raised protein-to-creatinine ratio, indicative of mild preeclampsia, while a blood test showing mild derangements of liver and renal function tests confirms the diagnosis.

Ms AC is asymptomatic, and is allowed to go home, with twice-weekly follow-up organised. By 39/40 gestation, the antihypertensive labetalol is commenced (200 mg twice daily), and the decision is made to commence an induction of labour, as there is little to be gained from her baby staying in utero at 39/40 gestation.

After two 1 mg doses of per vagina dinoprostone gel, she progresses quickly to a normal vaginal delivery of a 3.2 kg healthy baby girl. Her blood pressure normalises postpartum, such that her GP can cease her labetalol at her 6-week check-up.

Source: Acknowledgments to Dr Alison Bryant-Smith, MRCOG (personal communication).

- dinoprost, a $PGF_2\alpha$ analogue, for intractable PPH, or termination of first- or second-trimester pregnancy, by intravaginal or intrauterine administration
- misoprostol, a PGE_1 analogue, orally or buccally, for prevention and treatment of PPH, and for management of miscarriage or termination of pregnancy. For early medical termination (at less than 63 days gestational age), oral mifepristone 200 mg (RU486, an antiprogestogen) followed 36–48 hours later by misoprostol self-administered at home has been shown to be a safe and effective treatment option.

PG analogues are used in obstetrics only where gynaecological care is available. They are also used to prevent dyspepsia and peptic ulceration induced by NSAIDs, in the treatment of erectile dysfunction in men and topically as eyedrops to treat glaucoma (Drug Monograph 40.1).

Tocolytics (inhibitors of premature labour)

Preterm labour, occurring before the 37th week of pregnancy, is a problem in 10–15% of all pregnancies. Premature birth increases the possibility of neonatal morbidity and mortality. Drugs that relax the uterus, and hence delay labour or inhibit threatened miscarriage, are described as **tocolytics**. Delaying labour by 1–2 days allows time for transport of the mother to a specialist centre for delivery of a significantly preterm infant or for administration of corticosteroids to the mother to facilitate fetal production of lung surfactant.

Tocolytics are not used when prolongation of pregnancy is hazardous for the fetus or mother. Most tocolytics effectively delay labour for 2–3 days, but they do not improve perinatal outcomes (mortality, respiratory distress syndrome) or decrease the rate of preterm delivery. Responses of both fetus and mother (heart rate, glycaemia) must be carefully monitored.

Nifedipine and salbutamol

The main drugs used as tocolytics are the calcium channel blocker nifedipine or the β_2-adrenoceptor agonist salbutamol. Other drugs that may relax uterine smooth muscle include progestogens, general anaesthetics, alcohol, magnesium sulfate, direct vasodilators and NSAIDs (by inhibiting PG synthesis).

The preferred drug for delaying labour is the antihypertensive/vasodilator nifedipine. In threatened preterm labour up to 34 weeks, standard 20 mg tablets can be given every 3–8 hours until contractions cease or labour becomes too well established to stop.

Salbutamol (a bronchodilator; Ch 15, Drug Monograph 15.2) is administered as a tocolytic for management of uncomplicated preterm labour (24–34 weeks' gestation). It is infused IV at a slowly increasing rate up to 45 micrograms/minute until contractions cease, maintained for 1 hour, then gradually reduced, for a maximum duration of 48 hours.

Drugs during lactation

Drugs taken by a breastfeeding mother may affect lactation, and can be absorbed by the infant in sufficient amounts to cause pharmacological or toxic effects. However, it is essential for the welfare of both mother and baby that the mother's health be maintained, so drug therapy may be required.

Lactation promoters and inhibitors

Lactation – that is, production of milk from the mammary glands (breasts) – is initiated and maintained by the anterior pituitary hormone prolactin (Ch 26). Lactation begins when levels of progesterone and estradiol drop rapidly after birth. Suckling at the breast by the infant increases secretion of prolactin by neural reflexes, which act via the hypothalamus and pituitary gland, and triggers the milk let-down reflex, with oxytocin as a mediator. Prolactin release is inhibited by the hypothalamic prolactin release-inhibitory factor, the neurotransmitter dopamine.

Suckling or mechanical stimulation of the nipple are the best stimulators of prolactin secretion. The dopamine antagonists domperidone and metoclopramide, normally prescribed as antiemetics or to stimulate motility of the upper GIT, have been used to stimulate lactation by inhibiting prolactin release-inhibitory factor; however, there are safety concerns. Dopamine antagonists such as the phenothiazine psychotropic agents may cause gynaecomastia and galactorrhoea (Clinical Focus Box 26.2).

It may be necessary, for clearly defined medical reasons, to inhibit lactation – for example, if the mother must take essential drugs that would be harmful to the infant when ingested in breast milk, or if the infant has died. Dopamine agonists cabergoline and bromocriptine inhibit release of prolactin from the anterior pituitary gland, resulting in suppression of lactation.

Estrogens in combination contraceptive pill formulations also inhibit lactation; hence, estrogens are not used in OC formulations in breastfeeding women; they are no longer indicated to treat postpartum breast engorgement. Conservative measures such as breast binding and ice-packs are effective, with analgesics.

Passage of drugs into breast milk

Almost all drugs in maternal circulation can be readily transferred to the colostrum (milk produced in the first week after birth) and breast milk; exceptions are large molecules such as heparin and insulin. In general, the proven benefits of continuing breastfeeding must be weighed on an individual basis against the risks of exposure of the infant to maternal medications, and risks to the mother from ceasing essential drugs.

The mammary alveolar epithelium is more permeable to drugs during the colostrum stage of milk production; transfer of a drug or its metabolites into milk occurs predominantly by passive diffusion. Drug factors that enhance drug excretion into milk are dose and frequency, high maternal plasma drug concentration, low maternal plasma protein binding, low molecular weight (< 200) and greater lipid solubility. CNS-active drugs, being lipid-soluble, are likely to partition into breast milk, and hence need caution in prescribing. CNS depressants may sedate the baby and depress suckling. Antidepressants may be needed to treat postpartum depression; sertraline and paroxetine appear to be the safest.

Pharmacokinetics in infants

Data on pharmacokinetics in infants are scant and conflicting (see detailed discussion in Ch 7). It is believed that absorptive processes in the infant's GIT and drug distribution are similar to those in the adult and that lipid-soluble drugs are well absorbed. A single measurement of a drug in human milk will not accurately reflect the total dose an infant receives. The infant's actual dose depends largely on the volume of milk consumed, which is on average 0.15 L/kg/day. The dose received via milk is generally much less than known safe doses given to an infant.

The following factors are also relevant:

- If the drug is fat-soluble, it may be more highly concentrated in breast milk at the end of feeding (hindmilk), which contains more fat than at commencement of feeding.
- Because the infant's plasma protein concentration is lower compared with an adult's, more free drug may be available to act.
- Metabolic reactions in the infant's liver are slower than in an older child's; hence, drug metabolism may be delayed.
- Drug excretion via the kidneys is delayed in the neonate, since glomerular filtration and tubular functioning remain immature for months.

Drugs and breastfeeding guidelines

It is often necessary to know how a drug affects lactation and whether it is safe for a breastfeeding mother and child. Guidelines have been drawn up based on clinical experience (see Hotham & Hotham 2015 and *Pregnancy and Breastfeeding Medicines Guide*, The Royal Women's Hospital, Melbourne, in 'Online resources'), with advice on specific drugs. In general, the following is suggested:

- Benefits of breastfeeding to both infant and mother are important.
- Optimising the mother's health is in the best interests of mother and infant.
- Only essential drugs should be taken by breastfeeding women.
- Most commonly used drugs are relatively safe for breastfed babies.
- Older drugs that appear safe should be prescribed in preference to new drugs with which there is little clinical experience.
- Many oral drugs reach maximum plasma concentrations within 2–3 hours, and babies tend to feed at 4–6-hour intervals, so the mother taking a dose of drug immediately after a feed and before the infant's longest sleep period usually minimises intake by the baby.
- If possible, surgery should be postponed; breastfeeding mothers requiring surgery generally can continue to breastfeed, provided adequate hydration is maintained and the first quantity of milk after surgery is discarded.
- Local administration minimises dose and systemic absorption of a drug; hence, it minimises transfer into milk.
- Feeding can be withheld (or expressed milk given) if a one-off drug is needed – for example, a diagnostic agent.
- The milk-to-plasma ratio has been determined for some drugs; if this is high – for example, with antidepressants, some β-blockers and some NSAIDs – the drug may not be recommended, or recommended only with caution and monitoring of the infant.

Breastfeeding is contraindicated:

- if any diagnostic radioisotope testing is scheduled (breastfeeding is interrupted until all the radioactive substance is absent from milk samples)
- when the drug is so toxic that minute amounts may profoundly affect the infant
- when the drug has high allergenic potential
- when the mother's renal function deteriorates (which augments drug excretion into breast milk)
- when serious pathological conditions require prolonged administration of high doses of drugs (e.g. cancer chemotherapy; antithyroid drugs).

Examples of drugs to be avoided while breastfeeding are listed in Box 30.1.

KEY POINTS

Drugs in pregnancy, childbirth and lactation

- During pregnancy, hormones secreted by the mother and placenta interact and maintain pregnancy.

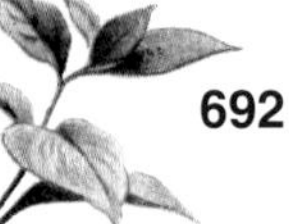

BOX 30.1 examples of drugs that should be avoided during breastfeeding

Alcohol (delay drinking until after a feed)
Amiodarone
Anthracyclines (e.g. doxorubicin)
Antineoplastic agents
Aspirin (high dose)
Atenolol
Chloramphenicol
Ciclosporin
Cocaine
Combined oral contraceptives
Cyclophosphamide
Diazepam
Dopamine agonists
Doxorubicin
Ephedrine hydrochloride
Gold salts (e.g. auranofin, aurothiomalate)
Heroin
Iodine
Lamotrigine
Lithium
Marijuana
Methadone
Methotrexate
Estrogens
Phenobarbital (phenobarbitone)
Propylthiouracil
Radiopharmaceuticals
Retinoids
Smoking (nicotine replacement is preferable)
Sotalol
Tetracyclines
Theophylline
Vigabatrin

Sources: Australian Medicines Handbook 2021; Hotham & Hotham 2015. Consult specialist pregnancy drug information centres for comprehensive advice.

- Drugs taken by the mother pass across into the fetal circulation and may cause adverse pharmacological effects in the fetus. Drugs are used cautiously during pregnancy, and guidelines as to relative safety of drugs in pregnancy should be observed.
- The Australian categorisation system for prescribing medicines in pregnancy has seven categories (A, B1, B2, B3, C, D and X) to indicate the level of risk to the fetus of drugs used at the recommended therapeutic doses.
- Drugs affecting uterine smooth muscle activity include those that induce labour (oxytocics) and prevent postpartum haemorrhage, such as oxytocin and ergometrine. Tocolytics inhibit premature labour and include nifedipine and salbutamol.
- Drug factors that enhance drug excretion into milk are low maternal plasma protein binding, higher maternal plasma drug concentration, low molecular weight (< 200) and greater lipid solubility.
- Lactation can be affected by drug therapy of the mother, as can the infant if drugs are excreted in breast milk. Guidelines for use of drugs by lactating mothers are described, including careful drug use and dosing just after breastfeeding to minimise drug concentrations in milk.

Menopause and hormone replacement therapy

Menopause

Menopause is loosely defined as the transitional period at the end of the reproductive period of a woman's life when ovulation and menstruation cease. The timing varies with ethnicity, geographical regions, socioeconomic status, extremes of bodyweight, smoking status, amount of heavy exercise and a woman's menstrual, gynaecological and surgical history. The term 'climacteric' refers to the signs, symptoms and consequences of the period around menopause.

Menopause can occur over a wide age range – from 42 to 58 years of age, with the average age of the last menstrual period for Australian and New Zealand women being around 51. This age has not changed significantly in recorded history (except that it is earlier in women who smoke), despite increasingly younger onset of menarche and improved living conditions and nutrition. Until about 1900, the median survival age for females was only 45 years (with many dying in childhood or childbirth); hence, a large proportion of females never reached menopause. The average life span of women in developed countries is now over 80, so most women can expect to spend one-third of their lives after menopause.

Physiological changes

Changes occurring during menopause are due to depletion of the stock of ova and follicles (estimated to be 0.2–2 million at birth) by decades of ovulation and atresia. Gonadotrophins are still released, but there is a relatively sudden decrease in secretion of estrogens and progesterone despite high levels of FSH; ovulation and menstruation cease, genital organs and breasts may atrophy, and protein anabolism is reduced. There is still some production of estrone, testosterone and androstenedione, and libido and sexual performance are not necessarily decreased.

Many women suffer unpleasant symptoms during early years of menopause: hot flushes (sudden rise in temperature and excessive sweating, thought to coincide with bursts of GnRH), nausea, insomnia, vaginitis, palpitations, increased risk of ischaemic heart disease, fatigue, depression, breast tenderness and osteoporosis. For many women, menopause is a relief from decades of menstruation and the risk of unplanned pregnancies.

Hormone replacement therapy

In some women, menopausal symptoms are severe and need treatment. Postmenopausal **hormone replacement therapy** involves daily low doses of a natural estrogen (e.g. estradiol), possibly for many years. In women with an intact uterus (who have not undergone surgical hysterectomy), a progestogen must also be given 10–12 days per month to prevent endometrial hyperplasia and endometrial cancer; this is 'opposed' therapy. Adverse reactions, drug interactions and contraindications are generally as for the constituent estrogen and progestogen, but doses are considerably lower than in OC preparations to reduce adverse reactions.

Controversies and conclusions

The Women's Health Initiative was a 15-year research program set up in 1991 by the US Department of Health and Human Services to study the health status of 161,808 women, most many years after onset of menopause. Clinical trials tested the effects of HRT (estrogen-plus-progestogen in women with a uterus and estrogen-alone in women without a uterus), diet modification and calcium and vitamin D supplements on heart disease, bone fractures and breast and colorectal cancer. Important results were disseminated widely (see Women's Health Initiative under 'Online resources').

Results initially appeared to show increased risk of coronary heart disease and breast cancer, which led to an abrupt decrease in the use of HRT. Subsequent reanalysis of data and new meta-analyses consistently show reductions in heart disease, mortality, symptoms of menopause and risk of osteoporotic fractures or colon cancer and improved quality of life when HRT is initiated soon after menopause (Lobo 2017). Risk of breast or ovarian cancer may be increased.

HRT formulations and administration

Natural estrogens are preferred because of lower potency and fewer adverse reactions; oral administration is convenient and cheap. Oral estrogens used are estradiol valerate (Drug Monograph 30.1, earlier), conjugated estrogens and estriol. A low dose is taken daily – for example, estradiol 1–2 mg orally. Oral progestogens used for 10–14 days/month in HRT are MPA, norethisterone, drospirenone or dydrogesterone. Various combination packs are available. A new combination formulation contains conjugated estrogens with the SERM bazedoxifene to oppose estrogenic effects on the endometrium.

Non-oral HRT formulations

Non-oral formulations are indicated for women intolerant of oral estrogens or who prefer not to take daily tablets.

Transdermal estrogen bypasses the liver, avoids first-pass metabolism and is considered more physiological in terms of the estradiol:estrone ratio. The patches are more expensive and many women (10–20%) suffer unpleasant skin reactions (redness, irritation, itchiness). Combination patch formulations contain estradiol with/without norethisterone to mimic the natural menstrual cycle.

Other formulation types are transdermal gel, vaginal cream, pessaries and the levonorgestrel IUD. Vaginal estrogens appear to offer no protection against osteoporosis. As there are many types and formulations of HRT available, subject to frequent changes, a current reference such as *Australian Medicines Handbook* should be consulted for specific guidelines.

Other menopause therapies

Tibolone

Tibolone is an interesting steroidal drug for treating menopausal symptoms, protecting against bone resorption, and elevating mood and libido. It is neither estrogen nor SERM but is classified as a 'gonadomimetic', with estrogenic, anti-estrogenic, progestogenic and androgenic effects. After oral administration it has active metabolites with estrogenic effects in vagina, bone and thermoregulatory centre, progestogenic and anti-estrogenic actions in breast and endometrium and androgenic effects on lipid metabolism.

Tibolone (2.5 mg/day) is useful for menopausal symptoms of hot flushes and vaginal dryness, and in preventing reduced bone mineral density. Mild adverse reactions include bloating, vaginal discharge, excess hair growth and acne. In older women, stroke risk and recurrence of breast cancer were increased. Precautions are required in women with a history of hormone-dependent tumours, cardiovascular or hepatic diseases.

Phytoestrogens as SERMs

Phytoestrogens (non-steroidal plant compounds with estrogenic activity) are of interest for menopausal symptoms, and are advertised as being more 'natural' than synthetic drugs. They are phenolic isoflavones, coumestans and lignans occurring in some plants and seeds, especially in clovers and soybeans.[7] Chemically, they are related to both estrogens and the coumarin anticoagulants. Pharmacologically, they are SERMs, binding to ERs causing varying agonist and antagonist actions in estrogen-responsive tissues plus enzyme-modulating and antioxidant activities. Clinical trials so far have shown little if any benefit over placebo in females; vaginal dryness and frequency of hot flushes may be reduced. In men, soy foods and isoflavone supplements have no deleterious effects on testosterone or sperm concentrations. In Australian Indigenous medicine, berries of the 'kangaroo apple' (*Solanum aviculare*) have

7 Japanese women have a low rate of breast cancer, attributed to high intakes of phytoestrogens in soybean paste soup. Genistein, a phytoestrogen in Australian subterranean clover, has been held responsible for low fertility and high abortion rates in sheep grazing on these pastures. In a fine vein of anthropomorphism, it has been hypothesised that some plants produce anti-estrogenic constituents in order to reduce the fertility of animals that eat them.

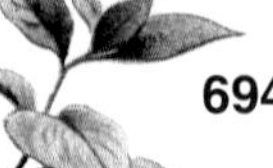

been used for contraception. Active extracts contain steroids, alkaloids and solasodine, and have been used in the synthesis of OCs and cortisone.

Non-hormonal therapies

Useful lifestyle modifications in menopause include regular light exercise, reducing stress, wearing layered clothing and practising 'sleep hygiene' (Ch 20). Smoking and excessive caffeine, alcohol and spicy foods should be avoided.

Antidepressants of the selective serotonin or noradrenaline reuptake inhibitor types have a small effect in reducing hot flushes. (5-HT is involved in emotions and mood, control of body temperature, endocrine regulation and sleep.) High doses of gabapentin, an anticonvulsant, also reduce hot flushes by approximately two per day. Clonidine, a partial agonist at β_2-adrenoceptors and a centrally acting antihypertensive agent, also reduces frequency of hot flushes; the mechanism of this action is unclear.

KEY POINTS

Drugs in menopause

- Cessation of menstruation at menopause may be associated with symptoms of low estrogen levels and increased risk of cardiovascular disease and osteoporosis.
- Hormone replacement therapy – that is, regular use of low-dose natural estrogen with/without cyclical progesterone – suppresses menopausal symptoms and protects against some cancers and bone disease. HRT may be administered orally, transdermally or with an IUD.
- Long-term use of HRT may cause slightly increased risk of some conditions (e.g. stroke, breast cancer, VTE) and reduced risk of others (osteoporotic fractures, colorectal cancer, dementia and diabetes).

DRUGS AT A GLANCE

PHARMACOLOGICAL GROUP AND EFFECT	KEY EXAMPLES	CLINICAL USE
Gonadotrophin-releasing hormones • Initially increases synthesis of FSH and LH • With high continuous use, decreases FSH and LH	Nafarelin	• Endometriosis • Controlled ovarian stimulation for IVF
Gonadotrophins • Each recombinant gonadotrophic mimics the respective endogenous gonadotrophin	Recombinant FSH Recombinant LH hCG (mimics LH)	• Female infertility • Treat hypogonadism
Estrogens • Mimic the action of endogenous estradiol	Estradiol valerate, ethinylestradiol (EE)	• Hormone replacement therapy (HRT) • Estrogen deficiency symptoms • COC (see below)
Selective estrogen receptor modulators (SERMs) • Estrogen agonist actions on bone and cardiovascular system • Estrogen antagonist effects on breast and uterus tissue	Raloxifene	• Protect against menopausal osteoporosis • Decrease risk of breast cancer
Anti-estrogens • Inhibits estrogen binding in the hypothalamus, pituitary; increases LH release, FSH estrogen	Clomifene	• Anovulatory infertility
Progestogens • Mimic the action of endogenous progesterone • Increase progesterone; the body will not ovulate	Levonorgestrel, norethisterone	• Contraception • Endometriosis • HRT (to oppose actions of estrogen) • Assisted reproduction technologies
Progesterone antagonists • Block LH surge prevents implantation	Mifepristone	• Early termination of pregnancy (mifepristone)
Selective progesterone receptor modulators (SPRMs) • Partial agonists (both agonist and antagonist activity) at the progesterone receptor	Ulipristal	• Emergency contraceptive pill • Management of uterine fibroids
Contraceptives		
Combined oral contraceptives (COCs) • Inhibit GnRH • Inhibit both LH and FSH • Disrupt the mid-cycle LH surge • Prevent ovulation	Various combinations of EE, estradiol or mestranol with levonorgestrel, norethisterone or other progestogen	• Prevent unwanted pregnancy

Progesterone-only • Increase progesterone; the body will not ovulate	Progesterone-only (oral) Progesterone-only (depot) Intrauterine devices (IUDs)	• Prevent unwanted pregnancy
Oxytocics		
Oxytocin analogue • Mimics the effect of oxytocin	Carbetocin	• Stimulates contractions • Induces labour
Ergot alkaloids • α-1A adrenergic receptor agonist • Cause arterial vasoconstriction	Ergometrine	• Stimulate uterine contractions • Prevent postpartum haemorrhage
Prostaglandin analogues • Prostaglandin E_2 agonists • Cause myometrial stimulation	Dinoprostone	• Induce labour
Tocolytics		
β-adrenoceptor agonists • Stimulate β-adrenoceptors in smooth muscle of the uterus = relaxation	Salbutamol	• Stop contractions of premature labour
Calcium channel blockers • Block calcium in the uterus, promote smooth muscle relaxation	Nifedipine	• Delay threatened preterm labour
Hormone replacement therapy (HRT)		
Estrogens, progestogens • Mimic actions of endogenous estrogens, progestogens	Various combinations of estradiol, estriol and conjugated estrogens mestranol with norethisterone, dydrogesterone or other progestogens	• Relieve symptoms caused by decreasing endogenous estrogens • Progestogens decrease risky health outcomes from unopposed estrogens
Gonadomimetics • Synthetic steroid with estrogenic and progestogenic activity	Tibolone	• Relieve symptoms caused by decreasing endogenous estrogens

REVIEW EXERCISES

1. Mrs SO, a 35-year-old woman with a long history of smoking, presented to her GP for a routine check-up. Her GP ceased her combined oral contraceptive pill. Discuss why the GP ceased the COC and discuss suitable contraception options for this person.
2. Ms PH, a 23-year-old woman (BMI = 31) presented to her local pharmacy and asked for the emergency contraceptive pill. Describe the different types of emergency contraception available and how they work. What would be the most appropriate emergency contraceptive pill for Ms PH? Why?
3. Ms IE is a 33-year-old primiparous women who is 40 weeks' pregnant. Her obstetrician prescribes dinoprostone 2 mg administered into the vagina to induce labour. Describe how dinoprostone works to induce labour. Discuss the other oxytocins that could have been prescribed and how they work.
4. Ms BI, a 33-year-old primiparous women, presents to the emergency department as she has gone into premature labour at 32 weeks' gestation. She is prescribed nifedipine 20 mg orally stat. As her contractions did not stop, she is prescribed another 20 mg orally at 30-minute intervals for another two doses. In this time, Ms BI is transferred by ambulance to a hospital with neonatal facilities. Describe how nifedipine works to prevent preterm labour. What other tocolytics are available to delay delivery of a newborn?

REFERENCES

Abreu, AP and UB Kaiser. Pubertal development and regulation. The Lancet Diabetes & Endocrinology, 2016. 4(3): 254–264.

Australian Medicines Handbook 2021. Australian Medicines Handbook. Adelaide: AMH

Brown J, Farquhar C: An overview of treatments for endometriosis, JAMA: The Journal of the American Medical Association 313(3):296–297, 2015.

Bryant–Smith, AC, Lethaby, A, Farquhar, C, et al. Antifibrinolytics for heavy menstrual bleeding. Cochrane Database of Systematic Reviews, 2018(4).

Chrousos, GP, B Katzung, and A Trevor. Basic and clinical pharmacology. Adrenocorticosteroids & Adrenocortical Antagonists, 13th ed.; McGraw-Hill Medical: New York, NY, USA, 2015.

Ellis, AJ, Hendrick, VM, Williams, R, et al. Selective estrogen receptor modulators in clinical practice: a safety overview. Expert Opinion on Drug Safety, 2015 14(6): 921–934.

Endocrinology Expert Group. Therapeutic Guidelines: endocrinology. Version 5. 2014.

Frost, JJ, JE Darroch, and L Remez, Improving contraceptive use in the United States. Issues in brief (Alan Guttmacher Institute), 2008(1): 1–8.

Hofmeister, S and S Bodden, Premenstrual syndrome and premenstrual dysphoric disorder. American Family Physician, 2016. 94(3): 236–240.

Hotham, N and E Hotham, Drugs in breastfeeding. Australian Prescriber, 2015. 38(5): 156.

Katzung BG: Basic and clinical pharmacology, ed 12, New York, 2012, McGraw-Hill.

Kennedy, D, Classifying drugs in pregnancy. Australian Prescriber, 2014. 37: 38–40.

Lobo, RA, Hormone-replacement therapy: current thinking. Nature Reviews Endocrinology, 2017. 13(4): 220–231.

Lu, CL and C Herndon. New roles for neuronal estrogen receptors. Neurogastroenterology & Motility, 2017. 29(7): e13121.

Moore KL, Persaud TVN, Torchia M: The developing human: clinically oriented embryology, ed 10, Philadelphia, PA, 2016, Saunders/Elsevier

Salerno E: Pharmacology for health professionals, St Louis, MO, 1999, Mosby.

Stewart, M and K Black, Choosing a combined oral contraceptive pill. Australian Prescriber, 2015. 38(1): 6–11.

Wagenfeld, A, Saunders, PTK, Whitaker, L, et al. Selective progesterone receptor modulators (SPRMs): progesterone receptor action, mode of action on the endometrium and treatment options in gynecological therapies. Expert Opinion on Therapeutic Targets, 2016. 20(9): 1045–1054.

ONLINE RESOURCES

Australian College of Midwives: https://www.midwives.org.au/ (accessed 15 September 2021)

Australasian Menopause Society: https://www.menopause.org.au/ (accessed 15 September 2021)

Drugs in pregnancy database: https://www.tga.gov.au/prescribing-medicines-pregnancy-database/ (accessed 15 September 2021)

Endometriosis Australia: https://www.endometriosisaustralia.org/ (accessed 15 September 2021)

Jean Hailes Foundation for Women's Health: https://jeanhailes.org.au/ (accessed 15 September 2021)

RANZCOG – College statements and guidelines: https://www.ranzcog.edu.au/Statements-Guidelines/ (accessed 15 September 2021)

Therapeutic Goods Administration – goods exempt from pregnancy categorisation: https://www.tga.gov.au/therapeutic-goods-exempted-pregnancy-categorisation/ (accessed 15 September 2021)

The Royal Women's Hospital (Melbourne) – Contraception guide: https://www.thewomens.org.au/health-information/contraception/ (accessed 15 September 2021)

The Royal Women's Hospital (Melbourne) – Pregnancy and breastfeeding medicines guide: https://thewomenspbmg.org.au/ (accessed 15 September 2021) [This resource requires a subscription]

The Royal Women's Hospital (Melbourne) information website: https://www.thewomens.org.au/health-information (accessed 15 September 2021)

Women's Health Initiative (US Department of Health and Human Services): https://www.nhlbi.nih.gov/science/womens-health-initiative-whi (accessed 15 September 2021)

World Health Organization publications on sexual and reproductive health: https://www.who.int/reproductivehealth/publications/en/ (accessed 15 September 2021)

More weblinks at: http://evolve.elsevier.com/AU/Knights/pharmacology/.

— CHAPTER 31 —

DRUGS AFFECTING THE MALE REPRODUCTIVE SYSTEM

Mary Bushell

KEY ABBREVIATIONS

AR	androgen receptor
BPH	benign prostatic hyperplasia (or hypertrophy)
DHT	dihydrotestosterone
FSH	follicle-stimulating hormone
GnRH	gonadotrophin-releasing hormone
ICSH	interstitial cell-stimulating hormone
SARM	selective androgen receptor modulator

KEY TERMS

Chapter Focus

Androgens, primarily testosterone and its ester derivatives, are male sex hormones with physiological actions in male sexual maturation and functions and development of male secondary sexual characteristics. They are used for replacement therapy in androgen deficiency and for treating advanced stages of breast cancer. (Androgenic anabolic steroids are abused in sport for their muscle-building effects.) Anti-androgens such as flutamide, and continuous administration of gonadotrophin-releasing hormone analogues, are used for prostate cancer.

Benign prostatic hyperplasia is a common disorder in older men. The use of α_1-adrenoceptor antagonists and 5α-reductase inhibitors for treating this condition is discussed. Erectile dysfunction is another problem, commonly treated with phosphodiesterase 5 inhibitors.

Common causes of infertility in men and the drugs used to treat infertility are discussed. Methods of contraception for men are described, and their relative advantages, disadvantages, rates of use and failure are compared. Many drugs can enhance or reduce sexual desire or functioning.

KEY DRUG GROUPS

Androgens:
- **Testosterone** (Drug Monograph 31.1)

ANTI-ANDROGENS:
- **Cyproterone**, **flutamide**, **SARMs**

Drugs that affect sexual functioning:
- Antihypertensives, CNS depressants, social drugs, vasodilators

Drugs for benign prostatic hypertrophy:
- α_1-adrenoceptor antagonists: **prazosin**, **terazosin**
- 5α-reductase inhibitors: **dutasteride** (Drug Monograph 31.2), **finasteride**

Drugs for erectile dysfunction:
- Drug for premature ejaculation: SSRI: **dapoxetine**
- Phosphodiesterase 5 inhibitors: **sildenafil** (Drug Monograph 31.3), **tadalafil**, **vardenafil**
- Prostaglandins: **alprostadil**
- Smooth muscle relaxants: **papaverine**

Gonadotrophin-releasing hormone analogues:
- **Goserelin**, **leuprorelin**

Gonadotrophins:
- **Interstitial cell-stimulating hormone**

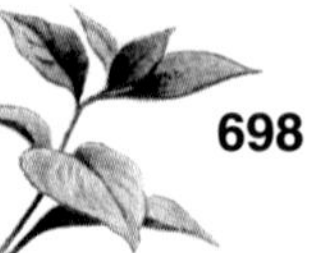

CRITICAL THINKING SCENARIO

Anthony has been taking the drug sildenafil for his erectile dysfunction for approximately a decade. Recently, Anthony presented to the emergency department with severe chest pain, shortness of breath and pain in his left arm, jaw and neck. Anthony is subsequently diagnosed with stable angina and prescribed atenolol 50 mg daily and isosorbide mononitrate modified release 60 mg daily to prevent his angina. He is also prescribed sublingual glyceryl trinitrate spray (a short-acting nitrate) to be administered at the onset of an angina attack. The prescriber ceases his sildenafil and prescribes alprostadil as a replacement medicine for his erectile dysfunction.

1. **Discuss the mechanism of action of both sildenafil and alprostadil.**
2. **What are some common side effects of both medicines?**
3. **For what reason would the prescriber have ceased sildenafil?**
4. **Discuss how alprostadil is administered.**

Introduction: Male reproductive system controls and hormones

The hypothalamic and pituitary controls of the male reproductive organs (the testes, seminal vesicles, prostate gland, bulbourethral glands and penis) are described in Chapter 26, and shown diagrammatically in Figure 30.1. To summarise in the context of male reproductive functions:

- The hypothalamus secretes gonadotrophin-releasing hormone (GnRH), which stimulates the anterior pituitary gland to release the **gonadotrophins**, the pituitary hormones involved in the male reproductive system – follicle-stimulating hormone (FSH) and **interstitial cell-stimulating hormone** (ICSH) (known in the female as luteinising hormone, LH).
- FSH stimulates the seminiferous tubules in the testes to increase production of spermatozoa, while ICSH stimulates the interstitial cells to increase secretion of androgens, the male sex hormones, mainly testosterone; production of androgens is not cyclical.
- Androgens are also produced in the adrenal cortex, stimulated by adrenocorticotrophic hormone.
- ICSH is down-regulated (activity is *reduced*) by hypothalamic GnRH when given *continuously*; this effect is exploited as 'chemical castration' in treating prostate cancer.
- In some cells (e.g. in the seminal vesicles and prostate gland), testosterone is converted to a more potent metabolite, dihydrotestosterone (DHT).
- A high level of circulating androgens will inhibit the release of FSH and ICSH from the pituitary by typical negative-feedback mechanisms.

Puberty in males

Puberty is the development stage during which reproductive capacity is attained. In girls it is clearly marked by the onset of the first menstrual period (menarche); in boys it is less easily defined. In both sexes the timing of puberty varies greatly, and the specific genes controlling the onset of puberty are not known. There is increasing pulsatile secretion of hypothalamic GnRH stimulating the release of pituitary gonadotrophins and in turn gonadal activity; other hormones including leptin, ghrelin, kisspeptins,[1] neurokinin B, inhibin B and insulin-factor 3 are also involved (Abreu & Kaiser 2016). In boys, testicular growth is dependent on gonadotrophins, while androgens stimulate 'virilisation'.

If puberty is long delayed in a boy, there is a risk of his failing to achieve target height and bone mass, plus delayed sexual and social integration in peer groups and associated adverse psychological and educational problems. In mild cases, no treatment may be required; however, short courses of low-dose testosterone are effective.

1 Newly described regulators of reproductive function are the neuropeptides called 'kisspeptins', which along with the receptor KISS1R have fundamental roles in initiating the onset of puberty. Formerly known as metastatin, kisspeptin was appropriately renamed by the team of scientists who discovered the gene when working in Hershey, Pennsylvania, USA, famous for its chocolates named 'Hershey's Kisses'.

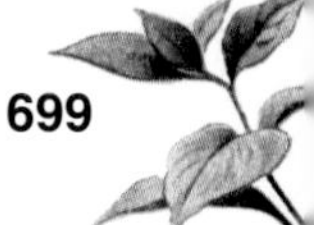

Drugs used in male reproductive disorders

Gonadotrophin-releasing hormone, analogues and antagonists

Gonadotrophin-releasing hormone (gonadorelin) is a 10-amino-acid peptide that stimulates release of FSH and ICSH from the anterior pituitary gland.

Gonadorelin analogues (i.e. GnRH agonists; see Table 30.1 in Ch 30) have been developed to have longer half-lives and hence more useful activities when administered. Leuprorelin, goserelin and triptorelin are all indicated for continuous administration in palliative treatment of prostate cancer. The GnRH analogues cause initial stimulation of the gonads (and possibly a 'flare-up' of cancer symptoms), then suppression of testicular steroidogenesis and thus reduction in tumour growth and atrophy of the reproductive organs. (As their main indications for use in men are in treatment of cancers, these drugs are considered in more detail in Ch 32.)

The GnRH antagonist, degarelix, inhibits gonadorelin production and thus reduces androgen production in the testes; it is used to treat prostate cancer.

Gonadal hormones and antagonists

Male sex hormones: androgens

Synthesis and metabolism

Androgens, primarily **testosterone**, are the steroidal male sex hormones necessary for the normal development and maintenance of male sex functions and characteristics. Testosterone is produced in the Leydig (interstitial) cells of the testes, from precursors dehydroepiandrosterone and androstenedione synthesised in the adrenal cortex. Some of the testosterone acts in the seminiferous tubules in production of sperm, and the rest is secreted into the bloodstream where it circulates, bound to steroid-binding proteins, to target tissues where its effects are exerted.

The actions of androgens are mediated in cells in androgen-sensitive tissues after conversion of testosterone (a steroid) by the 5α-reductase enzyme to the more active metabolite 5α-DHT. Androgens can also be converted to estrogenic metabolites by the aromatase enzyme, which 'aromatises' the A ring of the steroid structure to an aromatic benzene ring as in estradiol. Chemicals that selectively inhibit these enzymes and thus reduce levels of hormones are used to treat hormone-dependent disorders: 5α-reductase inhibitors indicated for benign prostatic hypertrophy (BPH; see later), and aromatase inhibitors for postmenopausal breast cancer. Another enzyme essential in the synthesis of testosterone is the cytochrome P450 enzyme CYP17A1, which has both 17-α-hydroxylase and $C_{17,20}$-lyase activity. A drug designed specifically to inhibit this enzyme, abiraterone acetate, has been approved in advanced prostate cancer.

Mechanisms and actions

Androgen receptors

Testosterone and DHT act via binding to specific high-affinity androgen receptors (ARs), widely distributed in reproductive organs, cardiovascular, musculoskeletal, immune, neural and haemopoietic tissues. Binding by ligand (androgen) induces a conformational change in the AR, allowing translocation into the nucleus, phosphorylation and formation of dimers, which activate and regulate expression of androgen-responsive genes by binding to response elements in their regulatory regions, hence altering protein synthesis. (ARs are being targeted in the search for new drugs in the treatment of prostate cancer.)

Androgens can also exert rapid effects not mediated via genomic/transcriptional mechanisms. For example, via activation of a membrane receptor associated with sex hormone-binding globulin and a G-protein, second messenger activation of protein kinases or adenylate cyclase causes cellular effects such as smooth muscle relaxation, neurotransmission across the neuromuscular junction and neuronal plasticity (Davey & Grossmann 2016).

Androgen actions

Androgenic effects can be summarised into four main groups:

- before birth – masculinisation of the reproductive tract and external genitalia; descent of the testes into the scrotum
- reproduction-related effects – growth and sexual maturation at puberty; spermatogenesis; maintenance of the reproductive tract; feedback control of gonadotrophin secretion
- development of male secondary sexual characteristics (deep voice, male-pattern hair growth, muscle growth and male body shape) and behaviours, and maintenance of male accessory sex organs, such as the prostate gland, seminal vesicles, penis and bulbourethral glands
- non-reproductive functions – anabolic effects on bone and skeletal muscle, neuroprotective effects in the central and peripheral nervous systems, bone protection (possibly after aromatisation to estrogens) and stimulation of vascular cell adhesion molecules in endothelial cells.

Pharmacokinetic and pharmaceutical aspects

Testosterone has a high first-pass effect when given orally as a drug, being rapidly metabolised in the liver

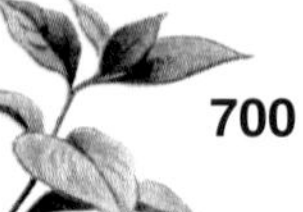

Drug Monograph 31.1
Testosterone undecanoate depot injection

Testosterone undecanoate has long-acting androgenic and anabolic actions.

Indications
It is indicated for treatment of primary and secondary androgen deficiency, such as testicular failure caused by cryptorchidism, orchitis or orchiectomy, or pituitary–hypothalamic insufficiency.

Mechanism and actions
See text under 'Androgen receptors' and 'Androgen actions'. Testosterone increases body lean mass and muscle strength and may improve sexual function and mood.

Pharmacokinetics
After IM injection, the ester is cleaved to testosterone and undecanoic acid. Maximum levels are reached after 7–14 days, then decline with a half-life of about 53 days. Testosterone circulates 98% bound to globulins, is metabolised in the liver and is excreted 90% as conjugates by the kidneys.

Drug interactions
Significant drug interactions have been reported when testosterone was given concurrently with oral anticoagulants (warfarin), leading to enhanced anticoagulant effects, or with antidiabetic agents (enhanced hypoglycaemic effects). Drugs that induce microsomal enzymes may enhance clearance of testosterone.

Adverse reactions
Common adverse reactions reported after IM injection are acne and injection site pain; urinary urgency, breast swelling or tenderness (gynaecomastia), frequent or continuous erections, testicular atrophy, prostate enlargement and impaired spermatogenesis can occur.

Contraindications and precautions
Testosterone is contraindicated in women and children (except for boys with delayed puberty), and in men with androgen-dependent cancers, liver tumours or hypersensitivity to androgens. Anabolic androgenic steroids are banned in sport.

Dosage and administration
Testosterone undecanoate is formulated for slow depot IM injection. For male hypogonadism, the maintenance IM dosage is usually 1 g every 10–14 weeks.

to androstenedione, excreted via the urine, with a half-life of only 5–20 minutes. To prolong its duration of action it is formulated as ester compounds, which are hydrolysed in the body to the active drug form. Examples are:

- testosterone undecanoate, administered intramuscularly (IM) every 10–14 weeks (Drug Monograph 31.1)
- testosterone enanthate, an oily solution for depot IM injection, usually administered once every 2–3 weeks
- other testosterone esters are formulated for injection, and other synthetic androgens include mesterolone and nandrolone
- transdermal testosterone systems are available for application to the skin as a gel (1%), cream (1%, 2%, 5%), patches (5 mg), all applied once daily; care must be taken to avoid transferring the drug to other people by skin contact.

Because androgens are used for replacement therapy in conditions of chronic androgen deficiency, lifelong therapy may be required – hence the importance of long-acting derivatives and depot preparations.

Androgen replacement therapy

Testosterone, its derivatives and synthetic analogues are commonly used as replacement therapy in cases of deficiency, analogous to estrogen/progestogen hormone replacement therapy in postmenopausal women. This has beneficial effects on visceral obesity, insulin sensitivity, glycaemic control and lipid profiles, body contour, voice and other secondary sex characteristics, as well as improving mood, sexual function and quality of life, in men with diagnosed hypogonadism and testosterone concentrations less than 300–500 ng/dL (Perry-Keene 2014).

Androgen replacement therapy is contraindicated in men with prostate cancer, and used only with caution in older men and those with cardiovascular, renal or blood disorders, or in elite athletes subject to drug testing.

Androgen deficiencies

Androgen deficiency is relatively common (one in 200 men) and may be due to disorders of the hypothalamus, pituitary or testis, or to androgen-receptor defects, when 5α-reductase is deficient, and in men with obesity and associated metabolic syndrome, insulin resistance or type 2 diabetes. In obese males, aromatase enzymes in excess fat tissue convert the androgens to estrogenic hormones, leading to male hypogonadism, possible erectile dysfunction and gynaecomastia. Excess aromatase activity can also occur in men with liver disease, thyrotoxicosis or neoplasia of the testes, liver or adrenal glands.

'Andropause'

In the later stages of male adult life, gonadal function and androgen production decrease, leading to partial androgen deficiency; this has been termed the male climacteric, or andropause. (However, there is no close analogy to the sudden cessation of menstruation, at menopause, in women.) There may be loss of muscle mass, **hypogonadism**, decline in sexual functions, psychological changes and increased risk of bone fractures, atherosclerosis, ischaemic heart disease, metabolic syndrome and type 2 diabetes. Low circulating levels of androgens have also been associated with infertility, declining cognitive performance and increased levels of β-amyloid protein, and as a risk factor for Alzheimer's disease.

Although androgen replacement therapy may slow down deterioration in bone and muscle function, there is no general recommendation for androgen replacement in ageing men unless there is clinical evidence of androgen deficiency (Yeap et al. 2016).

Women need testosterone, too

Women do naturally synthesise testosterone, with circulating levels of total testosterone approximately 1/15 of those in adult men. (However, low levels are notoriously difficult to measure accurately and reproducibly.) Androgen deficiency has been demonstrated in women with hypopituitarism, after adrenalectomy or oophorectomy and in some women on oral estrogen therapy. Symptoms include fatigue and low mood and libido (sexual interest). The symptoms are alleviated with low doses of testosterone or dehydroepiandrosterone; a cream formulation of testosterone 1% is available, with 0.5 mL (5 mg dose) to be applied to the inner aspect of the forearm or upper thigh. Apply to clean dry skin of the upper outer thigh and buttock. Adverse reactions in a minority of women are typical androgenic effects: mild acne and hirsutism.

Androgens are also used in breast cancer in women and (in conjunction with an estrogen) to treat severe osteoporosis in women.

Anti-androgens and SARMs

Orally active anti-androgens act by inhibiting androgen uptake or binding to receptors. Flutamide and analogues (bicalutamide) are used in advanced prostatic cancer. Other drugs with **anti-androgen** activity may block androgen receptors, decrease the release of gonadotrophins, physiologically antagonise androgenic effects or inhibit enzymes for androgen synthesis.

- Cyproterone has weak anti-androgen activity and has progestogenic activity, hence its use in some oral contraceptives and hormone replacement therapy products.
- Spironolactone, best known as an aldosterone antagonist used as a potassium-sparing diuretic, is a weak competitive anti-androgen used to treat androgenisation in women.
- Continuous administration of GnRH decreases gonadotrophin release and so is used to treat prostate cancer.
- Estrogens and progesterone, by negative-feedback loops, suppress gonadotrophin secretion and hence reduce endogenous production of sex hormones.

Clinical uses

Anti-androgen agents have the following uses: low doses: acne, hirsutism in women; medium doses: hypersexuality in men; high doses: prostatic cancer. They have also been tested as male contraceptives. They are contraindicated in pregnant women as they can cause feminisation of a male fetus. All carry the risks of impotence, osteoporosis, gynaecomastia, increased cardiovascular risk and decreased libido.

Selective androgen receptor modulators

Analogous to the rationale of selective estrogen receptor modulators (SERMs) being useful in female endocrine disorders, there has been a search for drugs that would selectively act as agonists on some ARs, but antagonists on others – that is, selective androgen receptor modulators (SARMs). SARMs with anabolic actions in muscle and bone, but without androgenic actions in causing prostate enlargement and polycythaemia, could potentially be especially useful in treating prostate cancer, breast cancer, osteoporosis and muscle wasting (Narayanan et al. 2018).

Androgen disruptors

Just as environmental chemicals such as in pesticides, plastics and packaging materials can be endocrine-disrupting chemicals (EDCs) in females due to their estrogenic actions,

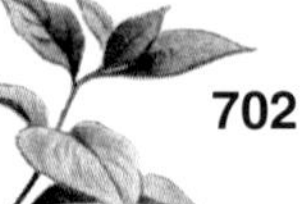

CLINICAL FOCUS BOX 31.1

A famous survivor of male breast cancer

Breast cancer can occur in men, accounting for less than 1% of all cancers in men and less than 1% of all breast cancers. In Australia the incidence is about 0.7 per 100,000 men, and rising.

Risk factors for men developing breast cancer include increasing age (average age at diagnosis is 69 years), known mutation in BRCA1 and 2 genes, strong family history, past radiation to the chest area, higher than normal estrogen levels caused by obesity, environmental hormones and 'androgen disrupters', long-term liver disorders or genetic conditions such as Klinefelter's syndrome. About 85% of male breast cancers are (o)estrogen-receptor (ER) positive, and 70% are progesterone-receptor positive. Most men survive with treatment, with a 5-year survival rate of 86% (Cancer Australia 2022).

Treatment is initially surgical, then possibly radiotherapy, chemotherapy and/or hormone therapy. Antineoplastic drugs indicated include those commonly used in female breast cancers. Hormone therapies include the SERM tamoxifen for ER-positive cancers, aromatase inhibitors to inhibit synthesis of estrogens and fulvestrant (an anti-estrogen). Drugs targeting receptors for prolactin and androgens are being trialled.

Issues in men with breast cancer include sexual and hormonal adverse effects of therapies, and unique psychosocial impacts of having a condition commonly associated with women. A famous survivor of male breast cancer is the rock-and-roll legend Peter Criss, the co-founder and original drummer with the hard rock band Kiss. Criss was diagnosed in 2008 at the age of 63 and underwent successful surgery but kept quiet about his condition for a year, saying 'I was freaked out ... men don't get breast cancer' and finding it 'embarrassing to talk about, because it's not a man thing'. However, realising that there were no prominent figures raising awareness of the disease, he decided to speak out about the importance of early detection and treatment. Criss was honoured in 2013 by the American Cancer Society as Humanitarian of the Year. He hopes his heavy-metal credentials will help reduce the stigma surrounding breast cancer in men.

Sources: Cancer Australia; Fentiman 2016; www.petercriss.net.

so they can be metabolic and androgen disruptors. Exposure to EDCs during early stages of development and differentiation of male tissues can lead to problems in adulthood: reduced sperm counts, misshapen and low-quality sperm, infertility and testicular and prostate diseases. Rising levels of EDCs (phthalates, bisphenol A and parabens) in the environment have been linked to the increasing prevalence of obesity metabolic syndrome, type 2 diabetes and male breast and testicular cancers (Giulivo et al. 2016) (Clinical Focus Box 31.1).

Anabolic steroids

'Anabolism' refers to metabolic processes in which small molecules are combined to form larger molecules – for example, amino acids to proteins, or simple sugars to polysaccharides. This definition is extended to imply generalised building up of tissues and, in the context of pharmacology, to drugs that increase the bulk of the body, particularly muscle mass.

Androgenic steroids are potent **anabolic agents**, stimulating formation and maintenance of muscular and skeletal protein. Those used particularly for their anabolic effects include nandrolone, oxandrolone and stanozolol.[2]

2 One of the few drugs with a name ending in '-olol' that is not a β-blocker; it is a veterinary steroid often abused by (human) weight-lifters and banned in sport. Other groups of drugs may have anabolic activity, notably the β_2-adrenoceptor agonists such as salbutamol and salmeterol, which increase lean body mass (muscle) and decrease fat by metabolic actions. The β_2-agonists are sympathomimetics similar to catecholamines in structure, so by definition are not anabolic steroids. They are banned in sport as anabolics but are permitted for use as inhaled bronchodilators by people with notified asthma.

They have been used clinically to treat cachexia (generalised wasting) – for example, after long chronic illness – and for improving appetite, wellbeing and libido in people with wasting conditions such as osteoporosis, anaemia, adverse effects of corticosteroid therapy and terminal cancers. Given the lack of proof of efficacy and the availability of safer drugs with more specific actions, they are no longer recommended for such indications and not marketed in Australia

Adverse reactions are those of excessive androgenic actions), including fluid retention and weight gain, testicular atrophy, sterility, gynaecomastia, increased risk of coronary heart disease, liver disease, mood swings and aggressiveness ('steroid rage') and induction of psychotic disorders. (Women run the additional risks of virilisation, including irreversible deep voice changes.)

Abuse in sport

Athletes have used anabolic androgenic steroids to increase weight, musculature and muscle strength, especially for endurance events requiring stamina (and to improve the 'macho' image). Anabolic androgenic steroids and related chemicals are banned in sports. 'Designer steroids' such as trenbolone are produced with the intention of avoiding detection by drug-control laboratories, and to maximise anabolic actions (in bone and muscle) and reduce androgenic effects (in testes, prostate and seminal vesicles). They are also used in veterinary medicine and in meat production in animals (Christou et al. 2017).

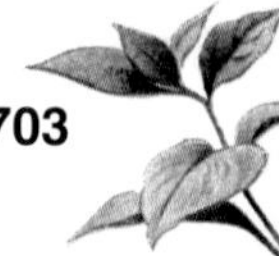

KEY POINTS

Male sex hormones

- Reproductive functions in the male are regulated by pituitary gonadotrophins and androgens from the testes; GnRH analogues are used by continuous administration in treating prostate cancer.
- Testosterone is the male sex hormone (androgen) necessary for the normal development and maintenance of male reproduction and sex characteristics.
- Testosterone is indicated for hormonal replacement therapy in males with androgen deficiency and to treat advanced breast carcinoma. Testosterone is usually administered as one of its ester derivatives in depot formulations or for transdermal administration.
- Androgens are anabolic steroids and are sometimes abused by athletes in endurance sports.
- The adverse reactions to androgens include cardiovascular disease, gynaecomastia in males and virilism in females.
- Anti-androgens such as cyproterone or flutamide are used in conjunction with other therapies in prostatic cancer.

Benign prostatic hyperplasia

Pathology

Testicular androgens are believed to have a permissive role in the development of **benign prostatic hyperplasia**, excessive growth of tissue in the prostate gland surrounding the urethra and increase in smooth muscle tone. This is a normal age-related change beginning around age 40 in men; by age 80, about 36.8% of men will develop BPH (Lee et al. 2017).

BPH obstructs the bladder neck and compresses the urethra, resulting in urinary retention, increasing the risk of bacteriuria, hydroureter (dilation of the ureter), hydronephrosis (swelling of a kidney due to a build-up of urine) and renal failure. The symptoms of BPH include hesitancy (difficulty starting the urinary stream), decrease in the urine stream, post-void dribbling, frequency and nocturia. Mild BPH does not require immediate treatment and benefits from watchful waiting. BPH does not cause prostate cancer, but both types of hypertrophy are stimulated by androgens. Surgical treatment (transurethral resection of the prostate) reduces the size of the prostate gland and is recommended for severe BPH.

Drugs exacerbating BPH

BPH is exacerbated by anabolic agents and androgens, particularly DHT in the prostate gland. Alpha-adrenoceptor agonists can also have a long-term trophic effect on smooth muscle; in the prostate this can lead to proliferation and the symptoms described.

Pharmacological treatment

Alpha-blockers

Because the pathophysiology of BPH may include increased smooth muscle tone in the bladder outlet and the prostate, mediated by α_1-adrenergic receptors, pharmacological treatment of BPH with selective α_1-adrenoceptor blockers has been tried (Chs 8, 13). The antihypertensive drugs prazosin (Drug Monograph 9.2), terazosin (registered for use in NZ only), tamsulosin and alfuzosin (less likely to cause orthostatic hypotension) are used for their smooth muscle relaxant actions in BPH and can improve urine flow rate; if effective, long-term therapy is required.

Common adverse effects are those typical of vasodilators – that is, headaches, dizziness and orthostatic hypotension – and abnormal ejaculation during intercourse.

5α-reductase inhibitors

5α-reductase inhibitors act by a very different mechanism: they specifically inhibit 5α-reductase enzyme type II, which in the prostate gland metabolises the conversion of testosterone to DHT, a more potent androgen responsible for prostate gland growth. Dutasteride (Drug Monograph 31.2) and finasteride reduce levels of DHT in the bloodstream and in the prostate, reducing hypertrophy of the gland and resistance to urinary outflow. They do not impair synthesis of testosterone and so do not have anti-androgenic actions. They appear most effective in men with large prostates and may take 6 months of treatment for clinical improvement.

Male infertility

Infertility is defined as the absence of conception by a couple after more than 1 year of regular sexual intercourse without contraception. It affects 10–15% of all cohabiting couples, and is attributed to male factors in about 40% of cases. Diagnosis of the cause of infertility in a particular couple and its treatment are highly specialised areas of medicine.

Many cases of male infertility are due to abnormalities of sperm production, duct obstruction, hypothalamic or pituitary dysfunction, disorders of ejaculation or exposure to radiation. Other causes are endocrine-disrupting chemicals (see earlier discussion), cadmium, smoking and drugs including androgens and anabolic steroids (which via negative feedback switch off the hypothalamic–pituitary–gonadal axis), cytotoxics, sulfasalazine, cyproterone acetate, opioids, tramadol, GnRH analogues and sartans (Semet et al. 2017).

Treatment of male infertility

Endocrine causes such as hyper- or hyposecretion by pituitary, thyroid or adrenal glands usually respond to

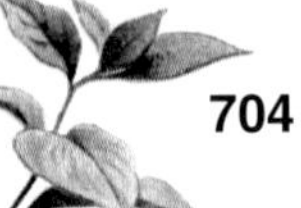

Drug Monograph 31.2
Dutasteride

Mechanism and actions

Dutasteride is an inhibitor of both 5α-reductase isoenzymes, thus inhibits the conversion of testosterone to the more active dihydro-metabolite DHT. With chronic administration it reduces prostate size, alleviates symptoms of BPH, improves urinary flow and reduces need for surgery.

Indications

Dutasteride is indicated for mild to moderate symptoms of BPH with clinically demonstrated prostatomegaly, when surgical treatment is contraindicated or refused. It may be co-administered with an α-blocker such as tamsulosin.

Pharmacokinetics

Dutasteride has a long half-life, so it takes 3–6 months to reach steady-state levels and full treatment effect. It is well absorbed after oral administration, with maximum plasma concentrations being reached in about 2 hours; about 99.5% is bound to plasma proteins. Dutasteride is extensively metabolised in the liver, and five metabolites are excreted in the faeces, with an elimination half-life of 3–5 weeks. No dosage adjustments are required for elderly people or those with renal disease; however, use should be avoided in men with liver disease.

Drug interactions

No significant drug interactions have been reported, although the drug is a known substrate for enzyme CYP3A4. Co-administration with an α-blocker showed no evidence of pharmacokinetic or pharmacodynamics drug interactions.

Adverse reactions

These include decreased libido, impotence, decreased sperm count and amount of ejaculate, gynaecomastia and allergic reactions. There is a possible association with increased risk of male breast cancer or prostate cancer, so changes in breast tissue or signs of prostate cancer should be monitored. When co-administered with an α-blocker, combined adverse effects include hypotension and syncope.

Warnings and contraindications

Use should be avoided in those with liver disease, obstructive uropathy or dutasteride hypersensitivity. Dutasteride is not indicated for use in women or children; women of childbearing age should not handle broken or crushed tablets, as it is categorised X in terms of pregnancy safety. Dutasteride reduces serum levels of prostate-specific antigen (PSA), so may interfere with diagnosis of prostate cancer; PSA levels should be monitored. Men treated with dutasteride should not donate blood for at least 6 months after the last dose, to obviate the risk of dutasteride being passed to a female recipient.

Dosage and administration

The drug is administered orally, 1 capsule 500 micrograms daily. Clinically useful effects may take at least 6 months to develop. Dutasteride is also formulated in a combination product, 500 micrograms with 400 micrograms controlled-release tamsulosin.

appropriate hormone therapy. The 'biological clock' ticks for men as well as women: men aged over 40 are at higher risk of having a child with autism or birth defects. The average time to pregnancy by men under 25 is about 4.5 months, but in men over 40 is nearly 2 years (Clinical Focus Box 30.2). As the average age for first-time fathers in Australia increases, fertility experts advise men to pay more attention to their 'fertility clocks'.

Combinations of androgens, anti-estrogens and antioxidants have been tried. Erectile dysfunction may also require treatment, and drugs that impair sexual functioning need to be avoided.

Gonadotrophins

In gonadotrophin-deficient men who have been treated with androgens, gonadotrophin therapy can re-establish the hypothalamic–pituitary–gonadal axis and induce spermatogenesis. Human chorionic gonadotrophin (hCG, which has mainly ICSH activity in males) is given two to three times weekly for several months; then, if necessary, FSH is added for several months. Semen analysis is used to assess sperm numbers, and pregnancy is often achieved despite oligospermia (Ohlander et al. 2016).

KEY POINTS

Drugs for male reproductive disorders

- BPH is a common condition in older men; it can be treated by surgery or by α-blockers (prazosin, terazosin [NZ only]) or 5α-reductase inhibitors (dutasteride).
- Infertility is a common problem, with many possible causes. Male infertility is treated with gonadotrophins (if the cause is hypogonadal).

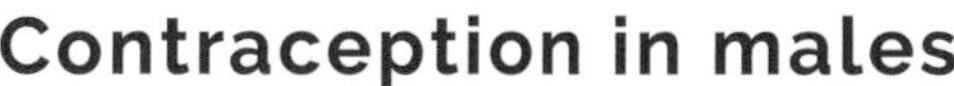

Contraception in males

For many sexually active men and women, an ongoing problem is not inability to conceive, but the desire to prevent conception and pregnancy after sexual intercourse – that is, **contraception**. An ideal contraceptive technique should be safe, 100% effective, immediately functional, easy to use, rapidly reversible after discontinuation and should not interfere with sex life. (Methods in females are discussed in Ch 30.)

Contraceptive methods in males

With the rapidly increasing world population, especially in developing countries, it is desirable to find a simple, safe, cheap, effective and reversible male contraceptive. Currently, the main options for male contraception are surgical methods such as vasectomy (most vasectomies can be surgical reversed), barrier methods such as condoms or penile withdrawal (coitus interruptus). Drugs and other chemicals that impair male fertility usually have too many adverse effects to be useful as contraceptives. While no products are on the market, the search for a hormonal oral contraceptive, the 'male pill', continues.

Non-drug contraception

Non-drug methods (except for condoms) generally have much lower success rates than hormonal methods in preventing pregnancies (see Table 30.3 in Ch 30 for failure rates).

Barrier methods

Barrier methods impose a physical barrier between sperm ejaculated by the man during sexual intercourse and an oocyte in the woman's uterine tube. Some barrier methods or occlusive devices have the advantage of offering protection against sexually transmissible infections and cervical cancer; condoms are especially effective.

Condoms (male) – thin rubber sheaths stretched over the erect penis before intercourse – prevent sperm from entering the vagina and effectively protect against both pregnancy and most sexually transmissible infections. They are safe and inexpensive and have been widely used throughout history. When used properly and regularly, they are 97% effective as contraceptives.

'Natural' methods

The 'natural' methods of family planning or contraception include total abstinence from sexual activity, periodic abstinence to avoid the most fertile days of a woman's cycle ('rhythm methods') or withdrawal of the penis before ejaculation ('coitus interruptus'). Other physical methods used in men rely on the fact that higher temperatures than those normally reached in the scrotum lead to reversible germ cell apoptosis and inactivation of sperm. The thermal effects of hot water, microwaves, ultrasound and infrared heat have been trialled to produce azoospermia (absence of viable sperm).

Sterilisation

Sterilisation is virtually 100% effective as a contraceptive method and is the most widely used form of contraception in the world. Vasectomy involves surgical interruption of the vas deferens to prevent transport of sperm to the ejaculatory duct and through the penis, from which semen (sperm and seminal vesicle secretions) is ejaculated during sexual intercourse. (Thus, a vasectomy is effective because it interrupts the passage of sperm, which are still produced, but they degenerate and are resorbed by phagocytes. Because blood vessels are not cut, gonadotrophins continue to stimulate testosterone production, so libido and sexual performance are not impaired.) Severe complications are rare. Approximately 6% of men who have a vasectomy will later have a vasovasostomy (surgical vasectomy reversal). Most are successful, with approximately 80% of men having sperm in their ejaculate and over half achieving a pregnancy post vasovastomy (Namekawa et al. 2018).

Future innovations and potential targets

The worldwide need for safe, effective, reversible contraception methods, combined with the enormous potential market for such products, and the fact that all current methods have some disadvantages, means that research is needed in this area. Potential targets or new methods for contraception in men include:

- adjudin, an indazole-carboxylic acid derivative
- compound JQI, a complex chlorinated diazepine bromodomain inhibitor originally developed as an anticancer drug, which targets the cell-division process in sperm
- enzymes controlling vitamin A metabolism in the testis
- compounds that inhibit EPPIN, an epididymal protease inhibitor essential for sperm motility
- isoform 4 of the plasma membrane calcium ATPase, expressed in spermatozoa where it functions in sperm motility
- implants of 7-alpha-methyl-19-nortestosterone (a SARM)
- vaccines against various hormones, and against components of the reproductive tract or of spermatozoa
- injection into the vas deferens of a positively charged polymer gel that inactivates negatively charged sperm.

KEY POINTS

Contraception in males

- Current male contraceptive methods are non-pharmacological: condoms, vasectomy or 'natural methods'. Researchers are seeking a safe and effective hormonal 'male pill'.

Drugs that affect sexual functioning (male and female)

Many factors are involved in sexual functioning: general health, partner availability, appropriate environment, self-esteem, religious beliefs, society's standards and lifestyle factors. Many have physiological, psychological and social ramifications that are beyond the scope of this discussion.

Various conditions and drugs can produce adverse effects on sexual function, such as:

- low levels of testosterone, which is normally present in both sexes and enhances libido, or sexual drive
- higher or lower levels of estrogen
- clinical depression, which may limit interest in or response to sexual stimuli
- autonomic nervous system blockade, which may interfere with lubrication, erection or ejaculation.

Hormonal aspects of female reproductive physiology and sexual responses are described in the previous chapter; male aspects are summarised briefly below.

Neuronal controls

Central nervous system

An embryo is characteristically female initially and a male fetus does not differentiate until fetal androgens begin to masculinise tissues (between the 7th and 12th weeks of pregnancy; Fig 30.6). Hence, mature organs function in analogous ways and can be influenced by hormones of both sexes. Female hormones generally increase sexual functions in women and decrease them in men, and vice versa. Central nervous system (CNS) involvement in sexual functioning includes both behavioural and endocrine effects, with stimuli integrated via nuclei in the thalamus and hypothalamus. Many drugs that affect dopaminergic transmission have effects on hypothalamic–pituitary pathways, and any drugs with CNS-depressant effects may depress sexual interest or functions.

Autonomic nervous system

The male sexual response

Penile erection is partly a parasympathetic response that occurs during the phase of sexual excitement. Acetylcholine acting through muscarinic receptors causes dilation of the arteries and arterioles in the penis, which compresses the veins in this area; the cavernous tissue of the penis becomes engorged with blood and erection occurs; at the same time, mucus is secreted by the associated glands, and sperm and secretions (semen) from the genital ducts are moved to the prostatic urethra. Orgasm, the climax of the sexual act, moves the semen through the ejaculatory ducts. Drugs that interfere with parasympathetic neurotransmission, such as atropinic anticholinergic drugs and drugs with atropinic side effects, commonly cause erectile dysfunction.

Sympathetic (adrenergic) impulses in the male produce emission and ejaculation by causing contraction of the vas deferens and seminal vesicles and rapid muscular contractions, with expulsion of semen and simultaneous cardiovascular stimulation that increases heart rate and blood pressure and constricts arterioles, leading to waning of the erection. **Impotence** is the inability of a man to achieve or maintain a penile erection to allow sexual intercourse; it may be caused by drugs that block adrenergic impulses. Androgens are required for normal seminal fluid content and volume, and play important roles in libido and erections and responsiveness to erotic stimuli.

Drugs that may enhance male sexual functioning

Treatment of erectile dysfunction

Erectile dysfunction in men, or impotence, is the condition in which a man is unable to attain or maintain an erection long enough for sexual intercourse, or is unable to ejaculate. It is estimated that 25% of men over 55 years of age are impotent; the proportion is much higher in men who have smoked regularly. Very few, however, present for treatment because of embarrassment or denial. There are many possible causes of erectile dysfunction:

- medical (diabetes mellitus, arterial disease, hypertension, renal failure, abnormalities of the reproductive system, infections such as syphilis)
- surgical causes (pelvic surgery, especially radical prostatectomy)
- psychogenic (stress, fear of pregnancy or infection, religious or social inhibitions)
- neurogenic (autonomic dysfunction)
- hypogonadal (endocrine deficiencies)
- iatrogenic (especially antihypertensives, antipsychotics, antidepressants and anti-androgens; see also below under 'Drugs That Decrease Sexual Functioning')
- lifestyle factors (long-term smoking, excess alcohol)
- idiopathic (no obvious cause).

Attention to psychological factors and treatment of any underlying disorder are important in all cases, as well as specific pharmacotherapies.

Phosphodiesterase 5 inhibitors

The first **phosphodiesterase 5 (PDE5) inhibitor** (1998) was sildenafil, which rapidly became renowned worldwide by its trade name Viagra (Drug Monograph 31.3, Fig 31.2); related drugs are avanafil, tadalafil and vardenafil. Tadalafil has a significantly longer half-life (17.5 hours compared with 3–5 hours) and duration of action (24–36 hours compared with 4–6 hours).

Mechanism and actions

Sexual stimulation releases nitric oxide from nitrergic nerves, activating guanylate cyclase which increases cyclic guanosine monophosphate (cGMP) levels, enhancing vasodilation and penile erection. cGMP is inactivated by the enzyme PDE5, found primarily in the penis; hence, inhibiting this enzyme prolongs actions of cGMP to maintain erection. Thus, PGE5 inhibitors enhance nitric oxide functions (Fig 31.1). They have little effect in the absence of sexual stimulation.

Precautions

Common side effects of PDE5 inhibitors are found in Figure 31.2. Post-marketing surveillance has disclosed adverse reactions and several reports of fatality possibly associated with PDE5 use. There is now a warning that PDE5 inhibitors should not be taken concomitantly with an organic nitrate vasodilator by any route, as the combination causes severe hypotension and possibly decreased coronary perfusion and myocardial infarction. Men need advice as to treatment of priapism (prolonged erection) if it occurs: if the erection lasts more than 2 hours, a sympathomimetic vasoconstrictor such as phenylephrine is useful; more than 4 hours becomes a medical emergency.

Other drugs used to treat erectile dysfunction

Second-line drugs used to treat erectile dysfunction are testosterone derivatives, prostaglandins and papaverine.

Drug Monograph 31.3
Sildenafil

Sildenafil (Viagra) is a selective inhibitor of cGMP-specific PDE5. After oral administration, it is active particularly in the penis, where it potentiates the vasodilator actions of nitrates released during sexual excitement.

Indications

Sildenafil is indicated for erectile dysfunction in men, except for those taking nitrates or other antihypertensive drugs, or for whom sexual intercourse is inadvisable.

Pharmacokinetics

Sildenafil is rapidly absorbed after oral administration, and peak blood concentrations are reached after about 60 minutes; bioavailability is around 40%. Absorption is delayed by a high-fat meal. Metabolism is by CYP3A4 (and CYP2C9) enzymes. The drug and its major metabolite (also active as a PDE5 inhibitor) are highly protein-bound and widely distributed in tissues. Metabolites are mainly excreted in faeces, with a terminal half-life of 3–5 hours. Clearance is reduced in people with severe liver or kidney disease, and in elderly men.

Drug interactions

Sildenafil should not be used with other vasodilators, especially nitrate preparations and selective α-blockers, as the hypotensive vasodilator effects are synergistic. There may be interactions with all other drugs that inhibit or induce CYP3A4 enzymes, including many anticonvulsants, corticosteroids, hypoglycaemic agents, antibiotics, antivirals, antifungals, warfarin and grapefruit juice. (Reference lists should be consulted for specific interactions and doses varied accordingly.) Food may delay the onset of action.

Adverse reactions

See Figure 31.2.

Warnings and contraindications

Use with caution in those with cardiovascular, renal or hepatic diseases, bleeding disorders, retinal disorders, Peyronie's disease (an anatomical abnormality of the penis) or conditions that predispose to priapism, such as multiple myeloma, leukaemia and sickle cell anaemia. Avoid use in men with sildenafil hypersensitivity or concurrent use of organic nitrates (see 'Precautions').

Dosage and administration

The usual adult dose is 50–100 mg (25 mg in the elderly, or those with renal or hepatic impairment), taken about 1 hour before sexual activity, to a maximum of 100 mg in any day.

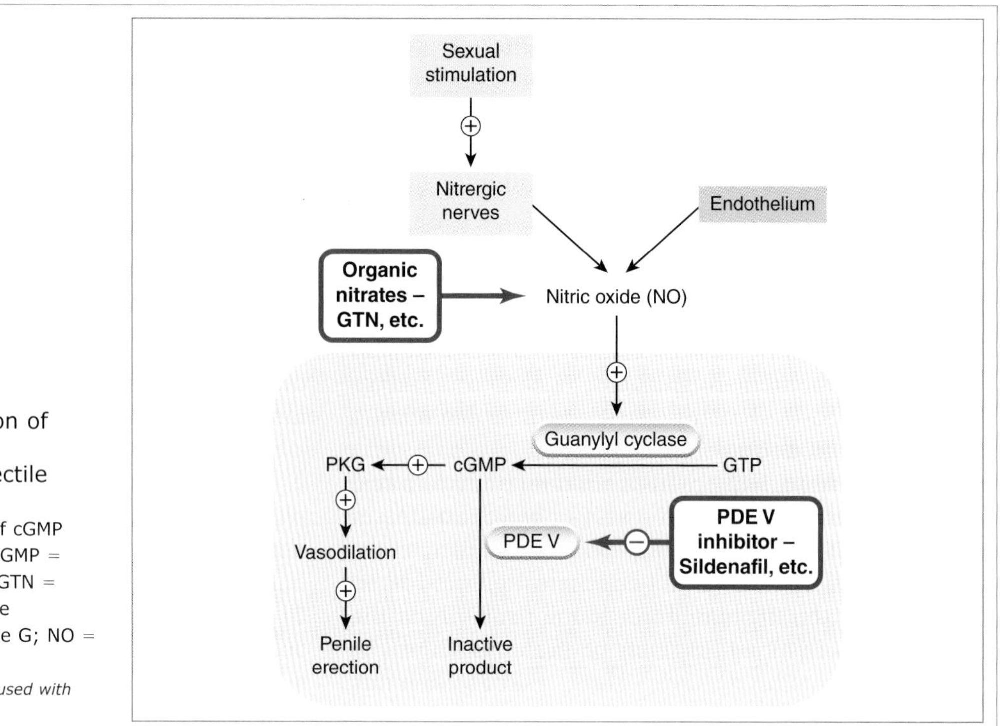

FIGURE 31.1 Mechanism of action of phosphodiesterase 5 (PDE5) inhibitors in treatment of erectile dysfunction

Inhibition of PDE5 allows buildup of cGMP and maintenance of vasodilation. cGMP = cyclic guanosine monophosphate; GTN = glyceryl trinitrate; GTP = guanosine triphosphate; PKG = phosphokinase G; NO = nitric oxide

Source: Ritter et al. 2019, Figure 35.6; used with permission.

These are generally given by injection or locally; hence the major advantage of oral PDE5 inhibitors.

- Alprostadil, a synthetic form of prostaglandin E_1 (PGE_1), is given by penile injection (10 or 20 micrograms, into the corpora cavernosa); it dilates the cavernosal arteries and thus assists erectile function. Testosterone IM depot injections, implants and patches or transdermal gels are tried if the dysfunction is due to androgen deficiency (Drug Monograph 31.1); however, the role of testosterone in the human erectile response is not well defined.
- Papaverine, a smooth muscle relaxant, is given by intracavernosal injection; it relaxes all vascular components of the penile erectile system.
- Bromocriptine or cabergoline is indicated in people in whom the cause of erectile dysfunction is hyperprolactinaemia (Clinical Focus Box 31.2).

Drugs for premature ejaculation

When ejaculation of semen during sexual intercourse consistently occurs before desired, this can lead to distress or interpersonal difficulties for the male. As well as the following drugs, therapies tried include surgical procedures and prosthetic devices.

Dapoxetine

Dapoxetine is a short-acting selective serotonin reuptake inhibitor (SSRI) used to treat premature ejaculation; it increases time to ejaculation by 1–2 minutes. It is also perceived to enhance sexual performance. Adverse effects are common, including sexual and cardiovascular dysfunctions. Numerous drug interactions occur as for SSRIs, and men are advised to avoid taking dapoxetine in combination with other drugs which can affect serotonin such as antidepressants, sedatives or recreational drugs.

Drugs to increase libido

Substances that will increase **libido** (sexual potency or drive) have been sought throughout history. Inscriptions in the ruins of ancient cultures have described the preparation of 'erotic potions', and an endless number of 'aphrodisiacs' have been hopefully described since then.

In contemporary society, many drugs and chemicals that temporarily modify physiological responsiveness and subjective sexual enjoyment are claimed to have aphrodisiac properties, but few drugs specifically enhance libido or performance. Some agents are considered briefly in this section; most are of psycho- or ethno-pharmacological interest only and are not available clinically.

Vasodilators

As well as the PDE5 inhibitors, other drugs with vasodilator activity may enhance the sexual response:

- Yohimbine, an alkaloid from the West African tree *Coryanthe yohimbe*, related chemically to the ergot

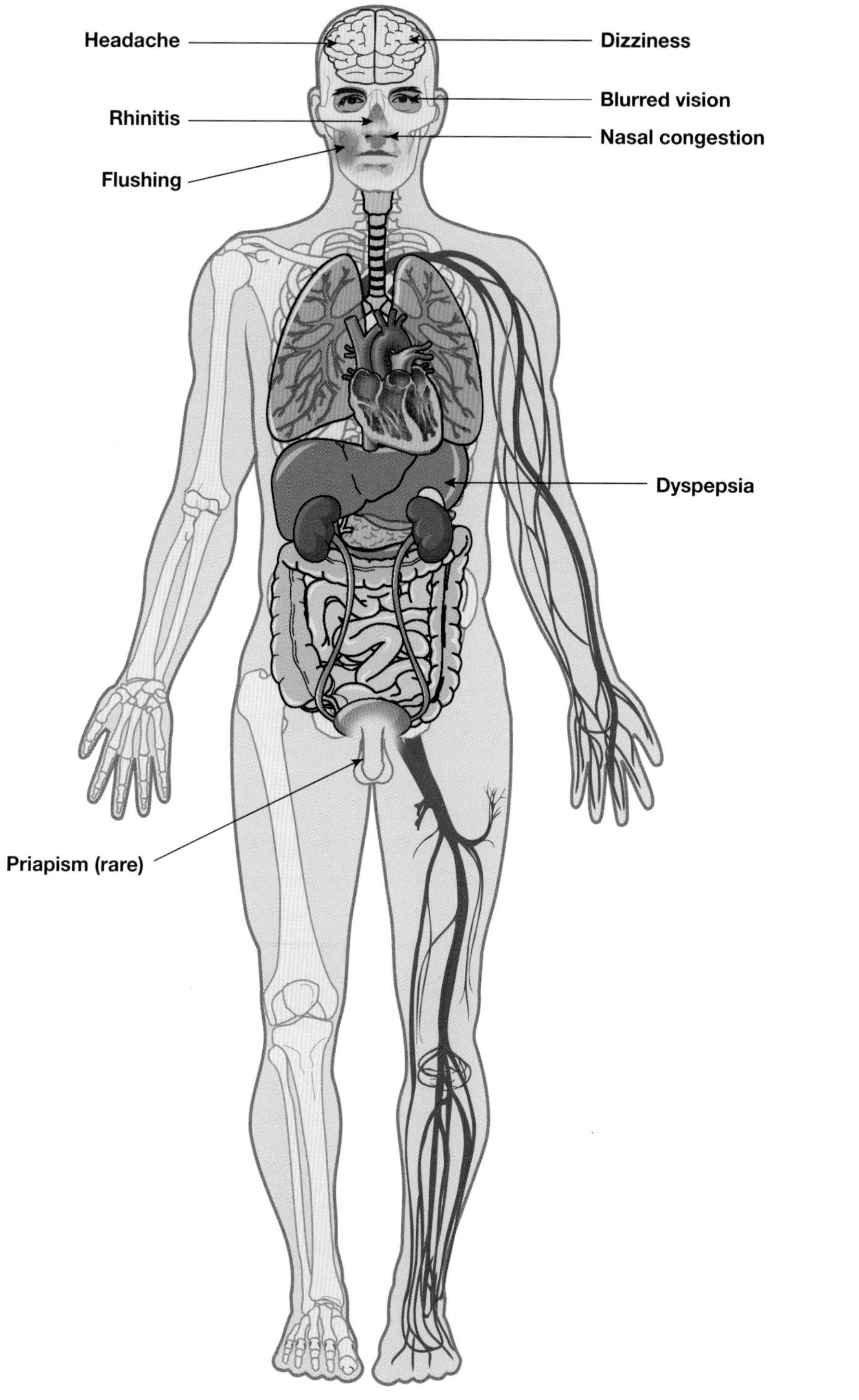

Headache
Dizziness
Blurred vision
Rhinitis
Nasal congestion
Flushing
Dyspepsia
Priapism (rare)

FIGURE 31.2 Common adverse effects of phosphodiesterase-5 (PDE5) inhibitors

alkaloids, produces a competitive α-adrenergic block, leading to vasodilation, enhanced erection and increased ejaculatory reflexes.

- Organic nitrates (glyceryl trinitrate, isosorbide mononitrate, amyl nitrate) have non-specific vasodilator actions, causing headaches, hypotension and fainting, which would be counterproductive.

Social drugs

The use of social drugs such as heroin, cocaine, alcohol, marijuana, LSD, amphetamines and 'designer drugs' in the hope of aphrodisiac actions has become widespread in contemporary society (Ch 25). These agents may enhance the enjoyment of the sexual experience, depending on the user's state of mind, the amount of

CLINICAL FOCUS BOX 31.2
Male infertility and androgen deficiency

A 44-year-old man and his 39-year-old wife presented to an infertility specialist having been unable to conceive in their relationship of 2 years. He had a laparoscopic banding procedure for obesity 2 years before and had lost 20 kg in weight. Over the previous 2 years he noted increasing difficulty with sexual performance, particularly with collecting semen for testing. Treatment with sildenafil was effective, so the couple had intercourse twice a week. He had a varicocele operated on when in his 20s. She was overweight but otherwise well and had regular ovulatory cycles. Physical examination showed a pale obese man with reduced secondary sex hair, mild gynaecomastia without galactorrhoea and normal-sized testes. Investigations showed a low volume of semen 0.7 mL (normal > 1.5 mL) with a few sperm 0.2 million/mL (normal > 14), an elevated serum prolactin level 1140–1720 mU/L (normal < 375), low testosterone 1.7 nmol/L (normal > 9) and a pituitary microadenoma about 5 mm diameter in the left side on magnetic resonance imaging.

Treatment with cabergoline 0.25 mg weekly improved libido and sexual performance, reduced the prolactin levels to normal in 1 month and testosterone levels increased to normal by 4 months. Semen tests improved but remained subnormal, and his FSH level increased, suggesting that there was an additional primary seminiferous tubule disorder. Four attempts with intracytoplasmic sperm injection over the next 2 years were unsuccessful mainly because only 1–3 oocytes could be collected each time. Despite these problems and their ages, the couple conceived naturally in the third year and had a daughter. He continues well on treatment and the microadenoma has not changed in size.

Source: Contributed by Dr Gordon Baker, Professorial Fellow, The University of Melbourne; acknowledged with thanks.

drug(s) consumed and the surrounding company and environment. Many act on the CNS to weaken inhibitions, which are often the cause of sexual problems. More commonly, however, sexual drive and function decrease.

Effects of some common social drugs on sexual functioning are summarised below:

- Opioids such as morphine and heroin are general CNS depressants, causing disorientation and mental confusion; habitual users have low libido and impaired potency.
- Marijuana (cannabis) is considered a sexual stimulant, through causing relaxation, release from inhibitions and the illusion that sexual climax is prolonged. However, marijuana smokers have a high incidence of decreased libido, potency and fertility, possibly because of its estrogenic-type effects, decreased levels of gonadotrophins and testosterone and reduced prolactin and ovulation in women.
- LSD is an agonist at central serotonin (5-HT) receptors, facilitating sensory input, altered sensations and improved mood. Although sometimes considered an aphrodisiac, repeated use of LSD may produce serious psychological problems that could adversely affect sexual interest or functions.
- Amphetamines ('speed') have powerful central stimulant actions and peripheral sympathomimetic effects, leading to wakefulness, increased motor and speech activity, euphoria and decreased fatigue. Effects on sexual performance are inconsistent, possibly due to reduced feelings of inadequacy or to delaying sleep.
- Nicotine is a CNS stimulant with complex peripheral effects at acetylcholine nicotinic receptors in autonomic ganglia and skeletal muscle. Long-term smoking impairs cardiovascular functions and causes impotence in men.

Other drugs that may improve sexual performance

Appropriate hormones and neurotransmitters may enhance sexual performance, as follows:

- Hormones involved in the reproductive systems affect sexual functions; thus, estrogens and androgens may increase sexual activity in people of the appropriate sex. Oxytocin appears to have roles in mating and parenting behaviours.
- Levodopa, used in parkinsonism to enhance dopamine transmission, is reported to increase libido and incidence of penile erections, and has caused priapism, possibly reflecting partial recovery of sexual functions impaired by Parkinson's disease.

Drugs that decrease sexual functioning

As described earlier, effective sexual activity depends on optimal central and autonomic nervous system and endocrine system functions, as well as behavioural, social and lifestyle aspects. Not surprisingly, many drugs can impair sexual functioning, libido or gratification in men and women. In particular, drugs that depress the central and autonomic nervous systems, and reproductive hormone antagonists, are likely to have adverse effects; these are summarised below.

Antihypertensives

Early antihypertensive agents, especially ganglion blockers and adrenergic neuron-blocking agents, had such deleterious effects on sexual functions in men (by blocking both parasympathetic and sympathetic nervous systems) that compliance with the therapy was often very poor. More specific modern drugs cause fewer problems.

Effects of antihypertensive drugs on sexual functioning include the following:

- β-blockers, calcium channel blockers, centrally acting α_2-agonists and angiotensin-converting enzyme inhibitors can cause impotence and sexual dysfunction.
- The thiazide diuretic hydrochlorothiazide may induce sexual dysfunction through its hypotensive and vasodilator actions.

CNS-active agents

Many centrally acting agents affect sexual functions directly and indirectly. Neuroleptics (antipsychotics), antidepressants, benzodiazepines and barbiturates are often associated with adverse sexual dysfunctions, as summarised below:

- Antipsychotic agents inhibit dopaminergic transmission in the CNS, stimulating prolactin release and causing gynaecomastia (in men) or galactorrhoea (in women). They decrease release of pituitary gonadotrophins and of sex hormones, causing priapism and ejaculatory disorders or impaired menstruation and ovulation. They also block α-receptors (causing hypotension and ejaculatory disorders) and cholinergic receptors (causing erectile dysfunction). Atypical neuroleptics, clozapine and olanzapine, appear to be less problematic in these respects.
- Antidepressant drugs (tricyclics, monoamine oxidase inhibitors and SSRIs) elevate mood and thus may facilitate sexuality; however, antidepressants can cause impotence, menstrual disorders, ejaculatory disturbances/failure or gynaecomastia.
- Benzodiazepines are commonly prescribed as antianxiety medications, sedatives and skeletal muscle relaxants; they may cause decreased sexual activity, anorgasmia in men and women and ejaculation failure; or may reduce anxiety about sexual performance.
- Barbiturates such as phenobarbital (phenobarbitone) and thiopentone are used as antiepileptics, sedatives or induction anaesthetics; they depress various bodily functions, including sexual performance and ability.
- First-generation H_1-antihistamines (competitive inhibitors at H_1-receptor sites) are used as antiemetics, mild sedatives and to control allergies; most cause anticholinergic effects such as dry mouth, urinary retention and constipation, and can interfere with sexual activity. The histamine H_2-receptor antagonists, used to treat peptic ulcers, have been reported to cause gynaecomastia and impotence in men in high doses.
- Ethyl alcohol (ethanol) is, for its effects on human sexual function and behaviour, a drug of unique notoriety (Ch 25, Drug Monograph 25.2). It may appear to enhance sexual activity by reducing anxieties and inhibitions. Continued consumption depresses cerebral functions, slows reflexes, dilates blood vessels, produces a potent diuretic effect and diminishes sexual functions. A male chronic alcoholic experiences delayed ejaculation and impotence, caused by vascular changes, peripheral neuropathy and lower testosterone levels, all compounded by testicular atrophy, 'beer gut' and gynaecomastia. In the often-quoted words of Shakespeare (*Macbeth*, Act II, Scene III), Macduff asks: 'What three things does drink especially provoke?' to which the porter at the gate replies: 'Lechery, sir, it provokes and it unprovokes: it provokes the desire, but it takes away the performance'.

Hormones and derivatives

Not surprisingly, many hormones adversely affect sexual functioning.

- Sex hormones influence reproductive functions, sexual behaviours and mood; thus, female hormones may produce the mood changes associated with premenstrual syndrome, whereas male hormones are associated with aggression and increased sexual interest.
- Anabolic steroids are related to testosterone (Drug Monograph 31.1), and are misused to promote muscle growth and endurance. In women, these drugs cause virilisation, hirsutism, libido changes and clitoral enlargement, while in men they cause testicular atrophy, impotence, chronic priapism and oligospermia.
- Anti-androgens (e.g. cyproterone) have been used to reduce sexual drive in overaggressive men and sexual offenders.
- Spironolactone, an aldosterone antagonist, has both diuretic and endocrine effects and is associated with impotence, gynaecomastia and a decrease in libido.

Other drugs

Many of the drugs described earlier as reputedly having aphrodisiac or sexual stimulating actions, including opioids, marijuana, LSD, nitrates and cantharidin, are more likely to cause sexual dysfunction, and so could be included in this section.

KEY POINTS

Drugs affecting male sexual functioning

- Sexual response in males is under hormonal, neuronal and psychological controls. The sexual response involves initially parasympathetic stimulation of erectile tissue, leading to engorgement of the penis, and sympathetic stimulation leading to ejaculation and muscular, respiratory and cardiovascular responses.
- Erectile dysfunction (impotence) in men is a common and distressing disorder. The most effective drug treatments are the oral PDE5 inhibitors such as sildenafil (Clinical Focus Box 31.3); other drugs used to treat erectile dysfunction include injected alprostadil or papaverine.
- Dapoxetine, an SSRI, is indicated to treat premature ejaculation.
- Although many drugs have been postulated or tried as sexual stimulants (aphrodisiacs), very few are effective, and none are prescribed for this purpose. Psychoactive agents, including social drugs and hallucinogens, tend merely to suppress inhibitions or alter sensations.
- Many groups of drugs impair sexual functioning, including antihypertensives, diuretics, antihistamines, antipsychotics, antidepressants, hormones and CNS depressants, including alcohol.

CLINICAL FOCUS BOX 31.3

Sex, serendipity, sildenafil and share prices

Sildenafil was discovered serendipitously: it was being tested as a vasodilator treatment for angina but was not significantly effective. However, many men taking the active drug in the clinical trial reported an unexpected effect, experiencing better erections during sexual intercourse. This effect was followed up and the mechanism was elucidated: inhibition of PDE5 in the penis, leading to improved erectile function.

Other interesting facts to emerge from the clinical trials of sildenafil were that many of the men in the group taking the active drug were reluctant to return leftover tablets after the trial, and that 25% of the men in the placebo group also reported improved sexual function (compared with 62% on low-dose sildenafil).

Sildenafil was fast-tracked through drug-regulating agencies in the United States, as demand for the drug was expected to be high. Sildenafil had one of the fastest uptakes in pharmacology, with sales rapidly reaching billions of US dollars. Share prices for the drug company Pfizer increased dramatically when rumours about the drug spread on Wall Street.

DRUGS AT A GLANCE

Drugs affecting the male reproductive system

PHARMACOLOGICAL GROUP AND EFFECT	KEY EXAMPLES	CLINICAL USE
GnRH agonists • Initially increase synthesis of FSH and LH, increase testosterone • High continuous use decreases FSH and LH, then decreases testosterone • Inhibit growth of steroid dependent tumours	Leuprorelin, goserelin, triptorelin	Prostate cancer
Androgens (anabolic steroids) • Bind to androgen receptors to induce gene expression that regulates the response of masculine sexual characteristics	Testosterone	Androgen deficiency Male delayed puberty
α_1-adrenoceptor antagonists • Block α_1-adrenoceptors • Then decrease smooth muscle tone in the bladder outlet and prostate • Improve urine flow rates	Prazosin, terazosin, tamsulosin	Symptomatic relief of benign prostatic hyperplasia (BPH)
5α-reductase inhibitors • Inhibit 5α-reductase enzyme in the prostate gland • Inhibit conversion of testosterone to DHT (potent androgen responsible for prostate gland growth) • Decrease DHT hypertrophy	Dutasteride, finasteride	Treatment of BPH
ICSH activity	hCG	Spermatogenesis stimulant
Phosphodiesterase 5 inhibitors • Block breakdown of cyclic guanosine monophosphate = prolongation of the action of nitric oxide as mediators of vasodilation • Cause vasodilation in the penis	Sildenafil, tadalafil	Erectile dysfunction

Prostaglandin agonists • Synthetic prostaglandin E_1 analogue activates prostaglandin receptors, increasing cAMP • Relaxes corpus cavernosum smooth muscle	Alprostadil	Erectile dysfunction
Selective serotonin reuptake inhibitor • Inhibits reuptake of serotonin at the transporter • Increases concentration of serotonin in synaptic cleft that can bind to receptors and exert effect	Dapoxetine	Premature ejaculation

REVIEW QUESTIONS

1 Mr TO presents to his GP with the symptoms of a constant urge to urinate, urinating more than eight times a day and nocturia. On examination his prostate is enlarged. Mr TO is subsequently diagnosed with benign prostatic hyperplasia. He is initially prescribed the α-adrenoceptor antagonist tamsulosin. On a visit back to his GP 6 months later, as he was still experiencing symptoms, he is prescribed a fixed dose combination therapy with tamsulosin and dutasteride. Describe the mechanism of action of both active ingredients in the combination therapy. How long does it take for dutasteride to have its full effect? Explain why. What benefits does the combination therapy have when compared with the tamsulosin monotherapy?

2 Mr LA, a 43-year-old otherwise healthy builder, presents to his GP. He describes the signs of premature ejaculation and psychological distress it is causing him. His GP recommends psychological therapy and the SSRI dapoxetine 30 mg, to be taken 1 to 3 hours before intercourse. What drugs should be avoided to reduce Mr LA's risk of serotonin toxicity? Describe some other adverse effects of this medicine.

3 Mr CH, an 82-year-old retired picture framer, is diagnosed with advanced prostate cancer and is prescribed the GnRH agonist, leuprorelin. It is administered by depot injection every 3 months. Describe the mode of action of leuprorelin and some of the more common adverse effects of this medicine.

REFERENCES

Abreu, A.P. and U.B. Kaiser, Pubertal development and regulation. The Lancet Diabetes & Endocrinology, 2016. 4(3): 254–264.

Cancer Australia 2022. Breast cancer in Australia statistics. Online. https://www.canceraustralia.gov.au/cancer-types/breast-cancer/statistics

Christou, M.A., Christou, P.A., Markozannes, G., et al., Effects of anabolic androgenic steroids on the reproductive system of athletes and recreational users: a systematic review and meta-analysis. Sports Medicine, 2017. 47(9): 1869–1883.

Davey, R.A. and M. Grossmann, Androgen receptor structure, function and biology: from bench to bedside. Clin Biochem Rev, 2016. 37(1): 3–15.

Fentiman, I.S., Male breast cancer is not congruent with the female disease. Critical Reviews in Oncology/Hematology, 2016. 101: 119–124.

Giulivo, M., Lopez de Alda, M., Capri, E., et al., Human exposure to endocrine disrupting compounds: Their role in reproductive systems, metabolic syndrome and breast cancer. A review. Environmental Research, 2016. 151: 251–264.

Lee, S.W.H., E.M.C. Chan, and Y.K. Lai, The global burden of lower urinary tract symptoms suggestive of benign prostatic hyperplasia: a systematic review and meta-analysis. Scientific Reports, 2017. 7(1): 1–10.

Namekawa, T., Imamoto, T., Kato, M., et al., Vasovasostomy and vasoepididymostomy: Review of the procedures, outcomes, and predictors of patency and pregnancy over the last decade. Reproductive Medicine and Biology, 2018. 17(4): 343–355.

Narayanan, R., C.C. Coss, and J.T. Dalton, Development of selective androgen receptor modulators (SARMs). Molecular and Cellular Endocrinology, 2018. 465: 134–142.

Ohlander, S.J., M.C. Lindgren, and L.I. Lipshultz, Testosterone and Male Infertility. Urologic Clinics of North America, 2016. 43(2): 195–202.

Perry-Keene, D., Low testosterone in men. Australian Prescriber, 2014. 37: 196–200.

Ritter, J., Flower, R., Henderson G., et al., Rang and Dale's pharmacology. 2019.

Semet, M., Paci, M., J Saïas-Magnan, J., et al., The impact of drugs on male fertility: a review. Andrology, 2017. 5(4): 640–663.

Yeap, B.B., Grossmann, M., McLachlan, R.I., et al., Endocrine Society of Australia position statement on male hypogonadism (part 1): assessment and indications for testosterone therapy. Medical Journal of Australia, 2016. 205(4): 173–178.

ONLINE RESOURCES

Healthy Male (Andrology Australia) – What every man should know: https://www.healthymale.org.au/ (accessed 21 September 2021)

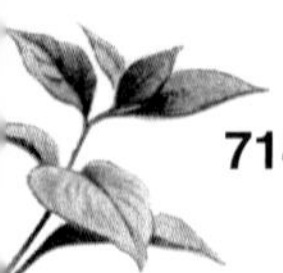

Cancer Council – Breast cancer in men: https://www.cancer.org.au/cancer-information/types-of-cancer/breast-cancer-in-men (accessed 21 September 2021)

New Zealand Medicines and Medical Devices Safety Authority: https://www.medsafe.govt.nz/ (accessed 21 September 2021)

Prostate Cancer Foundation of Australia: https://www.prostate.org.au/ (accessed 21 September 2021)

More weblinks at: http://evolve.elsevier.com/AU/Knights/pharmacology/.

CHAPTER 32

PRINCIPLES OF CANCER THERAPY

Andrew Rowland

KEY ABBREVIATIONS

CDK	cyclin-dependent kinase
DNA	deoxyribonucleic acid
EGF	epithelial growth factor
MTD	maximum tolerated dose
RNA	ribonucleic acid
TNF	tumour necrosis factor
VEGF	vascular endothelial growth factor

KEY TERMS

Chapter Focus

This chapter presents an overview of the pathways involved in the development of cancer, including the cell cycle, with an emphasis on regulation and the phases at which checkpoints and antineoplastic drugs act. Principles of antineoplastic chemotherapy and clinical aspects of oncology (age-related considerations, combination chemotherapy, drug resistance, safe handling of cytotoxics, toxicity and treatment regimens) are described.

CRITICAL THINKING SCENARIO

Samantha (a 38-year-old mother with two young children) and her 72-year-old dad, Frank, are diagnosed with cancer 2 weeks apart. Samantha is diagnosed with stage 1 breast cancer and is otherwise healthy, while Frank is diagnosed with stage 4 pancreatic cancer. Frank has a history of significant cardiovascular, liver and renal diseases. While both people are diagnosed with cancer, their prognoses and goals of treatment are very different. How will you account for each of these factors when designing a treatment plan for these two people?

Introduction

Neoplasia refers to the uncontrolled proliferation and spread of abnormal cells of the body. This growth is uncoordinated and persists after the stimulus provoking the growth ends. Other characteristics of tumours are that their presence is not useful; there may be de-differentiation of cells leading to loss of organ function; and characteristics of abnormal cells are inherited indefinitely by successive generations. Benign tumours may cause problems by their excessive growth and may kill by putting pressure on critical adjacent organs. The biological capabilities acquired by human cells during development of cancer have been termed 'cancer hallmarks'. Six hallmark capabilities were summarised by Hanahan and Weinberg (2000); two emerging hallmark capabilities and two enabling characteristics were subsequently added (Hanahan & Weinberg 2011). They are:

1. sustaining proliferative signalling
2. evading growth suppressors
3. activating invasion and metastasis
4. enabling replicative immortality
5. inducing angiogenesis
6. resisting cell death
7. dysregulating cellular energetics – emerging hallmarks
8. avoiding immune destruction – emerging hallmarks
9. genome instability and mutation – enabling characteristics
10. tumour-promoting inflammation – enabling characteristics.

These hallmark capabilities are based on aspects of tumour biology and serve as key targets for many drugs used in the treatment of cancer (Fig 32.1). As such, some understanding of key components of tumour biology, such as the cell cycle and regulators of this cycle, provides an important basis for understanding the mechanisms of antineoplastic drugs.

Treatment of cancer

The three main treatment modalities in cancer are surgery, radiation therapy and drug therapy. If it is possible to remove all of a cancer surgically, then this is the first choice and may be curative. In cases of a large inoperable tumour in a vital organ, a tumour difficult to access, metastatic disease or non-solid organ tumours such as leukaemias or lymphomas, then radiation and/or drugs are used. Antineoplastic drugs can be distinguished based on four broad strategies (Sun et al. 2017):

- non-selectively blocking the cell cycle (cytotoxic drugs)
- targeting hormone sensitive pathways (hormonal drugs)
- targeting mutated pathway regulators (non-cytotoxic drugs)
- enhancing the immune response to cancer (immunomodulatory drugs).

Non-selectively blocking the cell cycle (cytotoxic drugs)

Cytotoxic drugs act by inhibiting the synthesis of nucleic acids, deoxyribonucleic acid (DNA), ribonucleic acid (RNA) or proteins that are required in order for the cell cycle to proceed. Cytotoxic drugs may have more than one site of action in pathways of nucleic acids, DNA, RNA or proteins synthesis.

The cell cycle

Controlled cell division and growth is essential for normal tissue size, physiological function, replacement of cells as required and development of complex organs such as the brain and kidney. Uncontrolled cellular replication is a fundamental defect that occurs in cancer. When a cell divides, two daughter cells are produced with identical chromosomes to those of the parent cell. This process of division and proliferation, known as the cell cycle, is

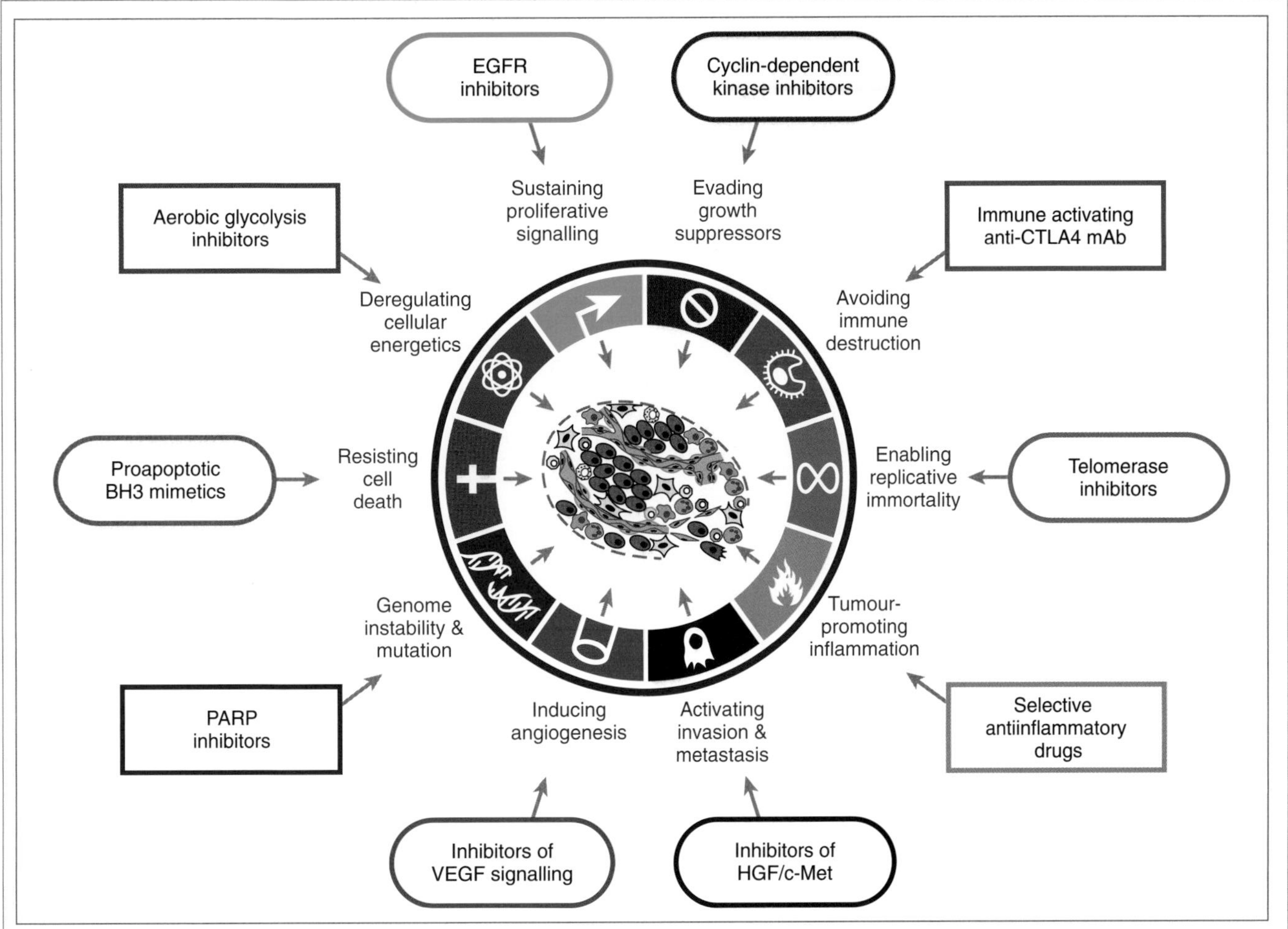

FIGURE 32.1 Therapeutic targeting of cancer hallmarks
Drugs that interfere with each of the acquired capabilities necessary for cancer growth and progression have been developed and are in clinical trials or, in some cases, approved for clinical use.
Source: Hanahan & Weinberg 2011, Figure 6; used with permission.

described in phases. Cytotoxic drugs non-discriminately interfere with basic functions at one or more phases of the cell cycle, blocking replication in all cell types (Fig 32.2):

- Pre-synthesis gap phase (G1): synthesis of RNA and protein occurs and the cell prepares for passing the first checkpoint into the DNA synthesis phase.
- DNA synthesis phase (S): genetic material, DNA in chromosomes, is duplicated in preparation for cell division.
- Pre-mitotic gap phase (G2): DNA synthesis ceases, but RNA and protein synthesis continues, to prepare the cell for mitosis, spindle formation and cell division.
- Mitosis phase (M): cells divide into two new 'daughter' cells that may leave the cell cycle and differentiate into specialised cells or become either temporarily or permanently non-proliferative (G0 phase).
- Resting phase (G0): a 'neutral gear', cells may be recruited later to re-enter the cell cycle or may mature and die.

The duration of the cell cycle for a rapidly replicating human cell type is about 24 hours and is mainly determined by time spent in the S phase. As tumour cells replicate rapidly they are particularly susceptible to damage by cytotoxic drugs. However, because this process is essentially the same in normal and cancer cells, rapidly replicating non-tumour cells are also damaged to a similar extent. Damage to these cells causes a common set of toxicities including myelosuppression (impaired bone marrow production of blood cells), alopecia, gastrointestinal tract (GIT) irritation and infertility that are associated with the use of most cytotoxic drugs.

Synthesis of proteins and nucleic acids

For cells to proliferate, the DNA must be replicated once every cell cycle. DNA is composed of four kinds of

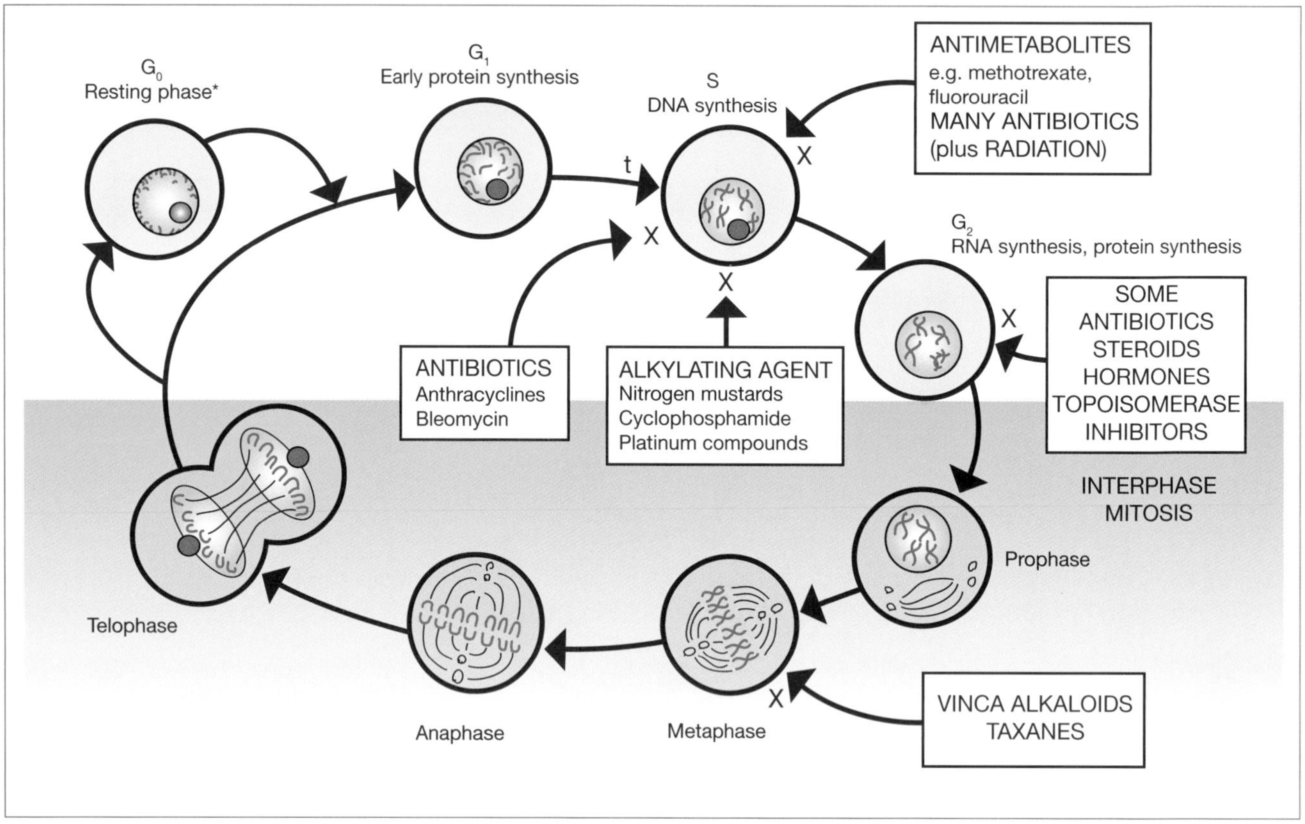

FIGURE 32.2 Phases of the cell cycle

Drugs (in boxes) are identified, showing the main sites at which they act.

* = Commitment to cell division: leads to cell enlargement, DNA replication and mitosis; † = first checkpoint: if damaged DNA cannot be repaired, cell undergoes apoptosis; G_0 = resting phase, cells not cycling; G_1 = first gap, between previous nuclear division and beginning of DNA synthesis (duration highly variable, about 9 hours in rapidly replicating cells); G_2 = second gap, between DNA replication and nuclear division (about 4.5 hours); M = mitosis (about 30 minutes); S = period of DNA synthesis (8–20 hours)

Source: Adapted from Beare & Myers 1998.

serially repeating nucleotide bases: pyrimidines (cytosine and thymine) and purines (adenine and guanine), linked via sugar and phosphate groups (Fig 32.3). Particular nucleotide sequences make up the genes, the biological units of inheritance that occupy precise positions on a chromosome. When genes are expressed, DNA is 'transcribed' into messenger RNA copies, which are transported out of the nucleus into the cytoplasm and they act as templates to direct the amino acid sequence (translation) in the synthesis of proteins such as enzymes and structural proteins. Folic acid antagonists are an example of a class of cytotoxic antineoplastic drugs that interfere with these processes; these drugs inhibit nucleic acid synthesis.

DNA replication and topoisomerases

Packaging of DNA into chromosomes involves 'supercoiling' of DNA fragments – that is, regions where the double-stranded DNA helix is twisted on itself. This requires actions of topoisomerase enzymes. Topoisomerases control the number and amount of twist in the supercoils, by cutting one or both strands, twisting them about each other and resealing the ends. These actions are essential in replication of DNA and controlled growth of cells. Camptothecins (topoisomerase I) and podophyllotoxins (topoisomerase II), which selectively inhibit these enzymes, have become useful classes of antineoplastic drugs.

Chromosome duplication and telomerase

Normal cells are only able to undergo a limited number of divisions because a small fragment of non-coding DNA (called a telomere) is shaved off the end of part of the chromosome each time replication occurs. In normal adult cells, the daughter DNA strand is normally shortened at each cell division, leading to chromosomal instability and contributing to tissue ageing.

An enzyme called telomerase (telomere terminal transferase) can re-form telomeres, thus preventing the shortening of the chromosome. The gene for telomerase

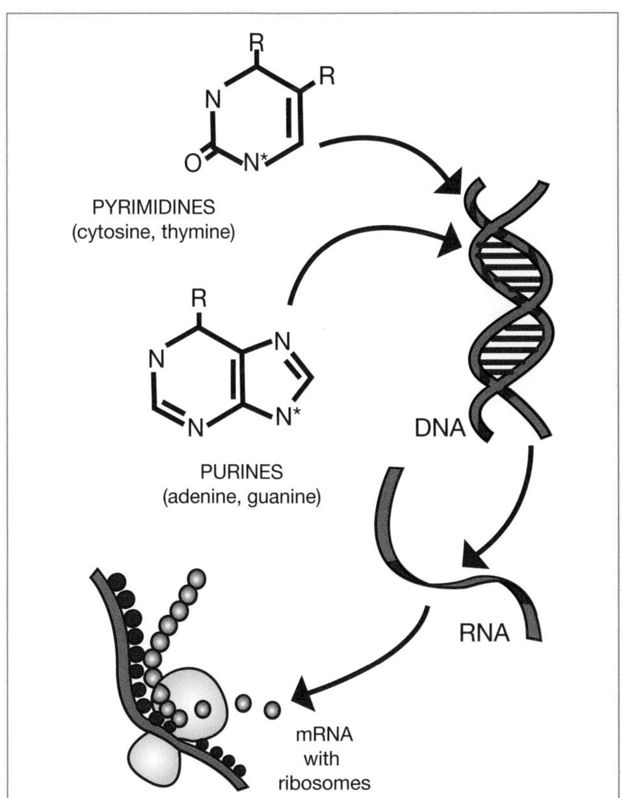

FIGURE 32.3 Synthesis of nucleic acids and proteins
In the general structures shown for the purine and pyrimidine bases, R stands for an oxygen (=O) or amine ($-NH_2$) group. In the polymers of DNA or RNA, each base is linked via the N* nitrogen atom to a sugar molecule (deoxyribose or ribose), and the sugar molecules are linked via phosphate groups to form long chains. In DNA, two complementary strands are twisted into the famous double-helix shape.
Source: Salerno 1999; used with permission.

and its associated RNA are active in germ cells and stem cells but are usually switched off in fully differentiated cells of adult tissues. However, this enzyme is present in about 90% of human cancers and may contribute to the immortality of cancer cells. The prognosis for neuroblastoma, a paediatric tumour of the peripheral nervous system, can be estimated by measuring levels of telomerase activity; high telomerase levels predict a poor response to therapy. Telomerase inhibition is being evaluated as the target for antineoplastic drugs, with imetelstat undergoing phase II/III clinical trials in myelodysplastic syndromes and myelofibrosis.

Targeting hormone-sensitive pathways (hormonal drugs)

Growth of some tumours depends on stimulation of neoplastic cells by particular hormones; for example, breast cancer is stimulated by estrogens, prostate cancer by androgens and thyroid cancer by thyroid-stimulating hormone. These cancers may be effectively suppressed by antihormones such as tamoxifen (an antiestrogen; Drug Monograph 33.4), drugs that suppress synthesis or secretion of the hormone, or by surgical removal or irradiation of the gland producing the hormone.

Targeting mutated pathways (non-cytotoxic drugs)

Also commonly referred to as 'targeted therapies', these drugs can be either small molecules (i.e. chemicals with a molecular weight less than 1 kD) or therapeutic proteins (e.g. monoclonal antibodies). They typically inhibit specific pathological (i.e. mutated) pathways that contribute to the dysregulation of the tumour cell cycle or tumour cell functions, and include:

- tyrosine kinase inhibitors (e.g. imatinib)
- cyclin-dependent kinase inhibitors (e.g. palbociclib)
- serine threonine kinase inhibitors (e.g. everolimus)
- histone deacetylase inhibitors (e.g. vorinostat)
- replication checkpoint inhibitors (e.g. olaparib)
- monoclonal antibodies that block interaction of growth factors or their receptors (e.g. bevacizumab).

Regulatory factors determine the orderly progression of cells through the cycle by activating receptors on the cell membrane followed by signal transduction, by which growth stimulatory signals are integrated and passed on to the nucleus in cascades of biochemical reactions, where they trigger activation or repression of genes required for DNA replication, cell division and proliferation. Regulatory factors that, when mutated, have been implicated in tumour development, proliferation or metastatic dissemination include cyclins, growth factors, tyrosine kinases, serine-threonine kinases, PI3 kinases, mitotic regulators, checkpoints and tumour suppressor genes and proteins. These factors contribute to various cancer hallmark capabilities and are targets for non-cytotoxic antineoplastic drugs (Fig 32.1).

Cyclins

Cyclins are the regulatory sub-units of protein kinases; they control mitosis and regulate activities of many transcription and replication factors, structural proteins and proteins involved in mitosis and chromosome formation. The catalytic parts of these phosphorylating enzymes are called cyclin-dependent kinases (CDKs); they activate or inhibit proteins at specific regulatory sites at the appropriate time, and thus govern progression through the cell cycle. Elevated levels of cyclins are found in many tumours. CDKs that are improperly regulated can cause unscheduled proliferation and genomic and chromosomal instability. Selective CDK inhibition is an important emerging target, with several drugs in this class already approved.

Growth factors

Growth factors involved in signal transduction pathways include epidermal growth factor (EGF), fibroblast growth factor and insulin-like growth factor, each with its related receptor. Sustaining proliferative signalling and altering cellular energy metabolism are hallmarks of cancer cells. EGF stimulates proliferation of many types of epithelial cells, including those lining the GIT and ducts in the mammary glands of women. In many cancers, tumour cells produce raised levels of an EGF receptor called HER2, making cells hypersensitive to EGF and stimulating growth of tumour cells. Biopsy of cancerous tissue can determine the level of expression of HER2, and likely sensitivity to trastuzumab, a monoclonal antibody specific against HER2 that is used to treat breast cancer.

Tyrosine kinases

Kinase receptors contain an intracellular catalytic domain that functions as a phosphorylating enzyme. Phosphorylation is an essential biochemical reaction in nearly all cell functions. These receptors are involved in regulating signalling pathways and help mediate metabolism, transcription, cell-cycle progression, differentiation, cell movement, apoptosis and immunological functions. Tyrosine kinases add phosphate groups to tyrosine residues in proteins. These kinases are involved in the signalling of growth factors and thus help regulate the passage of cells through the cell cycle.

Many tyrosine kinases can activate the RAS protein pathway. RAS is a small intracellular G-protein that promotes formation of signal transduction complexes and thence a cascade of kinase enzymes that activate target proteins. Mutations in tyrosine kinases, RAS proteins or RAS kinase enzymes are found in almost all tumour cell types. HER2 is a membrane-associated tyrosine kinase that acts as an oncogene; it is overexpressed in many cancers, where it provides proliferative and antiapoptotic signals, leading to aggressive subtypes of cancer. Inhibitors of specific tyrosine kinases (the -tinib group of drugs) are useful antineoplastic drugs.

Serine-threonine kinases

A serine/threonine kinase that is important in ageing and cancer is the mammalian target of rapamycin (mTOR). The main functions of mTOR are as a sensor of cellular nutrient and energy levels and oxidation status, in regulating cell growth and controlling protein synthesis, angiogenesis and the cytoskeleton. Rapamycin is a natural bacterial product that can inhibit mTOR. The mTOR pathway is often aberrantly activated in cancers. Drugs that inhibit mTOR activity are used in treatment of cancer (e.g. everolimus) and of transplant rejection, and may prove useful in treating some age-related diseases.

Another important family of serine-threonine kinases are the RAF/ERK kinases, which are encoded by the BRAF gene. The BRAF gene is involved in a signalling pathway affecting cell division, differentiation and secretion. It is mutated in approximately 8% of all human cancers, notably in melanomas and thyroid and colorectal carcinomas, which have been difficult to treat. Levels of expression of BRAF mutations (e.g. BRAF V600E) in tumours can be measured, and can be used to guide treatment with selective inhibitors such as dabrafenib and vemurafenib that target this protein.

PI3 kinases

Phosphoinositide 3-kinases (PI3Ks) are a family of intracellular kinases. PI3Ks are involved in cell growth, proliferation, differentiation and survival. Mutations in some PI3Ks activate enzymes and contribute to cellular transformation and cancer. Early broad inhibitors of the enzymes were so general that they are too toxic to be useful; however, the specific inhibitor against the delta isoform (PI3Kδ), idelalisib, has demonstrated success in treating haematological malignancies, including chronic lymphocytic leukaemia, follicular B-cell non-Hodgkin lymphoma and small lymphocytic lymphoma.

Mitotic regulators

Many cancer cell types have the hallmark of 'replicative immortality' because the carcinogenic mutations are inherited indefinitely by daughter cells during mitosis. Regulators of mitosis include two groups of serine-threonine kinases, the aurora kinases and polo-like kinases, and the kinesin spindle proteins, which have roles in the formation of the spindle. Current cytotoxic antimitotic drugs such as the vinca alkaloids and the taxanes are 'spindle poisons', targeting microtubules during mitosis.

Checkpoints

Checkpoints are additional surveillance mechanisms that control cell-cycle events at particular stages to ensure exact duplication of chromosomes from parent cell to daughter cells during cell division, and completion of each stage before transition to the next. Checks at the G1/S transition, S phase, G2/M transition or at the spindle-assembly checkpoint during mitosis ensure that any damaged DNA can be blocked and mitotic division of mutated chromosomes inhibited, leading to apoptosis of mutated cells. Mechanisms of checking are mainly through control of activation of cyclin–CDKs. For example, at the intra-S-phase checkpoint, activation of CDK1 is inhibited if DNA synthesis is not yet complete. Mutations that impair checkpoint signalling molecules or DNA repair genes (e.g. BRCA1 and 2) occur frequently in cancers, allowing the hallmark characteristics of instability of genome and ability to resist cell death. Cells with defective BRCA1 and 2 may be more sensitive to antineoplastic drugs; targeting the poly (ADP-ribose) polymerase (PARP) checkpoint with drugs such as olaparib in people with BRCA mutant breast cancer is an example of this strategy.

Tumour suppressors

The ability to evade growth suppressors is a hallmark of cancer cells. The transforming growth factor β (TGFβ) superfamily contains extracellular signalling molecules with widespread roles in regulating development; examples are the bone morphogenetic proteins. The TGFβ-1 isoforms all potently prevent proliferation by inducing synthesis of proteins that inhibit the cell cycle and thus act as tumour suppressors in early stages. Mutations that impair receptors or proteins in the TGFβ pathway cause enhanced cell proliferation in many human cancers, including retinoblastoma, colon, pancreatic and gastric cancers, hepatoma, and some T- and B-cell malignancies.

Angiogenesis

Ability to induce angiogenesis is another hallmark of cancer cells. Members of the TGFβ family, particularly vascular endothelial growth factors (VEGF), are involved in tumour angiogenesis. Angiogenesis inhibitors can slow growth and **metastasis** of cancers by reducing their blood supply. Antibodies against VEGF (e.g. bevacizumab) and small molecules that inhibit its receptor (VEGFR inhibitors; e.g. sunitinib) are important drugs for treating multiple solid organ tumours, including breast, colorectal, gastrointestinal, renal and thyroid cancers.

p53 protein

The p53 family of genes and their associated isoform proteins are involved in a wide variety of functions, including reproduction, metabolic regulation, longevity and development of the nervous and immune systems, and skin. p53 is a phosphoprotein with molecular weight 53 kDa and is a major regulator of the G1 checkpoint in response to cellular stress. If DNA damage is severe, p53 protein activates expression of genes leading to enhanced apoptosis, which normally prevents accumulation of damaged DNA. Mutations in the p53 gene impair normal 'braking mechanisms', allowing cancer cells to evade immune destruction and lead to uncontrolled proliferation of altered cells. p53 has important checkpoint roles as a tumour suppressor, explaining why mutations in the p53 gene and decline in p53 activity are commonly associated with cancers, especially in older people.

Tumour suppressor genes

Tumour suppressor genes direct synthesis of regulatory proteins that inhibit cyclins and halt the cell cycle at checkpoints. Examples include p53 (described above) and the following:

- The retinoblastoma family proteins (pRb) act as an 'emergency brake' to prevent cell-cycle progression. Mutations that inactivate the Rb function allow unscheduled progression of cells from G1 to S phase, and occur in nearly every type of adult cancer. Inheritance of a mutant allele of the Rb gene by a human fetus most frequently happens in the retina, leading to highly malignant retinoblastomas which usually manifest very early in infancy.
- The repressor protein encoded by the Wilms' tumour gene (WT1) is expressed preferentially in the developing kidney. Children who inherit two mutated WT1 genes produce no functional repressor WT1 protein, and inevitably develop kidney tumours.
- The PTEN gene is deleted in many advanced human cancers, allowing abnormal cells to proliferate. Cells lacking the PTEN gene have elevated levels of PI3K and protein kinase B activity, and reduced ability to undergo apoptosis. Restoring PTEN functions is another potential mechanism for cancer therapy.

Apoptosis

A damaged cell normally undergoes programmed cell death, or apoptosis, a useful process that eliminates abnormal cells via genetically programmed biochemical reactions causing rounding up of the cell, shrinkage, then fragmentation and digestion. Apoptosis is probably the 'fall-back' position, automatically triggered at cell-cycle checkpoints unless inhibited by factors necessary for cell cycling and survival.

Many neoplastic cells have the ability to evade apoptosis, normally induced by cytokines known as tumour necrosis factors (TNF). The first member of the family, TNF-α, is a monocyte-derived cytotoxin implicated in tumour regression. TNF-related apoptosis-inducing ligand is a protein that activates two death receptors (DR4 and DR5) mediating apoptosis. While it is believed that drugs targeting these receptors may enhance apoptosis of damaged and mutated cells, in clinical trials only a small proportion of people respond to drugs targeting DR4 or DR5.

The Bcl-2 family proteins have opposing functions: some are antiapoptotic, thus allowing survival of tumour cells, and others are pro-apoptotic, neutralising damaged cells. Damage to the Bcl-2 gene is a cause of a number of cancers, and of resistance to cancer treatments. Agents that mimic the pro-apoptotic useful proteins, particularly the Bcl-2 homology 3 domains, known as BH3 mimetics, are proving useful as anticancer drugs, as are Bcl-2 inhibitors.

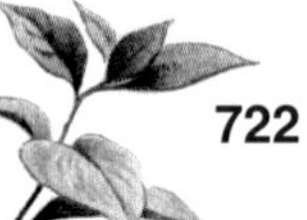

Enhancing immune response to cancer (immunomodulatory drugs)

The immune system plays an important role in protecting the body from cancer. Mutated DNA often causes the production of abnormal proteins known as tumour antigens. Tumour antigens on the cell surface mark mutated cells as 'non-self', targeting them for destruction by immune cells; the immune system eliminates mutated cells on a daily basis. However, a hallmark capability of cancer cells is the ability to avoid immune destruction, in particular by T and B lymphocytes, macrophages and natural killer cells. When the immune system loses the ability to detect and remove tumour cells, these cells are able to form a tumour. Proposed mechanisms by which cancer cells avoid immune destruction include:

- reducing expression of tumour antigens on their surface
- expressing proteins on their surface that induce immune cell inactivation
- inducing cells in the tumour microenvironment to release substances that suppress immune responses.

The therapeutic potential of enhancing the immune response to cancer has been recognised for many years, and many specific therapeutic strategies have been developed:

- immune checkpoint modulators (e.g. pembrolizumab)
- antineoplastic antibodies (e.g. trastuzumab)
- immune system modulators (e.g. interferon alpha)
- immune cell therapy (e.g. tumour-infiltrating lymphocytes)
- cancer vaccines (e.g. Gardasil).

The success of non-specific immunomodulatory drugs such as interferon alpha (IFN-α) as therapeutic options for the treatment of cancer has been limited by frequent and severe toxicities associated with systemic immunostimulation, and attempts to develop cancer vaccines have been challenging. The recent development of **immune checkpoint** modulators and antineoplastic antibodies that specifically target pathways modified in cancer (e.g. overexpression of PD-1) has advanced the capacity to enhance immune response to cancer. Important issues that will further advance the use of immunomodulatory drugs for the treatment of cancer include:

- understanding why immunotherapy works in some people but not others
- expanding the range of immunotherapy drugs to target more types of cancer
- increasing the effectiveness of immunotherapy by combining it with other types of cancer treatment.

Inflammation and cancer

Inflammation itself does not cause cancers, but an environment rich in inflammatory cells, growth factors, activated cell stroma and DNA-damaging agents increases the risk of **neoplasia**. Sites of chronic irritation or inflammation, and inflammation associated with a tumour, produce many inflammatory cells and mediators such as cytokines, interleukins, interferons, reactive oxygen species, angiogenic growth factors, TNF-α and protease enzymes, many of which can enhance growth of cells, act as cancer promoters and promote angiogenesis. Later, inflammation may actually be protective against neoplastic growth, by enhancing apoptosis and immune responses. Tumour cells can also use adhesion molecules, chemokines and receptors to enhance migration and metastasis to distant tissues. Cancers associated with inflammation include those caused by viruses such as human papillomavirus, hepatitis B virus and Epstein-Barr virus; gastric carcinoma is associated with peptic ulcers and infection by *Helicobacter pylori*. Cancers associated with chronic inflammatory conditions include colon cancer with ulcerative colitis and Crohn's disease, and liver carcinoma with hepatitis C.

KEY POINTS

Treatment of cancer

- Cytotoxic drugs generally have antiproliferative effects by impairing nucleic acid or protein synthesis (antimetabolites, alkylating agents, antitumour antibiotics) or by disrupting mitosis (vinca alkaloids, taxanes).
- Tumours that depend on hormones for growth may be treated with antihormonal drugs or by suppressing secretion of the trophic hormone.
- Non-cytotoxic drugs target specific enzymes, proteins, receptors, growth factors, genes and cytokines in relevant neoplastic pathways.
- Enhancing immune response to cancer, particularly through approaches that specifically overcome a tumour's ability to avoid immune cells, is emerging as an important therapeutic strategy in the treatment of cancer.

Clinical aspects of treating cancer

In treating cancer, the term 'cure' is used differently from the way it is understood for acute conditions that can be totally healed or eradicated. A cancer cure is defined as the disappearance of any evidence of the tumour for several years, with a high probability of a normal life span. This definition, referring to a probability, acknowledges the difficulty of removing every malignant cell and recognises the possibility of recurrence. The person may go into remission after a course of **chemotherapy** when the tumour and signs and symptoms are no longer detectable, then relapse some months or years later. Medical oncology is a medical specialty that primarily deals with drug-based treatment of cancer. The primary goal of treatment is governed by a range of factors relating to the cancer and the person:

- location of the primary tumour
- extent (or stage) of disease
- molecular characteristics of the tumour or person
- person's physical performance status
- person's mental status
- person's age
- person's preferences/wishes.

In some circumstances, other factors such as gender, ethnicity and access to medicines may also influence decisions around treatment, although the latter is rarely an issue in Australia. Characteristics of the tumour may be particularly useful as prognostic markers (i.e. markers that indicate the person's likely progression) or predictive markers (i.e. markers defining the likelihood that a person will benefit from a particular treatment). Predictive markers are particularly useful, as they help to direct treatment decisions.

Treatment guidelines and protocols

Because of the diversity of cancer subtypes even within tumours originating from the same tissue, and the array of potential treatment interventions, more so than other medical disciplines, the treatment of cancer is highly protocol driven. International treatment guidelines such as the National Comprehensive Cancer Network (NCCN) clinical practice guidelines in oncology and European Society of Medical Oncologists (ESMO) oncology clinical practice guidelines provide recommendations by site relating to:

- clinical presentation
- workup
- findings
- primary treatment
- pathological stage
- adjunct treatments
- surveillance
- survivorship.

Recommendations presented in these guidelines are based on high-quality data from phase III trials and meta-analyses. Similarly, the Evidence and Quality (eviQ) cancer treatment protocols make more formal recommendations relating to:

- assessment
- cancer genetics
- chemotherapy protocols
- clinical procedures
- radiation protocols
- supportive therapy.

These resources are updated regularly to reflect changes in understanding and best practice. In addition to providing guidance for health professionals, the resources are also a useful source of evidence-based patient information. In addition to these national and international resources, many medical oncology departments operate within a framework of local protocols defined by the local health service or network.

Pathological staging

Tumours are not homogeneous, even tumours of the same cell type in the same organ. They may vary in cell-cycling time, proportion of cells cycling, their vascularity, susceptibility or resistance to actions of particular drugs and in their size and extent of spread. Tumours are commonly 'staged' by the 'TNM' method to indicate the size of the primary tumour and extent of spread to lymph nodes and distant metastases. In some cases, growth of the tumour can be monitored by measuring levels of surrogate marker, such as prostate-specific antigen (PSA) for prostate cancers or monoclonal immunoglobulins for multiple myeloma. The extent (or stage) of disease is an important determinant of the treatment plan.

Roles of antineoplastic drugs

Removing large, localised tumours by surgery reduces the tumour burden; subsequent courses of radiation or drug therapy aim to remove residual cancer cells to levels that can be controlled by the person's immune system. This reduction in tumour burden may produce remission, but if further therapies are not instituted or the immune system response is inadequate, the remaining cancer cells may multiply and grow into another detectable tumour – that is, recurrence and relapse. In this setting, antineoplastic drugs play two roles:

- as neoadjuvant therapy: where a drug is given as a first step to shrink a tumour before the primary treatment, usually surgery, to make the treatment more effective
- as **adjuvant therapy**: where surgery is followed by drug (or radiation) therapy to help decrease the risk of the cancer recurring.

The use of antineoplastic drugs alone can cure certain types of cancer – in particular, haematological malignancies such as leukaemias, lymphomas, germ cell tumours and choriocarcinoma. However, many solid organ cancers are 'chemotherapy insensitive'. While these cancers have been treated with improved outcomes in recent years with the development of non-cytotoxic drugs, interventions are rarely curative and the primary objective is to slow disease progression. The success of an antineoplastic drug in this setting is evaluated based on its ability to:

- achieve a response: stabilise disease progression or reduce tumour burden
- extend survival – both progression-free (PFS) and overall (OS)
- manage symptoms: improve quality of life.

Patients are likely to have many questions about their treatment (Clinical Focus Box 32.1), and it is important for all health professionals to be able to respond appropriately.

Treatment regimens

A treatment regimen defines the drug or drugs to be used, their dosage, the frequency and duration of treatments, as well as other considerations. Treatment regimens are often complicated, with people being administered two to four **cytotoxic agents** on various days for 2–3 weeks, followed by a drug-free period (to allow white blood cells to recover), then another course of treatment, possibly also with surgery and/or radiation therapy. Regimens are designed for optimum efficacy in specific cancers and take into account potential drug interactions. Adjuvant drugs may also be given to treat adverse effects, and fluids administered to rehydrate the person and 'flush out' the kidneys, where cytotoxic agents may concentrate.

In modern oncology, many regimens combine several drugs as combination therapy. These combination regimens are often designated by acronyms or initialisms that identify the agents used in the combination (Table 32.1). The use of multiple drugs in combination is based on the philosophy that by having drugs that work through different mechanisms, it is possible for the drugs to work together to achieve a synergistic outcome. Combinations with different dose-limiting adverse effects are typically the most effective, as each drug can be given in the combination at a full dose. The following principles are used to select drugs for combination therapy:

1. Each drug when used alone should be active against the specific cancer.
2. Each drug should have different mechanisms of action.

CLINICAL FOCUS BOX 32.1
What people want to know

The information people want or need to know about any prescribed drug can be summed up in three questions. In the context of antineoplastic agents, the following sample answers may help provide information and counselling.

1. What is it for?
   - Anticancer drugs slow or stop the growth and spread of tumours.
   - Very few cancer drugs cure the disease; many control or slow symptoms or may help you feel better.
   - Some extra drugs may be given to control side effects of cancer drugs; for example, antiemetics help prevent vomiting.
2. What will it do to me?
   - Not everyone who takes a cancer drug will benefit from doing so.
   - The drugs may slow down or stop the tumour growth and help relieve symptoms.
   - Some side effects may occur, such as allergies and rashes, infections, vomiting, sore mouth or throat, bleeding, hair loss or temporary or permanent sterility.
3. How do I use it?
   - Usually these drugs are injected while you are in a hospital or clinic, but some can be taken by mouth at home.
   - Often there are complicated 'courses' of treatment, with several drugs taken over weeks or months.
   - If you take them at home, it is important that the drugs be taken exactly as prescribed by your doctor.
   - Avoid going out into the sun without sunscreen and protective clothing.
   - Avoid use of over-the-counter or complementary medicines, unless your doctor has approved them.
   - You may be asked to come for regular tests to check how you are progressing.
   - Use effective contraception and/or avoid breastfeeding while taking these drugs.

TABLE 32.1 Examples of combination chemotherapeutic regimens

CANCER	ABBREVIATION	DRUGS
Breast	CMF(P)	Cyclophosphamide, methotrexate, fluorouracil (+/− prednisolone)
	CFPT	Cyclophosphamide, fluorouracil, prednisone, tamoxifen
Colon	FOLFOX6	Leucovorin, fluorouracil (2 dose levels), oxaliplatin
	FOLFIRI	Leucovorin, fluorouracil (2 dose levels), irinotecan (+/− bevacizumab)
Lung	CAV	Cyclophosphamide, doxorubicin, vincristine
	CE	Cyclophosphamide, etoposide
Stomach	ECF	Epirubicin, cisplatin, fluorouracil
	EOX	Epirubicin, oxaliplatin, capecitabine
Hodgkin's disease	MOPP	Carmustine, vincristine, procarbazine, prednisone
	ABVD	Doxorubicin, bleomycin, vinblastine, dacarbazine

3. Each drug should have different organ toxicities or, if similar, at different times after drug administration.

The response rates for individual agents versus a combination therapy for the treatment of advanced Hodgkin's disease using mustine, Oncovin (vincristine), procarbazine and prednisone (MOPP) are a good illustration:

- M (mustine) – complete response rate (CR) 20%
- (vincristine) – CR < 10%
- P (procarbazine) – CR < 10%
- P (prednisone) – CR < 5%
- MOPP combination – CR 80%.

Mustine (now superseded by carmustine and lomustine) is an alkylating agent that impairs DNA. Vincristine inhibits mitosis by interfering with the mitotic spindle. Procarbazine inhibits synthesis of DNA, RNA and protein, and interferes with mitosis. Prednisone has lympholytic properties so is useful in white-cell tumours, and may produce an antifibrotic effect useful in metastases surrounded by fibrous materials; it also improves appetite and general feelings of wellbeing.

The third principle, that of different organ toxicity or toxicities that occur at different times, has also been substantiated for the MOPP combination. Both mustine and procarbazine cause dose-limiting toxicity bone marrow suppression, but the nadir (lowest point) occurs after about 10 days for mustine and 21 days for procarbazine, thus largely avoiding additive myelosuppression. Vincristine does not suppress bone marrow but does exhibit a dose-limiting neurotoxicity. Prednisone may be immunosuppressant, but its other adverse effects are very different from cytotoxic drugs.

When considering chemotherapy regimens, the phase of treatment is also an important consideration. 'Induction regimens' are used for the initial treatment of a disease, while 'maintenance regimens' consist of ongoing treatments to reduce the chances of a cancer recurring or to prevent an existing cancer from continuing to progress.

Molecular markers

As the molecular and genetic changes associated with the development of neoplastic cells have become better understood, altered genes and proteins are being identified as diagnostic 'biomarkers' of particular cancers or pathway mutations. These markers improve personalised treatment with drugs targeting specific aberrant mechanisms, and may define a tumour's sensitivity to a treatment or indicate the emergence of resistance to a treatment (Table 32.2). Testing for other markers such as PSA in prostate cancer, beta-human chorionic gonadotrophin in testicular cancer and faecal occult blood in colorectal cancer may assist in diagnosing the cancer at an earlier stage.

Dosing

Due to the low therapeutic index of many antineoplastic drugs, there is a fine line between minimum effective dose and maximum tolerated dose. Several methods are used to determine correct dosage for a person, while there is some overlap (e.g. dosing by maximum tolerated dose; MTD) these approaches are generally different between cytotoxic and non-cytotoxic drugs.

Fixed dose

Standard practice for orally administered non-cytotoxic drugs such as small molecule kinase inhibitors is to administer the same fixed dose (tablet) to all people. This dose is often defined as the population MTD, or one step down from the MTD determined in early clinical trials. The use of MTD here differs from the practice of specifically dosing based on MTD (below), as the MTD here is a population average. Due to inter-individual variability in exposure, it is likely that this dose may not reflect the actual MTD in an individual being administered the drug.

Body surface area dosing

Highly toxic intravenous cytotoxic drugs are frequently dosed in units of mg drug/m^2 body surface area, rather

TABLE 32.2 Examples of molecular markers that define response to cancer treatments

MARKER	CANCER	TREATMENT	IMPLICATION
BCR-ABL fusion protein (Philadelphia chromosome) expression	Chronic myeloid leukaemia	Bosutinib Dasatinib Imatinib Nilotinib Ponatinib	Confers sensitivity
BCR-ABL T315I mutation	Chronic myeloid leukaemia	Imatinib	Confers resistance
BRAF V600E mutation	Melanoma	Dabrafenib Vemurafenib	Confers sensitivity
BRCA1 mutation	Breast cancer	Olaparib	Confers sensitivity
c-KIT overexpression	Gastrointestinal stromal tumours	Imatinib	Confers sensitivity
EGFR del19 mutation	Non-small cell lung cancer	Afatinib Erlotinib Gefitinib Osimertinib	Confers sensitivity
EGFR T790M mutation	Non-small cell lung cancer	Afatinib Erlotinib Gefitinib	Confers resistance
ER/PR overexpression	Breast cancer	Hormonal drugs	Confers sensitivity
HER2 overexpression	Breast cancer	Lapatinib Trastuzumab	Confers sensitivity
KRAS exon 2 mutations	Colorectal cancer	Cetuximab Panitumumab	Confers resistance
MSI-High or dMMR	Multiple cancers	Pembrolizumab	Confers sensitivity

than the more common mg drug/kg body weight. This approach has been used for more than 50 years and is based on the principle that the surface area of cells in the target tumour relates more closely to the person's body surface area (BSA) than to their weight. Drug clearance is also related to BSA. BSA can be estimated from nomograms; for example, an adult weighing 80 kg with height 180 cm is estimated to have a BSA of 2.00 m^2. While this approach accounts for some sources of variability, large inter-patient variability in drug clearance and response still occurs.

Maximum tolerated dose

Traditionally, the dose of cytotoxic drugs has been considered to be the maximum dose that an individual can take before intolerable adverse effects occurred (MTD) such as life-threatening depression of the bone marrow or unbearable vomiting. This approach is the foundation of the concept of grade 3 or 4 'dose-limiting toxicities'. With non-cytotoxic drugs such as monoclonal antibodies and small kinase inhibitors, the MTD may be greater than the required therapeutic dose.

Concentration guided dosing

With the emergence of non-cytotoxic drugs, the need to account for variability in drug exposure that is not addressed by fixed dosing has become more prominent. The simplest and most direct way to account for variability in drug exposure is by measuring how much drug is in a person's blood using an approach known as therapeutic drug monitoring (TDM). This approach is based on the principle that people with exposure above a defined concentration threshold are more likely to obtain a benefit than those that fail to reach that concentration threshold. There are several examples of non-cytotoxic drugs where concentration thresholds associated with better outcomes have been established – in particular, small molecule kinase inhibitors: erlotinib, gefitinib, imatinib, pazopanib and sunitinib (Mueller-Schoell et al. 2021).

Pharmacogenetic guided dosing

Genetic differences in tumour markers and drug metabolising enzymes help explain pharmacokinetic and dynamic variabilities. Pharmacogenetic studies thus allow personalisation of dosing, especially thiopurines, methotrexate, cisplatin, vincristine and anthracyclines. For example, levels of thiopurine methyltransferase can predict the metabolism and potential toxicity of mercaptopurine in acute lymphoblastic leukaemia in children. Like most areas of medicine, the use of pharmacogenetic guided dosing in oncology is limited to a few key examples.

Adverse drug reactions

Adverse drug reactions are often dose-limiting and may be common to most antineoplastic drugs, at least within a broad class, or specific to particular drugs. The target of most cytotoxic drugs is cell proliferation, so most body tissues are also vulnerable, especially the most rapidly dividing cells in bone marrow, hair follicles, skin and GIT.

The most common adverse effects are alopecia (hair loss), gastrointestinal toxicities (anorexia, diarrhoea, mucositis, nausea, stomatitis, ulceration and vomiting) and myelosuppression.

Long-term toxicities also need to be monitored, as cytotoxic agents impair cell division and proliferation; they may thus cause infertility or possibly be mutagenic, carcinogenic or teratogenic. Immunosuppression and mutagenicity can lead to high incidences of secondary tumours: there is a 20% chance of developing a second cancer within 20 years of MOPP treatment. People need to be warned of these potential dangers, as do health professionals handling the drugs or people's excreta, since the drugs may be absorbed through the skin (Clinical Focus Box 32.2).

Nausea and vomiting

Cytotoxic-induced nausea and vomiting can become dangerous and discourage the person from continuing with chemotherapy. The propensity of a drug to cause nausea and vomiting is described as its emetic potential (Table 32.3). For cytotoxics with high emetogenic potential, antiemetic drugs such as dexamethasone with a 5-HT_3 antagonist (e.g. ondansetron) or aprepitant may be required for both prophylaxis and symptom relief.

Myelosuppression

Bone marrow suppression (myelosuppression) is the dose-limiting adverse reaction most often encountered: suppression of white cells (leucopenia or neutropenia) or of platelets (thrombocytopenia) can lead to life-threatening infections and haemorrhage, respectively. Cytotoxic agents are usually dosed to the limit of tolerance, with subsequent drug-free periods to allow recovery of white cell functions.

Tumour lysis syndrome

Tumour lysis syndrome refers to the massive release of breakdown products from tumour cells killed by chemotherapeutic agents; it occurs most commonly in leukaemias and lymphomas. In particular, urate may accumulate and precipitate in renal distal tubules and joints. To prevent this, urine may be alkalinised and/or hydration increased and allopurinol administered prophylactically. Hyperkalaemia, hyperphosphataemia and hypocalcaemia also occur.

CLINICAL FOCUS BOX 32.2
Safe handling of cytotoxic drugs

Cytotoxic drugs are inherently toxic and, if lipid-soluble, may be readily absorbed through the skin of people contacting the drug. Safe handling guidelines have been developed to protect pharmacists, doctors and nurses, patients and their families and carers. Suggested precautions include:

- Drugs are prepared and dispensed in a cytotoxic drug safety cabinet, a dedicated space with exhaust air filtered before being vented to the atmosphere.
- Staff handling the drug use protective clothing and equipment, including masks, gloves, head and shoe coverings and respiratory protective equipment.
- Excess drug, waste secretions and contaminated equipment are disposed of by high-temperature incineration.
- Health of staff is monitored by blood tests, and tests for liver and kidney functions.
- Labelling of equipment and solutions, containment and transport of drugs before and after dispensing and administration, both within hospitals and at home, must be carefully controlled.
- After administration of cytotoxic drugs, the person's body fluids are treated as mutagenic.
- Extra precautions apply to handling of radiopharmaceuticals.

Treatment of adverse drug reactions

Most adverse effects are treated symptomatically – for example, nausea with antiemetics, infections with

TABLE 32.3 Emetic potential of cytotoxic antineoplastic drugs

EMETIC POTENTIAL	DRUGS
High	Dacarbazine
Moderate-to-high (depending on dose)	Carmustine, cisplatin, cyclophosphamide
Moderate	Arsenic trioxide, azacitidine, carboplatin, clofarabine, dactinomycin, daunorubicin, doxorubicin, epirubicin, idarubicin, ifosfamide, irinotecan, methotrexate ($>$ 250 mg/m^2), oxaliplatin, raltitrexed
Moderate-to-low (depending on dose)	Cytarabine
Low	Busulfan, etoposide, fluorouracil, gemcitabine, methotrexate (50–250 mg/m^2), mitomycin, taxanes, thiotepa, topotecan
Minimal	Asparaginase, bleomycin, bortezomib, cladribine, fludarabine, methotrexate ($<$ 50 mg/m^2), monoclonal antibodies, temsirolimus, vinca alkaloids

Note: Emetic potential may depend on doses administered, route of administration, other concurrent drugs and patient history.

Source: Adapted from Australian Medicines Handbook 2021.

appropriate antimicrobial agents, mouth ulcers with mouthwashes, and zinc solutions and fever with antipyretic analgesics. Many people find loss of hair most distressing; this can be helped with sensitive encouragement and use of hairpieces, wigs and scarves; usually hair regrows after cessation of cytotoxic chemotherapy. Adjunct therapies used to treat specific adverse drug reactions are discussed in Chapter 35.

Development of drug resistance

Tumour cells have the potential to develop resistance to an antineoplastic drug and pass this acquired characteristic on to daughter cells. When this occurs, the cancer then becomes resistant to specific drugs, with declining therapeutic benefits in successive treatment cycles.

Mechanisms of drug resistance

Some of the mechanisms by which cells develop resistance are:

- defective activation of the drug – for example, cyclophosphamide and methotrexate are prodrugs that are activated in tumour cells
- enhanced inactivation of the drug – for example, highly reactive compounds may be 'scavenged' by cell-protective mechanisms
- decreased uptake of the drug into cells
- increased removal of the drug from cells – for example, by a drug efflux transporter such as p-glycoprotein and breast cancer resistant protein
- altered DNA repair – for example, DNA damaged by cytotoxic agents is partly repaired
- defective checkpoints – for example, the spindle assembly checkpoint
- increased synthesis of precursor molecules – for example, of purine or pyrimidine bases to circumvent the incorporation of antimetabolites into DNA
- altered expression of the drug target – for example, an enzyme less sensitive to drug, or an alternative pathway less dependent on an inhibited enzyme.

Overcoming drug resistance

Optimising antineoplastic drug usage helps minimise development of resistance. Methods include use of the most specific drugs targeting the particular cancer, using drugs in rotation or cycles and use of combinations acting at different stages of the cell cycle. Inhibitors of drug-efflux pumps are an emerging group of potentially useful agents; strategies to overcome cells' resistance to apoptosis are also being studied.

Age-related considerations

Cancer in children

Cancer in children under 15 years is relatively uncommon, with about 5% of childhood deaths due to cancer. The most common cancers in children in Australia are leukaemias and lymphomas, followed by brain and central nervous system cancers. Carcinomas (malignant tumours of epithelial tissues such as breast, GIT, lung and skin) are rare in children, while sarcomas (malignant tumours of connective tissues such as bone and muscle) are more common in children. Because tumours in children grow rapidly, cancers are generally more responsive to treatment than in adults; children also tend to tolerate acute adverse effects of chemotherapy better than adults. Of all children with cancer, more than 80% become long-term survivors or are cured.

Cancer in those of reproductive age

Antineoplastic drugs may have deleterious effects on reproduction. At different stages of life, factors to be considered are:

- Children treated with cytotoxic agents, especially alkylating agents, may show infertility in later years.
- Alkylating agents administered to adults may cause lowered sperm count in men and infertility due to ovarian failure in women.
- Most cytotoxic agents are mutagenic and potentially teratogenic, and should not be taken during pregnancy. Effective contraception should be practised if either partner is being administered antineoplastic agents.
- Most antineoplastic drugs can be secreted into breast milk and are likely to be toxic to a baby. Breastfeeding should be avoided unless indicated safe by the oncologist.

The importance of preserving fertility in both children and young adults, male and female, requiring drug or radiation therapy for cancer is recognised, especially as most children now survive cancer to reproductive age. For those at significant risk of later infertility, cryopreservation of sperm or ovarian tissue may be considered.

Cancer in older adults

The incidence of cancer increases with age, with about 70% of new cancers occurring in people aged 60 and older. Cancer risk is related to duration of exposure to exogenous carcinogens, such as cigarette smoke, radiation or chemicals, or endogenous mutations; older people are most likely to have accumulated mutations causing cell transformation and cancer. Older people also generally have more concurrent illnesses and less compensatory

capacity compared with younger cancer patients, making them more vulnerable to effects of cancer or of antineoplastic drugs. There is increased possibility of impaired liver or kidney functions reducing drug clearance, polypharmacy and interactions with many drugs, reduced independence and income and loss of friends and family support. Efficacy of chemotherapy is not age-dependent, so dose reduction based on age alone is not always appropriate. Treatment approaches should be based on physiological parameters in the person and the specific cancer.

Clinical trials of anticancer drugs

Because of their potential for severe toxicity, antineoplastic drugs may be fast-tracked through phase I healthy volunteer trials into phase II clinical trials, in a small number of people with the condition to be treated, starting with low doses and regular monitoring for safety and efficacy. People are often invited to participate in multi-centre clinical trials, as cooperation between clinicians and researchers in several oncology units will increase the rate of participant recruitment and thus reduce time taken for trials to be completed, results published and new therapies implemented.

Special access schemes

A Special Access Scheme is administered in Australia by the Therapeutic Goods Administration. It covers importation or supply of an unapproved therapeutic drug or device for a single person on a case-by-case basis. The medical practitioner must provide details of the participant, product and prescriber, and give clinical justification for the application. The Special Access Scheme may be applied in the case of seriously ill people who may benefit from a new antineoplastic drug that is being used overseas but has not yet been approved for general use in Australia.

Orphan drugs

Many antineoplastic drugs are considered 'orphan drugs' and are subsidised under the Pharmaceutical Benefits Scheme's PBS-S100 initiative, despite being expensive or rarely used. These drugs include antineoplastic monoclonal antibodies, kinase inhibitors, taxanes and vinca alkaloids.

KEY POINTS

Clinical aspects of treating cancer

- Treatment guidelines and protocols provide useful recommendations relating to clinical presentation, workup, findings, primary treatment, pathological stage, adjunct treatments, surveillance and survivorship.
- Treatment regimens usually combine drugs that act by different mechanisms, with different specific adverse effects; this minimises toxicity and development of drug resistance.
- Adverse drug reactions common to cytotoxic drugs include damage to other rapidly dividing cells (bone marrow, hair, skin, gastrointestinal mucosa), nausea and vomiting, kidney tubule damage and hyperuricaemia.
- Long-term adverse effects include the risks of sterility or mutagenic, carcinogenic and teratogenic actions (hence the importance of safe handling of cytotoxic agents) and the development of drug resistance.

REVIEW EXERCISES

1. Mr AH has presented to you with a positive faecal occult blood test and is concerned that he may have cancer. Consult an international cancer treatment guideline (e.g. NCCN or ESMO), and formulate an intervention plan for this patient.
2. Ms SB has been diagnosed with colon cancer and is starting chemotherapy with a FOLFOX6 regimen. Discuss the three considerations used to select drugs for combination antineoplastic chemotherapy and identify how this regimen addresses the principles.
3. Ms AF is about to begin chemotherapy with CMFP for breast cancer and is worried about the adverse effects that she may experience. Identify the common set of adverse reactions caused by most cytotoxic drugs and discuss the physiological basis and potential clinical consequences of these adverse reactions.

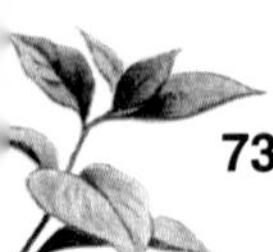

REFERENCES

Australian Medicines Handbook 2021. Australian medicines handbook, Adelaide, AMH.

Beare PG, Myers JL: Adult health nursing, ed 3, St Louis, MO, 1998, Mosby.

Hanahan D, Weinberg RA: Hallmarks of cancer: the next generation. Cell 144:646–674, 2011.

Hanahan D, Weinberg RA: The hallmarks of cancer. Cell 100:57–70, 2000.

Mueller-Schoell A, Groenland SL, Scherf-Clavel O, et al: Therapeutic drug monitoring of oral targeted antineoplastic drugs. European Journal of Clinical Pharmacology 77: 441–464, 2021.

Salerno E: Pharmacology for health professionals, St Louis, MO, 1999, Mosby.

Sun J, Wei Q, Zhou Y, et al: A systematic analysis of FDA-approved anticancer drugs. BMC Systems Biology 11, 87, 2017.

— CHAPTER 33 —

ANTINEOPLASTIC DRUGS

Andrew Rowland

KEY ABBREVIATIONS

ER estrogen receptor
KI kinase inhibitor
mAb monoclonal antibody
mTOR mammalian target of rapamycin

KEY TERMS

alkylating agents 732
antimetabolites 732
cytotoxic agents 732
immunomodulatory drugs 748
kinase inhibitor 744
monoclonal antibodies 744
non-cytotoxic 743

Chapter Focus

Antineoplastic drugs are used along with surgery and radiation therapy to treat cancer. An understanding of molecular biology is particularly important for identifying the pathways underlying the development of cancers and the mechanisms of antineoplastic drugs. In this chapter, the actions and clinical uses of cytotoxic and non-cytotoxic antineoplastics, hormonal antineoplastics and immunomodulatory drugs will be described. Cancer chemotherapy requires supportive adjunctive therapy, with modalities including antiemetic and analgesic drugs; these are also described.

KEY DRUG GROUPS

Cytotoxic antineoplastics:

- Alkylating agents: carboplatin, cisplatin, **cyclophosphamide**, dacarbazine, lomustine, lomustine, temozolomide
- Antimetabolites: capecitabine, **fluorouracil**, gemcitabine, mercaptopurine, **methotrexate**
- Cytotoxic antibiotics: bleomycin, doxorubicin, epirubicin
- Mitotic inhibitors: docetaxel, paclitaxel, vincristine
- Topoisomerase inhibitors: etoposide, irinotecan, topotecan
- Proteasome inhibitors: bortezomib

Hormonal antineoplastics:

- Antiandrogens: enzalutamide, flutamide
- Antiestrogens: fulvestrant, raloxifene, **tamoxifen**
- Aromatase inhibitors: anastrozole, exemestane
- Gonadotrophin-releasing hormone analogues: goserelin, leuprorelin

Immunomodulatory drugs:

- Colony-stimulating factors: filgrastim, pegfilgrastim
- Immune checkpoint inhibitors: ipilimumab, nivolumab, pembrolizumab
- Interferons: interferon alpha, interferon gamma

Non-cytotoxic antineoplastics:

- Monoclonal antibodies: bevacizumab, cetuximab, rituximab, trastuzumab
- mTOR inhibitors: everolimus, temsirolimus
- PARP inhibitors: olaparib
- Small molecule kinase inhibitors: axitinib, dabrafenib, erlotinib, gefitinib, lapatinib, imatinib, pazopanib, sorafenib, sunitinib, trametinib

CRITICAL THINKING SCENARIO

Bill, a 62-year-old male, has been diagnosed with lung cancer and is about to start treatment. There is a range of new cancer medicines that can be used to treat lung cancer, and before his doctor decides which treatment to prescribe Bill he orders a range of tests that includes a tumour mutation profile. Why is understanding tumour mutations important when selecting a treatment protocol, particularly for newer cancer medicines?

Cytotoxic antineoplastic drugs

Cytotoxic antineoplastic drugs act by interfering with cell proliferation or replication. They are divided into classes based on major mechanisms of action; the phases of the cell cycle where many classes of cytotoxic antineoplastics act. Adverse effects tend to be specific for individual drugs but can be common to a class of drugs. All antiproliferative agents impair rapidly dividing cells, and so are likely to cause myelosuppression (impaired bone marrow production of blood cells), alopecia, gastrointestinal tract (GIT) irritation, infertility, possible secondary malignancies and tissue damage after inadvertent extravasation. Febrile neutropenia resulting from myelosuppression is a major dose-limiting toxicity for most **cytotoxic agents** (Clinical Focus Box 33.1). While these drugs remain a mainstay of many protocols, their use is being phased out with the increasing development and regulatory approval of newer targeted cancer medicines (Lasala et al. 2020).

Alkylating agents

Alkylating agents were the first class of drugs applied clinically in the modern era of antineoplastic drug therapy (Table 33.1). They are still commonly used. Alkylating agents contain highly reactive alkyl (e.g. methyl, ethyl) groups that bind to nitrogen atoms in guanine bases of deoxyribonucleic acid (DNA), forming strong bonds. Most alkylating agents are bifunctional in that they contain two alkyl groups that can either bind twice to one strand of DNA forming an intra-strand link along the DNA strand, or once to each strand of DNA forming a crosslink across the two DNA strands (Fig 33.1). These links between guanine bases cause breakage of the DNA strand when the cell initiates repair or replication, which leads to apoptosis (programmed cell death). The cell cycle is blocked mainly at the S phase before the G2 phase, and cell proliferation is slowed or stopped. Various types of alkylating agents are available. The main drug classes are the nitrogen mustard analogues, nitrosoureas and platinum-based agents. Other important drugs are busulfan (alkyl sulfonate), dacarbazine and temozolomide (triazenes), and procarbazine.

Nitrogen mustards

Nitrogen mustards, in particular cyclophosphamide (Drug Monograph 33.1), remain a core component of many chemotherapy regimens, particularly those used to treat haematological malignancies. The nitrogen mustard analogue chlormethine (mustine) was the prototypic alkylating agent and the first drug to demonstrate clinical efficacy as an anticancer medicine. This drug is now rarely used because it causes excessive toxicity.

Nitrosoureas

Nitrosoureas are highly lipophilic alkylating agents that readily cross the blood–brain barrier so are useful in treating primary brain tumours. In practice, carmustine and lomustine are used to treat brain cancers including high-grade gliomas such as anaplastic astrocytoma and glioblastoma multiforme.

Platinum compounds

Cisplatin, carboplatin and oxaliplatin are sometimes considered alkylating agents because they have similar mechanisms of action. In cisplatin, the platinum atom is bonded to two amine groups, which cross-link between DNA strands. Cisplatin is particularly emetogenic, and most likely to cause nephrotoxicity and neurotoxicity. The three platinum compounds have different indications, contraindications, adverse drug reactions and dosage and administration guidelines, so specialist oncology protocols should be consulted.

Antimetabolites

Antimetabolites impair the use of endogenous chemicals involved in metabolic processes. These drugs are typically similar in structure to the endogenous chemical.

CLINICAL FOCUS BOX 33.1
Febrile neutropenia caused by cytotoxic chemotherapy

Myelosuppression caused by cytotoxic antineoplastic drugs often results in a marked reduction in the number of neutrophils present in the blood. This reduction in neutrophil count (neutropenia) markedly increases a cancer patient's risk of contracting an infection and reduces their ability to fight off the infection. Febrile neutropenia is the development of fever (often with other signs of infection) in a person with neutropenia, and is a time-critical and potentially life-threatening complication of cytotoxic chemotherapy that people with cancer and all health professionals, including those working in community, prehospital and acute hospital settings, need to be able to recognise and respond to quickly.

People with cancer who present with febrile neutropenia should be treated with empirical antibiotics until their absolute neutrophil count has recovered to greater than 500/mm^3 and the fever has abated. If the neutrophil count does not improve, treatment may need to continue for 2 or more weeks. The latest guidelines from the Infectious Diseases Society of America, updated in 2010, recommend using different antibiotic combinations in specific settings; low-risk people can be treated with a combination of oral amoxicillin–clavulanic acid and ciprofloxacin, while more severe cases require the use of cefepime, carbapenems (meropenem and imipenem/cilastatin) or piperacillin/tazobactam. People who do not fulfil the criteria of low-risk patients should be admitted to hospital and treated as high-risk patients. In cases of recurrent or persistent fevers, addition of an antifungal agent may be considered.

TABLE 33.1 Overview of major alkylating agents

DRUG	EXAMPLE INDICATIONS[a]	COMMON TOXICITIES[b]
Nitrogen mustards		
Bendamustine	Chronic lymphocytic leukaemia, non-Hodgkin lymphomas	Infusion reactions, hepatotoxicity, hypokalaemia
Chlorambucil	Chronic lymphocytic leukaemia, lymphoma, Waldenstrom macroglobulinaemia	
Cyclophosphamide	See Drug Monograph 33.1	Haemorrhagic cystitis, nasal congestion (with rapid injection)
Ifosfamide	Sarcomas, testicular cancer, lymphomas	Haemorrhagic cystitis, nephrotoxicity, neurotoxicity
Nitrosoureas		
Carmustine	Gliomas (including anaplastic astrocytoma, glioblastoma multiforme), multiple myeloma	*Injection*: pulmonary fibrosis and/or infiltrates, burning at injection site *Implant*: cerebrospinal leakage, intracranial infection, oedema, seizure, subdural fluid collection *Topical*: dermatitis, erythema, hyperpigmentation, pain, telangiectasia
Fotemustine	Malignant melanoma	Hepatotoxicity, neurotoxicity
Lomustine	Glioma, Hodgkin's lymphoma, medulloblastoma	
Platinum compounds		
Carboplatin	Ovarian cancer, small cell and non-small cell lung cancer, squamous cell head and neck cancer	Arthralgia, electrolyte disturbance, hypersensitivity reactions including anaphylaxis, myalgia, nephrotoxicity, ototoxicity, peripheral neuropathy, taste disturbance, weakness
Cisplatin	Bladder cancer, cervical cancer, gastric cancer, germ cell tumours, mesothelioma, oesophageal cancer, osteosarcoma, ovarian cancer, small cell and non-small cell lung cancer, squamous cell head and neck cancer	Electrolyte disturbance, hypersensitivity reactions including anaphylaxis, local phlebitis, myasthenia-like syndrome, nephrotoxicity, ototoxicity, peripheral neuropathy
Oxaliplatin	Colorectal cancer, gastric cancer, oesophageal cancer	Arthralgia, cough, electrolyte disturbance, dysphagia, dyspnoea, hypersensitivity reactions including anaphylaxis, metabolic acidosis, myalgia, nephrotoxicity, peripheral neuropathy, taste disturbance, weakness
Others		
Busulfan	Chronic myeloid leukaemia, myelofibrosis	Hepatotoxicity, neurotoxicity including seizures, rash, tachycardia
Dacarbazine	Hodgkin lymphoma, metastatic malignant melanoma, soft tissue sarcoma	Flu-like syndrome, flushing, neurotoxicity, pain along injected vein
Procarbazine	Hodgkin lymphoma, glioma	Neurotoxicity
Temozolomide	Gliomas (including anaplastic astrocytoma, glioblastoma multiforme), metastatic malignant melanoma	Dyspnoea, fever, headache, malaise, pain, rigors, weight loss

Australian Medicines Handbook (2017); eviQ cancer treatment protocols.
[a] May be included in various other treatment protocols.
[b] In addition to alopecia, GIT disorders (including abdominal pain, anorexia, bleeding, diarrhoea, nausea, oral mucositis and vomiting) and myelosuppression.
Sources: eviQ cancer treatment protocols.

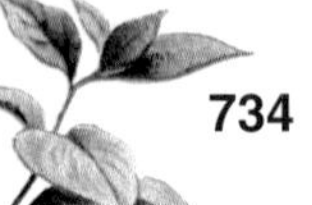

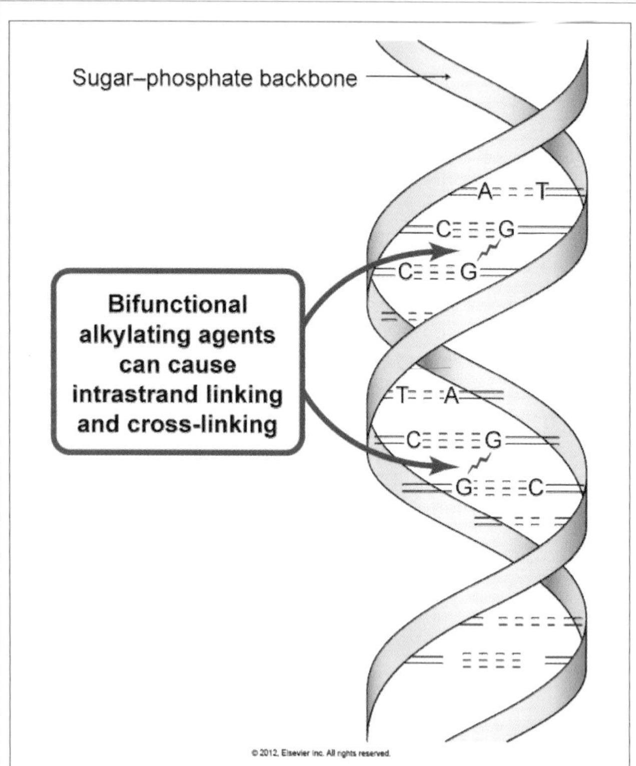

FIGURE 33.1 The effects of bifunctional alkylating agents on DNA
A = adenine; C = cytosine; G = guanine; T = thymine
Source: Rang et al. 2012, Figure 55.3; reproduced with permission from Elsevier.

Drug Monograph 33.1
Cyclophosphamide

Cyclophosphamide is an alkylating agent that interferes with cellular replication by forming intra-strand links along, or cross-links between, DNA strands.

Indications

A component of chemotherapy treatment protocols for multiple haematological and solid organ cancers including acute lymphoblastic leukaemia, breast cancer, chronic lymphocytic leukaemia, lymphoma, multiple myeloma, sarcoma and Waldenstrom macroglobulinaemia.

Pharmacokinetics

Cyclophosphamide may be administered orally or intravenously. Cyclophosphamide is rapidly absorbed following oral administration with a bioavailability of approximately 75%. Peak cyclophosphamide concentrations occur at around 1 hour after oral dosing, although the onset of action is a little slower at 2–3 hours as the drug requires cytochrome P450 (CYP)-mediated metabolic activation. Cyclophosphamide distributes throughout the body, including the brain and cerebrospinal fluid and has a volume of distribution of approximately 50 L. The elimination half-life is 4–6 hours.

Drug interactions

Increased bone marrow depression may occur when cyclophosphamide is co-administered with immunosuppressant drugs, increasing the risk of infections and secondary neoplasia. Drugs that induce CYP2B6 or CYP3A4 increase the metabolic activation of cyclophosphamide, and may enhance the therapeutic and toxic effects of this drug.

Adverse reactions

Cyclophosphamide commonly causes alopecia, anorexia, haemorrhagic cystitis, myelosuppression and nasal congestion. Myelosuppression is the major dose-limiting toxicity, with neutrophil nadir occurring 7–14 days after dosing with recovery over 1–2 weeks; thrombocytopenia and anaemia are less common. Haemorrhagic cystitis occurs with high doses or prolonged low doses, due to accumulation of metabolites in the bladder.

Dosage and administration

Cyclophosphamide is formulated as 50 mg tablets and powder (500 mg, 1 g or 2 g) for injection. Dosing differs between treatment protocols.

Antimetabolites used to treat cancer are analogues of folic acid, purine or pyrimidine (Table 33.2). They inhibit enzymes involved in pathways for nucleic acid synthesis and/or act as false 'building blocks', causing damaged polymers of nucleic acids to be built up into impaired DNA and ribonucleic acid (RNA). Hydroxyurea inhibits DNA synthesis by interfering with conversion of ribonucleotides to deoxyribonucleotides; it is also considered an antimetabolite.

Folic acid antagonists

Folic acid is an essential co-factor for the synthesis of purines nucleotides and thymidylate, which in turn are essential for DNA synthesis and cellular replication. The anticancer effects of folic acid antagonists are primarily achieved by interfering with thymidylate synthesis. Methotrexate (Drug Monograph 33.2) is the main drug in this class, and is one of the most commonly used antimetabolites. As shown in Figure 33.2, methotrexate competes with dihydrofolate for binding to the active site of the enzyme dihydrofolate reductase (DHFR). In doing so, methotrexate blocks the synthesis of tetrahydrofolate, which is the essential co-factor for thymidylate synthesis by the enzyme thymidylate synthetase.

Purine and pyrimidine antagonists

Purine and pyrimidine base analogues such as mercaptopurine and fluorouracil (Drug Monograph 33.3)

TABLE 33.2 Overview of major classes of antimetabolites

DRUG	EXAMPLE INDICATIONS[a]	COMMON TOXICITIES[b]
Folic acid antagonists		
Methotrexate	See Drug Monograph 33.2	Hepatotoxicity, neurotoxicity, photosensitivity, pulmonary toxicity, rash, urticaria
Pemetrexed	Malignant mesothelioma, non-squamous NSCLC	Conjunctivitis, desquamation, fever, hepatotoxicity, hypersensitivity (rarely anaphylaxis), nephrotoxicity, oedema, peripheral neuropathy, pharyngitis, rash, taste disturbance
Raltitrexed	Colorectal cancer	Fever, flu-like symptoms, hepatotoxicity, rash, weakness
Purine antagonists		
Cladribine	Chronic lymphocytic leukaemia, hairy cell leukaemia, Waldenstrom macroglobulinaemia	Arthralgia, cough, fever, infusion site reactions, myalgia, neurotoxicity, oedema, rash, trunk pain, tachycardia, weakness
Clofarabine	Acute lymphoblastic leukaemia	Arthralgia, bleeding, cytokine release, fever, flushing, hand–foot syndrome, hepatotoxicity, hypersensitivity, hypokalaemia, hypotension, myalgia, nephrotoxicity, oedema, neurotoxicity, tachycardia
Fludarabine	Acute myeloid leukaemia, chronic lymphocytic leukaemia, non-Hodgkin lymphoma, Waldenstrom macroglobulinaemia	Chills, fever, hepatotoxicity, hyperglycaemia, malaise, neurotoxicity, oedema, paraesthesia, rash
Mercaptopurine	Acute lymphoblastic leukaemia, acute promyelocytic leukaemia, lymphoblastic lymphoma	Hepatotoxicity
Thioguanine	Acute lymphoblastic leukaemia, acute myeloid leukaemia	Hepatotoxicity
Pyrimidine antagonists		
Azacitidine	Acute myeloid leukaemia, chronic myelomonocytic leukaemia, myelodysplastic syndromes	Anorexia, bleeding, dyspnoea, erythema, fever, hypokalaemia, injection site reactions, neurotoxicity, rash
Capecitabine	Breast cancer, colorectal cancer, gastric cancer, oesophageal cancer	Anorexia, cardiotoxicity, conjunctivitis, hand–foot syndrome, hepatotoxicity, nephrotoxicity, neurotoxicity, rash, skin pigmentation, taste disturbance, weakness
Cytarabine	Acute lymphoblastic leukaemia, acute myeloid leukaemia, chronic myeloid leukaemia, lymphomas, meningeal leukaemia	Anorexia, neurotoxicity, ocular toxicity, pulmonary toxicity
Fluorouracil	See Drug Monograph 33.3	Cardiotoxicity, hand–foot syndrome, rash
Gemcitabine	Bladder cancer, breast cancer, lymphomas, nasopharyngeal cancer, NSCLC, ovarian cancer, pancreatic cancer	Fever, flu-like symptoms, haematuria, hepatotoxicity, peripheral oedema, phlebitis, proteinuria, pulmonary toxicity, rash

[a] May be included in various other treatment protocols.
[b] In addition to alopecia, GIT disorders (including abdominal pain, bleeding, diarrhoea, nausea, oral mucositis and vomiting) and myelosuppression.
NSCLC = non-small cell lung cancer
Sources: eviQ cancer treatment protocols.

can be incorporated into DNA strands in place of the true bases, forming permanently modified DNA and leading to improper base pairing and improper transcription to RNA. They may also act as specific inhibitors of enzymes involved in DNA synthesis (Fig 33.3). These drugs act particularly at the S phase of the cell cycle.

Capecitabine is a prodrug for 5-fluorouracil. It was rationally designed to be 'tumour-activated' after oral administration. It is metabolised in three stages, the last of which involves thymidine phosphorylase, an enzyme more active in liver and tumour cells than in normal cells. This strategy results in 2.5-fold higher exposure to fluorouracil in tumour cells compared with adjacent tissue, thus facilitating more selective toxicity. Capecitabine is particularly effective in treating breast, gastric and colorectal cancers.

Colaspase

Colaspase is a form of asparaginase produced from cultures of *Escherichia coli* that may be classed as an antimetabolite, as it exploits differences between metabolic pathways in normal and neoplastic cells. The enzyme asparaginase hydrolyses the amino acid l-asparagine to l-aspartic acid and ammonia. Asparagine is necessary for cell survival; normal cells can synthesise adequate supplies, so they are unaffected by asparagine deficiency. Cancer cells that are unable to synthesise asparagine are vulnerable to administration of asparaginase. Due to the risk of allergic reactions, including anaphylaxis, colaspase should only be administered in a hospital setting after a subcutaneous test dose.

Drug Monograph 33.2
Methotrexate

Methotrexate is a folic acid antagonist that inhibits DNA synthesis and cell replication by competitively inhibiting the conversion of folic acid to folinic acid.

Indications

Methotrexate is used in treatment protocols for multiple cancers including breast cancer, bladder cancer, squamous cell cancer of head and neck, gestational trophoblastic disease, acute leukaemias, non-Hodgkin lymphomas, osteosarcoma and brain tumours.

Pharmacokinetics

Methotrexate may be administered orally or intravenously. Low-dose methotrexate has an oral bioavailability of approximately 60%, which increases at higher doses, possibly due to saturation of intestinal efflux pathways. Its volume of distribution is 15–20 L following a single dose, increasing to around 40 L with steady-state dosing. Methotrexate undergoes hepatic and intracellular metabolism to polyglutamate forms, which can be converted back to methotrexate by hydrolase enzymes. Methotrexate's elimination half-life of 3–10 hours.

Drug interactions

Co-administration with hepatotoxic drugs increases the risk of hepatotoxicity and should be avoided; when this is not possible, monitoring of liver enzymes is recommended. High-dose aspirin and other non-steroidal anti-inflammatory drugs (NSAIDs) cause additive platelet inhibition and should be avoided. Low-dose aspirin may be used concurrently. Probenecid and salicylates reduce methotrexate excretion and increase the risk of toxicity.

Adverse reactions

Methotrexate causes neutropenia, thrombocytopenia and anaemia. Methotrexate commonly causes transient and asymptomatic increases in aminotransferases. Chronic hepatotoxicity generally only occurs with long-term treatment. Pulmonary toxicity can develop rapidly and be fatal. Toxicities may also commonly affect the GIT system (oral mucositis, nausea and vomiting), central nervous system (meningitis, encephalopathy, leukoencephalopathy) and skin (itch, photosensitivity, rash, urticaria).

Dosage and administration

Methotrexate may be administered orally, by intramuscular, intravenous, subcutaneous or intrathecal injection, or by intravenous infusion. Dose depends on the indication, and specific treatment guidelines should be consulted.

Cytotoxic antibiotics

Anthracyclines are the main class of cytotoxic antibiotics, but there are a number of other individual drugs: dactinomycin, bleomycin and mitomycin (Table 33.3). Cytotoxic antibiotics are defined as antibiotics because they are isolated from a microorganism (usually fungi) and act against another organism (neoplastic cells).

Anthracyclines

Anthracyclines are complex polycyclic molecules derived from *Streptomyces* bacteria. These drugs mainly exert their antitumour activity by:

- directly binding to DNA (intercalating), thus inhibiting DNA and RNA synthesis
- stabilising the DNA-topoisomerase II complex, preventing relaxation of supercoiled DNA
- producing reactive free radicals that damage tumour cells.

In addition to the standard toxicities that are associated with the use of cytotoxic drugs, potential irreversible cardiac toxicity may occur with all drugs in this class. This toxicity may be acute, chronic or delayed. Acute ECG changes and arrhythmias (acute toxicity) occur during or immediately after infusion and are not dose-related. These changes are usually transient but may cause myopericarditis and cardiac failure in rare circumstances. Cardiomyopathy and heart failure (chronic toxicities) usually occur within a year of finishing treatment and are related to the cumulative exposure (i.e. the dose and duration of treatment). Delayed toxicities including arrhythmia, conduction disturbance, heart failure or ventricular dysfunction can occur years, or even decades, after treatment and are thought to be dose-related. The risk of cardiac toxicity is exacerbated by the use of other cardiotoxic drugs, including trastuzumab, and in people with pre-existing cardiac disease. Typically, clinicians will check cardiovascular function by echocardiogram prior to initiating treatment with an anthracycline.

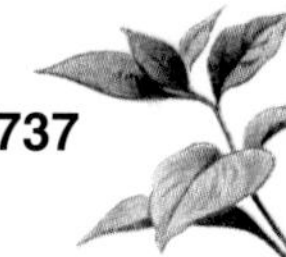

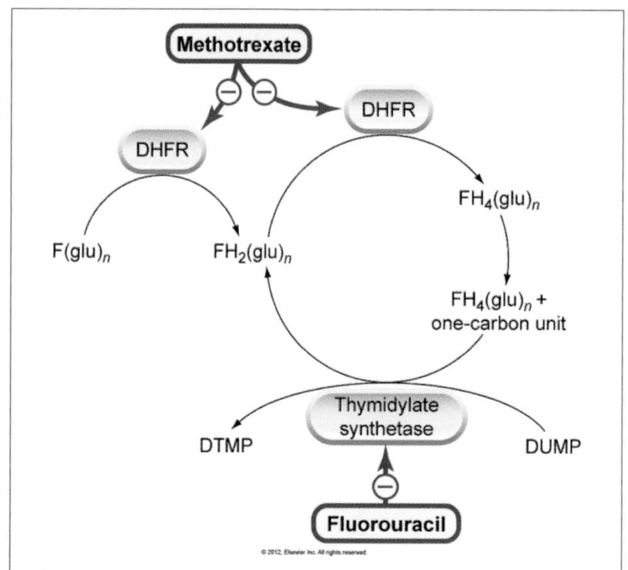

FIGURE 33.2 Simplified diagram of the actions of methotrexate and fluorouracil on thymidylate synthesis

Tetrahydrofolate polyglutamate $FH_4(glu)n$ functions as a carrier of a one-carbon unit, providing the methyl group necessary for the conversion of 2′-deoxyuridylate (DUMP) to 2′-deoxythymidylate (DTMP) by thymidylate synthetase. This one-carbon transfer results in the oxidation of $FH_4(glu)n$ to $FH_2(glu)_n$. Fluorouracil is converted to FDUMP, which inhibits thymidylate synthetase. DHFR = dihydrofolate reductase

Source: Rang et al. 2012, Figure 55.6; reproduced with permission from Elsevier.

Dactinomycin

Dactinomycin (also known as actinomycin-D) is a complex polypeptide antibiotic isolated from *Streptomyces* soil bacteria. This drug is an intercalating agent and topoisomerase II inhibitor; it interferes with DNA-dependent RNA synthesis and is an immunosuppressant.

Bleomycin and mitomycin

Bleomycin antibiotics, isolated from a *Streptomyces* species, have complex glycopeptide structures; family members differ in substituents on the tail of the molecule. 'Bleomycin' is a mixture mainly of bleomycins A_2 and B_2. Bleomycin antibiotics have cytotoxic and mutagenic actions; they chelate metal ions, generate reactive free radicals, degrade preformed DNA into fragmented chains and block incorporation of thymidine into DNA. They cause little bone marrow suppression or immunosuppression but can cause pulmonary fibrosis in up to 50% of people. Mitomycin has actions similar to bleomycin and alkylating agents.

Mitotic inhibitors

Taxanes and vinca alkaloids are antineoplastic agents isolated from plants. During the metaphase stage of mitotic division, replicated chromosomes line up on a spindle formed by microtubules. Vinca alkaloids and taxanes bind to tubulin, a constituent of microtubules, which inhibits its polymerisation into microtubules and disrupts spindle formation. This activates the

Drug Monograph 33.3
Fluorouracil

Fluorouracil (also called 5-FU) undergoes intracellular conversion to active metabolites that inhibit thymidylate synthase and interfere with DNA and RNA synthesis.

Indications

Fluorouracil is used in treatment protocols for solid organ malignancies including anal, breast, colorectal, gastric, head and neck, oesophageal and pancreatic cancer.

Pharmacokinetics

Fluorouracil is minimally (~10%) bound to plasma proteins and exhibits modest distribution throughout the body, including the intestinal mucosa, bone marrow, liver, cerebrospinal fluid and brain tissue, with a small volume of distribution of approximately 20 L. Around 5–20% of the parent drug is excreted unchanged in the urine. The remaining drug is metabolised in the liver, primarily by CYP enzymes. Fluorouracil's elimination half-life is dose-dependent, increasing from 8 to 20 minutes.

Drug interactions

Fluorouracil should not be administered to people receiving drugs known to modulate dihydropyrimidine dehydrogenase. Allopurinol reduces fluorouracil efficacy; this interaction can be exploited to minimise the oral mucositis caused by fluorouracil through the use of allopurinol mouthwash.

Adverse reactions

Severe diarrhoea may be dose-limiting, particularly when given with calcium folinate. Other gastrointestinal effects including nausea, vomiting and oral mucositis are also common. Myelosuppression - including neutropenia, thrombocytopenia and anaemia - occurs more commonly with bolus. Cardiotoxicity usually occurs during, or shortly after, the first round of treatment and is thought to be due to coronary vasospasm. The most common symptom is angina-like chest pain with or without ECG changes. Skin toxicities including hand–foot syndrome, itch and maculopapular rash are also common.

Dosage and administration

Fluorouracil should be administered by slow intravenous infusion over 4 hours or by continuous infusion over 24 hours or longer. Dose depends on the indication, and specific treatment guidelines should be consulted.

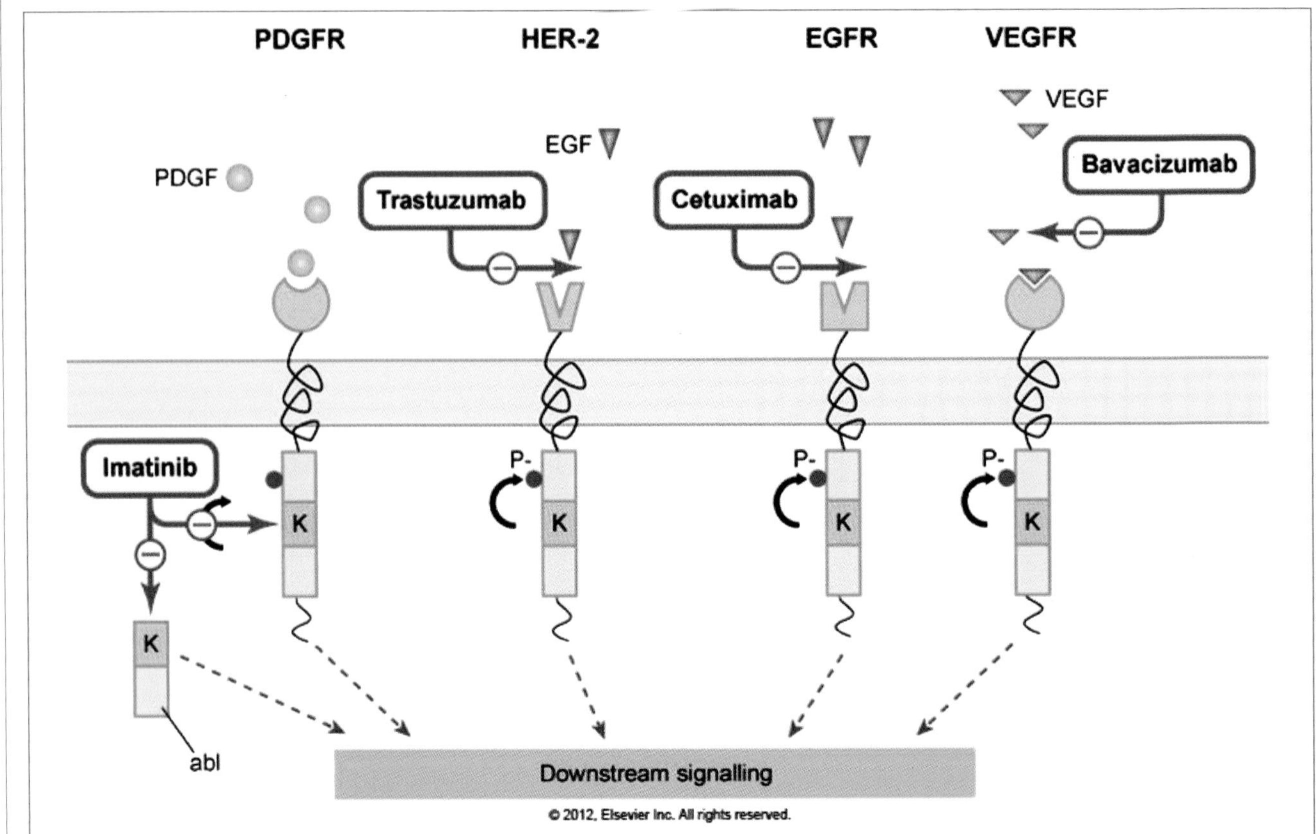

FIGURE 33.3 Molecular targets and mechanism of action of antineoplastic monoclonal antibodies and small molecule kinase inhibitors

Source: Rang et al. 2012, Figure 55.8; reproduced with permission from Elsevier.

TABLE 33.3 Overview of cytotoxic antibiotics

DRUG	EXAMPLE INDICATIONS[a]	COMMON TOXICITIES[b,c]
Anthracyclines		
Daunorubicin	Acute lymphoblastic leukaemia, acute myeloid leukaemia	Phlebitis, thrombophlebitis
Doxorubicin	Acute lymphoblastic leukaemia, bladder cancer, breast cancer, lymphomas, multiple myeloma, neuroblastoma, sarcomas, Wilms' tumour	Infusion reactions, rash
Doxorubicin (pegylated)	Breast cancer, Kaposi's sarcoma, ovarian cancer, multiple myeloma	Allergy, fever, hand–foot syndrome, infusion reactions, paraesthesia, rash
Epirubicin	Bladder cancer, breast cancer, gastric cancer	Local erythema, facial flushing
Mitozantrone	Acute myeloid leukaemia, non-Hodgkin lymphoma, prostate cancer	Rash
Others		
Bleomycin	Germ cell tumours, Hodgkin lymphoma	Chills, fevers, nail changes, pulmonary toxicity, Raynaud's phenomenon, skin reactions
Dactinomycin	Gestational trophoblastic disease, rhabdomyosarcoma, Wilms' tumour	Acne, fever, malaise, myalgia, pharyngitis, rash

[a] May be included in various other treatment protocols.
[b] In addition to alopecia, GIT disorders (including abdominal pain, bleeding, diarrhoea, nausea, oral mucositis and vomiting) and myelosuppression.
[c] As a class, anthracyclines also commonly cause cardiac toxicity (may be acute, chronic or delayed), extravascularisation and secondary malignancies.

Sources: eviQ cancer treatment protocols.

spindle-assembly checkpoint and arrests the cell cycle in mitosis. Mitotic inhibitors generally also have other actions contributing to their cytotoxic effects; for example, the vinca alkaloids impair uridine incorporation into mRNA. Unfortunately, resistance to these drugs develops readily.

Taxanes

Cabazitaxel, docetaxel and paclitaxel (Table 33.4) have antimitotic and immunostimulatory effects; they stabilise microtubules, inhibit mitosis and initiate apoptosis. They also stimulate immune responses and regulate lymphocyte activation. Dexamethasone is usually given before the taxane drug to minimise the risk of oedema and allergic reactions.

Vinca alkaloids

Vincristine and vinblastine, isolated from *Catharanthus roseus* (also called *Vinca rosea*), and the related semi-synthetic alkaloids vinorelbine and vinflunine have varying therapeutic indications and adverse effects (Table 33.4). Neurotoxicity is a common and major dose-limiting toxicity for vincristine and, to a lesser extent, the other vinca alkaloids. Severity is related to the total cumulative and single dose exposures and often presents as autonomic (e.g. orthostatic hypotension, paralytic ileus and urinary retention) or peripheral neuropathy (e.g. paraesthesia, paralysis). In severe cases, motor function may be impaired, and temporary or permanent vestibular and auditory nerve damage may result in deafness, dizziness, nystagmus or vertigo.

Epothilones

Natural epothilones are extracted from the myxobacterium *Sorangium cellulosum*. Their actions are generally similar to those of taxanes, but early trials suggest that epothilones may have better efficacy and milder adverse effects. The prototypic drug in this class, ixabepilone, is used to treat metastatic breast cancer in the United States. The only drug in this class approved in Australia is eribulin, which is indicated for breast cancer and liposarcoma.

Topoisomerase inhibitors

Topoisomerase inhibitors are a class of drugs that impair the ability of topoisomerase I or II to regulate changes in DNA structure during the cell cycle.

Camptothecins (topoisomerase I inhibitors)

Irinotecan and topotecan are derivatives of camptothecin, which is isolated from the plant *Camptotheca acuminata*. These drugs inhibit topoisomerase I enzymes, which are involved in untwisting, nicking and resealing of DNA strands during DNA duplication, which causes breaks in double-stranded DNA, blocking macromolecular synthesis leading to tumour cell death.

Irinotecan, which is activated by hydrolysis to SN-38, is used to treat metastatic colorectal cancer and small cell lung cancer that has progressed after treatment with other cytotoxics. In addition to severe myelosuppression, nausea and vomiting, irinotecan also commonly causes a cholinergic syndrome, which often presents as severe

TABLE 33.4 Overview of mitotic inhibitors

DRUG	EXAMPLE INDICATIONS[a]	COMMON TOXICITIES[b,c]
Taxanes		
Cabazitaxel	Prostate cancer	Arrhythmia, cough, dyspnoea, haematuria, hypersensitivity, nephrotoxicity, taste disturbance
Docetaxel	Breast cancer, gastric cancer, non-small cell lung cancer, ovarian cancer, prostate cancer, squamous cell head and neck cancer	Fluid retention, hand–foot syndrome, hypersensitivity, lacrimal duct obstruction, rash, taste disturbance
Paclitaxel	Breast cancer, cervical cancer, endometrial cancer, germ cell cancer, Kaposi's sarcoma, non-small cell lung cancer, ovarian cancer	Bradycardia, hepatotoxicity, hypersensitivity, hypotension
Vinca alkaloids		
Vinblastine	Bladder cancer, germ cell tumours, Hodgkin lymphoma, non-small cell lung cancer	Neurotoxicity
Vincristine	Acute lymphoblastic leukaemia, brain tumours, lymphomas, multiple myeloma, neuroblastoma, sarcoma, Wilms' tumour	Anaphylaxis, chest pain, neurotoxicity
Vinflunine	Bladder cancer	Hyponatraemia, myalgia, neurotoxicity
Vinorelbine	Breast cancer, non-small cell lung cancer	Injection site reactions, neurotoxicity, phlebitis

[a] May be included in various other treatment protocols.
[b] In addition to alopecia, GIT disorders (including abdominal pain, bleeding, diarrhoea, nausea, oral mucositis and vomiting) and myelo-suppression.
Sources: eviQ cancer treatment protocols.

diarrhoea, but may also involve abdominal cramps, lacrimation, miosis, rhinitis, salivation or sweating. This toxicity requires immediate treatment with atropine or loperamide. Topotecan is used to treat relapsed or refractory cervical, ovarian and small cell lung cancers. Like many cytotoxic drugs, neutropenia is the major dose-limiting toxicity for topotecan; however, alopecia, anaemia, dyspnoea, GIT disturbances, headache, neuromuscular pain, thrombocytopenia and tiredness also occur commonly.

Podophyllotoxins (topoisomerase II inhibitors)

The podophyllin-type compounds etoposide and teniposide inhibit topoisomerase II, resulting in DNA strand breaks and inhibition of cell division in the late S and G2 phases of the cell cycle. They are sometimes called mitotic inhibitors as they cause metaphase arrest. These drugs are mainly used to treat leukaemias and lymphomas but may also be used to treat lung, ovarian and testicular cancers (etoposide) and neuroblastoma (teniposide). Podophyllotoxins cause many of the common toxicities associated with the use of cytotoxic antineoplastic drugs: alopecia, anorexia, diarrhoea, hypersensitivity reactions, myelosuppression, nausea and vomiting and oral mucositis.

Proteasome inhibitors

Proteasomes are large protease-containing complexes in cells in which ubiquitinated proteins are degraded. There are hundreds of ubiquitin-protein ligases by which chains of poly-ubiquitinated proteins can be formed and proteins targeted for destruction by proteolysis in proteasomes. Complete inhibition of proteasome functions kills cells, so researchers are seeking small molecule specific inhibitors for regulatory proteins in the proteasome complex.

Bortezomib is the first proteasome inhibitor used in humans; it can be classed with cytotoxic agents. Bortezomib disrupts various cell signalling pathways, leading to cell cycle arrest, apoptosis and inhibition of angiogenesis. It inhibits nuclear factor (NF)-kappa B, a protein that mediates cell survival in some cancers, so reduces tumour growth and angiogenesis, and enhances cytotoxic effects of radiation and chemotherapy. It is used to treat mantle cell lymphoma and multiple myeloma.

Topical cytotoxic agents

The number of skin cancers treated each year in Australia – melanomas, squamous cell carcinomas (SCC) and basal cell carcinomas (BCC) – exceeds that of all other cancers combined. Most skin cancers are removed surgically or with cryotherapy, or can be treated with radiotherapy. Topical formulations of antineoplastic agents have been developed for application to skin lesions; these may be equally effective for removal of SCCs and BCCs, with less facial scarring. Fluorouracil and imiquimod are administered topically, intentionally to cause a severe inflammatory reaction over a period of days or weeks; as the inflammatory reaction heals, cancerous and precancerous cells are cleared by the body's natural defences. Anti-inflammatory agents should not be used during the process, and sun exposure should be avoided.

Fluorouracil cream 5%

Fluorouracil is a pyrimidine antimetabolite, long used systemically to treat many cancers, including breast, gastrointestinal and head and neck cancers. The cream is applied topically to treat actinic keratoses and Bowen's disease (intra-epidermal SCC) twice daily for 3–4 weeks. There is little risk of systemic adverse effects; however, fluorouracil is contraindicated in pregnancy.

Methyl aminolevulinate hydrochloride

A cream formulation of this photosensitising drug is used in photodynamic therapy. In treating BCCs, Bowen's disease and solar keratoses, the cream is applied, then 3 hours later a special red light is applied that produces reactive oxygen radicals that selectively destroy tumour cells. The burning pain produced may require oral analgesics or local anaesthetic.

KEY POINTS

Cytotoxic antineoplastics

- Use of cytotoxic agents in cancer treatment is based on the effects of the drug in inhibiting regulation of replication or macromolecular synthesis in the cell cycle. These drugs are classified according to their potential mechanisms of action: alkylating agents, antimetabolites, antibiotic antitumour agents and mitotic inhibitors.
- Alkylating agents such as cyclophosphamide contain reactive alkyl groups that bind strongly to bases in DNA, thus impairing DNA replication and transcription of RNA.
- Antimetabolites are chemically related to folic acid (e.g. methotrexate) or to a purine or pyrimidine base (mercaptopurine, fluorouracil). They cause copying errors during DNA synthesis or inhibit enzymes in pathways to macromolecules DNA, RNA and proteins.

- Antibiotic antitumour agents include the anthracycline, bleomycin and actinomycin groups. These may bind to DNA, intercalate between DNA strands or inhibit topoisomerase II enzymes.
- Mitotic inhibitors such as vinca alkaloids and taxanes are M phase-specific agents.
- Cytotoxic drugs are usually non-selective, with antiproliferative actions on all rapidly dividing cells, commonly causing mouth ulceration, GIT dysfunction, bone marrow suppression and alopecia.

Hormonal antineoplastic drugs

Hormonal drugs are used to treat neoplasia that is sensitive to hormonal growth. For example, growth of prostate cancer is stimulated by androgens, breast cancers by estrogens and thyroid cancer by thyrotrophin. Hormones used in cancer treatments are not specifically antiproliferative in neoplastic cells, but have their usual hormonal actions, so are often more selective and less toxic than cytotoxic antineoplastics. Hormonal antineoplastic drugs include corticosteroids, androgens and antiandrogens, estrogens and antiestrogens, progestogens, hormone synthesis inhibitors and analogues of gonadotrophin-releasing hormone (GnRH) (Table 33.5). Often there are several options for treating hormone-sensitive cancers. For example, prostate cancer may be treated by:

- surgical removal of prostate and/or testes
- radiation
- administration of antiandrogenic drugs:
  - estrogenic hormones
  - GnRH analogues
  - GnRH antagonists
- administration of cytotoxic agents such as docetaxel.

TABLE 33.5 Overview of hormonal antineoplastic drugs

DRUGS	MAIN INDICATION	COMMON ADVERSE EFFECTS
Antiandrogens		
Non-steroidal: Bicalutamide Enzalutamide Flutamide Nilutamide *Steroidal:* Cyproterone	Prostate cancer	Body hair loss, breast pain, gynaecomastia, headache, hot flushes, impotence, itch, mood changes, reduced libido, sweating, weight changes
Selective estrogen receptor modulators		
Tamoxifen Toremifene	Hormone receptor-positive breast cancer	Hepatotoxicity, hot flushes, nausea, oedema, sweating, uterine polyps, vaginal discharge
Antiestrogens		
Fulvestrant Raloxifene	Hormone receptor-positive breast cancer	Anorexia, diarrhoea, headache, hepatotoxicity, hot flushes, injection site reactions, nausea, musculoskeletal pain, peripheral oedema, pharyngitis, rash, urinary tract infection, vomiting, weakness
Aromatase inhibitors		
Anastrozole Exemestane Letrozole	Hormone receptor-positive breast cancer	Alopecia, arthralgia, diarrhoea, fractures, headache, hot flushes, myalgia, nausea, peripheral oedema, rash, reduced bone density, vaginal dryness, vomiting, weakness
Gonadotrophin-releasing hormone analogues		
Goserelin Leuprorelin Riptorelin	Breast cancer, prostate cancer	*Males:* altered glucose tolerance, anaemia, diabetes, increased body fat, loss of body hair, muscle atrophy, weight gain *Females:* abdominal pain, decreased libido, dysmenorrhoea, headache, hot flushes, hypertension
Gonadotrophin-releasing hormone antagonists		
Degarelix	Prostate cancer	Anaemia, arthralgia, chills, constipation, erectile dysfunction, gynaecomastia, hepatotoxicity, hot flushes, injection site reactions, loss of libido, nausea, neurotoxicity, sweating, testicular atrophy, weight gain
Somatostatin analogues		
Lanreotide Octreotide	Gastroenteropancreatic neuroendocrine tumours	Abdominal pain, bradycardia, diarrhoea, fatigue, flatulence, gallstones, hair loss, hyperglycaemia, hypoglycaemia, injection site reactions, nausea, vomiting
Note: In addition, estrogens can be used in treatment of prostate cancers, and androgens in breast cancers.		

Androgens and antiandrogens

Androgens

Androgens such as testosterone are used to treat advanced breast cancer if surgery, radiation and other therapies are inappropriate or ineffective.

Antiandrogens

Antiandrogens inhibit uptake or binding of androgens at their target cells or receptors. Cyproterone (a partial agonist) is a steroidal antiandrogen, while bicalutamide, flutamide and nilutamide are non-steroidal antiandrogens. These drugs suppress ovarian and testicular steroidogenesis, thus inducing a 'medical castration', and are indicated in combination with surgery and a GnRH analogue in advanced prostate cancer.

Androgen synthesis inhibitors

Abiraterone is an orally active potent inhibitor of the CYP17 enzyme essential for synthesis of testosterone from cholesterol. Treatment with abiraterone causes rapid, complete inhibition of androgen synthesis, reducing residual androgens (after surgical or medical castration) and improving survival in men with castration-resistant metastatic prostate cancer. Abiraterone can cause fluid retention, secondary hyperaldosteronism with hypokalaemia and hypertension, so prednisolone should be given concurrently.

Estrogens and antiestrogens

Estrogens

Estrogens may be used to treat advanced breast carcinoma in postmenopausal women. They may also be used occasionally in breast cancer to 'recruit' resting cells from the G0 phase into active cell cycling again (G1 phase), so the cells will be sensitive to cytotoxic agents. Estrogens, including diethylstilboestrol and ethinylestradiol, have been used as antiandrogens to treat advanced prostatic carcinoma; however, they are now rarely used for this indication due to adverse cardiovascular and estrogenic effects.

Antiestrogens

Antiestrogens are drugs of first choice in postmenopausal breast cancers that are estrogen receptor (ER)-positive – that is, tumours that contain high concentrations of ERs. Antiestrogen therapy is less useful in premenopausal women because the effects are swamped by high levels of estrogens produced by the ovaries. Raloxifene is used to prevent postmenopausal osteoporosis, as it has estrogenic effects in bone, but antiestrogenic effects in uterus and breast tissues. It significantly reduces invasive cancer in women at increased risk of breast cancer. Fulvestrant, another antiestrogen, is used to treat hormone receptor-positive metastatic breast cancer in postmenopausal women with disease progression following other therapy.

Selective estrogen receptor modulators

Selective ER modulators were designed to block ERs in breast cancers but maintain ER agonist actions in tissues such as bone and the cardiovascular system where estrogen has protective actions. The main drugs in this class are tamoxifen (Drug Monograph 33.4) and toremifene. Tamoxifen is a synthetic non-steroidal antiestrogen with both agonist and antagonist effects; it is a partial agonist at ERs in breast cancer cells where it competitively inhibits estrogen. It is an estrogen agonist in the liver, with positive effects on plasma lipids, and helps to preserve bone mineral density and decrease osteoporosis risk in postmenopausal women. Toremifene has activity and adverse effects profiles that are similar to that of tamoxifen.

Aromatase inhibitors

In the biochemical synthesis of estrogens, a critical stage is 'aromatisation' of the steroid A ring, from testosterone to estradiol. In postmenopausal women, the main endogenous source of estrogens is from androgens via aromatase enzyme actions in peripheral (non-ovary) tissues. Compounds that inhibit aromatase include anastrozole, exemestane and letrozole. They are indicated for use in women with natural or induced postmenopausal status, whose breast cancer has progressed despite antiestrogen therapy. Aromatase inhibitors do not block synthesis of glucocorticoids or mineralocorticoids.

Gonadotrophin-releasing hormone analogues and antagonist

GnRH analogues

Synthetic GnRH peptide analogues such as goserelin, leuprorelin and triptorelin, when administered on a continuous basis, effectively suppress production of gonadotrophins from the pituitary gland, and thus have indirect antiandrogenic and antiestrogenic effects. They are used for gonadal suppression in precocious puberty, endometriosis, polycystic ovary syndrome and prostatic and premenopausal breast cancer.

Goserelin is used as a palliative agent in advanced prostate carcinoma. With chronic administration there is an initial surge in gonadotrophin release, causing a 'flare' in prostatic cancer growth that may exacerbate symptoms such as bone pain and obstruction to bladder outflow. Concentrations of testosterone drop to levels seen in surgically castrated men within 2–4 weeks. A 3.6-mg

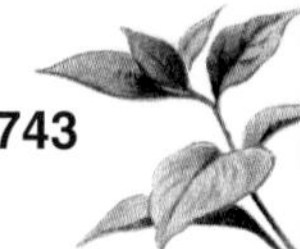

Drug Monograph 33.4
Tamoxifen

Tamoxifen acts as an antagonist at estrogen receptors in breast tissue, inhibiting tumour growth. It also has estrogen agonist activity on endometrium, bone and lipids, and can cause suppression of other growth factors and cytokines.

Indications

Tamoxifen is indicated for treating postmenopausal estrogen receptor positive breast cancer, and for prophylaxis in women at high risk.

Pharmacokinetics

Tamoxifen is administered orally and absorbed slowly, with peak concentrations observed 3–6 hours after administration. The drug is widely distributed throughout the body (apparent volume of distribution ~3500 L), including the ovaries and uterus. It is highly (> 99%) bound to plasma proteins and to estrogen receptors in target tissues. Tamoxifen is extensively metabolised in the liver and eliminated in the faeces. It has a long half-life of 4–11 days.

Drug interactions

Tamoxifen is a prodrug that is metabolised by CYP3A4 and CYP2D6 to active metabolites. Drugs that induce CYP2D6 or CYP3A4 increase the metabolic activation of tamoxifen and may enhance the therapeutic and toxic effects. Tamoxifen increases the anticoagulant effects of warfarin; international normalised ratio should be monitored and the dose of warfarin may require reduction.

Adverse reactions

Abnormal gynaecological reactions such as vaginal bleeding and hot flushes are common, and endometrial changes such as polyps and cancer can develop. Other common adverse reactions include alopecia and leg cramps.

Dosage and administration

Usual dose is 20 mg/day; in advanced breast cancer, the dose may be increased to 40 mg/day.

dose as a prolonged-release formulation is implanted subcutaneously in the anterior abdominal wall every 28 days.

GnRH antagonist

'Chemical castration' can also be induced with the GnRH antagonist degarelix. It blocks pituitary receptors, thus reducing testosterone levels (without the surge caused by GnRH agonists) and causing regression of prostate cancer and lowered prostate-specific antigen.

Somatostatin analogues

Analogues of somatostatin are used to treat cancers of the pituitary gland that produce excess growth hormone (causing acromegaly) and in carcinoid tumours of the GIT that secrete excess 5-hydroxytryptamine. The analogues are octreotide and lanreotide; adverse reactions in the GIT are common (Table 33.5).

Corticosteroids

Glucocorticoids retard lymphocytic proliferation by suppressing white cell production; hence, they are used in lymphocytic leukaemias and lymphomas. Prednisone and dexamethasone are also used as adjuncts with radiation therapy to decrease oedema in critical areas such as the brain and spinal cord, and in conjunction with antiemetic drugs and as supportive therapy for their general metabolic, anti-inflammatory and euphoric effects.

KEY POINTS

Hormonal antineoplastics

- Growth of hormone-dependent tumours can be inhibited by depriving the tumour of its hormone (by surgery, radiation or suppression of synthesis or release) or by use of an antagonistic hormone.
- Prostate cancers may be treated pharmacologically with antiandrogens (e.g. flutamide) or GnRH agonists or antagonists.
- Breast cancers may be treated with antiestrogens (tamoxifen), selective estrogen receptor modulators or aromatase inhibitors.

Non-cytotoxic antineoplastic drugs

Also commonly referred to as 'targeted therapies', the distinction between the broad classes of cytotoxic (or untargeted) and **non-cytotoxic** (targeted) antineoplastic

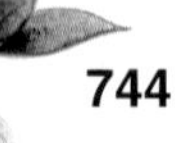

drugs is sometimes unclear. In general, the two main classes of non-cytotoxic antineoplastic drugs are the small molecule **kinase inhibitors** (KIs) and antineoplastic **monoclonal antibodies** (mAbs). These drugs mainly act on families of membrane-bound kinase-linked receptors, in particular:

- platelet-derived growth factor receptor (PDGFR)
- human epidermal growth factor receptor (HER)
- epidermal growth factor receptor (EGFR)
- vascular endothelial growth factor receptor (VEGFR).

KIs target an intracellular (i.e. inside the cell) domain of cell surface kinase-linked receptors. Monoclonal antibodies are too large to readily enter cells; as such, these agents target the extracellular domain of these receptors (Fig 33.3). These drugs are relatively more selective because they specifically block signal transduction pathways that impair tumour growth and metastatic dissemination and are typically better tolerated than cytotoxic drugs; however, their use is still routinely associated with severe and potentially life-threatening toxicities (Rowland et al. 2017).

Small molecule kinase inhibitors

The first small molecule KI, imatinib, was approved in 2001. Since then a further 61 KIs have been approved by the United States Food and Drug Administration (FDA) for treating various cancers (Roskoski 2021). Examples of drugs of each of the key classes are shown in Table 33.6. KIs are potent inhibitors of pathways that regulate cellular functions such as growth, differentiation and survival. These pathways are activated by a superfamily of membrane-bound cell surface kinase receptors that comprises more than 500 members. Receptor families of particular importance to developing malignancy are EGFR, PDGFR and VEGFR and their associated signalling pathways, such as the mitogen-activated protein kinase (MAPK) pathway, which incorporate families of signalling proteins, including RAS, RAF, MEK, MAPK, ERK and c-KIT.

TABLE 33.6 Molecular targets and indications for small molecule kinase inhibitors

CLASS	DRUG	INDICATIONS	MOLECULAR TARGETS
VEGFR inhibitors	Axitinib	RCC	KIT, PDGFRβ, VEGFR1–3
	Cabozantinib	MTC	FLT3, c-KIT, c-MET, RET, VEGFR2
	Lenvatinib	TC	VEGFR1–3, FGFR1–4, RET, KIT, PDGFRα
	Pazopanib	RCC	VEGFR1–3, PDGFRα/β, c-KIT, FGFGR2
	Regorafenib	CRC, GIST	c-KIT, PDGFRβ, RAF, RET, VEGFR1–3
	Sorafenib	HCC, RCC, TC	VEGFR2/3, PDGFRβ, FLT3, FGFR1, c-KIT, RAF, RET
	Sunitinib	GIST, pNET, RCC	VEGFR1–3, c-KIT, PDGFRα/β, FLT3, RET
	Vandetanib	MTC	EGFR, RET, VEGFR2
EGFR inhibitors	Afatinib	NSCLC (EGFR MUT)	EGFR, HER2, HER4
	Erlotinib	NSCLC, PC	EGFR
	Gefitinib	NSCLC (EGFR MUT)	EGFR
	Lapatinib	BC (HER2+)	EGFR, HER2
	Osimertinib	NSCLC (EGFR MUT)	EGFR
ALK inhibitors	Alectinib	NSCLC (ALK MUT)	ALK
	Ceritinib	NSCLC (ALK MUT)	ALK, IGF-1, ROS1, InsR
	Crizotinib	NSCLC (ALK MUT)	ALK, c-MET
BRAF/MEK inhibitors	Cobimetinib	MEL (BRAF MUT)	MEK1–2
	Dabrafenib	MEL (BRAF MUT)	BRAF
	Trametinib	MEL (BRAF MUT)	MEK1–2
	Vemurafenib	MEL (BRAF MUT)	BRAF
BCR–ABL inhibitors	Bosutinib	CML (Ph+)	ABL, SRC
	Dasatinib	ALL(Ph+), CML (Ph+)	BCR–ABL, SRC, c-KIT, PDGFRα/β, EphA2
	Imatinib	ALL (Ph+), CML (Ph+), DFSP, GIST (KIT+)	c-KIT, PDGFRα/β, BCR-ABL
	Nilotinib	CML (Ph+)	KIT, PDGFRα/β, BCR–ABL
	Ponatinib	ALL (Ph+), CML (Ph+)	BCR–ABL, FGFR1–3, FLT3, VEGFR2, c-KIT, RET, PDGFRα

ALL = acute lymphoblastic leukaemia; BC = breast cancer; CLL = chronic lymphocytic leukaemia; CML = chronic myelogenous leukaemia; CRC = colorectal cancer; DFSP = dermatofibrosarcoma protuberans; FNHL = follicular B-cell non-Hodgkin lymphoma; GIST = gastrointestinal stromal tumours; HCC = hepatocellular carcinoma; MCL = mantle cell lymphoma; MEL = melanoma; MTC = medullary thyroid cancer; NSCLC = non-small cell lung cancer; PC = pancreatic cancer; Ph+ = Philadelphia chromosome positive; pNET = pancreatic neuroendocrine tumours; RCC = renal cell carcinoma; SLL = small lymphocytic lymphoma; TC = thyroid cancer; WM = Waldenstrom's macroglobulinaemia

Impaired regulation of kinase activity, either through mutation of the kinase receptor or downstream proteins, causes constitutive pathway activation, uncontrolled cell proliferation and malignancy. Many KIs such as EGFR and VEGFR inhibitors act directly on the membrane-bound cell surface kinase receptor, while other KIs such as BRAF and MEK inhibitors act on downstream proteins. Almost all KIs inhibit the ATP binding site of the intracellular catalytic domain of the kinase receptor. Consistent with this common mechanism of action, there are similarities in the physiochemical properties between most, but not all, KIs that also translate to common pharmacokinetic characteristics and potential for drug interactions. KIs differ in terms of their target selectivities and mechanism of inhibition and, therefore, are effective in treating a variety of malignancies, with some KIs effective in treating multiple malignancies. Dosing of KIs can be challenging, with growing evidence that a one-size-fits-all approach is not effective, but an individualised approach may be costly (van Dyk et al. 2021).

VEGFR inhibitors

In cancers including hepatocellular, renal cell and thyroid carcinomas, activation of VEGF-mediated angiogenesis plays a critical role in tumour growth and metastasis. By inhibiting the intracellular catalytic domain of VEGF receptors, small molecule VEGFR inhibitors (Table 33.6) block VEGF-mediated angiogenesis and impair the tumour's capacity to access the nutrients required for growth. Pharmacokinetic parameters describing exposure to VEGFR inhibitors are reported in Table 33.7.

EGFR inhibitors

Activating mutations in exons 18, 19 and 21 of the EGFR are present in approximately 30% of non-small cell lung cancer (NSCLC) tumours. These mutations confer sensitivity to EGFR inhibitors (Table 33.6). Currently, there are four EGFR inhibitors approved for treating EGFR activating mutation positive NCSLC; afatinib, erlotinib (Drug Monograph 33.5) and gefitinib are first-line options, while osimertinib is a second-line option for tumours that develop resistance to afatinib, erlotinib and gefitinib. In approximately 50% of people, resistance to first-line EGFR inhibitors occurs through acquisition of the T790M mutation in exon 20 of EGFR (Nikolaou et al. 2018); unlike first-line options, osimertinib retains activity against T790M positive tumours. Lapatinib is a dual KI with activity against HER2 and EGFR pathways. Unlike other EGFR inhibitors, it is mainly used to treat HER2-positive breast cancer. Pharmacokinetic parameters describing exposure to EGFR inhibitors are reported in Table 33.8.

TABLE 33.7 Pharmacokinetics of VEGF inhibitors

DRUG	HALF-LIFE (HR)	VOLUME OF DISTRIBUTION (L)	CLEARANCE (L/HR)
Axitinib	3.3	180	38
Cabozantinib	28	349	11
Lenvatinib	35	336	6.7
Nintedanib	9.5	1050	83.4
Pazopanib	31	25	0.6
Regorafenib	36	88	1.7
Sorafenib	37	216	8.1
Sunitinib	60	2230	34
Vandetanib	220	4048	14

Drug Monograph 33.5
Erlotinib

Erlotinib is a small molecule KI that binds to the ATP binding site on the intracellular kinase domain of the EGFR. By inhibiting EGFR mediated MAPK signalling, erlotinib slows tumour growth and prevents metastatic dissemination.

Indications

Erlotinib is indicated for treating EGFR, activating mutation positive NSCLC and pancreatic cancer.

Pharmacokinetics

Erlotinib has a bioavailability of approximately 60%, which is substantially increased by the consumption of acidic foods and beverages to almost 100%. Peak plasma concentrations occur at 4 hours after dosing. Following absorption, erlotinib is approximately 93% protein bound to plasma proteins. Erlotinib has a large apparent volume of distribution of 232 L. It is primarily cleared by CYP3A4, and to a lesser extent CYP1A2, catalysed hepatic metabolism. Following oral dosing, more than 85% of the drug is recovered in the faeces, and less than 15% in urine. The elimination half-life of erlotinib is approximately 36 hours.

Adverse reactions

Erlotinib commonly causes a papulopustular rash that mainly affects the face and upper body within the first 2–4 weeks of treatment. There is some evidence that the occurrence and/or severity of the rash may be associated with improved response or survival. Other skin toxicities include itch, dry skin and fissures. Paronychia, nail disorders and abnormal hair growth become apparent after 1–2 months of treatment. Erlotinib also commonly causes a range of gastrointestinal toxicity, including diarrhoea, nausea, vomiting, anorexia, oral mucositis, abdominal pain and gastrointestinal bleeding.

Dosage and administration

Erlotinib is administered orally; the standard dose for NSCLC is 150 mg/day and the standard dose for pancreatic cancer is 100 mg/day. Erlotinib should be taken on an empty stomach at least 1 hour before or 2 hours after food.

TABLE 33.8 Pharmacokinetics of EGFR inhibitors

DRUG	HALF-LIFE (HR)	VOLUME OF DISTRIBUTION (L)	CLEARANCE (L/HR)
Afatinib	34	2520	83
Erlotinib	36	232	5.3
Gefitinib	48	1400	36
Lapatinib	24	> 2200	28
Osimertinib	48	986	14

BRAF/MEK inhibitors

BRAF is a member of the RAF family of serine/threonine kinases that are related to retroviral oncogenes. Mitogen-activated protein kinase kinase (MEK) is the protein that phosphorylates MAPK. BRAF and MEK are two regulatory proteins in the signalling cascade known as MAPK/ERK (extracellular signal-regulated kinase), which affects cell division and differentiation. When BRAF and/or MEK is inhibited, cell proliferation is blocked and apoptosis is induced. Mutations in the BRAF gene, particularly at residue 600, are associated with various cancers, including colorectal, lung, melanoma and thyroid. Vemurafenib and dabrafenib are BRAF inhibitors approved for treating unresectable or metastatic BRAF V600E-positive melanoma. In order to maximise therapeutic effect, BRAF inhibitors are often used in combination with a MEK inhibitor, cobimetinib (with vemurafenib) or trametinib (with dabrafenib).

BCR–ABL inhibitors

The BCR–ABL fusion gene results from a rearrangement of genetic material between chromosomes 9 and 22 (the Philadelphia chromosome). This fusion gene, which is the ABL1 gene from chromosome 9 translocation onto the BCR gene from chromosome 22, codes for a hybrid BCR–ABL tyrosine kinase that is always 'switched on', causing cells to divide uncontrollably. BCR–ABL is highly prevalent in chronic myeloid and acute lymphoblastic leukaemias, and targeting of BCR–ABL by the prototypic KI, imatinib, is widely regarded as one of the greatest advances in cancer treatment.

Other kinase inhibitors

In addition to VEGFR, EGFR, BRAF/MEK and BCR–ABL, a number of other kinases have been implicated in the development and progression of cancer. In recent years, inhibitors of anaplastic lymphoma kinase (ALK; alectinib, ceritinib, crizotinib), Bruton's tyrosine kinase (BTK; ibrutinib), phosphoinositide 3-kinase (PI3K; idelalisib) and cyclin-dependent kinase (CDK; palbociclib) have emerged as effective drugs for treating solid organ tumours including breast cancer and NSCLC, and various forms of leukaemia (Table 33.6).

PARP inhibitors

BRCA1 and 2 are proteins that repair double-strand DNA breaks by a process called homologous recombination repair. Mutations in the BRCA1 or 2 lead to errors in DNA repair that can eventually cause breast or ovarian cancer. PARP1 is an enzyme that repairs single-strand breaks or 'nicks' in DNA. In breast cancer caused by defects in BRCA1 or 2, if these nicks are not repaired by the time the DNA is replicated, then the replication process causes double strand breaks. PARP inhibitors cause multiple double strand breaks to form in this way, and in tumours with BRCA1 or 2 mutations, these breaks cannot be repaired, and thus lead to cell death. Due to a poor understanding of this mechanism and poor trial design, several potentially useful PARP inhibitors have failed in clinical trials. Currently, olaparib is the only approved PARP inhibitor in Australia or New Zealand, although there are a number of additional drugs close to approval.

mTOR inhibitors

The mTOR is a central serine/threonine kinase that regulates metabolism and physiology. Everolimus and temsirolimus indirectly inhibit the mTOR pathway by binding to the intracellular protein FKBP-12. The protein–drug complex blocks the activity of mTOR kinase, inhibiting angiogenesis and tumour cell proliferation, growth and survival. Everolimus is used to treat renal cell cancer, pancreatic neuroendocrine tumour and breast cancer, while temsirolimus is used to treat renal cell cancer and mantle cell lymphoma. Given the important function of mTOR as a regulator of metabolism and physiology, these drugs commonly cause electrolyte disturbance (hypokalaemia and hypophosphataemia) and metabolic disturbance (hyperglycaemia, hypercholesterolaemia and hypertriglyceridaemia). Other common serious adverse effects include anaemia, hepatotoxicity, lymphopenia, nephrotoxicity, neutropenia, pneumonitis and thrombocytopenia.

Histone deacetylase inhibitors

Histone deacetylase inhibitors have been used for many years to treat psychological and neurological disorders. In recent years, there has been considerable interest in their role as cancer treatments or adjuncts. These drugs induce expression of cyclin-dependent KI1 (p21), a regulator of the tumour suppressor p53. Histone deacetylase inhibitors that are widely approved for treating cancer include romidepsin and vorinostat to treat cutaneous T-cell lymphoma, belinostat for treating peripheral T-cell lymphoma and panobinostat for treating multiple myeloma. The commonly used anticonvulsant and mood stabiliser valproic acid has also completed phase III trials in cervical and ovarian cancers.

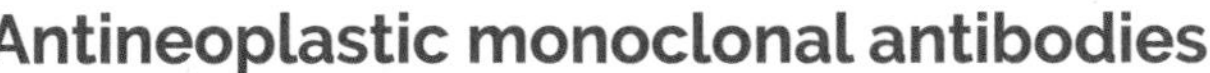

Antineoplastic monoclonal antibodies

Antineoplastic monoclonal antibodies (mAbs) are antibodies that are synthetically produced from a single clone of immune cells; the clone produces antibodies against the specific antigen, such as tumour-associated antigens or growth factors. Binding of a mAb to the antigen usually inactivates the antigen and/or causes cell lysis, leading to various antineoplastic actions including inhibition of signal transductions, induction of apoptosis or inhibition of angiogenesis. As mAbs are large proteins, they must be administered parenterally. The convention for the generic naming of therapeutic antibodies is based on five components:

- prefix that carries no special meaning, but that should be unique for each drug and contribute to a well-sounding name (e.g. TRAS-)
- sub-stem defining the target (e.g. -TU-; tumour)
- sub-stem defining the source (e.g. -ZU-; humanised)
- stem defining whether the drug is mono- or poly-clonal (e.g. –MAB)
- additional word indicating that another substance is attached (e.g. EMTANSINE).

In this example, TRAS-TU-ZU-MAB EMTANSINE is a humanised monoclonal antibody used against a tumour that is conjugated to the cytotoxic microtubule inhibitor emtansine. A summary of all antineoplastic mAbs approved in Australia and New Zealand is provided in Table 33.9.

Anti-CD20 mAbs

Rituximab was the first genetically engineered monoclonal antibody for clinical use in oncology; it is specific against antigen CD20 located on the surface of normal and malignant B-lymphocytes. Binding triggers an immune response that lyses B-cells. The CD20 antigen governs early steps in cell-cycle initiation and differentiation, and is found in more than 90% of B-cell non-Hodgkin lymphomas. While there are numerous drugs in development, obinutuzumab, ofatumumab and rituximab are the approved mAbs with this target. Rituximab is usually administered with the CHOP chemotherapy regimen: cyclophosphamide, doxorubicin, vincristine and prednisone.

Anti-EGFR mAbs

Cetuximab and panitumumab are antibodies against EGFR, which is overexpressed in many colorectal and in squamous cell head and neck tumours. By inhibiting EGFR, these mAbs inhibit cell growth and production of some cytokines and growth factors and induce apoptosis. Because constitutive activation of the EGFR-regulated MAPK pathway can occur if there are mutations in downstream proteins such as RAS (K-RAS, N-RAS and H-RAS), anti-EGFR mAbs are only useful in treating RAS wild-type cancers. Skin-related toxicity is common, due to impairment of EGF actions; other serious adverse effects include infusion-related reactions, thromboembolism and hypomagnesaemia.

Anti-HER2 mAbs

Trastuzumab is a monoclonal antibody targeting a receptor for EGF, encoded by an oncogene (HER2) that is overexpressed in about 30% of women with breast cancer, and in other cancers such as gastric and colorectal. By

TABLE 33.9 Representative approved antineoplastic antibodies

MAB	EXAMPLE INDICATIONS[a]	TARGET	SOURCE
Alemtuzumab	B-cell chronic lymphocytic leukaemia	CD52 on B- and T-lymphocytes	Humanised (from rat)
Bevacizumab	Breast, cervical, colorectal, non-squamous non-small cell lung, ovarian and renal cell cancer	VEGF-A	Humanised (from mouse)
Blinatumomab	B-cell acute lymphoblastic leukaemia	CD3 on T-cells and CD19 on B-cells	Mouse
Brentuximab vedotin	Anaplastic large cell lymphoma, CD30-positive Hodgkin lymphoma	CD30 on tumour cells	Chimeric (mouse/human)
Cetuximab	RAS wild-type colorectal cancer, squamous cell head and neck cancer	EGFR	Chimeric (mouse/human)
Obinutuzumab	Chronic lymphocytic leukaemia, follicular lymphoma	CD20 on B-lymphocytes	Humanised (from mouse)
Ofatumumab	Chronic lymphocytic leukaemia	CD20 on B-lymphocytes	Human
Panitumumab	RAS wild-type colorectal cancer	EGFR	Human
Pertuzumab	HER2-positive breast cancer	HER2/neu	Humanised (from mouse)
Rituximab	Chronic lymphocytic leukaemia, CD20-positive B-cell non-Hodgkin lymphoma	CD20 on B-lymphocytes	Chimeric (mouse/human)
Trastuzumab emtansine	HER2-positive breast cancer	HER2/neu	Humanised (from mouse)

[a] May be included in various other treatment protocols.
Sources: eviQ cancer treatment protocols.

blocking the HER2 receptor, trastuzumab slows breast cancer progression and reduces tumours in women with this altered gene. It is used as monotherapy or for synergistic effects in combination chemotherapy regimens with paclitaxel or an antitumour antibiotic and cyclophosphamide. Trastuzumab can also be used in combination with a second anti-HER2 mAb (pertuzumab) and docetaxel for treating metastatic HER2-positive breast cancer. Trastuzumab's epitope on HER2 is the domain where HER2 binds to another HER2 protein, while the epitope for pertuzumab is the domain of HER2 where it binds to HER3. When administered together, the two mAbs act synergistically to prevent HER2 from functioning.

Anti-VEGF mAb

Bevacizumab slows the growth of new blood vessels supplying a tumour by binding to circulating VEGF, and is sometimes called an angiogenesis inhibitor or antiangiogenic drug. Consistent with the therapeutic effect of this drug, the main adverse effects are hypertension and cardiovascular toxicity. Infusion-related reactions can also occur and there are precautions about potentially life-threatening necrotising fasciitis.

Immunomodulatory drugs

The immune system comprises three layers of defence that protect the body against illness caused by pathogenic organisms (Wahid et al. 2021). Initially, physical barriers prevent pathogens from entering the body. If a pathogen breaches these barriers, the innate immune system mounts an immediate but non-specific response. If a pathogen evades this non-specific response, the adaptive immune system mounts a response tailored to the specific pathogen or pathogen-infected cells. The function of the immune system in people with cancer is important because:

- cancer and cancer treatments can weaken the immune system, predisposing people to potentially life-threatening infections
- the immune system may be harnessed to help fight certain types of cancer.

Immune checkpoint inhibitors

Immune checkpoints are molecules that modulate the duration and amplitude of immune responses to minimise collateral tissue damage. Many cancers protect themselves from the immune system by using these checkpoints to inhibit T-cell signalling. These checkpoints emerged as exciting new targets for cancer immunotherapies due to the impressive effectiveness of two classes of checkpoint inhibitors for advanced melanoma. While still effective across a range of cancers, and typically more so than existing drugs, immune checkpoint inhibitors have unfortunately demonstrated poorer efficacy in treating other cancers compared with the initial results seen with melanoma. Additionally, these drugs are often only effective in a subset of people who are difficult to identify prior to treatment using existing markers.

CTLA4 inhibitors

Ipilimumab is a mAb that inhibits cytotoxic T-lymphocyte associated antigen 4 (CTLA4), an inhibitory checkpoint that blocks the cytotoxic reaction mounted by T-cells against a tumour. By blocking the inhibitory checkpoint, ipilimumab activates the protective T-cells to destroy cancer cells. This has been described as 'releasing the brakes on the immune system'. Ipilimumab is approved in Australia and New Zealand to treat metastatic melanoma; it is also being trialled against lung, head and neck, bowel, prostate and kidney cancers. Adverse effects are mainly due to excess immunological activation in the GIT and skin, causing enterocolitis, hepatitis, dermatitis and neuropathies.

PD-1/PD-L1 inhibitors

Programmed cell death receptor 1 (PD-1) is a cell surface receptor that plays an important role in mediating the immune system by suppressing or co-stimulating T-cell activity. Binding of the cell surface proteins programmed death ligand 1 (PD-L1) or 2 (PD-L2) to PD-1 suppresses T-cell activation. Several cancers overexpress the ligand for PD-1 (PDL-1) as a mechanism for avoiding immune destruction. Monoclonal antibodies that block the interaction of PDL-1 with PD-1 enhance T-cell-mediated destruction of cancer cells and are important emerging therapies for several forms of cancer.

Nivolumab and pembrolizumab (Drug Monograph 33.6) are anti-PD-1 mAbs that bind to and inhibit PD-1. Both drugs are approved for treating metastatic melanoma and NSCLC. Nivolumab is also approved for renal cell carcinoma. These drugs are being trialled for a large number of other cancers, particularly those that have high expression of PD-L1 or a high degree of mismatch repair deficiency, termed 'microsatellite instability high (MSI-high)' and are changing the paradigm of FDA cancer medicine approvals.

The development and approval of PD-L1 inhibitors has been slightly behind that of PD-1 inhibitors, although three mAbs – atezolizumab, avelumab and durvalumab – have received FDA approval in recent years; avelumab for Merkel-cell carcinoma and NSCLC, atezolizumab for bladder and NSCLCs and durvalumab for bladder cancer.

Interferons

Interferons are naturally occurring small protein molecules with antiproliferative and immunostimulating

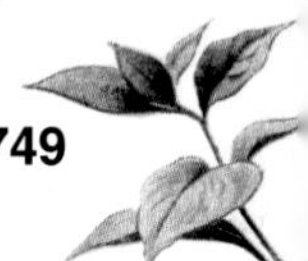

Drug Monograph 33.6
Pembrolizumab

Pembrolizumab is a monoclonal antibody immune checkpoint inhibitor that binds to the programmed death receptor (PD-1) on the surface of T-cells and pro-B-cells.

Indications

Pembrolizumab is indicated for treating people with metastatic melanoma and people with metastatic NSCLC whose tumours have high PD-L1 expression.

Pharmacokinetics

Pembrolizumab is administered intravenously and has limited extravascular distribution, with a volume of distribution at steady state approximately equal to blood volume of 7.5 L. As an antibody, pembrolizumab does not bind to plasma proteins. The drug is catabolised via non-specific pathways, and metabolism does not contribute to clearance. The systemic clearance of pembrolizumab is 0.2 L/day and the elimination half-life is 26 days.

Drug interactions

Pembrolizumab may decrease the effectiveness of immunosuppressant drugs, worsening the underlying disease or increasing the risk of organ rejection. Immunosuppressant drugs may also reduce the effectiveness of pembrolizumab.

Adverse reactions

Immune-related adverse reactions to pembrolizumab are common and often occur during treatment but may be delayed for weeks to months afterwards. Reactions may involve any organ, including endocrine (e.g. hyperthyroidism, type 1 diabetes), GIT (e.g. diarrhoea, microscopic colitis), liver (e.g. increased aminotransferases, hepatitis), kidneys (e.g. nephritis) and skin (e.g. rash or severe skin reactions). Infusion-related reactions, including chills, itch, fever, flushing, hypotension rash, rigors and wheezing, are rarely severe. Other common adverse reactions to pembrolizumab include anaemia, decreased appetite, constipation, cough, dyspnoea, headache, nausea and peripheral oedema.

Dosage and administration

In adults, the standard dose of pembrolizumab is 200 mg every 3 weeks administered by intravenous infusion over 30 minutes via an in-line 0.45 micrometre filter. Treatment protocols should be consulted for specific populations.

actions. Defects in interferon responses occur in many cancer-initiating cells. Interferons produced by recombinant technology have effects similar to endogenous interferon subtypes. Two synthetic interferons are used to treat cancer: interferon alpha (IFN-α) for its cytotoxic properties, and interferon gamma (IFNγ) for its immunostimulatory properties, which increase granulocyte, platelet and haemoglobin levels.

There are two forms of IFN-α: 2a and 2b. IFN-α-2a is used to treat malignant melanoma, mycosis fungoides, myeloproliferative disorders, renal cell cancer and Sézary syndrome; IFN-α-2b is used to treat multiple myeloma. Both forms of IFN-α may be used to treat chronic myeloid leukaemia, follicular lymphoma and hairy cell leukaemia. Adverse effects include a flu-like syndrome with fever, chills, muscle pain, loss of appetite and lethargy. At higher doses, cardiotoxicity, myelosuppression, nausea and vomiting and neurotoxicity can occur. IFNγ-1b is used as an adjunct to reduce serious infections in chronic granulomatous disease.

Levamisole

Levamisole was initially used clinically as a treatment for intestinal worm infestations, and was found to have useful immunostimulant effects, enhancing T-cell-mediated immunity and macrophage actions. Levamisole is used in combination with 5-fluorouracil to treat colorectal carcinoma. The combination lengthens survival time and lowers risk of cancer recurrence. Levamisole can be administered orally, and adverse effects are usually mild; reversible bone marrow suppression and a flu-like syndrome can occur.

Aldesleukin

Aldesleukin, a recombinant version of human interleukin-2 (IL-2), is another immunostimulatory lymphokine. It stimulates T-cell proliferation, is a co-factor in enhancing growth of natural and lymphokine-activated killer cells and increases production of interferons. Aldesleukin is indicated in metastatic renal cell carcinoma, melanoma and thymoma, and after bone marrow transplant. Adverse effects include oedema, anaemia, thrombocytopenia and hypotension. It is not generally available in Australia, but may be obtained via the Therapeutic Goods Administration's Special Access Scheme.

Granulocyte colony-stimulating factors (G-CSFs)

Filgrastim, lenograstim and pegfilgrastim are recombinant versions of bone marrow-stimulating factors with

immunomodulatory actions. Administered after myelosuppressant cytotoxic chemotherapy or bone marrow transplant, these granulocyte colony-stimulating factors (G-CSFs) stimulate neutrophil precursor cells to produce phagocytes, reducing duration of neutropenia and risk of infections. They should not be administered within 24 hours before or after chemotherapy, as rapidly dividing cells (i.e. those stimulated by the G-CSF) are most sensitive to cytotoxics.

Non-vaccine Bacillus Calmette-Guérin therapy

Bacille Calmette-Guérin (BCG) is the main intravesical immunotherapy used to treat early-stage bladder cancer. BCG is live, attenuated *Mycobacterium bovis* that produces a local inflammatory reaction resulting in elimination or reduction of superficial bladder tumour lesions. BCG is a microbe that is related to bacterium that causes tuberculosis, but it doesn't usually cause serious disease. BCG is put directly into the bladder through a catheter. Immunocompromised people are at risk of systemic tuberculosis infection; other adverse effects include urinary tract pain and dysfunction, fever and malaise.

Thalidomide and lenalidomide

Thalidomide is the drug infamous for having caused thousands of deaths or congenital malformations during the late 1950s and 1960s in babies whose mothers took it as a supposedly safe sedative in early pregnancy. It was banned from use for many years but is undergoing re-evaluation for limited specific uses, in treatment of leprosy, and as adjunctive therapy in some AIDS-associated infections and tumours. It has immunostimulatory actions and inhibits TNF, and is being trialled as an antiangiogenic agent in cancers including multiple myeloma, renal cell carcinoma and glioblastoma. In Australia, it is tightly controlled because of its teratogenicity; patients must give prior written informed consent.

A related analogue, lenalidomide, is indicated in multiple myeloma. It has direct cytotoxic effects via induction of apoptosis, production of T-cells, IL-2 and IFNγ and inhibition of TNF-α, IL-6 and angiogenesis. It enhances survival rate when added to dexamethasone therapy. Serious adverse effects include venous thromboembolism, leucopenias, GIT disturbances and teratogenicity.

Tumour vaccines

Immune surveillance by T-cells against non-self cells means that the body can usually mount an immune response against antigens expressed on the surface of tumour cells and destroy them. Only when the immune system is depressed, and/or the load of mutated tumour cells becomes too great, do cancers continue to develop. A notable recent vaccine against the human papillomavirus (HPV) is the non-live vaccine (Gardasil) developed in Australia. It is already in large-scale use in teenage girls and young women (and young men) in many countries and provides effective protection against various strains of HPV.

KEY POINTS

Non-cytotoxic antineoplastics and immunomodulators

- Small molecule KIs and monoclonal antibodies inhibit the interaction of kinase receptors with their endogenous ligand.
- Small molecule KIs typically bind to the ATP binding site of the intracellular catalytic (or kinase) domain.
- Monoclonal antibodies can either bind to the extracellular domain of the kinase receptor (e.g. the anti-EGFR mAb cetuximab) or to the receptor ligand (e.g. the anti-VEGF mAb bevacizumab).
- Immune checkpoint inhibitors are a class of monoclonal antibodies that stimulate T-cell-mediated immune response against a tumour.
- Immune responses against a tumour can also be enhanced using interferons, other cytokines, colony-stimulating factors and BCG (non-vaccine).

Adjunct therapies

Adjunct therapies are additional treatments used together with the primary treatment to assist or overcome limitations of the primary treatment. When treating cancer, antineoplastic drugs may be used as adjunct therapies to primary treatments such as surgery to minimise the risk of tumour reoccurrence or to 'mop-up' residual circulating tumour cells. Here, we describe the roles of other drugs and drug classes as means of supporting the benefit or overcoming the toxicities caused by antineoplastic drugs.

Treatment of adverse drug reactions

Cytotoxic drugs damage rapidly dividing cells, especially in the hair, skin, GIT mucosa and bone marrow, and are usually concentrated in and excreted via kidneys, so kidney tubules are vulnerable. Particular drugs may cause other specific reactions; for example, anthracycline antibiotics cause cardiomyopathy and sex hormone inhibitors may reduce libido. Adverse effects may be sufficiently severe as to require acute or prophylactic treatment. Adverse reactions may be treated symptomatically – for example, infections due to myelosuppression with specific antimicrobial agents and fever with antipyretic drugs.

Treatment of nausea and vomiting

The chemoreceptor trigger zone in the medulla oblongata is sensitive to chemical stimuli, including emetogenic substances produced by cytotoxics and endogenous substances produced in radiation sickness and tumour lysis syndrome. Cytotoxic drugs can be compared in terms of their emetogenic potential.

Nausea and vomiting are treated with antiemetic drugs, preferably prophylactically. For cytotoxic drugs with low emetogenic potential, metoclopramide is given when necessary; for intermediate-potential drugs, intravenous or oral metoclopramide with dexamethasone may be given. Drugs with high emetic potential require dexamethasone before chemotherapy with a stronger antiemetic such as an oral 5-HT_3 antagonist (ondansetron or tropisetron, which can be given as sublingual formulations for faster onset of action). Palonosetron is a new 5-HT_3 antagonist administered 30 minutes before cytotoxic chemotherapy; its long elimination half-life prolongs antiemetic actions. Phenothiazine antiemetics (e.g. prochlorperazine) and antianxiety agents may also be helpful.

Aprepitant is a newer antiemetic that inhibits substance P-mediated vomiting by selectively antagonising the neurokinin-1 receptor. It is recommended for use only with highly emetogenic cytotoxics such as high-dose cisplatin or cyclophosphamide plus an anthracycline. Fosaprepitant, a prodrug, is an intravenous formulation producing higher concentrations; it is effective in stopping delayed emesis. Ondansetron and metoclopramide are carried by paramedics and can be administered for the immediate out-of-hospital treatment of severe nausea and vomiting induced by cytotoxic agents. Severe delayed emesis ($>$ 24 hours after chemotherapy) may require intravenous antiemetics for 2–4 days.

Treatment of myelosuppression

Bone marrow depression (myelosuppression) is usually the limiting factor in clinical use of cytotoxics, causing treatment delays and dose reductions. White cells and platelets are first affected, leading to immunosuppression, infections, bruising and bleeding. Neutrophil counts and platelet counts are monitored to indicate when, after cessation of chemotherapy, levels have risen back enough for another cycle to begin. Thrombocytopenia (low platelet count) may cause haemorrhage; it is treated or prevented with infusions of platelets or haemostatic agents. Anaemia associated with chemotherapy is treated with blood transfusions or, where transfusion is inappropriate, with erythropoietin. Bone marrow suppression may be overcome by subcutaneous administration of a recombinant G-CSF such as, filgrastim (see 'Immunomodulatory drugs'), and calcium folinate.

Folinic acid rescue

Folinic acid (leucovorin) is the active form of folic acid. It is used for 'folinic acid rescue therapy' following high doses of parenteral methotrexate. Folinic acid is essential for DNA and RNA synthesis. By acting as a folic acid antagonist, methotrexate prevents the reduction of folic acid to folinic acid. Administration of folinic acid bypasses this inhibition, restoring the capacity DNA/RNA synthesis, and helping to prevent much of the bone marrow toxicity caused by methotrexate without reversing the antineoplastic effects in cancer cells. It also enhances the cytotoxicity of 5-fluorouracil by further inhibiting thymidylate synthetase.

Cytoprotective agents

Phosphamide (cyclophosphamide, ifosfamide) and platinum-containing (cisplatin, oxaliplatin) alkylating agents are specifically toxic in the renal epithelium, causing haemorrhagic cystitis. This toxicity may be prevented or reduced by prior administration of a sulfur-donating cytoprotective agent such as mesna or amifostine.

Ifosfamide is used to treat germ cell testicular tumours, but haemorrhagic cystitis limits its usefulness. Mesna, a thiol donor in the kidneys, acts as a specific antidote. Using them in combination allows more aggressive therapy while reducing the dose-limiting adverse effects of ifosfamide. Amifostine is a cytoprotective agent administered before platinum-containing or other alkylating agents to reduce their renal toxicity. It is a prodrug activated to free thiol groups that protect normal cells against radiation and DNA-binding agents. It also reduces xerostomia (excessively dry mouth) caused by radiotherapy to the head and neck.

Hydration therapy and treatment of tumour lysis syndrome

Tumour lysis syndrome occurs due to release of cell breakdown products from large tumour masses (especially leukaemias and lymphomas) treated with chemotherapy, overwhelming normal homeostatic mechanisms. It manifests as hyperuricaemia, hyperkalaemia, hyperphosphataemia and hypocalcaemia.

Rasburicase is a recombinant form of an enzyme that catalyses the conversion of uric acid to a more soluble metabolite. It is given for prophylaxis and treatment of hyperuricaemia associated with cytotoxic chemotherapy of haematological malignancies. Rehydration therapy to prevent renal tubular damage or hyperuricaemia requires vigorous intravenous fluid infusion. During therapy with high-dose cisplatin, for example, about 2.5 L of fluids (saline, mannitol and/or glucose) are infused before chemotherapy over 2–3 hours; then, after chemotherapy, 2 L of fluids are given over the next 10 hours.

Treatment of oral mucositis

Mucositis is a painful inflammation and ulceration of the mucous membranes lining the GIT; oral mucositis refers specifically to inflammation and ulceration of the mouth. The symptoms of oral mucositis can be minimised by practices such as maintaining good oral hygiene, drinking plenty of water and avoiding alcohol. These practices can be supported by the use of antiseptic and anaesthetic mouthwashes such as chlorhexidine gluconate with benzydamine hydrochloride (e.g. Difflam) or lidocaine (lignocaine) viscous solution. For more serious cases, palifermin may be used.

Oral thrush is a common complication of oral mucositis in people with cancer due to the lesions and the person's reduced immune function. Mild to moderate disease can be treated with oral nystatin, while more serious infection may require the use of amphotericin lozenges or oral fluconazole.

Treatment of problems due to bony metastases

Bisphosphonates including pamidronate, zoledronic acid, ibandronic acid and sodium clodronate bind to hydroxyapatite in bone and specifically inhibit osteoclast-mediated bone resorption. They are used to improve bone mineral density in osteoporosis and Paget's disease of bone, and to prevent corticosteroid-induced osteoporosis. In cancers, they are used to reduce skeletal morbidity that occurs with bony metastases and reduce tumour-induced hypercalcaemia. The radioisotopes strontium-89 and samarium-153 are also used for palliation of bone pain in osteoblastic skeletal metastases (secondary cancers in the bone).

Palliative care

Palliative care at the end of life aims to treat all aspects of a person's suffering – physical, psychological, social and spiritual – with a multidisciplinary approach and to include the person's family and close friends. Traditionally, palliative care was only employed when anticancer treatment had failed and active medical treatment of related problems ceased. It is now recognised that palliative care is most successful when introduced at an earlier stage with other therapeutic modalities.

Optimal care acknowledges that suffering includes many aspects: the person's responses to diagnosis of a life-threatening illness; the person's choice to transfer from curative to palliative care; deterioration to a terminal stage; optimal ways to answer questions put by people and their families; ethical issues related to withdrawal of treatment and life-support; support for completing essential life-tasks; discussion (or not) of death and dying; and later bereavement and grief of family and friends.

The team aims to provide specialist palliative care services coordinated by one member, and may include the person's general practitioner, a palliative care nurse, palliative medicine specialist, other specialist doctors (e.g. oncologist, radiologist, neurologist), clinical pharmacist, social worker, counsellor, chaplain, nutritionist, other allied health professionals, an after-hours phone service, volunteer carer and patient support group representative.

Advance care plans

Palliative Care Australia recommends that everyone – not just those facing the end of life – should plan in advance for the type of care they prefer to have, and flag their preferences to family, carers and health professionals. Facilitating such discussions and planning is the responsibility of all members of a person's care team. Written advance care directives can later guide carers about the type and level of medical (and other) care needed. No standard 'pro forma' care plan is published, but several aspects to consider are:

- how illness or injuries affect the person
- likely effects of any treatments needed
- the person's own attitudes to illness and medical treatments
- the person's goals and priorities
- situations where the person might prefer to be kept comfortable and allowed to die naturally, as distinct from treatment to prolong life
- relevant religious and legal aspects of terminal care and patient consent.

As well as drugs used to treat the patient's conditions, many other drugs may improve quality of life and comfort, such as analgesics for pain and dyspnoea and drugs to treat side effects of the primary drugs (e.g. antiemetics, immunostimulants, hydration, laxatives). Decisions may need to be made about continuance with drugs administered for concurrent chronic conditions such as diabetes mellitus, hypertension, arthritis or asthma. The following drugs are commonly administered in palliative care situations:

- analgesics: paracetamol, NSAIDs, opioids
- analgesic adjuvants: antiepileptic agents for neuropathic pain, antidepressants, antianxiety drugs and sedatives, corticosteroids

- laxatives and antiemetics
- skeletal and/or smooth muscle relaxants.

Analgesics in palliative care

For many people, pain is the most feared symptom in advanced cancer. Adequate pain control is an important issue in palliative care – for example, in people with bony metastases from cancer. Pain may exacerbate anxiety, depression and social, cultural and spiritual problems. People need reassurance that satisfactory pain control can be achieved for more than 90% of people, and that they are unlikely to become dependent on opioid analgesics.

Analgesics need to be chosen appropriately and given in adequate doses and frequency to keep the person pain-free, with instructions for extra dosing for 'breakthrough' pain and treatments for adverse effects such as constipation. The stepwise 'ladder' approach is used: non-opioids first (paracetamol), then mild opioids (codeine), then strong opioids. Fentanyl patches provide sustained analgesia; sufentanil, a fentanyl analogue, may be available through the Pharmaceutical Benefits Scheme's Special Access Scheme. Corticosteroids are useful adjuncts in situations of spinal cord compression, superior vena cava obstruction, raised intracranial pressure and bowel obstruction.

Breakthrough pain

Breakthrough pain occurs between regular doses of an analgesic that normally controls the person's pain. It is important that this pain be controlled effectively, usually with an extra dose of the person's regular opioid. The breakthrough dose is determined by consideration of the person's 24-hour analgesic dose equivalent, one-sixth of which is given every 4 hours (for immediate-release formulations). The breakthrough dose may be 50–100% of the regular 4-hourly dose, at intervals not less than 30 minutes, for up to three doses. The normal dose should then be given at the regular time. The number of breakthrough doses required over a 24-hour period is an indication of the need to increase the regular dose. Fentanyl lozenges, which allow absorption through buccal membranes, are especially useful for breakthrough pain. Particularly careful dosing of opioids is required in elderly people, those with renal or severe liver impairment and when changing between formulations (oral to parenteral or transdermal, or immediate- to sustained-release) or between opioids (morphine to fentanyl).

Treatment of opioid-induced constipation

Constipation is an adverse effect of opioid analgesic use, and may be so severe as to deter usage. This should be pre-empted by a high-fibre diet (fruit, bran, prunes) and prophylactic use of laxatives such as coloxyl with senna. Methylnaltrexone, a peripherally acting μ-opioid receptor antagonist, is indicated in refractory opioid-induced constipation in people with advanced illness such as cancer. It can be administered subcutaneously once every 2 days, and stimulates bowel movement in most people within 4 hours. Pain relief is generally undiminished, as the drug preferentially blocks peripheral opioid receptors due to low transfer across the blood–brain barrier.

KEY POINTS

Adjunct therapies and palliative care

- Serious adverse reactions to antineoplastic agents are treated with specific methods or drugs – for example, with powerful antiemetics or bone marrow-supportive drugs.
- Other adjunctive and supportive therapies include drugs to relieve pain, prevent vomiting or constipation, reduce uric acid load or minimise bone resorption.
- Palliative care involves attention to all needs of the person with cancer, including medical, physical, psychological, social and spiritual aspects, with a multidisciplinary approach.

DRUGS AT A GLANCE

Antineoplastic drugs

PHARMACOLOGICAL GROUP AND EFFECT	KEY EXAMPLES	CLINICAL USE
Alkylating agents	Cyclophosphamide	Various haematological and solid organ malignancies
	Dacarbazine	
	Lomustine	
	Temozolomide	

Platinum compounds	Carboplatin	Various solid organ malignancies
	Cisplatin	
	Oxaliplatin	
Antimetabolites	Capecitabine	Various haematological and solid organ malignancies
	Fluorouracil	
	Gemcitabine	
	Mercaptopurine	
	Methotrexate	
Cytotoxic antibiotics	Bleomycin	Various haematological and solid organ malignancies
	Doxorubicin	
	Epirubicin	
Mitotic inhibitors	Docetaxel	Various haematological and solid organ malignancies
	Paclitaxel	
	Vincristine	
Topoisomerase inhibitors	Etoposide	Various solid organ malignancies
	Irinotecan	
	Teniposide	
	Topotecan	
Proteasome inhibitors	Bortezomib	Various haematological malignancies
Androgens	Testosterone	Breast cancer
Antiandrogens	Enzalutamide	Prostate cancer
	Flutamide	
Antiestrogens / selective estrogen receptor modulators	Fulvestrant	Breast cancer
	Raloxifene	
	Tamoxifen	
Aromatase inhibitors	Anastrozole	Breast cancer
	Exemestane	
Gonadotrophin-releasing hormone analogues	Goserelin	Breast and prostate cancer
	Leuprorelin	
Gonadotrophin-releasing hormone antagonist	Degarelix	Prostate cancer
Somatostatin analogues	Lanreotide	Neuroendocrine cancers
	Octreotide	
Small molecule kinase inhibitors	Axitinib	Various haematological and solid organ malignancies
	Dabrafenib	
	Erlotinib	
	Gefitinib	
	Lapatinib	
	Imatinib	
	Pazopanib	
	Sorafenib	
	Sunitinib	
	Trametinib	
mTOR inhibitors	Everolimus	Various solid organ malignancies
	Temsirolimus	
PARP inhibitors	Olaparib	Breast and ovarian cancer
Monoclonal antibodies	Bevacizumab	Various solid organ malignancies
	Cetuximab	
	Rituximab	
	Trastuzumab	
Immune checkpoint inhibitors	Ipilimumab	Various solid organ malignancies
	Nivolumab	
	Pembrolizumab	
Interferons	Interferon alpha	Various haematological and solid organ malignancies
	Interferon gamma	
Tumour vaccines	HPV vaccine	HPV

REVIEW EXERCISES

1. Mr DE has been diagnosed with advanced NSCLC. Molecular testing reveals that the cancer cells contain an EGFR-activating mutation. Based on this information, what is the most appropriate treatment for the person, and how does this treatment work?
2. Ms SL is a 31-year-old mother of two who has just been diagnosed with metastatic breast cancer. Referring to an appropriate treatment guideline/protocol, discuss the potential treatment options for this person and identify the diagnostic tests that may be used to inform this decision.
3. Mr TP has recently been diagnosed with metastatic bladder cancer, which is being treated with a regimen of gemcitabine (1000 mg/m^2) and cisplatin (70 mg/m^2). He presents short of breath, complaining of chills, with a temperature of 39.5°C. His last round of chemotherapy was 7 days ago. What may be wrong with him, and how should he be managed by a professional in your field?

REFERENCES

Lasala, R., Logreco, A., Romagnoli, A. et al; Cancer drugs for solid tumors approved by the EMA since 2014: an overview of pivotal clinical trials. European Journal of Clinical Pharmacology 76, 843–850 (2020).

Nikolaou M, Pavlopoulou A, Georgakilas AG. et al; The challenge of drug resistance in cancer treatment: a current overview. Clinical & Experimental Metastasis. 35, 309–318, 2018.

Rang HP, Dale MM, Ritter JM, et al: Rang and Dale's pharmacology, ed 7, Edinburgh, 2012, Churchill Livingstone.

Roskoski R Jr. Properties of FDA-approved small molecule protein kinase inhibitors: A 2021 update. Pharmacological Research. 165:105463, 2021.

Rowland A, van Dyk M, Mangoni AA, et al; Kinase inhibitor pharmacokinetics: comprehensive summary and roadmap for addressing inter-individual variability in exposure. Expert Opinion on Drug Metabolism & Toxicology. 13 :31–49, 2017.

van Dyk M, Bulamu N, Boylan C, et al. Cost-effectiveness of oral anticancer drugs and associated individualised dosing approaches in patients with cancer: protocol for a systematic review. BMJ Open; 11: e047173, 2021.

Wahid B, Ali A, Rafique S, et al; An overview of cancer immunotherapeutic strategies. Immunotherapy. 10: 999–1010, 2021.

CHAPTER 34

ANTI-INFLAMMATORY AND IMMUNOMODULATING DRUGS

Kathleen Knights

KEY ABBREVIATIONS

COX	cyclo-oxygenase
DMARDs	disease-modifying antirheumatic drugs
Ig	immunoglobulin
IL	interleukin
LT	leukotrienes
mTOR	mammalian target of rapamycin
NFAT	nuclear factor of activated T-cells
NSAIDs	non-steroidal anti-inflammatory drugs
PG	prostaglandin
RA	rheumatoid arthritis
TNF	tumour necrosis factor
XO	xanthine oxidase

KEY TERMS

disease-modifying antirheumatic drugs 765
gout 778
histamine 758
hyperuricaemia 778
immunostimulating drug 775
immunosuppressant drug 770
non-steroidal anti-inflammatory drugs 760

Chapter Focus

This chapter reviews the uses of anti-inflammatory and immunomodulating drugs. They include the non-steroidal anti-inflammatory drugs, which are among the most widely prescribed drugs in the world; disease-modifying antirheumatic drugs, used as first-line treatment for rheumatoid arthritis; immunosuppressant drugs, crucial in treating multiple diseases and to the success of organ transplantation; antihistamines, which are widely used for motion sickness, vertigo and skin and allergic disorders; and drugs used to treat gout, a disorder of uric acid metabolism.

KEY DRUG GROUPS

Disease-modifying antirheumatic drugs:

- **Auranofin**, **hydroxychloroquine**, **penicillamine**, **sulfasalazine**
- Cytokine modulators: **abatacept**, **anakinra**, **baricitinib**, **rituximab**, **tocilizumab**, **tofacitinib**, **upadacitinib**
- TNF-α antagonists: **adalimumab**, **certolizumab**, **etanercept**, **golimumab**, **infliximab**

Drugs used for the treatment of gout:

- **Allopurinol** (Drug Monograph 34.2), **colchicine**, **febuxostat**, **probenecid**

Histamine$_1$-antihistamines:

- **Loratadine**, promethazine

Immunostimulant drugs:

- interferons

Immunosuppressant drugs:

- **Azathioprine**, **basiliximab**, **ciclosporin** (Drug Monograph 34.1), **everolimus**, **leflunomide**, **sirolimus**, tacrolimus

Non-steroidal anti-inflammatory drugs:

- COX-2 selective: **celecoxib**, **etoricoxib**, **meloxicam,** parecoxib
- Non-selective: **diclofenac**, **ibuprofen**, **ketoprofen**, **naproxen**, **piroxicam**

CRITICAL THINKING SCENARIO

Katherine, a 69-year-old woman, has been diagnosed with osteoarthritis and has been prescribed the NSAID ibuprofen 200 mg three times daily. Several weeks later, she presents with gastrointestinal adverse effects and requests that the drug be changed for 'Naprosyn' (naproxen), the same as her friend.

1. Explain why she has developed gastrointestinal adverse effects.
2. Will changing to naproxen decrease these effects?
3. What alternative drug/NSAID could you consider and explain why?

Introduction

The immune system is composed of cells and organs that mount defensive responses against pathogens (e.g. microbes, toxins and chemicals) and cancer cells and, in some cases, unfortunately, against normal body tissues (autoimmune diseases). The body's resistance to disease is both non-specific (e.g. physical and chemical barriers that offer immediate protection) and specific (i.e. an acquired resistance or immunity that develops more slowly). The lymphatic system is responsible for eliciting highly specific immune responses and comprises the lymph system, red bone marrow, thymus gland, spleen and tonsils. These organs and tissues are collectively responsible for the production and maturation of the immunocompetent cells and for facilitating the immune response.

Inflammation

The initial lines of defence for the body are the skin, the mucous membranes of the respiratory and gastrointestinal (GI) tracts and chemical secretions such as saliva and gastric acid. Penetration of these barriers by pathogens results in the mobilisation of natural killer cells, which are lymphocytes that are of neither B- nor T-cell type, and phagocytic neutrophils and macrophages. If cells are damaged by bacteria or viruses, physical trauma (e.g. a surgery, radiation), foreign bodies or chemical substances, the body will elicit an inflammatory response.

The four characteristic signs of inflammation are swelling (oedema), redness (erythema), pain and heat, which are accounted for by three basic events: (1) blood vessel vasodilation and increased capillary permeability, (2) cellular infiltration and (3) tissue repair. These processes involve a variety of chemical mediators that modify and contribute to the inflammatory response. For example, cells will release **histamine** (a product of mast cells and basophils), prostaglandins (generated from arachidonic acid), leukotrienes (LTs), kinins and complement into the tissue, forming a chemotactic gradient, and fluids and cells will begin to accumulate in the area. Blood vessels dilate (primarily because of the action of histamine and kinins) within 30 minutes of the insult, which allows an increase in blood flow and exudation of fluid, due to increased capillary permeability, in the injured tissues. The exudate includes protein-rich fluids high in fibrinogen that will attract other substances to the area, such as complement, antibodies and leucocytes. Fluid collection in the area results in oedema, which generally occurs within 4 hours of the injury.

If the injury is due to a foreign substance or bacteria, the monocytes will transform into wandering macrophages, which are more powerful phagocytes than the neutrophils and engulf and destroy the foreign material (phagocytosis). The resulting debris is removed by the macrophages and neutrophils, thus resolving the inflammatory reaction.

The complement system

The complement system is composed of plasma proteins (at least 18 distinct proteins and their cleavage products) present in the blood in the form of inactive proteases. Activation of the protein called complement 1 (C1) by proteolytic cleavage is the initial step in this cascading pathway that mediates destruction of invading pathogens. The system is divided into two pathways: the 'classical pathway', which is activated by an antigen–antibody complex; and the 'alternative pathway', which is antibody-independent and involves protein factors B, D and P (properidin) and activation of the complement cascade at C3 (Fig 34.1). Complement is essential in the response to an acute inflammatory reaction caused by bacteria, some viruses and immune complex diseases. Complement

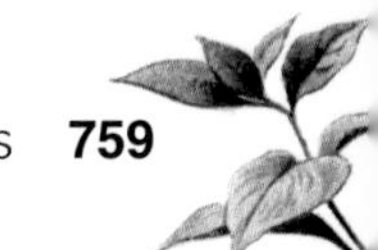

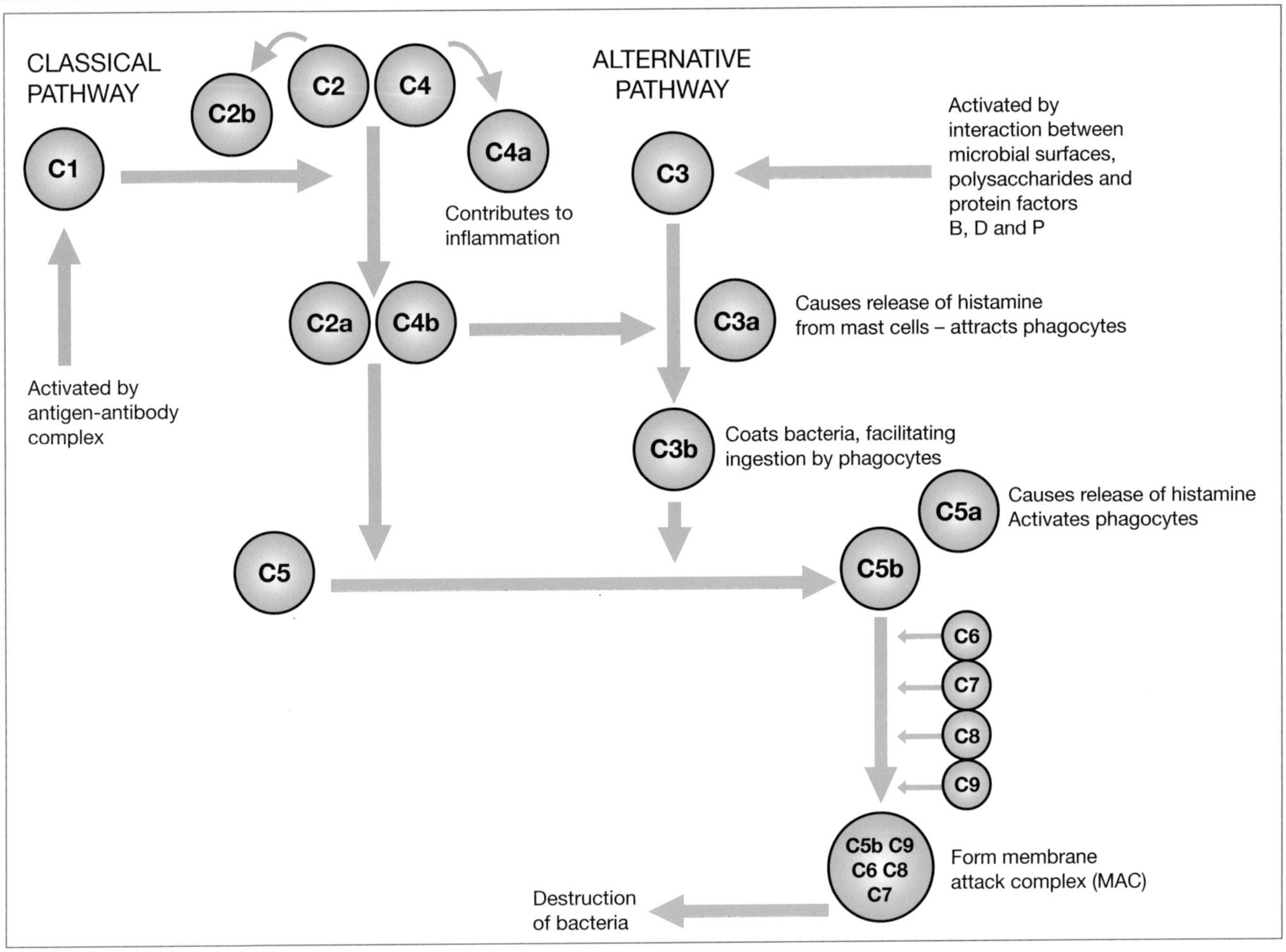

CLASSICAL PATHWAY
C1
C2b
C2
C4
C4a
Contributes to inflammation
ALTERNATIVE PATHWAY
C3
Activated by interaction between microbial surfaces, polysaccharides and protein factors B, D and P
C2a
C4b
C3a
Causes release of histamine from mast cells – attracts phagocytes
Activated by antigen-antibody complex
C3b
Coats bacteria, facilitating ingestion by phagocytes
C5a
Causes release of histamine Activates phagocytes
C5
C5b
C6
C7
C8
C9
C5b C9 C6 C8 C7
Form membrane attack complex (MAC)
Destruction of bacteria

FIGURE 34.1 The complement system
Complement protein C1, activated by an antigen–antibody complex, initiates the classical pathway. The alternative pathway is initiated at C3 by an interaction between the microbe and factors B, D and P.

enhances chemotaxis, increases blood vessel permeability and eventually causes cell lysis.

Immunoglobulins

Antibodies (immunoglobulins) are gamma globulins (a type of protein) that are produced by lymphoid tissue in response to antigens and consist of four polypeptide chains: two heavy (H) and two light (L) chains that can form either a T or a Y shape. Differences in the constant region of the H chains provide the basis for the five classes of antibodies that have been identified: IgG, IgM, IgA, IgD and IgE. ('Ig' stands for immunoglobulin; the other letter designates the class.)

IgG is the main immunoglobulin in the blood and enters tissue spaces, coating microorganisms and activating the complement system, thus accelerating phagocytosis.

IgM is produced first during an immune response. It is located primarily in the bloodstream, and it activates complement and can destroy foreign invaders during the initial antigen exposure. Its level decreases over 2 weeks, while IgG levels are progressively increasing.

IgA is located primarily in saliva, sweat, tears, mucus, bile and colostrum – and it is found in respiratory tract mucosa and in plasma. It provides a defence against antigens on exposed surfaces and antigens that enter the respiratory and GI tracts.

IgD is located in blood and on lymphocyte surfaces together with IgM. IgD is involved in activation of B-cells. Levels are elevated in chronic infections.

IgE binds to histamine-containing mast cells and basophils. It is involved in allergic and hypersensitivity reactions and can mediate the release of histamine in response to parasites (helminths). Concentrations are low in the plasma because the antibody is firmly fixed on tissue surfaces. Once activated by an antigen, it will trigger the release of the mast cell granules, resulting in the signs and symptoms of allergy and anaphylaxis.

Allergic (hypersensitivity) reactions

There are four different types:

- *Type I: immediate, or anaphylactic, reaction* occurs within minutes of exposure to the antigenic material (e.g. pollen, dust, animal dander, some drugs or food) in a previously sensitised person. This reaction is mediated by IgE antibodies that fix to the surfaces of mast cells and basophils, releasing histamine and cytokines. The most dramatic form of anaphylaxis is sudden, severe bronchospasm, vasospasm, severe hypotension and rapid death. Signs and symptoms are largely caused by contraction of smooth muscles, mucosal oedema and increased vascular permeability, and may begin with irritability, extreme weakness, nausea and vomiting, and then proceed to dyspnoea, cyanosis, convulsions and cardiac arrest. Some drugs are associated with this type of reaction (e.g. penicillin).
- *Type II: antibody-dependent cytotoxic reaction* involves IgG- or IgM-directed complement activation and lysis of normal cells; it has sometimes been called an autoimmune response. This reaction may manifest as systemic lupus erythematosus and other autoimmune diseases, as haemolytic anaemia after incompatible blood transfusion or as agranulocytosis.
- *Type III: Arthus, or complex-mediated, reaction* is sometimes called serum sickness. With this reaction, the antigen forms a complex with IgG antibodies, often in small blood vessels, resulting in fever, swollen lymph nodes (lymphadenopathy) and splenomegaly in about 1–3 weeks.
- *Type IV: cell-mediated, or delayed hypersensitivity, reaction* is the basis for most skin rashes, such as contact dermatitis from poison ivy and reactions to insect bites. Direct skin contact between sensitised cells results in an inflammatory reaction and cell-mediated immune response involving sensitised T-lymphocytes ($CD4^+$ cells).

KEY POINTS

Inflammation

- The body's resistance to disease is both non-specific, which offers immediate protection, and specific – that is, an acquired specific resistance or immunity that develops more slowly.
- The initial lines of defence for the body are the skin, the mucous membranes of the respiratory and GI tracts and chemical secretions such as saliva and gastric acid.
- Damage to cells by bacteria or viruses, physical trauma (e.g. a cut), foreign bodies, chemical substances and so on will elicit an inflammatory response.
- The four characteristic signs of inflammation are swelling (oedema), redness (erythema), pain and heat, which are accounted for by three basic events: (1) blood vessel vasodilation and increased capillary permeability, (2) cellular infiltration and (3) tissue repair.
- Mediators of inflammation include the complement system and local hormones such as histamine, prostaglandins and cytokines.
- Antibodies are gamma globulins (a type of protein), called immunoglobulins, that are specific for particular antigens. Five classes of antibodies have been identified: IgG, IgM, IgA, IgD and IgE.
- The four different types of allergic or hypersensitivity reactions are type I (immediate or anaphylactic), type II (antibody-dependent), type III (complex-mediated) and type IV (delayed hypersensitivity).

Non-steroidal anti-inflammatory drugs

Non-steroidal anti-inflammatory drugs (NSAIDs) are one of the most commonly used groups of drugs worldwide. Generally, NSAIDs are either prescribed or purchased over the counter (OTC) for their analgesic, anti-inflammatory and antipyretic properties.

Around 12 different NSAIDs are available in Australasia and, although aspirin is also a NSAID, this term commonly refers to the aspirin-like substitutes on the market. Despite diversity in their chemical structures (Table 34.1), all the NSAIDs possess the same therapeutic properties – analgesic, antipyretic and anti-inflammatory effects. Unfortunately, they share to varying degrees the same adverse reactions. This is because inhibition of prostaglandin (PG) synthesis, which accounts for all of the therapeutic effects (e.g. antipyretic/anti-inflammatory), also accounts for the adverse renal and GI effects (Fig 34.2).

Cyclo-oxygenase enzymes and prostaglandin synthesis

Cyclo-oxygenase (COX) catalyses the oxygenation of arachidonic acid, which is a 20-carbon fatty acid esterified

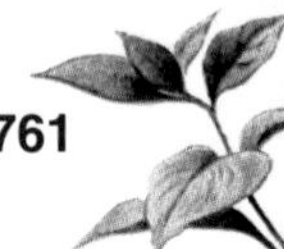

TABLE 34.1 The main chemical classes of NSAIDs

ACETIC ACIDS	FENAMATES	PROPIONIC ACIDS	OXICAMS	SALICYLATES	COXIBS
Diclofenac	Mefenamic acid	Ibuprofen	Meloxicam	Aspirin	Celecoxib
Indometacin		Ketoprofen	Piroxicam		Etoricoxib
Ketorolac		Naproxen			Parecoxib

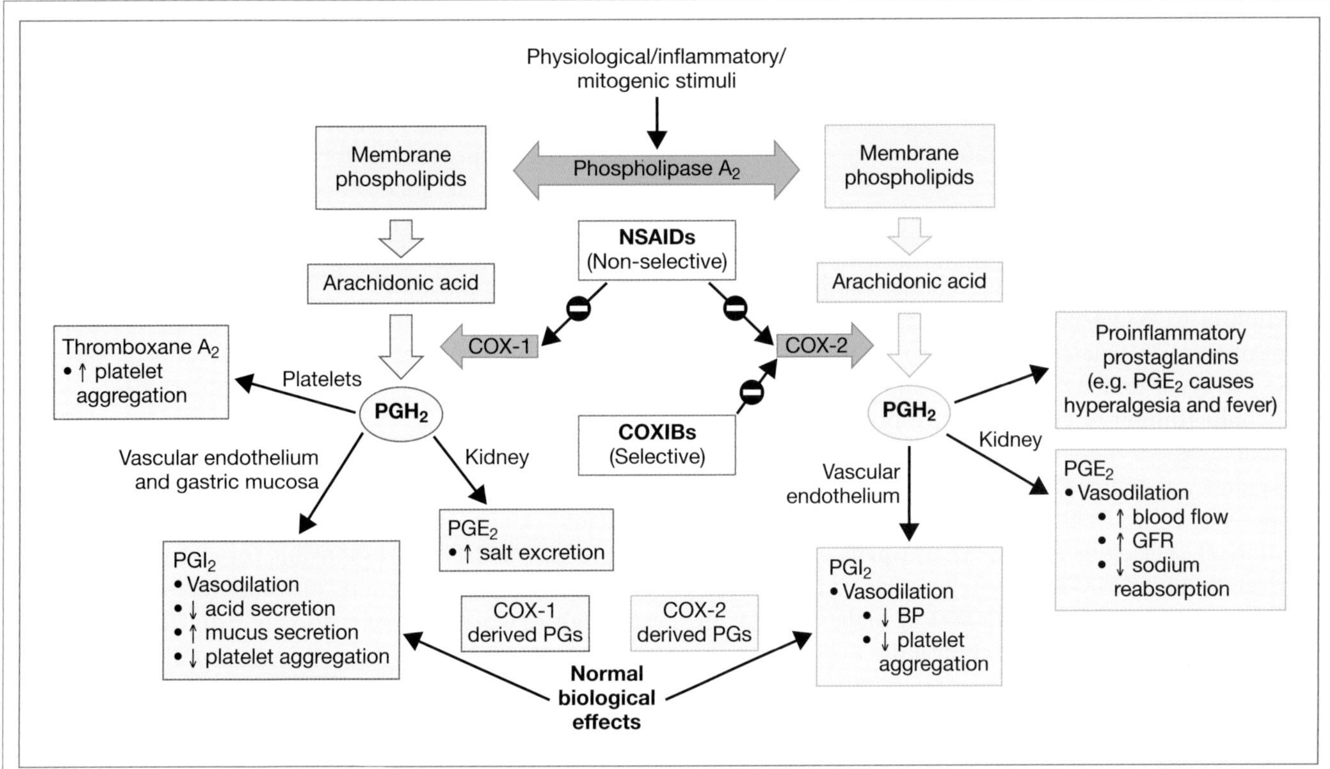

FIGURE 34.2 Inhibition of COX-1/2 by non-selective and selective NSAIDs
Following chemical/physical stimuli arachidonic acid is released from phospholipid membranes by the action of phospholipase A_2. COX-1 and COX-2 then catalyse the metabolism of arachidonic acid to PGH_2. Subsequent metabolism to the eicosanoids (e.g. thromboxane A_2 and PGI_2, PGE_2) differs in different cells/organs.
PGs = prostaglandins; (−) = inhibition by NSAIDs; green arrows denote enzymes

to phospholipids of cell membranes. Arachidonic acid is released from the cell membrane by a variety of physical, chemical and hormonal stimuli through the action of acylhydrolases, principally phospholipase A_2 (Fig 34.2). Once released, arachidonic acid is metabolised principally to PGs and LTs. At the time, this single enzyme was thought to be responsible for the synthesis of all PGs, which fall into several main classes, designated by letters and distinguished by substitutions on the cyclopentane ring (e.g. PGE_1, PGE_2, PGI_2).

PGs are synthesised by most cells in the body and bind to a number of PG receptors. With regard to PGE_2, there are currently four subtypes of EP receptors, EP1–EP4. PGE_2 is the main PG that contributes to inflammatory erythema and pain. It does not cause pain directly but appears to potentiate the pain induced by mediators such as bradykinin or histamine by sensitising nociceptors on sensory nerve terminals to painful stimulation. This property of hyperalgesia is also shared by PGI_2. Both of these PGs are found in the synovial fluid of arthritic patients. PGE_2 also causes fever. Following its release by inflammatory mediators from endothelial cells in blood vessels of the hypothalamus, PGE_2 binds to EP3 receptors in a specialised region of the hypothalamus, interfering with temperature control and thus producing a pyretic effect.

In the kidney, PGE_2 and PGI_2 play an important role (especially in older people) in maintaining glomerular filtration, acting as vasodilators increasing renal blood flow, inhibiting sodium reabsorption and stimulating renin release. Within the GI tract, PGE_2 (acting on EP3 receptors) and PGI_2 (acting on prostacyclin receptors) reduce the secretion of gastric acid and, through a vasodilator action, increase gastric mucosal blood flow. In addition, PGE_2 stimulates production of a viscous mucus that plays a major role in protecting the gastric mucosa against gastric acid-induced damage.

By 1990, a second COX enzyme (COX-2) had been identified. It was soon established that COX-1 (the original enzyme identified) is expressed in most tissues and, in particular, catalyses the synthesis of protective mucosal PGs in the GI tract and vasodilatory PGs in the kidneys. COX-2 is constitutively expressed in many tissues – for example, brain, kidney, placenta and GI tract (often at low levels) – and is upregulated in cancer tissues and by inflammatory cytokines, laminar shear stress and various growth factors.

Mechanism of action

Aspirin and the older NSAIDs (e.g. the -profens) inhibit both COX-1 and COX-2 and it was thought at the time that inhibition of COX-2 accounted for the anti-inflammatory actions of NSAIDs, whereas inhibition of COX-1 explained the GI and renal toxicity. This led to the search for drugs that would inhibit COX-2 selectively (the -coxibs). Celecoxib was the first COX-2 selective drug approved (1998), and was followed soon after by rofecoxib, which was marketed in 1999 (withdrawn 2004). With the exception of celecoxib, etoricoxib and parecoxib, which selectively inhibit COX-2, and meloxicam, which inhibits COX-2 at normal doses (also COX-1 at higher doses), all of the other NSAIDs in current clinical use non-selectively inhibit both COX-1 and COX-2.

In addition to inhibition of COX, the non-selective NSAIDs also reduce synthesis of superoxide radicals, inhibit expression of adhesion molecules, reduce the activity of nitric oxide synthase, induce apoptosis, modify lymphocyte activity and cell membrane function and decrease activity of proinflammatory cytokines. All of these actions may contribute variously to the anti-inflammatory action of NSAIDs, but this remains to be established. In general, by interfering with PG synthesis, NSAIDs tend to reduce the inflammatory process and ultimately provide pain relief.

Clinical Uses of NSAIDs

- Treatment of rheumatoid arthritis, osteoarthritis, ankylosing spondylitis and other rheumatic diseases
- Mild to moderate pain, especially when the anti-inflammatory effect is also desirable (e.g. after dental procedures, obstetric and orthopaedic surgery and soft-tissue athletic injuries)
- Gout
- Fever
- Non-rheumatic inflammation (e.g. dysmenorrhoea, renal colic, headache, migraine)

The choice between the various drugs in the group comes down to a clinical decision based on pharmacokinetic properties (especially short versus long half-life). Table 34.2 lists important properties of the commonly used NSAIDs, grouped together under chemical class where possible. Some NSAIDs are available OTC, and the differences between the prescription and OTC NSAIDs are usually in the strengths of the products and the indications for which they are recommended.

Pharmacokinetics

For specific NSAID pharmacokinetics, the usual adult dose and comments, see Table 34.2. Oral absorption of these drugs is very good. Food may delay absorption, but it has not been proven to significantly change the total amount of drug absorbed. Plasma protein binding is high ($\geq$ 90%) and most of these drugs are metabolised to varying degrees by the liver and the metabolites excreted by the kidneys. Parecoxib is a prodrug and is converted by the liver to the active metabolite valdecoxib.

Adverse reactions

Although NSAIDs are commonly used and readily available, there has been a long history of adverse reactions. NSAIDs are responsible for almost one-quarter of all adverse drug reactions officially reported in the UK and feature worldwide in reports of drug-related deaths.

Gastrointestinal

Adverse reactions of concern are gastric pain, distress and/or ulceration, GI bleeding and perforation. The risk of GI effects appears to be higher with ketoprofen and piroxicam, and lower with ibuprofen and diclofenac. The beneficial effect of the latter two drugs is lost when the dose is increased. Virtually every person taking NSAIDs has some gastric damage, which may be unnoticeable or can develop into frank ulceration and haemorrhage. In attempts to lessen the risk, NSAIDs, including aspirin, have been formulated in enteric-coated forms to minimise the presence of drug in the stomach. This has been unsuccessful, however, because the effect is not only a local one but occurs also due to decreased synthesis of mucosal protective PGs by systemically absorbed NSAIDs. Treatment of NSAID-induced peptic ulcers includes misoprostol (a PG analogue) and proton pump inhibitors (Ch 16). The incidence of gastroduodenal ulceration appears to be lower with the COX-2-selective drugs, but ulcer healing rates may be impaired in people with preexisting ulceration.

Renal

Adverse renal effects of NSAIDs occur consistently in a small percentage (1–5%) of patients. The most common adverse effects include fluid retention, electrolyte disturbances (e.g. hyponatraemia, hyperkalaemia) and an

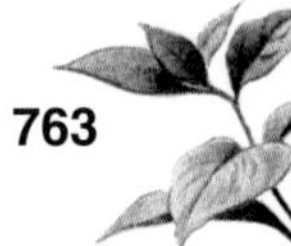

TABLE 34.2 Pharmacokinetics and dosing of NSAIDs

NSAID	HALF-LIFE (h)	USUAL ADULT ORAL DOSE (mg)	DOSES/DAY	COMMENTS
Acetic acids				
Diclofenac	1.2–2	25–50 (max. 200)[a]	2–3	Non-selective Used to treat arthritis, pain, primary dysmenorrhoea Cardiovascular toxicity appears high
Indometacin	4.5–6	25–50 (max 200)[a]	2–4	Non-selective Higher risk for GI effects and renal dysfunction than other agents Used for arthritis, acute gout attacks and pain
Ketorolac	4–6	10 (max 40)[a]	4–6	Non-selective Should not be given by any route for longer than 5 days Risks of GI bleeding and other severe effects increase with duration of treatment Do not give preoperatively or intraoperatively if bleeding control is necessary
Coxibs				
Celecoxib	4–15	100 (max. 200 short term use)[a]	1–2	Selective COX-2 Ulcer-related complications can occur Similar to conventional NSAIDs, causes adverse renal effects in some patients Cardiovascular toxicity increases with dose
Etoricoxib	22	30–60 (osteoarthritis) 120 (acute gout)	1 1	Selective COX-2 Contraindicated in patients with heart failure (NYHA II–IV) and inadequately controlled hypertension Increases blood pressure to greater extent than other NSAIDs Contraindicated in coronary artery disease, cerebrovascular or peripheral arterial disease
Parecoxib	3.5–4 (6.5–7[b])	IM/IV route only	1	Selective COX-2 Indicated for postoperative pain in adults (single dose only)
Fenamates				
Mefenamic acid	3–4	500	3	Non-selective; Can prolong prothrombin time Used for short-term treatment of pain and dysmenorrhoea
Oxicams				
Piroxicam	30–50	10–20 (no longer than 14 days)	1	Non-selective Contraindicated in patients with renal impairment May cause flu-like syndrome May accumulate in the elderly
Meloxicam	20	7.5–15	1	COX-2 selectivity is dose-dependent Higher frequency of adverse GI effects with 15 mg dose
Propionic acids				
Ibuprofen	2–2.5	200–400 (max. 2400)[a]	3–4	Non-selective Available in tablets, liquid and OTC Can reduce cardioprotective effect of low-dose aspirin by reducing antiplatelet activity
Ketoprofen	1.5–2	200	1[c]	Can cause fluid retention and rise in creatinine concentration, especially in patients receiving diuretics and in the elderly Monitor renal function closely
Naproxen	12–15	Conventional product 250–500 (max. 1250)[a]	2	Available as conventional tablets and controlled-release tablets
		Controlled release product 750–1000 mg (max. 1250)[a]	1[c]	Gluten-free formulations available

[a] 'Max.' refers to maximum daily dose
[b] Active metabolite
[c] Controlled-release form
Source: Australian Medicines Handbook 2021, pp. 711–718. Verify adult dose range using up-to-date drug/product information sources.

increase in blood pressure. Additionally, as a consequence of fluid retention, NSAIDs may worsen congestive heart failure and, in a small percentage (< 1%) of at-risk people (e.g. the elderly or those with volume depletion, renal insufficiency, heart failure or diabetes), NSAIDs cause acute renal failure due to inhibition of synthesis of vasodilator PGs. Rarely, NSAIDs can cause acute tubulointerstitial nephritis or acute papillary necrosis. The adverse renal effects appear to be comparable for the selective and non-selective NSAIDs. Importantly, it has been recognised that a combination of an angiotensin-converting-enzyme (ACE) inhibitor/angiotensin receptor antagonist, a diuretic and an NSAID results in an adverse renal outcome.

Cardiovascular

Cardiovascular toxicity has been reported with both non-selective NSAIDs and COX-2 inhibitors. Unlike aspirin, the COX-2 inhibitors do not reduce platelet aggregation, and in many studies prothrombotic activity manifests, leading to a higher risk of myocardial infarction and stroke.

Other adverse reactions

Other common adverse reactions to NSAIDs include skin reactions (rashes, urticaria). All NSAIDs, especially aspirin, can precipitate asthma attacks in sensitive people, and in some people NSAIDs may cause specific adverse reactions; for example, salicylates generally can cause tinnitus, impaired haemostasis and acid–base imbalances.

Use NSAIDs with caution in the elderly and in people with compromised cardiac function and/or hypertension. Avoid use in persons with a history of hypersensitivity or a severe allergic reaction to aspirin (or to other NSAIDs), asthma, severe renal or liver disease, active ulcer disease or GI bleeding.

Drug interactions with NSAIDs

In view of the widespread use of NSAIDs, both prescribed and OTC preparations, it is important to be aware of drug interactions that can occur with this drug group. Generally speaking, NSAIDs have the potential to interact with other drugs that affect inflammatory responses, kidney or liver function, blood pressure, blood coagulation, acid–base balance and hearing. With the exception of aspirin, most non-selective NSAIDs are metabolised to varying degrees by CYP2C9 and, as such, are subject to few drug–drug interactions. In contrast, etoricoxib is metabolised by CYP3A4 and, to a lesser extent, by CYP2C9, CYP2D6 and CYP1A2. Inhibitors of CYP3A4 (e.g. miconazole and voriconazole) increase the plasma concentration of etoricoxib, while CYP3A4 inducers such as rifampicin (rifampin) decrease the plasma concentration of etoricoxib. Ibuprofen is a racemate and R-ibuprofen is metabolised by CYP2C8 and S-ibuprofen by CYP2C8 and CYP2C9. Fluconazole and voriconazole are known inhibitors of CYP2C9, and both drugs inhibit the metabolism of ibuprofen, increasing the risk of adverse effects. Examples of important interactions are detailed in Drug Interactions 34.1.

DRUG INTERACTIONS 34.1
NSAIDs

DRUG	POSSIBLE EFFECTS AND MANAGEMENT
Antihypertensives, diuretics	Monitor blood pressure closely if an NSAID is used concurrently, as reduction in renal function may reduce the antihypertensive effect
Colestyramine	Colestyramine, a bile acid-binding resin, reduces the absorption of diclofenac, meloxicam and piroxicam and reduces efficacy. Separating administration may not prevent the interaction and the combination is not recommended
Ciclosporin and other nephrotoxic drugs	Concurrent use with NSAIDs may result in higher plasma concentration of ciclosporin, increasing potential for nephrotoxicity. Concurrent use of nephrotoxic drugs and NSAIDs may also increase the risk for nephrotoxicity. Monitor closely during concurrent drug use
Lithium	All NSAIDs may decrease excretion of lithium, which may result in higher plasma lithium concentration and toxicity. Monitor lithium plasma concentration and clinical symptoms
Methotrexate	Concurrent use of methotrexate with low-to-moderate doses of a NSAID may result in methotrexate toxicity due to reduced renal excretion of methotrexate. Avoid combination
Probenecid	May result in higher plasma concentration of the NSAIDs and increased risk of toxicity. Concurrent use with ketorolac is not recommended. If probenecid is given with a NSAID, monitor closely, as a decrease in NSAID dosage may be indicated
Warfarin	May increase the risk of GI ulcers or haemorrhage. Monitor closely. Warfarin may be displaced from protein-binding sites, resulting in a higher risk of bleeding episodes. Monitor international normalised ratio closely. Platelet inhibition may be dangerous in people receiving anticoagulant or thrombolytic agents. Avoid concurrent drug administration if possible

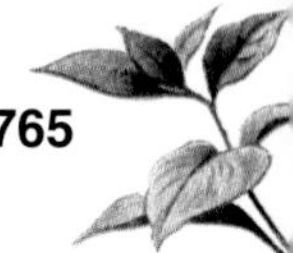

KEY POINTS

NSAIDs

- Despite chemical diversity, all the NSAIDs possess the same therapeutic properties - analgesic, antipyretic and anti-inflammatory effects.
- NSAIDs include non-selective COX-1/COX-2 inhibitors (e.g. ibuprofen) and COX-2 selective inhibitors (e.g. celecoxib).
- NSAIDs also share, to varying degrees, the same adverse reactions because inhibition of COX-1, and hence PG formation, accounts for all of the therapeutic effects as well as the renal and GI toxicity.

Disease-modifying antirheumatic drugs

Rheumatoid arthritis (RA) affects millions of people worldwide, with women three times more likely to have RA than men. The onset and clinical course of RA varies, and the incidence increases with age. The traditional approach for many years involved the prescribing of NSAIDs as first-line therapy, but this approach has been superseded, and **disease-modifying antirheumatic drugs** (DMARDs) are now prescribed much earlier. Use of DMARDs has substantially improved the control of RA and the long-term quality of life of the person. In many instances, combinations of DMARDs may be used.

DMARDs comprise a group of drugs with diverse chemical structures, and their mechanisms of action in many cases are largely unknown (Fig 34.3). The main antirheumatic drugs are:

- methotrexate (discussed in Drug Monograph 33.2)
- the gold salt auranofin
- hydroxychloroquine, penicillamine and sulfasalazine
- the TNF-α antagonists adalimumab, certolizumab, etanercept, golimumab and infliximab
- the cytokine modulators abatacept, anakinra, baricitinib, rituximab, tocilizumab, tofacitinib and upadacitinib
- the immunosuppressants azathioprine, ciclosporin and leflunomide.

Auranofin

Formulations in which gold is attached to sulfur (to increase solubility) are used to treat RA. Although the exact anti-inflammatory mechanism of action is unknown, auranofin appears to suppress the synovitis of the acute stage of RA. Proposed mechanisms of action include inhibition of sulfhydryl systems and various enzyme systems, suppression of phagocytic action of macrophages and leucocytes and alteration of the immune response. Auranofin is indicated for treating RA.

The onset of action after oral administration of auranofin occurs in 3–4 months and the plasma half-life is highly variable and may be as short as 1 week with a low dose, increasing to weeks and months with chronic therapy. In some people, gold can still be found in the liver and skin years after therapy has ceased. Auranofin is predominantly excreted in faeces.

Auranofin should be used with caution in people with inflammatory bowel disease, skin rash, diabetes or heart failure and avoided in people with known gold drug hypersensitivity, blood dyscrasias, severe haematological disease, a history of bone marrow toxicity, renal or hepatic impairment, chronic skin disorders or systemic lupus erythematosus. Concurrent use of gold compounds with penicillamine (see below) will increase the risk of serious blood dyscrasias and/or renal toxicity.

Efficacy and toxicity are positively related when it comes to the use of auranofin. Not surprisingly, a significant number of people manifest adverse drug reactions, most commonly involving the skin (allergic reactions) and mucous membranes (sore, irritated tongue or gums; mouth ulcers) or fungal infections. Additional adverse drug reactions include abdominal distress or pain, diarrhoea, nausea and vomiting.

Hydroxychloroquine

The quinoline drugs, which included chloroquine and hydroxychloroquine, were originally developed as antimalarial drugs. Although primarily used as an antimalarial (Ch 38), hydroxychloroquine also possesses anti-inflammatory activity and is used to treat mild RA. The mechanism of action is not well understood, but hydroxychloroquine inhibits the release of lysosomal enzymes, PML chemotaxis, interleukin-1 (IL-1) release and the action of phospholipase A_2, thus decreasing the formation of inflammatory mediators (Fig 34.3). The onset of action is delayed; it takes several weeks to a month or more before a reduction in joint swelling is observed. Hydroxychloroquine is less effective than other DMARDs but is better tolerated, with a lower incidence of toxicity.

People commonly experience nausea, diarrhoea, abdominal cramps and anorexia. Hydroxychloroquine has a lower incidence of ocular toxicity (retinopathy) than the older drug chloroquine but can cause severe haematological reactions, including agranulocytosis, aplastic anaemia and thrombocytopenia. In people with haematological disorders, hydroxychloroquine may cause

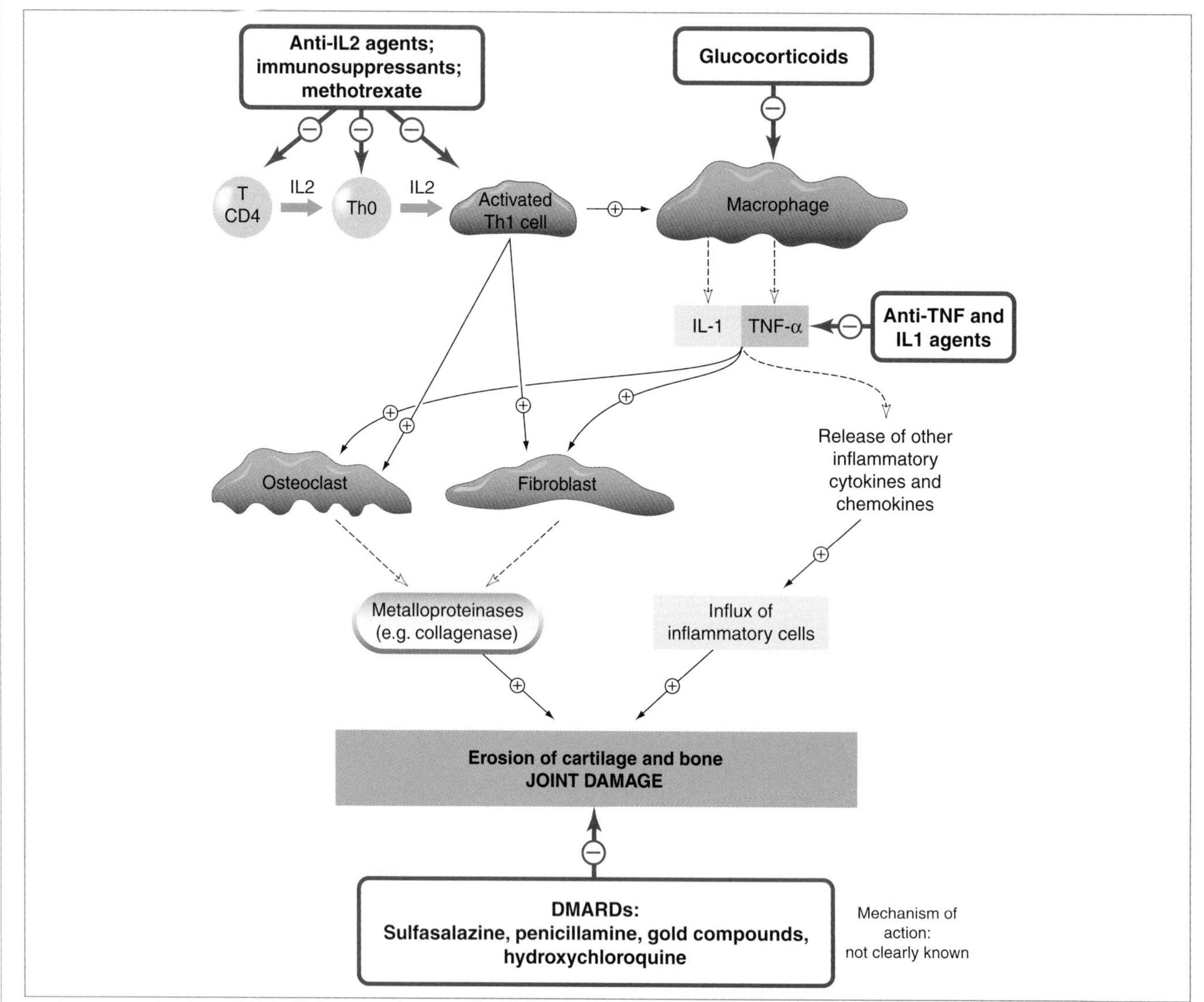

FIGURE 34.3 A schematic diagram of the cells and mediators involved in the pathogenesis of rheumatoid joint damage, indicating the sites of action of antirheumatoid drugs

DMARD = disease-modifying antirheumatic drug. See text for details of individual drugs.

Source: Adapted from Rang et al. 2012, Figure 26.4; used with permission.

further myelosuppression and exacerbate porphyria; in addition, it may exacerbate the symptoms of myasthenia gravis and psoriasis, and is not used in pregnant women because of the risk of neurological disturbances in the fetus.

Penicillamine

Penicillamine chelates heavy metals such as mercury, lead, copper and iron. Knowledge of its metal-chelating properties has led to its use in Wilson's disease (characterised by an excess of copper) and heavy-metal intoxications. After chelation by penicillamine, the metals are more water soluble and are readily excreted by the kidneys. Penicillamine is metabolised extensively in the liver, and the metabolites are excreted in both urine and faeces.

The mechanism of action of penicillamine as an antirheumatic agent is unknown, although lymphocyte function is improved, and concentrations of IgM rheumatoid factor and immune complexes located in blood and synovial fluids are reduced. The relationship of these effects to RA is unknown.

Penicillamine is indicated for the prophylaxis and treatment of Wilson's disease and for treating RA (especially for people with moderate-to-severe arthritis who have not responded to other therapies), juvenile chronic arthritis and cystinuria. The onset of action in Wilson's disease is 1–3 months, and in RA 2–3 months.

Penicillamine may impair renal and haematological function; hence its concurrent use with gold compounds may result in serious blood dyscrasias and/or renal toxicity. Also, use in people with renal impairment or blood dyscrasias should be avoided. Adverse reactions include anorexia, diarrhoea, loss of taste, nausea, vomiting, abdominal pain, allergic reactions and stomatitis. Use penicillamine with caution in people with Goodpasture's syndrome or myasthenia gravis, and avoid use in pregnancy, with the exception of those with Wilson's disease and certain people with cystinuria. Women receiving penicillamine should not breastfeed.

Sulfasalazine

Sulfasalazine consists of the sulfonamide antibiotic sulfapyridine linked to the anti-inflammatory salicylate mesalazine. Sulfasalazine is poorly absorbed, and in the colon, it is split by bacteria into sulfapyridine and mesalazine, which is the active component. This drug is indicated for treating RA, and is also used in treating inflammatory bowel disorders (Ch 16).

Most adverse reactions are dose-dependent and related to the sulfonamide moiety. Common adverse reactions include nausea, anorexia, rashes, tinnitus, dizziness and headache. Of a more serious nature are the haematological effects, which include haemolytic anaemia, agranulocytosis and thrombocytopenia. Sulfasalazine is contraindicated in people with haematological disorders or with a known sensitivity to sulfonamide derivatives. Close monitoring is required in people with renal or hepatic impairment.

TNF-α antagonists

Tumour necrosis factor alpha (TNF-α), produced by macrophages, is a cytokine that plays an important role in normal inflammatory and immune responses. It is also a proinflammatory mediator that stimulates accumulation of neutrophils and macrophages at sites of inflammation, induces vascular adhesion molecules and matrix metalloproteinases, causes an acute phase response and stimulates macrophages to produce IL-1, which is a co-stimulator of T- and B-cell proliferation. TNF-α binds to the type 1 TNF receptor (TNFRI) and the type 2 TNF receptor (TNFRII). It clearly plays a complex role in RA, and current strategies have been to develop drugs that inhibit TNF-α production or release, to neutralise TNF-α on the cell surface or to block the TNF-α receptor or its downstream signal transduction pathway (Fig 34.3).

Contraindications for use of TNF-α antagonists because of a worsening of the underlying condition include heart failure, history of blood dyscrasias, lupus-like syndrome, multiple sclerosis, psoriasis and respiratory disease. Additionally, these drugs are contraindicated in serious or untreated infections such as sepsis, hepatitis B and active tuberculosis (Clinical Focus Box 34.1). Evidence is also accumulating that TNF-α antagonists are implicated in the development of malignancies.

CLINICAL FOCUS BOX 34.1
TNF-α antagonists and infections

TNF-α is important for immune responses and host defence. Not surprisingly, the use of TNF-α antagonists predisposes people to a range of infections, especially in the first 2 years of anti-TNF-α therapy. The risk appears greater with infliximab than etanercept. Most infections are minor, but there is concern about reactivation of latent tuberculosis. Current recommendations include a chest X-ray and Mantoux test and, if required, commencing treatment of tuberculosis prior to starting on a TNF-α antagonist (Murdaca et al. 2015). Careful evaluation should be made of risk factors for *Pneumocystis jirovecii*, hepatitis B and C infections and herpes zoster, and health professionals should remain vigilant for the development of opportunistic infections during TNF-α treatment.

Clinical Uses of TNF-α Antagonists

- Ankylosing spondylitis
- Crohn's disease (infliximab)
- Psoriatic arthritis
- Plaque psoriasis
- Rheumatoid arthritis

Adalimumab

Adalimumab is a recombinant human monoclonal antibody that binds to TNF-α with high affinity, thus impairing binding to its receptors. This results in lysis of cells expressing TNF-α receptors on their surface.

It is administered subcutaneously once every 2 weeks. In view of the predisposition to serious infection with this drug, including tuberculosis and other opportunistic infections, signs of infection such as persistent fever should be reported immediately to the treating health professional.

Certolizumab

Certolizumab is the antibody Fab fragment (does not contain the Fc portion) of a humanised monoclonal antibody against TNF-α. It is conjugated to polyethylene glycol (pegylated), which increases the plasma half-life such that it is comparable to that of the whole antibody TNF-α inhibitors such as adalimumab. Certolizumab binds to both soluble and membrane-bound TNF-α, inhibiting the proinflammatory actions of TNF-α. Bioavailability is about 80% after subcutaneous injection and the terminal elimination half-life is 14 days. Some people develop certolizumab antibodies that increase clearance of the drug from plasma, thus reducing the clinical effectiveness. Adverse reactions include injection-site reactions and a higher incidence of infections, including respiratory tract infections and tuberculosis.

Etanercept

Etanercept is a bioengineered fusion protein comprising two tumour necrosis factor receptors coupled with a portion of human IgG, which binds to TNF-α and blocks its activity (Fig 34.3).

Etanercept has been shown to be effective when used as monotherapy in RA. It is absorbed slowly, and peak plasma concentrations occur at approximately 50 hours; the half-life is in the order of 4–5 days. It is administered subcutaneously either once or twice a week. In view of suppression of the activity of TNF-α, oral vaccines (e.g. polio vaccine) should not be administered to people receiving etanercept, and medical advice should be sought if a person is exposed to chickenpox or shingles during therapy. Contraindications to its use include hypersensitivity to etanercept and sepsis. Adverse reactions have included fatal pancytopenia and aplastic anaemia.

Golimumab

Golimumab is a fully humanised anti-TNF IgG monoclonal antibody that has high affinity for both soluble and membrane-bound TNF-α. It is indicated for moderate-to-severe RA and psoriatic arthritis refractory to other DMARDs. Maximum serum concentration is achieved within 2–6 days and the elimination half-life is 11–14 days. Administered subcutaneously once a month, clinical response is seen within 12 weeks. The most common adverse effect is nausea. In addition to the usual adverse effects of TNF-α antagonists, golimumab also causes an increase in liver enzymes, and routine monitoring of liver function is recommended.

Infliximab

Infliximab is an antibody against TNF-α and comprises the antigen-binding region of the mouse antibody and the constant region of human IgG_1. It binds to soluble and membrane-bound TNF-α, preventing TNF-α from binding to its receptor and hence initiating inflammatory cell actions in chronic conditions such as RA. Like etanercept, infliximab should be used with great caution as it may reactivate latent tuberculosis, worsen heart failure, exacerbate or induce a lupus-like syndrome and worsen multiple sclerosis. It is administered intravenously at a dose of 3 mg/kg (for RA), repeated every 2–6 weeks and then at 8-week intervals. Common adverse reactions include, but are not limited to, abdominal pain, cough, dizziness, headache, itching, fatigue and nausea.

Cytokine modulators

Clinical Uses of Cytokine Modulators

- Giant cell arteritis (tocilizumab)
- Polyarticular juvenile idiopathic arthritis
- Psoriatic arthritis
- Rheumatoid arthritis
- Ulcerative colitis (tofacitinib)

Abatacept

Abatacept is an engineered drug comprising the extracellular portion of CTLA-4 conjugated to the Fc portion of IgG_1. It binds to CD80 and CD86 on antigen-presenting cells, which modulates a key co-stimulatory signal required for activation of T-lymphocytes expressing CD28. This results in a reduction in cytokine synthesis and inflammation. It is currently indicated for use with methotrexate in people who have an inadequate clinical response to methotrexate or TNF-α antagonists. Given as an intravenous infusion at 0, 2 and 4 weeks, and then at 4-week intervals, the most significant adverse effects are infusion-related reactions (e.g. headache, dizziness and hypertension usually within 1 hour of the start of infusion) and infections. The latter precludes use in serious infections, including active tuberculosis.

Anakinra

Multiple mediators are involved in inflammatory processes, and one such mediator is IL-1. IL-1 is produced in a variety of cells, including monocytes, macrophages and specialised cells in the synovial lining of joints. It is a proinflammatory cytokine, and suppression of its activity by antagonists that bind to the IL-1 receptor tends to reduce the inflammatory response (Fig 34.3).

Anakinra is a recombinant form of the endogenous IL-1 receptor antagonist and inhibits the action of IL-1 by competitively blocking the binding of IL-1 to IL-1 receptors on IL-1 responsive target cells. Due to its relatively short half-life (3–6 hours), it is administered daily (at the same time) by the subcutaneous route.

Contraindications, adverse reactions and predisposition to infection are similar to those of the other cytokine blockers. As there are no data, the use of anakinra should be avoided in pregnancy.

Baricitinib

Dysregulation of cytokine signalling pathways including Janus kinase (JAK) is a key feature of RA. Stimulation of intracellular signal transduction by cytokines leads to changes in cell activation, proliferation and survival (Choy et al. 2019). JAK is a family of cytoplasmic protein tyrosine kinases comprising JAK1–3 and tyrosine kinase 2. JAK1/JAK2 are widely expressed in people with RA and they mediate the signalling of IL-6, IL-23, G-CSF, GM-CSF and interferons.

Baricitinib is a small molecule chemical inhibitor of JAK1/JAK2. It competitively inhibits adenosine triphosphate (ATP) kinase, which blocks signalling by certain cytokines (e.g. IL-6) by preventing the transfer of a phosphate group from ATP to JAK1/JAK2 hence preventing JAK activation. Inhibition of JAK activation decreases the inflammatory/immune response in RA.

Administered orally baricitinib reaches peak plasma concentration in 1.5 hours and the long half-life of about 14 hours allows once daily dosing. Predominantly renally excreted as unchanged drug (~64%), dose reduction is recommended in people with compromised renal function. Adverse effects include serious and opportunistic infections, hypercholesterolaemia and a range of GI effects (e.g. nausea, abdominal pain, vomiting).

Rituximab

Rituximab is a genetically engineered chimeric (mouse–human) IgG_1-kappa monoclonal antibody that targets the CD20 antigen found on the surface of malignant and normal B-lymphocytes. It depletes $CD20^+$ B-cells through a combination of complement-dependent cytotoxicity, antibody-dependent cellular cytotoxicity and induction of apoptosis. As a consequence of B-cell depletion, antibody production, cytokine networks, B-cell-mediated antigen presentation and activation of T-cell and macrophages are all affected. Rituximab causes lymphopenia in most people, typically lasting 6 months, and a full recovery of B-lymphocytes in the peripheral blood is usually seen 9–12 months after therapy, as CD20 is not expressed on haematopoietic stem cells. It is indicated for treating severe RA in people who are refractory to or intolerant of TNF-α antagonists. Given as an intravenous infusion (1 g for two doses 2 weeks apart) the most significant adverse effect is infusion-related reactions (e.g. headache, back pain, limb pain, heat sensations, pruritus and rash) and, rarely, anaphylaxis. The severity and frequency of infusion-related reactions can be controlled by the administration of paracetamol and an antihistamine 30–60 minutes prior to the infusion and intravenous methylprednisolone 30 minutes before the infusion (Australian Medicines Handbook 2021).

Tocilizumab

The recombinant humanised monoclonal IgG_1 antibody tocilizumab binds to soluble and membrane-bound IL-6 receptors, thus inhibiting the binding of IL-6. IL-6, which is produced by a variety of cell types in response to infection, trauma and immunological challenge, plays a significant role in disease processes and has both proinflammatory and anti-inflammatory characteristics. Tocilizumab inhibits the inflammatory and immunological responses mediated by IL-6. It is used in people who have an inadequate response to other antirheumatic drugs. Tocilizumab has non-linear pharmacokinetics and with increasing doses clearance decreases and half-life increases (~240 hours) indicating saturable elimination processes. It is administered by intravenous infusion once a month.

Tofacitinib

Tofacitinib is a preferential JAK3 inhibitor. JAK3 is a member of the tyrosine kinase group of enzymes and is expressed on haematopoietic cells. It is crucial for the signal transduction of ILs that are integral to lymphocyte activation and proliferation. Hence, tofacitinib blocks cytokine pathways that lead to lymphocyte activation. It is indicated for treating RA in people who are either intolerant of or with inadequate response to methotrexate.

Administered orally, it reaches steady state in 24–48 hours, but the maximal effect on lymphocytes is not achieved for 8–10 weeks. Tofacitinib is metabolised by CYP3A4 (~70%) and the remainder excreted in urine as unchanged drug (~30%). It is contraindicated in severe hepatic impairment, and drug interactions are likely with inducers and inhibitors of CYP3A4.

Tofacitinib increases the risk of serious infections (e.g. cellulitis, pneumonia), and live vaccines should not be administered. In addition, this drug increases plasma cholesterol and should not be used in pregnancy, lactating women or those contemplating pregnancy.

Upadacitinib

Upadacitinib is a small molecule chemical inhibitor that was specifically engineered to be selective inhibitor of JAK1 (Tanaka 2020). JAK1 was targeted because of its key role in signalling downstream of the proinflammatory cytokines. Clinical studies have reported a significant improvement in both functional and clinical outcomes compared with methotrexate in people with RA. Upadacitinib is well absorbed after oral administration

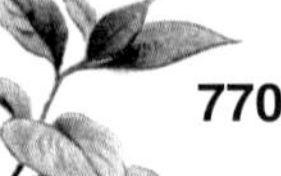

and the maximal plasma concentration occurs in about 4 hours. The long half-life of around 15 hours allows once daily dosing. The drug is metabolised by CYP3A4 and 16–21% is excreted as unchanged drug in urine (Mohamed 2020). Coadministration of strong inhibitors (e.g. ketoconazole) or inducers (e.g. rifampicin (rifampin)) of CYP3A4 with upadacitinib are contraindicated. Adverse effects include headache and upper respiratory tract symptoms (e.g. cough, loss of voice, nasal congestion, sore throat).

KEY POINTS

DMARDs

- Inflammatory disorders such as RA require lifelong therapy, and the choice of drugs is often weighed against the risk of adverse effects.
- DMARDs comprise a group of drugs with diverse chemical structures, and their mechanisms of action in many cases are largely unknown.
- Drugs include methotrexate, auranofin, TNF-α antagonists (e.g. certolizumab), cytokine modulators (e.g. abatacept), immunosuppressants (e.g. leflunomide) and hydroxychloroquine, penicillamine and sulfasalazine.
- Use of DMARDs has substantially improved the control of RA and long-term quality of life. In many instances, combinations of DMARDs may be used.

Immunosuppressant drugs

In Australasia each year, around 1500 people receive organ transplants. The rejection of allogenic transplants led to the development of **immunosuppressant drugs**, which are crucial to the success of organ transplantation. An organ transplant activates an immune response by the release of macrophages to phagocytose and process the foreign tissue. In addition, IL-1 production increases, which activates helper T-lymphocytes that have a surface CD3 receptor. The activated T-cells stimulate production of killer, or cytotoxic, T-lymphocytes and B-lymphocytes, in part by producing IL-2. T-cells are necessary for cellular immunity, while B-cells are responsible for humoral immunity (production of antibodies). The primary sites of action of the immunosuppressant drugs are illustrated in Figure 34.4.

Immunodeficiency or immunosuppression may also occur because of a genetic or an acquired disorder of the immune system. Acquired immune deficiency may be induced by a variety of drugs such as chemotherapeutic and immunosuppressant agents, by radiation therapy or through viral infections. Not surprisingly, much research has been directed towards developing either immunosuppressant or immunostimulating drugs.

There are several classes of immunosuppressant drugs:

- corticosteroids (discussed in Ch 29)
- calcineurin inhibitors – ciclosporin and tacrolimus
- mammalian target of rapamycin (mTOR) inhibitors – everolimus, sirolimus
- cytotoxic immunosuppressants – azathioprine, methotrexate, cyclophosphamide and mercaptopurine (discussed in Ch 33)
- immunosuppressant antibodies – antithymocyte globulins, basiliximab
- other immunosuppressant drugs – mycophenolate and leflunomide.

Calcineurin inhibitors

Complete T-cell activation involves translocation of the nuclear factor of activated T-cells (NFAT) to the nucleus, where transactivation of genes that control synthesis of cytokines such as IL-2 occurs. IL-2 stimulates T-cell proliferation and generation of cytotoxic T-lymphocytes. Calcineurin is the enzyme that removes phosphate groups from NFAT, which then allows its nuclear translocation. If calcineurin is inhibited, NFAT does not enter the nucleus, gene transcription does not proceed and the T-lymphocyte does not respond to specific antigenic stimulation. The two calcineurin inhibitors in clinical use are ciclosporin and tacrolimus.

Ciclosporin

See Drug Monograph 34.1 for the pharmacology of ciclosporin.

Tacrolimus

Tacrolimus, in conjunction with corticosteroids, is indicated for the prophylaxis of organ rejection. It inhibits activation of T-lymphocytes and is believed to bind to cyclophilin or FKBP-12 protein, forming a complex with calcineurin that prevents T-cell activation.

Oral and parenteral formulations of tacrolimus are available. Oral absorption is variable, blood concentrations are reached in 0.5–4 hours and the elimination half-life is 11–40 hours. Tacrolimus is metabolised in the liver (primarily by CYP3A4/5) to a range of metabolites, including 13-*O*-demethyl-tacrolimus. Less than 1% is excreted in the urine as unchanged drug. In view of its metabolism by CYP3A4, the plasma tacrolimus concentration may be reduced by inducers and increased by inhibitors of the enzyme.

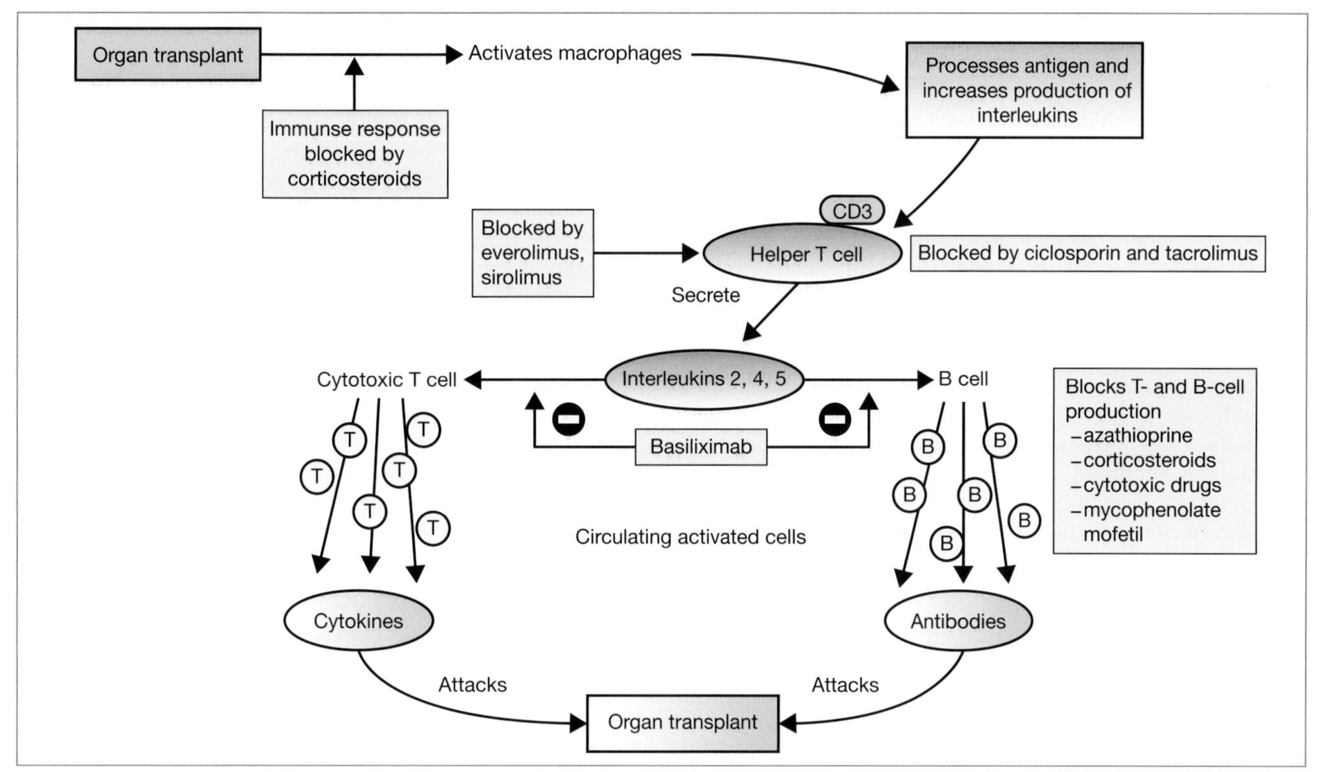

FIGURE 34.4 Sites of action of immunosuppressant drugs
(−) = inhibition

Drug Monograph 34.1
Ciclosporin

Ciclosporin is a potent immunosuppressant drug used to prevent organ transplant rejection and to induce or maintain remission in people with immune or inflammatory disorders. It is usually administered in combination with corticosteroids. Both calcineurin inhibitors (ciclosporin and tacrolimus) form a complex with cyclophilin that blocks the action of calcineurin in activated T-cells. This prevents cytokine production and subsequent cell proliferation and differentiation. Calcineurin inhibitors do not cause significant myelosuppression or bone marrow depression.

Pharmacokinetics

Ciclosporin is available in oral and parenteral dosage forms. After oral administration, its bioavailability is variable (~30%), and may improve with increasing doses and chronic administration. Absorption may decrease after a liver transplant or in people with liver impairment or GI dysfunction such as diarrhoea or vomiting. It has a half-life of about 7 hours in children and 19 hours in adults; orally, it reaches peak plasma concentration in 3.5 hours. Ciclosporin is extensively metabolised (99.9%) in the liver by CYP3A4 and is subject to many drug interactions. The metabolites are eliminated principally via the faeces, with approximately 6% excreted in urine.

Adverse reactions

These are dose-related and include:

- hirsutism
- gingival hyperplasia (swollen, bleeding gums) – this is a common problem and is generally reversible about 6 months after ciclosporin is discontinued
- nephrotoxicity, hyperkalaemia, hepatotoxicity
- hypertension, hypercholesterolaemia.

The incidence of lymphomas, skin malignancies and other lymphoproliferative-type disorders increases as the extent and duration of immunosuppression increases.

Drug interactions

Therapeutic drug monitoring plays a major role in preventing both ciclosporin toxicity and sub-therapeutic dosing, both of which can be potentially catastrophic. The effect on the plasma ciclosporin concentration of adding, removing or changing any drug should be monitored. Multiple drug interactions have been described and current drug information sources should be consulted. Examples include the following:

- Calcium channel blockers, macrolide antibiotics, azole antifungals – may result in higher plasma concentration of ciclosporin due to decreased hepatic metabolism, increasing the potential risk for hepatotoxicity and nephrotoxicity. If drugs must be administered concurrently, use extreme caution and monitor closely.
- Potassium-sparing diuretics, potassium supplements, ACE inhibitors – may increase the risk of hyperkalaemia. Use with caution and monitor ciclosporin plasma concentration and signs and symptoms of hyperkalaemia.
- Grapefruit juice – inhibits metabolism of ciclosporin by CYP3A4 in the GI tract, leading to increased bioavailability. Avoid.
- Statins – may increase the risk of developing rhabdomyolysis and acute renal failure. Monitor closely if concurrent therapy is necessary.
- Nephrotoxic drugs (e.g. NSAIDs, aminoglycosides) – risk of additive renal toxicity. Avoid combinations.
- St John's wort – induces metabolism of ciclosporin and the efflux transporter P-glycoprotein, leading to lower ciclosporin plasma drug concentration. Avoid combination.

Warnings and contraindications

Use with caution in people with renal impairment or recent surgery. Avoid use in people with ciclosporin hypersensitivity; recent chickenpox, herpes zoster or measles infections; and in severe liver or kidney function impairment.

Dosage and administration

Regimens may vary in different transplant centres. Children may require a higher dose per kilogram because they metabolise this drug rapidly. The intravenous dose is approximately one-third of the total daily oral dose.

Drug interactions with tacrolimus are similar to those of ciclosporin and include the statin class of drugs, which lead to an increase in the statin plasma drug concentration and increased incidence of rhabdomyolysis, and the protease inhibitors (e.g. ritonavir, saquinavir), which result in an increased plasma concentration of tacrolimus and increased incidence of tacrolimus neurotoxicity. The absorption of tacrolimus is reduced by aluminium hydroxide gel, resulting in decreased bioavailability. Administration of the aluminium gel should be avoided for at least 3 hours either side of dosing with tacrolimus.

Adverse reactions are numerous and commonly dose-related. They include opportunistic infections, diabetes, hyperglycaemia, hyperkalaemia, hypomagnesaemia, nephrotoxicity, neurotoxicity, headaches, tremors, confusion, paraesthesia and hypertension.

In view of the range of adverse reactions, tacrolimus is used with caution in people with diabetes mellitus, liver or neurological dysfunction, hepatitis B or C infection or hyperkalaemia. Its use is avoided in people with hypersensitivity to tacrolimus or polyoxyl 60 hydrogenated castor oil (the solubiliser in the intravenous preparation), current cancer, chickenpox, herpes zoster infection or kidney function impairment. The last is particularly important, as tacrolimus may cause permanent renal damage.

mTOR inhibitors

mTOR, also called FK506 binding protein, is a protein kinase that belongs to the phosphoinositide-3-kinase-related protein kinase (PIKK) family. The mTOR linked pathways (mTORC1 and mTORC2) control cell growth and catabolic processes in response to multiple signal inputs, including energy, nutrients and growth, and environmental factors. Dysregulation of mTOR signalling pathways has been implicated in cancer and cardiovascular and metabolic diseases. Inhibitors of mTOR are used to prevent transplant rejection and to inhibit a variety of autoimmune diseases.

Sirolimus and everolimus

Both of these drugs act by complexing with cyclophilin or FKBP-12, in the same manner as ciclosporin and tacrolimus. Unlike the ciclosporin–FKBP-12 complex, which then inhibits calcineurin, the sirolimus/everolimus–FKBP-12 complex inhibits the protein kinase mTOR, which is crucial to cell cycle progression and cytokine-induced B- and T-cell proliferation. Sirolimus is one of the drugs used in drug-eluting stents to reduce proliferation of smooth muscle cells and neointimal hyperplasia. Everolimus is indicated for the prevention of kidney, heart or liver transplant rejection, while sirolimus tends to be used in cases of renal transplant rejection.

Both drugs are administered orally, and peak blood concentrations occur within 1–2 hours. A high-fat meal decreases the peak concentration of both drugs, and it is recommended that these drugs be taken at the same time each day with the same type of food or fluid. This is important, because the plasma concentrations of these drugs are routinely monitored, and dosage adjustments may be made based on the result obtained.

Everolimus and sirolimus are metabolised by CYP3A4 and are substrates for P-glycoprotein. Not surprisingly, both are subject to many drug interactions, and concomitant administration of an inhibitor of CYP3A4 will increase plasma concentration, while administration of an inducer of CYP3A4 will decrease the plasma drug concentration.

Multiple drug interactions (Drug Interactions 34.2) may occur with either everolimus or sirolimus. In addition, due to the involvement of CYP3A4, consumption of grapefruit should be avoided, as it may increase the risk of toxicity with either of these drugs.

The use of everolimus and sirolimus is associated with a dose-dependent rise in triglycerides and cholesterol. This may warrant either a dose reduction or treatment with a statin. Limited data are available, and use should be avoided in pregnancy. Contraception is recommended during treatment and for 2–3 months after the last dose.

Common adverse reactions include hypertriglyceridaemia, hypercholesterolaemia and various haematological disorders – for example, leucopenia, neutropenia, thrombocytopenia and raised plasma creatinine (with ciclosporin).

Cytotoxic immunosuppressant drugs

The cytotoxic immunosuppressant drugs include azathioprine, methotrexate, cyclophosphamide and 6-mercaptopurine; the last three are discussed in Chapter 33.

Azathioprine

Azathioprine is indicated as an adjunct medication to prevent rejection in organ transplantation, and for severe active RA in people who have not responded to other therapies. The mechanism of action involves alterations in purine synthesis that primarily suppress T- and B-cell production, cell-mediated hypersensitivity and antibody production. In combination with steroids, azathioprine appears to have a steroid-conserving effect, and a lower dose of steroid may be used to treat chronic inflammatory processes when given with azathioprine.

Azathioprine is available in oral and parenteral dosage forms. When given orally, it is well absorbed from the intestinal tract. It has a half-life of 5 hours, with an onset of action of 6–8 weeks in RA and approximately 4–8 weeks in other inflammatory disease states. It is metabolised in the liver to active metabolites (6-mercaptopurine and 6-thioinosinic acid), with further metabolism by xanthine oxidase (XO). It is primarily excreted via the biliary system.

Drug interactions occur with:

- *Allopurinol:* inhibits XO, resulting in higher concentration of 6-mercaptopurine and potential bone marrow toxicity. Avoid, or a potentially serious drug interaction may occur. If it is absolutely necessary to give both drugs concurrently, reduce the dose of azathioprine to one-quarter to one-third of the usually prescribed dose; monitor closely and adjust dosage as needed.
- *Other immunosuppressant agents* (glucocorticoids, cyclophosphamide, ciclosporin): may increase the risk of developing infections and/or neoplasms. Avoid, or a potentially serious drug interaction may occur.
- *Vaccines, live virus:* immunisation with live vaccines should be postponed in people receiving azathioprine, and in close family members. The use of a live virus vaccine in immunosuppressed people may result in increased replication of the vaccine virus, may increase adverse reactions to the vaccine virus, and may cause a decrease in antibody response to the vaccine. Avoid, or a potentially serious drug interaction may occur.

DRUG INTERACTIONS 34.2
Everolimus/sirolimus

DRUG	POSSIBLE EFFECTS AND MANAGEMENT
Ciclosporin	Increases the plasma concentration of everolimus, and plasma monitoring of everolimus concentration is necessary when adjusting ciclosporin dose.
Erythromycin	May inhibit the metabolism of both mTOR inhibitors, leading to increased plasma concentrations and possible toxicity. Monitor and decrease dose if necessary.
Itraconazole	May inhibit metabolism of both drugs, increasing plasma concentrations and risk of toxicity. Avoid combination or monitor plasma concentration of everolimus and sirolimus.
Rifampicin	May increase metabolism of everolimus and sirolimus, reducing plasma drug concentration and therapeutic effect. Monitor closely if this combination is used.

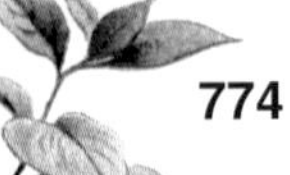

Adverse reactions are often observed and include anorexia, nausea, vomiting, leucopenia or infection, megaloblastic anaemia (the person may be asymptomatic but may also have fever, chills, cough, low-back or side pain, pain on urination or increased weakness), hepatitis (infrequent), thrombocytopenia, hypersensitivity, pancreatitis, pneumonitis, sores in the mouth and on the lips and skin rash. The risk of hepatotoxicity is greater when the dosage of azathioprine exceeds 2.5 mg/kg daily.

Due to its immunosuppressant actions, azathioprine is used with caution in people with pancreatitis or hepatic, renal or bone marrow impairment. It is also contraindicated in people with neoplastic disorders, uncontrolled infection or recent exposure to varicella virus infections.

Immunosuppressant antibodies

Antibodies directed against cell-surface antigens on T-lymphocytes have been in clinical practice for decades and are widely used for preventing organ transplant rejection. Currently available immunosuppressant antibodies include antithymocyte globulins and basiliximab.

Antithymocyte globulins

The available polyclonal antithymocyte globulins include a horse antibody directed against human thymocyte cell surface markers and a rabbit antibody raised against human T lymphoblast cell surface markers. Both of these antibodies bind to cell-surface receptors (e.g. CD2–CD4 antigens, HLA class I and II molecules) on the surface of human T-lymphocytes. Once bound, these antibodies are cytotoxic and hence deplete the number of circulating lymphocytes and block lymphocyte function. Both products (horse and rabbit) contain small concentrations of antibodies that will cross-react with other blood components, and they are not interchangeable. It is usual to perform a skin test for allergy before administration, and these globulins are contraindicated in people who manifest an allergic response to the test dose.

Antithymocyte globulins are used to prevent and treat organ transplant rejection. They are administered intravenously (infusion), and the dosage is calculated on a per-kilogram basis. Common adverse reactions include fever, chills, dyspnoea, chest pain, hypotension, diarrhoea, nausea and vomiting, and a variety of haematological complications (e.g. leucopenia and thrombocytopenia), which are all related to a cytokine release syndrome. As many people develop anti-antibodies (e.g. anti-rabbit antibodies), this limits the possibility of repeated doses. As would be expected with chronic immunosuppression, these antithymocyte globulins are associated with the development of lymphoproliferative disorders.

Basiliximab

Basiliximab is a purified monoclonal antibody that is used in combination with ciclosporin and corticosteroids to prevent acute rejection of transplanted kidneys. This drug is an IL-2-receptor antagonist, binding to the IL-2 receptor complex, and thus inhibiting IL-2 binding. This inhibition results in a decreased activation of lymphocytes and an impaired immune system response to antigens. The drug is administered parenterally and has an elimination half-life of approximately 7–10 days.

Unlike the antithymocyte globulins, which produce several adverse reactions related to a cytokine release syndrome, basiliximab appears to be relatively free of adverse reactions other than those that would be expected to be observed in transplant patients on multiple therapies. Rarely, a hypersensitivity reaction (e.g. anaphylaxis, hypotension, tachycardia) has been reported. Long-term adverse effects are unknown, but currently the drug appears not to increase the incidence of opportunistic infections or lymphoproliferative disorders (compared with baseline) in immunosuppressed people.

Pregnancy should be prevented when using this drug and contraception continued for at least 2 months after the last dose.

Other immunosuppressants

Leflunomide

Leflunomide is an oral DMARD that inhibits pyrimidine synthesis, thus limiting the available pool of pyrimidine precursors needed for proliferation of cells, including T-cells in the inflammatory response. It is highly protein-bound and undergoes continuous enterohepatic recirculation. In the liver, leflunomide is converted (95%) to the primary active metabolite teriflunomide (also referred to as A77 1726). Teriflunomide is excreted slowly in urine (about 30%) and faeces (about 70%) and has a long half-life of 2–3 weeks. As teriflunomide undergoes extensive enterohepatic recirculation, it may take up to 2 years for the drug concentration to decrease to an undetectable level in plasma. (Teriflunomide is used for the treatment of relapsing forms of multiple sclerosis.)

Common adverse reactions with leflunomide include diarrhoea, nausea, rashes and alopecia. Serious reactions such as pancytopenia and skin reactions of the toxic epidermal necrolysis type have been reported. In addition, there is increasing evidence of a spectrum of severe lung toxicity, including pneumonitis and pulmonary fibrosis. As clinical presentation of interstitial lung disease has occurred at varying times after starting leflunomide therapy, patients should be monitored closely for evidence of a decline in pulmonary function, worsening of a cough or dyspnoea.

Mycophenolate

Mycophenolate mofetil and mycophenolate sodium, used in conjunction with ciclosporin and corticosteroids, are indicated for the prophylaxis of renal transplant rejection. Both drugs are metabolised to mycophenolic acid, an active metabolite that inhibits the responses of T- and B-lymphocytes to mitogenic and allospecific stimulation. It also suppresses antibody formation by B-cells and may inhibit the influx of leucocytes into inflammatory and graft rejection sites.

Available orally, mycophenolate is rapidly metabolised to the active metabolite mycophenolic acid and an inactive metabolite, a phenolic glucuronide. The half-life of mycophenolic acid is 18 hours, with excretion primarily as the phenolic glucuronide in urine (~85%).

Adverse reactions are dose-related and include GI tract disturbances (e.g. diarrhoea, nausea, vomiting) and haematological effects (e.g. anaemia, leucopenia, thrombocytopenia) and gingival hyperplasia, gingivitis and oral moniliasis.

Mycophenolate is used with caution in people with delayed post-transplant renal graft function, and dose reduction may be necessary. The drug should be avoided in people with active GI disease or severe kidney function impairment.

KEY POINTS

Immunosuppressant drugs

- The rejection of kidney, liver and heart allogenic transplants has led to the development of immunosuppressant drugs, or agents that decrease or prevent an immune response.
- There are several classes of immunosuppressant drugs: the corticosteroids (discussed in Ch 29); the calcineurin inhibitors, (e.g. ciclosporin); the mTOR inhibitors (e.g. everolimus); the cytotoxic immunosuppressants (e.g. azathioprine); the immunosuppressant antibodies, including the antithymocyte globulins and basiliximab; and other immunosuppressants, including mycophenolate and leflunomide.

Immunostimulant drugs

Advances in biotechnology have allowed the development of new agents that can either activate the body's immune defences or modify a response to an unwanted stimulus, such as an antitumour response. These agents are called biological response modifiers; when the immune system is activated, they are commonly referred to as **immunostimulating drugs**. Common immunostimulants include vaccines, colony-stimulating factors (refer to Ch 14) and the interferons. Interferons (alpha, beta, gamma) bind to specific cell-surface receptors that are linked through to the inner networks of the cell that control functions such as enzyme activity, cell proliferation and enhancement of immune activity.

Lymphokines (IL-1 and IL-2), interferons (primarily alpha-interferon) and granulocyte or granulocyte–macrophage colony-stimulating factors (G-CSF or GM-CSF-leukine) are used as immunostimulants. Lymphokines are protein substances released by sensitised lymphocytes when in contact with specific antigens. They activate macrophages to stimulate humoral and cellular immunity for the host. ILs have been called the chemical messengers of immune cell communication. IL-2 is believed to be a T-cell growth factor that promotes the long-term survival and growth and proliferation of T-lymphocytes, which is necessary for the continuation of the immune response and is also involved in the rejection of transplanted organs. Although some people have been helped with these therapies, major problems are limited effectiveness or extreme systemic toxicity. The currently available immune stimulants are listed in Table 34.3.

Histamine and H_1-antihistamines

Distribution of histamine

Histamine, a chemical mediator, is present in highest concentration in the skin, lung and GI tract and, when liberated from cells, plays an early transient role in the inflammatory process. The chief site of production and storage of histamine is the cytoplasmic granules of the mast cell – or, in the case of blood, the basophil, which closely resembles the mast cell in function. Mast cells are small ovoid structures especially abundant in small blood

TABLE 34.3 Immunostimulants

DRUG	USE(S)	COMMON ADVERSE REACTIONS
Interferon alpha-2a (IFN-α-2a)	Renal cell carcinoma, myeloproliferative disorders, follicular lymphoma, chronic myeloid leukaemia, hairy cell leukaemia	Flu-like symptoms (dose-related), anaemia, anorexia, abdominal pain, alopecia, nausea, diarrhoea, weight loss, palpitations, muscle aches
Interferon gamma (IFN-γ)	To reduce serious infections in chronic granulomatous disease	Flu-like symptoms; commonly, nausea and vomiting

vessels and in bronchial smooth muscle, which appears to have the highest concentration of mast cells of any organ in the body. The mast cells and basophils make up the mast-cell histamine pool. A second major site of histamine production is known as the non-mast-cell pool, where the histamine is stored in the cells of the epidermis, GI mucosa and the central nervous system. Although histamine is present in various foods and is synthesised by intestinal flora, the amount absorbed does not contribute to the body's stores of this amine.

Actions

The reactions mediated by histamine are attributable to binding to four distinct populations of G-protein coupled receptors: H_1, H_2, H_3 and H_4 receptors. Current drugs are targeted at H_1 and H_2 receptors, while the development of drugs targeted at H_3 and H_4 receptors continues. The principal actions of histamine are listed in Table 34.4.

Vascular effects

In arterioles, capillaries and venules, the liberation of histamine has been shown to involve both the H_1 and the H_2 receptors. Stimulation of these receptors dilates the capillaries and venules, producing increased localised blood flow, increased capillary permeability, erythema and oedema. Activation of H_1 and H_2 receptors on the smooth muscles of the arterioles causes vasodilation, which can result in a profound fall in blood pressure.

Smooth muscle effects

Although histamine relaxes smooth muscle of the arterioles, it causes contraction of the smooth muscles of many non-vascular organs, such as the bronchi and GI tract. In sensitised people, activation of the H_1 receptors of the lungs can cause marked bronchoconstriction that often progresses to dyspnoea and airway obstruction.

TABLE 34.4 Histamine receptor-mediating effects

STRUCTURE	HISTAMINE RECEPTORS	EFFECTS
Vascular system		
Capillary (microcirculation)	H_1 and H_2	Dilation, increased permeability
Arteriole (smooth muscle)	H_1 and H_2	Dilation
Smooth muscle		
Bronchial, bronchiolar	H_1	Contraction
Gastrointestinal	H_1	Contraction
Exocrine glands		
Gastric	H_2	Gastric acid secretion (HCl)
Epidermis	H_1	Triple response (flush, flare, weal)
Adrenal medulla	H_1	Adrenaline and noradrenaline release
Central nervous system	H_1	Motion sickness

Exocrine glandular effects

Although histamine stimulates gastric, salivary, pancreatic and lacrimal glands, the main effect is seen on the gastric glands. Stimulation of H_2 receptors in the exocrine glands of the stomach increases production of gastric acid secretions. The high hydrochloric acid concentration is attributed to the activity of the parietal cells of the stomach and is implicated in the development of peptic ulcers (Ch 16).

Central nervous system effect

Histamine is known to be present throughout the tissues of the brain. Its effects seem to involve both H_1 and H_2 receptor mediation. The activation of H_1 receptors of the semicircular canals is associated with motion sickness.

Inflammatory effects

Although four different types of hypersensitivity responses to immunological injury exist, the type I anaphylactic reaction is the one associated with the release of histamine (see 'Introduction').

People with type I-mediated hypersensitivity develop allergies as a result of sensitisation to an allergen (e.g. pollens, grasses and weeds, house dust, feathers, moulds and other similar substances) that may be ingested, inhaled or injected. Hypersensitivity to a variety of foods such as shellfish or strawberries requires ingestion of the antigen. Insects such as bees or wasps, and even drugs (particularly penicillin), also possess allergenic properties that may induce a severe response in hypersensitive people.

The mechanism of type I anaphylactic reaction involves the attachment of an antigen (Ag) to an antibody, specifically IgE, and this complex in turn becomes fixed to the mast cell. The pathological manifestations of Ag–IgE interaction are caused by mast cell degranulation, resulting in the release of histamine and other mediators responsible for producing the allergic symptoms. The type I anaphylactic reaction is responsible for various disorders, such as urticaria, atopy (allergic rhinitis and hay fever), food allergies, bronchial asthma and systemic anaphylaxis.

Urticaria

Urticaria is characterised by immediate formation of a weal and flare accompanied by severe itching resulting from the release of histamine from the mast cells in the skin. The local vasodilation produces the red flare, and the increased permeability of the capillaries leads to tissue swelling. These swellings are often called hives. Antihistamines administered before exposure to the antigen will prevent this response.

Atopy

Atopy occurs in susceptible people and is usually caused by seasonal pollen that manifests as allergic rhinitis (hay

fever). After the interaction of Ag–IgE antibody on the surface of the bronchial mast cells, histamine is released, producing local vascular dilation and increased capillary permeability. This change produces a rapid fluid leakage into the tissues of the nose, resulting in swelling of the nasal linings. In some people, antihistaminic therapy can prevent the oedematous reaction if the drug is administered before antigen exposure.

Bronchial asthma

When an inhaled antigen combines with IgE, stimulation of the mast cells triggers the release of mediators in the lower respiratory tract, usually in the bronchi and bronchioles. Histamine plays a role in the early asthma response, but administration of antihistaminic drugs actually does not help to relieve bronchoconstriction because more potent chemical mediators than histamine are responsible for causing the reaction (Ch 26).

Systemic anaphylaxis

Anaphylaxis is a generalised reaction manifested as a life-threatening systemic condition. The Ag–IgE mediator response involves the basophils of the blood and the mast cells in the connective tissue. The most common precipitating causes of this response are drugs (particularly penicillin), insect stings (wasps and bees) and, occasionally, certain foods. The release of massive amounts of histamine into the circulation causes widespread vasodilation, resulting in a profound fall in blood pressure. The excessive dilation also allows plasma leakage from capillaries and a loss of circulatory volume ensues. When the reaction is fatal, death is usually caused not only by shock but also by laryngeal oedema. The symptoms of the latter condition include bronchoconstriction and pharyngeal oedema, which usually leads to asphyxiation.

Antihistamines

Many H_1-antihistamines are available OTC and are widely used for motion sickness, vertigo and skin and allergic disorders. Antihistamines are divided according to actions on H_1- and H_2-receptors. H_2-receptor antagonists, which includes ranitidine, are discussed in Chapter 16. This section reviews the sedating and newer, less sedating antihistamines.

H_1-antihistamines

H_1-antihistamines have the greatest therapeutic effect on nasal allergies. They relieve symptoms better at the beginning of the hay fever season than during its height but fail to relieve the asthma that often accompanies hay fever. These preparations are palliative and do not protect against allergic reactions. Dozens of antihistamines are available. They generally differ from one another in potency, duration of action and incidence of adverse reactions, particularly sedation. In general, they fall into two categories: the older, sedating drugs and the newer, non-sedating antihistamines.

Indications

The sedating antihistamines are indicated for treating allergies, skin disorders, vertigo, motion sickness and nausea, and for sedation. Generally, their oral absorption pattern is good, with most having an onset of action within 15–60 minutes. The newer, non-sedating antihistamines are primarily used for allergic disorders. They have a reduced incidence of anticholinergic effects and sedation and are generally better tolerated. Individual response to antihistamines varies, and nearly all of these drugs are recommended for short-term treatment. Antihistamines are primarily metabolised in the liver and the metabolites excreted in urine. Concurrent use with alcohol should be avoided.

Adverse reactions/warnings and contraindications

See Figure 34.5. Avoid using these drugs in people with specific antihistamine hypersensitivity, hypokalaemia, liver function impairment (phenothiazine-type), prostatic hypertrophy or urinary retention. The elderly may be more sensitive to adverse effects such as hypotension and dizziness; lower doses are preferable in this age group.

Dosage and administration

The dosage varies for each drug and among adults, children and infants. The newer agents released are generally longer acting drugs with fewer sedative effects. Loratadine, for example, is taken once a day and has few, if any, sedative and anticholinergic effects. Fexofenadine is a metabolite of terfenadine. Manufacture of terfenadine has ceased because of the serious and potentially fatal cardiovascular drug interactions associated with its use. The likelihood of serious cardiac dysrhythmias with fexofenadine is low, but care should still be exercised in persons with prolonged QT interval. The available dosage forms and sedating effects are noted in Table 34.5.

KEY POINTS

Antihistamines

- Histamine is a natural chemical found in the skin, lung and GI tract, principally in cytoplasmic granules of mast cells.
- Histamine release plays an early transient role in inflammatory processes and has been implicated in a range of conditions such as urticaria, atopy, bronchial asthma and systemic anaphylaxis.

- Antihistamines prevent the actions of histamine principally at the H_1 receptor.
- The older antihistamines tend to produce a greater degree of sedation; the newer agents, such as loratadine, have reduced sedating effects.

Drugs used for the treatment of gout

Gout is a chronic inflammatory condition characterised by **hyperuricaemia** (a high concentration of uric acid in the blood) (Dalbeth et al. 2021). It predominantly affects men, and its onset is usually during middle age. In some

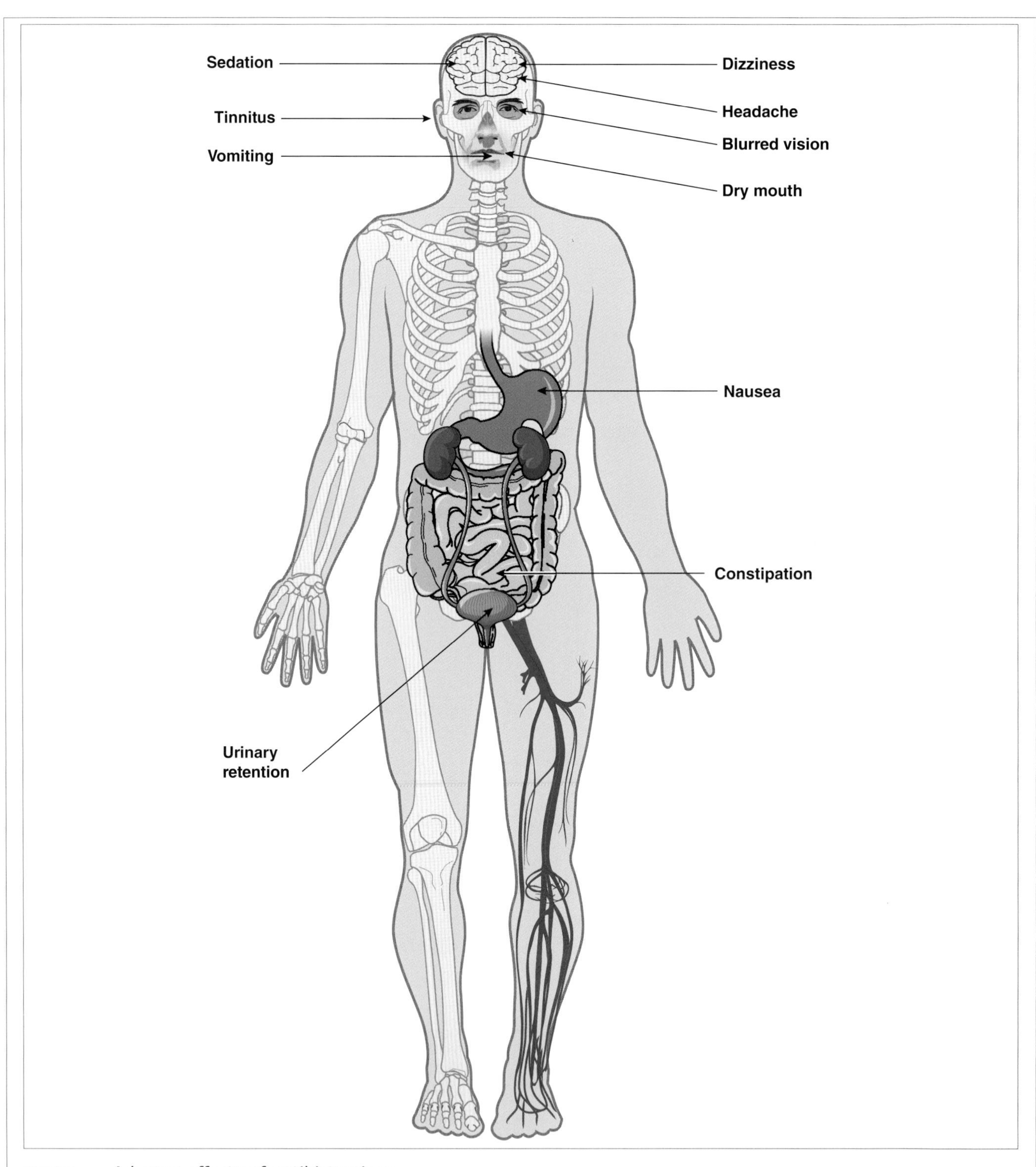

FIGURE 34.5 Adverse effects of antihistamines

TABLE 34.5 Antihistamines: available dosage forms and sedating effect

DRUG	FORMULATION	COMMENT
Sedating		
Cyclizine	Tablet, injection	Slight sedative effects, antiemetic
Cyproheptadine	Tablet	Moderately sedating, may increase weight
Dexchloropheniramine	Tablet, oral liquid	Moderate sedation and anticholinergic effects
Dimenhydrinate	Tablet	Significant sedation and anticholinergic effects, available only in combination with hyoscine hydrobromide
Diphenhydramine	Tablet, capsule, oral liquid	Significant sedation and anticholinergic effects
Doxylamine	Tablet, capsule	Significant sedation and anticholinergic effects. Short-term use for insomnia
Pheniramine	Tablet	Moderate sedation and anticholinergic effects
Promethazine	Tablet, oral liquid, injection	Significant sedation and anticholinergic effects
Less sedating		
Cetirizine	Tablet, oral liquid, oral drops	Less sedation and anticholinergic effects. Increased risk of sedation in elderly
Desloratadine	Tablet, oral liquid	Metabolite of loratadine; similar effects
Fexofenadine	Tablet, oral liquid	Least likely to cause sedation in elderly
Loratadine	Tablet, chewable tablet, oral liquid	Increased risk of sedation in elderly

Source: Australian Medicines Handbook 2021. Verify formulation information using up-to-date drug/product information sources.

people, hyperuricaemia may occur as a result of under-excretion of uric acid by the kidneys. Recurrent gouty arthritis is painful, and uric acid crystal deposits can occur throughout the body, including the kidneys, which results in an inflammatory response.

Gout is characterised by defective purine metabolism and manifests itself by attacks of acute pain, swelling and tenderness of joints, such as those of the big toe, ankle, instep, knee and elbow. The amount of uric acid in the blood becomes elevated and tophi (deposits of uric acid or urates) form in the cartilage of various parts of the body. Chronic arthritis, nephritis and premature sclerosis of blood vessels may develop if gout is uncontrolled.

Before treatment, causes of hyperuricaemia should be excluded. These include secondary hyperuricaemia as a result of increased cell breakdown in neoplastic diseases, psoriasis, Paget's disease, chronic renal disease and metabolic syndrome. Lifestyle factors that may also cause hyperuricaemia include high intake of purine-rich foods (e.g. seafood and red meat), obesity, hypertension and excess alcohol consumption (especially purine-rich beers). Many drugs have also been reported to increase uric acid concentrations, including cancer chemotherapeutic drugs, ciclosporin and thiazide diuretics. Asymptomatic hyperuricaemia in an elderly person may or may not be drug-induced and often is not treated because of potential adverse drug reactions.

Treatment goals for gout include:

- ending an acute gout attack as soon as possible
- preventing a recurrence of acute gouty arthritis
- preventing the formation of uric acid stones in the kidneys
- reducing or preventing disease complications that result from sodium urate deposits in joints and kidneys.

Management strategies include the initial use of specific drugs for the acute attack, lifestyle modifications and drugs for preventing recurrent gout.

Drugs used to treat an acute gout attack include:

- NSAIDs
- intra-articular corticosteroids
- colchicine (when indicated).

NSAIDs (except aspirin) are primarily used to treat the acute inflammation and associated pain (all appear to be equally effective), but they have no effect on the underlying metabolic problem. They are often prescribed to relieve an acute gout attack, while colchicine, because of its potentially toxic effects, is reserved for people who are not responsive to these agents or those who cannot tolerate them.

Drugs to treat chronic gouty arthritis or to prevent recurrent gout attacks include:

- allopurinol (drug of choice, Drug Monograph 34.2)
- febuxostat (second line)
- probenecid (if allopurinol is not tolerated, Fig 34.5).

Colchicine

Colchicine is a plant alkaloid from the autumn crocus and was introduced for treating gout in 1763. It is remarkably effective during an acute attack but is of little benefit when used as a prophylactic drug.

Mechanism of action

The mechanism of action of colchicine in gout is unknown. It is thought to inhibit neutrophil migration,

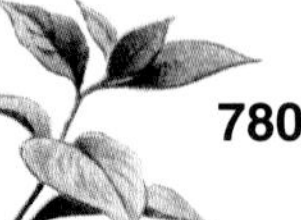

Drug Monograph 34.2
Allopurinol

Allopurinol decreases the production of uric acid by inhibiting XO, the enzyme necessary to convert hypoxanthine to xanthine, and xanthine to uric acid (Fig 34.6). It also increases the reuse of both hypoxanthine and xanthine for nucleic acid synthesis, thus resulting in feedback inhibition of purine synthesis. The result is a decrease in uric acid concentration in both the plasma and the urine that prevents or decreases urate deposits, thus preventing or reducing both gouty arthritis and urate nephropathy. The reduction in urinary urate concentration prevents the formation of uric acid or calcium oxalate calculi in the kidneys.

Indications

This drug is indicated for treating chronic gout, urate nephrolithiasis and acute uric acid nephropathy. It is also used for treating hyperuricaemia (due to high levels of cell breakdown) secondary to disease, chemotherapy and radiotherapy.

Pharmacokinetics

Allopurinol is well absorbed orally and about 60% of a dose is metabolised in the liver to an active metabolite, oxypurinol, which also inhibits XO. The plasma half-life of allopurinol is 1–2 hours, while that of oxypurinol is 18–30 hours. The onset of action in reducing plasma uric acid concentration is 2–3 days, and a fall in uric acid concentration to within the normal range occurs in 1–3 weeks. A decrease in frequency of acute gout attacks may require several months of drug therapy. Approximately 20% of the drug is excreted in faeces and the remainder is excreted via the kidneys (20–30% as unchanged drug in urine).

Warnings and contraindications

Avoid use in people with renal disease, as accumulation of the active metabolite (oxypurinol) may cause toxicity. Dosage reduction may be necessary in persons with hepatic or renal impairment. Avoid use in people with known allopurinol hypersensitivity.

Drug interactions

The following effects may occur when allopurinol is given with the drugs listed:

WARNING

Allopurinol reduces metabolism of azathioprine and mercaptopurine. This increases the risk of severe bone marrow toxicity and concurrent administration should be avoided or reduce dose of azathioprine or mercaptopurine to one quarter/one third of normal.

- *Theophylline:* high-dose allopurinol increases the plasma concentration of theophylline and the risk of adverse reactions. Monitor plasma theophylline concentration and adjust dose of theophylline if indicated.

Adverse reactions

These include:

- flare of acute gout, rash (common)
- diarrhoea, abdominal distress, vomiting
- rarely, bone marrow depression, hepatotoxicity, a hypersensitivity syndrome.

Dosage and administration

The adult oral dose is 100 mg daily initially, increased by 50–100 mg/day at monthly intervals if necessary. The maintenance dosage is 300–600 mg (maximum 900 mg) daily. For maintenance therapy, adjust the dose according to plasma uric acid concentration, which is analysed 2–5 weeks after the initiation of allopurinol and periodically thereafter.

decrease the release of a glycoprotein produced during phagocytosis of urate crystals and block the release of chemotactic factors and inflammatory mediators. These actions result in a decrease in urate deposits and inflammation, even though the drug does not affect uric acid production or excretion. Colchicine is used in low doses for treating acute gout when NSAIDs or corticosteroids are inappropriate.

Pharmacokinetics

Colchicine is rapidly but poorly absorbed after oral administration and concentrates in white blood cells. In acute gouty arthritis, it has an onset of action within 18 hours of oral administration. The peak effect for relief of pain and inflammation is reached in 1–2 days, but reduced swelling may require 3 days or more. Colchicine is partly metabolised in the liver and undergoes extensive

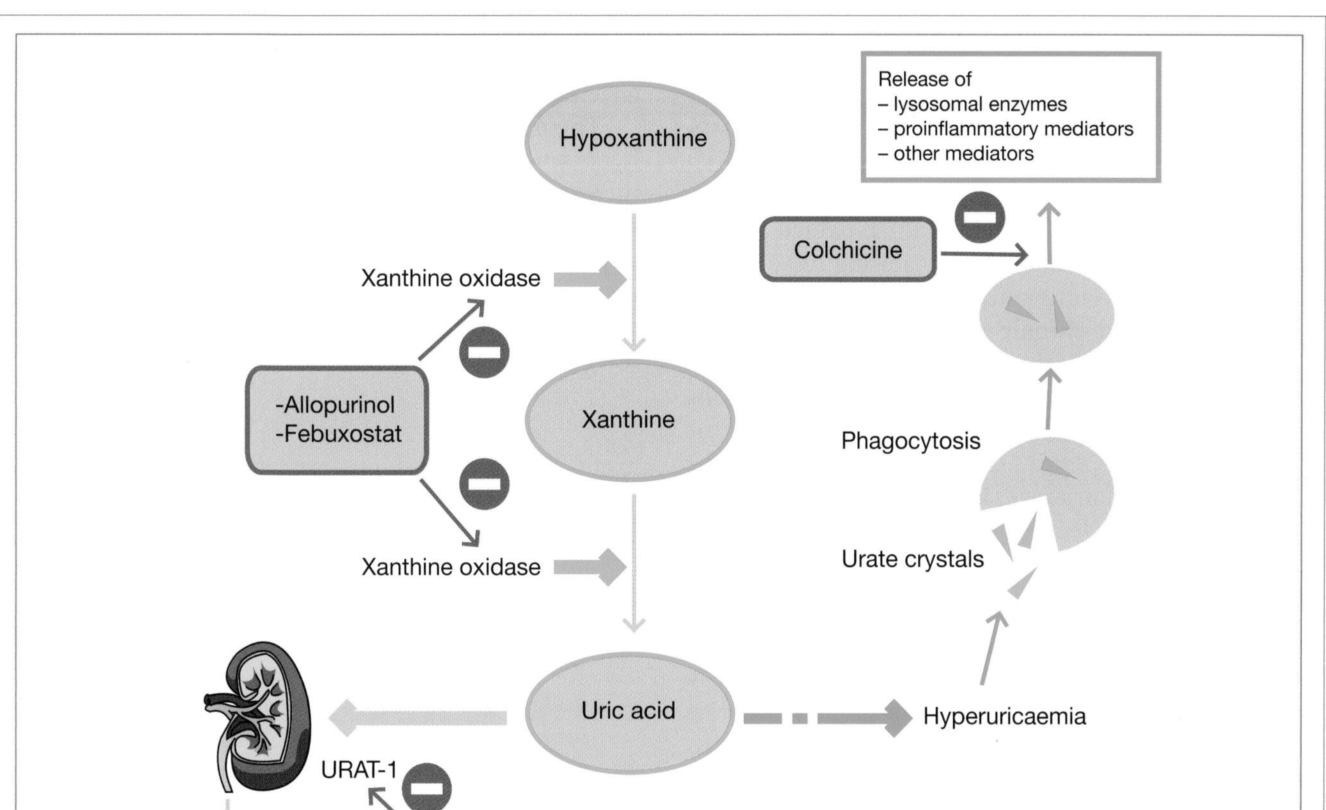

FIGURE 34.6 Uric acid production and the sites of action of drugs used for the treatment of hyperuricaemia
(−) = inhibition

enterohepatic recirculation, with most of the inactive metabolites eliminated in the faeces. Only 10–20% of unchanged drug is excreted in urine.

Adverse reactions

Common adverse reactions to colchicine include diarrhoea, nausea, vomiting, abdominal pain, anorexia and, with chronic therapy, alopecia. Rare adverse reactions include hypersensitivity reactions, blood dyscrasias, neuropathy, myopathy and bone marrow suppression. Due to the inherent toxicity of colchicine, it is used with caution in people with moderate-to-severe liver and kidney impairment and GI disorders, and avoided in people with known colchicine hypersensitivity, a history of blood dyscrasias and pregnancy.

Febuxostat

Mechanism of action

Febuxostat is a non-purine selective inhibitor of XO inhibiting both oxidised and reduced XO. Unlike allopurinol, it does not inhibit enzymes in the purine and pyrimidine synthetic pathways. A second-line drug, it is used in persons with chronic symptomatic gout with limited response to allopurinol.

Pharmacokinetics

Following oral administration, the drug is well absorbed (~85%). It is metabolised in the liver primarily by glucuronidation involving UGT 1A1, 1A3, 1A9 and 2B7, with the majority of metabolites appearing in urine and faeces. The half-life of febuxostat is in the order of 5–8 hours.

Adverse reactions

The most common adverse reactions are diarrhoea, nausea and headache. Febuxostat is contraindicated in people with ischaemic heart disease or congestive heart failure (increased risk of myocardial infarction, stroke and cardiovascular death).

WARNING

Febuxostat reduces metabolism of azathioprine and mercaptopurine. This increases the risk of severe bone marrow toxicity and concurrent administration should be avoided.

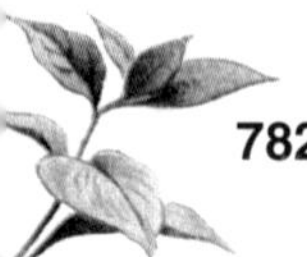

Probenecid

Mechanism of action

Probenecid was developed during the late 1940s specifically to retard the renal elimination of penicillin. It competitively inhibits the secretion of penicillin and the some of the cephalosporins, at both the proximal and the distal renal tubules consequently raising the plasma concentration of the antibiotic. It is indicated for treating hyperuricaemia and chronic gouty arthritis, and as an adjunct to antibiotic therapy. It lowers the serum concentration of uric acid by competitively inhibiting the reabsorption of urate at the proximal renal tubule by the organic anion transporter URAT-1, thus increasing the urinary excretion of uric acid. It has no anti-inflammatory action or analgesic effect.

Pharmacokinetics

Probenecid is well absorbed orally and is highly bound to plasma proteins, especially to albumin. The peak uricosuric effect is reached within 30 minutes, whereas peak suppression of penicillin excretion is noted in 2 hours and lasts nearly 8 hours. Probenecid is metabolised in the liver and excreted by the kidneys. Important drug interactions are detailed in Drug Interactions 34.3.

Adverse reactions

Adverse reactions to probenecid include headaches, anorexia, mild nausea or vomiting, sore gums, pain and/or blood on urination, lower back pain, frequent urge to urinate, renal stones, dermatitis and, rarely, anaphylaxis, anaemia, leucopenia and nephrotic syndrome.

This drug should be avoided in people with probenecid hypersensitivity; in those with any conditions that may increase uric acid formation, such as a history of renal stones; in moderate-to-severe kidney function impairment; or in anyone undergoing treatment that may increase uric acid formation, such as cancer chemotherapy or radiation therapy and in those with a history of blood disorders.

KEY POINTS

Drugs for gout

- Gout is a metabolic disorder of uric acid metabolism that is characterised by hyperuricaemia.
- The primary goals of therapy for gout are to end the acute attack as soon as possible, to prevent a recurrence, to prevent the formation of uric acid stones in the kidneys and to prevent or minimise the complications of sodium urate deposits in the joints.
- The primary medications used for these purposes are colchicine, the XO inhibitors allopurinol and febuxostat, and probenecid – an inhibitor of the organic anion transporter URAT-1.

DRUG INTERACTIONS 34.3
Probenecid

DRUG	POSSIBLE EFFECTS AND MANAGEMENT
Aspirin or salicylates	Not recommended, because aspirin or salicylates in moderate-to-high doses given chronically will inhibit the effectiveness of probenecid.
Cephalosporins, penicillins	Probenecid decreases the renal tubular secretion of penicillin and selected cephalosporins, which may result in higher plasma concentration and prolonged duration of action of the antibiotic.
Methotrexate	Probenecid may decrease the tubular secretion of methotrexate, which may increase the risk of serious toxicity with methotrexate. Avoid combination or, if used concurrently, administer a lower dose of methotrexate and monitor closely for toxicity.
NSAIDs: indometacin, ketorolac	Probenecid decreases excretion of weak acids such as NSAIDs, which leads to higher plasma concentrations and increased potential for NSAID toxicity. The daily dose of NSAID may need to be adjusted.
Zidovudine	Concurrent drug administration may lead to inhibition of zidovudine metabolism and secretion, resulting in elevated plasma concentration and an increased risk of zidovudine toxicity. Avoid combination or monitor for adverse effects.

DRUGS AT A GLANCE

Antiinflammatory and immunomodulating drugs

PHARMACOLOGICAL GROUP AND EFFECT	KEY EXAMPLES	CLINICAL USE
Non-steroidal anti-inflammatory drugs (NSAIDs) *Non-selective cyclo-oxygenase (COX-1/2) inhibitors* • Competitive inhibitors of COX-1/2 • Inhibition of PG synthesis results in anti-inflammatory, analgesic and antipyretic effects • ↓PG synthesis results in impaired gastric cytoprotection, antiplatelet effects and renal dysfunction *Selective COX-2 inhibitors* • Inhibition of COX-2 at therapeutic doses • Inhibition of PG synthesis results in anti-inflammatory and analgesic effects • Impaired gastric ulcer healing	diclofenac ibuprofen ketoprofen naproxen piroxicam tenoxicam[NZ] celecoxib etoricoxib meloxicam	• Pain due to inflammatory arthropathies (e.g. RA, osteoarthritis, gout, ankylosing spondylitis) • Pain due to inflammation or tissue damage (e.g. bone metastases, headache, migraine, dysmenorrhea, pericarditis, renal colic, post-operative pain).
Disease-modifying antirheumatic drugs (DMARDs) *Gold salt* • Exact mechanism of action is unknown • Thought to inhibit various enzyme systems, suppress phagocytic function and alter immune response	auranofin	• Rheumatoid arthritis (RA)
TNF-α antagonists • TNF-α plays an important role in inflammation and immune responses • Bind to TNF-α and block its activity	adalimumab certolizumab etanercept	• Ankylosing spondylitis • Plaque psoriasis • Psoriatic arthritis • RA
	golimumab	• All of the above • Ulcerative colitis
	infliximab	• All of the above • Crohn's disease • Ulcerative colitis
Cytokine modulators • Binds to CD80/86 on antigen presenting cells which modulates co-stimulatory signal preventing activation of CD28 lymphocytes. • ↓ cytokine synthesis and inflammation	abatacept	• RA • Psoriatic arthritis • Juvenile idiopathic arthritis (JIA)
• Inhibits action of IL-1 by blocking binding of IL-1 to IL-1 receptors on target cells	anakinra	• RA • JIA • Cryopyrin-associated periodic syndromes
• Janus kinases 1 and 2 inhibitor suppressing immune response	baracitinib[AUS]	• RA
• Binds to CD20 on lymphocytes • Suppresses inflammation and immune responses	rituximab	• Severe RA
• Inhibits binding of IL-6 and prevents inflammatory and immunological actions of Il-6	tocilizumab	• RA • JIA • Giant cell arteritis
• Janus kinases 1 and 2 inhibitor suppressing immune response	tofacitinib	• RA • Psoriatic arthritis • Ulcerative colitis
• Inhibits Janus kinase 1	upadacitinib	• RA
Immunosuppressant drugs *Calcineurin inhibitors* • Form complex with cyclophilin that blocks action of calcineurin in activated T cells • Prevents cytokine production and cell proliferation and differentiation	ciclosporin	• Severe atopic dermatitis • Severe RA • Severe psoriasis • Prevention of transplant rejection
	tacrolimus	• Prevention of transplant rejection
Cytotoxic immunosuppressant • Interferes with purine synthesis • Suppresses T- and B- cell and antibody production	azathioprine	• Prevention of transplant rejection • Severe RA • Inflammatory bowel disease • SLE

Immunosuppressant antibody • IL-2 receptor antagonist • ↓ activation of T lymphocytes and response to antigens	basiliximab	• Prevention acute kidney transplant rejection
mTOR inhibitors • Block mTOR kinase linked pathways	everolimus	• Prevention transplant rejection e.g. heart, liver and kidney
• Prevent cell growth and catabolic processes	sirolimus	• Prevention kidney transplant rejection
Other immunosuppressant drugs • Inhibits pyrimidine synthesis • ↓ availability of pyrimidine precursors for cell proliferation	leflunomide	• RA • Psoriatic arthritis
• Inhibits response of T and B lymphocytes to mitogenic and allospecific stimulation • ↓ antibody formation by B cells	mycophenolate	• Prevention kidney transplant rejection in adults and children
Drugs for gout *Xanthine oxidase inhibitors* • Inhibits xanthine oxidase	allopurinol	• Symptomatic hyperuricaemia
• ↓ production of uric acid lowers plasma uric acid concentration	febuxostat	• Symptomatic hyperuricaemia (second line)
Other drugs for gout • Inhibits neutrophil migration • Blocks release of chemotactic factors and inflammatory mediators	colchicine	• Pain relief in acute gout
• ↓ Inhibits renal URAT-1 transporter • ↓ reabsorption of urate in PCT • ↑ uric acid excretion	probenecid	• Gout • Adjunct to beta- lactam therapy

AUS = Australia only
NZ = New Zealand only

REVIEW EXERCISES

1 Anna, a 15-year-old, has been suffering from severe rhinitis for which she is taking loratadine, 10 mg once daily. She has complained on several occasions to her mother that since starting on loratadine her mouth is slightly dry and she feels 'jumpy'. Explain in terms of the pharmacology of loratadine why Anna is experiencing these symptoms.

2 Following a routine blood test, Mr GH, an 81-year-old, was found to have a high uric acid concentration (0.5 mmol/L). The doctor has decided to treat his gout with allopurinol, as Mr GH is symptomatic. Mr GH is commenced initially on 50 mg on alternate days, and he is advised to notify the clinic if he develops a rash or swollen lips/mouth. Discuss the mechanism of action of allopurinol. Why has Mr GH has been commenced on a low dose? Why he has been advised to monitor for a rash or swollen lips/mouth?

REFERENCES

Australian Medicines Handbook 2021: Australian Medicines Handbook, Adelaide, 2021, AMH.

Choy EHS, Miceli-Richard C, Gonzalez-Gay MA, et al. The effect of JAK1/JAK2 inhibition in rheumatoid arthritis: efficacy and safety of baricitinib. Clinical and Experimental Rheumatology 2019; 37:694–704.

Dalbeth N, Gosling AL, Gaffo A, et al. Gout. Lancet 2021;397:1843–55.

Mohamed M-EF, Klünder B, Othman AA. Clinical pharmacokinetics of upadacitinib: Review of data relevant to the rheumatoid arthritis indication. Clinical Pharmacokinetics 2020;59:531–44.

Murdaca G, Spano F, Contatore M, et al. Infection risk associated with anti-TNF-α agents: A review. Expert Opinion in Drug Safety 2015;14:571–82.

Rang HP, Dale MM, Ritter JM, et al: Rang and Dale's pharmacology, ed 7, Edinburgh, 2012, Elsevier Churchill Livingstone.

Tanaka Y. A review of upadacitinib in rheumatoid arthritis, Modern Rheumatology 2020;30:779–87.

ONLINE RESOURCES

Arthritis Australia: https://arthritisaustralia.com.au/ (accessed 14 March 2022)

Arthritis New Zealand: https://www.arthritis.org.nz/ (accessed 14 March 2022)

More weblinks at: http://evolve.elsevier.com/AU/Knights/pharmacology/.

CHAPTER 35

OVERVIEW OF ANTIMICROBIAL CHEMOTHERAPY AND ANTIBIOTIC RESISTANCE

Andrew Rowland

KEY ABBREVIATIONS

ESBL	extended spectrum β-lactamases
MIC	minimum inhibitory concentration
MRSA	methicillin-resistant *Staphylococcus aureus*
PBP	penicillin-binding proteins

KEY TERMS

acquired resistance 789
bactericidal agents 788
bacteriostatic agents 788
Gram stain 786
intrinsic resistance 789
selective toxicity 788
superinfection 792

Chapter Focus

The development of antimicrobial drugs over the past century has had an enormous effect on the health and wellbeing of humans. Since the mass production of penicillin in 1943, the number of antibiotics has continued to grow. Unfortunately, the use of antimicrobial drugs has been followed by the emergence of resistant organisms. The challenge to health professionals now includes not only the prudent use of antimicrobial drugs but the need to develop new agents and to curtail the continued emergence of resistant 'superbugs'.

CRITICAL THINKING SCENARIO

Tammi is a 7-year-old girl who visits her GP with her mum complaining of a runny nose, general aches and pains and feeling tired. The GP determines that Tammi has an infection that is definitely viral. Tammi's mum insists that the GP give her antibiotics to treat her infection. What would be the likely benefits and harms of giving Tammi antibiotics?

Introduction

Infectious diseases encompass a broad range of illnesses caused by pathogenic microorganisms. Some common pathogens and their likely sites of infection in the body are listed in Table 35.1. These pathogens can cause conditions such as pneumonia, urinary tract infections, respiratory tract infections and gastroenteritis, to name a few. An infection involves the invasion and multiplication of pathogenic microorganisms that cause disease either by local cellular injury or by secretion of a toxin or by antigen–antibody reaction. Infections can be classified primarily as local or systemic. A localised infection involves the skin or a single internal organ but may progress to a systemic infection if the pathogen spreads. A systemic infection involves the whole body rather than a localised area.

Microorganisms are divided into several groups: bacteria, mycoplasma, spirochaetes, fungi and viruses. Bacteria are classified according to their shape, such as bacilli, spirilla and cocci, and their capacity to be stained. Specific identification of bacteria requires a Gram stain and culture with chemical testing. A **Gram stain** is a sequential procedure involving crystal violet and iodine solutions followed by alcohol that allows the rapid classification of organisms into groups such as Gram-positive or Gram-negative bacilli (rods) or cocci. The culture procedures identify specific organisms, but they require 24–48 hours for completion.

Often, initial antibiotic selection is empiric and based on the prescriber's clinical impression. Once the results of culture and sensitivity testing are available, the antibiotic may be changed. This is referred to as directed therapy.

TABLE 35.1 Common infectious microorganisms and sites of infection

ORGANISM	INFECTION SITE
Gram-positive cocci	
Staphylococcus aureus	Burns, skin infections, decubital and surgical wounds, paranasal sinus and middle ear (chronic sinusitis and otitis), lungs, lung abscess, pleura, endocardium, bone (osteomyelitis), joints
Non-penicillinase-producing	
Penicillinase-producing	
Staphylococcus epidermidis	
Non-penicillinase-producing	
Penicillinase-producing	
Methicillin-resistant	
Streptococcus pneumoniae	Paranasal sinus and middle ear, lungs, pleura
Streptococcus pyogenes (group A β-haemolytic)	Burns, skin infections, decubital and surgical wounds, paranasal sinus and middle ear, throat, bone (osteomyelitis), joints
Streptococcus viridans group	Endocardium
Gram-positive bacilli	
Clostridium tetani (anaerobe)	Puncture wounds, lacerations and crush injuries; toxins affecting nervous system
Corynebacterium diphtheriae	Throat, upper part of the respiratory tract
Gram-negative cocci	
Neisseria gonorrhoeae	Urethra, prostate, epididymis and testes, joints
Neisseria meningitidis	Meninges
Enteric Gram-negative bacilli	
Bacteroides, *Enterobacter*, *Escherichia coli*, *Klebsiella pneumoniae*, *Proteus mirabilis*, other *Proteus*, *Salmonella*, *Serratia*, *Shigella*	Peritoneum, biliary tract, kidney and bladder, prostate, decubital and surgical wounds, bone

TABLE 35.1 Common infectious microorganisms and sites of infection—cont'd

ORGANISM	INFECTION SITE
Bacteroides	Brain abscess, lung abscess, throat, peritoneum
Enterobacter	Peritoneum, biliary tract, kidney and bladder, endocardium
Escherichia coli	Peritoneum, biliary tract, kidney and bladder
Klebsiella pneumoniae	Lungs, lung abscess
Other Gram-negative bacilli	
Burkholderia cepacia, Burkholderia gladioli, Burkholderia pseudomallei	Respiratory tract, sputum
Haemophilus influenzae	Meninges, paranasal sinus and middle ear, lungs, pleura
Pseudomonas aeruginosa	Burns, paranasal sinus and middle ear (chronic otitis media), decubital and surgical wounds, lungs, joints
Acid-fast bacilli	
Mycobacterium tuberculosis, Mycobacterium avium	Lungs, pleura, peritoneum, meninges, kidney and bladder, testes, bone, joints
Miscellaneous	
Chlamydia trachomatis	Genitalia, endocervical, rectum, eyes (neonates)
Mycoplasma pneumoniae	Lungs
Spirochaetes	
Treponema pallidum (syphilis)	Any tissue or vascular organ of the body
Fungi	
Aspergillus	Paranasal sinus and middle ear, lungs
Candida species	Skin infections, throat, lungs, endocardium, kidney and bladder, vagina
Cryptococcus	Lungs
Pneumocystis jirovecii	Lungs
Viruses	
Cytomegalovirus (CMV)	Saliva, urine or other body fluids
Enterovirus, mumps virus and others	Meninges, epididymis, testes
Herpes virus or varicella zoster virus	Skin infections (herpes simplex or zoster)
Respiratory viruses (including Epstein-Barr virus)	Throat, lungs
Anaerobes	
Gram-positive	Deep wounds, gut
Clostridium difficile	
Clostridium perfringens	
Peptococcus species	
Peptostreptococcus species	
Gram-negative	
Bacteroides fragilis	
Fusobacterium species	

Antimicrobial therapy

The treatment of an infectious disease depends on the microorganism responsible, and different groups of antimicrobial drugs are used to treat different groups of microorganisms. Antimicrobial drugs can help cure or control most infections caused by microorganisms but alone do not necessarily produce the cure. They are often adjuncts to methods such as surgical incision and drainage, and wound debridement for removal of non-viable infected tissue.

The first major class of antimicrobial drugs was the sulfonamides, which were introduced into clinical practice in 1933. These drugs were so successful in treating staphylococcal septicaemia that Gerhard Domagk was awarded the Nobel Prize for Medicine in 1939 for this discovery. The authorities in Germany at that time forced him to decline the award, but he later received the diploma and medal. The second major group of antimicrobial drugs was the penicillins (introduced in the 1940s).

Antibiotics are natural substances derived from certain organisms (bacteria, fungi and others) that can suppress growth of or destroy microorganisms. There are now thousands of natural, synthetic and semisynthetic antibacterial drugs that are all commonly referred to as antibiotics. Other antimicrobial agents include antifungal and antiviral drugs. These drugs differ markedly in their physicochemical characteristics, mechanisms of action, pharmacological properties and antimicrobial activity.

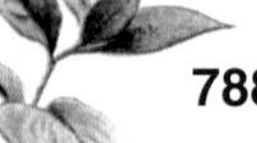

Pharmacokinetics and pharmacodynamics

The goal of antimicrobial therapy is to destroy or suppress the growth of infecting microorganisms so that normal host defences and other supporting mechanisms can control the infection, resulting in a cure. One important aspect of all antimicrobial drugs is their **selective toxicity**. What this means is that an antimicrobial drug has to be selectively toxic to the microbe but to have minimal or no toxicity to human cells. An increase in selective toxicity of a drug is achieved by targeting sites in the microbe that do not exist in human cells. A very good example is the penicillin antibiotics that inhibit bacterial cell wall synthesis by inhibiting peptidoglycan cross-linking. The high selective toxicity of penicillins towards bacteria and not human cells occurs because human cells do not have a cell wall (they have cell membranes) and nor do we have peptidoglycan in our cell membranes.

Another important pharmacodynamic aspect with regard to antibiotics is the relationship between the concentration of the antibiotic and its antimicrobial efficacy. This relationship is influenced by the pharmacokinetic profile of the drug; the latter includes absorption (if administered orally), distribution, metabolism and excretion. Ultimately, the success of antimicrobial therapy depends on:

- achieving a sufficient concentration of drug at the site of infection
- the bacterial load
- the phase of the bacterial growth
- the minimum inhibitory concentration (MIC) of the antimicrobial drug.

In pharmacokinetic terms, this translates to:

- the time (T) that the plasma concentration of the drug remains above the MIC over the dosing period – that is, T > MIC
- the ratio of the maximum plasma drug concentration (C_{max}) to the MIC – that is, C_{max}:MIC
- the area under the concentration time curve (AUC) over a 24-hour period divided by the MIC ($AUC_{0–24}$ / MIC).

The varying relationships between T, C_{max}, MIC and $AUC_{0–24}$ have been shown to correlate with antimicrobial efficacy, bacterial eradication and a reduction in the development of resistance. In simple terms, antimicrobial drugs can display concentration-dependent kill characteristics and/or time-dependent effects. For example, depending on the bacteria, a high ciprofloxacin C_{max}:MIC ratio (~10) assists bacterial killing, while a high $AUC_{0–24}$/MIC (> 125) predicts better clinical outcomes for infections caused by Gram-negative organisms. Similarly, aminoglycosides exhibit concentration-dependent kill characteristics, and suboptimal dosing may lead to adaptive resistance because of reduced drug uptake by the bacteria. In contrast, the β-lactam antibiotics exhibit time-dependent killing: their efficacy is related to the time that the concentration of the β-lactam exceeds the MIC of the bacteria – that is, T > MIC. Current data suggest that for penicillin the plasma drug concentration should be above the MIC for about 50% of the dosing interval, 60–70% for cephalosporins and 40% for carbapenems. It is apparent that achieving the pharmacodynamic target for antibiotic exposure is essential both for clinical efficacy and for reducing the emergence of resistant microbial strains.

Mechanism of action

To exert its effects, an antimicrobial agent must first gain access to the target site. Specific antibiotics or antimicrobial agents in certain circumstances (e.g. changes in permeability of the blood–brain barrier with meningitis) are capable of penetrating the site of infection and exerting a pharmacological effect on the bacteria. Sometimes, as in the case of infections of the skin and eyes, local application to the infected area is necessary. Once the drug has reached its site of action, it can exert either bactericidal or bacteriostatic effects, depending on its mechanism of action.

Bacteriostatic agents inhibit bacterial growth, allowing intact and active host defence systems time to remove the invading microorganisms. **Bactericidal agents**, on the other hand, cause bacterial cell death and lysis and eradicate the infection, which is especially important in situations of impaired host defences. Antimicrobial agents can be divided into bacteriostatic and bactericidal categories; the sulfonamides are an example of the former and the penicillins of the latter. Such categorisation is not always valid or reliable because the same antimicrobial agent might have either effect depending on the dose administered and the concentration achieved at its site of action. Tetracyclines, for example, are generally bacteriostatic but may be bactericidal in high concentrations. Chloramphenicol, which is often listed as a bacteriostatic drug, has bactericidal effects against *Streptococcus pneumoniae* and *Haemophilus influenzae* in the cerebrospinal fluid. Antimicrobial drugs exert their bacteriostatic or bactericidal effects in one of four main ways:

- Inhibition of bacterial cell wall synthesis: unlike host cells, bacteria are not isotonic with body fluids, so their contents are under high osmotic pressure and their viability depends on the integrity of their cell walls. Any compound that inhibits any step in the synthesis of the cell wall weakens it and causes the cell to lyse. Antimicrobial agents with this mechanism of action are bactericidal.

- Disruption or alteration of membrane permeability: this process results in leakage of essential bacterial metabolic substrates. Agents causing these effects can be either bacteriostatic or bactericidal.
- Inhibition of protein synthesis: some antimicrobial agents induce the formation of defective protein molecules; such agents are bactericidal in their action. Antimicrobial agents that inhibit specific steps in protein synthesis are bacteriostatic.
- Inhibition of synthesis of essential metabolites: antimicrobial agents that work in this manner structurally resemble normal intracellular chemicals and act as competitive inhibitors in a metabolic pathway. Generally, they are bacteriostatic agents.

KEY POINTS

Antimicrobial therapy

- Infectious diseases comprise a wide spectrum of illnesses caused by pathogenic microorganisms including bacteria, mycoplasma, spirochaetes, fungi and viruses.
- Antimicrobial therapy may include either bacteriostatic (inhibiting bacterial growth) or bactericidal (causing bacterial cell death and lysis) drugs, or drugs that have both effects, depending on the concentration at the site of action.
- The goal of antimicrobial therapy is to destroy, or suppress the growth of, infecting microorganisms so that normal host defences and other supporting mechanisms can control the infection, resulting in its cure.

Antibiotic resistance

The emergence of antibiotic-resistant organisms continues to be a major problem in high-dependency healthcare settings (e.g. intensive care units), in hospitals in general and in other healthcare arenas (e.g. aged-care facilities). When resistance to antibiotics causes these drugs to become ineffective, we will lose the ability to treat some infections, which will lead to increases in healthcare costs related to treating chronically ill patients (Dadgostarb 2019). Although recent evidence suggests that many types of resistance mechanisms and resistant bacteria were present long before humans began to use antimicrobial drugs, it is overwhelmingly accepted that the main driver of **acquired resistance** is the prescribing of antimicrobial drugs (Reygaert 2018). Not surprisingly, resistance is most prevalent in countries where antibiotic use is considered heavy – for example, Spain, Portugal, Luxembourg and Italy. It is estimated that about 70% of the bacteria implicated in hospital-acquired infections in the United States are resistant to one or more antibiotics. A major concern for all health professionals is that, in this era of increasing drug-resistant pathogens, the development of antimicrobial drugs has slowed dramatically as pharmaceutical companies pursue more lucrative areas of drug development. Between 1998 and 2002, the United States Food and Drug Administration (FDA) approved 225 new drugs of which seven were antibiotics; during 2003–04, two antibiotics were approved; and in 2010 the FDA approved ceftaroline fosamil, an injectable cephalosporin antibiotic for the treatment of methicillin-resistant *Staphylococcus aureus* (MRSA) and multidrug-resistant *Streptococcus pneumonia*. Ceftaroline and the newer macrolide antibiotic fidaxomicin (approved by the FDA in 2011) used to treat *Clostridium difficile* were approved for use in Australia in 2013.

In general, when using antibiotics, if the concentration of the antibiotic at the site of infection inhibits the pathogen and is below the concentration that is toxic to human cells, the pathogen is considered 'susceptible'. If, however, the concentration of the antibiotic exceeds what is considered 'safe' for human cells, the pathogen is considered to be 'resistant' to the drug. Resistance can be either intrinsic or acquired. **Intrinsic resistance** refers to the organism's 'innate chromosomal (genetic) makeup' that predictably specifies the resistance. For example, all streptococci are intrinsically resistant to aminoglycosides because their inherent genetic composition results in a cell wall that does not permit penetration of this class of antibiotics to its site of action at the ribosome. In contrast, acquired resistance 'arises in an organism because of a change (mutation) in its genetic makeup or because of the acquisition of new genetic information (new DNA) specifying a new mechanism of resistance that the organism did not previously possess' (Mulvey & Simor 2009). Mutations occur infrequently, but invariably result in development of resistant bacteria that were susceptible initially to an antibiotic. From a historical perspective, with each cycle of introduction of new antibiotics, there has been an accompanying cycle of emerging resistance to the drugs. This 'selective pressure consistently results in the survival and spread of resistant bacteria' (Barbosa & Levy 2000). In 2013, the US Centers for Disease Control and Prevention published a report outlining the 18 biggest drug-resistant microorganism threats, which were categorised as 'urgent', 'serious' or 'concerning' based on level of risk and burden (Table 35.2).

The threat level criteria specified by the US Centers for Disease Control and Prevention are:

- *Urgent:* High-consequence antibiotic-resistant threats because of significant risks identified across several

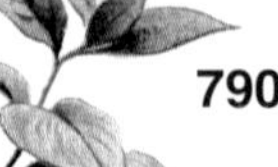

TABLE 35.2 Most important drug-resistant microorganism threats

THREAT LEVEL	MICROORGANISMS
Urgent	Carbapenem-resistant *Enterobacteriaceae* (CRE)
	Drug-resistant *Clostridium difficile* (CDIFF)
	Drug-resistant *Neisseria gonorrhoeae*
Serious	Multidrug-resistant *Acinetobacter*
	Drug-resistant *Campylobacter*
	Fluconazole-resistant *Candida*
	Extended-spectrum β-lactamase-producing *Enterobacteriaceae* (ESBL)
	Vancomycin-resistant *Enterococcus* (VRE)
	Multidrug-resistant *Pseudomonas aeruginosa*
	Drug-resistant non-typhoidal *Salmonella*
	Drug-resistant *Salmonella* serotype *typhi*
	Drug-resistant *Shigella*
	Methicillin-resistant *Staphylococcus aureus* (MRSA)
	Drug-resistant *Streptococcus pneumoniae*
	Drug-resistant *Tuberculosis*
Concerning	Vancomycin-resistant *Staphylococcus aureus*
	Erythromycin-resistant Group A *Streptococcus*
	Clindamycin-resistant Group B *Streptococcus*

criteria. May not be currently widespread but have the potential to become so and require urgent public health attention to identify infections and to limit transmission.

- *Serious:* Significant antibiotic-resistant threats for several reasons (e.g. low or declining domestic incidence or reasonable availability of therapeutic agents). They are not considered urgent, but these threats will worsen and may become urgent without ongoing public health monitoring and prevention activities.
- *Concerning:* Bacteria for which the threat of antibiotic resistance is low and/or there are multiple therapeutic options for resistant infections. Bacterial pathogens that cause severe illness.

Mechanisms of antimicrobial drug resistance

There are seven major mechanisms by which antibiotic resistance can occur (Fig 35.1). They involve the following four broad categories (Walsh 2000):

1. Intracellular concentration of the antimicrobial agent can be reduced. Some organisms, such as *Pseudomonas*, form a protective membrane (a glycocalyx [biofilm] or slime) that prevents the antibiotic from reaching the cell wall. In addition, Gram-negative bacteria produce porins (outer membrane proteins) that allow diffusion of molecules including antibiotics into the cytoplasm. Mutations in these porins change their structure and impede antibiotic access. An example is tobramycin-resistant *Pseudomonas aeruginosa*. Alternatively, the drug may be actively pumped out of the bacterial cell by an efflux pump. These pumps are found in both Gram-positive and Gram-negative bacteria. An example is tetracycline-resistant *Staphylococcus aureus*.
2. Drug may be inactivated. Examples of these enzymes are the β-lactamases, which cleave the β-lactam ring on penicillins, cephalosporins and carbapenems. There are hundreds of β-lactamases; some are chromosomal, whereas others are located on plasmids (extrachromosomal pieces of DNA) or transposons (a small DNA sequence that is transferred from one bacterial cell to another). Extended-spectrum β-lactamases (ESBLs) have arisen in the past decade, and have led to bacteria that are cross-resistant to penicillins and cephalosporins. Often these bacteria are also resistant to other antibiotic classes – for example, fluoroquinolones and aminoglycosides. Broad-spectrum β-lactamases called carbapenemases degrade carbapenem antibiotics. More recently, *Klebsiella pneumoniae* carbapenemases have been identified that can inactivate all β-lactam antibiotics, including the carbapenems.
3. The site of action can be altered. Penicillin-binding proteins (PBPs) are membrane-associated enzymes that are present in the cell wall of peptidoglycan-containing organisms. They are divided into two classes: class A PBPs catalyse both polymerisation of the polysaccharide chains and transpepidation (cross-linking) of the chains; while the class B PBPs catalyse only cross-linking (Ch 37). To date, 430 class A and 350 class B PBPs have been identified and each class is further subdivided. There are two main forms of the class A PBPs and four main groups of class B PBPs. Changes in these PBPs can explain the development of antibiotic resistance. For example, the resistance of *Staphylococcus aureus* to β-lactam antibiotics occurs as a result of the development of a highly resistant class B enzyme called PBP2a. In contrast, *Streptococcus pneumoniae* exhibits low-level β-lactam resistance due to mutations in the class B PBPs, PBP2x and PBP2b, and high-level resistance from a further mutation in the class A enzyme PBP1a (Macheboeuf et al. 2006).
4. The inhibited steps can be bypassed or the target enzyme can be overproduced. This can be achieved by developing bypass pathways that compensate for the loss of function due to the antibiotic (e.g. resistance to sulfonamides).

Resistance can also develop as a result of horizontal gene transfer – that is, the acquisition of foreign DNA from another organism. This can occur when two organisms populate the same host at the same time.

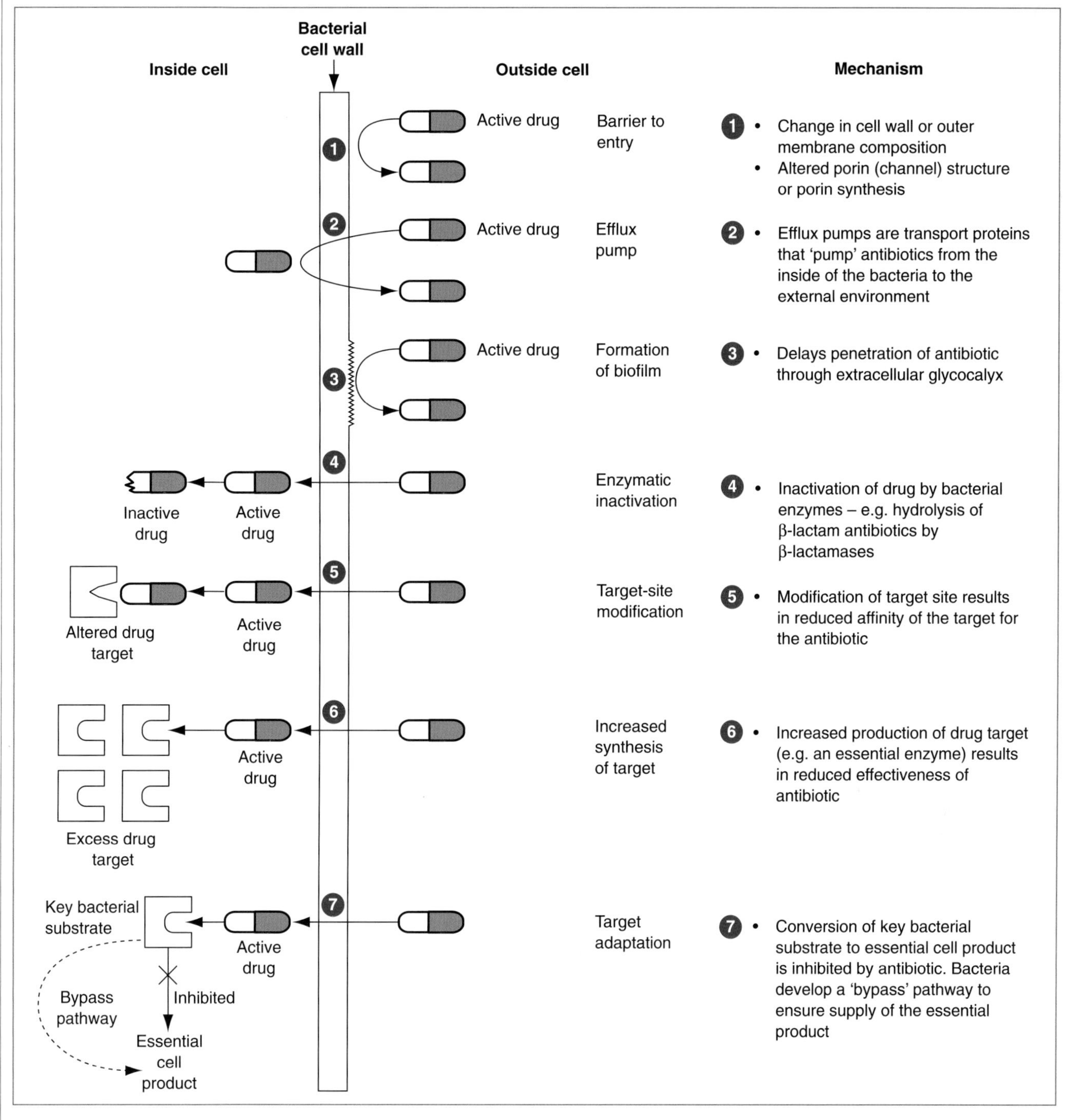

FIGURE 35.1 Seven mechanisms of antibiotic resistance

KEY POINTS

Antimicrobial resistance

- Resistance can be either intrinsic or acquired. From a historical perspective, with each cycle of introduction of new antibiotics, there has been an accompanying cycle of emerging resistance to the drugs.
- Resistance is a worldwide problem, but it is not a new one; resistant microorganisms were present in our environment before the introduction of antibiotics into clinical medicine.

Combating antimicrobial drug resistance

Many resistant strains of bacteria exist in Australia and New Zealand. One major and ongoing problem is MRSA in hospital outpatients and inpatients. Resistance is not just an antibacterial problem; almost all parasitic microorganisms are known to have either partial or full resistance to some drug classes. Examples of other non-bacterial drug-resistant microbial diseases include:

- multidrug-resistant influenza virus
- multidrug-resistant tuberculosis
- azole-resistant thrush
- imatinib-resistant chronic myeloid leukaemia.

The adverse consequences of increasing antimicrobial drug resistance will inevitably be increases in rates of hospitalisation, duration of hospital stay and rates of mortality. To assist in combating these problems, cooperative relationships have developed between health professionals. Variously called antibiotic management programs, antibiotic vigilance programs and antibiotic management strategies, they are more frequently referred to as antimicrobial stewardship programs. These programs focus on:

- making proper and judicious use of antimicrobial drugs
- providing the best possible patient outcomes
- reducing the risk of adverse effects
- preventing/reducing antimicrobial resistance
- promoting cost-effectiveness.

Such programs require long-term commitment and a willingness to invest resources and a process of evaluation to determine their benefit. Other strategies to combat antimicrobial drug resistance include:

- optimal and judicious use of antimicrobials, including limiting use of drugs such as vancomycin, teicoplanin imipenem unless advised by a specialist microbiologist
- selective control, restriction or removal of antimicrobial agents or classes – recent data from Israel clearly highlight that a reduction in the use of quinolone antibiotics resulted in a significant increase in the susceptibility of *Escherichia coli* urine isolates to quinolones
- use of antimicrobial drugs in rotation or cyclical patterns
- use of combinations of antimicrobial drugs in certain circumstances to prevent the emergence of resistance
- improved knowledge of the relationship between the pharmacokinetics of the drug and its anti-infective ability to prevent selection pressure – for example, administering the highest recommended dose to maximise antibiotic exposure.

Superinfection

Superinfection is an infection that occurs during antimicrobial therapy delivered for therapeutic or prophylactic reasons. Most antibiotics reduce or eradicate the normal microbial flora of the body, which are then replaced by resistant exogenous or endogenous bacteria. If the number of these replacement organisms is large and the host conditions favourable, clinical superinfection can occur.

Around 2% of people treated with antibiotics contract superinfections. The risk is greater when large doses of antibiotics are given, when more than one antibiotic is administered concurrently and when broad-spectrum drugs are used. Some specific antimicrobials are more commonly associated with superinfection than others. For example, *Pseudomonas* organisms frequently colonise and infect individuals taking cephalosporins. In a similar manner, people taking tetracyclines may become infected with *Candida albicans*. Generally, superinfections are caused by microorganisms that are resistant to the drug the person is receiving. In the past, penicillinase-producing staphylococci were the most common cause of superinfection. *Staphylococcus aureus* and *Staphylococcus epidermidis* superinfections, especially with methicillin-resistant strains, are again on the rise. Gram-negative enteric bacilli and fungi are the most common offenders (Sekyere & Asante 2018). The proper management of superinfections includes discontinuing the drug being given or replacing it with another drug to which the organism is sensitive, culturing the suspected infected area and administering an antimicrobial agent effective against the new offending organism.

General guidelines for using antibiotics

When treating an infection, the first question that should be posed is whether an antimicrobial drug is needed (Clinical Focus Box 35.1). Several important principles, however, guide the judicious and optimal use of the antibiotics. These include:

- Never treat a viral infection with an antibiotic.
- Use an antibacterial drug only when there is clear evidence that spontaneous resolution is unlikely.
- Identify the infecting microorganism.
- Determine susceptibility of the microorganism.
- Use a drug with the narrowest spectrum of activity for the known or likely organism.
- Use a single drug unless combination therapy is specifically indicated to ensure efficacy or reduce the emergence of resistance.
- Use a dose of drug that is high enough to ensure efficacy with minimal toxicity and reduces the likelihood of resistance.

CLINICAL FOCUS BOX 35.1
The antimicrobial creed

M	microbiology guides therapy wherever possible
I	indication should be evidence-based
N	narrowest spectrum required
D	dosage appropriate to the site and type of infection
M	minimise duration of therapy
E	ensure monotherapy in most situations

Source: Antibiotic Expert Group 2019.

- Use a short duration of treatment unless evidence indicates that a longer duration is required.

As most antimicrobial agents have a specific effect on a limited range of microorganisms, the prescriber must formulate a specific diagnosis about the potential pathogens or organisms causing the infection. The drug most likely to be specifically effective against the suspected microorganism can then be selected (empirical therapy). It is known, for example, that microorganisms commonly isolated in acute adult infections of the lung include pneumococci, *Haemophilus*-strain streptococci and staphylococci. Antimicrobial agents specifically toxic to those organisms may be administered temporarily. The drugs can then be changed, if necessary, after laboratory reports have been received.

Identification of the microorganism is most reliably accomplished by obtaining specimens from the infected area if possible (e.g. urine, sputum or wound drainage) or by obtaining venous blood samples and sending them to the laboratory for identification of the causative organism. It is desirable to receive laboratory reports before initiating antimicrobial therapy. Once the organism has been identified, the appropriate drug can be administered (directed therapy).

In some situations, however, it is not practical to wait for laboratory results. For example, antimicrobial therapy must be initiated without delay in acute, life-threatening situations such as peritonitis, septicaemia or pneumonia. In such situations, the choice of antimicrobial agent for initial use may be based on a tentative identification of the pathogen.

Some infections are most effectively treated with only one antibiotic. In other situations, combined antimicrobial drug therapy may be indicated. Indications for simultaneously using two or more antimicrobial agents include:

- treating mixed infections, in which each drug acts on a separate organism of a complex of microbial flora
- needing to delay the rapid emergence of bacteria that is resistant to one drug
- needing to reduce the incidence or intensity of adverse reactions by decreasing the dose of a potentially toxic drug.

Indiscriminate use of combined antimicrobial drug therapy should be avoided because of expense, toxicity and the higher incidence of superinfections and resistance.

Dosage and duration of therapy

Administering antimicrobial drugs for therapeutic purposes in adequate dosage and for long enough periods is an important principle of infectious disease therapy (Roberts et al. 2008). Fortunately, plasma concentrations of some of the more potent antibiotics (e.g. aminoglycosides) can be monitored to prevent or minimise the risk of toxicity. Failure of antimicrobial therapy is frequently the result of drug doses being too low or being given for too short a period of time. Follow-up laboratory tests should be undertaken if necessary to assess the effectiveness of therapy.

Inadequate drug therapy may lead to remissions and exacerbations of the infectious process and can contribute to the development of resistance. When antibiotics are used prophylactically, they are usually given for short periods to enhance host defence mechanisms. For example, with perioperative antibiotics, a loading dose is given immediately before surgery and continued for 48 hours after surgery.

Many antimicrobial agents are currently in use, and health professionals should be familiar with the general characteristics of each drug group or category and with one or two prototype drugs in each group. Because the dosage for any given antibiotic varies with the type of infection, the site of infection and the age and health status of the person, only general dosages or dose ranges are given in this text. The manufacturer's package insert or a hospital formulary or pharmacy should be consulted for specific dosages.

KEY POINTS

Combating antimicrobial resistance

- Strategies to combat antimicrobial drug resistance include encouraging optimal use of antimicrobials; selective control, restriction or removal of antimicrobial agents or classes; use of antimicrobial drugs in rotation or cyclic patterns; and use of combinations of antimicrobial drugs to prevent emergence of resistance.
- Superinfection is an infection that occurs during antimicrobial therapy delivered for therapeutic or prophylactic reasons.

- Guidelines have been developed for the prudent use of antibiotics. They include: using an antibacterial drug only when indicated; identifying the infecting microorganism; determining the susceptibility of the microorganism; using a drug with the narrowest spectrum of activity for the known or likely organism; using a single drug unless combination therapy is specifically indicated to ensure efficacy or reduce the emergence of resistance; using a dose of drug that is high enough to ensure efficacy with minimal toxicity and reduces the likelihood of resistance; and using a short duration of treatment (e.g. 1 week) unless evidence indicates that a longer duration is required.

REVIEW EXERCISES

1. Mr JR has been treated with amoxicillin for the past 6 weeks. Initially his infection appeared to be responding to the drug, but more recently the MIC determined in the lab has increased and his clinical symptoms appear to be worsening leading the treating team to suspect that the patient has developed a superinfection. Providing examples, describe what is meant by the term 'superinfection'.
2. Mr CM is unresponsive to the narrow-spectrum penicillins and it is concluded that he has a resistant strain of *Staphylococcus aureus.* Discuss the mechanisms by which *Staphylococcus aureus* can develop drug resistance. Which antibiotics are now available for the treating health professional to use?
3. Mrs ST has presented to hospital with a high fever and rash and is diagnosed with a systemic bacterial infection. In determining a treatment plan for Mrs ST, outline the general guidelines for the prudent use of antibiotics.

REFERENCES

Antibiotic Expert Group: Therapeutic guidelines: antibiotics 2019, Melbourne, 2019, Therapeutic Guidelines Limited.

Barbosa TM, Levy SB: The impact of antibiotic use on resistance development and persistence, Drug Resistance Update 3: 303–311, 2000.

Dadgostarb P: Antimicrobial Resistance: Implications and Costs. Infection and drug resistance 12: 3903–3910, 2019

Macheboeuf P, Contreras-Martel C, Job V, et al: Penicillin binding proteins: key players in bacterial cell cycle and drug resistance processes, Federation of European Microbiological Societies Microbiology Reviews 30:673–691, 2006.

Mulvey MR, Simor AE: Antimicrobial resistance in hospitals: how concerned should we be?, Canadian Medical Association Journal 180:408–415, 2009.

Reygaert WC: An overview of the antimicrobial resistance mechanisms of bacteria. AIMS Microbiology 4: 482–501, 2018

Roberts JA, Kruger P, Paterson DL, et al: Antibiotic resistance – what's dosing got to do with it?, Critical Care Medicine 36:2433–2440, 2008.

Sekyere JO, Asante J: Emerging mechanisms of antimicrobial resistance in bacteria and fungi: advances in the era of genomics. Future Microbiology 13: 241–262, 2018.

Walsh C: Molecular mechanisms that confer antibacterial drug resistance, Nature 406:775–781, 2000.

CHAPTER 36

ANTIBACTERIAL DRUGS

Andrew Rowland

KEY ABBREVIATIONS

MRSA methicillin-resistant *Staphylococcus aureus*
MRSE methicillin-resistant *Staphylococcus epidermis*
UTI urinary tract infection

KEY TERMS

aminoglycosides 802
antibiotics 796
carbapenems 798
cephalosporins 800
macrolide antibiotics 805
penicillins 796
quinolones 807
tetracyclines 806

Chapter Focus

The discovery of sulfonamides and penicillin in the 1940s revolutionised the treatment of infectious diseases. The multiplicity of infectious organisms and the success of the early drugs spurred the development of numerous classes of antimicrobial drugs. Although many infections have been controlled with antimicrobial drugs, during the past 20 years drug-resistant strains of microorganisms have steadily increased, and this has necessitated the continued development of new antimicrobial drugs (Butler & Paterson 2020). The challenge facing health professionals is the continued and prudent use of antimicrobial drugs.

KEY DRUG GROUPS

Inhibitors of bacterial cell wall synthesis:

- Amoxicillin, ampicillin, aztreonam, benzathine penicillin, benzylpenicillin, cefaclor, cefalotin, cefepime, cefotaxime, cefoxitin, ceftazidime, ceftriaxone, cefuroxime, cefalexin, cefazolin, dicloxacillin, ertapenem, flucloxacillin, imipenem with cilastin, meropenem, phenoxymethylpenicillin, **piperacillin with tazobactam**, teicoplanin, vancomycin

Inhibitors of bacterial DNA synthesis:

- Amikacin, azithromycin, chloramphenicol, clarithromycin, clindamycin, doxycycline, erythromycin, **gentamicin**, lincomycin, minocycline, neomycin, roxithromycin, tigecycline, tobramycin

Inhibitors of bacterial protein synthesis:

- Ciprofloxacin, moxifloxacin, norfloxacin

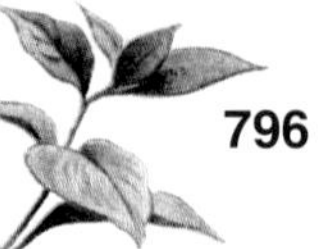

CRITICAL THINKING SCENARIO

Ben, a 28-year-old male, has a bacterial middle ear infection and requires antibiotics to treat his infection. His GP is considering giving him ampicillin to treat the infection, but Ben tells him that he had an allergic reaction to penicillin when he was young. The GP instead decides to prescribe cefalexin to Ben.

1. Compared with ampicillin, is it likely cefalexin will be effective in treating Ben's infection?
2. How likely is it that Ben will have an allergic reaction to this drug?

Introduction

Antibiotics are chemical substances produced from various microorganisms (bacteria and fungi) that kill or suppress the growth of other microorganisms. This term is also commonly used to describe synthetic antimicrobial agents such as sulfonamides and quinolones that are not products of microorganisms. Hundreds of antibiotics are available that vary in antibacterial spectrum, mechanism of action, potency, toxicity and pharmacokinetic properties.

Inhibitors of bacterial cell wall synthesis

Penicillins

Penicillins are antibiotics derived from several strains of common moulds often seen on bread or fruit. Introduced in the 1940s, penicillin and related antibiotics constitute a large group of antimicrobial agents that remain the most effective and least toxic of all available antimicrobial drugs. The common chemical feature of penicillins, cephalosporins, monobactams and carbapenems is a β-lactam ring that is essential to activity of the drug but is also the site of attack by resistant bacteria that possess β-lactamase enzymes that render the antibiotic inactive. Penicillin hypersensitivity (Clinical Focus Box 36.1) is among the most commonly described drug hypersensitivities.

Mechanism of action

The bacterial cell wall is a rigid, lattice-like structure of peptidoglycan composed of cross-linked glycan chains comprising alternating molecules of the amino sugars *N*-acetylglucosamine and *N*-acetylmuramic acid. Peptidoglycan is essential for the normal growth and development of bacteria. The thickness of the cell wall varies: in Gram-positive bacteria it is 50–100 molecules thick, whereas in Gram-negative bacteria it is 1–2 molecules thick. Penicillin-binding proteins (PBPs) are membrane-associated enzymes that are present in the cell wall of peptidoglycan-containing organisms. They are divided into two classes: class A PBPs catalyse both polymerisation of the polysaccharide chains and transpeptidation (cross-linking) of the chains, whereas the class B PBPs catalyse only cross-linking. There are two main forms of the class A PBPs and four main groups of class B PBPs. Penicillins weaken the cell wall by binding to the PBPs, thus inhibiting the transpeptidase activity responsible for cross-linking the glycan strands; this results in cell lysis and death (Fig 36.1). Penicillins are considered to be bactericidal time-dependent drugs because they kill susceptible bacteria, but their effectiveness can be influenced by the presence of, or resistance to, certain β-lactamase enzymes and their combination with β-lactamase inhibitors.

Certain antibiotics are combined with β-lactamase inhibitors such as clavulanate or tazobactam. This extends the spectra of their antibacterial activity and improves their effectiveness but increases the cost. Although most penicillins are much more active against Gram-positive than Gram-negative bacteria, ticarcillin, aztreonam, imipenem and the combination of penicillins with β-lactamase inhibitors are more effective against Gram-negative bacteria (*Escherichia coli*, *Klebsiella pneumoniae* and others). Penicillins are divided into the following categories.

Narrow-spectrum penicillins

These include penicillin G (also known as benzylpenicillin) and penicillin V (also called phenoxymethylpenicillin). Penicillin G and penicillin V are comparable therapeutically, but penicillin V is more stable in stomach acid and is available as an oral preparation. Penicillin G is available in various salt formulations – benzylpenicillin sodium, which may be administered intramuscularly or intravenously (IM/IV), and procaine benzylpenicillin (procaine penicillin) and benzathine benzylpenicillin tetrahydrate,

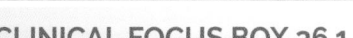

CLINICAL FOCUS BOX 36.1
Penicillin rash and anaphylaxis

Penicillins are among the most widely prescribed and safest antimicrobial drugs. However, hypersensitivity (allergy) to penicillin is one of the adverse drug reactions most people have an awareness of, either through personal experience or through knowledge of someone who has experienced a reaction. In fact, hypersensitivity is the most commonly reported adverse effect of penicillins with a rate that varies from 1% to 10%. The rate of life-threatening allergic reaction (anaphylaxis) is in the order of 0.01–0.05%, and about 0.001% die as a result. No single penicillin is the obvious sole culprit. Penicillins and other structurally related drugs are metabolised (> 95%) to benzylpenicilloyl, which is a stable allergenic metabolite that binds to proteins forming an immunogenic hapten complex. Formation of this hapten complex is the major determinant of penicillin allergy. Unfortunately, many people who report having an 'allergy' to penicillin may in fact not have an allergy but rather experience a viral rash or gastrointestinal symptoms of the infection that coincide with, in particular, treatment with amoxicillin, leading to the conclusion of an 'allergy'. In fact, it is estimated that 90% of reports cannot be substantiated by follow-up blood or skin prick testing. If a true allergy is established, complete avoidance of all penicillins is warranted.

True allergic reactions are mediated by either antibodies or immune cells. As the allergic reaction involves degranulation of mast cells with the release of histamine and other vasoactive substances, the clinical manifestations are easily recognised. These may include urticaria, laryngeal oedema, bronchospasm, hypotension, local swelling and angio-oedema typically occurring within 72 hours. A reaction can occur with any dosage and in the absence of prior knowledge of exposure, which often occurs as a result of ingestion of food of animal origin where antibiotics may have been used in animal feed, or through ingestion of fungi-producing penicillin. Severe allergic reactions most often occur after parenteral administration but have been reported after ingestion of small doses and even after a minute intradermal injection to test for penicillin sensitivity (Lagace-Wiens & Rubinstein 2012).

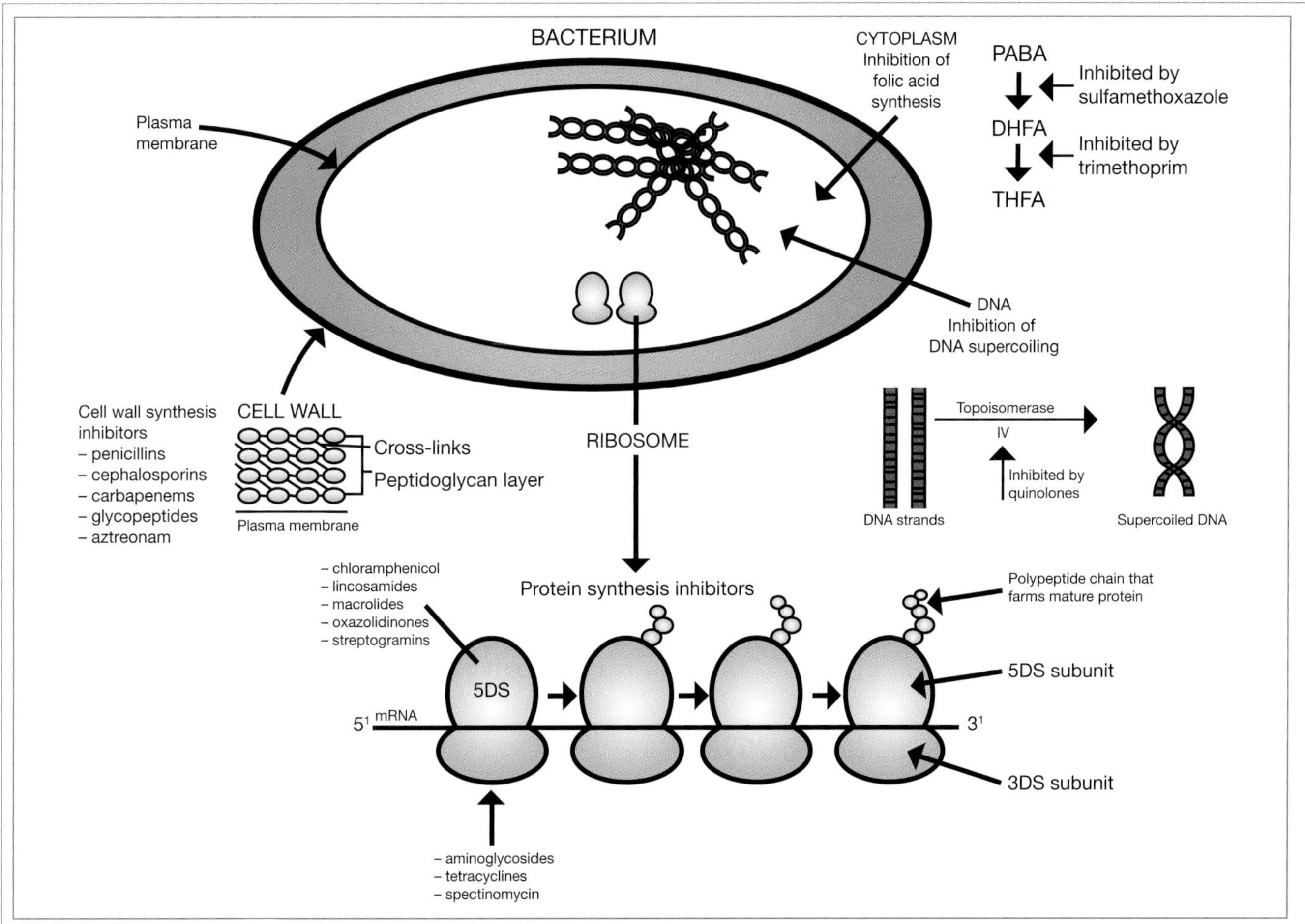

FIGURE 36.1 Sites of action of antimicrobial drugs

TABLE 36.1 Bacterial susceptibility to narrow-spectrum penicillins

	DRUG		
ORGANISM	PENICILLIN G	PENICILLIN V	PROCAINE PENICILLIN
Gram-negative			
Escherichia coli	R	R	R
Haemophilus influenzae	S	R	R
Klebsiella spp.	R	R	R
Neisseria meningitidis	S	S	S
Pseudomonas aeruginosa	R	R	R
Gram-positive			
Enterococcus faecalis	S[a]	R	R
Staphylococcus aureus	R	R	R
Streptococcus pneumoniae	S	S	S
Anaerobes			
Clostridium perfringens	S	S	S
Clostridium difficile	R	R	R

R = resistant; S = sensitive.
[a] Must be used with a synergistic drug (e.g. gentamicin).
Source: Australian Medicines Handbook 2021.

CLINICAL FOCUS BOX 36.2

Prehospital treatment of meningococcal infection

Meningococcal infection often presents as either septicaemia or meningitis. Both meningococcal septicaemia and meningococcal meningitis are time-critical infections, causing death in as little as a few hours. As such, timely administration of antibacterial drugs is critical and should be given immediately on suspicion of invasive meningococcal infection.

While third-generation cephalosporins (e.g. ceftriaxone) are the preferred choice for meningococcal infection, practical limitations mean that paramedic services in many Australian states including South Australia treat with benzylpenicillin. A proportion of people will report an allergy to penicillin, many of whom do not have such a history and can safely be given benzylpenicillin. This creates a clinical conundrum whereby the potential consequences of failing to treat a potentially life-threatening and time-critical infection need to be weighed up against the risk of inducing anaphylaxis in a hypersensitive person. Benzylpenicillin should not be used if the person has a history of anaphylactic or immediate penicillin hypersensitivity reaction (e.g. difficulty breathing, angio-oedema or generalised urticarial rash).

which are only administered IM. The active substance in all these formulations is penicillin G (benzylpenicillin). Examples of susceptible and resistant bacteria are shown in Table 36.1. In combination with ceftriaxone, benzylpenicillin is an important drug in the treatment of time-critical meningococcal infection (Clinical Focus Box 36.2).

Narrow-spectrum penicillinase-resistant penicillins

These are penicillins with antistaphylococcal activity, and include dicloxacillin and flucloxacillin. A chemical alteration of the penicillin structure resulted in penicillins resistant to β-lactamase inactivation; thus they are used against penicillinase-producing staphylococci. These antibiotics are not, however, effective against methicillin-resistant bacteria.

Moderate-spectrum β-lactamase-sensitive aminopenicillins

These include amoxicillin (one of the most widely prescribed antibiotics in the world) and ampicillin. Although these antibiotics have a similar spectrum of activity to that of penicillin, they have greater efficacy against selected Gram-negative bacteria (e.g. *Haemophilus influenzae*) but are usually not very effective against *Staphylococcus aureus* and *Escherichia coli* (β-lactamase-producing bacteria) unless combined with clavulanic acid (e.g. amoxicillin with clavulanic acid).

Broad- and extended-spectrum (antipseudomonal) penicillins

This group includes piperacillin with tazobactam (Drug Monograph 36.1). These antibiotics have a broader spectrum of antimicrobial activity, but only piperacillin (as the single drug) is effective against *Pseudomonas aeruginosa*. Health professionals should be aware that antibiotic therapy may provide an environment that is conducive to the unrestrained growth of undesirable microorganisms, such as bacteria or fungi that would ordinarily have been controlled by the normal body flora. Table 36.2 lists penicillin pharmacokinetics, and Table 36.3 describes the effect of food on oral penicillin absorption.

Carbapenems

Ertapenem, imipenem and meropenem are members of a class of antibiotics called **carbapenems**, which are related to the β-lactam antibiotics but differ from them in having another 5-membered ring in their chemical structure. They bind to the penicillin-binding proteins, thus

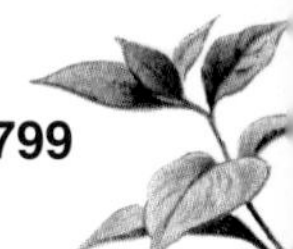

Drug Monograph 36.1
Piperacillin with tazobactam

Piperacillin with tazobactam is an extended-spectrum combination penicillin antibiotic. Tazobactam is a β-lactamase inhibitor that extends piperacillin's spectrum of activity. This drug has activity against Gram-positive and Gram-negative pathogens, including many that produce β-lactamase, and *Pseudomonas aeruginosa*.

Indications

Piperacillin with tazobactam is indicated for treating febrile neutropenia and moderate-to-severe aerobic and anaerobic infections, especially *Pseudomonas aeruginosa*.

Pharmacokinetics

Peak plasma concentrations of piperacillin and tazobactam are attained immediately after completing an IV infusion. Both drugs are approximately 30% bound to plasma proteins and distribute extensively into tissue. The half-life of piperacillin and of tazobactam is approximately 1 hour; both drugs are primarily eliminated in the urine.

Drug interactions

Probenecid decreases piperacillin excretion by competitive renal tubule secretion, prolonging its activity. Large doses of piperacillin may inhibit platelet aggregation, prolonging bleeding time; administration with drugs that affect the clotting process may result in an increased risk of bleeding.

Adverse reactions

Piperacillin with tazobactam is generally well tolerated. The most common adverse reactions include allergy, diarrhoea, nausea, pain and inflammation at injection site. Transient increases in liver enzymes and bilirubin and cholestatic jaundice occur rarely.

Dosage and administration

Piperacillin with tazobactam is administered by slow IV infusion over 30 minutes. The usual total daily dose in adults is 3.375 g every 6 hours, totalling 13.5 g (12.0 g piperacillin / 1.5 g tazobactam) daily. For the initial presumptive treatment of people with nosocomial pneumonia, a higher dose of 4.5 g every 6 hours plus an aminoglycoside, totalling 18.0 g (16.0 g piperacillin / 2.0 g tazobactam) daily. Treatment with the aminoglycoside should be continued in people from whom *Pseudomonas aeruginosa* is isolated. If *Pseudomonas aeruginosa* is not isolated, the aminoglycoside may be discontinued at the discretion of the treating doctor.

TABLE 36.2 Penicillins pharmacokinetics

CLASSIFICATION	ORAL ABSORPTION (%)	TIME TO PEAK PLASMA CONCENTRATION (HR)	RENAL EXCRETION[a] (%)
Narrow-spectrum			
Penicillin G (IM/IV)	–	0.5–1	60–90
Penicillin V (oral)	Up to 60	0.5–1	20–40
Procaine benzylpenicillin (procaine penicillin) (IM)	–	1–3	60–90
Narrow-spectrum penicillinase-resistant			
Dicloxacillin (oral)	37–50; 50–94 if fasting	0.5–2	50–70
Flucloxacillin (oral)	> 80	0.5–1	40–70
Moderate-spectrum β-lactamase-sensitive aminopenicillins			
Amoxicillin (oral) (IM/IV)	75–90	1–2	60–75
	–	1	60–75
Ampicillin (IM/IV)	–	1	75–90
Broad- and extended-spectrum (antipseudomonal activity)			
Amoxicillin–clavulanate (oral dose is based on amoxicillin component)	90	1–2	50–78
Piperacillin–tazobactam (IV)	–	E of I	68

E of I = end of infusion
[a] Renal excretion = % excreted unchanged.
Source: Australian Medicines Handbook 2021.

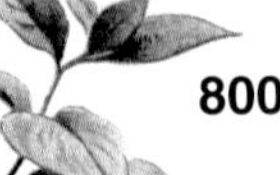

TABLE 36.3 Effect of food on oral penicillin absorption[a]

DRUG	FOOD EFFECT	DRUG	FOOD EFFECT
Amoxicillin	None	Dicloxacillin	Decreased
Amoxicillin–clavulanate	None	Flucloxacillin	Decreased
Ampicillin	Decreased	Phenoxymethylpenicillin potassium	Decreased slightly

[a] Penicillins whose absorption decreases after food intake are generally acid-labile; therefore, administer with a full glass of water on an empty stomach 1 hour before or 2 hours after meals.

Source: Brody et al. 1998; used with permission.

inhibiting bacterial cell wall synthesis. Carbapenems have the broadest spectrum of activity of all the antimicrobials against Gram-positive and Gram-negative aerobic and anaerobic organisms. All of these drugs are inactive against methicillin-resistant *Staphylococcus aureus* (MRSA) and *Enterococcus faecium*, while ertapenem is inactive against *Enterococcus faecalis*, *Pseudomonas aeruginosa* and *Acinetobacter*. Increasingly, *Enterobacteriaceae* resistant to carbapenems have been identified. Imipenem is degraded by renal dehydropeptidase-1 (DHP-1) and is combined with the DHP-1 inhibitor cilastatin, which inhibits renal DHP-1 and also blocks the tubular secretion of imipenem, thus preventing renal metabolism of this drug. Meropenem and ertapenem are more resistant to renal dehydropeptidase-1 degradation and are given without cilastatin. These drugs are expensive and are generally reserved for nosocomial and life-threatening infections when other antibiotics are contraindicated or inappropriate. Meropenem is used for treating meningitis, whereas imipenem is contraindicated because of the high incidence of seizures. This is likely to apply also to ertapenem, which is likewise associated with seizures.

When carbapenems are administered IV, peak plasma concentration is achieved rapidly. The half-life of imipenem is 2–3 hours, about 1 hour for meropenem and about 4 hours for ertapenem. These drugs are excreted to varying degrees as unchanged drug in urine within 10 hours. Dosage adjustment is required in people with significant renal impairment. Imipenem and meropenem should not be given with probenecid, as renal secretion of the carbapenems is inhibited, increasing the risk of toxicity.

Cephalosporins

Cephalosporins were originally isolated from sea fungus found near a sewerage outlet off the Sardinian coast in 1948. Since then, chemical modification of the central active component, 7-aminocephalosporanic acid, and the addition of side chains, have created compounds with different and greater antimicrobial activities. To classify easily the differences in antimicrobial activity, cephalosporins are divided into first, second, third and fourth generations. While there are some common traits, the chemical modifications that alter antimicrobial activity also give individual drugs their distinct pharmacokinetic characteristics (Table 36.4).

Mechanism of action

Like penicillin, cephalosporins inhibit bacterial cell wall synthesis and are also bactericidal (Fig 36.1). They are effective in numerous situations, but with only a few exceptions they are rarely the drugs of first choice. The first-generation cephalosporins (e.g. cefalexin) are primarily active against Gram-positive bacteria, whereas the second-generation drugs (e.g. cefaclor) have increased activity against Gram-negative microorganisms. The third-generation drugs are more active against Gram-negative bacteria (e.g. ceftazidime is also effective against *Pseudomonas aeruginosa*) and β-lactamase-producing microbial strains but less effective against Gram-positive cocci. Cefepime is a fourth-generation cephalosporin with antimicrobial effects comparable to those of third-generation cephalosporins and is also more resistant to some β-lactamases. Specific examples of bacteria susceptibility to commonly used cephalosporins are shown in Table 36.5.

TABLE 36.4 Cephalosporins pharmacokinetics

DRUG	ORAL ABSORPTION (%)	TIME TO PEAK PLASMA CONCENTRATION (HR)	RENAL EXCRETION (%)[a]
First-generation			
Cefazolin	–[b]	IM: 1–2	56–89
	–	IV: E of I	80–100
Cefalexin	95	PO: 1	80
Cefalotin (cefalothin)	–	IV: 0.5	60–70
Second-generation			
Cefaclor	95	PO: 0.5–1	60–85
Cefoxitin	–	IM: 0.3–0.5 IV: E of I	85
Cefuroxime	52	PO: 2–3.6	32–48
Third-generation			
Cefotaxime	–	IM: 0.5 IV: E of I	60
Ceftazidime	–	IM: 1 IV: E of I	80–90
Ceftriaxone	–	IM: 2–3 IV: E of I	33–67
Fourth-generation			
Cefepime	–	IM: 1–2 IV: E of I	80

E of I = end of infusion; PO = by mouth
[a] Renal excretion = % excreted unchanged.
[b] Not given orally.

Source: Australian Medicines Handbook 2021.

TABLE 36.5 Bacterial susceptibility to cephalosporins

ORGANISM	DRUG			
	CEFALEXIN	CEFACLOR	CEFOXITIN	CEFTRIAXONE
Gram-negative				
Escherichia coli	S	S	S	S
Haemophilus influenzae	R	S	S	S
Klebsiella species	S	S	S	S
Neisseria meningitidis	R	S	S	S
Pseudomonas aeruginosa	R	R	R	R
Gram-positive				
Enterococcus faecalis	R	R	R	R
Staphylococcus aureus	S	[a]	[a]	[a]
Streptococcus pneumoniae	S	S	S	S
Anaerobes				
Clostridium perfringens	S	S	S	S
Clostridium difficile	R	R	R	R

R = resistant; S = sensitive.
[a] No data on drug; not recommended.

Source: Australian Medicines Handbook 2021.

Cephalosporin antibiotics may be considered for those allergic to penicillin. However, the possibility of a cross-reaction is 5–15%, and cephalosporins should not be used if a person reports a history of a serious reaction or anaphylaxis to penicillin (Campagna et al. 2012). If use is critical, specialist advice should always be sought prior to administration.

Glycopeptides

Vancomycin and teicoplanin are complex glycopeptide antibiotics. Vancomycin was isolated from the soil actinomycete *Streptococcus orientalis*, while teicoplanin was isolated from *Actinoplanes teichomyceticus*. Both drugs inhibit bacterial wall synthesis and are primarily active against Gram-positive bacteria. Due to increasing problems with resistance, Australia has adopted the guidelines for glycopeptide use from the United States Centers for Disease Control Hospital Infection Control Practices Advisory Committee controlling the use of these drugs.

Vancomycin absorption from the intestinal tract is poor; hence, it is usually administered slowly via the IV route and never IM. In contrast, teicoplanin is usually administered IV but can be administered IM. An oral formulation of vancomycin is available but is only ever used for the treatment of pseudomembranous colitis. Parenteral vancomycin has an elimination half-life of 4–6 hours in adults and about 2–3 hours in children, whereas it is close to 100 hours for teicoplanin. Both are excreted primarily by the kidneys, and dosage adjustment is crucial in people with compromised renal function. Routine therapeutic plasma drug concentration monitoring is undertaken for vancomycin in circumstances such as during concomitant aminoglycoside administration, in people on haemodialysis and during high-dose prolonged treatment in people with unstable or impaired renal function. Examples of potential drug interactions with vancomycin and teicoplanin and possible outcomes are listed in Drug Interactions 36.1.

DRUG INTERACTIONS 36.1
Vancomycin or teicoplanin

DRUG	POSSIBLE EFFECTS AND MANAGEMENT
Aminoglycosides	Increased potential for ototoxicity and nephrotoxicity with vancomycin and teicoplanin. Monitor renal function and plasma drug concentrations; adjust dose if necessary.
Bile acid-binding resins (colestipol or colestyramine)	When given concurrently with the oral dosage form, a reduction in vancomycin antibacterial activity is reported. Avoid this combination if possible. If not, give oral vancomycin several hours apart from the other medications.
Muscle relaxants and general anaesthetics	Vancomycin may potentiate the neuromuscular blockade produced by non-depolarising muscle relaxants and suxamethonium. Vancomycin infusion should be completed before induction of general anaesthesia because of increased risk of vancomycin-related adverse reactions (e.g. hypotension).

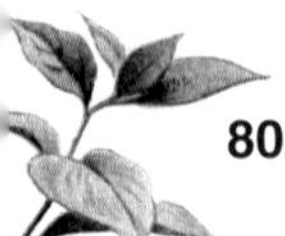

Adverse reactions are much more common with rapid IV infusions and include rash, itching, chills and fever. Rarely, the 'red-neck' or 'red-man' syndrome is reported after bolus or too rapid drug injection with vancomycin (less often with teicoplanin), which results in histamine release and chills, fever, tachycardia, pruritus, rash or red face, neck, upper body, back and arms. The dosage of either drug depends on age, renal function and indication, and relevant drug information sources should be consulted prior to administration.

Monobactams

Aztreonam, the first drug in the monobactam class of antibiotics, is a synthetic bactericidal antibiotic with a similar mechanism of action to that of penicillin. It binds to penicillin-binding proteins, resulting in inhibition of bacterial cell wall synthesis, cell lysis and death. It is active only against Gram-negative aerobic organisms (e.g. *Pseudomonas aeruginosa*). It is reserved for treatment of infections when other antibacterial drugs are contraindicated and for urinary tract, bronchitis, intra-abdominal, gynaecological and skin infections. Aztreonam is highly resistant to most β-lactamase enzymes.

Aztreonam is not given orally, as it is not absorbed from the gastrointestinal tract. After IM injection, peak plasma concentration occurs in 0.6–1.3 hours. The half-life in adults with normal renal function is 1.4–2.2 hours, and 60–70% of the drug is eliminated in the urine within 8 hours. No significant drug interaction has been reported at this stage.

Adverse reactions include gastric distress, diarrhoea, nausea, vomiting, hypersensitivity and thrombophlebitis at the site of injection. Rarely, anaphylaxis, hepatitis, jaundice, thrombocytopenia and prolonged bleeding time have been reported. Use aztreonam with caution in people receiving anticoagulant therapy. A low risk of allergic reaction exists in those allergic to penicillins or cephalosporins, but people who are allergic to ceftazidime may develop cross-reactivity. Dose reduction is required in moderate and severe renal impairment.

KEY POINTS

Inhibitors of bacterial cell wall synthesis

- Penicillins can be broadly divided into the following groups: narrow-spectrum penicillins; narrow-spectrum penicillinase-resistant penicillins with antistaphylococcal activity; moderate-spectrum β-lactamase-sensitive aminopenicillins; and the broad- and extended-spectrum (antipseudomonal activity) penicillins.
- Ertapenem, imipenem and meropenem are members of the class of antibiotics called carbapenems, which are related to the β-lactam antibiotics. They have a wide spectrum of activity against Gram-positive and Gram-negative aerobic and anaerobic organisms.
- There are now four generations of cephalosporins. Modification of the central β-lactam ring has resulted in many drugs with different microbiological and pharmacological activities.
- Vancomycin is reserved for treatment of serious infections that are resistant to penicillins – methicillin-resistant *Staphylococcus aureus* (MRSA) and methicillin-resistant *Staphylococcus epidermis* (MRSE).

Inhibitors of bacterial protein synthesis

Aminoglycosides

Aminoglycosides are potent bactericidal antibiotics usually reserved for serious or life-threatening infections. They are very effective against many Gram-negative bacteria but as monotherapy they have limited activity against Gram-positive bacteria. Safer and less toxic agents are available to treat most Gram-positive infections but combinations of aminoglycosides with β-lactam antibiotics provide a synergistic effect against *Listeria* spp. and *Staphylococcus aureus*. Currently, available drugs include amikacin, gentamicin (Drug Monograph 36.2), tobramycin and neomycin (Hutchings et al. 2019).

The mechanism of action of aminoglycosides involves irreversible binding to the 30S ribosomal sub-unit of susceptible bacteria, thus inhibiting protein synthesis, leading to eventual cell death. They are used with penicillins, cephalosporins or vancomycin for their synergistic effects and are especially useful for the treatment of Gram-negative infections such as those caused by *Pseudomonas* spp., *Escherichia coli*, *Proteus* spp., *Klebsiella* spp., *Serratia* spp. and others.

Aminoglycosides are poorly absorbed (< 1%) from the intestinal tract but are rapidly absorbed IM, with peak plasma concentrations occurring 30–90 minutes after injection. As the aminoglycosides are strongly polar molecules, they do not distribute to the central nervous system (CNS), and tissue concentrations are low. They are almost entirely eliminated by the kidneys and, in people with normal renal function, the plasma half-life is in the range of 2–3 hours. Monitoring aminoglycoside plasma concentrations is essential to ensuring that therapeutic concentrations are achieved without the risk of adverse reactions due to high plasma concentrations. Monitoring the plasma concentration is generally not undertaken if the course of treatment is shorter than 48 hours. If it is

Drug Monograph 36.2
Gentamicin

Gentamicin is a parenterally administered aminoglycoside that possesses potent bactericidal antibiotics. It is usually reserved for serious or life-threatening infections.

Indications

Gentamicin is used as an empirical treatment for serious Gram-negative infections, serious systemic enterococcal infections (with β-lactams or vancomycin), serious infections due to sensitive organisms that are resistant to other antibacterial drugs including *Pseudomonas aeruginosa* and brucellosis, surgical prophylaxis and eye infections.

Pharmacokinetics

Following IV/IM dosing, peak plasma concentrations are attained within 1 hour. Gentamicin is approximately 10% bound to plasma proteins but has limited tissue distribution. The half-life of gentamicin is 2 hours; this drug is more than 90% eliminated unchanged in the urine.

Drug interactions

Administration with other drugs that are ototoxic or nephrotoxic may increase risk of these adverse effects, especially in people with renal impairment. Additive neuromuscular blocking effects occur with parenteral administration of magnesium sulfate.

Adverse reactions

Nephrotoxicity occurs commonly but is usually reversible and can be anticipated if treatment lasts more than 7–10 days. Vestibular ototoxicity (nausea, vomiting, vertigo, nystagmus, difficulties with gait) and cochlear ototoxicity (noticeable hearing loss, tinnitus, feeling of fullness in ear) occur in 2–4% of treated people. Ototoxicity is irreversible in about 50% of people; permanent deafness may occur. Neuromuscular blockade may result in respiratory depression, which can usually be reversed with prompt administration of IV calcium gluconate.

Dosage and administration

Doses less than 120 mg may be given as an IV injection over 3–5 minutes; otherwise, the dose should be infused over 15–30 minutes. Treatment for under 48 hours in adults with normal renal function does not require gentamicin concentration monitoring; the standard dose is 5–7 mg/kg once daily. Higher mg/kg doses are used in children and young adults, while lower doses are used in the elderly and for surgical prophylaxis.

The preferred, but most complex, method for monitoring gentamicin is based on target area under the plasma concentration time curve (AUC). This approach requires two samples collected about 30 minutes apart, then 6–14 hours after completing the infusion.

longer, monitoring of plasma concentration and renal function determines the dosage regimen. Local diagnostic laboratory services should be contacted for specialist information. Drug Interactions 36.2 lists those effects that may occur when aminoglycosides are given with the drugs listed.

Chloramphenicol

Chloramphenicol, a broad-spectrum antibiotic, potently inhibits bacterial protein synthesis by binding to the 50S sub-unit of the bacterial ribosome. It is a bacteriostatic agent used for a wide variety of Gram-negative and Gram-positive organisms and anaerobes; however, because it has the potential to be seriously toxic to bone marrow (aplasia leading to aplastic anaemia and possibly death), its use has declined but local application (ophthalmic use) is still prevalent. It is indicated for treating *Haemophilus influenzae*, *Streptococcus pneumoniae* and *Neisseria meningitidis* because it may be bactericidal to these organisms.

Chloramphenicol has good oral and parenteral bioavailability, with the highest concentrations reported in the liver and kidneys. Concentrations up to 50% of those in plasma have been noted in cerebrospinal fluid. Chloramphenicol is metabolised in the liver to an inactive glucuronide, 75–90% of which is excreted in the urine over a 24-hour period. In neonates, chloramphenicol causes 'grey baby syndrome': a blue–grey skin discolouration, hypothermia, irregular breathing, coma and cardiovascular collapse. This occurs because of lack of maturation of UDP-glucuronosyltransferase enzymes in the liver during the first 3–4 weeks of life and inadequate renal capacity to excrete unchanged drug. The potential effects of giving chloramphenicol with the drugs listed are listed in Drug Interactions 36.3.

Extreme caution is required when using chloramphenicol in people who have recently had antineoplastic chemotherapy or radiation therapy. Chloramphenicol is contraindicated in people with pre-existing bone marrow

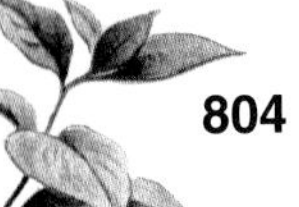

DRUG INTERACTIONS 36.2

Aminoglycosides

DRUG	POSSIBLE EFFECTS AND MANAGEMENT
Aminoglycosides (two or more concurrently)	Potential for ototoxicity, nephrotoxicity and neuromuscular blockade is enhanced. Hearing loss may progress to deafness even after the drug is stopped. In some cases, hearing loss may be reversed. Avoid, or a potentially serious drug interaction may occur.
Loop diuretics	Increased risk of irreversible hearing loss. Avoid prolonged use of high doses of aminoglycosides.
Muscle relaxants	Aminoglycosides may potentiate the neuromuscular-blocking effect of non-depolarising muscle relaxants and suxamethonium.
Non-steroidal anti-inflammatory drugs	NSAID-induced reduction in renal function may lead to increased plasma concentration of aminoglycoside. Monitor drug concentration and renal function, and adjust dose if necessary.
Penicillins and cephalosporins	Antibacterial action of aminoglycoside may be enhanced as a result of greater penetration. Do not mix aminoglycosides with penicillins and cephalosporins, as the parenteral solutions are incompatible.

Source: Australian Medicines Handbook 2021.

DRUG INTERACTIONS 36.3

Chloramphenicol

DRUG	POSSIBLE EFFECTS AND MANAGEMENT
Phenytoin	Impaired phenytoin metabolism and increased risk of toxicity. Monitor phenytoin concentration, and reduce dose if required.
Tacrolimus	Increased plasma concentration of tacrolimus when administered concurrently with chloramphenicol. Monitor plasma concentration of tacrolimus and decrease tacrolimus dose if necessary to avoid toxicity.

Source: Australian Medicines Handbook 2021.

suppression and/or blood dyscrasias. Specialist advice should be sought before prescribing to infants and children.

Lincosamides

The lincosamides include lincomycin and clindamycin. Lincomycin inhibits protein synthesis by binding to the bacterial 50S ribosomal sub-unit and preventing peptide bond formation. It is primarily bacteriostatic, although it may be bactericidal in high doses with selected organisms. It is used to treat serious streptococcal and staphylococcal infections, but clindamycin is preferred as it has better oral absorption and is more potent than lincomycin. Clindamycin, which is a semisynthetic derivative of lincomycin, has a similar mechanism of action to that of lincomycin but is more effective. It is indicated for treating bone and joint, pelvic (female), intra-abdominal and skin and soft tissue infections, bacterial septicaemia and pneumonia caused by susceptible bacteria.

Oral clindamycin is well absorbed and should be administered with food or with a full glass of water. It is rapidly distributed to most body fluids and tissues, with the exception of cerebrospinal fluid; the highest concentrations are noted in bone, bile and urine. The half-life of clindamycin in adults is 2–3 hours. It reaches peak blood concentrations within 0.75–1 hour of oral administration in adults, within 1 hour in children and within 3 hours of IM injection. It is metabolised in the liver and excreted primarily in bile, with only a small proportion (6–10%) excreted as unchanged drug in urine.

A significant adverse and limiting effect for both drugs is antibiotic-associated pseudomembranous colitis in which the normal bacterial flora within the colon are disturbed, facilitating the growth of *Clostridium difficile* or other bacteria. With overgrowth of the bacteria, potent bacterial toxins are released causing inflammation of the colon. People at risk include the elderly, those with a compromised immune system and those with pre-existing inflammatory bowel disease. Use these drugs with caution in people with gastrointestinal disorders, especially ulcerative colitis, antibiotic-induced colitis and regional enteritis.

Macrolide antibiotics

Macrolides are antibiotics that contain a many-membered lactone ring that has one or more sugar molecules attached. They inhibit bacterial RNA-dependent protein synthesis by binding to the 50S ribosomal sub-unit (Fig 36.1). Macrolides are bacteriostatic: that is, they inhibit growth of microorganisms and, in high concentrations with selected organisms, may be bactericidal. The **macrolide antibiotics** include azithromycin, clarithromycin, erythromycin and roxithromycin. Erythromycin was the first macrolide and is the key drug from this group.

These agents have similar antimicrobial action against Gram-positive and some Gram-negative microorganisms and are used for respiratory, gastrointestinal, skin and soft tissue infections when β-lactam antibiotics are contraindicated because of allergy. Clarithromycin is used in conjunction with amoxicillin and the proton pump inhibitor esomeprazole for the eradication of *Helicobacter pylori*. Macrolide pharmacokinetics are described in Table 36.6.

Macrolides inhibit hepatic CYP3A4 and, as a consequence, are subject to numerous drug interactions. In general, they inhibit the metabolism of other drugs, leading to increased plasma concentration and the risk of toxicity. The potential for drug interactions is greatest with erythromycin > clarithromycin > roxithromycin > azithromycin. Drug Interactions 36.4 lists some of the more significant drug interactions, but it is not complete and reference should be made to appropriate drug information sources if uncertain about a specific drug.

Use macrolide antibiotics with caution in people with severe liver function impairment. In addition, use erythromycin cautiously in people with hearing loss, and clarithromycin cautiously in people with severe kidney function impairment. Avoid use of erythromycin in those with cardiac dysrhythmias.

Oxazolidinones

The only drug available in this class is linezolid, a novel compound with a broad spectrum of activity against community and hospital-acquired Gram-positive organisms (e.g. MRSA). Unlike chloramphenicol, which binds to the 50S ribosomal sub-unit and inhibits bacterial protein synthesis, the site of action of linezolid is proximal to the 50S sub-unit. At that specific site, linezolid inhibits protein synthesis by interfering with the formation of a complex that is essential for protein translation. It was anticipated that the site and mechanism of action of linezolid would reduce the likelihood of cross-resistance between Gram-positive bacterial strains; however, enterococci and MRSA resistant to linezolid have now been isolated.

Linezolid is indicated for treating serious infections due to Gram-positive organisms where other drugs are either contraindicated or not appropriate. It is available in both oral and IV formulations. After oral administration, linezolid is well absorbed (~100% bioavailability), and peak plasma concentrations occur in 1–1.5 hours. It is metabolised by the liver to inactive metabolites, and

TABLE 36.6 Macrolide antibiotic pharmacokinetics

DRUG	ORAL ABSORPTION (%)	TIME TO PEAK PLASMA CONCENTRATION (HR)	EXCRETION
Azithromycin	Good	2–4	Biliary (72%)
Clarithromycin	Good	2–3	Urine (20–30%)
Erythromycin	30–65	2–4	Biliary (high)
Roxithromycin	50	1–2	Faecal (about 53%)

Source: Australian Medicines Handbook 2021.

DRUG INTERACTIONS 36.4
Macrolide antibiotics

DRUG	POSSIBLE OUTCOMES	MANAGEMENT
Benzodiazepines	Increased/prolonged sedation	Avoid combined use with erythromycin. Exercise caution with other macrolides.
Carbamazepine	Neurotoxicity	Decrease dose of carbamazepine if necessary.
Cyclosporin, tacrolimus	Nephrotoxicity, neurotoxicity	Adjust doses of cyclosporin and tacrolimus if necessary.
Digoxin	May cause digoxin toxicity	Monitor plasma digoxin concentration.
Theophylline	Theophylline toxicity	Monitor plasma theophylline concentration. Use alternative agent.
Warfarin	Increased risk of bleeding	Monitor INR; decrease or cease warfarin. Use alternative antibiotic.

Source: Australian Medicines Handbook 2021.

approximately 30% of the drug is excreted unchanged in urine. The half-life is in the order of 4.5–5.5 hours, and dose adjustment is generally not necessary in the elderly or in the presence of renal or hepatic dysfunction.

The predominant adverse reactions include nausea, diarrhoea and headache. As linezolid may cause thrombocytopenia, leucopenia, eosinophilia and neutropenia, full blood count should be monitored before treatment and weekly during therapy. Linezolid is a weak inhibitor of monoamine oxidase and hence has the potential to interact with adrenergic (e.g. adrenaline [epinephrine] and salbutamol) and serotonergic (e.g. SSRI) drugs. Counselling should be provided on foods to be avoided during linezolid treatment.

Tetracyclines

Tetracyclines were the first broad-spectrum antibiotics developed after a systematic search for antibiotic-producing microorganisms in soil. The first drug produced was chlortetracycline, which was released in 1948. This group now includes a number of drugs that have a common basic structure and similar chemical activity: doxycycline, minocycline and tetracycline. Minocycline is not as well tolerated as doxycycline, producing vestibular and CNS adverse effects, hepatitis and serum sickness during long-term use for acne.

Tetracyclines are bacteriostatic towards many Gram-negative and Gram-positive organisms; they exhibit cross-sensitivity and cross-resistance. Tetracyclines inhibit protein synthesis by reversibly blocking the 30S sub-unit of the ribosome and preventing access of tRNA to the mRNA–ribosome complex (Fig 36.1). These drugs have been commonly used to treat many infections, such as acne vulgaris, actinomycosis, anthrax, bacterial urinary tract infections (UTIs), bronchitis and numerous systemic bacterial infections.

Oral tetracyclines are well absorbed and are distributed in most body fluids. Concentration in cerebrospinal fluid varies and can range from 10% to 25% of the plasma drug concentration after parenteral administration. Tetracyclines localise in teeth, liver, spleen, tumours and bone. Doxycycline can reach clinical concentrations in the eye and prostate, whereas minocycline reaches high levels in saliva, sputum and tears. Doxycycline and minocycline are metabolised in the liver, but most tetracyclines are excreted via the kidneys.

Adverse reactions include dizziness (minocycline), oesophagitis (doxycycline), ataxia, gastrointestinal distress, photosensitivity (doxycycline, depends on dose and extent of sun exposure), discolouration of infants' or children's teeth (do not give to children under 8 years), skin and mucous membrane pigmentation (minocycline), dark or discoloured tongue, rectal or genital fungal overgrowth; rarely, hepatotoxicity, pancreatitis and benign intracranial hypertension. Minocycline and doxycycline only may be taken with food or milk to reduce gastric adverse effects, as interactions with food and milk are less problematic in comparison to tetracycline. Tetracyclines are not recommended in people with renal impairment, but doxycycline and minocycline may be used. These drugs are contraindicated in pregnant women after week 18 and in children less than 8 years of age, as they cause discolouration of teeth and enamel dysplasia.

Tigecycline is a derivative of minocycline and, like minocycline, binds to the 30S ribosomal sub-unit blocking protein synthesis. However, in tigecycline the addition of an *N*,*N*-dimethylglycylamido group to the minocycline molecule results in a more than fivefold increase in the affinity of tigecycline for the ribosomal target when compared to minocycline or tetracycline. This increased affinity explains the expanded spectrum of activity against tetracyclineresistant organisms such as penicillin-resistant *Streptococcus pneumoniae*, MRSA, MRSE and vancomycin-resistant enterococci species. Resistance has been documented in Australian isolates of *Acinetobacter baumanni*, and acquired resistance has been reported in *Klebsiella pneumoniae*, *Enterobacter aerogenes*, *Enterobacter cloacae* and *Enterococcus faecalis*. Tigecycline is approved for treating complicated skin and soft tissue infections and complicated intra-abdominal infections caused by susceptible organisms.

KEY POINTS

Inhibitors of bacterial protein synthesis

- Include the aminoglycosides, lincosamides, macrolides, oxazolidinones and tetracyclines.
- The aminoglycosides are very potent bactericidal antibiotics that are primarily indicated for serious or life-threatening infections.
- Therapeutic drug monitoring plays a major role in ensuring that a therapeutic aminoglycoside plasma concentration is achieved and the risk of toxicity is minimised.
- The lincosamides, such as clindamycin, are primarily bacteriostatic and are used to treat serious streptococcal and staphylococcal infections.
- The macrolide antibiotics, typified by erythromycin, are bacteriostatic agents that inhibit protein synthesis and, at high concentrations, are bactericidal for selected microorganisms.
- The tetracyclines (minocycline, doxycycline and tigecycline) are bacteriostatic.

Inhibitors of DNA synthesis

Fluoroquinolones

The **quinolones** (including fluoroquinolones) are synthetic, broad-spectrum agents with bactericidal activity. They interfere with bacterial topoisomerase II (DNA gyrase) and topoisomerase IV, the enzymes involved in the supercoiling of DNA that is necessary for the duplication, transcription and repair of bacterial DNA (Fig 36.1). An equivalent topoisomerase II enzyme exists in eukaryotic cells, but this enzyme is inhibited by fluoroquinolones only at much higher concentrations. Examples of fluoroquinolones include ciprofloxacin, moxifloxacin, norfloxacin and ofloxacin, which is available through the Special Access Scheme as a second-line drug for the treatment of leprosy and as eyedrops for severe conjunctivitis and bacterial keratitis. The quinolones are effective against *Pseudomonas aeruginosa* and are reserved for infections when alternative drugs are either contraindicated or ineffective. These include bone and joint infection, *Legionella pneumonia*, epididymo-orchitis, prostatitis and complicated UTIs. Individual quinolones may vary in their spectrum of activity. Unfortunately, bacterial resistance to the quinolones is increasing worldwide, and appropriate use is needed to extend their clinical life. The pharmacokinetics of flouroquinolones are described in Table 36.7. Quinolones interact with a number of drugs (Drug Interactions 36.5), and the effects shown may occur when quinolones are given with the drugs listed.

Adverse reactions include dizziness, drowsiness, restlessness, stomach distress, diarrhoea, nausea, vomiting and photosensitivity; rarely, CNS stimulation (psychosis, confusion, hallucinations, tremors), hypersensitivity (skin rash, redness, Stevens-Johnson syndrome, face or neck swelling, shortness of breath) and interstitial nephritis. Additionally, young athletes participating in extensive training are also at risk of tendon adverse effects. These drugs should be ceased at the first sign of tendon pain or inflammation. Use quinolones with caution in people with CNS disorders, including epilepsy and seizures.

Miscellaneous antibiotics

Metronidazole and tinidazole

Metronidazole and tinidazole are reduced intracellularly in anaerobic microorganisms or anoxic or hypoxic cells to a short-acting cytotoxic agent that interacts with DNA, inhibiting bacterial synthesis and causing cell death. They are selectively toxic to many anaerobic bacteria and protozoa. Both are indicated for the treatment of amoebiasis (intestinal and extraintestinal), bone infections, brain abscesses, CNS infections, bacterial endocarditis, genitourinary tract infections, septicaemia, trichomoniasis and other infections caused by organisms susceptible to metronidazole.

Oral metronidazole is well absorbed and distributed throughout the body, penetrating many tissues, including

TABLE 36.7 Fluoroquinolone pharmacokinetics

DRUG	ORAL BIOAVAILABILITY (%)	HALF-LIFE (HR)	RENAL EXCRETION (%)
Ciprofloxacin	50–70	4	45–55
Moxifloxacin	86	~15	20–25
Norfloxacin	30–40	3–4	~30
Ofloxacin	95–100	4–7	> 70

DRUG INTERACTIONS 36.5

Tetracyclines

DRUG	POSSIBLE OUTCOMES AND MANAGEMENT
Antacids, calcium, iron or magnesium supplements	May result in a non-absorbable complex, reducing the absorption and plasma levels of the antibiotic. Also, antacids may raise gastric pH, which decreases the absorption of tetracyclines and reduces antibacterial effectiveness. If given concurrently, separate medications by 2–3 hours from the oral tetracyclines.
Colestipol and colestyramine	May bind oral tetracyclines, decreasing their absorption. Separate drugs by at least 2 hours.
Estrogen-containing oral contraceptives	Concurrent long-term therapy may reduce contraceptive effectiveness and may also result in breakthrough bleeding. Avoid concurrent drug usage or increase contraceptive cover.

vaginal secretions, seminal fluid, saliva and breast milk. It reaches peak plasma concentration within 1–2 hours and has a half-life of 8 hours. It is metabolised in the liver (~50%), and both unchanged metronidazole and metabolites are excreted by the kidneys. Tinidazole has a longer half-life and is given once daily.

Adverse reactions include dizziness, headache, gastric distress, diarrhoea, anorexia, nausea, vomiting, dry mouth, taste alterations, dark urine, peripheral neuropathy, CNS toxicity, hypersensitivity, leucopenia, thrombophlebitis, vaginal candidiasis and convulsions (with high drug doses). Use with caution in people with renal disease and hepatic impairment. Avoid use in those with metronidazole hypersensitivity, blood dyscrasias, severe liver disease or active organic CNS disease. Dosage regimens vary according to the infection being treated, and relevant sources should be consulted for information.

Trimethoprim–sulfamethoxazole (co-trimoxazole)

The use of sulfonamides has declined substantially because of widespread bacterial resistance. These agents are primarily bacteriostatic, rather than bactericidal, in concentrations that are normally useful in controlling infections in humans. All the sulfonamides used therapeutically are synthetically produced and, because they are structurally similar to para-aminobenzoic acid (PABA), they competitively inhibit the bacterial enzyme dihydropteroate synthase, necessary for incorporating PABA into dihydrofolic acid (Fig 36.1). The blocking of dihydrofolic acid synthesis results in a decrease in tetrahydrofolic acid, which interferes with the synthesis of purines, thymidine and DNA in the microorganism. Susceptible bacteria are particularly sensitive to sulfonamides because bacteria need to synthesise their own folic acid. The combination with trimethoprim (trimethoprim–sulfamethoxazole) is synergistic, as this agent blocks a further step in the synthesis of folic acid. The combination often has no advantage over the use of trimethoprim as monotherapy but is associated with a greater incidence of adverse reactions. Trimethoprim alone is indicated for uncomplicated UTIs, epididymo-orchitis and prostatitis.

After oral administration of trimethoprim–sulfamethoxazole, the absorption of trimethoprim is more rapid than that of sulfamethoxazole. Peak concentration occurs within 2 hours for trimethoprim and 4 hours for sulfamethoxazole. Trimethoprim distributes into tissues, while sulfamethoxazole distributes in extracellular fluids. About 60% of the trimethoprim and 25–50% of the sulfamethoxazole is excreted by the kidneys in 24 hours.

Urinary tract antimicrobials

UTIs rank as one of the problems most commonly reported to general practitioners in Australia. UTIs are broadly classified as acute uncomplicated UTI, acute uncomplicated pyelonephritis, complicated UTI and acute complicated pyelonephritis. The term 'uncomplicated' usually applies to non-pregnant women without underlying abnormalities (functional or anatomical) of the urinary tract. The incidence of UTIs increases in institutional settings, up to as much as 50% of the population in extended-stay hospitals. Risk factors for UTIs include indwelling catheters (~65%) and pregnancy (4–10%).

UTIs are primarily caused by bacteria. In community-acquired infections, 75–90% of uncomplicated UTIs are caused by *Escherichia coli*. It has been reported that *Escherichia coli* may cause up to 90% of all community-acquired uncomplicated UTIs. Hospital-acquired infections are often complicated and difficult to treat. Organisms involved include *Pseudomonas aeruginosa*, *Serratia* spp., *Enterobacter* spp. and other Gram-negative microorganisms.

Drug therapies for lower UTIs are often started before culture and sensitivity reports are available. Treatment guidelines for the various types of UTIs can be found in the Therapeutic Guidelines: Antibiotic (Antibiotic Expert Group 2019); depending on the circumstances, drug regimens may involve monotherapy (e.g. trimethoprim or cefalexin or amoxicillin–clavulanate for the treatment of acute uncomplicated UTI) or combination therapy. Drugs that may be used include ampicillin, amoxicillin–clavulanate, cefalexin, ciprofloxacin, nitrofurantoin, norfloxacin, trimethoprim, trimethoprim–sulfamethoxazole or, in severe infections, gentamicin. Many of these drugs have been covered in preceding sections; the remaining drugs indicated for treating UTIs are discussed below. Current guidelines recommend treating febrile UTI or acute pyelonephritis with antimicrobials for at least 14 days.

Methenamine (hexamine) hippurate

Methenamine (hexamine) hippurate, which is used to treat UTIs, combines the action of hexamine with hippurate. Its effectiveness depends on the release of formaldehyde, which requires an acid medium. The acids released from hippurate salts contribute to this acidity and, if sulfonamides are co-administered, this may result in crystalluria from precipitation of the formaldehyde with the sulfonamide. Formaldehyde may be bactericidal or bacteriostatic and its effects are believed to be the result of denaturation of bacterial protein. The drug is ineffective in alkaline urine as alkalinity inhibits the conversion of hexamine to formaldehyde. Because of its fairly wide bacterial spectrum, low toxicity and low incidence of resistance, hexamine has often been the drug of choice in the long-term suppression of infections.

DRUG INTERACTIONS 36.6
Quinolones

DRUG	POSSIBLE EFFECTS AND MANAGEMENT
Antacids, ferrous sulfate or sucralfate	May decrease absorption of ciprofloxacin, reducing drug effectiveness. Administer quinolone at least 2 hours before these medications.
Nitrofurantoin	Antibacterial effect of quinolones is antagonised. Avoid combination.
Theophylline and other xanthines	Ciprofloxacin and norfloxacin may inhibit theophylline metabolism, resulting in increased theophylline plasma concentration and toxicity. Monitor theophylline plasma concentration closely, as dosage adjustments may be necessary.
Warfarin	May result in increased anticoagulant effect and potential for bleeding. While not currently reported with all quinolones, it is recommended that the INR be monitored closely whenever these drugs are administered concurrently. Reduce warfarin dose if necessary.

Methenamine (hexamine) hippurate is absorbed orally and takes 0.5–2 hours to reach peak urinary formaldehyde concentration at a urinary pH of 5.6. Excretion is via the kidneys. Use hexamine with caution in severely dehydrated people. Avoid use in people with severe kidney impairment, as renal tubule concentration will be inadequate to achieve a response. For prophylaxis of recurrent UTIs, the adult oral dose is 1 g 12-hourly, and that for children aged 6–12 years is 500–1000 mg every 12 hours.

Nitrofurantoin

Nitrofurantoin is a broad-spectrum bactericidal agent that can be prescribed by endorsed/authorised midwives (Clinical Focus Box 36.3). Its mechanism of action is not fully understood, but it is reduced by bacteria to reactive substances that inactivate or alter cell wall synthesis, bacterial ribosomal proteins and DNA and RNA function. It is indicated for treating acute UTIs caused by organisms such as *Escherichia coli* and *Staphylococcus aureus*, and for prophylaxis of recurrent UTIs.

After oral administration, nitrofurantoin is well absorbed and has a half-life of 20–60 minutes. About 65% of the drug is excreted, mainly as unchanged drug in the urine. Alkalisation of urine is not recommended because it reduces antimicrobial activity. Antacids decrease absorption while probenecid inhibits tubular secretion of nitrofurantoin, leading to increased plasma concentration and possible toxicity. Combination with quinolones is contraindicated because they antagonise the bacterial action of nitrofurantoin (Drug Interactions 36.6). Use nitrofurantoin with caution in people with G6PD deficiency. Acute allergic pneumonitis may occur within days of initiation of treatment and presents as fever, chills, cough, dyspnoea, chest pain and often a rash. It is more common in women aged 40–50 years. Rarely, chronic irreversible interstitial pulmonary fibrosis can occur in older people following chronic treatment (> 6 months). The mechanism is unclear but is thought to involve the production of oxygen radicals within the lung. Nitrofurantoin should not be used in women at/near term because of risk of haemolytic anaemia in the neonate. Additionally, this drug may turn urine a brownish colour and stain soft (hydrogel) contact lenses. Avoid use in those with nitrofurantoin hypersensitivity, peripheral neuropathy, lung disease or moderate-to-severe renal impairment.

DRUGS AT A GLANCE
Antimicrobial drugs

PHARMACOLOGICAL GROUP AND EFFECT	KEY EXAMPLES	CLINICAL USE
Narrow spectrum penicillins • Inhibitors of bacterial cell wall synthesis	Benzylpenicillin	Community acquired pneumonia, staphylococcal skin infections
	Benzathine benzylpenicillin tetrahydrate	
	Dicloxacillin	
	Flucloxacillin	
	Phenoxymethylpenicillin	
Moderate spectrum penicillins • Inhibitors of bacterial cell wall synthesis	Amoxicillin	UTI, community-acquired pneumonia
	Ampicillin	
Broad spectrum penicillins • Inhibitors of bacterial cell wall synthesis	Piperacillin with tazobactam	Mixed (aerobic and anaerobic) infections, febrile neutropenia

Carbapenems • Inhibitors of bacterial cell wall synthesis	Ertapenem Imipenem with cilastin Meropenem	Life-threatening infections, febrile neutropenia
Cephalosporins • Inhibitors of bacterial cell wall synthesis	Cefaclor Cefalexin Cefazolin Cefepime Cefotaxime Cefoxitin Ceftazidime Ceftriaxone Cefuroxime	Staphylococcal and streptococcal infections, UTI, gonococcal infection
Glycopeptides • Inhibitors of bacterial cell wall synthesis	Teicoplanin Vancomycin	Endocarditis, MRSA infections
Aminoglycosides • Bacterial protein synthesis inhibitors	Amikacin Gentamicin Neomycin Tobramycin	*Pseudomonas aeruginosa* infections, serious systemic enterococcal infections
Macrolides • Bacterial protein synthesis inhibitors	Azithromycin Clarithromycin Erythromycin Roxithromycin	Community-acquired pneumonia, upper and lower respiratory tract infections
Lincosamides • Bacterial protein synthesis inhibitors	Clindamycin Lincomycin	Malaria, anaerobic infections
Tetracyclines • Bacterial protein synthesis inhibitors	Doxycycline Minocycline Tetracycline Tigecycline	Acne, prophylaxis of malaria, Q fever
Fluoroquinolone • Inhibitors of bacterial DNA synthesis	Ciprofloxacin Moxifloxacin Norfloxacin	Community-acquired pneumonia, complicated UTIs
Other antibiotics	Chloramphenicol Methenamine (hexamine) hippurate Metronidazole Nitrofurantoin Sulfamethoxazole Trimethoprim	UTIs, eradication of *Helicobacter pylori*, anaerobic bacterial infections, bacterial conjunctivitis

REVIEW EXERCISES

1. Mr GB, a 52-year-old male, has presented with a UTI and advises you that, when he was in his 20s, he thinks he had an allergic reaction to penicillin. His description of the reaction is not very informative, but he thought it was a mild reaction. You have a choice of three antibiotics: cefalexin, ciprofloxacin and trimethoprim. Which antibiotic would you administer? Discuss the reasons for your choice.
2. Discuss the mechanism of action of the macrolides and the aminoglycosides. Why are they relatively selective inhibitors of ribosomal function in bacteria and not human cells?
3. While in hospital, Mrs AM is administered gentamicin as a prophylactic measure following a surgical procedure. Each day, 1 hour after administering the drug, a nurse collects a blood sample to measure the drug concentration. Explain why monitoring of gentamicin blood concentration is performed.

REFERENCES

Antibiotic Expert Group. Therapeutic guidelines: antibiotic, Melbourne, 2019, Therapeutic Guidelines.

Australian Medicines Handbook 2021, Australian medicines handbook, Adelaide, AMH.

Brody TM, Larner J, Minneman KP: Human pharmacology: molecular to clinical, ed 3, St Louis, MO, 1998, Mosby.

Butler MS, Paterson DL: Antibiotics in the clinical pipeline in October 2019. Journal of Antibiotics 73, 329–364, 2020.

Campagna JD, Bond MC, Schabelman E, et al: The use of cephalosporins in penicillin-allergic patients. Journal of Emergency Medicine 42:612–620, 2012.

Hutchings MI, Truman AW, Wilkinson B: Antibiotics: past, present and future. Current Opinion on Microbiology 51: 72–80, 2019.

Lagace-Wiens P, Rubinstein E: Adverse reactions to β-lactam antimicrobials. Expert Opinion in Drug Safety 11:381–399, 2012.

CHAPTER 37
ANTIFUNGAL AND ANTIVIRAL DRUGS

Andrew Rowland

KEY ABBREVIATIONS

AIDS	acquired immunodeficiency syndrome
CMV	cytomegalovirus
DAA	direct-acting antiviral
HBV	hepatitis B
HCV	hepatitis C
HIV	human immunodeficiency virus
HSV	herpes simplex virus
NNRTI	non-nucleoside reverse transcriptase inhibitor
NRTI	nucleoside/nucleotide reverse transcriptase inhibitor
PI	protease inhibitor
VZV	varicella zoster virus

KEY TERMS

candidiasis 813
DNA polymerase 818
fungistatic agent 816
mycoses 813
neuraminidase inhibitor 819
nucleoside analogue 817
polymerase inhibitor 817
protease inhibitors 821
retroviruses 817
reverse transcriptase inhibitor 820

Chapter Focus

Over the past 30 years, the number of immunocompromised people has risen dramatically as a result of the spread of HIV and the use of immunosuppressant drugs in organ transplant recipients and chemotherapy for neoplastic diseases. These factors have contributed to a substantial rise in the incidence of severe fungal infections and the use of antifungal drugs. Similarly, viral infections (e.g. influenza and hepatitis) continue to exist globally, necessitating the continued development of effective antiviral drugs. The development of antiretroviral drugs has also evolved in concert with our knowledge of HIV and the need for multiple drug therapy to combat the devastating consequences of AIDS.

KEY DRUG GROUPS

Antifungal drugs:

- Azoles: fluconazole, itraconazole, miconazole, posaconazole, voriconazole
- Echinocandins: anidulafungin, caspofungin

Antiviral drugs:

- Nucleoside DNA polymerase inhibitors: **aciclovir**, cidofovir, ganciclovir, penciclovir
- Non-nucleoside DNA polymerase inhibitors: foscarnet
- Nucleoside reverse transcriptase inhibitors: abacavir, didanosine, emtricitabine, lamivudine, stavudine, tenofovir, zidovudine
- Non-nucleoside reverse transcriptase inhibitors: **efavirenz**, etravirine, nevirapine, rilpivirine
- Neuramidase inhibitors: oseltamivir, zanamivir
- NS3/4A Protease inhibitors: grazoprevir, paritaprevir, simeprevir
- NS5A Inhibitors: daclatasvir, elbasvir, ledipasvir, ombitasvir, velpatasvir
- NS5B RNA-dependent RNA protease inhibitors: dasabuvir, sofosbuvir
- Protease inhibitors: atazanavir, darunavir, fosamprenavir, indinavir, lopinavir, ritonavir, saquinavir, tipranavir

CRITICAL THINKING SCENARIO

Elise, a 56-year-old female, has been diagnosed with COVID-19 and is considered a high risk of serious complications because she has several underlying health issues including chronic obstructive pulmonary disease, for which she takes several medicines. Elise's GP decides that because of her risk of severe complications, it is appropriate to prescribe her Paxlovid to help minimise her COVID-19 symptoms. When deciding to prescribe Paxlovid to Elise, what should her GP consider in terms of the existing medicines Elise is currently taking?

Treating fungal infections

Fungal infections can be caused by any of about 50 species of plant-like, parasitic microorganisms. These simple organisms, lacking chlorophyll, cannot make their own food and so depend on other life forms. Infections by fungi, termed **mycoses**, can range from mild and superficial to severe and life-threatening. Infecting organisms can be ingested orally, become implanted under the skin after injury or be inhaled if the fungal spores are airborne. One species of fungus, *Candida albicans*, is usually part of the normal flora of the skin, mouth, intestines and vagina, and overgrowth and systemic infection from it can result from antibiotic, antineoplastic and corticosteroid drug therapy. This is often referred to as an opportunistic infection. Oral **candidiasis** (thrush) is common in newborn infants and immunocompromised people, whereas vaginal candidiasis is more common in pregnant women, women with diabetes mellitus and women who take oral contraceptives.

Azole antifungals

Azole antifungals used in Australia and New Zealand are fluconazole, itraconazole, miconazole, posaconazole and voriconazole. Those that contain two nitrogens in the azole ring are called imidazoles (e.g. miconazole), and those with three nitrogens are called triazoles (e.g. itraconazole, fluconazole, posaconazole and voriconazole). These agents are fungistatic and affect the biosynthesis of fungal ergosterols by interfering with the cytochrome P450 (CYP)-dependent enzyme lanosterol demethylase (also called 14α-sterol demethylase) that catalyses ergosterol formation (Fig 37.1). Ergosterol is a major

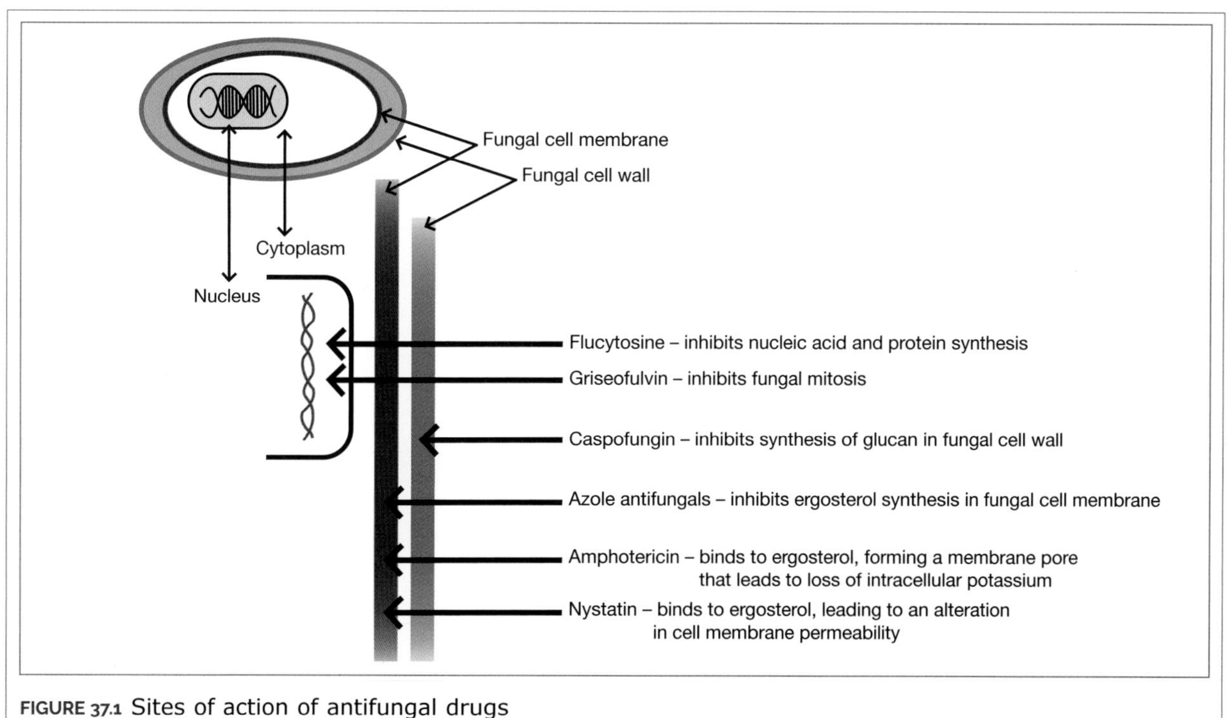

FIGURE 37.1 Sites of action of antifungal drugs

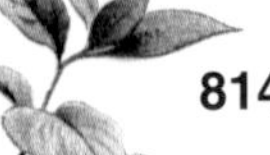

component of the fungal cell membrane, and the azoles cause depletion of ergosterol and accumulation of 14α-methylated sterols. This results in inhibition of fungal growth, interference in nutrient transport and, ultimately, cell leakage and death. At therapeutic concentrations, the azoles have a greater affinity for the fungal 14α-sterol demethylase than for the human liver equivalent CYP 14α-sterol demethylase. This selective toxicity allows for the use of these drugs in humans.

Azole antifungals are administered orally; fluconazole and voriconazole may also be administered IV. Absorption rates are good if fluconazole is administered to a fasting person, while itraconazole should be administered with food and voriconazole administered at least 1 hour before or 1 hour after a meal. Fluconazole and posaconazole are excreted predominantly as unchanged drug (> 75%); itraconazole and voriconazole are extensively metabolised by CYP enzymes. Pharmacokinetic parameters describing exposure and standard adult dosages of azole antifungals are shown in Table 37.1.

Drug interactions and adverse reactions

Azoles are clinically relevant inhibitors of CYP-mediated metabolism (Table 37.2), although interactions rarely occur with miconazole (moderate inhibitor of CYP2C9 only). Drug Interactions 37.1 lists the drugs that can interact with azole antifungal agents, and the possible outcomes and management. Up-to-date drug interaction sources should always be consulted before administering any of the azoles.

Common adverse reactions associated with the use of azole antifungals include nausea, vomiting, stomach distress, diarrhoea, flushing, drowsiness, dizziness, headache and hypersensitivity (fever, chills and rash). Voriconazole can cause redness, swelling or pain at the injection site. Other rare effects include liver toxicity, anaemia, agranulocytosis and exfoliative skin disorders such as Stevens-Johnson syndrome (for fluconazole) and thrombocytopenia (for fluconazole and miconazole). Voriconazole is associated with visual abnormalities, including altered visual perception, blurred vision and colour changes. These effects are dose-related and are in general reversible.

Echinocandins

Anidulafungin and caspofungin

Anidulafungin and caspofungin are the first drugs in the echinocandins class of antifungals. They have significant activity against *Candida* spp. and *Aspergillus* spp. They act by inhibiting the fungal enzyme glucan synthase and hence the synthesis of glucan, a vital component of the

TABLE 37.1 Pharmacokinetics and standard adult doses for azole antifungal drugs

	PHARMACOKINETICS		
DRUG	TIME TO PEAK CONCENTRATION (H)	HALF-LIFE (H)[a]	STANDARD ADULT DOSE
Fluconazole	1–2	Adults: 30 Children: 14–20	50–400 mg orally/IV daily
Itraconazole	3–4	Single dose: 21 Steady state: 64	Capsule 100–200 mg orally daily
Miconazole	2–4	20–25	½ teaspoon (i.e. 62 mg) oral gel 6-hourly for 7–14 days
Posaconazole	3–5	20–66	400 mg 12-hourly
Voriconazole	1–2	~6[b]	Consult relevant sources for IV/oral loading and maintenance doses

[a] Half-life for normal renal function.
[b] Varies depending on dose because of non-linear (saturable) metabolism.
Source: Dosages in Australian Medicines Handbook 2021.

TABLE 37.2 FDA guidance regarding azole antifungals as inhibitors of hepatic CYPs

CYP	FLUCONAZOLE	ITRACONAZOLE	POSACONAZOLE	VORICONAZOLE
CYP2B6				Weak
CYP2C9	Moderate			Weak
CYP2C19	Strong			Weak
CYP3A4	Moderate	Strong	Strong	Strong

Strong inhibitors increase the AUC of sensitive index substrates of a given metabolic pathway ≥ 5-fold (≥ 10-fold for CYP3A4).
Moderate inhibitors increase the AUC of sensitive index substrates of a given metabolic pathway ≥ 2 to < 5-fold.
Weak inhibitors increase the AUC of sensitive index substrates of a given metabolic pathway ≥ 1.25 to < 2-fold.

DRUG INTERACTIONS 37.1
Azole antifungals

DRUG	POSSIBLE OUTCOMES	MANAGEMENT
Amphotericin	Antagonistic effect, reduced antifungal activity	Avoid concurrent use.
Carbamazepine	Decreased metabolism of carbamazepine and increased risk of toxicity	Reduce dose of carbamazepine if required.
Ciclosporin, tacrolimus	Increased plasma concentrations	Monitor renal function and ciclosporin/tacrolimus plasma concentrations.
H_2 antagonists, proton pump inhibitors, antacids	Reduced absorption, reduced antifungal effect	Avoid combination with H_2 antagonists and proton pump inhibitors. Give 2 hours apart from antacids.
Indinavir	Itraconazole decreases metabolism of indinavir, which increases plasma concentration of indinavir	Reduce dose of indinavir.
Phenytoin	Voriconazole increases phenytoin concentration and risk of toxicity Phenytoin increases metabolism of voriconazole, decreasing its efficacy	Monitor plasma concentration of phenytoin and reduce dose if necessary. Increase voriconazole dose.
Thiazolidinediones	Reduced metabolism increases risk of hypoglycaemia	Monitor blood glucose, reduce dose of thiazolidinediones if necessary.
Triazolam	Itraconazole inhibits metabolism increasing the risk of sedation and adverse effects	Avoid combination or reduce dose of triazolam.
Warfarin	Reduced metabolism increases risk of bleeding	Monitor international normalised ratio and reduce warfarin dose if necessary.

Source: Australian Medicines Handbook 2021.

fungal cell wall. Anidulafungin, which was marketed after caspofungin, is poorly absorbed orally and is administered daily as an intravenous (IV) infusion. It is not metabolised but degrades slowly over time. Dosage adjustment is not required for those with hepatic or renal impairment. Available only for IV administration, caspofungin is highly protein-bound (97%) and is slowly metabolised by hydrolysis and N-acetylation, with less than 2% excreted as unchanged drug in urine. Dosage adjustment is not necessary in people with mild renal or mild hepatic impairment, but dose reduction is required in those who have moderate hepatic impairment, and this drug should not be used in the presence of severe hepatic impairment. As the site of action of caspofungin is unique to fungi, the drug is reasonably well tolerated.

Other antifungal drugs

Amphotericin B

Amphotericin B (amphotericin) is the premier drug for treating severe systemic mycoses. It binds to ergosterol in the fungal cell membrane; this binding results in pores or channels forming that alter cell permeability and results in a loss of potassium and other elements from the cell (Fig 37.1). Ergosterol is a major component of fungal cell membranes. It not only provides the structure, but is also involved in nutrient transport. Amphotericin B is effective for treating aspergillosis, blastomycosis, candidiasis (moniliasis), coccidioidomycosis, cryptococcosis, fungal endocarditis, histoplasmosis, cryptococcal meningitis, fungal septicaemia and many other severe systemic fungal infections.

Amphotericin B is widely distributed in the body after parenteral administration. After oral administration, little or no absorption occurs from the gastrointestinal tract (GIT). It has an initial half-life in adults of 24 hours and a terminal half-life of about 15 days. Caution should be exercised in people with renal impairment, as IV amphotericin alters renal function. The drug is contraindicated in people with amphotericin B hypersensitivity unless no alternative exists.

Flucytosine

Flucytosine enters fungal cells, where it is converted to fluorouracil, an antimetabolite (Fig 37.1). It interferes with pyrimidine metabolism, thus preventing nucleic acid and protein synthesis. It has selective toxicity against susceptible strains of fungi because human cells do not convert significant quantities of this drug into fluorouracil. Flucytosine is indicated for treating fungal endocarditis (caused by *Candida* spp.), fungal meningitis (caused by *Cryptococcus* spp.) and fungal pneumonia, septicaemia or urinary infections caused by *Candida* or *Cryptococcus* spp. As resistance develops rapidly, combined use with another antifungal is recommended.

Griseofulvin

Griseofulvin is a **fungistatic agent** that inhibits fungal cell mitosis during metaphase. It is also deposited in the keratin precursor cells in skin, hair and nails, thus inhibiting fungal invasion of the keratin. When infested keratin is shed, healthy keratin will replace it. Griseofulvin is indicated for treating susceptible organisms for onychomycosis (nail fungus), tinea barbae (fungal infection of the bearded section of face and neck), tinea capitis (fungal infection of the scalp; ringworm), tinea corporis (fungal infection of non-hairy skin), tinea cruris (fungal infection in the groin) and tinea pedis (fungal infection of the foot; athlete's foot).

Nystatin

Nystatin is an antibiotic with antifungal activity and is used to treat cutaneous or mucocutaneous infections caused by the monilial organism *Candida albicans*. It has both fungistatic and fungicidal effects and is also used to suppress intestinal candidiasis. Nystatin adheres to sterols in the fungal cell membrane, altering cell membrane permeability, which results in loss of essential intracellular contents. Nystatin is poorly absorbed from the GIT and is not absorbed when applied topically to skin or mucous membranes. It produces a local antifungal effect. Nystatin is not metabolised, and most of the unabsorbed nystatin is excreted in the faeces. No drug interaction has been documented. Adverse reactions are uncommon and the drug is well tolerated by all ages. Large doses may cause gastric distress.

Terbinafine

Terbinafine is an orally and topically active allylamine antifungal agent and is indicated for severe ringworm unresponsive to topical treatment, onychomycoses (tinea unguium) and dermatophyte skin infections (tinea corporis, tinea cruris and tinea pedis). It inhibits squalene epoxidase, thereby inhibiting formation of lanosterol, an essential component of fungal cell membranes.

KEY POINTS

Antifungal drugs

- Systemic fungal and viral infections can be serious (even life-threatening).
- Antifungal drugs are potent and potentially toxic medications. They include amphotericin B, anidulafungin, caspofungin, fluconazole, flucytosine, griseofulvin, itraconazole, miconazole, nystatin, posaconazole, terbinafine and voriconazole.
- Drugs that are systemic fungistatic or fungicidal agents are used to treat a wide variety of mycotic infections.

Treating viral infections

Drugs for treating viral infections have been more limited than for bacterial infection because the development and clinical application of antiviral drugs is more difficult (Portugal & Raboni 2017). For many viral infections the replication of the virus in the body reaches its peak before any clinical symptoms are visible, meaning that by the time the infection is apparent, multiplication of the virus is maximal and the subsequent course of the illness has been determined. In most cases, to alter the course of the infection an antiviral drug must be administered prophylactically, before symptoms of infection appear. Historically, a major limitation has been that drugs that inhibit virus replication often also perturb replication within the host cell, making the drugs too toxic at the concentrations required to 'cure' infection.

Viruses

Physically, viruses are simply genetic material (DNA or RNA) contained within a protein coating known as the capsid. This structure is known as the virus particle or virion. Viruses lack their own metabolic activity, making them true parasites as they replicate within mammalian cells using the host's metabolic machinery. The Baltimore classification system is used to sort viruses into seven groups based on their type of genetic material (DNA or RNA) and mechanism of replication.

DNA viruses

DNA viruses belong to Group I, Group II or Group VII of the Baltimore classification system. These viruses have DNA as their genetic material and usually replicate within the nucleus of the host by producing and utilising a DNA-dependent polymerase enzyme. DNA viruses generally do not incorporate into the host's chromosomal DNA.

RNA viruses

RNA viruses belong to Group III, Group IV, Group V or Group VI of the Baltimore classification system. They typically have a single strand of RNA as the genetic material and adopt different reproduction strategies depending on the directionality of that RNA (sense or antisense). For viruses with RNA in the sense orientation, the RNA serves as mRNA; whereas for RNA viruses with RNA in the antisense orientation, the RNA is transcribed into mRNA by an RNA-dependent RNA polymerase. Depending on specific features of the virus, DNA and RNA viruses may be effectively treated using different types of typical (non-antiretroviral) antiviral drugs.

Retroviruses

Retroviruses are a special class of RNA virus that replicate in a host cell via the enzyme reverse transcriptase. These viruses produce DNA from the RNA genome, then replicate as part of the host cell's DNA. This replication mechanism makes **retroviruses** particularly difficult to treat. Indeed, retroviruses cannot be treated effectively using typical antiviral drugs and require a separate class of medicines known as antiretroviral drugs.

Treating herpesviruses

Herpesviruses are large enveloped, double-stranded DNA viruses. Their genomes encode around 35 proteins. Infection with herpesviruses is lifelong and characterised by latency following initial acute exposure with relapses later in life (especially when a person is immunocompromised). The major herpesviruses that are widespread in humans are herpes simplex virus 1 and 2 (HSV-1 and HSV-2), varicella zoster virus (VZV; causes chickenpox and shingles), Epstein-Barr virus and cytomegalovirus (CMV); more than 90% of adults are infected with at least one of these viruses. Each virus is antigenically different. Antiviral drugs used to treat herpesviruses are:

- nucleoside DNA polymerase inhibitors – aciclovir, cidofovir, ganciclovir, penciclovir
- non-nucleoside DNA polymerase inhibitors – foscarnet.

Nucleoside DNA polymerase inhibitors

Aciclovir, ganciclovir and penciclovir are **nucleoside analogues**. Cidofovir is more explicitly a nucleotide analogue, where a nucleotide is a nucleoside with a phosphate group; as such, cidofovir can also be broadly considered as a nucleoside analogue. In virally infected cells, a viral thymidine kinase adds a phosphate group to the nucleoside analogue. Host kinases then add an additional two phosphate groups (one, in the case of cidofovir), producing an active tri- (di- for cidofovir) phosphorylated nucleoside analogue that inactivates viral DNA polymerases preventing viral DNA synthesis. Selective toxicity is achieved as the affinity for viral thymidine kinase is 200-fold greater than for the analogous host enzyme.

Aciclovir and valaciclovir

Aciclovir (Drug Monograph 37.1) is the prototypical DNA **polymerase inhibitor** and the first to be approved for treating herpes simplex virus (HSV) and VZV. Valaciclovir is a prodrug that is converted to aciclovir by first-pass intestinal and liver metabolism. It is indicated for treating herpes simplex infections, varicella zoster

Drug Monograph 37.1
Aciclovir

Aciclovir is selectively taken up by HSV-infected cells and is converted to an active triphosphate form. This active form inhibits viral DNA synthesis by preventing the incorporation of the normal deoxyguanosine into viral DNA by the viral DNA polymerase and causing irreversible termination of viral DNA synthesis.

Indications

Aciclovir is used in the prophylaxis and treatment of herpes simplex infections including genital herpes, shingles, chickenpox and in herpetic eye infections.

Pharmacokinetics

The oral dose form is poorly absorbed (15–30%), but plasma concentrations achieved are therapeutic. It is widely distributed to various body fluids and tissues. Concentrations in CSF are around 50% of the plasma drug concentration. The half-life is about 2.5 hours in people with normal renal function but prolonged in people with renal dysfunction. Aciclovir is minimally metabolised and is excreted predominantly as unchanged drug in urine.

Drug interactions

Concurrent use of aciclovir with probenecid will result in high plasma concentration of aciclovir and the risk of adverse neurological effects. During concomitant administration with theophylline, the plasma concentration of theophylline may increase and a decrease in theophylline dose may be necessary.

Adverse reactions

Adverse reactions with the oral dosage form include gastric distress, headache, dizziness, nausea, diarrhoea and vomiting. With the parenteral form, phlebitis at the injection site, acute renal failure with rapid injection or, rarely, encephalopathic alterations such as confusion, hallucinations, convulsions, tremors and coma can occur.

Dosage and administration

Aciclovir is available as oral, topical and IV formulations. The usual oral adult dose for an initial genital herpes infection is 200 mg every 4 hours during waking hours (five times daily) for 10 days. For prophylaxis of recurrent infection, the dose is 200 mg orally two to three times daily for up to 6 months. The parenteral adult dosage for HSV encephalitis and varicella zoster in immunocompromised people is 10 mg/kg IV 8-hourly. For other dosage recommendations, consult current drug information sources.

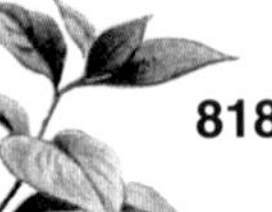

infections, for primary and recurring genital HSV and for preventing CMV disease following organ transplantation.

Cidofovir

Cidofovir has almost exclusively been used to treat CMV retinitis in acquired immunodeficiency syndrome (AIDS). The diphosphate active metabolite selectively inhibits viral DNA polymerase and prevents DNA synthesis. Cidofovir is administered IV with oral probenecid, which blocks active renal tubule secretion and hence reduces the renal clearance of the drug. Cidofovir also has efficacy against aciclovir-resistant HSV infections and is believed to have efficacy against smallpox, meaning that it could be used in the event of a bioterrorism incident involving this virus.

Ganciclovir and valganciclovir

In the presence of CMV, ganciclovir is rapidly phosphorylated to ganciclovir triphosphate. Ganciclovir is carcinogenic, and appropriate cytotoxic handling procedures should be adopted. It is used for CMV pneumonitis in bone marrow and renal transplant recipients and for sight-threatening CMV retinitis in severely immunocompromised people (Australian Medicines Handbook 2021). Ganciclovir is excreted unchanged, primarily by the kidneys, and the half-life is substantially prolonged in people with renal impairment.

Valganciclovir is a prodrug of ganciclovir. It is indicated for prophylaxis of CMV disease after organ transplant. As valganciclovir is quickly metabolised to the active component ganciclovir, the pharmacodynamics and pharmacokinetics of valganciclovir are the same as those of ganciclovir. Ganciclovir and valganciclovir are contraindicated in pregnancy and lactation because of potential embryotoxic and teratogenic effects. The adverse reactions of valganciclovir are similar to those of ganciclovir. Drug Interactions 37.2 provides examples of interactions that can occur with ganciclovir or valganciclovir if given with the drugs listed.

Famciclovir

Famciclovir is active against HSV (types 1 and 2) and VZV. It is indicated for treating acute herpes zoster (shingles) infections and recurrent genital herpes. Administered orally, famciclovir is well absorbed and converted in the intestinal wall to the active antiviral penciclovir, which is primarily excreted as unchanged drug in urine and faeces. Adverse reactions include headaches, weakness, gastric distress (nausea, vomiting and diarrhoea) and fatigue. Famciclovir should not be used in lactating women. Dosing is based on renal function, and current drug information sources should be consulted.

Non-nucleoside DNA polymerase inhibitors

Foscarnet

Foscarnet is a virustatic agent that inhibits viral replication of all the major species of herpesviruses that are widespread in humans. It acts by selective inhibition at the pyrophosphate binding site of viral **DNA polymerase**. If the drug is discontinued, viral replication will resume. It is particularly used to treat CMV retinitis in people with AIDS and can be used to treat nucleoside analogue treatment-experienced people with HIV as part of salvage therapy.

One common mechanism of resistance to nucleoside analogue DNA polymerase inhibitors involves developing mutant thymidine kinases that do not phosphorylate these drugs. Unlike the nucleoside analogues, foscarnet is not activated by viral kinases, making it potentially useful in aciclovir- or ganciclovir-resistant HSV and CMV infections. However, resistance to aciclovir or ganciclovir may also occur through mutation of the DNA polymerase, in which case the virus may also be resistant to foscarnet.

DRUG INTERACTIONS 37.2
Ganciclovir/valganciclovir

DRUG	POSSIBLE EFFECTS AND MANAGEMENT
Bone marrow depressant drugs	Concurrent use can result in increased bone marrow-suppressant effects. Monitor blood closely for neutropenia and thrombocytopenia.
Foscarnet	Synergistic antiviral effects but increased haematological and renal toxicity. Monitor blood count and electrolytes.
Imipenem	Avoid combined use because of increased risk of seizures.
Probenecid	Inhibits renal secretion of ganciclovir, increasing the concentration and risk of toxicity. Avoid combination.
Zidovudine (AZT)	Can result in severe haematological toxicity. Withhold zidovudine or change to another antiretroviral drug.

Treating influenza and viral respiratory infection

Influenza virus is the most common of the orthomyxoviruses, which are large, enveloped RNA viruses with anti-sense single-stranded RNA. Influenza virus is spread by droplets and fomite contact, and hence infection control precautions (e.g. hand hygiene) are important in minimising the spread of infection. Use of drugs to treat influenza is prioritised for people with risk factors for poor outcomes such as pregnant women, the elderly (> 65 years), the very young (< 5 years), people who are morbidly obese or suffer from chronic diseases (especially asthma and respiratory diseases) and immunosuppressed people (transplant recipients). Two classes of drugs are used to treat influenza:

- **neuraminidase inhibitors** – oseltamivir and zanamivir
- amantadines – amantadine.

Respiratory syncytial virus (RSV) is a syncytial virus and a major cause of lower respiratory tract infections requiring hospitalisation in infants and children. Palivizumab is a monoclonal antibody that can be used as a prophylactic to prevent RSV in preterm infants, or infants with congenital heart defects or bronchopulmonary dysplasia or congenital airway malformations.

Neuraminidase inhibitors

Influenza A and B viruses contain two main antigens: haemagglutinin and neuraminidase. Haemagglutinin binds to sialic acid residues on the surface of epithelial cells in the respiratory tract of a host. After viral replication, the progeny virion is still bound to the host cell via these sialic acid residues. Viral neuraminidases cleave the sialic acid groups, allowing the progeny virion to bind to new cells and undergo further rounds of replication. As sialic acid analogues, oseltamivir and zanamivir competitively inhibit viral neuraminidase enzymes on the surface of influenza A and B viruses, block release of progeny virion from infected cells and prevent further rounds of infection (Liu et al. 2021).

Oseltamivir

Oseltamivir is a prodrug that is well absorbed following oral administration and undergoes ester hydrolysis (~75%) in the GIT and liver to the active carboxylate metabolite. It is indicated for treating influenza A and B in adults and children aged over 1 year. Metabolic drug interactions are unlikely because oseltamivir is not metabolised by typical hepatic drug-metabolising enzymes.

Zanamivir

Similar to oseltamivir, zanamivir is indicated for treating influenza A and B in adults and children older than 5 years old within 48 hours of the onset of symptoms. Administration is via oral inhalation, and approximately 10–20% of the dose is systemically available. After inhalation, zanamivir is widely deposited within the respiratory tract. It is not metabolised and is excreted as unchanged drug in the urine. Zanamivir is generally well tolerated, and in clinical trials the frequency of adverse reactions is similar to that for placebo. Rarely, an allergic reaction has been reported (facial and oropharyngeal oedema), as have bronchospasm and dyspnoea.

Amantadines

Amantadine and rimantadine are closely related compounds. These drugs are only active against influenza A, and widespread emergence of adamantine-resistant strains of influenza A limits their use. Their selective efficacy is because the influenza A, but not influenza B, virion contains a proton selective ion channel within the envelope (the Matrix-2 [M2] protein). This pump enables hydrogen ions to enter the virion from the host cell and by doing so lowers the pH inside of the virion, which facilitates dissociation of the viral matrix protein from the ribonucleoprotein. Amantadine and rimantadine bind to the transmembrane region of the M2 protein, sterically blocking this channel. This prevents uncoating of the virion and stops the virus from taking over the host respiratory epithelial cells. Within the host, amantadine also increases dopamine release and inhibits the reuptake of dopamine and noradrenaline (norepinephrine) centrally. It is also indicated for treating Parkinson's disease (Ch 17) and drug-induced extrapyramidal reactions.

Amantadine is rapidly absorbed after oral administration; it is distributed in saliva and nasal secretions and crosses the blood–brain barrier. It has a half-life of 11–15 hours, reaching peak plasma concentration within 2–4 hours. It is excreted mostly unchanged by the kidneys, and the half-life is prolonged in people with renal impairment.

Palivizumab

Palivizumab is a humanised monoclonal antibody directed against a protein of the surface of RSV. Once bound to the virus, palivizumab inhibits RSV replication. It is indicated for serious lower respiratory tract diseases caused by RSV in infants and children at high risk of RSV disease. These include infants born at 32–35 weeks' gestation, or with bronchopulmonary dysplasia or significant congenital heart disease (Australian Medicines Handbook 2021). Determination of the pharmacokinetics of monoclonal antibodies is difficult, and considerable individual variation in palivizumab plasma concentration has been reported. To date, the metabolism of palivizumab has not been determined and drug interactions have not been

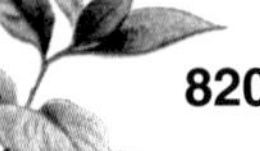

described. Adverse reactions include fever, rash, wheeze, cough and, rarely, hypersensitivity including anaphylaxis.

Treating hepatitis B

Hepatitis B virus (HBV) is a double-stranded DNA virus. HBV infection is a global public health problem, with an estimated 250 million HBV carriers, approximately 600,000 of whom die annually from HBV-related disease. Despite the availability of HBV vaccines, the rate of HBV-related hospitalisations and deaths continues to rise at an alarming rate. Like many chronic viral infections, the mainstay of treating HBV involves the use of nucleoside analogues that inhibit viral protease, viral DNA polymerase or viral reverse transcriptase. The nucleoside **reverse transcriptase inhibitors** used to treat HBV are lamivudine and tenofovir; these drugs are also used to treat human immunodeficiency virus (HIV). (See treatment of HIV later in this chapter for a full description of these drugs.) In addition to nucleoside analogues, the immunomodulatory interferon peginterferon alpha-2a is used to treat HBV (Ch 40). Recently, the re-emergence of HBV in hepatitis C (HCV) patients treated with new direct-acting antivirals (DAAs) has led to safety concerns regarding the use of these drugs (Clinical Focus Box 37.1).

CLINICAL FOCUS BOX 37.1

Reactivation of HBV in people treated with direct-acting antivirals

In December 2016, the United States Food and Drug Administration (FDA) and Health Canada issued warnings about the risk of HBV reactivation in people treated for HCV using some DAA, who had a current or previous HBV infection. In some of the reported cases, reactivation of HBV resulted in serious liver problems or death; HBV reactivation was usually observed within 4–8 weeks after starting DAA treatment. As a result, the FDA and Health Canada have required that the information describing the risk of reactivation be added to DAA drug labels.

Health professionals have further been advised to screen all patients for evidence of current or prior HBV infection before prescribing a DAA for the first time and to regularly perform tests to check for HBV flare-ups or reactivation during DAA treatment and following treatment. Patients are advised against stopping treatment with DAA without first talking to a health professional but to contact them immediately if they develop fatigue, weakness, loss of appetite, nausea and vomiting, discolouration of the eyes or skin or light-coloured stools, as these may be signs of serious liver problems.

Nucleoside analogues

Adefovir

Adefovir dipivoxil is rapidly absorbed and metabolised by esterases to the active drug adefovir. In the host cell, enzymes phosphorylate adefovir (an analogue of adenosine) to adefovir diphosphate, which then inhibits viral polymerase, resulting in termination of viral DNA synthesis. The half-life after oral administration is 5–7 hours, and approximately 60% of the drug is eliminated unchanged by the kidney. To date, dose-related nephrotoxicity has been reported but other adverse reactions may not yet be fully known.

Entecavir

Entecavir is a deoxyguanosine nucleoside analogue with selective activity towards HBV and little or no activity against other viral pathogens. The active form of entecavir is the triphosphate, which inhibits HBV DNA replication at three stages: (1) priming of the HBV DNA polymerase, (2) at the reverse transcription stage and (3) at the synthesis stage of the positive strand of HBV DNA. Entecavir is indicated for chronic HBV in the presence of liver inflammation and especially if there is evidence of lamivudine resistance.

Entecavir is well absorbed on an empty stomach and bioavailability is 100%. Entecavir does not undergo extensive metabolism and is not an inducer or inhibitor of CYP enzymes. It is primarily excreted as unchanged drug (62–73%) in urine. The elimination half-life is 128–149 hours and dosage adjustment is required in people with creatinine clearance of less than 50 mL/minute.

Telbivudine

Telbivudine is a synthetic nucleoside analogue of thymidine, which has significant activity against HBV. Intracellularly, it is phosphorylated by cellular kinases to form the active metabolite telbivudine triphosphate. The active metabolite then competitively inhibits viral DNA polymerase. Consequently, DNA synthesis is terminated and viral replication inhibited. Fortunately, telbivudine triphosphate does not inhibit human DNA polymerase at clinically relevant plasma drug concentrations.

Administered orally, the elimination half-life is in the order of 40–49 hours and steady state is reached after 5–7 days. As the drug is excreted unchanged in urine, dosage adjustment is required in situations of renal impairment. Common adverse effects include diarrhoea, dizziness, fatigue, headache, rash and muscle-related problems such as myalgia and myopathy. Similar to other antiviral drugs, resistance is a problem and cross-resistance with lamivudine is limiting its role in treating chronic HBV.

Treating hepatitis C

HCV is an enveloped virus containing positive polarity single-stranded RNA. The viral genome encodes a single polypeptide, and the virion has no viral polymerase. Transmission occurs through exposure to infected blood. HVC has seven major genotypes, which are referred to as genotypes one to seven. In Australia, like many Western countries including the United States and much of Europe, the HCV genotype 1 is most common. Each of the different HCV genotypes has different sensitivity to antiviral drugs. Historically, treating chronic HCV involved administering a combination of peginterferon alfa (Ch 40) and ribavirin. Some of the most important therapeutic advances in recent history have related to developing new antiviral drugs for treating HCV. While these drugs have substantially changed the treatment landscape for HCV, including the potential to cure this infection, their use is associated with a significant financial burden (Zhang et al. 2016). These drugs, which are commonly used in combinations to maximise treatment benefit, include:

- NS3/4A protease inhibitors: grazoprevir, paritaprevir, simeprevir
- NS5A inhibitors: daclatasvir, elbasvir, ledipasvir, ombitasvir, velpatasvir
- NS5B RNA-dependent RNA protease inhibitors: dasabuvir, sofosbuvir.

NS3/4A protease inhibitors

The NS3/4A serine protease is an enzyme involved in post-translational processing and replication of HCV. NS3/4A **protease inhibitors** (PIs) disrupt HCV by blocking the NS3 catalytic site or the NS3/NS4A interaction. In addition to its role in viral processing, the NS3/NS4A protease also impairs induction of interferons, blocking viral elimination. Thus, inhibition of the NS3/4A protease is believed to contribute to antiviral activity through two mechanisms.

Telaprevir and boceprevir were the first NS3/4A PIs, as well as the first DAA used to treat HCV. Recently, the introduction of newer and better-tolerated agents has negated the clinical importance of these drugs because of their complicated administration, serious adverse effects and low barrier to resistance.

Grazoprevir

Grazoprevir is a second-generation NS3/4A PI that is only available as a fixed-dose combination with the NS5A inhibitor elbasvir (described later). This combination has good activity against a range of HCV genotypes. Grazoprevir is metabolised in the liver by CYP3A4 and is transported by OATP1B1 and 1B3. Drugs that alter the activity of these proteins are known to alter exposure to grazoprevir.

Paritaprevir

Paritaprevir is given with low-dose ritonavir (also a PI but does not have activity against HCV) for a pharmacological boosting effect. Paritaprevir and ritonavir are administered in a fixed-dose combination with NS5A PI ombitasvir, usually with dasabuvir (combination described later). Especially when used in combination with other antivirals, resistance to paritaprevir is uncommon because of the importance of the site that this drug binds to on the NS3/4A protein.

Simeprevir

Simeprevir was the first of the second-generation PIs. It is used in combination with sofosbuvir, and with peginterferon and ribavirin. To minimise the risk of resistance, simeprevir should not be used without other antiviral agents, and the dose of simeprevir should not be decreased. Simeprevir is mainly cleared by the liver and should not be used in people with moderate or severe liver disease because these conditions increase in exposure by two- to fivefold.

The most common serious adverse effects reported with simeprevir use are photosensitivity and rash. Patients should be cautioned about this risk and counselled on sun protective measures and limiting sun exposure.

NS5A inhibitors

The NS5A protein has important, but currently uncertain, functions in the replication and assembly of the hepatitis C virion. NS5A inhibitors are generally effective drugs for treating HCV, but they have a low barrier to resistance and can be quite toxic to the host. NS5A inhibitors are rarely used as sole agents, but have been shown to significantly reduce HCV infection and enhance response when given in conjunction with peginterferon, ribavirin or other DAA.

Daclatasvir

Daclatasvir is a NS5A inhibitor that is used mainly in combination with sofosbuvir. It is listed by the World Health Organization among its Essential Medicines, which are the most effective and safe medicines needed in a health system.

Daclatasvir is generally well tolerated, although the use of daclatasvir-containing regimens is commonly associated with mild to moderate headache, fatigue and nausea. Daclatasvir is given orally with or without food and is only used in combination with other DAA agents. No dose adjustments are required for renal or hepatic impairment. As daclatasvir is primarily cleared by CYP3A metabolism, dose modifications are warranted when used in combination with drugs that alter CYP3A4 activity. For example, daclatasvir dose should be halved when administered with CYP3A4 inhibitors such as ritonavir-boosted atazanavir,

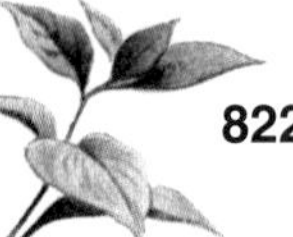

azole antifungals and clarithromycin. On the other hand, the daclatasvir dose should be increased by 50% when used with moderate or strong CYP3A4 inducers such as efavirenz, etravirine, dexamethasone and nafcillin.

Elbasvir

As elbasvir has only been used or tested in combination with other antiviral drugs such as grazoprevir, its antiviral effectiveness as a sole agent remains unclear. In saying this, combinations including elbasvir are among the most successful regimens at curing HCV. Elbasvir is hepatically cleared, primarily by CYP3A4. Co-administration of drugs that inhibit/induce CYP3A4 activity can alter exposure to elbasvir, which can affect efficacy and tolerability.

Ledipasvir

Ledipasvir was the first NS5A inhibitor; it is used in fixed-dose combination with the NS5B inhibitor sofosbuvir. Ledipasvir is generally rapidly absorbed, although its solubility is pH-dependent, meaning that co-administration with antacids, proton pump inhibitors and H_2-receptor antagonists can decrease absorption. Ledipasvir is primarily cleared by biliary excretion, with most of the drug recovered unchanged in the faeces. No dose adjustment is required in people with hepatic impairment.

Ombitasvir

Ombitasvir is only available as a fixed-dose combination with the NS3/4A PI paritaprevir with ritonavir (for a pharmacological boosting effect; described earlier), and is often used in combination with the NS5B inhibitor dasabuvir. Ombitasvir, paritaprevir and ritonavir are co-formulated in a single tablet. As for other DAA regimens, ritonavir does not directly treat HCV; rather, it is included to increase levels of paritaprevir through inhibition of CYP3A metabolism.

Given orally, this combination is formulated as a normal-release three-drug (ombitasvir, paritaprevir and ritonavir) tablet that is administered once daily with or without dasabuvir, which is administered twice daily. Alternatively, there is an extended-release four-drug tablet that contains ombitasvir, paritaprevir, ritonavir and dasabuvir, which is administered once daily. Both formulations should be given with food. The combination is generally well tolerated, but mild adverse effects – including asthenia, diarrhoea, insomnia, nausea and pruritus – are relatively common. Many of these effects are likely to have been caused by the ribavirin component of the combination.

Velpatasvir

The NS5A inhibitor velpatasvir is unique in that it is a pan-genotypic treatment for HCV, meaning that it is effective against all HVC genotypes. It is only available as a fixed-dose combination with the NS5B inhibitor sofosbuvir (described later).

NS5B protease inhibitors

NS5B is a key enzyme involved in post-translational processing, which is necessary for HCV replication. It is an RNA-dependent RNA polymerase that has an active site where nucleosides bind and at least four allosteric sites where non-nucleoside compound can bind. Because the enzyme is highly conserved across all HCV genotypes, NS5B inhibitors are effective drugs against all HCV genotypes.

Dasabuvir

Dasabuvir is the only non-nucleoside NS5B inhibitor that is currently approved for use. It is only administered in combination with ombitasvir, paritaprevir and ritonavir (described earlier). As a class, non-nucleoside NS5B inhibitors are less potent and more genotype-specific compared with nucleotide NS5B inhibitors. They also have a low to moderate barrier to resistance and variable toxicity profiles. Consequently, non-nucleoside NS5B inhibitors have only been studied as adjuncts to more potent drugs that have a higher barrier to resistance.

Sofosbuvir

Sofosbuvir (Drug Monograph 37.2) is a nucleotide NS5B inhibitor that is activated in the liver through a series of phosphorylation steps to a nucleoside triphosphate. Once activated, sofosbuvir triphosphate competitively inhibits the active site of HS5B causing chain termination during RNA replication of the viral genome.

NS5B PIs have moderate to high efficacy across all HCV genotypes and a very high barrier to resistance. However, this class has been plagued by unacceptable toxicity, with a number of drugs, including the non-nucleoside inhibitors deleobuvir and filibuvir, failing during late clinical development.

Ribavirin aerosol

Ribavirin is a virustatic drug that rapidly penetrates virus-infected cells and is believed to reduce intracellular guanosine triphosphate storage. It inhibits viral RNA and protein synthesis, thus inhibiting viral duplication and spread to other cells. Ribavirin is also indicated for serious viral pneumonia caused by RSV in children under 2 years of age.

After oral inhalation, ribavirin is well absorbed and rapidly distributed to plasma, respiratory tract secretions and erythrocytes. Its half-life is 9.5 hours after oral inhalation and around 40 days in erythrocytes. Ribavirin is metabolised in the liver to a triazole carboxamide, and both ribavirin and the metabolite are excreted primarily by the kidneys. Adverse reactions are uncommon and can

Drug Monograph 37.2
Sofosbuvir

Sofosbuvir is activated in the liver to a nucleoside triphosphate. Sofosbuvir triphosphate competitively inhibits the active site of the HS5B RNA-dependent RNA polymerase enzyme, causing chain termination during replication of the viral genome.

Indications

Sofosbuvir is used for treating chronic genotype 1, 2, 3 or 4 HCV as a component of a combination antiviral treatment regimen.

Pharmacokinetics

Sofosbuvir is well absorbed and rapidly converted to its active metabolite. Sofosbuvir is more than 80% eliminated by renal clearance, with the remainder excreted in the faeces, in both cases mainly as an inactive metabolite. No dose adjustment is required for people with mild or moderate renal dysfunction, although sofosbuvir exposure is increased in people with severe renal dysfunction, including those on dialysis.

Drug interactions

As sofosbuvir is a substrate for p-glycoprotein, drugs that induce this transporter may decrease sofosbuvir exposure. Caution is advised against co-administration of carbamazepine, oxcarbazepine, phenytoin, phenobarbitone (phenobarbital), rifampicin (ripampin), rifabutin, rifapentine, St John's wort or tipranavir/ritonavir.

Adverse reactions

Sofosbuvir is well tolerated with no major adverse effects. When used in combination with ribavirin, the most commonly reported adverse effects of sofosbuvir are anaemia, fatigue, headache, insomnia and nausea.

Dosage and administration

Sofosbuvir is orally administered as a single 400 mg tablet once daily with or without food. Sofosbuvir should always be used in combination with ribavirin or peginterferon and ribavirin, and the dose of sofosbuvir should never be decreased. For regimen-specific dosage recommendations, consult current drug information sources.

include skin rash or irritation (inhalation product), CNS effects (insomnia, headache and lethargy) with IV and oral dosages and gastric distress (anorexia and nausea) and anaemia (usually with higher doses). Health professionals or providers should use caution in administering this medication, as headache, itching, swelling and red eyes have been reported.

Treating coronavirus

Coronaviridae viruses are a family of enveloped, single-stranded positive-sense RNA viruses. They are grouped into four genera (alpha-, beta-, gamma- and delta-) that mainly infect birds and mammals, including humans. There are seven coronaviruses that are known to infect humans, and these are members of the alpha- and beta-genera. The emergence of the severe acute respiratory syndrome coronavirus 2 (SARS-CoV-2) in 2019 and resulting international pandemic (COVID-19) has resulted in an explosion in development of novel drugs and testing of existing antivirals to combat this virus. As of the start of 2021, there are more than 500 therapeutic candidates being investigated to reduce the severity of COVID-19, with more than 400 of these in human clinical trials (Hartenian et al. 2020). This includes some existing drugs but also a number of novel drugs that have been developed explicitly to treat COVID-19.

Repurposing existing drugs

Antiviral drugs including α-interferon, arabinol, chloroquine, hydroxychloroquine, lopinavir, remdesivir, ritonavir and anti-inflammatory drug regimens have been tested for their efficacy against COVID-19 in large-scale international randomised clinical trials. Unfortunately to date the results of these trials have consistently demonstrated that these existing antiviral drug regimens had little or no benefit in hospitalised people with COVID-19.

Novel drugs to treat coronavirus

Several novel monoclonal antibodies that target the coronavirus spike protein have been rapidly developed and received accelerated regulatory authorisation for treating COVID-19.

Bamlanivimab/etesevimab

Bamlanivimab and etesevimab are two investigational monoclonal antibodies that target the surface spike protein of SARS-CoV-2. These drugs are administered as a combination via IV infusion. This combination is authorised in the United States for treating mild-to-moderate COVID-19 in people 12 years or older. This drug is not currently authorised for use in Australia.

Sotrovimab

Sotrovimab is an investigational monoclonal antibody that targets the surface spike protein of SARS-CoV-2. In

May 2021 the FDA and European Medicines Agency (EMA) authorised the use of sotrovimab to treat mild-to-moderate COVID-19 in people 12 years or older. Sotrovimab was granted provisional approval by the Therapeutic Goods Administration (TGA) for treating COVID-19 in Australia, making it the first approved drug for treating COVID-19 in this country.

Tixagevimab/cilgavimab

Tixagevimab and cilgavimab are two investigational human monoclonal antibodies that target the surface spike protein of SARS-CoV-2. In October 2021 the EMA initiated a review of this combination. This combination has not currently received authorisation for treating COVID-19 by any regulatory agency.

Molnupiravir

Molnupiravir is a prodrug for the synthetic nucleoside N-hydroxycytidine, which is incorporated into viral RNA and causes copy errors during viral RNA replication. This results in the inhibition of SARS-CoV-2 replication. Molnupiravir is approved for treating COVID-19 in Australia for patients who are at risk of progressing to severe COVID-19.

Nirmatrelvir/ritonavir

Unlike most other treatments for SARS-CoV-2, nirmatrelvir is not a monoclonal antibody. This drug is an orally active 3C-like protease inhibitor. In November 2021 nirmatrelvir was licensed and approvedto treat COVID-19 in combination with ritonavir in 95 countries. As this combination contains ritonavir (a pharmacological booster that works by inhibiting CYP3A4), this product has a high drug interaction liability.

KEY POINTS

Antiviral drugs

- Chemotherapy for viral diseases has tended to be more limited than chemotherapy for bacterial diseases because the development and clinical application of antiviral drugs is more difficult.
- Antiviral drugs are primarily used prophylactically to prevent the onset of infection.
- Antiviral drugs discussed in this chapter are used to treat HBV and HCV, HSV, influenza virus and RSV.
- DAAs used to treat HCV have revolutionised the treatment of this virus, but at a high financial cost.
- To minimise the risk of resistance, drugs used to treat HCV are typically used in combinations.

Treating human immunodeficiency virus

HIV was discovered in 1983, and in 2015 was estimated to infect approximately 36.7 million people worldwide. Approximately 35 million people have died since the epidemic started. Since 1983 the development of antiviral drugs to combat HIV has continued at a furious pace because of the problem of HIV-resistant strains. Vaccines have always been used to control viral infections, but the prospect of an effective vaccine against HIV is still very remote.

There are two main families of HIV: HIV-1 and HIV-2. The latter predominates in Western Africa and is closely related to the simian immunodeficiency virus. The following drugs are used to treat HIV:

- nucleoside reverse transcriptase inhibitors (NRTIs): abacavir, didanosine, emtricitabine, lamivudine, stavudine, tenofovir, zidovudine, lopinavir
- non-nucleoside reverse transcriptase inhibitors (NNRTIs): efavirenz, etravirine, nevirapine, rilpivirine
- protease inhibitors: atazanavir, darunavir, fosamprenavir, indinavir, lopinavir with ritonavir, ritonavir, saquinavir, tipranavir
- other antiretrovirals: enfuvirtide, maraviroc, raltegravir.

Nucleoside reverse transcriptase inhibitors

All these drugs are nucleoside analogues with the exception of tenofovir, which is a nucleotide analogue. They are indicated for treating HIV infection (in adults and children) in combination with other retroviral drugs, for prophylaxis during pregnancy to prevent transmission to the fetus and for prophylaxis post-exposure to HIV. NRTIs are used in combination therapy with NNRTIs and PIs in people infected with HIV. The most effective regimens continue to be combinations of three or more drugs that include at least two different classes of antiretrovirals. Unfortunately, the problems faced in treating HIV continue to be rebound viral replication, development of resistance and inadequate drug potency.

All of these drugs are substrates for the viral reverse transcriptase enzyme (Fig 37.2), which converts viral RNA into proviral DNA before it becomes incorporated in the host cell chromosome. To do this, the drugs must first be phosphorylated in the cytoplasm to enable them to effectively compete with the normal host cell triphosphates. The phosphorylated drug, once incorporated in the growing viral DNA chain, causes chain termination. These drugs are thus effective only in susceptible cells but are ineffective in cells already infected with HIV.

Significant adverse reactions of the NRTIs include lipodystrophy (changes in cutaneous fat distribution: loss in the face, limbs and buttocks but accumulation in the

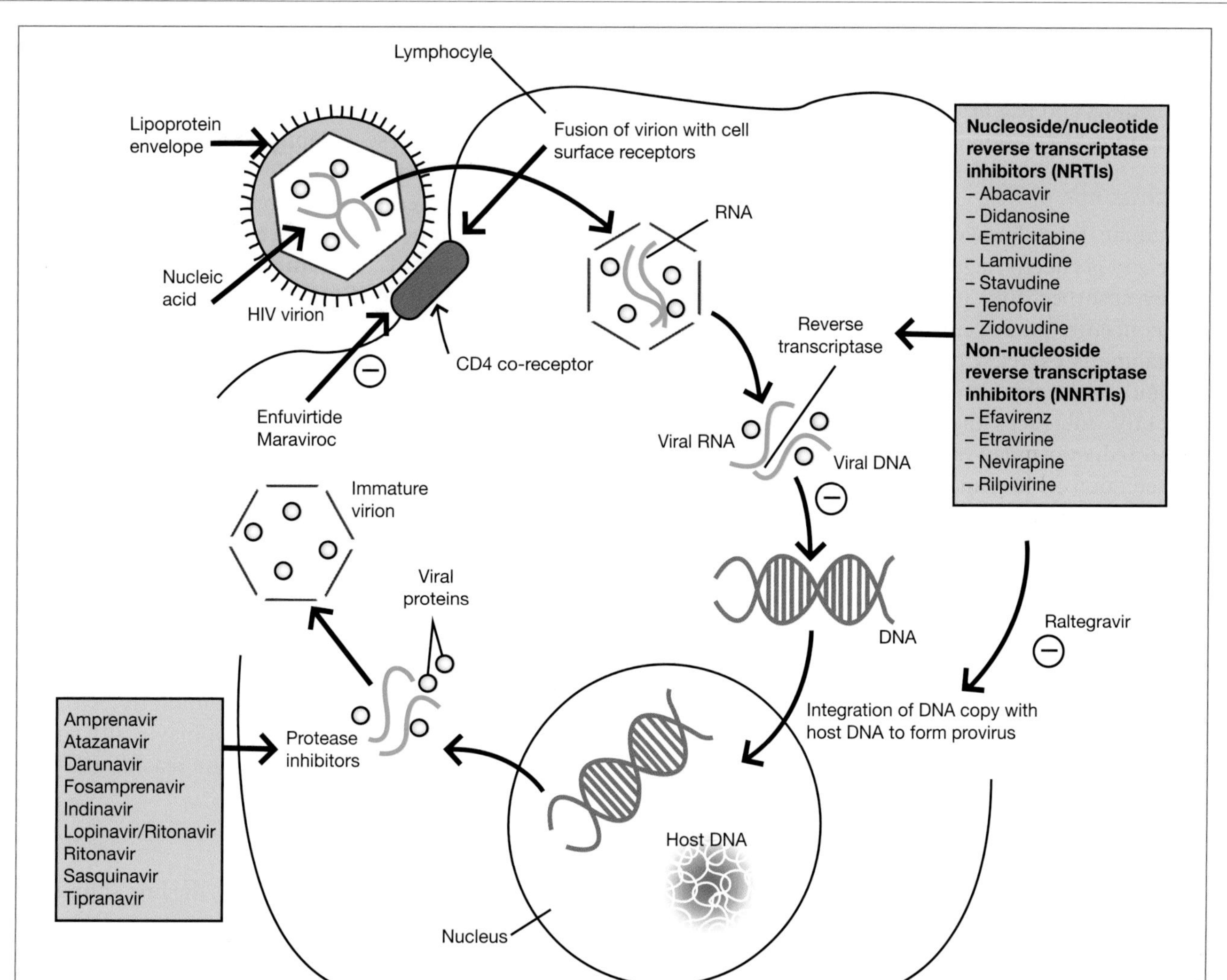

FIGURE 37.2 Inhibition sites for HIV replication
The HIV redundant genes are composed of RNA, which is translated to DNA by reverse transcriptase (RT) for viral reproduction. The RT inhibitors interfere with virus production at this site. When integrated DNA becomes part of the cell, the cell produces viral proteins requiring the protease enzyme for the production of new virions. The PIs block this enzyme to prevent the release of new viruses into the bloodstream. As a result, combination therapies can reduce the viral load of new HIV produced in the body.
(–) = inhibition.

abdominal, breast and dorsocervical region). Metabolic abnormalities may also occur, and these include insulin resistance and hyperlipidaemia. Many of the NRTIs are subject to numerous drug interactions, and current drug information sources should be consulted before starting therapy.

Abacavir

Abacavir, a guanosine analogue (also known as ABC), is selective against HIV-1 and HIV-2 and is indicated for treating HIV infection. It is administered orally; bioavailability is about 83%; the half-life is 1.5 hours; and the drug is widely distributed, including good penetration of the CSF. Abacavir is extensively metabolised in the liver by alcohol dehydrogenase to the 5'-carboxylic acid and by glucuronidation forming the 5'-glucuronide. Less than 2% is excreted as unchanged drug in urine.

Adverse reactions include a hypersensitivity reaction in at least 5% of people within 6 weeks. The severity of this reaction is such that the drug should be stopped immediately and never reintroduced as therapy, as fatalities have occurred on rechallenge.

Didanosine

Didanosine (also known as DDI) is converted intracellularly to its active form, DDA-triphosphate, which inhibits HIV DNA reverse transcriptase. Inhibition suppresses HIV replication. This product, which is available in oral dosage forms, is acid-labile. The oral

formulations are buffered to increase gastric pH to protect didanosine from gastric acid destruction. Didanosine crosses the blood–brain barrier, has a half-life of 1.5 hours in adults and reaches peak plasma concentration in 30–60 minutes. Excretion is primarily via the kidneys.

Emtricitabine

Emtricitabine (also known as FTC) is an analogue of cytosine and is effective against HIV-1, HIV-2 and HBV. It is rapidly absorbed after oral administration, with peak plasma concentrations occurring at 1–2 hours post-dose. Emtricitabine is excreted predominantly by the kidneys (86%) and in faeces (14%). Hence, renal impairment significantly influences the plasma drug concentration, and dose reduction may be necessary. The potential for drug interactions is low, and no clinically significant drug interactions have been noted with indinavir, zidovudine, stavudine or famciclovir.

Lamivudine

Lamivudine (also known as 3TC) is converted in the body to an active metabolite, lamivudine triphosphate (L-TP), which inhibits HIV (and HBV) reverse transcription by terminating the viral DNA chain. It also inhibits RNA- and DNA-dependent DNA polymerase functions of reverse transcriptase. Synergism of antiviral activity is achieved with a combination dosage form containing 150 mg lamivudine and 300 mg zidovudine.

Rapidly absorbed after oral administration, lamivudine reaches peak plasma concentration in 1 hour (fasting state) or 3.2 hours (with food). L-TP has an intracellular half-life of 10–15 hours and is excreted unchanged by the kidneys. The potential for drug interactions exists with IV pentamidine, which increases the risk of pancreatitis, and trimethoprim, which competes with lamivudine for renal excretion. This latter combination can result in increased lamivudine concentration, and the combination should be avoided in people with renal impairment. Use lamivudine with caution in people with pancreatitis or peripheral neuropathy, including people with a history of these conditions, and in diabetics, as 5 mL of oral solution contains 1 g sucrose.

Stavudine

Stavudine (also known as D4T) is converted to stavudine triphosphate, which competes with deoxythymidine triphosphate, resulting in inhibition of HIV replication and DNA synthesis. Oral stavudine is rapidly absorbed and reaches peak plasma concentration in 0.5–1.5 hours. It has a half-life of 1–1.6 hours and is excreted unchanged, primarily by the kidneys.

When administered with drugs that cause peripheral neuropathy, such as chloramphenicol, cisplatin, dapsone, didanosine, hydralazine, isoniazid, lithium, metronidazole, nitrofurantoin, phenytoin or vincristine, stavudine can cause peripheral neuropathy; whenever possible, avoid combination with other drugs that can cause peripheral neuropathy. When administered with ganciclovir or pentamidine (IV), stavudine increases the risk of pancreatitis, so these combinations should be avoided. Adverse reactions include dose-related peripheral neuropathy, increased liver enzymes and anaemia. Use with caution in people with liver function impairment or alcoholism. Avoid use in people with peripheral neuropathy or kidney function impairment.

Tenofovir

Tenofovir disoproxil fumarate is a prodrug that is converted to tenofovir, an analogue of the nucleotide adenosine. Similar to the NRTIs, tenofovir competitively inhibits the HIV reverse transcriptase and causes chain termination after its incorporation in DNA. Currently, it is indicated for use in combination with other antiretrovirals. Administered orally, the bioavailability of tenofovir is enhanced if taken with a high-fat meal. Tenofovir is excreted predominantly by the kidneys (70–80%) and can cause nephrotoxicity, which may be exacerbated if administered concomitantly with other nephrotoxic drugs. (For example, lopinavir with ritonavir increases tenofovir concentration, increasing the risk of nephrotoxicity.)

Zidovudine

Zidovudine (also known as AZT) was the first antiretroviral drug developed to target HIV infection. It was first used in 1987, and by the early 1990s it was evident that zidovudine slowed the rate of progression of AIDS. Survival rates, however, did not improve and it became apparent that resistant HIV strains had developed. By 1996, the use of combination therapy had emerged, with better results in retarding disease progression and decreasing mortality.

Zidovudine is an antiviral agent (virustatic) that intracellularly is converted by cellular enzymes to monophosphate, diphosphate and then to zidovudine triphosphate. The triphosphate form competitively inhibits the reverse transcriptase with respect to the incorporation of natural thymidine triphosphate in growing chains of viral DNA, thus inhibiting viral replication. It has a greater affinity for retroviral reverse transcriptase than for the human α-DNA polymerase; thus, it selectively inhibits viral replication.

Non-nucleoside reverse transcriptase inhibitors

Efavirenz, etravirine, nevirapine and rilpivirine are NNRTIs. These drugs block RNA-dependent and DNA-dependent DNA polymerases (Fig 37.2) and have antiviral activity against HIV-1, but not HIV-2. They are usually combined with two or more other drugs to suppress HIV viral replication because use as sole agents results in rapid emergence of viral resistance (can occur within 1 week). Many interactions occur with these drugs because of the involvement of specific CYP enzymes. Relevant drug information sources should be consulted for specific drug interactions, as some are life-threatening.

Efavirenz

Efavirenz (Drug Monograph 37.3) is used in combination with tenofovir and emtricitabine as one of the preferred NNRTI-based antiretroviral regimens for treating HIV. In combination with other antiretroviral agents, efavirenz is also used as post-exposure prophylaxis to reduce the risk of HIV infection in people exposed to a significant risk (e.g. needle stick).

Metabolism of efavirenz is complex, as this drug both induces its own metabolism and inhibits the metabolism of other drugs by hepatic CYP enzymes. Involvement of CYP3A4 in the metabolism of efavirenz increases the likelihood of drug interactions. The half-life is 40–55 hours, and less than 1% appears in urine as unchanged drug. Many drug interactions occur, and current information sources should be consulted.

Etravirine

Etravirine (also known as ETR and TMC125) is active against HIV-1 and is unique in that it is effective when mutations in the reverse transcriptase enzyme have developed that confer resistance to other NNRTIs. Metabolism-forming methyl- and dimethyl-hydroxylated metabolite is mediated by CYP3A4, CYP2C9 and CYP2C19, and virtually no unchanged drug is excreted in urine. As would be expected, etravirine is subject to multiple drug interactions. A rash may occur in the first few weeks of treatment and, if severe, liver function tests should be undertaken and the drug stopped immediately.

Nevirapine

Administered orally, nevirapine is well absorbed. Nevirapine is metabolised in the liver and is also an inducer of hepatic CYPs; thus, auto induction, or an increased clearance and a decrease in drug half-life, occurs within 2–4 weeks of therapy.

Adverse reactions include nausea, headache, diarrhoea, fever, hepatitis, ulcerative stomatitis and life-threatening skin reactions such as Stevens-Johnson syndrome. Nevirapine should be discontinued in people who develop a severe rash or a rash accompanied by symptoms such as fever, myalgia, fatigue, oral lesions and conjunctivitis.

Rilpivirine

Rilpivirine (also known as RPV and TMC278) is a diarylpyrimidine NNRTI effective against HIV-1. Administered orally, the absorption of rilpivirine is improved when taken with food or a high-fat meal, but

Drug Monograph 38.3
Efavirenz

Efavirenz is an NNRTI that blocks RNA- and DNA-dependent DNA polymerases, giving it antiviral activity against HIV-1, but not HIV-2.

Indications

Efavirenz is used in combination with other antiretroviral drugs for treating HIV-1 infection.

Pharmacokinetics

Under fasting conditions, efavirenz has a bioavailability of approximately 45%. It is extensively (> 99.5%) protein-bound and is primarily cleared by CYP2B6- and CYP3A4-mediated hepatic metabolism. When administered orally, efavirenz has an onset of action of 3–5 hours and a half-life of 40–55 hours. It is approximately two-thirds excreted in the faeces and one-third excreted in the urine.

Drug interactions

Co-administration of efavirenz can alter the concentrations of other drugs, and other drugs may alter the concentrations of efavirenz. The potential for drug–drug interactions must be considered before commencing and during therapy. Consult up-to-date drug information sources.

Adverse reactions

The most common adverse reactions associated with the use of efavirenz (> 5%, moderate–severe) are dizziness, fatigue, headache, insomnia, nausea, rash and vomiting.

Dosage and administration

Efavirenz is orally administered and should be taken once daily on an empty stomach, preferably at bedtime. The recommended initial adult dose is 600 mg. Therapeutic drug monitoring can be used to tailor dosing to optimise therapy once steady state has been achieved. Efavirenz is available as 200 and 600 mg tablets.

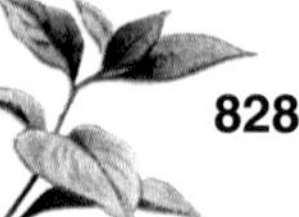

absolute bioavailability is unknown because of the lack of an IV formulation. The half-life of the drug is in the order of 50 hours. Rilpivirine is metabolised by CYP3A4, and to a lesser extent by CYP1A2 and CYP2C19, with 85% of the drug excreted in faeces of which 25% is unchanged drug. Minimal excretion occurs via urine (~6%), with less than 1% as unchanged drug. Potent inducers of CYP3A4 will decrease the plasma concentration of rilpivirine and reduce efficacy.

Protease inhibitors

The HIV protease, which is essential for viral infectivity, cleaves the viral precursor polypeptide into active viral enzymes and structural proteins. PIs prevent the protease from cleaving the polypeptide and hence block the subsequent maturation of the virus (Fig 37.2). PIs used to treat HIV include atazanavir, darunavir, fosamprenavir, indinavir, lopinavir, ritonavir, saquinavir and tipranavir. These drugs are the most potent antiviral agents available and have suppressed viral replication for up to a year in clinical trials. Administering them in combination therapies has decreased viral loads and increased CD4 counts. Various combinations of these agents and their effects on HIV infection and AIDS complications and disease progression are continually under investigation.

Adverse reactions are common and include headache, diarrhoea, nausea, vomiting, elevated liver enzymes and a variety of metabolic disorders (e.g. diabetes, hypertriglyceridaemia and hypercholesterolaemia). Like many of the other antiretroviral drugs, PIs are subject to multiple drug interactions and, in particular, their use is contraindicated with ergot alkaloids, midazolam and triazolam. Comparative data for atazanavir, darunavir and ritonavir are shown in Table 37.3.

Indinavir

Indinavir affects the replication cycle of HIV. It is active both in acute infection and in chronically infected cells, which are generally not affected by the nucleoside analogue reverse transcriptase inhibitors such as didanosine, lamivudine, stavudine and zidovudine. Thus, this drug has a virustatic effect.

Administered orally, indinavir reaches peak plasma concentration in about 1 hour. It is extensively metabolised in the liver by CYP3A4 and to a lesser extent by CYP2D6. The drug is primarily recovered in faeces as metabolites (~75%) and unchanged drug about 10%. The half-life of indinavir is about 2 hours, and co-administration with ritonavir or itraconazole potent inhibitors of CYP3A4 prolongs the half-life of indinavir significantly.

Lopinavir with ritonavir

Lopinavir is an inhibitor of HIV-1 and HIV-2 proteases, while ritonavir, which is also a PI, is an inhibitor of the lopinavir metabolism by CYP3A. The combination is formulated as soft capsules and as an oral liquid, and enhanced bioavailability occurs when both formulations are taken with food. Lopinavir is metabolised by hepatic CYP3A, and after multiple dosing less than 3% is excreted as unchanged drug in urine. Ritonavir is also metabolised by CYP3A and, although this was initially viewed as undesirable, it was later realised that this inhibitory action could be useful in allowing a lower dose of a PI to be given.

Drug interactions are to some extent predictable, and include rifampicin, corticosteroids, statins, St John's wort, azole antifungals, methadone, efavirenz and nevirapine. Adverse reactions include exacerbation of diabetes mellitus, increased bleeding, lipodystrophy, hyperlipidaemia and, rarely, pancreatitis.

Saquinavir

Administered orally, saquinavir undergoes extensive first-pass metabolism, is highly protein-bound and is metabolised in the liver by CYP3A4. Both saquinavir and its metabolites are excreted primarily in the faeces (> 95%), with minimal excretion (< 3%) via urine.

Adverse reactions are usually mild and include diarrhoea, abdominal distress, headache, weakness and, rarely, paraesthesia, skin rash, confusion, ataxia, Stevens-Johnson syndrome, seizures, thrombocytopenia, anaemia

TABLE 37.3 Comparative information on protease inhibitors

DRUG	HALF-LIFE (H)	METABOLISM	EXCRETION	ADVERSE REACTIONS
Atazanavir	6.5	Hepatic (CYP3A4)	Faecal and renal	Abdominal pain, depression, dizziness, fatigue, GIT disturbance, heart block, hyperbilirubinaemia, insomnia, rash, worsening cough
Darunavir	15	Hepatic (CYP3A4)	Faecal and renal	Hepatitis, decreased white cell count, hyperbilirubinaemia, rash
Ritonavir	3–5	Hepatic (CYP3A4)	Faecal	Abdominal pain, asthenia, diarrhoea, dizziness, insomnia, malaise, metabolic disturbance, nausea and vomiting, sweating, taste abnormality

and hepatotoxicity. Dosage reduction may be required in people with hepatic dysfunction.

Tipranavir

Tipranavir is a novel non-peptide PI that is used under specialist care in highly treatment-experienced people with HIV virus resistant to multiple PIs. Metabolised by CYP3A4, tipranavir is administered with low-dose ritonavir, which inhibits CYP3A4 and the intestinal P-gp efflux pump in order to achieve a therapeutic plasma concentration. Administration is contraindicated in the presence of moderate or severe hepatic impairment. Adverse effects include fatigue, myalgia and rash.

Other antiretroviral drugs

Enfuvirtide

Enfuvirtide is a novel antiretroviral drug termed a fusion (HIV entry) inhibitor. It is a synthetic 36-amino-acid peptide that binds to the gp41 sub-unit of a glycoprotein found in the viral envelope. This blocks viral fusion with the CD4 receptor of the host cell and prevents the conformational changes required to allow fusion. Currently, this drug is indicated for HIV-1 infection in people where other treatments have failed.

It is administered subcutaneously and, because it is a peptide, it is likely that it is catabolised to its constituent amino acids. Adverse reactions are common and include injection site reactions (e.g. pain, erythema, itch), which result in discontinuation in about 3% of people, peripheral neuropathy, insomnia, depression, respiratory symptoms (e.g. cough, dyspnoea) and loss of weight and appetite.

Maraviroc

It is essential for HIV to bind to the host cell in order to enter and then replicate and release new virions. Human $CD4^+$ cells express chemokine receptors CCR5 and CXCR4. Maraviroc competitively and selectively binds to CCR5, blocking the interaction between the HIV glycoprotein gp120 and CCR5. gp120 is responsible for exposing co-receptor binding sites that then bind to CCR5 and CXCR4 on the membrane of the host cell. Maraviroc is a substrate of CYP3A4 and P-gp, and hence it is susceptible to multiple drug interactions.

Administered orally, common adverse reactions include gastrointestinal toxicity (e.g. abdominal pain, constipation), rash, bronchospasm, infections and neurological symptoms (e.g. myalgia, muscle spasms, paraesthesia, dysaesthesia and disturbed sleep).

Raltegravir

Raltegravir is an HIV integrase inhibitor that inhibits the strand transfer reaction, which is essential for integration of the viral DNA into the host DNA, and hence its viral expression and replication. It is indicated for treating multi-drug-resistant HIV infection in people whose current therapy is failing. Raltegravir is rapidly absorbed and is metabolised principally by UGT1A1 to raltegravir glucuronide, which is excreted in faeces (51%) and urine (32%). Clinical data are currently limited and specialist sources of drug information should be consulted.

KEY POINTS

Antiretroviral drugs

- Antiretroviral drugs are mainly used to treat HIV and AIDS.
- These drugs include entry inhibitors, fusion inhibitors, integrase inhibitors, nucleoside and non-nucleoside reverse transcriptase inhibitors, reverse transcriptase inhibitors and protease inhibitors.
- Treating HIV typically involves a combination of drugs from different classes.

DRUGS AT A GLANCE

PHARMACOLOGICAL GROUP AND EFFECT	KEY EXAMPLES	CLINICAL USE
Azole antifungals	Fluconazole	Vulvovaginal candidiasis
	Itraconazole	Onychomycosis
	Miconazole	Fungal skin infections
	Posaconazole	Serious fungal infections
	Voriconazole	Invasive aspergillosis
Echinocandins	Anidulafungin	Invasive candidiasis
	Caspofungin	Oesophageal candidiasis

Other antifungals	Amphotericin B	Oral and perioral candidiasis
	Flucytosine	Cryptococcal infections
	Griseofulvin	Dermatophyte infection
	Nystatin	Oropharyngeal candidiasis
	Terbinafine	Onychomycosis
DNA polymerase inhibitors	Aciclovir	Herpes simplex infections
	Cidofovir	CMV retinitis in AIDS
	Famciclovir	Shingles
	Foscarnet	Aciclovir-resistant herpes simplex in HIV
	Ganciclovir	Sight-threatening CMV retinitis
	Valaciclovir	Herpes simplex infections
	Valganciclovir	Prevention of CMV disease after solid organ transplantation
Neuraminidase inhibitors	Oseltamivir	Influenza A and B
	Zanamivir	Influenza A and B
NS3/4A protease inhibitors	Grazoprevir	Not used in Australia
	Paritaprevir	Not used in Australia
	Simeprevir	Not used in Australia
NS5A inhibitors	Daclatasvir	Not used in Australia
	Elbasvir	Not used in Australia
	Ledipasvir	Chronic HCV
	Ombitasvir	Not used in Australia
	Velpatasvir	Chronic HCV
NS5B RNA-dependent RNA protease inhibitors	Dasabuvir	Not used in Australia
	Sofosbuvir	Chronic HCV
Other antiviral drugs	Adefovir	Chronic HBV
	Amantadine	Prevention of influenza type A
	Entecavir	Chronic HBV
	Ribavirin	Chronic hepatitis C
	Telbivudine	Not used in Australia
Nucleoside reverse transcriptase inhibitors (NRTIs)	Abacavir	HIV infection
	Didanosine	Not used in Australia
	Emtricitabine	HIV infection
	Lamivudine	HIV infection
	Stavudine	Not used in Australia
	Tenofovir	HIV infection
	Zidovudine	HIV infection
Non-nucleoside reverse transcriptase inhibitors (NNRTIs)	Efavirenz	HIV infection
	Etravirine	HIV infection
	Nevirapine	HIV infection
	Rilpivirine	HIV infection
Protease inhibitors	Atazanavir	HIV infection
	Darunavir	HIV infection
	Fosamprenavir	HIV infection
	Indinavir	Not used in Australia
	Lopinavir	HIV infection
	Ritonavir	HIV infection
	Saquinavir	HIV infection
	Tipranavir	HIV infection
Entry inhibitors	Enfuvirtide	HIV infection
	Maraviroc	HIV infection
Integrase inhibitor	Raltegravir	HIV infection

REVIEW EXERCISES

1. Mr SM is diagnosed with HSV and started on a course of aciclovir. What is the action of aciclovir in treating HSV? What are the primary drug interactions, adverse reactions and contraindications that a health professional should be aware of when using this drug?
2. Six weeks ago, Mrs KF was diagnosed with HCV and commenced on a course of ledipasvir and sofosbuvir. Initially, she appeared to be tolerating the combination well, but in the past week she has noticed that she has lost her appetite and has been feeling constantly sick. Her partner has also noticed that during this time her skin has developed a yellowish tint. Are these symptoms likely to relate to the drug? What tests and patient history might be useful to work out what is happening?
3. Mr VB has been prescribed saquinavir, in combination with ritonavir, for treating HIV. He asks you to explain to him why he has to have the ritonavir as well. Why is it absolutely necessary that he take both drugs? What could the clinical consequences be if he fails to take the ritonavir?

REFERENCES

Australian Medicines Handbook P/L, Australian medicines handbook 2021, Adelaide, 2021, AMH.

Hartenian E, Nandakumar D, Lari A, et al: The molecular virology of coronaviruses. Journal of Biological Chemistry 295: 12910–12934, 2020.

Liu J, Lin S, Wang L, et al: Comparison of antiviral agents for seasonal influenza outcomes in healthy adults and children: a systematic review and network meta-analysis. JAMA Network Open 4: e2119151, 2021.

Portugal MEG, Raboni SM; Antiviral drug review: a guide to clinicians. Revista de Biologia Tropical / International Journal of Tropical Biology and Conservation 46: 1–21, 2017.

Zhang J, Nguyen D, Ke-Qin Hu KQ: Chronic hepatitis C virus infection: a review of current direct-acting antiviral treatment strategies. North American Journal of Medical Sciences 9: 47–54, 2016.

CHAPTER 38

ANTIPROTOZOAL, ANTIMYCOBACTERIAL AND ANTHELMINTIC DRUGS

Andrew Rowland

KEY ABBREVIATIONS

MAC Mycobacterium avium complex
TB tuberculosis

KEY TERMS

Chapter Focus

Knowledge of the various drugs available alone and in combination to treat malaria, tuberculosis, leprosy, amoebiasis and helminthiasis is vital information for health professionals. This chapter reviews the drugs used to treat protozoal diseases such as malaria and amoebiasis, mycobacterial infections such as Mycobacterium avium complex, tuberculosis and leprosy and helminth infections. These diseases are prevalent throughout the world. Their control peaks and wanes, often due to factors such as availability of drugs, patient compliance with specific drug therapies and the development of drug-resistant strains. Control of these infections is important and challenging to health professionals, and in some instances a global approach has been adopted.

KEY DRUG GROUPS

Amoebicidal drug:

- Paromomycin

Anthelmintic drugs:

- Albendazole, ivermectin, mebendazole, praziquantel, pyrantel

Antimalarial drugs:

- Artemether with lumefantrine, atovaquone with proguanil, mefloquine, primaquine, quinine

Antimycobacterial drugs:

- Capreomycin, clofazimine, cycloserine, dapsone, ethambutol, **isoniazid** (Drug Monograph 38.2), pyrazinamide, rifabutin, **rifampicin**, streptomycin

Other antiprotozoal drugs:

- **Metronidazole**, pentamidine, pyrimethamine

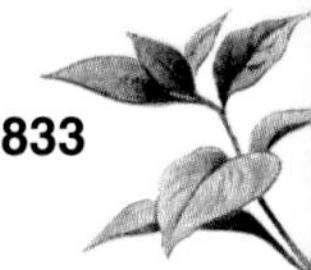

CRITICAL THINKING SCENARIO

Vivian, a 47-year-old mum, has recently returned from a family holiday to South America. Before leaving for the holiday, Vivian's GP had advised her to take a course of malaria prophylaxis. Despite filling the prescription Vivian became busy in the days prior to leaving and forgot to take the tablets. Vivian became ill while on holiday and upon returning to Australia has been diagnosed with malaria. What are your considerations for Vivian's treatment?

Protozoal infections

Malaria

In 2020 there were an estimated 242 million cases of **malaria** worldwide, resulting in 627,000 deaths. Malaria remains a prominent cause of mortality, particularly in sub-Saharan Africa, Southeast Asia, Latin America and the Middle East. While the incidence has been gradually decreasing since 2010, incidence of malaria spiked in these countries in 2020–21. The global incidence grew by 5%, and malaria mortality rates increased by 12% compared with 2019 (WHO 2021a). In Australia, malaria has largely been eradicated on the mainland, with only occasional cases in the Torres Strait Islands, although there are approximately 500 notifications of overseas-acquired malaria annually.

Plasmodium vivax (*P. vivax*) is the most common form of malaria; this infestation is usually mild, drug resistance is uncommon and it can easily be treated with antimalarial medications. The *P. falciparum* strain of malaria is less common but much more severe than the *P. vivax* form. Drug-resistant strains of *P. falciparum* exist, and the symptoms with this infestation occur at irregular intervals and can cause very serious complications. If untreated or if treatment is delayed, the disease may progress to irreversible cardiovascular shock and death.

Life cycle of the malarial parasite

To understand the treatment of malaria, it is essential to review the life cycle of the malarial parasite, the plasmodium. Figure 38.1 presents the cycle.

When a malaria-infected female Anopheles mosquito feeds, she inoculates sporozoites into a human host. When sporozoites are introduced into the systemic circulation of a human, they infect liver cells and mature into schizonts, which rupture and release merozoites (the exo-erythrocytic phase). Drugs affecting malarial parasites in the systemic circulation do not always destroy those in the exo-erythrocytic phase. After this initial replication in the liver, when merozoites are released into the blood, they infect erythrocytes (Fig 38.2) and multiply asexually (erythrocytic phase). During this phase, some parasites differentiate into male and female gametocytes (sexual forms of the parasite). Parasites in the blood are responsible for the clinical manifestations of malaria.

When a female Anopheles mosquito feeds on an infected host, she draws blood containing male and female gametocytes. In the stomach of the mosquito, the female gametocytes are fertilised by the male gametocytes to form zygotes, which undergo numerous cell divisions to develop into sporozoites. The formation of sporozoites in the mosquito completes the sexual cycle. Sporozoites then migrate to the salivary glands of the infected mosquito and are injected into the bloodstream of humans by the bite of the female insect.

Antimalarial drugs

The emergence of drug-resistant strains of malaria, particularly that caused by *P. falciparum*, poses a major public health problem throughout the world. Despite the combined efforts of many countries to eradicate malaria, it remains the most devastating infectious disease in the world because of the many lives lost and the economic burden it imposes. It is essential that travellers visiting areas where malaria is endemic be aware of the need to obtain information about measures for reducing exposure to the disease. Travellers should receive malaria chemoprophylaxis before entering these areas. Health professionals should refer people to current information, which can be obtained from several reputable sources, including:

- United States Centers for Disease Control and Prevention, Travellers Health yellow book website: https://wwwnc.cdc.gov/travel/page/yellowbook-home
- World Health Organization (WHO) travel advice website: https://www.who.int/travel-advice.

The choice of a drug for malaria prophylaxis or treatment is based on the particular malarial strain, especially drug-resistant strains of *P. falciparum*, and the

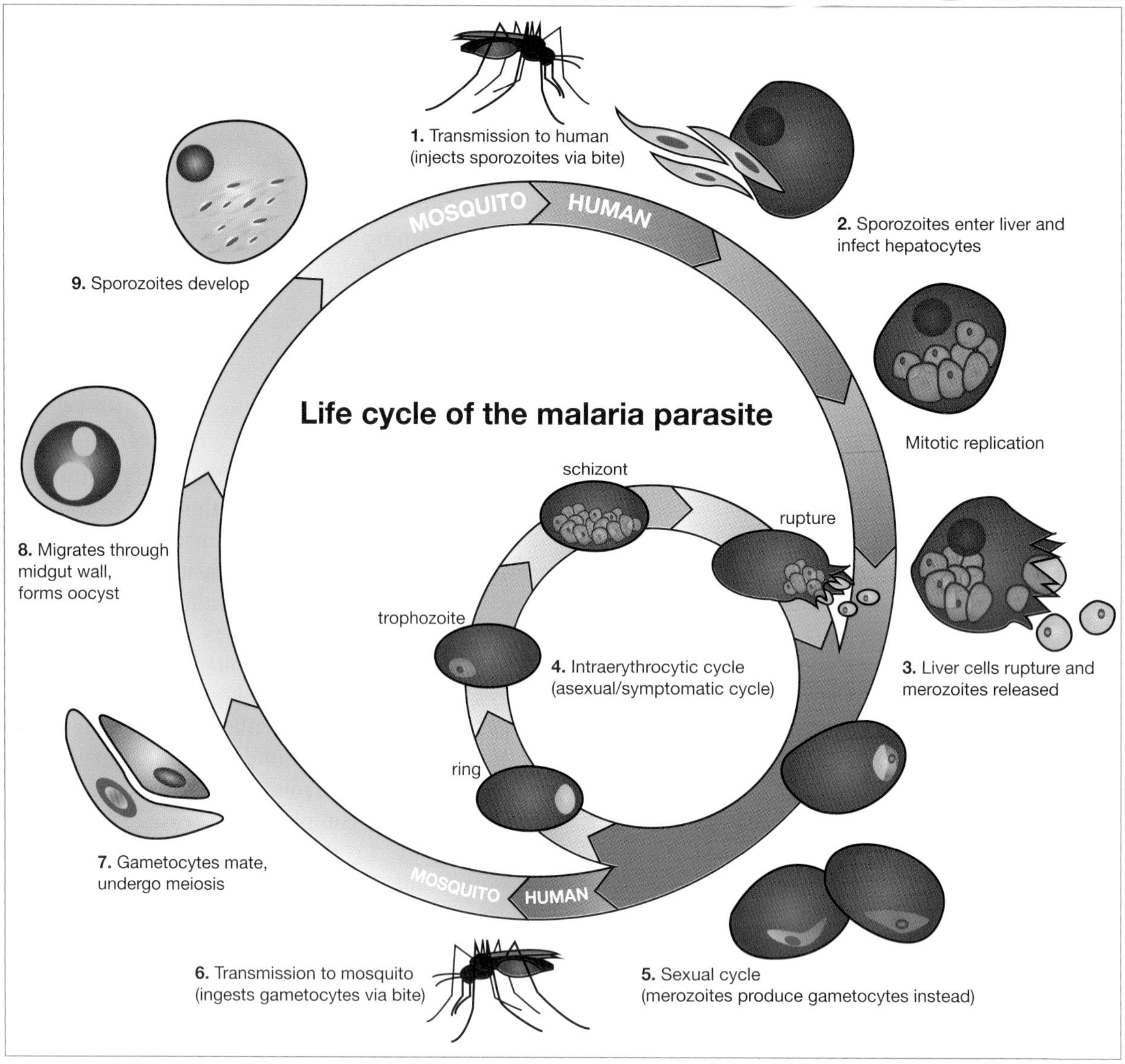

Life cycle of the malaria parasite

1. Transmission to human (injects sporozoites via bite)

2. Sporozoites enter liver and infect hepatocytes

Mitotic replication

3. Liver cells rupture and merozoites released

4. Intraerythrocytic cycle (asexual/symptomatic cycle)

schizont

rupture

trophozoite

ring

5. Sexual cycle (merozoites produce gametocytes instead)

6. Transmission to mosquito (ingests gametocytes via bite)

7. Gametocytes mate, undergo meiosis

8. Migrates through midgut wall, forms oocyst

9. Sporozoites develop

MOSQUITO

HUMAN

MOSQUITO

HUMAN

FIGURE 38.1 Life cycle of the malarial parasite

Source: Salerno 1999, Figure 53.1.

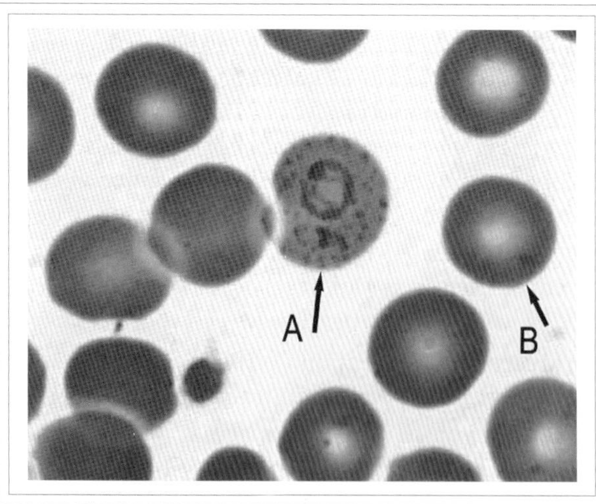

FIGURE 38.2 Peripheral blood film (magnification × 100) showing a normal red cell (B) and a red cell with a trophozoite of *P. vivax* displaying the typical signet ring form and Schüffner's stippling (A)

Source: Reproduced with kind permission of Ros Biebrick, Haematology, SA Pathology, Flinders Medical Centre, Adelaide.

stage of the plasmodium life cycle. Regimens are complex, and current health authorities and experts should be consulted and the risk of contracting the disease in a malarious area balanced against the potential efficacy and toxicity of the drug(s) to be used. These include a number of drugs such as doxycycline and clindamycin and those discussed below. Chloroquine prophylaxis is now used only in areas with chloroquine-susceptible malaria, such as Central America north of Panama. The drug should be commenced a week before entering the area and continued for 4 weeks after leaving it. Chloroquine is not marketed in Australia but may be available through the Special Access Scheme managed by the Therapeutic Goods Administration (TGA). If chloroquine is not available, hydroxychloroquine may be used as an alternative drug.

Mefloquine

Mefloquine prevents the replication of asexual erythrocytic parasites but has no effect on the gametocytes of *P. falciparum*. Its exact mechanism of action is unknown, but it is believed to inhibit protein synthesis (by binding plasmodial DNA), inhibit plasmodial haem polymerase and raise the intravascular pH of the acidic food vacuoles in the parasite. It is not effective in eliminating the exo-erythrocytic or intrahepatic stages of *P. vivax* or *P. ovale* infections.

Mefloquine is indicated for prophylaxis of chloroquine-resistant malaria and treatment of chloroquine-resistant *P. vivax*. It is a potent and fast-acting antimalarial drug that is well absorbed orally, widely distributed in the body and reaches peak plasma concentration in 2–12 hours. It undergoes extensive enterohepatic circulation and has a long elimination half-life of 13–33 days. It is extensively metabolised by the liver, with less than 10% of the drug excreted unchanged in the urine. Most of the drug is eliminated via bile and excreted in faeces.

Adverse reactions are generally dose-related and occur more commonly in therapeutic than in prophylactic drug regimens. Adverse effects include nausea, vomiting, headache, dizziness, insomnia, gastric distress, diarrhoea, visual disturbances and, rarely, bradycardia and central nervous system (CNS) toxicity (depression, hallucinations, convulsions, psychosis, anxiety and confusion). Use mefloquine with caution in people with cardiac disease or hepatic impairment. Avoid use in people with epilepsy, heart block (first- or second-degree) or a history of psychiatric problems (psychosis, hallucinations, anxiety or depression).

Primaquine

Primaquine is very effective in the exo-erythrocytic stages of *P. vivax* and *P. ovale* malaria and against the primary (exo-erythrocytic phase) of *P. falciparum* malaria. It is also effective against the sexual forms (gametocytes) of plasmodia (especially *P. falciparum*). Indications include preventing malaria relapses (radical cure) caused by *P. vivax* and *P. ovale*. It is also effective against gametocytes of *P. falciparum*. Primaquine is absorbed rapidly from the gastrointestinal tract (GIT) and reaches peak plasma concentrations within 2–3 hours. The drug undergoes extensive metabolism to the inactive metabolite, carboxyprimaquine. It has a half-life of about 6 hours, and the amount of unchanged drug excreted in urine is less than 4%.

The use of primaquine concurrently with other myelosuppressive drugs should be avoided because of the higher risk of myelosuppression. Use primaquine with caution in people with a history (personal or family) of acute haemolytic anaemia or a nicotinamide adenine dinucleotide methaemoglobin reductase deficiency. Avoid use in people with primaquine hypersensitivity or G6PD deficiency (primaquine may cause haemolytic anaemia, especially in people deficient in G6PD) and in children under 12 months old because of increased risk of methaemoglobinaemia.

Quinine

Quinine was the first drug used to treat malaria (Clinical Focus Box 38.1) and is now a second-line agent used for treating *P. falciparum*. As an antimalarial agent, it concentrates in parasitised erythrocytes causing accumulation of haem, which may be why it has selective toxicity during the erythrocytic phase of plasmodial infections and is ineffective during the exo-erythrocyte phase. It can also bind to plasmodial DNA, thus inhibiting RNA synthesis and DNA replication.

Quinine sulfate is indicated in combination with other drugs (doxycycline or clindamycin) for treating uncomplicated chloroquine-resistant malaria caused by *P. falciparum*. Additionally, the intravenous formulation quinine dihydrochloride is used to treat severe *P. falciparum* malaria. As quinine is metabolised by CYP3A4, inducers of this enzyme (e.g. nevirapine and rifampicin) may increase metabolism, thus reducing efficacy, while inhibitors (e.g. ritonavir) increase the plasma concentration of quinine causing toxicity.

Combination antimalarials

Two combination antimalarials are used in Australia: artemether with lumefantrine, and atovaquone with proguanil.

Artemether with lumefantrine

Artemether is a semisynthetic derivative of a natural antimalarial (artemisinin) extracted from a Chinese plant called qing hao. It acts rapidly on the asexual erythrocytic stages of *P. vivax* and chloroquine-sensitive/resistant and

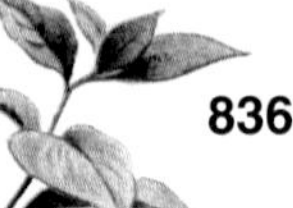

CLINICAL FOCUS BOX 38.1

Treating malaria with gin and tonic

Although malaria had been around since the first century CE, the first specific effective treatment was found in the 17th century, with bark of the cinchona trees (called 'quin' by the Incas) found in South America. This remedy was brought from Ecuador to Europe by returning Jesuit missionaries and became known as 'Jesuit's powder'. It quickly proved to be effective in Italy, Europe and England, and was highly prized.

The active principle was isolated in pure form in 1820 and named quinine; much effort went into procuring seeds and growing high-yield strains of the trees in Europe. Pharmacological studies on quinine led to the development of related drugs: chloroquine, mepacrine, primaquine and other aminoquinolines. Many strains of the plasmodium parasites, however, have developed resistance to these drugs, and chloroquine-resistant malaria is now a major problem worldwide. Quinine also proved to have useful skeletal muscle-relaxant properties and has been used in the past to treat muscle spasms.

Quinine has a very bitter taste, so a tradition was instituted by the British Raj rulers in India and the Far East of putting gin into their quinine mixtures ('tonic water') to disguise the taste. This became a habit and nowadays tonic water (containing quinine) is taken to enhance the flavour of gin! Bitter lemon drinks also have added quinine to enhance the bitter flavours. Tonic water now contains about 83 mg quinine per litre, and bitter lemon about 44 mg quinine per litre.

multidrug-resistant *P. falciparum*. Artemether is not suitable for prophylaxis because it does not affect either primary or latent tissue-stage parasites. Lumefantrine is structurally related to quinine and is very effective against *P. falciparum*. The combination of artemether with lumefantrine gives effectiveness greater than that of either drug alone. The currently available drug combination is a fixed ratio of one part artemether to six parts lumefantrine. Both drugs are thought to interfere with the conversion of haem to the malaria pigment haemozoin in the food vacuole of the malarial parasite. Additionally, both inhibit nucleic acid synthesis within the malarial parasite.

Administered orally, artemether is rapidly absorbed, with peak plasma concentration reached in approximately 2 hours. In contrast, lumefantrine is highly lipophilic and absorption is slow, with peak plasma concentration reached at about 6–8 hours after dosing. Absorption is improved if the tablets are taken with food. Both drugs are extensively (> 97%) bound to plasma proteins. Artemether as a prodrug is extensively metabolised to the active metabolite dihydroartemisinin, predominantly by CYP3A4. Because lumefantrine has a longer half-life than artemether, it is thought to clear any residual parasites that remain after combination treatment. Lumefantrine is a clinical significance CYP2D6 inhibitor; hence, drug interactions occur with other drugs (e.g. flecainide, metoprolol, clomipramine) metabolised by CYP2D6, resulting in increased plasma concentration of the co-administered drug. Relevant drug information sources should be consulted for potential drug interactions before administering artemether with lumefantrine.

Atovaquone with proguanil

Atovaquone is a hydroxynaphthoquinone drug that is used in combination with proguanil. Together, atovaquone with proguanil causes a synergistic antimalarial effect as a result of interference with the synthesis of pyrimidines, which are required for nucleic acid synthesis. Atovaquone inhibits mitochondrial electron transport in *P. falciparum*. In contrast, proguanil, through its active metabolite cycloguanil, inhibits dihydrofolate reductase and potentiates the ability of atovaquone to collapse the mitochondrial membrane potential. The combination is a fixed ratio of 2.5 parts atovaquone to 1 part proguanil, and it is used to treat uncomplicated *P. falciparum* malaria (second-line drug) and for prophylaxis of chloroquine- or mefloquine-resistant malaria. For the latter, treatment begins 1–2 days before entering an endemic area and is continued for 1 week after leaving the area.

The absorption of atovaquone is affected by dose and diet, which results in inconsistent oral bioavailability, while proguanil is rapidly and extensively absorbed regardless of diet. It is recommended that the drug be taken with food or a milky drink because dietary fat enhances absorption of atovaquone. Unlike proguanil, atovaquone is not metabolised, and more than 90% is excreted as unchanged drug in faeces, with very little excretion via urine. Proguanil is metabolised to polar metabolites which, along with unchanged drug (~40%), are excreted in urine. The elimination half-life of atovaquone is 2–3 days in adults (1–2 days in children), whereas the elimination half-life of proguanil is 12–15 hours. At therapeutic doses, common adverse GIT effects include nausea, vomiting and diarrhoea. The safety of the combination in human pregnancy has not been fully established.

Amoebiasis

Amoebiasis is an infection of the large intestine produced by a protozoan parasite, *Entamoeba histolytica*. This infestation is found worldwide but is prevalent and severe in tropical areas. Transmission is usually through ingestion of cysts (faecal to oral route) from contaminated food or water or from person-to-person contact. Poor personal hygiene can increase the spread of this parasite.

Life cycle of amoebae

This protozoan has two stages in its life cycle: the trophozoite (vegetative amoeba), which is the active, motile form; and the cyst, or inactive, drug-resistant form that appears in intestinal excretion. The trophozoite stage is capable of amoeboid motion and sexual activity. Because of its susceptibility to injury, it generally succumbs to an unfavourable environment. However, in certain circumstances, the trophozoite protects itself by entering the cystic stage. During this phase, the protozoan becomes inactive by surrounding itself with a resistant cell wall within which it can survive for a long time, even in an unsuitable environment.

The complete life cycle of the amoeba occurs in humans, the main host. It begins with ingestion of cysts that are present on hands, food or water contaminated by faeces. In the stomach, the hydrochloric acid does not destroy the swallowed cysts, which pass unharmed into the small intestine. The digestive juices penetrate the cystic walls and the trophozoites are released. The motile amoebae later pass into the colon, where they live and multiply for a time, feeding on the bacterial flora of the gut.

The presence of bacteria is essential to their survival. Finally, before excretion, the trophozoites move towards the terminal end of the bowel and again become encysted. After the cysts are eliminated in the faeces, they remain viable and infective. The cycle may begin again when the cysts appearing in faecal excretion are ingested through contamination of food or water.

Amoebicidal drugs

Drugs for treating amoebiasis are classified according to the site of amoebic action. Luminal amoebicides act primarily in the bowel lumen and are generally ineffective against parasites in the bowel wall or tissues. Tissue amoebicides are drugs that act primarily in the bowel wall, liver and other extra-intestinal tissues. No single drug is effective for both types of amoebiasis; therefore, a luminal and extraluminal (tissue) amoebicide or combination therapy is often prescribed. Drugs used for symptomatic intestinal or extra-intestinal amoebiasis include metronidazole and tinidazole (Ch 37), and for the eradication of cysts, paromomycin.

Paromomycin

Paromomycin is an aminoglycoside antibiotic with antibacterial properties similar to those of neomycin. It is effective as both an amoebicidal and an antibacterial agent. In Australia, paromomycin is only available through the TGA-managed Special Access Scheme. Paromomycin acts directly on intestinal amoebae and on bacteria such as *Salmonella* and *Shigella*. Because the drug is poorly absorbed from the GIT, it exerts no effect on systemic infections such as extra-intestinal amoebiasis, and most of the drug is excreted in the faeces. It is indicated for treating acute and chronic intestinal amoebiasis.

Miscellaneous antiprotozoal drugs

Metronidazole

Metronidazole (Drug Monograph 38.1) is the drug of choice for treating **trichomoniasis** and is usually administered as a single dose. Trichomoniasis is an infection of the vagina caused by the anaerobic protozoan *Trichomonas vaginalis*. Usually, both sexual partners are infected by this organism, which can be identified microscopically from semen, prostatic fluid or exudate from the vagina. Infections often recur, which indicates that the protozoans persist in extra-vaginal foci, the male urethra or the periurethral glands and ducts of both sexes. Treatment must be given simultaneously to both infected partners to effect a cure.

Pentamidine

Pentamidine is an aromatic diamine with a broad spectrum of activity against several species of pathogenic protozoa, including *Trypanosoma brucei gambiense* (sleeping sickness) and the ascomycetous fungus *Pneumocystis jiroveci* (formerly known as *Pneumocystis carinii*). It is indicated for treating *P. jiroveci* in people with AIDS and for trypanosomiasis excluding *Trypanosoma brucei rhodesiense*, which is refractory to pentamidine. The mechanism of action is unclear, but the sites of drug action include membrane phospholipids, intracellular enzymes and DNA and RNA. The drug is administered intravenously as pentamidine isethionate but can also be administered via inhalation using a specialised nebuliser. It is eliminated slowly over weeks to months.

Pyrimethamine

Toxoplasmosis is caused by an intracellular parasite, *Toxoplasma gondii*. This parasite is found worldwide in raw vegetables and the soil, and infests a variety of animals, including humans. Cats and other feline species are the natural hosts, and it is often harboured in the host with no evidence of the disease. Toxoplasmosis is contracted by ingesting cysts in inadequately cooked or raw meat, fish or vegetables, or by accidentally ingesting cysts from cat faeces.

Symptomatically, the individual may experience lymphadenopathy, fever and, occasionally, a rash on the palms and soles. The most serious complication of

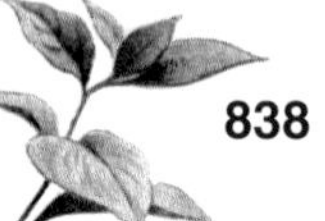

Drug Monograph 38.1
Metronidazole

Metronidazole is a prodrug that is metabolically activated by the infecting organism and is selectively toxic for anaerobic species.

Indications

Metronidazole is indicated for treating Gram-positive and Gram-negative anaerobic bacterial infections, protozoal infections including giardiasis, trichomoniasis, *Clostridium difficile*-associated disease, aspiration pneumonia, lung abscess and bacterial vaginosis.

Pharmacokinetics

Well absorbed after oral administration, metronidazole widely distributes into breast milk, cerebrospinal fluid, saliva, vaginal secretions and seminal fluid. It is excreted principally as metabolites in urine, with only 10% excreted as unchanged drug. The half-life of metronidazole is about 8 hours, while that of the hydroxylated metabolite, which has around 50% of the antitrichomonal activity of the parent drug, is in the order of 12 hours.

Drug interactions

Treatment with disulfiram may cause psychotic reactions; do not use metronidazole within 2 weeks of disulfiram. Avoid treatment with fluorouracil, as the combination increases fluorouracil toxicity.

Adverse reactions

Thrombophlebitis occurs commonly when metronidazole is administered intravenously. Rare adverse reactions include pancreatitis, hepatitis, optic neuritis, thrombocytopenia and *Clostridium difficile*-associated disease. High-dose and/or prolonged treatment may cause leucopenia or peripheral neuropathy, although both are usually reversible. CNS toxicity including seizures, encephalopathy and cerebellar toxicity are more likely with higher doses.

Warnings and contraindications

Metabolites may accumulate in severe impairment, possibly causing adverse effects, although dose adjustment is not usually necessary. There is a risk of accumulation and toxicity in severe impairment, especially if renal impairment is also present; reduce dose.

Dosage and administration

Metronidazole may be administered orally or intravenously as an infusion over 15–30 minutes. Dosing depends on the type and severity of infection, the age of the person and route of administration. Specific treatment guidelines should be consulted.

toxoplasmosis is meningoencephalitis, which is common in people with HIV. Pyrimethamine plus sulfadiazine is used as maintenance suppressive therapy against toxoplasmosis in HIV-positive people. Both drugs alter the folic acid cycle of the *Toxoplasma* organism, resulting in its death. Lifelong suppressive therapy is essential to prevent relapse, and inclusion of calcium folinate reduces bone marrow suppression.

Pyrimethamine is an antiprotozoal agent used to treat toxoplasmosis. It binds to and inhibits the protozoal enzyme dihydrofolate reductase, thus inhibiting the conversion of dihydrofolic acid to tetrahydrofolic acid. This results in a depletion of folate, which is essential for nucleic acid synthesis and protein production. Pyrimethamine is slowly absorbed after oral administration and is widely distributed in the body, although it concentrates mainly in blood cells, kidneys, liver and spleen. It reaches peak plasma concentrations in 2–6 hours and has a half-life of 35–175 hours. It is extensively metabolised in the liver, and approximately 30% is excreted in the urine over 40 days.

KEY POINTS

Antiprotozoal drugs

- The choice of antimalarial drugs is based on the particular malarial strain involved and the stage of the plasmodium life cycle.
- Travellers to endemic areas should receive malaria chemoprophylaxis starting 1–3 weeks before entering the area.
- Amoebiasis is an infection of the large intestine produced by a protozoan parasite, *Entamoeba histolytica*. This infestation is found worldwide but is prevalent and severe in tropical areas.

Mycobacterial infections

Mycobacterial infections in humans include *Mycobacterium avium* complex (MAC), **tuberculosis** (TB) and leprosy.

Mycobacterium Avium complex

MAC consists of two species: *Mycobacterium avium* and *Mycobacterium intracellulare*. *M. avium* accounts for most MAC infections in people with HIV, while *M. intracellulare* is responsible for 40% of MAC infections in immunocompetent people. These mycobacteria are found in fresh and salt water worldwide, and the common environmental sources of MAC include aerosolised water, household and hospital water supplies, house dust, soil, birds, farm animals and the various components that make up a cigarette.

MAC is transmitted via inhalation and oral ingestion. Following translocation across the mucosal epithelium, the bacteria infect macrophages and spread in the submucosal tissue. The mycobacteria are then spread via the lymphatic system and, in immunocompromised people, to the liver, spleen, bone marrow and other sites. Specialist advice should be sought regarding drug regimens for either HIV-negative or HIV-positive people. Drugs used include clarithromycin or azithromycin, plus ethambutol and rifampicin (rifampin) or amikacin and some of the drugs discussed below.

Tuberculosis

TB, a chronic granulomatous infection caused by the acid-fast bacillus *Mycobacterium tuberculosis*, is both a curable and a controllable infection that is transmitted from person to person.

In 2020, 10 million people were infected with TB, of whom 1.5 million died from the disease. More than 95% of deaths due to TB occur in developing countries, with India, Indonesia, China, Nigeria, Pakistan and South Africa accounting for 60% of the total cases of this disease. TB is the leading killer of HIV-infected people: in 2020, 214,000 people infected with HIV died as a result of TB infection. TB is the 13th leading cause of death annually and was the second leading cause of infectious death in 2020 (behind COVID-19). An estimated 66 million lives have been saved between 2000 and 2020 through the use of TB medicines (WHO 2021b).

Pathogenesis

TB most commonly affects the lungs, but other body areas can also be infected, such as bones, joints, skin, meninges or the genitourinary tract. *M. tuberculosis* is an aerobic bacillus that needs a highly oxygenated organ site for growth; thus the lungs, the growing ends of bones and the cerebral cortex are ideal sites. The bacilli can become inactive and be walled off by calcified and fibrous tissues, often for the lifetime of the person. If host defences break down, however, or if the individual receives an immunosuppressive drug, the bacilli may be reactivated.

Drug treatment regimens

Combination therapy is used to treat TB both to prevent the emergence of resistance and to shorten the duration of treatment. Drug selection is based on preventing the development of drug-resistant organisms and drug toxicity. General recommendations include the following:

- To avoid the development of drug-resistant organisms, all people in whom TB is diagnosed should have drug susceptibility tests on their first isolation.
- A four-drug combination provides an adequate cover that will be at least 95% effective, even in the presence of drug-resistant organisms.
    - In Australia, the preferred combination is isoniazid (Drug Monograph 38.2), rifampicin (Drug Monograph 38.3) and ethambutol.
    - This combination can be administered using different regimens (Table 38.1), with intensive and continuation phases to accommodate different scenarios.
- When drug susceptibility results are available, the drug regimen can be adjusted.
- Monitor the prescribed therapy regimen closely to support compliance, detect adverse reactions and register progress of the treatment program.

Antimycobacterial agents used for MAC and TB

Antimycobacterial agents used to treat MAC and TB are discussed in `alphabetical order below. Many are not marketed in Australia but may be available through the Special Access Scheme.

Capreomycin (TB)

Capreomycin is an antimycobacterial agent indicated in combination therapy for treating pulmonary TB after primary medications (isoniazid, rifampicin, pyrazinamide and ethambutol) fail, or when these medications cannot be used because of resistant bacilli or drug toxicity. Administered parenterally, capreomycin has a half-life of 3–6 hours and reaches peak plasma concentration in 1–2 hours after intramuscular administration. It is excreted by the kidneys primarily as unchanged drug.

When capreomycin is given with any of the drugs listed in Drug Interactions 38.1, very serious reactions may result. Avoid concurrent use if possible. Adverse reactions include nephrotoxicity, hypokalaemia, neuromuscular blockade, ototoxicity, hypersensitivity and pain, and soreness or hardness at the injection site. Use capreomycin with caution in dehydrated people.

DRUG INTERACTIONS 38.1
Capreomycin

DRUG	POSSIBLE EFFECTS AND MANAGEMENT
Aminoglycosides	Increased risk of developing ototoxicity, nephrotoxicity and neuromuscular blockade. Hearing loss may progress to deafness, even after the drug is stopped. This can be a very dangerous combination. Avoid concurrent drug administration.
Cisplatin, ciclosporin, ethacrynic acid, frusemide, paromomycin, streptomycin or vancomycin	Concurrent, or even sequential, use of capreomycin with any of these drugs can increase the risk of ototoxicity and nephrotoxicity. Hearing loss may occur and progress to deafness, even if drugs are stopped. Avoid if at all possible.
Neuromuscular-blocking agents	May result in increased neuromuscular-blocking effects, causing respiratory depression or paralysis. Monitor closely, especially during surgery or in the postoperative period. If possible, avoid this combination.

Cycloserine (MAC and TB)

This is a second-line broad-spectrum antibiotic that can be bacteriostatic or bactericidal, depending on drug concentration at the infection site and on organism susceptibility. Cycloserine is an antimycobacterial agent that interferes with bacterial cell wall synthesis. In combination with other drugs, it is indicated for treating TB or MAC after failure of first-line antitubercular medications.

Cycloserine is well absorbed orally and is widely distributed in body tissues and fluids. The peak plasma concentration occurs in 3–4 hours, and the drug has a half-life of 10 hours. Approximately 70% of unchanged drug is excreted in urine within 24 hours. See Drug Interactions 38.2 for drugs that interact with cycloserine and possible outcomes.

Ethambutol (MAC and TB)

This drug is bacteriostatic; it is believed to diffuse into the mycobacteria bacilli and suppress RNA synthesis. Ethambutol is effective only against actively dividing mycobacteria. It is indicated in combination with other drugs for the treatment and re-treatment of TB and MAC. There is an increased risk of neurotoxicity, such as optic and peripheral neuritis, when ethambutol is administered concurrently with other neurotoxic medications. Monitor closely if concurrent therapy is instituted.

DRUG INTERACTIONS 38.2
Cycloserine

DRUG	POSSIBLE EFFECTS AND MANAGEMENT
Alcohol	In chronic alcohol abusers, cycloserine may increase the risk of seizures. Avoid, or a potentially serious drug interaction may occur.
Isoniazid	May increase CNS adverse effects such as seizures. Monitor closely, as dosage adjustments may be necessary.

Ethambutol is absorbed after oral administration and distributed to most body tissues and fluids, with the exception of cerebrospinal fluid. High concentrations are found in the kidneys, lungs, saliva, urine and erythrocytes. Therapeutic plasma concentrations occur within 4 hours and the half-life is 3–4 hours. Ethambutol is partly metabolised (15%) in the liver, and 75% of the oral dose is excreted unchanged in urine and 10% in faeces.

Isoniazid (TB)

Isoniazid (Drug Monograph 38.2) is an antimycobacterial (bactericidal) agent that affects mycobacteria in the dividing phase. In combination with rifampicin, it is a core drug of the intensive (also with pyrazinamide and ethambutol) and continuation phases of the preferred first-line TB treatment regimen (Table 38.1).

Pyrazinamide (TB)

Pyrazinamide is an antimycobacterial agent that is metabolised to pyrazinoic acid within the mycobacterium. Pyrazinoic acid is believed to interfere with the synthesis of mycolic acid (essential for cell wall synthesis), alter intracellular pH by increasing acidity that enhances microbial death, and disrupt membrane transporters. Depending on its concentration at the site of action and susceptibility of the mycobacteria, this drug can be bacteriostatic or bactericidal. It is indicated in combination with other agents for treating TB. Pyrazinamide is well absorbed orally and is widely distributed in the body. The time to peak plasma concentration is 1–2 hours and the elimination half-life is 9–10 hours. Pyrazinamide is primarily metabolised in the liver to 5-hydroxy pyrazinoic acid that is excreted by the kidneys.

Rifabutin (MAC and TB)

Rifabutin is an antimycobacterial agent indicated for the prophylaxis of disseminated MAC in people with advanced HIV infection. It inhibits DNA-dependent RNA

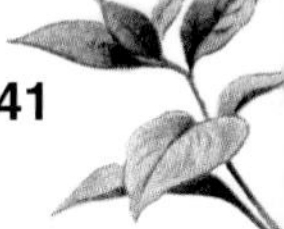

Drug Monograph 38.2
Isoniazid

Isoniazid is an antimycobacterial (bactericidal) agent that affects mycobacteria in the dividing phase. In the mycobacteria, isoniazid is converted to a toxic isonicotinoyl radical.

Indications

Isoniazid is indicated for the primary treatment, re-treatment and prophylaxis of TB.

Pharmacokinetics

Isoniazid is well absorbed orally and is widely distributed throughout the body. Metabolism in the liver by NAT2 is subject to genetic polymorphism in humans. Excretion is primarily via the urine, partly as unchanged drug and as the inactive acetylated form, *N*-acetyl-isoniazid.

Drug interactions

Daily alcohol consumption may increase isoniazid metabolism and the risk of hepatotoxicity. Monitor patients, as a drug dose adjustment may be necessary. Co-administration of disulfiram may increase the incidence of CNS adverse effects such as ataxia, irritability, dizziness or insomnia. Monitor closely for these symptoms, as dosage reduction, or even discontinuation of disulfiram, may be required. Hepatotoxic drugs may increase potential for hepatotoxicity. Avoid, or a potentially serious drug interaction may occur. In particular, use of isoniazid in combination with rifampicin may increase the potential for hepatotoxicity, especially in people with liver impairment and in fast acetylators of isoniazid. Monitor closely for hepatotoxicity, especially during the first 90 days of therapy.

Adverse reactions

These include gastric distress, anorexia, nausea, vomiting, tiredness, hepatitis, peripheral neuritis and, rarely, blood dyscrasias, hypersensitivity reactions and optic neuritis. Increases in plasma aminotransferases may occur in the first few months of treatment.

Warnings and contraindications

Use with caution in people with severe kidney disease and convulsive disorders. Avoid use in people with isoniazid, pyrazinamide, niacin or nicotinic acid hypersensitivity or liver function impairment, and in people addicted to alcohol.

Dosage and administration

The adult oral dose (daily regimen) of isoniazid is 5 mg/kg (max. 300 mg daily). When a thrice-weekly regimen is used, the dose is 15 mg/kg (max. 900 mg) thrice weekly. For children, the daily regimen is 10–15 mg/kg up to a maximum of 300 mg daily.

TABLE 38.1 Preferred tuberculosis treatment regimens

	INTENSIVE PHASE		CONTINUATION PHASE	
REGIMEN	DRUGS	INTERVAL AND DOSES	DRUGS	INTERVAL AND DOSES
One	Isoniazid Rifampicin Pyrazinamide Ethambutol	**Daily for 8 weeks** 7 days per week for 56 doses (8 weeks), or 5 days per week for 40 doses (8 weeks)	Isoniazid Rifampicin	7 days per week for 126 doses (18 weeks), or 5 days per week for 90 doses (18 weeks)
Two	Isoniazid Rifampicin Pyrazinamide Ethambutol	**Daily for 8 weeks** 7 days per week for 56 doses (8 weeks), or 5 days per week for 40 doses (8 weeks)	Isoniazid Rifampicin	Three times weekly for 54 doses (18 weeks)
Three	Isoniazid Rifampicin Pyrazinamide Ethambutol	**Three times weekly for 8 weeks** Three times weekly for 24 doses (8 weeks)	Isoniazid Rifampicin	Three times weekly for 54 doses (18 weeks)
Four	Isoniazid Rifampicin Pyrazinamide Ethambutol	**Daily for 2 weeks, then twice weekly for 6 weeks** 7 days per week for 14 doses (2 weeks), then twice weekly for 12 doses	Isoniazid Rifampicin	Twice weekly for 36 doses (18 weeks)

polymerase in susceptible *Escherichia coli* and *Bacillus subtilis*. It is used for the prophylaxis and treatment of MAC and the treatment of TB if rifampicin is unsuitable.

Rifabutin is absorbed from the GIT, reaches peak plasma concentration in 2–4 hours and has a terminal half-life of 45 hours. It is highly lipophilic and crosses the blood–brain barrier; cerebrospinal fluid levels are about 50% of the corresponding plasma concentration. Metabolism in the liver involves CYP3A; five metabolites have been identified, which are excreted primarily by the

Drug Monograph 38.3
Rifampicin

Rifampicin (rifampin) is a broad-spectrum bactericidal antibiotic (antimycobacterial) that binds to DNA-dependent RNA polymerase and blocks mycobacterial RNA transcription. It is indicated for treating TB and for asymptomatic carriers of *Neisseria meningitidis*.

Indications

Rifampicin is used to treat several types of bacterial infections, including TB, leprosy and Legionnaire's disease. It is almost always used along with other antibiotics, except when given to prevent *Haemophilus influenzae* type B and meningococcal disease in people who have been exposed to those bacteria. When used to treat TB, rifampicin is administered in combination with isoniazid, pyrazinamide and ethambutol.

Pharmacokinetics

Rifampicin is well absorbed orally and distributes widely in the body. As it is lipid-soluble, it reaches and kills intracellular and extracellular susceptible bacteria. Therapeutic plasma concentrations occur in 1.5–4 hours, and the elimination half-life is up to 5 hours. Rifampicin is metabolised in the liver by esterases to a range of metabolites, including an active metabolite 25-O-desacetylrifampicin. Excretion is primarily via bile into faeces.

Drug interactions

Rifampicin induces CYP 1A2, 2C9, 2C19 and 3A4, which results in increased clearance of drugs metabolised by these CYP enzymes, leading to reduced exposure and potential loss of efficacy. Of particular note, increased liver metabolism of estrogen may result in menstrual irregularities, spotting and unplanned pregnancies. Advise the person of the possible effects when these drugs are combined and suggest alternative contraception. Co-administration of hepatotoxic drugs increases the risk of hepatotoxicity. Avoid, or a potentially serious drug interaction may occur.

Adverse reactions

These include gastric distress, hypersensitivity, a flu-like syndrome, fungal overgrowth and, rarely, blood dyscrasias, hepatitis and interstitial nephritis.

Dosage and administration

The oral dosage of rifampicin for adults and children in combination with other agents (for TB) is 10 mg/kg to a maximum of 600 mg daily, or 15 mg/kg (max. 600 mg) three times a week.

kidneys. When used in combination with zidovudine, plasma zidovudine concentration may decrease; monitoring of zidovudine plasma concentrations should be performed when using the combination.

Rifampicin

Rifampicin (rifampin) (Drug Monograph 38.3) is used either orally or intravenously to treat several types of bacterial infections, although intravenous use can be logistically challenging when used to treat TB because rifampicin is administered daily for at least 6 months (Table 38.1). Rifampicin can be used in people with latent TB to prevent or delay the onset of active disease, as only small numbers of bacteria are present. A notable, but generally harmless, characteristic of treatment with rifampicin is that the drug often turns urine, sweat and tears a vibrant red or orange colour.

Streptomycin (TB)

Streptomycin is an aminoglycoside antibiotic that is poorly absorbed from the GIT; it is therefore given intramuscularly. One of the first effective agents used to treat TB, it is still an important agent in treating TB resistant to the first-line antitubercular drugs and of other non-TB mycobacteria when specialist advice is necessary. Like the other aminoglycosides, its major toxicities include ototoxicity and nephrotoxicity, especially when given to people with impaired renal function or with other medications with the same toxicities.

Leprosy

Leprosy, or Hansen's disease, is caused by *Mycobacterium leprae* in humans. In 2020, there were more than 127,000 new cases of leprosy worldwide. Leprosy is considered a rare disease in Australia, but it is yet to be eradicated; on average over the past 10 years there have been between 10 and 20 cases reported annually. Although the precise mode of transmission is unknown, the incubation period for leprosy is a few months to decades. Large numbers of leprosy bacilli are generally shed from skin ulcers, nasal secretions, the GIT and biting insects.

M. leprae is a bacillus that in humans first presents as a skin lesion: a large plaque or macule that is erythematous or hypopigmented in the centre. More numerous lesions, peripheral nerve trunk involvement and the common complications of plantar ulceration of the feet – footdrop, loss of hand function and corneal abrasions – may follow.

Drug therapy can cure leprosy, stop transmission of the disease and prevent the disfigurement that results in social exclusion and stigmatisation. Since 1982, WHO has recommended the use of multidrug therapy comprising dapsone, rifampicin (Drug Monograph 38.3) and clofazimine for multibacillary leprosy and rifampicin with dapsone for paucibacillary leprosy. This combination is bactericidal and prevents the occurrence of drug resistance.

Drugs used to treat leprosy

Clofazimine

The antileprotic mechanism of action of clofazimine is unknown; it has a bactericidal effect on *M. leprae*, inhibits mycobacterial growth and tends to bind preferentially to mycobacterial DNA. Oral absorption of clofazimine is variable and is increased in the presence of high-fat meals and decreased in the presence of antacids. It is distributed primarily in fatty tissues and cells. Macrophages accumulate the drug and further distribute it throughout the body. Its half-life is about 2–3 months with chronic therapy, and peak plasma concentrations occur 1–6 hours after dosing. It is excreted primarily in faeces.

Dapsone

Dapsone is an antibacterial agent that is bacteriostatic, with an action similar to that of sulfonamides. It is a competitive inhibitor of dihydropteroate synthase and thus interferes with folate metabolism. Dapsone is effective against *M. leprae* and is indicated for treating all types of leprosy and for dermatitis herpetiformis. Dapsone is absorbed following oral administration, distributed throughout the body and is found in body fluids and in all body tissues. Therapeutic plasma concentrations are achieved in 2–6 hours and the half-life is around 30 hours. The drug is acetylated by NAT2 in the liver; thus, slow acetylators are more likely than fast acetylators to develop higher plasma concentrations and adverse reactions. It is also metabolised by CYP2E1, forming dapsone hydroxylamine, which is taken up into erythrocytes resulting in methaemoglobin formation. The vast majority of the drug is excreted as glucuronide and sulfate conjugates in urine. Drug Interactions 38.3 identifies drugs that may interact with dapsone and possible outcomes.

DRUG INTERACTIONS 38.3
Dapsone

DRUG	POSSIBLE EFFECTS AND MANAGEMENT
Didanosine	Concurrent administration may reduce dapsone absorption. Administer dapsone a minimum of 2 hours before didanosine.
Trimethoprim, sulfamethoxazole	Decreased elimination of both dapsone and trimethoprim may occur. Monitor for increased incidence of adverse effects.

KEY POINTS

Antimycobacterial drugs

- The main mycobacterial infections in humans are MAC, TB and leprosy.
- WHO has recommended the Directly Observed Treatment – Short Course (DOTS) approach for controlling TB and has projected that using this system would result in curing 85% of all new cases.
- The recommended first-line drugs for TB are isoniazid, rifampicin, pyrazinamide and ethambutol.
- In developing countries, streptomycin is an important agent in treating TB resistant to the first-line antitubercular drugs and of other non-tuberculous mycobacteria when specialist advice is necessary.
- Leprosy, or Hansen's disease, is caused by *M. leprae* in humans. Today, the estimated number of infected people worldwide has fallen dramatically and many countries are now free of leprosy.
- Drug treatment of leprosy includes the use of dapsone and clofazimine.

Helminth infections

The disease-producing **helminths** (worms) are classified as metazoa, or multicellular animal parasites. Unlike the protozoa, they are large organisms with complex cellular structures and feed on host tissue. They may be present in the GIT, but several types also penetrate tissues and some undergo developmental changes, during which they move extensively in the host. Because most anthelmintics used today are highly effective against specific parasites, the organism must be accurately identified before treatment is started, usually by finding the parasite ova or larvae in the faeces, urine, blood, sputum or tissues of the host.

Parasitic infestations do not necessarily cause clinical manifestations, although they may be injurious for a variety of reasons:

- Worms may cause mechanical injury to the tissues and organs. Roundworms in large numbers may cause obstruction in the intestine, filariae may block lymphatic channels and cause massive oedema, and hookworms often cause extensive damage to the wall of the intestine and considerable loss of blood.
- Toxic substances produced by the parasite may be absorbed by the host.
- The tissues of the host may be damaged by the presence of the parasite and made more susceptible to bacterial infections.
- Heavy infestation with worms will deprive the host of food. This is particularly significant in children.

Helminths parasitic to humans are classified as: platyhelminths (flatworms), which include two subclasses, cestodes (tapeworms) and trematodes (flukes); or nematodes (roundworms).

Platyhelminths (flatworms)

Cestodes

Cestodes are tapeworms, of which there are four varieties: *Taenia saginata* (beef tapeworm), *Taenia solium* (pork tapeworm), *Diphyllobothrium latum* (fish tapeworm) and *Hymenolepis nana* (dwarf tapeworm). As indicated by the common name of the worm, the parasite enters the intestine by way of improperly cooked beef, pork or fish, or from contaminated food, as in the case of the dwarf tapeworm.

The cestodes are segmented flatworms with a head, or scolex, that has hooks or suckers used to attach to tissues and a number of segments, or proglottids, which in some cases may extend for 6–9 metres in the bowel. Drugs affecting the scolex allow expulsion of the organisms from the intestine. Each of the proglottids contains both male and female reproductive units. When filled with fertilised eggs, they are expelled from the worm into the environment. On ingestion, the infected larvae develop into adults in the small intestine of the human. The larvae may travel to extra-intestinal sites and enter other tissues, such as the liver, muscle and eye. The tapeworms, with the exception of the dwarf tapeworm, spend part of their life cycle in a host other than humans (pigs, fish or cattle). The dwarf tapeworm does not require any such intermediate host. The tapeworm has no digestive tract; it depends on the nutrients that are intended for the host. Subsequently, the victim suffers by eventually developing nutritional deficiency.

Trematodes

Trematodes, or flukes, are flat, non-segmented parasites with suckers that attach to and feed on host tissue. The life cycle begins with the egg, which is passed into fresh water after faecal excretion from the body of the human host. The egg containing the embryo forms into a ciliated organism, the miracidium. In the presence of water, the miracidium escapes from the egg and enters the intermediate host, the freshwater snail, which exists extensively in rice paddies and irrigation ditches. After entry, the fluke forms a cyst in the lungs of the snail. In the cyst, many organisms develop. They can penetrate other parts of the snail and grow into worms called cercariae. Eventually, the cercariae are released from the snail into the water, attaching themselves to blades of grass to encyst.

When encysted organisms in snails or fish and crabs are swallowed by humans, they develop into adult flukes in different structures of the body. The flukes are therefore classified according to the type of tissue they invade. After ingestion, the eggs of *Schistosoma haematobium* appear in the urinary bladder and cause inflammation of the urogenital system. This can result in chronic cystitis and haematuria. Infestations with *Schistosoma japonicum* and *Schistosoma mansoni* produce intestinal disturbance with resultant ulceration and necrosis of the rectum. *S. japonicum* is more concentrated in the veins of the small intestine. If the liver and spleen become infected, the disease is usually fatal. *S. mansoni* prefers the portal veins that drain the large intestine, particularly the sigmoid colon and rectum. Unlike the other parasites, the cercariae of *S. mansoni* are not ingested but burrow through the skin, especially between the toes of the human host who is standing in contaminated water. They then make their way to the portal system, where they mature into adult flukes. Schistosomiasis is endemic to Africa, Asia, South America and Caribbean islands. The disease can be controlled largely by eliminating the intermediate host, the snail. Travellers to these areas must avoid contact with contaminated water for drinking, bathing or swimming.

Nematodes (roundworms)

Nematodes are non-segmented cylindrical worms that consist of a mouth and complete digestive tract. The adults reside in the human intestinal tract; there is no intermediate host. Two types of nematode infection exist in the human: the egg form and the larval form.

Egg infective form

Ascaris lumbricoides is a large nematode (about 30 cm in length) and is known as the 'roundworm of humans'. The adult *Ascaris* usually resides in the upper end of the small intestine of the human, where it feeds on semidigested foods. The fertilised egg, when excreted with faeces, can survive in the soil for a long time. When inadvertently ingested by another host, the embryos escape from the eggs and mature into adults in the host. To prevent the disease, proper sanitary conditions and meticulous personal habits must be observed.

Infection with *Enterobius vermicularis*, or threadworm/pinworm, is highly prevalent among children and adults. Adult pinworms reside in the large intestine but the female migrates to the anus, depositing her eggs around the skin of the anal region. This causes intense itching and can be noted especially in children. Ingestion of excreted eggs can infect an individual. Eggs that contaminate clothing, bedding, furniture and other items may be responsible for continuing the reinfection of an individual and initiating the infection of others.

Larval infective form

Necator americanus (New World) or *Ancylostoma duodenale* (Old World) hookworms are somewhat similar in action. They reside in the small intestine of humans. When the eggs are excreted in the faeces, the larvae hatch in the soil. The larvae can penetrate the skin of humans, particularly through the soles of the feet, producing dermatitis (ground itch). On entry into the small intestine, they develop into adult worms. During the process, they extravasate blood from the intestinal vessels and cause a profound anaemia in the victim. The presence of eggs in the faeces indicates a positive test for hookworm disease. This infection can be avoided by wearing shoes.

Trichinella spiralis is a small pork roundworm that causes trichinosis. In humans, the disease begins by ingestion of insufficiently cooked pork meat. On entry of encysted meat into the small intestine, the larvae are released from the cysts. After maturation, the females develop eggs that later form into larvae. They then migrate via the bloodstream and lymphatic system to the skeletal muscles and encyst. Encapsulation and eventually calcification of the cysts occur. Diagnosis of trichinosis is made by muscle biopsy, whereby microscopic examination reveals the presence of larvae. The disease is prevented by thoroughly cooking pork meat before eating.

Anthelmintic drugs

Anthelmintics are among the most basic forms of drug therapy. The main class of anthelmintic drugs is the benzimidazoles, including albendazole and mebendazole. The other anthelmintics are ivermectin, praziquantel and pyrantel.

Benzimidazoles

The benzimidazoles cause degeneration of a parasite's cytoplasmic microtubules, which leads to blocking of glucose uptake in the helminth, and hence death of the parasite. They are indicated for treating *Trichuris* (whipworm), *Enterobius* (threadworm/pinworm), *Ascaris* (roundworm), *Ancylostoma* (common hookworm) and some tapeworms and liver flukes.

Albendazole

Albendazole is poorly absorbed and essentially remains within the GIT. However, absorption is significantly increased by consumption of a fatty meal. The small amount of drug absorbed is rapidly metabolised by hepatic CYP3A4 to an active sulfoxide metabolite that is thought to be the active drug against tissue infestation. The plasma half-life of albendazole sulfoxide is 8–9 hours; however, after release from cysts, low concentrations can be detected in plasma for several weeks. Elimination is principally via bile, with only small quantities detected in urine.

Adverse reactions occur with higher doses and extended dosing, and include headache, nausea, vomiting and diarrhoea. Rarely, allergic reactions, liver toxicity and haematological reactions occur. In people with hepatic impairment, dosage reduction may be necessary. Albendazole is contraindicated in pregnancy because of evidence of teratogenic effects in several animal species. It is minimally excreted in breast milk and may be used with caution.

Mebendazole

The oral absorption of mebendazole is poor but is increased if given with fatty foods. It is distributed to plasma, cyst fluid, liver, hepatic cysts and muscle tissues, with a half-life of 2.5–5.5 hours. It is metabolised in the liver to the primary metabolite 2-amino-5-benzoylbenzimidazole. Less than 2% is excreted via urine as unchanged drug, with the remainder excreted primarily in faeces as unchanged drug and the primary metabolite.

Other anthelmintics

Praziquantel

Praziquantel is an anthelmintic agent that penetrates cell membranes and increases cell permeability in susceptible worms. This results in an increased loss of intracellular calcium, contractions and muscle paralysis of the worm. The drug also disintegrates the schistosome tegument (covering). Subsequently, phagocytes are attracted to the worm and ultimately kill it. Praziquantel is indicated for treating schistosomiasis due to various blood flukes and for tapeworms but is ineffective against roundworms. Praziquantel is absorbed after oral administration and reaches a peak plasma concentration in 1–3 hours. Half-life is 0.8–1.5 hours for praziquantel and 4–6 hours for its metabolites. Approximately 70% of the administered dose is excreted as metabolites by the kidneys.

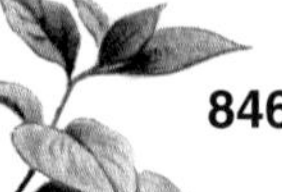

Pyrantel

Pyrantel is a depolarising neuromuscular-blocking anthelmintic agent; it causes contraction and then paralysis of the helminth's muscles. The helminths are dislodged and then expelled from the body by peristalsis. Pyrantel is indicated for treating *Ascaris lumbricoides* (roundworm), *Enterobius vermicularis* (threadworm) and hookworm, but is ineffective against whipworm. This product is poorly absorbed from the GIT. Pyrantel reaches peak plasma concentration in 1–3 hours and is primarily excreted in the faeces.

KEY POINTS

Anthelmintic drugs

- Anthelmintic drugs are used to rid the body of worms (helminths). It has been estimated that one-third of the world's population is infested with these parasites.
- The main class of anthelmintic drugs is the benzimidazoles, which include albendazole and mebendazole. Other anthelmintics include ivermectin, praziquantel and pyrantel.

DRUGS AT A GLANCE
Antiprotozoal, antimycobacterial and anthelmintic drugs

PHARMACOLOGICAL GROUP AND EFFECT	KEY EXAMPLES	CLINICAL USE
Antimalarials	Artemether with lumefantrine	Uncomplicated malaria
	Atovaquone with proguanil	Prophylaxis and treatment of uncomplicated malaria
	Mefloquine	Prophylaxis and treatment of malaria
	Primaquine	Radical cure of *P. vivax* and *P. ovale* malaria
	Quinine	Malaria
Amoebicidals	Paromomycin	Amoebiasis due to *E. histolytica*
Miscellaneous antiprotozoals	Metronidazole	Anaerobic bacterial infections; *C. difficile*-associated disease
	Pentamidine	Treatment of *Pneumocystis* pneumonia
	Pyrimethamine	Congenital or acquired toxoplasmosis
Drugs for treating MAC and TB	Capreomycin	Treatment of TB when some or all of the first-line agents cannot be used
	Cycloserine	Infections caused by multidrug-resistant strains of *M. tuberculosis* or MAC
	Ethambutol	Treatment of TB and MAC
	Isoniazid	Treatment of TB and latent TB
	Pyrazinamide	Treatment of TB
	Rifabutin	Treatment of TB
	Rifampicin	Treatment of TB; leprosy; MRSA infections
	Streptomycin	Infections due to *M. tuberculosis* and non-tuberculous mycobacteria
Antileprotic drugs	Clofazimine	Leprosy
	Dapsone	Leprosy
Benzimidazoles	Albendazole	Roundworm; threadworm; hookworm; whipworm; liver flukes
	Mebendazole	Roundworm; threadworm; hookworm; whipworm; liver flukes
Other anthelmintic drugs	Ivermectin	Onchocerciasis; strongyloidiasis; scabies; rosacea
	Praziquantel	Schistosomiasis
	Pyrantel	Roundworm; threadworm; hookworm

MAC = *Mycobacterium avium* complex; TB = tuberculosis

REVIEW EXERCISES

1 Mr RP has recently returned home from a holiday in Southeast Asia and presents with symptoms suspicious for TB. Discuss the general guidelines for selecting a drug regimen for treating TB.
2 Billy, a 6-year-old boy, presents with a worm infestation that has been identified as threadworm (*Enterobius vermicularis*). Discuss with his parents the drug options you have available to treat this infection, how the drugs actually work to rid the body of the infestation, and any specific advice they should adhere to in terms of administering the drug.
3 Ms AG is diagnosed with malaria and is commenced on a combination of drugs to treat this condition. Identify the two drug combinations that are used to treat malaria in Australia and discuss the rationale for using a drug combination in this setting.

REFERENCES

Salerno E: Pharmacology for health professionals, St Louis, MO, 1999, Mosby.

World Health Organization 2021a, Guidelines for the treatment of malaria. Geneva, WHO.

World Health Organization 2021b, Guidelines for the treatment of tuberculosis, Geneva, WHO.

CHAPTER 39
DRUGS AFFECTING THE SKIN

Mary Bushell

KEY ABBREVIATIONS

BCC/SCC	basal/squamous cell carcinoma
NMSC	non-melanocytic skin cancer
SPF	sun protection factor
UVR	ultraviolet radiation
UVA/B/C	UVR of wavelengths in the A, B or C region

KEY TERMS

acne vulgaris 866
antifungals 861
antimicrobials 860
burn 870
corticosteroids 863
dermatitis 863
eczema 864
formulation 854
nanoparticle 859
occlusive dressing 864
phototoxicity 856
pressure sore 872
psoriasis 865
retinoids 866
skin 850
sun protection factor 859
sunscreen 858
topical administration 852
transcutaneous absorption 852
ulcer (leg, foot) 873
ultraviolet radiation 857
vehicle 853

Chapter Focus

The skin serves as a barrier against the environment, protects underlying tissues, helps regulate body temperature and produces vitamin D. Drugs may be administered via topical and systemic routes for treating skin conditions, or may be applied to the skin intended for transcutaneous absorption and systemic actions. This chapter reviews the formulations and topical products available and indications for their use.

Drugs commonly applied to the skin include sunscreen preparations, antimicrobials, anti-inflammatory and immunosuppressant agents and drugs used to treat eczema, psoriasis, acne, burns, pressure sores and leg ulcers. Their pharmacological actions, clinical uses and adverse effects are described. Many hundreds of chemicals (including tattoos) applied to or contacting the skin can cause serious dermatological conditions such as dermatitis, Stevens-Johnson syndrome, fixed drug eruptions and phototoxicities.

KEY DRUG GROUPS

Anti-acne preparations:
- Keratolytics: **azelaic acid**
- Retinoids: **tretinoin** (Drug Monograph 39.2)

Anti-inflammatory and immunomodulating agents:
- Calcineurin inhibitors: **pimecrolimus**
- Corticosteroids: **betamethasone**, **hydrocortisone**
- TNF antagonists: **etanercept**

Burns treatments:
- **Silver sulfadiazine** (Drug Monograph 39.3)

Drugs for actinic keratoses:
- Diclofenac
- Fluorouracil

Sunscreens:
- Organics (absorbers): benzophenones, cinnamates
- Inorganics (reflectors): titanium dioxide, zinc oxide

Topical antimicrobials:
- Antibiotics: **mupirocin**
- Antifungals
- (Imid)azoles: **miconazole**
- **Amorolfine** (Drug Monograph 39.1), **terbinafine**

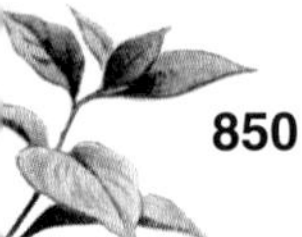

KEY DRUG GROUPS—cont'd

- Antiseptics: **chlorhexidine**
- Antivirals: **aciclovir**, **idoxuridine**
- For warts: **imiquimod**
- Ectoparasiticidals: **malathion** (maldison), **permethrin**

Topical formulations A–Z

Ulcer and pressure sore treatments:

- Debriding agents
- Medicated dressings

CRITICAL THINKING SCENARIO

Alexandra is a 5-year-old preschooler, who suffers from severe atopic dermatitis (eczema).

Alexandra's parents apply prescribed topical corticosteroids to the affected areas.

1. Describe the different formulations and potencies of the different types of topical corticosteroids that are available.
2. How are topical corticosteroids applied safely and for best effect?

Alexandra is also prescribed pimecrolimus 1% cream applied twice a day to her sensitive areas (face or genitals). Her doctor has advised against using occlusive dressings.

3. How does pimecrolimus 1% cream work to reduce the severity of Alexandra's atopic dermatitis?
4. Why has the doctor advised against the application of occlusive dressings?
5. What non-drug preventive measures should be performed to minimise the atopic dermatitis?

Several months later, Alexandra develops a bacterial skin infection secondary to her atopic dermatitis. Her GP prescribes mupirocin 2% ointment to be applied to the skin, twice daily for 5 days.

6. What type of drug is mupirocin? What is its mode of action? What is the difference between the ointment and cream formulation of this topically applied drug?

Introduction

Skin functions and disorders

The **skin** is the largest organ in the body. The main layers are the epidermis, consisting of epithelial cells and melanocytes, and the dermis (containing elastic and connective tissues, blood vessels, nerves, lymphatic tissue, sweat glands, sebaceous glands and hair follicles) (Fig 39.4 later).

Functions of the skin include:

- protection against microorganism invasion, chemicals, physical abrasion and loss of water and heat
- transfer of sensations such as heat, cold, touch, pressure and pain
- body temperature regulation – cooling occurs by dilation of dermal blood vessels and evaporative cooling of perspiration
- reservoir for blood
- excretion of fluid and electrolytes (via sweat glands)
- storage of fat and synthesis of vitamin D
- absorption of lipid-soluble drugs such as estrogens, corticosteroids, nicotine and fat-soluble vitamins (A, D, E and K)
- contributing to body image.

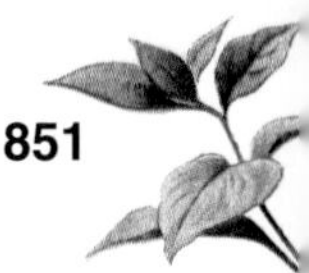

Protection and maintenance of skin integrity is an important part of professional nursing practice, notably in the treatment of burns, pressure sores and leg ulcers.

Signs and symptoms of skin disorders

Common dermatological disorders include acne vulgaris (cystic acne and acne scars), dermatitis (atopic, contact, seborrhoeic), eczema, folliculitis, fungal infections, herpes simplex, psoriasis, skin cancers, verrucae (warts) and vitiligo. Disorders of the skin are manifested by symptoms such as itching or pain, and by signs such as swelling, redness, papules, pustules, blisters and hives.

Dermatological diagnosis may require physical assessment, personal and family medical history, drug history including over-the-counter (OTC) medications and laboratory tests, cytodiagnosis and biopsy. When the nature of the lesion has been established, its characteristics are defined according to size, shape, surface and colour and distribution on the body.

Skin conditions vary over time. Acute conditions tend to show red, burning, blistered or weeping skin (such as from burns); thick ointments cannot be applied to these lesions. Subacute conditions may be oedematous, hot and chapped; creams and gels can be applied. Chronic skin conditions tend to be scaling, lichenified, crusting and dry; moisturising/emollient creams and ointments may soften such skin.

Causes of skin disorders

As the tissue most at risk of environmental damage, the skin often becomes infected, inflamed, burned, ulcerated or impaired by antigens, chemicals, mechanical injury or radiation. Disorders of the skin may be due to allergy, infection, sensitivity to drugs or other chemicals, emotional stress, genetic predisposition (e.g. atopic eczema or psoriasis), hormonal imbalances or degenerative disease. Sometimes the cause is unknown and the treatment is empirical.

Drug-induced skin disorders

A wide range of dermatological reactions can be caused by chemicals (including drugs). Skin reactions include:

- exfoliative dermatitis (inflamed, red and scaly skin which sloughs off; hyperkeratosis, pruritus and physiological dysfunctions; may take weeks or months to resolve; can be fatal)
- Stevens-Johnson syndrome (erythema multiforme): widespread skin lesions, may involve fever, haemorrhagic crusts, ocular lesions and multi-system involvement; can be life-threatening
- lupus erythematosus: autoimmune connective tissue disorder with red rash, joint swelling and pain, oral ulcers; renal, haematological, pulmonary and other systems may be affected; reversible when drug is stopped
- purpura: multiple small haemorrhages in the skin and mucous membranes
- urticaria: oedema and wheals due to vasodilation and increased capillary permeability; may be immune-mediated
- alopecia: lack or loss of hair from area where hair is normally present
- fixed drug eruptions: inflammatory skin lesion, often with itching or burning, that recurs at same site in response to administration of the drug, resolving after stopping the drug
- contact dermatitis or eczema: skin inflammation due to contact with a substance; may have allergic or irritant mechanism
- photosensitivity: abnormal response of skin to light at wavelengths 280–400 nm; it may be photoallergy or phototoxicity.

Some conditions can be life-threatening, with high fever, pharyngitis, neck stiffness and toxic epidermal necrolysis. Simply discontinuing a particular drug may resolve a complicated dermatological problem.

Chemicals causing skin disorders

Hundreds of chemicals have been implicated, including various plants, vegetables and fruits. Drug groups commonly involved are alkylating agents, androgenic hormones, anticoagulants, antiepileptic agents, antihistamines, antimetabolites, antiseptics, antitumour antibiotics, barbiturates, bismuth salts, cephalosporins, coal tars, corticosteroids, cosmetics, dyes, ergot alkaloids, gold salts, insulins, iodides, local anaesthetics, oils, opioids, oral contraceptives, penicillins, perfumes, phenothiazines, polyaromatic hydrocarbons (tattoo inks), porphyrins, psoralens, quinine antimalarials, salicylates, silver salts, sulfonamides, tetracyclines, thiazides, transdermal patches, tricyclic antidepressants and vaccines.

Application of drugs to the skin

Types of drugs used for the skin

The general objectives of treating skin disorders are to:

- identify and remove the cause of the skin disorder, if possible
- restore and maintain the normal structure and functions of the skin
- relieve symptoms that are produced by the disorder, such as itching, dryness, pain and inflammation.

So many dermatological products are available, both OTC and by prescription, that they cannot all be covered in this chapter. For the sake of simplicity, we discuss here specific dermatological products: sunscreens, topical antimicrobials and anti-inflammatories, retinoids and other drugs used to treat acne and agents used specifically for eczema, psoriasis, actinic keratoses, burns and wounds, ulcers and pressure sores.

The detailed pharmacology of some dermatological drugs has been discussed in previous chapters, as follows:

- corticosteroids in Chapters 29 and 34
- immunosuppressants, including calcineurin inhibitors, in Chapter 34
- vitamin D in Chapter 27
- antimicrobials in Chapters 36 and 37
- antineoplastic immunosuppressants in Chapter 33.

Other general dermatological products include astringents, cleansers, liniments, antiseptics, keratolytics, antiperspirants, antiseptics, antidandruff shampoos, bath oils and body washes, face washes for acne, freezing sprays (cryotherapy) for warts, skin lighteners and darkeners, filling agents for wrinkles and lips, medicated toothpastes, insect repellents, hair removers and hair restorers. (Strictly speaking, topical agents acting on mucous membranes could also be included, such as eyedrops and ointments, nasal drops and sprays, mouthwashes and even suppositories and enemas.)

Natural plant extracts and oils with some proven or claimed antiseptic properties include oils of melaleuca (tea tree), lemon, lemongrass, eucalyptus, clover leaf, thyme, pine, citronella and peppermint flowers and extract of aloe vera. Honey and pawpaw ointment are also used. Many of these products are available OTC in pharmacies and supermarkets.

Topical administration of drugs

Medications for most diseases are administered at a site distant from the target organ – for example, orally for systemic effects. In dermatology, medications can be administered:

- by **topical administration** directly to the target site (skin)
- systemically to treat skin disorders
- by application to the skin with the intention that lipid-soluble drugs will be absorbed into the systemic circulation to act at distant sites.

Drugs applied for local actions may be absorbed, and systemic effects and toxicity can occur.

How much to prescribe?

How much of a topical preparation is needed for one dose, or for 1 week's supply? This is less easy to estimate than the quantity of tablets or other solid dose forms. Current guidelines suggest that for a cream or ointment to cover an adult's face and neck would require about 1.25 g for one application, so twice-daily application for 10 days would require a 25–30 g tube of cream.

Some creams are provided in a tube with dose advised as centimetres of cream squeezed out; other prescribers might recommend 'enough to cover a 10-cent coin', or a 'fingertip unit' (Fig 39.1 and below).

Transcutaneous absorption of drugs

Most drugs are partially water-soluble (to dissolve readily in aqueous fluids such as blood plasma and extracellular fluids) and so do not readily penetrate unbroken skin; for a drug to be readily absorbed through the skin its lipid solubility must be high. Nicotine, hyoscine, estrogens, fentanyl and glyceryl trinitrate are lipid-soluble drugs formulated in ointments or patches for transdermal absorption; these are usually applied to soft skin such as on the inner arm or abdomen. Chemicals can also be absorbed unintentionally across the skin, with unexpected consequences.

Skin layers to be crossed

For **transcutaneous absorption** (also known as percutaneous absorption) of drugs into the bloodstream, the drugs must pass through the following layers of skin cells and membranes:

- surface layer of epidermis – passage across the stratum corneum, the outer and thickest layer, is the rate-limiting step
- dermis – anti-inflammatory agents, topical local anaesthetics and antipruritic (anti-itching) drugs act in these layers

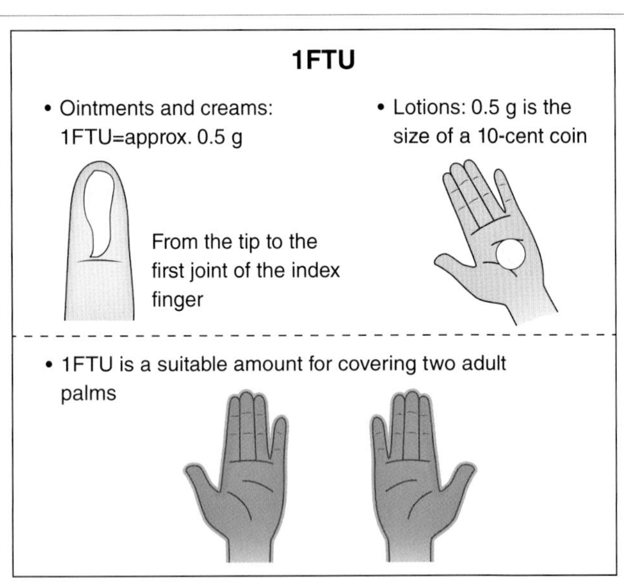

FIGURE 39.1 Topical corticosteroid application using the fingertip unit

- endothelial cells of skin blood vessels – very lipid-soluble drugs will pass through into the circulation.

Skin appendages (glands and hairs) can be affected by antiperspirants, depilatory agents (hair removers) and antimicrobials.

Factors affecting transcutaneous absorption

Absorption through the skin is slow, incomplete and variable (except for lipid-soluble agents). The extent of absorption depends on the following:

- *The person's age.* The skin of infants is very thin and delicate, and elderly people may also have thin, fragile skin; this can be both dangerous (fatalities have occurred after absorption of boric acid from baby powders) and advantageous (zinc can be absorbed from zinc cream to assist healing).
- *Lipid solubility.* Lipid-soluble drugs are better absorbed than water-soluble drugs.
- *The drug's molecular weight.* For passive absorption, MWt < 500 Da is necessary.
- *Skin condition and site.* The stratum corneum layers of the palms and soles are usually toughened and thickened so are not readily permeable; moistened, diseased or damaged skin is more permeable.
- *Hydration of skin.* Some medications are applied then covered with an occlusive dressing (e.g. plastic wrap, rubber gloves or shower cap; Fig 39.2) or administered in an occlusive vehicle (e.g. zinc cream or petroleum jelly); both will trap and prevent water loss from skin, enhancing blood circulation to the area and increasing its temperature and hydration.
- *Metabolism and circulation.* Wound healing is compromised, and ulcers may develop readily in people with poor peripheral circulation; 'rubbing in' a drug with a cream or ointment may enhance circulation to the area and penetration of the drug.
- *Vehicle in which the drug is administered.* The drug needs to leave the vehicle to be available for absorption; products with high alcohol content may be administered for drying and cooling effects after evaporation.

Permeation of larger and more water-soluble molecules is enhanced by physical methods such as iontophoresis, ultrasound and skin abrasion.

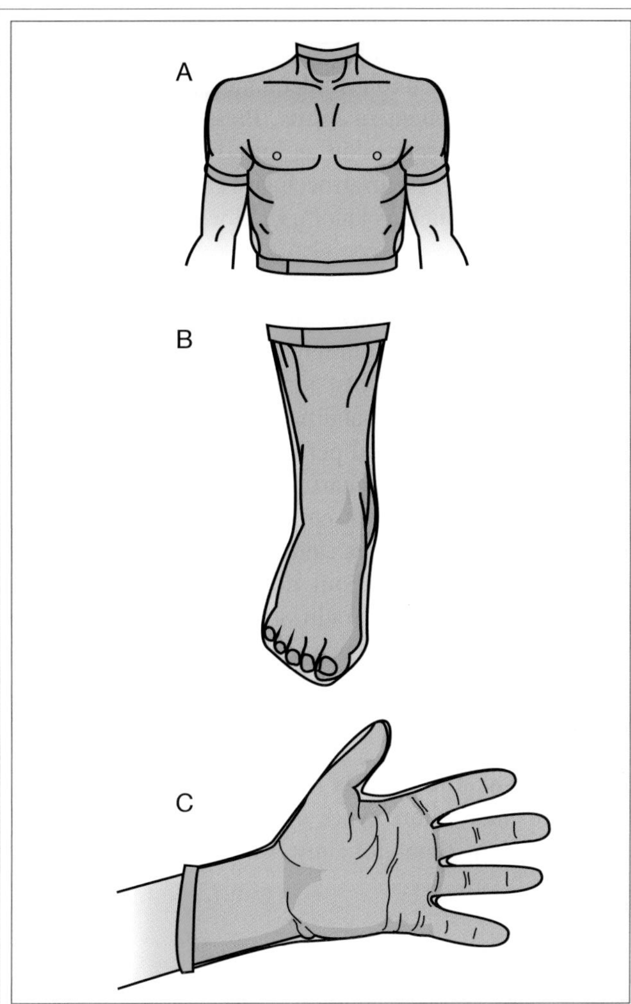

FIGURE 39.2 Examples of occlusive dressing to enhance hydration of particular areas of skin and transcutaneous absorption of drugs
A Plastic wrap applied to upper trunk. **B** Plastic wrap applied to foot. **C** Rubber glove applied to hand and sealed around wrist.

Formulations and medications for topical application

Vehicles and emulsions

The drug is dissolved or mixed into a **vehicle** – that is, the liquid or solid that carries the drug to the site of application on the skin. Many formulations are emulsions (liquid or semi-solid mixtures of aqueous and oily phases, with one phase as tiny droplets in the other).[1] A lipid-soluble drug such as estradiol (Drug Monograph 30.1), nicotine (Drug Monograph 25.4) or glyceryl trinitrate (Drug Monograph 11.1) distributes into the oily phase of an emulsion, whereas a water-soluble drug (diphenhydramine, lidocaine (lignocaine)) distributes into the aqueous phase. Microemulsions, with nanoparticle-sized droplets, are formulated to increase markedly the surface area for delivery of a drug to the skin.

Wet or dry preparations

Some topical formulations provide a useful effect without an active ingredient – simply rubbing in or dabbing on may

1 For example, milk is an oil-in-water emulsion. The tiny butterfat droplets distributed in water give milk its white colour. Don't believe a label that says low-fat milk is 'fat-free' – if it really were totally free of fat, it would look pale blue due to casein micelles.

have a warming or drying effect. Lesions heal better, with less scarring, when kept moist, so moist wound healing is encouraged – for example, under a medicated dressing (see later under 'Treatment of Burns, Pressure Sores and Leg Ulcers'). For dry, scaly skin as found in psoriasis or dry eczema, an ointment with an occlusive emollient (softening) effect is helpful, such as lanolin or zinc cream.

Multiple ingredients

Topical formulations may include a wide range of ingredients such as ointment or cream bases, water, preservatives, antioxidants, long-chain fatty acid esters and alcohols, plus suspending, thickening, emulsifying and colouring agents and perfumes, as well as the active drug: this is the field of pharmaceutics. For example, one commercial 'lip revitaliser' contains 38 listed ingredients plus flavours. (It has been said that calamine lotion may make a lot of mess without doing a lot of good. This could be true of many traditional topical preparations, which remain in pharmacopoeias without ever being subjected to controlled clinical trials of safety and efficacy.)

Formulations and agents A–Z

There are many more types of **formulations** for topical administration than for any other route; some are described below.

Antipruritic agents

Antipruritic (anti-itching) preparations include lotions and baths, containing calamine, phenol, menthol, pine tar, potassium permanganate, hydrocortisone, aluminium subacetate, boric acid, physiological saline, cornstarch or oatmeal. Local anaesthetics (benzocaine, lidocaine) can decrease pruritus but may induce allergic reactions; antihistamines are poorly absorbed topically. Water has antipruritic effects, and cools by evaporation.

Antiseptics

Antiseptics (skin disinfectants) reduce the skin's microbial flora; they are generally broad-spectrum but not active against spores (see later under 'Antimicrobials').

Astringents

Astringent solutions, applied topically, cause precipitation of proteins, vasoconstriction and reduced cell permeability – for example, aluminium acetate or calcium hydroxide solutions, calamine lotion, hamamelis (witch hazel), potassium permanganate and alcohol in aftershave lotions.

Cleansers

Soaps have cleansing and drying actions but are alkaline; soap-free cleansers are neutral or less alkaline so are less irritating for people with sensitive, dry or irritated skin.

'Cosmeceuticals'

These 'cosmetic' and 'pharmaceutical' preparations claim to reverse skin ageing. Preparations containing epidermal growth factors with antioxidants, skin conditioners and 'matrix-building agents' are sold at great expense, with little evidence of efficacy.

Creams and ointments

Creams and ointments are thick semi-solid preparations to be smoothed on to the skin; they have emollient and protective properties. They may be one phase (usually oily, as in ointments) or emulsions (creams). Water-in-oil (W/O) preparations, such as lanolin and cold cream, are greasy, occlusive and help retard water loss; they effectively deliver lipid-soluble drugs to the skin – for example, eye ointments containing antibiotics or anti-inflammatory agents. Oil-in-water (O/W) preparations, such as aqueous creams and vanishing creams, have cooling and moisturising effects, and are good vehicles for water-soluble drugs but are more easily washed off.

Emollients

Emollients are fatty or oily substances used to soften or soothe irritated skin or as a vehicle for other drugs; examples include lanolin, white soft paraffin (petroleum jelly, Vaseline), silicones, oils and sorbolene cream.

Gels

Gels are viscous, non-oily, water-miscible, semi-solid preparations containing gelling agents; they cool as the solvent evaporates leaving a film.

Glues

Skin glues (glue adhesives) are cyanoacrylate products (much like super glue) that are used to close short clean wounds not infected or under tension. They are typically used after vasectomy, laparoscopy and removal of benign skin lesions, and in children. Skin glues are safe, effective and cost-effective, being eventually sloughed off.

Keratolytics

Keratolytics (keratin dissolvers) such as salicylic acid (5–20%), resorcinol, alpha-hydroxy acids and urea soften skin squames (scales) and enhance penetration of other medicinal substances; they are used to treat psoriasis, eczema, ichthyosis, warts, corns, acne and dandruff. Newer formulations used to remove solar keratoses are diclofenac 3% gel, fluorouracil 5% cream or imiquimod 5% cream. In the treatment of dandruff (seborrhoeic dermatitis of the scalp), shampoos may contain pyrithione zinc, selenium sulfide and imidazole antifungals.

Keratoplastics

These stimulate the epidermis and thus cause thickening of the cornified layer; examples are coal tar and sulfur

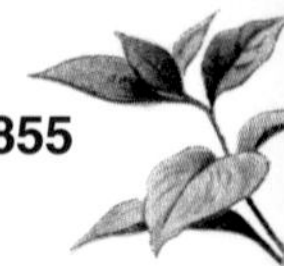

preparations, and low concentrations (1–2%) of salicylic acid.

Liniments and rubs

Liniments and rubs are applied to intact skin to relieve pain caused by muscle aches, neuralgia, arthritis and sprains. Simply massaging any oily substance into the skin has a rubefacient (reddening) effect by dilating skin blood vessels and may assist healing. Ingredients can include a counter-irritant (e.g. camphor or oil of cloves), antiseptic (chloroxylenol, eugenol, thymol), local anaesthetic (benzocaine) or anti-inflammatory analgesic (methyl salicylate, also known as oil of wintergreen).

Lotions and solutions

Liquid preparations used as wet dressings can be applied without pressure, producing soothing and cooling from evaporation. They may be mild acidic (boric acid) or alkaline (limewater) solutions. Aluminium acetate solution (Burow's solution) is a mild astringent that coagulates bacterial and serum protein. Calamine lotion is a suspension containing calamine (powdered mixture of zinc carbonate and ferric oxide), zinc oxide, bentonite (a suspending agent), phenol and glycerol in a sodium citrate solution; the insoluble powder is left on the skin as the solution dries. It is a soothing, mildly astringent lotion used for dermatitis caused by plants, insect bites, sunburn and prickly heat.

Moisturisers (humectants)

Moisturisers improve hydration of dry skin by retaining water, and are also used as vehicles to deliver drugs. They are similar to emollients, and include glycerin and glycols. Greasy moisturisers are more effective than aqueous bases.

Pastes

Pastes are very thick mixtures of solids in cream or ointment bases. Magnoplasm is a commercial magnesium sulfate and glycerin paste with high osmotic pressure, used to withdraw fluid from lesions such as boils.

Patches

A transdermal patch is an adhesive dressing with a reservoir of active drug incorporated behind a polymer membrane, designed to deliver potent lipid-soluble drugs such as glyceryl trinitrate (Drug Monograph 11.1), estradiol (Drug Monograph 30.2), fentanyl (Drug Monograph 19.2) or nicotine (Drug Monograph 25.4) at a specified rate. They eliminate variables affecting oral absorption, including ability to swallow, gastric emptying time, stomach acidity, presence of food and the first-pass effect and obviate the need for frequent oral dosing.

Powders

Powders are mixtures of finely divided drugs in a dry form; dusting powders based on talcum, zinc oxide or starch are intended for external application. They reduce friction and promote drying in body fold areas, and are used as vehicles for antimicrobial agents, especially antifungals for feet. Non-absorbable powders are also protectants; however, they adhere to wet surfaces and may have to be scraped off.

Preservatives

Preservatives are chemicals added to aqueous formulations to retard oxidation or microbial growth; common preservatives are hydroxybenzoates, alcohols, chlorocresol and benzalkonium chloride. They can frequently cause contact dermatitis.

Protectants

Skin protectants are soothing, cooling preparations that form a film on the skin, to coat minor skin irritations, protect the skin from chemical irritants and assist healing by preventing crusting and trauma. Examples are Compound Benzoin Tincture (see below) and collodion, a 5% solution of pyroxylin in a mixture of ether and alcohol; the solvents evaporate to leave a transparent film that adheres to skin.

Psoralens

Psoralens are plant constituents that induce pigmentation in skin. They are used to treat vitiligo (patchy whitening of the skin and hair). As photosensitising agents that absorb ultraviolet radiation (UVR), they are used to treat psoriasis. An example is methoxsalen (8-methoxypsoralen), given orally or applied as a lotion or wash, 1–2 hours before exposure to UVR in phototherapy procedures. Severe burning may result, and long-term adverse effects include premature skin ageing and skin cancers.

Rubefacients

'Rubefacient' means 'making red' – simply rubbing an inert lubricant into skin can cause a mild inflammatory response with vasodilation and warmth and thus acts as a counter-irritant to itch or pain.

Soaps

Ordinary soap, the sodium salt of palmitic, oleic or stearic acids, is made by saponifying fats or oils with alkalis. All soaps are relatively alkaline and are potential sources of skin irritation, as are added perfumes or antiseptics; they can be used in enemas.

Sprays

Sprays are fine mists or aerosols of drug in solution, often with a propellant gas. The vehicle evaporates and deposits drug on the skin or mucous membrane. Sprays are used commonly in the nose for administration of decongestants and antihistamines, and to administer drugs for systemic absorption, including hormones such as desmopressin (Drug Monograph 26.3).

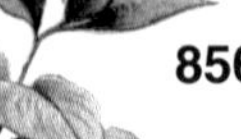

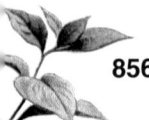

Tars

Extracts of coal tar, wood tar or bitumen – such as coal tar solution, dithranol and ichthammol – are old-fashioned dermatological remedies. They are mild irritants to the skin, suppress DNA synthesis and have antipruritic and antiseptic properties. They are used for dermatoses, including eczema, psoriasis and dandruff. Topically applied tars appear to be safe, whereas ingested or inhaled tars (from occupational exposure or cigarette smoking) can be carcinogenic. Tars should be kept away from sensitive areas such as the face, groin, eyes and mucous membranes; tar solutions stain the skin, hair and clothes, and may cause photosensitivity.

Tinctures

Tinctures are alcoholic solutions of chemicals or plant extracts; when applied, the alcohol evaporates. Alcohol has an astringent effect and can cause stinging on raw or damaged surfaces. Compound Tincture of Benzoin (Tinct Benz Co, Friar's Balsam) is an alcoholic solution of three balsams (dried plant exudates) and aloes. It is administered as a paint or spray for antiseptic, protective and styptic actions, and as an inhalation for upper respiratory tract infections.

Wet dressings

These include some of the preparations discussed under 'Lotions and solutions'. Wet or astringent, they are used to treat inflammations. Moist dressings impregnated with antiseptics, silver, collagen or honey are used to enhance wound healing (see later sections).

Zinc oxide

Zinc oxide has long been used in 'zinc cream' as a sunscreen; it is also useful for its astringent, soothing and protective properties in powders, ointments and lotions. Zinc is a required co-factor in healing, often effective in the treatment of mild inflammatory conditions, musculoskeletal pains, allergic reactions and nappy-rash in babies.

KEY POINTS

Application of drugs to the skin

- The main function of the skin is as a barrier to the external environment. It also contains sensory nerve endings, synthesises vitamin D and helps in body temperature regulation.
- The skin serves as the site for topical drug application for treating a variety of dermatological problems and can be used for administration of lipid-soluble drugs intended for transcutaneous absorption and systemic actions.
- Penetration of topical drugs into the skin, and absorption through the skin, are affected by the age, condition, hydration and site of the skin; the metabolism and skin circulation; the drug's molecular size and lipid solubility; and the vehicle in which the drug is formulated.
- A wide variety of pathological conditions affects the skin; most are due to infection, excessive inflammatory or immune responses, or reactions to sun exposure. Examples are fungal and viral infections, acne vulgaris, eczema and dermatitis, psoriasis, urticaria, sunburn and skin cancers.
- Drugs, given either topically or systemically, can cause adverse reactions in the skin, such as urticaria, purpura, fixed eruptions, dermatitis or eczema, and photosensitisation.
- There are numerous formulations for administration of drugs to the skin; they include creams and ointments, lotions and solutions, skin protectants and emollients, wet dressings and soaks, rubs and liniments, pastes, patches, powders and sprays. Many contain several ingredients and are available OTC.
- Therapeutic agents applied topically for actions on or in the skin include sunscreens, antimicrobials (antibiotics, antivirals, antifungals and ectoparasiticidal drugs), corticosteroids and other immunosuppressants, keratolytics, acne products, burn products, antipruritics and wound dressings and treatments for skin ulcers and pressure sores.

Sunscreen preparations

Skin damage from the sun

Phototoxicity and photoallergy reactions

Phototoxicity is an excessive response to solar radiation occurring in the presence of a photosensitising agent, such as chemicals (dyes, cosmetics), plants and drugs (sun-tanning preparations, tetracyclines, estrogens, sulfonamides, thiazides and phenothiazines), when the inducing agent in the skin is exposed to sunlight. The radiation energy produces a reactive molecule or free radical destructive to cell membranes or lysosomes. Exposed skin becomes red, painful or 'burning', with peak skin reaction reached within 24–48 hours. This reaction does not involve the immune system but resembles excessive sunburn.

Phytophotodermatitis is a common phototoxic inflammatory skin reaction resulting from contact with plant-derived sensitising psoralens followed by exposure to sunlight, especially UVA (long wavelength ultraviolet light). Plants implicated include parsley, celery, carrots, citrus species and figs.

A photoallergy reaction is less common; it requires prior exposure to a photosensitising agent that is activated to an allergen or hapten by UV radiation, causing a delayed hypersensitivity reaction presenting as pruritus and a rash that can spread to skin areas not exposed to sunlight.

Ultraviolet radiation damage

Extended exposure to the sun from sunbathing, outdoor occupation or lifestyle can cause sunburn, premature ageing of skin, immunosuppression and skin disorders including cancers. The damage is caused by solar **ultraviolet radiation**, comprising electromagnetic radiation with wavelengths shorter than those of visible light (at the violet end of the colour spectrum) and longer than those of x-rays. Very little UVR is blocked by cloud cover, although infrared radiation contributing to heating is reduced, giving a false sense of security against sunburn. The sun's rays can be reflected on to skin from water, concrete, snow and sand, but are deflected by the earth's atmosphere and by sweat; hence, sunburn is worse at high altitudes and in dry conditions.

Effects of UVR

UVR has useful effects in activating sterols to vitamin D compounds and has been used to treat acne and neonatal jaundice (and thus prevent kernicterus and permanent brain damage). UVR damages DNA strands by causing thymine bases to link in dimers, and causes mutations in the tumour-suppressor gene p53. Excessive exposure to UVR results in skin damage that progresses from minor irritations, blistering, skin darkening (tanning) and thickening, through severe sunburn to a precancerous skin condition and skin cancer later in life (Clinical Focus Box 39.1)).

CLINICAL FOCUS BOX 39.1
Sunburn, skin cancer and sun protection factors

Incidence

Skin cancers mainly comprise malignant melanomas (5%) and non-melanocytic (keratinocyte) skin cancers (NMSC): basal (BCC; 80%) and squamous cell (SCC; 15%) carcinomas. Skin cancer accounts for the largest number of cancers diagnosed in Australia each year: two out of three people who live their lives in Australia will require treatment for at least one skin cancer. Malignant melanoma has been associated with excessive sun exposure, especially during childhood, whereas large cumulative UVR over a lifetime increases incidence of NMSCs. There is a 10–20-year delay between UVR exposure (especially UVB) and the appearance of skin cancer.

Melanoma has been called the Australian cancer. Because of the largely fair-skinned populations, excessive sun exposure, our relatively clean air and lack of cloud cover, Australia and New Zealand have the highest rates of incidence and mortality from melanoma in the world. In the 15–24 age group in Australia, melanomas are the most common cancers. Most melanomas are cured through early detection and surgery, but more than 1600 Australians die of them each year.

Prevalence of NMSCs is less certain because they may be treated by GPs without numbers being notified to a central cancer registry. BCC and SCC are almost twice as common in men as in women, as they are associated with occupational sun exposure.

Actinic keratosis (solar keratosis) is a common condition of epidermal dysplasia appearing on skin chronically exposed to solar radiation, such as the head, scalp, face, forearms and backs of the hands, primarily in people with fair skin. In Australia, actinic keratosis is found in 40–50% of the Caucasian population over the age of 40 years.

Preventive measures

The primary method of protection is avoiding sunburns, especially in childhood and adolescence. Outdoor activities should be avoided when the sun is strongest ('from 11 to 3, stay under a tree'), protective clothing worn (broad-brimmed hat and long sleeves) and shade sought. A broad-spectrum sunscreen that blocks exposure to UVA and UVB (sun protection factor 30^{+} or 50^{+}) should be applied liberally and reapplied every 2 hours and after swimming, vigorous activity and towelling dry.

UVR can also increase the risk for cataracts and other eye disorders, and can suppress the immune system. Sunglasses that block 99–100% of UVR should be worn, especially by people with pale-coloured eyes.

Treatment measures

Treatment depends on the type, site, size and stage of skin tumour; the age and condition of the person; and facilities and skills of the doctor. Surgical excision is most common. NMSCs inaccessible by surgery may be treated with radiotherapy, curettage, cryotherapy and topical treatment with retinoids, antibiotics, powerful keratolytics and cytotoxic agents. Lifelong follow-up is required, as patients are at greater risk of recurrence and further primary tumours. BRAF inhibitors are showing promise in the treatment of melanomas (Ch 35). Actinic keratoses, which can potentially develop into SCCs, are sometimes treated topically with diclofenac 3% gel, fluorouracil or imiquimod 5% creams, methyl aminolevulinate 16% cream plus photodynamic therapy, 5-aminolevulinic acid patches.

Sources: Australian Medicines Handbook 2021; Melanoma Institute Australia – see 'Online resources'.

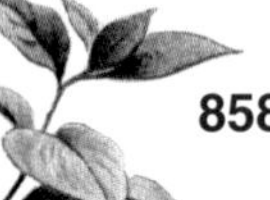

UVR spectrum: 'UVA ages, UVB burns'

UVA has long wavelengths (400–320 nm) and is closest to visible light; it can pass through glass and penetrate into the dermis (have you ever been sunburnt while driving long distances in a car?). It causes indirect DNA damage, produces darkening of preformed melanin in the epidermis, results in a light suntan, contributes to skin cancer via immunosuppression and is responsible for photo-ageing and many photosensitivity reactions. (This is the wavelength formerly used in commercial solariums.)

UVB has wavelengths of 320–290 nm. It is associated with vitamin D3 synthesis, causes erythema and sunburn, contributes to photo-ageing, directly damages DNA and is responsible for skin cancer induction. Around 90% of UVB has in the past been blocked by the earth's ozone layer; hence, worldwide concern that 'holes' in the ozone layer (caused by environmental pollutants and 'greenhouse gases' such as chlorofluorocarbons) will allow passage of more solar UVB and increase the incidence of skin cancers.

Most of the UVC from the sun (wavelength 290–200 nm) does not reach the earth's surface. Exposure to UVC is usually from artificial sources such as mercury lamps and arc-welding. UVC can cause retinal damage and erythema but will not stimulate tanning.

Why skin ages

UVA induces age-associated changes in skin via mitochondrial damage, oxygen free radicals and protein oxidation, reduction in transforming growth factor and DNA and collagen damage, leading to reduced elasticity. Clinical signs include dryness, irregular darkened pigmentation, deep furrows and leathery appearance. Eating foods rich in antioxidants may delay ageing processes, but creams and ointments merely plump up the outer layers of skin.

Sunscreens

Organics (absorbers) and inorganics (reflectors)

Sunscreen preparations are applied to absorb and/or to reflect UVR, to reduce the risks of photo-ageing, sunburn, actinic keratoses and skin cancers; they reduce p53 mutations and formation of reactive oxygen species. In this context, 'broad spectrum' refers to sunscreens that block both UVA and UVB.

Some *organic* chemicals (previously known as *absorbers*) absorb and block at least 85% of the UVB: examples are *p*-aminobenzoic acid (PABA) derivatives, benzophenones (which absorb both UVA and UVB), cinnamates, some salicylates, camphors and anthranilates (Yap et al. 2017) (see also Table 39.1). Some can cause allergic or irritant contact dermatitis.

Inorganics (reflectors) such as titanium dioxide and zinc oxide reflect and scatter UVB and UVA but do not absorb it. Normally opaque (e.g. zinc 'cream', actually thick white paste) unless in nanoparticle form,[2] they must be applied heavily to physically block out the UVR; thus, they are not readily cosmetically acceptable.

2 The term 'nanotechnology' refers to controlling matter at the nanometre (nm) level; a nanometre is one-billionth of a metre, 10^{-9} m. One nm is about 7 or 8 carbon-carbon bond lengths; a DNA double-helix has a diameter of about 2 nm; thus, nanotech concerns matter on the scale of atoms and molecules. Very different physical properties can be expected, as surface tension is more important than gravity and particles are small enough to pass readily into cells and even into the nucleus.

TABLE 39.1 Properties of some sunscreen agents

SUNSCREEN AGENT	RANGE OF PROTECTION	DIS/ADVANTAGES	SOLUBILITY	ALLERGY RISK
4-methylbenzylidene camphor	UVB	Endocrine (animals); systemic absorption	Ethanol	High
Bemotrizinol	UVA2, UVB	No endocrine effects	Oil	
Butyl methoxydibenzoyl methane	UVA1, UVA2, UVB	Low systemic bioavailability	N/A	High
Diethylaminohydroxy-benzoylhexyl-benzoate	UVA1		Oil	
Homosalate	UVB	Endocrine (animals)	Oil	Medium
Octocrylene	UVA2, UVB	High risk of photoallergy in children		High
Octyl methoxycinnamate	UVB	Endocrine (animals); systemic absorption	Oil	Low
Octyl salicylate	UVB	Low penetration through skin		Low
Octyl triazone	UVB	Strong UV absorber	Oil	Low
Oxybenzone	UVA2, UVB	Endocrine (animals); systemic absorption	Oil-in-water emulsion	High
Titanium dioxide	UVA2, UVB	Non-toxic, non-irritant, hypoallergenic	Hydro- and lipophilic	No
Zinc oxide	UVA, UVB	Non-toxic, non-irritant, hypoallergenic	Hydro- and lipophilic	No

UVR ranges: UVA1: 340–400 nm; UVA2: 320–340 nm; UVB: 290–320 nm; Endocrine (animals): some evidence of endocrine disrupting effects in animal studies.

Source: Yap, F.H., H.C. Chua, and C.P. Tait, Active sunscreen ingredients in Australia. Australasian Journal of Dermatology, 2017. 58(4): p. e160–e170.

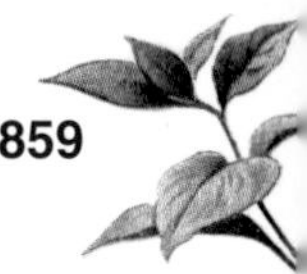

Many sunscreens contain multiple agents. For example, the Cancer Council of Australia's *Ultra Cooling Sunscreen SPF50+* contains: homosalate 100 mg/g, octyl salicylate 50 mg/g, butyl methoxydibenzoylmethane 40 mg/g and octocrylene 80 mg/g; it is advertised as providing 'broad spectrum UVA and UVB protection; 4 hours water resistant'.

Nanoparticles in sunscreens

Both types of agents (absorbers and reflectors) may also be formulated as nano-sized particles in sunscreens; 'micronised' products are less opaquely white, and hence are more cosmetically acceptable. Most studies show that insoluble **nanoparticles**, such as titanium and zinc oxides, do not penetrate human skin or hair follicles and are non-toxic, and that the known benefits clearly outweigh the risks. Consequently, the Australian Therapeutic Goods Administration (TGA) does not require that warnings about nanoparticles be placed on labels of such products.[3]

Sun protection factors

The **sun protection factor** (SPF) is a value given to a sunscreen preparation to indicate its effectiveness due to the included sunscreening agents. The SPF for a product is the ratio between the dose of UVR required to cause erythema (reddening) with and without the sunscreen. This is expressed as the minimal erythemal dose (MED): if a person experiences 1 MED with 25 units of UVR (in an unprotected state) and after application of a sunscreen requires 250 units of radiation to produce the same reddening, then this product has an SPF rating of 10. In Australia, sunscreens are regulated by the TGA and are assessed for safety, quality and efficacy. Current Australian regulatory guidelines (2021) classify SPF categories as low (SPF 4–10), medium (SPF 15–25), high (SPF 30–50) and very high (SPF 50+) (Therapeutic Goods Administration – see 'Online resources').

Water resistance of sunscreens

The efficacy of a sunscreen agent depends on its ability to remain effective during vigorous exercise, sweating and swimming. The test for water resistance excludes vigorous water jets or towelling-off, so water-resistance ratings may overstate effectiveness. Water resistance is largely dependent on the vehicle in the product – in particular, how water-soluble it is; thus oil-based lotions and creams are likely to remain on the skin longer while swimming or sweating than are O/W creams or lotions.

Choice and application of sunscreens

Sunscreen is chosen according to skin type, length of time in the sun, whether water resistance is important, the usual intensity of the sun's rays in the geographic area and the type of formulation preferred. The higher the SPF of product used, the longer a person takes to burn or develop a tan. However, real-life SPF does not necessarily mimic laboratory SPF, due to factors such as frequency, thickness and method of application; skin thickness, colour, type and anatomical site; individual sensitivity and vehicle in formulation. Dermatologists recommend that 'Consumers should select sunscreens that are broad spectrum SPF 50+, ... photostable and in a vehicle that improves compliance ... to protect us from photoageing and photocarcinogenesis' (Yap et al. 2017).

Generally, Australians do not use enough sunscreen: studies show that most people only apply one-quarter to one-half the recommended amount, hence the theoretical SPF is rarely achieved, and people get sunburnt despite applying sunscreen. Sunscreens are dated products and may lose efficacy if kept after their use-by date. There is now a 'SunSmart app' that can be consulted for advice on how much sunscreen is needed.

Sunscreens should be liberally applied to all exposed body areas (except eyelids) 30 minutes before exposure and reapplied every 2 hours, depending on factors such as the product used (the SPF and water resistance category), activity and sweating levels, time of day, cloud cover and reflections. Spray-on sunscreens, while seemingly easy to apply, cannot be applied near eyes, may blow away and are rarely applied in effective amounts. The Australian Cancer Council has ceased manufacture of its brand, and strongly recommends against relying on aerosol sunscreens.

It is recommended that people stay out of the sun when UVR is at its highest intensity (between 11 am and 3 pm daylight saving time). Infants should be kept out of the sun; children older than 6 months should always wear protective clothing, hats and sunscreens with high SPF. It has been projected that consistent use of medium–high SPF products from 6 months through to 18 years of age will result in about 80% reduction in the risk of skin cancer over a person's lifetime.

Sunscreens and low vitamin D

'There is a delicate line between balancing the beneficial effects of sunlight exposure while avoiding its damaging effects' (Stalgis-Bilinski et al. 2011), and this is particularly true for fair-skinned people in Australia. There is an increasing incidence of vitamin D deficiency in Australia and New Zealand (Ch 27). It is estimated that 30–48% of adults are vitamin D deficient (25(OH)D concentrations < 50 nmol/L). This is partly due to prevention of solar activation of vitamin D in the skin, by people wearing

3 In 2011, the TGA forced the manufacturer of a 'nanoparticle-free' sunscreen to withdraw advertising that implied its product was safer than rival sunscreens that contained 'potentially dangerous ingredients ... unsuitable for children'; the TGA said that the advertisement undermined the key message that people should select a broad-spectrum SPF 30+ sunscreen.

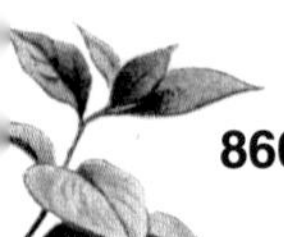

long covering clothing and veils, and using shade, hats and sunscreens. The prevalence of vitamin D deficiency is also high in institutionalised elderly people. The Dermatology Expert Group advises that 'fair-skinned Australians should be able to maintain adequate vitamin D concentrations with 10 minutes of sun exposure to the face, arms and hands on most days of the week during summer, and for 2–3 hours per week over winter … People who receive little sunlight should be investigated for vitamin D deficiency and when present, supplemental vitamin D should be offered.'

KEY POINTS

Sunscreen preparations

- Exposure to the sun – in particular, to UVR in the UVA and B wavelength ranges – causes major harm to the skin, ranging from sensitisation, allergies, ageing, reddening and burning through to benign and malignant skin cancers.
- Chemicals used in sunscreens may act by either absorbing particular UVR (e.g. organics: aminobenzoates and benzophenones) or reflecting UVR (inorganics: zinc and titanium oxides).
- Sunscreens are given SPF numbers, indicating their protective capacities; people who burn easily should use a non-aerosol product with SPF 30+ or 50+.

Topical antimicrobial agents

Antimicrobial therapy of skin infections

Antimicrobials used on the skin or to treat skin infections include antibacterial, antiviral, antifungal and antiparasitic agents. There is an increasing problem worldwide with organisms developing resistance to antimicrobials; hence, concerted efforts are being made to encourage the judicious prescribing of broad-spectrum antibiotics and only to use drugs against organisms sensitive to them.

Antimicrobials used topically are preferably not the same as those used systemically, both to minimise the risk of development of resistance and to use drugs that may be toxic systemically but not topically. In some severe infections – for example, fungal nail infections or acne resistant to topical treatment – systemic oral antimicrobials may be required.

(All antimicrobial drug groups [except those used to treat parasitic infestations, acne, nail infections and warts] have been covered in detail in Chs 35–38, so only summaries will be given here.)

Antibacterial agents

The common bacterial skin flora *Streptococcus pyogenes* and *Staphylococcus aureus* cause folliculitis, impetigo, furuncles and carbuncles (boils) and cellulitis. The following antibacterials are used topically:

- *mupirocin:* used to treat mild impetigo and the nasal carrier status caused by *S. aureus* and β-haemolytic streptococci; usually applied as a 2% cream or ointment to affected areas three times daily for up to 10 days
- *sodium fusidate:* 2% ointment for staphylococcal skin infections; preferably saved for oral use to reduce risk of resistance developing
- *silver sulfadiazine:* 1% cream, especially for burns (see later)
- *clindamycin:* 1% gel, liquid or lotion used in acne (see later)
- *gramicidin, metronidazole and erythromycin:* used in acne and other skin infections
- *chloramphenicol and aminoglycosides (framycetin, neomycin, gentamicin):* used in antibiotic eyedrops or eardrops (Ch 40)
- *retapamulin:* a new pleuromutilin antibiotic formulated as 1% ointment, indicated in treatment of impetigo and other infected dermatoses and wounds.

  (See Ch 36 for mechanisms and adverse effects.)

Antiseptics

Many topical preparations containing simple antiseptics are available OTC as first-aid products to help prevent infection in minor burns or injuries. Antiseptics (skin disinfectants) are solutions or creams of antimicrobial agents applied topically to the skin; they are effective as detergents or solubilising agents but are too toxic to be administered internally. Examples include benzalkonium chloride, triclosan, chlorhexidine, cetrimide, povidone–iodine and hypochlorite solutions. Plant products such as aloes, benzoin and oils of melaleuca, lemon, clove, thyme and lemongrass have mild antiseptic properties.

Antiviral agents

Only three antivirals are commonly used topically: aciclovir (5% cream; Drug Monograph 37.1), penciclovir (1% cream) and idoxuridine (0.5% cream with lidocaine 2%) are used to treat cutaneous herpes simplex infections of the lips ('cold sores'). In immunocompromised people, systemic antiviral treatment is more effective. The dosage is enough for adequate covering of the lesions with cream, from as early as possible in the infection, several times a day until the lesion disappears. Adverse reactions from topical application of aciclovir or idoxuridine include hypersensitivity reactions, pruritus and stinging (see Ch 37 for mechanisms).

Treatment of warts

Although warts are caused by a virus (human papillomavirus; HPV), they are not treated with specific antiviral drugs. Warts are usually overcome by the body's immune defences and resolve without treatment. In immunocompromised people, they can become extensive and may develop into SCCs.

- Anogenital warts in young people are predominantly transmitted by sexual intercourse. The condition can undergo malignant transformation, and in women there is a strong association with cervical cancer. There is now an effective vaccine against HPV (Ch 43).
- Cutaneous wart treatment depends on the site and extent of spread. Keratolytics, such as salicylic acid and trichloroacetic acid, and topical antimicrobials, including podophyllotoxin and glutaraldehyde, have been used.
- Non-pharmacological treatments include curettage, electrosurgery and cryotherapy with liquid nitrogen or solid carbon dioxide.
- Imiquimod is used for treating external genital and perianal warts; it acts via agonist activity at toll-like receptor-7 to enhance the body's immune response. (It has also been approved for topical use in solar keratoses and some NMSCs.) For anogenital warts, a 5% cream is applied topically at night and left on for 6–10 hours, 3 nights per week for a maximum of 16 weeks; severe inflammatory responses are possible.

Podophyllotoxin is also used to treat external genital and perianal warts; it acts by binding to tubulin, arresting mitosis and leading to cell death. It is applied twice a day for 3 days, followed by no treatment for 4 days. This process is repeated for up to five cycles.

Antifungal agents

Three pathogenic fungi (dermatophytes) can cause superficial fungal infections: *Microsporum*, *Trichophyton* and *Epidermophyton*; the yeast *Candida albicans* can also cause infections. (Systemic mycoses usually occur only in severely immunocompromised people.) Dermatophytes exist in moist, warm environments such as skin areas covered by shoes and socks (tinea pedis, or athlete's foot), or in the groin, scalp or trunk. The fungi invade the stratum corneum and cause inflammation and sensitivity. Spread of fungi via shed skin occurs by contact, commonly around swimming pools or bathrooms; hygiene measures such as wearing rubber thongs in communal change-rooms and showers, and drying skin well (especially between the toes), help reduce the risk of infection. Before starting treatment, skin or nail scrapings should be taken for microscopic identification of the causative organism. Treatment may be required for many months, and relapse after cessation is common. Systemic drug administration is required for widespread and unresponsive infections.

Foot infections are dangerous in people with diabetes, as fungal infections can lead to bacterial infections, gangrene and amputations (Ch 28). Onychomycoses (fungal infections of toenails) are particularly resistant to treatment by usual topical or oral formulations but are a predictor of foot ulcers, so early intervention and good foot care are critical. Medicated nail varnishes have been developed: amorolfine 5% and ciclopirox 8%.

Topical antifungals

The primary topical **antifungals** include the (imid)azole group (clotrimazole, ketoconazole, miconazole, etc.), terbinafine and amorolfine (Drug Monograph 39.1), and miscellaneous antifungal agents including undecenoic acid, benzoic, salicylic and propionic acid products, tolnaftate, the antibiotics nystatin and ciclopirox, povidone–iodine and a variety of antifungal combination creams, ointments, powders, sprays, liquids and paints.

Table 39.2 summarises the generic names, formulation type and strength and properties of some topical antifungals. Adverse reactions with the use of the topical antifungals are generally mild and include local irritation, pruritus, erythema and stinging. Systemic azole antifungals are infamous for causing drug interactions because they inhibit many cytochrome P450 enzymes and thereby inhibit the metabolism of many drugs metabolised in the liver. (See Ch 37 for individual mechanisms, interactions and adverse effects.)

Drugs against lice and mites

Ectoparasites are insects that live on the outer surface of the body. Ectoparasiticides are drugs used against these parasites. They include pediculicides (against lice) and scabicides or acaricides (against mites).

Treatment of pediculosis (lice infestation)

Pediculosis is a parasite infestation of lice on the skin. Lice are transmitted by close contact with infested people, clothing, combs and towels. They may infest the general body skin, pubic area or head and hair. Common findings in a person who is infested include pruritus (itching), nits (eggs of lice) on hair shafts and lice on skin or clothes (especially in seams in the axillae [armpits], beltline or collar regions).

Pediculicides

The drugs of choice are permethrin and malathion (maldison). Local public health officers or school nurses usually recommend the current treatment regimen,

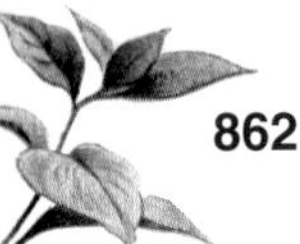

Drug Monograph 39.1
Amorolfine nail lacquer

Mechanism and actions
Amorolfine has fungistatic and fungicidal actions against a broad spectrum of yeasts, dermatophytes and other fungi and moulds. It impairs sterol synthesis in fungal cell membranes and is active both orally and topically (Ch 37).

Indications
Amorolfine nail varnish is indicated for topical treatment of onychomycoses; it alleviates or cures 70–80% of cases.

Pharmacokinetics
Amorolfine is very lipophilic but is virtually insoluble in intestinal fluids. After application to the nail, it penetrates and diffuses through the nail plate and can reach measurable levels in the blood.

Adverse reactions
Because fungal sterols are different from those in mammalian cells, there are few adverse effects. Occasionally, itching and burning sensations are felt; nail discolouration and allergic reactions are rare. In animal studies, high oral doses caused cataract formation.

Drug interactions
There are no known drug interactions; patients are advised not to use any other nail preparations (polishes, artificial nails) during treatment.

Warnings and contraindications
Amorolfine is contraindicated if a previous hypersensitivity to it has occurred. Users are warned not to apply the varnish to the skin beside the nails. There is little information on the use of this product in pregnant or lactating women or in children, so its use in these people is not recommended.

Dosage and administration
Amorolfine is supplied as a 5% solution in a 5 mL nail lacquer base; also included in the kit are cleaning pads, nail files and spatulas to be used in applying the varnish. The varnish is applied one to two times weekly after first cleaning the nail and filing it down (including the nail surface) to remove as much infected nail as possible. Before next application, remaining varnish is cleaned off and the nail filed down again. The process needs to be continued for about 6 months for fingernails and 12 months for toenails.

TABLE 39.2 Some topical antifungal agents

NAME	STRENGTH	FORMULATION[a]	SPECIAL COMMENTS
Azoles			
Bifonazole	1%	C	Broad-spectrum antifungal agent; also packaged with 40% urea ointment for nail infections
Clotrimazole	1%	C, L	Broad-spectrum antifungal agent; also 1% cream with hydrocortisone 1% for inflamed fungal infections
Econazole	1%	C, L	Broad-spectrum antifungal agent
Ketoconazole	1%, 2%	C, Sh	Broad-spectrum antifungal agent
Miconazole	2%	C, L, O, P, S, Sh, T	Used for tinea pedis (athlete's foot), tinea cruris, tinea corporis and tinea versicolor; also as cream with hydrocortisone (0.5%, 1%) or ointment with zinc oxide (15%)
Other antifungals			
Amorolfine	5%	NV	Fungicidal/static; onychomycoses (fungal nail infections)
Ciclopirox	1.5% (Sh); 8% (NV)	NV, Sh	Mechanism not well understood; impairs DNA repair, mitosis and transport processes in fungi; for seborrhoeic dermatitis/onychomycosis
Nystatin	100,000 U/g	C, O	Fungicidal/fungistatic antibiotic; for *Candida* infections
Selenium sulfide	1%, 2.5%		For tinea capitis and pityriasis versicolor
Terbinafine	1%	C, G, L, S	Fungicidal/static; tinea, *Candida* infections
Tolnaftate	0.07–1%	C, O, P, S	Used for fungal skin infections including tinea
Undecenoic acid/ zinc undecenoate	1%, 5%/25%	L, P	Antifungal and antibacterial agent for athlete's foot and ringworm (not on hairy sites); and for nappy rash, prickly heat, minor skin irritations, jock itch, excessive perspiration

[a] Formulations: C = cream; G = gel; L = lotion or liquid; NV = nail varnish; O = ointment; P = powder; S = spray; Sh = shampoo; T = tincture

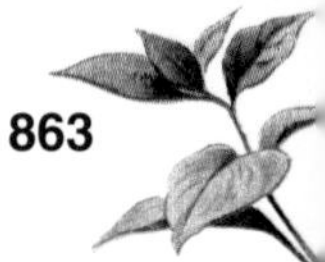

including using medicated shampoo and combing the hair with a fine-tooth comb to remove nits. Affected family members may also require treatment, and hairbrushes, hats, clothing and bedding require cleaning. Different regimens are needed to treat pubic lice.

Permethrin acts on the nerve cell membranes of lice, ticks, mites and fleas, disrupting sodium channel depolarisation, thus paralysing the parasites. It has a high cure rate (up to 99%) in treating head lice after application of 1% lotion or shampoo, left in for 10 minutes, then repeated after 1 week. The most common adverse reactions include pruritus, mild burning on application and transient erythema. Permethrin is also used to impregnate clothing and nets with repellent.

Malathion (maldison) is an organophosphate cholinesterase inhibitor for treating head lice and nits; it is relatively non-toxic to humans and usually effective within 24 hours. Malathion (maldison) lotion 0.5%/foam 1% is rubbed into the scalp and left for 12 hours/30 minutes; repeated after 7–10 days. Because the drug is flammable, the person must be warned to avoid open flames and smoking and not to use a hairdryer.

Older examples of pediculicides are benzyl alcohol, dimeticone, isopropyl myristate and the allethrins and natural pyrethrins found in chrysanthemum flowers (related to permethrin).

Treatment of scabies (mite infestation)

Scabies is a parasitic infestation caused by the itch mite *Sarcoptes scabiei*. It is an obligate parasite of humans and is transmitted by close contact with an infested person. It bores into the horny layers of the skin in cracks and folds (almost exclusively at night), causing irritation and pruritus. The infestation in adults is usually generalised over the body, especially in web spaces between fingers, wrists, elbows and buttocks.

Acaricides

The acaricide of choice is permethrin 5% cream or lotion, two applications 1 week apart (considered more effective than crotamiton or benzyl benzoate). Family members and close contacts should also be treated, and items such as bedding, clothes and soft toys sprayed. Benzyl benzoate is also used as an insect repellent; clothes or mosquito nets can be soaked in a solution and dried.

KEY POINTS

Topical antimicrobial agents

- Antimicrobials used topically for skin infections should be those that are not administered systemically.
- Antibacterial antibiotics frequently prescribed for topical use include clindamycin and mupirocin.
- For herpes simplex viral infections, aciclovir and idoxuridine are available topically.
- Fungal skin infections, particularly of moist areas of skin or of finger- and toenails, can be difficult to eradicate. Topical preparations of antifungals available include imidazoles, and terbinafine and amorolfine. Severe infections may require systemic antifungal therapy.
- Skin infestations with insects (lice and mites) cause severe itching; permethrin or malathion (maldison) can be applied as a shampoo, lotion or cream.

Anti-inflammatory and immunomodulating agents

Many conditions manifested in the skin involve inflammatory or autoimmune pathological processes, so drugs that modify these responses are widely used to target cytokines, receptors and inflammatory cells. Most commonly used topically are the corticosteroids; other topical immunosuppressants include newer 'immunobiological agents' such as pimecrolimus. For optimal efficacy, the drugs should penetrate into the deeper layers of the skin but not be absorbed into the systemic circulation, to avoid systemic adverse effects. In severe cases of inflammatory or autoimmune dermatological conditions, it may be necessary to administer ciclosporin, methotrexate, infliximab or etanercept systemically.

Corticosteroids

Actions and uses

Corticosteroids are used topically for their anti-inflammatory, antipruritic, vasoconstrictor, antiproliferative (antimitotic) and immunosuppressant actions in various types of **dermatitis** (eczema) and psoriasis, in skin reactions to insect bites and for sunburn. The mechanisms, actions, indications, adverse effects and interactions of these drugs are discussed in greater detail in Chapters 29 and 34.

Topical formulations and potencies

Corticosteroids are available in a wide range of topical formulations that are stable, easy to apply and rapid-acting, causing no pain, discolouration or odour on application. Combination preparations with antifungal or antibacterial antibiotics are also available for use in inflammatory dermatitis with infection.

The vehicle in which the corticosteroid is formulated can alter the therapeutic efficacy: penetration into skin is enhanced by (in decreasing order of effectiveness) ointments, gels, creams and lotions. Lotions, sprays and gels are suited to hairy areas or for lesions that are oozing and wet. Creams and ointments are suited to dry, scaling, thickened and pruritic areas. Inflamed or moist skin absorbs topical steroids to a greater degree than thick or lichenified skin. **Occlusive dressings** (Fig 39.1) increase drug penetration up to 100-fold, making systemic adverse effects more likely.

Fluorinated corticosteroids are particularly recommended for topical application to thickened skin and in severe inflammations because of their potency, lipid solubility (hence topical efficacy) and low tendency to cause sodium retention. In decreasing order of potency, some topical corticosteroids and typical formulations are:

- betamethasone[f], 0.02–0.1% cream or ointment
- clobetasone[f], 0.05% cream or shampoo; mometasone, 0.1% cream, ointment, gel or lotion; methylprednisolone, 0.1% cream, lotion or ointment
- triamcinolone[f], 0.02% cream or ointment; desonide[f], 0.05% lotion
- hydrocortisone, 0.5–1% cream, ointment, spray.

(Those marked [f] are fluorinated compounds; potencies can vary depending on the ester form and strength of formulation.)

Acute inflammatory eruptions usually respond to the medium- and low-potency steroids, whereas chronic hyperkeratotic lesions such as eczema and psoriasis require potent or highly potent drugs.

Dosage and adverse drug reactions

Topical corticosteroids should be applied 'sparingly'. There is a general rule of thumb, or should we say 'fingertip', to describe what is meant by this. To cover an area of skin the size of two adult hands (palm and digits), a fingertip unit (FTU) of corticosteroid should be applied. A fingertip unit is measured by squeezing out enough cream or ointment to cover from tip of the index finger to the first crease as shown in Fig 39.2. Educating patients to use this method prevents the application of both a subtherapeutic or an excessive dose (that may increase side effects). Additional guidance on the FTU method and application of topical corticosteroids in children can be found in the Australian Medicines Handbook 2021 and in their publicly available resources – see 'Online resources'. For most topical formulations, the dosage of corticosteroid is one or two applications daily, depending on the site and response to medication.

Local adverse reactions from topical corticosteroids include skin atrophy and striae, acneiform eruptions, burning sensations, dryness, itching, hypopigmentation, purpura and haemorrhage, hirsutism (usually facial), folliculitis, alopecia (usually of scalp) and masking or aggravation of fungal infections. Contact dermatitis can occur as an allergic reaction, which may be difficult to distinguish from the initial inflammatory condition.

If a significant amount of corticosteroid is absorbed, suppression of the hypothalamic–pituitary–adrenal axis and classical cushingoid effects can occur. Children are more susceptible, so only low-potency steroids should be used topically, for short periods. Use of very potent steroids during pregnancy is not advised.

In conditions resistant to milder treatment, intralesional injection of corticosteroids is used – for example, triamcinolone injected into the lesions of keloid scars, acne cysts or alopecia areata.

Immunomodulators

Other drugs used to modify immune responses in skin conditions (discussed in detail in Ch 34) include the following:

- Calcineurin inhibitors, which block T-cell activation and prevent release of inflammatory mediators. Pimecrolimus is indicated for short-term or intermittent treatment of psoriasis and eczema, applied twice daily as a cream. Adverse reactions are local stinging, erythema and secondary infections.
- Antagonists of tumour necrosis factor-alpha (TNF-α), an important regulator of inflammation. Etanercept is a TNF-α receptor fusion protein, while adalimumab, infliximab and golimumab are monoclonal antibodies against TNF. They are given by injection in treatment of moderate-to-severe chronic plaque psoriasis.
- Cytokine modulators: new anti-inflammatory drugs that reduce production of proinflammatory mediators such as interleukins include apremilast (a phosphodiesterase 4 inhibitor), secukinumab and ixekizumab (interleukin 17A inhibitors), and ustekinumab, guselkumab, tildrakizumab and risankizumab (inhibits interleukins -12 and -23).

Anti-inflammatories in eczema, psoriasis and urticaria

Eczema

Eczema, also known as atopic dermatitis, is an inflammatory condition with genetic predisposition in which skin becomes red, itchy, scaly, moist and blistered.

Emollient moisturisers help maintain skin hydration; tar preparations such as coal tar (gel, lotion, foam or shampoo, 0.5–3%) or ichthammol (cream 1%, or ointment 10%) are used for antipruritic effects, and once-daily topical corticosteroids for anti-inflammatory effects. Potent new immunosuppressants pimecrolimus and tacrolimus are second-line therapy. Antibiotics may be required for infected skin, and antihistamines, sedatives or analgesics for relief from itching UVR therapy and avoidance of triggering factors such as soaps, perfumes and preservatives are also useful. Strategies with no proven benefit include homoeopathy, Chinese herbs, dietary restrictions, hypno- or massage therapy, reduction of house dust and salt baths.

Eczema occurs in 10–20% of children under 10 years; itching and infections are likely. Prevention is best, with education of parents and avoidance of irritant triggers such as harsh, perfumed or coloured bath additives. Topical corticosteroids are used short term for flare-ups, and calcineurin inhibitors (e.g. pimecrolimus cream 1%) can be administered to children over 3 months old with severe disease (maximum 3 weeks' treatment for children up to 2 years old).

Psoriasis

Pathology

Psoriasis is a common skin disease (2–3% prevalence worldwide; peak onset in early adult years) characterised by abnormal immune response, silvery-red epidermal proliferation, with pain, itching and bleeding. Large areas of skin may be involved, commonly elbows, knees, buttocks and scalp. Thick plaque lesions packed with activated T-cells cause chronic inflammation and impaired skin functions. There appears to be an immunological cause; trigger factors include stress, injury, smoking, alcohol, infections and drugs including angiotensin-converting enzyme inhibitors, β-blockers, non-steroidal anti-inflammatory drugs (NSAIDs), quinine derivatives and lithium.

Antipsoriasis drugs

Drugs used in treatment include those administered for eczema (see above), plus:

- vitamin D analogues (calcipotriol, calcitriol), which act as antiproliferative agents in the keratinocytes
- retinoids (tazarotene)
- in severe cases, systemic administration of the immunosuppressants ciclosporin and methotrexate (in lower dose than used in anticancer chemotherapy; Drug Monograph 33.2)
- immunomodulators (described above) – can be administered orally (apremilast) or parentally administered (guselkumab, ixekizumab, risankizumab, secukinumab, tildrakizumab and ustekinumab).

Phototherapy with UVA or UVB has been tried in combination with many of the above agents.

Some TNF inhibitors, when used to treat autoimmune diseases such as rheumatoid arthritis and Crohn's disease, have induced psoriasis, a condition that they can be used to treat – this anomaly is being studied.

Psoriasis can occur in children; it is estimated that about 27% of cases occur before the age of 16 years. Topical treatment is usually with corticosteroids or calcipotriol; potent drugs such as methotrexate, acitretin and ciclosporin pose more risks of toxicity in children. Calcipotriol is not recommended for children under 18 years of age.

Urticaria

Urticaria, or hives, is a common skin condition in which there is transient itchiness, reddening and swelling of the dermis; angio-oedema may be associated. In about 20% of cases, some precipitating factor may be identifiable – for example, heat, cold, sun exposure, food (shellfish, fungi), drugs (penicillins, aspirin) or plants. Urticaria is treated not with topical agents but with systemic antihistamines, corticosteroids, NSAIDs, tricyclic antidepressants or various other drugs.

KEY POINTS

Anti-inflammatory and immunomodulating agents

- Many dermatological conditions such as dermatitis and urticaria have an inflammatory or immune component, so corticosteroids are commonly used topically for their anti-inflammatory and immunosuppressant effects, in ointments, creams and lotions.
- Fluorinated steroids such as betamethasone are particularly effective.
- Hydration of skin – for example, by use of occlusive dressings or ointments – markedly enhances absorption of corticosteroids, which improves actions but increases the risk of systemic adverse effects.
- New immunomodulators such as calcineurin inhibitors and TNF antagonists are being used to treat eczema and psoriasis.
- Severe psoriasis may require treatment with potent immunosuppressants, including the cytotoxic agents ciclosporin and methotrexate.

Retinoids and treatment of acne

Pathology

Acne vulgaris is a skin disease involving increased sebum production, excessive keratinisation leading to the formation of keratin plugs at the base of pilosebaceous follicles, proliferation of the bacterium *Propionibacterium acnes* and inflammation, possibly with comedones ('blackheads'), papules and pustules, abscesses, cysts and widespread scarring. It is the most common skin disorder in many Western countries, occurring at any age and affecting up to 90% of adolescents, and is associated with high androgen levels. There may be significant psychological and emotional trauma associated with disfigurement.

At the molecular level, increased fibroblast growth factor receptor-2 (FGFR-2) signalling may be involved in the pathogenesis, and many anti-acne agents act by downregulating FGFR-2. Other aetiological factors implicated in women are androgens, estrogens, growth hormone, insulin-like growth factor and association with polycystic ovary syndrome. Acne may be exacerbated by excessive skin washing causing skin irritation, oily cosmetics, exposure to industrial oils and many drugs (androgenic hormones, danazol, androgen-derived oral contraceptives, oral corticosteroids, phenytoin, isoniazid, iodides and lithium). Some people note increased skin oiliness and acne flare-ups after eating particular foods such as chocolate or high-fat dairy products.

Treatment of acne

The targets of acne therapy are reduction and removal of sebum and bacteria, improvement of the complexion, reduction in scarring and psychosocial benefits. There is no 'quick fix': improvement may not be seen for weeks, and most treatments need to be continued for many months for significant benefits, and even for years to prevent relapses. First-line treatment is with topical retinoids, possibly in conjunction with a different topical treatment (benzoyl peroxide, azelaic acid or an antibacterial) and oral (antibacterial, hormonal or retinoid) therapies.

Retinoids (vitamin A analogues)

Vitamin A: actions and mechanism

Vitamin A, or retinol, is a carotenoid substance formed from β-carotene pigments in fruit and vegetables, and present in some fish oils and animal foods. It is a fat-soluble vitamin, long known to be involved in skin physiology (Clinical Focus Box 39.2).

CLINICAL FOCUS BOX 39.2

Vitamin A deficiency and toxicity

The recommended intake of vitamin A in adults is 0.9 mg/day for men and 0.7 mg/day for women, with higher amounts needed by lactating women. Deficiency of vitamin A occurs during malnutrition, in people on diets deficient in fats and in people with disorders of fat absorption and storage. Signs of deficiency include night blindness, corneal opacity and damaged epithelium, with skin becoming dry and infected.

Over-dosage and toxicity can occur, particularly in children and elderly people being given herbal remedies laced with vitamin A or taking 'mega-doses' of supplements. Chronic overdose causes irritability, itchiness, hypertrophy of bone, increased incidence of metaplasia and neoplasia, and cardiotoxicity, whereas acute toxicity causes vomiting, peeling of skin, nose bleeds, eye disorders and raised intracranial pressure; deaths have occurred. High oral doses of retinoids are mutagenic and teratogenic and are contraindicated in pregnancy (Category X).

During the Australian Antarctic expeditions of 1911–14, Sir Douglas Mawson and his companion, Xavier Mertz, suffered from severe malnutrition after their sledge and supplies (and a third member of the team) were lost down a crevasse. Mawson and Mertz were forced to eat the meat from their husky dogs that had died. They became very ill, with layers of skin peeling off, severe diarrhoea, convulsions and headaches. Mertz succumbed, but Mawson survived after months of illness. They suffered from vitamin A toxicity from eating the livers and fat of the dogs, which had been fed fish and seal meat that had accumulated vitamin A from plankton in seawater. At the top of the food chain, the men received toxic overdoses of retinoids. In the northern hemisphere, Inuit and Arctic explorers knew from folklore that eating the livers of polar bears or seals was taboo; 100 g has been shown to contain toxic doses of vitamin A.

Retinoids have found important new medical uses in acne and psoriasis. Given orally or topically, retinoids act as keratolytics, enhance discharge and drainage of acne pustules and reduce epithelial proliferation in psoriasis. Retinoids have effective anticancer actions in some leukaemias and renal cancers. The mechanism of their antineoplastic action may be via inhibition of telomerase enzymes. Retinoid receptor ligands have potential therapeutic applications also in neurodegenerative, metabolic, ophthalmic, muscle and inflammatory disorders.

Source: Marchwicka et al. 2016

There are two main types of receptors for retinoids, constitutively present in cell nuclei: RA receptors (RAR; ligand retinol), and retinoid X receptors (RXR; ligand 9-*cis*-retinoic acid) (Fig 39.2). Activated receptors can interact directly with DNA, modifying gene transcription and mediating liberation of proteolytic enzymes, breakdown of cartilage, synthesis of mucopolysaccharides and steroids, morphogenesis, differentiation and proliferation of epithelial tissues, reproduction, bone and teeth formation, functions of retina, induction of neural growth factors, regulation of the immune system and development of the kidneys.

Clinical use of retinoids

Retinoids, analogues of retinol, are formulated for oral or topical administration in acne, psoriasis, hyperpigmentation and keratinisation disorders. Examples are tretinoin (all-trans retinoic acid; RA), isotretinoin (the 13-*cis*-RA form) and acitretin. In acne, retinoids facilitate the extrusion of fatty material from existing comedones, prevent the reblocking of plugs and formation of new lesions, have anti-inflammatory actions and reduce keratinisation (Leyden et al. 2017).

Topical retinoids

Topical retinoids are used for treating mild acne vulgaris: tretinoin creams 0.025–0.05% (Drug Monograph 39.2), adapalene cream and gel 0.1% and tazarotene creams 0.05% or 0.5%. Gels are preferred for oily skins, and creams for those with dry skin: a combination gel contains 0.1% adapalene and 2.5% benzoyl peroxide. These topical medications are contraindicated in pregnancy (Category D) because of the possibility of birth defects if absorbed.

Drug Monograph 39.2
Tretinoin creams

Tretinoin (all-trans RA) is the active metabolite of vitamin A. (For actions and mechanism, see text.) It stimulates epidermal cell turnover, causing skin peeling, reducing free fatty acids and horny cell adherence within the comedone.

Indications

Tretinoin cream is used to treat acne vulgaris in which comedones, pustules and papules predominate; also indicated for photo-ageing skin wrinkling and pigmentation (the first prescription drug in Australia with this indication).

Pharmacokinetics

Topical application of the tretinoin cream to normal skin does not lead to significant absorption of tretinoin, except after repeated application to inflamed skin.

Adverse reactions

Adverse reactions of topical tretinoin are all reversible: skin irritation with red and oedematous blisters; dry, crusted, stinging or peeling skin; alterations in pigmentation and increased sensitivity to sunlight.

Drug interactions

Concomitant topical use with other drying or peeling agents can result in excessive keratolytic and peeling effects. There are additive adverse effects if used with oral retinoids, other photosensitising agents or minoxidil, so these combinations should be avoided.

Warnings and contraindications

Use of tretinoin cream is contraindicated in eczematous or inflamed skin or if previous hypersensitivity reactions. Because of the risk of birth defects, topical use rates Pregnancy Safety Category D, and is contraindicated in pregnant women and those of childbearing age. Those using the cream should be warned about the risk of excessive sunburning effects and advised to use a sunscreen and protective clothing. Contact of the cream with mucous membranes and skin around the eyes and mouth should be avoided.

Dosage and administration

Tretinoin is available as 0.025% and 0.05% creams; 0.5 g of 0.05% cream is estimated to contain the equivalent of 250 micrograms of vitamin A activity as tretinoin. The lowest-strength cream should be tried first. The cream is applied (usually daily) to the affected areas before retiring at night, then a moisturiser is used in the morning. A slight exacerbation of the condition may occur at first, but improvement should be noted within 2–3 weeks. Treatment is prolonged for several months to achieve remission of acne. (Tretinoin is also available as 10 mg oral capsules [Pregnancy Safety Category X] for treating promyelocytic leukaemia.)

Oral retinoids

For treating severe cystic acne resistant to milder therapies, systemic drugs may be required; they can induce prolonged remissions. Isotretinoin 10 mg, 20 mg or 40 mg and acitretin 10 and 25 mg capsules are available. Acetretin is also used in psoriasis and as prophylactic therapy against skin cancers in transplant patients treated with immunosuppressant agents.

There are many common adverse effects of oral retinoids (Fig 39.3 and Clinical Focus Box 39.2). Women

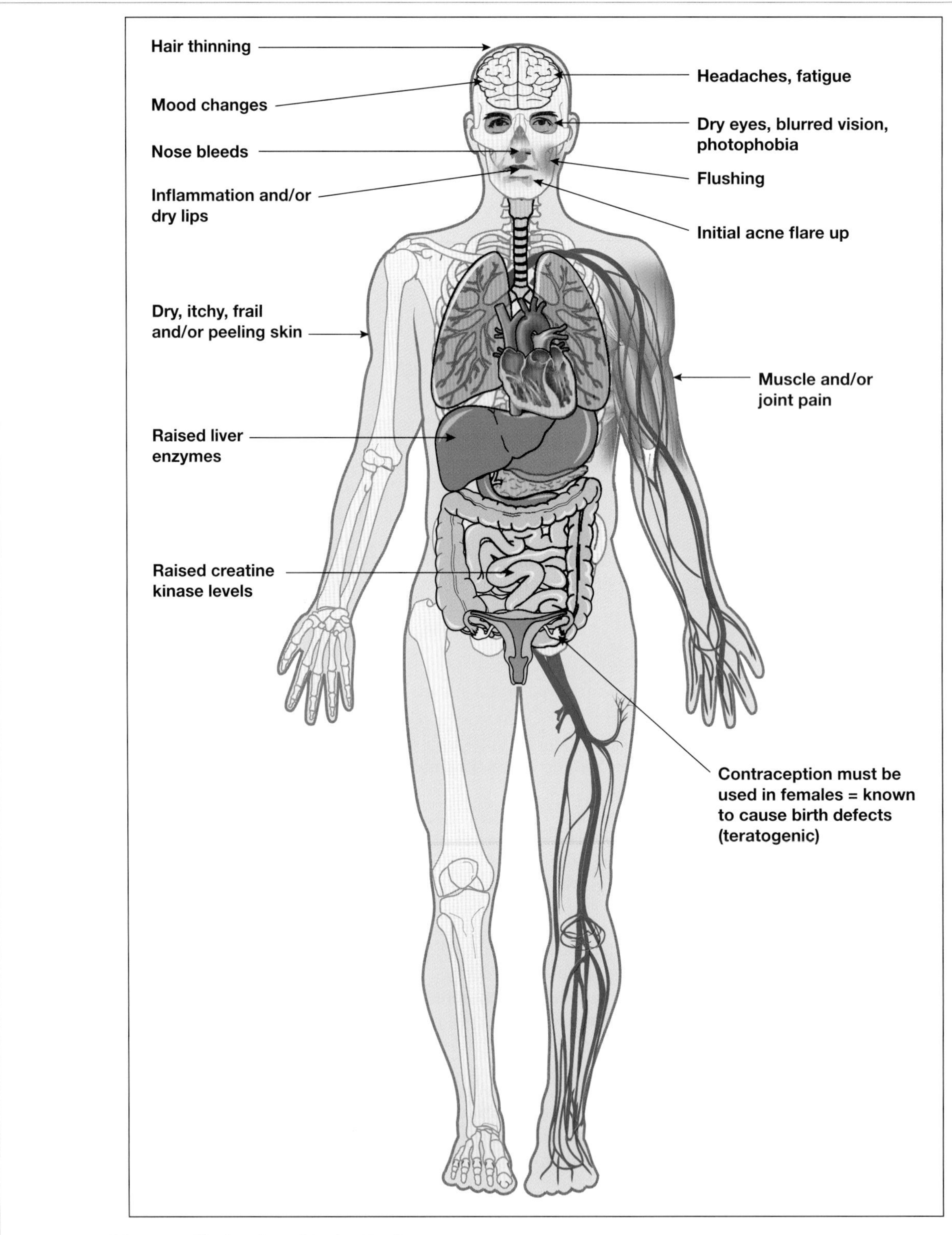

FIGURE 39.3 Adverse effects of oral isotretinoin.

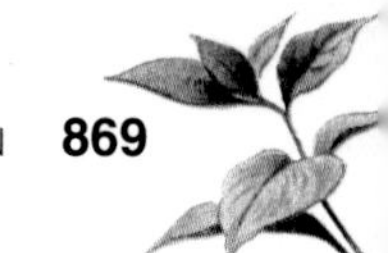

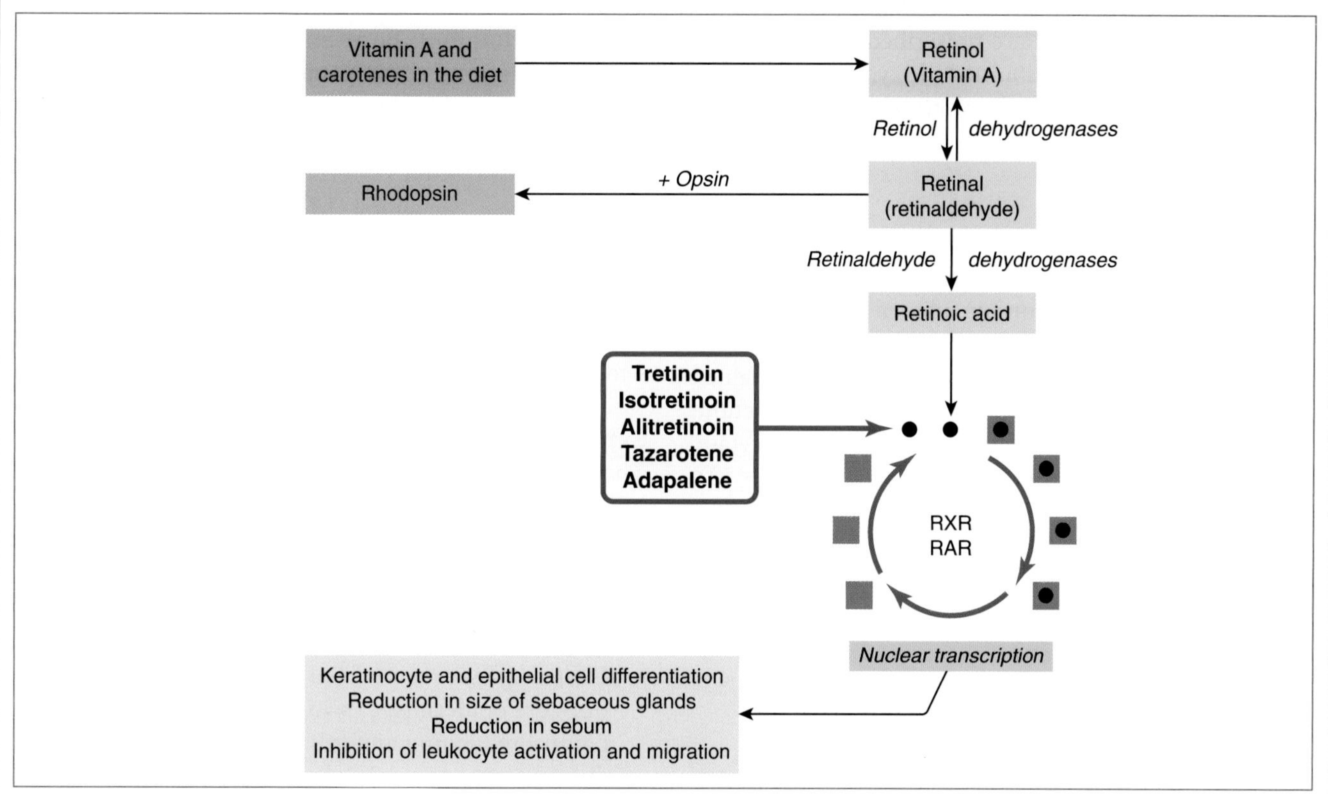

FIGURE 39.4 The retinoid pathway

Dietary vitamin A is converted to retinal, which may be utilised for the visual pigment rhodopsin, or oxidised to retinoic acid which interacts with nuclear RAR and RXR to modify gene transcription in many biochemical pathways. Synthetic retinoids acting via retinoid receptors have useful anti-acne and anti-inflammatory actions in skin disorders.

Source: Ritter et al. 2019; used with permission.

who are pregnant, are planning to or could possibly become pregnant should not use these oral preparations (Category X), which can cause spontaneous abortions or major abnormalities in the fetus (hydrocephalus, microcephalus and external ear and cardiovascular problems). Prescription of oral retinoids is restricted to specialist dermatologists and authorised doctors. Sexually active women of childbearing age who are prescribed these drugs must use efficient contraceptive methods for 1 month before starting the treatment, continuously during treatment and for 1 month (isotretinoin) or 2 years (acitretin) after cessation of treatment. Acitretin has a long half-life (> 2 days) and an active metabolite etretinate ($t_{1/2}$ > 4 months).

Other acne products

Other drugs used to treat acne are keratolytics, antimicrobials and hormones. Adjunctive measures include avoidance of oil- or alcohol-based cleansers, exfoliants, harsh soaps and vigorous scrubbing of skin, as these tend to increase oiliness. New treatments being trialled include topical dapsone, taurine bromamine, resveratrol or lauric acid. New formulations are microsponges, liposomes, nano-emulsions and aerosol foams.

Keratolytics and antimicrobials

In mild acne, topical keratolytics and antibacterials are the treatments of first choice. The following are examples:

- Azelaic acid (a straight-chain 9-carbon dicarboxylic acid) gel 15% or lotion 20% has antibacterial activity against *P. acnes*, reduces keratinisation and removes keratin plugs. It can cause burning, stinging or pruritus if applied to broken skin.
- Benzoyl peroxide creams or gels, 2.5–10%, liberate oxygen, which produce antibacterial, keratolytic and drying effects, reduce the growth of *P. acnes* and release fatty acids from sebum and shrinking pustules.
- Treatment 'kits', combining a keratolytic and an antiseptic cleanser, can help improve compliance with therapy.
- Antibiotics may decrease colonisation by *P. acnes* and the formation of sebaceous fatty acid byproducts and

new acne lesions. Topical clindamycin products (gel, liquid or lotion, all 1%) are prescribed for mild to moderate acne; oral antibiotics (doxycycline or erythromycin) are generally reserved for severe or unresponsive acne. Development of antibiotic resistance is common.

Hormones

Because acne in women is sometimes associated with excess androgen production or use of combined oral contraceptives containing an estrogen with significant androgenic activity, women with acne can be helped with anti-androgen agents, which reduce sebum secretion; anti-androgenic agents include cyproterone acetate, spironolactone and estrogens such as desogestrel (Ch 30).

KEY POINTS

Drug treatment of acne

- Acne vulgaris may be alleviated by topical treatment with skin cleansers, keratolytics and antibiotics, or topical retinoids such as isotretinoin.
- Severe cases of acne may require systemic hormones or oral retinoids, which carry the risk of teratogenesis and must not be prescribed in women of childbearing age without adequate contraception being assured.

Treatment of burns, pressure sores and skin ulcers

Burns, pressure sores, leg (and other skin) ulcers and open wounds from accidents have similar pathologies in their loss of skin, subcutaneous tissue and fluid, and consequent risk of infection, chronic pain and inflammation, and extension of necrosis into underlying tissues. Thus, the treatment methods, drugs and wound dressings used are often similar. Wound dressing is a specialised area of nursing; the types of dressings available change frequently. (There is a separate edition of *Therapeutic Guidelines* devoted to this area of healthcare: see 'Ulcer and wound management' in Vemuri 2019.)

Burns

Pathophysiology of burns

Burns can be caused by heat, chemical agents (strong acids or bases), electricity or friction (as in bicycle/motorcycle crashes when riders were not wearing protective clothing). Burn injuries range from mild and superficial lesions accompanied by pain, to very severe with extensive skin loss associated with systemic and metabolic derangements in multiple organ systems, inflammatory cascades and recurrent sepsis. People with burns have a sustained release of stress hormones, including corticosteroids and catecholamines, leading to a prolonged hypermetabolic state. The chief cause of death after burning is shock due to loss of plasma fluid, depleted blood volume, decreased cardiac output and widespread tissue anoxia.

Extent and depth of burns

The proportion of body surface area affected is estimated by the 'rule of nines' for adults (Fig 39.5A). If large areas of skin are burned (> 20% total body surface area), there is an increased risk of infection and mortality.

Burns are classified by degree, which is determined by the depth of skin involved within a local area (Fig 39.5B):

- First-degree, or superficial-thickness, burns involve only the epidermis, causing erythema with dry, painful reddening and inflammation (e.g. overexposure to sun).
- Second-degree, or partial-thickness, burns involve the epidermis and dermis and may be superficial or involve deep dermal necrosis; characterised by a moist, blistered, painful surface (e.g. flash or scald burns from liquids).
- Third-degree, or full-thickness, burns involve destruction of the entire epidermis and dermis and may go into the subcutaneous tissue. They are characterised by white, opaque, dry, leathery skin or coagulated, charred skin without sensation due to destruction of nerve endings with scarring (e.g. flame burns or hot viscous liquids).
- Fourth-degree burns extend deeply into subcutaneous tissues, and may damage underlying tendons, muscles, bone and nerves. They appear black and dry, and cause scarring.

Partial- or full-thickness burns are open wounds with the accompanying danger of infection from normal body flora (*Staphylococcus*, *Candida* and *Pseudomonas*) becoming pathogenic. If tissue becomes anoxic and necrotic, anaerobic organisms such as *Clostridium tetani* and *Clostridium perfringens* can grow. The immune system becomes suppressed from injury and shock, resulting in poor defence mechanisms.

Management of burns

First-aid treatment of burns

An important first-aid treatment for burns is to cool the wound immediately to decrease inflammation and

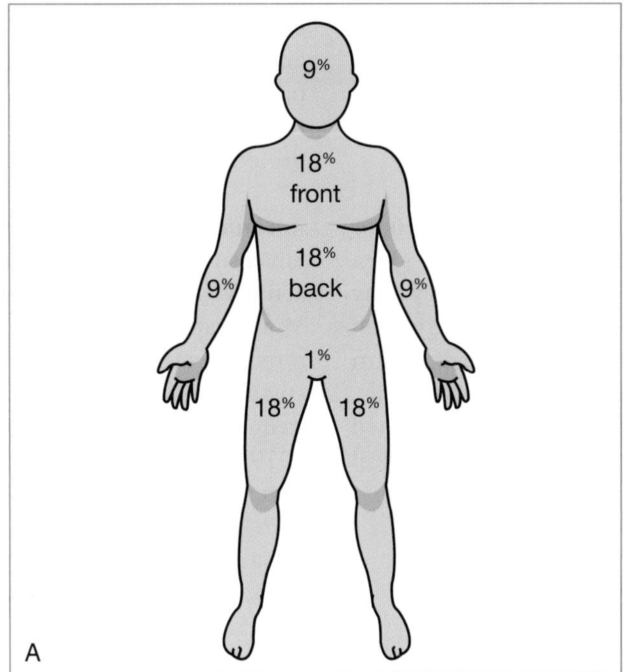

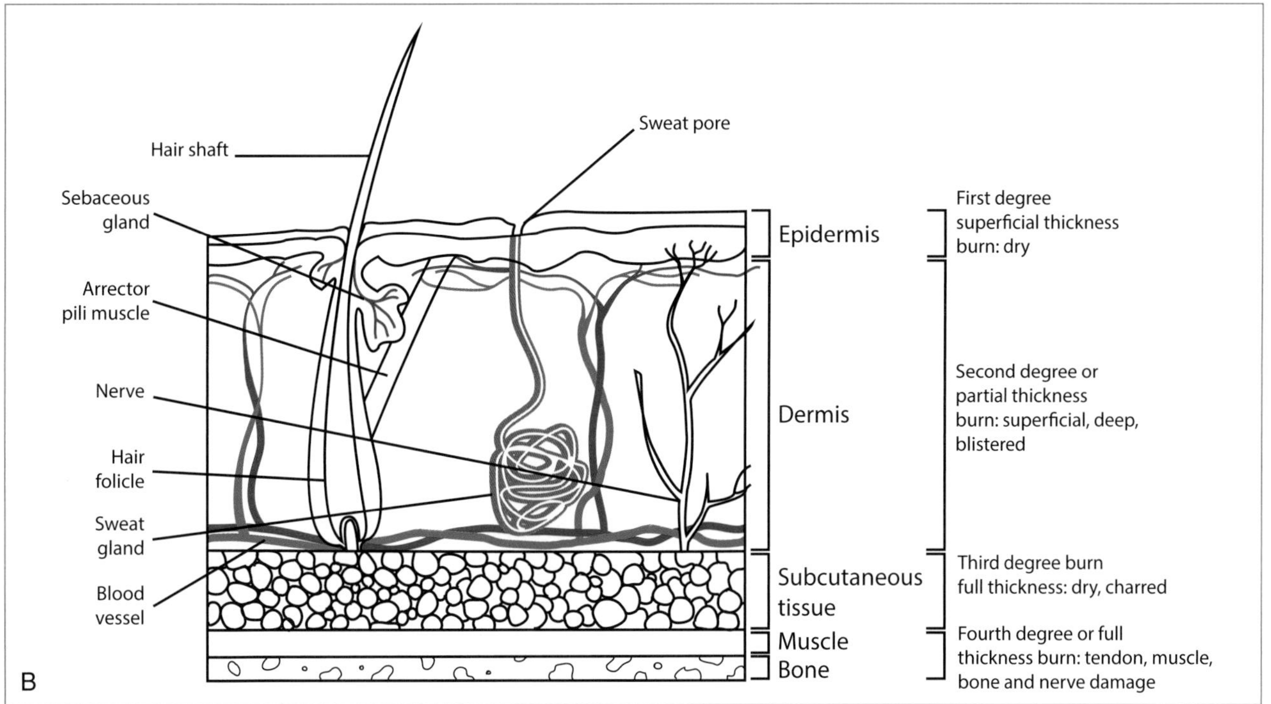

FIGURE 39.5 Extent of body burns: percentage and thickness
A The 'rule of nines' in describing percentage of adult body burned: the head (front and back) and the arms each count as 9%, the front and back of the trunk each count as 18%, each leg as 18%, and the groin area as the remaining 1% of body surface area.
B Diagram of layers of skin and subcutaneous tissue, showing definition of burn depth.

constrict blood vessels to reduce their permeability and minimise oedema, tissue damage, subsequent morbidity and need for surgery. The burned area and hot clothing should be flushed with cool running water (10–15°C) for 20–30 minutes. The burn can then be covered with cling wrap or sterile sheet until the person can be transported for medical attention. No greasy ointments, butter or dressings should be applied to serious burns, as these agents inhibit loss of heat from the burn, which increases discomfort and tissue damage. Fluids for intravenous rehydration of people suffering from burns, sepsis or anaphylactic shock are carried by ambulances; compound sodium lactate solution or normal saline is administered intravenously by paramedics. Major burns need referral to a burns unit (Clinical Focus Box 39.3).

Drugs used in managing people with burns

People with burns treated in an emergency department or burns unit are stabilised with intravenous fluids, given analgesics for pain and sedated if necessary; they may require immunisation against tetanus and catheterisation to measure urinary output. After stabilisation, the burn wound is cleaned with a mild soap and water, and a sterile, non-adherent dressing applied. Small, uncontaminated burns that can be adequately dressed do not require topical or oral antimicrobials.

> **CLINICAL FOCUS BOX 39.3**
> **Spray-on skin and scaffolding matrices**
>
> Dr Fiona Wood, Clinical Professor in the School of Paediatrics and Child Health at the University of Western Australia and plastic surgeon and Head of the Burns Unit of Royal Perth Hospital, came to prominence when a large proportion of the survivors of the 2002 Bali bombings arrived at Royal Perth Hospital. Professor Wood led a courageous and committed team to save 28 people suffering severe burns (from 2% to 92% of body surface area), life-threatening infections and delayed shock.
>
> In her research, Dr Wood had discovered that scarring after burns is markedly reduced if replacement skin can be provided within 10 days. With her colleague Dr Marie Stoner, Dr Wood developed techniques to culture a suspension of cells that could be sprayed on to the damaged area after only 5 days. Pressure bandaging is also important for protection and to reduce hypertrophy of subsequent scars.
>
> Her vision in having developed a plan to cope with large-scale disasters 5 years before the first Bali tragedy, and her exceptional leadership, research and surgical skills, led to Dr Wood being honoured as Australian of the Year for 2005.
>
> More recent techniques in the field of regenerative skin tissue engineering are based on the use of suitable scaffolds such as porous, fibrous, microsphere, hydrogel, composite and acellular matrices. These highly biocompatible scaffolds are either of natural biomaterials, such as collagen and chitosan, or synthetic materials such as polycaprolactone and polyethylene glycol. Scaffolds improve tensile strength for faster wound healing and effective skin tissue regeneration.
>
> *Source: www.australianoftheyear.org.au*

The hypermetabolic state increases requirements for energy, carbohydrates, proteins, fats, vitamins, minerals and antioxidants; these may have to be supplied by parenteral nutrition. β-blockers have been used to help reduce the catabolic effects of burn injury and reverse protein breakdown.

Antimicrobials

Silver sulfadiazine (SSD) has broad-spectrum antimicrobial activity and is easy to apply to a burned site (Drug Monograph 39.3). Dressings impregnated with silver provide faster healing, and are generally preferred to SSD creams because they don't need to be changed as frequently, minimising pain for the person (Nímia et al. 2019). There is some concern about potential toxicity of silver to various host (patient) cells. New formulations with nano-crystalline silver particles have stronger antimicrobial activity with reduced frequency of dressing changes, less pain and reduced infection rates and hospital stay. Silver nanoparticles are widely used in many fields (clothing, electronics, biosensors, paints, sunscreens, cosmetics, medical devices); they are detectable in blood and can be deposited in various organs; long-term toxicity is being studied.

Other antimicrobials used include povidone–iodine, which penetrates eschar (dead, separated, damaged skin) but causes pain on application and hardens the eschar area when dry. For superficial or partial thickness wounds, topical medical-grade honey promotes debridement and reduces time to healing and scar formation.

Other pharmacological management includes adequate pain relief, especially during dressing changes, and relief of severe itching in rehabilitating patients.

Pressure sores and skin ulcers

Pressure sores

A **pressure sore** (bedsore or decubitus ulcer) is a break in the skin and underlying subcutaneous and muscle tissue caused by abnormal, sustained pressure or friction exerted over bony prominences of the body; contributing factors are prolonged bed rest, local circulatory impairment, loss of sensation of pressure or pain, debilitation, muscle atrophy, motor paralysis, poor nutrition, obesity, infection, septicaemia and heat and moisture. It results in vascular insufficiency, ischaemic necrosis and infection with a wide range of bacterial flora. Chronic ulcers may be complicated by extension to bone, causing osteomyelitis and development of SCCs. In Australia and New Zealand, the prevalence of pressure ulcers is approximately 13% in acute care facilities (Rodgers et al. 2021). This increases to approximately 23% in nursing homes, and 33% in critical care patients

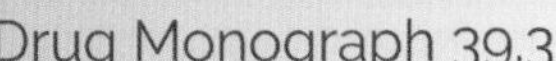

Drug Monograph 39.3
Silver sulfadiazine

SSD is the antimicrobial agent of choice in the treatment and prevention of infection in severe skin wounds, formulated 1% in an O/W cream.

Actions and mechanisms

SSD has broad antimicrobial activity against many Gram-negative and Gram-positive bacteria and some yeasts and anaerobic bacteria. It combines antibacterial actions of silver nitrate with those of sulfonamides through actions on cell membranes and cell walls, but appears not to inhibit folic acid synthesis. Resistance may develop during therapy.

Indications

SSD is used for prevention and treatment of infections associated with second- and third-degree burns, leg ulcers, pressure sores and other wounds with extensive denuded areas of skin. It softens eschar, facilitating its removal and preparation of the wound for grafting.

Pharmacokinetics

SSD in contact with exudates is slowly metabolised. When applied to extensive areas of the body, up to 10% of the drug may be absorbed, reaching therapeutic plasma concentrations and producing adverse reactions characteristic of both sulfonamides and silver.

Adverse reactions

Pain, burning, itching and skin discolouration occur infrequently. Hypersensitivity to sulfonamides can occur; if so, the drug should be discontinued. Renal function should be monitored, and adequate hydration supplied. Leukopenia can occur, and argyria if significant amounts of silver are absorbed.

Drug interactions

The cream should not be used concurrently with enzymatic debriding agents, which may be inactivated by silver. In large-area burns, there may be interactions with oral hypoglycaemic agents, phenytoin, cimetidine, oral anticoagulants, ciclosporin and other nephrotoxic agents.

Warnings and contraindications

Caution should be observed with extensive use in people with renal or liver impairment, or sensitive to sulfonamides. The cream (initially white) darkens on exposure to light. Sulfonamides can cause kernicterus in babies if used extensively by pregnant or lactating women or on infants, so SSD is in Pregnancy Safety Category C. It retards re-epithelialisation so should be discontinued after 3 days.

Dosage and administration

SSD 1% cream is applied topically to cleansed, debrided burn wounds once or twice daily, for 3 days after a burn; it is applied with a spatula or gloved hand to a thickness of about 3–5 mm. Burn wounds should be continuously covered with the cream; daily bathing and debriding are important.

and those with spinal injuries. In addition to the suffering of patients, the total cost to the healthcare system of treating such wounds is enormous.

Leg and foot ulcers

An ulcer is a defect in the surface of the skin, with loss of epidermis, and possibly dermis and subcutaneous tissue, due to sloughing of inflammatory necrotic tissue. Skin **ulcers** on the legs (and on the feet, particularly in people with diabetes) are slow to heal and may require prolonged nursing and podiatrist care; there is risk of developing necrosis and gangrene, and subsequent requirement for amputation.

Physical management

Pressure sores and leg ulcers are notoriously difficult to treat, and should be prevented by watchful nursing care with frequent turning of bedridden people and ambulation whenever possible. If ulcers do develop, maximum activity is even more essential to relieve pressure, stimulate circulation and optimise the muscle pump and venous return. Wound management has become a specialised area of nursing and podiatry, with many techniques and dressings available (see 'Ulcer and wound management' in Vemuri 2019).

A treatment plan takes into consideration four basic principles: interventions to improve the person's general health; reduction of pressure sites by repositioning or the use of supports; maintenance of a clean wound site, with dressings and topical antiseptics if necessary; and use of appropriate agents for debriding the wound or stimulation of new granulation tissue.

Physical therapies tried include electrical stimulation, infrared and UVR, laser therapy, hyperbaric oxygen, compression bandages or stockings, bio-engineered skin substitutes, negative pressure therapy and ultrasound. A person with a full-thickness loss of skin may require surgical intervention either to debride and cover the area or to stabilise the wound.

Pharmacological management

Systemic antibiotics are not usually indicated, as adequate drug levels are not reached in granulating wounds, but may be needed in difficult-to-treat infected pressure sores, for sepsis, osteomyelitis, bacteraemia and advancing cellulitis, and as an adjunct to surgical management. Antiseptics such as povidone–iodine, other iodophors, potassium permanganate and hydrogen peroxide are usually contraindicated because they may be cytotoxic to fibroblasts and thus interfere with the granulation process.

Medications used include:

- antimicrobials similar to those used in burns (SSD, medical-grade honey) and bacterial skin infections (mupirocin)
- metronidazole, an antibacterial agent used systemically to treat decubitus ulcers infected with anaerobic bacteria
- granulocyte colony-stimulating factors, oral pentoxifylline (a vasodilator) and prostanoids
- sterile saline solutions for cleaning
- debriding agents, for removal of eschar, or slough, which may be retarding healing and providing a medium for bacterial infection; possible preparations include ointments containing active peptidase enzymes such as collagenase or papain
- 'biosurgery': the use of living maggots (larvae of insects); when applied to the wound (e.g. in an upturned plastic container), they gently remove necrotic tissue, decreasing risk of infection and improving healing
- EMLA cream (lidocaine [lignocaine]–prilocaine) or inhaled methoxyflurane, as analgesics for pain relief during dressing changes
- finely powdered sterile gelatin, dusted into wounds, to stimulate growth of granulation tissue.

Dressings may be films, foams or 'bio-active', impregnated with antiseptics (iodine, povidone–iodine, chlorhexidine, silver, peroxides, propylene glycol, triclosan), adsorbents (alginates, carmellose, cadexomers, foam, hydro-colloids) or other medicaments (zinc oxide, glycerol, melaleuca oil, honey).

KEY POINTS

Drug treatment of burns, pressure sores and skin ulcers

- When large areas of skin are burned, there is severe risk of infection, shock and hypermetabolic syndrome; fluid replacement is critical.
- Topical SSD is the antibacterial agent of choice in the early stages of treatment. Scaffolding matrices provide support for new skin.
- The best treatment for pressure sores (decubitus ulcers) and ulcers (leg or foot) is prevention, as they are painful, may cause necrosis and osteomyelitis and may require prolonged extensive care.
- Wound dressings impregnated with antimicrobial agents or adsorbent particles are used, as are proteolytic enzyme preparations or insect larvae.

DRUGS AT A GLANCE
Drugs affecting the skin

PHARMACOLOGICAL GROUP AND EFFECT	KEY EXAMPLES	CLINICAL USE
Sunscreens	(Organics (UV absorbers) PABA derivatives, cinnamates Inorganics (UV reflectors) zinc oxide, titanium dioxide	• Prevent sunburn
Antibacterials (skin)	Mupirocin	• Impetigo
Antivirals (skin)	Aciclovir, idoxuridine	• Herpes simplex virus of the skin and lips
Wart treatments	Imiquimod, podophyllotoxin	• External genital and perianal warts

Imidazoles • Blocks synthesis of ergosterol, decreasing cell membrane-associated functions, inhibiting fungal growth; fungistatic	Clotrimazole, ketoconazole	• Fungal skin infections
Sterol synthesis inhibitors • Impairs sterol synthesis in fungal cell membranes, decreasing cell membrane-associated functions, fungistatic and fungicidal	Amorolfine	• Antifungal / Onychomycoses
Pediculocides • Irreversible cholinesterase inhibitor	Malathion	• Head and pubic lice
Acaricides • Binds to sodium channels on nerves, causing them to remain open and repetitively fire • Decreases repolarisation of neural cell membranes in lice, causing paralysis	Permethrin	Scabies treatment
Corticosteroids (topical) • Anti-inflammatory, antipruritic, immunosuppressive, antiproliferative, vasoconstrictive effect	Betamethasone, hydrocortisone	• Eczema • Psoriasis • Skin reactions to insect bites • Sunburn
Calcineurin inhibitors • Inhibits calcineurin; blocks T-cell proliferation and release of inflammatory cytokines • Anti-inflammatory	Pimecrolimus	• Eczema
TNF-α antagonists • Bind to TNF-α (cytokine) and inhibit its binding to cell membrane-bound receptors and activity; decrease inflammatory and immune effect	Etanercept, infliximab	• Psoriasis
Vitamin D analogues • Bind to vitamin D receptors • Suppress proliferation of keratinocytes	Calcipotriol	Psoriasis
Retinoids • Increase epithelial cell follicular turnover and decrease inflammation	Adapalene, isotretinoin, tretinoin	• Acne treatments
Silver sulfadiazine • Binds to bacterial cell membranes, bactericidal	Silver sulfadiazine creams impregnated dressings	• Burn and ulcer treatment

REVIEW QUESTIONS

1. Ms YR presents to you, the health professional, for advice about a rash. On inspection you can see that the rash is in the area under her breasts where the skin is moist and warm. The rash is red and inflamed and you identify that it has a fungal component.

   What treatments are available to reduce the rash and alleviate symptoms? What is their mechanism of action? How should they be applied?
2. The condition Ms YR (above) has developed is known as intertrigo (rash that affects the folds of the skin, caused by skin-to-skin friction, where it is often moist). What treatments can be used to prevent the development of the intertrigo?
3. Miss JE, a 17-year-old high school student, has severe cystic acne. Her dermatologist has prescribed isotretinoin 30 mg to be taken orally once daily. Her therapy is to start on the second day of the next menstrual period. Discuss the mechanism of action and common adverse effects of oral retinoids. Explain why the dermatologist is commencing therapy on the second day of Miss JE's period.

REFERENCES

Australian Medicines Handbook 2021. Australian Medicines Handbook. Adelaide, AMH.

Griffiths, CEM, Armstrong, AW, Gudjonsson, JE, et al., Psoriasis. The Lancet, 2021. 397(10281): 1301–15.

Landeck, L, Sabat, R, Ghoreschi, K, et al., Immunotherapy in psoriasis. Immunotherapy, 2021. 13(7): 605–19.

Leyden, J, L Stein-Gold, and J Weiss, Why topical retinoids are mainstay of therapy for acne. Dermatology and Therapy, 2017; 7(3): 293–304.

Marchwicka, A, Cunningham, A, Marcinkowskaet E, al., Therapeutic use of selective synthetic ligands for retinoic acid receptors: a patent review. Expert Opinion on Therapeutic Patents, 2016; 26(8): 957–71.

Nímia, HH, Carvalho, VF, Isaac, C, et al., Comparative study of Silver Sulfadiazine with other materials for healing and infection prevention in burns: a systematic review and meta-analysis. Burns, 2019; 45(2): 282–92.

Ritter, J, Flower, R, Henderson, G, et al., Rang and Dale's pharmacology. 2019.

Rodgers, K, J Sim, and R Clifton, Systematic review of pressure injury prevalence in Australian and New Zealand hospitals. Collegian, 2021; 28(3): 310–23.

Stalgis-Bilinski KL, Boyages J, Salisbury EL, et al. Burning daylight: balancing vitamin D requirements with sensible sun exposure. Medical Journal of Australia 2011; 194 (7): 345–48.

Vemuri, K, Therapeutic Guidelines: Ulcers and wound management. Version 2. Australian Prescriber, 2019; 42(6): 206.

Yap, FH, HC Chua, and CP Tait, Active sunscreen ingredients in Australia. Australasian Journal of Dermatology, 2017; 58(4): e160–70.

ONLINE RESOURCES

All About Acne: https://www.acne.org.au (accessed 23 September 2021)

Australasian College of Dermatologists: https://www.dermcoll.edu.au/atoz/dermatitis-eczema/ (accessed 24 September 2021)

Australian Institute of Health and Welfare (AIHW) – Skin cancer in Australia: https://www.aihw.gov.au/reports/cancer/skin-cancer-in-australia/contents/table-of-contents (accessed 23 September 2021)

Australian Medicines Handbook – public resources: https://resources.amh.net.au/public/fingertipunits.pdf (accessed 22 September 2021)

Australian & New Zealand Burn Association https://anzba.org.au/ (accessed 23 September 2021)

DermNet New Zealand https://dermnetnz.org/ (accessed 22 September 2021)

Melanoma Institute Australia: https://www.melanoma.org.au/ (accessed23 September 2021)

Therapeutic Goods Administration – Factsheet on sunscreens: https://www.tga.gov.au/sunscreens (accessed 23 September 2021)

More weblinks at: http://evolve.elsevier.com/AU/Knights/pharmacology/.

CHAPTER 40
DRUGS AFFECTING THE EYE AND EAR

Mary Bushell

KEY ABBREVIATIONS

ACh	acetylcholine
AMD	age-related macular degeneration
IOP	intraocular pressure
LA	local anaesthetic
NSAID	non-steroidal anti-inflammatory drug
POAG	primary open-angle glaucoma

KEY TERMS

Chapter Focus

Disorders that affect vision or hearing markedly impair a person's ability to function optimally and require early detection and treatment.

Drugs are used to treat ocular conditions such as acute and chronic glaucoma, macular degeneration, infections, inflammations and muscular dysfunction, and to assist in ocular examination, diagnosis and surgery. The major drug groups are: drugs used to treat glaucoma; drugs for macular degeneration; antimicrobial agents; anti-inflammatory and antiallergic agents; mydriatic and cycloplegic agents; and ocular local anaesthetics. (Most of these drugs are used systemically in other conditions, so detailed pharmacology is covered in other chapters.) The common route of administration of drugs for ocular effects is topical, via eyedrops or ointments. Drugs administered this way can be absorbed across the cornea and can have systemic effects. Adverse reactions may also be manifest in the eyes after ocular or systemic drug administration.

The most common ear disorders include infections of the ear (bacterial or fungal), ear wax accumulation, painful or inflammatory conditions, deafness and problems with balance. Many ear disorders are minor and self-limiting or easily treated; however, people with ear disorders may have ear pain, vertigo, tinnitus, deafness and difficulty with communication. Persistent untreated disorders can lead to hearing loss. The main pharmacological agents used to treat common ear disorders are antimicrobial and anti-inflammatory drugs; many systemic agents can affect the ear adversely, causing ototoxicity.

KEY DRUG GROUPS

For the eye:

- + Antiallergy agents:
- antihistamines: **azelastine**, **ketotifen** (Drug Monograph 40.2)
- cromones (mast cell stabilisers): **sodium cromoglycate**, **lodoxamide**
- + Anti-inflammatory agents:
- corticosteroids: **fluorometholone**, **prednisolone**
- non-steroidal anti-inflammatory drugs: **diclofenac**, **flurbiprofen**, **ketorolac**
- + Antimicrobial agents:
- antibacterials: **chloramphenicol**, **tobramycin**
- antivirals: **aciclovir**
- anti-amoeba agents: **propamidine**
- + Decongestants/vasoconstrictors (sympathomimetics): **naphazoline**

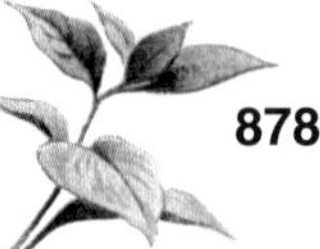

KEY DRUG GROUPS—cont'd

- + Drugs for dry eyes:
- ocular lubricants
- anti-inflammatory: ciclosporin
- + Drugs for glaucoma:
- prostaglandin agonists: **bimatoprost**, **latanoprost** (Drug Monograph 40.1), **travoprost**
- β-blockers: **betaxolol**, **timolol**
- α_2-adrenoceptor agonists: **apraclonidine**, **brimonidine**
- carbonic anhydrase inhibitors: **acetazolamide**, **dorzolamide**
- miotics; osmotic agents
- + Drugs for macular degeneration: **bevacizumab**, **ranibizumab**, **verteporfin**
- + Local anaesthetics: **tetracaine (amethocaine)**, **oxybuprocaine**, **proxymetacaine**
- + Miotics (muscarinic agonists): **pilocarpine**
- + Miscellaneous drugs:
- stains: **fluorescein**
- artificial tears, **botulinum toxin** (Drug Monograph 40.3), contact lens products
- + Mydriatics:
- anticholinergics (cycloplegics): **atropine**, **tropicamide**
- sympathomimetics: **phenylephrine**

For the ear:

- + Drugs for Ménière's disease: **betahistine**
- + Local anaesthetics: **benzocaine**
- + Miscellaneous drugs:
- for ear wax: cerumenolytics (oils, surfactants)
- for otitis media: paracetamol
- + Topical otic antimicrobials
- antibiotics: **ciprofloxacin**, **framycetin**
- antiseptics: **acetic acid**
- + Topical otic corticosteroids: **dexamethasone**, **flumetasone**, **triamcinolone**

CRITICAL THINKING SCENARIO

Trevor, a 70-year-old man, presents to the optometrist for a routine eye test. The optometrist identified that Trevor had raised intraocular pressure (27 mmHg) and structural signs of disease. He was subsequently referred to an ophthalmologist and diagnosed with open angle glaucoma. Trevor was prescribed latanoprost 0.005% once daily. Trevor has a history of type 2 diabetes and asthma. His current medications include metformin 500 mg three times a day, fluticasone propionate + salmeterol inhaler two puffs twice daily (preventer), and salbutamol inhaler (reliever) when required.

1. Discuss the mode of action of latanoprost, common side effects and contraindications to its use.

Several years later Trevor's ophthalmologist adds the eyedrop betaxolol 0.5% (topical β-blocker) to his medicines. The ophthalmologist counsels Trevor to continue to use his latanoprost as well as his new eyedrop.

2. There is a fixed dose combination eyedrop with latanoprost 0.005% and timolol 0.5%. Why did the ophthalmologist not prescribe this?
3. Describe how the topical β-blocker will help to reduce intraocular pressure.
4. Discuss how Trevor should administer his eyedrops for best effect and to reduce unwanted adverse effects.
5. Trevor experiences allergic conjunctivitis and in the past has been prescribed ocular corticosteroids. Given his glaucoma diagnosis, are ocular corticosteroids an appropriate treatment? Discuss alternative topical drugs that may be used to reduce the symptoms of allergic conjunctivitis.

Introduction

Disorders that affect vision or hearing markedly impair a person's ability to function optimally and require early detection and treatment. The cornea of the eye, and the outer ear (and middle and inner ear, if the eardrum is perforated) are open to the environment, and hence may suffer – as does the skin – from infections, inflammation and other damage. Thus, antimicrobial and anti-inflammatory agents are commonly administered to the eye or ear. In addition, there are conditions specific to each sensory organ that require appropriate drug treatment, notably glaucoma and macular degeneration in the eye, and otitis media and vertigo in the ear.

Drugs to treat such conditions are preferably administered directly to the affected part; thus, there are specialised formulations and techniques for administration.

Drugs affecting the eye

Administration of ocular drugs

Drugs intended to treat eye conditions may be administered in three ways: systemically, by injection to the eye or – most commonly – topically to the eye. Examples of systemic administration of drugs to act in the eye include oral or intravenous (IV) administration of acetazolamide to treat glaucoma, or of systemic antibiotics in eye infections. In some acute serious conditions, drugs may be administered by direct injection to the eye, either by a periocular route (subconjunctival or retrobulbar) – for example, antibiotics, corticosteroids or local anaesthetics; or by the intravitreal route (into the vitreous humour, the gel-like viscous fluid–collagen matrix which bathes the retina and comprises 80% of eye volume) – for example, antibiotics for a severe infection or ranibizumab in macular degeneration. Local anaesthetics may be required first to relieve the pain of the main injection.

Ocular administration

Most commonly, drugs intended to act in the eye are administered topically to the eye, usually directly onto the conjunctival surface as eyedrops or ointment. (The conjunctiva is the mucous membrane lining the anterior part of the sclera – the white fibrous envelope of the eye – and the inner surfaces of each eyelid; see Fig 40.1.) Ocular administration requires some dexterity and may be difficult with children.

Tears are secreted by lacrimal glands at the rate of about 1–2 microL/min and contain lysozyme, a mucolytic enzyme with bactericidal action; tears have lubricating and cleansing actions. Tear fluid is lost by evaporation and by draining into two small **nasolacrimal ducts** at the inner corners of the eyelids, and then into the throat and eventually the systemic circulation. Through these ducts,

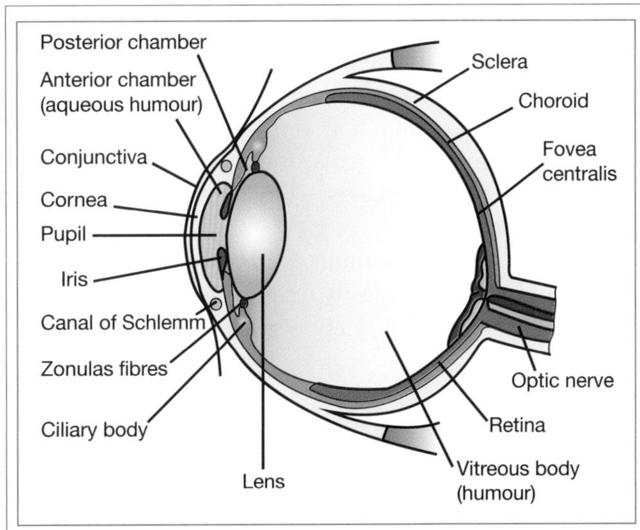

FIGURE 40.1 Cross-sectional anatomy of the eye (eyelid not shown)
Source: Salerno 1999.

drugs applied topically to the eye can cause systemic effects (and may be tasted).

The following are some general points to note:

- Most drugs used in the eye have marked effects elsewhere in the body when given systemically.
- Drugs applied topically to the conjunctival surfaces may then be absorbed through the cornea (the avascular transparent anterior covering of the eye) and diffused through the aqueous humour (the fluid bathing the anterior structures).
- Drugs need to be both water-soluble, to dissolve in body fluids and the cornea, and lipid-soluble, to pass cell membranes and the corneal epithelium.
- Non-polar, uncharged molecules penetrate the cornea most readily, leading to effective drug concentrations in the anterior segment (in front of the lens).
- Absorption is likely to be enhanced if the cornea is damaged, and topical administration is not generally used in open eye injuries.
- The drug (in eyedrops) is rapidly blinked or washed away; excess solution spills over or drains through the nasolacrimal ducts to the nasal mucosa.
- Reflex tear production rapidly dilutes the drug within 1–2 minutes after application to the eye, making it difficult to maintain a pharmacologically effective concentration in the eye.
- The vehicle and the formulation (i.e. solution in drops, ointment base, gel or plastic insert) can affect retention and absorption of the drug.

Ocular formulations

There are many eye formulations available, including eyedrops, eye ointments, eye lotions, irrigating solutions and inserts. The formulation of ocular preparations is a specialised branch of pharmaceutics, as the preparation must be sterile, buffered to body pH and isotonic with body solutions so that it is non-irritant, and stable in solution. Consequently, ocular formulations may contain buffers and pH adjusters (typically, phosphates or borates), preservatives (e.g. benzalkonium chloride, hydrogen peroxide, sodium perborate), antioxidants, agents to increase viscosity (e.g. polyvinyl alcohol or hypromellose) and salts, all of which may affect tissues or cause allergies.

Sterility and shelf-life

The cornea and lens are avascular – hence their transparency – so they have no immediate blood supply to provide immune defences and are at risk if infection or trauma occurs. Therefore, all drugs administered to the eye, particularly during operations or when there is tissue damage, must be provided in a sterile form if possible. The shelf-life of eye formulations is usually stated to be a maximum of 28 days after opening (in the home situation), or 7 days in a clinic situation. The date of first opening the container should be marked on it. Every effort must be made to avoid contaminating the preparation by touching the tip or lid of the dropper bottle or ointment tube onto any surface.

Drug intractions after ocular administration

A small amount of drug administered to the eye may be absorbed via the nasolacrimal ducts, and so potentially may exert systemic effects and interact with drugs already in the systemic circulation. For possible interactions between prostaglandin analogues and non-steroidal anti-inflammatory drugs (NSAIDs), see Drug Monograph 40.1, later; for other drugs groups, refer to Drug Interactions text and tables in the relevant chapter (e.g. for interactions with α_2-agonists: Ch 11; anticholinergics: Ch 8; antimicrobials: Chs 36–38; β-blockers: Ch 10; corticosteroids: Ch 34; and local anaesthetics: Ch 18).

Eyedrops

Eyedrops are drugs formulated in aqueous or oily solutions, dispensed in a small dropper bottle (usually 10–15 mL capacity) such that a small drop can be instilled into the conjunctival sac. Aqueous (watery) drops generally provide for quick absorption and effect, have a brief duration of action and produce little interference with eye examination. The response is variable because of spillage, tears or blinking away of the drop, and systemic effects are possible after absorption, without the drug having passed through the liver first. Oily or gel drops are less common because they interfere more with vision, but they provide longer retention time on the cornea, are more stable and are less likely to cause systemic toxicity.

Administering eyedrops

Technique is important: the person should be instructed to wash their hands, remove any contact lenses, shake the bottle gently, remove the cap (without contaminating it), gently pull down the lower lid, tilt head back and look up, instil one drop into the pouch formed between lid and eye, then close eyes and press on the inner corner of the eyelids against the nose for 2–3 minutes to minimise systemic absorption. If another eyedrop preparation is also being used, wait at least 3 minutes before instilling the next drop, and at least 15 minutes before inserting contact lenses. Fig 40.2 shows the 'traditional' (two-handed) method.

There is no point in trying to administer more than one drop because the volume of a drop is about 25–50 microL and the conjunctival sac's capacity is 10 microL. Excess solution will simply overflow, drain or be blinked away.

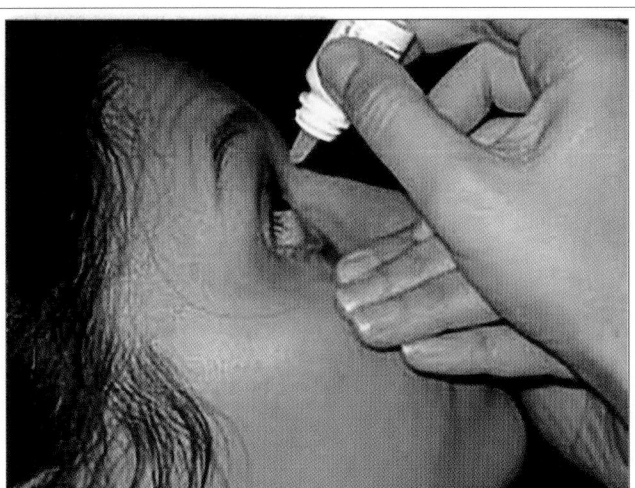

FIGURE 40.2 'Traditional' method of instilling eyedrops
Source: Steiner 2008; reproduced with permission from Australian Prescriber.

To minimise the risk of contamination and growth of microorganisms in solutions, some eyedrops are also produced in single-dose containers (e.g. the Minim brand in Australia). These come as a tiny pack (0.5 mL) for one use only and are then discarded. The advantages are: the drop is always sterile, the solution need contain no preservative, less waste is discarded and there is no risk of cross-contamination between eyes or patients.

Strength of solutions

The strength of drug solutions in eyedrops is usually expressed in percentage terms rather than as milligrams per millilitre or in molar units. Pilocarpine eyedrops, for example, are available in strengths ranging from 1% to 4%. Here, '%' refers to % weight in volume (% w/v) – that is, number of *grams of solid* dissolved in *100 mL of solution*. Thus, 1% means 1 g/100 mL, equating to 10 mg/mL.

Eye ointments and gels

Ointments are semisolid preparations intended for topical application to the skin or mucous membranes; the active drug is incorporated into an oily vehicle. **Eye ointments** are supplied in small (e.g. 5 g) tubes and have short shelf-lives similar to eyedrops. The advantages of eye ointments are:

- They are more stable than aqueous solutions.
- There is less absorption of drug into the lacrimal ducts.
- There is a longer retention time on the conjunctival surface.
- They are safer for home use with potent drugs.
- Due to the emollient (softening) effect of oily ointment bases, they are useful for protection and comfort at night.

However, eye ointments can be difficult to self-administer, they can cause blurred vision or interfere with ocular examination and the greasy base forms an oily film over a contact lens. Good hygiene is again important to minimise contamination.

Gels are thick liquid or semisolid suspensions, usually aqueous (like a jelly) rather than oily; they are less likely to blur vision than are ointments, yet retain the drug in contact with the corneal surface longer than do watery eyedrops. Timolol has been formulated in a gel eyedrop form, 0.25% or 0.5%, suitable for once-daily administration in glaucoma.

Other ocular formulations

Eye lotions, or irrigating solutions, are used to wash foreign materials from the eye. They should be sterile, at pH 6.6–9, and isotonic; in an emergency, normal saline, 0.9% sodium chloride, can be used (4.5 g of sodium chloride in 500 mL water – i.e. approximately 1 teaspoonful of salt in 2 cups of water). Buffered solutions of sodium hyaluronate and of salts are used during intraocular surgery.

Ocular inserts impregnated with drug can be applied to the conjunctival surface for prolonged administration of drug across the cornea; they may be difficult to insert and remove and may appear to become lost (temporarily) in the conjunctival sac. Absorbable gelatin implants are available for use in ocular surgery; there is an intravitreal implant containing dexamethasone 700 micrograms.

KEY POINTS

Administration of drugs to the eye

- Drugs to treat eye conditions may be administered systemically, locally by injection into the eye or topically to the cornea.
- Drugs administered topically are formulated as eyedrops, ointments, gels or via inserts for local effects.
- Some systemic absorption can occur via the nasolacrimal ducts; pressing on the inner corner of the eye can reduce systemic absorption.

Drugs for glaucoma

The part of the eye in front of the lens, the anterior segment, is bathed and nourished by **aqueous humour**, a fluid similar in composition to blood plasma. Formed continually by the ciliary body, it flows forwards between the lens and the iris and drains, through a trabecular meshwork called the canal of Schlemm located near the junction of the cornea and sclera, into the venous system of the eye (Fig 40.3). Equilibrium between formation and

POTENTIAL SITES OF INCREASED RESISTANCE TO AQUEOUS FLOW

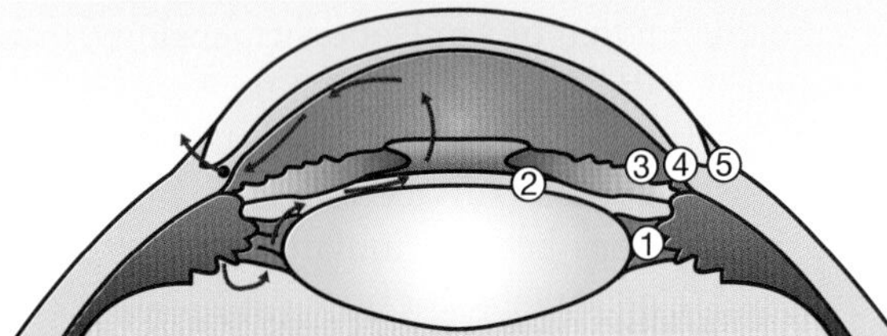

1 Ciliary body processes (when ciliary body swollen by congestion), fibrin debris, vitreous face against the lens equator
2 Pupillary block by anterior position of lens or swollen lens
3 Pretrabecular by neovascular or cellular membranes
4 Trabecular by abnormal accumulation of extracellular matrix
5 Post-trabecular by increased episcleral venous pressure

FIGURE 40.3 Potential sites of increased resistance to aqueous flow

Note: The 'angle' is the angle of the anterior chamber – effectively, the angle between the iris and the cornea; it is the main region of drainage of the aqueous chamber.

Source: Yanoff & Duker 2004, Figure 1-194; used with permission.

uveoscleral outflow of aqueous humour is critical for maintaining a constant **intraocular pressure** (IOP).

Glaucomas are a group of progressive optic neuropathies involving damage to the optic nerve, retinal cell death and changes in visual fields, with abnormally elevated IOP (> 21 mmHg), sometimes referred to as 'ocular hypertension', the third most common cause of blindness worldwide. The raised IOP may result from excessive production of aqueous humour or diminished outflow. About a third of the population has a familial tendency to raised IOP and so is predisposed to glaucoma. The global prevalence in people aged 40–80 years is about 3.5%.

Primary glaucoma includes two forms: about 90% is primary open-angle glaucoma (POAG; also known as chronic open-angle glaucoma), occurring in 2–3% of the population aged over 70 years. It is a familial condition, with gradual insidious onset. Acute closed-angle glaucoma is due to a physiological or anatomical predisposition to mechanical blockage of the trabecular network. This is a rare acute optical emergency, with severe pain and a rapid rise in IOP, threatening vision. Emergency drug therapy with IV acetazolamide or mannitol, oral glycerol or topical pilocarpine is needed, followed usually by surgery.

Secondary glaucoma may result from previous eye disease or cataract extraction, or may be secondary to inflammation (uveitis), trauma, tumour, adhesions (iritis) or drugs (corticosteroids, mydriatics, vasodilators, phenothiazines, antidepressants or anticholinergics). Therapy requires attention first to the primary cause and avoidance of precipitating factors, then antiglaucoma drugs.

Drug treatment of glaucomas

The goal of therapy is to lower IOP to preserve vision for the person's lifetime; medication is likely to be chronic. The main drugs are prostaglandin agonists, β-adrenoceptor antagonists (β-blockers), carbonic anhydrase (CA) inhibitors, sympathomimetics and miotics (cholinergics) (see Li et al. 2016 and Table 40.1); drug selection is determined by desired reduction in IOP, efficacy, safety, tolerability and compliance, which is often poor because the person may not feel any symptoms. Whenever possible, drugs are formulated as once-daily eyedrops. People with dark eyes may need higher doses, and it is important to teach people to minimise systemic absorption of drugs by pressing on the nasolacrimal ducts for 2–3 minutes after administration.

TABLE 40.1 Antiglaucoma agents: pharmacokinetics and dosing

DRUG	ONSET OF ACTION (H)	PEAK EFFECT (H)	DURATION OF ACTION (H)	USUAL ADULT DOSAGE
α_2-adrenoceptor agonists				
Apraclonidine	1	3–5	N/A ($t_{1/2}$ 8 h)	0.5%: 1 drop 2–3 times daily
Brimonidine	rapid	2	8–12	0.15%, 0.2%: 1 drop 2 times daily
β-blockers				
Betaxolol	0.5	2	12–18	0.5%: 1 drop 2 times daily
Timolol (also available in combinations)	0.5	1–2	Up to 24	0.5%: 1 drop 1 or 2 times daily gel 0.25% or 0.5%: 1 drop daily
Carbonic anhydrase inhibitors *Systemic* Acetazolamide				
Tablets IV injection	1–1.5 2 min	2–4 15 min	8–12 4–5	250 mg PO 1–4 times daily 250–1000 mg/24 hours IV
Eyedrops				
Brinzolamide Dorzolamide	<1 N/A	<1 2.5	8–12 8–12	1%: 1 drop 2 times daily 2%: 1 drop 3 times daily or 1 drop 2 times daily if used with timolol

TABLE 40.1 Antiglaucoma agents: pharmacokinetics and dosing—cont'd

DRUG	ONSET OF ACTION (H)	PEAK EFFECT (H)	DURATION OF ACTION (H)	USUAL ADULT DOSAGE
Prostaglandin agonists				
Bimatoprost	4	8–12	24–36	0.03%: 1 drop in the evening or 1 drop in the morning if used with timolol
Latanoprost	4	8–12	24–36	50 microgram/mL (0.005%): 1 drop in the evening
Travoprost	2	>12	24–36	0.004%: 1 drop in the evening
Miotics (muscarinic agonists)				
Pilocarpine	Up to 0.5	1–1.25	4–12	1%, 2%, 4%: 1 drop 3 or 4 times daily
Hyperosmotic agent				
Mannitol	Rapid (30 min)	6	1–2 g/kg IV over 30 min	

All are administered topically as eyedrops except acetazolamide and mannitol, used in acute glaucomas.
IV = intravenously; N/A = not available; PO = orally; $t_{1/2}$ = half-life

Initial treatment is usually with a prostaglandin agonist eyedrop. Most people eventually require one or more added drugs, commonly a β-blocker, α_2-agonist or CA inhibitor. (Meta-analysis has shown this is the order of descending efficacy in reducing IOP.) Some combination preparations are now available, such as eyedrops containing timolol plus a CA inhibitor/PG agonist/α_2-agonist, or brinzolamide plus brimonidine. Adding more drugs becomes decreasingly effective; tachyphylaxis develops to some drug groups, especially β-blockers.

Prostaglandin agonists

Latanoprost, bimatoprost, travoprost and tafluprost are synthetic prostaglandin F_2 agonists approved to treat POAG. They reduce IOP via actions on prostanoid receptors, increasing aqueous humour outflow (Drug Monograph 40.1 for mechanism of action, drug interactions and ADRs). They are generally well tolerated, and their long duration of action enhances compliance.

Beta-blockers (β-adrenoceptor antagonists)

The β-blockers used in glaucoma are betaxolol and timolol, as 0.25% and 0.5% drops, and timolol as 0.1% eye gel. The exact mechanism of action in glaucoma is uncertain; they block β-receptor-mediated stimulation of ciliary epithelium, leading to impaired aqueous humour formation (less effective during sleep hours). The advantages are their safety, duration of action (only requiring 1–2 doses per day) and lack of effect on pupil size or accommodation.

Betaxolol, a cardioselective (β_1) blocking agent, is indicated for the treatment of POAG and ocular hypertension, and may be preferred for people with airways disease, as it is less likely than non-cardioselective β-blockers to cause bronchoconstriction and asthma (Fig 40.4).

Adverse reactions are primarily local: burning, stinging or eye irritation. Rare effects include visual disturbances, pruritus or allergic reaction. Systemic absorption can lead to adverse effects, including hypotension, asthma and depression, and to drug interactions; precautions need to be taken in people with asthma or diabetes, and in the elderly and children (Fig 40.4).

Sympathomimetics (α_2-receptor agonists)

Stimulation of α-receptors increases aqueous humour outflow via vasoconstriction and may suppress aqueous humour formation. Old agents were adrenaline (epinephrine) and phenylephrine; newer sympathomimetics are α_2-receptor selective agonists apraclonidine and brimonidine, related to the antihypertensive clonidine (see Ch 10 for mechanism of action). They are indicated as adjunct therapy in POAG. Apraclonidine is indicated for short-term use only, for up to 3 months, due to allergies. Mild adverse drug reactions (ADRs) include eye irritation, taste disturbances and mydriasis. Effects of systemic absorption are those of α_2-adrenoceptor stimulation: palpitations, hypotension, tremors and light-headedness.

Carbonic anhydrase inhibitors

The enzyme carbonic anhydrase catalyses the interconversion of bicarbonate with carbon dioxide and water; its actions are necessary for the secretion of aqueous humour. Drugs that inhibit this enzyme are used in glaucoma, and as mild diuretic agents, to treat epilepsy and raised intracranial pressure. The most commonly used systemic CA inhibitor is acetazolamide; given PO or IV in glaucoma emergencies, it lowers IOP by decreasing aqueous production to about half its baseline amount.

CA inhibitors available as topical eyedrops are dorzolamide and brinzolamide (Table 40.1); the latter has a high affinity for the ocular enzyme and can be used twice daily. Some drug is absorbed systemically and binds to the CA enzyme in red blood cells, with a very long elimination half-life, but few significant adverse effects. Precautions

Drug Monograph 40.1
Latanoprost

Latanoprost is a prostaglandin $F_{2\alpha}$ analogue – that is, a selective prostanoid FP-receptor agonist. It can reduce IOP by 27–34%; no tolerance develops over at least 4 years.

Mechanism of action
Latanoprost binds to receptors on the ciliary body, upregulating metalloproteinases which remodel extracellular matrix, allowing increased uveoscleral outflow of aqueous humour.

Indications
Latanoprost is indicated for people with open-angle glaucoma, to reduce IOP in ocular hypertension and to prevent the risk of optic nerve damage.

Pharmacokinetics
Latanoprost is administered as eyedrops. Its onset of action is 3–4 hours, maximum effect occurs in 8–12 hours and duration of action is more than 24 hours. It is a prodrug, an ester hydrolysed to the active acid form during passage through the cornea; it is distributed to the anterior segment of the eye, conjunctiva and eyelids. Following ocular administration, approximately 45% is absorbed systemically; it is metabolised in the liver to inactive metabolites excreted in the urine. The elimination half-life is approximately 17 minutes.

Drug interactions
There are additive IOP effects with β-blockers, and the drug can be used effectively as adjunct therapy with most other antiglaucoma agents. Eyedrops containing NSAIDs (diclofenac, ketorolac) can reduce the effects of a prostaglandin eyedrop; IOP should be monitored if NSAID eyedrop is being used long term.

Adverse reactions
The most common adverse reactions are stinging, blurred vision, conjunctivitis, red eye, eyelash changes, itching and eye pain and a bitter taste. An unusual ADR is change in iris colour: people with hazel or yellow-brown eyes are particularly susceptible to darkening of the iris due to increased melanin, the effect usually starting within 8 months of commencing therapy.

Warnings and contraindications
Patients should be warned of the possible irreversible change in eye colour, especially if the drug is being applied only to one eye. Latanoprost should be used with caution in people with, or susceptible to, asthma or macular oedema. It is contraindicated if there is intraocular inflammation or known hypersensitivity to any ingredient; thus far, there are few data on use in children or during pregnancy or lactation. In people with a history of herpes simplex keratitis, there may be a recurrence.

Dosage and administration
One drop of latanoprost solution (0.005%) is administered to the eye daily, preferably in the evening; more frequent administration may decrease the IOP-lowering effect. Pressure should be applied to the tear duct to minimise systemic absorption. It is also available in a combination formulation with timolol (0.5%) for additive effects.

are needed for those who are allergic to sulfonamides. Important drug interactions can occur from systemically administered CA inhibitors, due to alkalinisation of the urine and hence decreased excretion of basic drugs such as amphetamines. High-dose aspirin, or renal impairment, can increase the toxicity of systemic acetazolamide.

Cholinergic agents (miotics)
Miotics (discussed earlier) contract the circular muscle of the iris, thus relieving obstruction to outflow of aqueous humour and reducing IOP in glaucoma. They are used less commonly since development of more specific drugs. Pilocarpine drops (1%, 2%, 4%) may impair driving, and make it difficult to adjust quickly to changes in illumination, especially for elderly people.

Osmotic agents
Osmotic agents are hyperosmotic solutions of chemicals that remain in the bloodstream and raise plasma osmotic pressure; they are given IV or orally to reduce IOP by dehydration of the vitreous body, decreased formation and increased resorption of aqueous humour. Mannitol 10% or 20% solution IV is rapid and effective in emergency treatment of acute glaucoma, before surgery for cataract and sometimes to reduce intracranial pressure; it may cause fluid and electrolyte shifts.

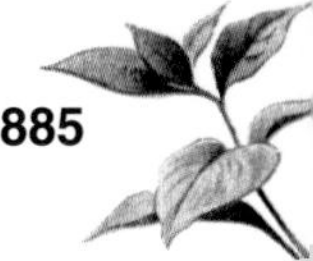

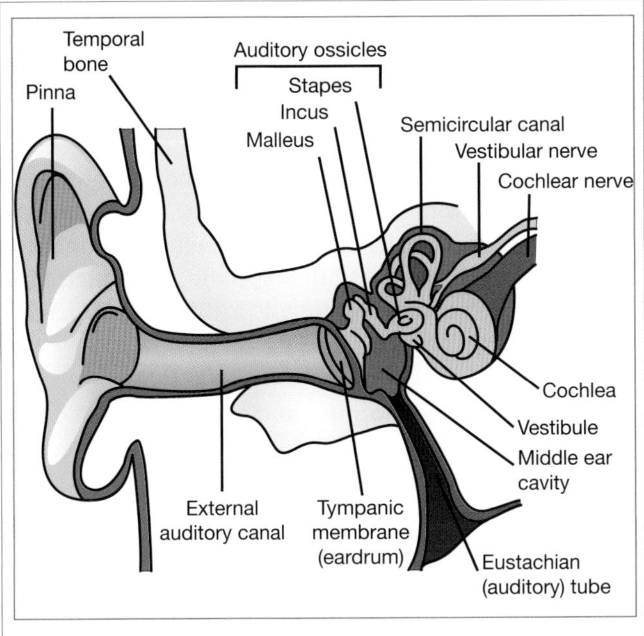

FIGURE 40.4 Anatomy of the ear
Source: Salerno 1999.

KEY POINTS

Drugs for glaucoma

- Glaucomas are a group of optic neuropathies that threaten vision; treatments aim to reduce the associated raised IOP.
- Topically applied drugs used to treat glaucoma are:
  - prostaglandin agonists (e.g. latanoprost; Drug Monograph 40.1)
  - β-blockers (betaxolol, timolol)
  - carbonic anhydrase inhibitors (topically: brinzolamide, dorzolamide; systemically: acetazolamide)
  - α_2-agonists (apraclonidine, brimonidine)
  - miotics (pilocarpine).
- Combinations of drugs are often required; various fixed-dose combination eyedrops are available.
- Systemically, the carbonic anhydrase inhibitor acetazolamide or osmotic agent mannitol are used.

Drugs for macular degeneration

Age-related macular degeneration (AMD) is the condition in elderly people where the most sensitive part of the retina degenerates, new blood vessels are formed and central vision is lost. It is the leading cause of irreversible blindness in Australia; major risk factors are smoking, obesity, positive family history and long-term (15–20 years) use of aspirin. AMD was previously treatable only by laser burns to seal the leaks into the retina; drugs are now available.

Monoclonal antibodies

Ranibizumab is a monoclonal antibody fragment against vascular endothelial growth factor A (VEGF-A); following monthly intravitreal injections (one eye each visit), it inhibits growth of new blood vessels under the macula of the retina and slows loss of vision. Potential adverse events include ocular irritation, infection or haemorrhage and raised IOP. Bevacizumab, a related drug used to treat colorectal cancer, is now frequently used 'off-label' as an alternative.

Aflibercept

Aflibercept also blocks VEGF-A but by a different mechanism: it blocks binding of VEGF-A to its receptor by acting as a soluble decoy receptor. It is administered by intravitreal injection, three times at monthly intervals then every 8 weeks. Safety, efficacy and adverse effects are similar to those of ranibizumab.

Verteporfin, a photosensitiser

Many chemical compounds can act as photosensitisers, absorbing energy from electromagnetic radiation or light and forming activated metabolites, such as oxygen free radicals, which damage cell constituents (see 'Phototoxicity' in Ch 41). This process can be exploited in photodynamic therapy, in which a photosensitiser plus light energy can be directed to ablate specific lesions.

Verteporfin is a porphyrin-type photosensitiser used to treat macular degeneration. It is a dark green-black powder, dissolved and administered as an IV infusion over 10 minutes. At 15 minutes, non-thermal red light from a laser source is focused on the macular lesion for about 80 seconds; reactive oxygen free radicals formed cause local damage and vessel occlusion. It is (rarely) used to treat AMD and choroidal neovascularisation due to other macular diseases. Adverse reactions include loss of visual acuity, field defects, haemorrhages, cataract, blepharitis and pain at the infusion site.

Anecortave

Anecortave acetate is a new steroidal drug for AMD. It and its desacetate derivative are effective inhibitors of pathological blood vessel growth in the eye; many mechanisms for the antiangiogenic actions have been proposed. Posterior juxtascleral depot injections are given by ophthalmic surgeons under local anaesthesia at 6-monthly intervals. Most common adverse events are decreased visual acuity, eye pain and hyperaemia.

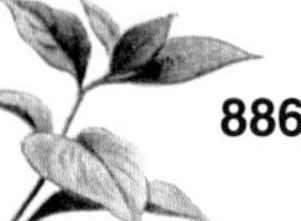

Antimicrobial agents

Because the conjunctival surface is open to the atmosphere and maintained in a moist condition, it is prone to infection. The body's natural defences cannot readily function in avascular tissues, so infections may damage the eye and impair vision. Eye infections require prompt treatment with antimicrobial agents; solutions (eyedrops) are preferred formulations because ointment bases tend to interfere with healing.

Common ocular infections

Conjunctivitis is an acute inflammation of the conjunctiva resulting from bacterial or viral infection, or of allergic or irritative origin; it is usually self-limiting. The infected eye should be protected from light; antibiotic eyedrops or ointment may be required. Gonococcal conjunctivitis in neonates is sight-threatening and requires IV antibiotics.

Blepharitis (inflammation of the eyelids) may result from bacterial or viral infection, inflammation or allergy. For seborrhoeic (dandruff-type) blepharitis, treatment is to wash lids gently with a mild soap (e.g. diluted 'baby shampoo' or 'baby soap') or sodium bicarbonate solution. If the infection is staphylococcal, the lids are cleansed, then antibiotic eye ointment (chloramphenicol) is applied.

Hordeolum (stye) is an acute localised infection of the eyelash follicles and the lid glands, forming a small abscess or cyst, treated by drainage. An internal hordeolum may also require oral anti-staphylococcal antibiotics such as dicloxacillin.

Keratitis is corneal inflammation caused by bacterial or viral infection. Adenoviral keratoconjunctivitis is contagious but usually resolves simply. Herpes simplex keratitis may cause corneal ulcers and scarring and requires treatment with an antiviral agent (aciclovir).

Infection with *Acanthamoeba* (a protozoon) can occur in wearers of soft contact lenses from contaminated water. It causes redness, pain and photophobia, and can lead to corneal scarring and loss of vision. It requires early diagnosis and aggressive antimicrobial therapy – for example, with an antiamoebic agent (propamidine) plus an antibacterial (neomycin) and possibly an antifungal to prevent secondary infections.

Trachoma is a type of chronic conjunctivitis caused by the bacterium *Chlamydia trachomatis*. If left untreated it can cause the person's eyelids to turn inwards, causing their eyelashes to rub the cornea and conjunctiva of the eye (trichiasis). This constant rubbing can lead to corneal scarring and even blindness. Trachoma is a serious world health problem, estimated to affect 500 million people, and the major cause of preventable blindness. It is common in northern parts of Australia, especially in children. Early detection, good public health education and effective compliance with therapy are critical. Antibiotic treatment is prescribed in adults and children with a single oral dose of the macrolide antibiotic azithromycin. In adults, the dosage is 1 g and in children 20 mg/kg up to 1 g.

Toxoplasmosis is an infection with the unicellular organism *Toxoplasma gondii*; it is commonly contracted before birth or from domestic cats. If the eye is affected, posterior uveitis can lead to loss of sight. Treatment is combination therapy with specific antimicrobials (clindamycin) plus corticosteroids to limit the damaging inflammatory response.

Common ocular pathogens and routes

Common ocular pathogens include bacteria (especially *Staphylococcus aureus*, streptococci and pneumococci), viruses (adenovirus, herpes simplex virus), *Chlamydia* and protozoa (acanthamoebae). The common routes of transmission of infection to the eye include:

- congenital, during passage of the infant down the birth canal if infection is present (e.g. ophthalmia neonatorum, a gonococcal infection)
- direct contact (e.g. herpes simplex transmitted by fingers from 'cold sore' lesions)
- airborne droplet transmission in aerosol (e.g. from coughing or sneezing)
- migration from other sites, especially from the nasopharynx
- trauma, especially penetrating eye injuries
- from infected contact lenses, instruments, water or contaminated ocular drug formulations.

Ocular antimicrobial chemotherapy

Selection of an antimicrobial to treat infection is based on clinical experience, the nature and sensitivity of the organisms likely to have caused the condition, the sensitivity and response of the person and laboratory results. (See Chs 35–38 for general aspects of antimicrobial drugs.)

Most antimicrobial agents do not easily penetrate the eye when applied. Some drugs will cross the blood–aqueous humour barrier if impaired or inflamed. Topically applied antimicrobials can cause sensitivity reactions (stinging, itching and dermatitis) and an unpleasant taste following nasolacrimal drainage; they can also interfere with normal flora and encourage other organisms. Severe eye infections may require systemic antimicrobials.

Antimicrobials used topically (in the eye or on the skin) should be different from those used systemically, to reduce development of resistance in the organisms or sensitisation in the person. Drugs that are too toxic systemically may be safe locally. In Australia, some topical antibiotics (ciprofloxacin, ofloxacin, gentamicin and tobramycin) are preferentially reserved for ophthalmologists' use.

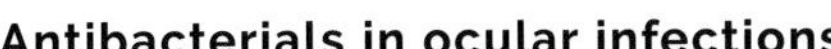

Antibacterials in ocular infections

Antibacterial antibiotics used in the eye include chloramphenicol, aminoglycosides, quinolones (ciprofloxacin and ofloxacin; both 0.3% drops) and propamidine (0.1% drops).

Chloramphenicol

A broad-spectrum bacteriostatic agent, chloramphenicol prevents peptide bond formation and protein synthesis in a wide variety of Gram-positive and Gram-negative organisms and has good penetration in eye infections. Formulated as 0.5% drops and 1% ointment, it can cause burning and stinging on administration.

Aminoglycosides

Aminoglycosides (gentamicin [Drug Monograph 36.2], framycetin and tobramycin) are used against a wide variety of Gram-negative organisms, including *Proteus* and *Klebsiella* organisms and *Escherichia coli*. Gentamicin and tobramycin are also active against *Pseudomonas* infections. Typical formulations are: framycetin eyedrops 0.5%, gentamicin eyedrops 0.3% and tobramycin eyedrops 0.3%, eye ointment 0.3%, applied two to four times daily.

The aminoglycosides are safer topically than systemically; ADRs include hypersensitivity, lid itching, swelling and conjunctival erythema (Gilissen et al. 2019). When topical and systemic aminoglycosides are used concurrently, the total plasma concentration should be monitored, as systemic toxicity (renal damage, ototoxicity and impaired neuromuscular transmission) may occur.

Quinolones

Quinolone antibiotics are bactericidal. They inhibit the bacterial enzymes, DNA gyrase and topoisomerase IV. This blocks DNA replication and inhibits bacterial DNA synthesis. Quinolones are broad spectrum antibiotics; they have excellent Gram-negative activity (e.g. *Escherichia coli*, *Pseudomonas*) and good Gram-positive (staphylococcus, *Streptococcus* spp.) activity. Topical quinolone drugs include ciprofloxacin and ofloxacin. They are indicated for keratitis (corneal inflammation) and conjunctivitis. They are reserved for ophthalmologist use, due to emerging bacterial resistance issues.

Antiviral in ocular infections

The only ophthalmic antiviral preparation available in Australia is aciclovir eye ointment, 3%, for treatment of herpes simplex keratitis. The dose is a 1-cm ribbon of ointment to the lower conjunctival sac, five times daily. Aciclovir (Drug Monograph 37.1) is well absorbed through the cornea into the aqueous humour. Adverse reactions include transient stinging, sensitivity reactions and occasionally superficial corneal damage. Use during pregnancy and breastfeeding is considered safe.

Antifungals in ocular infections

Eye infections due to fungi such as *Aspergillus* or *Candida* need treatment with an appropriate antifungal agent. No antifungal eye formulations are readily available in Australia; however, natamycin eyedrops 5% may be imported under the Special Access Scheme.

Antiseptics in ocular infections

Anti-amoeba agents

Propamidine (a mild antiseptic and skin disinfectant) and its dibromo-derivative are effective topically against *acanthamoebae*. Propamidine eyedrops (0.1%) are indicated for *acanthamoeba* protozoal keratitis and mild acute bacterial conjunctivitis. Protozoal keratitis, while rare, is associated with poor soft contact lens care.

KEY POINTS

Drugs for eye infections

- Eye infections are relatively common and usually self-limiting. Treatment with antimicrobials specific to the pathogenic organism can speed recovery time and prevent complications.
- Ocular infections may be caused by bacteria, viruses or protozoa.
- Antimicrobials that are not commonly used systemically are preferred for topical use.
- Antimicrobials formulated for use in the eye include antibacterials (chloramphenicol, aminoglycosides, quinolones), an antiviral (aciclovir) and anti-amoeba agent (propamidine).
- Azithromycin is indicated by oral route to treat trachoma, a common vision-threatening infection caused by the bacteria *Chlamydia*.

Anti-inflammatory and antiallergy agents

Treatment of ocular inflammations

Inflammation of the eyes, with reddening, tearing, itching and mild pain, is relatively common and may accompany infections, mechanical damage or allergies, or occur as an ocular ADR. Inflammatory conditions include uveitis (intraocular inflammation), episcleritis and scleritis, ranging from common and mild to severe vision-threatening conditions. Initial treatment is with normal saline wash, cold compresses and ocular lubricants; then topical antihistamines, oral or ocular NSAIDs and steroid drops if more severe. (Inflammatory mediators and anti-inflammatory drugs are covered in detail in Ch 34.)

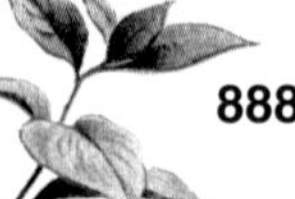

Ocular corticosteroids

Corticosteroids inhibit the inflammatory cascade and the functions of fibroblasts and keratocytes. Their anti-inflammatory and immunosuppressant effects are useful in many ocular inflammations (uveitis, conjunctivitis, scleritis and episcleritis), in dry eye disease, to prevent postoperative adhesions and in posterior segment diseases such as AMD, diabetic retinopathy and macular oedema, to reduce growth of new blood vessels (Gaballa et al. 2021).

Corticosteroids are available for ophthalmic use as topical solutions, suspensions or ointments (Table 40.2). They include dexamethasone, fluorometholone, hydrocortisone and prednisolone; prednisolone is also formulated as combination drops with the vasoconstrictor phenylephrine, and dexamethasone as an intravitreal implant for diabetic macular oedema. Corticosteroids are contraindicated in ocular infections (e.g. herpes simplex epithelial keratitis) and glaucoma, and in people predisposed to raised IOP. Given the serious nature of their adverse effects, which can threaten vision, ocular corticosteroids should only be used when there is close supervision by an ophthalmologist (Australian Medicines Handbook 2021).

Ocular non-steroidal anti-inflammatory drugs

Some NSAIDs are available in formulations for ocular use (early drugs such as aspirin were too irritant to the cornea). Diclofenac (0.1%), ketorolac (0.5%) or nepafenac (0.3%) drops are used with the following indications:

- to prevent and treat postoperative pain and inflammation after cataract surgery
- to treat conjunctivitis and seasonal allergic ophthalmic pruritus (itching associated with hay fever).

The most common ADRs after ocular use are transient stinging on application, irritation, allergies and delayed healing. Eyedrops containing NSAIDs can reduce the effects of a prostaglandin eyedrop (Drug Monograph 40.1); IOP should be monitored if both eyedrops are being used long term. If absorbed, NSAIDs may cause systemic effects. (See Ch 34 for mechanism of action, adverse effects and drug interactions.)

TABLE 40.2 Potency of ocular corticosteroids

STEROID FORMULATION	POTENCY	RELATIVE TENDENCY TO RAISE INTRAOCULAR PRESSURE
Hydrocortisone 1% ointment	Low	++
Prednisolone 0.5% drops	Mid	+++
Fluorometholone 0.1% suspension drops	Mid–high	+++
Dexamethasone 0.1% suspension drops	High	++++

Source: Adapted from Australian Medicines Handbook 2021.

Ocular antiallergy agents

Allergic reactions of the eyelid and conjunctiva, such as in hay fever, can lead to oedema, erythema, itching, crusting and contact dermatitis. Typical allergens are pollens, dust mites, bites and stings, food, cosmetics, contact lenses, animals and chemicals. Drugs known to cause ocular allergies include some antibiotics, preservatives, topical antihistamines (a paradoxical effect) and timolol.

Ocular antihistamines

Treatment of ocular allergies is first to eliminate the allergen (if possible); then cooling, saline lotions and oral NSAIDs may bring relief. Topical treatment is with eyedrops – for example, H_1-antihistamines such as azelastine 0.05%, levocabastine 0.05%, ketotifen 0.025% (Drug Monograph 40.2) or olopatadine 0.1%. (The last two also have useful mast-cell stabilising activity.) If allergy is severe, corticosteroids such as prednisolone 0.5% may be required.

Note that the combination of a sympathomimetic decongestant with an antihistamine often leads to rebound exacerbated conjunctivitis, so these combinations are no longer recommended.

Ocular mast-cell stabilisers (cromones, cromolyns)

Sodium cromoglycate 2% (cromolyn sodium) and lodoxamide 0.1% are used for allergic eye disorders (vernal and allergic keratoconjunctivitis, papillary conjunctivitis and keratitis) that have symptoms of itching, tearing, redness and discharge. Their mechanism of action is to inhibit degranulation of sensitised mast cells occurring after exposure to a specific antigen, preventing mediators of inflammation from actions. They have a delayed onset of action, so treatment should be started 1 month before hay-fever season. (See Ch 15 for prophylactic use in asthma.) Adverse reactions include stinging and burning sensation in the eyes.

KEY POINTS

Ocular anti-inflammatory and antiallergy agents

- Minor ocular inflammations may be self-limiting; however, severe or chronic inflammations can cause scarring or retinal detachment and require treatment with anti-inflammatory agents such as corticosteroids or NSAIDs.
- Allergic reactions in the eye are treated with antihistamines (e.g. ketotifen) or mast-cell stabilisers (sodium cromoglycate).

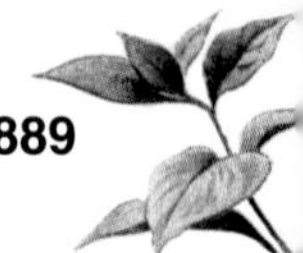

Drug Monograph 40.2
Ketotifen

Ketotifen is an antihistamine and mast-cell stabiliser formulated for ocular administration. It is indicated for prophylaxis and treatment of seasonal allergic conjunctivitis (hay-fever-associated itchy eyes).

Mechanism of action

Ketotifen is a histamine H_1-receptor antagonist (classical antihistamine), thus inhibiting type 1 anaphylactic reactions and capillary dilation. It also inhibits release of mediators including histamine, leukotrienes and prostaglandins from cells involved in immediate allergic reactions.

Pharmacokinetics

After 14 days of repeated topical ocular administration to volunteers, plasma levels of ketotifen were in most cases below level of detection. (After oral administration, ketotifen is eliminated biphasically with a terminal half-life of 21 hours, and is excreted in the urine mainly as inactive metabolites.)

Drug interactions

None known; if other ocular drugs are used concomitantly, at least 5 minutes should elapse between administrations.

Adverse reactions

Common ADRs include local ocular effects: eye irritation and pain, dry eyes, rarely punctate keratitis or corneal erosion, and paradoxical local and systemic allergic reactions.

Precautions and contraindications

The multi-dose formulation contains benzalkonium chloride as a preservative; this can cause eye irritation and discolour soft contact lenses, which should be removed before and for 15 minutes after use. Anyone experiencing blurred vision or sleepiness should not drive or operate machinery.

Dosage and administration

Ketotifen is provided as a 0.25 mg/mL solution, in either multi-dose 5 mL containers or single-dose 0.4 mL units. The dosage for adults and children over 3 years old is one drop into the conjunctival sac twice daily. Care must be taken not to contaminate the dropper tip. No dosage adjustment is required for geriatric people or those with renal or liver impairment, or in pregnant or breastfeeding women (Pregnancy Safety Category B1). The containers should be stored below 25°C; multi-dose containers must be discarded 4 weeks after opening, and single-use units immediately after use.

Drugs for dry eyes

Eyes can become excessively dry, irritated and scratchy in conditions of hot winds, dry air-conditioning or heating, or inadequate tear production; the medical term is keratoconjunctivitis sicca. Dry eye syndrome affects one in five adults and results from the excessive evaporation or insufficient production of tears. Most people have mild disease and require only simple treatment (ocular lubricants). Complex interventions in severe disease aim to prevent long-term complications (e.g. ulceration or scarring). It is common in older adults and contact lens users. It can also occur as an ADR, notably after anticholinergics such as cycloplegics, antihistamines, antidepressants and antipsychotics (see Australian Medicines Handbook 2021).

Ocular lubricants

Ocular lubricants, artificial tears and isotonic external irrigating solutions are used to provide moisture and lubrication, to cleanse and lubricate artificial eyes and contact lenses, to remove debris and to protect the cornea during procedures. These are available OTC as drops, irrigations and eye-washes. Such products may include a balanced salt solution, buffers to adjust pH (especially boric acid/sodium borate) and preservatives to reduce microbial growth. Preservatives can irritate the cornea; some preservative-free formulations are available. Agents to increase viscosity and extend eye contact time may also be present, such as hypromellose and carmellose, propylene glycol, carbomers, dextrans, polyvinyl alcohol, glycerol, mannitol, lecithin, povidone and triglycerides. (Similar chemicals are also used in some contact lens solutions and blood volume expanders.) These products are usually administered three or four times a day.

Ointment preparations containing paraffins are also used as ocular lubricants. They will help to protect and lubricate the eye – for example, during and after eye surgery. They are particularly valuable for people who have an impaired blink reflex and for night-time use.

Ciclosporin

Ciclosporin is indicated for treating moderate-to-severe dry eye syndrome when ocular lubricants are insufficient.

Ciclosporin is a calcineurin inhibitor immunosuppressant with anti-inflammatory properties. It complexes with cyclophilin after entering immune T-cells, inhibiting calcineurin phosphatase and halting activity of the NFATc transcription factor. This prevents the production of inflammatory cytokines (including IL-2 and IFN-γ) associated with dry eye syndrome, resulting in increased tear production (De Paiva et al. 2019). Ciclosporin increases the average number of conjunctival goblet cells within the eye (De Paiva et al. 2019). These cells act like lubricants to protect the eye by secreting mucus. One drop should be administered into each eye twice daily to relieve dry eye symptoms.

KEY POINTS

Drugs for dry eyes

- The most common drugs used to treat dry eye syndrome are ocular lubricants, also known as artificial tears.
- Ciclosporin is an anti-inflammatory ocular drug that is used when ocular lubricants are insufficient. Ciclosporin increases the number of conjunctival goblet cells that secret mucus, providing ocular lubrication.

Autonomic drugs in the eye

Autonomic innervation of ocular tissues

Many drugs used in the eye affect autonomic pathways; hence, it is important to review autonomic innervation of ocular tissues, the relevant neurotransmitters and receptors involved and drug groups affecting autonomic responses (see Unit 3, 'Drugs affecting the peripheral nervous system', tables in Chs 8 and 9, Table 40.1 and Table 40.3).

TABLE 40.3 Effects of autonomic stimulation on ocular tissues[a]

OCULAR TISSUE	SYMPATHETIC	PARASYMPATHETIC
Smooth muscle of iris	Dilator pupillae (radial muscle) (α_1) contraction causes mydriasis	Sphincter pupillae (circular muscle) (M_3) contraction causes miosis and regulation of IOP
Ciliary muscle (adjusts curvature of lens)	Relaxation (β_2) causes focus for distant vision	Contraction causes accommodation for near vision and increases filtration angle, so drains aqueous humour
Lacrimal gland		Secretion of tears
Blood vessels	Vasoconstriction (α_1) decreases formation of aqueous humour	
Muscle of upper lid	Contraction (α_1) widens eyes	

[a] The main effects of stimulation of autonomic pathways to ocular tissues are shown; sympathetic effects are mediated by actions of noradrenaline on α or β adrenoceptors, and parasympathetic effects are mediated by acetylcholine actions on muscarinic receptors.

Ocular uses of autonomic drugs

Mydriatic and cycloplegic agents

Mydriatics

Mydriatics are drugs that cause pupil dilation (mydriasis). They are primarily used to facilitate examination of the peripheral lens and retina in the diagnosis of ophthalmic disorders and to prevent or break down posterior synechiae (adhesions) in iridocyclitis. Mydriasis can be achieved either by blocking acetylcholine (ACh) effects on muscarinic receptors with anticholinergic agents, or by enhancing noradrenaline (norepinephrine) effects on α_1-adrenoceptors with sympathomimetics. Mydriatic agents evoke less of a response in people with heavily pigmented (dark) irises than in those with lighter-pigmented (blue) eyes, because the drug may bind to melanin.

Anticholinergics (antimuscarinics, atropinic agents)

Anticholinergics reversibly produce mydriasis and cycloplegia (paralysis of ciliary muscle). Contraction of the iris sphincter can lead to an increase in IOP; hence, glaucoma may be precipitated. Other adverse effects include increased glare, blurred vision and stinging (which may be relieved by prior administration of a local anaesthetic eyedrop). Patients should be advised to wear dark glasses afterwards. Systemic 'atropinic' effects may follow absorption via the nasolacrimal ducts: dry eyes, dry mouth, tachycardia, decreased gastrointestinal tract (GIT) functions and ataxia. Anticholinergic eyedrops should be used cautiously in people with head injury or glaucoma, and in children.

Commonly used anticholinergic agents include atropine, tropicamide and cyclopentolate (Table 40.4). Note that atropine eyedrops cause prolonged mydriasis and cycloplegia (for 7–14 days) and are too strong for routine use. Examples of systemic drugs with atropinic effects include some antihistamines, phenothiazines, antiparkinson agents and antidepressants (see Australian Medicines Handbook 2021); these may affect the eyes. Interactions with anticholinesterases will antagonise the anticholinergic effects.

Sympathomimetics (adrenergic agonists)

Topical **sympathomimetic drugs** mimic the α_1-receptor-mediated actions of noradrenaline on the dilator muscle of the iris. This results in mydriasis, vasoconstriction and decreased congestion of conjunctival blood vessels, a decrease in aqueous humour formation and an increase

TABLE 40.4 Ocular anticholinergic agents: pharmacokinetics and dosing

DRUG	TIME TO MAXIMAL MYDRIASIS (MIN)	RECOVERY	TIME TO MAXIMAL CYCLOPLEGIA	RECOVERY	USUAL ADULT DOSE
Atropine 1%	30–40	7–10 days	3–6 hours	7–14 days	1%: 1 drop
Cyclopentolate 0.5–1%	30–60	1 day	25–75 min	6–24 hours	0.5%, 1%: 1 drop
Tropicamide 0.5–1%	20–40	6 hours	30–40 min	2–6 hours	0.5%, 1%: 1 drop

Systemic adverse effects are most common with atropine and rare with tropicamide.
Source: Based on data in Australian Medicines Handbook 2021; MIMS Online.

in outflow and relaxation of the ciliary muscle. Sympathomimetics do not affect accommodation or the pupillary light reflex.

Adrenergic drugs are used to produce mydriasis for ocular examination, to treat wide-angle glaucoma and glaucoma secondary to uveitis and to relieve congestion and hyperaemia (red eyes). As a mydriatic, phenylephrine is generally used as an adjunct to anticholinergic mydriatics. Systemic absorption can lead to tachycardia and elevated blood pressure, brow ache, sweating, tremors and confusion; adverse effects are likely to be greater in children and in the elderly. Adverse drug interactions may occur with monoamine oxidase inhibitors and with α- or β-adrenoceptor antagonists.

The main adrenergic drugs used in ophthalmology include: phenylephrine, naphazoline and tetryzoline (tetrahydrozoline) (mild agents used as vasoconstrictors); and α_2-agonists used in glaucoma: apraclonidine and brimonidine (Table 40.1); note that strengths of solutions, and hence doses, vary widely depending on use (antiglaucoma, mydriatic or vasoconstrictor). Sympathomimetics are also formulated in combination drops with antihistamines or corticosteroids.

Cycloplegics

Cycloplegic drugs are agents that paralyse ciliary muscle, causing loss of accommodation. As explained earlier, cycloplegia is invariably accompanied by mydriasis. Cycloplegics are used to prevent accommodation during refraction, for pain relief in iridocyclitis or to induce chemical occlusion for treating amblyopia ('lazy eye').

Cycloplegic agents are the anticholinergics – that is, atropine (Drug Monograph 8.2), cyclopentolate and tropicamide; see again Table 40.4. Note that the same peripheral and central anticholinergic ADRs can occur; these agents are used only with great caution in children (particularly those with blue eyes), or people with disorders of the central nervous system (CNS) due to the risk of adverse effects.

Miotic agents

Miotic drugs constrict the pupil – that is, cause miosis; they are used to treat glaucoma (see later). Parasympathomimetic drugs act as miotics and cause accommodation for near vision; hence, they are likely to cause blurring of vision. Drugs can enhance parasympathetic effects either by acting as direct agonists on ACh_M receptors or by increasing the amount of ACh available to act, as do anticholinesterases.

Muscarinic agonists

Muscarinic agonists stimulate muscarinic receptors in the circular muscle of the iris, causing contraction and thus pupil constriction. Acetylcholine itself can be used; however, it is subject to rapid hydrolysis and inactivation by cholinesterase enzymes, so has a very brief action. It is occasionally used by injection (20 mg or 2 mL) into the anterior chamber for rapid miosis during surgery, as is carbachol.

Pilocarpine is a natural compound from various *Pilocarpus* species plants; it mimics the effects of ACh in the parasympathetic nervous system. Pilocarpine is an uncharged molecule and so is well absorbed and likely to have CNS adverse effects. It has little effect on the ciliary muscle and so does not markedly affect accommodation. It is an effective miotic, enhancing outflow of aqueous humour and decreasing IOP, hence its usefulness in glaucoma. To allow careful titration of doses and effects, pilocarpine eyedrops are available in a range of strengths (1%, 2%, 4%).

Ocular decongestants

Drugs that are vasoconstrictors have '**decongestant**' effects in the eye (and nose: see Ch 15). These drugs are sympathomimetics, and their mechanism of action is as α-adrenoceptor agonists. Vasoconstriction reduces hyperaemia and fluid exudation, and hence reduces reddening. Rebound hyperaemia may occur and lead to overuse. Vasoconstriction may also decrease the absorption of other drugs into the bloodstream.

Examples of drugs used as ocular decongestants are phenylephrine, naphazoline and tetryzoline (tetrahydrozoline) (Table 40.5); note that much lower doses are used for vasoconstrictor and decongestant effects than for mydriasis. Decongestants are often formulated as eyedrops together with an antihistamine (antazoline, pheniramine), to reduce itching and redness, or a corticosteroid, for anti-inflammatory effects.

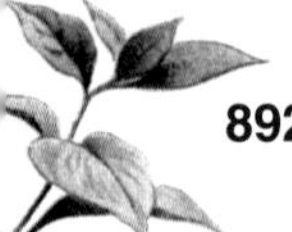

TABLE 40.5 Ocular adrenergic agents

DRUG	USES	USUAL ADULT DOSAGE
Naphazoline	V	0.012–0.1%: 1 drop every 3–4 hours as necessary
Phenylephrine	IOP, M V	2.5%, 10%: 1 drop as necessary 0.12%: 1 drop every 3–4 hours as necessary
Tetryzoline (tetrahydrozoline)	V	0.05%: 1 drop 2–4 times daily
Brimonidine	IOP	0.15%, 0.2%: 1 drop 2 times daily
Apraclonidine	IOP	0.5%: 1 drop 2–3 times daily

IOP = (reduction in) intraocular pressure; M = mydriasis; V = vasoconstriction

KEY POINTS

Autonomic ocular drugs

- Understanding autonomic effects in the eye is important: sympathetic innervation leads to mydriasis, focus for distant vision and vasoconstriction, whereas parasympathetic effects include miosis, reduced IOP, accommodation for near vision and secretion of tears.
- Drugs acting on the autonomic nervous system are frequently used in ocular conditions for the following purposes:
  - to achieve mydriasis in eye examinations (with sympathomimetics such as phenylephrine or anticholinergics such as atropine)
  - to achieve cycloplegia (paralysis of accommodation) for diagnostic refraction – that is, assessment of optical errors (with anticholinergics)
  - to achieve miosis (reduction in pupil size) and lowered IOP, with muscarinic agonists (parasympathomimetics such as pilocarpine); miotics are used to treat glaucoma or to reverse the effects of a mydriatic
  - to achieve vasoconstriction, useful for a decongestant effect (with sympathomimetics)
  - to decrease formation of aqueous humour in glaucoma (with α-2 agonists or β-blockers).

Local anaesthetics

Actions and indications

Local anaesthetics (LAs) temporarily block nerve conduction by reducing membrane permeability to sodium. (For mechanism, see Ch 18 and Fig 18.9.) LAs can be applied topically to the eye as drops to temporarily anaesthetise the conjunctival and corneal epithelium. LA solutions can also be injected subcutaneously or by retrobulbar technique, or for nerve block of the orbital or frontal nerve. LAs are particularly useful for ophthalmic surgery, in which the cooperation of the person may be required, and to relieve pain associated with drug administrations, foreign body removal, contact lens fitting, removal of sutures, some diagnostic procedures, irritations, stinging from other drops and in tonometry (measurement of IOP) and gonioscopy (examination of the interior of the eye).

Ocular LAs usually increase the penetration of other drugs (eyedrops) applied around the same time and commonly cause stinging and sometimes allergies. It is recommended that a person never be given LA drops to take home because the drops may be overused, abolishing normal protective reflexes and causing impaired healing and ulceration.

Ocular local anaesthetics

LAs available as eyedrops are tetracaine (amethocaine) (0.5%, 1%), oxybuprocaine (0.4%; aka benoxinate) and proxymetacaine (0.5%). They have onset of action within 10–20 seconds and duration of action about 20 minutes. Proxymetacaine has the advantages of remaining stable in solution, with rapid onset of action and short duration, while causing minimal mydriasis, irritation or other ADRs. Excessive use can cause allergic contact dermatitis, pupillary dilation, cycloplegia and damage to cornea and conjunctiva. It is more toxic if it enters the systemic circulation. Lidocaine (lignocaine; Drug Monograph 18.4) 4% is also formulated with fluorescein 0.25% in eyedrops, to reduce stinging (see 'Diagnostic aids: stains', below).

Diagnostic aids: stains

Stains rapidly provide useful diagnostic information due to their differential staining characteristics on cell constituents. The ideal properties of an ocular stain are as follows:

- It is water-soluble and readily reversed or washed away.
- It selectively stains certain cells while not staining skin, contact lenses, instruments or clothes.
- It does not interfere with vision or have other pharmacological effects.
- It is compatible with other drugs likely to be used concurrently.

The main stain used in the eye is fluorescein (for corneal staining); another is lissamine green for conjunctival staining.

Fluorescein

Fluorescein is a non-toxic, orange-red, water-soluble dye that fluoresces even when very dilute and colours the tear film. It is sensitive to changes in pH; areas of corneal abrasion show up intensely green. Fluorescein is very commonly used for tonometry (measurement of IOP), to show corneal abrasions, in location of a foreign body, in detection of retinopathy, in fitting hard contact lenses and to test whether the nasolacrimal drainage system is open.

Fluorescein solutions readily support growth of *Pseudomonas* colonies; however, the usual preservatives are incompatible with the dye, so it is formulated in single-dose packages as eyedrops (1%, 2%) and as 1 mg drug-impregnated paper strips. Drops combining fluorescein with lidocaine (lignocaine) are also available to reduce the stinging caused by fluorescein.

IV injection of a sterile solution of fluorescein (10% or 25%) is used in ophthalmic angiography. Possible ADRs after IV injection include nausea, headache, abdominal distress, vomiting, hypotension and hypersensitivity reactions.

KEY POINTS

Local anaesthetics and stains as diagnostic aids

- LAs temporarily block nerve conduction by reducing membrane permeability to sodium.
- LAs are used in the eye for ophthalmic surgery, to facilitate examinations and procedures and to treat pain. Proxymetacaine is particularly effective.
- The stains fluorescein, rose bengal and lissamine green are administered topically to show up areas of abrasion and cell damage.

Contact lens products

Types of contact lenses

Contact lenses are classified as hard (including 'rigid gas-permeable' lenses) or soft; some are now disposable after 1 day's wear, to obviate the need for cleaning and risk of contamination and infection. Soft contact lenses are made from hydrogels and silicone elastomers, and all contain more than 80% water. There are potential problems of chemicals (even systemically administered drugs) binding to lenses and staining them, and of microbial growth due to high water content. Hard lenses are generally manufactured from polymethylmethacrylate, and rigid gas-permeable lenses (permeable to oxygen) from silicone resins. They are more durable, less adsorbent of chemicals and better optically. If a person with contact lenses is prescribed eyedrops, it is recommended that the drops be instilled before lenses are inserted in the morning and again after removal in the evening. Oily drops or eye ointments may contaminate lenses and obscure vision.

Originally developed and prescribed to correct refractive errors, contact lenses are now being used as drug reservoirs, providing sustained release drug in chronic ocular conditions (Hui & Willcox 2016).

Products for use with contact lenses

Many products (in fact, a bewildering array in most pharmacies) are available for care of contact lenses; products are not interchangeable between soft and hard lenses. Solutions should be sterile (initially), non-harmful to the lens or eye, simple to use and with a reasonable shelf-life. Likely pathogens in solutions, lenses and lens cases include *Escherichia coli*, *Staphylococcus aureus*, *Pseudomonas aeruginosa*, *Serratia*, *Haemophilus influenzae*, *Bacillus* spp., fungi and acanthamoebae from tap water. Contact lens wearers are advised never to use saliva or tap water to clean their lenses; sterile saline solution is required.

Typical lens care protocols are as follows:

- After the lens is removed, it is cleansed by gentle rubbing with a few drops of cleaning solution, which may include detergents, surfactants or bactericidal disinfectants such as benzalkonium chloride, chlorhexidine or EDTA (ethylenediamine tetra-acetic acid).
- The lens is rinsed with normal saline solution and kept in storage solution in a lens case to maintain hydration in a bacteriostatic solution and help remove deposits; these contain disinfectants, buffers and salts to maintain isotonicity.
- Before insertion next morning, it may be rinsed again.
- To facilitate insertion and wearing, wetting solutions and 'comfort drops' may be used: these promote spreading of water across the lens, and include a surfactant (wetting agent) such as polyvinyl alcohol or methylcellulose, plus a disinfectant.
- Occasionally, lenses are soaked for a specified time in an enzymatic solution, reconstituted from tablets containing dried enzymes (non-specific lipases and/or proteases), to remove deposits of fat or protein.

Combination solutions for cleaning, wetting and storage are available. These simplify lens care and improve compliance.

Systemic diseases and drugs affecting the eye

Many systemic diseases can affect the eye; in general, the primary condition is treated first, then treatment for ocular manifestations may not be required. For example, antihypertensive agents reduce the risk of retinal artery damage, antihyperlipidaemic drugs reduce the risk of embolism from internal carotid arteries and treatment of

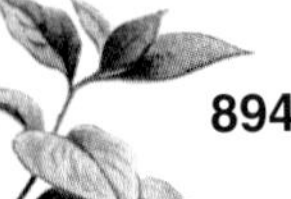

congestive heart failure reduces the risk of cerebral and ocular hypoxia.

Systemic diseases affecting the eye

Endocrine disorders

Thyrotoxicosis may cause exophthalmos, orbital pain, photophobia, ocular muscle weakness and blurred vision. Treatment is with thyroid surgery or antithyroid drugs such as carbimazole (Ch 27). Ocular manifestations of diabetes mellitus include retinopathy, haemorrhages, detachment and oedema; treatment is with insulin or oral hypoglycaemic drugs (Ch 28).

Collagen diseases

Rheumatoid arthritis, systemic lupus erythematosus and Sjögren's syndrome may cause dry eyes, scleritis, pain, uveitis, corneal opacity and retinopathy. Treatment is with ocular steroid drops and artificial tears, and systemic steroids, NSAIDs and other anti-inflammatory agents. Ocular ADRs from steroids and hydroxychloroquine require monitoring.

Muscular diseases

Myasthenia gravis involves autoimmune reactions to ACh receptors at the neuromuscular junction; usually ocular muscles are first affected, with ptosis and diplopia (Ch 24). Treatment is with anticholinesterases (neostigmine, pyridostigmine), which raise the concentration of ACh at remaining functional ACh receptors.

Adverse drug reactions affecting the eye

There are several possible scenarios:

- Drugs administered systemically to treat ocular conditions may have ADRs in the eye or elsewhere in the body.
- Drugs administered systemically to treat systemic conditions may have ADRs in the eye (Table 40.6).
- Drugs administered topically to the eye may have ADRs in the eye.[1]
- Drugs administered topically to the eye may have ADRs elsewhere in the body after nasolacrimal absorption (Fig 40.4, Clinical Focus Box 40.1, Table 40.7).

The most common ocular ADRs are decreased tolerance to contact lenses, dry eyes, stinging or irritation from eyedrops, development of cataract, diplopia, retinopathy, corneal irritation or conjunctivitis, raised IOP and impaired accommodation with or without mydriasis (Fraunfelder 2020). In the next section, drugs causing particular ocular pathologies or impairment of vision are grouped together.

1 Non-drugs mistakenly applied to the eye: a retrospective study of calls to the NSW Poisons Information Centre between 2004 and 2011 related to accidental ocular administration found about 900 cases of super glue being accidentally applied to the eye – possibly because both products are supplied in small dropper-type bottles, and usually kept in the refrigerator.

TABLE 40.6 Ocular adverse effects induced by some systemic medications

DRUG	POSSIBLE OCULAR ADVERSE EFFECT
Allopurinol	Retinal haemorrhage, exudative lesions
Anticholinergics	Dry eyes, mydriasis, glaucoma
Anticholinesterases	Cataracts
Antidepressants	Glaucoma
Aspirin	Allergic dermatitis, including keratitis and conjunctivitis
Busulfan	Cataracts
Cannabis, marijuana	Nystagmus, conjunctivitis, double vision, red eyes
Clomiphene citrate	Blurred vision, light flashes
Clonidine	Miosis
CNS depressants	Impaired vision, nystagmus, diplopia
Corticosteroids	Cataracts, raised IOP, papillo-oedema
Diazoxide	Oculogyric crisis
Digoxin	Scotomas, optic neuritis, changes in colour vision
Estrogens	Vessel occlusion
Ethambutol	Optic neuritis
Ethanol	Nystagmus
Glyceryl trinitrate	Transient elevation in IOP
Hydroxychloroquine	Lenticular and corneal opacity, retinopathy
Ibuprofen	Altered colour vision, blurred vision
Indometacin	Mydriasis, retinopathy
Isoniazid	Optic neuritis
Lithium carbonate	Exophthalmos
Opiates	Miosis, nystagmus
Oxygen	Retrolental hyperplasia, blindness (in newborns)
Phenothiazines	Corneal and conjunctival deposits, cataracts, retinopathy, oculogyric crisis
Phenytoin	Nystagmus
Quinine	Blurring of vision, optic neuritis, blindness (reversible)
Statins	Extraocular muscle disorders
Thiazide diuretics	Acute transient myopia, yellow colouring of vision
Vincristine	Ptosis, paresis of extraocular muscles
Vitamin A overdose	Papillo-oedema, increased IOP
Vitamin D toxicity	Calcium deposits in cornea

Retinopathies

- Methanol (as in methylated spirits) is highly toxic to the retina: as little as 10 g can cause blindness; toxicity is due to the metabolite formaldehyde (formalin), which inhibits cellular respiration and glycolysis in the retina.
- Chloroquine and related antimalarial and anti-inflammatory agents: chronic high doses accumulate in the retinal pigmentary epithelium and impair protein synthesis and vitamin A metabolism; total doses should be recorded, and all people monitored for retinal changes.

CLINICAL FOCUS BOX 40.1

Keep an eye out for systemic effects of ocular drops

Did you know that a single eyedrop can have systemic effects?

When a person instils an eyedrop, on average only 2–10% of the drug has a topical effect. The rest of the drug dose may be absorbed systemically by the several routes including drainage through the nasolacrimal duct (up to 80% of the drug), across the conjunctival vessels, via the GIT (ever tasted an eyedrop?) and across eyelid and cheek skin.

When an ocular drug is drained into the nasolacrimal duct, it is then absorbed directly into the systemic circulation via the highly vascular nasopharyngeal mucosa. The dose that is absorbed via this route does not undergo first-pass metabolism in the liver and can reach relatively high concentrations in the plasma. This can lead to unintended systemic effects; for example, ocular timolol (a non-selective β-blocker) can trigger bronchoconstriction (contraindicated in asthma) and bradycardia.

To prevent systemic absorption and promote medicine safety, health professionals should counsel on how to prevent systemic absorption of eyedrops using the 'double dot method' – that is, digital occlusion of the tear duct and the 'don't open' technique. In this technique, patients need to keep their eye closed and gently press on their tear duct for 2–5 minutes immediately after instilling an eyedrop. This will reduce drainage into the nasolacrimal duct and subsequent systemic absorption.

TABLE 40.7 Ophthalmic drugs: adverse systemic effects

OPHTHALMIC DRUG	REPORTED ADVERSE EFFECT
Antimicrobials	Secondary infections, drug resistance
Anticholinergics, atropine, cyclopentolate	Tachycardia, elevated temperature, fever, delirium, convulsions, hallucinations
Phenylephrine (10%)	Hypertension, arrhythmias, tremors
Antiglaucoma medications	
β-blocking agents (timolol, betaxolol)	Bradycardia, low blood pressure, asthma attack, hallucinations, depression, weakness (Fig 40.4)
Parasympathomimetics (pilocarpine)	Nausea, sweating, salivation, headache, bradycardia
α_2 agonists	Hypotension, palpitations

- Oxygen in high concentrations is retinotoxic in newborns: oxygen administered to prevent hypoxia can lead to permanent blindness, so levels provided must be restricted (Ch 15).
- Phenothiazine antipsychotic agents such as chlorpromazine (Drug Monograph 22.1) can bind to melanin and cause lens deposits; high doses are retinotoxic.
- Other drugs that can cause retinal damage include digoxin, corticosteroids, chloramphenicol, cocaine and interferon.

Cataracts

Many organic chemicals can induce development of cataracts (opacity in the crystalline lens) leading to blindness unless treated, including the following:

- Organophosphorus anticholinesterases (used to treat myasthenia gravis or Alzheimer's disease) can produce vacuoles behind the lens.
- Corticosteroids – people on chronic high doses of glucocorticoids have a high incidence of cataract; the mechanism is not well understood. Corticosteroids can also cause glaucoma and predispose to infections.
- Phenothiazines – high doses can lead to pigment deposition and polar cataract; the cause may be a metabolite.

Photosensitivity

Photosensitivity is a hypersensitivity reaction in which ultraviolet light energy stimulates production of a hapten–protein complex between the drug and a natural protein, leading to photoallergy or phototoxicity (Ch 39). The drugs most commonly implicated are sulfonamides, tetracyclines, phenothiazines and thiazide diuretics, also natural body porphyrins (see verteporphin, earlier). Note that mydriatics also increase the sensitivity of the eye to light.

Excessive tear formation

Lacrimators (more infamously known as 'tear gases') are chemicals that cause intense corneal and conjunctival irritation and pain, inducing reflex tear secretion, eyelid spasm, coughing and nausea. They are used as crowd controllers, 'harassing agents' and war gases; if used in confined spaces, their toxicity can cause blindness and death. Many are highly reactive organic chemicals with cyano groups (carbon and nitrogen linked in a triple bond). Others include bromoacetone, acrolein (a compound produced from overheated cooking fats) and the organic sulfides present in onions and garlic.

KEY POINTS

Diseases and drugs affecting the eye adversely

- The eye can be affected in many systemic diseases, particularly cardiovascular, endocrine and musculoskeletal conditions. The primary disease needs to be treated first, to minimise ocular complications.
- Many ADRs occur in the eye, such as ocular irritation, retinopathy, cataract, raised IOP and glaucoma, dry

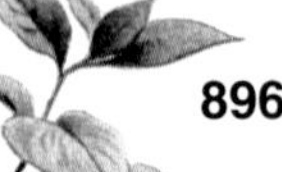

eye, photosensitivity and effects on contact lenses, from both ocular and systemically administered drugs.

- Drugs that commonly cause ocular adverse effects are anticholinergics, methanol, chloroquine, corticosteroids, phenothiazines, sulfonamides and oxygen in newborns. 'Tear gases' are used purposely to induce ocular irritation and pain.

Drugs affecting the ear

Common ear disorders

The most common ear disorders include infections (bacterial or fungal), ear wax accumulation, painful or inflammatory conditions, deafness and problems with balance. Many ear disorders are minor and self-limiting or easily treated; however, persistent untreated disorders can lead to hearing loss.

External ear disorders

The ear consists of three sections: the external ear, middle ear and inner ear (Fig 40.5). The external ear has two divisions: the outer ear, or pinna, and the external auditory canal, which leads to the tympanic membrane (eardrum), a thin transparent partition of tissue between the canal and the middle ear. The external ear receives sounds and transmits them to the eardrum, which then transmits sounds to the bones of the middle ear.

External ear disorders usually involve trauma and subsequent infections, such as from lacerations to the skin of the ear canal or infected water entering the canal. If the injury results in bleeding or a haematoma, referral to a doctor may be necessary. Localised infections of the hair follicles may result in boils (furuncles associated with *Staphylococcus aureus*); recurring boils may require surgical drainage and systemic antibiotics.

Cerumen (ear wax) impaction

Cerumen (ear wax) is the yellowish waxy substance secreted by glands in the external ear, consisting of long-chain fatty acids, alcohols, squalene and cholesterol, plus shed skin cells and hair. It has cleansing, antimicrobial and lubricating functions. Excess ear wax can block the external auditory canal or press against the tympanic membrane (eardrum), possibly causing hearing loss, and damage hearing aids. The type of wax produced is genetically determined: wet-type wax (yellow-brown) dominant and dry type (grey, flaky) recessive.

Ear wax gradually dries out and is naturally moved towards the outer ear by epithelial migration assisted by jaw movements. Excessive wax may be removed by cerum or by syringing with warm solutions, but NEVER by cotton buds, which only push the wax further in, nor by lit hollow 'ear candles', which can cause burns!

Cerumenolytics are ear preparations that aid the removal of ear wax by softening and dispersing the ear wax. They include carbamide peroxide (antibacterial agent that releases oxygen to help remove wax), ortho-dichlorobenzene with chlorobutanol, docusate and sodium bicarbonate. Oils (almond, arachis [peanut], olive, eucalyptus) can also be used. They can be used alone, or to prepare the ear for syringing.

Swimmer's ear

Swimmer's ear (otitis externa) is an infection of the ear canal associated with aquatic activities such as swimming or hair-washing. Bacteria may be introduced with water (especially if chlorination of pools is inadequate) and multiply in the warm moist ear canal, causing pain, swelling, sensation of fullness in the ear and impaired hearing. Prevention and treatment are assisted by excluding moisture from the canal (e.g. with ear plugs) and by desiccation and acidification of the canal with drying eardrops[2] containing acetic acid and/or isopropyl alcohol, propylene glycol or glycerol, and an astringent agent such as aluminium acetate.

Middle ear disorders

The middle ear is an air-filled cavity in the temporal bone containing three small auditory ossicles:[3] the malleus (hammer; attached to the surface of the tympanic membrane), incus (anvil) and stapes (stirrup). These bones amplify (about 10-fold) and transmit vibrations from sound waves to the inner ear. The middle ear is directly connected to the nasopharynx by the eustachian (auditory) tube, which equalises air pressure in the inner ear with atmospheric pressure to prevent rupture of the tympanic membrane. Middle ear disorders should not be home-treated with OTC medications because prescription-only treatment, such as antibiotics, may be required. Medical attention is necessary when perforated eardrum is suspected.

Otitis media

Middle ear inflammation, **otitis media**, is one of the commonest infections of childhood, especially in children between 6 and 12 months of age with viral upper

2 A DIY version of eardrops for swimmer's ear, recommended by a Melbourne ear, nose and throat specialist, can be readily made by mixing 1 volume (e.g. 5 mL) of methylated spirits with 2 volumes (10 mL) of white vinegar; as eardrops do not need to be sterile (assuming the eardrum is intact), these can be homemade provided attention is paid to hygiene.

3 These are in fact the smallest bones in the body, and the stapedius muscle, which dampens the vibrations of the stapes and thus protects the ear against loud noises, is the smallest skeletal muscle. At birth, these are fully grown and the sense of hearing is already well developed.

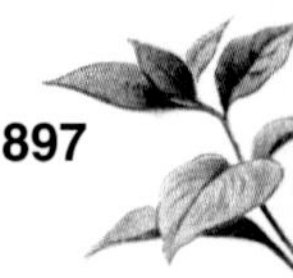

Dizziness, syncope
CNS effects
Depression, hallucinations
insomnia, memory loss
Bronchoconstriction,
exacerbation of asthma
Bradycardia
Cardiac arrhythmias
AV block, sinoatrial block
Hypotension
Irregular pulse

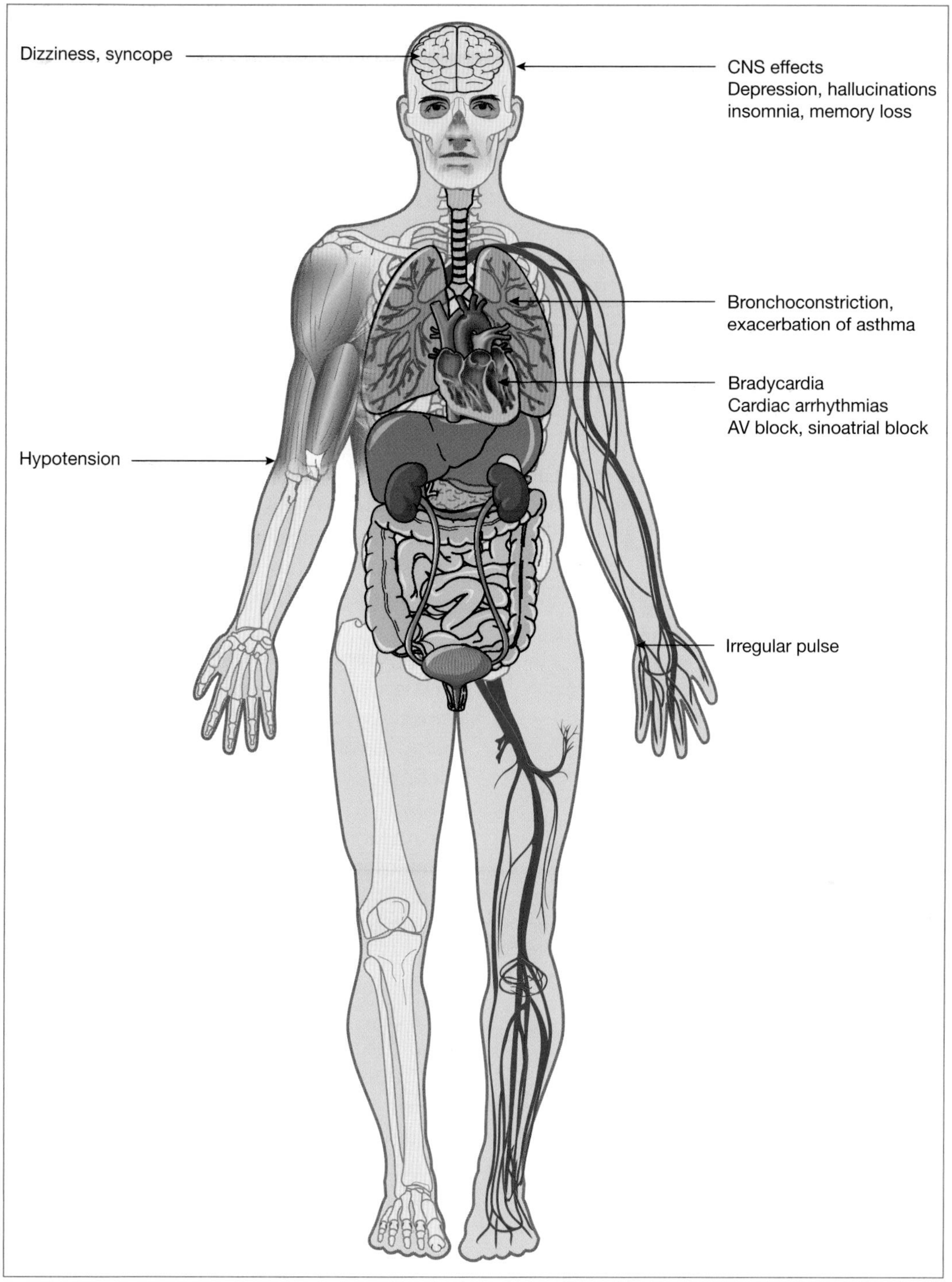

FIGURE 40.5 Adverse effects of nonselective ocular betablockers

respiratory tract infections (Clinical Focus Box 40.2). Other risk factors are passive smoking exposure, toddlers drinking bottles of milk or juice while lying down and babies using a dummy/pacifier overnight. Viruses picked up in childcare or playgroup situations are unfortunately often unavoidable. Otitis media can occur with or without perforation, effusion and suppuration (pus); symptoms are redness, pain, fever, malaise, a sensation of fullness in the ear and hearing loss. Common bacterial pathogens are *Streptococcus pneumoniae* and *Haemophilus influenzae*.

Otitis media is usually a mild condition resolving without treatment; parents may need reassurance during

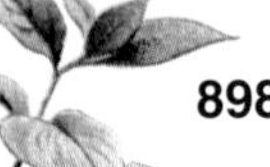

CLINICAL FOCUS BOX 40.2

Otitis media in a child

Middle ear inflections (otitis media) are common in children, with 75% of children having at least one infection before starting school. Most cases of otitis media respond spontaneously, and antibiotics should not be routinely recommended.

Case: A 20-month-old toddler is brought to the local family doctor after having a tonic–clonic seizure at home; the little girl has been grumpy and refusing food earlier that day, with two spikes of fever during the previous 24 hours. The girl has a history of three prior simple febrile convulsions but is otherwise in good general health. There is a family history of febrile convulsions during childhood, and penicillin allergy.

The doctor examines the child and diagnoses a left acute otitis media (bulging dull red tympanic membrane) with associated runny nose, inflamed pharynx, mildly enlarged cervical lymph nodes bilaterally and a dry cough. The GP explains to the mother why the child's symptoms indicate that a viral infection is much more likely than bacterial, and provides a printed handout explaining the many disadvantages of antibiotic use in simple otitis media. The doctor advises regular analgesia (oral paracetamol 20 mg/kg for three doses on the first day, then paracetamol 15 mg/kg every 6 hours as required). In addition, topical benzocaine/phenazone eardrops (2–3 drops per dose, repeated up to hourly until good analgesia is achieved) are prescribed, although the mother believes that administration may be difficult. The mother agrees to bring the child for review within 2 days if there is no improvement in her symptoms, and the doctor arranges a later appointment to screen for serous 'glue ear' otitis media, and to catch up on her overdue chickenpox immunisation.

Source: Acknowledgments to Dr Philippa Shilson, Paediatrician; personal communication.

a 'watchful waiting' period of 24 hours. Pain relief can be provided with paracetamol or ibuprofen, but systemic decongestants and antihistamines have no proven efficacy. Systemic antibiotics (amoxicillin, cefuroxime or cefaclor) may be required, especially in immunocompromised people and in Aboriginal and Torres Strait Islander children. Eardrops containing benzocaine (a local anaesthetic) and phenazone (a topical non-steroidal anti-inflammatory agent) may relieve pain.

Glue ear

Persistent effusion of fluid in the middle ear (glue ear) with pain and hearing loss may resolve after some weeks or may require relief by drainage with a ventilating tube (grommet). Chronic suppurative otitis media, in which the eardrum has become ruptured and purulent exudate (pus) appears in the external canal, can cause hearing loss, and may require surgical removal of the pus and treatment with topical combination eardrops containing an anti-inflammatory agent and antibiotics.

Inner ear disorders

The bony labyrinth consists of the vestibule, cochlea and semicircular canals, and the membranous labyrinth consists of a series of sacs and tubes within the bony labyrinth. The cochlea, through which pass fibres of the cochlear division of the acoustic nerve, is the primary organ of hearing, while the vestibular apparatus maintains equilibrium and balance.

Hearing and balance deficits may be caused by infections, genetic diseases or slowly progressive diseases such as otosclerosis or Ménière's disease. Some drugs, especially aminoglycoside antibiotics, platinum anticancer drugs and NSAIDs (aspirin), can cause impaired hearing – see later under 'Drug-induced ototoxicity'.

Vertigo and motion sickness

Vertigo, motion sickness and dizziness are thought to be caused by a disparity in the proprioceptive information being received from the two sides of the head – for example, when viewing outside stationary objects from within a moving vehicle. The aquaporins (water channels) and vasopressin receptors involved in homeostasis of water may play a crucial role in homeostasis of endolymph in the inner ear. Other causes of vertigo may be peripheral (rubella, mumps, acoustic neuroma, otitis media) or central (migraine, epilepsy, multiple sclerosis).

Acute episodes usually settle within 1–2 days. Drug treatment depends on the cause: vertigo due to inner ear balance disorders is treated with 'vestibular blocking agents', which may include anticholinergics, betahistine (Drug Monograph 40.3; see below), corticosteroids, antiemetics and benzodiazepines. Distressing vertigo may also be helped by manoeuvres in which the head is moved through different planes to attempt to remove fluid in the canals.

Ménière's disease

Ménière's disease (named after the French physician Prosper Ménière, 1799–1862) is a progressive, episodic inner ear disease caused by an increase in endolymph pressure and spontaneous bursts of activity within the labyrinth. It involves recurrent attacks of severe vertigo, nausea, tinnitus and hearing loss. Positioning manoeuvres, physical exercises and drugs as for vertigo can help; sometimes the only effective treatment is surgery.

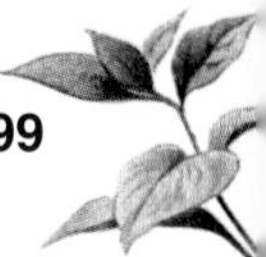

KEY POINTS

Common ear diseases

Conditions commonly affecting specific parts of the ear are:

- *external ear:* infections, swimmer's ear (treated with mildly acidic drops) and excessive ear wax (removed with cerumenolytics such as oils and surfactants)
- *middle ear:* otitis media (treated with analgesics, possibly a mild local anaesthetic, and systemic antibiotics if prolonged and serious); glue ear (may require surgery, antibiotics and anti-inflammatory agents)
- *inner ear:* vertigo, motion sickness, tinnitus, Ménière's disease (all difficult to treat; betahistine may be effective).

Drug treatment of ear disorders

Otic administration

Drugs are administered to the ear for local effects only and are not absorbed systemically (as they can be from the eye). The pharmaceutical aspects of eardrops and ear ointments are basically similar to the requirements for eyedrops and ointments; however, there is not the same sterility requirement, as substances cannot penetrate the middle or inner ear unless the eardrum is perforated, and tissues of the ear are well vascularised. Some drops are formulated for either eye or ear use.

Eardrops and sprays are commonly formulated with the active drug(s) dissolved in aqueous solvents (alcohols, glycols, saline solutions or glycerol), or oily solvents (arachis oil). Acetic acid 1–2% is used in eardrops to acidify the ear canal after swimming or bathing. Before otic administration, ear wax and debris should be gently removed. Dosage of eardrops is usually two or three drops, two to four times daily, or via a gauze wick in the external ear. Ointment is applied and the ear gently massaged two to three times daily.

Direct inner ear drug delivery

Systemically administered drugs do not readily enter inner ear fluids due to the blood – perilymph and middle ear barriers. Treatment of disorders of the inner ear that cause auditory or vestibular dysfunction is enhanced if the drug can be delivered directly. New methods are being developed, including miniaturised wearable implantable microsystems, for administration of corticosteroids, growth factors, antioxidants, antibodies and apoptosis inhibitors (El Kechai et al. 2015).

Intra-tympanic injections

Injections of drug can be made through the tympanic membrane (eardrum) into the middle ear cavity, from where it can diffuse into the inner ear via thin membranous 'windows'. This route is used for administration of aminoglycoside antibiotics (e.g. gentamicin; Drug Monograph 36.2) and corticosteroids for treatment of Ménière's disease and sudden sensorineural hearing loss. The aminoglycoside antibiotics themselves cause hearing loss, and it is thought that trans-tympanic administration of gentamicin damages hair cells, reducing vestibular function; the dose must be carefully judged so that hearing is not completely lost.

Intracochlear or intralabyrinthine administration

These routes are more invasive, but deliver a drug directly to the inner ear, via nanoparticle or microfluidic technologies. Drugs in minute nanoparticles can diffuse through membranes; this method is also studied as a possible route for gene therapy, to regenerate functions of the inner ear.

Antimicrobial otic formulations

Antimicrobials are applied topically for infections of the external auditory canal (otitis externa). For serious middle or inner ear infections, systemic antibiotics are indicated. Antibiotics preferred for topical use are those that are not used systemically (due to systemic toxicity or adverse pharmacokinetics), including the antibacterial gramicidin and the antifungals nystatin and clioquinol. (Antimicrobial drugs are covered in detail in Unit 13.) Antimicrobial eardrops are also formulated in combination with a corticosteroid.

Antimicrobials

The aminoglycoside antibiotics such as framycetin and neomycin have been used in eardrops, but these drugs are liable to cause ototoxicity, so aminoglycosides are used only with caution if the eardrum is perforated or ventilated (with a grommet). They should be ceased immediately the infection resolves or adverse effects appear. Framycetin (a component of neomycin, and also known as neomycin B) is available as eardrops (5 mg/mL), and combination eardrops 5 mg/mL with dexamethasone and gramicidin, both indicated for otitis externa.

The fluoroquinolone antibiotic ciprofloxacin, available as eardrops (0.3%), is not ototoxic so it is preferable in people with chronic suppurative otitis media infections with a perforated tympanic membrane or a patent grommet.

Corticosteroid/antimicrobial otic combinations

Corticosteroid anti-inflammatory agents used in the ear include triamcinolone, flumetasone, dexamethasone and hydrocortisone; they are usually formulated combined with antimicrobials. The corticosteroid is included for its anti-inflammatory, antipruritic and antiallergic effects (Ch 34), while the antibiotic treats infections. The antibiotic components are not usually absorbed through intact skin. Corticosteroids and neomycin may be absorbed, particularly if the skin is inflamed, and can cause mild systemic effects. Prolonged use can lead to hypersensitivity reactions, skin irritations and contact dermatitis; corticosteroids can cause delayed healing and secondary infections, especially fungal infections.

Drug treatment of Ménière's disease

There is no simple cure for Ménière's disease; many drugs have been tried.

Betahistine

The main drug used for long-term treatment is betahistine, an orally administered, centrally acting histamine analogue (Drug Monograph 40.3).

Other drugs

Other drugs tried include an anticholinergic antihistamine, such as promethazine or diphenhydramine, and a diuretic (hydrochlorothiazide) to reduce fluid load. Corticosteroids help reduce inflammation, and 'labyrinthine sedation' is attempted with phenothiazine antipsychotics such as prochlorperazine or a benzodiazepine. Trans-tympanic administration of a corticosteroid for anti-inflammatory effect, or of gentamicin for its ototoxic effect ('chemical labyrinthectomy'), may reduce vestibular function. Between attacks, restricted intake of salt, sugar, cigarettes, alcohol, chocolate, caffeine and other CNS stimulants may be prophylactic.

Over-the-counter otic preparations

As with eye conditions, people often self-medicate when they realise they have ear problems. Although most OTC otic preparations (summarised below) are considered safe and effective, patients should be advised to see a doctor if symptoms do not improve within 2–3 days of using these preparations or if an ADR occurs.

Antiseptics and emollients

OTC otic preparations often contain acetic or boric acid, benzalkonium chloride, aluminium acetate (Burow's solution),

Drug Monograph 40.3
Betahistine

Betahistine is a close chemical analogue of histamine, the chemical mediator and central neurotransmitter.

Indications

Betahistine is indicated in treatment of Ménière's disease (vertigo, hearing loss and tinnitus); it is not effective in preventing vertigo attacks.

Mechanism of action

The precise mechanism of betahistine's actions is unclear; it has antagonistic actions on histamine H_3 receptors, and is a weak agonist at H_1 receptors. In animal studies, it inhibits generation of spikes in vestibular nuclei. Its vasodilator activity (similar to histamines) presumably improves blood flow in the inner ear and brainstem.

Pharmacokinetics

After oral administration, betahistine is rapidly and completely absorbed, rapidly metabolised (to one major metabolite, 2-pyridylacetic acid) and 90% excreted within 24 hours. Plasma and urinary half-lives are about 3.5 hours.

Drug interactions

Co-administration of betahistine and monoamine oxidase inhibitors type B reduces metabolism of betahistine. Theoretically, interactions might occur with concurrent antihistamines; however, no significant problems have been reported.

Adverse reactions

Common ADRs include headache, nausea and dyspepsia. More rarely, hypersensitivity reactions (rash, pruritus, bronchospasm) and hypotension may occur.

Precautions and contraindications

Betahistine should be used with caution in people with asthma, urticaria, phaeochromocytoma or hypersensitivity to any components of tablets. Betahistine is contraindicated in people with active or history of peptic ulcer. Betahistine is classified in Pregnancy Safety Category B2: insufficient data available; it is contraindicated in pregnancy and lactation, and in children under 18.

Dosage and administration

Betahistine is provided as scored tablets, 16 mg. Dose is 8–16 mg taken three times daily. It should be taken with food to minimise risk of GIT upsets. Warn that it may take several weeks for beneficial effects to be noticed.

ichthammol (a coal-tar derivative), ethanol, isopropyl alcohol or propylene glycol, sodium bicarbonate and isotonic saline. Glycerol, mineral oil and olive oil are used as emollients to help relieve itching and burning in the ear.

Analgesics

Eardrops for relief of ear pain associated with otitis media may contain a NSAID (e.g. phenazone) and a local anaesthetic (benzocaine). There are precautions if the person has symptoms such as fever, dizziness, hearing loss or tinnitus, and the drops are contraindicated in perforated eardrums, ear discharge or known hypersensitivity to any ingredient. Minimal systemic absorption occurs, so adverse systemic effects or drug interactions are unlikely. Benzocaine is an ester-type local anaesthetic, so frequent use can cause contact dermatitis. If pain persists beyond 24 hours, medical assistance should be sought.

Drug-induced ototoxicity

Mechanisms and manifestations

Many medications potentially cause **ototoxicity**, affecting the person's hearing (auditory or cochlear function), balance (vestibular function) or both. The most common symptom reported is tinnitus, 'ringing in the ears'. Ototoxicity is usually bilateral and reversible but can become irreversible if the offending medications are not withdrawn. Cochlear ototoxicity causes progressive loss of high tones, then lower tones. Vestibular toxicity may start with a severe headache, followed by nausea, dizziness, ataxia, difficulty with equilibrium and vertigo.

Reactive oxygen and nitrogen species, including free radicals, have been implicated in ototoxicity: oxidative stress damages macromolecules and sensory hair cells in the inner ear (and cells of the proximal tubules in the kidneys). Treatments attempting to prevent or reverse ototoxicity include stem cells, curcumin, *N*-acetylcysteine, caffeic acid esters and nicotinamide adenine dinucleotide.

Those most at risk of ototoxicity are the elderly, those with impaired drug excretion processes (exacerbated by nephrotoxicity from the same drugs that cause ototoxicity), people working or living with high noise levels and those taking ototoxic agents in high doses or for prolonged duration.

Tinnitus

Tinnitus is a common distressing and enigmatic disorder. No clear aetiology or pathology is agreed; exposure to noise and salicylate drugs has been implicated. It is difficult to treat; attempts have been made with cognitive behaviour therapy, devices that mask the perceived buzzing/ringing noises, electrical or vibration stimulation, surgery and hearing aids. Drug therapies tried include local lidocaine (lignocaine) or botulinum toxin, or systemic corticosteroids, carbamazepine, antidepressants or benzodiazepines. Dietary supplements, complementary and alternative therapies, acupuncture and *Ginkgo biloba* extracts have proven to be little better than placebo. The most recent pharmacological treatment is with trans-tympanic perfusion of corticosteroids or gentamicin, as for vertigo.

Drugs implicated in ototoxicity

Irreversible ototoxicity is associated with the use of aminoglycoside antibiotics, vancomycin and platinum antineoplastic agents. Damage from erythromycin, azithromycin, salicylate anti-inflammatory agents, quinine antimalarials, loop diuretics and metronidazole is usually reversible after ceasing treatment (Lanvers-Kaminsky et al. 2017) (Clinical Focus Box 40.3).

Aminoglycoside antibiotics

The aminoglycoside antibiotics are commonly used to treat Gram-negative bacterial infections and mycobacterial diseases because of their high efficacy and low cost. They are readily absorbed into inner ear fluids and thence into sensory hair cells, and can cause irreversible ototoxicity. Streptomycin and gentamicin (Drug Monograph 36.2) are primarily vestibulotoxic, producing dizziness, ataxia and nystagmus, while amikacin, neomycin and tobramycin are cochleotoxic, causing permanent hearing loss.

> **CLINICAL FOCUS BOX 40.3**
> **Sudden hearing loss after metronidazole**
>
> Clinical case: A 30-year-old man presented to the emergency department of the Royal Victorian Eye and Ear Hospital, Melbourne, with bilateral profound deafness, tinnitus and headache associated with paraesthesias and myalgia. He had been taking metronidazole (400 mg tds) and amoxicillin (500 mg tds) for 4 days to treat gingivitis. Audiographic testing showed moderate–severe sensorineural hearing loss.
>
> Questioning revealed that an uncle had experienced identical symptoms while taking metronidazole. The drug was discontinued, and oral prednisolone (50 mg daily) administered, weaning off over 3 weeks. After 6 weeks, hearing was normal up to 2000 Hz, but high-frequency loss remained.
>
> The doctors involved speculated about the mechanism of the ototoxicity: free radical generation via NMDA receptors, impaired GABA-ergic transmission and RNA-binding; the familial link suggested a genetic susceptibility. Given the very widespread use of metronidazole (Drug Monograph 39.1) in bacterial and protozoal infections, the rare but potentially damaging effects on hearing should be promulgated to prescribers.
>
> *Source: Rotman et al. 2015.*

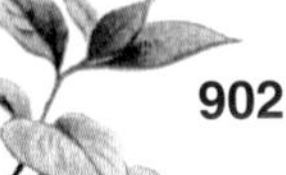

Mechanisms proposed for the ototoxic actions are inhibition of mitochondrial protein synthesis, free-radical cell damage from reactive oxygen species and activation of NMDA receptors. Susceptibility to ototoxicity is dose-related or idiosyncratic and genetically linked: carriers of a mutation in the mitochondrial 12S ribosomal RNA gene are predisposed.

The total aminoglycoside dosage should be noted, and both ototoxicity and nephrotoxicity monitored in clinical usage. Once-daily administration may be useful in increasing efficacy and reducing toxicity. Prophylactic treatment with antioxidants has been trialled.

Salicylates and other anti-inflammatories

Salicylates such as aspirin and methyl salicylate have long been known to cause auditory toxicity, especially after high doses (> 4 g/day aspirin). Tinnitus, loss of acoustic sensitivity and alterations of perceived sounds occur, particularly at high frequencies. Outer hair cells in the cochlea are damaged; the mechanisms are not well understood. It is not yet clear whether the very low antiplatelet doses of aspirin used long term to prevent ischaemia (75–100 mg/day) will have a cumulative toxic effect on hearing.

KEY POINTS

Drugs affecting the ear

- Drugs can be administered to the outer ear as eardrops or ear ointments, or to the middle or inner ear by direct techniques.
- Antimicrobials used topically are preferably those not used systemically: framycetin and ciprofloxacin. These are commonly used in combination formulations with corticosteroid anti-inflammatory agents such as triamcinolone, flumetasone, dexametasone and hydrocortisone.
- The main drug for Ménière's disease is betahistine, a histamine analogue.
- Products available OTC for self-medication include antiseptics, emollients, analgesics and cerumenolytics (wax removers).
- Drugs commonly causing ototoxicity include aminoglycoside antibiotics, vancomycin, platinum antineoplastic agents, erythromycin, azithromycin, salicylate anti-inflammatory agents, quinine antimalarials and loop diuretics; hearing loss can be severe and irreversible.

DRUGS AT A GLANCE
Drugs affecting the eye

PHARMACOLOGICAL GROUP AND EFFECT	KEY EXAMPLES	CLINCAL USE
Antiglaucoma drugs		
α_2-adrenoceptor agonists • Decrease aqueous humour production • Decrease intraocular pressure (IOP) • Increase uveoscleral outflow of aqueous humour	Apraclonidine, brimonidine	• Glaucoma
β-blockers • Block β receptors on the ciliary epithelium • Decrease aqueous humour production	Betaxolol, timolol	• Glaucoma • Ocular hypertension
Carbonic anhydrase inhibitors • Inhibit carbonic anhydrase • Decrease aqueous humour production	Acetazolamide (systemic) Dorzolamide, brinzolamide (topical)	• Glaucoma • Ocular hypertension
Prostaglandin agonists • Decrease IOP • Increase uveoscleral outflow of aqueous humour	Bimatoprost, latanoprost	• Glaucoma • Ocular hypertension
Muscarinic agonists (miotics) • Pupil constriction, increase uveoscleral outflow of aqueous humour • Decrease IOP	Pilocarpine	• Chronic open angle glaucoma • Acute angle-closure
Antimicrobial drugs		
Aminoglycosides • Inhibit bacterial protein synthesis • Mainly effective against Gram-Negative bacteria	Framycetin, gentamicin, tobramycin	• Bacterial conjunctivitis
Quinolones • Bactericidal • Inhibit bacterial DNA synthesis	Ciprofloxacin, ofloxacin	• Bacterial conjunctivitis • Corneal ulcers • Keratitis (corneal inflammation)

Chloramphenicol • Bacteriostatic (broad spectrum) • Inhibit peptide bond formation • Inhibit bacterial protein synthesis	Chloramphenicol	• Bacterial conjunctivitis • Blepharitis • Reserved for ophthalmologist use
Macrolide • Bacteriostatic • Inhibit bacterial protein synthesis • Immunomodulatory and inflammatory effects	Oral azithromycin	• Trachoma prevention and treatment
Antivirals • Purine nucleoside analogue • Inhibit viral DNA synthesis	Aciclovir	• Ocular herpes
Anti-inflammatory and antiallergy drugs		
Corticosteroids • Inhibit inflammatory cascade • Decrease prostaglandin-mediated inflammation • Immunosuppressive effects	Dexamethasone, fluorometholone, hydrocortisone, prednisolone	• Inflammatory conditions of lids, conjunctiva, cornea, iris, sclera and ciliary body • Postoperative inflammation • In dry eye disease, to prevent postoperative adhesions • Decrease macular oedema, to reduce growth of new blood vessels
Non-steroidal anti-inflammatory drugs • Inhibit cyclo-oxygenase (COX) enzymes • Decrease prostaglandin synthesis, decrease prostaglandin-mediated inflammation	Diclofenac, ketorolac	• Decrease postoperative pain after cataract surgery • Conjunctivitis • Seasonal and perennial allergic conjunctivitis
Antihistamines • Block histamine release	Azelastine, levocabastine, ketotifen, olopatadine	• Seasonal and perennial allergic conjunctivitis
Mast-cell stabilisers (cromones) • Inhibit degranulation of sensitised mast cells after exposure to a specific antigen • Decrease inflammation	Cromoglycate, lodoxamide	• Seasonal and perennial allergic conjunctivitis • Vernal keratoconjunctivitis
Drugs for ocular examinations, procedures and surgery		
Anticholinergics (antimuscarinics) • Block acetylcholine (ACh) receptors on the iris sphincter and ciliary muscle	Atropine, cyclopentolate, tropicamide	• Mydriasis (pupil dilation) and cycloplegia (paralysis of accommodation)
Sympathomimetics • α1-adrenoceptor agonists • Increase noradrenaline effects, dilator pupillae (radial muscle)	Phenylephrine (high-dose)	• Diagnostic mydriasis (pupil dilation)
Local anaesthetics • Reversibly block nerve conduction	Oxybuprocaine, proxymetacaine, lidocaine (lignocaine)	• Ocular anaesthesia e.g. for minor surgery, foreign body removal, initial ocular assessment for minor trauma

DRUGS AT A GLANCE
Drugs affecting the ear

PHARMACOLOGICAL GROUP AND EFFECT	KEY EXAMPLES (ALL AS EARDROPS)	CLINICAL USE
Acidifying/drying agents	Acetic acid, isopropyl alcohol	• Prevent 'swimmer's ear' otitis externa
Antibacterials	Ciprofloxacin, framycetin	• Chronic suppurative otitis media (ciproflaxin only) • Otitis externa
Antifungal	Nystatin	• Fungal otitis externa
Corticosteroids • Decrease prostaglandin-mediated inflammation	Triamcinolone, flumetasone	• Reduce pain and inflammation of otitis externa
H_1-receptor agonist • Vasodilator; increases blood flow to the inner ear	Betahistine (oral)	• Ménière's disease (vertigo, hearing loss, tinnitus)
Cerumenolytics • Soften and disperse ear cerumen	Carbamide peroxide	• Wax removal agents

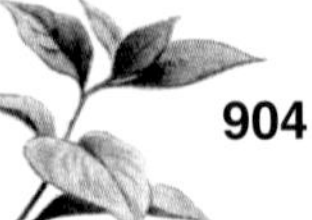

REVIEW QUESTIONS

1. Mrs PE, 65-year-old women, has primary open-angle glaucoma and is prescribed the muscarinic agonist, pilocarpine 1%. Describe the mode of action of pilocarpine. How long does it take for pilocarpine to have an effect after first use, what is its duration of action and how often are drops instilled? Discuss some counselling considerations for people taking pilocarpine. When might optometrists/ophthalmologists use pilocarpine in the diagnostic/acute care process?
2. Mrs JE suffers from seasonal allergic conjunctivitis; on examination her eyes are red and itchy. Mrs JE is recommended topical ketotifen. Describe the mode of action of this medicine. How often should ketotifen be applied for best effect? What other ocular histamines are available to prevent and treat allergic conjunctivitis? What are some general measures Mrs JE could take to reduce her symptoms?
3. Mr BI suffers allergic conjunctivitis and has been using levocabastine daily to reduce symptoms. His eyes are still very red, and he is getting married in 3 days. His pharmacist has recommended naphazoline 0.1% eyedrops, one drop every 6–12 hours. What is the mode of action of naphazoline? Why is it advised not to use these drops for longer than 5 days at a time?
4. Mr MI, a 32-year-old man, has recently been diagnosed with Ménière's disease, with episodes of vertigo and hearing problems. He is prescribed betahistine 16 mg three times a day with food. Discuss the mechanism of action of betahistine, common ADRs and precautions and contraindications for its use.

REFERENCES

Australian Medicines Handbook 2021. Australian Medicines Handbook. Adeleide, AMH.

De Paiva CS, Pflugfelder SC, Ng SM, et al., Topical cyclosporine A therapy for dry eye syndrome. Cochrane Database of Systematic Reviews, 2019; Sep 13;9(9):CD010051.

El Kechai N, Agnely F, Mamelie E, et al., Recent advances in local drug delivery to the inner ear. International Journal of Pharmaceutics, 2015. 494(1): 83–101.

Fraunfelder F, Drug-induced ocular side effects: clinical ocular toxicology,. 8 ed. 2020, Philadelphia: Elsevier

Gaballa SA, Kompella UB, Elgarhy O, et al., Corticosteroids in ophthalmology: Drug delivery innovations, pharmacology, clinical applications, and future perspectives. Drug Delivery and Translational Research, 2021. 11(3): 866–893.

Gilissen L, De Decker L, Hulshagen T, et al., Allergic contact dermatitis caused by topical ophthalmic medications: Keep an eye on it! Contact Dermatitis, 2019. 80(5): 291–297.

Hui A, Willcox M. In vivo studies evaluating the use of contact lenses for drug delivery. Optometry and Vision Science, 2016. 93(4): 367–376.

Lanvers-Kaminsky C, Zehnhoff-Dinnesen AA, Parfitt R, et al., Drug-induced ototoxicity: mechanisms, pharmacogenetics, and protective strategies. Clinical Pharmacology & Therapeutics, 2017. 101(4): 491–500.

Li T. Lindsley K, Rouse B, et al., Comparative effectiveness of first-line medications for primary open-angle glaucoma: a systematic review and network meta-analysis. Ophthalmology, 2016. 123(1): 129–140.

Rotman A, Michael P, Tykocinski M, et al., Sudden sensorineural hearing loss secondary to metronidazole ototoxicity. Medical Journal of Australia, 2015. 203(6): 253.

Salerno E. Pharmacology for health professionals, St Louis, MO, 1999, Mosby.

Steiner M. On the correct use of eye drops, Australian Prescriber 31:16–17, 2008.

Yanoff M, Duker JS: Ophthalmology, ed 2, St Louis, MO, 2004, Mosby.

ONLINE RESOURCES

Australian Tinnitus Association: http://www.tinnitus.asn.au/ (accessed 8 September 2021)

Medsafe: http://www.medsafe.govt.nz/ (accessed 8 September 2021)

Ménière's disease: https://brainfoundation.org.au/disorders/menieres-disease (accessed 8 September 2021)

More weblinks at: http://evolve.elsevier.com/AU/Knights/pharmacology/.

CHAPTER 41
DRUGS IN AGED CARE
Kathleen Knights

KEY ABBREVIATIONS

ADRs	adverse drug reactions
DBI	drug burden index
FRIDs	fall risk-increasing drugs
PIMS	potentially inappropriate medications
QUM	quality use of medicines
RACF	residential aged care facility
RMMR	Residential Medication Management Review

KEY TERMS

Chapter Focus

A significant proportion of the Australasian population are aged 65 years or older. Although many live independently and lead healthy and productive lives, increasing disease burden and/or physical/cognitive impairment often results in a move to residential aged care facilities. Those living in aged care in general have a greater number of comorbidities and experience a higher incidence of polypharmacy and drug-related harms. The latter often results in increasing risk of falls, hospitalisation and/or death. Multiple drug groups are implicated in increasing falls risk. Residential Medication Management Review and the process of deprescribing play a role in addressing/reducing inappropriate polypharmacy and the harms associated with multiple drug use in older adults.

KEY DRUG GROUPS

Anticholinergics

Antipsychotics

Benzodiazepines

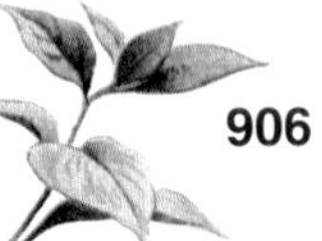

CRITICAL THINKING SCENARIO

Kitty, an 84-year-old, lives in a residential aged care facility and has multiple health issues including hypertension, diabetes and Parkinson's disease. Staff at the facility have asked for a Residential Medication Management Review because they have noticed a deterioration in Kitty's health including episodes of dizziness, confusion, memory impairment and increasing drowsiness. For her Parkinson's disease Kitty has been taking benzatropine 5 mg daily for the past 2 years.

1. Discuss the relationship between benzatropine and her current clinical symptoms.
2. What age-related factors may have contributed to developing her current symptoms?
3. What actions could be taken at this stage to improve her clinical condition?

Introduction

> *'Population ageing is a human success story, a reason to celebrate the triumph of public health, medical advancements, and economic and social development over diseases, injuries and early deaths that have limited human life spans throughout history.'*
>
> United Nations 2019

In 2019 approximately 10% (703 million) of the world's population were aged 65 years or older. This is expected to double to 1.5 billion people by 2050, which equates to one in every six people being older adults (65 years or older) (Australian Bureau of Statistics 2017). In Australia, one in seven people were aged 65 years or older in 2011, and one in six in 2016. This is expected to rise to one in five by 2031. With a total population of 5,122,600 15.9% of the New Zealand population (June 2021; 819,100 people) were aged 65 years or older, and the proportion of people aged 85 years or older is projected to double by 2063 (Stats NZ 2021). Australians and New Zealanders can, on average, expect to live long (80–85 years) and relatively healthy lives. However, the continued rise in the proportion of aged people in the population has placed, and will continue to place, increased pressure on support systems. This is not limited to just the support provided by the family but more broadly the vast array of aged-care services funded by government and private providers. The long-term goal for any ageing person should be the ability to balance age-related changes in their physical and psychological health with a healthy, productive and socially inclusive lifestyle. However, for many people a decline in their physical and/or mental health necessitates a change to their living environment.

In 2020, 189,954 people, of which 50% were aged between 80 and 89 years, lived in residential aged care facilities (RACFs) in Australia (Australian Institute of Health and Welfare 2021). In 2017–18, 31,600 New Zealanders lived in RACFs, of which about 25% were aged 85 years or older. The need for cultural inclusivity in New Zealand RACFs is evident from the fact that around 5% of residents identified as Māori and 2% as Pacific Islanders (Stats NZ 2021). Throughout Australasia, RACFs are divided into three categories:

- self-care retirement villages (low-level care)
- hostels (intermediate-level care)
- nursing homes (high-level care).

Clearly many factors will impact on both the quality of life of and the level of care of an aged person in an RACF. Not surprisingly these factors include long-term health conditions (Clinical Focus Box 41.1), physical limitations/disabilities (e.g. incomplete use of arms or legs), cognitive issues and medication use. It is estimated that about 75% of aged care residents have between five and 10 long-term health conditions. In addition, 53% of residents in Australian RACFs have dementia including Alzheimer's disease (Australian Institute of Health and Welfare 2020).

Changes in pharmacodynamics and pharmacokinetics with ageing

Pharmacotherapy in the older population is challenging because this group in general:

- often have multiple comorbidities
- take a high proportion of prescribed drugs and over-the-counter medications
- take three times more drugs than younger people
- frequently take multiple medications (four to five prescription drugs at any one time)

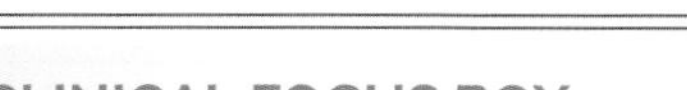

CLINICAL FOCUS BOX 41.1

Examples of long-term health conditions in older adults

Anxiety
Arthritis
Atrial fibrillation
Cerebrovascular disease
Chronic obstructive pulmonary disease
Congestive heart failure
Dementia
Depression
Diabetes
Hyperlipidaemia
Hypertension
Insomnia
Migraine
Osteoporosis
Partial/complete deafness
Peripheral vascular disease
Stroke
Vision impairment

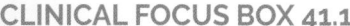

- experience drug interactions and adverse drug reactions (ADRs) more frequently than younger adults.

The pattern of drug use also varies depending on the setting; for example, in the community, use of analgesics and cardiovascular drugs (e.g. antihypertensive, statins, anticoagulants) is common, while in RACFs there is also a tendency for greater use of sedative-hypnotics and antipsychotics (see later sections). Without a doubt many drugs are beneficial (e.g. antihypertensives, oral hypoglycaemic agents, antibiotics), and appropriate prescribing in older adults is very much a balance between benefits and harms. Unfortunately, the incidence of **polypharmacy** (commonly defined as the concomitant use of five or more drugs) is high, and this can impact negatively on the quality of life of older people by increasing the incidence of ADRs. Drug interactions and ADRs may then contribute to a reduction in daily physical/social activities and increase mortality. In addition to polypharmacy, other medication-related issues that can affect the quality of life of older people are age-related alterations in pharmacodynamics and pharmacokinetics.

Pharmacodynamic changes with ageing

Changes in target-organ or receptor sensitivity in older adults may result in either a greater or a lesser drug effect than normal. The reason for this alteration is often unknown, but it may be due to either a decrease in the number of receptors at the target site or an altered receptor response (second-messenger effect) subsequent to drug binding. Older people often have a decreased response to β-adrenoceptor agonists (e.g. salbutamol) and β-adrenoceptor antagonists (e.g. propranolol), but they have a greater response (e.g. central nervous system [CNS] depression) to diazepam. It has also been reported that the muscarinic receptor density in the cortex tends to decrease with ageing, so older adults are often very sensitive to anticholinergic drugs.

Pharmacokinetic changes with ageing

It has been estimated that 70–80% of all ADRs in the older population are dose-related. As physiological changes (Fig 41.1) may alter the pharmacokinetics of a drug, this can lead to higher blood and tissue concentrations of drugs and/or their metabolites, thus increasing the incidence of ADRs.

Absorption and distribution

Pharmacokinetics of a drug may be altered in old age because of reduced gastric acid secretion and slowed gastric motility, resulting in unpredictable rates of dissolution and absorption of drugs. Changes in absorption may occur when gastric acid production decreases, altering the absorption of weakly acidic drugs such as barbiturates. However, few studies of drug absorption have shown clinically significant changes occurring with advanced age.

Changes in body composition, such as an increased proportion of body fat and decreased total body water, plasma volume and extracellular fluid, have been noted in the older population. The increased proportion of body fat increases the volume of distribution of some lipid-soluble drugs (e.g. benzodiazepines), prolonging half-life. The half-life of diazepam increases from 20 hours in a 20-year-old to 90 hours in people in their 80s because of the increase in volume of distribution in the latter. The loss in total body water and lean body mass (decreased volume of drug distribution) in many older people may require initiation of therapy at a lower adult dose or re-evaluation of dosages of polar drugs already in use because the risk of toxicity with hydrophilic (water-soluble) drugs increases as total body water decreases. Digoxin, theophylline, lithium and gentamicin are examples of hydrophilic drugs that may accumulate, causing adverse effects.

In older adults, the criterion for dosage should be shifted from age to weight, as some older people weigh no more than the average large child and some weigh a lot less, yet they are often prescribed the 'normal' adult doses.

Metabolism

Hepatic drug metabolism is also affected by ageing. For drugs with a high extraction ratio, the clearance is rate-limited by blood flow and hence, with an age-related

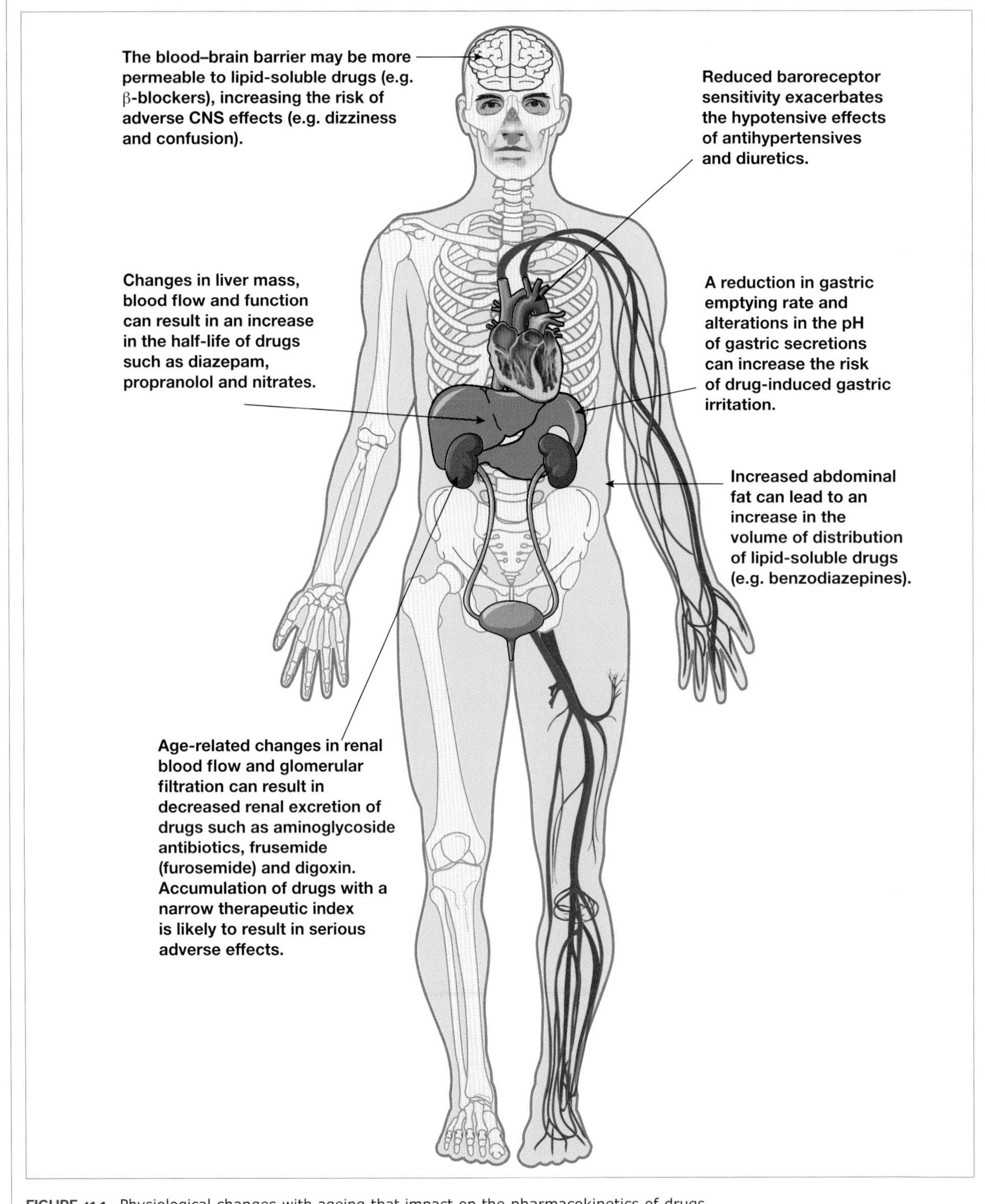

The blood–brain barrier may be more permeable to lipid-soluble drugs (e.g. β-blockers), increasing the risk of adverse CNS effects (e.g. dizziness and confusion).
Reduced baroreceptor sensitivity exacerbates the hypotensive effects of antihypertensives and diuretics.
Changes in liver mass, blood flow and function can result in an increase in the half-life of drugs such as diazepam, propranolol and nitrates.
A reduction in gastric emptying rate and alterations in the pH of gastric secretions can increase the risk of drug-induced gastric irritation.
Increased abdominal fat can lead to an increase in the volume of distribution of lipid-soluble drugs (e.g. benzodiazepines).
Age-related changes in renal blood flow and glomerular filtration can result in decreased renal excretion of drugs such as aminoglycoside antibiotics, frusemide (furosemide) and digoxin. Accumulation of drugs with a narrow therapeutic index is likely to result in serious adverse effects.

FIGURE 41.1 Physiological changes with ageing that impact on the pharmacokinetics of drugs.
Source: Figure 8.1 from the 5th edition. Goodman RM, Gorlin RJ. Atlas of the face in genetic disorders, ed 2 St louis, MO, 1977, Mosby

decrease in liver blood flow, the hepatic extraction of high clearance drugs will be affected (Ch 6). Drugs that are metabolised by functionalisation reactions (e.g. oxidation, hydroxylation or demethylation) may have a decreased metabolism, while conjugative metabolism (e.g. glucuronidation) appears not to be affected by ageing (Ch 4). Disorders common to the older population, such as congestive heart failure, may impact on liver function and decrease the metabolism of drugs, increasing the risk of drug accumulation and toxicity.

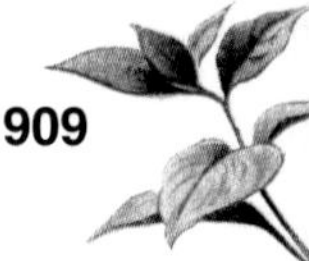

Renal excretion

For drugs primarily excreted by the kidneys, reduced renal function may result in drug accumulation and toxicity because a significant proportion of older adults have some degree of renal dysfunction. Renal function may be impaired because of loss of nephrons, decreased renal blood flow and decreased glomerular filtration rate. A reduction in renal function is also secondary to heart failure. Decreased renal clearance may cause increased plasma drug concentrations and longer half-lives of drugs and active metabolites excreted by the kidney.

A 2015 Australian study identified inappropriate prescribing of renally cleared drugs in older residents in both the community and RACFs. The drugs inappropriately prescribed included alendronate, fenofibrate, glibenclamide, olmesartan, metformin, perindopril and the gliptins (Khanal et al. 2015). When compromised renal function is suspected, determination of creatinine clearance and the use of therapeutic drug monitoring will help optimise dosing in this group.

KEY POINTS

Changes in drug disposition with ageing

- Age-related changes in target-organ or receptor sensitivity can result in enhanced or diminished drug response (e.g. increased CNS depression with diazepam but reduced response to salbutamol and propranolol).
- Pharmacokinetics of a drug in older adults can be altered by a reduction in gastric acid secretion, slowed gastric motility, changes in body composition (e.g. increased body fat and decreased total body water, plasma volume and extracellular fluid).
- Changes in body fat increases the volume of distribution of lipid-soluble drugs (e.g. benzodiazepines), increasing half-life.
- Reduction in total body water decreases the volume of distribution of hydrophilic (water-soluble) drugs, necessitating a reduction in dose.
- Weight-related changes in older adults should be taken into consideration when initiating drug therapy.

Drug treatment for older adults

Drug treatment in older adults is often a challenging process because of changes in physiology, the impact of acute and chronic disease states and alterations in drug pharmacodynamics and pharmacokinetics that occur with ageing. Some factors for consideration when considering drug treatment in this group include:

- balancing the risks and benefits for the person
- referring to evidence-based guidelines and treating comorbid diseases as appropriate
- optimising polypharmacy, using the simplest drug regimen and avoiding over/under treatment
- using the lowest dose to achieve the desired clinical outcome
- considering any new symptoms as possible drug interactions or ADRs
- providing simple written and verbal instructions to the client and all people (e.g. RACF staff, carers, family members) involved in medication management
- undertaking regular Residential Medication Management Reviews (see later section)
- deprescribing drug(s) (see later section).

Beers Criteria

Developed by Mark H Beers in 1991 (updated 2003, 2012, 2015 and 2020), the evidence-based **Beers Criteria** is a tool widely used to guide prescribers on the drugs that should be:

(1) avoided in most older people
(2) avoided in older adults with certain conditions
(3) used with caution when the benefit outweighs the risk
(4) avoided in people with cognitive impairment or dementia (American Geriatrics Society 2015; Croke 2020).

Prescribing of potentially inappropriate medications (PIMs) according to the Beers Criteria in RACFs has been shown to increase the risk of hospitalisation and death (Lau et al. 2005). Table 41.1 lists examples of potentially inappropriate drug groups used in older people (independent of diagnoses), Beers Criteria and adverse effects.

Drug Burden Index

Unlike the Beers Criteria that provides a list of inappropriate drugs the **Drug Burden Index** (DBI) 'calculates individuals' exposure to anticholinergic and sedative drugs utilising dose-response and cumulative effect parameters' (Harrison et al. 2018). Calculation of the DBI takes into account:

- the daily dose of each anticholinergic or sedative drug taken by a person
- the minimum recommended daily dose registered with the Australian Therapeutic Goods Administration that achieves 50% of the maximum anticholinergic/sedative effect of the particular drug.

DBI ranges from 0 to 1, and a value of 0.5 indicates exposure of the person at the minimum recommended

TABLE 41.1 Examples of potentially inappropriate drug groups used in the older population, Beers Criteria and adverse effects

DRUG GROUP[a,b]	BEERS CRITERIA	ADVERSE EFFECTS
Anticholinergics (first-generation antihistamines)	Avoid	Blurred vision, dry mouth, constipation, confusion, urinary retention, nausea, delirium, orthostatic hypotension
Antidepressants (tricyclics)	Avoid	Sedation, agitation, delirium, dry mouth, blurred vision, confusion, cardiac dysrhythmias, dizziness, insomnia, tachycardia
Antipsychotics	Avoid (exceptions: schizophrenia, bipolar disorder or short-term use as antiemetic)	Increased risk of stroke, orthostatic hypotension, sedation, agitation, anxiety, blurred vision, cognitive impairment, extrapyramidal effects, mortality, hospitalisation
Barbiturates	Avoid	Physical dependence, sedation, confusion, cognitive impairment, altered mood and behaviour, paradoxical insomnia
Benzodiazepines	Avoid	Older adults have increased sensitivity (oversedation), ataxia, cognitive impairment, delirium, falls
Central α-blockers	Avoid	CNS effects, bradycardia, orthostatic hypotension
Digoxin	Avoid as first-line therapy for atrial fibrillation	Nausea, vomiting, cardiac dysrhythmias, visual disorders, mental status changes, hallucinations
NSAIDs	Avoid chronic use if possible	Gastritis, gastrointestinal bleeding, ulceration

[a] Drug group independent of diagnoses
[b] See American Geriatrics Society 2015 for details of individual drugs in each group.
Sources: Gnjidic et al. 2012; Adapted from American Geriatrics Society 2015.

daily dose. It has been demonstrated that in the older population a higher DBI score is associated with impaired physical functioning (Harrison et al. 2018), a lower quality of life (Hasan et al. 2020) and frailty (Australian Medicines Handbook 2021).

The impact of drugs on functional outcomes in older adults

Antipsychotics

Of particular concern is the use of antipsychotics to manage behavioural and psychological symptoms commonly associated with dementia. These symptoms fluctuate over time, occur episodically, negatively impact on the quality of life of the affected person, and are distressing for the family and other people living/working in the RACF. The use of antipsychotics in older people is complicated; in Lewy body dementia these drugs can worsen behaviours, increase agitation and further impair cognitive and motor function (Gnjidic et al. 2012). In addition, older drugs like haloperidol can increase the risk of stroke and death in older people. In Australia, risperidone is the only drug indicated for use in Alzheimer's disease to control severe behavioural and psychological symptoms, but use is not recommended beyond 12 weeks (Gnjidic et al. 2012).

Various programs to reduce the use of antipsychotics in RACFs have been implemented. These include in-house educational programs, pharmacist-driven regular medication reviews and involvement of multidisciplinary teams (pharmacists, doctors, nurses, RACF support staff) with a view to reducing antipsychotic drug use.

In recent times an emphasis has been placed on non-pharmacological approaches including personalised interventions that focus on distraction and reassurance rather than resorting in the first instance to antipsychotics to control behavioural and psychological issues (Aged Care Quality and Safety Commission 2020).

For more on antipsychotics, see Chapter 22.

Benzodiazepines

Insomnia is a common problem in the older population, manifesting in earlier bed and rise times, difficulty falling asleep, easy arousability, brief awakenings and in general lighter and less sleep. Consequently, an older insomniac experiences increased daytime cognitive and attentional impairment that may be misconstrued as early symptoms of dementia. Chronic sleep deprivation also increases the risk of cancer, stroke, heart disease, depression, anxiety, suicide and falls (Abad & Guilleminault 2018).

Non-drug strategies should always be first-line. These include:

- avoiding daytime naps, caffeine-containing drinks and alcohol consumption late in the day
- cognitive behaviour therapy, relaxation therapy, mindfulness interventions
- combinations of psychological and behavioural therapy.

In addition, rescheduling and adjusting the dose of medications that cause CNS stimulation and insomnia to morning or early afternoon (e.g. adrenoceptor agonists, anticholinesterases, β-blockers, glucocorticoids, selective serotonin reuptake inhibitors) is advised.

Older people are more susceptible to the effects of benzodiazepines because of the increased volume of distribution and prolonged half-life. If adhering to the Beers Criteria, benzodiazepines should not be prescribed in this group because of the increased risk of ataxia, falls/fractures, excessive sedation, delirium and impaired cognition. However, benzodiazepines are widely prescribed in old age to treat anxiety and insomnia, but long-term use is not recommended (Aged Care Quality and Safety Commission 2020). The short-acting agents (e.g. temazepam, oxazepam) are preferred, while the long-acting benzodiazepines (e.g. diazepam, nitrazepam) should be avoided. Tolerance develops rapidly, and rebound insomnia is highly variable and occurs even with intermittent dosing. In general, benzodiazepines are not the drug of choice for the routine management of insomnia in older adults.

For more on benzodiazepines, see Chapter 20.

Drugs that increase the risk of falls

Falls in general can result in soft tissue injuries, fractures and short/long-term physical impairment. In the older population, falls contribute to loss of quality of life and an increase in morbidity and mortality. Not surprisingly, many studies have reported a high risk of falls in RACF residents who are either of an advanced age, have balance disorders, are frail, have diminished cognition, have physical impairments or who are taking psychotropic drugs or drugs known to cause orthostatic hypotension (Fig 41.2). Preventing falls is paramount, and all modifiable risk factors should be addressed including, for example, removing tripping hazards (e.g. loose floor mats) and reviewing the drugs administered.

In 2010 the Swedish National Board of Health and Welfare published a list of fall risk-increasing drugs (FRIDs) classifying them into two main categories

- drugs increasing the risk of falls
- drugs implicated in causing/worsening orthostatic hypotension (Clinical Focus Box 41.2).

CLINICAL FOCUS BOX 41.2
Examples of falls risk-increasing drugs

Drugs increasing falls risk

Antiarrhythmics
Antidepressants
Antipsychotics (excluding lithium)
Anxiolytics
Cardiac glycosides
Hypnotics and sedatives
Opioids

Drugs causing/worsening orthostatic hypotension

α-Adrenoceptor antagonists
Antidepressants
Antihypertensives
Antipsychotics (excluding lithium)
β-Blockers
Calcium channel blockers
Diuretics
Dopaminergic drugs
Renin–angiotensin–aldosterone system inhibitors

Sources: Beunza-Sola et al. 2018; Wang et al. 2021.

Lower falls risk
• Walks unaided
• No gait/balance issues
• Independent lifestyle/low care
• Physically active
• No major sensory deficits
• No falls history
• No major cognitive issues
• Low disease burden
• Limited drug therapy
• No PIMs/FRIDs
Higher falls risk
• Needs assistance with walking (e.g. cane/walker)
• Gait/balance issues
• High level of care
• Limited physical activity
• Vision/hearing impairment
• Falls history
• Cognitive issues
• Multiple chronic conditions
• Polypharmacy
• ↑ likelihood of PIMs/FRIDs

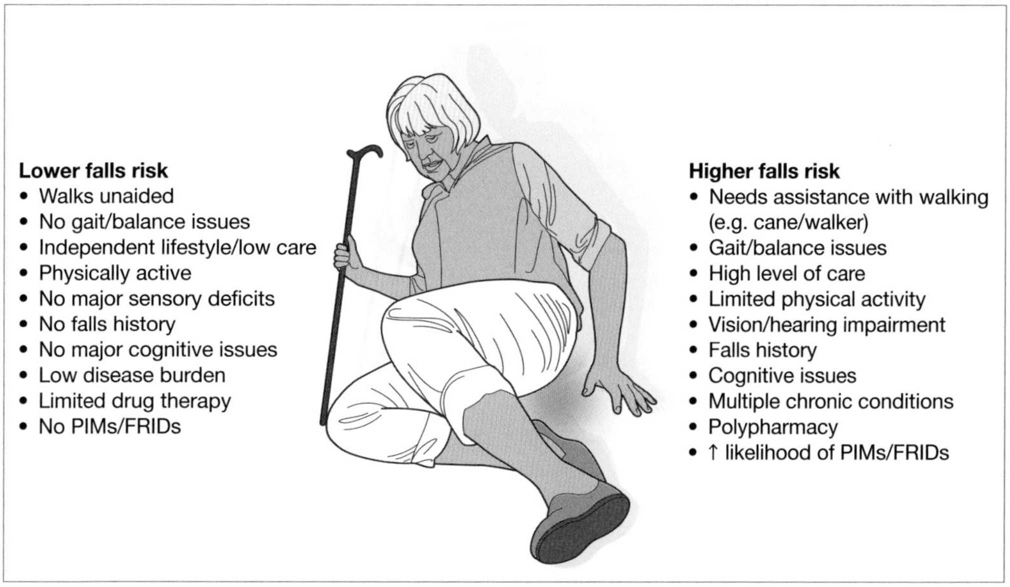

FIGURE 41.2 Examples of factors that can either lower or increase the risk of falls in older adults

Not prescribing a FRID in the first instance or ceasing or reducing the dose of a FRID would appear to be an important strategy to prevent the risk of either a fall or fall-related injuries in at-risk people.

KEY POINTS

Impact of drugs on functional outcomes

- The Beers Criteria and the DBI are tools used to guide prescribing in older adults. The former provides information on potentially inappropriate medications, while the latter is an indication of exposure to anticholinergic and sedative drugs.
- Antipsychotics are administered to manage behavioural and psychological symptoms commonly associated with dementia.
- These drugs can worsen behaviours, increase agitation and further impair cognitive and motor function. In addition, they can increase the risk of stroke and death in older people.
- Risperidone is the only drug indicated for use in Alzheimer's disease to control severe behavioural and psychological symptoms, but use is not recommended beyond 12 weeks.
- Managing insomnia in the older population should involve non-drug strategies and rescheduling of drugs that may exacerbate insomnia.
- Short-acting benzodiazepines (e.g. temazepam, oxazepam) are preferred but are not the drug of choice for routine management of insomnia in older age.
- Falls contribute to a loss of quality of life and an increase in morbidity and mortality.
- FRIDs are classified into those that increase the risk of falls (e.g. antipsychotics, hypnotics, sedatives) or those drugs that cause/worsen orthostatic hypotension (e.g. antihypertensives, antidepressants).

Medication reviews and deprescribing

Medication reviews

The Guiding Principles for Medication Management in Residential Aged Care Facilities (see Australian Government Department of Health – 'Online resources') has at its core the principles of quality use of medicines (QUM) and is intended to guide RACFs in developing a framework to assist both residents and carers in safe and effective medication management. This is as simple as either providing informative, accurate, easily read medicines information to both staff and residents, or assisting residents to self-administer their drugs safely, which helps maintain a degree of independence and control over their health.

Similarly in New Zealand, the Medicines Management Guide for Community Residential and Facility-based Respite Services – Disability, Mental Health and Addiction (NZ Ministry of Health – 'Online resources') outlines policies and procedures for medication management with the central focus that 'the person who is taking the medicine is the focus of the medicines management system'. This guide further details the responsibilities of the person taking the drug, the staff and support staff administering the drug, the authorised prescriber and the pharmacist. The latter two have multiple responsibilities in line with QUM principles.

Polypharmacy is highly prevalent in RACFs, and medication reviews are common practice. Medication reviews have been shown worldwide to reduce the rate of potentially inappropriate prescribing. In Australia, the Residential Medication Management Review (RMMR) program is a national government-funded review service that has been in place since 1997. The main aims of an RMMR are to optimise medication use, to improve clinical outcomes and to ensure adherence to the tenets of QUM. If requested by a GP or family physician, an RACF resident is entitled to have their medications reviewed by a clinical pharmacist every 2 years, or more frequently if required. A report is then provided by the clinical pharmacist to the requesting health professional who is then responsible for consulting with the resident, carer or RACF staff about implementing the recommendations. A 2018 study found that RMMRs identified a range of '2.7–3.9 medication-related problems per resident' and that 45–84% of recommendations to resolve a problem were accepted by GPs highlighting the valuable role of pharmacists and GPs working together to support QUM in RACFs (Chen et al. 2019).

Deprescribing

Effective use of drugs in the older population is problematic, with numerous reports of overprescribing, inappropriate prescribing and ADRs resulting in hospitalisations. **Deprescribing** is one strategy to either reduce or address inappropriate polypharmacy and the harms associated with it in older adults. However, to date, data on the effectiveness of deprescribing and the benefit in terms of clinical outcomes in this group are limited. Value can be seen in terms of linking medication reviews with the ethos of deprescribing, but clearly there are enablers and barriers to the process. Enabling reflects the concerns of the prescriber/pharmacist/RACF staff in reducing harms, while barriers include both the person concerned and their reluctance to 'stop' their drugs, and the concerns of family and staff who must deal with the deprescribing process, the likelihood of withdrawal symptoms and possible worsening of clinical symptoms.

It is crucial that the older person taking the drug is at the centre of any decision and that all parties involved (e.g. RACF staff/carer, family, GP, community pharmacist) are involved in the decision when attempting to deprescribe a particular drug(s). Clinical evidence has indicated that initially deprescribing a drug with no noticeable withdrawal effects is a good strategy because it alleviates any perceived concerns about 'stopping' a drug. Similarly, it is essential to choose carefully which drugs are stopped, as drugs with overlapping indications may make it difficult to ascertain which drug may be causing withdrawal effects (Liacos et al. 2020). Other factors for consideration include a gradual reduction in drug dose to mitigate withdrawal effects (e.g. benzodiazepines) and trialling discontinuation with reinstatement of the drug at a lower dose if symptoms reoccur (e.g. antihypertensives).

Clearly, deprescribing is a complex process and is only one tool for managing inappropriate polypharmacy in older adults. The main aims are to reduce harm and improve quality of life. To date, there are limited data on the clinical and cost-effectiveness of deprescribing and the impact of deprescribing on quality of life (e.g. psychosocial functioning, cognitive ability or physical functioning). Similarly, there are limited guidelines to assist in the deprescribing process and to mitigate against withdrawal symptoms. Clearly comprehensive guides to assist health professionals in the deprescribing process for individual drugs would be valuable.

KEY POINTS

Medication management in older adults

- Safe and effective medication management is a cornerstone of QUM.
- Use of drugs in older adults is problematic, with numerous reports of overprescribing, inappropriate prescribing and ADRs resulting in hospitalisations.
- Regular medication reviews optimise medication use, improve clinical outcomes and ensure adherence to the tenets of QUM.
- Deprescribing is one strategy to either reduce or address inappropriate polypharmacy and the harms associated with it in the older population.
- There are limited data on the clinical and cost-effectiveness of deprescribing and the impact of deprescribing on quality of life (e.g. psychosocial functioning, cognitive ability or physical functioning).
- To date, comprehensive guidelines for individual drugs to aid in the deprescribing process are limited.

REVIEW EXERCISES

1. Mrs BC, an active 76-year-old woman, lives in an RACF and regularly enjoys social outings. She has been treated for the past 6 years with warfarin for atrial fibrillation. Although her international normalised ratio is usually 2–3, her most recent result was 1. She reluctantly advises you that she bought a 'little pick-me-up' from the local pharmacy without speaking to the pharmacist. You immediately recognise that she has bought St John's wort, which she has been taking for 3 weeks. Discuss the mechanistic interaction between warfarin and St John's wort.
2. Mr OD, an 87-year-old resident of Sunny View Aged Care, recently complained of persistent dizziness and fell while going to the bathroom. Because he has been prescribed multiple drugs to treat a variety of disorders, an RMMR was undertaken. The pharmacist in his report noted that Mr OD had been taking a combination of amlodipine (5 mg), valsartan (160 mg) and hydrochlorothiazide (12.5 mg) that had recently been increased to 10 mg/320 mg/25 mg by a visiting GP. Discuss the pharmacology of the three drugs and provide an explanation as to his recent persistent dizziness. What action should be taken to address his dizziness?
3. Mrs DP has recently celebrated her 96th birthday. Over the past 6 months her general health, both mental and physical, has deteriorated and her care team, along with her family, have decided to trial deprescribing alendronate, ibuprofen and pantoprazole. Explain why these three drugs have been selected. Is she likely to experience any withdrawal symptoms?

REFERENCES

Abad VC, Guilleminault C. Insomnia in elderly patients: Recommendations for pharmacological management. Drugs and Ageing 2018;35:791–817.

Aged Care Quality and Safety Commission 2020. Psychotropic medications used in Australia information for aged care. Online. Available: https://www.agedcarequality.gov.au/sites/default/files/media/acqsc_psychotropic_medications_v10_hr.pdf

American Geriatrics Society 2015. Updated Beers Criteria for potentially inappropriate medication use in older adults. Journal of the American Geriatrics Society 2015;63:2227–46.

Australian Bureau of Statistics 2017, Census of Population and Housing: Reflecting Australia – Stories from the Census, 2016. Online: https://www.abs.gov.au/ausstats/abs@.nsf/Lookup/by%20Subject/2071.0~2016~Main%20Features~Ageing%20Population~14

Australian Institute of Health and Welfare 2020. GEN dashboard 2018–19: People using aged care 2018–19. Canberra: AIHW.

Australian Institute of Health and Welfare 2021. GEN fact sheet 2019–20 People using aged care. Canberra: AIHW. https://www.gen-agedcaredata.gov.au/www_aihwgen/media/2020-factsheets-and-infographics/People-using-aged-care-Factsheet_2020.pdf

Australian Medicines Handbook. Australian Medicines Handbook Pty Ltd. Adelaide: 2021.

Beunza-Sola M, Hidalgo-Ovejero AM, et al. Study of fall risk-increasing drugs in elderly patients before and after bone fracture. Postgrad Med J 2018;94:76–80.

Chen EYH, Wang KN, Sluggett JK, et al. Process, impact and outcomes of medication review in Australian residential aged care facilities: a systematic review. Australasian Journal of Ageing 2019;38(Suppl. 2):9–25.

Croke L. Beers Criteria for inappropriate medication use in older patients: an update from the AGS. American Family Physician 2020;101:56–7.

Gnjidic D, Le Couteur DG, Abernethy DR, et al. Drug burden index and Beers Criteria: Impact on functional outcomes in older people living in self-care retirement villages. Journal of Clinical Pharmacology 2012;52:253–65.

Goodman RM, Gorlin RJ: Atlas of the face in genetic disorders, ed 2, St Louis, MO, 1977, Mosby.

Harrison SL, O'Donnell LK, Bradley CE, et al. Association between the Drug Burden Index, potentially inappropriate medications and quality of life in residential aged care. Drugs Ageing 2018;35:83–91.

Hasan SS, Chang SH, Thiruchelvam K, et al.. Drug burden index, polypharmacy and patient health outcomes in cognitively intact older residents of aged care facilities in Malaysia. Journal of Pharmacy Practice and Research 2020;50:13–21.

Khanal A, Peterson GM, Castelino RL, et al. Potentially inappropriate prescribing of renally cleared drugs in elderly patients in community and aged care settings. Drugs Aging 2015;32:391–400.

Lau DT, Kasper JD, Potter DE, et al. Hospitalization and death associated with potentially inappropriate medication prescriptions among elderly nursing home residents. Arch Intern Med 2005;165:68–74.

Liacos M, Page AT, Etherton-Beer C. Deprescribing in older people. Australian Prescriber 2020;43:114–120.

Stats NZ 2021. https://www.stats.govt.nz/

United Nations 2019. World population ageing 2019: highlights (ST/ESA/SER.A/430). Department of Economic and Social Affairs, Population Division. Online: https://www.un.org/en/development/desa/population/publications/pdf/ageing/WorldPopulationAgeing2019-Highlights.pdf

Wang KN, Bell JS, Gilmartin-Thomas JFM, et al. Use of falls risk increasing drugs in residents at high and low falls risk in aged care services. Journal of Applied Gerontology 2021;40:77–86.

ONLINE RESOURCES

Australian Government Department of Health – Medication Management Reviews: https://www1.health.gov.au/internet/main/publishing.nsf/Content/medication_management_reviews.htm (accessed 24 January 2022)

Australian Government Department of Health – Guiding principles for medication management in residential aged care facilities: https://www1.health.gov.au/internet/main/publishing.nsf/Content/EEA5B39AA0A63F18CA257BF0001DAE08/$File/Guiding%20principles%20for%20medication%20management%20in%20residential%20aged%20care%20facilities.pdf (accessed 24 January 2022)

New Zealand Ministry of Health – Medicines Management Guide for Community Residential and Facility-based Respite Services – Disability, Mental Health and Addiction: https://www.health.govt.nz/publication/medicines-management-guide-community-residential-and-facility-based-services-disability-mental (accessed 24 January 2022)

More weblinks at: http://evolve.elsevier.com/AU/Knights/pharmacology/.

CHAPTER 42
PHARMACOTHERAPY OF OBESITY
Kathleen Knights

KEY ABBREVIATIONS

BMI body mass index
CCK cholecystokinin
FTO fat mass and obesity-associated gene
GLP-1 glucagon-like peptide-1
WHR waist:hip ratio

KEY TERMS

body mass index 916
cholecystokinin 919
glucagon-like peptide-1 921
incretins 921
leptin 919
pancreatic lipase 921
waist:hip ratio 917

Chapter Focus

The incidence of obesity is increasing in both Australian and New Zealand residents. Overweight (body mass index [BMI] of $\geq$ 25.0 kg/m^2) and obese (BMI $\geq$ 30.0 kg/m^2) people have a higher long-term risk of morbidity and mortality. A wide range of interacting biopsychological factors contribute to obesity. Alterations in diet, increased physical activity and behaviour modification are central to preventing and treating obesity. Continued advances in understanding the pathophysiology of obesity are aiding in the development of newer anti-obesity drugs.

KEY DRUG GROUPS

Drugs inhibiting nutrient absorption:
- **Orlistat** (Drug Monograph 42.1)

Glucagon-like peptide 1 analogue:
- **Liraglutide**

Noradrenergic drug:
- **Phentermine**

Anorexiant:
- **Naltrexone/bupropion**

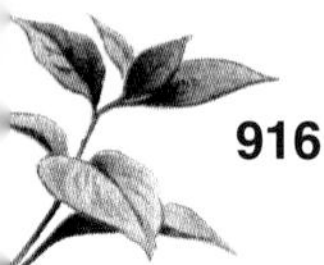

CRITICAL THINKING SCENARIO

Kaylee, a 24-year-old administrative assistant, has always been described as a 'perfectionist' by her work colleagues. At one stage, due to emotional stress, her perfectionist tendencies (the need to always tidy her desk) caused her considerable anxiety. She was treated successfully with fluoxetine for 6 months until her life became less stressful and her compulsive tidying habits were controlled. Kaylee noticed that when she was taking the drug, she lost weight because her appetite was reduced. Admitting that her current weight (BMI 29.9 kg/m^2) is causing her some concern and she fears her 'tidying habits' may worsen, she asks if you could prescribe the same drug again to help with her weight.

1. What is the mechanism of weight loss with fluoxetine?
2. Why is this class of drug not recommended for treating obesity?

Introduction

The prevalence of obesity has reached epidemic proportions across the globe, bringing with it increased risks of cancer, cardiovascular disease, diabetes mellitus, dyslipidaemia, hypertension and sleep apnoea. In the past three decades, self-interest in our weight and body shape has maintained a billion-dollar industry that ranges from glossy magazines to the sale of diet foods, fitness regimens and sojourns at health resorts. Unfortunately, a significant proportion of adult Australians (31.3%) and adult New Zealanders (32%) are considered obese. How do we define underweight, normal weight, overweight and obesity?

It is recognised that simply weighing a person does not provide an indication of either weight distribution or of risk factors. The measurement most frequently relied on is the **body mass index** (BMI). However, BMI is highly variable: it does not account for high body mass due to muscle rather than fat; it is unreliable in young people and the elderly; and it reflects intra-abdominal fat poorly, which is related to the metabolic syndrome and cardiovascular risk.

The BMI is calculated from the following equation:

BMI (kg/m^2) = weight (kg) divided by height^2 (m^2)

For example, for a 120 kg person who is 1.67 m tall, their BMI is $120 \div 1.67^2 = 120 \div 2.79 = 43.0$ kg/m^2. According to World Health Organization guidelines, this person would be considered obese Class III (Table 42.1).

With the BMI used as the main indicator, in 2017–18, 67% of adult Australians aged over 18 years were either overweight (36%) or obese (31%). This equated to 12.5 million adults (Australian Institute of Health and Welfare 2020). In New Zealand, the 2019–20 Health Survey reported that approximately one in three adults aged 15 years or older were obese (30.9%). The prevalence of obesity differed with ethnicity, with the highest prevalence in those of Pacific (63.4%), followed by Māori (47.9%), European/other (29.3%) and Asian (15.9%) heritage (New Zealand Ministry of Health 2020).

Obesity is not unique to Australasia; it is a global health problem, and the number of obese adults has trebled since 1975, with around 1.9 billion adults now classed as either overweight or obese.

TABLE 42.1 Body mass index: international classification

CLASSIFICATION	BMI (KG/M^2)
Underweight	< 18.5
Normal weight	18.5–24.9
Overweight (pre-obese)	25.0–29.9
Obese Class I	30.0–34.9
Obese Class II	35.0–39.9
Obese Class III	≥ 40.0

Source: World Health Organization – see www.who.int

Health risks associated with obesity

Obesity is well recognised as a disease in its own right. Health risks associated with obesity are numerous, and overweight people have a higher mortality rate than people with a normal BMI. Each year, around 2.8 million people die as a result of being overweight or obese. It has been well documented that obese people have a greater risk of the diseases noted in Clinical Focus Box 42.1.

The distribution of fat is also important in relation to disease risk. A high proportion of visceral (e.g. abdominal)

CLINICAL FOCUS BOX 42.1
Diseases associated with obesity

• Breast cancer • Cardiovascular disease • Colon cancer • Gall bladder cancer • Gallstones • Hirsutism • Hypercholesterolaemia • Hyperinsulinaemia • Hypertension • Hypertriglyceridaemia • Hyperuricaemia (gout)	• Hypogonadism • Infertility • Insulin resistance • Ischaemic heart disease • Osteoarthritis • Ovarian and uterine cancer • Prostate cancer • Sleep apnoea • Stroke • Type 2 diabetes mellitus • Varicose veins

fat carries a greater risk of morbidity and mortality than does a peripheral distribution. Although large studies that have measured concomitantly body weight and glucose and insulin concentrations are rare, a strong association exists between abdominal adiposity, blood glucose concentration, insulin resistance and developing type 2 diabetes. In Australia, the higher prevalence of obesity has been identified as a major contributing factor to the increasing incidence of diabetes, specifically type 2 diabetes. A simple measurement of visceral fat is the **waist:hip ratio** (WHR), which is calculated from the following equation:

$$\text{WHR} = \frac{\text{waist circumference (cm)}}{\text{hip circumference (cm)}}$$

The WHR should be under 0.9 in men and under 0.85 in women. Although there is no standard cutoff for waist circumference that provides an indication of greater risk, the World Health Organization suggests that a waist measurement over 94 cm in men and over 80 cm in women indicates some risk, and a waist circumference over 102 cm in men and over 88 cm in women indicates a substantially increased risk of health problems. These waist circumference measurement guidelines have been developed for Caucasians; similar guidelines have yet to be fully established for other populations.

The need for prevention and intervention to reduce obesity has been recognised in both Australia and New Zealand. A range of strategies has been developed, including guidelines for food and nutrition in schools and national approaches aimed at encouraging people to participate in physical activity. Both the National Health and Medical Research Council of Australia (2013) and the Ministry of Health, New Zealand (2017) have developed clinical guidelines for managing weight problems. To understand the complexities of obesity and to develop management strategies, it is essential to appreciate the pathophysiology of the disorder.

Pathophysiology of obesity

Obesity is a complex multifactorial disorder involving changes in energy balance (intake and expenditure), genetic factors, environmental factors (dietary and physical activity) and psychosocial factors (Fig 42.1). The complexity of these interacting forces has made the management of obesity difficult, and some people have resorted to surgical procedures such as gastric bypass and banded gastroplasty.

Primary obesity rarely results from endocrine disorders (e.g. Cushing's syndrome, hypothyroidism or hypogonadism) or from neurological disorders or drug treatment. From the simplest viewpoint, obesity, which is manifest by increased fat storage, is a consequence of an imbalance between increased energy (food) intake and decreased energy expenditure. Although on the surface this is a simple relationship, various factors can modify the balance between energy intake and expenditure. However, it is likely that the most successful approach is to prevent weight gain from the outset. In the current environment the challenge is to maintain 'a healthy body weight ... match energy intake with energy expenditure and to overcome biological tendencies to overeat and under exercise' (Hill et al. 2012).

Energy balance: integration involving the periphery and the hypothalamus

The control of food intake is complex and not fully understood. It is regulated by a system of interacting monoamine and peptide neurotransmitters, involving both peripheral and central hypothalamic pathways that either promote or suppress food intake. The involvement of the sympathetic nervous system (and its neurotransmitter noradrenaline) in regulating energy expenditure has been well documented scientifically, and it is popularly accepted that obese people have 'slow metabolism' and lean people have 'high metabolism'. Stimulation of α-adrenoceptors by noradrenaline decreases food intake via an action in the feeding centre in the hypothalamus and increases energy expenditure via stimulation of peripheral β-adrenoceptors. Similarly, activation of central 5-hydroxytryptamine (5-HT, serotonin) receptors by an excess of 5-HT inhibits food intake (Fig 42.2).

In addition to these monoamine transmitters, many central and peripheral peptide neurotransmitters are involved. These are classed as orexigenic (increasing food intake, such as neuropeptide Y) or anorexigenic (decreasing food intake, such as cholecystokinin [CCK]). Interest has focused more recently on the role of peripherally released leptin and CCK, and anti-obesity drugs targeted at these sites are being developed.

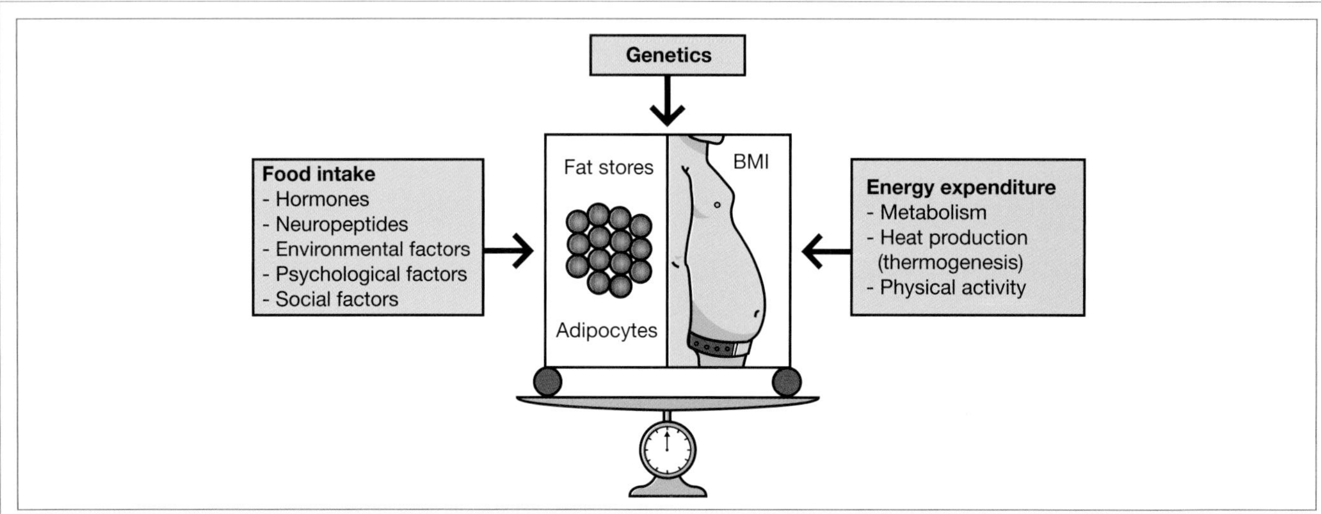

FIGURE 42.1 Energy balance: factors influencing energy intake and energy expenditure

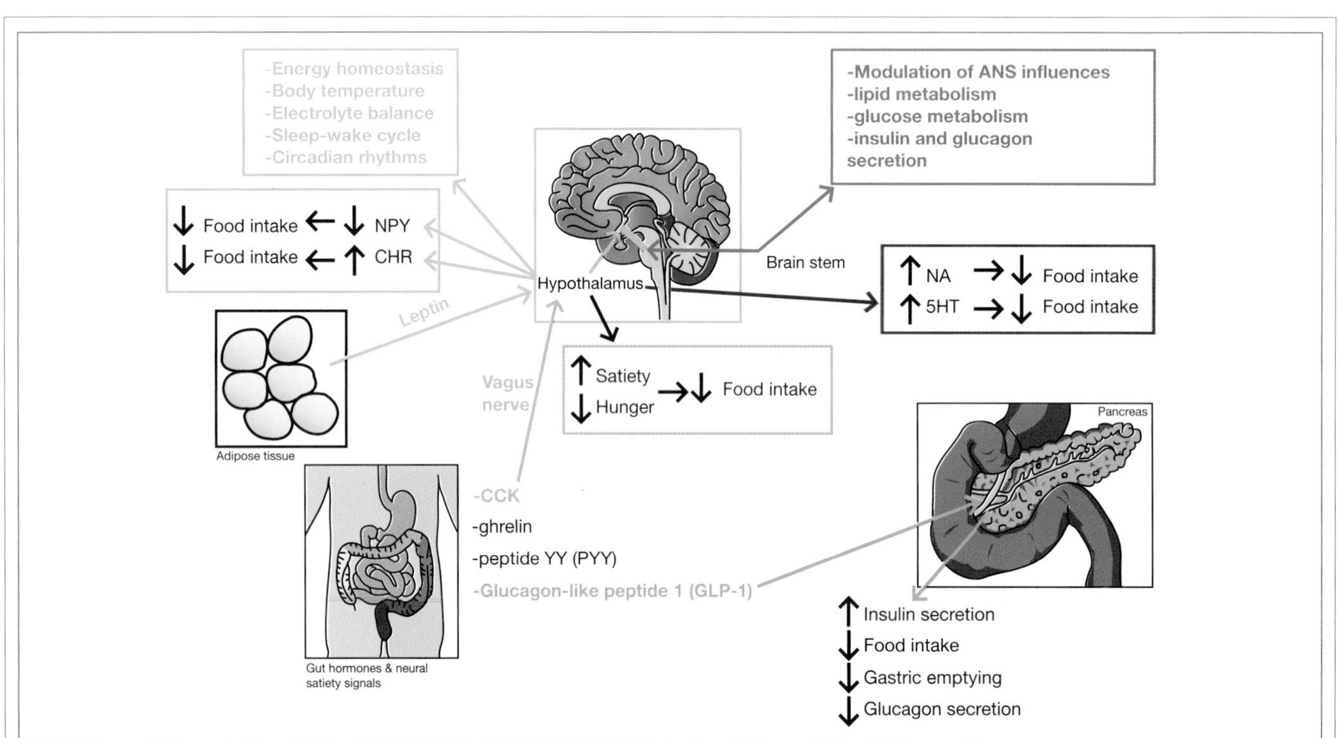

FIGURE 42.2 Schematic representation of food-regulating pathways

The hypothalamus regulates a number of key body processes, including energy homeostasis. The long-term regulation of food intake involves the leptin system, which causes a reduction in food intake by decreasing hypothalamic neuropeptide Y (NPY) synthesis and release and increasing the release of corticotrophin-releasing hormone (CRH). Short-term control involves cholecystokinin (CCK) released from the duodenum; CCK stimulates receptors on the vagus nerve to signal the hypothalamus of reduced feelings of hunger and satiety. Signals are also received by the hypothalamus from the peripheral nervous system and various gut hormones. GLP-1 stimulates insulin secretion and decreases food intake, gastric emptying and glucagon secretion. Specialised nuclei in the hypothalamus integrate the various signals and modulate the release of neurotransmitters (e.g. noradrenaline and 5-HT) that affect food intake. Additionally, the hypothalamus activates neurons in the brainstem that modulate the autonomic nervous system and energy expenditure.

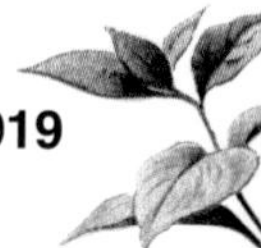

Leptin

Leptin (derived from the Greek word *leptos*, meaning 'thin') is the protein product of the obesity (*ob*) gene. This protein is released from adipocytes (fat cells) and via an action on leptin receptors on hypothalamic neurons signals the brain about the fat stores of the body. It is also a gut peptide that stimulates leptin receptors on vagal afferents. Generation of leptin is increased by estrogen, glucocorticoids and possibly by insulin, and is reduced by β-adrenoceptor agonists. On reaching the brain, leptin reduces the production of neuropeptide Y, which normally stimulates food intake and causes a reduction in energy expenditure. In contrast, fasting or weight loss results in a decrease in leptin concentration that triggers an increase in energy intake. Leptin also stimulates the production of corticotrophin-releasing hormone, which reduces food intake (Fig 42.2). In a small proportion of obese people, alterations in leptin synthesis, secretion and/or signalling may be associated with an intense desire to overeat (van der Klaauw & Farooqi 2015). Additionally, leptin influences energy balance in humans through modulation of melanocortin-dependent and -independent pathways in the hypothalamus.

Cholecystokinin

Cholecystokinin is a hormone secreted from the duodenum in the presence of food. It inhibits gastric emptying, pyloric sphincter contraction and stimulation of pancreatic exocrine secretions, and significantly reduces feelings of hunger and increases satiety (feeling of fullness) (Fig 42.2). Stimulation of CCK-A receptors on the vagus nerve sends signals to the hypothalamus, and the an interaction appears to occur between leptin and CCK. This interaction may play a role in both the short- and the long-term regulation of body weight. Other peripheral and central pathways may also be involved in the regulation of food intake and energy storage, and our knowledge is still advancing (Page et al. 2012).

Genetic factors

There is now widespread acceptance of a genetic component to obesity. Studies with adopted children have shown that their weight is related to that of their biological parents and not to that of their adopted parents. Estimates of a contribution of genetic effects to obesity range from 40% to 70%, and these findings have undoubtedly given credibility to the widely held perception that overweight parents have overweight kids.

It has long been recognised that many people with diabetes are obese, but a link between the two disorders has been difficult to establish. In a hallmark study using mice, a team of researchers has shown a link between diabetes and a protein called resistin, which is produced in adipocytes. Their studies established that diabetic mice have higher resistin levels, and these are linked to both diet-induced and genetic obesity (Steppan et al. 2001). Recent data on genetic linkage with obesity-related traits come from the fat mass and obesity-associated (*FTO*) gene. A number of variant alleles of *FTO* have been demonstrated, and people who are homozygous for the high-risk alleles weigh on average 3 kg more than those with the low-risk allele. This gene encodes for an enzyme in the hypothalamic nuclei that is involved in regulating energy balance (Gerken et al. 2007). Further research has identified mutations in melanocortin-4 receptors, which are associated with hypothalamic neural circuits involved in energy balance (Heymsfield & Wadden 2017).

Environmental factors

The availability of 'fast foods' and foods high in fat is an ever-present problem, coupled with changing lifestyles and a tendency for more sedentary pursuits. The tendency for us to obtain our daily energy from bread, milk drinks and potatoes (mashed potato or hot chips) does not fit with a 'healthy' diet. Strategies are aimed at increasing the consumption of vegetables, fruit, grains and cereals in an attempt to control the pandemic of obesity. Increased physical activity is also being encouraged, again attempting to redress the imbalance between high dietary fat intake and reduced energy expenditure.

KEY POINTS

Obesity

- Obesity is a complex multifactorial disorder involving changes in energy balance, genetic factors, environmental factors and psychosocial factors.
- The estimates of genetic component to obesity range from 40% to 70%.
- BMI is highly correlated with body fat and is calculated by dividing a person's body mass (kg) by the square of the height in metres (m^2).
- People with a BMI over 25 kg/m^2 are considered overweight, and those with a BMI over 30 kg/m^2 are considered obese.
- A WHR over 0.9 for men and over 0.85 for women indicates significant visceral fat distribution, which is associated with a greater risk of morbidity and mortality.
- The control of food intake is regulated by a complex system of interacting central and peripheral pathways.
- Interest has more recently focused on the role of peripheral modulators, which include leptin and CCK.

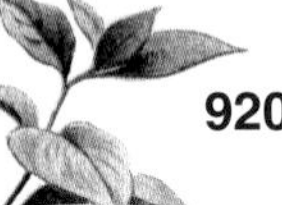

Management of obesity

Obesity is a complex disorder, and a complete understanding of all the interacting factors that lead to obesity is still to come. Management is difficult, and a person's compliance with one or all aspects of a program may vary enormously. Regulation of weight and the adoption of a healthy lifestyle are the main issues for many people, including those whose genes predispose them to obesity. There is often initial difficulty in losing weight, and further difficulties in maintaining the weight reduction. Strategies include dietary modification (low-fat diet), exercise programs and behaviour modification. Obesity is a lifelong problem for many people and too often the obese person is stigmatised as lacking the discipline to eat less and exercise more. Pharmacological agents may play an important role as knowledge of the biochemical and genetic factors contributing to obesity improves. Although drugs may produce an initial weight loss, maintaining the weight loss is still the key issue, and many anti-obesity drugs have failed in clinical practice because of severe and unacceptable psychiatric and/or cardiovascular effects.

Drug therapy

Safe and effective drugs free of adverse effects for treating obesity are not yet available, but multiple drugs targeted at specific sites are in development. Previously, the main drugs used for treating obesity were the centrally acting appetite suppressants that mimic the actions of noradrenaline.

Noradrenergic drugs

Mechanism of action

Deamfetamine was introduced during the 1930s to treat narcolepsy (desire to sleep) and was found to produce weight loss. It was later established that the anorectic effect of amphetamine is mediated via release of noradrenaline in the hypothalamus, which enhances sympathetic neurotransmission, resulting in appetite suppression and increased energy expenditure.

Because of its actions on central dopaminergic pathways, which produce central excitatory effects, amphetamine unfortunately has very high addictive and abuse potential. Other noradrenergic amphetamine-like drugs developed specifically as appetite suppressants were designed with the aim of reducing the potential for drug abuse. These included benzphetamine, diethylpropion, phentermine, methamphetamine and phendimetrazine. Phentermine is the only noradrenergic drug currently available in Australia and New Zealand (not funded by Pharmac), and its role in treating obesity should adhere to good prescribing practice. This drug increases catecholamine concentration, making it unsuitable for use in obese people with cardio- or cerebrovascular disease. Phentermine may be used for short-term treatment of obesity (maximum of 12 weeks) in conjunction with a management plan of caloric restriction, an exercise program and behaviour modification. Tolerance to the anorectic effect of this drug develops at varying times and, as it is subject to abuse, long-term usefulness is limited. Common adverse effects include headache, insomnia, irritability, palpitations and nervousness.

Drugs acting via 5-HT

Dexfenfluramine and fenfluramine are drugs that enhance 5-HT release and inhibit neuronal reuptake of 5-HT. This leads to an increase in 5-HT concentration in the hypothalamus and a subsequent decrease in food intake. Both drugs have minimal effect on sympathetic and dopaminergic neurotransmission. These agents were often used in combination with phentermine but were found to cause pulmonary hypertension and thickening of cardiac valves, requiring valve replacement in some women. Both drugs were withdrawn voluntarily from the market.

Fluoxetine, a selective serotonin reuptake inhibitor used to treat depression, produces a dose-related decrease in body weight, but the effect is not long term, lasting approximately 6 months in spite of continued use of the drug. Fluoxetine has not been approved for treating obesity.

Inhibition of nutrient absorption

Orlistat is synthesised from lipstatin, a natural product of *Streptomyces toxytricini*, and was approved for use in Australia in 2000 (Drug Monograph 42.1). Many clinical trials have demonstrated that use of orlistat results in a reduction in waist circumference and improvement in cardiovascular risk factors – for example, reduction in total and LDL-C, blood pressure and blood glucose concentration and insulin resistance. Weight loss generally occurs within 2 weeks of commencing drug therapy and is maintained with continued use. However, the value of orlistat in treating obese adolescents (12–16 years) is unclear, and further studies are required to determine its efficacy and safety for this purpose.

Orlistat (120 mg) is available as a Schedule 4 (Prescription Only) drug, while the 60 mg tablets are available through a pharmacy (Schedule 3, Pharmacist Only) in both Australia and New Zealand. Availability over the counter was based on the outcome of clinical trials that indicated reasonable efficacy for weight reduction and a low incidence of adverse effects. It also recognised the role of pharmacists in providing high-quality advice on managing obesity.

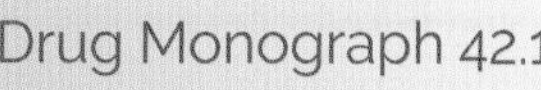

Drug Monograph 42.1
Orlistat

Mechanism of action

Orlistat is a reversible inhibitor of gastric and **pancreatic lipase**. It binds to the active site of the enzyme. Inhibition of the action of the lipases prevents the breakdown of dietary triglycerides (fat) and inhibits the absorption of cholesterol and lipid-soluble vitamins. Orlistat decreases the absorption of dietary fat by approximately 30% and promotes a modest reduction in body weight and plasma cholesterol.

Pharmacokinetics

Orlistat undergoes minimal systemic absorption and is essentially retained within the gastrointestinal tract. Plasma concentrations of the drug are either not detectable or exceedingly low (< 2 microgram/L). Metabolism occurs within the gastrointestinal wall, and five major metabolites have been identified. Less than 2% of orlistat is excreted in urine; most of the drug is eliminated in faeces ($> 96\%$), with unchanged drug accounting for 83% of the total dose excreted.

Drug interactions

Co-administration of orlistat and ciclosporin may result in reduced plasma concentration of ciclosporin.

Orlistat may reduce absorption of the fat-soluble vitamins (A, D, E) and vitamin K. People taking warfarin should be monitored for changes in coagulation parameters due to possible decrease in vitamin K absorption.

Additional contraceptive precautions are recommended when taking combined oral contraceptives and orlistat concurrently because of reports of breakthrough bleeding and contraceptive failure.

Adverse reactions

Common adverse reactions include headache and nausea, dyspepsia, fatty or oily stools, oily spotting, flatulence, liquid stools, abdominal pain and faecal incontinence and urgency.

Warnings and contraindications

Current drug information sources should be consulted regarding warnings and contraindications. Orlistat should be used with caution in people with active peptic ulcer disease or significant cardiac, gastrointestinal, renal, hepatic or endocrine disorders.

Use in people with cholestasis, chronic pancreatitis or pancreatic enzyme deficiency or chronic malabsorption syndrome is contraindicated.

Its safety in pregnant women has not been established and, generally, use of weight-loss drugs during pregnancy is inappropriate.

Dosage and administration

No advantage has been observed with doses greater than 120 mg three times daily with food. Orlistat should be taken either with each main meal which contains some fat or up to 1 hour after each meal.

Glucagon-like peptide-1 analogue

Incretins are gut hormones secreted from enteroendocrine cells into the blood in response to food. **Glucagon-like peptide-1** (GLP-1), an appetite suppressant, binds to GLP-1R receptors on pancreatic β-cells stimulating insulin secretion, decreasing food intake, inhibiting both gastric emptying and glucagon secretion and reducing the rate of production of endogenous glucose.

Liraglutide was approved by the Therapeutic Goods Administration in May 2016 for treating obesity (BMI > 30 kg/m^2) in people with at least one weight-related comorbidity. It is not subsidised by the Pharmaceutical Benefits Scheme and the cost is around $400 a month for a private prescription. It is an analogue of GLP-1 and mimics the action of GLP-1, hence exerting an insulinotropic effect. In addition to its role in managing obesity, liraglutide is used to treat type 2 diabetes (Ch 28). Similar to endogenous GLP-1, liraglutide is completely metabolised by dipeptidyl peptidase-IV, a neutral endopeptidase, but at a much slower rate, hence prolonging its duration of action.

Liraglutide is administered subcutaneously once daily, increasing at intervals of at least 1 week from an initial dose of 0.6 mg to a maximum of 3 mg daily. Its effect on weight is dose-dependent, and treatment is stopped after 12 weeks if weight loss is less than 5% of the person's initial weight. Adverse effects principally relate to the gastrointestinal tract – for example, diarrhoea, constipation, dyspepsia, nausea and/or vomiting. Long-term (> 1 year) safety data are lacking, but there are emerging concerns at the incidence of acute pancreatitis. Liraglutide is not recommended in pregnancy.

Naltrexone with bupropion

In 2014 the United States Food and Drug Administration (FDA) approved the combination of naltrexone with

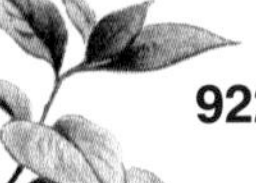

CLINICAL FOCUS BOX 42.2
Naltrexone with bupropion

- Used in adults with a BMI over 30 kg/m^2 and in adults with a BMI over 27 kg/m^2 and cardiovascular risk factors, and as an adjunct to lifestyle modifications.
- If weight loss is less than 5% of initial body weight, treatment is ceased after 16 weeks.
- Should not be administered to adults receiving chronic opiate therapy (due to the naltrexone component).
- Is subject to multiple drug interactions, and relevant drug information sources should be consulted.
- Blood pressure and pulse should be regularly monitored (may increase blood pressure).
- Long-term efficacy and safety has not been established.
- Due to its modified release formulation, tablets should be taken whole – not chewed, cut or crushed.

bupropion. Bupropion is an antidepressant but is mainly indicated as an aid for smoking cessation and nicotine dependence. Its mechanism of action is not fully understood but it is thought to be a non-selective inhibitor of transporters involved in the reuptake of dopamine and noradrenaline. It produces very modest weight loss. Naltrexone (Ch 19), an opioid receptor antagonist, is indicated for treating alcohol dependence and maintaining opioid abstinence and is generally devoid of weight-loss properties. Both drugs when used as monotherapy produced little in the way of weight loss. However, the combination produces an anorectic response thought to be mediated by pro-opiomelanocortin neurons in the brain that release a melanocyte-stimulating hormone that decreases hunger and induces satiety. The most common adverse effects include nausea, constipation, headache, vomiting, dizziness, insomnia, dry mouth and diarrhoea.

In clinical studies the combination is effective in sustaining weight loss and improving cardiometabolic parameters including a reduction in waist measurement and an improvement in lipid profiles. The combination drug was approved for use in Australia in 2019 and in New Zealand in 2020 (Clinical Focus Box 42.2).

KEY POINTS

Drugs for obesity

- Drugs for treating obesity are limited.
- Phentermine, orlistat, liraglutide and naltrexone with bupropion are indicated for treating overweight (BMI > 25 kg/m^2) or obesity (BMI > 30 kg/m^2) in people with at least one weight-related comorbidity – for example, cardiovascular risk factors.
- Phentermine is a centrally acting noradrenergic appetite suppressant subject to misuse and is indicated for short-term use.
- Tolerance to the anorectic effect of the noradrenergic drugs limits their usefulness.
- Orlistat is a lipase inhibitor that prevents the absorption of dietary fat. Weight loss is modest (2–3 kg over several years).
- Liraglutide is an analogue of GLP-1 and exerts an insulinotropic effect. It delays gastric emptying and decreases appetite. Treatment is stopped after 12 weeks if weight loss is less than 5% of the person's initial weight.
- Naltrexone with bupropion is an anorexiant with mixed opioid receptor antagonist and noradrenaline dopamine reuptake inhibitor properties. Treatment is ceased after 16 weeks if weight loss is less than 5% of the person's initial weight.

The future

Weight gain after discontinuing drug therapy is common. Maintaining a desirable and realistic weight on a long-term basis is a difficult, confidence-destroying task for many people. Currently, orlistat is the only drug available for the long-term treatment of obesity; however, a similar drug, cetilistat, which is thought to have fewer gastrointestinal adverse effects, was approved in 2008 for sale in Japanese pharmacies. Investigations of the effectiveness of the leptin analogue, metreleptin, the neuropeptide Y5 antagonist velneperit, the dual neuropeptide Y2/Y4 receptor agonist obinepitide, the amylin mimetic davalintide and the serotonin/dopamine/noradrenaline reuptake inhibitor tesofensine are ongoing.

Lorcaserin, a selective 5-HT$_{2C}$ agonist with 15–100-fold greater selectivity for 5-HT$_{2C}$ receptors than 5-HT$_{2A}$ and 5-HT$_{2B}$ was approved by the FDA in June 2012 for treating select populations of obese people. Data indicates that the weight loss with lorcaserin is not as great as that seen with other drugs under development. However, concerns have been raised regarding the possibility of increased malignancies in animal studies. The drug has not been approved for use in Europe, and studies are ongoing to evaluate its safety and efficacy. There is already evidence of central nervous system adverse effects including headache, dizziness, nausea, memory problems and attention difficulties.

In 2012, the FDA also approved a combination of phentermine and topiramate (an antiepileptic drug that is known to induce weight loss) for obese people (BMI ≥ 30 kg/m^2) with at least one weight-related comorbidity such as hypertension, type 2 diabetes or dyslipidaemia. Adverse cardiovascular effects have already been reported, as have the common central nervous system adverse effects of topiramate, which include depression and decreased attention, concentration and memory. In addition, because obesity is a problem for many young women, there are concerns regarding the teratogenic potential of topiramate. The European Medicines Agency has twice rejected marketing approval for the drug because of ongoing concerns over cardiovascular toxicity, teratogenicity and psychiatric and cognitive effects and the potential for misuse by recipients.

The search for safe and effective drugs continues, but it is unlikely that there will ever be a drug that produces weight loss if a person's increased food intake and reduced physical activity persist.

DRUGS AT A GLANCE
Anti-obesity drugs

PHARMACOLOGICAL GROUP AND EFFECT	KEY EXAMPLES	CLINICAL USE
Sympathomimetic anorexiants • Increase release of noradrenaline in hypothalamus • Increase sympathetic transmission • Decrease appetite • Increase energy expenditure	Phentermine	• Adjunct to lifestyle modifications in obese adults BMI > 30 kg/m^2 or in adults with BMI > 27 kg/m^2 with cardiovascular risk factors
Lipase inhibitors • Reversible inhibitor of gastric and pancreatic lipase • Decrease breakdown of dietary triglycerides • Inhibit absorption of cholesterol and lipid-soluble vitamins	Orlistat	• Adjunct to lifestyle modifications in obese adults BMI > 30kg/m^2 or in adults with BMI > 27kg/m^2 with cardiovascular risk factors
GLP-1 analogues • Bind GLP-1 receptors on pancreatic β-cells • Stimulate insulin secretion • Decrease food intake • Suppress glucagon secretion	Liraglutide	• Adjunct to lifestyle modifications in obese adults BMI > 30 kg/m^2 or in adults with BMI > 27 kg/m^2 with one or more weight-related comorbidity
Anorexiants (mixed action) • Act in the appetite regulatory centre in the hypothalamus • Combined opioid receptor antagonist with inhibitor of dopamine and noradrenaline transporters	Naltrexone with bupropion	• Adjunct to lifestyle modifications in obese adults BMI > 30 kg/m^2 or in adults with BMI > 27 kg/m^2 with cardiovascular risk factors

REVIEW EXERCISES

1 Ms BG, a 28-year-old office employee, was overweight throughout her childhood and is now obese (Class III, BMI 42.4 kg/m^2). She has sought your advice regarding any drug that would help her lose weight. On a previous visit her blood pressure was 139/85. She admits that she 'loves' food and 'hates' exercise and says she doesn't have time to do anything about her weight. Considering her lifestyle factors, discuss your approach to managing a weight reduction program for her. At this stage, which drug therapy would you consider?

2 Mr BD, a 31-year-old builder, has presented to the local GP practice complaining of intense dyspepsia, loose oily stools and persistent flatulence. You asked his height while weighing him and a quick calculation indicated he had a BMI of 43 kg/m^2. He told you that he was getting married in a month's time and his fiancée was keen for him to lose some weight before the wedding. When asking about his symptoms he volunteered that he had been taking six capsules daily for the past week of 'Alli' (orlistat 60 mg), which he had bought from his local pharmacy because he wanted to lose weight quickly. Discuss the pharmacological relationship between his symptoms and the dose of orlistat he has been taking daily.

REFERENCES

Australian Institute of Health and Welfare 2020. Australia's Health 2020: Overweight and obesity. Online. Available: https://www.aihw.gov.au/reports/australias-health/overweight-and-obesity (accessed 22 March 2021).

Gerken T, Girard CA, Tung YC, et al. The obesity-associated FTO gene encodes a 2-oxoglutarate-dependent nucleic acid demethylase. Science 2007;318:1469-72.

Heymsfield SB, Wadden TA. Mechanisms, pathophysiology, and management of obesity. The New England Journal of Medicine 2017;376:254-66.

Hill JO, Wyatt HR, Peters JC. Energy balance and obesity. Circulation 2012;126:126-32. https://www.health.govt.nz/publication/annual-update-key-results-2019-20-new-zealand-health-survey (accessed 22 March 2021).

National Health and Medical Research Council 2013: Clinical practice guidelines for the management of overweight and obesity in adults, adolescents and children in Australia. Online. Available: https://www.nhmrc.gov.au/about-us/publications/clinical-practice-guidelines-management-overweight-and-obesity (accessed 22 March 2021).

New Zealand Ministry of Health 2020. Annual update of key results 2019/20: New Zealand Health Survey. Online. Available:

New Zealand Ministry of Health 2017. Clinical Guidelines for Weight Management in New Zealand Adults. Wellington: Ministry of Health. Online. Available: https://www.health.govt.nz/system/files/documents/publications/clinical-guidelines-for-weight-management-in-new-zealand-adultsv2.pdf (accessed 22 March 2021).

Page AJ, Symonds E, Peiris M, et al. Peripheral neural targets in obesity. British Journal of Pharmacology 2012;166:1537-58.

Steppan CM, Bailey ST, Bhat S, et al. The hormone resistin links obesity to diabetes, Nature 2001;409:307-12.

van der Klaauw AA, Farooqi S. The hunger genes: pathways to obesity, Cell 2015;161:119-32.

ONLINE RESOURCES

Australian Chronic Disease Prevention Alliance (ACDPA) – The National Obesity Strategy 2022–2032: https://www.health.gov.au/resources/publications/national-obesity-strategy-2022-2032 (accessed 14 March 2022)

Ministry of Health Manat≈´ Hauora – Obesity: https://www.health.govt.nz/our-work/diseases-and-conditions/obesity (accessed 14 March 2022)

More weblinks at: http://evolve.elsevier.com/AU/Knights/pharmacology/.

CHAPTER 43

VACCINATIONS

Mary Bushell

KEY ABBREVIATIONS

DNA	deoxyribonucleic acid
DTPa	diphtheria-tetanus acellular pertussis vaccine (paediatric formulation)
dTpa	diphtheria-tetanus vaccine acellular pertussis vaccine (reduced antigen formulation)
Hib	*Haemophilus influenzae* type b
HPV	human papillomavirus
Ig	immunoglobulin
IM	intramuscular
IPV	inactivated poliovirus
mRNA	messenger ribonucleic acid
RNA	ribonucleic acid
SARS-CoV-2	severe acute respiratory syndrome coronavirus 2
SC	subcutaneous
VLP	virus-like particle

KEY TERMS

adjuvant 933
adsorbed vaccine 933
antibody 927
antigen 927
cell-mediated immunity 927
conjugate polysaccharide vaccine 935
humoral immunity 927
live attenuated vaccine 932
primary series 935
pure polysaccharide vaccine 935
recombinant vaccine 935
toxoid 935

Chapter Focus

A vaccine is a biological preparation that contains antigens (or ANTIbody GENerating substances) that are derived from a disease-causing microorganism. When introduced into the body a vaccine confers acquired immunity to a specific disease.

Vaccines are considered one of the greatest achievements in modern medicine. Globally, it is estimated that each year they prevent more than 3 million deaths. All health professionals play a vital role in vaccine advocacy and education. Appropriately trained and qualified health professionals, such as nurses, pharmacists and medical doctors, may administer vaccines.

This chapter provides an overview of the immune system, passive and active immunisation, vaccine immunology and clinical considerations. It outlines the different types of vaccines and how they work to elicit an immune response. Understanding how the different types of vaccines work enables health professionals to appreciate the rationale behind vaccine schedules (e.g. number of primary and booster doses), contraindications and common adverse effects following immunisation.

KEY DRUG GROUPS

Whole pathogen:

- Live attenuated vaccines

Measles, mumps, rubella

- Inactivated or killed vaccines
- Whole cell

Pertussis

- Split virion

Influenza

Subunit vaccines (pieces of pathogen):

- Recombinant vaccines
- Protein

Hepatitis B

- Virus-like particles

Human papillomavirus vaccine

- Polysaccharide vaccines
- Pure polysaccharide
- Conjugate vaccines

Meningococcal vaccines

- Toxoid vaccines

Diphtheria, tetanus vaccines

- Nucleic acid vaccines
- mRNA vaccines

COVID-19 vaccine

- Viral vector vaccines

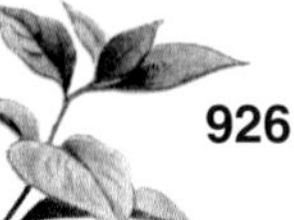

CRITICAL THINKING SCENARIO

Paola recently gave birth to her first child, Isaiah. Before being discharged from the maternity ward, Isaiah was administered the hepatitis B vaccine. Today, 2 months on, Paola is attending an appointment with her son at the community health centre, where the community nurse will administer the recommended vaccines. Isaiah is given two injections and one vaccine orally. One injection contained antigens to protect against six infections (diphtheria, tetanus, pertussis, hepatitis B, polio and *Haemophilus influenzae* type b). The other injection protected against pneumococcal, while the oral vaccine provided protection against rotavirus. The injections were administered into the mid anterolateral thigh (vastus lateralis muscle).

1. How do the vaccines work to protect Isaiah from the natural infections? How long before Isaiah develops antibodies to the antigens present in the vaccines?
2. Describe and explain the different types of vaccines Isaiah had administered.
3. To improve immunogenicity, which vaccines contained adjuvants? What is meant by a conjugated vaccine? Which vaccine administered is conjugated?
4. Describe which vaccines are part of a primary series and what vaccines will require booster doses to maintain protection.
5. Discuss some of the common side effects of vaccines. Why might they occur?

Introduction

A vaccine is a biological preparation that confers acquired immunity to an infectious disease when introduced into the body. The first vaccine, Dr Edward Jenner's smallpox vaccine, was introduced in 1796. Today, 29 infectious diseases can be prevented through vaccination, including cholera, COVID-19, dengue fever, diphtheria, Ebola virus, *Haemophilus influenzae* type b (Hib), hepatitis A, B and E, herpes zoster (shingles), human papillomavirus (HPV) infection, influenza, Japanese encephalitis, malaria, measles, meningococcal disease, mumps, pneumococcal disease, pertussis, poliomyelitis, Q fever, rabies, rotavirus, rubella (German measles), varicella (chickenpox) and yellow fever.

Calculating the exact number of deaths that vaccines have prevented is impossible. However, the World Health Organization estimates that, each year, vaccination prevents 3 million deaths globally. Because of vaccination, smallpox, a highly infectious disease that killed one-third of those infected and left those who survived with permanent scarring, was declared globally eradicated in 1980. Today, once common childhood diseases such as measles and poliomyelitis are controlled in most parts of the world, and the global COVID-19 pandemic that was responsible for the death of more than 5 million people is coming to an end.

Most vaccines are administered intramuscularly (IM) via an injection; however, they can also be administered subcutaneously (SC), intradermally, intranasally and orally. There is a range of vaccine types, and broadly they can be divided into whole cell and subunit vaccines. Whole cell vaccines contain the whole pathogen (bacteria or virus) and include live attenuated and whole cell killed or inactivated vaccines. Subunit vaccines contain only a piece or multiple pieces of the pathogen and include toxoid, pure polysaccharide, conjugated polysaccharide, recombinant protein, virus-like particle, nucleic acid and viral vector vaccines. The different types of vaccines work differently to elicit an immune response in the vaccinated person. When an immune response is stimulated and sufficient antibodies and memory have been produced, it is said that the person is immunised.

Immune system

Our bodies are exposed to millions of potential pathogens (disease-causing microorganisms such as bacteria, viruses and fungi) each day. When a pathogen is introduced into the body, the immune system responds.

Broadly the immune system is classified into two subtypes:

- innate immune system (or natural, non-specific)
- adaptive immune system (or acquired, specific).

The immune system is also divided into first-, second- and third-line defences. The first and second line of defence are part of the innate immune system, while the third line of defence is part of the adaptive immune system.

Innate immunity

Innate immunity comprises the body's first two lines of defence. It is rapid, non-specific and has no memory. The body's first lines of defence are barriers or broad external defences that prevent pathogens from gaining entry. It includes physical barriers (e.g. skin and mucous membranes, hairs, cilia and tears), chemical barriers (e.g. acidic pH, enzymes) and reflexes (e.g. airway defences such as the sneeze and cough). If the pathogen breaks through the first line of defence it encounters the second line of defence. The second line of defence includes physiological (fever, inflammation), protein (interferon, complement, acute-phase protein) and cellular defences (e.g. granulocytes [neutrophils, basophils, eosinophils, mast cells], natural killer cells, macrophages). The second line works quickly to prevent the spread of pathogens in the body and fight infection.

The innate response may eradicate the pathogens independently or it may call in the adaptive immune response for assistance using antigen-presenting cells (macrophages and dendritic cells). Together, both arms of the immune system will now work to remove pathogens from the body and restore health.

Adaptive immunity

Adaptive immunity, also known as acquired immunity, is specific to a particular pathogen. Pathogens have unique **antigens** (proteins, peptides or polysaccharides) usually on their surface. Simply put, an antigen is any substance that causes the immune system to GENerate ANTIbodies (also known as immunoglobulins) against it.

There are two main types of adaptive immunity: humoral and cellular immunity.

Humoral immunity

As the name suggests, **humoral immunity**, also known as antibody-mediated immunity, deals with antigens that are circulating freely in the humors (or body fluid – blood, plasma, lymph).

On first exposure to an antigen, the antigen-presenting cells (macrophages, dendritic cells) of the innate immune system will engulf, break down and process the antigen and 'present' a component of it on a structure on the surface of the antigen-presenting cells known as the major histocompatibility complex II (MHC-II).

Presenting the antigen on the MHC-II complex is like the cell flying a flag saying, 'I'm infected with antigen! Help!'. Enter the T-helper cell. On the surface of T-helper cells is a T-cell receptor. T-cell receptors can recognise and bind to a corresponding antigen presented on the MHC-II. If the T-cell has never seen the pathogen before, it is called a naïve T-helper cell. When the processed antigen on the MHC-II binds with a corresponding T-cell receptor, the T-helper cell is activated and becomes an effector cell. T-helper cells are characterised by a CD4 marker or co-receptor on their surface; for this reason you may see them referred to as CD4 cells, $CD4^+$ T-cells or T4 cells. T-helper cells make up approximately 13% of circulating white blood cells.

T-helper cells coordinate both the humoral and the cellular immune response (Fig 43.1). Specifically, on first exposure to an antigen, in humoral immunity T-helper cells stimulate and enable naïve B-cells to differentiate into plasma B-cells (the effector cell). Plasma B-cells are antibody factories, and once activated they produce antigen-specific antibodies. Antibodies are Y-shaped proteins that bind to antigens and neutralise, agglutinate (clump together) and trigger their destruction (by lysin or phagocytosis). Antibodies are antigen-specific, much like a lock and key. For each antigen (key), there is only one type of **antibody** (lock) – they are highly specific. The location of the antigen that binds to the antibody is known as the epitope or antigenic determinant.

The humoral immune response cannot destroy antigen that has already entered and infected host cells (i.e. the antigen is no longer in the humors).

Cell-mediated immunity

Cell-mediated immunity does not involve antibodies; instead, it activates the production of antigen-specific T-cytotoxic cells and enables the destruction of infected host cells. On first exposure to an antigen, the activated T-helper cells release cytokines (signalling molecules) that lead to naïve T-cells binding to the infected cell's MHC antigen complex, enabling the T-cell to differentiate into either T-cytotoxic or T-helper cells.

As the name suggests, T-cytotoxic cells kill infected cells; they do this via a process known as lysis (disintegration or rupture of the cell). The T-helper cells generated will secrete more cytokines that attract neutrophils and macrophages, which further assist in destroying the pathogen. Both memory T-helper and memory T-cytotoxic cells are generated after exposure to an antigen (Fig 43.1). These antigen-specific memory cells locate themselves in lymph nodes and spleen. On subsequent exposure, these cells proliferate rapidly,

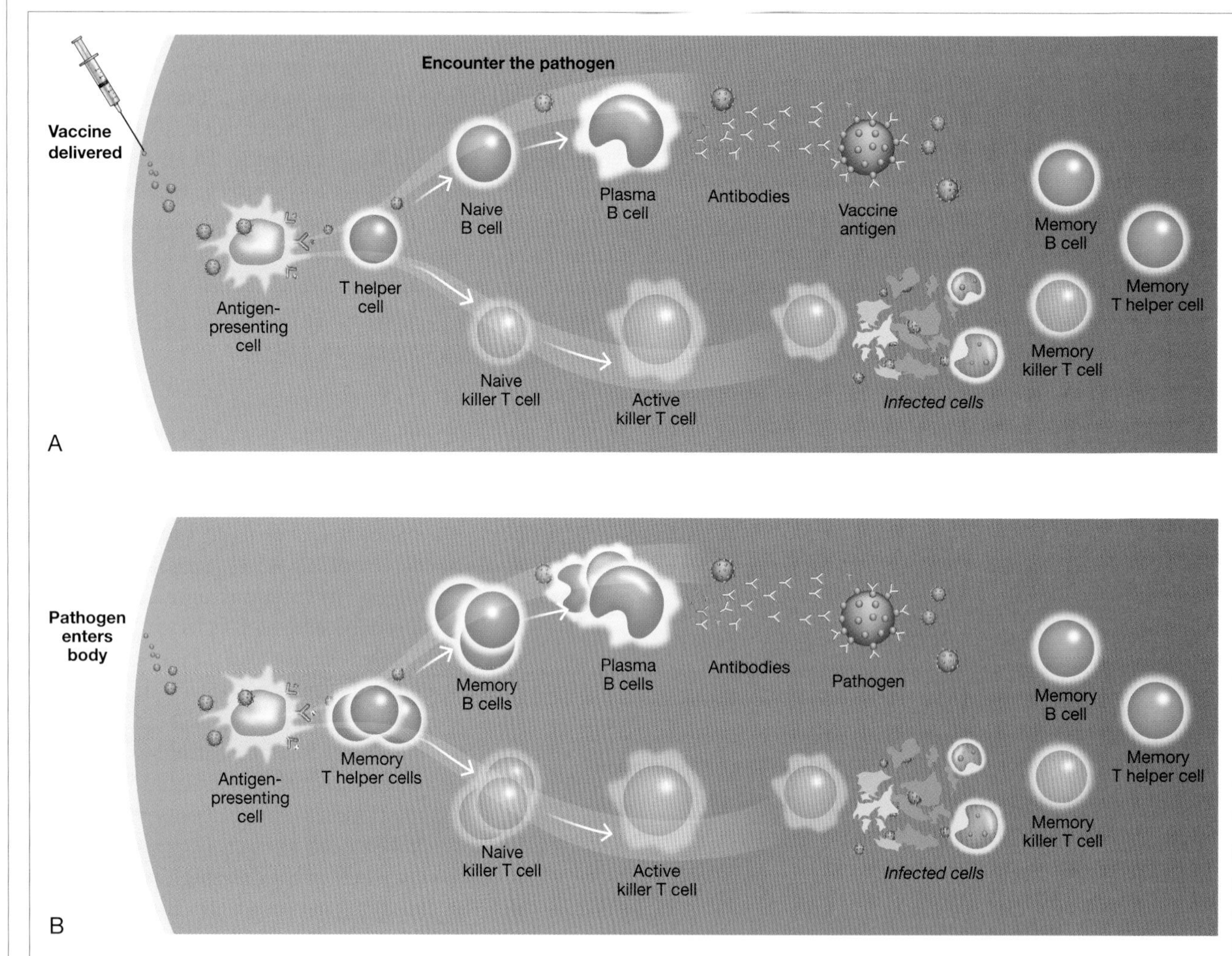

FIGURE 43.1 **A** Immune response following first exposure to an antigen; **B** Immune response following subsequent exposure to an antigen

enabling a more immediate and robust immune response to the antigen.

Primary immune response and immunological memory

When the body is exposed to an antigen (i.e. pathogen) for the first time, the primary immune response, or primary immunisation, occurs. This response is slow and limited (Fig 43.2). Depending on the type of pathogen, the primary infection can take up to 14 days to resolve, after which immunological memory has developed. On subsequent exposure to the same antigen, the existence of antigen-specific lymphocytes (T and B memory cells) created during the primary immune response enables the immune system to respond rapidly and effectively. The hallmark of the adaptive immune response is the clonal expansion of antigen-specific lymphocytes (Adams et al. 2020). Clonal expansion is the rapid proliferation of T- and B-cells from a few clonal cells to millions in a short time. Each T- and B-cell clone is specific for the same antigen as the original clone (parent cell). Memory cells are also specific for a particular antigen and are long-lasting. Memory cells are what sustain the adaptive immune response long term, and they form the biological basis of vaccination.

Secondary immune response

On successive exposure to a pathogen the immune pathways are pre-existing (there is immunological memory). Reactivation of the immune pathway is immediate, and specific antibodies (predominantly immunoglobulins [Ig] G and M) are rapidly produced, neutralising the antigen, often with the absence of symptoms.

Active vs artificially acquired immunity

Active immunity occurs when the person develops antibodies and memory to a specific disease. This is

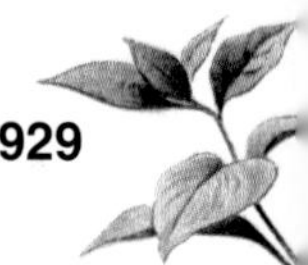

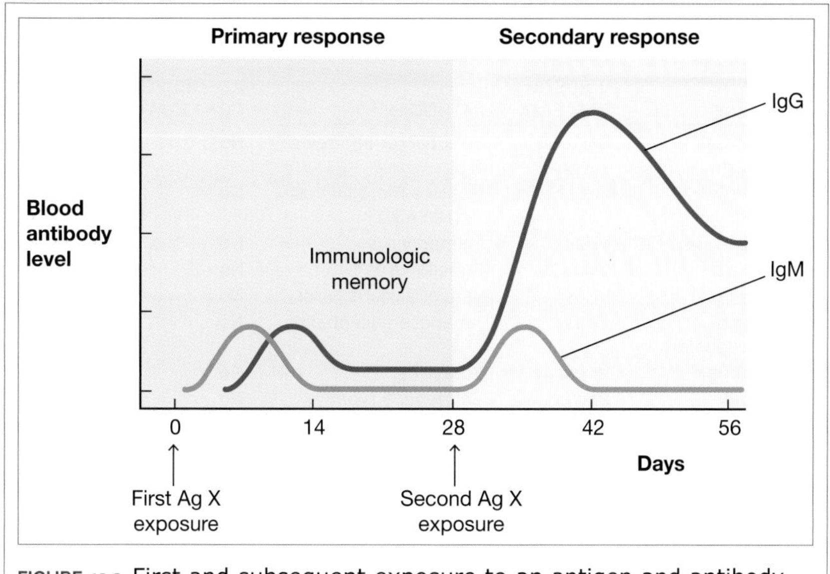

FIGURE 43.2 First and subsequent exposure to an antigen and antibody concentration

different from passive immunity, which is when the antibodies themselves (natural or synthetic) are administered. Passive immunity provides short-term protection, and immunological memory is not developed – for example, the transfer of maternal antibodies in breastmilk to the feeding baby, or the parental administration of monoclonal antibodies (e.g. sotrovimab) to treat and prevent COVID-19.

Active immunity can be naturally acquired (caused by the disease itself) or artificially acquired through vaccination. The principle behind vaccination is to intentionally introduce an antigen, derived from or synthetically designed to mimic an antigenic component of a disease-causing microorganism. The antigenic component should stimulate the adaptive immune system and immunological memory, but not cause disease. New vaccine technologies (e.g. mRNA; see section below) introduce genetic material that codes for an antigen, so the host essentially makes the vaccine (the antigen) in situ. The artificially acquired immunity is the body's first exposure to the pathogen, so on subsequent exposure the body already has memory. Memory cells are not generated immediately after the administration of a vaccine. That is why patients should receive vaccines in advance of, and no less than 10 days before, travelling to areas where vaccine-preventable diseases are endemic – for example, yellow fever, cholera and tuberculosis. Antigen-specific memory cells are usually at their highest approximately 1 month after vaccination. How long artificial immunity lasts depends on the vaccine type, the type of immune response stimulated (humoral and/or cell mediated) and host factors.

KEY POINTS

The immune system

- The immune system can be divided into two subsystems: the innate (non-specific) and the adaptive system (specific). Both systems continually interact with each other to elicit an immune response.
- There are two main types of adaptive immunity: humoral (B-cells) and cell-mediated immunity (T-cells). Humoral immunity is antibody-mediated. Cell-mediated immunity does not involve antibodies; instead, it activates cytotoxic T-cells to kill infected cells.
- An important outcome of the adaptive immune response is the development of immunological memory. Whether via natural or artificial infection (vaccination), people exposed to an antigen acquire long-term protection from the disease. This state of protection is due to immunological memory.

Types of vaccines

Not all vaccines use the same technology to stimulate an immune response, hence there are different types of vaccines. Conventional vaccine types include live attenuated vaccines, inactivated (killed whole antigen) and subunit (purified antigen) vaccines (Table 43.1). Over recent decades, a better understanding of the genomes of pathogens, coupled with enhanced laboratory and computer technologies, has led to new types of vaccines. New vaccine types include nucleic acid vaccines

TABLE 43.1 Types of vaccines

	VACCINE TYPE	VACCINE	VIRUS/ BACTERIA	PATHOGEN	ADSORBED OR CONJUGATED	PRIMARY SERIES BOOSTER	ROUTE
Whole cell	Live attenuated	Bacille Calmette-Guérin	Bacteria	*Mycobacterium bovis*	No	No	Intracutaneously or ID
		Measles	Virus	Measles morbillivirus (DM 43.1)	No	Booster	SC or IM
		Mumps	Virus	Mumps virus	No	Booster	SC or IM
		Rubella	Virus	Rubella virus	No	Booster	SC or IM
		Varicella	Virus	Varicella zoster virus	No	Booster	SC or IM
		Japanese encephalitis	Virus	Japanese encephalitis	No	No	Imojev SC
		Rotavirus	Virus	Rotavirus	No	No	Oral
		Typhoid	Bacteria	*Salmonella typhi*	No	No	Vivotif Oral
		Yellow fever	Virus	Yellow fever virus	No	No	SC or IM
		Zoster	Virus	Herpes virus	No	No	
Whole cell	Inactivated (inactivated bacteria are also called killed antigen vaccines – viruses that were never alive to begin with)	Cholera	Bacteria	*Vibrio cholerae*	No	Primary series + booster	Oral
		Hepatitis A	Virus	Hepatitis A virus	Adsorbed	Primary series + booster	IM
		Q fever (killed)	Bacteria	*Coxiella burnetii*	No	Single dose (do not revaccinate)	SC
		Influenza	Virus	Influenza A or B	Adsorbed	Annual	IM
		Japanese encephalitis (IM)	Virus	Japanese encephalitis	Adsorbed	Primary series + booster	JEspect IM
		Poliomyelitis (IPV)	Virus	Poliovirus	No	Primary series + booster	SC
		Rabies	Virus	*Rabies lyssavirus*	No	Primary series + booster	IM
Subunit	Toxoid (inactivated toxin)	Diphtheria	Bacteria	*Corynebacterium diphtheriae* secretes diphtheria toxin	Adsorbed	Primary series + booster	IM
		Tetanus	Bacteria	*Clostridium tetani* secretes tetanospasmin, a neurotoxin	Adsorbed	Primary series + booster	IM
Subunit	Recombinant subunit	COVID-19	Virus	Severe acute respiratory syndrome coronavirus 2	Adsorbed	Primary series + booster Primary series + booster	IM
		Pertussis (acellular) (Drug Monograph 43.2)	Bacteria	*Bordetella pertussis*	Combination only dTPa (Clinical Focus Box 43.1)	Primary series	IM
		Hepatitis B (recombinant DNA hepatitis b surface antigen)	Virus	Hepatitis B virus	Adsorbed	Primary series	IM
		Meningococcal B (recombinant)	Bacteria	*Neisseria meningitidis*	Adsorbed not conjugated	Primary series	IM
Subunit	Virus-like particles (VLPs)	HPV (recombinant HPV capsid [L1] protein)	Virus	HPV Malaria	Adsorbed	Primary series	IM
Subunit	Conjugate/ polysaccharide	Hib	Bacteria	Hib	Conjugated	Primary series	IM IM
		Meningococcal C	Bacteria	*Neisseria meningitidis*	Conjugated		IM
		Meningococcal ACWY	Bacteria	*Neisseria meningitidis*	Conjugated		IM
		Pneumococcal 13vPCV	Bacteria	*Streptococcus pneumoniae*	Conjugated		IM
		Pneumococcal 23vPPV (not conjugated)	Bacteria	*Streptococcus pneumoniae*	Not conjugated		IM or SC
		Typhoid	Bacteria	*Salmonella typhi*	Conjugated		Typhim Vi IM
Nucleic acid	Messenger ribonucleic acid (mRNA)	COVID-19	Virus	Severe acute respiratory syndrome coronavirus 2	No	Primary series + booster	IM
Vector	Viral vector	COVID-19	Virus	Severe acute respiratory syndrome coronavirus 2	No	Primary series + booster	IM

Drug Monograph 43.1
Measles vaccine

Measles is a live attenuated vaccine. Measles is not available as a single-antigen vaccine. It is only available in combination with mumps and rubella virus (MMR) or measles, mumps and varicella virus (MMRV).

Indications

Children should be vaccinated against measles according to the National Immunisation Program Schedule and should receive a two-dose primary series (12, 18 months). Due to gaps in past immunisation policies, there is a group of adults who are at risk of measles. In Australia, the second dose of the measles vaccine was not routinely given until the 1990s. People born between 1966 and 1994 may not be fully protected against measles. Those born before 1966 were likely to have been infected with the measles virus itself and are low risk.

Pharmacokinetics immunogenicity

Antibodies for the measles virus appear several days following vaccination, with the greatest protection after 2 or 3 weeks. One dose of measles-containing vaccine provides long-term immunity in approximately 95% of people. After a second vaccine dose, about 99% of people have seroconverted and are protected against measles. The minimum interval between the first and second dose of a measles-containing vaccine is 4 weeks (28 days). After two doses the person should have lifelong immunity.

Drug interactions

- Because it is a live attenuated vaccine, it should be given 1 month before or after administration of other vaccines.
- People who have received or are receiving immunoglobulin or a blood product should wait 3–11 months before vaccine administration.
- People who are taking high doses of corticosteroid should wait $>$ 1 month before vaccine administration.

Adverse reaction

Local reactions are common (17–30%) – for example, pain and tenderness at the injection site (usually resolves within 3 days). Systemic reactions may also occur (5–15% of vaccine recipients), usually between days 7 and 12, and last 1 or 2 days. A generalised rash that lasts for about 2 days occurs in 2–5% of people.

Warnings and contraindications

History of anaphylaxis following a previous dose of measles-mumps-rubella vaccine or to any vaccine component. It should not be given to pregnant or immunocompromised people. It should not be given to someone who is febrile, or who has active untreated tuberculosis. Precaution should be taken in people with a history of low blood platelet count.

Dosage and administration

The measles vaccine should be administered via IM or SC injection. See specific vaccine product information.

Drug Monograph 43.2
Pertussis vaccine

The pertussis vaccine is an acellular vaccine. It contains various pertussis antigens (subunits) including pertussis filamentous haemagglutinin (adherence protein), pertussis fimbriae 2 + 3 and pertussis toxoid. It is not available as a single antigen vaccine. It comes in combination with diphtheria and tetanus toxoids, with or without other antigens such as hepatitis B, inactivated poliomyelitis and Hib.

Indications

To reduce the risk of being infected with pertussis, a highly contagious respiratory infection caused by the bacterium *Bordetella pertussis*, in both children and adults.

Children should be vaccinated against pertussis according to the National Immunisation Program Schedule and receive a three-dose primary series (at 2, 4 and 6 months). This is followed by two booster doses (at 18 months and 4 years), which contain the same amount of antigen as the primary series. Adolescents are administered one reduced antigen pertussis-containing vaccine; however, the age of administration differs between jurisdictions. Women who are pregnant should be vaccinated when they are between 20- and 32-weeks' gestation. Vaccination with dTpa (Clinical Focus Box 43.1) is recommended for any adult who wishes to reduce the risk of being infected with pertussis, particularly people (family, carers) who are around newborn babies.

Pharmacokinetics immunogenicity

The three-dose vaccine DTPa primary series at (2, 4 and 6 months of age) results in 84% protective efficacy against severe pertussis. Natural infection with pertussis or a primary series of pertussis vaccination does not confer lifelong protection against reinfection. Protective immunity after pertussis vaccination wanes after 4–6 years, while naturally acquired immunity wanes after 4–20 years. Booster doses of pertussis are needed to increase antibodies and combat waning pertussis immunity.

Drug interactions

Immunosuppressant medicines such as corticosteroids, chemotherapy alkylating agents, antimetabolites and radiation may reduce the effectiveness of the vaccine. The pertussis vaccine can be given at the same time as other vaccines.

Adverse reaction

Local reactions are common and include pain and tenderness at the injection site. Irritability and drowsiness are also common.

Warnings and contraindications

History of anaphylaxis following a previous dose of a pertussis-containing vaccine or to any vaccine component.

Dosage and administration

The dose of all pertussis-containing vaccines is 0.5 mL administered by IM injection.

CLINICAL FOCUS BOX 43.1

Diphtheria, tetanus and pertussis vaccine terminology

To ensure patient safety, it is important that health professionals understand and use the correct capitalisation and terminology when referring to diphtheria, tetanus and pertussis vaccines. The initialism DTPa (using capital letters) signifies a paediatric formulation of diphtheria, tetanus and acellular pertussis (D = diphtheria, T = tetanus, P = pertussis and 'a' is lower case for acellular). Paediatric formulations contain between three and five times more diphtheria toxoid than adult (booster) formulations.

The initialism 'dTpa' (i.e. using lower case letters) refers to an adult or booster formulation. This formulation contains substantially less diphtheria toxoid and pertussis antigens than the paediatric (DTPa-containing) formulations. The amount of tetanus toxoid in both the paediatric and the adult formulations is the same, so 'T' remains capitalised in both abbreviations.

(e.g. mRNA) and viral vector vaccines. The COVID-19 global pandemic, and the urgent need for the widespread use of an effective vaccine, resulted in the novel vaccine types used extensively in humans for the first time (Iwasaki & Omer 2020).

Types of vaccine include:

- whole cell
- live attenuated vaccines
  - viral
  - bacterial
- inactivated vaccines
  - split
- viral vector vaccines
- subunit (fractional) vaccines
  - protein-based
  - recombinant protein
    - DNA recombinant
    - virus-like particles (VLPs)
  - toxoid
  - polysaccharide (sugars)
    - pure
    - conjugate
  - nucleic acid vaccines (genetically engineered)
    - mRNA
    - DNA.

Whole-cell vaccines

Live attenuated vaccines

Live attenuated vaccines contain a weakened or altered version of the whole pathogen (virus or bacteria). Weakening, but not killing, the pathogen means that while it can replicate, it has lost significant pathogenicity, and cannot cause serious disease in people with a healthy immune system. Live attenuated vaccines that can replicate in the human host provide continuous antigenic stimulation and confer longer and stronger immunity than most other types of vaccines. They activate both humoral (B-cells) and cellular immunity (T-cells). Examples of live attenuated vaccines include bacille Calmette-Guérin (tuberculosis), measles, mumps, rubella, varicella (chickenpox), poliomyelitis, yellow fever, rotavirus, rabies, herpes zoster (shingles), Japanese encephalitis and influenza (intranasal formulation only). The first vaccine that provided protection against smallpox was also a live vaccine. Smallpox is now globally eradicated because of a successful immunisation campaign; it is no longer manufactured. It remains the only infectious disease to be eradicated in humans.

Several methods can be used to attenuate pathogens to be used as vaccines. One method is to pass the original 'wild' live virus through foreign host cells (e.g. cell or tissue culture, embryonated chicken eggs or live animals) many, many times in a process known as serial passage. As the virus is passed through the foreign host, it develops mutations. The virus may be passed through more than 200 chick embryo cell or tissue cultures in the attenuation process. The mutations result in the virus being significantly different from the original virus. The result is a live attenuated virus that, while not pathogenic like the original wild virus, can still trigger an immune response and generate disease-specific antibodies in the human host. Live attenuated vaccines do not generally contain an adjuvant (Table 43.1). This is in comparison with most subunit vaccines that usually contain an adjuvant to improve the immune response.

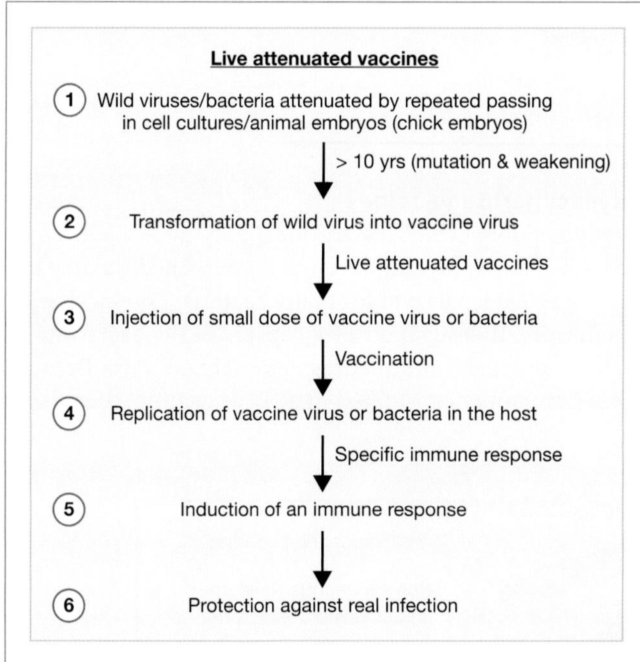

Dinesh K Yadav, Satyendra Mohan Paul Khurana, in Animal Biotechnology, 2014 Request use of this image

Live attenuated vaccines are generally contraindicated in pregnant women due to a theoretical risk of harm to the fetus. Women should avoid conceiving for 28 days after having a live attenuated vaccine. Live vaccines are also contraindicated in immunocompromised people. That is, all people with congenital (e.g. congenital agammaglobulinaemia, congenital IgA deficiency), acquired (e.g. HIV/AIDS) and pharmacological (e.g. chemotherapy, radiotherapy, immunosuppressive therapy) immune-deficient states should not be given live attenuated vaccines. In such people, an attenuated vaccine pathogen may replicate too much, causing disease – the risks outweigh the benefits of the vaccine. Immunocompromised people rely on herd immunity to protect them from vaccine-preventable diseases.

Inactivated whole-cell vaccines

Inactivated vaccines are made from whole pathogens (e.g. virus, bacteria) that have been killed by chemicals, such as formalin, formaldehyde and β-Propiolactone, or inactivated through heat or radiation. The inactivated pathogens are then used to make vaccines. Many will contain an **adjuvant** (immune enhancer), a substance that helps elicit a more robust immune response (Table 43.1). When a vaccine contains an adjuvant, we say it is **adsorbed**. Because the pathogens used to make the vaccine are inactivated or dead, they cannot replicate, and they cannot cause disease. However, this also means that they cannot mount a strong, lasting immune response, and booster (multiple) doses are required. Examples of inactivated whole-cell killed vaccines include the inactivated poliovirus (IPV) vaccine, the inactivated influenza vaccine, adsorbed inactivated Japanese encephalitis virus and the inactivated whole-cell oral cholera vaccine.

They are safe in pregnant women and in immunocompromised people. However, an immunocompromised person may require additional doses of inactivated vaccine to mount an immune response comparable to that seen in a healthy person.

Split virus vaccines

Split virion vaccines are composed of whole-cell inactivated viruses (e.g. influenza vaccine) that have been 'split' with an ether and/or detergent.

Viral vector vaccines

Viral vector vaccines use the vaccinated person's own body cells to produce the antigen, which confers immunity. So how does this happen? The name of the vaccine tells us that this technology employs the use of 'viral vectors'. When most people think of a 'vector' they think of an animal such as a mosquito or tick that transmits a disease from one animal to another – for example, mosquitoes are vectors for malaria. Essentially, the vector is a 'host' or a 'delivery system' that enables the transmission of disease. We can extrapolate this logic to 'viral vector vaccines'. In this case, the vector (or the host that carries and enables the transfer of disease) is a live, harmless, modified virus. Its cargo is a piece of genetic material from another virus, the one that protection is sought from, that codes for an antigen.

It has long been known that viruses are non-living, and they must be taken into a host cell to replicate. Viral vector vaccines exploit this process, so both the vector and the genetic material (usually DNA) it is carrying are taken into the human cells. Because the viral vector is genetically modified, it cannot cause disease. Consistent with how viruses obtain entry to a human cell, the viral vector attaches to the host cell and injects the genetic material. The human cell then transcribes the DNA into mRNA, which generates the protein antigen. The antigens are then presented on the infected host cell's surface, eliciting a robust immune response that generates both humoral and cell-mediated immunity. Viral vectors can be categorised into replicating and non-replicating viral vectors.

The Ebola vaccine and the Oxford AstraZeneca COVID-19 vaccine (Vaxzevria) are viral vector vaccines. The viral vector used in Vaxzevria is an adenovirus, a chimpanzee common cold pathogen, ChAdOx1. The genetic material or DNA it carried inside the vector codes for the severe acute respiratory syndrome coronavirus 2 (SARS-CoV-2) protein spike, a key antigen of the COVID-19 virus. Because there is only a piece of the SARS-CoV-2 genetic material (only the code for the protein spike), it cannot assemble the entire SARS-CoV-2 virus, and therefore cannot cause COVID-19. Viral vector vaccines are safe in immunocompromised people and pregnant women.

One limitation of viral vector vaccines is that people may have already have pre-existing immunity to the vector. When this happens, the body will mount an immune response against the viral vector, clearing it from the body, before it has played its role and delivered the genetic material to the host cell that codes for an antigen. For this reason, the Oxford AstraZeneca COVID-19 vaccine used a chimpanzee common cold virus that was not a common infection in humans as the viral vector, improving the vaccine's efficacy.

Subunit vaccines

Subunit vaccines (sometimes called acellular vaccines) contain only the antigenic components/pieces of the pathogen (e.g. a surface antigen). Specifically, they contain the parts of the pathogen required to elicit an immune response. Because they are only 'parts' of the pathogen, they are not 'live'. Imagine if you chopped off part of a human such as the arm; the arm would not be 'live' so could not replicate on its own. So it is with subunit vaccines. All subunit vaccines are, by their nature, inactivated. When compared with live or nucleic acid vaccines, most subunit vaccines do not elicit strong immune responses. They generally require repeated doses initially (priming series) and boosters to maintain immunity. Adjuvants are often used in subunit vaccines (Table 43.1). Adjuvants are non-antigen vaccine components that are pro-inflammatory and increase the activity of antigen-presenting cells, which activate further innate (e.g. natural killer cells) and adaptive immune responses (B-cells and T-cells). Aluminium salts and toll-like receptor agonists are currently used in vaccines as adjuvants. A downside is that vaccines that contain adjuvants are associated with increased local reactions such as a sore arm.

There are several types of subunit vaccines:

- pure polysaccharide
- conjugate polysaccharide
- toxoid
- recombinant
- virus-like particles.

Polysaccharide vaccines

Capsular polysaccharides are long polymers made up of repeating units of simple sugars that encapsulate and provide an external layer for many bacteria. Polysaccharide vaccines use this sugar surface capsule of the bacterium to elicit a targeted immune response (Fig 43.3). Because viruses are not encapsulated in a sugar coating, there is no

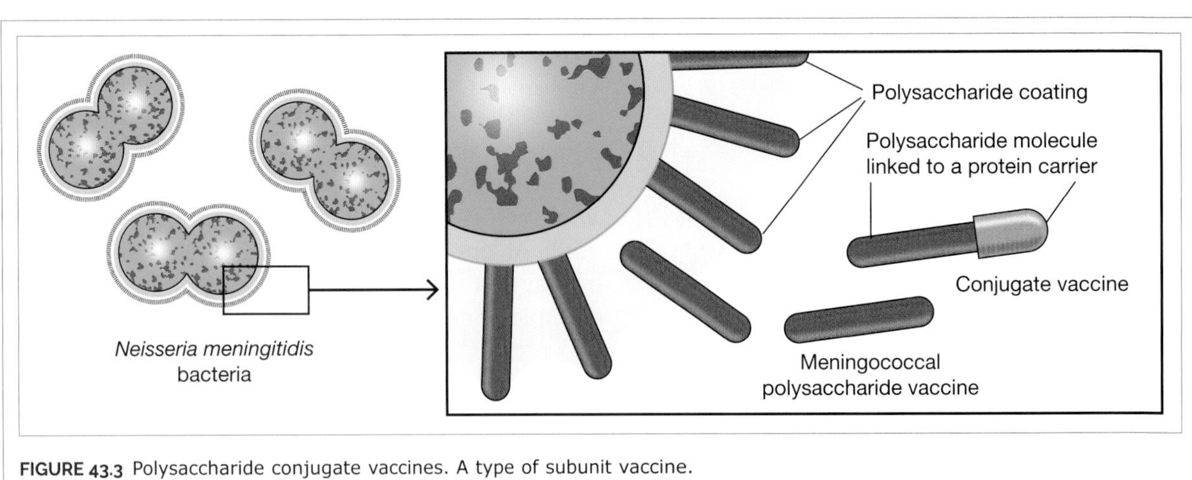

FIGURE 43.3 Polysaccharide conjugate vaccines. A type of subunit vaccine.

such thing as a polysaccharide viral vaccine. To date, there are polysaccharide vaccines for pneumococcal and meningococcal diseases, Hib and *Salmonella typhi*. **Pure polysaccharide vaccines** trigger a T-cell independent response and therefore cannot generate a robust and long-lasting immune response.

Conjugate vaccines

Polysaccharides can also be covalently linked (or chemically combined) to a protein carrier. This process results in a **conjugate polysaccharide vaccine** and greatly increases the immunogenicity of the polysaccharide vaccine. This is because conjugated polysaccharide vaccines can stimulate T-cell dependent immune responses, and subsequent T-cell memory. Most polysaccharide vaccines are conjugated (Table 43.1). For example, the Hib vaccine is conjugated with the tetanus toxoid. It is important to note that the carrier protein that the polysaccharide is conjugated with offers little to no protection against that pathogen. For example, the Hib vaccine is conjugated with the tetanus toxoid and does not confer or boost immunity to tetanus.

Toxoid vaccines

Some bacteria, such as diphtheria, tetanus, botulism and cholera, cause disease by secreting a toxin. **Toxoid** vaccines exploit this characteristic. For example, the tetanus toxoid vaccine is manufactured by growing the highly toxigenic strain *Clostridium tetani*. The *Clostridium tetani* bacteria secrete the toxin in the laboratory environment, in large quantities. The toxin is then chemically denatured by formaldehyde to produce a tetanus toxoid. The toxoid is physiochemically like the toxin, enabling the generation of antibodies and subsequent immunity; however, it is different enough to be non-toxigenic and unable to cause the disease itself. The other toxoid vaccines are produced in a similar way. They generally cannot mount a strong immune response unless given in multiple doses (**primary series**) and booster doses. To strengthen their immunogenicity, they contain adjuvants (i.e. they are adsorbed).

Recombinant protein vaccines

Recombinant vaccines use DNA technology in their manufacture. In the laboratory, a small piece of DNA is taken from a virus or bacterium that immunity is sought from. This small piece (subunit) of DNA is the gene or genetic code for an antigen. For example, the hepatitis B vaccine uses the DNA that codes for the hepatitis B surface antigen (HBsAg). This piece of DNA is then inserted into an expression vector (a harmless host such as yeast or bacteria). To produce the hepatitis B vaccine, the genetic code is inserted into a yeast cell, *Saccharomyces cerevisiae* (Table 43.2). Like virus-infected human cells, the transformed and infected yeast cell secretes high levels of HBsAg. The secreted HBsAg is then purified and used as the antigen (active ingredient) in the recombinant vaccine.

The first recombinant protein vaccine was the hepatitis B vaccine, first marketed in the late 1980s. To date, there are three recombinant vaccines that are marketed in Australia:

- hepatitis B vaccine (adsorbed recombinant DNA surface antigen)
- meningococcal B recombinant vaccines
- HPV vaccine (adsorbed recombinant HPV capsid [L1] protein). This vaccine is also known as a virus-like particle vaccine and is discussed in more detail below.

Virus-like particles

VLPs are assembled from viral proteins and are therefore structurally like viruses; however, they do not contain viral genetic material (DNA or RNA). Because they do not contain genetic material, they cannot replicate and therefore are not infectious when used as vaccines. The HPV vaccine is an example of a recombinant vaccine and a VLP vaccine.

The HPV vaccine uses the major capsid (outer protein shell) of the papillomavirus as the antigen. This capsid, known as the L1, is formed from a single viral protein and creates an icosahedral (20-sided) surface. The L1 capsule is produced using recombinant technology with *Saccharomyces cerevisiae* (yeast) as the host. Once released from the yeast cells, the VLPs are purified. The purified L1 used in the vaccine can re-form into the icosahedral shape without any genetic material enclosed. So, while it characteristically 'looks' like the real virus, it is not a virus; it is 'virus-like'.

TABLE 43.2 Recombinant vaccines

VACCINE	ANTIGEN	HOST CELL	ADJUVANT	TRADE NAME
Hepatitis B	Hepatitis B surface antigen (HBsAg)	*Saccharomyces cerevisiae* yeast	Aluminium	Engerix-B (Hep-B[Eng])
HPV Virus-like particle	L1 major capsid protein of HPV encodes for purified VLPs	*Saccharomyces cerevisiae* yeast	Aluminium	Gardasil Cervarix
Meningococcal B recombinant vaccines	Neisserial adhesin A, Neisserial heparin binding antigen, and factor H binding protein	*Escherichia coli*	Aluminium	Bexsero; Trumenba

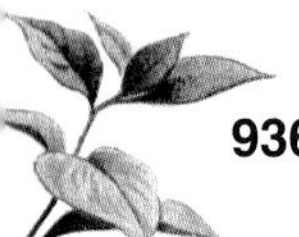

When the HPV VLPs are introduced into the body via vaccination, the body recognises them as foreign, triggering an immune response. Despite being a subunit vaccine, the VLPs used in the HPV vaccine are highly immunogenic and efficacious. They elicit a robust immune response and stimulate both the antibody and the cell-mediated arms of the adaptive immune system. Studies show that 98% of vaccinated people will develop antibodies against the HPV types in the vaccine, and they are close to 100% effective at preventing cervical cancer caused by the HPV strains included in the vaccine. On subsequent exposure to the real virus, the body mounts a strong and immediate secondary immune response. The new malaria vaccine uses VLPs in its formulation.

Nucleic acid vaccines

Although scientists had been working on nucleic acid vaccines since the late 1980s, the first nucleic acid vaccine was not approved for human use until 2020. It was a COVID-19 vaccine. There are two types of nucleic acid vaccines:

- mRNA vaccines
- plasmid DNA vaccines.

To date, outside clinical trials, no DNA vaccine has been approved for human use; however, several are approved for use in animals such as the horse vaccine against West Nile virus.

To understand how nucleic acid vaccines work, it is essential to understand the relationship between DNA, mRNA and protein synthesis. DNA is a complex molecule that contains all the instructions to build and maintain an organism. A *gene* is a length of DNA that codes for a specific protein. DNA cannot produce proteins directly. For a start, DNA cannot leave the nucleus of a cell, and ribosomes (where proteins are synthesised) are located in the cell's cytoplasm. This is where mRNA has a role. *It* serves as a 'messenger' between DNA and the ribosomes. The genetic code is first transcribed (or copied) from the DNA into mRNA. The mRNA then leaves the cell's nucleus and moves to the cytoplasm, where ribosomes are located. Ribosomes then read the mRNA and translate the code into an amino acid sequence that makes up a protein. In short, mRNA is essential for protein synthesis.

All pathogens (except viruses) are living things. All living things are made up of cells, which contain DNA. While viruses are considered non-living (i.e. they cannot replicate outside a host cell), they are still made up of either DNA or RNA. Therefore, all disease-causing pathogens have genetic material that codes for their own protein antigens. Nucleic acid vaccines use the genetic material of pathogens that code for these antigens to stimulate an immune response.

mRNA vaccines

Once the genome for a pathogen has been sequenced, mRNA vaccines can be chemically synthesised in a laboratory from a template. When producing the vaccine, there is no need for pathogen cells. The key immunogenic component of mRNA vaccines is the mRNA that encodes for the pathogen of interest's protein antigen. For example, the Pfizer/Biontech COVID-19 vaccine (Cominarty) contained the mRNA that encoded for the protein spike of the SARS-CoV-2 virus (Polack et al. 2020).

mRNA alone is very fragile and degrades easily when introduced into the body. It is also difficult for mRNA alone to enter into host cells because the cell membrane acts as a barrier. To stimulate an immune response, the mRNA must cross the host cell membrane to reach the cytoplasm. Therefore, to prevent degradation and enable entry into host cells, the mRNA is enclosed in a delivery system. Delivery systems include: lipid nanoparticles, polymers, cell-penetrating peptides and dendrimers. The most widely used delivery system are lipid nanoparticles (Reichmuth et al. 2016).

Lipid nanoparticles are carriers that protect the mRNA from degradation and enable the structure (lipid nanoparticle + mRNA) to adhere to host cells. By a process known as endocytosis, the lipid nanoparticle with the enclosed mRNA is taken into host cell cytoplasm. The mRNA is read at the ribosomes and results in the synthesis of translated protein antigens. The host has effectively created the 'vaccine' in situ. The antigens that have been produced are then displayed on the cell membrane, triggering an immune response. Because the antigen has been taken into the host cells, it activates both humoral and cellular immunity (Sahin 2020). The result is a robust immune response. Because mRNA does not enter the host cell's nucleus, it cannot integrate into the host cell genome (and cannot alter human DNA). The mRNA is transiently expressed and eventually destroyed by the host cell.

Cutting out the middleman (because the human host creates the vaccine in situ), mRNA vaccines are quicker, easier and cheaper to produce than more traditional vaccine technologies. They can also be modified easily to provide protection against rapidly mutating pathogens.

DNA vaccines

Once a pathogen's genome has been sequenced, DNA vaccines can be chemically synthesised in a laboratory from a template, much like mRNA vaccines can.

The naked DNA that codes for the target antigen is then inserted into a plasmid, hence the name plasmid DNA vaccines. A plasmid is a small, circular piece of DNA found in bacteria and some other cells. Plasmids can replicate independently, making them ideal vectors. The plasmid with the inserted DNA makes up the vaccine and is injected into the host.

The process of artificially introducing nucleic acids (DNA or RNA) into host cells is known as transinfection. The DNA is taken up by host cells, where it enters the cell cytoplasm; from there, it needs to get into nucleus, where it is read and transcribed to mRNA and produces the protein antigen. These host cells may be engulfed by antigen-presenting cells. Once the DNA is taken into the host antigen-presenting cells, it is processed and presented, triggering both arms of the adaptive immune response. Like the mRNA vaccine, DNA vaccines create the antigen in situ (in the human host). It is anticipated that DNA vaccines will be used in humans soon.

How do DNA vaccines differ from recombinant DNA vaccines?

Recombinant DNA vaccines such as the meningococcal B and hepatitis B vaccines are not the same as the DNA vaccines that have just been described. The notable difference is that recombinant DNA vaccines, including the antigenic protein, are produced in a laboratory using host cells (using recombinant DNA technology) and then administered to people. Recombinant DNA vaccines themselves are not made up of DNA. In contrast, a DNA vaccine contains only the 'genetic material' that encodes for a protein. When administered, the introduced genetic material is taken up by the host cells, and the antigen is generated by the cells of the host (human or animal). DNA vaccines are made in situ in the host; recombinant DNA vaccines are not.

Vaccine schedules

Vaccine schedules are based on an understanding of how the different types of vaccine work and epidemiological research. Schedules are constantly being reviewed by immunisation experts to ensure people are protected against vaccine-preventable diseases. The National Immunisation Program Schedule (Australia) and the New Zealand Immunisation Schedule (New Zealand) outlines the vaccines that should be given at specific times across the lifespan. Both countries offer these vaccines free to citizens.

When examining the vaccine schedules, it is evident that some vaccines are given as a primary series, and then in booster doses.

Primary series

A 'primary series' is when a series of vaccine doses (usually 2–4) are required to achieve full vaccine effectiveness. For example, in New Zealand the diphtheria, tetanus, pertussis, polio, hepatitis B and Hib are all given at the age of 6 weeks, 3 months and 5 months. In Australia, these vaccines are given at 2, 4 and 6 months of age. Both schedules are examples of a primary series.

Boosters

Excluding several live attenuated vaccines, most vaccines will require booster doses to ensure protection (Table 43.1). Booster doses are those given months or years after the primary dose/series. They 'boost' the immune system and protect against waning immunity. For example, two booster doses are recommended for diphtheria, tetanus and whooping cough in childhood. The first booster is given at 18 months of age and the second at 4 years of age. Another booster is given in adolescence at roughly 12–13 years and is then recommended for adults who wish to reduce their risk of becoming ill or transmitting the infection to others (e.g. people caring for a newborn).

Annual influenza vaccine

Influenza is a highly contagious acute respiratory infection caused by an influenza virus. In Australia in 2019 (pre-pandemic) there were 313,033 laboratory-confirmed cases and 902 influenza deaths. It is estimated that globally influenza causes 389,000 deaths (uncertainty range 294,000–518,000) each year (Paget et al. 2019). Mitigation strategies, such as the use of social distancing, lockdowns, quarantines and use of protective personal equipment such as face masks, significantly reduced influenza transmission in 2020 and 2021. To reduce the risk of influenza and its complications, the influenza vaccine is recommended to all people aged 6 months or older. It is the only vaccine recommended to be given annually, and the vaccine composition (i.e. the included influenza strains) also changes annually. The reason for this is the gradual 'drift' and occasional 'shift' in the circulating influenza viruses.

There are three influenza virus types that infect humans: A, B and C. Influenza A and B are the most common and are included in influenza vaccines. Influenza A is a responsible for pandemics and is a great threat to human health. History tells us that there have been nine severe influenza pandemics in the past 300 years. The 'Spanish flu' of 1918 was the last devasting influenza A pandemic, and it is estimated to have killed more than 50 million people globally. To understand why influenza A pandemics like this are so deadly, we first must understand the virus itself. The influenza virus is made up of eight distinct RNA segments that are packaged together in an envelope. The virus has two surface proteins: haemagglutinin (HA) and neuraminidase (NA). HA enables the virus to attach or bind to host cells, while NA enables the influenza virus to leave the infected host cell and thereby go on and infect other cells. There are 18 HA subtypes and 11 NA subtypes. Many different combinations of HA and NA are possible, resulting in many kinds of influenza A such as H3N2, H1N1 and H5N1. While influenza A infects humans, it also infects

other animals such as birds (avian flu) and pigs (swine flu). Antigenic shift happens when two or more differing influenza viruses (e.g. a human and an animal influenza virus) co-infect a host cell and the segmented RNA of both viruses intermix. This leads to the generation of a new influenza virus strain that no human has pre-existing immunity to and subsequent widespread infection, morbidity and mortality ensues.

Influenza B virus is categorised based on lineage and spreads almost exclusively in humans. While influenza B is responsible for many hospital admissions and can be life-threatening, it does not cause pandemics and results in less mortality than influenza A. Both influenza A and influenza B viruses are constantly evolving in a process known as antigenic drift, which occurs when there is an accumulation of genetic mutations as viruses replicate over time. In influenza A, the changes in the genetic material of the virus can lead to changes in the antigenic surface proteins HA and NA. While the virus is evolving gradually, the population usually has 'cross-protection' from a previous influenza virus. However, changes may accumulate over time, and it may result in antigens that humans no longer recognise, leading to subsequent infections.

Influenza vaccine composition

Influenza viruses are constantly evolving and changing, and different strains can circulate in the population. This is the rationale behind changing the influenza vaccine composition each year. To provide the greatest protection, the vaccine should contain viruses that are a 'match' or are antigenically like those currently circulating. Each year, the World Health Organization recommends the strains to be included in influenza vaccines. This recommendation is based on knowledge of the circulating strains in the opposite hemisphere's influenza season (usually winter). That is, the southern hemisphere looks to the northern hemisphere (and vice versa) to inform vaccine composition. The influenza vaccine comes in both quadrivalent (two influenza A subtypes and two influenza B lineages) and trivalent (two influenza A subtypes and one influenza B lineage) formulations.

For example, based on circulating strains in the northern hemisphere's influenza season, the World Health Organization has recommended that quadrivalent vaccines for use in the 2022 southern hemisphere flu season (e.g. Australia and New Zealand) include:

- egg-based vaccines
  - an A/Victoria/2570/2019 (H1N1)pdm09-like virus
  - an A/Darwin/9/2021 (H3N2)-like virus
  - a B/Austria/1359417/2021 (B/Victoria lineage)-like virus
  - a B/Phuket/3073/2013 (B/Yamagata lineage)-like virus
- cell- or recombinant-based vaccines
  - an A/Wisconsin/588/2019 (H1N1)pdm09-like virus
  - an A/Darwin/6/2021 (H3N2)-like virus
  - a B/Austria/1359417/2021 (B/Victoria lineage)-like virus
  - a B/Phuket/3073/2013 (B/Yamagata lineage)-like virus.

Trivalent vaccines contain all strains excluding the B/Phuket/3073/2013 (B/Yamagata lineage)-like virus.

Naming influenza viruses

To understand the strains that are included in the influenza vaccines, it helps to know the internationally accepted naming convention.

In order from left to right is the:

- influenza virus type (e.g. A, B, C)
- host of origin (e.g. swine, avian): for human-origin viruses, the host origin is omitted – for example:
  - (duck-origin example): A/duck/Alberta/35/76
  - (human-origin example): A/Darwin/6/2021 (H3N2)-like virus
- place the virus was first isolated (e.g. Victoria, Darwin, Wisconsin)
- strain number (e.g. 35, 6)
- year of isolation (e.g. 2019, 2021).

For influenza A viruses, the HA and NA antigen is usually given in parentheses – for example, '(H3N2)'.

Vaccine efficacy of the influenza vaccine varies by year but is generally less than 60% in healthy adults, well below the efficacy of other vaccines. This is, in part, attributed to the difficulty of predicting the circulated strains.

There are two types of influenza vaccine: the live attenuated (LAIV) and the inactivated (IIV). In Australia, however, the LAIV is yet to be marketed. There are two types of IIV split-virion or subunit vaccines (see above). Split-virion influenza vaccines report a greater vaccine efficacy than subunit vaccines (Talbot et al. 2015).

Herd immunity

Vaccines have both an individual and a collective benefit. The person who is administered a vaccine is likely to go on to develop immunity and individual protection against the vaccine-preventable disease. The collective benefit arises when a significant number of people (often called the critical mass threshold) within the population have developed immunity either naturally or by vaccination, reducing the number of susceptible hosts and the spread of the disease. This provides protection to those without individual immunity (e.g. unvaccinated). The critical proportion of the population that must be immune to provide herd immunity varies by the disease. For example, to provide adequate measles protection for the whole population, approximately 95% of the population needs to have active immunity. Given that measles is a live attenuated vaccine, and is contradicted in people who are immunocompromised, such people rely on the 'herd' to get vaccinated to protect them. With such a high critical mass threshold, there have been several sporadic and small outbreaks of measles in Australia in recent times. Vaccines are also victims of their own success. Because people do not have a lived experience of the morbidity and mortality that the now vaccine-preventable diseases caused, they become more concerned about vaccine safety. Vaccine hesitancy or reduced vaccine uptake is a barrier to achieving herd immunity, leaving those who cannot be or choose not to be vaccinated at greater risk.

Clinical considerations

Vaccine cold chain

Vaccines are temperature-sensitive. To ensure potency, they must be stored in a predetermined cold chain from initial manufacture, during transportation and storage through to administration. This process is known as 'cold chain management'. Breaches in the vaccine cold chain may result in the administration of vaccines that cannot elicit an immune response and therefore may leave the person and community at risk of vaccine-preventable diseases. Most vaccines need to be stored between 2°C and 8°C, and exposure to freezing temperatures is likely to cause irreversible loss of vaccine potency. However, the new mRNA vaccines (e.g. COVID-19) need to be stored at ultra-cold temperatures during initial transport and storage (between –90°C and –60°C). Keeping mRNA vaccines at such ultra-low temperatures was one of the great logistical challenges during the COVID-19 vaccine rollout. It is important that health professionals ensure vaccines are maintained within the cold chain at all times and that suspected or actual breaches in vaccine cold chain are reported.

Vaccine administration technique

It is important that vaccinators use the correct injection site, technique and equipment when vaccinating. This includes selecting the correct gauge (needle thickness) and needle length. The smaller the gauge the greater the thickness of the needle. For example, an 18G needle (commonly referred to as a blunt drawing up needle) has a wider bore or width than a 22G needle. Needles used for IM injections generally have a lower gauge (i.e. wider) than those used for SC injections. A needle with a wider bore helps to dissipate the vaccine over a wider area, reducing localised inflammation at the injection site. IM injections need to go deeper into the body tissues than SC injections, and therefore IM needles are longer (usually 25 mm) and inserted at a 90° angle. SC vaccines are inserted on a 45° angle (Fig 43.4). Interestingly, while administered deeper into the body tissues, IM vaccines tend to cause fewer local reactions such as irritation and inflammation than SC injections.

Vaccines that are administered IM deposit the antigen into the muscle fascia, which has an abundant blood supply. In comparison, the SC layer does not have a rich blood supply. Administering a vaccine into the SC layer, when is it is intended for the muscle fascia, may delay the presentation of the antigen to the immune cells and result in a reduction in immunogenicity or even vaccine failure.

Using body landmarks to administer intramuscular vaccines

There are two anatomical sites that are routinely used to administer vaccines: the anterolateral thigh and the deltoid (upper arm) muscle. The ventrogluteal (side of hip) area may also be used as an alternative. The anatomical site selected for vaccine administration depends on the patient's age. In general, infants up to 12 months of age will receive vaccines in the anterolateral thigh, and people aged over 12 months will have vaccines administered into the deltoid. Vaccinators should use anatomical markers or landmarking techniques when administering vaccines to ensure appropriate vaccine administration. Common landmarking techniques are described below. Further information can be found in the *Australian Immunisation Handbook* (see 'Online resources').

Administering a vaccine into the vastus lateralis (anterolateral thigh)

The vastus lateralis (VL) or anterolateral thigh muscle is the preferred anatomical site for vaccines in infants aged under 12 months. Vaccines should be administered into the outer side of the middle third of the VL muscle. To locate the site of the injection, the vaccinator should landmark the femur (greater trochanter) and the knee (patella) and draw an imaginary line between the two landmarks down the front of the thigh (dividing the thigh into sides). Then they should draw two imaginary lines dividing the thigh across into thirds. The vaccines should be administered in the middle third and on the outer side. It is recommended to remove the infant's nappy to locate the anatomical landmarks and administer the vaccine. If two vaccines are to be administered at the one appointment, both VLs should be used. When more than two vaccines are to be administered, up to two vaccines may be administered into a single VL; however, they should be spaced 2.5 cm apart.

Administering a vaccine into the deltoid

The deltoid is a triangular shaped muscle located on the upper arm (Fig 43.5). It sits on top of the clavicle, scapular and humerus bones. IM vaccines should be administered into the middle (or bulkiest part) of the deltoid. The

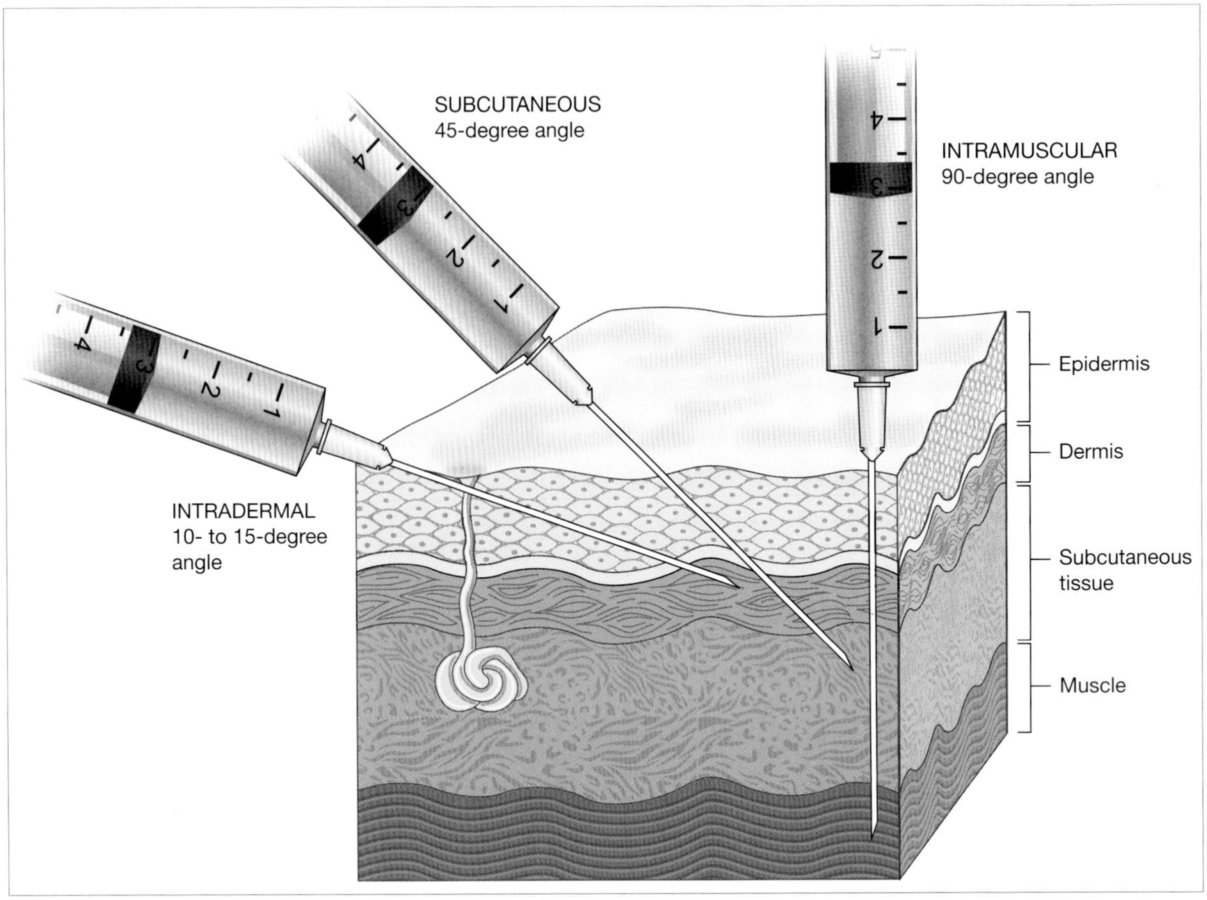

SUBCUTANEOUS
45-degree angle
INTRAMUSCULAR
90-degree angle
INTRADERMAL
10- to 15-degree angle
Epidermis
Dermis
Subcutaneous tissue
Muscle

FIGURE 43.4 Routes of vaccine administration and insertion angles

Acromion
Subdeltoid bursa
Deltoid muscle
Deltoid tuberosity
Brachial artery
Radial nerve
X

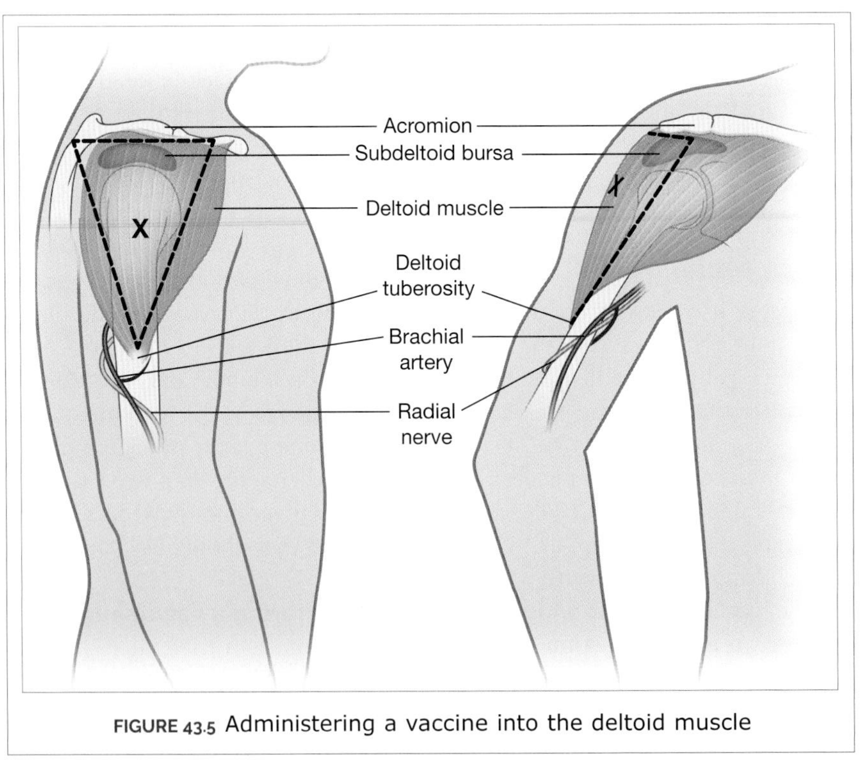

FIGURE 43.5 Administering a vaccine into the deltoid muscle

Australian Immunisation Handbook recommends vaccinators landmark using both the acromion process (shoulder tip) and the deltoid tuberosity (deltoid muscle insertion point roughly in the middle of the humerus bone). The vaccinator should measure two to three fingerbreadths below the acromion process; the fingers form the top of an imaginary inverted triangle, preventing the vaccine being injected into the shoulder bursae. Anywhere within this inverted triangle area is an appropriate site for IM vaccination (Clinical Focus Box 43.2).

When administering an IM injection, the vaccinator should:

- use a needle 22–25 in gauge
- for infants (> 2 months), children or adults, use a needle 25 mm in length
- insert the needle on a 90° angle to the skin

CLINICAL FOCUS BOX 43.2
Shoulder injury related to vaccine administration

A shoulder injury related to vaccine administration (SIRVA) is a very rare, preventable complication that occurs when a vaccine is administered incorrectly. It can occur when a vaccine is administered too high into the shoulder joint (into the shoulder bursae, filled with synovial fluid), too low or too far to the side, causing damage to the radial nerve or axillary nerve respectively. Damage can be caused by the direct trauma of the needle itself or from the inflammatory response that is triggered by the introduction of the antigen. Damage to the radial or axillary nerve can result in an immediate burning and neuropathic pain, and can lead to paralysis.

To ensure patient safety, it is imperative that vaccinators use correct vaccination technique every time. Vaccines administered in the arm should be administered in the middle of the deltoid muscle. When administering a vaccine, vaccinators should get the patient to expose their complete deltoid (upper arm muscle) when vaccinating and avoid partially rolling up or down a shirt to administer a vaccine.

Vaccinators should use appropriate landmarking techniques, helping to identify key anatomical landmarks to determine a safe injecting zone. The *Australian Immunisation Handbook* recommends the inverted triangle method. In this method the vaccinator uses the acromion process and deltoid tuberosity as anatomical markers. Another common technique used is palpation of the acromion process, with the injection site being two or three fingerbreadths below (two for someone with large fingers; three for small fingers). This method uses the vaccinator's fingers to cover the shoulder bursae, preventing the vaccine being administered too high and into the shoulder joint. These landmarking techniques promote vaccine delivery to the middle of the deltoid, where there is maximum muscle bulk.

- insert the needle all the way to the hub
- withdraw the needle on the same angle as it was inserted (i.e. 90° angle).

When administering a vaccine to an obese or very large person, a 38 mm needle may be used to ensure the antigen is delivered into the muscle layer. Using a needle this length on a small or thin person may result in the needle 'hitting the bone' and may cause osteonecrosis. Therefore, it is important the vaccinator uses a needle of an appropriate length.

When administering an SC injection, the vaccinator should:

- use a needle 25–27 in gauge
- use a needle 16 mm in length
- insert the needle on a 45° angle to the skin plane
- insert the needle all the way to the hub
- withdraw the needle on the same angle as it was inserted (i.e. 45° angle).

Reporting vaccinations to national registers

In Australia, health professionals should upload the details of every vaccine administered to the Australian Immunisation Register at the time of vaccination. This enables an accurate real-time vaccination record to be kept for individuals. It also enables vaccination coverage to be determined at the population level. Health professionals can view a person's vaccination history to recommend vaccines to be administered. Some vaccines should not be given more than once (e.g. Q fever). In this case, revaccination to a person who is already immune can cause a serious hypersensitivity reaction. During the COVID-19 pandemic, people needed a record of their vaccination status (vaccination passport) to move freely about the country and enjoy international travel.

As outlined in section 48A(2) of Poisons and Therapeutic Goods Regulation 2008, details that should be uploaded to the Australian Immunisation Register include:

- the person's name, address, date of birth and contact details
- the name and contact details of the person's primary medical practitioner
- the brand, batch number and expiry date of the vaccine
- the part of the body to which the vaccine was administered
- the date on which the vaccine was administered
- the authorised immuniser's name and contact details and his or her certificate of accreditation number
- the address of the place at which the vaccination was administered

- a unique reference number for the supply and administration.

Vaccine side effects

While vaccines have an excellent safety profile, all vaccines have side effects (Dudley et al. 2020). By their mechanism of action, vaccines stimulate an immune response, and thereby it is not surprising that many people experience the signs and symptoms of inflammation such as pain, redness and swelling at the injection site. This could be interpreted as a good thing because it is an indication that the vaccine has stimulated an immune response. Vaccines can also have systemic adverse effects such as fever, headache, myalgia, rash or fatigue (Hervé et al. 2019). Common adverse events following vaccination are shown in Figure 43.6. Other very rare adverse events

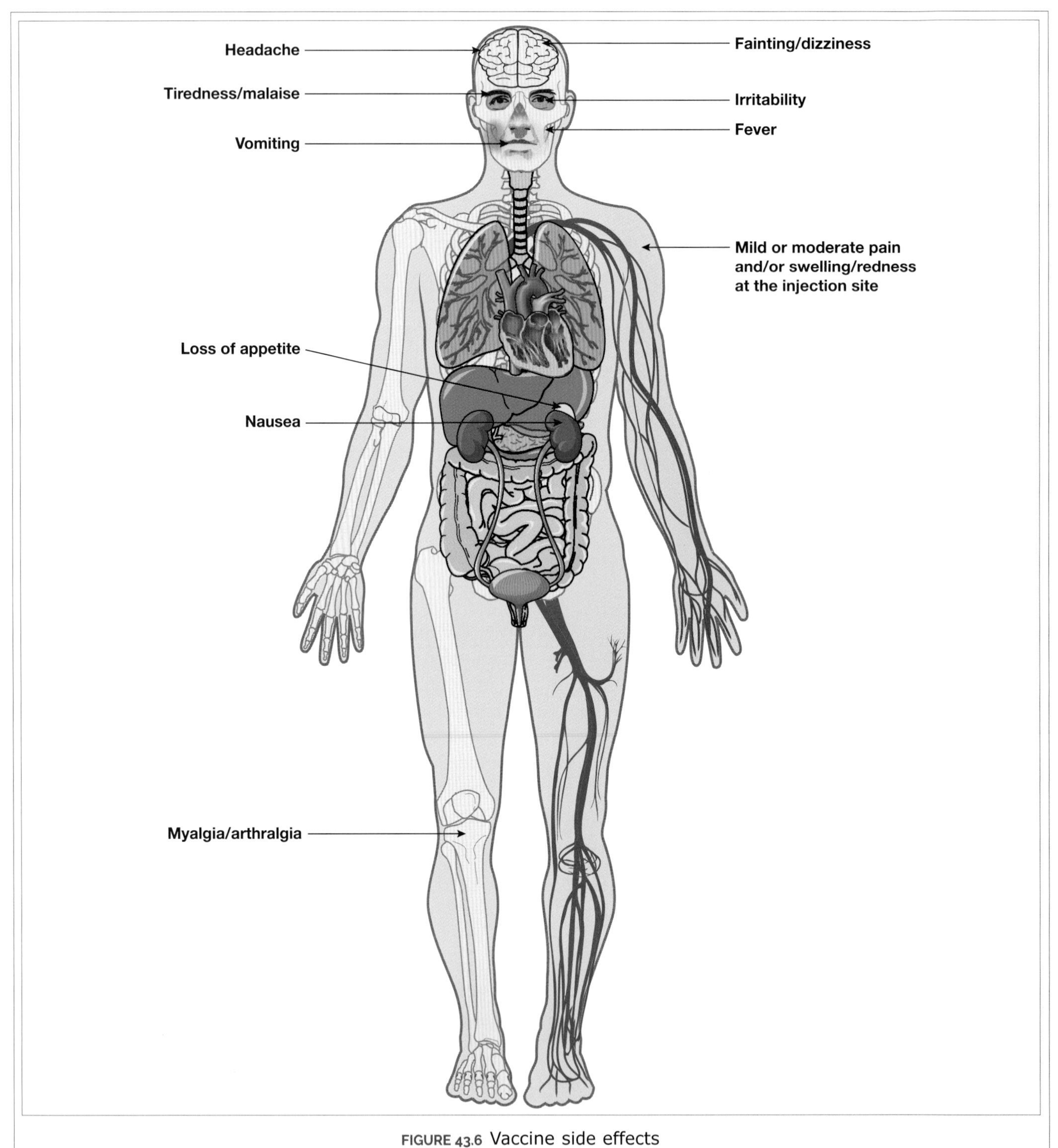

FIGURE 43.6 Vaccine side effects

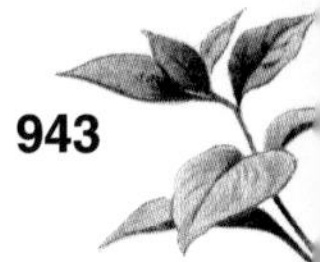

include mild acute arthralgia or arthritis, encephalitis, febrile seizures, Guillain-Barré syndrome, herpes zoster, immune thrombocytopenic purpura, meningitis and syncope. Such adverse events are estimated to occur in less than 0.01% of vaccines administered. The incidence of vaccine-associated anaphylaxis is less than one in 1,000,000 doses for most vaccines. All health professionals should be trained to administer adrenaline and manage this life-threatening event.

All suspected adverse events following immunisation should be reported. In Australia, this is via a National Adverse Events Following Immunisation reporting form submitted to the Therapeutic Goods Administration (see 'Online resources').

Future of vaccines

When the deadly COVID-19 pandemic hit, the world needed a vaccine, and scientists across the globe put efforts into vaccine development. More than 500 vaccines entered clinical trials. Some vaccines used traditional (e.g. protein subunit, inactivated), and some used new vaccine technology (e.g. mRNA, viral vector). Prior to COVID-19, no nucleic acid vaccine had been licensed for human use. However, the first vaccine for COVID-19 that was developed and approved was an mRNA vaccine. So how did this happen? Well, for a start the technology had been 30 years in the making and there were safe and effective DNA vaccines for veterinary use.

When comparing the production of more traditional vaccines where the antigens need to be inactivated or attenuated or created through recombination, producing nucleic acid vaccines is faster, easier and safer. Once the genetic code for the COVID-19 virus was known, it took less than 2 months to design and create an mRNA vaccine. Now with billions of mRNA vaccines administered, there is a plethora of evidence to show that mRNA vaccines are safe and effective. It is expected that the future of vaccine technology will continue to gain momentum in this area.

KEY POINTS

Vaccines

- Vaccines are temperature-sensitive and must be stored in a predetermined cold chain from initial manufacture, during transportation and storage through to administration.
- Using the correct administration technique for the given vaccine helps to optimise immunogenicity and reduce the local side effects.
- IM injections are inserted on a 90° angle to the skin plane. SC vaccines are inserted on a 45° angle.
- The anterolateral thigh and the deltoid muscle are the most common anatomical sites for vaccine administration.
- All vaccinations should be recorded and information uploaded to the national immunisation register.

DRUGS AT A GLANCE
Vaccinations

PHARMACOLOGICAL GROUP AND EFFECT	KEY EXAMPLES	CLINICAL USE
Live attenuated vaccines • Stimulate cell-mediated and humoral immunity	Measles Mumps Rubella Varicella Rotavirus	• Stimulate an immune response against the antigen introduced into the body – confer immunity against the vaccine-preventable disease
Whole-cell inactivated • Use a whole cell (killed) or inactivated antigen to stimulate an immune response; usually requires booster	Hepatitis A Q fever (killed) Poliomyelitis (IPV)	• Stimulate an immune response against the antigen introduced into the body – confer immunity against the vaccine-preventable disease
Viral vector vaccines • Use a carrier virus to deliver genetic material that codes for the antigen of a pathogen to human cells • The vaccine is made 'in situ' and stimulates an immune response	Ebola vaccine COVID-19 vaccine (AstraZeneca)	• Stimulate an immune response against the antigen introduced into the body – confer immunity against the vaccine-preventable disease
Toxoid vaccines • Uses inactivated toxins as the vaccine antigen to elicit an immune response	Diphtheria Tetanus	• Stimulate an immune response against the antigen introduced into the body – confer immunity against the vaccine-preventable disease

Polysaccharide vaccines • Uses the sugar capsule of the bacteria as the antigen to elicit an immune response • Vaccines may be conjugated to a carrier protein to elicit a more robust immune response	Meningococcal Pneumococcal Hib	• Stimulate an immune response against the antigen introduced into the body – confer immunity against the vaccine-preventable disease
Nucleic acid vaccines • mRNA	mRNA COVID-19 vaccines	• Stimulate an immune response against the antigen introduced into the body – confer immunity against the vaccine-preventable disease
Recombinant protein • Uses DNA recombinant technology to proliferate the protein antigen (subunit), which is used to stimulate an immune response	Hepatitis B HPV	• Stimulate an immune response against the antigen introduced into the body – confer immunity against the vaccine-preventable disease

REVIEW EXERCISES

1. Mr SM, a healthy middle-aged police officer, is eligible to have his COVID-19 booster vaccine. What is the difference in the mode of action between the mRNA and viral vector COVID-19 vaccines? Which is more effective and why? What are the common local and systemic side effects associated with each of the vaccines?
2. Mrs SJ, a 70-year-old retiree, at her last visit to her GP was administered the Prevenar 13 (pneumococcal 13-valent conjugate vaccine) and Zostavax (shingles, herpes zoster) vaccines. What is the difference between the pure polysaccharide pneumococcal vaccine and the polysaccharide pneumococcal conjugate vaccine? What type of vaccine is Zostavax (shingles, herpes zoster)? Was it safe and appropriate for both vaccines to be co-administrated on the same day? Give an example of when two vaccines would not be co-administrated on the same day.
3. Mrs HA is examining her son's immunisation history statement alongside her own. She can see that her son received the inactivated poliovirus vaccine at 2 months, 4 months, 6 months and 4 years of age. Mrs HA notes that she received the live oral poliomyelitis vaccine in the 1980s. What is the difference between the two vaccines?

REFERENCES

Adams NM, S Grassmann and JC Sun, Clonal expansion of innate and adaptive lymphocytes. Nature Reviews Immunology, 2020. 20(11): 694–707.

Dudley MZ, Halsey NA, Omer SB, et al. The state of vaccine safety science: systematic reviews of the evidence. The Lancet Infectious Diseases. 2020 May 1;20(5):e80–9.

Hervé C, Laupèze B, Del Giudice G, et al. The how's and what's of vaccine reactogenicity. npj Vaccines. 2019 Sep 24;4(1):1.

Iwasaki A and SB Omer, Why and how vaccines work. Cell, 2020. 183(2): 290–295.

Paget J, Spreeuwenberg P, Charu V, et al. Global mortality associated with seasonal influenza epidemics: new burden estimates and predictors from the GLaMOR Project. Journal of Global Health, 2019. 9(2): 020421.

Polack FP, Thomas SJ, Kitchin N et al. Safety and efficacy of the BNT162b2 mRNA Covid-19 vaccine. The New England Journal of Medicine, 2020. 383(27): 2603–2615.

Reichmuth AM, Oberli MA, Jaklenec A, et al. mRNA vaccine delivery using lipid nanoparticles. Therapeutic Delivery, 2016. 7(5): 319–334.

Sahin U, Muik A, Derhovanessian E, et al. COVID-19 vaccine BNT162b1 elicits human antibody and TH1 T cell responses. Nature, 2020. 586(7830): 594–599.

Talbot HK, Nian H, Zhu Y, et al. Clinical effectiveness of split-virion versus subunit trivalent influenza vaccines in older adults. Clinical Infectious Diseases: an official publication of the Infectious Diseases Society of America, 2015. 60(8): 1170–1175.

ONLINE RESOURCES

Australian Immunisation Handbook: https://immunisationhandbook.health.gov.au/ (accessed 1 November 2021)

Australian Immunisation Register for health professionals: https://www.servicesaustralia.gov.au/australian-immunisation-register-for-health-professionals (accessed 1 November 2021)

National Centre for Immunisation Research and Surveillance (NCIRS): https://www.ncirs.org.au/health-professionals (accessed 1 November 2021)

National Immunisation Program Schedule: https://www.health.gov.au/health-topics/immunisation/when-to-get-vaccinated/national-immunisation-program-schedule (accessed 1 November 2021)

NSW Health immunisation programs: https://www.health.nsw.gov.au/immunisation/Pages/default.aspx (accessed 1 November 2021)

World Health Organization – Vaccines and immunization: https://www.who.int/health-topics/vaccines-and-immunization (accessed 1 November 2021)

More weblinks at: http://evolve.elsevier.com/AU/Knights/pharmacology/.

CHAPTER 44
COMPLEMENTARY MEDICINES
Mary Bushell

KEY ABBREVIATIONS

ADR adverse drug reaction
CAM complementary and alternative medicine
EBM evidence-based medicine
OTC over-the-counter
TCM traditional Chinese medicine
TGA Therapeutic Goods Administration

KEY TERMS

Chapter Focus

An increasing number of people are turning to complementary and alternative medicines to prevent and treat medical conditions. The term complementary medicine is broad and includes vitamins, minerals, herbs, aromatherapy, traditional Chinese and Indian medicines and homeopathic preparations. Because they are perceived to be more 'natural', people often believe complementary medicines are safer than conventional or Western medicines. However, by our definition, they are still drugs: 'substances used to modify or explore physiological systems or pathological states for the benefit of the recipient'. Complementary medicines can have pharmacological action, adverse effects and interact with other medicines.

This chapter reviews the regulation of complementary medicines as well as the benefits and risks associated with their use.

KEY DRUG GROUPS

Complementary and alternative medicine products:

- Herbal remedies (Clinical Focus Box 44.3): cranberry (Drug Monograph 44.1)
- Indigenous remedies
- Traditional Chinese medicines: *Scutellaria / huang qin* (Drug Monograph 44.2)

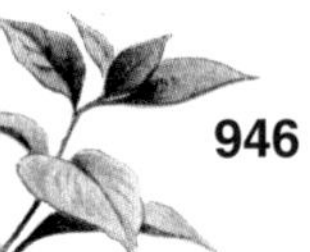

CRITICAL THINKING SCENARIO

Jeremiah visits you, the health professional, for a regular checkup. You ask him if he is taking any medicines. He informs you that he is taking atorvastatin 40 mg daily, ramipril 10 mg daily, aspirin 100 mg daily and escitalopram 20 mg daily. You ask specifically if he is taking any complementary medicines. He replies, 'I don't know what you mean by complementary medicines'.

1. How would you explain to Jeremiah what complementary medicines are?

Jeremiah then tells you he is taking fish oil (for his heart), a men's multivitamin (general wellbeing), Caruso's Prostate EZE Max (for frequent night-time urination) and St John's wort (for depression). He states that he never thought of these preparations as 'drugs' because he has never needed a prescription to purchase them and suggests that they are natural and therefore safe.

2. Looking at Jeremiah's complementary medicines list, describe the current evidence for each.
3. Are there any adverse effects associated with his current complementary therapies?
4. Is there potential for drug interactions between Jeremiah's prescribed medicines and complementary medicines?

Introduction

As well as medicines prescribed by doctors and other health professionals, people often take or use substances they can access themselves – whether bought over the counter in pharmacies, supermarkets, health food stores or online, provided by traditional healers or even harvested from gardens – to treat or prevent medical conditions. These substances can still have pharmacological action, adverse drug reactions and interactions with other medicines.

Complementary and alternative therapies

What is 'complementary and alternative medicine'?

The term '**complementary and alternative medicine**' (CAM) refers to healthcare practices not usually taught or practised in the local mainstream scientific (Western) medicine. Although the terms 'alternative' and 'complementary' are often used interchangeably, there may be a distinction between them. 'Complementary' indicates that some scientific validation exists, the practice is accepted and it may complement mainstream healthcare practice; whereas 'alternative' generally refers to practices that are either scientifically unfounded or lacking in supporting evidence. Complementary therapies include specialised diets, traditional Chinese medicine (TCM), exercise, osteopathic/chiropractic treatment, counselling, biofeedback, massage therapy, relaxation, herbal therapy, acupuncture and hypnosis. Under the 'alternative' label come modalities such as homeopathy, iridology, aromatherapy and macrobiotics. 'Integrative medicine' implies integrating CAM modalities into comprehensive treatment plans alongside evidence-based medicine (EBM) practice; the term has been criticised as merely a rebranding and whitewashing of alternative medicine practices.

Some practitioners now are regulated by the Australian Health Practitioner Regulation Agency (Ahpra), notably via the Chinese Medicine Board, Osteopathy Board and Chiropractic Board, and some treatments may be covered by health insurance schemes.

Types of CAM therapies

There is a very wide range of modalities, outside the scope of conventional scientific medicine, for which therapeutic claims are made. The range includes:

- psychological methods (including counselling, hypnotherapy, music therapy, cognitive behaviour therapy, prayer, faith healing, homeopathy, relaxation, meditation, humour and laughter therapy and 12-step self-help programs such as that of Alcoholics Anonymous)

- dietary changes (megavitamins, vegetarian/veganism, other specialised diets)
- physical methods (Alexander technique, massage, chiropractic, dance therapy, osteopathy, yoga, acupuncture, biofeedback, Pilates, Qi Gong, tai chi, reflexology and electromagnetic applications)
- pharmacological means (herbal medicines, other supplements, traditional ethnic medicines, essential oils, chelation therapy, some aromatherapy, Bach flower remedies and homeopathic preparations).

Some CAM modalities are grouped under the umbrella of 'naturopathy', which focuses on self-healing and disease prevention through natural products and changes in lifestyle, and there are other eclectic practitioners who apply various methods in holistic therapy – for example, mind–body medicine. There is no clearcut distinction between mainstream and CAM therapies; for example, there is much overlap between physiotherapy, chiropractic, osteopathy, Pilates and massage therapy; and many 'Western' drugs originate from traditional herbal remedies.

To discuss the different types of CAMs is beyond the scope of a pharmacology textbook, so we will concentrate on the pharmacological group, particularly herbal remedies.

Use of CAM

Prevalence

The World Health Organization (2019) estimates that 80% of the world's population use herbal preparations from non-Western medicine for some of their health care. Spending on CAMs has more than doubled since the mid-1990s and continues to increase. In the past 30 years, there has been an increasing interest in CAMs, resulting in a vast proliferation of alternative healers, health food stores, natural products, organic fruits and vegetables, and the use of herbal remedies. In fact, it has evolved into a multibillion-dollar industry that is not limited to specific age, cultural or ethnic groups.

In the UK, 20–39% of the population uses CAMs (World Health Organization 2019). The most popular CAM therapies are Ayurvedic medicine, herbalism, aromatherapy, homeopathy, chiropractic, acupuncture/acupressure, massage, reflexology, TCM and Unani medicine. In other European countries, 20–50% of residents report using complementary and alternative therapies; herbal remedies and homeopathy are particularly popular in German-speaking countries.

In Australia

About 63% of the Australian population use at least one complementary or alternative therapy each year (not counting minerals such as calcium, fluoride or iron, or prescribed vitamins), and 36% visit an alternative practitioner (Steel et al. 2018). The groups most commonly using complementary medicines are:

- tertiary-educated young women
- people with chronic conditions such as diabetes, musculoskeletal disorders, cancer, chronic pain or mental illness
- older women with menopausal symptoms
- women in the second half of pregnancy
- people with HIV attending specialist clinics.

The forms of CAM most frequently used by elderly Australians are clinical nutrition, chiropractic, massage therapy, meditation and herbal medicine. Some of the most used CAM products are fish oil (Clinical Focus Box 44.2), glucosamine, aloe vera, garlic, green tea, chamomile, echinacea (in winter), ginger, cranberry (Drug Monograph 44.1, later), peppermint, ginseng, glucosamine, *Ginkgo biloba* and St John's wort as an antidepressant. Fewer than half of CAM users inform their doctor, even when asked.

The number of CAM providers continues to increase in Australia to meet the public's desire to integrate CAM with other medicine. Data from the Australian Institute of Health and Welfare reported that in 2019 there were 950 acupuncture, 2486 chiropractic, 235 homeopathy, 2982 naturopathy, 2631 natural remedy, 776 osteopathy, 481 TCM and 8199 massage therapy providers. According to 2021 data from Ahpra, there were 5561 practising chiropractors and 4901 TCM practitioners registered in Australia.

In New Zealand

In New Zealand, it is estimated that there are at least 10,000 CAM practitioners nationally; most CAM professions are not regulated. About half the population take dietary and health supplements, and approximately one in five adults visits a CAM practitioner annually (Lee et al. 2021). There is a consistent demand for products for arthritis, women's health issues, gut health and brain health. CAM users are likely to be female, rich, well-educated, middle-aged and of European descent. The natural products industry contributes an estimated NZ$1.4 billion to the economy annually. Osteopaths, chiropractors and acupuncturists can register with the Accident Compensation Corporation. Osteopathy and chiropractic are regulated professions under the *Health Practitioners Competence Assurance Act 2003*.

Many conventional GPs practise some form of CAM, mainly acupuncture, hypnosis and chiropractic, and feel that information about CAM should be included in medical education.

Reasons for use

CAM therapies are used in a wide variety of disorders, for both prevention and treatment. This interest in CAM may have been encouraged by numerous warnings issued on

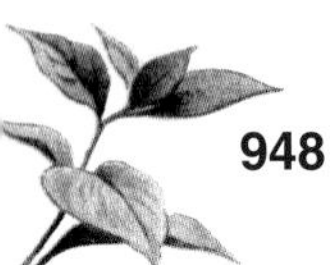

Drug Monograph 44.1
Cranberry

Cranberry juice is an extract of the fruit of plants of *Vaccinium* spp.; these were traditionally used by North American Indian people as a food and treatment for kidney diseases. The juice is high in flavonols, including proanthocyanidins, plus catechin, glycosides, fructose, organic acids and vitamin C; it is quite acidic and usually sweetened with significant amounts of sugar (or artificial sweetener). Its main actions are bacteriostatic and antioxidant, and possibly also cardioprotective by reducing levels of HDL cholesterol. The fruit is also available in dried form.

Mechanism of action

Cranberry inhibits the action of bacterial fimbriae (adherence 'hairs'), thus reducing adherence of bacteria to urinary tract epithelial linings. There is no significant change in urinary pH. The flavonol glycosides have free radical scavenging activity comparable to that of vitamin E.

Indications

Cranberry juice has proven efficacy in prophylaxis of urinary tract infections (UTI), especially in women with recurrent UTIs, and in spinal cord injury patients with catheter-associated UTIs. There is no reliable evidence of efficacy in treating established UTIs as a sole medicine, or in gout, type 2 diabetes or *Helicobacter pylori* infection in stomach ulcers.

Pharmacokinetics

Studies of the bioavailability and metabolism of bioactive components of cranberry juice show marked variation in the plasma and urinary concentrations and rates of reaching C_{max}; metabolites found were sinapic acid, homovanillic acid, protocatechuic acid, myricetin, kaempferol and quercetin. Results suggest that phenolic constituents of cranberry juice are absorbed at different sites in the gastrointestinal tract (GIT) and that phenolic acids and flavonoids are bioavailable to act in the urinary tract. Evidence from users drinking one to two glasses of cranberry juice daily suggests that it takes 4–8 weeks to take effect.

Drug interactions

Co-administration (not recommended) of cranberry and warfarin may alter blood coagulation status: monitor for changes in bleeding times.

There is potential for interaction between cranberry juice and proton pump inhibitors, affecting absorption of vitamin B12.

Adverse reactions

The acidity of cranberry juice can lead to kidney stones; people with a history of oxalate stones should limit their intake.

Consumption of high doses (3 L or more per day!) causes GIT discomfort and diarrhoea.

Precautions and contraindications

Cranberry should be used with caution in people with diabetes (due to high sugar content) or a history of kidney stones. There is little direct evidence of safety or harm in pregnant or breastfeeding women.

Dosage and administration

Cranberry is available as juice (may be already diluted or sweetened) and in tablets and capsules; constituents and strengths vary: capsules may contain from 250 mg to 30,000 mg (30 g). Doses quoted for adults are: 30–300 mL/day or 400 mg capsule/day; children: 15 mL/kg/day up to 300 mL/day. However, much higher doses, equivalent of up to 50 g fresh fruit per day, are sometimes taken for quicker results.

Cranberry juice is readily available; tablets and capsules may be **listed medicines** by the Therapeutic Goods Administration (TGA).

Source: Braun & Cohen 2017.

'chemicals' (food additives, preservatives) said to be cancer-producing substances. Other reasons given by users and practitioners of complementary and alternative therapies include:

- the belief that natural methods are better and safer than scientific methods and products
- the perception that only complementary and alternative therapies treat the whole person (holistic medicine)
- endorsement of a method by a celebrity,[2] despite minimal scientific justification
- dissatisfaction with conventional medicine if found to be hard to access or too technologically oriented

2 Celebrities including Prince Charles, Olivia Newton-John and David Beckham have recommended 'treatments' such as homeopathic 'vaccinations', digestive enzymes, plant tonics, silicone bracelets with holograms, and unprotected sex. A spokesman for the Sense About Science group said he'd like to see more celebrities checking out the science before they send the wrong message worldwide via the internet.

- attempts to prevent illness such as colds, whereas conventional medicine is seen as useful only for treating symptoms
- perceived lower cost if scientific medicine is unaffordable
- offer of comfort for those with a poor prognosis in a severe condition, or a disorder with a major psychological component
- desire to participate in therapy, leading to self-empowerment.

Regulation of CAM

More than 100 years ago in Australia there were concerns about the widespread promotion and purchase of dangerous and useless medicines; a wide-ranging inquiry reported problems with secret trafficking in drugs, drug sellers not being subject to licensing or examination, ingredients not being openly declared and misleading advertising. This inquiry may well have been the forerunner of the TGA, which now regulates all therapeutic goods to ensure their quality, safety, **efficacy** and timely availability. (Separate state and territory legislation may also apply – as discussed in Ch 2.)

Regulation in Australia

The TGA defines complementary medicines as 'a therapeutic good consisting principally of one or more designated active ingredients ... [with] a clearly established identity and traditional use'; 14 types of ingredients are listed, including amino acids, charcoal, choline salt, plant or herbal material, microorganisms (except vaccines), minerals, mucopolysaccharides, non-human animal materials, lipids, a substance produced by or obtained from bees, a sugar, polysaccharide or carbohydrates, vitamins and homeopathic preparations.

Through its Advisory Committee on Complementary Medicines, the TGA has the responsibility, with respect to CAM medicines, to:

- allocate licences to manufacture and to ensure manufacturing complies with the relevant standards for Good Manufacturing Practice
- carry out pre-market assessment of risks related to toxicity, dosage, indications, adverse effects and interactions
- determine whether products are to be 'listed' (either listed or assessed listed) or 'registered'
- list allowable ingredients and evaluate their safety
- monitor safety and efficacy post-marketing, with regular and random audits
- have effective recall procedures
- audit and control advertising
- ensure safety and quality of exported medicines.

The TGA advises consumers not to order CAM medicines over the internet unless they are very sure about the legality and content of the product.

An overview of the regulatory guidelines for complementary medicines in Australia is shown on the TGA website (see 'Online resources').

Listed/registered complementary medicines

In Australia there are three types of complementary medicines available to the public: listed (AUST L), assessed listed (AUST L(A)) and **registered** (AUST R). The assessed listed category was introduced in 2018.

Listed complementary medicines have low-risk ingredients (they do not contain ingredients that are scheduled in the *Poisons Standard*) and are not assessed by the TGA for efficacy. They are for use in low-risk indications only – for example, health enhancement and maintenance, prevention of dietary deficiency and self-limiting conditions. Most CAMs are listed.

Assessed listed complementary medicines (Fig 44.1), as the title suggests, have been assessed by the TGA and shown to have evidence of efficacy (they work). They are used for intermediate-level indications; for example, the product may prevent, cure or alleviate a non-serious form of a medical condition. To date, there are two AUST L(A) complementary medicines. In May 2021, Caruso's Prostate EZE Max was the first product to receive AUST L(A) listing. The product is indicated 'For the relief of frequent night-time urination associated with medically diagnosed benign prostatic hypertrophy' and contains herbal extracts of pygeum, saw palmetto, willowherb, pumpkin seed oil and lycopene. However, the AUST L(A) listing has been criticised by medical experts who have highlighted that there is only one published study about the herbal product, a randomised controlled trial with a small sample size and at best further studies should be conducted to determine efficacy. Assessed listed medicines can display the TGA assessed symbol and/or statement on their product.

Registered complementary medicines are also assessed for efficacy by the TGA, and they are used for high-level indications; that is, they may prevent, alleviate or cure a serious form of a medical condition. For example, various preparations that contain ferrous fumarate (a type of iron) are indicated for treating and preventing iron deficiency and iron deficiency anaemias.

Registered complementary medicines can also display the TGA assessed symbol and/or statement to let consumers know the product is supported by scientific evidence.

Regulation in New Zealand

Despite attempts, there is no specific legislation regulating natural health products in New Zealand. Until legislation is developed, a natural health product, if its main

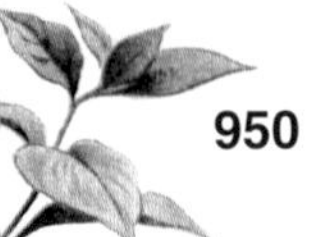

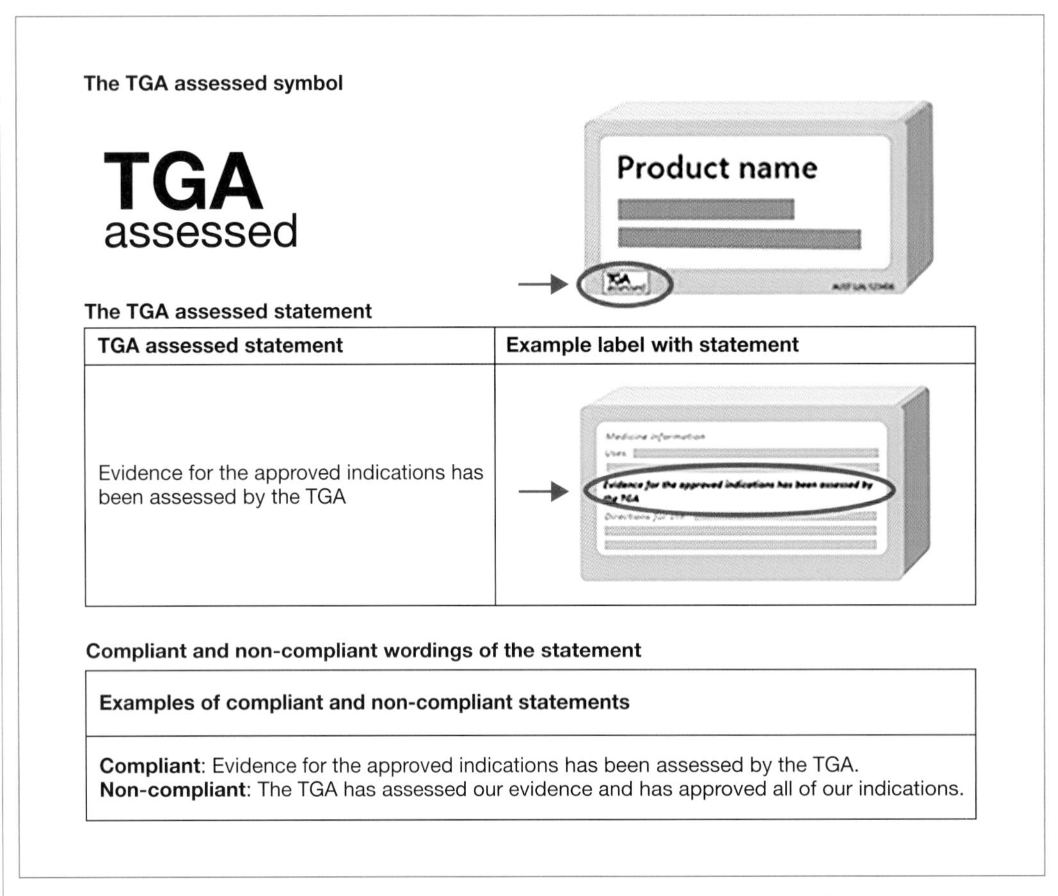

FIGURE 44.1 The 'TGA assessed' symbol and/or statement can be displayed on complementary medicines that have been deemed by the TGA to have scientific evidence of efficacy.

indication is therapeutic, is considered a medicine under the *Medicines Act 1981*. Dietary supplements (vitamin and minerals) are regulated under the Dietary Supplements Regulations 1985 (under the *Food Act 1981*). CAMs derived from animal products are regulated under the *Animal Products Act 1999*.

Natural Products NZ describes itself as the voice of the natural products industry, it says New Zealand has a track record of identifying and exploiting the medicinal uses of local natural products such as manuka honey.

Pharmacological CAM

The primary pharmacological modality in CAM therapies is the administration of herbal products; use dates back to early civilisations, when it was believed that herbal extracts, minerals or folk medicines could treat or cure many illnesses. Table 44.1 lists some common remedies still in use today, available from the kitchen; some of these might now be termed 'functional foods'– for example, active yoghurts, enriched breakfast cereals, iodised salt and sports drinks. Other 'kitchen' ingredients for which medicinal properties are claimed include spices such as cinnamon, cloves and ginger, and herbs such as rosemary, sage, thyme and turmeric.

Herbal remedies

Herbal remedies – that is, using parts or extracts of plants for treatment of illness – have been used for millennia, as described in Chapter 1 in the section on the history of medicine (Table 1.2). Many active prescription drugs in current use were originally discovered from plants such as digitalis glycosides from foxglove, vinca alkaloids from periwinkle and ephedra (ephedrine) from ma huang. Today a wide range of herbal remedies (usually partially purified extracts) are commonly used (Table 44.2).

The principal outlets for sale of herbal products in Australia are health food stores, dispensaries of CAM practitioners and the internet; pharmacies and supermarkets may also carry these products. As an example, relevant information on cranberry is summarised in Drug Monograph 44.1 in our usual format; however, it will be noted that detailed pharmacodynamic and pharmacokinetic information is often unavailable for herbal products. (The definitive textbooks in this field are Braun and Cohen's *Herbs and Natural Supplements* [2017] and Evans' *Pharmacognosy* [2009] – see 'References'.)

Figure 44.2 shows some Australian plants from which herbal medicines are extracted.

TABLE 44.1 Common kitchen or folk remedies and their proposed benefits

REMEDY	POTENTIAL USES OR INDICATIONS	COMMENTS
Celery (*Apium graveolens*)	Anti-inflammatory; to lower serum cholesterol; chemoprotection against cancers	High in sodium; contains coumarins and flavonoids; potential interactions with warfarin
Cocoa (*Theobroma cacao*)	Many actions: antioxidant, central nervous system and cardiovascular stimulant, diuretic, antiplatelet; a highly nutritive food source; may protect against cardiovascular disease and premenstrual syndrome	Chocolate is made from cocoa beans dried, roasted, crushed, alkalinised, then homogenised with sugar, cocoa butter and milk; contains methylxanthines plus many other phenols, amines and minerals
Cranberry (various *Vaccinium* spp.)	Bacteriostatic, antioxidant	Prevention and treatment of UTIs (Drug Monograph 44.2, below)
Fish oils	Antiarrhythmic, lower cholesterol levels and high blood pressure, antithrombotic, anti-inflammatory, neuroprotective, chemoprotective against cancers	Contain two polyunsaturated fatty acids, also various vitamins (Bs, E) and minerals (Clinical Focus Box 44.2)
Garlic (*Allium sativum*)	Antimicrobial, antiplatelet, coronary artery disease, lowers high blood cholesterol, hypertension, antitumour, antioxidant	Garlic contains alliin, which converted to allicin is responsible for garlic odour and potential antibacterial effects; ajoene may be responsible for antithrombotic and antiplatelet effects, and sulfenic acid for free radical scavenging and immunostimulant effects
Green tea (*Camellia sinensis*)	Antioxidant, antimicrobial, anticancer; protection against cardiovascular disease	Green tea is made from leaves that have not been oxidised; it contains flavonoid polyphenols, caffeine and other methylxanthines
Honey	Antibacterial, antiseptic; used in burns and to enhance wound healing (Clinical Focus Box 41.7 in Ch 41)	Constituents depend largely on nectar from which it is derived; may include many acids, esters, flavonoids, enzymes and beeswax
Horseradish (*Armoracia rusticana*)	Irritant to mucous membranes; circulatory and digestive stimulant	Roots contain peroxidase enzymes, volatile oils, glycosides, coumarins, acids
Licorice (liquorice; root of the plant *Glycyrrhiza glabra*)	Has mineralocorticoid and expectorant actions; extract is used as a flavouring agent and in cough mixtures	As a sweet it is compounded with sugars; main saponin is glycyrrhizin; many other ingredients including flavonoids, sterols, coumarins, amines, sugars and oils
Mussels, New Zealand green-lipped (*Perna canaliculus*)	Anti-inflammatory, especially in rheumatoid and osteoarthritis	Bivalve molluscs contain many proteins (especially pernin) and lipids; inhibits synthesis of leukotrienes, hence anti-inflammatory; glycosaminoglycans enhance joint functions
Oats and oatmeal	Lipid-lowering actions, also antihypertensive and hypoglycaemic	Contain soluble fibre, saponins, alkaloids, starch, proteins, coumarins, flavonoids, plus minerals and vitamins
Soy (beans, sauce, tofu; from *Glycine max*)	Selective estrogen receptor actions useful in menopausal symptoms and against cardiovascular disease, osteoporosis and some cancers	Includes isoflavones genistein and daidzein; may have phytoestrogenic and antioxidant activities, and improve cognitive functions
Yoghurt (active strains of *Lactobacillus acidophilus*, *Bifidobacteria bifidum*, etc.)	After diarrhoea, or after oral administration of antibiotics, may enhance immune response, improve digestive processes; may protect against irritable/ inflammatory bowel, peptic ulcers, allergic reactions	'Probiotics'; probably do not survive stomach acid to colonise the GIT, but may assist in re-establishing normal gut flora conditions

Note that 'kitchen remedies' also include various herbs and spices (Table 44.3).
Source: Braun & Cohen 2017, inter alia.

Essential oils and aromatherapy

Essential oils and plant extracts used in aromatherapy, Bach flower products and scented candles provide volatile oils, esters, alcohols and other plant chemicals (Fig 1.3; Table 1.4), which contribute aromas to affect the senses and body functions. Aromatherapy with wildflower essences is used in some hospitals for stress and pain management. Tea-tree oil is a commonly used natural remedy in Australia, and its popularity has spread internationally. It is the essential oil from *Melaleuca alternifolia* and contains terpenes such as cineole. Its main proven actions are antifungal, antibacterial and antiviral (against *Herpes simplex*); it is used particularly in skin infections and inflammations, in podiatry and in cosmetics. It is currently being investigated to treat scabies in Australian Aboriginal children (Thomas et al. 2018).

Non-herbal supplements

Non-herbal supplements include the following:

- 'Biochemicals': Many natural compounds known to have useful biochemical actions also have medicinal properties claimed for them; these include chemicals such as carnitine, creatine, coenzyme Q10, folate (also considered a B vitamin, B9), L-glutamine, lutein, lycopene, L-lysine and policosanol. These can be administered as drugs for their normal actions.
- Animal products: Some other natural supplements with useful actions are animal products such as colostrum, chitosan, chondroitin, fish oils (Clinical Focus Box 44.2), glucosamine and shark cartilage. People who are strict vegetarians may refuse to use these products, and indeed may also refuse hormones produced from animal sources such as conjugated (equine) estrogens and bovine insulin.

TABLE 44.2 Some commonly used herbal remedies

HERB (SCIENTIFIC NAME)	PART USED	CLAIMED ACTIONS AND USES	COMMENTS
Aloes (*Aloe vera*)	Leaves produce resin and gel	Orally, for constipation; topically, heals external wounds and burns; also promoted as a hypoglycaemic agent, anti-inflammatory and for dozens of other uses (Clinical Focus Box 41.2)	Use of aloes to treat burns dates back to ancient Egypt (Cleopatra). A preparation of fresh aloes is effective topically for burns (sunburn, radiation burns) and wound healing; orally, it is a potent laxative
Dandelion (*Taraxacum officinale*)	Leaves, root	Tonic, gastrointestinal distress, mild diuretic, mild laxative	Old native American remedy and food; good source of vitamin A; used to make wine and roasted roots as coffee substitute
Echinacea (*Echinacea* spp.)	Root and leaf	Antiseptic, stimulates immune system, used in respiratory tract infections; anti-inflammatory	Commonly recommended for respiratory tract infections
Evening primrose (*Oenothera* spp.)	Whole plant, oil from seeds	Anti-inflammatory, antithrombotic, speeds wound healing; for cough, sedation, atopic eczema, mastalgia; premenstrual syndrome	Also used in hypertension and diabetes
Feverfew (*Tanacetum parthenium*)	Leaves	Relaxes smooth muscle; anti-inflammatory, analgesic; prophylaxis of migraine	Inhibits serotonin (5-HT) release and blocks receptors
Ginger (*Zingiber officinale*)	Rhizome	Soothes the GIT; prevention of motion sickness	Antiemetic, commonly used in nausea of pregnancy or seasickness
Ginseng, Chinese or Korean (*Panax ginseng*)	Root	Ginsengs are adaptogens, i.e. help the person adapt to physical and mental stress, fatigue and cold Immunostimulant, panacea for many illnesses including adrenal disorders, debility, stress; claimed to provide chemoprotection against cancers	There are claims that ginseng is abused in the West where it is taken as a tonic instead of a medicine (i.e. it should not be taken for more than 6 weeks)
Maidenhair tree (*Ginkgo biloba*)	Mucilage from leaves, seeds	Has antioxidant, vasodilator and antiplatelet actions; alters many CNS transmitters; for circulatory insufficiencies and cognitive impairment	Used for many varied indications, including as a tea for asthma and bronchitis
Noni (kura in Fijian; *Morinda citrifolia*)	All parts	Many actions claimed: analgesic, anti-inflammatory, antioxidant, anticancer, antimicrobial, antihypertensive	Popular medicine in Indian and Pacific cultures; contains alkaloids, terpenes, glycosides, carotene, coumarin, acids; little hard evidence from clinical trials
Saw palmetto (*Serenoa serrulata* or *S. repens*)	Fruit	Diuretic, urinary antiseptic, endocrine and anabolic effects; treatment of prostatic enlargement	Inhibits 5α-reductase and binding of androgens to receptors
Slippery elm (*Ulmus fulva*)	Bark	Gastrointestinal distress, cough, sore throat; topically as a lubricant and poultice for boils and splinters	Has demulcent properties, soothes irritated surfaces such as the GIT and throat
St John's wort (*Hypericum perforatum*)	Herb, flowers	Sedative, astringent for wound healing; neuroses, depression	Many pharmacological actions; enhances many CNS neurotransmitters (Ch 15)
Valerian (*Valeriana officinalis*)	Dried root	Tranquilliser, antispasmodic	Used in insomnia and anxiety

Note: 'Herbal remedies' could also include mainstream drugs originating from plants such as digoxin, morphine, atropine and paclitaxel; also social drugs such as caffeine, nicotine, alcohols and kava kava, and plants listed in Table 44.1.
CNS = central nervous system
Source: Braun & Cohen 2017; inter alia.

Drug Monograph 44.2
Scutellaria / huang qin / Chinese skullcap

This herb is the root from *Scutellaria baicalensis*; it is a component of a popular Chinese and Japanese herbal mixture, Minor Bupleurum Combination, also known as *Xiao Chai Hu Tang* (Mandarin). For simplicity, it will be referred to as *Scutellaria*. The main active constituents are flavonoids baicalin, baicalein and wogonin; melatonin is also present. Medicinal actions are: antibacterial, antiviral, anti-inflammatory, hepatoprotective, antifibrotic, antioxidant, antiallergic and diuretic; other actions claimed include antiemetic, antiplatelet, neuroprotective, anxiolytic, reducing cholesterol, antidiabetic, antiepileptic and as an adjunct in chemotherapy of cancers.

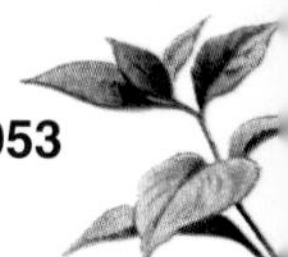

Mechanism of action

Scutellaria reduces the biological activities of pro-inflammatory chemokines; it inhibits the enzymes COX-2, 5-lipoxygenase and nitric oxide synthase, and inhibits NF-κB.

Indications

Scutellaria is indicated in TCM to 'clear heat and dry dampness' (fever, cough, diarrhoea, painful urination); in Western terms, it is indicated for infections and inflammations of the respiratory, intestinal and urinary systems.

Pharmacokinetics

Few details are available; baicalin itself is poorly absorbed from the gut and is hydrolysed to the aglycone. When *Scutellaria* is taken for acute conditions, effects should appear within a few days.

Drug interactions

- Co-administration of *Scutellaria* and interferons in chronic hepatitis is contraindicated.
- *Scutellaria* inhibits CYP1A2 and 2E1, so interactions with drugs metabolised by these enzymes are possible.
- *Scutellaria* may reduce levels of co-administered ciclosporin and increase bleeding with warfarin.

Adverse reactions

Scutellaria is reported to have very low acute and sub-chronic toxicity; however, cases of interstitial pneumonia have been reported.

Precautions and contraindications

Safety in pregnancy is not confirmed; however, the herb is used in TCM to protect the fetus.

Dosage and administration

Scutellaria is administered orally or intravenously. Dosage of dried herb is 6–15 g/day; of the liquid extract (1:2): 30–60 mL/week in divided doses.

Note: A systematic review of randomised controlled trials of intravenous *Scutellaria* (in combination with forsythia) for acute respiratory infections found that it 'may have potential effect on relieving some symptoms such as fever, cough and sore throat'; however, due to the methodological weaknesses of trials, the authors 'cannot make any definite conclusions regarding the clinical effectiveness'.

Source: Zhang et al. 2013.

Homeopathy

Homeopathy is a form of treatment in which diseases are treated by administering minute amounts of substances (minerals, plant extracts, chemicals or microorganisms) that in sufficient amounts would produce a similar set of symptoms in healthy people. It is based on the teachings of a German physician–pharmacist Samuel Hahnemann (1755–1843).

Homeopaths are said to encourage the body's own healing by a 'vital force' – by administering an extract of fresh natural product, a process known as 'proving' the drug. The mother tincture is then diluted thousands of times,[4] with vigorous shaking and tapping (succussion), which is said to increase the 'power' of the medicine. Contaminating the preparation could affect its 'potency'. Formulations include tablets, drops, tinctures and powders.

The lack of scientific rationale for homeopathic principles, in particular the total negation of proven dose–response relationships, and the lack of scientifically acceptable and repeatable evidence for clinical efficacy in randomised controlled double-blind trials, make this modality anathema to pharmacologists trained in pharmacodynamic principles. The lack of scientific validity is exemplified by a homeopathic preparation of Berlin Wall dust, which is claimed to cure every condition from indescribable evil to pushy parents, including both narcolepsy (excessive sleepiness) and insomnia (see 'Online resources').

A meta-analysis systematically reviewed all relevant papers for and against homeopathy, using the Cochrane Database as the source of reviews. The author, himself the Director of Complementary Medicine at the Medical School of the University of Exeter, UK, concluded that 'the most reliable evidence … fails to demonstrate that homeopathic medicines have effects beyond placebo' (Ernst 2010). Recent high-level government investigations of homeopathy in both the UK and Australia have concluded that there is no reliable evidence that homeopathy is effective. It is nonetheless widely practised in Europe and followed by many influential people, including royalty. In Australia, homeopathic preparations are exempt from listing on the Australian Register of Therapeutic Goods by the TGA unless they contain ingredients of human or animal origin, but labels must state that they are not approved by the TGA and cannot claim to cure serious illnesses.

4 In fact, so many times that the dilution goes well below Avogadro's number – that is, less than one in 10^{26}. As a professor of chemistry asked at a seminar on homeopathy: 'By my back-of-tram-ticket calculations, you have a solution with a concentration about equivalent to one molecule in the whole Pacific Ocean. How do you know that you've captured it in your bottle?'

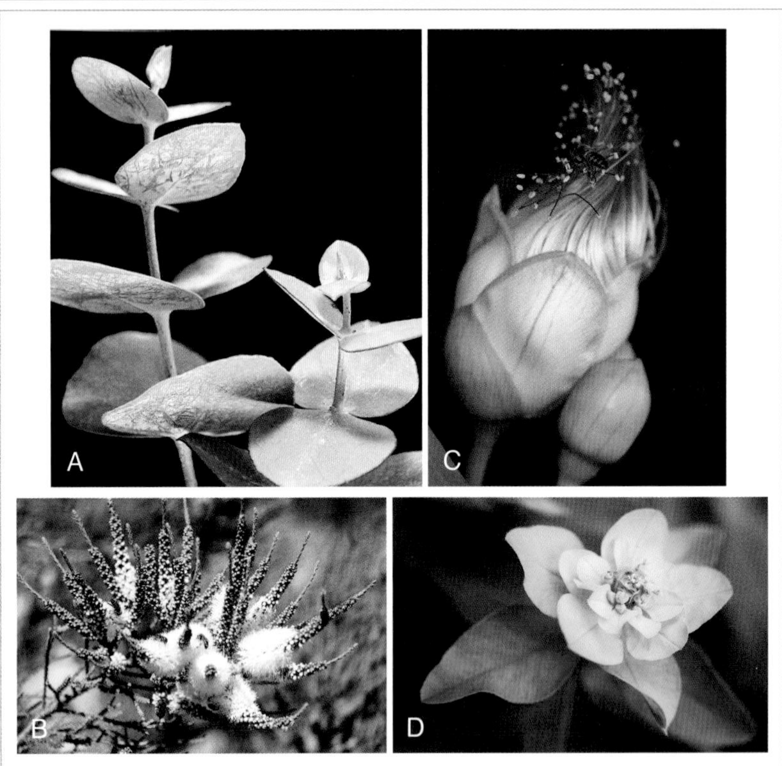

FIGURE 44.2 Some Australian plants from which herbal medicines are extracted

A Eucalyptus (gum trees); **B** *Melaleuca alternifolia*; **C** *Barringtonia asiatica*; **D** *Euphorbia peplus*; **E** St John's wort

A–D iStockphoto/ivanastar; Dreamstime/Alison Underwood; Dreamstime/18042011e; Dreamstime/Mihai-bogdan Lazar; gmayfield10/ under CC BY-SA 2.0; E 'Hypericum perforatum COMMON ST. JOHN'S WORT' by gmayfield10 is licensed under CC BY-SA 2.0. St John's Wort https://www.flickr.com/photos/33397993@N05/3348599281

CLINICAL FOCUS BOX 44.1

What vitamins should I take?

Health professionals are frequently asked – often by 'worried well' people – for advice as to what vitamins should be taken. There are several issues to consider:

- Medical advice may teach that vitamin supplements are a waste of money for people on a good diet.
- Vitamin supplements (e.g. folic acid in pregnancy) can prevent some serious clinical conditions.
- The diet of many people is far from ideal, relying on 'fast foods' and 'junk foods'.
- Vitamins are 'pushed' by the health food industry for profit, with supermarket and pharmacy shelves groaning under the weight of all the products.
- Fragmentation of product types based on gender, age and stage is usually unnecessary.
- 'Bonus ingredients' such as 'power herbs', 'super fruits' and 'power nutrients' are often in such minute doses as to be ineffective.
- Labels are often confusing as to names and quantities present.
- Multivitamin tablets for children – even when packaged with pictures of princesses or superheroes – cannot solve problems of obesity, lack of dietary fibre or saturated fat-filled foods.
- A vitamin pill is no substitute for a healthy lifestyle or diet and cannot begin to compensate for the risks associated with smoking, obesity or inactivity.

Few good randomised controlled clinical trials have been carried out to provide proof of efficacy for multivitamin products, and results from many trials conflict, especially on risks of cancer or heart disease. Most studies confirm there is little or no benefit from supplementation in healthy adults.

CLINICAL FOCUS BOX 44.2

Fish oils and heart disease protection: Truth or a fishy tale?

A great debate rages about fish oils – are they the best way to prevent heart disease? Or the quickest way to waste money in a health food store?

The initial enthusiasm for fish-rich diets came from the observation that Inuit people ('Eskimos') in North America have low rates of heart disease. An association linked this with their high intake of fish, and the assumption was made that omega-3 fatty acids were the active moieties in fish. Theories developed that fish oils will reduce risks of cardiovascular, neurocognitive, ophthalmic, inflammatory, metabolic, behavioural, respiratory and skin disorders.

Omega-3 fatty acids are essential polyunsaturated fatty acids found in seafood, with lesser amounts in eggs and meat; the plant source is less effective. The long-chain omega-3s most important for human health are docosahexaenoic acid (DHA) and eicosapentaenoic acid (EPA); a standard 1000 mg fish oil capsule will usually contain 300 mg DHA+EPA. Recommended intakes vary: suggested DHA+EPA intakes by health foundations are about 610 mg/day for men, and 430 mg/day for women; for arthritis pain relief 3000 mg/day is recommended (10 average capsules, which would tend to cause very 'fishy burps'!). Foods especially high in DHA and EPA are oily fish (e.g. sardines, salmon, caviar and trout); there is no strong evidence that krill oil is more effective than fish oil.

A recent meta-analysis of published trials showed that supplementation reduced total coronary heart disease (clogged arteries), death from coronary heart disease, myocardial infarction, cardiovascular disease and deaths attributed to cardiovascular disease (Hu et al. 2019).

Omega-3s can interact with drugs, especially anticoagulants such as warfarin, making bleeding more likely. Chemical analysis of many fish oil supplements in New Zealand showed that almost 70% contained less than two-thirds of the claimed content of omega-3s and that 50% of samples exceeded recommended levels of oxidised (potentially toxic) fatty acids.

Traditional medicine practices

With the major influxes into Australian society of immigrants from Asian countries, including Vietnam, Korea, China (and Hong Kong) and Indonesia, and in New Zealand from Pacific islands, there is increased interest in and usage of traditional medical practices. The concepts of 'holistic medicine' – that is, considering the whole person – and of public health measures and prevention, are combining various medical philosophies into 'integrative medicine'.

Australian Indigenous medicine

The traditional Indigenous Australian beliefs about causation of illness emphasise social and spiritual dysfunction as the main causes, with supernatural intervention causing serious illness. A large part of maintaining health was eating the right foods, and some quite sophisticated 'bush medicine' methods were developed.

Bush medicine usage predates Western medicine by many millennia and is still preserved and implemented today. Active constituents of plants, such as tannins, oils, mucilages, latex and gums, vary in strength seasonally and geographically. Traditionally, plants were used as fresh preparations in a range of ways: for inhalation of aromatic oil vapour or of crushed leaves, drinking an infusion of leaves or bark, as 'kinos' (resins and gums), and crushed plants for topical administration as poultices or ointments.

Plants commonly used as 'Aboriginal bush medicines' include:

- tea-tree oil (from *Melaleuca* spp.) – crushed leaves and oil used for antiseptic actions
- eucalyptus oil, from infused leaves, in mouthwashes, throat lozenges and inhalants
- Kakadu plum/Billy goat plum (*Terminalia ferdinandiana*), a major source of food and vitamin C
- Gumbi Gumbi (*Pittosporum angustifolium*) for coughs, colds and dermatitis, and to induce lactation
- desert mushrooms (*Pycnoporus* spp.) to cure a sore mouth or oral thrush
- emu bush (*Eremophila* spp.) – antibiotic activity used as an oral antiseptic and gargle
- witchetty grub (*Endoxyla leucomochla*) – bush tucker, and as a paste to treat burns
- snake vine (*Tinospora smilacina*) for headaches and inflammatory conditions
- sandpaper fig (*Ficus opposita*) and stinking passionflower (*Passiflora foetida*) – combination to relieve itching and treat fungal infections
- kangaroo apple (*Solanum laciniatum* and *S. aviculare*) – fruit used as a poultice (contains a steroid useful in production of cortisone)
- goat's foot (*Ipomoea pes-caprae*) – crushed leaves applied to stings.

The knowledge of preparation and use of medicinal plants has largely been inherited through oral tradition and singing/dancing ceremonies. Traditional tribal healers are identified early and given special training by older healers, often the grandmothers in the tribe. Unfortunately, these practices are becoming more infrequent as people are displaced from their lands, family structures change and the number of tribal elders with such knowledge diminishes, and there is therefore concern that much of this invaluable information may be lost.

Traditional Māori medicine: rongoā māori

Rongoā is the Māori term for medicines produced from New Zealand native plants – their use has prevented and treated many sicknesses. Diagnosis involved a holistic approach that included *mauri* (spark or life force), *wairua* (spirit), *tapu* (natural law) and *whakapapa* or genealogy. Tohunga, the medical practitioners of the world, passed their knowledge down through the generations; they were skilled in the use of healing plants, made *rongoā* or tonics and preparations and used massage, incantations and steam and heat applications. Many of these concepts and practices are used by modern Māori healers (see Rongoā Māori – 'Online resources').

Indigenous Māori medicinal plants

Plants must be collected properly, taking care not to damage trees, before preparing the medicines according to custom. Some traditional remedies are now produced commercially. Some common New Zealand plants used for *rongoā* are:

- *harakeke* (New Zealand flax) – sticky gum used topically for wounds and burns; leaves used to bind broken bones, juice as an antiseptic and the root for intestinal problems
- *koromiko* – leaves used to treat diarrhoea and dysentery, ulcers, sores, headaches, kidney and bladder problems
- *kowhai* – all plant parts used, but contains toxic alkaloids so care is required; used to treat internal ailments, colds and sore throats and skin wounds
- *pohutukawa* (New Zealand Christmas bush) – extracts made by the *tohunga* had *tapu* (sacred) status; bark extracts used to treat diarrhoea and dysentery; nectar (honey) from flowers used to treat sore throats; essential oils extracted from bark.

Other traditional medicine practices

Traditional Chinese medicine

In **traditional Chinese medicine** (TCM), maintaining an energy balance in the body is most important for good health: a balance between yin (negative) and yang (positive) forces. Chinese physicians may prescribe a variety of interventions such as herbal therapy (Drug Monograph 44.2: *Scutellaria*), acupuncture (shallow insertion of fine sterile needles into specific points on the body), moxibustion (burning the herb moxa [*Artemisia vulgaris*] to warm and stimulate painful parts), diet changes, exercise (tai chi) and meditation.

Chinese herbal remedies

In TCM, herbs are described by their properties – for example, heat-clearing herbs, *Qi*-regulating herbs; they are taken orally or applied externally. Texts describe the philosophy and techniques for harvesting, production and application of the materials. A typical TCM herbal formula may contain eight to 15 herbs; it is believed that herbal preparations are much more effective when used in a balanced formula (see example in Clinical Focus Box 44.3, below); however, there is little scientific evidence for this.

African traditional medicine

Traditional medicine practitioners in many African countries include herbalists, midwives, bone-setters, faith healers and spiritualists. Disease is considered to arise not only from physical and psychological causes but also from astral, spiritual and other esoteric causes. Traditional practices may include herbal, mineral and animal remedies, administered orally as liquids, topically as powders, ointments or balsams, or by inhalation; also diets and fasting, hydrotherapy or dry heat therapy, surgical operations, bloodletting, spinal manipulation, faith healing and occultism.

African remedies have provided several important drugs: physostigmine (an anticholinesterase), yohimbine (an α-receptor antagonist), reserpine (an antihypertensive and neuroleptic agent) and ouabain (a cardiac glycoside). Other potentially valuable indigenous plants, including *Pelargonium* spp., *Harpagophytum* and 'devil's claw', are being assessed for pharmacological activity.

Ayurvedic medicine

Ayurveda, the indigenous healing system of India, has been practised there for more than 5000 years, focusing on prevention and self-care to restore health balance. It incorporates exercise, diet, life activities, psychotherapeutic methods, massage and botanical medicine. Herbal mixtures and preparations known as *rasayanas* are used, along with common spices including:

- turmeric (curcumin) in wound healing, rheumatic disorders, rhinitis, gastrointestinal disorders, worm infestations, decreasing DNA damage and reducing tumour formation
- fenugreek seeds in reducing blood glucose and lipid levels.

Garlic, onions and ginger have all been shown to impair the process of carcinogenesis.

CLINICAL FOCUS BOX 44.3
Herbal products: use and risks in Australia

Four pharmacologists based in universities in Adelaide and Perth have recently studied the usage of herbal products in Australia (Byard et al. 2017) and examined the range of problems encountered from both raw materials and processed products. Here are some of their findings:

- Herbal medicines may appear to have few adverse effects reported, but this may be simply due to lack of systematic observations.
- Products have been found adulterated with pharmaceutical drugs to increase their apparent efficacy; ostensibly herbal products have been found containing antiepileptic drugs, antibiotics, antihistamines, corticosteroids, benzodiazepines, anti-inflammatories and antidiabetic agents.
- Adulteration poses risks of allergies, toxicities and drug interactions.
- Cheaper plants have been substituted for rare or expensive plants, either deliberately or due to errors.
- Contaminants that are hepatotoxic have caused severe liver disease requiring transplantation.
- Poisonous toad venoms have been knowingly added to preparations to increase their 'potency' by stimulating the heart.
- Heavy metals such as arsenic, lead and thallium are essential components of some traditional medicines, and toxic levels have been found.
- Depending on their method of preparation and storage, herbal products may also contain pesticides, herbicides, microorganisms and insects.

Byard and colleagues (2017) noted that 'a major area of concern is the potential interaction of herbal medicines with conventional drugs, both prescribed and over-the-counter products'. Drug–herbal interactions are particularly common with St John's wort, and also with ginseng, evening primrose oil and garlic. They quote recommendations from the American Society of Anesthesiologists that 'herbal medicines should not be taken for at least 2 weeks before surgery' because of possible interactions, especially from herbs affecting blood coagulation, cardiovascular stability and sedation.

In Australia, the sale of herbal products is very profitable: they are advertised and strongly advocated in popular media but not balanced with warnings as to possible problems and adverse effects.

Source: Byard et al. 2017.

Traditional medicine in the Pacific region

In the southwest Pacific region – from Palau in the west, through Vanuatu, Fiji, Samoa and Tonga, to the Cook Islands and Kiribati in the east – waves of settlements with Pacific peoples and European colonists brought many plants found useful for medicinal purposes, plus traditional remedies, leading to a rich mixture of medicine practices. Vulnerable populations were devastated by European contact, which brought new epidemics such as measles, smallpox, cholera and venereal diseases. As Western lifestyles develop, now non-communicable diseases are the main public health problems: obesity, diabetes and cardiovascular disease.

Fijian traditional remedies

In Fiji, diseases were traditionally considered to be *mate vayano* – illnesses from accidental circumstances, such as coughs, headache and injuries – or *mate ni vanua* – diseases of the land caused by magic, behaviour or sorcerers. The *dauvakatevoro* (people who could control evil spirits) might use herbs, secretions of the victim or *yagona* (kava preparations). Traditional plant remedies were used as 'tonics', emetics, inhalations, ointments and poultices to treat infections, wounds, infertility, menstrual problems, respiratory disorders and so on. The chemical properties and pharmacological activities of many have been verified. The best-known Pacific herbal product is of course *kava* (*yagona*, or 'grog'), an extract of powdered root and stem of *Piper methysticum*, used in social and religious ceremonies (Ch 25), and as a diuretic, a panacea for various complaints, a contraceptive and applied to wounds. It is also widely known that heavy use leads to a condition called kava dermopathy (or scaly skin).

Some other examples of traditional Fijian remedies are:

- *davui* (*Datura candida*), containing hyoscine (leaves smoked for asthma)
- *niu* (*Cocos nucifera*), the coconut – as a vermifuge, for pains, as an emetic and purgative, and for kidney troubles, headache and to treat fish poisoning
- kura (*Morinda citrifolia*), known in Indian communities as *noni* – multiple uses (Table 44.2 above).

Issues related to CAM

Potential problems related to the use of CAM therapies are much the same as those related to the clinical use of any drugs – see Figure 2.2: 'Questions to ask and answer when prescribing a drug'. In addition, there are extra

issues due to the lack of objective scientific scrutiny of most CAM products.

Evidence-based complementary medicine?

To be officially approved, Western therapies are required to be based on sound scientific principles of safety and efficacy (and cost-effectiveness), with objective reproducible evidence published in peer-reviewed scientific journals (**evidence-based medicine**, EBM). CAM therapies, however, are often based on 'anecdotal evidence', personal experiences and time-honoured practices, possibly never submitted to randomised controlled clinical trials. Practitioners of CAM therapies often argue that their treatments are not conducive to scientific testing but are individualised to each person. Consequently, statistically valid scientific evidence concerning the safety and efficacy of many alternative medicine methods is usually lacking.

CAMs for which good supporting evidence at the EBM standard exists include fish oil, coenzyme Q10, St John's wort, *Ginkgo biloba*, glucosamine, echinacea, ginger, kava, peppermint, tea-tree oil and valerian.

Lack of evidence of efficacy

Consumers tend to assume that if products are allowed on the market, they must be effective and safe. However, while thousands of CAM 'remedies' are listed by the TGA, very few are in fact registered or listed (assessed) products that have been tested for efficacy. For example, while some echinacea products may be effective in adults, echinacea has been shown to be ineffective in treating children with colds. Many CAM products are 'prescribed' by practitioners without any evidence of their efficacy (see case study, Clinical Focus Box 44.4).

The placebo effect

Edzard Ernst, Professor of CAM at the University of Exeter in the UK, has carried out rigorous clinical trials and meta-analyses of hundreds of CAM treatments, ranging from acupuncture and herbal remedies to crystal healing and reflexology. His group's definitive *Desktop Guide to Complementary and Alternative Medicine* (Ernst et al. 2001) concludes that around 95% of the treatments tested are statistically indistinguishable from placebos (known ineffective methods such as a 'sugar pill' or sham procedure). The placebo effect is strongest for disorders with subjective and emotional components, such as pain and depression. Professor Ernst acknowledges the therapeutic value of 'the placebo effect', especially as CAM practitioners often have time to spend with patients and are passionate about their treatments. However, placebos can waste money and time, and those taking them can also complain of adverse effects.

CLINICAL FOCUS BOX 44.4
Toxic herbs

A female was brought into an emergency department with possible atypical pneumonia, plus post-viral fatigue after severe glandular fever and Epstein-Barr virus infections. Recently, she had been taking 30 (repeat: *30*) herbal tablets prescribed by a local TCM practitioner each day. Each tablet allegedly contained seven herbs in minute amounts (9–25 mg), plus various other natural products.

The concerned emergency department doctors did a quick search through reference sources to determine whether any of the ingredients might be potentially effective or toxic. They found that:

- *Prunella vulgaris* is used at a dose of 10–15 g to clear liver fire and phlegm fire.
- *Scrophularia nodosa* (10–15 g) is used for sore throat, boils, goitre and fevers.
- *Angelica polymorpha* is a stimulating expectorant, used to raise blood glucose levels.
- *Mentha haplocalyx*, 'mint' (2–10 g), is used to clear the head and liver, and as a mild antiseptic and anticolic agent.
- *Citrus aurantium*, sweet orange fruit (3–10 g), is used for liver, spleen, cough and as a flavouring agent.
- *Rheum palmatum*, rhubarb, is a laxative and astringent.
- *Fritillaria thunbergii* is distasteful and poisonous.

It was quickly realised that, while some of the herbs were possibly useful in respiratory infections, the 'doses' in the tablets were far too low to be effective, even if 30 tablets were taken daily. On the other hand, *Fritillaria thunbergii* is potentially poisonous. The person was advised to cease taking the herbal tablets and, after ceasing and then treatment with appropriate antibiotics, made a full recovery.

Source: Personal communication from Dr Philippa Shilson, Geelong; acknowledged with thanks.

Lack of evidence of safety

It has been stated that any medicine powerful enough to do some good is also powerful enough to do some harm; many natural products are indeed toxic, and some CAM procedures are dangerous (see below, under 'Adverse reactions'). Long-term trials may be needed to show up adverse effects.

Lack of pharmacodynamic or pharmacokinetic data

Drug companies seeking product approval by government bodies such as the TGA in Australia or the FDA in the United States must submit results of many years' testing in vitro, in animals and in humans, with detailed information as to the drug's actions and mechanisms of action (pharmacodynamics) and fate in the body (pharmacokinetics); this is not required of companies seeking marketing approval for CAM products. Pharmacokinetic studies on CAM preparations are complicated, as preparations vary widely in number and strength of constituents. Some common CAM medicines have been subjected to pharmacokinetic analysis – for example, St John's wort, echinacea, milk thistle, ginseng, ginkgo and ginger.

Lack of a full drug history

Health professionals taking a medication history should always ask about the person's use of **over-the-counter (OTC) medicines**, health food store therapies and herbal products, which are often not considered by the consumer to be drugs or medications and therefore not reported; however, they can interact with prescribed medicines and with food. Caution with respect to CAM therapies should in particular be exercised by women who are pregnant or breastfeeding, and by people with serious medical conditions.

Potential risks

The potential risks of CAM have been neatly summarised as follows:

- direct harm, such as adverse reactions and interactions (e.g. liver impairment from black cohosh and chaparral)
- indirect harm, from delay in obtaining effective treatment due to misinformation about the effectiveness of a CAM method (e.g. laetrile touted as a cancer cure)
- economic harm (e.g. people wasting money and governments committing funds to regulation, investigation and subsidisation of ineffective 'treatments', and money spent by companies on marketing and advertising).

Some more examples of risks with CAM products will be given briefly below; see also Chapter 7: 'Adverse drug reactions and drug interactions'.

Adverse reactions

Just as prescribed and synthetic drugs can cause adverse reactions, so many natural products can cause harm,[6] depending on the herb itself, the quantity consumed, whether the correct plant or part of the plant is present in the product, the presence of contaminants and other factors. Some serious problems have been reported in the medical literature (Table 44.3). Other examples are:

- Chaparral, promoted as a blood purifier and cancer cure, has caused serious liver damage, even requiring liver transplant after 10 months of use.
- Echinacea, one of the most popular CAMs, has caused asthma, rashes, aching muscles, GIT upsets and ocular adverse effects, and is contraindicated in people prone to allergies or with autoimmune disorders.
- Carp gall bladder contains 5-α-cyprinol sulfate, which is toxic to the liver and kidneys.
- Common plants known to be toxic include wisteria, agapanthus, daffodil and jonquil, lantana, oleander, poinsettia, primula, Angel's trumpet, privet, peach and apricot kernels, rhubarb leaves, some lilies and green potatoes.

CAM therapies other than herbal or animal products have also caused serious adverse effects such as:

- cervical manipulations causing cerebrovascular accidents (strokes)
- acupuncture leading to infections, trauma and pneumothorax
- homeopathic preparations containing toxic concentrations of heavy metals.

Drug interactions

Just as prescribed and OTC drugs can interact by various mechanisms – pharmaceutical, pharmacokinetic and pharmacodynamic (Ch 7) – so, too, can CAM drugs interact with each other, with food and with other drugs the person is taking. Natural or herbal products may contain unidentified ingredients that cause serious drug interactions or interfere with results of laboratory tests. The risk of interactions rises exponentially with the number of medicines a person takes.

Most commonly used herbal remedies have some potentially serious drug interactions related to their use, so reference lists should be consulted before advising their use and particularly if adverse effects or interactions are suspected (Braun & Cohen 2017). Some examples are as follows:

- Significant interactions involving evening primrose oil, garlic, ginkgo, glucosamine, hawthorn, kava, St John's wort and valerian; drugs most likely to be affected were warfarin, insulin, aspirin, digoxin, ticlopidine, oral contraceptives, antihypertensives, anticonvulsants and other central nervous system drugs.
- Many herbal compounds (capsaicin from chili peppers, sulfones in garlic, methysticins in kava, and resveratrol in grapes) are inhibitors of CYP450

6 There is a widespread belief that 'if it's natural, it can't harm you', whereas drugs made into tablets, ointments, injections and so on must be viewed as dangerous. A cursory consideration of a few natural substances such as arsenic, strychnine, thallium, atropine, digoxin, opium, deadly nightshade, tobacco and uranium will soon show this belief to be naive and unfounded.

TABLE 44.3 Some herbal preparations with a potential for toxicity

BOTANICAL NAME	COMMON NAMES	TOXICITY AND COMMENTS
Aconitum spp.	Monkshood	Various alkaloids may be cardiotoxic and cause convulsions
Aesculus spp.	Buckeyes, horse chestnut, aesculus	Coumarin glycosides may interfere with normal blood clotting
Amanita spp.	Mushrooms	Alkaloids including muscarine and muscimol have powerful cholinergic effects; can be fatal
Areca catechu	Betel nut and leaf	Chewed in many cultures as a euphoriant and intoxicant; users have a high incidence of mouth cancers
Aristolochia spp.	Birthwort, serpentary	Aristolochic acids in *Aristolochia* species are metabolised by CYP1A1/2 to highly reactive charged ions, which can activate oncogenes, cause mutations in renal cells and eventually kidney cancers
Arnica montana	Arnica flowers, wolfsbane, mountain tobacco	Extremely irritating and can induce toxic gastroenteritis, nervous system disturbances, extreme muscle weakness, cardiovascular collapse and even death
Artemisia absinthium	Wormwood, absinthe, madderwort, mugwort	Contains a narcotic poison (oil of wormwood); can cause nervous system damage and mental impairment
Atropa belladonna (also *Brugmansia* spp.)	Belladonna, deadly nightshade (Angel's trumpet)	Contain the toxic alkaloids atropine, hyoscyamine and hyoscine. Anticholinergic symptoms range from blurred vision, dry mouth and inability to urinate, to unusual behaviours and hallucinations
Conium maculatum	Hemlock, conium, spotted parsley, St Bennet's herb, spotted cowbane	Contains the toxic alkaloid coniine and other related alkaloids; the poison that killed Socrates
Datura stramonium	Thornapple	Formerly used in witches' brews and initiatory rites; source of hyoscyamine and atropine (see 'Atropa', above)
Digitalis purpurea	Purple foxglove	Contains digitalis and related cardiac glycosides; can cause dysrhythmias and hypotension
Ephedra sinica	Ma huang, ephedra	Contains sympathomimetics ephedrine and possibly pseudoephedrine; can raise blood pressure and heart rate; used to make methamphetamine ('speed') and as an alternative to 'ecstasy', illegal street drugs
Glycyrrhiza spp.	Licorice	Has mineralocorticoid actions; may cause hypertension
Lobelia inflata	Lobelia, Indian tobacco, asthma weed, emetic weed	Contains lobeline plus other alkaloids; excessive use causes severe vomiting, pain, sweating, paralysis, low temperature, coma and death
Panax ginseng (and others)	Ginseng	Estrogenic effects, hypoglycaemia, hypertension
Prunus armeniaca	Apricot	Kernels contain amygdalin and release cyanide: acute poisoning causes severe GIT toxicity, chronic toxicity causes neurological damage, in pregnant women can cause fetal cretinism
Symphytum spp.	Comfrey	Pyrrolizidine alkaloids, which are hepatotoxic
Vinca major, *Vinca minor*	Periwinkle, vinca	Alkaloids (vinblastine, vincristine) are cytotoxic (used to treat cancer) and may cause liver, kidney and neurological damage

drug-metabolising enzymes and so can cause potentially adverse interactions with prescribed and OTC drugs.

- Supplements containing antioxidants and estrogenic compounds may antagonise cancer therapies rather than 'complement' them.
- The TGA issues alerts about complementary medicines on its website; alerts have included warnings of interactions between many prescription medicines and St John's wort, which appears to act as a P-glycoprotein (P-gp) drug efflux transport system inducer.

Contaminated products

Regulation in Australia by the TGA requires that therapeutic goods be manufactured, prepared and standardised according to the standards of Good Manufacturing Practice; however, adulterated, contaminated or poor-quality products are sold by unscrupulous practitioners. Contaminants (adulterants) are frequently found in natural products; such **contamination** is potentially dangerous if the person is taking the 'natural' products in addition to prescribed drugs or is allergic to any of the unexpected ingredients. Contaminants may be natural, such as the heavy metals lead, arsenic, mercury and thallium found in some imported preparations or remaining in homeopathic solutions as they are successively diluted. In other cases, synthetic drugs have been found in supposed natural products; documented cases include:

- synthetic non-steroidal anti-inflammatory drugs found in supposed 'herbal' preparations for treating inflammation
- synthetic oral hypoglycaemic agents in 'herbs' used to treat diabetes
- animal products (including parts of the critically endangered Asiatic black bear) in imported Chinese medicines

- Chinese medicines containing aristolochic acid (carcinogenic, a banned product) in *Asarum* plant material
- a product claiming to contain 100% antelope horn powder that actually also contained goat and sheep DNA
- products containing up to 30 chemicals, some highly allergenic, but not shown on labels
- 'herbal' slimming and weight loss products found to contain prescription drugs (propranolol, nifedipine and ephedrine) as well as dangerous drugs withdrawn from the Australian market (sibutramine, fenfluramine and phenolphthalein)
- supposedly all-natural 'vitamin pills' targeting women with low libido, found to contain sildenafil (Viagra) used to treat male impotence
- 'do-it-yourself' injectable cosmetic kits containing dermal fillers and Botox-type products, which have caused severe facial scarring and allergic reactions.

People are particularly warned against purchasing unknown products online; the products most marketed fraudulently on the internet are treatments for hair loss, impotence and obesity.

False or misleading advertising

Post-marketing compliance reviews of TGA-listed products have shown that up to 90% of products reviewed were noncompliant with government regulations, most commonly in the areas of misleading labelling and inadequate evidence to substantiate claims made for safety and efficacy. Some producers are labelling products as 'food for special medical purposes', which allows them to circumvent the TGA's advertising code for therapeutic goods. 'Statistics' are perpetuated despite absence of proof; and labelling of remedies is often inadequate, with insufficient information as to dose, storage, contraindications, likely adverse effects and interactions, antidotes or instructions for use.

Other issues

Thus the main issues with respect to the use of complementary and alternative therapies relate to: the lack of scientific evidence available to prove safety and efficacy; the variability between preparations of the same herb in purity and strength; and the belief that natural methods and substances are harmless. Other aspects of the use of CAM therapies that may result in problems include:

- practitioner qualifications in some fields not being subject to regulation and substantiation
- a wide range of treatments often being recommended, with little agreement between practitioners as to the remedy of first choice in a particular condition
- CAM therapies being used for conditions in which they are contraindicated or dangerous
- issues related to costs – people, governments and health insurers may waste money on useless 'remedies'
- health policymakers being subjected to pressure from proponents of CAM therapies and neglecting the need for clinical trials
- patients with serious illnesses (especially cancer) relying on CAM therapies and denying their need for effective 'Western' medicine
- combination products in which ingredients have very different half-lives, or doses that cannot be adjusted to suit individual patients
- people rarely being warned to use the remedies only for short periods.

KEY POINTS

Complementary and alternative medicine products

- A wide range of CAM therapies are available for use, including psychological, physical, dietary and pharmacological modalities.
- Only registered and listed (assessed) complementary medicines are assessed by the TGA for efficacy. Most CAMs are listed and therefore consumers and health professionals need to use such products with caution and be responsible for detecting any unusual or adverse reactions with listed products.
- A thorough medication history requires noting all medicines being taken, including prescribed, OTC and CAM products; close monitoring is recommended.
- Traditional medical practices among indigenous populations in Australasian, Asian, Pacific Island and African countries may differ in philosophies and ranges of treatments from Western scientific medicine; combinations of types of medical treatments are commonly used.
- The main issues related to the increasing use of CAM therapies are the frequent absence of proof of safety and efficacy; the potential for adverse effects and drug interactions; inadequate information as to strength, purity, pharmacodynamic or pharmacokinetic properties or administration; contamination and adulteration; false advertising; costs; and delay in effective treatment of serious conditions.

REVIEW QUESTIONS

1. Mr TO, a patient, asks you if the fish oil (omega-3 fatty acid) that he bought from the supermarket is 'any good', and if it is 'any good', can he stop taking his heart medicines from his doctor? Discuss your answer to Mr TO.
2. You are taking a medication history for one of your female patients. She presents you with a plastic container of all of her medicines. You note that some of the complementary medicines have an AUST R number, some an AUST L number and some an AUST L(A) number. Describe the difference in the three different categories of complementary medicines.
3. As a health professional you would like to look up the pharmacokinetic and pharmacodynamic data related to several complementary medicines your patient is taking. When you conduct your search, you find there is limited data. Why might this be the case?

REFERENCES

Braun, L., Cohen, M. Essential herbs and natural supplements. 2017: Elsevier.

Byard, RW, Musgrave, I, Maker, G, et al., What risks do herbal products pose to the Australian community? Medical Journal of Australia, 2017. 206(2): 86–90.

Ernst, E, Homeopathy: what does the "best" evidence tell us? Medical Journal of Australia, 2010. 192(8): 458–460.

Ernst, E, Pittler MH, Stevinson C, et al, editors. The desktop guide to complementary and alternative medicine: an evidence-based approach. 2001: Mosby International Ltd, St Louis.

Evans, WC. Trease and Evans' pharmacognosy E-book. 2009: Elsevier Health Sciences.

Hu, Y, Hu, FB, Manson, JE. Marine omega-3 supplementation and cardiovascular disease: an updated meta-analysis of 13 randomized controlled trials involving 127 477 participants. Journal of the American Heart Association, 2019. 8(19): e013543.

Lee, EL, J Harrison, and J Barnes, Mapping prevalence and patterns of use of, and expenditure on, traditional, complementary and alternative medicine in New Zealand: a scoping review of qualitative and quantitative studies. The New Zealand Medical Journal (Online), 2021. 134(1541): 57–74.

Steel, A, McIntyre, E, Harnett, J, et al., Complementary medicine use in the Australian population: results of a nationally representative cross-sectional survey. Scientific Reports, 2018. 8(1): 1–7.

Thomas, J, Davey, R, Peterson, GM, et al., Treatment of scabies using a tea tree oil-based gel formulation in Australian Aboriginal children: protocol for a randomised controlled trial. BMJ Open, 2018. 8(5): e018507.

World Health Organization. WHO global report on traditional and complementary medicine 2019. 2019: World Health Organization.

Zhang, H, Cen, Q, Zhou, W, et al., Chinese medicine injection shuanghuanglian for treatment of acute upper respiratory tract infection: a systematic review of randomized controlled trials. Evidence-Based Complementary and Alternative Medicine, 2013. 2013. Article ID 987326.

ONLINE RESOURCES

Bush Medijina – What is bush medicine?: https://bushmedijina.com.au/pages/bush-medicine (accessed 5 November 2021)

National Health and Medical Research Council – Complementary medicines: https://www.nhmrc.gov.au/health-advice/all-topics/complementary-medicines (accessed 5 November 2021)

New Zealand Ministry of Health – Natural health products: https://www.health.govt.nz/our-work/regulation-health-and-disability-system/natural-health-and-supplementary-products (accessed 5 November 2021)

New Zealand Ministry of Health – Rongoā Māori: https://www.health.govt.nz/our-work/populations/maori-health/rongoa-maori-traditional-maori-healing (accessed 5 November 2021)

Therapeutic Goods Administration – Advisory Committee on Complementary Medicines: https://www.tga.gov.au/committee/advisory-committee-complementary-medicines-accm (accessed 5 November 2021)

Therapeutic Goods Administration – Complementary medicines: https://www.tga.gov.au/complementary-medicines (accessed 5 November 2021)

More weblinks at: http://evolve.elsevier.com/AU/Knights/pharmacology/.

APPENDIX 1

ABBREVIATIONS

5-HT	5-hydroxytryptamine (serotonin)
ABC	ATP binding cassette
ACE	angiotensin-converting enzyme
ACh	acetylcholine
AChE	acetylcholinesterase
ACTH	adrenocorticotrophic hormone (corticotrophin)
ADH	antidiuretic hormone (argipressin)
ADHD	attention deficit hyperactivity disorder
ADP	adenosine diphosphate
ADR	adverse drug reaction
AED	antiepileptic drug
Ahpra	Australian Health Practitioners Regulation Agency
AIDS	acquired immunodeficiency syndrome
AMD	age-related macular degeneration
AMH	*Australian Medicines Handbook*
ANP	atrial natriuretic peptide
ANS	autonomic nervous system
APF	*Australian Pharmaceutical Formulary and Handbook*
aPTT	activated partial thromboplastin time
AR	androgen receptor
ARB	angiotensin receptor blocker
ATP	adenosine triphosphate
AUC	area under the plasma concentration versus time curve
AV	atrioventricular
BCC/SCC	basal/squamous cell carcinoma
BGL	blood glucose level
BMI	body mass index
BNP	B-type natriuretic peptide
BP	British Pharmacopoeia
BPH	benign prostatic hyperplasia (or hypertrophy)
CA	carbonic anhydrase
CAD	coronary artery disease
CAM	complementary and alternative medicine
cAMP	cyclic 3,5-adenosine monophosphate
CF	cystic fibrosis
COPD	chronic obstructive pulmonary disease
DPI	dry powder inhaler
GMP	guanosine monophosphate
cAMP	cyclic adenosine monophosphate
CCK	cholecystokinin
CDK	cyclin-dependent kinase
cGMP	cyclic guanosine monophosphate
CKD	chronic kidney disease
CL	clearance
CL_S	systemic clearance
CMI	consumer medicine information
CMV	cytomegalovirus
CNP	C-type natriuretic peptide
CNS	central nervous system
CO	cardiac output
COC	combined oral contraceptive
COMT	catechol-*O*-methyltransferase
COX	cyclo-oxygenase
CrCl	creatinine clearance
CRF	corticotrophin-releasing factor
CSF	cerebrospinal fluid
CSF	colony-stimulating factor
C_{SS}	steady-state plasma drug concentration
Cth	Commonwealth
CTN	Clinical Trial Notification
CTZ	chemoreceptor trigger zone
CYP	cytochrome P450
DA	dopamine
DAA	direct-acting antiviral
DBI	drug burden index
DDC	dopa decarboxylase
DDCI	dopa decarboxylase inhibitor
DDI	drug–drug interaction
DHT	dihydrotestosterone
DMARDs	disease-modifying antirheumatic drugs
DNA	deoxyribonucleic acid
DOPA	dihydroxyphenylalanine
DOR	δ-opioid receptor
DPP4	dipeptidyl peptidase-4
DTPa	diphtheria-tetanus acellular pertussis vaccine (paediatric formulation)
dTpa	diphtheria-tetanus vaccine acellular pertussis vaccine (reduced antigen formulation)

DUE	drug use evaluation
EAA	excitatory amino acids
EBM	evidence-based medicine
EBM/P	evidence-based medicine/practice
ECT	electroconvulsive therapy
EE	ethinylestradiol
EEG	electroencephalograph
EGF	epithelial growth factor
eGFR	estimated glomerular filtration rate
E_H	hepatic extraction ratio
EM	extensive metaboliser
EMLA	eutectic mixture for local anaesthesia
eNOS	endothelium nitric oxide synthase
ENT	extraneuronal transporter
EO	endogenous opioids
EPO	erythropoietin
ER	estrogen receptor
ESBL	extended spectrum β-lactamases
F	bioavailability
FDA	US Food and Drug Administration
FRIDs	fall risk-increasing drugs
FSH	follicle-stimulating hormone
FTO	fat mass and obesity-associated gene
GA	general anaesthesia
GABA	gamma-aminobutyric acid
G-CSF	granulocyte colony-stimulating factor
GDP	guanosine diphosphate
GFR	glomerular filtration rate
GH	growth hormone (somatotropin)
GHB	gamma-hydroxybutyrate
GHRIF	growth hormone release-inhibiting factor
GIT	gastrointestinal tract
GLP	glucagon-like peptide
GLP-1	glucagon-like peptide-1
GnRH	gonadotrophin-releasing hormone
GORD	gastro-oesophageal reflux disease
GPCR	G-protein-coupled receptors
GR	glucocorticoid receptor
GRE	glucocorticoid response elements
GTN	glyceryl trinitrate
GTP	guanosine triphosphate
HBV	hepatitis B
hCG	human chorionic gonadotrophin
HCV	hepatitis C
HDL	high-density lipoproteins
Hib	*Haemophilus influenzae* type b
HIV	human immunodeficiency virus
HLA	human leucocyte antigen
HMG-CoA	3-hydroxy-3-methylglutaryl coenzyme A
HPA	hypothalamic–pituitary–adrenal (axis)
HPV	human papillomavirus
HR	heart rate
HRT	hormone replacement therapy
HSV	herpes simplex virus
IBS	irritable bowel syndrome
ICS	inhaled corticosteroids
IgE	immunoglobulin E
LABAs	long-acting β_2-agonists
LAMAs	long-acting muscarinic antagonists
MDI	metered-dose inhaler
$PaCO_2$	partial pressure of carbon dioxide in arterial blood
PaO_2	partial pressure of oxygen in arterial blood
PGs	prostaglandins
pMDI	pressurised metered-dose inhaler
SABAs	short-acting β_2-agonists
ICSH	interstitial cell-stimulating hormone
IDL	intermediate-density lipoproteins
Ig	immunoglobulin
IGF-1	insulin-like growth factor 1
IL	interleukin
IM	intramuscular
INN	International Non-proprietary Name
INR	international normalised ratio
IOP	intraocular pressure
IPV	inactivated poliovirus
ISA	intrinsic sympathomimetic activity
IU	International Units
IUD	intrauterine device
IV	intravenous
KGF	keratinocyte growth factor
KI	kinase inhibitor
KOR	κ-opioid receptor
LA	local anaesthetic
LARC	long-acting reversible contraceptives
LDL	low-density lipoproteins
LH	luteinising hormone
LMWHs	low-molecular-weight heparins
LPL	lipoprotein lipase
LSD	lysergic acid diethylamide
LT	leukotrienes
M6G	morphine-6-glucuronide
mAb	monoclonal antibody
MAC	minimum alveolar concentration (for anaesthesia)
MAC	*Mycobacterium avium* complex
mAChRs	muscarinic acetylcholine receptors
MAO	monoamine oxidase
MAOI	monoamine oxidase inhibitor
MDMA	3,4-methylenedioxymethamphetamine
Medsafe	Medicines and Medical Devices Safety Authority (NZ)

MIC	minimum inhibitory concentration
MOR	μ-opioid receptor
mRNA	messenger ribonucleic acid
MRP	multidrug resistance protein
MRSA	methicillin-resistant *Staphylococcus aureus*
MRSE	methicillin-resistant *Staphylococcus epidermis*
MTD	maximum tolerated dose
mTOR	mammalian target of rapamycin
mV	millivolts
NA	noradrenaline
nAChRs	nicotinic acetylcholine receptors
NERD	non-erosive reflux disease
NET	noradrenaline (norepinephrine) uptake transporter
NFAT	nuclear factor of activated T-cells
NKCC	Na^+–K^+–2 Cl^- co-transporter
NM	neuromuscular
NMDA	*N*-methyl-D-aspartate
NMJ	neuromuscular junction
NMSC	non-melanocytic skin cancer
NNRTI	non-nucleoside reverse transcriptase inhibitor
NO	nitric oxide
NOACs	new oral anticoagulants
NP	nurse practitioner
NPH	neutral protamine Hagedorn
NPS	National Prescribing Service
NRTI	nucleoside/nucleotide reverse transcriptase inhibitor
NSAID	non-steroidal anti-inflammatory drug
NZF	*New Zealand Formulary*
OAB	overactive bladder
OC	oral contraceptive
OHA	oral hypoglycaemic agent
OR	opioid receptor
OTC	over-the-counter
PABA	*p*-aminobenzoic acid
PBP	penicillin-binding proteins
PBS	Pharmaceutical Benefits Scheme
PCSK	proprotein convertase subtilisin/kexin
PEG	polyethylene glycol
PG	prostaglandin
PHARMAC	Pharmaceutical Management Agency (NZ)
PI	protease inhibitor
PIMS	potentially inappropriate medications
PM	poor metaboliser
PNS	peripheral nervous system
POAG	primary open-angle glaucoma
PPAR	peroxisome proliferator activated receptor
PPI	proton pump inhibitor
PRIF	prolactin release-inhibiting factor
PT	prothrombin time
PTH	parathyroid hormone
QUM	quality use of medicines
RA	rheumatoid arthritis
RAAS	renin–angiotensin–aldosterone system
RACF	residential aged care facility
RANKL	receptor activator of nuclear factor-kappa B ligand
RAS	reticular activating system
RBCs	red blood cells
RCCT	randomised controlled clinical trial
REM	rapid eye movement
RIMA	reversible inhibitor of MAO-A
RMMR	Residential Medication Management Review
RNA	ribonucleic acid
SA	sinoatrial
SAMAs	short-acting muscarinic antagonists
SARM	selective androgen receptor modulator
SARS-CoV-2	severe acute respiratory syndrome coronavirus 2
SC	subcutaneous
SCr	serum creatinine
SERM	selective estrogen receptor modulator
SGLT2	sodium-glucose co-transporter 2
SLC	solute carrier
SNP	single nucleotide polymorphism
SNRI	serotonin noradrenaline (norepinephrine) reuptake inhibitor
SPF	sun protection factor
SPRM	selective progesterone receptor modulator
SSRI	selective serotonin reuptake inhibitor
SUSMP	*Standard for the Uniform Scheduling of Medicines and Poisons*
SV	stroke volume
$t_{1/2}$	half-life
T_3	tri-iodothyronine (liothyronine)
T_4	tetra-iodothyronine (thyroxine)
TALH	thick ascending limb of the loop of Henle
TB	tuberculosis
TCA	tricyclic antidepressant
TCM	traditional Chinese medicine
TDM	therapeutic drug monitoring
TGA	Therapeutic Goods Administration
THC	tetrahydrocannabinol
TIVA	total intravenous anaesthesia
TNF	tumour necrosis factor
TPMT	thiopurine methyltransferase

TRH	thyrotrophin-releasing hormone
TSH	thyroid-stimulating hormone (thyrotrophin)
UGT	UDP-glucuronosyltransferase
UN	United Nations
UNODC	United Nations Office on Drugs and Crime
URM	ultra-rapid metaboliser
UTI	urinary tract infection
UVA/B/C	UVR of wavelengths in the A, B or C region
UVR	ultraviolet radiation
V_D	volume of distribution
VEGF	vascular endothelial growth factor
VLDL	very-low-density lipoproteins
VLP	virus-like particle
VMA	vanillylmandelic acid
VMAT2	vesicular monoamine transporter 2
VZV	varicella zoster virus
WBCs	white blood cells
WHO	World Health Organization
WHR	waist:hip ratio
XO	xanthine oxidase

APPENDIX 2

GLOSSARY

5-HT (serotonin) a monoamine neurotransmitter synthesised in central or peripheral neurons and chromaffin cells in the intestine by enzymatic action on tryptophan. It has many physiological actions, including action as a central neurotransmitter and contraction of smooth muscle.

5α-reductase inhibitors drugs that inhibit 5α-reductase, the enzyme that converts testosterone to the more active metabolite 5α-dihydrotestosterone.

α-adrenoceptor a receptor stimulated by adrenaline and noradrenaline, part of the sympathetic nervous system and which is a G-protein-coupled receptor. There are two subtypes: α_1 and α_2.

α-adrenoceptor agonists drugs designed to directly stimulate alpha(α)-adrenoceptors, producing actions similar to those of sympathetic stimulation (e.g. vasoconstriction of coronary arteries and other effects).

α-adrenoceptor antagonists drugs that competitively block the actions of catecholamines at alpha(α)-adrenoceptors.

α-blockers also known as alpha-blocker or antagonist, these are drugs that competitively block the actions of catecholamines on α-adrenoreceptors.

absence seizure a type of generalised non-motor (petit mal) seizure characterised by brief, sudden lapses of consciousness.

absorption the process by which unchanged drug proceeds from the site of administration into the blood.

acetylcholine a cholinergic neurotransmitter released by parasympathetic and somatic neurons and all preganglionic fibres of the autonomic nervous system. It is synthesised from choline and acetyl-CoA via the enzyme choline acetyltransferase and acts at muscarinic and nicotinic receptors.

acetylcholinesterase the enzyme that is responsible for breaking down acetylcholine to choline and acetate. It is found in the central nervous system, in red blood cells and the motor endplates of skeletal muscle.

acne vulgaris a chronic inflammatory disease of the pilosebaceous follicles of the skin, involving increased sebum production and excessive keratinisation.

acquired resistance when an organism (often a microorganism) obtains the ability to resist the activity of an intervention (e.g. drugs) to which it was previously susceptible.

active ingredient chemical in a medicine that has an effect in the body. Active ingredient prescribing uses the standardised International Non-proprietary Names.

acute pain pain of short onset and severe but with short duration.

addiction a behavioural pattern of drug abuse with overwhelming involvement in procurement and use of the drug and a high tendency to relapse back into dependence.

Addison's disease a deficiency of corticosteroids.

adenohypophysis the anterior part of the pituitary gland.

adherence (with therapy) the extent to which a person's behaviour corresponds with agreed recommendations from a healthcare provider.

adjuvant a substance that enhances the immunogenicity to a vaccine.

adjuvant analgesic drugs with a primary indication other than pain that have analgesic properties. Examples include some antidepressants and antiepileptics.

adjuvant therapy a treatment that is given in addition to the primary intervention to help achieve the ultimate goal.

adrenaline also known as epinephrine; a hormone and neurotransmitter released from the adrenal medulla and adrenergic neurons, respectively. It activates α- and β-adrenergic receptors.

adsorbed vaccine a vaccine containing an adjuvant, which assists to retain the antigen at the site of injection and increase its immunogenicity.

adverse drug event (ADE) injury resulting from medical intervention related to a drug but not necessarily due to the drug. Examples of ADEs include under- or overmedication resulting from misuse or malfunction of infusion pumps or devices; aspiration pneumonia resulting from drug overdose; and errors in ordering, dispensing or administration.

adverse drug reaction unintended and undesirable response to a drug.

aerosol a suspension of particles dispersed in air or gas.

affective disorders psychiatric disorders, also called mood disorders. The main types of affective disorders are depression, bipolar disorder and anxiety disorder.

affinity how well a drug can bind to a target/protein.

afterload the pressure that must be overcome before the ventricles can eject the blood; one of the factors that regulates stroke volume.

agonist a drug that binds to (occupies) and activates the receptor, producing the same response as the endogenous ligand. Some drugs may be considered partial agonists because they produce less than the maximal effect even when all receptors are occupied.

akinesia loss or impairment of voluntary movement.

alcohol a hydrocarbon derivative in which one or more of the hydrogen atoms has been replaced by a hydroxyl group; in a medical or social context, the term usually refers to ethanol (ethyl alcohol).

alcoholism physical or psychological dependence on alcohol, with a compulsion to consume despite adverse effects.

aldosterone a mineralocorticoid steroid hormone produced by the adrenal cortex; increases sodium and water reabsorption in renal tubule and promotes potassium excretion

alkylating agents agents that introduce an alkyl group into a molecule; they combine with DNA bases, altering their chemical structure, thus impairing synthesis of DNA and RNA; usually anticancer drugs.

allele variant form of a gene.

allergic rhinitis also known as hay fever; an irritation of the nose due to allergic/immune reactions to allergens in the air. Symptoms include itching and runny nose.

allosteric modulator a drug that indirectly influences (modulates) the effects of a primary ligand.

Alzheimer's disease named after the German physiologist Alois Alzheimer, this is a chronic neurodegenerative disease characterised by loss of cholinergic neurons and subsequent loss of intellectual function.

aminoglycosides potent bactericidal antibiotics that are usually reserved for serious or life-threatening infections.

amoebiasis an infection caused by any of the amoebas of the *Entamoeba* group.

amphetamine a sympathomimetic amine that has a stimulating effect on the central and peripheral nervous systems.

amyloid a protein deposited in organs in certain diseases.

anabolic agents agents that promote build-up of tissues; drugs that treat debilitating states; they are abused to build muscle mass.

anaemia a condition of reduced oxygen-carrying capacity of the blood.

anaesthesia the loss of the sensations of pain, pressure, temperature or touch, in a part or the whole of the body.

analeptics central nervous system stimulants that stimulate respiration.

analgesic a drug that relieves pain.

androgens male sex hormones, primarily testosterone and its ester derivatives, with physiological actions in male sexual maturation and functions and development of male secondary sexual characteristics.

angina pectoris a temporary interference with coronary blood flow that reduces oxygen and nutrient supply to heart muscle.

angiotensin II a potent vasoconstrictor that causes the release of aldosterone from the adrenal cortex.

angiotensin-converting enzyme inhibitors drugs that competitively inhibit angiotensin converting enzyme and hence formation of angiotensin II.

anorectics appetite suppressants.

antagonist a drug that binds to the receptor and blocks access of the endogenous ligand, thus diminishing the normal response; drugs may act as competitive (reversible) or irreversible antagonists. (Drugs that are antagonists are commonly called blockers.)

anterograde amnesic effect a drug effect that decreases the patient's memory for a period following an event (anterograde amnesia).

antiandrogens drugs that act by inhibiting androgen uptake or binding to androgen receptors.

antianxiety (anxiolytic) agents drugs that reduce anxiety.

antibiotics natural substances derived from certain organisms (bacteria, fungi and others) that can either suppress the growth of or destroy microorganisms.

antibody a Y-shaped protein produced by B-cells (plasma cells). They bind to and neutralise, agglutinate (clump together) and trigger the destruction of antigen.

anticholinergics drugs that block the parasympathetic and somatic nervous system effects by blocking postjunctional muscarinic and nicotinic receptors, respectively.

anticholinergic effect effects of drugs that block the parasympathetic and somatic nervous system by blocking postjunctional muscarinic and nicotinic receptors, respectively. Anticholinergic (muscarinic effects) include dry mouth, dry eyes, urinary retention, constipation, blurred vision and cognitive defects. Nicotinic effects include skeletal muscle paralysis.

anticholinesterase agents drugs that block the enzyme acetylcholinesterase and thereby produce an increase in the effects of acetylcholine.

anticoagulant drugs drugs that prevent the blood from coagulating; anticoagulation is primarily prophylactic because these agents act by preventing fibrin deposits, extension of a thrombus and thromboembolic complications.

antidepressants drugs that relieve depression; includes serotonin selective reuptake inhibitors, tricyclic antidepressants and monoamine oxidase inhibitors.

antidiarrhoeals relates to relieving symptoms of rapid passage of loose faeces, and the prevention of fluid and electrolyte loss.

antiemetics substances that prevent or alleviate nausea or vomiting.

antiepileptic (anticonvulsant) drugs drugs that combat epilepsy; include sodium channel blockers and GABA receptor agonists.

antiepileptic hypersensitivity syndrome syndrome in which there is a delayed adverse drug reaction associated with the use of drugs such as phenytoin, carbamazepine and phenobarbital.

antifibrinolytic drugs drugs that hasten clot formation and reduce bleeding.

antifungals drugs that destroy or suppress the growth of fungi (microorganisms that lack chlorophyll and reproduce through spores); effective against fungal infections.

antigen ANTIbody GENerating substance.

antiglycaemic drugs drugs that, by their mechanism of action, reduce blood glucose levels and are indicated to treat diabetes.

antimetabolites drugs that are analogues of folic acid or of the purine and pyrimidine bases, and inhibit metabolic pathways in microorganisms or neoplastic cells.

antimicrobials drugs that destroy or suppress the growth of microorganisms.

antiplatelet drugs used to treat arterial thrombosis; they include aspirin, dipyridamole and abciximab.

antipsychotics drugs that are effective in the treatment of psychosis.

anxiety emotional state that may include a physiological response to real or perceived danger.

apolipoproteins proteins carried on the surface of lipoproteins; functions include serving as ligands for cell receptors, activating enzymes involved in lipoprotein metabolism and providing structure of the lipoprotein.

approved name the name of a chemical approved by a drug-regulating authority, as distinct from the proprietary name (trade name or brand name) under which a drug is marketed commercially.

aqueous humour a fluid similar in composition to blood plasma; formed continually by the ciliary body, it bathes and nourishes the anterior segment of the eye, in front of the lens.

area under the plasma concentration versus time curve (AUC) the total area under the plasma concentration versus time curve that describes the concentration of the drug in the systemic circulation as a function of time (from zero until infinity).

argipressin (also known as arginine vasopressin (AVP) and antidiuretic hormone (ADH), previously known in Australia as vasopressin); increases tubular reabsorption of water and is a vasoconstrictor (increases blood pressure). Indicated for diabetes insipidus.

assay the analysis of the purity, amount or effectiveness of a drug or other substance, including laboratory and clinical measurements.

atherosclerosis a disorder involving large- and medium-sized arteries characterised by cholesterol deposits in the arterial wall.

asthma a disease characterised by airways inflammation, spasm of smooth muscle, bronchoconstriction and wheezing.

attention deficit hyperactivity disorder (ADHD) a neurodevelopmental disorder with a recognised and persistent pattern of behaviour including difficulties avoiding distraction and impulsivity.

atypical antipsychotics newer, second-generation antipsychotics used to treat psychotic disorders; includes clozapine and olanzapine.

Australian categorisation system for prescribing medicines in pregnancy a system with seven categories to indicate the level of risk to the fetus of drugs used in the mother at recommended therapeutic doses.

automaticity the ability to spontaneously initiate an electrical impulse; automaticity is a property of cells and fibres of the conduction system that normally controls heart rhythm.

autonomic ganglion a cluster of nerve cell bodies in both the sympathetic and parasympathetic nervous systems.

autonomic nervous system a major division of the peripheral nervous system, including parasympathetic and sympathetic divisions.

β-adrenoceptor a receptor stimulated by adrenaline and noradrenaline, part of the sympathetic nervous system and which is a G-protein-coupled receptor. It is present on smooth and cardiac muscle and in glandular tissue, and is classified into three subgroups: β_1, β_2 and β_3.

β-adrenoceptor agonists drugs designed to directly stimulate beta(β)-adrenoceptors, producing actions similar to those of β-sympathetic stimulation, such as increased cardiac output, dilation of coronary arterioles, bronchial dilation and a variety of other effects.

β-adrenoceptor antagonists drugs that competitively block the actions of the catecholamines on β-adrenoceptors.

bacteriostatic agents agents that inhibit bacterial growth, allowing host defence mechanisms additional time to remove the invading microorganisms.

balanced anaesthesia the use of a combination of agents to achieve unconsciousness, analgesia, muscle relaxation and amnesia. Premedication may include an antianxiety agent and glycopyrrolate to suppress secretions. Antiemetics and opioids are used for postoperative nausea and pain.

basal ganglia a group of subcortical nuclei responsible primarily for motor control.

basal release (related to insulin) the low rate of continuous insulin supply by the pancreas, to enable glucose utilisation.

Beers Criteria a tool developed to guide prescribers on the use of drugs in older people.

benign prostatic hyperplasia excessive growth of tissue in the prostate gland surrounding the urethra, with increase in smooth muscle tone leading to urinary retention.

benzodiazepines minor tranquillisers that act at allosteric sites on GABA receptors, facilitating the binding of GABA and leading to decreased neuronal activity in the central nervous system.

bioassay a biological test method to measure the amount of a pharmacologically active substance in a preparation (tissue extract or pharmaceutical formulation).

bioavailability the proportion of the administered dose that reaches the systemic circulation intact.

bipolar affective disorder a mood disorder, previously known as manic depression, in which there are severe mood swings.

bisphosphonates analogues of pyrophosphate with the general structure P-C-P.

blood–brain barrier a highly selective semipermeable membrane separating the blood from the cerebrospinal fluid. The endothelial cells form tight junctions allowing only small molecules, fat-soluble molecules and some gases to pass freely.

blood glucose level a measurement of the concentration of glucose in the blood plasma; normal range is below 11.1 mmol/L.

body mass index (BMI) a person's body mass in kilograms divided by the square of their height in metres; BMI is highly correlated with the proportion of body fat.

bone morphogenic proteins cytokines that are essential for bone and cartilage formation, embryonic skeletal development and bone repair following fracture.

bradykinesia slowness of movement and one of the symptoms of Parkinson's disease.

bronchoconstriction constriction of the airway's lumen due to contraction of the smooth muscle.

bronchodilator drug that relaxes smooth muscle thereby dilating the lumen of the airways.

burn injury to tissues caused by contact with heat, corrosive chemicals, electricity, friction or radiant energy.

calcitonin hormone secreted by thyroid C-cells, an antagonist of actions of parathyroid hormone and vitamin D.

calcium channel blockers block inward current of calcium through slow channels of the cell membranes of cardiac and smooth muscle cells.

candidiasis fungal infection caused by candida that often affects the skin or mucous membranes.

carbapenems highly effective class of antibiotics used to treat severe or high-risk bacterial infections.

carbonic anhydrase an enzyme that aids in converting carbon dioxide to carbonic acid and bicarbonate ions and the reverse process. It is important in maintaining acid–base balance in the blood.

carrier-mediated transport the movement of a drug from one side of a membrane to the other, mediated by a transmembrane carrier protein.

catecholamine any one of a group of sympathomimetic compounds composed of a catechol moiety and the aliphatic portion of an amine. There are three naturally occurring catecholamines in the body: dopamine, noradrenaline and adrenaline.

cell-mediated immunity an adaptive immune response that leads to the activation of cytotoxic T-lymphocytes to a specific antigen. It enables the destruction of antigen within host cells. It does not involve antibodies.

centrally acting adrenergic inhibitors drugs that act as agonists at central α_2 adrenoceptors and/or central I_1 imidazoline receptors thereby reducing sympathetic tone and hence blood pressure.

central nervous system (CNS) one of the two main divisions of the nervous system, consisting of the brain and the spinal cord. The CNS processes information to and from the peripheral nervous system and is the main network of coordination and control for the entire body.

cephalosporins antibacterial drugs that inhibit cell wall synthesis similarly to penicillin and are also bactericidal.

cestodes tapeworms.

chemical name the unique, precise description of the chemical composition and molecular structure of a chemical substance.

chemotherapy drug treatment of disease, typically used in the context of cancer or microbial infection.

cholecystokinin a hormone secreted from the duodenum.

choline esters drugs such as bethanecol and carbachol that act as agonists at muscarinic receptors.

cholinergic neurons neurons that release acetylcholine and are found in both the central and peripheral nervous systems.

cholinomimetic alkaloids naturally occurring plant-based chemicals (alkaloids) having an action similar to that of acetylcholine. Also called parasympathomimetic, they include arecoline, pilocarpine and muscarine.

cholinomimetics drugs having an action similar to that of acetylcholine. Also called parasympathomimetics.

chronic kidney disease defined by eGFR < 60 mL/min/1.73 m^2 or renal dysfunction (e.g. proteinuria for more than 3 months.

chronic pain pain of moderate or severe intensity lasting 3 months or more.

chronotropic effect a significant increase (positive chronotropic effect) or decrease (negative chronotropic effect) in cardiac rate occurring as a result of increased or decreased rate of membrane depolarisation in the pacemaker cells in the sinoatrial node.

clearance the rate at which a drug is removed from the blood; it determines the maintenance dose rate required to achieve the target plasma concentration at steady state.

clinical pharmacology concerns the drug treatment of patients; the study of drugs 'at the bedside'.

clinical trial a prospective study carried out in humans to determine whether a treatment that is believed to benefit a patient actually does provide a benefit.

colony-stimulating factors cytokines that regulate cell proliferation, differentiation and growth through an action on progenitor cells.

combined oral contraceptive a formulation with both estrogenic and progestogenic hormones, in a dose regimen to optimise contraceptive activity, taken by mouth.

complementary and alternative medicine healthcare practices not usually taught or practised in mainstream scientific (Western) medicine.

conjugate polysaccharide vaccine contains a polysaccharide (outer sugar coating of a bacteria) that is chemically combined (attached) with a protein to increase the immunogenicity of the vaccine (e.g. pneumococcal and meningococcal conjugate vaccines).

Conn's syndrome excess of mineralocorticoids.

constipation a condition in which bowel movements are infrequent or hard to pass.

contamination a condition of being soiled, stained, touched or otherwise exposed to harmful agents, making an object potentially unsafe for use as intended or without barrier techniques.

contraception prevention of pregnancy after sexual intercourse.

contraindication a factor that makes dangerous or undesirable the administration of a drug or the performance of an act or procedure in the care of a specific patient.

controlled drugs drugs that may produce addiction or dependence, deemed 'controlled drugs' in Australia and New Zealand, and subject to tight restrictions as to availability, usage and storage.

controller drug used to treat the inflammation associated with asthma or long-acting β-adrenoceptor agonist.

conventional antipsychotic first-generation antipsychotics. They are also called neuroleptics, and are mainly used to treat the symptoms of psychotic disorders.

corticosteroids glucocorticoids and mineralocorticoids; steroidal hormones that are synthesised in and released from the adrenal cortex.

cough suppressant (antitussive) drug that suppresses the intensity and frequency of cough (e.g. opioids that act on opioid receptors and depress the medullary cough centre).

Crohn's disease an inflammatory bowel disease causing inflammation of the full thickness of the bowel wall and in any part of the digestive tract from the mouth to the anus.

cromones a group of structurally related compounds that inhibit the release of histamine from mast cells and inflammation in a number of allergen-mediated diseases including asthma and allergic rhinitis.

Cushing's syndrome excess of glucocorticoids.

cyclooxygenase a rate limiting enzyme responsible for converting arachidonic acid to the prostaglandins and thromboxane. There are two isoforms of the enzyme: COX-1 and COX-2.

cycloplegic drugs drugs that paralyse the ciliary muscle, causing loss of accommodation.

cytoprotective agents substances that protect cells from damage.

decongestants drugs used to relieve nasal congestion in the upper respiratory tract.

delirium a disturbance in mental abilities that results in confused thinking and reduced awareness of the environment.

dementia a general term for a decline in mental ability severe enough to interfere with daily life.

dependence the condition in which administration of a drug is compulsively sought in the absence of a therapeutic indication and despite adverse psychological, social or physical effects.

depolarising drug a nicotinic-receptor agonist that maintains the depolarised state of the motor endplate, thus preventing transmission of another action potential.

depolarising neuromuscular blocker a drug that stimulates nicotinic receptors on the motor endplate, causing an action potential that spreads through the skeletal muscle fibre and prevents transmission of another action potential.

deprescribing the process of intentionally ceasing a drug or reducing its dosage, or reducing the number of drugs, to improve the person's health or reduce adverse effects.

depression a mood disorder characterised by feelings of sadness, flat or low mood.

dermatitis an inflammatory condition in which skin may become red, itchy, scaly, moist and blistered.

designer drugs semi/synthetic drugs designed to mimic the actions of cannabis or amphetamines, with the aim of keeping a step ahead of drug policymakers and law-enforcement officers.

diabetes mellitus a chronic disorder of carbohydrate and lipid metabolism affecting about 2% of the population, characterised by polyuria associated with and an inappropriate rise in glucose level in the blood, due to a relative or absolute lack of insulin.

diarrhoea frequent passing of watery and unformed faeces.

disease-modifying antirheumatic drugs a group of drugs with diverse chemical structures and mechanisms of action that modify the course of rheumatoid arthritis and improve quality of life.

distribution the process of reversible transfer of a drug between one location and another (one of which is usually blood) in the body.

diuretics drugs that modify renal function and induce diuresis (increased rate of urine flow) and natriuresis (enhanced excretion of sodium).

DNA polymerase family of enzymes that synthesise DNA from deoxyribonucleotides.

dopa decarboxylase the enzyme responsible for the synthesis of dopamine and serotonin from L-DOPA and L-5-hydroxytryptophan, respectively.

dopamine an important neurotransmitter that is the precursor for adrenaline and noradrenaline.

dose the quantity of drug to be administered at one time; the amount determined by experience as likely to be effective in most people.

dose form/formulation the form in which the drug is administered – for example, as a tablet, injection, eyedrop or ointment.

dromotropic effect effect of a drug in increasing (positive dromotropic effect) or decreasing (negative dromotropic effect) the rate of atrioventricular conduction; the effect may also occur in conduction abnormalities. Dromotropic drugs affect conduction velocity through specialised conducting tissues.

drug a substance that is used to modify or explore physiological systems or pathological states for the benefit of the recipient.

drug abuse/misuse self-administration of a drug in chronically excessive quantities, in a manner that deviates from approved medical or social patterns in a given culture, resulting in physical or psychological harm.

Drug Burden Index an indication of a person's exposure to anticholinergic and sedative drugs.

drug development the stages in bringing a new drug to market, from initial idea through screening for effects, preclinical studies, clinical trials, formulation studies and registration.

drug–drug interaction the interaction of two drugs whereby the exposure, efficacy or tolerability of one drug (the interaction victim) is altered by the other (the interaction perpetrator).

drug interaction an effect on the responses of an individual to a drug with any other drug taken, including non-prescribed over-the-counter drugs and complementary and alternative medicines, as well as other ingested compounds such as food and drinks.

drug offences actions related to drugs that are considered illegal under relevant local laws. In Australia, Commonwealth, state or territory laws may apply.

drug schedule an Australian categorisation system whereby 'poisons' (i.e. drugs and other chemicals) are subject to varying levels of controls on labels, containers, storage, disposal, record-keeping, sale, supply, possession and use, and advertising of the scheduled substances.

drug-seeking behaviour the scenario in which dependent people 'shop around' among prescribers to obtain prescriptions, particularly seeking narcotic analgesics, amphetamines, benzodiazepines and antipsychotics.

drug use evaluation a process of obtaining information related to drug use problems to ensure standards of care, control drug costs, prevent problems related to medications, or evaluate outcomes of drug therapy.

dyskinesia rapid, involuntary, and uncontrollable movements of the limbs, trunk and face.

dysmenorrhoea painful menstruation due to spasms of uterine muscles.

dysrhythmia any deviation from normal rhythm of the heartbeat

dystonia a neurological disorder affecting movement by causing skeletal muscles in the body to contract or spasm involuntarily.

eardrops, eyedrops a formulation in which drugs are dispensed in aqueous or oily solutions, in a small dropper bottle (usually 10–15-mL capacity) such that a small drop can be instilled into the ear or eye.

eclampsia the onset of seizures in a woman with preeclampsia, a condition in which there is high blood pressure in pregnancy and either proteinuria or other organ dysfunction.

eczema a type of dermatitis with genetic predisposition.

efficacy the ability of a drug to achieve the desired therapeutic effect.

electroconvulsive therapy a procedure used to relieve severe depressive and psychotic symptoms by passing a carefully controlled electrical current through the brain.

elimination the irreversible loss of drug from the body by the processes of metabolism and excretion.

emergency contraception administration of a hormone formulation to prevent pregnancy within 72 hours after unprotected sexual intercourse.

embolus mass of undissolved matter that breaks off from the thrombus.

endocrine gland organs in the body that secrete into the bloodstream hormones that act on distant tissues.

endogenous opioids opioid peptides produced by neurons including β-endorphin, the met- and leu-enkephalins, and the dynorphins.

endometriosis a chronic condition of endometrial tissue at unusual (ectopic) locations, leading to hormone imbalances, dysmenorrhoea and chronic inflammation.

endorphin endogenous opioid neuropeptide or peptide hormone synthesised in the central nervous system and that acts at opioid receptors.

enkephalins naturally occurring pentapeptides and endogenous opioids that act at opioid receptors.

epidural anaesthesia an injection of local anaesthetic into the space between the dura mater and the ligamentum flavum, at spinal cord levels C7–T10. This 'space' is actually filled with loose adipose tissue and lymphatic and blood vessels; the solution tends to remain localised at the level where it is injected.

epilepsy a common, long-term brain condition characterised by repeated seizures.

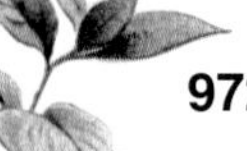

equianalgesic dose a dose of one analgesic that is equivalent in pain-relieving effects to a dose of another analgesic. This equivalence permits substitution of medications to prevent possible adverse reactions to one of the drugs.

erectile dysfunction the condition in which a man cannot attain or maintain an erection long enough for sexual intercourse, or is unable to ejaculate.

erythropoietin a hormone synthesised in the kidney that stimulates the division and differentiation of erythroid progenitors in the bone marrow that regulate erythrocyte production.

estrogen receptor nuclear receptor class 1-type receptors of α- and β-subtypes, mainly in nuclei of cells in the uterus, vagina and breast, with 17β-estradiol as the main endogenous ligand.

estrogens steroidal hormones secreted by mainly ovarian follicles, responsible for female reproductive and sexual functions and characteristics.

ethanol ethyl alcohol.

evidence-based medicine the conscientious, explicit and judicious use of current best evidence in making decisions about the medical care of individual patients.

excretion (of drug) irreversible loss of chemically unchanged drug from the body (e.g. in urine, bile, expired air or faeces).

expectorants drugs that loosen mucus in the airways and enable it to be coughed up more easily.

extrapyramidal effects drug-induced movement dysfunction including side effects such as akathisia, dystonias and parkinsonism. They are usually due to blockade of dopamine receptors in the central nervous system.

extrapyramidal tracts a series of indirect motor pathways located in the central nervous system that are outside the main motor pathways that traverse the pyramids in the thalamus. The name embraces many pathways or tracts, which innervate mainly muscles in the limbs, head and eyes. This system is associated with coordination of muscle-group movements and posture.

eye ointments thick semisolid drug formulations, usually oily, to be applied to the eye; they have soothing and protective properties.

ferritin iron compound stored in organs (e.g. liver, spleen) and bone marrow that is available for incorporation into haemoglobin.

first-pass effect the amount of an orally administered drug that is 'extracted' by the liver before the drug reaches the systemic circulation (absorbed drugs travel first through the portal system and the liver before entering the systemic circulation). Often only a small fraction of the dose is available for distribution and to produce a pharmacological effect. For such medications, the oral drug dose is calculated to compensate for this variable first-pass effect.

focal seizure type of seizure that affects initially only one hemisphere of the brain; also called partial or localised seizure.

formulary similar to a pharmacopoeia but may include information on drug actions, adverse effects, general medical information, guidelines for pharmacists dispensing medicines and the 'recipes' for formulation or production of different medicines.

formulation the way the drug is presented, including dose form and active and inactive ingredients.

fungistatic agent a drug that is capable of inhibiting the growth and reproduction of fungi without destroying them.

gamma-aminobutyric acid the main inhibitory neurotransmitter in the central nervous system that reduces neuronal excitability.

gastrin a peptide hormone released by G-cells and that stimulates secretion of gastric acid (HCl) by the parietal cells of the stomach as well as promoting gastric motility.

gastritis inflammation, erosion or irritation of the stomach lining. It may be acute or chronic.

gastrointestinal tract a hollow, muscular tube or passageway from the mouth to the anus through which food passes and is digested and excreted. It is part of the gastrointestinal system.

gate control theory a theory that proposes that a mechanism in the dorsal horn of the spinal cord (the spinal 'gate') can modify the transmission of painful sensations from the peripheral nerve fibres to the thalamus and cortex of the brain, where the sensations are recognised as pain.

general anaesthesia/anaesthetic a state of unconsciousness and general loss of sensation, with varying amounts of analgesia, muscle relaxation and loss of reflexes; a drug used to achieve this state.

generalised seizure a seizure affecting both cerebral hemispheres and producing loss of consciousness, either briefly or for a longer period. They are sub-categorised into several main types that include motor (tonic–clonic and atonic) or non-motor (absence).

generic name strictly speaking, this refers to a group name – for example, the penicillins, the salicylates or the β-blockers; however, it has come to be used interchangeably with the term 'approved name'.

genetic polymorphism any variation in a DNA sequence that is common in the population.

glaucoma a group of progressive optic neuropathies involving damage to the optic nerve, retinal cell death and changes in visual fields, with abnormally elevated intraocular pressure.

glomerular filtration the ultrafiltration of water and solutes through pores of the glomerular capillaries into the capsular space of the Bowman's capsule.

glucagon a 29-amino-acid polypeptide hormone secreted by α cells of the pancreatic islets of Langerhans in response to hypoglycaemia and high-protein meals, and stimulated by exercise, stress and infections; it has 'fuel-mobilising' activities.

glucagon-like peptide-1 an appetite suppressant that binds GLP-1R receptors on pancreatic beta cells stimulating insulin secretion.

goitre enlargement of the thyroid gland resulting from any one of a number of factors such as hyper/hypothyroidism and multiple cystic nodules.

gonadotrophin-releasing hormone a factor secreted from the hypothalamus that stimulates the anterior pituitary gland to release gonadotrophic hormones.

gonadotrophins glycoprotein hormones responsible for the development and maintenance of gonadal functions.

gout a condition characterised by deposition of uric acid crystals in joints and non-articular structures.

Gram stain a method used to distinguish and classify bacterial species.

granulocyte colony-stimulating factor a haematopoietic growth factor of the granulocyte lineage controlling the development of neutrophils.
growth factor a naturally occurring protein or steroid hormone that can stimulate cellular growth, proliferation and cellular differentiation (e.g. growth hormone and insulin-like growth factor 1).
growth hormone (and somatotropin) a 191-amino-acid protein, secreted from the anterior pituitary gland, that promotes skeletal, visceral and general growth.
gustation the act or sensation of tasting.

H_2-receptor antagonists drugs that reduce the amount of acid produced by the parietal cells in the stomach by blocking histamine H_2 receptor subtypes. They include cimetidine and ranitidine.
haematinics agents used to treat anaemias such as folic acid, iron and vitamin B_{12}.
haemosiderin degraded form of ferritin iron.
haemostasis the physiological process that stops bleeding. It involves blood vessel constriction, platelet plug formation and blood coagulation.
haemostatic drugs agents that enhance haemostasis – that is, hasten clot formation and reduce bleeding. The purpose of these agents is to control rapid loss of blood.
heart failure characterised by reduced cardiac output and the consequential failure to provide adequate perfusion to meet the metabolic requirements of the body.
half-life the time taken for the blood or plasma concentration of a drug to fall by one-half (50%).
hallucinogen a drug that produces auditory or visual hallucinations, such as LSD or ecstasy.
harm minimisation policies and procedures that aim to reduce problems and damage to individuals and society caused by drug dependence.
headache pain in any region of the head.
Helicobacter pylori bacteria commonly known as *H. pylori* that colonises the stomach and can cause peptic ulcers and gastritis.
helminths commonly known as parasitic worms; large multicellular parasites.
herbal remedies using parts or extracts of plants to treat illness.
high-density lipoproteins one of three primary classes of lipoproteins found in the blood of fasting individuals.
histamine a local hormone and neurotransmitter involved in immune responses and physiological actions respectively by agonist action at histamine receptors.
histamine (H_2) receptors G-protein-coupled receptors located on parietal cells, in the heart and vascular smooth muscle and cells of the immune system. Stimulation of H_2 receptors primarily causes gastric acid secretion and vasodilation.
HMG-CoA reductase 3-hydroxy-3-methylglutaryl coenzyme A is the rate-limiting enzyme in the synthesis of cholesterol.
homeostasis the ability of an organism to maintain a constant internal environment owing to a coordinated response to a stimulus.
hormone a natural chemical secreted into the bloodstream from an endocrine gland that initiates or regulates the activity of an organ or group of cells in another part of the body, with specific physiological effects on metabolism, growth, homeostasis and integration of bodily functions.
hormone replacement therapy in the context of alleviation of symptoms in postmenopausal women: administration of daily low doses of a natural estrogen; additionally, in women with an intact uterus a progestogen is given 10–12 days per month.
humoral immunity the adaptive immune response which facilitates the formation of B lymphocytes (B-cells) into plasma cells that produce and secrete antibodies to a specific antigen.
hypercalcaemia greater than normal concentration of calcium in the blood.
hypercapnia a condition arising from too much carbon dioxide in the blood, often caused by hypoventilation or disordered breathing.
hyperglycaemia high levels of glucose in the bloodstream (casual $>$ 11.1 mmol/L, fasting $>$ 7.0 mmol/L).
hyperparathyroidism hyperactivity of parathyroid glands with excessive secretion of parathyroid hormone.
hyperuricaemia a high concentration of uric acid in the blood.
hypnotics drugs used to induce sleep.
hypoglycaemia low level of glucose in the blood ($<$ 3.5 mmol/L).
hypogonadism a condition resulting from abnormally decreased gonadal function, resulting in retardation of growth, sexual development and secondary sexual characteristics.
hypoparathyroidism diminished secretion of the parathyroid glands.
hypothalamic factor a factor from the hypothalamus that stimulates or inhibits the release of hormones from the anterior pituitary gland.
hypothalamic–pituitary–adrenal axis linked functions of the hypothalamus, the anterior pituitary gland and the adrenal cortex.
hypothyroidism decreased activity of the thyroid gland.
hypoxia (hypoxemia) reduction in the partial pressure of oxygen dissolved in arterial blood.

illicit drugs drugs that are deemed illegal outside of approved medical use on prescription in a particular jurisdiction, such as ecstasy, heroin, cocaine, 'ice', cannabis or LSD.
immune checkpoint regulators of immune activation that play a key role in maintaining immune homeostasis and preventing autoimmunity.
immunomodulating drugs agents that can either activate the body's immune defences or modify a response to an unwanted stimulus, such as an antitumour response.
immunostimulating drug an agent that activates the immune system.
impotence the inability of a man to achieve or maintain a penile erection to allow sexual intercourse.
incretins glucose-dependent peptide hormones that are secreted from the digestive tract into the circulation in response to food, thus stimulating insulin release from the pancreas.
indication an illness or disorder for which a drug has a documented specific usefulness.
infertility the absence of conception after more than one year of regular sexual intercourse without contraception.
infiltration anaesthesia the use of local anaesthetics in an area that circles the operative field; it is produced by injecting dilute solutions of the agent into the skin and subcutaneously into the region to be anaesthetised.
inflammatory bowel disease a disorder that encompasses diseases involving chronic inflammation of the digestive tract. Types of IBD include ulcerative colitis and Crohn's disease.

inhalation anaesthetic inhalation, or volatile, anaesthetics are gases or volatile liquids that can be administered by inhalation when mixed with oxygen.
inhibitory transmitter a neurotransmitter (e.g. GABA) that inhibits the generation of an action potential in the receiving neuron.
inotropic effect something that increases or decreases the force of muscular contractions, particularly the heartbeat.
insomnia a sleep disorder, also known as sleeplessness, where there may be difficulty falling asleep or staying asleep.
insulin a protein hormone consisting of two polypeptide chains joined by disulfide bridges, synthesised in the B-cells of the pancreas and released in response to increased glucose levels in the blood.
interstitial cell-stimulating hormone a glycoprotein gonadotrophic hormone (known in females as luteinising hormone) produced by the anterior pituitary gland, which in males stimulates the interstitial cells in the testes to increase secretion of androgens, the male sex hormones.
intraocular pressure the pressure of the fluid (aqueous humour) within the interior of the eye, normally less than 21 mmHg.
intrauterine device a small plastic or metal appliance inserted into the uterus to prevent conception and pregnancy.
intravenous regional anaesthesia (Bier's block) a specialised technique for anaesthetising the upper limb. A tourniquet is applied to occlude the arterial flow, then the local anaesthetic is injected intravenously distal to the cuff.
intrinsic resistance the innate ability of a bacterial species to resist activity of a particular antimicrobial agent.
intrinsic sympathomimetic activity characterised by drugs that, by their chemical structure, are both β-blockers and partial receptor agonists.
irritable bowel syndrome a common problem affecting the colon or large bowel; symptoms include abdominal pain, cramps, bloating and bouts of diarrhoea or constipation.

ketoacidosis acidosis accompanied by an accumulation of ketones in the body, resulting from extensive breakdown of fats because of faulty carbohydrate metabolism, as in diabetes or starvation.
key, or prototype, drug an important drug in a class, to which other drugs in the class can be compared.
kinase inhibitor a drug (small molecule of monoclonal antibody) that elicits its therapeutic effect by inhibition of a kinase receptor.

lactation production of milk from the mammary glands (breasts) by a woman after giving birth.
laxatives drugs that loosen the stools and promote bowel movements.
'legal highs' new psychoactive substances, semi/synthetic drugs designed to mimic the actions of cannabis or amphetamines and to keep a step ahead of drug policymakers and old laws covering the misuse of drugs.
leptin the protein product of the obesity (ob) gene (derived from the Greek word *leptos*, meaning 'thin').
leukotriene-receptor antagonists drugs that block the action of leukotrienes in the inflammatory pathways of the airways. They are classified as preventers in treating asthma.
libido sexual interest, potency or drive.
lipoprotein lipase catalyses the breakdown of triglycerides present in chylomicrons and VLDL releasing fatty acids.
listed medicines products considered by the Australian Therapeutic Goods Administration to be of low risk, containing only permitted ingredients, and allowed to be self-assessed by the proposer, who must have documentation to back up any claims of efficacy.
live attenuated vaccine contains a weakened whole, living pathogen (bacteria or virus) that replicates within the host and induces immunity.
local anaesthesia/anaesthetic absence of pain due to blocked sensory nerve conduction in a body region or localised area; an agent used to achieve this.
long-acting β_2-agonists drugs used to relieve bronchoconstriction by activating β receptors in airway smooth muscle. Due to their chemical structure and binding to receptors, their duration of action may be as long as 12 hours.
long-acting muscarinic antagonists drugs used to relieve bronchoconstriction by blocking muscarinic receptors in airway smooth muscle. Due to their chemical structure and binding to receptors their duration of action may be 12–24 hours.
low-density lipoproteins one of three primary classes of lipoproteins found in the blood of fasting individuals.
low-molecular-weight heparins fragments that are approximately one-third the size of standard heparin and are prepared by enzymatic or chemical cleavage of unfractionated heparin.

macro/microvascular disease disorders of the blood vessels occurring in diabetes: macrovascular disease causing atherosclerosis and thrombosis of larger vessels, and microvascular disease leading to ischaemia, neuropathies, nephropathy and diabetic retinopathy.
macrolide antibiotics antibiotics that contain a many-membered lactone ring attached to deoxy sugars.
malaria infectious disease caused by *plasmodium* parasites that is transmitted by mosquitoes.
malignant hyperthermia rare, but potentially fatal, condition of rapidly developing high body temperature occurring in susceptible patients with an inherited abnormality in muscle membranes. It appears to be precipitated by the combination of a depolarising neuromuscular-blocking agent (e.g. suxamethonium) with a general anaesthetic agent.
mania a facet of bipolar disorder marked by periods of euphoria, delusions and overactivity.
mast-cell stabilisers drugs that block mast cell degranulation, thereby preventing the release of histamine and other inflammatory mediators.
medical ethics the principles and values that guide the decisions of medical practitioners, and by extension apply to all health practitioners; usually listed as non-maleficence, beneficence, justice, veracity, confidentiality and autonomy of the patient.
medication a drug or medicine, possibly dispensed in a formulation to allow appropriate administration.
medicine drug(s) given for therapeutic purposes; possibly a mixture of drug plus other substances to provide stability in the formulation; also, the branch of science devoted to the study, prevention and treatment of disease.
Medsafe the New Zealand Medicines and Medical Devices Safety Authority.
melatonin a neurohormone released from the pineal gland and important in the sleep–wake cycle.

menarche the first menstrual period in a girl, signalling the onset of puberty.

Ménière's disease dysfunction of the semicircular canals of the inner ear, leading to recurrent bouts of vertigo, tinnitus and deafness.

menopause the transitional period at the end of the reproductive period of a woman's life when ovulation and menstruation cease.

menstrual cycle the physiological changes in the female uterus leading to regular menstruation, recurring at approximately 28-day intervals.

mental health a state of emotional, psychological and social wellbeing.

metabolism the enzymatic conversion of a drug (substrate) to a metabolite (product) that is typically less biologically active and more water soluble (i.e. more readily excreted in the urine).

metastasis a secondary malignant growth at a distance from a primary site of cancer.

methadone a synthetic opioid agonist indicated for opioid dependence and pain. It is primarily a primarily a μ-receptor agonist. It is administered orally (tablet, oral liquid) or parentally.

methylxanthines methylated xanthine derivatives, including caffeine, theobromine and theophylline, which are stimulants. Theophylline is used to treat asthma and chronic obstructive pulmonary disease.

micturition the act of emptying the bladder, which can be stopped voluntarily because of control exerted at the level of the cerebral cortex.

migraine a type of severe headache that includes a throbbing sensation and may include associated aura, sensitivity to light and sound, and nausea and vomiting.

mineralocorticoids steroid hormones from the adrenal cortex that act in the kidneys to cause reabsorption of sodium and water, and enhance the excretion of potassium and hydrogen.

minimum alveolar concentration the alveolar (or end-expiratory) concentration for an inhaled anaesthetic at which 50% of patients will not show a motor response to a standardised surgical incision.

minipill a low-dosage, progestogen-only, oral contraceptive formulation developed for women who are unable to take estrogens.

miotic drugs drugs that constrict the pupil – that is, cause miosis. Their clinical uses are to reverse mydriatic effects and in the treatment of glaucoma.

monoamine oxidase inhibitors a class of drugs that block the enzymes monoamine oxidase A and monoamine oxidase B, responsible for the catalysis of monoamines such as dopamine, noradrenaline and serotonin. Known as MAO inhibitors, they are antidepressants.

monoamines compounds that have a single amine group and that include the neurotransmitters such as dopamine, noradrenaline and serotonin.

monoclonal antibodies antibodies that are made by identical immune cells that are all clones of a unique parent cell.

motor neurone disease a neurodegenerative disease affecting motor neurons and that causes muscle weakness.

mucociliary transport cilia or hair-like structures lining the epithelium of the airways that beat continuously and move mucus and other particles up and out of the airways.

mucolytics drugs that help break up mucus.

multiple sclerosis a neurodegenerative disorder in which neurons in the brain and spinal cord are demyelinated, interfering with nerve function.

muscarinic receptors G-protein-coupled receptors found on cardiac and smooth muscle and in glandular tissue and which are innervated by the parasympathetic nervous system. They are also present in the central nervous system.

myasthenia gravis neurodegenerative disorder in which there is an autoimmune destruction of nicotinic receptors at the neuromuscular junction leading to progressive muscle weakness.

mycoses any disease caused by a fungus.

mydriatics drugs that cause pupil dilation (mydriasis); they are primarily used to facilitate examination of the peripheral lens and retina in the diagnosis of ophthalmic disorders.

myoclonic seizure a type of generalised onset seizure involving brief, shock-like jerks of a muscle or a group of muscles.

nanoparticle a minute piece of matter at the nanometre (nm) level; a nanometre is one-billionth of a metre, 10^{-9} m.

narcolepsy neurological disorder affecting the sleep–wake cycle, characterised by symptoms such as excessive sleepiness, sleep paralysis and hallucinations.

narcotic a drug causing sleep; an illicit or proscribed drug, likely to cause addiction.

nasolacrimal duct the passage in the eye that conveys tears from the lacrimal sac into the inferior nasal meatus.

National Prescribing Service an independent, not-for-profit organisation, set up in 1998 by the Australian Government to improve the way health technologies, medicines and medical tests are prescribed and used.

natriuresis the enhanced excretion of sodium chloride.

nebuliser a pump that uses compressed air or oxygen or ultrasonic energy to produce a fine mist of drug in aerosol form from a solution; useful for delivering large doses to the airways for long periods.

negative feedback when some function of the output of a system acts back in a way that tends to reduce fluctuations in the output; generally promotes stability in the system and a reversion to equilibrium.

neoplasia the presence or formation of new, abnormal growth of tissue.

nerve block injection of a local anaesthetic into the vicinity of a nerve trunk, thus inhibiting the conduction of impulses to and from the area supplied by that nerve, the region of the operative site. The injection may be made at some distance from the surgical site.

neuraminidase inhibitor class of antiviral drugs that block the viral neuraminidase enzyme.

neurochemical transmission the process whereby a chemical messenger enables the transmission of nerve impulses across synapses or neuromuscular junctions. It involves the fundamental steps of synthesis, storage, release and interaction of the transmitter with receptors on the effector cell membrane and the associated change in the effector cell. It also involves breakdown or reuptake of neurotransmitters.

neuroeffector junction the synapse between a neuron (presynaptic site) and an effector cell other than another neuron.

neurohypophysis the posterior part of the pituitary gland; its hormones, vasopressin and oxytocin are released from nerve endings in response to neural stimuli.

neuroleptics drugs used to treat psychosis; also known as antipsychotics or minor tranquillisers.
neuromuscular blocking drugs drugs that interfere locally with the transmission or reception of impulses from motor nerves to skeletal muscles.
neuromuscular junction chemical synapse formed by the contact between a motor neuron and a skeletal muscle fibre.
neuron the basic unit of the brain and nervous system; also known as a nerve cell or neurone.
neuropathic pain pain due to neurological disease that affects a sensory pathway.
neuroses disorders characterised by anxiety, fear or depression.
neurotransmitter a chemical messenger enabling the transmission of nerve impulses across synapses or neuromuscular junctions. Of the many chemicals proposed as neurotransmitters in the central nervous system, the most important are acetylcholine, the catecholamines (dopamine, noradrenaline and adrenaline), 5-hydroxytryptamine, some amino acids and neuroactive peptides.
nociceptive pain pain arising from stimulation of superficial or deep nociceptors (pain receptors) by noxious stimuli such as tissue injury or inflammation.
non-depolarising drug a neuromuscular-blocking drug that blocks the action of acetylcholine at the motor endplate without first depolarising the cell membrane.
non-depolarising neuromuscular blocker a drug that blocks nicotinic receptors on the motor endplate, preventing transmission of another action potential.
non-linear pharmacokinetics also referred to as dose-dependent, it is usually due to saturation in active renal transport, hepatic metabolism or protein binding.
non–rapid eye movement (non-REM) sleep the stage of sleep in which there is no eye movement or muscle paralysis.
non-steroidal anti-inflammatory drugs (NSAIDs) a group of drugs having antipyretic, analgesic and anti-inflammatory effects; they bear no structural similarity to the corticosteroids.
noradrenaline a neurotransmitter released from sympathetic nerves and a hormone released from the adrenal medulla.
nucleoside analogue typically refers to antiviral drugs that can be incorporated into DNA and block natural maturation processes.

occlusive dressing a treatment that closes off the pores of the skin – for example, a type of ointment (e.g. petroleum jelly) or plastic wrapping – to trap and prevent water loss (sweat) from the skin, thus increasing hydration of the epidermis.
on–off syndrome associated with Parkinson's disease and levodopa treatment; the 'on–off' refers to the switch between phases of mobility (on) and immobility (off).
opioid pertaining to natural and synthetic chemicals that have morphine-like effects.
opioid analgesic drug derived from opium and which is used to treat pain.
opioid receptor G-protein-coupled receptor of ¬μ, δ or κ (mu, delta or kappa) subtypes, activated by opioids such as morphine, and which are widely distributed throughout the central nervous system and periphery.
opium narcotic analgesic derived from the seed pod of the opium poppy *Papaver somniferum*.
oral contraceptive female hormone taken by mouth to prevent conception and pregnancy.
orexin hypothalamic neuropeptide involved in regulating the sleep and arousal states.
orphan drug drug used to treat, prevent or diagnose rare diseases. It is recognised that, although such drugs might not be commercially viable, patients with rare conditions have as much right as all others to access drugs that are safe and effective.
osteoporosis pathological disorder characterised by loss of bone density and changes in bone microstructure with increased risk of fractures.
otitis media inflammation of the middle ear.
ototoxicity impairment of a person's ear functions, either hearing (auditory or cochlear function) and/or balance (vestibular function).
overactive bladder characterised by the urgency and increased frequency of voiding and nocturia.
over-the-counter (OTC) drug/medicine a drug that is considered safe for treating minor illnesses, which can be made available to the public without requiring a prescription or regular supervision of a licensed health professional.
oxygen free radicals an oxygen atom containing an unpaired electron, making it highly reactive and thereby able to damage all macromolecules.
oxytocics agents that stimulate contraction of the smooth muscle of the uterus, resulting in contractions and labour.
oxytocin a nine-amino-acid peptide hormone produced by the posterior pituitary gland, the main function of which is to contract uterine smooth muscle.

Paget's disease a disorder of bone remodelling, with focal areas of increased bone turnover and disorganised remodelling, leading to soft, poorly mineralised bone. The aetiology is unknown.
pain an unpleasant sensory and emotional experience associated with actual or potential tissue damage.
pancreatic lipase enzyme that breaks down dietary triglycerides.
parasympathetic nervous system one of three divisions of the autonomic nervous system. Sometimes called the rest and digest system, it innervates muscarinic receptors. The main neurotransmitter is acetylcholine.
parasympatholytics drugs such as muscarinic receptor blockers that block the action of the parasympathetic nervous system.
parasympathomimetic pertaining to a substance producing effects similar to those caused by stimulation of a parasympathetic nerve.
parenteral administration the administration of drugs by injection (literally: other than via the gastrointestinal tract).
parietal cells cells in the gastric glands located in the stomach that release hydrochloric acid and intrinsic factor.
Parkinson's disease a degenerative neurological disorder; named after the English physician James Parkinson, it affects the initiation, coordination and control of motor movement.
patient-controlled analgesia a delivery system whereby the patient can administer analgesia as required.
penicillins antibiotics related chemically to the original penicillin G, a product of the mould *Penicillium notatum*; they contain a β-lactam ring.
pepsin an enzyme secreted in the stomach that breaks down proteins.
peripheral vascular disease an abnormal condition affecting peripheral blood vessels that results in coolness or numbness of the extremities.

perinatal period the period around childbirth, defined as lasting from week 28 of pregnancy to the end of the first week of the infant's life.
peristalsis wave-like involuntary movements of the smooth muscle of the gastrointestinal tract that move food down the tract.
pharmaceutical a medicine, possibly dispensed in a formulation to allow appropriate administration of the active drug.
pharmaceutics the science of formulation of drugs into different types of preparation – for example, tablets, ointments, injectable solutions or eyedrops; it also includes study of the ways in which various drug forms influence pharmacokinetic and pharmacodynamic activities of the active drug.
pharmacist a health scientist who is qualified and licensed to prepare, dispense, provide and sell drugs and medicines, and to counsel about the use of drugs.
pharmacodynamics the study of the interaction between a drug and its molecular target, and the pharmacological response; 'what the drug does to the body'.
pharmacogenetics the study of genetic differences that can alter a person's response to a drug.
pharmacokinetics the study of how a drug is altered during the processes of absorption, distribution, metabolism and excretion; 'what the body does to the drug'.
pharmacologist a medical scientist who works in the discovery, development, chemistry, use and effects of drugs.
pharmacology the study of the discovery, development, chemistry, use and effects of drugs.
pharmacopoeia a reference book listing standards for drugs approved in a particular country; it may also include details of standard formulations and prescribing guidelines (a formulary).
pharmacovigilance post-marketing surveillance of medicines and medical devices in use.
pharmacy the branch of science dealing with preparing and dispensing drugs; also, the place where a pharmacist carries out these roles.
phenothiazines a class of typical antipsychotics that act as dopamine antagonists and includes chlorpromazine.
phenotype observable characteristics of a person that result from the interaction of their genotype with their environment.
phosphodiesterase 5 inhibitors drugs that inhibit the enzyme phosphodiesterase-5, the enzyme that inactivates cyclic GMP in the *corpus cavernosum* of the penis; used to treat erectile dysfunction.
phototoxicity an adverse drug reaction that occurs when the inducing agent is present on the skin in sufficient amounts and is also exposed to particular sunlight wavelengths.
phytoestrogens plant compounds with estrogenic activity.
pituitary gland a small endocrine body at the base of the skull, attached to the hypothalamus from which it receives hormonal and neural stimuli; it consists of two main lobes: anterior (adenohypophysis) and posterior (neurohypophysis).
placebo a Latin word literally meaning 'I will please'. In the pharmacological context, it refers to a harmless inactive preparation prescribed to satisfy a patient who does not require an active drug; in a clinical trial, it is formulated to look identical to the active drug under trial, to maintain 'double blinding', so that neither subject nor clinician knows which treatment group the subject is in.
polymerase inhibitors class of antiviral drugs that block the viral polymerase enzymes.
polypharmacy the concurrent use of multiple medications; in the clinical context, it has the connotation of implying over-prescription and use of too many or unnecessary drugs, often at frequencies greater than therapeutically essential.
potassium channel activators drugs that relax smooth muscle by acting on ATP-sensitive potassium channels; by antagonising action of ATP they prevent closure of the channel, which results in hyperpolarisation and relaxation of vascular smooth muscle.
potency the amount of drug required to produce 50% of that drug's maximal effect; the more potent the drug, the lower the dose required for a given effect.
precision medicine healthcare model where medical decisions, treatments, practices or products are tailored to an individual patient.
pregnancy the condition in a woman of having a developing embryo or fetus in the body, after implantation of a fertilised ovum.
preload the degree of stretch of heart fibres before contraction; the greater the preload, the greater the stretch.
premedication medication given before anaesthesia that may alleviate pain, reduce anxiety or promote sedation.
prescription a written direction for preparing and administering a drug for a specified person, containing the names and quantities of the active ingredients.
Prescription-Only drug a drug that can only be obtained after issuing a legally valid prescription; in Australia, a Schedule 4 or 8 drug.
pressure sore a bedsore or decubitus ulcer; a break in the skin and underlying subcutaneous and muscle tissue caused by abnormal, sustained pressure or friction exerted over bony prominences of the body.
pressurised metered-dose inhaler a device that releases aerosolised medication in specific dosages to the airways.
preventer a drug that prevents the onset of asthma symptoms by reducing inflammation in the airways. The drugs include corticosteroids and leukotriene antagonists.
primary, or idiopathic, epilepsy a form of epilepsy with no known cause and known as generalised epilepsy.
primary series the initial series of vaccinations that are administered to give a primary antibody response.
prodysrhythmogenic precipitating or producing dysrhythmias.
progestogen a hormone or drug with actions similar to progesterone, the steroidal hormone produced in the female mainly by the *corpus luteum*, with main functions to promote breast development and maintain pregnancy.
prolactin a protein hormone (198 amino acids) secreted by the anterior pituitary gland, involved in the proliferation and secretion of the mammary glands of mammals.
proprietary, or trade, name when a drug company markets a particular drug product, it selects and copyrights a proprietary, or trade, name for the drug. This copyright restricts the use of the name to only the individual drug company and refers only to that formulation of the drug (cf. generic name).
proprotein convertase subtilisin/kexin type 9 (PCSK9) an enzyme that up or down regulates LDL receptors by 'tagging' them and facilitating degradation by lysosomes.
proscribed drug prohibited drug.
prostaglandin lipid autocoids or hormone-like substances that have diverse functions in the body.

protease inhibitors a group of substances that block the activity of proteases, such as in viruses.

pseudoallergic reaction a condition that presents similarly to a true allergic reaction but that occurs through a non-immune mediated mechanism.

psoriasis a common skin disease, probably with an immunological cause, characterised by abnormal immune response, silvery-red epidermal proliferation, with thick plaque lesions, pain, itching and bleeding.

psycholeptics psychoactive drugs that act on the central nervous system and have a sedating effect.

psychoses mental disorders characterised by loss of contact with reality.

psychotropics drugs that affect the mind; may be used to treat neuroses and psychoses.

puffer alternative name for pressurised metered dose inhaler used in respiratory conditions such as asthma.

pure polysaccharide vaccine vaccine that uses the outer polysaccharide (sugar) coating from bacteria as the antigen (e.g. pneumococcal, and meningococcal polysaccharide vaccines).

Quality Use of Medicines optimisation of drug usage involving selecting management options wisely, choosing suitable medicines and using them safely and effectively.

quinolones a large group of broad-spectrum bactericidal drugs that share a bicyclic core structure related to the compound 4-quinolone.

randomised controlled clinical trial large-scale testing in humans of a drug or other medical therapy, which is administered to numerous patients under the guidance of experienced clinical investigators to ascertain whether, under defined conditions, the therapy shows statistically valid clinical benefit for the disease state, with an acceptably low rate of adverse reactions.

rapid eye movement (REM) sleep stage of sleep in which there is rapid eye movement and muscle paralysis.

receptors a large group of proteins that are the molecular targets for drugs; they are cellular macromolecules directly concerned with chemical signalling that initiates a change in cell function.

recombinant vaccine a vaccine produced using recombinant technology (e.g. enables DNA from two or more sources to be combined). A segment of DNA is taken from the virus or bacterium that we are wanting to protection against. This segment is then inserted into the manufacturing cells (e.g. yeast cells). The manufacturing cells produce the antigen in large quantities, which is purified then purified laboratory and used in the vaccine to elicit an immune response.

refractoriness cardiac tissue is non-responsive to stimulation during the initial phase of systole (contraction). This is known as refractoriness, and it determines how closely together two action potentials can occur.

regional anaesthesia the injecting of a local anaesthetic drug near a peripheral nerve trunk (nerve block) or around the spinal column to anaesthetise spinal nerve roots (epidural or subarachnoid techniques).

registered medicines products considered by the Australian Therapeutic Goods Administration to be of potentially high risk, thus requiring regulation.

reinforcement (in behavioural science) the presentation of a stimulus following a response, which increases the frequency of subsequent responses; a way of influencing behaviour through rewards or punishments.

releasing factor/hormone a peptide hormone released from the hypothalamus to the anterior pituitary gland that stimulates secretion of the relevant pituitary hormone.

reliever drug used to treat respiratory conditions that relaxes airway smooth muscle, causing bronchodilation.

renin-angiotensin-aldosterone system a system of renal secretions that regulate electrolyte and fluid balance and blood pressure. The major effector molecules are renin, angiotensin II and the mineralocorticoid aldosterone.

replacement therapy dosing back to physiological levels of a hormone to replace that not produced by a malfunctioning endocrine gland.

respiration the process of inhaling and exhaling air in order to exchange oxygen for carbon dioxide.

restless legs syndrome a neurological disorder causing unpleasant or uncomfortable sensations in the legs and an urge to move them.

retinoids synthetic analogues of retinol (vitamin A) used to treat acne.

retroviruses single-stranded positive-sense RNA viruses that form a DNA intermediate.

reverse transcriptase inhibitor class of antiretroviral drugs used to treat HIV infection that inhibit the activity of viral reverse transcriptase.

reversible inhibitors of MAO-A also known as RIMAs, they are antidepressants that selectively block monoamine oxidase, an enzyme, preventing the breakdown of monoamines.

rhinitis irritation and inflammation of the mucosa of the nasal passages.

rickets a condition seen in infancy and childhood caused by a deficiency of vitamin D and characterised by marked defects in bone mineralisation, with bone weakness, bending and distortion.

route the pathway by which a drug is administered to the body (e.g. oral route: drug is taken by mouth and swallowed).

salicylate a product of the bark of willow trees, and a derivate of salicylic acid.

schizophrenia a mental disorder causing altered experience of reality and involving delusions and hallucinations.

secondary epilepsy epilepsy of a known cause such as alteration in brain structure or chemistry.

sedatives drugs that reduce alertness, consciousness, nervousness or excitability by producing a calming or soothing effect.

selective serotonin reuptake inhibitors antidepressants whose action involves blocking the uptake of serotonin into the nerve terminal via transporters.

selective toxicity a therapy designed to select for differences between healthy human cells and other cells such as cancer cells or microorganisms.

selectivity the property of a drug that acts on a narrow range of receptors, cellular processes or tissues.

self-medication choosing and administering a drug to oneself, without recourse to a health professional.

serotonin noradrenaline (norepinephrine) reuptake inhibitors antidepressants whose action involves blocking the uptake of serotonin and noradrenaline into the nerve terminal.

serotonin syndrome serious clinical condition due to excess serotonin in the central nervous system and periphery.

short-acting β_2 agonists agonists that stimulate β_2 receptors in the airways causing bronchodilation for 4–6 hours.

short-acting muscarinic antagonists antagonists that competitively block M3 receptors in the airways causing bronchodilation and inhibition of mucus secretion for 4–6 hours.

side effects drug effects that are not necessarily the primary purpose for giving the drug in the particular condition. This term has been virtually superseded by the term 'adverse drug reactions'.

single nucleotide polymorphism a variation in a single nucleotide that occurs at a specific position in the genome.

six rights the optimal administration of a drug, with the right patient, drug/form, dose, route, frequency and clinical situation.

skeletal muscle relaxant drug that relaxes skeletal muscle due to central nervous system or direct action and used to treat spasticity or musculoskeletal conditions.

skin the outer layer covering the body, with the main layers being the epidermis and dermis.

sleep hygiene habits that help maximise the number of hours spent sleeping.

somatic nervous system part of the peripheral nervous system involved in motor movement and reflexes.

spacer a holding chamber used, in respiratory conditions, to increase the ease of administering aerosolised medication from a metered-dose inhaler.

spasms sudden involuntary muscular contractions or convulsive movements.

spasticity hypertonic state of skeletal muscles in which the muscles are continuously contracted.

specificity a term that is used loosely, such as 'selectivity', to refer to the narrowness of actions of a drug; the property of a drug that acts at one site, producing one effect.

spinal (subarachnoid) anaesthesia in spinal anaesthesia (also called subarachnoid, intradural or intrathecal block): injection of the local anaesthetic into the cerebrospinal fluid in the subarachnoid space, below the level of termination of the spinal cord – for example, at L3–4 or L4–5; it affects the lower part of the spinal cord and nerve roots.

standardisation the process of assaying the activity of a drug preparation to compare it to that of a model preparation.

status epilepticus one unremitting seizure lasting longer than 5 minutes, or recurrent seizures without gaining consciousness between seizures for greater than 5 minutes; status epilepticus is a clinical emergency.

steady state the situation in which the rate of drug administration equals the rate of elimination and the plasma drug concentration remains constant. Clearance determines the maintenance dose rate required to achieve the target plasma concentration at steady state.

stepwise management of pain 'ladder' for the use of analgesics, starting with non-opioid analgesics and moving to opioid and adjuvant analgesics according to the intensity and severity of pain.

stress incontinence the failure to prevent urine loss due to increased intraabdominal pressure.

stroke a blockage of blood flow or rupture of an artery in the brain, which causes the sudden death of brain cells due to lack of oxygen.

stroke volume volume of blood ejected by ventricle during contraction.

structure–activity studies experiments in which the activities of pharmacologically active substances are determined and related to their chemical structures.

substance P a peptide of the tachykinin family and a neurotransmitter with a wide range of effects, including facilitation of nociception.

substrate a molecule (e.g. drug) upon which an enzyme acts.

sun protection factor a value given to a sunscreen preparation to indicate its effectiveness due to the included sunscreening agents; the factor is the ratio between the dose of ultraviolet radiation required to cause erythema (reddening) with and without the sunscreen.

sunscreen a preparation applied to the skin to absorb and/or to reflect ultraviolet radiation in order to reduce the risks of photo-ageing, sunburn, actinic keratoses and skin cancers.

superinfection an infection that occurs during the course of antimicrobial therapy delivered for either therapeutic or prophylactic reasons.

surfactant a surface-active agent that reduces surface tension and increases wettability; in the airways, a phospholipid–glycoprotein–lipoprotein mixture secreted in alveolar cells and present in the secretions lining the alveoli.

sustained release release of active drug from a tablet or capsule, the rate of which is slowed by pharmaceutical processing, allowing prolonged drug actions.

sympatholytic drugs drugs that block the action of the sympathetic nervous system; includes β and α receptor blockers.

sympathomimetic drugs pharmacological agents that mimic the effects of stimulating organs by the sympathetic nervous system.

synapse a specialised junction between a neuron transmitting a chemical or electrical signal to another neuron or between a neuron and an effector organ.

systole period of contraction during cardiac cycle.

tablets solid disc-shaped compressed mixtures of active drug with various other chemicals, called excipients, which assist in the formulation.

tardive dyskinesia neurological disorder caused by long-term use of conventional antipsychotics, which involves repetitive involuntary muscle movements.

teratogen a substance that causes transient or permanent physical or functional disorders in a fetus, without causing toxicity in the mother.

testosterone the main male sex hormone, a steroid produced in the Leydig (interstitial) cells of the testes, with physiological actions in normal development and maintenance of male sex functions and characteristics.

tetracyclines the first broad-spectrum antibiotics, developed after a systematic search for antibiotic-producing microorganisms in soil.

therapeutic drug monitoring branch of chemical pathology and clinical pharmacology that specialises in measuring drug concentrations in blood.

Therapeutic Goods Administration a division of the Australian Commonwealth Department of Health that evaluates drugs, medical devices, diagnostic devices and biological entities pre-marketing for quality, safety, efficacy and cost-effectiveness, and access for the public.
thrombocytopenia a condition characterised by a reduced number of platelets; the most common cause of bleeding disorders.
thrombolytic (fibrinolytic) drugs drugs used to treat acute thromboembolic disorders; unlike anticoagulants, they dissolve clots.
thrombus an aggregation of platelets, fibrin, clotting factors and the cellular elements of blood that attaches to the inner wall of blood vessels.
thyroglobulin a glycoprotein synthesised in thyroid follicle cells.
thyroid-stimulating hormone substance secreted by the anterior pituitary gland that controls the release of thyroid hormone.
thyrotrophin-releasing hormone substance released from the hypothalamus that stimulates the release of thyroid-stimulating hormone from the anterior pituitary.
thyroxine hormone secreted by the thyroid gland.
tinnitus the sensation of 'ringing in the ears'.
tocolytics drugs that relax the uterus and hence delay labour or inhibit threatened abortion.
tolerance a phenomenon by which the body becomes increasingly resistant to a drug or other substance through continued exposure to the substance.
tonic–clonic seizure a seizure that affects the whole central nervous system and involves violent muscle contractions; also known as a generalised or grand mal seizure.
topical administration application of a drug to the surface of the skin.
total intravenous anaesthesia a general anaesthesic technique in which a combination of anaesthetics is given via the intravenous route alone.
toxoid a bacterial toxin that has been inactivated and used in a vaccine to induce immunity (e.g. tetanus toxoid).
toxoplasmosis infectious disease caused by infection with *Toxoplasma gondii*.
traditional Chinese medicine a style of medicine based on more than 2500 years of Chinese medical practice, including various forms of herbal medicine, acupuncture, massage, exercise and dietary therapies.
tranquilliser a drug that alleviates anxiety and causes sedation.
transcutaneous absorption uptake into the bloodstream of a drug or other chemical through the layers of the skin.
trichomoniasis sexually transmitted disease caused by infection with *Trichomonas vaginali*.
tricyclic antidepressants antidepressants, named after their three-ringed chemical structure, that block the reuptake of noradrenaline and serotonin.
tri-iodothyronine an active thyroid hormone that influences all bodily processes including gene expression.
tuberculosis potentially serious bacterial infection that mainly affects the lungs.
tubular reabsorption a selective reabsorptive process that occurs throughout the nephron.
tubular secretion movement of substances from capillaries into renal tubular cells and then into the tubular lumen.
type 1/type 2 diabetes diabetes mellitus (see earlier definition) due to an absolute (type 1) or relative (type 2) lack of insulin.
typical antipsychotics first-generation antipsychotics that block dopamine receptors and include the phenothiazines.
tyramine reaction hypertensive crisis occurring if monoamine oxidase inhibitors are given in combination with foods containing high doses of tyramine.

ulcer (leg, foot) a break or excavation in the skin or an organ due to sloughing of inflammatory necrotic tissue.
ulcerative colitis chronic inflammation of the large intestine.
urge incontinence the involuntary leakage of urine with the feeling of urgency to urinate.
ultraviolet radiation electromagnetic radiation with wavelengths (400–200 nm) shorter than those of visible light (at the violet end of the colour spectrum) and longer than those of x-rays.

vasodilator drugs drugs that produce vasodilation by relaxing smooth muscle in the blood vessel walls by either a direct or indirect action.
vehicle the formulation in which a drug is administered (e.g. the ointment base or injection solution); the drug needs to leave the vehicle to be available for absorption.
vertigo an illusory sensation that either the environment or one's own body is revolving.
very-low-density lipoproteins one of three primary classes of lipoproteins found in the blood of fasting individuals.
volume of distribution (V_D) the volume in which the amount of drug in the body would need to be uniformly distributed to produce the observed concentration in blood.

waist:hip ratio waist circumference (cm) divided by hip circumference (cm).
withdrawal syndrome physiological disturbances when administration of a drug ceases.
xanthine derivatives drugs that resemble the purine xanthine and include the plant-derived compounds caffeine, theobromine and theophylline. Drugs such as theophylline are used as bronchodilators in treating asthma.

Z-drugs drugs, including zolpidem and zopiclone, used as non-benzodiazepine hypnotics.

Some definitions adapted from: Youngson RM: *Collins dictionary of medicine: medicine defined and explained*, Glasgow, 2005, HarperCollins.
See also: Harris P, Nagy S, Vardaxis N (eds): *Mosby's dictionary of medicine, nursing and health professions*, ed 3, Sydney, 2014, Elsevier Australia.

APPENDIX 3
COMMON ABBREVIATIONS AND SYMBOLS USED IN PRESCRIPTIONS

ABBREVIATION	UNABBREVIATED FORM	MEANING
*ac	Ante cibum	Before meals
ad lib	Ad libitum	Freely
am	Ante meridiem	Morning
*aq	Aqua	Water, aqueous
*bd, bid	Bis die, bis in die	Twice each day
c	Cum	With
*cap	Capsule	Capsule
CR	Controlled/continuous release	Controlled/continuous release
D5W	Dextrose 5% water	5% Dextrose in water (5 g/100 mL)
DW	Distilled water	Water purified by condensation from steam
EC	Enteric-coated	Tablet or capsule formulation whose coating prevents dissolution until reaching the small intestine
elix	Elixir	Elixir
*g, gm	Gram	1000 milligrams
gtt	Gutta	Drop
h, hr	Hora	Hour
hs	Hora somni	At bedtime (may be confused with 'half-strength')
IA	Intra-arterial	Into an artery or arteriole
ID	Intradermal	Into the skin
*IM	Intramuscular	Into muscle
*inj	Injection	Injection
IT	Intrathecal	Into the subarachnoid space
IU	International Unit	Unit of pharmacological activity for a particular drug, as defined by an international convention (but easily confused with IV; better spelled out in full)
*IV	Intravenous	Into a vein
IVPB	IV piggyback	Secondary IV line
kg	Kilogram	1000 grams
KVO	Keep vein open	Very slow infusion rate
L	Litre	Litre (1000 cm^3)
M	Mitte	Send, supply
*mane	Morning	In the morning
mcg, microg	Microgram	One-millionth of a gram #
MDI	Metered dose inhaler	Metered dose inhaler
*mg	Milligram	One-thousandth of a gram
mEq	Milliequivalent	One-thousandth of the gram equivalent weight of a solute in an electrolyte solution
mist	Mistura	Mixture
*mL	Millilitre	One-thousandth of a litre, 1 cm^3
neb	Nebulised	Nebulised
NG	Nasogastric	Into the stomach via the nose
*nocte	At night	At night
NS	Normal saline	0.9% sodium chloride solution
Ō	Oral	Oral
oc	Oculorum	Eye

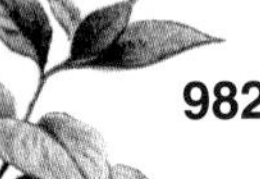

ABBREVIATION	UNABBREVIATED FORM	MEANING
os	Os	Mouth
OTC	Over-the-counter	Non-prescription drug
otic	Otikos	The ear
*pc	Post cibum	After meals
PCA	Patient-controlled analgesia	Patient-controlled analgesia
pess	Pessary	Pessary; small solid-dose form to be inserted into the vagina
PICC	Peripherally inserted central catheter	Peripherally inserted central catheter
pm	Post meridiem	After noon
PO or O	Per os	By mouth, orally
PR	Per rectum	Into the rectum
*prn	Pro re nata	When required (literally for the thing [i.e. need] having arisen)
PV	Per vagina	Into the vagina
q	Quaque	Every
*qid	Quater in die	Four times a day (may be confused with 'every day')
qh	Quaque hora	Every hour
q4h, qqh	Quaque quarta hora	Every 4 hours
qs	Quantum satis	Sufficient quantity
Rx	Receipt, recipe	Take (or dispense, provide)
s	Sine	Without
SC (subcut preferable)	Subcutaneous	Into subcutaneous tissue (may be misread as SL)
Sig.	Signature	Label, instructions
SL (subling preferable)	Sub linguam	Under the tongue (may be misread as SC)
SOS	Si opus sit	If necessary
SR	Sustained release	Sustained release
ss	Semis	A half
*stat	Statim	At once
supp	Suppository	Suppository; small solid-dose form to be inserted into the rectum
*tab	Tablet	Tablet
tbsp	Tablespoon	Tablespoon (15 mL)
*tid or tds	Ter in die, ter die sumendum	Three times a day
TO	Telephone order	Order received over the telephone
top	Topically	Applied to the skin
tsp	Teaspoon	Teaspoon (4 or 5 mL)
U	Unit	A dose measure of activity for natural products such as insulin, heparin
ung	Unguentum	Ointment (probably understood only by Latin scholars)
VO	Verbal order	Order received verbally
X	Times	(As in two times a week)

*Only the abbreviations marked with an asterisk are approved by the *Australian Medicines Handbook*.
#microgram should not be abbreviated to μg (the Greek letter m, mu). If the Greek/symbol font reverts to a normal font, it becomes mg, i.e. milligram, a 1000-fold greater amount!
An abbreviation such as 6/24 should not be used, as it may be read as 'every 6 hours' or as '6 times per day'.
If there is any possibility of confusion, words should be written in full: 'If in doubt, write it out!'

APPENDIX 4

DOSE CALCULATION EXAMPLES

Abbreviations used in these examples

WYW what you want WYH what you have WICI what it comes in

1 Calculation for oral administration of liquids

A child has been prescribed the antibiotic erythromycin 250 mg orally every 12 hours as prophylaxis for rheumatic fever. The stock liquid suspension contains 200 mg/5 mL.

What volume of the mixture should be given every 12 hours?

Estimate: the child is going to need a bit more than 5 mL each dose.

Step 1 Conversion is not required because in this example both prescribed dose and stock suspension strength involve the same unit of weight, mg. The strength of the stock suspension is 200/5 mg/mL = 40 mg/mL.

Step 2

WYW = 250 mg dose every 12 hours
WYH = 200 mg
WICI = 5 mL

To calculate the volume of suspension required, apply the formula:

$$\text{Volume required} = \frac{\text{WYW}}{\text{WYH}} \times \text{WICI}$$
$$= \frac{250\text{ mg}}{200\text{ mg}} \times 5\text{ mL}$$
$$= 6.25\text{ mL}$$

The child should be given 6.25 mL twice daily. (Check: yes, this is a bit more than 5 mL.)

2 Calculation for oral administration of tablets or capsules

The prescriber orders paracetamol 1 g orally every 6 hours for a patient with a high temperature. The label on the package states that each tablet contains 500 mg paracetamol. How many tablets do you administer to the patient every 6 hours?

Step 1 Convert both weights to the same unit of weight – in this case, milligrams.

$$\text{Prescribed dosage} = 1\text{g} \times 1000\text{ mg/g}$$
$$= 1000\text{ mg 6-hourly}$$

Step 2

WYW = 1 g dose every 6 hours = 1000 mg
WYH = 500 mg
WICI = 1 tablet

To calculate the number of tablets required, apply the formula:

$$\text{Tablets required} = \frac{\text{WYW}}{\text{WYH}} \times \text{WICI}$$
$$= \frac{1000\text{ mg}}{500\text{ mg}} \times 1\text{ tablet}$$
$$= 2\text{ tablets}$$

The patient should take 2 tablets every 6 hours.

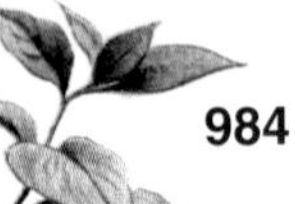

3 Calculation of dosage based on body weight

A child has been prescribed the antibiotic ampicillin and the recommended dosage is 10 mg/kg every 6 hours. What will be the size of a single dose for a child weighing 30 kg?

Method 1 Calculation by formula:

Step 1 Conversion is not required because, in this example, the body weight of the child and that in the recommended dosage are in the same units, kg.

Step 2 To calculate the size of a single dose, apply the formula:

$$\begin{aligned}\text{Prescribed dosage} &= \text{recommended dose (mg/kg)} \\ &\quad \times \text{body weight (kg)} \\ &= 10\text{ mg/kg} \times 30\text{ kg} \\ &= 300\text{ mg}\end{aligned}$$

The child should be given 300 mg every 6 hours.

Method 2 Calculation by simple proportion:

For 1 kg body weight, prescribe a 10 mg dose.

So, for 30 kg body weight, prescribe 10 mg/1 kg × 30 kg

$$\begin{aligned}&= \frac{10 \times 30\text{ mg}}{1} \\ &= 300\text{ mg (as before).}\end{aligned}$$

4 Calculation for safe maximum dose of a local anaesthetic

The safe maximum dose (SMD) of lidocaine (lignocaine) as a local anaesthetic in adults is set at 3 mg/kg body weight. You (a dentist) are provided with 5 mL ampoules of lidocaine injection 2%. What is the maximum number of ampoules you would expect to require for an average-sized adult patient before a dental extraction?

Step 1 Assuming a mean adult body weight of 70 kg,

$$\begin{aligned}\text{SMD} &= 70\text{ kg} \times 3\text{ mg/kg} \\ &= 210\text{ mg}\end{aligned}$$

Step 2 2% solution means 2 g lidocaine per 100 mL solution; that is, 2000 mg are present in 100 mL.

WYW = 210 mg = SMD
WYH = 2000 mg
WICI = 100 mL

$$\begin{aligned}\text{Dose required} &= \frac{\text{WYW}}{\text{WYH}} \times \text{WICI} \\ &= \frac{210\text{ mg}}{2000\text{ mg}} \times 100\text{ mL} \\ &= 10.5\text{ mL}\end{aligned}$$

So, the safe maximum dose will be present in 10.5 mL solution and, as the ampoules provided contain 5 mL, two ampoules (approximately 10 mL) will probably be adequate.

5 Calculation of divided doses

A child is to be given the antiprotozoal drug metronidazole to treat giardiasis. The recommended dosage is 30 mg/kg/day in three divided doses (i.e. 8-hourly). What is the size of a single dose if the child's weight is 18 kg?

Step 1 Conversion is not required because, in this example, the body weight of the child and that in the recommended dosage are in the same units, kg.

Step 2 To calculate the total daily dose, apply the formula:

$$\begin{aligned}\text{Prescribed dosage} &= \text{recommended dosage (mg/kg/day)} \\ &\quad \times \text{body weight (kg)} \\ &= 30\text{ mg/kg/day} \times 18\text{ kg} \\ &= 540\text{ mg/day total dose}\end{aligned}$$

Step 3 To calculate the size of a single dose, apply the formula:

$$\begin{aligned}\text{Single dose (mg)} &= \frac{\text{total dose (mg)}}{\text{number of doses}} \\ &= \frac{540\text{ mg}}{3} \\ &= 180\text{ mg}\end{aligned}$$

The child should be administered 180 mg every 8 hours.

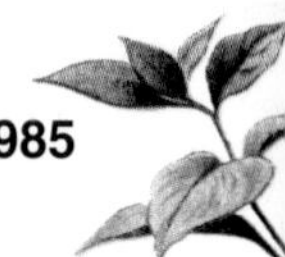

6 Conversion between weight units

An elderly patient is prescribed 0.125 mg digoxin once daily, which is available in your care facility pharmacy only as a 250-microgram tablet. How many tablets do you administer daily?

Method 1

Step 1 Convert both weights to the same unit of weight – in this case, micrograms.

$$\text{Prescribed dosage} = 0.125\ \text{mg} \times 1000\ \text{micrograms/mg} = 125\ \text{micrograms daily}$$

Now **estimate**: one tablet contains 250 micrograms, so the patient needs less than one tablet (actually, of course, one-half).

Step 2 To calculate the number of tablets required, apply the formula:

$$\text{Tablets required} = \frac{\text{prescribed dose}}{\text{tablets strength}} = \frac{125\ \text{micrograms}}{250\ \text{micrograms}} = 0.5\ \text{tablet}$$

The patient should take half a tablet once a day.

Method 2

WYW = 0.125 mg = 125 micrograms daily dose
WYH = 250 micrograms
WICI = 1 tablet

$$\text{Daily dosage} = \frac{125\ \text{micrograms}}{250\ \text{micrograms}} \times 1\ \text{tablet} = 0.5\ \text{tablet}$$

Helpful hints for Example 6:
Never use less than half a tablet, and preferably use a smaller-dose tablet if one is available; here, 2 × 62.5 microgram tablets would be preferable.

Exercise care, as some tablets or capsules should never be broken, especially enteric-coated or sustained-release preparations, unless otherwise indicated as safe to break.

Take care when converting from milligrams to micrograms. Always write in full or use the abbreviation 'microg' and not the Greek symbol μ. (If, by chance, the computer loses its fonts, the μg would become mg, a 1000 times overdose that would likely kill the patient!)

7 Calculation of dosage based on surface area

In some circumstances (e.g. critical-care situations, cancer chemotherapy), dosages of some drugs are calculated in terms of body surface area (see Ch 7). These calculations usually involve a nomogram that relates height (or length), weight and surface area.

A woman is to be administered epirubicin for treatment of cancer. The prescribed dosage is 100 mg/m^2 and her body surface area has been determined as 1.5 m^2. The stock solution of epirubicin is 2 mg/mL. What volume should be drawn up for infusion?

Conversion is not required because, in this example, the body surface area of the patient and that in the prescribed dosage are in the same units, m^2.

Step 1 To calculate the total dosage, apply the formula:

$$\text{Prescribed dosage} = \text{recommended dosage}\ (\text{mg/m}^2) \times \text{body surface area}\ (\text{m}^2) = 100\ \text{mg/m}^2 \times 1.5\ \text{m}^2 = 150\ \text{mg}$$

Step 2

WYW = 150 mg
WYH = 2 mg
WICI = 1 mL

To calculate the volume to be drawn up for infusion, apply the formula:

$$\text{Volume required} = \frac{\text{WYW}}{\text{WYH}} \times \text{WICI} = \frac{150\ \text{mg}}{2\ \text{mg}} \times 1\ \text{mL} = 75\ \text{mL}$$

The volume to be drawn up for infusion is 75 mL. Note that this drug is available for infusion in several pack sizes, ranging from 10 mg/5 mL to 50 mg/25 mL.

8 Calculation of drug dosage for intravenous infusion (by drip rate)

A patient has been ordered an infusion of sodium chloride and glucose, 500 mL over 24 hours. The IV infusion (giving) set delivers 20 drops/mL. At what rate (in drops/minute) should the giving set drip?

Method 1 Calculation by formula:

Step 1 Convert time to the same units, minutes:

$$24 \text{ hours} = 24 \times 60 \text{ minutes}$$
$$= 1440 \text{ minutes}$$

Step 2 To calculate the drip rate, apply the formula:

$$\text{Rate (drops/minute)} = \frac{\text{volume to be delivered} \times \text{drops/mL}}{\text{time (minutes)}}$$
$$= \frac{500 \text{ mL} \times 20 \text{ drops/mL}}{1440 \text{ minutes}}$$
$$= 6.9 \text{ drops/minute}$$
$$= 7 \text{ drops/minute (rounding off to next whole number)}$$

The giving set should be adjusted to a drip rate of 7 drops/minute.

Method 2 Calculation by simple proportion:

The patient needs, in 1 day, 500 mL solution – that is, in 1440 min needs 500 mL (as before), so in 1 min needs 500/1440 × 1 mL.

Each 1 mL contains 20 drops, so 500/1440 mL is contained in 20/1 × 500/1440 drops,

= (approx) 7 drops.

Therefore, the set should be adjusted to approximately 7 drops per minute.

Method 3 Calculation by converting to drops:

Step 1 is the same as above.

Step 2 Convert the dose to the same units (drops):

WYW = 500 mL
WYH = 1 mL
WICI = 20 drops

$$\text{Dosage} = \frac{500 \text{ mL} \times 20 \text{ drops}}{1 \text{ mL}}$$
$$= 10{,}000 \text{ drops}$$

Set needs to deliver 10,000 drops over 1440 minutes.

$$\text{Rate} = \frac{10{,}000 \text{ drops}}{1440 \text{ minutes}}$$
$$= 7 \text{ drops/minute}$$

9 Calculation of drug dosage for injection

A patient has been ordered 75 mg pethidine for pain relief. The ampoules available to you contain 100 mg in 2 mL. What volume is required for injection?

Method 1

Step 1 Conversion is not required because, in this example, the units of weight are the same, mg.

The strength of the solution in the ampoules is 100/2 mg/mL = 50 mg/mL.

Step 2 To calculate the volume to be drawn up for injection, apply the formula:

$$\text{Volume required} = \frac{\text{prescribed dosage}}{\text{strength of stock suspension}}$$
$$= \frac{75 \text{ mg}}{50 \text{ mg/mL}}$$
$$= 1.5 \text{ mL}$$

The volume to be drawn up for injection is 1.5 mL from the 2 mL ampoule.

Method 2

WYW = 75 mg
WYH = 100 mg
WICI = 2 mL

$$\text{Volume required} = \frac{75 \text{ mg} \times 2 \text{ mL}}{100 \text{ mg}}$$
$$= 1.5 \text{ mL}$$

Helpful hints for Example 9:

Measuring drug dosages for injection is important, as too high a dose may be dangerous and too low a dose may be ineffective. Always check your calculation with another qualified health professional if you have any doubts at all.

For drugs administered by injection, the number of decimal places in an answer should match the graduations on the syringe. For less than 1 mL, calculate then round off to two decimal places (e.g. 0.75 mL, 0.25 mL, 0.64 mL), as syringes are often graduated in hundredths of a mL – that is, 0.01 mL graduations. For more than 1 mL, calculate then round off to one decimal place (e.g. 1.8 mL, 8.7 mL, 12.5 mL), as syringes may be graduated in either fifths (0.2 mL graduations) or tenths (0.1 mL graduations).

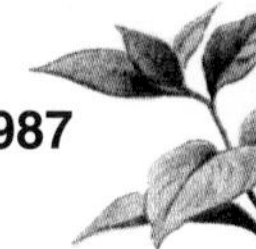

10 Bolus doses from infusion pumps

A palliative care patient is self-administering patient-controlled analgesia via an SC syringe pump, from a solution of fentanyl 300 micrograms/30 mL normal saline, set for bolus doses of 1 mL.

(a) What amount of fentanyl does she receive in each bolus dose?

(b) If she administers 6 bolus doses in an hour, what is the fentanyl dose rate in micrograms/minute?

(c) If the pump is re-set to deliver 5 mL per hour, what dose rate will she receive?

(d) At what rate should the pump be set to deliver an approximately equivalent dose to a 75 micrograms/h patch?

Method 1

(a) Solution contains 300 micrograms fentanyl in 30 mL, so in 1 mL (bolus dose) there are 300/30 × 1 micrograms = 10 micrograms – that is,

10 micrograms fentanyl in 1 mL bolus dose.

(b) If 1 bolus contains 10 micrograms fentanyl, then 6 boluses contain 60 micrograms fentanyl.

So, 6 doses in 1 hour means 60 micrograms/h – that is, in 60 min she receives 60 micrograms – so in 1 min she receives 60/60 × 1 micrograms = 1 microgram.

Fentanyl dose rate is 1 microgram/min.

(c) If the pump delivers 5 mL per hour – that is,

5 × 10 micrograms/60 min – in 60 min it delivers 50 micrograms, so in 1 min it delivers 50/60 × 1 micrograms = 0.83 micrograms.

Dose rate is 0.83 micrograms/min.

(d) Assume that fentanyl delivered by SC syringe has the same bioavailability as a dose absorbed from a 75-micrograms/h patch – that is, require the pump to deliver 75 micrograms/h.

Solution contains 10 micrograms/mL.

That is, 75 micrograms in 1/10 × 75 mL = 7.5 mL.

So, the dose rate required is 7.5 mL/h.

Method 2

(a) and **(b)** are the same as above.

(c) Convert the pump rate to the same units (minutes):

$$5 \text{ mL/hour} = 5/60 \text{ mL/minute}$$

$$\begin{aligned}\text{Dose delivered} &= \text{concentration} \times \text{volume}\\ &= 10 \text{ micrograms/mL} \times 5/60 \text{ mL minute}\\ &= 50/60 \text{ micrograms/minute}\\ &= 0.83 \text{ micrograms/minute}\end{aligned}$$

(d) If the pump delivers 75 micrograms/hour, dose/hour = 75 micrograms = WYW

WYH = 10 micrograms

WICI = 1 mL

$$\text{Dose/hour} = \frac{75 \text{ micrograms}}{10 \text{ micrograms}} \times 1 \text{ mL} = 7.5 \text{ mL/hour}$$

11 Calculation of drug dosage for intravenous infusion (by infusion pump)

Example 11(a)

For the same patient as in Example 8, an infusion pump becomes available. At what rate should the pump be set to deliver the sodium chloride/glucose solution?

The calculation here is much simpler, and can be done by simple proportions, as we know that 500 mL need to be delivered over 24 hours.

Thus: in 24 hours, deliver 500 mL

$$\text{so in 1 hour, deliver} \quad \frac{500 \text{ mL} \times 1 \text{ h}}{24 \text{ h}} = 20.8 \text{ mL}$$

The infusion pump should be set to deliver approximately 21 mL/hour.

Example 11(b)

The patient (a man weighing 80 kg) is prescribed gentamicin 3 mg/kg/day in 3 doses/day by IV infusion, given every 8 hours over a 2-hour period. Each dose is to be diluted in 100 mL sterile normal saline. How should the infusion pump be set?

Method 1 Calculation by first principles:

$$\begin{aligned}\text{Total daily dosage} &= 3 \text{ mg/kg/day} \times 80 \text{ kg}\\ &= 240 \text{ mg/day}\\ \text{divided into 3 equal doses} &= 240/3 \text{ mg/dose}\\ &= 80 \text{ mg/dose}\end{aligned}$$

Dose is to be diluted in 100 mL saline. Gentamicin Injection BP is provided as vials containing 80 mg/2 mL, so 1 vial contains 1 dose.

For each dose, contents of 1 vial are diluted to 100 mL in normal saline, giving 80 mg/100 mL – that is, 0.8 mg/mL.

Solution is to be run in IV over 2 hours – that is, 100 mL/2 h – so the pump is set at an infusion rate of 50 mL/h.

Method 2 Calculation by formula:

$$\text{Infusion rate (mL/h)} = \frac{\text{Drug required (mg/h)} \times \text{volume (mL)}}{\text{Total amount (mg)}}$$

From Method 1, each dose = 80 mg over 2 h = 40 mg/h, in a volume of 100 mL for a dose of 80 mg.

$$\text{Hence, infusion rate} = \frac{40 \text{ mg/h} \times 100 \text{ mL}}{80 \text{ mg}} = \frac{4000 \text{ mg} \cdot \text{mL}}{80 \text{ mg} \cdot \text{h}} = 50 \text{ mL/h}$$

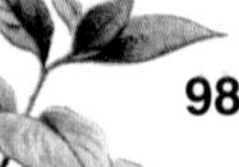

12 Calculation using strength of a solution

An ophthalmologist has prescribed timolol eye-drops 5 mg/mL, 1 drop in the affected eye twice daily. You (a pharmacist) have available timolol drops in 0.25% strength or 0.5% strength. What do you dispense?

Method 1 Check out the 0.25% drops:

Step 1 Convert the concentration of the stock solution to mg/mL:

0.25% solution means 0.25 g/100 mL.

Step 2 To calculate mg/mL, apply the formula:

$$\begin{aligned}\text{mg/mL} &= \frac{\text{g} \times 100}{\text{volume (mL)}}\\ &= \frac{0.25\ \text{g} \times 1000}{100\ \text{mL}}\\ &= 2.5\ \text{mg/mL}\end{aligned}$$

Step 3 To calculate the number of drops required, apply the formula:

$$\begin{aligned}\text{Number of drops} &= \frac{\text{prescribed dose}}{\text{strength of stock solution}} \times \text{number of drops prescribed}\\ &= \frac{5\ \text{mg/mL}}{2.5\ \text{mg/mL}} \times 1\ \text{drop}\\ &= 2\ \text{drops}\end{aligned}$$

The patient would have to instil 2 drops in the affected eye twice daily; however, note that 2 drops do not usually fit in the conjunctival sac (as discussed in Ch 18), so check the 0.5% solution.

Alternative approaches:

Step 2 Estimate, by simple proportion: if the solution provided is half the strength of that prescribed, then twice the volume prescribed will be required; that is, 2 drops of 0.25% solution (2.5 mg/mL) contains the same amount of drug as 1 drop of 0.5% solution (5 mg/mL).

Step 3 Using an algebraic method, assume 1 drop contains d mL.

$$\begin{aligned}\text{Dose required} &= \text{d mL of 5 mg/mL solution}\\ \text{Amount (mass) in d mL} &= \text{concentration} \times \text{volume}\\ &= 5\ \text{mg/mL} \times \text{d mL}\\ &= 5\text{d mg}\end{aligned}$$

WYW = 5d mg
WYH = 2.5 mg
WICI = 1 mL

$$\begin{aligned}\text{Volume required} &= \frac{5\text{d mg}}{0.5\ \text{mg}} \times 1\ \text{mL}\\ &= 2\text{d mL}\\ &= 2\ \text{drops}\end{aligned}$$

Method 2 Check out the 0.5% drops:

0.5% strength means 0.5 g per 100 mL,

that is, 500 mg/100 mL,

which equals 5 mg/mL

This is the strength prescribed by the doctor, so you dispense this strength and label the bottle as directed.

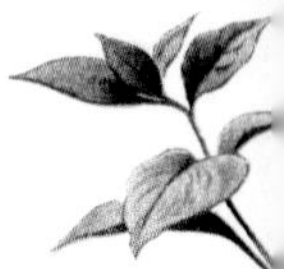

FURTHER READINGS

Chapter 1

Oprea TI, Bologa CG, Brunak S, et al., Unexplored therapeutic opportunities in the human genome. Nature Reviews Drug Discovery, 2018. 17(5): p. 317-332.

PHARMAC. Year in Review: Top 20 community medicines by number of funded prescriptions dispensed. 2020; Available from: https://pharmac.govt.nz/about/what-we-do/accountability-information/year-in-review/top-20-medicines-groups-by-prescription-volume/.

PHARMAC. Year in Review: Top 20 therapeutic groups by gross spend. 2020; Available from: https://pharmac.govt.nz/about/what-we-do/accountability-information/year-in-review/top-20-therapeutic-groups-by-gross-spend/.

Pharmaceutical Society of Australia, Australian pharmaceutical formulary and handbook. 25 ed, ed. Sansom LN. 2021, Canberra: Pharmaceutical Society of Australia.

Martindale: The Complete Drug Reference. 40 ed, ed. R. Buckingham. 2020, London, UK: Pharmaceutical Press.

Reilly, T., Jackson, W., Berger, V., et al., Accuracy and completeness of drug information in Wikipedia medication monographs. Journal of the American Pharmacists Association, 2017. 57(2): p. 193-196. e1.

Chapter 2

No further reading.

Chapter 3

Alexander SPH, Christopoulos A, Davenport AP, et al: The concise guide to pharmacology 2019/20: G protein-coupled receptors, British Journal of Pharmacology 176: s21-s141, 2019.

Alexander SPH, Fabbro D, Kelly E, et al: The concise guide to pharmacology 2019/20: catalytic receptors, British Journal of Pharmacology 176: s247-s296, 2019.

Alexander SPH, Fabbro D, Kelly E, et al: The concise guide to pharmacology 2019/20: enzymes, British Journal of Pharmacology 176: s297-s396, 2019.

Harding SD, Sharman JL, Faccenda E, et al: The IUPHAR/BPS guide to pharmacology 2018: updates and expansion to encompass the new guide to immunopharmacology, Nucleic Acids Research 46: D1091-D1106, 2018.

Santos R, Ursu O, Gaulton A, et al: A comprehensive map of molecular drug targets, Nature Reviews Drug Discovery 16: 19-34, 2017.

Chapter 4

Giacomini KM, Galetin A, Huang SM. The International Transporter Consortium: Summarizing advances in the role of transporters in drug development. Clinical Pharmacology and Therapeutics 104: 766-771, 2018.

Koren G, Pariente G. Pregnancy-associated changes in pharmacokinetics and their clinical implications. Pharmaceutical Research 35: 61, 2018.

Rowland M, Tozer TN: Clinical pharmacokinetics: concepts and applications, 5th ed, Philadelphia, 2019, Lea & Febiger.

Chapter 5

Barras M, Legg A. Drug dosing in obese adults. Australian Prescriber, 40, 189-193, 2017.

Begg EJ: Instant clinical pharmacokinetics, 2nd Ed, Oxford, UK, 2007, Wiley-Blackwell Publishing.

Birkett DJ: Pharmacokinetics made easy, 2nd Ed, Sydney, 2010, McGraw-Hill.

Notari RE: Biopharmaceutics and clinical pharmacokinetics: an introduction, 4th Ed, Boca Raton, 2017

Chapter 6

Carranza-Leon D, Dickson AL, Gaedigk A, et al: CYP2D6 genotype and reduced codeine analgesic effect in real-world clinical practice. Pharmacogenomics Journal 21: 484-490, 2021.

Goetz MP, Sangkuhl K, Guchelaar, HJ, et al: Clinical Pharmacogenetics Implementation Consortium (CPIC) Guideline for CYP2D6 and Tamoxifen Therapy. Clinical Pharmacology and Therapeutics, 103: 770-777, 2018.

Hopkins AM, Menz BD, Wiese MD, et al: Nuances to precision dosing strategies of targeted cancer medicines. Pharmacology Research and Perspectives 8: e00625, 2020.

Mueller-Schoell A., Groenland SL, Scherf-Clavel O. et al: Therapeutic drug monitoring of oral targeted antineoplastic drugs. European Journal of Clinical Pharmacology 77: 441-464, 2021.

Rodrigues AD, Rowland: From endogenous compounds as biomarkers to plasma-derived nanovesicles as liquid biopsy; Has the golden age of translational PK-ADME-DDI science finally arrived? Clinical Pharmacology and Therapeutics, 105: 1407-1420, 2019.

Venter JC, Adams MD, Myers EW, et al: The sequence of the human genome, Science 291:1304-1351, 2001.

Chapter 7

Bailey DG: Fruit juice inhibition of uptake transport: a new type of food–drug interaction, British Journal of Clinical Pharmacology 70:645-655, 2010.

Deng, J., Zhu, X., Chen, Z. et al. A review of food–drug interactions on oral drug absorption. Drugs 77, 1833-1855, 2017.

Edwards IR, Aronson JK: Adverse drug reactions: definitions, diagnosis, and management, Lancet 356:1255-1259, 2000.

Niu, J., Straubinger, R.M., Mager, D.E. (2019), Pharmacodynamic Drug–Drug Interactions. Clinical Pharmacology & Therapeutics, 105: 1395-1406, 2019

Chapter 8

Alexander SP, Peters JA, Kelly E, et al. The concise guide to pharmacology 2017/18: Ligand-gated ion channels. British Journal of Pharmacology. 2017; Dec;174 Suppl 1(Suppl 1):S130-S159. doi: 10.1111/bph.13879. PMID: 29055038; PMCID: PMC5650660.

Birdsall NJM, Bradley S, Brown A, et al. Acetylcholine receptors (muscarinic) (version 2019.4) in the IUPHAR/BPS Guide to Pharmacology Database. IUPHAR/BPS Guide to Pharmacology CITE. 2019; 2019(4). Available from: https://doi.org/10.2218/gtopdb/F2/2019.4

Brown JH, Brandl KA, Wess J: Muscarinic receptor agonists and antagonists. In Brunton LL, Chabner B, Knollman B, editors: Goodman & Gilman's The Pharmacological Basis of Therapeutics, ed 13, New York, 2017, McGraw-Hill.

Hibbs RE, Zambon AC. Nicotine and agents acting at the neuromuscular junction and autonomic ganglia. In: Brunton LL, Hilal-Dandan R, Knollmann BC. eds. Goodman & Gilman's: The pharmacological basis of therapeutics, 13e. McGraw Hill; 2017.

Hulse EJ, Haslam JD, Emmett SR, et al. Organophosphorus nerve agent poisoning: managing the poisoned patient. British Journal of Anaesthesia. 2019; Oct;123(4):457-463. doi: 10.1016/j.bja.2019.04.061. Epub 2019 Jun 24. PMID: 31248646.

Lilienfeld S: Galantamine – a novel cholinergic drug with a unique dual mode of action for the treatment of patients with Alzheimer's disease, CNS Drug Reviews 8:159-176, 2002.

Pirazzini M, Rossetto O, Eleopra R, et al. Botulinum neurotoxins: biology, pharmacology, and toxicology. Pharmacological Reviews. 2017 Apr;69(2):200-235. doi: 10.1124/pr.116.012658. PMID: 28356439; PMCID: PMC5394922.

Szinicz L: History of chemical and biological warfare agents, Toxicology 214:167-181, 2005.

Taylor P (2017). Anticholinesterase agents. In: Brunton L.L., & Hilal-Dandan R, & Knollmann B.C.(Eds.), Goodman & Gilman's: The pharmacological basis of therapeutics, 13e. McGraw Hill.

Therapeutic Goods Administration (TGA). 2021. Changes to adrenaline and noradrenaline labels [online] Available at: <https://www.tga.gov.au/changes-adrenaline-and-noradrenaline-labels> [Accessed 9 Oct 2021].

Westfall T.C., & Macarthur H, Westfall D.P. (2017). Neurotransmission: the autonomic and somatic motor nervous systems. In: Brunton L.L., & Hilal-Dandan R, & Knollmann B.C.(Eds.), Goodman & Gilman's: The pharmacological basis of therapeutics, 13e. McGraw Hill.

Chapter 9

Altosaar K, Balaji P, Bond RA, et al. Adrenoceptors (version 2019.4) in the IUPHAR/BPS Guide to Pharmacology Database. IUPHAR/BPS Guide to Pharmacology CITE. 2019; 2019(4). Available from: https://doi.org/10.2218/gtopdb/F4/2019.4

Chapter 10

Eschenhagen T. Therapy of heart failure. In: Brunton LL, Hilal-Dandan R, Knollmann BC, editors. Goodman & Gilman's The pharmacological basis of therapeutics. 13th ed. New York: McGraw Hill; 2018, pp. 527-546.

KnollmannBC, Roden DM. Antiarrhythmic drugs. In: Brunton LL, Hilal-Dandan R, Knollmann BC, editors. Goodman & Gilman's The pharmacological basis of therapeutics. 13th ed. New York: McGraw Hill; 2018, pp. 547-572.

Ponikowski P, Voors AA, Anker SD, Bueno H, Cleland JGF et al. ESC Guidelines for the diagnosis and treatment of acute and chronic heart failure: The Task Force for the diagnosis and treatment of acute and chronic heart failure of the European Society of Cardiology (ESC). Developed with the special contribution of the Heart Failure Association (HFA) of the ESC. European Heart Journal 2016; 37:2129-200.

Chapter 11

Hunter PG, Chapman FA, Dhaun N. Hypertension: Current trends and future perspectives. British Journal of Clinical Pharmacology 2021;1-16.

Chapter 12

Manniello M, Pisano M. Alirocumab (Praluent): first in the new class of PCSK9 inhibitors, Pharmacology & Therapeutics 2016;41(1):28-53.

Sabatine MS, Giugliano RP, Keech AC, Honarpour N, Wiviott SD, Murphy SA et al. Evolocumab and clinical outcomes in patients with cardiovascular disease, The New England Journal of Medicine 2017;376:1713-22.

Chapter 13

Australian Prescriber: Idarucizumab, Australian Prescriber 2016;39:183.

Chin PKL, Doogue MP: Long-term prescribing of new oral anticoagulants, Australian Prescriber 2016; 39:200-04.

Hogg K, Weitz JI. Blood coagulation and anticoagulant, fibrinolytic, and antiplatelet drugs. In: Brunton LL, Hilal-Dandan R, Knollmann BC, editor. Goodman and Gilman's The pharmacological basis of therapeutics. New York: McGraw Hill; 13th edn, 2018, p. 585-603.

Siegal DM, Curnutte JT, Connolly SJ. Andexanet alfa for the reversal of Factor Xa inhibitor activity. The New England Journal of Medicine 2015;37:2413-24.

Chapter 14

Kaushansky K, Kipps TJ: Hematopoietic agents: Growth factors, minerals and vitamins. In Brunton LL, Hilal-Dandan R, Knollman BC, editors: Goodman & Gilman's The pharmacological basis of therapeutics, 13th ed, New York, 2018, McGraw-Hill, Chapter 41 p.751-767.

Metcalf D. The colony-stimulating factors and cancer. Cancer Immunology Research 2013;1:351-56.

Wang LI, Baser O, Kutikova L, et al. The impact of primary prophylaxis with granulocyte-colony-stimulating factors on febrile neutropenia during chemotherapy: A systematic review and meta-analysis of randomized controlled trials. Support Care Cancer 2015;23:3131-40.

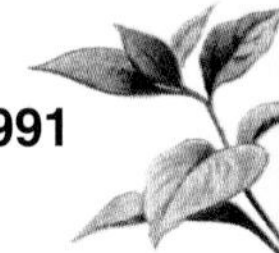

Chapter 15

Barnes PJ. Glucocorticosteroids. Handbook of Experimental Pharmacology. 2017; 237:93-115. doi: 10.1007/164_2016_62. PMID: 27796513

Cazzola M, Rogliani P, Matera MG. Ultra-LABAs for the treatment of asthma. Respiratory Medicine. 2019 Sep; 156:47-52. doi: 10.1016/j.rmed.2019.08.005. Epub 2019 Aug 12. PMID: 31425937.

Cho EY, Kim SY, Kim MJ, et al. Comparison of clinical efficacy between ultra-LABAs and ultra-LAMAs in COPD: a systemic review with meta-analysis of randomized controlled trials. The Journal of Thoracic Disease 2018 Dec;10(12):6522-6530. doi: 10.21037/jtd.2018.11.50. PMID: 30746196; PMCID: PMC6344669.

Doty RL. Treatments for smell and taste disorders: A critical review. The Handbook of Clinical Neurology 2019; 164:455-479. doi: 10.1016/B978-0-444-63855-7.00025-3. PMID: 31604562.

Jia X, Zhou S, Luo D, et al. Effect of pharmacist-led interventions on medication adherence and inhalation technique in adult patients with asthma or COPD: A systematic review and meta-analysis. Journal of Clinical Pharmacy and Therapeutics 2020 Oct;45(5):904-917. doi: 10.1111/jcpt.13126. Epub 2020 Feb 27. PMID: 32107837.

Lim A, Hussainy SY, Abramson MJ: Asthma drugs in pregnancy and lactation, Australian Prescriber. 2013; 36(5):150-153, 2013.Reddel H: Rational prescribing for asthma in adults – written asthma action plans, Aust Presc. 2012; 35(3):78-81, 2012.

Reddel HK. Updated Australian guidelines for mild asthma: what's changed and why? Australian Prescriber 2020; Dec;43(6):220-224. doi: 10.18773/austprescr.2020.076. Epub 2020 Dec 1. PMID: 33363311; PMCID: PMC7738702.

Respiratory Expert Group: Therapeutic guidelines: respiratory, ed 6, Melbourne, 2020, Therapeutic Guidelines Limited.

Rodrigo GJ, Price D, Anzueto A, et al. LABA/LAMA combinations versus LAMA monotherapy or LABA/ICS in COPD: a systematic review and meta-analysis. Int J Chron Obstruct Pulmon Dis. 2017; Mar 17; 12:907-922. doi: 10.2147/COPD.S130482. PMID: 28360514; PMCID: PMC5364009.

Scichilone N, Barnes PJ, Battaglia S, et al. The Hidden Burden of Severe Asthma: From Patient Perspective to New Opportunities for Clinicians. Journal of Clinical Medicine 2020 Jul 27;9(8): 2397. doi: 10.3390/jcm9082397. PMID: 32727032; PMCID: PMC7463666.

Sung V, Cranswick N: Cough and cold remedies for children, Australian Prescriber 2009; 32(5):122-124, 2009.

Chapter 16

No further reading.

Chapter 17

El-Zawahry A. Combination pharmacotherapy for treatment of overactive bladder (OAB). Current Urology Reports 2019:21:33.

Chapter 18

Australian Medicines Handbook P/L: Australian medicines handbook 2021, Adelaide, 2021, AMH.

Boron WF, Boulpaep EL: Medical physiology: a cellular and molecular approach, Updated ed, Philadephia, PA, 2005, Elsevier Saunders.

Bowman WC, Rand MJ: Chapters 7, 16. Textbook of pharmacology, ed 2, Oxford, 1980, Blackwell.

Brown EN, Pavone KJ, Naranjo M. Multimodal General Anesthesia: Theory and Practice. Anesth Analg. 2018 Nov;127(5):1246-1258. doi: 10.1213/ANE. 0000000000003668. PMID: 30252709; PMCID: PMC6203428.

Dong X. Current Strategies for Brain Drug Delivery. Theranostics. 2018 Feb 5;8(6):1481-1493. doi: 10.7150/ thno.21254. PMacute neurological disorders (217, 697) and neurodegeneration ID: 29556336; PMCID: PMC5858162.

Hoyer D, Bartfai T: Neuropeptides and neuropeptide receptors: drug targets, and peptides and non-peptide ligands: a tribute to Prof. Dieter Seebach, Chemistry and Biodiversity 9(11):2367-2387, 2012.

Hudson AE, Hemmings HC: Are anaesthetics toxic to the brain? British Journal of Anaesthesia 107(1):30-37, 2011.

Kim DG, Bynoe MS: A2A adenosine receptor modulates drug efflux transporter P-glycoprotein at the blood–brain barrier, The Journal of Clinical Investigation 126(5):1717-1733, 2016.

Oberoi G, Phillips G: Anaesthesia and emergency situations: a management guide, Sydney, 2000, McGraw-Hill.

Patton, K., Borshoff, D.C. 2018 Adverse drug reactions. Anaesthesia, 73 Suppl 1, pp. 76-84. doi: 10.1111/anae.14143.

Salerno E: Pharmacology for health professionals, St Louis, 1999, Mosby.

Speight TM, Holford NHG, editors: Avery's drug treatment, ed 4, Auckland, 1997, Adis.

Sweeney MD, Zhao Z, Montagne A, Nelson AR, Zlokovic BV. Blood-brain barrier: from physiology to disease and back. Physiological Reviews 2019;99(1):21-78. doi:10.1152/ physrev.00050.2017

Tosi G, Duskey JT, Kreuter J. Nanoparticles as carriers for drug delivery of macromolecules across the blood-brain barrier. Expert Opinion on Drug Delivery 2020 Jan;17(1):23-32. doi: 10.1080/17425247.2020.1698544. Epub 2019 Dec 3. PMID: 31774000.Copy

Zhang TT, Li W, Meng G, et al: Strategies for transporting nanoparticles across the blood–brain barrier, Biomaterials Science 4(2):219-229, 2016.

Chapter 19

Argoff C: Mechanisms of pain transmission and pharmacologic management, Current Medical Research and Opinion 27(10):2019-2031, 2011.

Borsodi A, Bruchas M, Caló G, et al. Opioid receptors (version 2019.4) in the IUPHAR/BPS Guide to Pharmacology Database. IUPHAR/BPS Guide to Pharmacology CITE. 2019; 2019(4). Available from: https://doi.org/10.2218/gtopdb/F50/2019.4.

Carr DB, Jacox AK, Chapman CR, et al: Acute pain management: operative or medical procedures and trauma. Clinical practice guideline. AHCPR Pub. No. 92-0032. Rockville, MD: Agency for Health Care Policy and Research, Public Health Service, US Department of Health and Human Services, 1992.
Iedema J: Cautions with codeine, Australian Prescriber 34(5):133-135, 2011.
Kennedy D: Analgesics and pain relief in pregnancy and breastfeeding, Australian Prescriber 34(1):8-10, 2011.
Price HR, Collier AC. Analgesics in pregnancy: an update on use, safety and pharmacokinetic changes in drug disposition. Current Pharmaceutical Design 2017;23(40):6098-6114. doi: 10.2174/1381612823666170825123754. PMID: 28847300.
McCaffery M, Pasero C: Pain: clinical manual, St Louis, MO, 1999, Mosby.
McDonough M: Safe prescribing of opioids for persistent non-cancer pain, Australian Prescriber 35(1):20-24, 2012.
Melzack R, Wall PD: Pain mechanisms: a new theory, Science 150:971-979, 1965.
Ministry of Health. 2019. Annual Data Explorer 2018/19: New Zealand Health Survey [Data File]. URL: https://minhealthnz.shinyapps.io/nz-health-survey-2018-19-annual-data-explorer/
Pollack A, Harrison C, Henderson J, et al: Neuropathic pain, Australian Family Physician 42(3):91, 2013.
Prommer E, Ficek B: Management of pain in the elderly at the end of life, Drugs and Aging 29(4):285-305, 2012.
Rang HP, Dale MM, Ritter JM, et al: Pharmacology, ed 6, Edinburgh, 2007, Churchill Livingstone.
Roberts LJ: Managing acute pain in patients with an opioid abuse or dependence disorder, Australian Prescriber 31:136, 2008.
Salerno E: Pharmacology for health professionals, St Louis, MO, 1999, Mosby.
Salerno E, Willens JS: Pain management handbook, St Louis, MO, 1996, Mosby.
Wong D, Hockenberry-Eaton M, Wilson D, et al: Wong's essentials of pediatric nursing, ed 6, St Louis, MO, 2001, Mosby.
Valentino, R.J., Volkow, N. Untangling the complexity of opioid receptor function. Neuropsychopharmacol 43, 2514-2520 (2018). https://doi.org/10.1038/s41386-018-0225-3
Wang C, Meng Q. Global Research Trends of Herbal Medicine for Pain in Three Decades (1990-2019): A Bibliometric Analysis. J Pain Res. 2021;14:1611-1626. Published 2021 Jun 4. doi:10.2147/JPR.S311311bhade

Chapter 20

Asnis GM, Thomas M, Henderson MA: Pharmacotherapy treatment options for insomnia: a primer for clinicians, International Journal of Molecular Science 17:50, 2016.
Australian Medicines Handbook P/L: Australian medicines handbook 2020, 2017. Adelaide: AMH.
Chua HC, Chebib M: GABA receptors and the diversity in their structure and pharmacology, Advances in Pharmacology 79:1-34, 2017.
Dubey AK, Handu SS, Mediratta PK: Suvorexant: the first orexin receptor antagonist to treat insomnia, Journal of Pharmacology & Pharmacotherapeutics. 2015; 6(2):118-121,
Engin E, Benham RS, Rudolph U. An Emerging Circuit Pharmacology of GABAA Receptors. Trends in Pharmacological Sciences 2018;39(8):710-732. doi:10.1016/j.tips.2018.04.003
Ettcheto M, Olloquequi J, Sánchez-López E, Busquets O, Cano A, Manzine PR, et.al. Benzodiazepines and related drugs as a risk factor in Alzheimer's disease dementia. Frontiers in Aging Neuroscience 2020 Jan 8; 11:344. doi: 10.3389/fnagi.2019.00344. PMID: 31969812; PMCID: PMC6960222.
Fulde G, Preisz P: Managing aggressive and violent patients, Australian Prescriber. 2011; 34(4):115-118
Hoyer D, Gee CE, Mang GM, et al: Orexin 2 receptor antagonism induces sleep: a novel series of orexin receptor antagonists with distinct effects on sleep architecture, Proceedings of Australasian Society of Clinical and Experimental Pharmacologists and Toxicologists. 2013.;82: abstract 313
Huang AR, Mallet L, Rochefort CM, et al: Medication-related falls in the elderly: causative factors and preventive strategies, Drugs Aging. 2012; 29(5):359-376
Mieda MI: The roles of orexins in sleep/wake regulation. Journal of Neuroscience Research. 2017; 118:56-65
Olson LG: Hypnotic hazards: adverse effects of zolpidem and other Z-drugs, Australian Prescriber. 2008; 31(6):146-149
Psychotropic Expert Group: Therapeutic guidelines: psychotropics, version 7, Melbourne, 2013, Therapeutic Guidelines Limited.
Salerno E: Pharmacology for health professionals, St Louis, 1999, Mosby.
Sartori SB, Singewald N. Novel pharmacological targets in drug development for the treatment of anxiety and anxiety-related disorders. Pharmacology & Therapeutics 2019 Dec; 204:107402. doi: 10.1016/j.pharmthera.2019.107402.
Slade T, Johnston A, Oakley Browne MA, et al: 2007 National Survey of Mental Health and Wellbeing: methods and key findings, Australian and New Zealand Journal of Psychiatry 43(7):594-605, 2009.
Westaway K, Blacker N, Shute R, Allin R, Elgebaly Z, Frank O, et al. Combination psychotropic medicine use in older adults and risk of hip fracture. Australian Prescriber 2019; 42:93-6. https://doi.org/10.18773/austprescr.2019.01.

Chapter 21

Billington M, Kandalaft OR, Aisiku IP: Adult status epilepticus: a review of the prehospital and emergency department management. Brophy GM, Vespa PM, eds, Journal of Clinical Medicine 5(9):74, 2016.
Lander C: Antiepileptic drugs in pregnancy and lactation, Australian Prescriber 31(3):70-72, 2008.
Meador KJ, Baker GA, Browning N, et al: Fetal antiepileptic drug exposure and cognitive outcomes at age 6 years (NEAD study): a prospective observational study, The Lancet. Neurology 12(3):244-252, 2013.
Patsalos (2020) Therapeutic drug monitoring of antiepileptic drugs: current status and future prospects, Expert Opinion on Drug Metabolism & Toxicology, 16:3, 227-238, DOI: 10.1080/17425255.2020.1724956
Perucca P, Scheffer IE, Kiley M. The management of epilepsy in children and adults. Medical Journal of Australia 2018 Mar 19;208(5):226-233. doi: 10.5694/mja17.00951. PMID: 29540143.

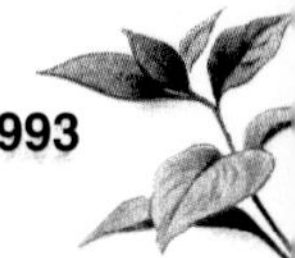

Rang HP, Dale MM, Ritter JM, et al: Rang & Dale's pharmacology, ed 8, Edinburgh, 2016, Churchill Livingstone.

Reimers A, Brodtkorb E: Second-generation antiepileptic drugs and pregnancy: a guide for clinicians, Expert Review of Neurotherapeutics 12(6):707-717, 2012.

Richens A, Dunlop A: Serum-phenytoin levels in management of epilepsy, Lancet 2:247-248, 1975.

Tomson T, Battino D, Perucca E. Teratogenicity of antiepileptic drugs. Current Opinion in Neurology 2019 Apr;32(2): 246-252. doi: 10.1097/WCO.0000000000000659. PMID: 30664067.

Wlodarczyk BJ, Palacios AM, George TM, et al: Antiepileptic drugs and pregnancy outcomes, American Journal of Medical Genetics. Part A 158A (8):2071-2090, 2012.

Chapter 22

Anderson KN, Lind JN, Simeone RM, et al. Maternal Use of specific antidepressant medications during early pregnancy and the risk of selected birth defects. JAMA Psychiatry. 2020 Dec 1;77(12):1246-1255. doi: 10.1001/jamapsychiatry. 2020.2453. PMID: 32777011; PMCID: PMC7407327.

Betcher HK, Wisner KL. Psychotropic treatment during pregnancy: research synthesis and clinical care principles. Journal of Women's Health 2020 Mar;29(3):310-318. doi: 10.1089/jwh.2019.7781. Epub 2019 Dec 3. PMID: 31800350; PMCID: PMC7207058.

Bousman CA, Forbes M, Jayaram M, et al: Antidepressant prescribing in the precision medicine era: a prescriber's primer on pharmacogenetic tools, BMC Psychiatry 17:60, 2017.

Braun L, Cohen M: Herbs and natural supplements: an evidence-based guide, 4th ed, Sydney, 2014, Elsevier Mosby.

Cade JF: Lithium salts in the treatment of psychotic excitement, Medical Journal of Australia 2(10):349-352, 1949.

Cipriani A, Furukawa TA, Salanti G, et al. Comparative efficacy and acceptability of 21 antidepressant drugs for the acute treatment of adults with major depressive disorder: a systematic review and network meta-analysis. Lancet. 2018;391(10128):1357-1366.

Chisolm MS, Payne JL: Management of psychotropic drugs during pregnancy, British Medical Journal 351:h5918, 2016.

Cioltan H, Alshehri S, Howe C, et al: Variation in use of antipsychotic medications in nursing homes in the United States: a systematic review, BMC Geriatrics 17:32, 2017.

Gartlehner G, Wagner G, Matyas N, et al. Pharmacological and non-pharmacological treatments for major depressive disorder: review of systematic reviews. BMJ Open. 2017;7(6):e014912. Published 2017 Jun 14. doi:10.1136/bmjopen-2016-014912

Hasnain MW, Victor RV, Hollett B: Weight gain and glucose dysregulation with second-generation antipsychotics and antidepressants: a review for primary care physicians, Postgraduate Medicine 124(4):154-167, 2012.

Kulkarni J, Storch A, Baraniuk A, et al. Antipsychotic use in pregnancy. Expert Opin Pharmacother. 2015 Jun;16(9):1335-45. doi: 10.1517/14656566.2015.1041501. PMID: 26001182.

Malhi GS, Tanious M, Bargh D, et al: Safe and effective use of lithium, Australian Prescriber 36(1):18-21, 2013.

McCutcheon RA, Reis Marques T, Howes OD. Schizophrenia—An Overview. JAMA Psychiatry. 2020;77(2):201-210. doi:10.1001/jamapsychiatry.2019.3360

McClellan J. Psychosis in children and adolescents. Journal of the American Academy of Child and Adolescent Psychiatry. 2018 May;57(5):308-312. doi: 10.1016/j.jaac.2018.01.021. Epub 2018 Mar 13. PMID: 29706159.

McKnight RF, Adida M, Budge K, et al: Lithium toxicity profile: a systematic review and meta-analysis, Lancet 379(9817):721-728, 2012.

Mitchell PB: Bipolar disorder, Australian Family Physician 42(9):616-619, 2013.

Moran SP, Maksymetz J, Conn PJ. Targeting muscarinic acetylcholine receptors for the treatment of psychiatric and neurological disorders. Trends in Pharmacological Sciences 2019 Dec;40(12):1006-1020. doi: 10.1016/j.tips.2019. 10.007. Epub 2019 Nov 8. PMID: 31711626; PMCID: PMC6941416.

Nabavi B, Mitchell AJ, Nutt D: A lifetime prevalence of comorbidity between bipolar affective disorder and anxiety disorders: a meta-analysis of 52 interview-based studies of psychiatric population, EBioMedicine 2(10):1405-1419, 2015.

National Prescribing Service: Depression: challenges in primary care, NPS News 74:3, 2011.

National Prescribing Service: Balancing benefits and harms of antipsychotic therapy, NPS News 78:1-4, 2012.

Wolf PL: If clinical chemistry had existed then, Clinical Chemistry 40:328-335, 1994.

Yohn CN, Gergues M, Samuels BA: The role of 5-HT receptors in depression, Molecular Brain 10:2, 2017.

Zohar J, Stahl S, Moller HJ, et al: A review of the current nomenclature for psychotropic agents and an introduction to the neuroscience-based nomenclature, European Journal of Neuropsychopharmacology 25(12):2318-2325, 2015.

Chapter 23

Australian Medicines Handbook P/L: Australian medicines handbook 2021, Adelaide, 2021, AMH.

Heckman MA, Weil J, Gonzalez de Mejia E: Caffeine (1, 3, 7-trimethylxanthine) in foods: a comprehensive review on consumption, functionality, safety, and regulatory matters, Journal of Food Science. 2010; 75(3): R77-R87,

Jones SC, Barrie L, Berry N: Why (not) alcohol energy drinks? A qualitative study with Australian university students, Drug & Alcohol Review 31(3):281-287, 2012.

Mazanov J, Dunn M, Connor J, et al: Substance use to enhance academic performance among Australian university students, Performance Enhancement and Health. 2013; 2(3):110-118,

Monteiro JP, Alves MG, Oliveira PF, Silva BM. Structure-bioactivity relationships of methylxanthines: Trying to make sense of all the promises and the drawbacks. Molecules. 2016;21(8):974. Published 2016 Jul 27. doi:10.3390/molecules21080974

Chapter 24

Chakraborty S, Lennon JC, Malkaram SA, et al. Serotonergic system, cognition, and BPSD in Alzheimer's disease. Neuroscience Letters 2019;704:36-44. doi: 10.1016/j.neulet.2019.03.050

Correale J, Gaitán MI, Ysrraelit MC, et al: Progressive multiple sclerosis: from pathogenic mechanisms to treatment, Brain: A Journal of Neurology 140(3):527-546, 2017.

Ferrero H, Solas M, Francis PT, et al. Serotonin 5-HT6 receptor antagonists in Alzheimer's disease: therapeutic rationale and current development status. CNS Drugs. 2017; Jan;31(1): 19-32. doi: 10.1007/s40263-016-0399-3. PMID: 27914038.

Howes O, McCutcheon R, Stone J. Glutamate and dopamine in schizophrenia: an update for the 21st century. Journal of Psychopharmacology 2015;29(2):97-115

Hung SY, Fu WM: Drug candidates in clinical trials for Alzheimer's disease. Journal of Biomedical Science 2017; 24(1):47.

Mittal R, Debs LH, Patel AP, et al. Neurotransmitters: the critical modulators regulating gut-brain axis. Journal of Cellular Physiology 2017; Sep;232(9):2359-2372. doi: 10.1002/jcp.25518. Epub 2017 Apr 10. PMID: 27512962; PMCID: PMC5772764.

Jankovic J, Tan EK. Parkinson's disease: etiopathogenesis and treatment. Journal of Neurology, Neurosurgery, and Psychiatry 2020; Aug;91(8):795-808. doi: 10.1136/jnnp-2019-322338. Epub 2020 Jun 23. PMID: 32576618.

Mann J: Murder, magic and medicine, Oxford, 1992, Oxford University Press.

National Prescribing Service: Headache: diagnosis, management and prevention, NPS News 2012; 79:1-4,

Reich DS, Lucchinetti CF, Calabresi PA. Multiple sclerosis. The New England Journal of Medicine 2018;378(2):169-180. doi:10.1056/NEJMra1401483.

Smith K, Flicker L, Dwyer A, et al: Factors associated with dementia in Aboriginal Australians, Australian and New Zealand Journal of Psychiatry. 2010; 44(10):888-893.

Thom RP, Mock CK, Teslyar P: Delirium in hospitalized patients: risks and benefits of antipsychotics, Cleveland Clinic Journal of Medicine 2017; 84(8):616-622.

Szeto JY, Lewis SJ: Current treatment options for Alzheimer's disease and Parkinson's disease dementia, Current Neuropharmacology 2016; 14(4):326-338,

Winkelman JW, Armstrong MJ, Allen RP, et al: Practice guideline summary: treatment of restless legs syndrome in adults: report of the Guideline Development, Dissemination, and Implementation Subcommittee of the American Academy of Neurology. Neurology. 2016; 87(24):2585-2593.

Chapter 25

Australasian College for Emergency Medicine, Alcohol and Methamphetamine Harm in Emergency Departments: Findings from the 2019 Snapshot Survey. 2020, ACEM: Melbourne

Barrett, M.J., F.E. Babl, Alcohol-based hand sanitiser: a potentially fatal toy. Medical Journal of Australia, 2015. 203(1): p. 43-44.

Cairns, R., Svhaffer, A.L., Brown, J.A., et al., Codeine use and harms in Australia: evaluating the effects of re-scheduling. Addiction, 2020. 115(3): p. 451-459.

Crowley, P., Long-term drug treatment of patients with alcohol dependence. Australian Prescriber, 2015. 38(2): p. 41-43.

Dobbin, M., Liew, D.F. Real-time prescription monitoring: helping people at risk of harm. Australian Prescriber, 2020. 43(5): p. 164.

Egerton-Warburton, D., Gosbell, A., Wadsworth, A., et al., Survey of alcohol-related presentations to Australasian emergency departments. Medical Journal of Australia, 2014. 201(10): p. 584-587.

Jauncey, M.E., Nielsen S., Community use of naloxone for opioid overdose. Australian Prescriber, 2017. 40(4): p. 137.

St John, A.L., Choi, H.W., Walker, Q.D., et al., Novel mucosal adjuvant, mastoparan-7, improves cocaine vaccine efficacy. NPJ Vaccines, 2020. 5(1): p. 1-9.

Ubaldi M, Cannella N, Ciccocioppo R, Emerging targets for addiction neuropharmacology: from mechanisms to therapeutics. Progress in Brain Research, 2016. 224: p. 251-284.

White, V.M., et al., Long-term impact of plain packaging of cigarettes with larger graphic health warnings: findings from cross-sectional surveys of Australian adolescents between 2011 and 2017. Tobacco Control, 2019. 28(e1): p. e77.

Chapter 26

No further reading.

Chapter 27

Loftley AE. Clinician's review of thyroid and parathyroid disease. Journal of Diabetes and Clinical Research 2020;2:37-44.

Tu KN, Lie JD, Wan CKV, et al. Osteoporosis: A review of treatment options. Pharmacy & Therapeutics 2018;43:92-104.

Chapter 28

Australian Medicines Handbook. Adelaide: Endrocrine Drugs, Australian Medicines Handbook Pty Ltd, 2021.

Boron WF, Boulpaep EL: Medical physiology: a cellular and molecular approach, ed 3, Philadelphia, 2017, Elsevier.

Endocrinology Expert Group: Therapeutic guidelines: diabetes, Melbourne, 2021, Therapeutic Guidelines Limited.

Padhi, S., Nayak A.K, Behera A., et al. 2020. Type II diabetes mellitus: a review on recent drug based therapeutics. Biomedicine & Pharmacotherapy 131: 110708.

Chapter 29

Barnes PJ. Glucocorticoids: current and future directions. British Journal of Pharmacology 2011;163:29-43.

Ciriaco M, Ventrice P, Russo G, et al. Corticosteroid-related central nervous system side effects. Journal of Pharmacology & Pharmacotherapeutics 2013; Suppl 1:S94-8. doi: 10.4103/0976-500X.120975.

Strehl C, Spies CM, Buttgereit F. Pharmacodynamics of glucocorticoids. Clinical and Experimental Rheumatology 2011; 29: S13-8.

Vandevyver S, Dejager L, Liebert C. Comprehensive overview of the structure and regulation of the glucocorticoid receptor. Endocrine Reviews 2014;35:671-93.

Chapter 30

Amer MR, Cipriano GC, Venci JV, et al: Safety of popular herbal supplements in lactating women, Journal of Human Lactation 31(3):348-353, 2015.

Anonymous: Vitamin supplementation in pregnancy, British Medical Journal, Drug & Therapeutics Bulletin 54(7):61-64, 2016.

Australian Medicines Handbook P/L: Australian medicines handbook 2017, Adelaide, 2017, AMH.

Braun L, Cohen M: Herbs and natural supplements: an evidence-based guide, ed 4, Sydney, 2015, Elsevier Mosby.

Brucker MC, King TL: The 2015 US Food and Drug Administration Pregnancy and Lactation Labeling Rule, Journal of Midwifery and Women's Health 62(3):308-316, 2017.

Hammarberg K: Endocrine disrupting chemicals and fertility, Vicdoc October/November 2017:28-29, 2017.

Hynes EF, Handasyde KA, Shaw G, et al: Levonorgestrel, not etonogestrel, provides contraception in free-ranging koalas, Reproduction, Fertility and Development 22(6):913-919, 2010.

McParlin C, O'Donnell A, Robson SC, et al: Treatments for hyperemesis gravidarum and nausea and vomiting in pregnancy: a systematic review, JAMA: The Journal of the American Medical Association 316(13):1392-1401, 2016.

Marcus DM, Snodgrass WR: Do no harm: avoidance of herbal medicines during pregnancy, Obstetrical and Gynecological Survey 105(5):1119-1122, 2005.

Mazza D, Harrison C, Taft A, et al: Emergency contraception in Australia: the desired source of information versus the actual source of information, Medical Journal of Australia 200(7):414-415, 2014.

Mittal S: Emergency contraception: which is the best?, Minerva Ginecologica 68(6):687-699, 2016.

Murji A, Whitaker L, Chow TL, et al: Selective progesterone receptor modulators (SPRMs) for uterine fibroids, Cochrane Database of Systematic Reviews (4):CD010770, 2017.

Onda K, Tong S, Beard S, et al: Proton pump inhibitors decrease soluble FMS-like tyrosine kinase-1 and soluble endoglin secretion, decrease hypertension, and rescue endothelial dysfunction, Hypertension 69(3):457-468, 2017.

Taylor T: Treatment of nausea and vomiting in pregnancy, Australian Prescriber 37(2):42-45, 2014.

Chapter 31

No further reading.

Chapter 32

No further reading.

Chapter 33

No further reading.

Chapter 34

Aletaha D, Smolen JS. Diagnosis and management of rheumatoid arthritis: A review. JAMA 2018; 320:1360-72.

Grosser T, Smyth EM, Fitzgerald GA. Pharmacotherapy of inflammation, fever, pain and gout. In Brunton LL, Hilal-Dandan R, Knollman BC, editors: Goodman & Gilman's The pharmacological basis of therapeutics, 13th ed, New York, 2018, McGraw-Hill, Chapter 38 pp. 685-709.

Skidgel R. Histamine, bradykinin, and their antgonists. In Brunton LL, Hilal-Dandan R, Knollman BC, editors: Goodman & Gilman's The pharmacological basis of therapeutics, 13th ed, New York, 2018, McGraw-Hill, Chapter 39 pp.711-226.

Chapter 35

No further reading.

Chapter 36

Yelin I, Kishony R: Antibiotic Resistance. Cell 22: 1136, 2018.

Chapter 37

WHO Solidarity Trial Consortium; Repurposed antiviral drugs for Covid-19 – Interim WHO solidarity trial results. The New England Journal of Medicine 384: 497-511, 2021.

Chapter 38

Antibiotic Expert Group: Therapeutic guidelines: antibiotic, Melbourne, 2019, Therapeutic Guidelines.

Australian Medicines Handbook P/L: Australian medicines handbook, Adelaide, 2021, AMH.

Bhatt S, Weiss DJ, Cameron E, et al: The effect of malaria control on *Plasmodium falciparum* in Africa between 2000 and 2015, Nature 526:207-211, 2015.

Chapter 39

Yap, F.H., H.C. Chua, C.P. Tait, Active sunscreen ingredients in Australia. Australasian Journal of Dermatology, 2017. 58(4): p. e160-e170.

Buckley, N., Australian Medicines Handbook 2021. 2021: Australian Medicines Handbook.

Vemuri, K., Therapeutic Guidelines: Ulcers and wound management. Version 2. Australian Prescriber, 2019. 42(6): 206.

Nímia, H.H., et al., Comparative study of Silver Sulfadiazine with other materials for healing and infection prevention in burns: A systematic review and meta-analysis. Burns, 2019. 45(2): p. 282-292.

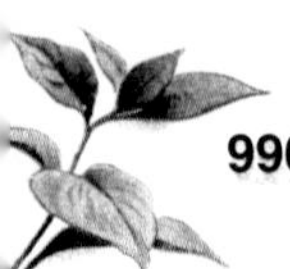

Rodgers, K., J. Sim, R. Clifton, Systematic review of pressure injury prevalence in Australian and New Zealand hospitals. Collegian, 2021. 28(3): p. 310-323.

Ritter, J., et al., Rang and Dale's pharmacology. 2019.

Chapter 40

No further reading.

Chapter 41

Ervin K, Finlayson S, Cross M. The management of behavioural problems associated with dementia in rural aged care. Collegian 2021;19:85-95.

Jackson S, Jansen P, Mangoni A. Prescribing for elderly patients. Chichester: Wiley-Blackwell; 2009.

Shrestha S, Poudel A, Steadman K, Nissen L. Outcomes of deprescribing interventions in older patients with life-limiting illness and limited life expectancy: A systematic review. British Journal of Clinical Pharmacology. 2020;86:1931-1945.

Westaway K, Sluggett J, Alderman C, et al. The extent of antipsychotic use in Australian residential aged care facilities and interventions shown to be effective in reducing antipsychotic use: A literature review. Dementia 2020;19:1189-1202.

Chapter 42

No further reading.

Chapter 43

No further reading.

Chapter 44

No further reading.

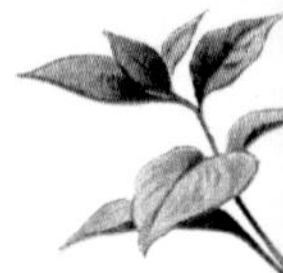

FIGURE LIST

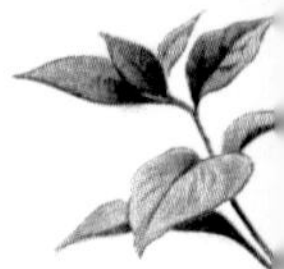

CLINICAL FOCUS BOX LIST

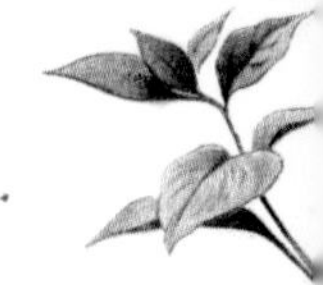

DRUG MONOGRAPH LIST

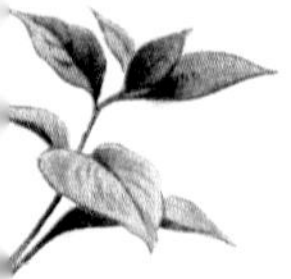

FIGURE AND PICTURE CREDITS

Figure 1.1 **B** *Lithograph by Pierre Roche Vigneron,* **C&D:** *Wellcome Library no. 4213i, CC BY 4.0.*

Figure 1.2 **A–D:** *iStockphoto/habari1; iStockphoto/kannika2013; iStockphoto/Petegar; iStockphoto/AtWaG*

Figure 1.6 *Source: Adapted from Therapeutic Goods Administration <https://www.tga.gov.au/sites/default/files/blue-card-adverse-reaction-reporting-form.pdf.>*

Figure 2.2 *Source: Adapted from Sweeney 1990; used with permission.*

Figure 2.3 *Source: Services Australia 2021; reproduced with permission.*

Figure 3.1 *Source: Katzung et al. 2012, Figure 2-11; reproduced with permission of The McGraw-Hill Companies.*

Figure 3.2 *Source: Rang HP, Dale MM, Ritter JM, et al: Pharmacology, Edinburgh, 2012, Elsevier.*

Figure 4.2 *Source: Salerno 1999, Figure 4-2; used with permission.*

Figure 4.5 *Source: Birkett 2010, Figure 5.1; reproduced with permission from McGraw-Hill.*

Figure 4.6 *Source: Birkett et al. 1979, Figure 2; reproduced with permission.*

Figure 4.7 *Source: Salerno 1999, Figure 4-6; used with permission.*

Figure 5.1 *Source: Adapted from Salerno 1999, Figure 4-7; used with permission.*

Figure 5.8 *Source: Rang et al. 2012, Figure 10.9; reproduced with permission from Elsevier.*

Figure 8.2 *Source: Adapted from Salerno 1999, Figure 14.3; used with permission.*

Figure 8.3 *Source: Adapted from Salerno 1999, Figure 14.2; used with permission.*

Figure 8.4 *Source: Adapted from Salerno 1999, Figure 14.4; used with permission.*

Figure 10.2 *Source: Adapted from Salerno 1999, Figure 18.3; used with permission.*

Figure 10.3 *Source: Adapted from Noble 1975; reproduced with permission from Rang 2012, Figure 21.1.*

Figure 10.5 *Source: Adapted from Salerno 1999, Figure 19.1; used with permission.*

Figure 11.1 *Source: Adapted from Rang et al. 2012, Figure 22.1; used with permission.*

Figure 12.1 *Source: Adapted from Rang et al. 2012, Figure 23.1; used with permission.*

Figure 12.3 *Source: Page & Watts 2016; reproduced with permission.*

Figure 13.2 *Source: Adapted from Rang et al 2012, Figure 24.10; reproduced with permission.*

Figure 13.4 *Source: Adapted from Rang et al 2012, Figure 24.7; reproduced with permission.*

Figure 14.2 *Source: Rang et al. 2016, Chapter 25, Figure 25.1; used with permission.*

Figure 15.1 *Source: ©2022 Medtronic. All rights reserved. Used with the permission of Medtronic*

Figure 15.2 *Source: Salerno 1999; used with permission.*

Figure 15.3 *Sources:* **A, C** *and* **D:** *courtesy GlaxoSmithKline, Australia; used with permission;* **E:** *Dreamstime/Podius;* **F:** *istock/Hulldude30*

Figure 15.4 *Source: Adapted from Rang et al. 2003; used with permission.*

Figure 15.5 *Source: Netter Images; used with permission.*

Figure 15.7 *Source: National Asthma Council Australia 2022.*

Figure 16.1 *Source: Salerno 1999, Figure 34.1.*

Figure 16.3 *Source: Adapted from Rang et al. 2012, Figure 29.2; used with permission.*

Figure 16.4 *Source: Adapted from Salerno 1999, Figure 35.1.*

Figure 16.5 *Source: Adapted from Salerno 1999, Figure 3.1.*

Figure 17.2 *Source: Data from Greger 2000, reproduced from Rang et al. 2012, Figure 29.4.*

Figure 18.1 *Source: Salerno 1999, Figure 11.1; used with permission.*

Figure 18.2 *Source: Salerno 1999, Figure 11.2; used with permission.*

Figure 18.3 *Source: Salerno 1999, Figure 11.3; used with permission.*

Figure 18.4 *Source: netterimages.com; used with permission.*

Figure 18.5 *Source: Boron & Boulpaep 2005; used with permission.*

Figure 18.7 *Sources: Data from Speight & Holford 1997; Oberoi & Phillips 2000.*

Figure 18.8 *Source: Bowman & Rand 1980; used with permission.*

Figure 18.10 *Source: Bowman & Rand 1980; used with permission.*

Figure 19.1 *Source: Developed by McCaffery & Pasero 1999; from Salerno 1999.*

Figure 19.2 *Sources:* **I:** *Adapted from Salerno 1999;* **II:** *Adapted from Carr et al. 1992;* **III.** *Adapted from Wong et al. 2001; reproduced with permission.*

Figure 19.3 *Sources: Adapted from Anekar et al. 2021; Salerno & Willens 1996; Therapeutic Guidelines Limited 2021.*

Figure 19.4 *Sources: Adapted from Argoff 2011; Rang et al. 2007; used with permission.*

Figure 20.1 *Source: Adapted from Salerno 1999; used with permission.*

Figure 21.1 *Sources: Adapted from Rang et al. 2016; Dale & Rang 2007, inter alia.*

Figure 21.2 *Source: Fisher et al. 2017a; with permission of John Wiley & Sons.*

Figure 21.3 *Source: Adapted from Fisher et al. 2017a.*

Figure 23.1 *Source: Figure adapted from Andrew Herxheimer, in Laurence 1973.*
Figure 25.1 *Source: Noever et al. 1995; used with permission.*
Figure 25.2 *Source: Rang et al. 2016, Figure 49-2.*
Figure 26.1 *Source: Salerno 1999; used with permission.*
Figure 26.3 *Source: Salerno 1999; used with permission.*
Figure 27.1 *Source: Getty Images/Stocktrek Images.*
Figure 27.2 *Source: Adapted from Rang et al. 2012, Figure 33-1; reproduced with permission from Elsevier Churchill Livingstone.*
Figure 27.5 *Source: Boron & Boulpaep 2012, Figure 49-7; reproduced with permission from Elsevier Saunders.*
Figure 27.7 *Source: Boron & Boulpaep 2012, Figure 52-4; reproduced with permission from Elsevier Saunders.*
Figure 28.1 *Source: Adapted from Heile & Schneider 2012.*
Figure 30.2 *Source: Adapted from Salerno 1999; used with permission.*
Figure 30.4 *Source: Merck Sharp & Dohme (Australia) Pty Ltd; reproduced with permission.*
Figure 30.6 *Source: Moore et al. 2016, Figure 20-15; reproduced with permission from Elsevier.*
Figure 31.1 *Source: Ritter et al. 2019, Figure 35.6; used with permission.*
Figure 32.1 *Source: Hanahan & Weinberg 2011, Figure 6; used with permission.*
Figure 32.2 *Source: Adapted from Beare & Myers 1998.*
Figure 32.3 *Source: Salerno 1999; used with permission.*
Figure 33.1 *Source: Rang et al. 2012, Figure 55.3; reproduced with permission from Elsevier.*
Figure 33.2 *Source: Rang et al. 2012, Figure 55.6; reproduced with permission from Elsevier.*
Figure 33.3 *Source: Rang et al. 2012, Figure 55.8; reproduced with permission from Elsevier.*
Figure 34.2 *PGs = prostaglandins; (–) = inhibition by NSAIDs; green arrows denote enzymes*
Figure 34.3 *Source: Adapted from Rang et al. 2012, Figure 26.4; used with permission.*
Figure 38.1 *Source: Salerno 1999, Figure 53.1.*
Figure 38.2 *Source: Reproduced with kind permission of Ros Biebrick, Haematology, SA Pathology, Flinders Medical Centre, Adelaide.*
Figure 39.4 *Source: Ritter et al. 2019; used with permission.*
Figure 40.1 *Source: Salerno 1999.*
Figure 40.2 *Source: Steiner 2008; reproduced with permission from Australian Prescriber.*
Figure 40.3 *Source: Yanoff & Duker 2004, Figure 1-194; used with permission.*
Figure 40.4 *Source: Salerno 1999.*
Figure 41.1 *Source: Figure 8.1 from the 5th edition. Goodman RM, Gorlin RJ. Atlas of the face in genetic disorders, ed 2 St louis, MO, 1977, Mosby*
Figure 44.2 **A–D** *iStockphoto/ivanastar; Dreamstime/Alison Underwood; Dreamstime/18042011e; Dreamstime/ Mihai-bogdan Lazar; gmayfield10/ under CC BY-SA 2.0;* **E** *'Hypericum perforatum COMMON ST. JOHN'S WORT' by gmayfield10 is licensed under CC BY-SA 2.0. St John's Wort https://www.flickr.com/photos/33397993@ N05/3348599281*

INDEX

A

C

D

E

F

G

H

I

J

K

L

M

N

P

Q

R

S

T

U

X

Y

Z